PATHOPHYSIOLOGY
Concepts of Altered Health States

PATHOPHYSIOLOGY
Concepts of Altered Health States
FOURTH EDITION

Carol Mattson Porth
R.N., M.S.N., PH.D. (Physiology)

Professor, School of Nursing
University of Wisconsin–Milwaukee
Milwaukee, Wisconsin

With 24 Contributors

Illustrated by Carole Russell Hilmer C.M.I., and Others

J.B. Lippincott Company   Philadelphia

Sponsoring Editor: Diana Intenzo
Project Editor: Tom Gibbons
Indexer: Maria Coughlin
Design Coordinator: Kathy Kelley-Luedtke
Interior Designer: Maria Karkucinski

Cover Designer: Lou Fuiano
Production Manager: Helen Ewan
Production Coordinator: Kathryn Rule
Compositor: Circle Graphics
Printer/Binder: Courier Book Company/Westford

4th Edition

Library of Congress Cataloging in Publications Data

Porth, Carol.
    Pathophysiology : concepts of altered health states / Carol
Mattson Porth; with 24 contributors; illustrated by Carole Russell
Hilmer and others.—4th ed.
        p.   cm.
    Includes bibliographical references and index.
    ISBN 0-397-54961-X
    1. Physiology, Pathological.   2. Nursing.   I. Title.
    [DNLM: 1. Disease—nurses' instruction.   2. Pathology—nurses'
instruction.   3. Physiology—nurses' instruction.   QZ 4 P851p 1994]
    RB113.P67   1994
    616.07—dc20
    DNLM/DLC
    for Library of Congress   93-30115
                                                        CIP

Any procedure or practice described in this book should be applied by the healthcare practitioner under appropriate supervision in accordance with professional standards of care used with regard to the unique circumstances that apply in each practice situation. Care has been taken to confirm the accuracy of information presented and to describe generally accepted practices. However, the authors, editor, and publisher cannot accept any responsibility for errors or omissions or for any consequences from application of the information in this book and make no warranty express or implied, with respect to the contents of the book.

Every effort has been made to ensure drug selections and dosages are in accordance with current recommendations and practice. Because of ongoing research, changes in government regulations and the constant flow of information on drug therapy, reactions and interactions, the reader is cautioned to check the package insert for each drug for indications, dosages, warnings and precautions, particularly if the drug is new or infrequently used.

CONTRIBUTORS

Debra A. Bancroft, R.N., B.S.N.
Specialty Coordinator–Rheumatology
Columbia Arthritis Center
Columbia Hospital
Milwaukee, Wisconsin

Laura J. Burke, R.N., M.S.N.
Research Project Coordinator/
Cardiovascular Clinical Nurse Specialist
Saint Luke's Medical Center
Milwaukee, Wisconsin

Edward W. Carroll, B.S., M.S., PH.D.
Assistant Professor
Department of Basic Health Sciences
Marquette University
School of Dentistry
Milwaukee, Wisconsin

Robin L. Curtis, PH.D.
Adjunct Professor
Department of Cellular Biology and Anatomy
Department of Physical Medicine and Rehabilitation
Department of Neurosurgery
The Medical College of Wisconsin
Department of Basic Sciences
School of Dentistry
Marquette University
Milwaukee, Wisconsin

Sheila M. Curtis, R.N., M.S.
Senior Lecturer
School of Nursing
University of Wisconsin–Milwaukee
Doctoral Candidate
Marquette University
Milwaukee, Wisconsin

Susan E. Dietz, R.N., M.S.
Chief, Community Education Section
Division of STD/HIV Prevention
Centers for Disease Control and Prevention
Atlanta, Georgia

Wm. Michael Dunne, Jr., PH.D.
Associate Professor of Pathology and Pediatrics
Baylor College of Medicine
Houston, Texas

Susan Gallagher-Lepak, R.N., M.S.N.
Former Transplant Clinical Nurse Specialist
Froedtert Memorial Lutheran Hospital
Milwaukee, Wisconsin
Current Doctoral Student
University of Wisconsin–Madison
Madison, Wisconsin

Kathryn J. Gaspard, PH.D.
Lecturer
University of Wisconsin–Milwaukee
School of Nursing
Milwaukee, Wisconsin

Kathleen E. Gunta, M.S.N., R.N., O.N.C.
Clinical Nurse Specialist
Saint Luke's Medical Center
Milwaukee, Wisconsin

Linda S. Hurwitz, R.N., B.S., M.S.
Vice President for Nursing
Babies Hospital/Sloane Hospital for Women
The Presbyterian Hospital in New York
New York, New York

Mary Kay Jiricka, R.N., M.S.N., C.C.R.N.
Clinical Nurse Specialist, Critical Care
Milwaukee County Medical Complex
Milwaukee, Wisconsin

Mark LaRocco, PH.D.
Director of Clinical Microbiology
Department of Pathology
Saint Luke's Episcopal Hospital
Houston, Texas

Judy Wright Lott, R.N. N.N.P., D.S.N.
Director, Neonatal Nurse Practitioner Program
Children's Hospital Medical Center
Cincinnati, Ohio

Sylvia Eichner McDonald, R.N., M.S.
Clinical Nurse Specialist–Spinal Cord Injury
Froedtert Memorial Lutheran Hospital
Milwaukee, Wisconsin

Patricia McCowen Mehring, R.N.C., M.S.N.
OB-GYN Nurse Practitioner
Private Practice
Women Care
Waukesha, Wisconsin

Janice Smith Pigg, B.S.N., R.N., M.S.
Director, Program Development and Research
Columbia Musculoskeletal Institute
Nurse Consultant, Rheumatology
Columbia Arthritis Center
Columbia Hospital
Milwaukee, Wisconsin

Janice Kuiper Pikna, M.S.N., R.N., C.S.
Clinical Nurse Specialist–Gerontology
Senior Health Program
Froedtert Memorial Lutheran Hospital
Milwaukee, Wisconsin

Joan Pleuss, M.S., R.D., C.D.E.
Senior Research Dietitian
Clinical Research Center
Medical College of Wisconsin
Milwaukee, Wisconsin

Marianne Sigda, R.N., M.N.
Neonatal Nurse Practitioner
Children's Hospital Medical Center
Cincinnati, Ohio

Gladys Simandl, R.N., PH.D.
Assistant Professor
College of Nursing
Marquette University
Milwaukee, Wisconsin

Stephanie Stewart, R.N., PH.D.
Associate Professor
Department of Nursing
University of Wisconsin–Oshkosh
Oshkosh, Wisconsin

Nancie Urban, R.N., M.S.N., C.C.R.N.
Manager, Clinical Practice and Research
Saint Joseph's Hospital
Milwaukee, Wisconsin

Patrick R. Walsh, M.D., PH.D.
Professor, Department of Neurosurgery
Medical College of Wisconsin
Milwaukee, Wisconsin

PREFACE

The meaning of pathophysiology, or physiology of altered health, reflects not so much the pathologic processes that take place but the physiologic changes and responses that produce signs and symptoms. These changes determine, to a large extent, how the disease impacts on functional status.

As a nurse-physiologist, my major aim in the fourth edition of *Pathophysiology: Concepts of Altered Health States*, as in previous editions, is to relate normal body functioning to the physiologic changes that participate in disease production and occur as a result of illness, as well as the body's remarkable ability to compensate for these changes. The beauty of physiology is that it integrates all of the aspects of the individual cells and organs of the human body into a total functional whole that can be used to explain both the physical and psychological aspects of altered health. Indeed, it has been my intent to capture the beauty of the human body and to emphasize that in disease as in health, there is more "going right" in the body than is "going wrong." It is hoped that readers will learn to appreciate this marvelous potential, incorporating it into their own beliefs and sharing it with their clients.

My second aim has been to present the content in a logical manner so it could be easily understood and incorporated into the reader's frame of reference. Concepts from physiology, biochemistry, physics, and other sciences are reviewed as deemed appropriate.

Learning aids and design features have been structured to assist the reader in assimilating the information presented:

- A *content outline* and *learning objectives* appear at the beginning of each chapter.
- *Summary paragraphs* appear at the end of each major area of content.

- *Headings* have been arranged for clarity and ease of reading.
- *Diagrams* to aid in visualizing contents and *tables* to aid in identifying and summarizing essential information have been included throughout the text.

A conceptual model that integrates developmental and preventive aspects of health has been used. Selection of content was based on common health problems, including the special health needs of children and elderly persons. The book provides the rationale but not the "how to's" of health care, including such particulars as diagnostic methods and drug therapies. It is assumed that the reader will have access to more complete reference sources in these areas than this book could provide.

The content of the book addresses three areas of focus based on the health–illness continuum: (1) control of normal body function; (2) pathophysiology, or alterations in body function; and (3) system or organ failure, regardless of pathologic state (*e.g.*, heart failure and renal failure). In some sections, separate chapters have been devoted to each of these areas; in others, the content has been integrated within a single chapter.

The book is organized into several units. Unit I deals with the cellular aspects of disease. Unit II covers developmental considerations with chapters devoted to altered health in children and older adults. Unit III addresses disruptions in integrated body function, whereas Unit IV examines the dynamics of body defenses. The remaining units deal with alterations in specific organ and system functions.

This fourth edition has been greatly expanded. Content has been updated and reorganized and new figures have been added. New content and chapters reflect contemporary health care issues. In particular, information on the health care needs of children and older adults has been augmented and presented in a new unit entitled *Developmental Aspects of Altered Health*. Another new unit, *Alterations in Integrated Body Function*, has been created to include the chapter on stress and adaptation and a new chapter on alterations in activity tolerance.

As with the previous editions, every effort has been taken to make the text as accurate and up to date as possible. This was accomplished through an extensive review of the literature and through the use of critiques provided by students, faculty, and content specialists. As this vast amount of information was processed, inaccuracies or omissions may have occurred. Readers are encouraged to contact me about such errors. Such feedback is essential to the continued development of the book.

Carol Mattson Porth, R.N., M.S.N., PH.D.

ACKNOWLEDGMENTS

As with previous editions, many persons contributed to the development of this edition.

Carole Russell Hilmer, medical illustrator, deserves a special commendation for her tireless effort in creating the illustrations for this edition as well as previous editions of the book.

The students in my classes deserve a special commendation, because their questions, comments, and enthusiasm provided the motivation needed for a task such as this.

A number of people were kind enough to review part of the text and make helpful suggestions: Ms. Octavia Brown; Mary A. Carvalho, RN, BNS, CCRN; Edmund H. Duthie, Jr., MD; Laurie Dziadulewicz, RN, BSN, CCRN; Molly Erickson, RN, BSN; Mary Chris Lynch, RN, BSN; Rita Lang, RN, MSN, CCRN; Regina Maibusch, RN, MSN; Ms. Annie Faye Prescott; Polly Ryan, RN, PhD; Dr. Ron Valdiserri; Larry Wadzinski, RN, MSN; Karen Yust, RN, MSN; and Darwin Zellmer, PhD. In addition, a number of persons who reviewed the text for the publisher, but who are unknown to the author, made valuable comments and are to be commended.

The contributing authors deserve a special mention, for they worked long hours to supply essential content. Darlene Thornhill and Eileen Sherburne were not able to contribute to this edition. Their contributions to the previous edition greatly facilitated the preparation of this edition.

Several other persons deserve special recognition. Georgianne Heymann, RN, BSN, assisted in editing selected parts of the manuscript. As with the previous edition, she provided not only excellent editorial services but encouragement and support when the tasks associated with manuscript preparation became most dismal. Katherine Gaspard, PhD, assisted with reading chapters and galley proofs. She too provided excellent editorial services as well as support and encouragement. I also want to thank Jennie Berndt, nursing student, who assisted in library research.

The editorial staff at JB Lippincott also deserves recognition and special thanks. They helped keep me on target and patiently acknowledged my requests for extension of deadlines and changes in book format.

CONTENTS

PATHOPHYSIOLOGY
Concepts of Altered Health States

ALTERATIONS IN CELL FUNCTION AND GROWTH

CHAPTER 1

CELL AND TISSUE CHARACTERISTICS

CAROL MATTSON PORTH
ROBIN L. CURTIS

**Functional Components
of the Cell**
The Nucleus
**The Cytoplasm and Its
Organelles**
The Cell Membrane
Membrane Transport
Diffusion, Osmosis, and Transport
Endocytosis and Exocytosis

Membrane Potentials
Diffusion Potentials
Resting Membrane Potentials
Action Potentials
**Alterations in Membrane
Excitability**
Cellular Energy Metabolism
Anaerobic Metabolism
Aerobic Metabolism

Tissue Types
Epithelial Tissue
Connective Tissue
Loose Connective Tissue
Hematopoietic Tissue
Strong Supporting Connective
Tissue
Muscle Tissue

■ OBJECTIVES

After you have studied this chapter, you should be able to meet the following objectives:

■ List the components of the cell nucleus and cytoplasm and state their functions.

■ State four functions of the cell membrane.

■ State the mechanisms of membrane transport.

■ State the function of cell differentiation.

■ Explain the relationship between membrane permeability and membrane potential.

■ Differentiate hypo- and hyperpolarization.

■ Define *absolute* and *relative refractory periods*.

■ Explain why the basic tissue types are described in terms of their embryonic origin.

■ Characterize the three types of epithelium.

■ Explain the function of the intercellular junctions.

■ State the function of each of the three types of connective tissue.

■ Describe the properties of muscle tissue.

■ Differentiate between the calcium movement during action potentials in skeletal and smooth muscle.

To understand the functioning of the human body in health and disease, it is necessary to understand how the individual cells of the body are structured and how they function. The *cell* is the smallest functional unit that an organism can be divided into and still retain the characteristics necessary for life. Cells, in turn, are organized into larger functional units called *tissue*. Tissues form body structures and organs. Although the cells of different tissues and organs vary in structure and function, certain characteristics are common to all cells. Cells are remarkably similar in their ability to exchange materials with their immediate environment, to obtain energy from organic nutrients, to synthesize complex molecules, and to du-

Carol Mattson Porth: PATHOPHYSIOLOGY: CONCEPTS OF
ALTERED HEALTH STATES, 4th ed. © 1994, 1990, 1986, 1982
J.B. Lippincott Company

plicate themselves. It is at the level of the cell that most disease processes exert their effects. Some diseases affect the cells of a single organ, others affect the cells of a particular tissue type, and still others affect the cells of the entire organism.

The substances that make up the cells of living organisms are collectively referred to as *protoplasm*. Protoplasm is composed of water, proteins, lipids, carbohydrates, and electrolytes. Water makes up 70% to 85% of the cell's protoplasm. The second most abundant constituent (10% to 20%) of protoplasm is the cell proteins, which form cell structures and the enzymes necessary for cellular reactions. Lipids constitute 2% to 3% of most cells and are insoluble in water. They serve as a cellular storage form for nutrients and combine with proteins to form the membranes that separate the various compartments of the cell. Only small amounts of carbohydrates are found in the cell, and these are used primarily for fuel. The major intracellular electrolytes are potassium, magnesium, phosphate, sulfate, and bicarbonate. There are also smaller quantities of sodium, chloride, and calcium. These electrolytes facilitate the generation and transmission of electrochemical impulses in nerve and muscle cells. Intracellular electrolytes participate in reactions that are necessary for cellular metabolism. This chapter discusses the functional components of the cell, cellular energy metabolism, tissue types, and membrane potentials.

■ FUNCTIONAL COMPONENTS OF THE CELL

Although diverse in their organization, all cells have common structures that perform unique functions. When seen under a light microscope, three major components of the cell become evident: the nucleus, the cytoplasm, and the cell membrane (Fig. 1-1).

THE NUCLEUS

The nucleus is the control center for the cell. It contains the individual units of inheritance—the *genes*, which are strung along the chromosomes. In the mature or nondividing cell nucleus, darkly stained granules represent inactive regions of chromosomal material. Regions of active genes do not stain. Chemically, each chromosome is an extremely long double-stranded helical molecule of deoxyribonucleic acid (DNA) containing variable sequences of four nitrogenous bases (see Chapter 3). These bases form the genetic code. The double-stranded DNA molecule is periodically coiled about basic proteins called *histones*. Other nonhistone proteins are also bound to it. The complex structure of DNA and DNA-associated proteins dispersed in the nuclear matrix is called *chromatin*.

Genes control cellular activity by determining the type of proteins that are being synthesized in the cytoplasm of the cell. These proteins include enzymes that are used to synthesize other substances including carbohydrates and lipids made by the cell. Chromatin is also the site of ribonucleic acid (RNA) synthesis. There are three kinds of RNA: messenger RNA (mRNA), which copies and carries the DNA instructions for protein synthesis to the cytoplasm; ribosomal RNA (rRNA), which moves to the cytoplasm where it becomes the site of protein synthesis; and transfer RNA (tRNA), which transfers amino acids to the elongating protein as it is being synthesized. In addition to chromatin, the nucleus contains one or more darkly stained round bodies called *nucle-*

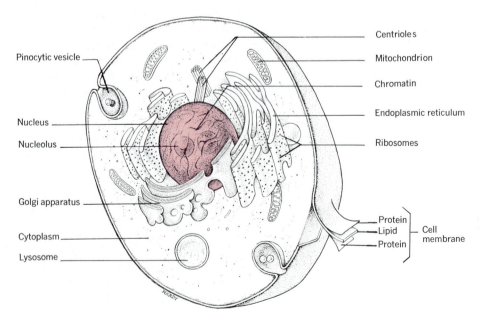

Pinocytic vesicle

Nucleus

Nucleolus

Golgi apparatus

Cytoplasm

Lysosome

Centrioles

Mitochondrion

Chromatin

Endoplasmic reticulum

Ribosomes

Protein
Lipid — Cell
Protein — membrane

FIG. 1-1. Composite cell designed to show, in one cell, all of the various components of the nucleus and cytoplasm. (Chaffee, E. E., & Greisheimer, E. M. [1974]. *Basic physiology and anatomy* [3rd ed.]. Philadelphia: J.B. Lippincott)

oli. They contain the regions of several chromosomes, each with part of the genetic code that is needed for the synthesis of rRNA.

The nuclear contents are surrounded by a doubled membrane called the *nuclear envelope*. This structure has many circular *pores* where the two membranes fuse to form a gap filled with a thin protein diaphragm. There is evidence to suggest that many classes of molecules, including fluids, electrolytes, RNA, some proteins, and perhaps some hormones, can move in both directions across the nuclear pores. The nuclear pore structure apparently regulates which molecules pass from the cytoplasm to the nucleus and vice versa.

THE CYTOPLASM AND ITS ORGANELLES

The cytoplasm surrounds the nucleus, and it is here that the work of the cell takes place. The cytoplasm is essentially a colloidal solution that contains water, electrolytes, suspended proteins, neutral fats, and glycogen molecules. Although they do not contribute to the cell's function, pigments may also accumulate in the cytoplasm. Some pigments, such as melanin, which gives skin its color, are normal constituents of the cell. Bilirubin is a normal major pigment of bile. Excess accumulation of bilirubin within cells is abnormal; it is evidenced clinically by a yellowish discoloration of the skin and sclera, a condition called *jaundice*.

Embedded in the cytoplasm are the *organelles*, or inner organs of the cell. These include the ribosomes, endoplasmic reticulum (ER), Golgi complex, mitochondria, lysosomes, microtubules, and filaments.

Ribosomes.   The ribosomes serve as sites of protein synthesis in the cell. They are small particles of nucleoproteins (rRNA and proteins) that can be found attached to the wall of endoplasmic reticulum or as free ribosomes (Fig. 1-2). The free ribosomes are scattered singly in the cytoplasm or joined to form functional units called *polyribosomes*. The free ribosomes are involved in the synthesis of proteins, such as intracellular enzymes, that are used within the cell. The ribosomes that are attached to the ER synthesize proteins that are exported from the cell.

Endoplasmic Reticulum.   The endoplasmic reticulum (ER) is an extensive system of paired membranes and flat vesicles that connects various parts of the inner cell (see Fig. 1-2). The fluid-filled space (matrix) between the paired ER membrane layers is connected with the space between the two membranes of the double-layered nuclear membrane, the cell membrane, and various cytoplasmic organelles. It functions as a tubular communication system

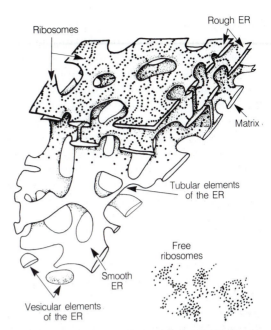

FIG. 1-2. Three-dimensional view of the rough endoplasmic reticulum (ER) with its attached ribosomal RNA and the smooth endoplasmic reticulum.

through which substances can be transported from one part of the cell to another. The large surface area and multiple enzyme systems attached to the ER membranes also provide the machinery for a major share of the metabolic functions of the cell.[1]

There are two types of ER—rough and smooth. The rough ER is studded with ribosomes. The ribosomes of the rough ER synthesize proteins. The rough ER segregates these proteins from other components of the cytoplasm and modifies their structure for a specific function. For example, the synthesis of digestive enzymes by the acinar cells in the pancreas and production of plasma protein by liver cells take place in the rough ER. All cells require rough ER for the synthesis of lysosomal enzymes.

The smooth ER is free of ribosomes and is continuous with the rough ER. The smooth ER contains enzymes involved in the synthesis of lipid molecules, regulation of intracellular calcium, and detoxification of drugs. It is the site of lipid, lipoprotein, and steroid hormone synthesis. The sarcoplasmic reticulum of skeletal and cardiac muscle cells is a form of smooth ER. Calcium ions needed for muscle contraction are stored and released from cisterns located in the sarcoplasmic reticulum of these cells.

In the liver, the smooth ER is involved in glycogen storage and metabolism of lipid-soluble drugs. An interesting form of adaptation occurs in the smooth ER of the liver cells responsible for metabolizing certain drugs such as phenobarbital. Repeated administration of phenobarbital leads to a state of increased tolerance to the drug, such that the same dose no longer produces the same degree of sedation. This response has been traced to increased drug metabolism due to increased synthesis of drug-metabolizing enzymes by the smooth ER of the cells. This enzyme system is sometimes called the *microsomal system* because the ER can be fragmented in the laboratory; when this is done, small vesicles called *microsomes* are formed. The microsomal enzyme system responsible for metabolizing phenobarbital has a crossover effect that influences the metabolism of other drugs that use the same metabolic pathway.

Golgi Complex. The Golgi complex (Golgi appartus) functions in association with the ER and consists of stacks of four or more thin, flat membranous sacs lying near the nucleus. Substances produced in the ER are carried to the Golgi complex in small membrane-covered transfer vesicles. Many cells synthesize proteins that are larger than the active product. Insulin, for example, is synthesized as a larger inactive proinsulin molecule that is cut apart to produce a smaller active insulin molecule in the Golgi complex of the beta cells of the pancreas. The Golgi complex modifies these substances and packages them into secretory granules. After an appropriate signal, the secretory granules move out of the Golgi complex into the cytoplasm and fuse to the inner side of the membrane where they release their contents into the extracellular fluid. Figure 1-3 is a diagram of the synthesis and movement of a hormone through the ER and Golgi complex. In addition to its function in producing secretory granules, the Golgi complex is thought to produce some of the larger carbohydrate molecules that combine with proteins in the rough ER to form glycoproteins.

Mitochondria. The mitochondria are literally the "power plants" of the cell, because it is here that the energy-rich compound adenosine triphosphate (ATP), which powers the various cellular activities, is generated. Only the mitochondria contain the enzymes needed for oxidative metabolism, which is necessary for capturing the energy in foodstuffs and converting it into the high-energy bonds of ATP.

Mitochondria are encased in double membranes. An outer membrane encloses the periphery of the mitochondria, and an inner membrane is enfolded to form the cristae, which aid in the production and temporary storage of ATP (Fig. 1-4). The mitochondria are located close to the site of energy consumption in the cell (*e.g.*, near the myofibrils in muscle cells). The number of mitochondria in a given cell type is largely determined by the type of activity the cell performs and the amount of energy needed to perform this activity.

Lysosomes and Peroxisomes. The lysosomes can be viewed as the digestive system of the cell. They consist of small membrane-enclosed vesicles or sacs that contain many types of hydrolytic enzymes including acid phosphatases and proenzymes that are capable of breaking down worn-out cell parts so they can be recycled. They also break down foreign substances such as bacteria that have been taken into the cell.

The lysosomal enzymes are synthesized in the rough ER and packaged into vesicles in the Golgi complex. Lysosomes that contain hydrolytic enzymes and have not entered into the digestive process are called *primary lysosomes. Secondary lysosomes* are those in which the hydrolytic enzymes have been

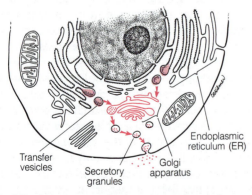

FIG. 1-3. Hormone synthesis and secretion. In hormone secretion, the hormone is synthesized by the ribosomes attached to the rough endoplasmic reticulum (ER). it moves from the rough ER to the Golgi complex where it is stored in the form of secretory granules. These leave the Golgi complex and are stored within the cytoplasm until released from the cell in response to an appropriate signal.

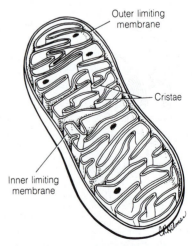

FIG. 1-4. Mitochondrion. The inner membrane forms transverse folds called cristae where the enzymes needed for the final step in adenosine triphosphate (ATP) production (oxidative phosphorylation) are located.

activated and the chemical degradation process has begun. They form when primary lysosomes fuse with material that needs to be digested. Secondary lysosomes can be formed in one of two ways—heterophagy or autophagy (Fig. 1-5). *Heterophagocytosis* refers to the uptake of material from outside the cell. External materials are taken into the cell by an infolding of the cell membrane to form a surrounding phagocytic vesicle or *phagosome*. Primary lysosomes fuse with phagosomes to form secondary lysosomes. Heterophagocytosis is most common in phagocytic white blood cells such as neutrophils and macrophages. *Autophagocytosis* involves the removal of individual cell organelles, such as mitochondria or ER, that have been damaged and must be removed if the cell's normal function is to continue. It is most pronounced in cells undergoing atrophy.

Although the enzymes in the secondary lysosomes are capable of breaking down most proteins, carbohydrates, and lipids to their basic constituents that diffuse through the lysosomal membrane into the cytoplasm, some materials remain undigested. Secondary lysosomes containing undigested material may remain as *residual bodies*, or their contents may be extruded from the cell. In some long-lived cells (neurons and heart muscle), large quantities of residual bodies accumulate as lipofuscin or age pigment. Other indigestible pigments, such as inhaled carbon particles in the lung and tattoo pigments in the skin, also accumulate and persist in residual bodies of macrophages for decades.[2]

The enzymes contained in the lysosomes are so powerful that the lysosomes are sometimes called "suicide bags," because under abnormal conditions

their enzymes can be released, causing massive destruction of cellular contents. This process is called *autolysis*. Under other conditions, primary lysosomes may release their contents into the extracellular spaces, destroying the surrounding cells. The release of lysosomal enzymes from bacteria-laden neutrophils is thought to be a contributing factor in the massive tissue destruction that characterizes purulent (pus-forming) inflammatory lesions.[2]

Lysosomes play an important role in the normal metabolism of certain substances in the body. In some inherited diseases known as *lysosomal storage diseases*, a specific lysosomal enzyme is absent or inactive, in which case the digestion of certain cellular substances (cerebrosides, gangliosides, sphingomyelin, and so forth) does not occur. As a result, these substances accumulate in the cell. In Tay-Sachs disease, an autosomal recessive disorder, the lysosomal enzyme needed for degrading the GM_2 ganglioside is missing. Although the GM_2 ganglioside accumulates in many tissues (*e.g.*, heart, liver, spleen), its accumulation in the nervous system and retina of the eye causes the most damage. Infants born with the disorder are normal at birth but soon begin to develop motor and mental deterioration and blindness as the GM_2 gangliosides accumulate in the nervous system. The course of the disease is rapid and relentless, and death usually occurs in the second or third year of life.

Even smaller than the lysosomes, spherical membrane-bound organelles, called *peroxisomes*, contain a special enzyme that degrades peroxides (*e.g.*, hydrogen peroxide). The peroxisomes function in the control of free radicals (see Chapter 2). Unless degraded, these highly unstable chemical species would otherwise damage other cytoplasmic molecules. Peroxisomes also contain the enzymes involved in breaking down very long chain fatty acids, which are ineffectively degraded by mitochondrial enzymes. In liver cells, enzymes of peroxisomes are involved in the formation of the bile acids.

Microtubules. The microtubules are slender tubular structures composed of globular proteins called *tubulin*. Because they control cell shape and movement, these structures are a major component of the structural elements called the *cytoskeleton*. Microtubules function in a number of ways, including: (1) development and maintenance of cell form; (2) participation in intracellular transport mechanisms, including axoplasmic transport in neurons, and melanin dispersion in pigment cells of the skin; and (3) formation of the basic structure for several complex cytoplasmic organelles, including the centrioles, cilia, and flagella. The *centrioles* are cylindrical structures composed of highly organized microtubules

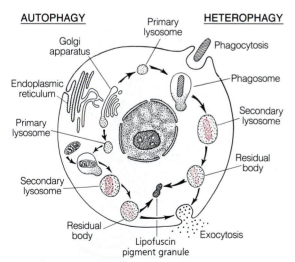

FIG. 1-5. The process of autophagy and heterophagy, showing the primary and secondary lysosomes, residual bodies, extrusion of residual body contents from the cell, and lipofuscin-containing residual bodies.

(see Fig. 1-1). In dividing cells, they form the mitotic spindle that aids in the separation and movement of the chromosomes. *Cilia* and *flagella* are hairlike processes extending from the cell membrane that are capable of sweeping and flailing movements, which can either move surrounding fluids or move the cell through fluid media. They contain a highly organized core of microtubules anchored to a basal body similar to the centrioles. Cilia are found on the wet surface of the epithelial lining of certain body cavities or passages such as the upper respiratory system. Flagella are tail-like structures that provide motility for sperm.

Abnormalities of the cytoskeletal system may contribute to alterations in cell mobility and function. For example, proper functioning of the microtubules is essential for various stages of leukocyte migration. In certain disease conditions, such as diabetes mellitus, alterations in leukocyte mobility and migration may interfere with the chemotaxis and phagocytosis of the inflammatory response and predispose toward the development of bacterial infection.

Microtubules can be rapidly assembled and disassembled according to the needs of the cell. The assembly of microtubules is halted by the action of the plant alkaloid *colchicine*. This compound stops cell mitosis by interfering with formation of the mitotic spindle and is used for cytogenetic (chromosome) studies. It is also used as a drug for treating gout. It is thought that the drug's ability to reduce the inflammatory reaction associated with this condition stems from its ability to interfere with leukocyte microtubular function and migration into the area.[2]

Filaments. The filaments are thin threadlike cytoplasmic structures. There are three classes of filaments: (1) microfilaments, which are equivalent to the thin actin filaments in muscle; (2) intermediate filaments, which are a heterogenous group of filaments with diameter sizes between the thick and thin filaments; and (3) thick myosin filaments, which are present in muscle cells, but may also exist temporarily in other cells as well. Muscle contraction depends on the interaction between the thin actin filaments and thick myosin filaments. Microfilaments are present in the superficial zone of the cytoplasm in almost all cells. Contractile activities involving the microfilaments and associated thick myosin filaments contribute to associated movement of the cytoplasm and cell membrane during endocytosis and exocytosis. Microfilaments are also present in the microvilli of the intestine. The intermediate filaments aid in supporting and maintaining the asymmetric shape of cells. Examples of intermediate filaments are the keratin filaments that are found anchored to the cell membrane of epidermal keratinocytes of the skin and the glial filaments that are found in astrocytes and other glial cells of the nervous system.

THE CELL MEMBRANE

The cell is enclosed in a thin membrane that separates the intracellular contents from the extracellular environment. To distinguish it from the other cell membranes, such as the mitochondrial or nuclear membranes, the cell membrane is often called the *plasma membrane*. In many respects, the plasma membrane is one of the most important parts of the cell. It acts as a semipermeable structure that separates the intracellular and extracellular environments, provides receptors for hormones and other biologically active substances, participates in the electrical events that occur in nerve and muscle cells, and aids in the regulation of cell growth and proliferation. It is also thought that the cell membrane may play an important role in the behavior of cancer cells, which will be discussed in Chapter 5.

The cell membrane consists of an organized arrangement of lipids, carbohydrates, and proteins (Fig. 1-6). The lipids form a bilayer structure that is essentially impermeable to all but lipid-soluble substances. Globular proteins embedded in this lipid bilayer participate in the transport of lipid-insoluble particles through the plasma membrane. Some of the globular proteins move within the membrane structure acting as carriers, some are attached to either side of the membrane, and others pass directly through the membrane and communicate with both the inside and the outside of the cell. It is probable that these latter proteins form channels that permit passage of substances such as water and ions such as sodium, hydrogen, and chloride. Different ions have different membrane channels; for example, one set of channels, called the *sodium channels*, are selectively permeable to sodium.

The cell surface is surrounded by a fuzzy-looking layer called the *cell coat*, or *glycocalyx*. This layer is made up of long complex carbohydrate chains that are attached to protein molecules that penetrate the outside half of the membrane (glycoproteins) and outward facing membrane lipids (glycolipids). The cell coat participates in cell-to-cell recognition and adhesion, and it contains tissue-transplant antigens that label cells as self or nonself. The ABO blood group antigens are contained in the cell coat of red blood cells. There is an intimate relationship between the cell membrane and the cell coat. If the cell coat is enzymatically removed, the cell remains viable and will generate a new cell coat, but damage to the cell membrane usually results in cell death.[1]

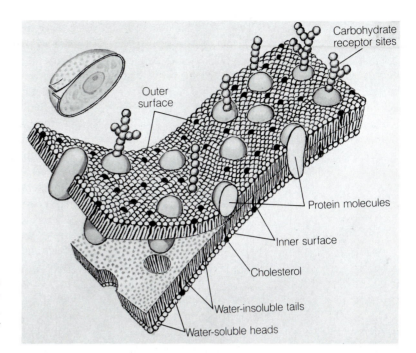

FIG. 1-6. Cell membrane. The right end is intact, but the left end has been split along the plane of the lipid tails. (Chaffee, E. E., & Lytle, I. M. [1980]. *Basic physiology and anatomy* [4th ed.]. Philadelphia: J.B. Lippincott)

In summary, the cell is a remarkably autonomous structure that functions in a manner strikingly similar to that of the total organism. The cell nucleus controls cell function and is the mastermind of the cell, whereas the cytoplasm contains the cell's inner organs and is the cell's work site. The ribosomes serve as sites for protein synthesis in the cell; the ER functions as a tubular communication system through which substances can be transported from one part of the cell to another and as the site of protein (rough ER), carbohydrate, and lipid (smooth ER) synthesis; and the Golgi complex modifies these substances and packages them into secretory granules for export from the cell. The mitochondria serve as power plants for the cell as they transform food energy into ATP, which is used to power cell activities. The lysosomes, which can be viewed as the digestive system of the cell, contain enzymes that digest worn-out cell parts and foreign materials. The microtubules are slender, stiff, tubular structures that influence cell shape, provide a means of moving organelles through the cytoplasm, and affect movement of the cilia and of chromosomes during cell division. Several types of threadlike filaments, including the actin and myosin filaments, participate in muscle contraction. The *plasma membrane* serves as the skin that surrounds the cell and separates it from its surrounding external environment. The cell surface is surrounded by a fuzzy-looking layer called the *cell coat*, which contains tissue antigens and participates in cell-to-cell recognition and adhesion.

■ MEMBRANE TRANSPORT

There is a constant movement of molecules and ions across the cell membrane. This movement is facilitated by diffusion, osmosis, facilitated diffusion, active transport, pinocytosis, phagocytosis, and exocytosis (Fig. 1-7).

DIFFUSION, OSMOSIS, AND TRANSPORT

Diffusion refers to process whereby molecules and other particles in a solution become widely dispersed and reach a uniform concentration due their spontaneous movement. Molecules of gases in solution and other substances move from an area of higher to an area of lower concentration as they diffuse and become evenly distributed across the cell membrane. Lipid-soluble molecules such as oxygen, carbon dioxide, alcohol, and fatty acids become dissolved in the lipid matrix of the cell membrane and diffuse through the membrane in the same manner that diffusion occurs in water. Other substances diffuse through fluid in minute pores of the cell membrane.

Most cell membranes are semipermeable in that they are permeable to water but not all solute particles. *Osmosis* is the passage of water across a semipermeable membrane. It is regulated by the concentration of nondiffusible particles on either side of the membrane. For example, when different concentrations of particles are present on the two sides of a semipermeable membrane, water will move from the side that has the lesser number of particles to the side with the greater number of particles. This movement of water will continue until the solute particles on both sides of the membrane are equally diluted or until the hydrostatic pressure created by the movement of water opposes its flow.

Facilitated diffusion involves a carrier system. Some substances, such as glucose, cannot pass through the cell membrane because they are not

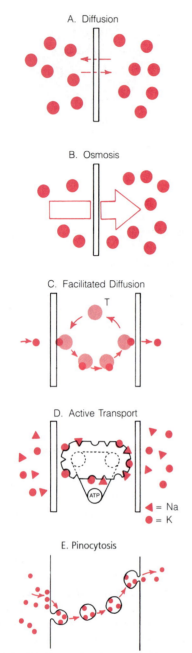

FIG. 1-7. Mechanisms of membrane transport. (**A**) Diffusion, in which particles move to become equally distributed across the membrane. (**B**) The osmotically active particles regulate the flow of water. (**C**) Facilitated diffusion uses a carrier system. (**D**) In active transport, selected molecules are transported across the membrane using the energy-driven (ATP) pump. (**E**) The membrane forms a vesicle that engulfs the particle and transports it across the membrane, where it is released. This is called pinocytosis.

lipid-soluble or are too large to pass through the membrane's pores. These substances combine with a special lipid-soluble carrier at the membrane's outer surface, are carried across the membrane attached to the carrier, and are released. In facilitated diffusion, a substance can move only from an area of higher

concentration to an area of lower concentration. The rate at which a substance moves across the membrane as a result of facilitated diffusion depends on the difference in concentration between the two sides of the membrane, the amount of carrier that is available for transport, and the rapidity with which the carrier can bind and release the substance. It is thought that insulin, which increases glucose transport, may increase either the amount of carrier that is present or the rate at which the reactions between glucose and the carrier take place.

Whereas diffusion and facilitated diffusion describe the movement of substances from an area of higher concentration to one of lower concentration, active transport is the movement of substances across the cell membrane against a concentration gradient (*i.e.*, from a lower to a higher concentration). Active transport requires expenditure of energy from the hydrolysis of ATP. The sodium and potassium membrane transport system, some times called the *sodium–potassium pump*, is an example of active transport. The sodium–potassium pump moves sodium from the inside to the outside of the cell, where its concentration is about 14 times greater than inside, and returns potassium to the inside, where its concentration is about 35 times greater than it is outside the cell. Were it not for the activity of the sodium–potassium pump, the osmotically active sodium particles would accumulate within the cell, causing cellular swelling due to an accompanying influx of water (see Chapter 2).

ENDOCYTOSIS AND EXOCYTOSIS

Endocytosis is the process whereby cells engulf materials from their surroundings. It includes pinocytosis and phagocytosis. Pinocytosis involves the ingestion of small amounts of extracellular fluid and dissolved particles by engulfing them into small membrane-surrounded vesicles for movement into the cytoplasm; it is important in the transport of proteins and strong solutions of electrolytes.

Phagocytosis involves the engulfment and killing or degradation of microorganisms and other particulate matter. During phagocytosis, a particle comes in contact with cell surface, is surrounded on all sides by the cell membrane, and forms a phagocytic vesicle. Once formed, the vesicle breaks away from the cell membrane and moves into the cytoplasm, where its contents are eventually freed by the action of lysosomes or other cytoplasmic enzymes. Blood neutrophils and macrophages are phagocytic cells (see Chapter 13).

Exocytosis is the mechanism for the secretion of intracellular substances into the extracellular spaces.

It is the reverse of endocytosis in that a secretory granule fuses to the inner side of the cell membrane and an opening occurs to the outside of the cell surface. This opening allows the contents of the granule to be released into the extracellular fluid. Exocytosis is important in removing cellular debris and releasing substances, such as hormones, that have been synthesized in the cell.

■ MEMBRANE POTENTIALS

The human body runs off a system of self-generated electricity in which cell membranes function like batteries. Electrical potentials exist across the membranes of most, if not all, cells in the body. Because these potentials occur at the level of the cell membrane, they are called *membrane potentials*. In excitable tissues, such as nerve or muscle cells, changes in the membrane potential are necessary for generation and conduction of nerve impulses and muscle contraction. In other types of cells, such as glandular cells, changes in the membrane potential contribute to hormone secretion and other functions.

An electrical potential, measured in volts (V), describes the ability of separated electrical charges of opposite polarity (+ and −) to do work. The potential difference is the difference between the separated charges. The terms *potential difference* and *voltage* are synonymous. Voltage is always measured with respect to two points in a system. For example, the voltage in a car battery (6 or 12 V) is the potential difference between the two battery terminals. Because the total amount of charge that can be separated by a biologic membrane is small, the potential differences are small and are measured in *millivolts* (1/1000 of a volt). The voltage or potential difference between the inside and the outside of a cell can be measured in the laboratory by inserting a very fine electrode into the cell and another into the extracellular fluid surrounding the cell and connecting the two electrodes to a voltmeter (Fig. 1-8). The movement of charge between two points is called *current*; it occurs when a potential difference has been established and a connection is made so that the charged particles are able to move between the two points.

Both extracellular and intracellular fluids are electrolyte solutions containing about 150 to 160 mmol/L of positively charged ions and an equal concentration of negatively charged ions; these are the *current-carrying ions* responsible for generating and conducting membrane potentials. Generally, there is a small excess of charged ions outside the cell membrane. This is represented as positive charges on the outside of the membrane and equal numbers of negative charges on the inside. Because of the extreme thinness of the

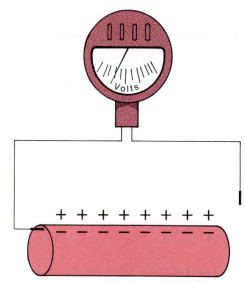

FIG. 1-8. *Alignment of charge along the cell membrane. The electrical potential is negative on the inside of the cell membrane in relation to the outside.*

cell membrane, these ions accumulate on either side of the membrane, contributing to the establishment of a membrane potential.

DIFFUSION POTENTIALS

A diffusion potential describes the voltage that is generated by ions that diffuse across the membrane. Two conditions are necessary for a membrane potential to occur as a result of diffusion: (1) the membrane must be selectively permeable, allowing a single type of ion to diffuse through membrane pores, and (2) the concentration of the diffusible ion must be greater on one side of the membrane than on the other. In the resting or unexcited state when the membrane is highly permeable to potassium, the concentration of potassium ions inside of the cell is about 35 times that on the outside of the cell. Because of the large concentration gradient from inside to outside, there is a strong tendency for the potassium ions to diffuse outward. As they do so, they carry their positive charges with them, thus the inside becomes negative in relation to the outside. This new potential difference repels further outward movement of the positively charged potassium ions. The same phenomenon occurs during an action potential when the membrane is highly permeable to sodium. The sodium ions move to the inside of the membrane, creating a membrane potential of the opposite polarity. An *equilibrium potential* is one in which there is no net movement of ions because the diffusion and electrical forces are exactly balanced. The following equation, known as the *Nernst equation*, can be used to calculate the equilibrium potential (electromotive force; EMF) of an univalent ion at a body temperature of 37°C.

$$EMF \text{ (millivolts)} = -61 \times \log \frac{\text{ion concentration inside}}{\text{ion concentration outside}}$$

For example, if the concentration of an ion inside the membrane was 100 mM and the concentration outside was 10 mM, the equilibrium potential for that ion would be $-61 \log (100/10 = 10$ and the log of 10 is 1). That is, it would take 61 mV of charge on the inside of the membrane to balance the diffusion potential created by the concentration difference across the membrane for this ion.

If the membrane were permeable only to potassium and there was no pumping of ions across the membrane, the equilibrium potential for the potassium ion, using normal intracellular (140 mM) and extracellular (4 mM) concentrations, would be -94 mV ($-61 \times \log 140$ mM/4 mM). This value approximates the -70 mV to -90 mV resting membrane potential for nerve fibers that has been measured in laboratory studies. Likewise, the equilibrium potential for sodium (intracellular 14 mM and extracellular 140 mM) would be about $+61$ mV ($-61 \times \log 14$ mM/140 mM) during the fraction of a second that occurs at the peak of the action potential when the membrane is much more permeable to the sodium ion than to the potassium ion. Again, this value is similar to the $+45$ mV value that has been measured experimentally in nerve fibers. When the membrane is permeable to several different ions, the diffusion potential reflects the sum of the diffusion potentials for the different ions.

RESTING MEMBRANE POTENTIALS

The resting membrane potential is the EMF that exists when a nerve or muscle is not transmitting an electrical impulse. The resting membrane potential is characterized by the relatively low permeability of the membrane to the rapid flow of charged ions. During this phase, there is about 70 to 90 mV less charge on the inside of the membrane (-70 to 90 mV) than on the outside. This difference in concentration of charge is necessary for the establishment of current flow once the membrane becomes permeable to the flow of charged ions. The membrane is said to be polarized during this phase because of the large negative membrane potential that is present and because charges of opposite polarity ($+$ and $-$) are aligned across the membrane.

Three factors contribute to the establishment of the resting membrane potential: (1) the presence of large numbers of nondiffusible negatively charged

intracellular anions, such as protein ions, sulfate ions, and phosphate ions; (2) the selective permeability of the resting membrane to the potassium ion; and (3) the sodium–potassium pump (Fig. 1-9). In the resting state, most excitable membranes are 50 to 100 times more permeable to potassium ions than to sodium ions. Despite this enhanced permeability, the positively charged potassium ions remain inside the membrane, attracted by the nondiffusible intracellular anions and repelled by the positively charged extracellular sodium ions. Although the cell membrane is relatively impermeable to the sodium ion, some sodium ions do cross the membrane and are subsequently extruded by the sodium–potassium membrane pump. In the process of removing sodium ions from inside the membrane, the sodium–potassium pump extrudes three positively charged sodium ions for every two positively charged potassium ions that are returned to the inside of the membrane; this results in a net removal of positive

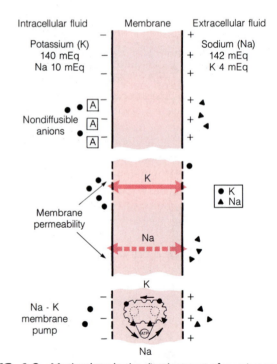

FIG. 1-9. Mechanisms in the development of membrane potentials. Three factors contribute to the difference in electrical potential (negative on the inside and positive on the outside) and Na^+ and K^+ concentration across the cell membrane: (1) the presence of nondiffusible anions on the inside of the embrane, which attract the positively charged K^+ ions; (2) selective permeability of the resting membrane to Na^+ and K^+ (the resting membrane is 100 times more permeable to K^+ than to Na^+) so that K^+ diffuses and remains inside the membrane and Na^+ remains outside; and (3) the Na^+–K^+ membrane pump, which extrudes three Na^+ ions for every two K^+ ions admitted, resulting in a net removals of positive charge from inside the membrane.

charges so that the inside becomes more negative than the outside.

ACTION POTENTIALS

Action potentials are abrupt, pulselike changes in the membrane potential that last a few ten thousandths to a few thousandths of a second. In a nerve fiber, an action potential can be elicited by any factor that suddenly increases the permeability of the membrane to the sodium ion. There are pores or channels in the cell membrane through which the current-carrying ions flow. These membrane channels are guarded by electrically operated "gates" that open and close with changes in the membrane potential (Fig. 1-10). The sodium and potassium ions use different channels as they move through the membrane, allowing the membrane to change its permeability during different phases of the action potential. Many tissues have similar channels for the calcium ion.

The *threshold potential* (about −60 mV) represents the membrane potential at which neurons or other excitable tissue are stimulated to fire. Stimuli that excite a neuron produce marked increases in membrane permeability and an increased flow of sodium ions across the membrane, causing it to become less negative and moving it toward the threshold potential. When the threshold potential is reached, the sodium channel gates swing open and there is a rapid inflow of positively charged sodium ions across the membrane. Once a neuron reaches the minimal threshold for excitation, it is committed to fire and its response will be maximal. This is called the *all-or-none law*.

Action potentials can be divided into three phases—the resting or polarized state, depolarization, and repolarization (Fig. 1-11).

The *resting phase* represents the period before the action potential begins. The membrane is said to be polarized during this phase because of the very large negative potential that is present.

Depolarization is the phase of the action potential during which the membrane is highly permeable to sodium ions. During this phase, the sodium gates are open and there is reversal of the membrane potential; the inside of the membrane becomes positive (about +30 to +45 mV). In neurons, the sodium ion gate remains open for only about a quarter of a millisecond and closes quickly.

Repolarization is the phase during which the polarity of the resting membrane potential is reestablished. This is accomplished as sodium channels

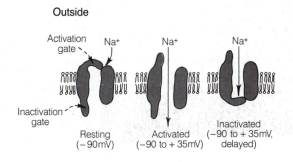

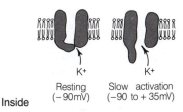

FIG. 1-10. Voltage-gated sodium and potassium channels, showing activation and inactivation of the sodium channel but activation of the potassium channels only when the membrane potential is changed from the normal negative resting value to a positive value. (Guyton, A. [1991]. *Textbook of medical physiology* [8th ed., p. 56]. Philadelphia: W.B. Saunders)

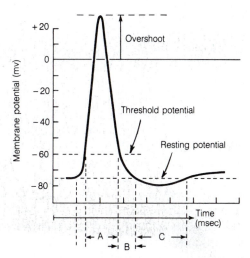

A = Absolute refractory period (active potential and partial recovery)
B = Relative refractory period
C = Positive relative refractory period

FIG. 10-11. Time course of the action potential recorded at one point of an axon with one electrode inside and one on the outside of the plasma membrane. The rising part of the action potential is called the spike. The rising phase plus approximately the first half of the repolarization phase is equal to the absolute refractory period (A). The portion of the repolarization phase that extends from the threshold to the resting membrane potential represents the relative refractory period (B). The remaining portion of the repolarization phase to the resting membrane potential is equal to the negative after potential (C). Hyperpolarization is equal to the positive relative refractory period.

close and sodium permeability decreases while potassium permeability increases. The outflow of positively charged potassium ions returns the membrane potential to negativity. The sodium–potassium pump gradually reestablishes the resting ionic concentrations on each side of the membrane.

The membrane of an excitable cell must be sufficiently repolarized before it can be reexcited. In the process of repolarization, the membrane remains refractory (will not fire) until the repolarization is about one third complete. This period, which lasts about half a millisecond, is called the *absolute refractory period*. There is an additional portion of the recovery period during which the membrane can be excited, but only by a stronger-than-normal stimulus. This period is called the *relative refractory period*.

ALTERATIONS IN MEMBRANE EXCITABILITY

Two main factors alter membrane excitability: (1) changes in the resting membrane potential and (2) changes in the permeability of the membrane.

The excitability of a neuron or muscle fiber depends on the amount of change in membrane potential that is needed to initiate an action potential. When the resting membrane potential becomes extremely negative, the membrane is said to be *hyperpolarized*. When this happens, reexcitation becomes more difficult or does not occur. *Hypopolarization*, on the other hand, represents the situation in which the resting membrane potential *becomes less negative*. When the resting membrane potential approaches the threshold potential, the membrane becomes extremely excitable and may undergo spontaneous depolarization.

Serum levels of potassium exert a strong influence on the repolarization (and resting membrane potential) of excitable tissue. When serum levels of potassium decrease, the resting membrane potential becomes more negative, and nerve and muscle fibers become hyperpolarized, sometimes to the extent that they cannot be reexcited. *Familial periodic paralysis* is a hereditary condition in which extracellular potassium levels periodically fall to low levels, causing muscle paralysis (see Chapter 29). An increase in serum potassium, on the other hand, causes the resting membrane potential to become hypopolarized as it moves closer to threshold. When this happens, the amplitude of the action potential is decreased because the membrane has not been fully repolarized. Should the resting potential be reduced so that it approaches zero, the membrane will remain depolarized and unexcitable. This situation is similar to what happens when a car battery goes dead and

needs to be recharged. Elevations in serum potassium exert their greatest effect on the conduction system of the heart. The force of cardiac contractions becomes weaker until, eventually, repolarization is inadequate to maintain excitability, and the heart stops beating.

Neural excitability is markedly altered by changes in membrane permeability. Calcium ions decrease membrane permeability to sodium ions. If there are not enough calcium ions available, the permeability of the membrane to sodium increases and, as a result, membrane excitability increases—sometimes to the extent that spontaneous muscle movements (tetany) occur. *Local anesthetic agents* (such as procaine or cocaine) act directly on neural membranes to decrease their permeability to sodium.

In summary, body cells generate their own electricity. Electrical potentials (negative on the inside and positive on the outside) exist across the membranes of most cells in the body. These electrical potentials result from the selective permeability of the cell membrane to Na^+ and K^+, the presence of nondiffusible anions inside the cell membrane, and the activity of the sodium–potassium membrane pump, which extrudes Na^+ from the inside of the membrane and returns K^+ to the inside. In the resting state, there is no net flow of electrically charged ions across the cell membranes in excitable tissues. An action potential is an abrupt, pulselike change in the membrane potential. It consists of a depolarization phase during which the membrane is permeable to the rapid inflow of charged ions, causing reversal (positive on the inside and negative on the outside) of the membrane potential, and a repolarization phase during which the resting membrane potential is reestablished. The threshold potential is the change in membrane potential that is sufficient to produce an action potential. The refractory period represents the time during the repolarization period when a cell absolutely cannot be reexcited (absolute refractory period) or requires a stronger than normal stimulus. Hyperpolarization refers to the situation in which the resting membrane potential becomes extremely negative, and hypopolarization refers to the situation in which it becomes less negative.

■ CELLULAR ENERGY METABOLISM

Energy is defined as the ability to do work. Cells use oxygen and the breakdown products of the foods we eat to produce the energy needed for muscle contraction, transport of ions and molecules, and the synthesis of enzymes, hormones, and other macromolecules. *Energy metabolism* refers to the processes by which fats, proteins, and carbohydrates from the foods we eat are converted into energy or complex energy sources in the cell. There are two phases of metabolism, *catabolism* and *anabolism*. Catabolism consists of the breaking down of stored nutrients and body tissues to produce energy. Anabolism is a build-

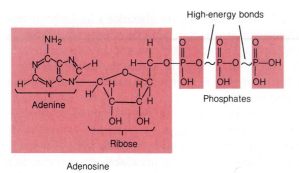

FIG. 1-12. Structure of the adenosine triphosphate (ATP) molecule.

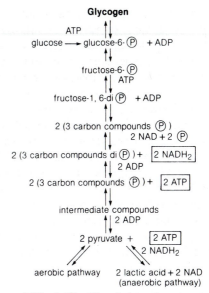

FIG. 1-13. Glycolytic pathway.

ing-up process in which more complex molecules are formed from simpler ones.

The special carrier for cellular energy is ATP. The ATP molecule consists of adenosine, a nitrogenous base; ribose, a five-carbon sugar; and three phosphate groups (Fig. 1-12). The phosphate groups are attached by two high-energy bonds. Large amounts of free energy are released when ATP is hydrolyzed to form adenosine diphosphate (ADP), an adenosine molecule that contains two phosphate groups. The free energy liberated from the hydrolysis of ATP is used to drive reactions that require free energy, such as muscle contraction. In turn, energy from foodstuffs is used to convert ADP back to ATP. ATP is often referred to as the "energy currency" of the cell; energy can be "saved or spent" using ATP as an exchange currency.

There are two sites of energy production in the cell: (1) the anaerobic (without oxygen) glycolytic pathway, which is located in the cytoplasm, and (2) the aerobic (with oxygen) pathways in the mitochondria. The glycolytic pathway serves as the prelude to the aerobic pathways.

ANAEROBIC METABOLISM

Glycolysis is the process by which energy is liberated from glucose (Fig. 1-13). Glycolysis is an important energy provider for cells that lack mitochondria, the cell structure in which aerobic metabolism occurs. The process also provides energy in situations when delivery of oxygen to the cell is either delayed or impaired. The process involves a sequence of reactions that converts glucose to pyruvate with the concomitant production of ATP from ADP. The net gain of energy from the glycolysis of one molecule of glucose is two ATP molecules. Although relatively inefficient in terms of energy yield, the glycolytic pathway is important during periods of decreased oxygen delivery, such as occurs in skeletal muscle during the first few minutes of exercise.

Glycolysis requires the presence of nicotinamide-adenine dinucleotide (NAD^+), a hydrogen carrier. The end-products of glycolysis are pyruvate and NADH. When oxygen is present, pyruvate moves into the aerobic mitochondrial pathway and NADH subsequently enters into oxidative chemical reactions that remove the hydrogen atoms. The transfer of hydrogen from NADH during the oxidative reactions allows the glycolytic process to continue by facilitating the regeneration of NAD^+. Under anaerobic conditions, such as cardiac arrest or circulatory shock, the majority of pyruvate is converted to lactic acid, which diffuses out of the cells into the extracellular fluid. The conversion of pyruvate to lactic acid is reversible, so that, once the oxygen supply has been restored, lactic acid is either converted back to pyruvate or used to synthesize glucose.

Heart cells are particularly efficient in converting lactic acid to pyruvic acid and using this as a fuel source. This is a particularly important source of fuel for the heart during heavy exercise when the skeletal muscles are producing large amounts of lactic acid and releasing it into the bloodstream.[1]

AEROBIC METABOLISM

Aerobic metabolism occurs in the cell's mitochondria and involves the citric acid cycle and oxidative phosphoration. It is here that hydrogen and carbon molecules from the fats, proteins, and carbohydrates in our diet are broken down and combined with molecular oxygen to form carbon dioxide and water as energy is released. Unlike lactic acid, which is an end-product of anaerobic metabolism, carbon dioxide and water are relatively harmless and easily eliminated from the body. In a 24-hour period, oxidative metabolism supplies the body with 300 to 500 ml of water.

The citric acid cycle, sometimes called the *tricarboxylic acid* or *Krebs' cycle*, provides the final common pathway for the metabolism of nutrients (Fig. 1-14). In the citric acid cycle, an activated two-carbon molecule of acetyl coenzyme A (acetyl-CoA) condenses with a four-carbon molecule of oxaloacetic acid and moves through a series of enzyme-mediated steps in which hydrogen and carbon dioxide are formed. As hydrogen is generated, it combines with one of two special carriers, NAD^+ or flavin adenine dinucleotide (FAD), as a means of transfer to the electron transport system. The carbon dioxide molecule that is formed is carried to the lungs and exhaled. In the citric acid cycle, each of the two pyruvate molecules that were formed in the cytoplasm from one molecule of glucose yields another molecule of ATP along with two molecules of carbon dioxide and eight hydrogen atoms. These hydrogen molecules are transferred to the electron transport system on the inner mitochondrial membrane for oxidation. In addition to pyruvate from the glycolysis of glucose, products of amino acid and fatty acid degradation enter the citric acid cycle.

Oxidative metabolism, which supplies 90% of the body's energy needs, is the process whereby hydrogen that is generated during the citric acid cycle combines with oxygen to form ATP and water. It is accomplished by a series of enzymatically catalyzed reactions that split each hydrogen atom into a hydrogen ion and an electron. During the process of ionization, the electrons that are removed from the hydrogen atoms enter an electron transport chain that is part of the inner membrane of the mitochrondion. This electron transport chain consists of electron acceptors that can be reversibly reduced or oxidized by accepting or giving up electrons. Each electron is shuttled from one acceptor to another until it reaches the end of the chain where its final two electrons are used to reduce elemental oxygen so that it can combine with the hydrogen ions to form water. As the electrons move along the electron transport chain, large amounts of energy are released. This energy is used to convert ADP to ATP. Because the formation of ATP involves the addition of a high-energy phosphate bond to ADP, the process is sometimes called *oxidative phosphorylation*. Cyanide causes death by poisoning the enzymes needed for one of the final steps in the oxidative phosphorylation sequence.

In summary, cellular energy metabolism is the process whereby the carbohydrates, fats, and proteins from the foods we eat are broken down and converted into energy that is stored in the form of ATP's high-energy bonds. There are two sites of energy metabolism in cells: the mitochondria and the cytoplasmic matrix. The most efficient of these pathways are the aerobic pathways located in the mitochondria. These pathways require oxygen and produce carbon dioxide and water as end-products. The glycolytic pathway, which is located in the cytoplasm, involves the breakdown of glucose to form ATP. It requires the presence of NAD^+ as a hydrogen acceptor. The end-products of glycolysis are pyruvate and NADH (hydrogen atoms attached to NAD^+). When oxygen is not available, NADH transfers its hydrogen atoms to pyruvate with the resultant formation of lactic acid.

■ TISSUE TYPES

In the preceding sections, we discussed the individual cell and its metabolic processes. Although cells are similar, their structure and function vary according to the needs of the tissues. There are four categories of specialized tissue: epithelium, connective tissue, muscle, and nerve. This section provides a brief overview of these tissue types as preparation for understanding the subsequent chapters in this and other units.

CELL DIFFERENTIATION

The formation of different types of cells and the disposition of these cells into tissue types is called *cell differentiation*. After conception, the fertilized ovum divides and subdivides and ultimately forms over a hundred different cell types. The process of cell differentiation normally moves forward and is irreversible, producing cells that are more specialized than their predecessors. This means that, once differentiation has occurred, the tissue type does not move

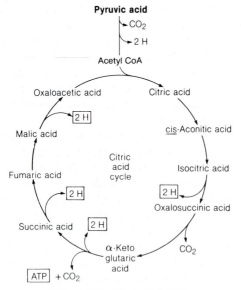

FIG. 1-14. Citric acid cycle.

backward to an earlier stage of differentiation. Usually, a highly differentiated cell loses its ability to undergo cell division.

Although most cells proceed through differentiation into specialized cell types, many tissues contain a few cells that apparently are only partially differentiated. These cells are still capable of cell division and serve as a stem cell, or reserve source, for continued production of specialized cells throughout the life of the organism. This is one of the major processes that make regeneration possible in some tissues. The gastrointestinal mucosal tissue, for example, has undifferentiated cells that allow for regeneration, whereas skeletal muscle tissue lacks undifferentiated cells and has limited regenerative capacity. Cancer cells are thought to originate from undifferentiated stem cells (see Chapter 5).

EMBRYONIC ORIGIN OF TISSUE TYPES

The four basic tissue types are often described in terms of embryonic origin. The very young embryo is essentially a three-layered tubular structure (Fig. 1-15). The outer layer of the tube is called the *ectoderm;* the middle layer is called the *mesoderm;* and the inner layer is called the *endoderm*. All of the adult body tissues originate from these three cellular layers. Epithelium has its origin in all three embryonic layers, connective tissue and muscle develop from the mesoderm, and nervous tissue develops from the ectoderm. Mesenchymal tissue is a precursor to connective tissue and has its origin in the mesoderm. The epithelial lining of the gut, the respiratory tract, and much of the urinary system is derived from the endoderm.

All of the more than 100 different types of body cells can be classified under four basic or primary tissue types: epithelial, connective, muscle, and nervous (Table 1-1). Nervous tissue, a specialized form of tissue designed for communication, is discussed in Chapter 47.

EPITHELIAL TISSUE

Epithelial tissue covers the body's outer surface, lines the internal surface, and forms the glandular tissue. The epithelium protects (skin and mucous membranes), secretes (glandular tissue and goblet cells), absorbs (intestinal mucosa), and filters (renal glomeruli). The epithelial cells are avascular (*i.e.,* they have no blood vessels of their own and must receive oxygen and nutrients from the capillaries of the connective tissue on which the epithelium rests; Fig. 1-16). To survive, the epithelial cells must be kept moist. Even the seemingly dry skin epithelium is kept moist by a nonvitalized waterproof layer of superficial skin cells filled with intermediate diameter filaments of tough protein called *keratin*, which prevents evaporation of moisture from the deeper living cells. Epithelium is able to regenerate quickly when injured.

Epithelial cells that cover the body or line body cavities are classified into three types according to the shape of the cells and the number of layers that are present: *simple, stratified*, and *pseudostratified*. The terms *squamous* (thin and flat), *cuboidal* (cube-shaped), and *columnar* (resembling a column) refer to the cell shapes (Fig. 1-17).

Simple epithelium contains a single layer of cells. Simple squamous epithelium is adapted for filtration; it is found lining the blood vessels, lymph nodes, and alveoli of the lungs. The single layer of squamous epithelium that lines the inside of the heart and blood vessels is known as the *endothelium*. A similar type of layer, called the *mesothelium*, is found in the serous membranes that line the pleura and the pericardial and peritoneal cavities. *Simple cuboidal epithelium* is found on the surface of the ovary and in the thyroid. *Simple columnar epithelium* lines the intestine. One form of simple columnar epithelium has hairlike projections called *cilia*, and another produces mucus and is called a *goblet* cell.

Stratified epithelium contains more than one layer of cells and is designed to protect the body surface. *Keratin* is a tough, fibrous protein in the form of filaments within the outer cells of skin epithelium. The outermost cells become totally filled with keratin and die, to be sloughed off and replaced by similar cells generated deeper in the stratified epithelium. Stratified squamous keratinized epithelium makes up the epidermis of the skin, and nonkeratinized cells are found on wet surfaces such as the mouth and tongue. *Pseudostratified epithelium* is a form of strati-

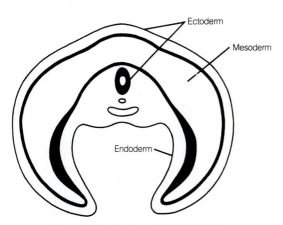

FIG. 1-15. Embryonic tissue layers.

TABLE 1-1. CLASSIFICATION OF TISSUE TYPES

TISSUE TYPE	LOCATION*
Epithelial	
Covering and Lining of Body Surfaces	
Simple epithelium	
Squamous	Lining of blood vessels and body cavities
Cuboidal	Covering of ovaries and thyroid gland
Columnar	Lining of intestine and gallbladder
Pseudostratified epithelium	Trachea and respiratory passages
Stratified epithelium	
Squamous keratinized	Skin
Squamous nonkeratinized	Mucous membranes of mouth, esophagus, and vagina
Transitional	Bladder
Glandular	
Endocrine	Pituitary, thyroid, adrenal, others
Exocrine	Sweat glands and glands in gastrointestinal tract
Connective	
Loose	Fibroblasts, adipose tissue, endothelial vessel lining
Hematopoietic	Blood cells, myeloid tissue (bone marrow), lymphoid tissue
Supporting tissues	Connective tissue and cartilage, bone and joint structures
Muscle	
Skeletal	Skeletal muscles
Cardiac	Myocardium
Smooth	Gastrointestinal tract, blood vessels, bronchi, bladder, others
Nervous	
Neurons	Central and peripheral neurons and nerve fibers
Supporting cells	Glial and ependymal cells in central nervous system, Schwann and satellite cells in peripheral nervous system

* Not inclusive.

fied epithelium in which all of the cells are in contact with the underlying intercellular matrix, but some do not extend the surface. Pseudostratified columnar ciliated epithelium with goblet cells forms the lining of most of the upper respiratory tract. All of the tall cells reaching the surface of this type of epithelium are ciliated cells or goblet cells. The basal cells that do not reach the surface serve as stem cells for the ciliated cells and goblet cells.[3]

Transitional epithelium is similar to stratified keratinized epithelium with the exception that its surface cells can change shape and become thinner when the tissue is stretched. Such tissue can be stretched without pulling the superficial cells apart. Transitional epithelium is well adapted for the lining of organs that are constantly changing their volume, such as the bladder.

Glandular epithelium can be divided into two types: exocrine and endocrine. The *exocrine glands* have ducts and discharge their secretions directly onto the epithelial surface where they are located. Sweat glands and alveolar glands are examples of exocrine glands. The *endocrine glands* produce secretions that move directly into the bloodstream.

CELL JUNCTIONS

Epithelial cells are held together by the intercellular adhesions that connect the membranes of adjacent cells. There are at least three types of intercellular junctions: tight junctions, adhering junctions, and gap junctions (Fig. 1-18). Often the cells in epithelial tissue are joined by all three types of junctions.

Tight or *occluding junctions*, which are found only

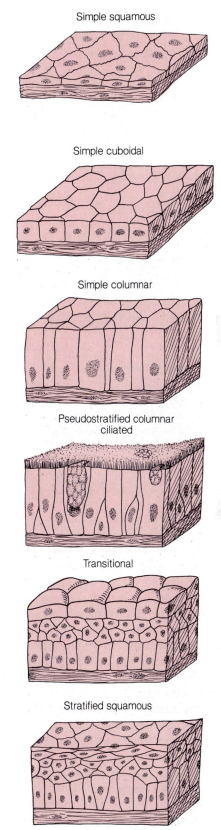

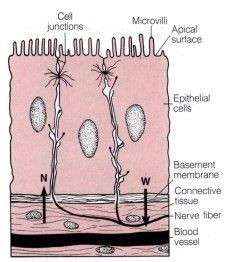

Simple squamous

Simple cuboidal

Simple columnar

Pseudostratified columnar ciliated

Transitional

Stratified squamous

FIG. 1-16. Typical arrangement of epithelial cells in relation to underlying tissues and blood supply. Epithelial tissue has no blood supply of its own but relies on the blood vessels in the underlying connective tissue for nutrition (*N*) and elimination of wastes (*W*).

in epithelial tissue, actually seal the surface membranes of adjacent cells together. This type of intercellular junction prevents materials such as macromolecules present in the intestinal contents from entering the intercellular space.

Adhering junctions represent a site of strong adhesion between cells. The primary role of adhering junctions appears to be that of preventing cell separation. Adhering junctions are not restricted to epithelial tissue; they provide adherence between adjacent cardiac muscle cells as well. There are two types of adhering junctions: continuous beltlike adhesive junctions and scattered spotlike adhesive junctions, called *desmosomes*.

Gap junctions, or *nexus*, involve the close adherence of adjoining cell membranes with the formation of channels that link the cytoplasm of the two cells. Again, the gap junctions are not unique to epithelial tissue; they are also present in heart tissue. Gap junctions play an essential role in cell-to-cell communication. Because they are low-resistance channels, gap junctions are important in cell-to-cell conduction of electrical signals such as between adjacent cardiac muscle cells or in sheets of smooth muscle cells. These multiple communication channels also enable ions and small molecules to pass directly from one cell to another.

CONNECTIVE TISSUE

Connective tissue is the most abundant tissue in the body. As its name indicates, it connects and holds tissues together. Connective tissue is unique in that it

FIG. 1-17. *Representation of the various epithelial tissue types.*

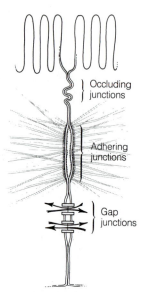

FIG. 1-18. Intercellular junctions. The tight occluding junctions (*top*) form a tight seal between adjacent cells, adhering junctions (*middle*) form a adhesive bond between adjacent cells, and gap junctions or nexus (*bottom*) form communicating channels that link the cytoplasm of adjoining cells.

includes nonliving forms of intracellular substances, such as collagen fibers and the tissue gel that fills the intercellular spaces. Connective tissue can be divided into three types: (1) *loose connective* tissue, (2) *hematopoietic* types of connective tissue, and (3) *strong supporting* types of tissue.

LOOSE CONNECTIVE TISSUE

Loose connective tissue is soft and pliable and contains large amounts of intercellular substance (Fig. 1-19). Loose connective tissue supports the epithelial tissues and provides the means by which these tissues are nourished. In an organ containing both functioning epithelial tissue and supporting connective tissue, the term *parenchymal tissue* is used to describe the functioning epithelium in contradistinction to the connective tissue framework. Cells of loose connective tissue include: fibroblasts, mast cells, adipose or fat cells, and the endothelial cells that line blood vessels.

The fibroblasts secrete substances that form the intercellular matrix that supports and connects body cells. These intercellular substances are of two types: the fibrous type (collagen, elastin, and reticular fibers), which holds cells together, and the amorphous type, which fills the tissue spaces. *Collagen* is the most common protein in the body; it is a tough, nonliving white fiber that serves as the structural framework for skin, ligaments, tendons, and nu-

merous other structures. *Elastin* acts like a rubber band; it can be stretched and then return to its original form. Elastin fibers are abundant in structures that are subjected to frequent stretching, such as the aorta. *Reticular fibers* are extremely thin fibers that create a flexible network in organs that are subjected to changes in form or volume, such as the spleen, liver, uterus, or intestinal muscle layer. The amorphous (nonliving) intercellular ground substance that fills the tissue spaces has a gel-like consistency and is sometimes referred to as *tissue gel*. Hyaluronic acid, which is one of the main components of tissue gel, has the ability to hold vast amounts of water; it facilitates the even dispersion of intercellular fluids and aids in the exchange of cellular nutrients and metabolites. In certain physiologic or pathologic conditions, a condition called *edema* develops in which there is an excess accumulation of water in the tissue gel of the intercellular matrix (see Chapter 29).

The *basement membrane* or basal lamina is a special type of intercellular matrix that is present where connective tissue comes in contact with the tissue it supports. A basement membrane is found along the interface between connective tissue and muscle fibers, on Schwann's cells of the peripheral nervous system, on the basal surface of endothelial cells, and on fat cells. These basement membranes bond cells to the underlying or surrounding connective tissues, serve as selective filters for particles that pass between connective tissue and other cells, and contribute to cell regeneration and repair.[3]

HEMATOPOIETIC TISSUE

The hematopoietic types of connective tissue include the blood cells, bone marrow, and lymphatic tissue. The role of the hematopoietic system in inflammation and immunity is discussed in Chapter 13; the reticulocyte, or red blood cell, is discussed in Chapter 18.

STRONG SUPPORTING CONNECTIVE TISSUE

The third form of connective tissue—the strong supporting form—consists of dense connective tissue, cartilage, and bone. The dense connective tissues are rich in collagen and form the tendons and ligaments that join muscle to bones and bones to bones. A layer of dense connective tissue also forms a capsule for many organs and body structures such as the kidney and heart. Dense connective tissue does not require many capillaries because it is composed largely of nonliving collagen fibers. Cartilage and bone are discussed in Chapter 55.

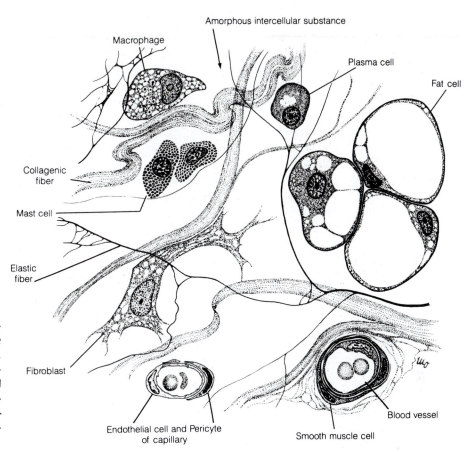

FIG. 1-19. Diagrammatic representation of cells that may be seen in loose connective tissue. The cells lie in an intercellular matrix that is bathed in tissue fluid that originates in capillaries. (Cormack, D. H. [1987]. *Ham's histology* [9th ed., p. 170]. Philadelphia: J.B. Lippincott)

MUSCLE TISSUE

There are three types of muscle tissue: *skeletal*, *cardiac*, and *smooth*. Skeletal and cardiac muscles are striated muscles. The actin and myosin filaments are arranged in large parallel arrays in bundles, giving the muscle fibers a striped or striated appearance when they are viewed through a microscope.

Skeletal muscle is the largest tissue in the body, accounting for 40% to 45% of the total body weight. Most skeletal muscle is attached to bones, and its contraction is responsible for movement of the skeleton. It differs from cardiac and smooth muscle in that it is innervated by the somatic rather than the autonomic nervous system.

Cardiac muscle, found in the myocardium, is designed to pump blood continuously. It has inherent properties of automaticity, rhythmicity, and conductivity. The pumping action of the heart is controlled by impulses originating in the cardiac conduction system and is modified by bloodborne neural mediators and impulses from the autonomic nervous system.

Smooth muscle is found in many organs, including the blood vessels, the iris of the eye, and in tubes that connect many internal organs, such as the ureters and bile ducts.

Neither skeletal nor cardiac muscle is able to undergo the mitotic activity needed to replace injured cells. Smooth muscle, however, may proliferate and undergo mitotic activity. Some increases in smooth muscle are physiologic, such as occurs in the uterus during pregnancy. Others, such as the increase in smooth muscle that occurs in the arteries of persons with chronic hypertension, are pathologic.

Although the three types of muscle tissue differ significantly in structure, contractile properties, and control mechanisms, they have many similarities. In the following section, the structural properties of skeletal muscle are presented as the prototype of muscle tissue. Smooth muscle and the ways in which it differs from skeletal muscle are discussed. Cardiac muscle is described in Chapter 22.

STRUCTURAL PROPERTIES

Muscle tissue is highly specialized for contractility and producing movement of internal and external body structures. Most muscle cells are long and narrow, a characteristic that allows the two ends of the cell to shorten and pull closer together during contraction. Because of their length, muscle cells are called *fibers* (Fig. 1-20). The cell membrane of a muscle fiber is called the *sarcolemma*, and the cytoplasm is referred to as the *sarcoplasm*. Embedded in the sarcoplasm are the contractile elements, *actin* and *myosin*. The *sarcoplasmic reticulum*, which is comparable to the ER, is composed of longitudinal tubules that run parallel to the muscle fiber and surround each bundle of actin and myosin filaments. The sarcoplasmic reticulum ends in enlarged, saclike regions called the *lateral sacs*, or *terminal cisternae*. The lateral sacs store calcium to be released during muscle contraction. A second system of tubules consists of the *transverse*, or *T-tubules*, which run perpendicular to the muscle fiber. The hollow part or lumen of the transverse tubule is continuous with the extracellular fluid compartment; and the membrane of the T-tubule is able to propagate action potentials, which are rapidly conducted over the surface of the muscle fiber and into the sarcoplasmic reticulum. As the action potential moves through the lateral sacs, the sacs release calcium, which initiates muscle contraction. The membrane of the sarcoplasmic reticulum also has an active transport mechanism for pumping the calcium ions back into the reticulum as a means of removing them from the vicinity of the actin and myosin interactions on termination of muscle contraction.

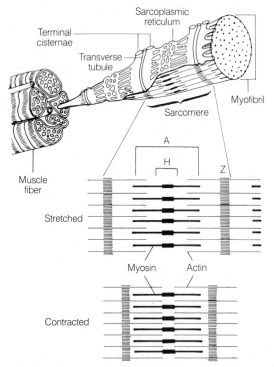

FIG. 1-20. Muscle fiber, structures of the myofibril, and the relationship between actin and myosin filaments when the muscle is stretched or contracted.

MOLECULAR MECHANISMS OF CONTRACTION

In striated muscle, the thin, lighter filaments and the thick, darker filaments are arranged in bundles (myofibrils), and these are further aligned parallel to each other through the diameter of the cell, giving skeletal muscle cells (muscle fibers) a striped appearance. Although the striated pattern appears to be continuous across a single muscle fiber, the muscle is actually composed of a number of independent cylindrical elements called *myofibrils* (see Fig. 1-20). The myofibril, in turn, consists of smaller filaments that form a regular repeating pattern along the length of the myofibril; each of these units is called a *sarcomere*. The sarcomeres, which contain the thin actin and thick myosin filaments, are the functional units of the contractile system in muscle. A sarcomere extends from one Z line to another Z line. The dark A bands contain the thick myosin filaments, and the lighter I bands contain the thin actin filaments. The Z lines consist of short elements that interconnect and provide the thin filaments from two adjoining sarcomeres with an anchoring point. The H zone in the center of the sarcomere corresponds to the space between the thin filaments; only thick filaments are found in this area. In the center of the H zone is a thin, dark band known as the *M line*, which is produced by linkages between the thick filaments.

During muscle contraction, the thick myosin and thin actin filaments slide over each other, causing shortening of the muscle fiber, whereas the length of the individual thick and thin filaments remains unchanged. The structures that produce the sliding of the filaments are the myosin heads that form cross-bridges with the thin actin filaments (Fig. 1-21). When activated by ATP, the cross-bridges swivel in a fixed arc, much like the oars of a boat, as they become attached to the actin filament. During contraction, each cross-bridge undergoes its own cycle of movement, forming a bridge attachment and releasing it, and moving to another site where the same sequence of movement occurs. This has the effect of pulling the thin and thick filaments past each other.

Myosin is the chief constituent of the thick filament; it consists of a thin tail, which provides the structural backbone for the filament, and a globular head. Each globular head contains a binding site able to bind to a complementary site on the actin molecule. In addition to the binding site for actin, each myosin head has a separate active site that catalyzes the breakdown of ATP to provide the energy needed to activate the myosin head so that it can form a cross-bridge with actin. Following contraction, myosin also binds ATP as a means of breaking the linkage between actin and myosin. The myosin molecules are

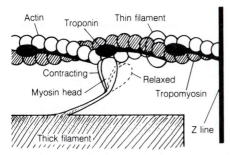

FIG. 1-21. Molecular structure of the thin actin filament and the thicker myosin filament of striated muscle. The thin filament is a double-stranded helix of actin molecules with tropomyosin and troponin molecules lying along the grooves of the actin strands. During muscle contraction, the ATP-activated heads of the thick myosin filament swivel into position, much like the oars on a boat, form a cross-bridge with a reactive site on tropomyosin and then pull the actin filament forward. During muscle relaxation the troponin molecules cover the reactive sites on tropomyosin.

bundled together side by side in the thick filaments so that half have their heads toward one end of the filament and their tails toward the other end, whereas the other half are arranged in the opposite manner.

The thin filaments are composed mainly of actin, a globular protein that is lined up in two rows that coil around each other to form a long helical strand. Associated with each actin filament are two regulatory proteins, tropomyosin and troponin (see Fig. 1-21). *Tropomyosin*, which lies in grooves of the actin strand, provides the site for attachment of the globular heads of the myosin filament. In the noncontractile state, *troponin* covers the tropomyosin binding sites and prevents formation of cross-bridges between the actin and myosin. During an action potential, calcium ions that are released from the sarcoplasmic reticulum diffuse to the adjacent myofibrils where they bind to troponin. The binding of calcium to troponin uncovers the tropomyosin binding sites so that the myosin heads can attach and form cross-bridges. Energy from ATP is used to break the actin and myosin cross-bridges and terminate muscle contraction. After breaking of the linkage between actin and myosin, the concentration of calcium around the myofibrils decreases as calcium is actively transported into the sarcoplasmic reticulum by a membrane pump that uses energy derived from ATP.

SMOOTH MUSCLE

Smooth muscle is often called *involuntary muscle* because its activity arises either spontaneously or through activity of the autonomic nervous system. On the whole, smooth muscle contraction tends to be slower and more sustained than skeletal or cardiac muscle contraction. Smooth muscle cells are spindle-shaped and considerably smaller than skeletal muscle fibers. There are no Z or M lines in smooth muscle fibers, and the cross-striations are absent because the bundles of filaments are not parallel or criss-cross obliquely through the cell. The contractile filaments of actin and myosin are scattered throughout the cytoplasm. The lack of Z lines and regular overlapping of the contractile elements provide for a greater range of tension development. This is important in hollow organs that undergo changes in volume, with consequent changes in the length of the smooth muscle fibers in their walls. Even at large increases in volume, the smooth muscle fiber retains some ability to develop tension, whereas such distention would have stretched skeletal muscle beyond the area where the thick and thin filaments overlap. Smooth muscle is generally arranged in sheets or bundles. In hollow organs, such as the intestines, the bundles are organized into two layers—an outer, longitudinal layer and an inner, circular layer. In blood vessels, the bundles are arranged in a circular or helical manner around the vessel wall.

Smooth muscle differs from skeletal muscle in the way its cross-bridges are formed. In smooth muscle, calcium binds to a cytoplasmic protein, called *calmodulin*. The calcium–calmodulin complex binds to and activates the myosin-containing thick filaments, which interact with actin. The sarcoplasmic reticulum is less well developed in smooth muscle than in skeletal muscle, and there are no transverse tubules connected to the cell membrane. Thus, smooth muscle relies on the entrance of extracellular calcium across the cell membrane as well as the release of calcium from the sarcoplasmic reticulum for muscle contraction. This dependence on movement of extracellular calcium across the cell membrane during muscle contraction is the basis for the action of calcium-blocking drugs that are used in treatment of cardiovascular disease.

Smooth muscle may be divided into two broad categories according to the mode of activation: multiunit and single-unit smooth muscle. In *multiunit* smooth muscle, each unit operates almost entirely independent of the others and is often innervated by a single nerve such as occurs in skeletal muscle. It has little, if any, inherent activity and depends on the autonomic nervous system for its activation. Smooth muscle of this type is found in the iris, in the walls of the vas deferens, and attached to hairs in the skin. The fibers in single-unit smooth muscle are in close contact with each other and are able to contract spontaneously in the absence of either nerve or hormonal stimulation. Normally, a large number of muscle fibers contract synchronously, hence the term *single-*

unit. Some single-unit smooth muscle, such as that found in the gastrointestinal tract, is self-excitable. This is usually associated with a basic slow wave rhythm that is transmitted from cell to cell by nexus (gap junctions) formed by the fusion of adjacent cell membranes. The cause of this slow wave is unknown. The intensity of contraction increases with the frequency of the action potential. Certain hormones, other agents, and local factors can modify smooth muscle activity by either depolarizing or hyperpolarizing the membrane. In addition to the gastrointestinal tract, the smooth muscle of the uterus and small-diameter blood vessels is single-unit smooth muscle.

In summary, body cells are organized into four basic tissue types: epithelial, connective, muscle, and nervous. The epithelium covers the body surfaces and forms the functional components of the glandular structures. Epithelial tissue is classified into three types according to the shape of the cells and the number of layers that are present: simple, stratified, and pseudostratified. The cells in epithelial tissue are held together by three types of intercellular junctions—tight junction, adhering junctions, and gap junctions. Connective tissue supports and connects body structures; it forms the bones and skeletal system, the joint structures, the blood cells, and the intercellular substances. Muscle tissue is a specialized tissue that is designed for contractility. There are three types of muscle tissue: skeletal, cardiac, and smooth. Actin and myosin filaments interact to produce muscle shortening, a process activated by the presence of calcium. In skeletal muscle, calcium is released from the sarcoplasmic reticulum in response to an action potential. Smooth muscle is often referred to as *involuntary muscle* because its activity arises either spontaneously or through activity of the autonomic nervous system. It differs from skeletal muscle in that it has a less well-defined sarcoplasmic reticulum and depends on entry of extracellular calcium ions for muscle contraction. Nervous tissue is designed for communication purposes and includes the neurons, the supporting neural structures, and the ependymal cells that line the ventricles of the brain and the spinal canal.

■ **REFERENCES**

1. Guyton, A. (1991). *Medical physiology* (8th ed., pp. 12, 751). Philadelphia: W.B. Saunders.
2. Cotran, S.L., Kumar, R.S., & Robbins, S.L. (1989). *Robbins' pathologic basis of disease* (4th ed., pp. 28, 100, 110). Philadelphia: W.B. Saunders.
3. Cormack, D.H. (1987). *Ham's histology* (9th ed., pp. 140, 165–168). Philadelphia: J.B. Lippincott.

CHAPTER 2

CELLULAR ADAPTATION/INJURY AND WOUND HEALING/REPAIR

Cellular Adaptation
Atrophy
Hypertrophy
Hyperplasia
Metaplasia
Dysplasia

Cell Injury
Mechanisms of Cell Injury
Reversible Cell Injury
Irreversible Cell Injury and Cell
   Death
Intracellular Accumulations

**Tissue Repair and Wound
   Healing**
Regeneration
Connective Tissue Repair
Factors That Affect Wound
   Healing

■ OBJECTIVES

After you have studied this chapter, you should be able to meet the following objectives:

■ Cite the general purpose of changes in cell structure and function that occur as the result of normal adaptive processes.

■ Describe cell changes that occur with atrophy, hypertrophy, hyperplasia, metaplasia, and dysplasia, and state general conditions under which the changes occur.

■ Describe three types of reversible cell changes that can occur with cell injury.

■ Compare the outcomes of intracellular accumulations due to systemic disorders and those due to inborn errors of metabolism.

■ Cite the reasons for the changes that occur with the wet and dry forms of gangrene.

■ Describe cell changes that occur with hypoxia, electrical injury, and thermal injury.

■ Define *free radical*.

■ Relate free-radical formation to cell injury and death.

■ Explain how injurious effects of biologic agents differ from those produced by physical and chemical agents.

■ Differentiate between the effects of ionizing and nonionizing radiation in terms of their ability to cause cell injury.

■ State how nutritional imbalances contribute to cell injury.

■ Define *parenchymal* and *stromal* as they relate to the tissues of an organ.

■ Compare labile, stable, and permanent cell types in terms of their capacity for regeneration.

■ Describe healing by primary and secondary intention.

■ Trace the wound-healing process through the inflammatory, proliferative, and remodeling phases.

■ Explain the effect of malnutrition; ischemia and oxygen deprivation; impaired immune and inflammatory responses; and infection, wound separation, and foreign bodies on wound healing.

■ Discuss the effect of age on wound healing.

Carol Mattson Porth: PATHOPHYSIOLOGY: CONCEPTS OF
ALTERED HEALTH STATES, 4th ed. © 1994, 1990, 1986, 1982
J.B. Lippincott Company

When confronted with stresses that tend to disrupt its normal structure and function, the cell undergoes adaptive changes that permit survival and maintenance of function. It is only when the stress is overwhelming or adaptation is ineffective that cell injury and death occur. This chapter focuses on cellular adaptation, cell injury and death, and wound healing.

■ CELLULAR ADAPTATION

Cells adapt to changes in the internal environment just as the total organism adapts to changes in the external environment. Cells may adapt by undergoing changes in size, number, and type. These changes, occurring singly or in combination, may lead to atrophy, hypertrophy, hyperplasia, metaplasia, and dysplasia. Whether adaptive cellular changes are normal or abnormal depends on whether the response was mediated by an appropriate stimulus. Normal adaptive responses occur in response to need and an appropriate stimulus. Once the need has been removed, the adaptive response ceases.

ATROPHY

When confronted with a decrease in work demands or adverse environmental conditions, most cells are able to revert to a smaller size and a lower and more efficient level of functioning that is compatible with survival. This decrease in cell size is called *atrophy*. Cell size, particularly in muscle tissue, is related to work load. As the work load of a cell diminishes, there is a general decrease in oxygen consumption and protein synthesis. Cells that are atrophied reduce their oxygen consumption and other cellular functions by decreasing the number and size of their organelles and other structures. There are fewer mitochondria, myofilaments, and lesser amounts of endoplasmic reticulum. When a sufficient number of cells are involved, the entire tissue or muscle atrophies.

The general causes of atrophy can be grouped into five categories: (1) disuse, (2) denervation, (3) lack of endocrine stimulation, (4) decreased nutrition, and (5) ischemia or a decrease in blood flow. Disuse atrophy occurs when there is a reduction in skeletal muscle use. An extreme example of disuse atrophy is seen in the muscles of extremities that have been encased in plaster casts. Because atrophy is adaptive and reversible, muscle size is restored once the cast is removed and muscle use is resumed. Denervation atrophy is a form of disuse atrophy that occurs in the muscles of paralyzed limbs. Likewise, lack of endocrine stimulation produces a form of

disuse atrophy. In women, the absence of estrogen stimulation during menopause results in atrophic changes in the reproductive organs. With both malnutrition and decreased blood flow, cells decrease their size and energy requirements as a means of survival.

In some cases, atrophy is accompanied by the presence of a yellow-brown intracellular pigment called *lipofuscin*. This form of atrophy is referred to as *brown atrophy*. The discoloration represents the accumulation of indigestible residues resulting from destruction of cell components (*e.g.*, mitochondria and endoplasmic reticulum). The accumulation of lipofuscin increases with age, and it is sometimes referred to as the wear-and-tear pigment. It is seen more commonly in heart, nerve, and liver cells than in other types of tissue. Lipofuscin is not injurious to cell structure or function.[1]

HYPERTROPHY

Hypertrophy represents an increase in cell size and with it an increase in the amount of functioning tissue mass. It results from an increased work load imposed on an organ or body part and is commonly seen in cardiac and skeletal muscle tissue, which cannot adapt to an increase in work load by mitotic division and formation of more cells. In hypertrophy, there is an increase in the functional components of the cell that allows it to achieve an equilibrium between demand and functional capacity. For example, as muscle cells hypertrophy, additional actin and myosin filaments, cell enzymes, and adenosine triphosphate (ATP) are synthesized. The precise signal for hypertrophy is unknown. It may be related to ATP depletion, stretching of muscle fibers, activation of cell degradation products, or hormonal factors.[1] Whatever the mechanism, a limit is eventually reached beyond which further enlargement of the tissue mass is no longer able to compensate for the increased work demands. The limiting factors for continued hypertrophy may be related to limitations in blood flow.[1] In hypertension, the progressive increase in left ventricular muscle mass that develops because of the work load imposed on the heart as it pumps blood against an elevated arterial pressure is no longer able to compensate for the increased burden, and heart failure ensues.

Hypertrophy may occur as the result of either normal physiologic or abnormal pathologic conditions. The increase in muscle mass associated with exercise is an example of physiologic hypertrophy. Pathologic hypertrophy occurs as the result of disease condition and may be adaptive or compensatory. Examples of adaptive hypertrophy are the thickening of the urinary bladder due to long-continued obstruction of urinary outflow and the myocardial hypertrophy that results from valvular heart disease or hypertension. Compensatory hypertrophy is the enlargement of a remaining organ or tissue after a portion has been surgically removed or rendered inactive. For instance, if one kidney is removed, the remaining kidney enlarges to compensate for the loss.

HYPERPLASIA

An increase in the number of cells in an organ or tissue is called *hyperplasia*. Hyperplasia occurs in tissues with cells that are capable of mitotic division, such as the epidermis, intestinal epithelium, and glandular tissue. Nerve cells and skeletal and cardiac muscle do not divide and, therefore, have no capacity for hyperplastic growth. As with other normal adaptive cellular responses, hyperplasia is a controlled process that occurs in response to an appropriate stimulus and ceases once the stimulus has been removed.

The stimuli that induce hyperplasia may be either physiologic or nonphysiologic. There are two common types of physiologic hyperplasia: hormonal and compensatory. Breast and uterine enlargement during pregnancy are examples of a physiologic hyperplasia that is due to estrogen stimulation. The regeneration of the liver that occurs after partial hepatectomy (partial removal of the liver) is an example of compensatory hyperplasia. Nonphysiologic hyperplasia occurs in response to abnormal hormonal stimulation of target cells. Excessive estrogen production can cause endometrial hyperplasia and abnormal menstrual bleeding.

Although hypertrophy and hyperplasia are two distinct processes, they may occur together and are often triggered by the same mechanism.[1] For example, the pregnant uterus undergoes both hypertrophy and hyperplasia as the result of estrogen stimulation. Hyperplasia is also an important response of connective tissue in wound healing, during which proliferating fibroblasts and blood vessels contribute to wound repair.

METAPLASIA

Metaplasia represents the conversion from one adult cell type to another adult cell type. It usually occurs in response to chronic irritation and inflammation and allows for substitution of cells that are better able to survive under circumstances in which a more fragile cell type might succumb. However, the conversion of cell types never oversteps the boundaries of the primary groups of tissue (*e.g.*, one type of epithelial cell may be converted to another type of epithelial cell but not to a connective tissue cell). An example of metaplasia is the adaptive substitution of stratified squamous epithelial cells for the ciliated columnar epithelial cells in the trachea and large airways of a habitual cigarette smoker. A vitamin A deficiency also induces squamous metaplasia of the respiratory tract. Although the squamous epithelium is better able to survive in these situations, the protective function that the ciliated epithelium provides for the respiratory tract is lost. Furthermore, the continued exposure to the influences that cause metaplasia may predispose to cancerous transformation in the metaplastic epithelium. The most common form of cancer of the respiratory tract is composed of squamous cells.[1]

DYSPLASIA

Dysplasia is characterized by deranged cell growth of a specific tissue that results in cells that vary in size, shape, and appearance. Minor degrees of dysplasia occur in association with chronic irritation or inflammation. It is most frequently encountered in metaplastic squamous epithelium of the respiratory tract and uterine cervix. Although dysplasia is abnormal, it is adaptive in that it is potentially reversible once the irritating cause has been found and removed. Dysplasia is strongly implicated as a precursor of cancer. In both cancer of respiratory tract and cancer of uterine cervix, dysplastic changes have been found adjacent to the foci of cancerous transformation. Through the use of the Papanicolaou (Pap) smear, it has been documented that cancer of uterine cervix develops in a series of incremental epithelial changes ranging from severe dysplasia to invasive cancer.

In summary, cells adapt to changes in their environment and in their work demands by changing their size, number, and characteristics. When confronted with a decrease in work demands or adverse environmental conditions, cells *atrophy* or reduce their size and revert to a lower and more efficient level of functioning. *Hypertrophy* represents an increase in tissue size brought about by an increase in cell size and functional components within the cell. An increase in the number of cells in an organ or tissue that is still capable of mitotic division is called *hyperplasia*. *Metaplasia* occurs in response to chronic irritation and represents the substitution of cells of a type that are better able to survive under circumstances in which a more fragile cell type might succumb. *Dysplasia* is characterized by deranged cell growth of a specific tissue that results in cells that vary in size, shape, and appearance. It is a precursor of cancer. Normal adaptive changes are consistent with the needs of the cell and occur in response to an appropriate stimulus. The changes are usually reversed once the stimulus has been withdrawn.

■ CELL INJURY

Cells can be injured in many ways. The extent to which any injurious agent can cause cell injury and death depends, in large measure, on the intensity and duration of the injury and the type of cell that is involved. When cells are injured or the need to adapt becomes overwhelming, degenerative changes begin to appear.

Degeneration is a process in which there is a cellular deterioration along with changes in both the chemical structure and microscopic appearance of the cell. Degeneration can follow many paths that eventually lead to cell changes, some of which may be reversible and others irreversible. Irreversible changes consist of necrosis (cell death) and tissue dissolution. Whether a specific stress causes irreversible or reversible cell injury depends not only on the severity of the insult, but on many variables related to the cells, including their particular vulnerability, blood supply, nutritional status, and previous reserves and state of functioning.

MECHANISMS OF CELL INJURY

Cell damage can occur in many ways. Some agents, such as heat, produce direct cell injury; other factors, such as genetic derangements, produce their effects indirectly by predisposing to metabolic disturbances and altered immune responses. For purposes of discussion, the mechanisms by which cells are injured have been grouped into seven categories: (1) free-radical injury, (2) hypoxic cell injury, (3) cell injury due to physical agents, (4) radiation injury, (5) chemical injury, (6) injury due to biologic agents, and (7) injury associated with nutritional imbalances.

FREE-RADICAL INJURY

Many injurious agents exert their damaging effects through a reactive chemical species called a *free radical*.[2-4] In fact, free-radical injury is rapidly emerging as a final common pathway for tissue damage by many injurious agents.

In most atoms, the outer electron orbits are filled with paired electrons moving in opposite directions to balance their spin. A free radical is a highly reactive chemical species that has one or more unpaired electrons in its outer orbit. In this state, the radical is highly unstable and will enter into reactions with cellular constituents, particularly key molecules in cell membranes and nucleic acids. Moreover, free radicals can establish chain reactions, sometimes thousands of events long, as the molecules they react with form free radicals. Uncontrolled free-radical production causes damage to cell membranes, cross-linking of cell proteins, inactivation of enzyme systems, and nucleic acid interaction that damages deoxyribonucleic acid (DNA). Although free radicals can be damaging to cell structures, they are also the main mechanism for killing microbes in phagocytic cells.

The sites of free-radical generation include all of the cellular constituents including mitochondria, lysosome, and nuclear, endoplasmic reticular, and plasma membranes as well as sites within the cytosol. Oxygen, with its two unpaired outer electrons, is the most frequent source of free radicals. During the course of normal cell metabolism, cells process energy-producing oxygen into water; in some reactions, a superoxide radical is formed. Exogenous sources of free radicals include tobacco smoke, certain pollutants and organic solvents, hyperoxic environments, pesticides, and radiation. Some of these compounds as well as certain medications are metabolized to free-radical intermediates that cause oxidative damage to target tissues.

Under normal conditions, most cells have chemical mechanisms that protect them from the injurious effects of free radicals. These mechanisms commonly break down when the cell is deprived of oxygen or exposed to certain chemical agents, radiation, or other injurious agents. Free-radical formation is a particular threat to tissues in which the blood flow has been interrupted and then restored. During the period of interrupted flow, the intracellular mechanisms that control free radicals are inactivated or damaged. When blood flow is restored, the cell is suddenly confronted with an excess of free radicals that it cannot control. Scientists continue to investigate the use of free-radical scavengers that would protect against cell injury during periods when protective cellular mechanisms are impaired. Defenses against free radicals include vitamin E, vitamin C, and β-carotene.[5] Vitamin E is the major lipid-soluble antioxidant present in all cellular membranes. Vitamin C is an important water-soluble cytosolic chain-breaking antioxidant; it acts directly with superoxide and singlet oxygen radicals. β-Carotene, a pigment found in most plants, reacts with singlet oxygen and can also function as an antioxidant.

HYPOXIC CELL INJURY

Hypoxia deprives the cell of oxygen and interrupts oxidative metabolism and the generation of ATP. The actual time necessary to produce irreversible cell damage depends on the degree of oxygen deprivation and the metabolic needs of the cell. Well-differentiated cells such as those in the heart, brain, and kidney require large amounts of oxygen to provide energy for their special functions. Brain cells, for example, begin to undergo permanent damage after 4 to 6 minutes of oxygen deprivation. Furthermore, there is often a fine margin between the time involved in reversible and irreversible cell damage. In one study, it was found that the epithelial cells of the proximal tubule of the kidney in the rat could survive 20 but not 30 minutes of ischemia.[6]

Hypoxia can result from an inadequate amount of oxygen in the air, respiratory disease, ischemia (decreased blood flow due to circulatory disorders), anemia, edema, or inability of the cells to use oxygen. In ischemia, there is both impaired oxygen delivery and impaired removal of metabolic end-products such as lactic acid. In contrast to pure hypoxia, which affects the oxygen content of the blood and affects all of the cells in the body, ischemia commonly affects blood flow through small numbers of blood vessels and produces local tissue injury. In edema, the distance for diffusion of oxygen may become a limiting factor. In hypermetabolic states, the cells may require more oxygen than can be supplied by normal respiratory function and oxygen transport. Hypoxia also serves as the ultimate cause of cell death in other injuries. For example, toxins from certain microorganisms interfere with cellular utilization of oxygen, and a physical agent such as cold causes severe vasoconstriction and impairs blood flow.

Hypoxia literally causes a power failure within the cell with widespread effects on the cell's functional and structural components. As oxygen tension within the cell falls, oxidative metabolism ceases and the cell reverts to anaerobic metabolism, using the cell's limited glycogen stores in an attempt to maintain vital cell functions. Cellular pH falls as lactic acid accumulates within the cell. This reduction in pH can have profound effects on intracellular structures. Clumping of the nuclear chromatin occurs, and myelin figures, which derive from destructive changes in cell membranes and intracellular structures, are seen within the cytoplasm and extracellular spaces.

One of the earliest effects of reduced ATP is acute cellular swelling caused by failure of the energy-dependent sodium–potassium membrane pump, which extrudes sodium and returns potassium to the cell. With impaired function of this pump, intracellular potassium levels decrease, and sodium and water accumulate within the cell. The movement of fluid and ions into the cell is associated with dilatation of the endoplasmic reticulum, increased membrane permeability, and decreased mitochondrial function.[1]

To this point, the cellular changes are reversible if oxygenation is restored. If the oxygen supply is not restored, however, there is a continued loss of essential enzymes, proteins, and ribonucleic acid through the hyperpermeable membrane of the cell. Injury to the lysosomal membranes results in leakage of de-structive lysosomal enzymes into the cytoplasm of the cell and enzymatic digestion of cell components. The leakage of intracellular enzymes through the permeable cell membrane into the extracellular fluid is used as an important clinical indicator of cell injury and death. These enzymes enter the blood and can be measured by laboratory tests. For example, heart muscle liberates glutamine-oxaloacetic transaminase (GOT), creatine phosphokinase (CPK), and lactate dehydrogenase (LDH) when injured. Because different types of tissue have different enzymes, the presence of elevated levels of specific enzymes provides information about the location of tissue injury due to hypoxia.

INJURY DUE TO PHYSICAL AGENTS

Physical agents responsible for cell and tissue injury include mechanical forces, extremes of temperature, and electrical forces.

Injury due to mechanical forces occurs as the result of body impact with another object. Either the body or the mass can be in motion, or, as sometimes happens, both can be in motion at the time of impact. These types of injuries split and tear tissue, fracture bones, injure blood vessels, and disrupt blood flow.

Extremes of Temperature. Extremes of heat and cold cause damage to the cell, its organelles, and its enzyme systems. Exposure to low-intensity heat (43° to 46°C), such as occurs with partial-thickness burns and severe heat stroke, causes cell injury by inducing vascular injury, accelerating cell metabolism, inactivating temperature-sensitive enzymes, and disrupting the cell membrane. With more intense heat, coagulation of blood vessels and tissue proteins occurs.

Exposure to cold induces vasoconstriction by direct action on blood vessels and also by reflex activity of the sympathetic nervous system. The resultant decrease in blood flow may lead to hypoxic tissue injury, depending on the degree and duration of cold exposure. Injury due to freezing is probably a combination of ice-crystal formation and vasoconstriction. The decreased blood flow leads to capillary stasis and arteriolar and capillary thrombosis. Edema results from increased capillary permeability.

Electrical Injuries. Electrical injuries can affect the body in two ways—through extensive tissue injury and disruption of neural and cardiac impulses. The effect of electricity on the body is mainly determined by (1) the type of current (direct or alternating), (2) its voltage, (3) its amperage, (4) the resistance of the intervening tissue, (5) the pathway of the current, and (6) the duration of exposure.[5]

Alternating current (AC) is usually more dangerous than direct current (DC) because it causes violent muscle contractions, preventing release of the electrical source and sometimes resulting in fractures and dislocations. In electrical injuries, the body acts as a conductor of the electrical current (*i.e.*, the current enters the body from an electrical source such as an exposed wire and passes through the body and exits to another conductor, such as the moisture on the ground or a piece of metal the person is holding). The pathway that a current takes is of critical importance because the electrical energy disrupts impulses in excitable tissues. Current flow through the brain may interrupt impulses from respiratory centers in the brain stem, and current flow through the chest may cause fatal cardiac arrhythmias.

In electrical circuits, resistance to the flow of current transforms electrical energy into heat. This is why the elements in electrical heating devices are made of highly resistive metals. Much of the tissue damage produced by electrical injuries is due to heat production in tissues that have the highest electrical resistance. Resistance to electrical current varies from the greatest to the least as follows: bone, fat, tendons, skin, muscles, blood, and nerves. The most severe tissue injury usually occurs at the skin sites where the current enters and leaves the body. After electricity has penetrated the skin, it passes rapidly through the body along the lines of least resistance—through body fluids and nerves. Degeneration of vessel walls may occur, and thrombi may form as current flows along the blood vessels. This can cause extensive muscle and deep tissue injury. Thick, dry skin is more resistant to the flow of electricity than thin, wet skin. It is generally believed that the greater the skin resistance, the greater the amount of local skin burn; the less the resistance, the greater the deep and systemic effects.

RADIATION INJURY

Electromagnetic radiation comprises a wide spectrum of wave-propagated energy ranging from ionizing gamma rays to radio-frequency waves (Fig. 2-1). A photon is a particle of radiation energy. Radiation energy above the visible ultraviolet range is called *ionizing radiation* because the photons have enough energy to knock electrons off atoms and molecules. Radiation energy at frequencies below that of visible light is often referred to as *nonionizing radiation*. Ultraviolet radiation represents the portion of the spectrum of electromagnetic radiation just above the visible range. It contains increasingly energetic rays that are powerful enough to disrupt intracellular bonds and cause sunburn.

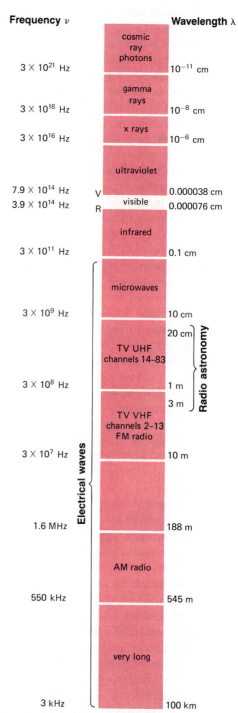

FIG. 2-1. The electromagnetic spectrum. The frequencies are shown on the left side of the diagram, and the corresponding wavelengths appear on the right. The frequencies and wavelengths are related by $C = \nu\lambda$, where C = the speed of light in free space (3×10^8 m/sec) and is the same for all wavelengths of the electromagnetic spectrum. (Hooper, H. O., & Gwynne, P. [1980]. *Physics and the physical perspectives.* New York: Harper & Row)

Ionizing Radiation. The spectrum of ionizing radiation includes two distinct forms of energy propagation: electromagnetic waves and fast-moving particles. Gamma waves and x-rays are similar in their interaction with body tissues but differ in their origin; x-rays are machine-generated, and gamma rays are emitted from the spontaneous decay of radioactive materials. Both of these forms of radiation are energetic and extremely penetrating, and they assume characteristics of both waves and particles.

Particulate radiation involves particles of definite mass and charge given off by both naturally occurring and artificially produced radioactive elements, processes of fission (atomic reactors), and particle accelerators. Naturally occurring radioactive substances (*e.g.*, radium) and artificially produced radioisotopes undergo spontaneous decay, during which they emit radiant energy. This rate of decay varies greatly and is expressed in terms of the half-life of the product, or the time necessary to reduce its radioactivity to one half its initial value. The half-life of a radioisotope may be as short as a fraction of a second, or it may be as long as 1638 years (radium).[7]

Ionizing radiation affects cells by causing ionization of molecules and atoms within the cells either by directly hitting the target molecules or by producing free radicals that interact with critical cell components. It can immediately kill cells, interrupt cell replication, or cause a variety of mutations, which may or may not be lethal. The cell's initial response to radiation exposure is characterized by swelling, disruption of the mitochondria and other organelles, alterations in the cell membrane, and marked changes in the nucleus. Because of inhibition of DNA synthesis and interference with the mitotic process, rapidly dividing cells such as those of the bone marrow and gastrointestinal epithelium are more susceptible to radiation injury than nondividing cells. Cancer cells are rapidly proliferating cells; therefore, radiation therapy is often used in treating cancer (see Chapter 5).

Dose-dependent vascular changes occur in all irradiated tissues. During the immediate postirradiation period, only vessel dilatation takes place (*e.g.*, the initial erythema of the skin after radiotherapy). Later, or with higher levels of radiation, destructive changes occur in small blood vessels such as the capillaries and venules.

At relatively low doses, both normal cells and cancer cells are able to repair radiation damage. If, however, cell recovery is not complete at the time of the next exposure, there may be additional damage. The importance of cell repair in protecting against radiation injury is evidenced by the vulnerability of people who lack enzymes to repair ultraviolet-induced defects in DNA replication. In a genetic disorder called *xeroderma pigmentosum*, an enzyme needed to repair sunlight-induced defects in DNA replication is lacking, and this predisposes to skin cancer at a very early age.

Nonionizing Radiation Nonionizing radiation includes infrared light, ultrasound, microwaves, and laser energy. Unlike ionizing radiation, which can directly break chemical bonds, nonionizing radiation exerts its effects by causing vibrations and rotations of atoms and molecules. All of this vibrational and rotational energy is eventually converted to thermal energy. Because all of these types of radiation are finding increasing usage for industrial, domestic, and medical purposes, there is increasing concern about the safety and long-term effects of exposure to these types of radiation. In laboratory animals, for example, cataracts and lymphocyte dysfunction have been associated with exposure to microwave radiation.[8] Unquestionably, much of this damage was due to local and general hyperthermia.[9] A number of epidemiologic studies on the ocular effects of occupational exposure have not found an increase in lens opacity in humans.[4]

CHEMICAL INJURY

Chemical agents can injure the cell membrane and other cell structures, block enzymatic pathways, coagulate cell proteins, and disrupt the osmotic and ionic balance of the cell. There are many injurious chemicals—even excessive amounts of simple table salt (sodium chloride) can cause cell damage by disrupting the cell's osmotic and ionic homeostasis. Chemicals can destroy cells at the site of contact. Corrosive substances such as strong acids and bases destroy cells as they come into contact with the body. Other chemicals may injure cells in the process of metabolism or elimination. Carbon tetrachloride (CCl_4), for example, causes little damage until it is metabolized by liver enzymes to a highly reactive free radical ($CCl_3^{\cdot}$). Carbon tetrachloride is extremely toxic to liver cells. Still other types of chemicals are selective in their sites of action. Carbon monoxide has a special affinity for the hemoglobin molecule.

INJURY DUE TO BIOLOGIC AGENTS

Biologic agents differ from other injurious agents in that they are able to replicate and thus can continue to produce their injurious effects. These agents range from submicroscopic viruses to the larger parasites. Biologic agents cause cell injury by a number of diverse mechanisms. Viruses enter the cell and become incorporated into its synthetic machinery. Certain bacteria elaborate exotoxins that interfere with cellular production of ATP. Other bacteria, such as the gram-negative bacilli, release endotoxins that cause cell injury and increased capillary permeability. Still other microorganisms produce their effects through inflammatory or immune mechanisms. Infectious processes are discussed in Chapter 12.

INJURY ASSOCIATED WITH NUTRITIONAL IMBALANCES

Both nutritional excesses and nutritional deficiencies predispose to cell injury. Obesity and diets high in saturated fats are thought to predispose to atherosclerosis. The body requires more than 60 organic and inorganic substances, in amounts ranging from micrograms to grams. These nutrients include minerals, vitamins, certain fatty acids, and specific amino acids. Dietary deficiencies can occur in the form of starvation, in which there is a deficiency of all nutrients and vitamins, or because of a selective deficiency of a single nutrient or vitamin. Iron-deficiency anemia, scurvy, beriberi, and pellagra are examples of injury caused by the lack of specific vitamins or minerals. The protein and calorie deficiencies that occur with starvation cause widespread tissue damage.

REVERSIBLE CELL INJURY

Reversible cell injury, while impairing cell function, does not result in cell death. Two patterns of reversible cell injury can be observed under the microscope: cellular swelling and fatty change. As previously described, cellular swelling occurs when there is impairment of the energy-dependent sodium–potassium membrane pump usually as the result of hypoxic cell injury.

Fatty changes are linked to intracellular accumulation of fat. When fatty changes occur, small vacuoles of fat disperse throughout the cytoplasm. The process is usually more ominous than cloudy swelling, and, although it is reversible, its presence usually indicates severe injury. These fatty changes may occur because normal cells are presented with an increased fat load or because injured cells are unable to metabolize the fat properly. In obesity, fatty infiltrates often occur within and between the cells of the liver and heart because of an increased fat load. Pathways for fat metabolism may be impaired during cell injury, and fat may accumulate within the cell as production exceeds use and export. The liver, where most fats are synthesized and metabolized, is particularly susceptible to fatty change, but fatty change may also occur in the kidney, the heart, and other organs.

IRREVERSIBLE CELL INJURY AND CELL DEATH

Necrosis means death of a cell, organ, or tissue that is still a part of the body. Widespread necrosis can occur without somatic (body) death. With cell death, there are marked changes in the appearance of both the cytoplasmic contents and the nucleus. These changes are often not visible, even under the microscope, for hours after cell death. The dissolution of the necrotic cell or tissue can follow several paths: (1) the cell can undergo liquefaction (liquefaction necrosis); (2) it can be transformed to a gray, firm mass (coagulation necrosis); (3) or it can be converted to a cheesy material by infiltration of fatlike substances (caseous necrosis).

Liquefaction necrosis occurs when some of the cells die but their catalytic enzymes are not destroyed. An example of liquefaction necrosis is the softening of the center of an abscess with discharge of its contents. During *coagulation necrosis*, acidosis develops and denatures the enzymatic and structural proteins of the cell. This type of necrosis is characteristic of hypoxic injury and is seen in infarcted areas. *Infarction* (tissue death) occurs when an artery supplying an organ or part of the body becomes occluded and no other source of blood supply exists. As a rule, the infarct is conical in shape and corresponds to the distribution of the artery and its branches. An artery may be occluded by an embolus, a thrombus, disease of the arterial wall, or pressure from outside the vessel. *Caseous necrosis* (so called because it has a soft, cheeselike center) is a distinctive form of coagulation necrosis. It is most commonly associated with tubercular lesions and is thought to result from immune mechanisms.

GANGRENE

The term *gangrene* is applied when a considerable mass of tissue undergoes necrosis. Gangrene may be classified as either dry or moist. In dry gangrene, the part becomes dry and shrinks, the skin wrinkles, and its color changes to dark brown or black. The spread of dry gangrene is slow, and its symptoms are not as marked as those of wet gangrene. The irritation caused by the dead tissue produces a line of inflammatory reaction (line of demarcation) between the dead tissue of the gangrenous area and the healthy tissue (Fig. 2-2). Dry gangrene is usually due to interference with arterial blood supply to a part without interference with venous return and is a form of coagulation necrosis.

In moist or wet gangrene, the area is cold, swollen, and pulseless. The skin is moist, black, and under tension. Blebs form on the surface, liquefaction

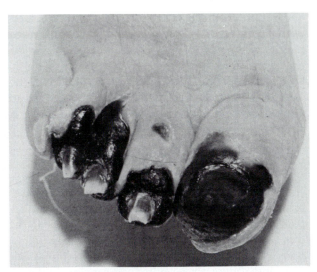

FIG. 2-2. Photograph of a foot with dry gangrene of the first four toes. Note the sharp line of demarcation between the normal and necrotic tissue. (Courtesy of M. Wagner, M.D., the Anatomy Department, Medical College of Wisconsin, Milwaukee, Wisconsin)

occurs, and a foul odor (due to bacterial action) is present. There is no line of demarcation between the normal and diseased tissues, and the spread of tissue damage is rapid. Systemic symptoms are usually severe, and death may occur unless the condition can be arrested. Moist, or wet, gangrene is primarily due to interference with the venous return from the part. Bacterial invasion plays an important role in the development of wet gangrene and is responsible for many of its prominent symptoms.

Dry gangrene is confined almost exclusively to the extremities, whereas moist gangrene may affect either the internal organs or the extremities. If bacteria invade the necrotic tissue, dry gangrene may be converted to wet gangrene.

Gas gangrene is a special type of gangrene that is due to infection of devitalized tissues by one of several *Clostridium* bacteria. The anaerobic and spore-forming organisms are widespread in nature, particularly in soil; thus, gas gangrene is prone to occur in trauma and compound fractures in which dirt and debris are embedded. Some species have been isolated in the stomach, gallbladder, intestine, vagina, and skin of healthy people. The bacteria produce toxins that dissolve the cell membranes causing death of muscle cells, massive spreading edema, hemolysis of red blood cells, hemolytic anemia, hemoglobinuria, and renal toxicity.[10] Characteristic of this disorder are the bubbles of hydrogen sulfide gas that form in the muscle. Gas gangrene is a serious and potentially fatal disease. Because the organism is anaerobic, oxygen is sometimes administered in a hyperbaric chamber.

INTRACELLULAR ACCUMULATIONS

Under certain conditions, various substances may accumulate in both normal and abnormal cells. Intracellular accumulation can be grouped into three categories: (1) normal cellular constituents, such as lipids, proteins, and carbohydrates, which are present in large amounts; (2) abnormal substances, such as those resulting from inborn errors of metabolism; and (3) products of excessive intracellular synthesis. The previously described fatty changes are an example of intracellular accumulation of a normal cell constituent.

The intracellular accumulation of abnormal substances can result from genetic disorders that disrupt the metabolism of selected substances. A normal enzyme may be replaced with an abnormal one, resulting in the formation of a substance that cannot be used or eliminated from the cell; or an enzyme may be missing, so that an intermediate product accumulates within the cell. For example, there are at least ten inborn errors of glycogen metabolism, most of which lead to the accumulation of intracellular glycogen stores. In the most common form of this disorder, von Gierke's disease, large amounts of glycogen accumulate in the liver and kidneys because of a deficiency of the enzyme glucose-phosphatase. Without this enzyme, glucose-6-phosphase, stored in the form of glycogen, cannot be broken down to form glucose that can be used by the cell or released into the bloodstream. In a similar manner, other enzyme defects lead to the accumulation of other substances.

Pigments are colored substances that may accumulate within cells. They can be either endogenous (arising from within the body) or exogenous (arising from outside the body) in origin. Icterus, or jaundice, is a yellow discoloration of tissue caused by the retention of bilirubin, an endogenous bile pigment. This condition may result from increased bilirubin production due to red blood cell destruction, obstruction of bile passage into the intestine, or toxic diseases that affect the liver's ability to remove bilirubin from the blood. One of the most common exogenous pigments is carbon in the form of coal dust. In coal miners or people exposed to heavily polluted environments, the accumulation of carbon dust blackens the lung tissue and may cause serious lung disease. The formation of a blue lead line along the margins of the gum is one of the diagnostic features of lead poisoning.

Whatever the nature or cause of the abnormal accumulation, it implies storage of some substance by a cell. If the accumulation is due to a correctable systemic disorder such as hyperbilirubinemia, which causes jaundice, the accumulation is reversible. If the disorder cannot be corrected, as often occurs in many inborn errors of metabolism, the cells become overloaded, causing cell injury and death.

In summary, cell injury can be caused by a number of agents. The injury may produce sublethal and reversible cellular damage or may lead to irreversible cell injury and death. Partially reduced oxygen species (free radicals) are important mediators of cell injury in many pathologic conditions. They are an important cause of cell injury in hypoxia and after exposure to radiation and certain chemical agents. Lack of oxygen underlies the pathogenesis of cell injury in hypoxia and ischemia. Hypoxia can result from inadequate oxygen in the air, cardiorespiratory disease, anemia, or the inability of the cells to use oxygen. Among the physical agents that produce cell injury are mechanical forces that produce tissue trauma, extremes of temperature, electricity, and radiation. Chemical agents can cause cell injury through several mechanisms; they can block enzymatic pathways, cause coagulation of tissues, or disrupt the osmotic or ionic balance of the cell. Biologic agents differ from other injurious agents in that they are able to replicate and continue to produce injury. Among the nutritional factors that contribute to cell injury are excesses and deficiencies of nutrients, vitamins, and minerals.

Necrosis refers to cell death. There are three forms of cell necrosis: (1) liquefaction necrosis, which occurs when cell death does not result in inactivation of intracellular enzymes; (2) coagulation necrosis, which occurs with ischemia; and (3) caseous necrosis, which is associated with tubercular lesions. Necrosis of large areas of tissue leads to gangrene. Gangrene can be classified as dry or wet gangrene. Dry gangrene is essentially a form of coagulation necrosis, and wet gangrene is due to bacterial invasion of the necrotic area.

Under some circumstances, normal cells may accumulate abnormal amounts of various substances. If the accumulation is due to a correctable systemic disorder such as hyperbilirubinemia, which causes jaundice, the accumulation is reversible. If the disorder cannot be corrected, as often occurs in many inborn errors of metabolism, the cells become overloaded, causing cell injury and death.

■ TISSUE REPAIR AND WOUND HEALING

Body organs and structures contain two types of tissues: parenchymal and stromal. The parenchymal (from the Greek for anything poured in) tissues contain the functioning cells of an organ or body part (*e.g.*, hepatocytes, renal tubular cells). The stromal tissues (from the Greek for something laid out to lie on) consist of the supporting connective tissues, blood vessels, and nerve fibers.

Injured tissues are repaired in two ways: (1) by regeneration of parenchymal cells or (2) by connective tissue repair in which scar tissue is substituted for the parenchymal cells of the injured tissue. The primary objective of the healing process is to fill the gap created by tissue destruction and to restore the structural continuity of the injured part. When regeneration cannot occur, healing by replacement with a connective scar tissue provides the means for maintaining this continuity. Although scar tissue fills the gap created by tissue death, it does not repair the structure with functioning parenchymal cells. Because the regenerative capabilities of most tissues are limited, wound healing usually involves some connective tissue repair.

Considerable research has contributed to the understanding of chemical mediators and growth factors that orchestrate the healing process.[11–13] These chemical mediators and growth factors are released in an orderly manner from many of the cells that participate in the healing process. Some growth factors act as chemoattractants, enhancing the migration of white blood cells and fibroblasts to the wound site, and others act as mitogens causing increased proliferation of cells that participate in the healing process. For example, platelet-derived growth factor, which is released from activated platelets, serves to attract white blood cells and acts as a growth factor for blood vessels and fibroblasts. Many of the cytokines (see Chapter 13) are growth factors.

REGENERATION

Regeneration involves replacement of the injured tissue with cells of the same parenchymal type leaving little, if any, evidence of the previous injury. The ability to regenerate varies with tissue and cell type. Body cells are divided into three types according to their ability to undergo regeneration: (1) labile, (2) stable, or (3) permanent.

Labile cells continue to divide and replicate throughout life, replacing cells that are continually being destroyed. Labile cells can be found in tissues that have a daily turnover of cells. They include the surface epithelial cells of the skin, the oral cavity, vagina, and cervix; the columnar epithelium of the gastrointestinal tract, uterus, and fallopian tubes; the transitional epithelium of the urinary tract; and bone marrow cells.[1]

Stable cells are those that normally stop dividing when growth ceases. These cells are capable, however, of undergoing regeneration when confronted with an appropriate stimulus. For stable cells to regenerate and restore tissues to their original state, the supporting stromal framework must be present. When this framework has been destroyed, the replacement of tissues will be haphazard. The hepatocytes of the liver are one form of stable cell, and the importance of the supporting framework to regeneration is evidenced by two forms of liver disease. In some types of viral hepatitis, for example, there is selective destruction of the parenchymal liver cells, whereas the cells of the supporting tissue remain unharmed. Consequently, once the disease has subsided, the injured cells regenerate and liver function returns to normal. In cirrhosis of the liver, fibrous bands of tissue form and replace the normal supporting tissues of the liver, causing disordered replacement of liver cells and disturbance of liver function.

Permanent or fixed cells are those that cannot undergo mitotic division. The fixed cells include nerve cells, as well as skeletal and cardiac muscle cells. These cells cannot regenerate; once destroyed, they are replaced with fibrous scar tissue that lacks the functional characteristics of the destroyed tissue. For example, the scar tissue that develops in the heart after a heart attack cannot conduct impulses nor can it contract to pump blood.

CONNECTIVE TISSUE REPAIR

Connective tissue replacement is an important process in the repair of tissue. It allows replacement of nonregenerated parenchymal cells by a connective tissue scar. Depending on the extent of tissue loss, wound closure and healing occur by either *primary* or *secondary intention* (Fig. 2-3). A sutured surgical incision is an example of healing by primary intention. Larger wounds (*e.g.*, burns and large surface wounds) that have a greater loss of tissue and contamination, heal by secondary intention. Healing by secondary intention is slower than healing by pri-

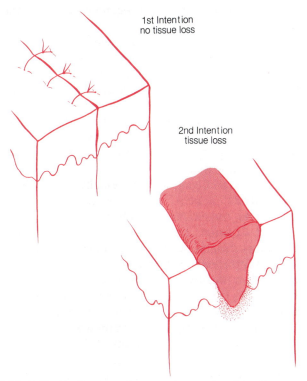

1st Intention
no tissue loss

2nd Intention
tissue loss

FIG. 2-3. *Healing by primary and secondary intention.*

mary intention and results in the formation of larger amounts of scar tissue. A wound that might otherwise have healed by primary intention may become infected and heal by secondary intention.

Wound healing is commonly divided into three phases: (1) the inflammatory phase, (2) the proliferative phase, and (3) the maturational or remodeling phase.[14, 15] In wounds healing by primary intention, the duration of the phases is fairly predictable. In wounds healing by secondary intention, the process is more variable depending on the extent of injury and the healing environment.

INFLAMMATORY PHASE

The inflammatory phase of wound healing begins at the time of injury and is a critical period because it prepares the wound environment for healing. It includes hemostasis (Chapter 17) and the vascular and cellular phases of inflammation (Chapter 13). Hemostatic processes are activated immediately at the time of injury. There is constriction of injured blood vessel and initiation of blood clotting by way of platelet activation and aggregation. After a brief period of constriction, these same vessels dilate and capillaries increase their permeability, allowing plasma and blood components to leak into the injured area. In small surface wounds, the clot loses fluid and becomes a hard, desiccated scab that serves to protect the area.

The cellular phase of inflammation follows and is evidenced by the migration of phagocytic white blood cells that digest and remove invading organisms, fibrin, extracellular debris, and other foreign matter. The polymorphonuclear cells (PMNs) are the first cells to arrive and are usually gone by day three or four. They ingest bacteria and cellular debris. About 24 hours after arrival of the PMNs, a larger and less specific phagocytic cell, called a *macrophage*, enters the wound area and remains for an extended period of time. This cell, arising from blood monocytes, is an essential cell in the healing process. Its functions include phagocytosis and release of growth factors that stimulate epithelial cell growth, angiogenesis (growth of new blood vessels), and attraction of fibroblasts. When a large defect occurs in deeper tissues, PMNs and macrophages are required to remove the debris and facilitate wound closure. Although a wound may heal in the absence of PMNs, it will not heal in the absence of macrophages.

PROLIFERATIVE PHASE

The proliferative phase of healing usually begins within 2 to 3 days of injury and may last as long as 3 weeks in wounds healing by primary intention.

The primary processes during this time focus on the building of new tissue to fill the wound space. The key cell during this phase is the fibroblast. The fibroblast is a connective-tissue cell that synthesizes and secretes collagen and other intercellular elements needed for wound healing. Fibroblasts also produce a family of growth factors that induce new blood vessel formation (angiogenesis) and endothelial cell proliferation and migration.

As early as 24 to 48 hours after injury, fibroblasts and vascular endothelial cells begin proliferating to form a specialized type of soft, pink granular tissue called *granulation tissue* that serves as the foundation for scar tissue development (Fig. 2-4). This tissue is fragile and bleeds easily because of the numerous, newly developed capillary buds. Wounds that heal by secondary intention have more necrotic debris and exudate that must be removed, and they involve larger amounts of granulation tissue. The newly formed blood vessels are leaky and allow plasma proteins and white blood cells to leak into the tissues. At about the same time, epithelial cells at the margin of the wound begin to regenerate and move toward the center of the wound, forming a new surface layer that is similar to that destroyed by the injury. In wounds that heal by primary intention, these epidermal cells proliferate and seal the wound within 24 to 48 hours.[16] When a scab has formed on the wound, the epithelial cells migrate between it and the under-lying viable tissue; when a significant portion of the wound has been covered with epithelial tissue, the scab lifts off. At times, excessive granulation tissue, sometimes referred to as "proud flesh," may form and extend above the edges of wound, preventing reepithelialization from taking place. Surgical removal or chemical cauterization of the defect allows healing to proceed.

As the proliferative phase progresses, there is continued accumulation of collagen and proliferation of fibroblasts. Collagen synthesis reaches a peak within 5 to 7 days and continues for several weeks depending on wound size. By the second week, the white blood cells have largely left the area, the edema has diminished, and the wound begins to blanch as the small blood vessels become thrombosed and degenerate.

REMODELING PHASE

The third phase of wound healing, the remodeling process, begins approximately 3 weeks after injury and can continue for 6 months to 2 years, depending on the extent of the wound. As the term implies, there is continued remodeling of scar tissue due to simultaneous synthesis of collagen by fibroblasts and lysis by collagenase enzymes. As a result of these two processes, the architecture of the scar becomes reoriented to increase the tensile strength of the wound.

Most wounds do not regain the full tensile strength of unwounded skin once healing is completed. Carefully sutured wounds immediately after surgery have approximately 70% of the strength of unwounded skin, due largely to the placement of the sutures. This allows people to move about freely after surgery without fear of wound separation. When the sutures are removed, usually at the end of the first week, wound strength is approximately 10%. It increases rapidly over the next 4 weeks and then slows, reaching a plateau of about 70% to 80% of the tensile strength of unwounded skin at the end of 3 months.[1]

An injury that heals by secondary intention undergoes wound contraction during the proliferative and remodeling phases. As a result, the scar that is formed is considerably smaller than the original wound. Cosmetically, this may be desirable because it reduces the size of the visible defect. On the other hand, contraction of scar tissue over joints and other body structures tends to limit movement and cause deformities. As a result of loss of elasticity, scar tissue that is stretched fails to return to its original length.

An abnormality in healing by scar tissue repair is *keloid* formation. Keloids are tumorlike masses due to excess production of scar tissue. The tendency to develop keloids is more common in African Americans and seems to have a genetic basis.

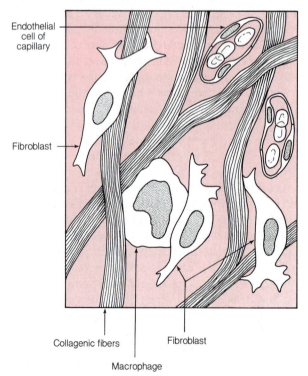

Endothelial cell of capillary

Fibroblast

Collagenic fibers

Fibroblast

Macrophage

FIG. 2-4. *Cells involved in the development of granulation tissue.*

FACTORS THAT AFFECT WOUND HEALING

Many factors, both local and systemic, influence wound healing. Science has not found any way to hasten the normal process of wound repair, but there are many factors that impair healing. Among the causes of impaired wound healing are: (1) malnutrition; (2) impaired blood flow and oxygen delivery; (3) impaired inflammatory and immune responses; (4) infection, wound separation, and foreign bodies; and (5) age effects.

MALNUTRITION

Successful wound healing depends, in part, on the presence of adequate nutritional stores of proteins, carbohydrates, fats, vitamins, and minerals. It is well recognized that malnutrition slows the healing process, causing wounds to heal inadequately or incompletely.[18, 19]

Protein deficiencies prolong the inflammatory phase of healing and impair fibroblast proliferation, collagen and protein matrix synthesis, angiogenesis, and wound remodeling. Although all amino acids influence the healing process, it is possible to single out at least one, methionine, that is essential to healing. Methionine is converted to cystine, which is a cofactor in enzyme systems responsible for collagen synthesis.[19] Carbohydrates are needed as an energy source for white cells. Carbohydrates also have a protein-sparing effect and help to prevent the use of amino acids for fuel when they are needed for the healing process. Fats are essential constituents of cell membranes and are needed for the synthesis of new cells.

Although all vitamins are essential cofactors for daily functions of the body, vitamins A and C play an essential role in the healing process. Vitamin C is needed for collagen synthesis. In a vitamin C deficiency, an improper sequencing of amino acids occurs, proper linking of amino acids does not take place, the by-products of collagen synthesis are not removed from the cell, new wounds do not heal properly, and old wounds may fall apart. Administration of vitamin C rapidly restores the healing process to normal. Vitamin A functions in stimulating and supporting epithelialization, capillary formation, and collagen synthesis. Vitamin A has also been shown to counteract the antiinflammatory effects of corticosteroid drugs and can be used to reverse these effects in people who are on chronic steroid therapy. The B vitamins are important cofactors in enzymatic reactions that contribute to the wound-healing process. All are water soluble, and, with the exception of vitamin B_{12}, which is stored in the liver, almost all must be replaced daily. Vitamin K plays an indirect role in wound healing by preventing bleeding disorders that contribute to hematoma formation and subsequent infection.

The role of minerals in wound healing is less clearly defined. The macrominerals, including sodium, potassium, calcium, and phosphorus, as well as the microminerals such as copper and zinc must be present for normal cell function. Zinc is a cofactor in a variety of enzyme systems responsible for cell proliferation. In animal studies, zinc has been found to aid in reepithelialization. Although a zinc deficiency tends to impair healing, zinc therapy does not seem to improve healing.[20]

BLOOD FLOW AND OXYGEN DELIVERY

For healing to occur, wounds must have adequate blood flow to supply the necessary nutrients and to remove the resulting waste, local toxins, bacteria, and other debris. Impaired wound healing due to poor blood flow may occur as a result of wound conditions (*e.g.*, swelling) or by preexisting health problems. Arterial disease and venous pathology are well-documented causes of impaired wound healing. In situations of trauma, a decrease in blood volume may cause a reduction in blood flow to injured tissues.

Molecular oxygen is required for collagen synthesis. It has been shown that even a temporary lack of oxygen can result in the formation of less stable collagen.[21, 22] Wounds in ischemic tissue become infected more frequently than wounds in well-vascularized tissue. Both PMNs and macrophages require oxygen for destruction of microorganisms that have invaded the area. Although these cells can accomplish phagocytosis in a relatively anoxic environment, they cannot digest bacteria.

IMPAIRED INFLAMMATORY AND IMMUNE RESPONSES

Both inflammatory and immune mechanisms function in wound healing. Inflammation is essential to the first phase of wound healing, and immune mechanisms prevent infections that impair wound healing. Among the conditions that impair inflammation and immune function are disorders of phagocytic function, diabetes mellitus, and therapeutic administration of corticosteroid drugs.

Phagocytic disorders may be divided into extrinsic and intrinsic defects. Extrinsic disorders are those that: (1) impair attraction of phagocytic cells to the wound site, (2) prepare bacteria and foreign agents for engulfment by the phagocytic cells (called *opsonization*), or (3) cause suppression in the total number of phagocytic cells (*e.g.*, immunosuppressive agents). Intrinsic phagocytic disorders are the result of enzymatic deficiencies within the metabolic pathway for destroying the ingested bacteria by the phagocytic cell. The intrinsic phagocytic disorders include chronic granulomatous disease (discussed in Chapter 14), an X-linked inherited disease in which there is a deficiency of myeloperoxidase and nicotinamide-adenine dinucleotide peroxidase (NADPH)-dependent oxidase enzyme. Deficiencies of these compounds prevent generation of hydrogen superoxide and hydrogen peroxide needed for killing bacteria.

There is a well-recognized problem with wound healing among people with diabetes mellitus, particularly among those who have poorly controlled blood glucose levels. Studies have shown delayed wound healing, poor collagen formation, and poor tensile strength in diabetic animals. Of particular importance is the effect of hyperglycemia on phagocytic function. Neutrophils, for example, have diminished chemotaxic and phagocytic function, including engulfment and intracellular killing of bacteria when exposed to altered glucose levels. Small blood vessel disease is also common among people with diabetes, impairing the delivery of inflammatory cells, oxygen, and nutrients to the wound site.

The therapeutic administration of adrenal corticosteroids is known to produce a decrease in the inflammatory process and to delay healing. These hormones decrease capillary permeability during the early stages of inflammation, impair the phagocytic property of the leukocytes, and inhibit fibroblast proliferation and function.

INFECTION, WOUND SEPARATION, AND FOREIGN BODIES

Wound contamination, wound separation, and foreign bodies delay wound healing.

Infection impairs all dimensions of wound healing. It prolongs the inflammatory phase, impairs the formation of granulation tissue, and inhibits proliferation of fibroblasts and deposition of collagen fibers. All wounds are contaminated at the time of injury. Although body defenses can handle the invasion of microorganisms at the time of wounding, badly contaminated wounds can overwhelm host defenses. Also, trauma and existing impairment of host defenses can contribute to the development of wound infections.

Approximation of the wound edges (*i.e.*, suturing of an incision type of wound) greatly enhances healing and prevents infection. Epithelialization of a wound with closely approximated edges occurs within 1 to 2 days. Large gapping wounds tend to heal more slowly because it is often impossible to effect wound closure with this type of wound.

Foreign bodies tend to invite bacterial contamination and delay healing. Fragments of wood, steel, glass, and the like may have entered the wound at the site of injury and can be difficult to locate when the wound is treated. Sutures are also foreign bodies, and, although needed for the closure of surgical wounds, they are an impediment to healing. This is why sutures are removed as soon as possible after surgery. Wound infections are of special concern in people with implantation of foreign bodies such as orthopedic devices (*e.g.*, pins and stabilization devices), cardiac pacemakers, and shunt catheters. These infections are difficult to treat and may require removal of device.

EFFECT OF AGE

The effects of both immaturity and aging affect healing. The rate of skin replacement slows with aging.

Wound Healing in Neonates and Children. Wound healing in the pediatric population follows a similar course to that in the adult population.[23] The child has greater capacity for repair than the adult but may lack the reserves needed to ensure proper healing. Such lack is evidenced by an easily upset electrolyte balance, sudden elevation or lowering of temperature, and rapid spread of infection.

The neonate and small child may have an immature immune system with no antigenic experience with organisms that contaminate wounds. The younger the child, the more likely the development of immune depression.

Successful wound healing also depends on adequate nutrition. Children need sufficient calories to maintain both growth and wound healing. The premature infant is often born with immature organ systems and minimal energy stores but high metabolic requirements—a condition that predisposes to impaired wound healing.

Wound Healing in Aged Persons. There is a slowing in the rate of cell replacement in normal aging skin and in epithelialization of open wounds.[24] The skin is more fragile and easily wounded. There is a gradual decline in immune function in the elderly. Multiple illnesses, circulatory problems, and nutritional deficits compound the wound-healing process.

In summary, the ability of tissues to repair damage due to injury depends on the body's ability to replace the parenchymal cells and to organize them as they were originally. Regeneration describes the process by which tissue is replaced with cells of a similar type and function. Healing by regeneration is limited to tissue with cells that are able to divide and to replace the injured cells. Body cells are divided into types according to their ability to regenerate: (1) labile cells, such as the epithelial cells of the skin and gastrointestinal tract, which continue to regenerate throughout life; (2) stable cells, such as those in the liver, which normally do not divide but which are capable of regeneration when confronted with an appropriate stimulus; and (3) permanent or fixed cells, such as nerve cells, which are unable to regenerate. Scar-tissue repair involves the substitution of fibrous connective tissue for injured tissue that cannot be repaired by regeneration.

Tissue injury is followed almost immediately by bleeding into the area and the development of a blood clot that contains fibrin and blood cells. Within several hours, the surface of the clot loses fluid and becomes a hard, dehydrated scab that serves to protect the area. At about the same time, inflammatory cells enter the injured area and begin to break down and remove the inflammatory debris.

■ REFERENCES

1. Cotran, R.S., Kumar, V., & Robbins, S.L. (1989). *Robbins' pathologic basis of disease* (4th ed., pp. 5, 25, 32–34, 54, 71, 501). Philadelphia: W.B. Saunders.
2. American Heart Association. (1987). Oxygen free radicals: When a good element goes bad. *Cardiovascular Research Report*, Summer, 12.
3. Dart, R.C., & Sanders, A.B. (1988). Oxygen free radicals and myocardial reperfusion injury. *Annals of Emergency Medicine, 17*, 53.
4. Sinclair, A.J., Barnett, H., & Lunec, J. (1990). Free radicals and antioxidant systems in health and disease. *British Journal of Hospital Medicine, 43*(2), 334–344.
5. Machlin, L.J., & Bendich, A. (1987). Free radical tissue damage: Protective role of antioxidant nutrients. *FASEB Journal, 1*, 441–445.
6. Vogt, M.T., & Farber, E. (1968). On the molecular pathology of ischemic renal cell death: Reversible and irreversible cellular and mitochondrial metabolic alterations. *American Journal of Pathology, 53*, 1.
7. Robbins, S.L., Cotran, R.S., & Kumar, V. (1979). *Pathologic basis of disease* (2nd ed., p. 551). Philadelphia: W.B. Saunders.
8. Erwin, D.N. (1983). An overview of the biological effects of radiofrequency radiation. *Military Medicine, 148*(2), 113–117.
9. Djordjevic, Z., Kolak, A., Djokovic, V., et al. (1983). Results of our 15-year study on biological effects of microwave exposure. *Aviation Space and Environmental Medicine, 54*(6), 539–542.
10. Corry, M., & Montoya, L. (1990). Gas gangrene: Certain diagnosis or certain death. *Critical Care Nursing, 9*(10), 30–38.
11. Pessa, M.E., Bland, K.I., & Copeland, E.M., III. (1987). Growth factors and determinants of wound repair. *Journal of Surgical Research, 42*, 207–217.
12. Sporn, M.B., & Roberts, A.B. (1986). Peptide growth factors and inflammation, tissue repair, and cancer. *Journal of Clinical Investigation, 78*, 329–332.
13. Brown, G.L., Nanney, L.B., & Griffen, J. (1989). Enhancement of wound healing by topical treatment with epidermal growth factor. *New England Journal of Medicine, 321*, 76–79.
14. Norris, S.O., Provo, B., & Stotts, N.A. (1990). Physiology of wound healing and risk factors that impede the healing process. *Clinical Issues in Critical Care Nursing, 1*, 545–552.
15. Cooper, D.M. (1990). Optimizing wound healing. *Nursing Clinics of North America, 25*, 165–171.
16. Orgill, D., & Deming, H.R. (1988). Current concepts and approaches to healing. *Critical Care Medicine, 16*, 899–908.
17. Young, M.E. (1988). Malnutrition and wound healing. *Heart and Lung, 17*, 6067.
18. Stotts, N.A., & Washington, D. (1990). Nutrition: A critical component of wound healing. *Clinical Issues in Critical Care Nursing, 1*, 585–592.
19. Ruberg, R.L. (1984). Role of nutrition in wound healing. *Surgical Clinics of North America, 64*(4), 795–814.
20. Neldner, K.H., & Hambridge, K.M. (1974). Zinc therapy. *New England Journal of Medicine, 292*, 879.
21. Whitney, J.D. (1989). Physiologic effects of tissue oxygenation on wound healing. *Heart and Lung, 18*, 466–474.
22. Whitney, J.D. (1990). The influence of tissue oxygenation and perfusion on wound healing. *Clinical Issues in Critical Care Nursing, 1*, 578–584.
23. Garvin, G. (1990). Wound healing in pediatrics. *Nursing Clinics of North America, 25*, 181–191.
24. Jones, P., & Millman, A. (1990). Wound healing and the aged patient. *Nursing Clinics of North America, 25*, 263–277.

CHAPTER 3

GENETIC CONTROL OF CELL FUNCTION AND INHERITANCE

■ OBJECTIVES

After you have studied this chapter, you should be able to meet the following objectives:

■ Describe the structure of a gene.
■ Explain the mechanisms whereby genes control cell function.
■ Explain how genetic information is transferred from one generation to another generation.
■ Compare the functions of messenger RNA, transfer RNA, and ribosomal RNA.
■ Describe the concept of induction and repression in terms of gene function.
■ Define *gene locus* and *allele*.
■ Describe the pathogenesis of gene mutation.

■ Explain how gene expressivity and penetrance determine the effects of a mutant gene that codes for the production of an essential enzyme.
■ List the steps in constructing a karyotype using cytogenetic studies.
■ Construct a hypothetical pedigree for a recessive and dominant trait according to Mendel's law.
■ Contrast genotype and phenotype.
■ Define *genomic mapping*.
■ Briefly describe the methods used in linkage studies, dosage studies, and hybridization studies.

The word *gene* is defined as the *fundamental unit of information storage*. This information is stored in the structure of *deoxyribonucleic acid (DNA)*, an extremely stable macromolecule within the nucleus of each cell. Because of the stable structure of DNA, the genetic information is able to survive the many processes of reduction division of the gametes (ovum and sperm), fertilization, and the many cell divisions involved in the formation of a new organism from the single-celled zygote.

Genes determine the types of proteins and enzymes that are made by the cell and hence control not only inheritance but the day-to-day function of all the cells in the body. For example, genes control the type and quantity of hormones that a cell produces, the antigens and receptors that are present on the cell

Carol Mattson Porth: PATHOPHYSIOLOGY: CONCEPTS OF ALTERED HEALTH STATES, 4th ed. © 1994, 1990, 1986, 1982 J.B. Lippincott Company

membrane, and the synthesis of enzymes needed for metabolism. Of the estimated 50,000 to 100,000 genes that humans possess, about 5,000 have been identified and about 2,300 have been localized to a particular chromosome. With few exceptions, each gene provides the instructions for the synthesis of a single protein. This chapter includes discussions of genetic regulation of cell function, chromosomal structure, patterns of inheritance, and gene technology.

■ GENETIC CONTROL OF CELL FUNCTION

The genetic information needed for protein synthesis is inscribed on the DNA contained in the cell nucleus. A second type of nucleic acid, *ribonucleic acid (RNA)*, is involved in the actual synthesis of cellular enzymes and proteins. Cells contain several types of RNA: messenger RNA, transfer RNA, and ribosomal RNA. *Messenger RNA* transcribes the instructions for protein synthesis from the DNA molecule and carries them into the cytoplasm. Transcription is followed by translation, the synthesis of proteins according to the instructions carried by messenger RNA. *Ribosomal RNA* provides the machinery needed for protein synthesis. *Transfer RNA* reads the instructions and delivers the appropriate amino acids to the ribosome, where they are incorporated into the protein being synthesized. The mechanism for genetic control of cell function is illustrated in Figure 3-1.

The nuclei of all the cells in an organism all contain the same accumulation of genes derived from the gametes of the two parents. This means that liver cells contain the same genetic information as skin and muscle cells. For this to be true, the molecular code must be duplicated prior to each succeeding cell division, or mitosis. Theoretically, although not yet achieved in humans, any of the highly differentiated cells of an organism could be used to produce a complete, genetically identical organism, or clone. Each particular tissue uses only some of the information stored in the genetic code. Although information required for the function of other types of tissues is still present, it is repressed.

GENE STRUCTURE

The structure that stores the genetic information within the nucleus is a long, double-stranded, helical molecule of DNA. The DNA molecule is composed of nucleotides, which consist of (1) phosphoric acid, (2) a five-carbon sugar called *deoxyribose*, and (3) one of four nitrogenous bases. The nitrogenous bases carry the genetic information. These four bases can be divided into two groups: the purine bases, *adenine* and

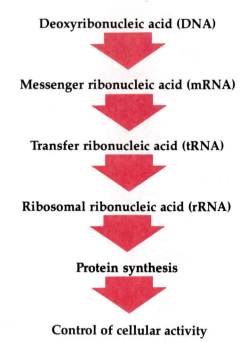

FIG. 3-1. DNA-directed control of cellular activity through synthesis of cellular proteins. Messenger RNA carries the transcribed message, which directs protein synthesis, from the nucleus to the cytoplasm. Transfer RNA selects the appropriate amino acids and carries them to ribosomal RNA, where assembly of the proteins takes place.

guanine, which have two nitrogen ring structures, and the pyrimidine bases, *thymine* and *cytosine*, which have one ring. Alternating groups of sugar and phosphoric acid form the backbone of the molecule, with the paired bases projecting inward from the sides of the sugar molecule. The entire chain is like a spiral staircase, with the paired bases representing the steps (Fig. 3-2C).

There is a precise complementary pairing of purine and pyrimidine bases in the double-stranded DNA molecule. Adenine is paired with thymine, and guanine is paired with cytosine (Fig. 3-3). Each nucleotide in a pair is on one strand of the DNA molecule, with the bases of the pair loosely bound by a hydrogen bond. Because of the looseness of the bond, the two strands can pull apart with ease so that the genetic information can be duplicated or transcribed (see Fig. 3-2A).

A gene can be regarded as being represented by several hundred to almost a million base pairs, the size being proportional to the protein product it encodes. Of the two DNA strands, only one is used in transcribing the information for the cell's polypeptide-building machinery. If the genetic information of one strand is meaningful, the complementary code of the other strand will not make sense and will be ignored. Both strands, however, are involved in DNA duplication. Prior to cell division, the two strands of the

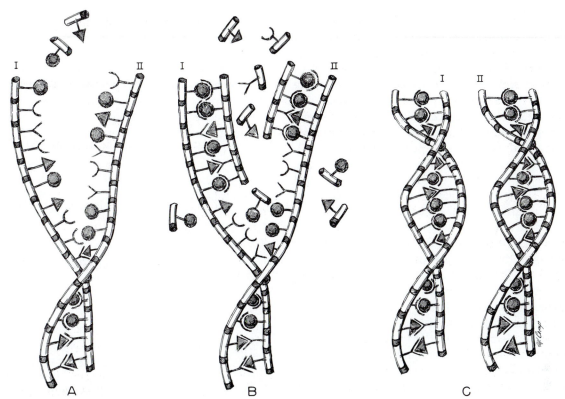

FIG. 3-2. Schematic representation of the replication of DNA. (**A**) Before cell division, the bonds between the nitrogenous bases are broken, the two strands separate, and each strand takes with it the bases attached to its side. (**B**) The bases attached to each single strand attract free-floating nucleotide units and pair off in the usual way: adenine with thymine, guanine with cytosine. (**C**) The end result is two exact replicas of the original DNA molecule, and the cell is ready to undergo division. (Chaffee, E. E., & Lytle, I. M. [1980]. *Basic physiology and anatomy* [4th ed.]. Philadelphia: J.B. Lippincott)

helix separate and a complementary molecule is organized next to each original strand. Thus, two strands become four strands (see Fig. 3-2*B*). During cell division, the newly duplicated double-stranded molecules are separated and placed in each daughter cell by the mechanics of mitosis. As a result, each of the daughter cells again contains the meaningful strand and the complementary strand joined in the form of a double helix. Replication of DNA has been termed *semiconservative* because each new daughter molecule contains one parental strand.

The DNA molecule is combined with several types of protein and small amounts of RNA into a complex known as *chromatin*. Chromatin is the more readily stainable portion of the cell nucleus. Some of these proteins form binding sites for repressor molecules and hormones that regulate genetic transcription. Other proteins may block genetic transcription by preventing access of nucleotides to the surface of the DNA molecule. A specific group of proteins called *histones* are thought to control the folding of the DNA strands.

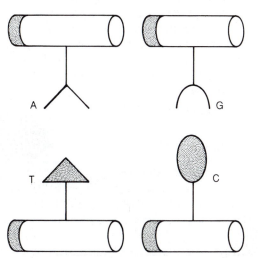

FIG. 3-3. Pairing of the nucleotides in DNA. Thymine pairs with adenine, and cytosine pairs with guanine.

GENETIC CODE

The four bases, guanine, adenine, cytosine, and thymine (uracil is substituted for thymine in RNA), make up the alphabet of the genetic code. A sequence of three of these bases constitutes the fundamental triplet code used in transmitting the genetic information needed for protein synthesis; this triplet code is called a *codon* (Table 3-1). An example is the nucleotide sequence GCU (guanine, cytosine, and uracil), which is the triplet RNA code for the amino acid alanine. The genetic code is a universal language used by almost all living cells (*i.e.*, the code for the amino acid tryptophan is the same in a bacterium, a plant, and a human being). There are also stop codes, which signal the end of a protein molecule. Mathematically, the four bases can be arranged in 64 different combinations ($4 \times 4 \times 4 = 64$). Sixty-one triplets correspond to particular amino acids, whereas three are stop signals. Because there are only 20 amino acids that can be used in protein synthesis, there may be several codes for the same amino acid. AUG is a part of the initiation or start signal as well as the codon for the amino acid methionine. Codons that specify the same amino acid are called synonyms. Synonyms usually have the same first two bases but differ in the third base.

PROTEIN SYNTHESIS

Although DNA determines the type of biochemical product that the cell synthesizes, the transmission and decoding of information needed for protein synthesis are carried out by RNA, the formation of which is directed by DNA. The general structure of RNA differs from DNA in three respects: (1) RNA is a single rather than a double-stranded molecule; (2) the sugar in each nucleotide of RNA is ribose instead of deoxyribose; and (3) the pyrimidine base thymine in DNA is replaced by uracil in RNA. As previously mentioned, there are three types of RNA: messenger RNA (mRNA), transfer RNA (tRNA), and ribosomal RNA (rRNA). All three types are synthesized in the nucleus by RNA polymerase enzymes that take directions from DNA.

MESSENGER RNA

Messenger RNA is the template for protein synthesis. It is a long molecule containing several hundred to several thousand nucleotides, which are codons that are exactly complementary to code words on the genes. Messenger RNA is formed by a process called *transcription*, in which the weak hydrogen bonds of the DNA are broken so that free RNA nucleotides can

TABLE 3-1. RNA CODONS FOR THE DIFFERENT AMINO ACIDS AND FOR START AND STOP

AMINO ACID	RNA CODONS					
Alanine	GCU	GCC	GCA	GCG		
Arginine	CGU	CGC	CGA	CGG	AGA	AGG
Asparagine	AAU	AAC				
Aspartic acid	GAU	GAC				
Cysteine	UGU	UGC				
Glutamic acid	GAA	GAG				
Glutamine	CAA	CAG				
Glycine	GGU	GGC	GGA	GGG		
Histidine	CAU	CAC				
Isoleucine	AUU	AUC	AUA			
Leucine	CUU	CUC	CUA	CUG	UUA	UUG
Lysine	AAA	AAG				
Methionine	AUG					
Phenylalanine	UUU	UUC				
Proline	CCU	CCC	CCA	CCG		
Serine	UCU	UCC	UCA	UCG	AGC	AGU
Threonine	ACU	ACC	ACA	ACG		
Tryptophan	UGG					
Tyrosine	UAU	UAC				
Valine	GUU	GUC	GUA	GUG		
Start (CI)	AUG					
Stop (CT)	UAA	UAG	UGA			

(Guyton, A. [1991]. *Textbook of medical physiology* [8th ed., p. 27]. Philadelphia: W.B. Saunders)

pair with their exposed DNA counterparts on the meaningful strand of the DNA molecule. As with the base pairing of the DNA strands, complementary RNA bases pair with the DNA bases (uracil, which replaces thymine in RNA, pairs with adenine).

During transcription, a specialized nuclear enzyme, called *RNA polymerase*, recognizes the beginning or start sequence of a gene, attaches to the double-stranded DNA, and proceeds to copy the meaningful strand into a single strand of RNA as it travels along the length of the gene. Upon reaching the stop signal, the enzyme leaves the gene and releases the RNA strand. The RNA strand is processed. Processing involves the addition of certain nucleic acids at the ends of the RNA strand and cutting and splicing of certain internal sequences. Splicing often involves the removal of stretches of RNA. Because of the splicing process, matured RNA differs in sequence from the original DNA template. RNA sequences that are retained are called *exons*, and those that are excised are called *introns*. The functions of the introns are not yet known. They are thought to be involved in the activation or deactivation of genes during various stages of development.

Splicing permits a cell to produce different RNA molecules from a single gene by splicing segments of the initial RNA differently. For example, in a muscle cell, the original tropomyocin RNA transcriptase is spliced in as many as ten different ways, yielding distinctly different protein products. This permits different proteins to be expressed from a single gene and compresses the amount of DNA that must be contained in the genome.[1]

TRANSFER RNA

Transfer RNA carries amino acids in the activated form to protein molecules as they are being synthesized in the ribosomes. It is clover shaped and contains about 80 nucleotides, making it the smallest RNA molecule. There are at least 20 different types of tRNA, each of which recognizes and binds to only one type of amino acid. Each tRNA has two recognition sites: one for the mRNA codon and a second for the amino acid itself. Each type of tRNA carries its own specific amino acid to the ribosomes where protein synthesis is taking place; there it recognizes the appropriate codon on the mRNA and delivers the amino acid to the newly forming protein molecule.

RIBOSOMAL RNA

The ribosome is the physical structure in the cytoplasm where protein synthesis takes place. Ribosomal RNA constitutes 60% of the ribosome, with the remainder of the ribosome being structural proteins and enzymes needed for protein synthesis. As with the other types of RNA, rRNA is synthesized in the nucleus. As the rRNA is synthesized, it collects in a specialized nuclear structure, called the *nucleolus*, which lies adjacent to the chromosomes. It combines with ribosomal proteins in the nucleus and is then transported into the cytoplasm. During protein synthesis, most ribosomes become attached to the endoplasmic reticulum. There is no specificity of ribosomes for synthesis of a particular protein; a particular mRNA can direct protein synthesis in any ribosome.

Proteins are made from a standard set of amino acids, which are joined end to end to form the long polypeptide chains of protein molecules. Each polypeptide chain may have as many as 100 to more than 300 amino acids in it. The process of protein synthesis is called *translation* because the genetic code is translated into the production language needed for protein assembly. In addition to rRNA, translation requires the coordinated actions of mRNA and tRNA. Transfer RNA transports amino acids to the ribosome for incorporation into the developing protein molecule. Messenger RNA provides the information needed for placing the amino acids in their proper order for each specific type of protein. During protein synthesis, mRNA comes in contact with and passes through the ribosome reading the directions for protein synthesis, in much the same way that a tape is read as it passes through a tape player.[2] As mRNA passes through the ribosome, tRNA delivers the appropriate amino acids for attachment to the growing polypeptide chain. The long mRNA molecule usually travels through and directs protein synthesis in more than one ribosome at a time. As the first part of the mRNA is read by the first ribosome, it moves on to a second, and a third; as a result, ribosomes that are actively involved in protein synthesis are often found in clusters called *polyribosomes*. The process of protein synthesis is depicted in Figure 3-4.

REGULATION OF GENE EXPRESSION

Although all cells contain the same genes, not all genes are active all of the time, nor are the same genes active in all cell types. On the contrary, only a small, select group of genes is active in directing protein synthesis in the cell, and this group varies from one cell type to another. For different types of cells to develop in the various organs and tissues of the body as a result of cell differentiation, the protein synthesis in some cells must be different from that in others. Furthermore, to adapt to an ever-changing environment, certain cells may need to produce varying amounts and types of proteins. In addition, there are certain enzymes, such as carbonic an-

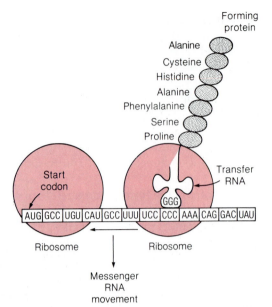

FIG. 3-4. Postulated mechanism by which a protein molecule is formed in ribosomes in association with messenger RNA and ribosomal RNA. (Guyton, A. [1991]. *Medical physiology* [8th ed.]. Philadelphia: W.B. Saunders)

hydrase, that all cells must synthesize for the fundamental metabolic process on which life depends.

The degree to which a gene or particular group of genes is active is referred to as *gene expression*. A phenomenon termed *induction* is an important process whereby gene expression is increased. Except in early embryonic development, induction is produced by some external influence. Gene *repression* is the process whereby a regulatory gene acts to reduce or prevent gene expression. Some genes are normally dormant and can be activated by inducer substances, and other genes are naturally active and can be inhibited by repressor substances.

Genetic mechanisms for the control of protein synthesis are much better understood in microorganisms than in humans. It can be assumed, however, that many of the same principles apply. The mechanism that has been most extensively studied is the one by which the synthesis of particular proteins can be turned on and off. In *Escherichia coli (E. coli)* grown in a nutrient medium containing the disaccharide lactose, an enzyme (galactosidase) can be isolated that catalyzes the splitting of lactose into a molecule of glucose and a molecule of galactose; this is necessary if lactose is to be metabolized by *E. coli*. On the other hand, if the *E. coli* is grown in a medium that does not contain lactose, very little of the enzyme is produced. From these and other studies, it is theorized that the synthesis of a particular protein, such as galactosidase, requires a series of reactions, each of which is catalyzed by a specific enzyme.

There are believed to be at least two types of genes that control protein synthesis: (1) structural genes that specify the amino acid sequence of a polypeptide chain and (2) regulator genes that serve a regulatory function without stipulating the structure of protein molecules. The regulation of protein synthesis is controlled by a sequence of genes, called an *operon*, located on adjacent sites on the same chromosome (Fig. 3-5).[2] An operon consists of a set of structural genes that code for enzymes used in the synthesis of a particular product and promoter site that binds RNA polymerase and initiates transcription of the structural genes. The function of the operon is further regulated by an activator operator and a repressor operator, which induce or repress the function of the promoter. The activator and repressor sites commonly monitor levels of the synthesized product and regulate the activity of the operon in a negative feedback manner; whenever product levels decrease, the function of the operon is activated, and, when levels increase, its function is repressed. Regulatory genes located elsewhere in the genetic complex can exert control over an operon through activator or repressor substances. Not all genes are subject to induction and repression.

GENE MUTATIONS

Rarely, accidental errors in duplication of DNA occur. These errors are called *mutations*. Mutations result from the substitution of one base pair for another, the loss or addition of one or more base pairs, or rearrangements of base pairs. Many of these mutations occur spontaneously; others are caused by environmental agents, chemicals, and radiation.

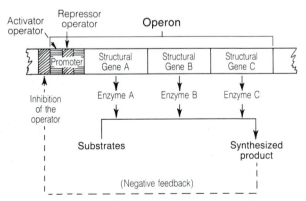

FIG. 3-5. Function of the operon to control biosynthesis. Note the synthesized product exerts a negative feedback to inhibit function of the operon, in this way automatically controlling the concentration of the product itself. (Guyton, A. [1991]. *Medical physiology* [8th ed.]. Philadelphia: W.B. Saunders)

Mutations may arise in either somatic cells or in germ cells. Only those DNA changes that occur in germ cells can be inherited. A somatic mutation affects a cell line that differentiates into one or more of the many tissues of the body and is not transmissible to the next generation. Somatic mutations that do not have an impact on the health or functioning of a person are called *polymorphisms*. Occasionally, a person is born with one brown eye and one blue eye as a result of a somatic mutation. The change or loss of gene information is just as likely to affect the fundamental processes of cell function or organ differentiation. Such somatic mutations in the early embryonic period can result in embryonic death or congenital malformations. Somatic mutations are important causes of cancer and other tumors in which cell differentiation and growth get out of hand. Fishermen, farmers, and others who are excessively exposed to the ultraviolet radiation of sunlight have an increased risk of developing skin cancer resulting from potential radiation damage to the genetic structure of the skin-forming cells.

In summary, genes are the fundamental unit of information storage in the cell. They determine the types of proteins and enzymes made by the cell and, therefore, control not only inheritance but day-to-day cell function. Genes store information in the form of a stable macromolecule called DNA. Genes transmit information in the form of a triplet code, which uses the nitrogenous bases of the four nucleotides (adenine, guanine, thymine (or uracil in RNA), and cytosine) of which the DNA molecule is composed. The transfer of stored information into production of cell products is accomplished through a second type of macromolecule called RNA. Messenger RNA transcribes the instructions for product synthesis from the DNA molecule and carries it into the cell's cytoplasm, where ribosomal RNA uses the information to direct product synthesis. Transfer RNA acts as a carrier system for delivering the appropriate amino acids to the ribosomes, where the synthesis of cell products occurs. Although all cells contain the same genes, only a small, select group of genes is active in a given cell type. In all cells, some genetic information is repressed whereas other information is expressed. Gene mutations represent accidental errors in duplication, rearrangements, or deletion of parts of the genetic code.

■ CHROMOSOMES

The genetic information of a cell is organized, stored, and retrieved in the form of small cellular structures called *chromosomes* (Fig. 3-6). Although the chromosomes are visible only in dividing cells, they retain their integrity between cell divisions.

The chromosomes are arranged in pairs; one member of the pair is inherited from the father, the other from the mother. Each species has a character-

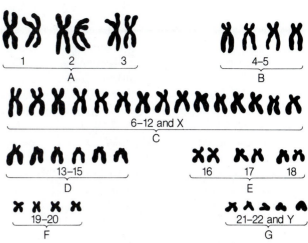

FIG. 3-6. Normal male karyotype. The first 22 pairs of chromosomes are the autosomes, and the last two chromosomes are the sex chromosomes, in this case, an X and Y chromosome. (Singer, S. [1978]. *Human genetics.* San Francisco: W.H. Freeman)

istic number of chromosomes. There are 46 single or 23 pairs of human chromosomes. Of the 23 pairs of human chromosomes, there are 22 pairs called the *autosomes* that are alike in males and females. Each of the 22 pairs of autosomes has the same appearance in all individuals, and each has been given a numeric designation for classification purposes (see Fig. 3-6).

The sex chromosomes constitute the 23rd pair of chromosomes. There are two sex chromosomes that determine the sex of a person. All males have an X and Y chromosome (an X chromosome from the mother and a Y chromosome from the father), and all females have two X chromosomes (one from each parent). It is believed that, of the two X chromosomes in the female, only one is active in controlling the expression of genetic traits. Both X chromosomes are involved, however, in transmission to the offspring. In the female, the active X chromosome is invisible, whereas the inactive X chromosome can be demonstrated, on appropriate nuclear staining, as the *chromatin mass* or *Barr body*. The genetic sex of a child can be determined by microscopic study of cell or tissue samples. The total number of X chromosomes is equal to the number of Barr bodies plus one (an inactive plus an active X chromosome). For example, the cells of a normal female have one Barr body and, therefore, a total of two X chromosomes. A male has no Barr bodies. In the female, whether the X chromosome derived from the mother or that derived from the father is active is determined within a few days after conception; the selection is random for each postmitotic cell line. This is called the Lyon principle (after Mary Lyon, the British geneticist who developed it).

CELL DIVISION

There are two types of cell division—meiosis and mitosis. *Meiosis* is limited to replicating germ cells and only takes place once in a cell line. It results in the formation of gametes or reproductive cells (ovum and sperm), each of which has only a single set of 23 chromosomes.

Mitosis is the process by which somatic or body cells effect growth and tissue repair. It results in the formation of 23 pairs of chromosomes. Mitosis is subdivided into four stages: prophase, metaphase, anaphase, and telophase (Fig. 3-7). During *prophase*, the centrioles in the cytoplasm separate and move toward opposite sides of the cell, the chromosomes become shorter and thicker, and the nuclear membrane breaks up so that there is no longer a barrier between the chromosomes and the cytoplasm. *Metaphase* involves the organization of the chromosome pairs in the midline of the cell and the formation of a mitotic spindle composed of the microtubules. *Anaphase* is the period during which splitting of the chromosome pairs occurs, with the microtubules pulling each set of 46 chromosomes toward the opposite cell pole in preparation for cell separation. Cell division is completed during *telophase*, when the mitotic spindles vanish and a new nuclear membrane develops and encloses each of the sets of chromosomes.

CHROMOSOME STUDIES

Cytogenetics is the study of the structure and numeric characteristics of the cell's chromosomes. Chromosome studies can be done on any tissue or cell that grows and divides in culture. The lymphocytes from venous blood are frequently used for this purpose. Once the cells have been cultured, a drug called *colchicine* is used to arrest mitosis in metaphase. A chromosome spread is prepared by fixing and spreading the chromosomes on a slide and using a staining technique to demonstrate chromosomal banding patterns so they can be identified. The chromosomes are photographed, and the photomicrograph of each chromosome is cut out and arranged in pairs according to a standard classification system. The completed picture is called a *karyotype*, and the procedure for preparing the picture is called *karyotyping*. The uniform system of chromosome classification was originally formulated at the 1971 Paris Chromosome Conference[3] and was later revised to describe the chromosomes as seen in more elongated prophase and prometaphase preparation.[4]

In the metaphase spread, each chromosome takes the form of chromatids to form an X or "wishbone" configuration. Human chromosomes are divided into three types according to centromere (central constriction) position (Fig. 3-8). If the centromere

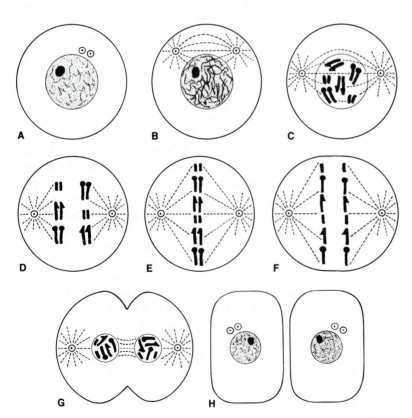

FIG. 3-7. Cell mitosis. *A* and *H* represent the nondividing cell; *B, C,* and *D* represent prophase; *E* represents anaphase; and *G* represents telophase. (Chaffee, E. E., & Greisheimer, E. M. [1974]. *Basic physiology and anatomy* [3rd ed.]. Philadelphia: J.B. Lippincott)

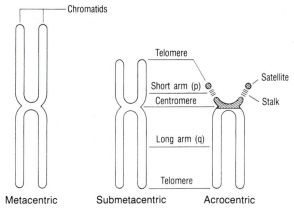

FIG. 3-8. Chromosome types and landmarks. (Thompson, M., Roderick, R., McInnes, R., & Huntington, F. W. [1991]. *Genetics in medicine* [5th ed.]. Philadelphia: W.B. Saunders)

is in the center and the arms are of approximately the same length, the chromosome is said to be *metacentric*; if it is off-center but the arms are of clearly different lengths, it is *submetacentric*; and, if it is near one end, it is *acrocentric*. The short arm of the chromosome is designated "p" for petite, and the long arm is designated "q" for no other reason than it is the next letter of the alphabet. Arms of the chromosome are indicated by the chromosome number followed by the *p* or *q* designation. Chromosomes 13, 14, 15, 21, and 22 have small masses of chromatin called *satellites* attached to their short arms by narrow stalks.

In summary, the genetic information in a cell is organized, stored, and retrieved in the form of small cellular structures called chromosomes. There are 46 chromosomes arranged in 23 pairs. Twenty-two of these pairs are autosomes. The 23rd pair is the sex chromosomes, which determine the sex of a person. There are two kinds of cell division—meiosis and mitosis. Meiosis is limited to replicating germ cells and results in the formation of gametes or reproductive cells (ovum and sperm) each of which has only a single set of 23 chromosomes. Mitotic division occurs in somatic cells and results in the formation of 23 pairs of chromosomes. A karyotype is a photograph of a person's chromosomes. It is prepared by special laboratory techniques in which body cells are cultured, fixed, stained to demonstrate identifiable banding patterns, and photographed.

■ PATTERNS OF INHERITANCE

The characteristics that are inherited from one's parents are inscribed in gene pairs located along the length of the chromosomes. Alternate forms of the same gene are possible (one inherited from the mother and the other from the father), and each may produce a different aspect of a trait.

DEFINITIONS

Genetics has its own set of definitions. The *genotype* of a person is the genetic information stored in the base sequence triplet code. The *phenotype* refers to the recognizable traits, physical or biochemical, associated with a specific genotype. In many instances, the genotype is not evident by available detection methods. Thus, more than one genotype may have the same phenotype. Some brown-eyed people are carriers of the code for blue eyes, and other brown-eyed persons are not. Phenotypically, these two types of brown-eyed people are the same, but genotypically they are different.

When it comes to a genetic disorder, not all people with a mutant gene are affected to the same extent. *Expressivity* refers to the expression of the gene in the phenotype, which can range from mild to severe. *Penetrance* means the ability of a gene to express its function. Seventy-five percent penetrance means that only 75% of the people of a particular genotype will demonstrate a recognizable phenotype.

The position of a gene on a chromosome is called *locus*, and alternate forms of a gene at the same locus are called *alleles*. When only one pair of genes is involved in the transmission of information, the term *single-gene* is used. Single-gene traits follow the mendelian laws of inheritance. *Polygenic* inheritance involves multiple genes at different loci, with each gene exerting a small additive effect in determining a trait. Most human traits are determined by multiple pairs of genes, many with alternate codes, accounting for some of the dissimilar forms that occur with certain genetic disorders. Polygenic traits are predictable, but less so than single-gene traits.

MENDEL'S LAW

The main feature of inheritance is predictability: given certain conditions, the likelihood of the occurrence or recurrence of a specific trait is remarkably predictable. The units of inheritance are the genes, and the pattern of single-gene expression can be predicted using Mendel's law, with some modification as the result of knowledge accumulated since 1865, the date of Mendel's publication.

Mendel discovered the basic pattern of inheritance by conducting carefully planned experiments with simple garden peas. From his experiments with wrinkled and round peas, Mendel proposed that inherited traits are transmitted from parents to offspring by means of independently inherited factors—now known as genes—and that these factors are transmitted as recessive and dominant traits. Mendel labeled dominant factors (his round peas)

CHART 3-1: POSSIBLE COMBINATIONS THAT CAN OCCUR WITH TRANSMISSION OF A SINGLE-GENE TRAIT

	A	a
A	AA	Aa
a	Aa	aa

''A'' and recessive (his wrinkled peas) ''a.'' Geneticists continue to use capital letters to designate dominant traits and lowercase letters to identify recessive traits. The possible combinations that can occur with transmission of single-gene dominant and recessive traits can be described by constructing a figure using capital and lowercase letters (Chart 3-1).

The observable traits are inherited from one's parents. During maturation, the germ cells (sperm and ovum) of both parents undergo meiosis, or reduction division, in which the number of chromosomes is divided in half (from 46 to 23). At this time, the two alleles from a gene locus separate so that each germ cell gets only one allele from each pair. According to Mendel's law, the alleles from the different gene loci segregate independently and recombine in a random fashion in the zygote formed by the union of the two germ cells. People in whom the two alleles of a given pair are the same (AA or aa) are called *homozygotes. Heterozygotes* have different (Aa) alleles at a gene locus.

A *recessive trait* is one that is expressed only in a homozygous pairing; a *dominant trait* is one that is expressed in either a homozygous or a heterozygous pairing. All persons with a dominant allele inherit that trait. A *carrier* is a person who is heterozygous for a recessive trait and does not manifest the trait. For example, if the genes for blond hair were determined to be recessive and those for brunette hair were dominant, then only persons with a genotype with two alleles for blond hair would be blond, and all persons with either one or two brunette alleles would have dark hair.

PEDIGREE

A pedigree is a graphic method for portraying a family history of an inherited trait. It is constructed from a carefully obtained family history and is useful for tracing the pattern of inheritance for a particular trait.

In summary, inheritance represents the likelihood of the occurrence or recurrence of a specific genetic trait. The genotype refers to information stored in the genetic code of a person. The phenotype represents the recognizable traits, physical and biochemical, associated with the genotype. Expressivity refers to the expression of a gene in the phenotype, and penetrance is the ability of a gene to express its function. The point on the DNA molecule that controls the inheritance of a particular trait is called a gene locus. Alternate codes at one gene locus are called alleles. According to Mendel's law, the two alleles at a gene locus can transmit recessive or dominant traits. A recessive trait is one that is expressed only when there is homozygous pairing of the alleles. A dominant trait is expressed with either homozygous or heterozygous pairing of the alleles. A pedigree is a graphic method for portraying a family history of an inherited trait.

■ GENE TECHNOLOGY

GENOMIC MAPPING

The genome is the gene complement of an organism. Genomic mapping is the assignment of genes to specific chromosomes or parts of the chromosome. Now underway is an international project to identify and localize all 50,000 to 100,000 genes in the human genome. The national effort toward genomic mapping is jointly coordinated by the National Institutes of Health and the Department of Energy. Organizers of the U.S. Human Genome Project hope to have the completed map by the year 2005.[5] It is anticipated that the project will reveal the chemical basis for as many as 4000 genetic diseases. It is also expected to provide tests for screening and diagnosing genetic disorders and provide the basis for new treatments.

There are two types of genomic maps: genetic maps and physical maps. Genetic maps are like highway maps. They use linkage studies (*e.g.*, dosage, hybridization) to estimate the distances between chromosomal landmarks (gene markers). Physical maps are similar to a surveyor's map. They measure the actual physical distance between chromosomal elements in biochemical units, the smallest being the nucleotide base.

Genetic maps and physical maps have been refined over the decades. The earliest mapping efforts localized genes on the X chromosome. The initial assignment of a gene to a particular chromosome was made in 1911 for the color blindness gene that was inherited from the mother (*i.e.*, followed the X-linked pattern of inheritance).[6] In 1968, the specific location of the Duffy blood group on the long arm of chromosome 1 was determined.[7] The locations of more than 2300 expressed human genes have been mapped to a specific chromosome and most of them to a specific region on the chromosome.[8] However, genetic mapping is proceeding so rapidly that these numbers are constantly being updated. Documentation of gene assignments to specific human chromosomes is updated almost daily in the *Online Mendelian Inheritance in Man (OMIM)*, an encyclopedia of expressed gene loci, and in the Genome Data Base, the central database for mapped genes and international repository for most mapping information.[5]

A number of methods have been used for developing genetic maps. The most important ones used are family linkage studies, gene dosage methods, and hybridization studies. Often, the specific assignment of a gene is made possible by the use of information from several mapping techniques.

LINKAGE STUDIES

Linkage studies assume that genes occur in a linear array along the chromosomes. During meiosis, the paired chromosomes of the diploid germ cell exchange genetic material in a phenomenon called *crossing over*. This exchange involves not single, but large blocks of genes, each accounting for a sizable fraction of the chromosome. Although the point at which one block separates from another occurs in a random fashion, the closer together two genes are on the same chromosome, the greater the chance they will be passed on together to the offspring. When two inherited traits occur together at a rate significantly greater than would occur by chance, they are said to be linked.

There are several methods of using the crossing over and recombination of genes to map a particular gene. In one method, any gene that is already assigned to a chromosome can be used as a marker to assign other linked genes. For example, it was found that both an extra-long chromosome 1 and the Duffy blood group were inherited as a dominant trait, placing the position of the blood group gene close to the extra material on chromosome 1. Color blindness has been linked to hemophilia A in some pedigrees, hemophilia has been linked to glucose-phosphatase deficiency in others, and color blindness has been linked to glucose-phosphatase deficiency in still others. Because the gene for color blindness is known to be located on the X chromosome, all three genes must be located in a small section of the X chromosome. Linkage analysis can be used clinically to identify affected persons in a family with a known genetic defect. Two autosomal recessive disorders successfully diagnosed prenatally (using amniocentesis) by linkage studies are congenital adrenal hyperplasia (due to 21-hydroxylase deficiency and linked to an immune response gene or HLA type) and hemophilia A (which is linked to glucose-phosphatase deficiency in some families). Postnatally, linkage studies have been used in diagnosing hemochromatosis, which is closely linked to another HLA type (see Chapter 13). People with this disorder are unable to metabolize iron, and it accumulates in the liver and other organs. It cannot be diagnosed by conventional means until irreversible damage has been done. Given a family history of the disorder, HLA typing can determine if the gene is present; if present, dietary restriction of iron intake may be used to prevent organ damage.

DOSAGE STUDIES

Dosage studies involve measuring enzyme activity. Autosomal genes are normally arranged in pairs, and normally both are expressed. If both alleles are present and both are expressed, the activity of the enzyme should be 100%. If one member of the gene pair is missing, only 50% of the enzyme activity will be present, reflecting the activity of the remaining normal allele.

HYBRIDIZATION STUDIES

One of the biologic discoveries in recent years is that two somatic cells from different species, when grown together in the same culture, occasionally fuse together to form new hybrid cell. Two types of hybridization methods are used in genomic studies: somatic cell hybridization and in situ hybridization.

Somatic cell hybridization involves the fusion of human somatic cells with those of a different species (typically, the mouse) to yield a cell containing the chromosomes of both species. Because these hybrid cells are unstable, they begin to lose chromosomes of both species during subsequent cell divisions. This makes it possible to obtain cells with different partial combinations of human chromosomes. By studying the enzymes that these cells produce, it is possible to determine that an enzyme is only produced when a certain chromosome is present; thus, the coding for that enzyme must be located on that chromosome.

In situ hybridization involves the use of a specific sequence of DNA or RNA to locate genes that do not express themselves in cell culture. Both DNA and RNA can be chemically tagged with radioactive or fluorescent markers. These chemically tagged DNA or RNA sequences are used as probes to determine gene location. The probe is added to a chromosome spread after the DNA strands have been separated. If the probe matches the complementary DNA of a chromosome segment, it hybridizes and remains at the precise location (hence the term in situ) on a chromosome. The radioactive or fluorescent markers are used to determine the location of the probe.

RECOMBINANT DNA TECHNOLOGY

During the past several decades, genetic engineering has provided the methods for manipulating nucleic acids and recombining genes (recombinant DNA) into hybrid molecules that can be inserted into unicellular organisms and reproduced many times over. Each hybrid molecule gives rise to a genetically identical population, called a *clone*, that reflects its common ancestor.

The techniques of gene isolation and cloning are based on the fact that the genes of all organisms, from bacteria through mammals, have a similar molecular organization. Gene cloning requires cutting a DNA molecule apart, modifying and reassembling its fragments, and producing copies of the modified DNA, its mRNA, and its gene product. The DNA molecule is cut apart through the use of a bacterial enzyme, called a *restriction enzyme*, that binds to DNA wherever a particular short sequence of base pairs is found and cleaves the molecule at a specific nucleotide site. In this way, a long DNA molecule can be broken down into smaller discrete fragments with the intent that one of the fragments contains the gene of interest. More than 100 restriction enzymes are commercially available that will cut DNA at different recognition sites.

The selected gene fragment is replicated through insertion into a unicellular organism, such as a bacterium. To do this, a cloning vector such as a bacterial virus or a small DNA circle that is found in most bacteria, called a *plasmid*, is used. Both viral and plasmid vectors replicate autonomously in the host bacterial cell. In the process of gene cloning, a bacterial vector and the DNA fragment are mixed together and joined by a special enzyme called a *DNA ligase*. The recombinant vectors are introduced into a suitable culture of bacteria, and the bacteria are allowed to replicate and express the recombinant vector gene. Sometimes mRNA taken from a tissue that expresses a high level of the gene is used to produce a complementary DNA molecule that can be used in the cloning process. Because the fragments of the entire DNA molecule are used in the cloning process, additional steps are taken to identify and separate the clone that contains the gene of interest.

In terms of biologic research and technology, cloning makes it possible to identify the DNA sequence in a gene and produce the protein product encoded by a gene. The specific nucleotide sequence of a cloned DNA fragment can often be identified by analyzing the amino acid sequence and mRNA codons of its protein product. It is also possible to synthesize short sequences of base pairs that can be radioactively labeled and used to identify their complementary sequence. In this way, it is possible to identify normal and abnormal gene structures.

Proteins that formerly were only available in small amounts can now be made in large quantities once their respective genes have been isolated. For example, genes encoding for insulin and growth hor-

mone have been cloned to produce these hormones for pharmacologic use. Although quite different from inserting genetic material into a unicellular organism such as bacteria, techniques are available for inserting genes into the genome of intact multicellular plants and animals. However, the introduction of the cloned gene into the multicellular organism can only influence the few cells that acquire the gene. An answer to this problem would be the insertion of the gene into a germ cell (sperm or ovum) in which the gene would be replicated in all of the differentiating cell types. Even so, techniques for cell insertion are limited. Not only are moral and ethical issues involved, but these techniques cannot direct the inserted DNA to attach to a particular chromosome nor can they supplant an existing gene by knocking it out of its place.

In summary, the genome is the gene complement of an organism. Genomic mapping is a method used to assign genes to particular chromosomes or parts of a chromosome. The most important ones used are family linkage studies, gene dosage methods, and hybridization studies. Often the specific assignment of a gene is made possible by the use of information from several mapping techniques. Linkage studies assign a chromosome location to genes based on their close association with other genes of known location. Recombinant DNA studies involve the extraction of specific types of messenger RNA used in synthesis of complementary DNA strands. The complementary DNA strands, labeled with a radioisotope, bind with the genes for which they are complementary and are used as gene probes. Now underway is an international project to identify and localize all 50,000 to 100,000 genes in the human genome. Genetic engineering has provided the methods for manipulating nucleic acids and recombining genes (recombinant DNA) into hybrid molecules that can be inserted into unicellular organisms and reproduced many times over. As a result, proteins that formerly were only available in small amounts can now be made in large quantities once their respective genes have been isolated.

■ REFERENCES

1. Behrman, R.E., Kliegman, R.M., Nelson, W., & Vaughan, V.C. III. (1991). *Nelson textbook of pediatrics* (14th ed., p. 264). Philadelphia: W.B. Saunders.
2. Guyton, A. (1991). *Textbook of medical physiology* (8th ed., pp. 29, 30). Philadelphia: W.B. Saunders.
3. International Committee on Human Cytogenic Nomenclature. (1981). An international system for human cytogenetic nomenclature—high resolution banding. *Birth Defects, 17*(5). New York: March of Dimes Foundation.
4. Thompson, M., McGinnes, R.R., & Willard, H.F. (1991). *Genetics in medicine*. Philadelphia: W.B. Saunders.
5. Erickson, D. (1992). Hacking the genome. *Scientific American, 264*(4), 128–137.
6. Wilson, E.B. (1911). The sex chromosomes. *Arch Mikrosc Anat, 77*, 249.
7. McKusick, V.A. (1981). The anatomy of the human genome. *Hospital Practice, 16*(4), 82–100.

8. McKusick, V.A. (1991). Genomic mapping and how it progressed. *Hospital Practice, 26*(10), 74–90.

■ BIBLIOGRAPHY

Gilbert, W. (1991). DNA sequencing today and tomorrow. *Hospital Practice, 26*(1), 165–174.

Ptashne, M. (1989). How gene activators work. *Scientific American, 260*(1), 41–47.

Watson, J.D. (1991). The human genome initiative: A statement of need. *Hospital Practice, 26*(10), 69–73.

White, R., & Lalouel, J. (1988). Chromosomal mapping with DNA markers. *Scientific American, 258*(2), 40–49.

GENETIC AND CONGENITAL DISORDERS

■ OBJECTIVES

After you have studied this chapter, you should be able to meet the following objectives:

- Define *congenital defect*.
- Describe three types of single-gene disorders.
- Contrast disorders due to multifactorial inheritance to those caused by single-gene inheritance.
- Describe two chromosomal abnormalities that demonstrate aneuploidy.
- Describe three patterns of chromosomal breakage and rearrangement.
- Relate maternal age and occurrence of Down's syndrome.
- Cite the most susceptible period of intrauterine life for development of defects due to environmental agents.

- State the cautions that should be observed when considering use of drugs during pregnancy.
- Describe the effects of alcohol and cocaine abuse on fetal development and birth outcomes.
- List four infectious agents that cause congenital defects.
- List types of information that are usually considered when doing assessment of genetic risk.
- Cite examples of fetal information that can be obtained with use of ultrasound, amniocentesis, chorionic villus sampling, percutaneous blood sampling.

Genetic and congenital defects are important at all levels of health care because they affect all age groups and can involve almost any of the body tissues and organs. Congenital defects, sometimes called *birth defects*, develop during prenatal life and are usually apparent at birth or shortly thereafter. Spinal bifida and cleft lip, for example, are apparent at birth, whereas other malformations, such as kidney and heart defects, may be present at birth but may not become apparent until they begin to produce symptoms. Not all genetic disorders are congenital; many are not expressed until later in life.

Congenital defects may be caused by genetic factors (single-gene or multifactorial inheritance or chromosomal aberrations), or they may be caused by environmental factors that occurred during embryonic or fetal development (maternal disease, infections, or drugs taken during pregnancy). In rare cases, congenital defects may be the result of intrauterine factors such as crowding, fetal positioning, or entanglement of fetal parts with the amnion. Birth defects occur in 1 of every 14 live births[1] and are associated with approximately 30% of all admissions to pediatric hospitals. A large prospective study showed that African Americans have higher overall rates of minor birth defects such as polydactly and supernumerary nipples, whereas whites have higher rates of major malformations.[2] Native Americans have the highest rate of fetal alcohol syndrome.[2] This chapter provides an overview of genetic and congenital disorders and is divided into three parts: (1) genetic and chromosomal disorders, (2) disorders due to environmental agents, and (3) diagnosis and counseling.

■ GENETIC AND CHROMOSOMAL DISORDERS

Genetic disorders involve a permanent change (or mutation) in the genome. A genetic disorder can involve a single-gene trait, multifactorial inheritance, or a chromosome disorder.

SINGLE-GENE DISORDERS

Single-gene disorders are caused by a single defective or mutant gene. The defective gene may be present on only one member of a gene pair (matched with a normal gene) or in both members of the pair. Single-gene defects follow the mendelian patterns of inheritance (see Chapter 3) and are often called mendelian disorders. At last count, there were more than 3000 single-gene disorders; although individually rare, they collectively account for approximately 1% of all adult and 5% of all pediatric hospital admissions.[3]

The genes on each chromosome are arranged in pairs and in strict order, with each gene occupying a specific location or locus. The two members of a gene pair, one inherited from the mother and the other from the father, are called *alleles*. If both members of a gene pair are identical (code the exact same gene product), the person is *homozygous* for the locus; if both members are different, the person is *heterozygous*. The genetic composition of a person is called a *genotype*, whereas the *phenotype* is the observable expression of a genotype in terms of a morphologic, biochemical, or molecular trait. If the trait is only expressed in the heterozygote, it is said to be *dominant*; if it is only expressed in the homozygote, it is *recessive*.

Although gene expression usually follows a dominant or recessive pattern, it is possible for both alleles (members) of a gene pair to be fully expressed in the heterozygote, a condition called *codominance*. Many genes have only one normal version, called a *"wild type"* allele. Other genes have more than one normal allele (alternate forms) at the same locus. This is called *polymorphism*. Blood group inheritance (AO, BO, AB) is an example of both codominance and polymorphism.

A single mutant gene may be expressed in many different parts of the body. Marfan's syndrome is a defect in connective tissue that has widespread effects involving skeletal, eye, and cardiovascular structures. In other single-gene disorders, the same defect can be caused by mutations at several different loci. Childhood deafness can result from 16 different types of autosomal recessive mutations.

Single-gene disorders are characterized by their patterns of transmission, which is usually obtained through a family genetic history. The patterns of inheritance depend on (1) whether the phenotype is dominant or recessive, and (2) whether the gene is located on an autosomal or sex chromosome. The most common types of single-gene disorders are autosomal dominant, autosomal recessive, and X-linked. Occasionally, a gene for an X-linked dominant disorder such as color blindness is present in both the father and mother, resulting in an X-linked recessive disorder. Disorders of the Y, or male, chromosome are extremely rare. Table 4-1 lists some of the common single-gene disorders and their significance. Many of these disorders are described in other parts of this book.

DISORDERS OF AUTOSOMAL INHERITANCE

The autosomes are represented on 22 homologous pairs of autosomal chromosomes. Disorders of autosomal inheritance include both autosomal dominant

TABLE 4-1. SOME DISORDERS OF MENDELIAN OR SINGLE-GENE INHERITANCE AND THEIR SIGNIFICANCE

DISORDER	SIGNIFICANCE
Autosomal Dominant	
Achondroplasia	Short-limb dwarfism
Adult polycystic kidney disease	Kidney failure
Huntington's chorea	Neurodegenerative disorder
Familial hypercholesterolemia	Premature atherosclerosis
Marfan's syndrome	Connective tissue disorder with abnormalities of skeletal, ocular, cardiovascular systems
Neurofibromatosis (NF)	Neurogenic tumors: fibromatous skin tumors, pigmented skin lesions, and ocular nodules in NF-1; bilateral acoustic neuromas in NF-2.
Osteogenesis imperfecta	Molecular defects of collagen
Spherocytosis	Disorder of red blood cells
von Willebrand's disease	Bleeding disorder
Autosomal Recessive	
Color blindness	Color blindness
Cystic fibrosis	Disorder of membrane transport of ions in exocrine glands causing lung and pancreatic disease
Glycogen storage diseases	Excess accumulation of glycogen in the liver and hypoglycemia (von Gierke's disease); glycogen accumulation in striated muscle in myopathic forms
Oculocutaneous albinism	Hypopigmentation of skin, hair, eyes as result of inability to synthesize melanin
Phenylketonuria (PKU)	Lack of phenylalanine hydroxylase with hyperphenylaninemia and impaired brain development
Sickle cell disease	Red blood cell defect
Tay-Sachs disease	Deficiency of hexosaminidase A; severe mental and physical deterioration beginning in infancy
X-Linked Recessive	
Bruton-type hypogammaglobulinemia	Immunodeficiency
Hemophilia A	Bleeding disorder
Duchenne's dystrophy	Muscular dystrophy
Fragile X syndrome	Mental retardation

and autosomal recessive traits. Among the approximate 4,500 single-gene disorders, more than half are autosomal dominant. Autosomal recessive phenotypes are less common, accounting for about one third of single-gene disorders.[4]

Autosomal Dominant Disorders. In autosomal dominant disorders, a single mutant allele from an affected parent is transmitted to an offspring regardless of sex. The affected person has a 50% chance of transmitting the disorder to each offspring (Fig. 4-1). The unaffected relatives of the parent or unaffected siblings of the offspring do not transmit the disorder.

In many conditions, the age of onset is delayed and the signs and symptoms of the disorder do not appear until later in life, as in Huntington's chorea (see Chapter 54).

Autosomal dominant disorders may also present as a new mutation. Whether the mutation is passed on to the next generation depends on the affected person's reproductive capacity. Many new autosomal dominant mutations are accompanied by reduced reproductive capacity; therefore, the defect is not perpetuated in future generations. If an autosomal defect is accompanied by a total inability to reproduce, essentially all new cases of the disorder

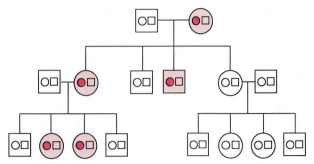

FIG. 4-1. Simple pedigree for inheritance of an autosomal dominant trait. The colored circle represents the mutant gene. An affected parent with an autosomal dominant trait has a 50% chance of passing the mutant gene on to each child regardless of sex.

will be due to new mutations. If the defect does not affect reproductive capacity, it is more likely to be inherited.

Although there is a 50% chance of inheriting a dominant genetic disorder, there can be wide variation in gene penetration and expression. When a person inherits a dominant mutant gene but fails to express it, the trait is described as having *reduced penetrance*. Penetrance is expressed in mathematical terms; a 50% penetrance indicates that a person who inherits the defective gene has a 50% chance of expressing the disorder. The person who has a mutant gene but does not express it is an important exception to the rule that unaffected persons do not transmit an autosomal dominant trait. These persons can transmit the gene to their descendants and so produce a skipped generation. Autosomal dominant disorders can also display *variable expressivity*, meaning that they can be expressed differently among individuals. Polydactyly or supernumerary digits, for example, may be expressed in either the fingers or the toes.

The gene products of autosomal dominant disorders are usually regulatory proteins involved in complex metabolic pathways, abnormal membrane-bound transport systems, or structural proteins. Two examples of autosomal dominant inheritance that are not discussed in other parts of this book are Marfan's syndrome and neurofibromatosis.

Marfan's syndrome is a connective tissue disorder that is manifested by changes in the skeleton, eyes, and cardiovascular system. There is a wide range of variation in expression of the disorder. Persons may have abnormalities of one or all three systems. The skeletal deformities, which are the most obvious features of the disorder, include a long thin body with exceptionally long extremities and long, tapering fingers (called *arachnodactyly* or *spider fingers*), hyperextensible joints, and a variety of spinal deformities including kyphoscoliosis. Chest deformity, either pectus excavatum (deeply depressed sternum) or pi-

geon chest deformity, is often present. The most common eye disorder is bilateral dislocation of the lens due to weakness of the suspensory ligaments. Myopia and predisposition to retinal detachment (see Chapter 52) are also common, the result of increased optic globe length due to altered connective tissue support of ocular structures. However, the most life-threatening aspects of the disorder are the cardiovascular defects, which include mitral valve prolapse, progressive dilation of the aortic valve ring, and weakness of aorta and other arteries. Dissection and rupture of the aorta often lead to premature death (see Chapter 20). The average age of death in persons with Marfan's syndrome is 30 to 40 years.

Neurofibromatosis (NF) is a condition involving neurogenic tumors that arise from Schwann cells and other elements of the peripheral nervous system.[5,6] It is a relatively common disorder with a frequency of 1 in 3000. Approximately 50% of cases have a family history of autosomal dominant transmission, and the remaining 50% appear to represent a new mutation. There are at least two genetically and clinically distinct forms of the disorder. Type 1 neurofibromatosis (NF-1), also known as *von Recklinghausen's disease*, and type 2 bilateral acoustic neurofibromatosis (NF-2). The gene for NF-1 has been mapped to chromosome 17, and the gene for NF-2 has been mapped to chromosome 22.

NF-1, which accounts for more than 90% of cases, is characterized by multiple hyperpigmented macular skin lesions, neurofibromatosis, and small, pigmented, tumor-like nodules (also called *Lisch* nodules) of the iris. The hyperpigmented skin lesions, known as *café-au-lait* spots, are large, flat lesions (usually 15 mm or more in diameter) of uniform light-brown color in whites and darker brown in African Americans, with sharply demarcated edges (Fig. 4-2). Although small single lesions may be found in normal children, the presence of larger lesions or six or more spots over 1.5 cm in diameter is suggestive of NF-1. The skin pigmentations become more evident with age as the melanosomes in the epidermal cells accumulate melanin. The Lisch nodules, which are specific for NF-1, are usually present after 6 years of age. They do not present any clinical problem but are useful in establishing a diagnosis.

The neurofibromas are of three types: cutaneous, subcutaneous, and plexiform. The cutaneous neurofibromas present as soft pedunculated lesions that project from the skin. They are the most common type, are often not apparent until puberty, and are present in greatest density over the trunk (Fig. 4-3). The subcutaneous neurofibromas become apparent toward the end of the first decade of life. When large numbers occur near the vertebral column, they may cause erosion of the spinal column

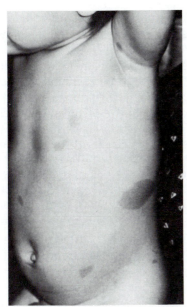

FIG. 4-2. Café-au-lait spot in a child with neurofibromatosis type 1. (Oski, F. A. [Ed.]. [1989]. *Principles and practices of pediatrics* [p. 1942]. Philadelphia: J.B. Lippincott)

with eventual spinal cord compression. The plexiform lesions are congenital and enlarge steadily with age. They are disfiguring multilobular masses that involve the subcutaneous tissue, are often hyperpigmented, and contain numerous tortuous thickened nerves.

In addition to the neurofibromatosis, persons with NF-1 have a variety of other associated lesions,

the most common being skeletal lesions such as scoliosis and erosive bone defects. Persons with NF-1 are also at increased risk for developing other nervous system tumors such as meningiomas, optic gliomas, and pheochromocytomas.

NF-2 is characterized by tumors of the acoustic nerves. Most often the disorder is asymptomatic through the first 15 years of life. The most frequent symptoms are headaches, hearing loss, and tinnitus (ringing in the ears). There may be associated intracranial and spinal meningiomas. The condition is made worse by pregnancy, and oral contraceptives may increase the growth and symptoms of tumors. Persons with the disorder should be warned that severe disorientation may occur during diving or swimming underwater and drowning may result. Surgery may be indicated for debulking or removal of the tumors.

Autosomal Recessive Disorders. Autosomal recessive disorders are manifested only when both members of the gene pair are mutant alleles. In this case, both parents may be unaffected but are carriers of the defective gene. Autosomal recessive disorders affect both sexes. The occurrence risk in each pregnancy is one in four for an affected child, two in four for a carrier child, and one in four for a normal (noncarrier, unaffected) homozygous child (Fig. 4-4).

With autosomal recessive disorders, the expression of the gene tends to be more uniform than with autosomal dominant disorders; the age of onset is frequently early in life; and, in many cases, enzyme proteins are affected by the mutation. These enzyme defects may result in any of the following: (1) deficiency of a metabolic end-product, (2) production of harmful intermediates or toxic by-products of metabolism, or (3) accumulation of destructive substances within the cell. Two examples of autosomal recessive

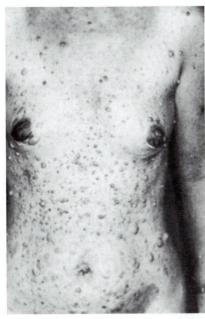

FIG. 4-3. Cutaneous neurofibromas are often not apparent until puberty and are present in highest density on the trunk. (Oski, F. A. [Ed.]. [1989]. *Principles and practices of pediatrics* [p. 1942]. Philadelphia: J.B. Lippincott)

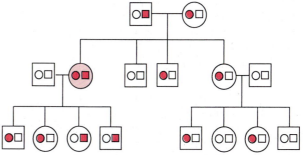

FIG. 4-4. Simple pedigree for inheritance of an autosomal recessive trait. The colored circle and square represent a mutant gene. When both parents are carriers of a mutant gene, there is a 25% chance of an affected child, a 50% chance of a carrier child, and a 25% chance of a nonaffected/noncarrier child regardless of sex. All children (100%) of an affected parent will be carriers.

disorders that are not covered elsewhere in the book are phenylketonuria and Tay-Sachs disease.

Phenylketonuria (PKU) is a genetically inherited enzyme defect. It is characterized by a deficiency of phenylalanine hydroxylase, the enzyme needed for conversion of phenylalanine to tyrosine, and, as a result of this deficiency, toxic levels of phenylalanine accumulate in the blood. Like other inborn errors of metabolism, PKU is inherited as a recessive trait and is manifested only in the homozygote. It is possible to identify carriers of the trait by subjecting them to a phenylalanine test in which a large dose of phenylalanine is administered orally and the rate at which it disappears from the bloodstream is measured. PKU occurs once in approximately 10,000 births, and damage to the developing brain almost always results when high concentrations of phenylalanine and other metabolites persist in the blood. Newborn infants are routinely screened for abnormal levels of serum phenylalanine. Infants with the disorder are treated with a special diet that restricts phenylalanine intake. Dietary treatment must be started early in neonatal life to prevent brain damage.

Tay-Sachs disease is caused by an accumulation of ganglioside GM_2 (a glycolipid) in body tissues due to an enzyme deficiency (hexosaminidase A), resulting in gangliosidosis. The disease is particularly prevalent among eastern European (Ashkenazi) Jews. Infants with Tay-Sachs appear normal at birth but begin to manifest neurologic signs at about 6 months of age. These neurologic manifestations eventually lead to muscle flaccidity, dementia, and finally death at about 2 to 3 years of age. Although there is no cure for the disease, analysis of the blood serum for a deficiency of hexosaminidase A allows for accurate identification of the genetic carriers for the disease.

DISORDERS OF SEX-LINKED INHERITANCE

Sex-linked disorders are almost always associated with the X, or female, chromosome, and inheritance is predominantly recessive. Because of a normal paired gene, heterozygous females rarely experience the effects of a defective gene. The common pattern of inheritance is one in which an unaffected mother carries one normal and one mutant allele on the X chromosome. This means that she has a 50% chance of transmitting the defective gene to her sons and that her female children have a 50% chance of being carriers of the mutant gene. When the affected male procreates, he transmits the defective gene to all of his daughters, who become carriers of the mutant gene. Because the genes of the Y chromosome are unaffected, the affected male does not transmit the defect to any of his sons and they will not be carriers

or transmit the disorder to their children. X-linked recessive disorders include glucose-6-phosphate dehydrogenase deficiency (see Chapter 18), hemophilia A (see Chapter 17), and Bruton's hypogammaglobulinemia (see Chapter 14).

The *fragile X syndrome* is an X-linked disorder associated with a fragile site on the X chromosome where the chromatin fails to condense during mitosis. It has a frequency of 1 in 1500 male births and is a common cause of mental retardation. Males with the disorder also have coarse facial features and macroorchidism. The basic defect responsible for this syndrome is unknown. The disorder cannot be categorized as a pure dominant or recessive trait because female carriers may or may not be retarded and may or may not reveal the fragile site on their chromosomes.

DISORDERS OF MULTIFACTORIAL INHERITANCE

Multifactorial (also called polygenic disorders) are caused by the multiple genes and, in many cases, environmental factors. The exact number of genes contributing to multifactorial traits is not known, and these traits do not follow a clear-cut pattern of inheritance as do single-gene disorders. Multifactorial inheritance has been described as a threshold phenomenon in which the factors contributing to the trait might be compared to water filling a glass.[7] Using this analogy, one might say that expression of the disorder occurs when the glass overflows. Disorders of multifactorial inheritance can be expressed during fetal life and be present at birth, or they may be expressed later in life. Congenital disorders that are thought to arise through multifactorial inheritance include: anencephaly, cleft lip or palate, clubfoot, congenital dislocation of the hip, congenital heart disease, hydrocephalus, myelomeningocele, pyloric stenosis, and urinary tract malformation. Environmental factors are thought to play a greater role in disorders of multifactorial inheritance that develop in adult life, such as coronary artery disease, diabetes mellitus, hypertension, cancer, as well as the common psychiatric disorders such as manic-depressive psychoses and schizophrenia.

Although multifactorial traits cannot be predicted with the same degree of accuracy as the mendelian single-gene mutations, characteristic patterns exist. First, multifactorial congenital malformations tend to involve a single organ or tissue derived from the same embryonic developmental field. Second, the risk of recurrence in future pregnancies is for the same or a similar defect. This means that parents of a child with cleft palate defect have an increased risk of having another child with a cleft palate, but not with spina bifida. Third, the increased risk (compared with the general population) among first-degree relatives of the affected person is 2% to 5%, and among second-degree relatives it is about one half that amount. Furthermore, the risk increases with increasing incidence of the defect among relatives. This means that the risk is greatly increased when a second child with the defect is born to a couple. The risk also increases with severity of the disorder and when the defect occurs in the sex not generally affected by the disorder.

CHROMOSOME DISORDERS

Chromosome disorders form a major category of genetic disease, accounting for a large proportion of reproductive wastage (early gestational abortions), congenital malformations, and mental retardation. At present, specific chromosomal abnormalities can be linked to over 60 identifiable syndromes that are present in 0.7% of all live births, 2% of all pregnancies in women over age 35 years, and 50% of all first-term abortions.[4]

During cell division in nongerm cells (mitosis), the chromosomes replicate so that each cell receives a full diploid number. In germ cells (sperm and ovum), a different form of division (meiosis) takes place. During meiosis, the double sets of 22 autosomes and the 2 sex chromosomes (normal diploid number) become reduced to single sets (haploid number) in each gamete. At the time of conception, the haploid number in the ovum and that in the sperm join and restore the diploid number of chromosomes. Chromosomal defects usually develop because of defective movement during meiosis or because of breakage of a chromosome with loss or translocation of genetic material.

ALTERATIONS IN CHROMOSOME DUPLICATION

Mosaicism is the presence in one individual of two or more cell lines characterized by distinctive karyotypes. This defect results from an accident during chromosomal duplication. Some times, mosaicism consists of an abnormal karyotype and a normal one, in which case the physical deformities caused by the abnormal cell line are usually less severe.

ALTERATIONS IN CHROMOSOME NUMBER

A change in chromosome number is called *aneuploidy*. Among the causes of aneuploidy is failure of the chromosomes to separate during oogenesis or spermatogenesis. This can occur in either the auto-

somes or the sex chromosomes and is called *nondisjunction*. Nondisjunction gives rise to germ cells that have an even number of chromosomes (22 or 24). The products of conception formed from this even number of chromosomes have an uneven number of chromosomes, either 45 or 47. *Monosomy* refers to the presence of only one member of a chromosome pair. The defects associated with monosomy of the autosomes are severe and usually cause abortion. Monosomy of the X chromosome (45,X/O), or Turner's syndrome, causes less severe defects. *Polysomy*, or the presence of more than two chromosomes to a set, occurs when a germ cell containing more than 23 chromosomes is involved in conception. This defect has been described for both the autosomes and the sex chromosomes. Trisomies of chromosomes 8, 13, 18, and 21 are the more common forms of polysomy of the autosomes. There are several forms of polysomy of the sex chromosomes in which extra X or Y chromosomes are present.

Trisomy 21 (Down's Syndrome). Trisomy 21, or Down's syndrome, is the most common form of chromosome disorder. It has an incidence of 1 in 600 to 800 births.[7] The condition is accompanied by varying levels of mental retardation.

The risk of having a baby with Down's syndrome is greater in women who are 35 years of age or older at the time of delivery (Table 4-2). Although the reason for the correlation between maternal age and nondisjunction is unknown, it is thought to be due to some aspect of aging of the oocyte. Although males continue to produce sperm throughout their reproductive life, females are born with all the oocytes they will ever have. These oocytes may change as a result of the aging process. Also, with increasing age, there is a greater chance of a woman having been exposed to damaging environmental agents such as drugs,

TABLE 4-2. THE RELATIONSHIP BETWEEN MATERNAL AGE AND THE RISK OF DOWN'S SYNDROME IN A NEWBORN CHILD

MATERNAL AGE (YEARS)	APPROXIMATE RISK OF OCCURRENCE
20–24	1 in 1350
25–29	1 in 1175
30–35	1 in 750
36–40	1 in 250
41–45	1 in 65
46–50	1 in 25(?)

(Wisniewski, L. P., & Hirschhorn, K. [1980]. *A guide to human chromosome defects* [2nd ed.]. White Plains: March of Dimes Birth Defects Foundation, BD: OAS XVI[6].)

chemicals, and radiation. However, recent evidence suggests that in approximately 5% of trisomy 21 the extra chromosome is of paternal origin.[8] Although 95% of Down's syndrome result from trisomy 21, other chromosomal aberrations can be involved, the most frequent being the robertsonian translocation (to be discussed). Unlike trisomy 21, the robertsonian translocation shows no relation to maternal age but has a relatively high recurrence risk in families when a parent, particularly the mother, is a carrier.

The physical features of a child with Down's syndrome are distinctive, and, therefore, the condition is usually apparent at birth. These features include a small and rather square head. There is upward slanting of the eyes, small and malformed ears, an open mouth, and a large, protruding tongue. The child's hands are usually short and stubby with fingers that curl inward, and there is usually only a single palmar (simian) crease. There are often accompanying congenital heart defects (Fig. 4-5). About 1% of persons with trisomy 21 Down's syndrome have mosaicism (*i.e.*, cell populations with both normal and trisomy 21); these persons may be less severely affected. Of particular concern is the much greater risk these children have for the development of acute leukemia—20 times greater than other children.[9]

Monosomy X (Turner's Syndrome). Turner's syndrome describes a monosomy of the X chromo-

some (45,X/O) with gonadal agenesis, or absence of the ovaries. This disorder is present in about 1 of every 2500 live births. There are variations in the syndrome, with abnormalities ranging from essentially none to webbing of the neck with redundant skin folds, nonpitting edema of the hands and feet, and congenital heart defects (particularly coarctation of the aorta). Characteristically, the female with Turner's syndrome is short in stature, but her body proportions are normal. She does not menstruate and shows no signs of secondary sex characteristics. Administration of the female sex hormones (estrogens) may cause the secondary sexual characteristics to develop and may produce additional skeletal growth. The infertility associated with Turner's syndrome cannot be reversed. When a mosaic cell line (45,X/O and 46,X/X or 45,X/O and 46,X/Y) is present, the manifestations associated with the chromosomal defect tend to be less severe.

Polysomy X (Klinefelter's Syndrome). Klinefelter's syndrome is characterized by an X-chromatin–positive (47,X/X/Y) male and is associated with testicular dysgenesis. In rare cases, there may be more than one extra X chromosome (*e.g.*, 47,X/X/X/Y). The incidence of Klinefelter's syndrome is about 1 in 600. The condition may not be detected in the newborn. The infant usually has normal male genitalia, with a small penis and small, firm testicles. Hypogonadism during puberty usually leads to a tall stature with abnormal body proportions in which the lower part of the body is longer than the upper part. Later in life, the body build may become heavy with a female distribution of subcutaneous fat and variable degrees of breast enlargement. There may be deficient secondary male sex characteristics, such as a voice that remains feminine in pitch and sparse beard and pubic hair. There may be sexual dysfunction, along with complete infertility and impotence. Personality problems may occur, but the intellect is usually normal. Replacement hormone therapy with testosterone is used to treat the disorder.

ALTERATIONS IN CHROMOSOME STRUCTURE

Aberrations in chromosome structure occur when there is a break in one or more of the chromosomes followed by rearrangement or deletion of the chromosome parts. Among the factors believed to cause chromosome breakage are the following: (1) exposure to radiation sources, such as x-rays; (2) influence of certain chemicals; (3) extreme changes in the cellular environment; and (4) viral infections.

A number of patterns of chromosome breakage and rearrangement can occur (Fig. 4-6). There can be

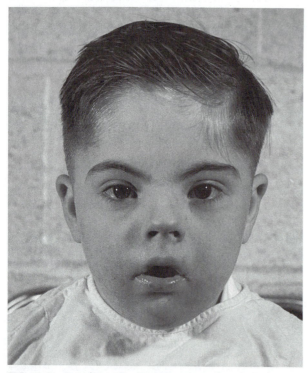

FIG. 4-5. A child with Down's syndrome. (Courtesy of March of Dimes, White Plains, NY)

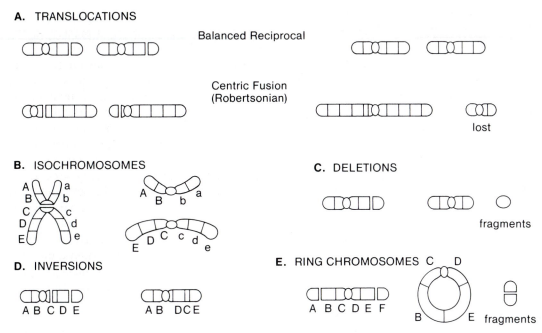

A. TRANSLOCATIONS

Balanced Reciprocal

Centric Fusion
(Robertsonian)

lost

B. ISOCHROMOSOMES

A   a
B   b
C   c
D   d
E   e

A   a
B   b

E D C c d e

C. DELETIONS

fragments

D. INVERSIONS

A B C D E   A B DCE

E. RING CHROMOSOMES   C   D

A B C D E F   B   E fragments

FIG. 4-6. Rearrangement after breaks in chromosome structures. (Robbins, S. L., & Kumar, V. [1987]. *Basic pathology* [4th ed., p. 120]. Philadelphia: W.B. Saunders)

a *deletion* of the broken portion of the chromosome. When one chromosome is involved, the broken parts may be *inverted*. *Isochromosome formation* occurs when the centromere, or central portion, of the chromosome separates horizontally instead of vertically. *Ring formation* results when deletion is followed by uniting of the chromatids to form a ring. *Translocation* occurs when there are simultaneous breaks in two chromosomes from different pairs with exchange of chromosome parts. With a balanced reciprocal translocation, no genetic information is lost; therefore, persons with translocations are generally normal. These persons are, however, translocation carriers and may have both normal and abnormal children. A special form of translocation called a *centric fusion* or *robertsonian translocation* involves two acrocentric chromosomes in which the centromere is near the end. Typically, the break occurs near the centromere affecting the short arm in one chromosome and the long arm in the other. Transfer of the chromosome fragments leads to one long and one extremely short chromosome (see Fig. 4-6). Often the short fragments are lost. In this case, the person has only 45 chromosomes, but the amount of genetic material that is lost is so small that it often goes unnoticed. Difficulty, however, arises during meiosis; the result is gametes with an unbalanced number of chromosomes. A rare form of Down's syndrome can occur in the offspring of persons in whom there has been a translocation involving the long arm of chromosome 21 q and the long arm of one of the acrocentric chro-

mosomes (most often 14 or 22). The translocation adds to the normal long arm of chromosome 21; therefore, the person with this type of Down's syndrome has 46 chromosomes, but essentially a trisomy of 21 q.[4]

The manifestations of aberrations in chromosome structure depend to a great extent on the amount of genetic material that is lost. Many cells suffering unrestored breaks are eliminated within the next few mitoses because of deficiencies that may, in themselves, be fatal. This is beneficial because it prevents the damaged cells from becoming a permanent part of the organism or, if it occurs in the gametes, from giving rise to grossly defective zygotes. Some altered chromosomes, such as those that occur with translocations, are passed on to the next generation.

In summary, genetic and congenital disorders affect all age groups and all body structures. Genetic disorders can affect a single gene (mendelian inheritance) or several genes (polygenic inheritance). Chromosome disorders result from a change in chromosome number or structure. A change in chromosome number is called aneuploidy. Monosomy involves the presence of only one member of a chromosome pair; it is seen in Turner's syndrome, in which there is monosomy of the X chromosome. Polysomy refers to the presence of more than two chromosomes in a set. Klinefelter's syndrome involves polysomy of the X chromosome. Trisomy 21 (Down's syndrome) is the most common form of chromosome disorder. Alterations in chromosome structure involve either deletion or addition of genetic material, which may involve a translocation of genetic material from one chromosome pair to another.

■ DISORDERS DUE TO ENVIRONMENTAL INFLUENCES

The developing embryo is subject to many nongenetic influences. After conception, development is influenced by the environmental factors that the embryo shares with the mother. The physiologic status of the mother—her hormone balance, her general state of health, her nutritional status, and the drugs she takes—undoubtedly influences the development of the unborn child. For example, diabetes mellitus is associated with increased risk of congenital anomalies. Smoking is associated with lower than normal neonatal weight. Alcohol, in the context of chronic alcoholism, is known to cause fetal abnormalities. Some agents cause early abortion. Measles and other infectious agents cause congenital malformations. Other agents, such as radiation, can cause chromosomal and genetic defects as well as developmental disorders.

Theoretically, an environmental agent can cause a birth defect in three ways: (1) by direct exposure of the pregnant woman and the embryo or fetus to a teratogenic agent; (2) through exposure of the soon-to-be-pregnant woman with an agent that has a slow clearance rate such that a teratogenic dose is retained during early pregnancy; or (3) as a result of mutagenic effects of an environmental agent that occur before pregnancy causing permanent damage to a woman's (or a man's) reproductive cells.[10]

PERIOD OF VULNERABILITY

The embryo's development is most easily disturbed during the period when differentiation and development of the organs are taking place. This time interval is often referred to as the period of *organogenesis;* it extends from day 15 to day 60 after conception. Environmental influences during the first 2 weeks after fertilization may interfere with implantation and result in abortion or early resorption of the products of conception. Each organ has a critical period during which it is highly susceptible to environmental derangements (Fig. 4-7). Often, the effect is expressed at the biochemical level just before the organ begins to develop. The same agent may affect different organ systems that are developing at the same time.

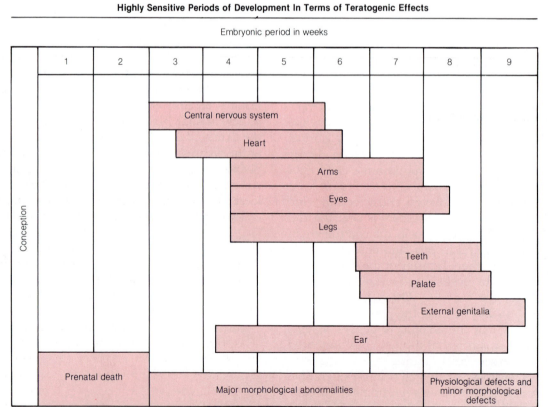

FIG. 4-7. Susceptible periods during embryologic development during which teratogenic agents are most likely to impair development of the various body structures. (Developed from information included in Moore, K. L. [1977]. *The developing human* [2nd ed.]. Philadelphia: W.B. Saunders)

TERATOGENIC AGENTS

A teratogenic agent is one that produces abnormalities during embryonic or fetal development. For discussion purposes, teratogenic agents have been divided into three groups: (1) irradiation, (2) drugs and chemical substances, and (3) infectious agents. Chart 4-1 lists commonly identified agents in each of these groups.

IRRADIATION

Heavy doses of ionizing radiation have been shown to cause microcephaly, skeletal malformations, and mental retardation. There is no evidence that diagnostic levels of radiation cause congenital abnormalities. Because the question of safety remains, however, many agencies require that the day of a woman's last menstrual period be noted on all radiologic requisitions. Other institutions may require a pregnancy test before any extensive diagnostic x-ray studies are performed. Radiation is not only teratogenic but also mutagenic, and there is the possibility of effecting inheritable changes in genetic materials. Administration of therapeutic doses of radioactive iodine (^{131}I) during the 13th week of gestation, the time when the fetal thyroid is beginning to concentrate iodine, has been shown to interfere with thyroid development.

CHART 4-1: TERATOGENIC AGENTS

Irradiation

Drugs and Chemical Substances

Alcohol
Anticoagulants
   Warfarin
Anticonvulsants
Cancer drugs
   Aminopterin
   Methotrexate
   6-mercaptopurine
Isotretinoin (Accutane)
Progestins and oral contraceptive drugs
Propylthiouracil
Tetracycline
Thalidomide

Infectious Agents

Viruses
   Cytomegalovirus
   Herpes simplex virus
   Measles (rubella)
   Mumps
   Chickenpox
Nonviral factors
   Syphilis
   Toxoplasmosis

CHEMICALS AND DRUGS

Both environmental chemicals and drugs can cross the placenta and cause damage to the developing embryo and fetus. It has been estimated that only 2% to 3% of developmental defects have a known drug or environmental origin.

Some of the best-documented environmental teratogens are the organic mercurials, which cause neurologic deficits and blindness. Sources of exposure to mercury include contaminated food (fish) and water. The precise mechanism by which chemicals and drugs exert their teratogenic effects is largely unknown. They may produce cytotoxic (cell killing), antimetabolic, or growth-inhibiting properties. Often their effects depend on the time of exposure (in terms of embryonic and fetal development) and extent of exposure (dosage). Drugs top the list of chemical teratogens, probably because they are regularly used at elevated doses. Although the placenta is virtually impermeable to compounds of molecular weight greater than 1000, most drugs have a molecular weight of less than 500.[11] Also, lipid-soluble drugs tend to cross the placenta more readily and enter the fetal circulation. Equilibration of a drug between the mother and the fetus ranges from 2 minutes to 2 hours. Fetal serum levels are generally 30% to 75% of the concentration in the mother's serum.[11]

A number of drugs are suspected of being teratogens, but only a few have been identified with certainty. Perhaps the best known of these drugs is thalidomide, which has been shown to give rise to a full range of malformations, including phocomelia (short, flipper-like appendages) of all four extremities. Other drugs known to cause fetal abnormalities are the antimetabolites used in the treatment of cancer, the anticoagulant drug warfarin, several of the anticonvulsant drugs, isotretinoin (Accutane) used in the treatment of cystic acne, ethyl alcohol, and cocaine. Some drugs affect a single developing structure; for example, propylthiouracil can impair thyroid development and tetracycline can interfere with the mineralization phase of tooth development. The progestins, which are included in many birth control pills, can cause virilization of a female fetus depending on their dosage and timing.

Because many drugs are suspected of causing fetal abnormalities, and even those that were once thought to be safe are now being viewed critically, it is recommended that women in their childbearing years avoid unnecessary use of drugs. This pertains to nonpregnant women as well as pregnant ones because many developmental defects occur early in pregnancy. As happened with thalidomide, the damage to the embryo often occurs before pregnancy is suspected or confirmed. Two drugs of particular importance are alcohol and cocaine.

Fetal Alcohol Syndrome. The fetal alcohol syndrome is rapidly becoming one of the leading causes of mental retardation in the United States. One out of 750 infants born in the United States manifests some characteristics of the syndrome.[12] Alcohol, which is lipid soluble and has a molecular weight between 600 and 1000, passes freely across the placental barrier; concentrations of alcohol in the fetus are at least as high as in the mother.[12] Unlike other teratogens, the harmful effects of alcohol are not restricted to the sensitive period of early gestation but extend throughout pregnancy.

Alcohol has widely variable effects on fetal development, ranging from minor abnormalities to a unique constellation of anomalies that has been termed the *fetal alcohol syndrome (FAS)*. Criteria for defining FAS were standardized by the Fetal Alcohol Study Group of the Research Society on Alcoholism in 1980,[13] and modifications were proposed in 1989 by Sokol and Clarren.[14] The proposed criteria are (1) prenatal and/or postnatal growth retardation (weight and/or length below the 10th percentile); (2) central nervous system involvement, including neurologic abnormalities, developmental delays, behavioral dysfunction, intellectual impairment, and skull and brain malformation; and (3) a characteristic face with short palpebral fissures (eye openings), a thin upper lip, and an elongated, flattened midface and philtrum (the groove in the middle of the upper lip). Each of these defects can vary in severity, which probably reflects the amount of alcohol consumed as well as hereditary and environmental influences. Sokol and Clarren suggested that the term *alcohol-related birth defects* be used to describe the anatomic and functional abnormalities associated with prenatal alcohol exposure.[14]

The amount of alcohol that can be safely consumed during pregnancy is unknown. Although clinical studies have focused on the consequences of chronic maternal alcoholism, there is inadequate information about the possible adverse effects of lower alcohol intake, including social drinking. One study showed that daily consumption of 10 g of alcohol (about one drink) in the week before recognition of pregnancy was related to a decrease in infant birth weight (independent of other factors), suggesting that the risk of decreased growth begins early in pregnancy.[15] In studies using pregnant monkeys, alcohol administration produced transient but marked collapse of the umbilical cord, causing severe hypoxia and acidosis in the fetus.[16] If this phenomenon occurs in humans, it could explain the teratogenicity of alcohol. Even in late gestation, the unborn child could be at risk for alcohol-induced hypoxia.

Cocaine Babies. Of recent concern is the increasing use of cocaine by pregnant women. Among the effects of cocaine use during pregnancy is a decrease in uteroplacental blood flow, maternal hypertension, stimulation of uterine contractions, and fetal vasoconstriction. The decrease in uteroplacental blood flow is associated with an increase in preterm births, lower birth weight, and delivery of small for gestational age infants.[17, 18] Maternal hypertension may increase the risk of abruptio placentae, particularly if it is accompanied by a decrease in uteroplacental blood flow.[17] Fetal vasoconstriction has been suggested as the cause of fetal anomalies, particularly limb reduction defects and urogenital tract defects such as hydronephrosis, hypospadias and undescended testicles, and ambiguous genitalia.[17, 19] Sudden infant death syndrome (SIDS) has also been more common in babies of mothers who have used cocaine during their pregnancy.[20] Other reported effects of maternal cocaine use on the infant are small head size, altered neonatal behavior patterns, and impaired neonatal brain stem auditory system development.[21] One study reported that 39% of 28 cocaine-exposed babies exhibited cerebral infarctions as documented on cranial ultrasound at birth.[22] Although the immediate effects of maternal cocaine use on infant behavior are being reported, the long-term effects are largely unknown.

Unfortunately, cocaine addiction often affects the behavior of the pregnant woman to the extent that the need to procure larger amounts of the drug overwhelms all other considerations of maternal and fetal well-being; hence, other factors such as malnutrition, use of other drugs and teratogens, and lack of prenatal care may also contribute to fetal disorders.

INFECTIOUS AGENTS

Many microorganisms cross the placenta and enter the fetal circulation, often producing multiple malformations. The acronym TORCH stands for *t*oxoplasmosis, *o*ther, *r*ubella, *c*ytomegalovirus, and *h*erpes, which are the agents most frequently implicated in fetal anomalies.[23] "Other" stands for type B hepatitis virus, coxsackie virus B, mumps, poliovirus, rubeola, varicella, listeria, gonorrhea, streptococcus, and treponema. Of these, hepatitis B poses the greatest threat to mother and infant. The TORCH screening test examines the infant's serum for the presence of antibodies to these agents. These infections tend to cause similar clinical manifestations, including microcephaly, hydrocephaly, defects of the eye, and hearing problems. Cytomegalovirus may cause mental retardation, and rubella virus may cause congenital heart defects.

Toxoplasmosis is a protozoal infection that can be contracted by eating raw or poorly cooked meat. The domestic cat also seems to carry the organism, excreting the protozoa in its stools. It has been suggested that pregnant women should avoid contact with the excrement from the family cat. *Rubella* (German measles) is a commonly recognized viral teratogen. About 15% to 20% of babies born to women who have had rubella during the first trimester have abnormalities.[24] The epidemiology of the *cytomegalovirus* is largely unknown. Some babies are severely affected at birth, and others, although having evidence of the infection, have no symptoms. In some symptom-free babies, brain damage becomes evident over a span of several years. There is also evidence that some babies contract the infection during the first year of life and in some of them the infection leads to retardation a year or two later. *Herpes simplex 2* is considered to be a genital infection and is usually transmitted through sexual contact. The infant acquires this infection either *in utero* or in passage through the birth canal.

In summary, a teratogenic agent is one that produces abnormalities during embryonic or fetal life. It is during the early part of pregnancy (15 to 60 days after conception) that environmental agents are most apt to produce their deleterious effects on the developing embryo. A number of environmental agents can be damaging to the unborn child, including radiation, drugs and chemicals, and infectious agents. The fetal alcohol syndrome is a recently recognized risk for infants of women who regularly consume alcohol during pregnancy. Of recent concern is the use of cocaine by pregnant women. Because many drugs have the potential for causing fetal abnormalities, often at an early stage of pregnancy, it is recommended that women of childbearing age avoid unnecessary use of drugs.

■ DIAGNOSIS AND COUNSELING

The birth of a defective child is a traumatic event in any parent's life. Usually two issues must be resolved. The first deals with the immediate and future care of the affected child, and the second with the possibility of future children in the family having a similar defect. Genetic assessment and counseling can help to determine whether the defect was inherited, as well as the risk of recurrence. Prenatal diagnosis provides a means of determining whether the unborn child has certain types of abnormalities.

GENETIC ASSESSMENT

Effective genetic counseling involves accurate diagnosis and communication of the findings and of the risks of recurrence, to the parents and other family members who need such information. Counseling may be provided after the birth of an affected child, or it may be offered to persons at risk for having defective children (siblings of persons with birth defects). A team of trained counselors can help the family to understand the problem and can support their decisions about having more children.

Assessment of genetic risk and prognosis is usually directed by a clinical geneticist, often with the aid of laboratory and clinical specialists. A detailed family history (pedigree), a pregnancy history, and detailed accounts of both the birth process and postnatal health and development are included. A careful physical examination of the affected child and often of the parents and siblings is usually needed. Laboratory work, including chromosomal analysis and biochemical studies, often precedes a definitive diagnosis.

The creases and dermal ridges on the palms and soles are examined in a genetic study called *dermatoglyphic analysis*. This is of value because the dermal ridges are formed by 16 weeks of gestation and any abnormalities document the time during which the developmental defect occurred. Dermatoglyphic analysis includes examination of the patterns of the arches on the fingertips, the flexion creases of the fifth finger, and the arch pattern of the base of the great toe.

PRENATAL DIAGNOSIS

The purpose of prenatal diagnosis is not just to detect fetal abnormalities. Rather, it has the following objectives: (1) to provide parents with information needed to make an informed choice at having a child with an abnormality; (2) to provide reassurance and reduce anxiety among high-risk groups; (3) to allow parents at risk for having a child with a specific defect, who might otherwise forgo having a children, to begin pregnancy with the assurance that knowledge about the presence or absence of the disorder in the fetus can be confirmed by testing.[4]

Among the methods used for fetal diagnosis are ultrasonography, amniocentesis, chorionic villus sampling, percutaneous umbilical fetal blood sampling, and laboratory methods to determine the biochemical and genetic makeup of the fetus. Alpha-fetoprotein screening is also used. Prenatal diagnosis is indicated in about 8% of pregnancies. Termination of pregnancy is only indicated in a small number of cases; in the rest, the fetus is normal and the procedure provides reassurance for the parents. Prenatal diagnosis can also provide the information needed for prescribing prenatal treatment for the fetus. For example, if congenital adrenal hyperplasia is diagnosed, the mother can be treated with adrenal cortical hormones to prevent masculinization of a female fetus.

ULTRASOUND

Ultrasound is a noninvasive diagnostic method that uses reflections of high-frequency sound waves to visualize soft tissue structures. Since its introduction in 1958, it has been used during pregnancy to determine fetal size, fetal position, and placental location. Improved resolution and real-time units have enhanced the ability of ultrasound scanners to detect congenital anomalies. With this more sophisticated equipment, it is possible to obtain information such as measurements of hourly urine output in a high-risk fetus.[25] Ultrasound makes possible the *in utero* diagnosis of hydrocephalus, spina bifida, facial defects, congenital heart defects, congenital diaphragmatic hernias, disorders of the gastrointestinal tract, and skeletal anomalies. Intrauterine diagnosis of congenital abnormalities permits planning of surgical correction shortly after birth, preterm delivery for early correction, selection of caesarean section to reduce fetal injury, and, in some cases, *in utero* therapy. Forty percent of obstetric practices in the United States have all of their patients undergo ultrasound scanning at least once during pregnancy.[25] When a congenital abnormality is suspected, a diagnosis made using ultrasound can generally be obtained by weeks 16 to 18 of gestation.

AMNIOCENTESIS

Amniocentesis involves the withdrawal of a sample of amniotic fluid from the pregnant uterus by means of a needle inserted through the abdominal wall (Fig. 4-8). The procedure is useful in women over age 35,

who have an increased risk of giving birth to a baby with Down's syndrome; in parents who have another child with chromosomal abnormalities; and in situations in which either parent is known to be a carrier of an inherited disease. Ultrasound is used to gain additional information and to guide the placement of the amniocentesis needle. Both the amniotic fluid and cells that have been shed by the fetus are studied. Usually, a determination of fetal status can be made by the 16th to 17th week of pregnancy. For chromosomal analysis, the fetal cells are grown in culture and the result is available in 2 to 3 weeks. To test for inborn errors of metabolism such as Tay-Sachs disease, the amniotic fluid cells are grown in culture for 4 to 6 weeks to provide sufficient cells to assay for the appropriate enzyme. The amniotic fluid can also be tested using various biochemical tests.

CHORIONIC VILLUS SAMPLING

Sampling of the chorionic villi from the fetus is performed at 8 to 12 weeks of gestation. The biopsy is taken through the cervix using a catheter and gentle suctioning under ultrasound guidance. Sometimes an abdominal approach is needed if the transcervical approach is inadequate or if a sample is required after the 12th week of gestation. The tissue that is obtained can be used for fetal chromosome studies, DNA analysis, and biochemical studies. The fetal tissue does

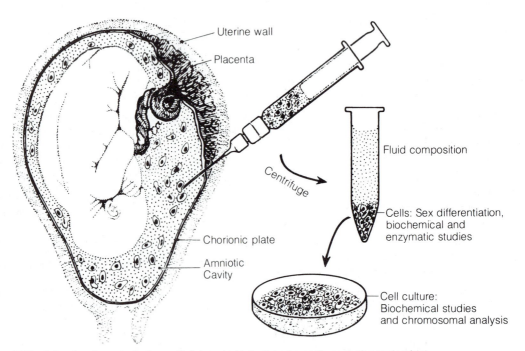

FIG. 4-8. Amniocentesis. A needle is inserted into the uterus through the abdominal wall, and a sample of amniotic fluid is withdrawn for chromosomal and biochemical studies. (Department of Health, Education and Welfare. [1977]. *What are the facts about genetic disease?* Washington, DC: DHEW)

not have to be cultured, and fetal chromosome analysis can be made available in 24 hours. DNA analysis and biochemical tests can be completed in 1 to 2 weeks.

PERCUTANEOUS UMBILICAL BLOOD SAMPLING

Percutaneous fetal blood sampling involves the transcutaneous insertion of a needle through the uterine wall and into the umbilical artery. It is performed under ultrasound guidance and can be done anytime after 16 weeks of gestation. It is used for prenatal diagnosis of hemoglobinopathies, coagulation disorders, metabolic and cytogenic disorders, and immunodeficiencies. Fetal infections such as rubella and toxoplasmosis can be detected through measurement of IgM antibodies or direct blood cultures.

CYTOGENETIC AND BIOCHEMICAL ANALYSES

Amniocentesis and chorionic villus sampling yield cells that can be used for cytogenetic and DNA analyses. Biochemical analyses can be used to detect abnormal levels of fetal proteins (alpha-fetoprotein) and abnormal biochemical products both in the maternal blood and in specimens of amniotic fluid and fetal blood.

Cytogenetic studies are used for fetal karyotyping to determine the chromosome makeup of the fetus. It is done to detect abnormalities of chromosome number and structure. Karyotyping also reveals the sex of the fetus. This may be useful when an inherited defect is known to affect only one sex.

DNA analysis is done on cells extracted from the amniotic fluid or obtained by chorionic villus sampling. It is done to detect genetic defects such as inborn errors of metabolism. The defect may be established through direct demonstration of the molecular defect or through methods that break the DNA into fragments so that the fragments may be studied to determine the presence of an abnormal gene. Direct demonstration of the molecular defect is done by growing the amniotic fluid cells in culture and measuring the enzymes that the cultured cells produce. Many of the enzymes are expressed in the chorionic villi; this permits earlier prenatal diagnosis because the cells do not need to be subjected to prior culture. DNA studies are used to detect genetic defects that cause inborn errors of metabolism such as Tay-Sachs disease, glycogen storage diseases, and familial hypercholesterolemia. Prenatal diagnoses are possible for more than 70 inborn errors of metabolism.

Alpha-Fetoprotein. Alpha-fetoprotein (AFP) is a major fetal plasma protein and has a structure similar to the albumin that is found in postnatal life. AFP is made initially by the yolk sac and later by the liver. It peaks at about 12 to 14 weeks in the fetus and falls thereafter.[26] AFP is found in the amniotic fluid at about one hundredth the concentration found in fetal serum. AFP reaches the maternal bloodstream and can be measured by laboratory methods. The normal maternal serum AFP rises from 13 weeks and peaks at 32 weeks gestation. In pregnancies where the fetus has a neural tube defect (anencephaly and open spina bifida) or certain other malformations such as an anterior abdominal wall defect, maternal and amniotic levels of AFP are elevated. Screening of maternal blood samples is usually done between weeks 16 and 20 of gestation. If the AFP is elevated, a second serum sample is taken and ultrasound studies are advised to check for a missed abortion or multiple pregnancy, both of which produce elevated AFP levels. When a second maternal blood sample is found to contain elevated levels of AFP, more extensive ultrasound and amniocentesis are advised.

In summary, genetic and prenatal diagnosis and counseling are done in an effort to determine the risk of having a child with a genetic or chromosomal disorder. They often involve a detailed family history (pedigree), examination of any affected and other family members, and laboratory studies including chromosomal analysis and biochemical studies. They are usually done by a genetic counselor and a specially prepared team of health care professionals. Both ultrasound and amniocentesis can be used to screen for congenital defects. Ultrasound is used for determination of fetal size and position and for the presence of structural anomalies. Amniocentesis and chorionic villus sampling are used to obtain specimens for cytogenetic and biochemical studies. They are used in the prenatal diagnosis of over 60 genetic disorders.

■   REFERENCES

1. *Birth defects.* (1992). White Plains, NY: March of Dimes.
2. Chavez, G.F., Cordero, J.F., & Becerra, J.E. (1988). Leading major congenital malformations among minority groups in the United States, 1981-86. *Morbidity and Mortality Weekly Reports (SS-3),* 17-24.
3. McKusick, V.A. (1983). *Mendelian inheritance in man: Catalogs of autosomal dominant, autosomal recessive, and X-linked phenotypes.* Baltimore: Johns Hopkins University Press.
4. Thompson, M.W., McInnes, R.R., Willard, H.F. (1991). *Thompson & Thompson genetics in medicine* (5th ed., pp. 59–66, 201, 411–425). Philadelphia: W.B. Saunders.
5. Oski, F.A. (Ed.). (1989). *Principles and practices of pediatrics* (pp. 1940–1945). Philadelphia: J.B. Lippincott.
6. Behrman, R.E. (Ed.). (1992). *Nelson textbook of pediatrics* (14th ed., pp. 1509–1510). Philadelphia: W.B. Saunders.
7. Riccardi, V.M. (1977). *The genetic approach to human disease* (pp. 92, 500). New York: Oxford University Press.
8. The Down Syndrome Collaborative Group. (1991). Par-

enteral origin of trisomy 21 as indicated by DNA polymorphisms. *New England Journal of Medicine, 324,* 872–876.

9. Hassold, T.J., & Jacobs, P.A. (1984). Trisomy in man. *Annual Review of Genetics, 18,* 69.

10. Janerich, D.T., & Polendnak, A.P. (1983). Epidemiology of birth defects. *Epidemiologic Reviews, 5,* 16–37.

11. Hill, L.M. (1984). Effects of drugs and chemicals on the fetus and newborn (first of two parts). *Mayo Clinic Proceedings, 59,* 7–16.

12. Streissguth, A., Landesman-Dwyer, S., Martin, J.C., et al.(1980). Teratogenic effects of alcohol in humans and laboratory animals. *Science, 209,* 353–361.

13. Rosett, H.L. (1980). A clinical perspective of the fetal alcohol syndrome. *Alcohol, Clinical and Experimental Research, 4,* 118.

14. Sokol, R.J., & Clarren, S.K. (1980). Guidelines for use of terminology describing the impact of prenatal alcohol on the offspring. *Alcohol, Clinical and Experimental Research, 13,* 587–589.

15. Little, R.E., Asker, R.L., Sampson, P.D., et al. Fetal growth and moderate drinking in early pregnancy. *American Journal of Epidemiology, 123,* 270–278.

16. Mukherjee, A.B., & Hodgen, G.D. (1982). Maternal alcohol exposure induces transient impairment of umbilical circulation and fetal hypoxia in monkeys. *Science, 218,* 700.

17. MacGregor, S.N., Keith, L.G., Chasnoff, I.J., Rosner, M.A., Chisnum, G.M., Shaw, P., & Minogue, J.P. (1987). Cocaine use during pregnancy: Adverse outcome. *American Journal of Obstetrics and Gynecology, 157*(3), 686.

18. Chasnoff, I.J., & Griffith, D.R. (1989). Cocaine: Clinical studies of pregnancy and the newborn. *Annals of the New York Academy of Sciences, 562,* 260.

19. Chasnoff, I.J., Chisum, G.M., & Kaplan, W.E. (1988). Maternal cocaine use and genitourinary malformations. *Teratology, 37,* 201.

20. Riley, J.B., Brodsky, N.L., & Porat, R. (1988). Risk of SIDS in infants with *in utero* cocaine exposure: A prospective study [Abstract]. *Pediatric Research, 23,* 454A.

21. Shih, B., Cone-Wesson, B., Reddix, B., & Wu, P.Y.K. (1988). Effects of maternal cocaine abuse on the neonatal auditory system [Abstract]. *Pediatric Research, 23,* 264A.

22. Dixon, S.D., & Bejar, R. (1988). Brain lesions in cocaine and methamphetamine-exposed neonates [Abstract]. *Pediatric Research, 23,* 405A.

23. DeVore, N.E., Jackson, V.M., & Piening, S.L. (1983). TORCH infections. *American Journal of Nursing, 83,* 1660.

24. Dudgeon, J.A. (1976). Infectious causes of human malformations. *British Medical Journal, 32,* 77.

25. Hill, L.M., Breckle, R., & Gehrking, R.T. (1983). The prenatal detection of congenital malformations by ultrasonography. *Mayo Clinic Proceedings, 58,* 805.

26. Connor, J.M., & Ferguson-Smith, M.A. (1987). *Essential medical genetics* (2nd ed., p. 191). London: Blackwell Scientific.

■ BIBLIOGRAPHY

Annas, G.J. (1987). Routine prenatal genetic screening. *New England Journal of Medicine, 317*(22), 1407.

Antonarakis, S.E. (1989). Diagnosis of genetic disorders at the DNA level. *New England Journal of Medicine, 320,* 153–162.

Buehler, B., Delimont, D., van Waes, M., et al. (1990). Prenatal prediction of fetal hydantoin syndrome. *New England Journal of Medicine, 322,* 1567–1572.

Cunningham, F.G., & Gilstrap, L.C. (1991). Maternal alpha-fetoprotein screening. *New England Journal of Medicine, 325,* 55–57.

Holtzman, N.A. (1991). What drives prenatal screening program. *New England Journal of Medicine, 325,* 802–804.

Humphreys, P., & Berkeley, D. (1987). Representing risks: Supporting genetic counseling. *March of Dimes: Original Article Series, 23,* 227–250.

Langlois, S. (1992). Genetic diagnosis based on molecular analysis. *Pediatric Clinics of North America, 39,* 91–105.

Lemons, P.K., & Brock, M.J. (1990). Prenatal diagnosis and congenital disease: Role of the clinical nurse specialist. *Neonatal Network, 9*(3), 15–22.

Little, B.B., Snell, L.M., Rosenfeld, C.R., et al. (1990). Failure to recognize fetal alcohol syndrome in newborn infants. *American Journal of Diseases of Children, 144,* 1142–1146.

Russell, M. (1991). Clinical implications of recent research in the fetal alcohol syndrome. *Bulletin of the New York Academy of Medicine, 67,* 207–221.

Seaver, L.H., & Hoyme, E. (1992). Teratology in pediatric practice. *Pediatric Clinics of North America, 39,* 111–134.

Shapiro, L.R. (1992). The fragile X-syndrome—a peculiar pattern of inheritance. *New England Journal of Medicine, 325,* 1736–1738.

Sokol, R.J., Martier, S.S., & Ager, J.W. (1989). The T-ACE questions: Practical prenatal detection of risk drinking. *American Journal of Obstetrics and Gynecology, 160,* 863–870.

Streissguth, A.P., Aase, J.M., Clarren, S.K., et al. (1991). Fetal alcohol syndrome in adolescents and adults. *Journal of the American Medical Association, 265,* 1961–1967.

Volpe, J.J. (1992). Effect of cocaine use on the fetus. *New England Journal of Medicine, 327,* 399–407.

Wexler, N.S. (1991). Disease gene identification: Ethical considerations. *Hospital Practice, 26*(1), 145–152.

ALTERATIONS IN CELL DIFFERENTIATION: NEOPLASIA

◼ OBJECTIVES

After you have studied this chapter, you should be able to meet the following objectives:

◼ Define *neoplasm* and explain how neoplastic growth differs from the normal adaptive changes seen in atrophy, hypertrophy, and hyperplasia.

◼ Distinguish between cell proliferation and differentiation.

◼ Describe the five phases of the cell cycle.

◼ Cite the method used for naming benign and malignant neoplasms.

◼ State at least six ways in which benign and malignant neoplasms differ.

◼ Relate the properties of cell differentiation to the development of a cancer cell line and the behavior of the tumor.

◼ Trace the pathway for hematologic spread of a metastatic cancer cell.

◼ Use the concepts of growth fraction and doubling time to explain the growth of cancerous tissue.

◼ Describe the general effects of cancer on body systems.

◼ Describe the role of proto-oncogenes and anti-oncogenes in the transformation of a normal life line to a cancer cell line.

◼ State how lifestyle can contribute to the cancer risk through increased exposure to carcinogenic agents.

◼ Relate the function of the immune system to prevention of cancer.

◼ Explain the mechanism by which radiation exerts its beneficial effects in the treatment of cancer.

◼ Describe the adverse effects of radiation therapy.

◼ Compare the action of cell-cycle–specific and cell-cycle–independent chemotherapeutic drugs.

◼ Describe the three mechanisms whereby biotherapy exerts its effects.

◼ Cite the early warning signs of cancer in children.

◼ State the tissue type involved in neuroblastoma, Wilms' tumor, and retinoblastoma, and list two manifestations of each of these types of cancer.

◼ Discuss possible concerns of adult survivors of childhood cancer.

Carol Mattson Porth: PATHOPHYSIOLOGY: CONCEPTS OF ALTERED HEALTH STATES, 4th ed. © 1994, 1990, 1986, 1982 J.B. Lippincott Company

Cancer is the second leading cause of death in the United States. The disease affects all age groups, causing more deaths in children 3 to 15 years of age than any other disease. The American Cancer Society has estimated that over 83 million Americans, or one out of every four alive today, will develop cancer during their lifetimes. In 1992, about 1,130,000 people were diagnosed as having cancer.[1] It has been estimated that with present methods of treatment, 51% of people who develop cancer each year will be alive 5 years later.

Cancers result from a process of altered cell growth called neoplasia. The term *neoplasm* comes from a Greek word meaning *new formation*. In contrast to the tissue growth that occurs with hypertrophy and hyperplasia, a neoplasm serves no useful purpose but tends to increase in size and persist at the expense of the rest of the body. Furthermore, neoplasms do not obey the laws of normal tissue growth. For example, they do not occur in response to an appropriate stimulus, and they continue to grow after the stimulus has ceased or the needs of the organism have been met.

Cancer is not a single disease; rather, the term describes almost all forms of malignant neoplasia. Cancer can originate in almost any organ, with the prostate being the most common site in men and the breast in women (Fig. 5-1). Cancers vary greatly in curability. Cancers such as acute lymphocytic leukemia, Hodgkin's disease, testicular and ovarian cancers, and osteogenic sarcoma, which only a few decades ago had a poor prognosis, are today cured in many cases. On the other hand, lung cancer, which is the leading cause of death in both men and women in the United States, is resistant to therapy, and although some progress has been made in its treatment, mortality remains high. This chapter is divided into five sections: (1) concepts of cell growth and differentiation, (2) characteristics of benign and malignant neoplasms, (3) carcinogenesis and causes of cancer, (4) diagnosis and treatment, and (5) childhood cancers. Specific forms of cancer are discussed elsewhere in this book.

■ CONCEPTS OF CELL GROWTH

Cell growth involves both cell proliferation and differentiation. Proliferation or cell division is an inherent adaptive mechanism for replacing body cells when old cells die or additional cells are needed. Differentiation is the process of specialization whereby new cells develop the structure and function of the cells they replace. When abnormal or mutant cells develop, either they are defective and incapable of survival or they are destroyed by the body's immune system. Defects in these two processes underlie the nature of neoplasia.

THE CELL CYCLE

The life of a cell is called the *cell cycle*. It consists of the interval between the midpoint of mitosis in a cell and the subsequent midpoint of mitosis in one or both daughter cells. *Mitosis* is the period of time when cell division is actually taking place.

The cell cycle is divided into five distinct phases, for which the *gap* or *G* terminology is used (Fig. 5-2). G_1, the first gap, is the postmitotic phase during which DNA synthesis ceases while RNA and protein synthesis and cell growth take place. Toward the end of G_1, some critical event occurs that commits the cell to continue through the phases of the gap cycle and enter mitosis. G_0 is a resting or dormant phase of G_1 during which the cell performs all activities except those related to proliferation. Cells can leave G_1 and enter G_0. The time spent in G_0 varies according to the cell type, and not all cells spend time in G_0. It is believed that some special growth signal is needed to move cells that have been dormant in G_0 back into the cell cycle. During the S phase, or synthesis phase, DNA replication occurs, giving rise to two separate sets of chromosomes, one for each daughter cell. G_2 is the premitotic phase. During this phase, as in G_1, DNA synthesis ceases whereas synthesis of RNA and protein continues. The cell cycle is completed during the M or mitosis phase when cell division occurs.

For rapidly reproducing cells, the entire cell cycle occupies about 16 hours. For others, such as liver cells, the cycle takes about 10,000 hours.[2] The durations of the G_2 period (8 hours), S period (2 hours), and mitosis (0.07 hours) are almost identical for all cell types. The time spent in G_1 and G_0 determines the length of the cell cycle.[2] When only a low rate of cell reproduction is needed to maintain health of tissues, the cells remain dormant in the G_0; when a more rapid rate of reproduction is needed, the G_0 dormant period is shortened.

CELL PROLIFERATION

The term *proliferation* refers to the process by which cells divide and bear offspring. In normal tissue, cell proliferation is regulated so that the number of cells actively dividing is equivalent to the number dying or being shed.

In terms of cell proliferation, the 100 or more cell types of the body can be divided into three large groups: (1) the well-differentiated neurons and cells of skeletal and cardiac muscle that are unable to divide and reproduce; (2) the parent, or progenitor

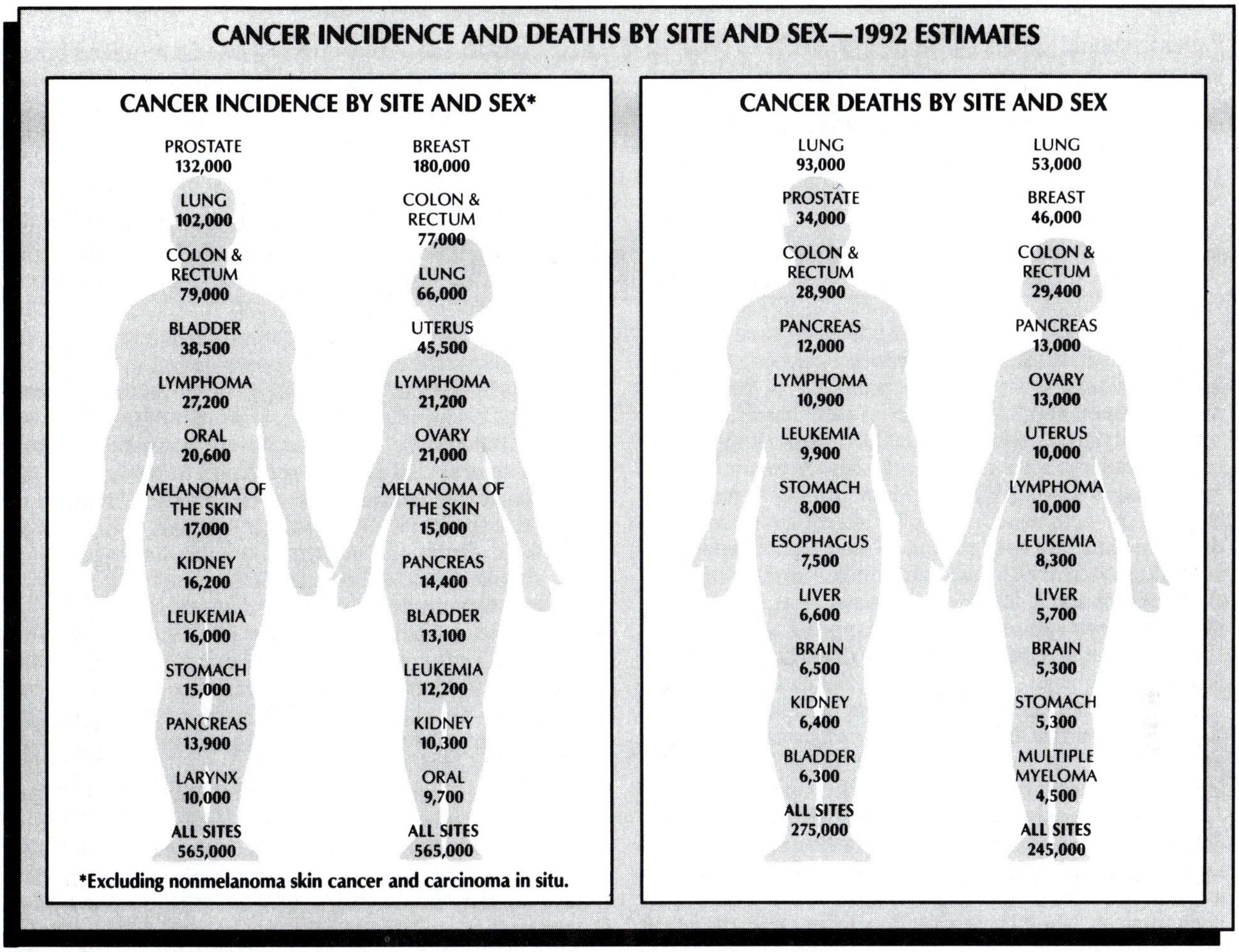

CANCER INCIDENCE AND DEATHS BY SITE AND SEX—1992 ESTIMATES

CANCER INCIDENCE BY SITE AND SEX*

PROSTATE 132,000	BREAST 180,000
LUNG 102,000	COLON & RECTUM 77,000
COLON & RECTUM 79,000	LUNG 66,000
BLADDER 38,500	UTERUS 45,500
LYMPHOMA 27,200	LYMPHOMA 21,200
ORAL 20,600	OVARY 21,000
MELANOMA OF THE SKIN 17,000	MELANOMA OF THE SKIN 15,000
KIDNEY 16,200	PANCREAS 14,400
LEUKEMIA 16,000	BLADDER 13,100
STOMACH 15,000	LEUKEMIA 12,200
PANCREAS 13,900	KIDNEY 10,300
LARYNX 10,000	ORAL 9,700
ALL SITES 565,000	ALL SITES 565,000

*Excluding nonmelanoma skin cancer and carcinoma in situ.

CANCER DEATHS BY SITE AND SEX

LUNG 93,000	LUNG 53,000
PROSTATE 34,000	BREAST 46,000
COLON & RECTUM 28,900	COLON & RECTUM 29,400
PANCREAS 12,000	PANCREAS 13,000
LYMPHOMA 10,900	OVARY 13,000
LEUKEMIA 9,900	UTERUS 10,000
STOMACH 8,000	LYMPHOMA 10,000
ESOPHAGUS 7,500	LEUKEMIA 8,300
LIVER 6,600	LIVER 5,700
BRAIN 6,500	BRAIN 5,300
KIDNEY 6,400	STOMACH 5,300
BLADDER 6,300	MULTIPLE MYELOMA 4,500
ALL SITES 275,000	ALL SITES 245,000

FIG. 5-1. Cancer incidence and deaths (1992 estimates) by site and sex. (*Cancer facts.* [1992]. New York: American Cancer Society.)

cells, that continue to divide and reproduce, such as blood cells, skin cells, and liver cells; (3) the undifferentiated stem cells that can be triggered to enter the cell cycle and produce large numbers of progenitor cells when the need arises. The rates of reproduction of these cells vary greatly. White blood cells and cells that line the gastrointestinal tract live several days and must be replaced constantly. In most tissues, the rate of cell reproduction is greatly increased when tissue is injured or lost. Bleeding, for example, stimulates the rapid reproduction of the blood-forming cells of the bone marrow. In some types of tissue, the genetic program for cell replication is normally repressed, but it can be resumed under certain conditions. The liver, as an example, has extensive regenerative capabilities under certain conditions.

CELL DIFFERENTIATION

Cell differentiation is the process whereby cells are transformed into different and more specialized cell types as they proliferate. Cell differentiation determines what a cell looks like, how it functions, and how long it will live. For example, a red blood cell is programmed to develop into a concave disk that functions as a vehicle for oxygen transport and lives 120 days.

All of the different cell types of the body originate from a single cell—the fertilized ovum. As the embryonic cells increase in number, they engage in an orderly process of differentiation that is necessary for the development of all the various organs of the body. What makes the cells of one organ different from those of another organ is the type of gene that is expressed. Although all cells have the same complement of genes, only a small number of these genes are expressed in postnatal life. When cells, such as those of the developing embryo, differentiate and give rise to committed cells of a particular tissue type, the appropriate genes are maintained in an active state whereas the rest become inactive. Normally, the rate of cell reproduction and the process of cell differentiation are precisely controlled in both prenatal and postnatal life so that both of these mechanisms

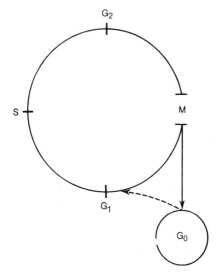

FIG. 5-2. Phases of the cell cycle. The cycle represents the interval from the midpoint of mitosis to the subsequent end point in mitosis in a daughter cell. G_1 is the postmitotic phase during which RNA and protein synthesis is increased and cell growth occurs. G_0 is the resting or dormant phase of the cell cycle. The S phase represents synthesis of nucleic acids with chromosome replication in preparation for cell mitosis. During G_2, RNA and protein synthesis occurs as in G_1.

cease once the appropriate numbers and types of cells are formed.

The process of differentiation occurs in orderly steps; with each progressive step, increased specialization is exchanged for a loss of ability to develop different cell characteristics and different cell lines. The more highly specialized a cell becomes, the more likely it is to lose its ability to undergo mitosis. Neurons, which are the most highly specialized cells in the body, lose their ability to divide and reproduce once development of the nervous system is complete. More importantly, there are no reserve or parent cells to direct their replacement. In other, less specialized tissues, such as the skin and mucosal lining, cell renewal continues throughout life.

But even in the continuously renewing cell populations, there are highly specialized cells that are similarly unable to divide. An alternative mechanism provides for their replacement. In this case, there are progenitor cells of the same lineage that have not yet differentiated to the extent that they have lost their ability to divide. These cells are sufficiently differentiated that their daughter cells are limited to the same cell line, but they are insufficiently differentiated to preclude the potential for active proliferation. As a result, these parent, or progenitor, cells are able to provide large numbers of replacement cells. The progenitor cells, however, have limited capacity for self-renewal and they become restricted to producing a single type of cell.

A third type of cell, called a *stem cell*, remains incompletely differentiated throughout life. Stem cells are reserve cells that remain quiescent until there is a need for cell replenishment, and then they divide to replenish or increase the progenitor cell population (Fig. 5-3). Stem cells are the main ingredient of bone marrow transplantation; the stem cells in the transplanted marrow reestablish the recipient's blood production and immune system.

In summary, the term *neoplasm* refers to a new growth. In contrast to normal cellular adaptive processes such as hypertrophy and hyperplasia, neoplasms do not obey the laws of normal cell growth. They serve no useful purpose, they do not occur in response to an appropriate stimulus, and they continue to grow at the expense of the host.

Cell proliferation is the process whereby cells divide and bear offspring; it is normally regulated so that the number of cells that are actively dividing is equal to the number dying or being shed.

The life of a cell is called the cell cycle. It is divided into five phases: (1) G_1 represents the postmitotic phase, during which RNA and protein synthesis occurs; (2) G_0 is the resting or dormant phase of the cell cycle; (3) the S phase is the synthesis phase, during which DNA replication occurs; (4) G_2 is the premitotic phase and is similar to G_1 in terms of RNA and protein synthesis; (5) the M phase is the phase during which cell mitosis occurs.

Cell differentiation is the process whereby cells are transformed into different and more specialized cell types as they proliferate. It determines the structure, function, and life span of a cell. There are three types of cells: (1) well-differentiated cells that are no longer able to divide, (2) progenitor or parent cells that continue to divide and bear offspring, and (3) undifferentiated stem cells that can be recruited to become progenitor cells when the need arises. As a cell line becomes more differentiated, it becomes more highly specialized in its function and less able to divide.

■ CHARACTERISTICS OF BENIGN AND MALIGNANT NEOPLASMS

Neoplasms are composed of two types of tissue: parenchymal tissue and the stroma or supporting tissue. The parenchymal cells represent the functional components of an organ. The supporting tissue consists of the connective tissue, blood vessels, and lymph structures. The parenchymal cells of a tumor determine its behavior and are the component for which a tumor is named. The supporting tissue carries the blood vessels and provides support for tumor survival and growth.

TERMINOLOGY

By definition, a *tumor* is a swelling that can be caused by a number of conditions, including inflammation and trauma. Although they are not synonymous, the

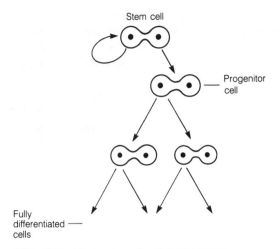

Stem cell

Progenitor cell

Fully differentiated — cells

FIG. 5-3. Mechanism of cell replacement.

terms *tumor* and *neoplasm* are often used interchangeably. There are two types of neoplasms: benign and malignant. The Latin word *malus* means bad; hence, a *malignant* tumor is a bad tumor. It usually causes suffering and death unless treated and controlled. A benign tumor is a *good tumor*. A benign tumor does not usually cause death unless by its location it interferes with vital functions.

Tumors are usually named by adding the suffix *-oma* to the parenchymal tissue type from which the growth originated. Thus, a benign tumor of glandular epithelial tissue is called an *adenoma*, and a benign tumor of bone tissue is called an *osteoma*. The term *carcinoma* is used to designate a malignant tumor of epithelial tissue origin. In the case of a malignant adenoma, the term *adenocarcinoma* is used. Malignant tumors of mesenchymal origin are called *sarcomas* (*e.g.*, osteosarcoma). Papillomas are benign microscopic or macroscopic fingerlike projections that grow on any surface. A polyp is growth that projects from a mucosal surface, such as the intestine. Although the term usually implies a benign neoplasm, some malignant tumors also appear as polyps.[3] *Oncology* is the study of tumors and their treatment. Table 5-1 lists the names of selected benign and malignant tumors according to tissue types.

BENIGN NEOPLASMS

Benign and malignant neoplasms are generally differentiated by their (1) cell characteristics, (2) manner of growth, (3) rate of growth, (4) potential for metastasizing or spreading to other parts of the body, (5) ability to produce generalized effects, (6) tendency to cause tissue destruction, and (7) capacity to

TABLE 5-1. NAMES OF SELECTED BENIGN AND MALIGNANT TUMORS ACCORDING TO TISSUE TYPES		
TISSUE TYPE	**BENIGN**	**MALIGNANT**
Epithelial Tumors		
Surface	Papilloma	Squamous cell carcinoma
Glandular	Adenoma	Adenocarcinoma
Connective Tissue Tumors		
Fibrous	Fibroma	Fibrosarcoma
Adipose	Lipoma	Liposarcoma
Cartilage	Chondroma	Chondrosarcoma
Bone	Osteoma	Osteosarcoma
Blood vessels	Hemangioma	Hemangiosarcoma
Lymph vessels	Lymphangioma	Lymphangiosarcoma
Muscle Tumors		
Smooth	Leiomyoma	Leiomyosarcoma
Striated	Rhabdomyoma	Rhabdomyosarcoma
Nerve Cell Tumors		
Nerve cell	Neuroma	
Glial tissue		Glioma
Nerve sheaths	Neurilemoma	Neurilemic sarcoma
Hematologic Tumors		
Granulocytic		Myelocytic leukemia
Erythrocytic		Erythroleukemia
Plasma cells		Multiple myeloma
Lymphoid		Lymphocytic leukemia

cause death. The characteristics of benign and malignant neoplasms are summarized in Table 5-2.

Benign tumors are characterized by a slow progressive rate of growth that may come to a standstill or regress, an expansive manner of growth, the presence of a well-defined fibrous capsule, and failure to metastasize to distant sites. Benign tumors are composed of well-differentiated cells that resemble their counterparts. For example, the cells of a uterine leiomyoma resemble uterine smooth muscle cells. For some unknown reason, benign tumors seem to have lost the ability to suppress the genetic program for cell replication but retain the program for normal cell differentiation. Benign tumors grow by expansion and are enclosed in a fibrous capsule. This is in sharp contrast to malignant neoplasms, which grow by infiltrating the surrounding tissue (Fig. 5-4). The presence of the capsule is responsible for a sharp line of demarcation between the benign tumor and the adjacent tissues, a factor that facilitates surgical removal. The formation of the capsule is thought to represent the reaction of the surrounding tissues to the tumor.

Benign tumors do not undergo degenerative changes as readily as malignant tumors, and they do not usually cause death unless by their location they interfere with vital functions. For instance, a benign

TABLE 5-2. CHARACTERISTICS OF BENIGN AND MALIGNANT NEOPLASMS

CHARACTERISTICS	BENIGN	MALIGNANT
Cell characteristics	Well-differentiated cells that resemble normal cells of the tissue from which the tumor originated	Cells are undifferentiated and often bear little resemblance to the normal cells of the tissue from which they arose
Mode of growth	Tumor grows by expansion and does not infiltrate the surrounding tissues; usually encapsulated	Grows at the periphery and sends out processes that infiltrate and destroy the surrounding tissues
Rate of growth	Rate of growth is usually slow	Rate of growth is variable and depends on level of differentiation; the more anaplastic the tumor, the more rapid the rate of growth
Metastasis	Does not spread by metastasis	Gains access to the blood and lymph channels and metastasizes to other areas of the body
General effects	Is usually a localized phenomenon that does not cause generalized effects unless by its location it interferes with vital functions	Often causes generalized effects such as anemia, weakness, and weight loss
Destruction of tissue	Does not usually cause tissue damage unless its location interferes with blood flow	Often causes extensive tissue damage as the tumor outgrows its blood supply or encroaches on blood flow to the area; may also produce substances that cause cell damage
Ability to cause death	Does not usually cause death unless by its location it interferes with vital functions	Will usually cause death unless growth can be controlled

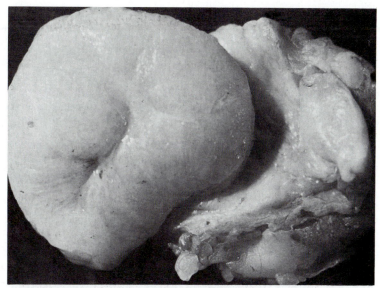

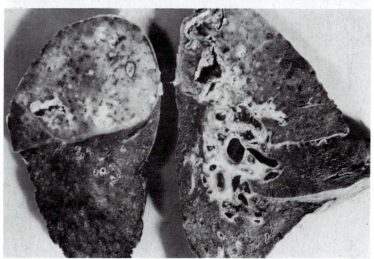

FIG. 5-4. Photograph of a benign encapsulated fibroadenoma of the breast at the top and a bronchogenic carcinoma of the lung at the bottom. Note that the fibroadenoma has sharply defined edges, whereas the bronchogenic carcinoma is diffuse and infiltrates the surrounding tissues.

tumor growing in the cranial cavity can eventually cause death by compressing brain structures. Benign tumors can also cause disturbances in the function of adjacent or distant structures by producing pressure on tissues, blood vessels, or nerves. Some benign tumors are also known for their ability to cause alterations in body function due to abnormal elaboration of hormones.

MALIGNANT NEOPLASMS

In contrast to benign tumors, malignant neoplasms tend to grow rapidly, spread widely, and kill regardless of their original location. Because of their rapid rate of growth, malignant tumors tend to compress blood vessels and outgrow their blood supply causing ischemia and tissue necrosis, to rob normal tissues of essential nutrients, and to liberate enzymes and toxins that destroy both tumor tissue and normal tissue. The destructive nature of malignant tumors is related to their lack of cell differentiation, cell characteristics, rate of growth, and ability to spread and metastasize.

There are two categories of cancer—solid tumors and hematologic cancers. Solid tumors initially are confined to a specific tissue or organ. As the growth of a solid tumor progresses, cells are shed from the original tumor mass and travel through the blood and lymph streams to produce metastasis in distant sites. Hematologic cancers involve the blood and lymph systems and hence are disseminated diseases from the beginning.

CANCER CELL CHARACTERISTICS

In tissues capable of regeneration, replacement cells usually derive from progenitor or undifferentiated stem cells. The process of cell differentiation involves changes in gene expression such that each step in the process is accomplished by expression of genes that produce more specialized cell functions. When a stem cell divides, one daughter cell retains the stem cell characteristics, and the other becomes a progenitor daughter cell. The progeny of each progenitor cell continues along the same genetic program, with the differentiating cells undergoing multiple mitotic divisions in the process of becoming a mature cell type and with each generation of cells becoming more specialized. In this way, a single stem cell can give rise to the many cells needed for normal tissue repair or blood cell responses. When the dividing cells become fully differentiated, they are no longer capable of mitosis. In the immune system, for example, appropriately stimulated B-lymphocytes become progressively more differentiated as they undergo successive mitotic divisions until they become mature plasma cells that can no longer divide but are capable of producing large amounts of antibody.

Cancer cells, as distinguished from normal cells, fail to undergo normal cell proliferation and differentiation. It is thought that cancer cells develop from mutations that occur during the differentiation process (Fig. 5-5). When the mutation occurs early in the process, the resulting tumor is poorly differentiated and highly malignant; when it occurs later in the process, more fully differentiated and less malignant tumors result.

The term *anaplasia* is used to describe the lack of cell differentiation in cancerous tissue. Undifferentiated cancer cells are altered in appearance and nuclear size and shape from the cells in the tissue where the cancer originated. As one descends the scale of differentiation, enzymes and specialized pathways of metabolism are lost and cells undergo functional simplification.[3] Highly anaplastic cancer cells, whatever their tissue origin, begin to resemble each other more than they do their tissue of origin. For example, when examined under the microscope, cancerous tissue that originated in the liver does not have the appearance of normal liver tissue. Some cancers display only slight anaplasia, and others display marked anaplasia.

Because cancer cells lack differentiation, they do not function properly and do not die on time. In some types of leukemia, for example, the lymphocytes do not follow the normal developmental process: they do not differentiate fully, they do not acquire the ability to destroy bacteria, and they do not die on schedule. Instead, these long-lived defective cells tend to crowd out normal blood cells, leaving the body less able to defend itself during infection.

Alterations in cell differentiation are also accompanied by changes in cell characteristics and cell function that distinguish cancer cells from their fully differentiated normal counterparts. These changes include alterations in contact inhibition; loss of cohesiveness and adhesion; impaired cell-to-cell communication; expression of altered tissue antigens; and elaboration of degradative enzymes that participate in invasion and metastatic spread.

Contact inhibition is the cessation of growth once a cell comes in contact with another cell. Contact inhibition usually switches off cell growth by blocking the synthesis of DNA, RNA, and protein. In wound healing, contact inhibition causes fibrous tissue growth to cease at the point where the edges of the wound come together. Cancer cells, on the other hand, tend to grow rampant without regard for other tissue. The reduced tendency of cancer cells to stick together (*cohesiveness* and *adhesiveness*) permits shedding of the tumor's surface cells; these cells appear in the surrounding body fluids or secretions and can often be detected using the Papanicolaou (Pap) test. Impaired *cell-to-cell* communication may interfere with formation of intercellular connections and responsiveness to membrane-derived signals.

Tissue antigens are coded by the genes of a cell. Many transformed cancer cells revert to earlier stages of gene expression and produce antigens that are immunologically distinct from the antigens that are

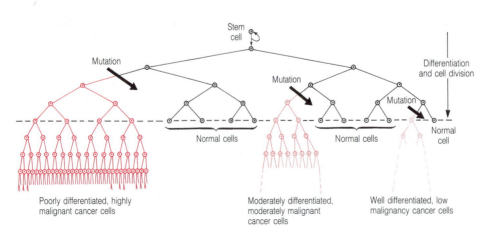

FIG. 5-5. Mutation of a cancer cell line. (Prescott, D. M., & Flexer, A. S. [1986]. *Cancer, the misguided cell.* Sunderland, MA: Sinauer Associates.)

expressed by cells of the well-differentiated tissue from which the cancer originated. Some cancers elaborate fetal antigens that are not produced by comparable cells in the adult. As is discussed later, tumor antigens may be used clinically as markers indicating the presence or progressive growth of a cancer.

Most cancers elaborate enzymes (proteases and glycosidases) that break down proteins and contribute to the invasiveness of the tumor. The production of *degradative enzymes* such as fibrinolysins contributes to the breakdown of the intercellular matrix and promotes cancer's invasive and metastatic properties. Cancers of nonendocrine tissues may assume hormone synthesis to produce so-called *ectopic hormones* (to be discussed under paraneoplastic syndrome).

INVASION AND METASTASIS

Cancer spreads by way of three pathways: (1) direct invasion and extension, (2) seeding of cancer cells within body cavities, and (3) metastatic spread through the blood or lymph pathways.

Unlike benign tumors, which grow by expansion and are usually surrounded by a capsule, cancers grow by extensive infiltration and invasion of the surrounding tissues. The word *cancer* is derived from the Latin word meaning crablike, because cancerous growth spreads by sending crablike projections into the surrounding tissues. The lack of a sharp line of demarcation separating them from the surrounding tissue makes the complete surgical removal of malignant tumors more difficult than removal of benign tumors. *Seeding* of cancer cells into body cavities occurs when a tumor erodes into these spaces. Most often the peritoneal cavity is involved, but other spaces such as the pleural cavity, pericardial cavity, and joint spaces may be involved. Seeding into the peritoneal cavity is particularly common with ovarian cancers.

The term *metastasis* is used to describe the development of a secondary tumor implant distant from the primary tumor. To a great extent, metastatic tumors retain many of the characteristics of the primary tumor from which they had their origin. Because of this, it is usually possible to determine the site of the primary tumor from the cellular characteristics of the metastatic tumor.

Some tumors tend to metastasize early in their course, whereas others do not metastasize until later. Occasionally, the metastatic tumor will be far advanced before the primary tumor becomes clinically detectable. Malignant tumors of the kidney, for example, may go completely undetected and be asymptomatic even when a metastatic lesion is found in the lung.

Metastasis occurs by way of the lymph channels (lymphatic spread) and/or blood vessels (hematogenic spread). In many types of cancer, the first evidence of disseminated disease is the presence of a mass in the lymph nodes that drain the tumor area. When metastasis occurs by way of the lymphatic channels, the tumor cells lodge first in the regional lymph nodes that receive drainage from the tumor site. Once in the lymph node, the cells may die because of the lack of a proper environment, grow into a discernible mass, or remain dormant for unknown reasons. All lymphatics empty into the venous system; the cancer cells that survive and grow eventually break loose and gain access to the venous system.

With hematogenic spread, the blood-borne cancer cells typically follow the venous flow that drains the site of the neoplasm. Before entering the general circulation, venous blood from the gastrointestinal tract, pancreas, and spleen is routed through the portal vein to the liver. The liver is therefore a common site for metastatic spread for cancers that originate in these organs. Although the site of hematologic spread is generally related to vascular drainage of the primary tumor, some tumors metastasize to distant and unrelated sites—the explanation being that cells of different tumors tend to "home" to specific target organs that can provide substances such as hormones or growth factors that are needed for their survival. For example, prostatic cancer preferentially spreads to bone, bronchiogenic cancer to the adrenal glands and brain, and neuroblastomas to the liver and bones. Even among tumors that arise in the lung and metastasize to the brain, different tumors selectively metastasize to distinct sites within the brain.[4] Certain organs such as the heart, skin, and skeletal muscle are rarely a site of metastasis despite ample blood flow capable of transporting metastatic cells to these tissues.

The selective nature of hematogenic spread indicates that metastasis is a finely orchestrated multistep process, and only a small select clone of cancer cells have the right combination of gene products to perform all of the steps needed for establishment of a secondary tumor. It has been estimated that fewer than 1 in 10,000 tumor cells that leave a primary tumor survives to start a secondary tumor.[5] To metastasize, a cancer cell must be able to: break loose from the primary tumor, invade the surrounding extracellular matrix and gain access to a blood vessel, survive its passage in the bloodstream, emerge from the bloodstream at a favorable location, and invade the surrounding tissue and begin to grow (Fig. 5-6). There is considerable evidence suggesting that cancer cells capable of metastasis secrete enzymes that break down the surrounding extracellular matrix, al-

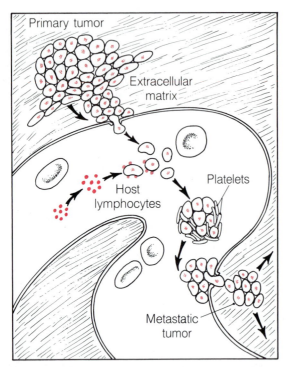

FIG. 5-6. Mechanism of hematogenic metastasis. (Adapted from Kumar, V., et al. [1992]. *Basic pathology* [6th ed., p. 196]. Philadelphia: W.B. Saunders)

lowing them to move through the degraded matrix and gain access to a blood vessel. Once in the circulation, the tumor cells are vulnerable to destruction by host immune cells. Some tumor cells gain protection from the antitumor host cells by aggregating and adhering to circulating blood components, particularly platelets, to form emboli. Tumor cells that survive their travel in the circulation must be able to halt their passage by adhering to the vessel wall. After that, they must be able to exit the vessel, move through the extracellular matrix of the target tissue, and subsequently establish growth of a secondary tumor. Once in the target tissue, the process of tumor development depends on the establishment of blood vessels (angiogenesis) and specific growth factors that promote proliferation of the tumor cells.

The selective nature of metastasis raises the question as to whether there are tumor genes that elicit or inhibit metastasis as their major function. If such genes were found to exist, their presence could be used to predict the likelihood of cancer metastasis and provide information that could be used in designing treatment protocols. To date, no single gene marker has been associated with metastasis in cancer cells. However, there has been interest in a tumor suppressor gene (nm23). In a series of human breast cancers, the nm23 lymph levels were highest in tumors that had spread to three or fewer nodes.[3] These findings are being investigated.

TUMOR GROWTH

The rate of tissue growth in both normal and cancerous tissue depends on three factors: (1) the number of cells that are actively dividing or moving through the cell cycle, (2) the cell-cycle time, and (3) the number of cells that are being lost. One of the reasons cancerous tumors often seem to grow so rapidly relates to the size of the cell pool that is actively engaged in cycling. It has been shown that the cell-cycle time of cancerous tissue cells is not necessarily shorter than that of normal cells; rather, cancer cells do not die on schedule. In addition, the growth factors that allow cells to enter G_0 when they are not needed for cell replacement is lacking; therefore, a greater percentage of cells are actively engaged in cycling than occurs in normal tissue.

The ratio of dividing cells to resting cells in a tissue mass is called the *growth factor*. The *doubling time* is the length of time it takes for the total mass of cells in a tumor to double. As the growth factor increases, the doubling time decreases. When normal tissues reach their adult size, an equilibrium between cell birth and cell death is reached. Cancer cells, however, continue to divide and multiply until limitations in blood supply and nutrients retard their growth. As this happens, the doubling time for cancer cells decreases.

Experimentally, it is possible to measure the cell-cycle time and the percentage of cells that are cycling during a given period and then to estimate the doubling time. From this information, it is possible to estimate the rate of cell increase per hour for the different types of tumors. Knowledge of cell-cycle time and the rate of cell increase is used in planning cancer therapy.

A tumor is generally undetectable until it has doubled 30 times and contains more than a billion (10^9) cells. At this point, it is about 1 cm in size (Fig. 5-7). After 35 doublings, the mass contains more than a trillion (10^{12}) cells, which is sufficient to kill the host.

Cancer in situ is a localized preinvasive lesion. Depending on its location, this type of lesion can usually be removed surgically or treated so that the chances of recurrence are small. For example, cancer in situ of the cervix is essentially 100% curable.

GENERAL EFFECTS

There is probably not a single body function left unaffected by the presence of cancer (Table 5-3). Because tumor cells replace normal functioning parenchymal tissue, the initial manifestations of cancer usually reflect the primary site of involvement.

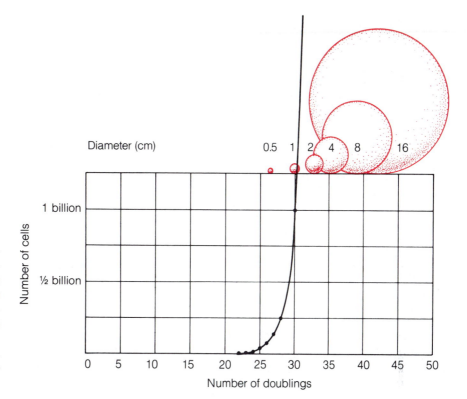

FIG. 5-7. Growth curve of a hypothetical tumor on arithmetic coordinates. Note the number of doubling times before the tumor reaches an appreciable size. (Adapted from Collins, V. P., et al. [1956]. Observations of growth rates of human tumors. *American Journal of Roentgenology, Radiation Therapy, and Nuclear Medicine, 76,* 988)

TABLE 5-3. GENERAL EFFECTS ON BODY FUNCTION ASSOCIATED WITH CANCER GROWTH

OVERALL EFFECT	RELATED TUMOR ACTION
Altered function of the involved tissue	Destruction and replacement of parenchymal tissue by neoplastic growth
Bleeding and hemorrhage	Compression of blood vessels, with ischemia and necrosis of tissue; or tumor may outgrow its blood supply
Ulceration, necrosis, and infection of tumor area	Ischemia associated with rapid growth, with subsequent bacterial invasion
Obstruction of hollow viscera or communication pathways	Expansive growth of tumor with compression and invasion of tissues
Effusion in serous cavities	Impaired lymph flow from the serous cavity or erosion of tumor into the cavity
Increased risk of vascular thrombosis	Abnormal production of coagulation factors by the tumor, obstruction of venous channels, and immobility
Anemia	Bleeding and depression of red blood cell production
Bone destruction	Metastatic invasion of bony structures
Hypercalcemia	Destruction of bone due to metastasis or production by the tumor of parathyroid-like hormone
Pain	Liberation of pain mediators by the tumor, compression, or ischemia of structures
Cachexia, weakness, wasting of tissues	Catabolic effect of the tumor on body metabolism along with selective trapping of nutrients by rapidly growing tumor cells
Inappropriate hormone production (*e.g.,* ADH or ACTH secretion by cancers such as bronchogenic carcinoma)	Production by the tumor of hormones or hormone-like substances that are not regulated by normal feedback mechanisms

For example, cancer of the lung initially produces impairment of respiratory function; as the tumor grows and metastasizes, other body structures become affected.

Cancer disrupts tissue integrity. As cancers grow, they compress and erode blood vessels, causing ulceration and necrosis along with frank bleeding and sometimes hemorrhage. One of the early warning signals of colorectal cancer is blood in the stool. Cancer cells may also produce enzymes and metabolic toxins that are destructive to the surrounding tissues. Usually, tissue damaged by cancerous growth does not heal normally. Instead, the damaged area persists and often continues to grow; hence, a sore that does not heal is a second warning signal of cancer. Furthermore, cancer has no regard for normal anatomic boundaries—as it grows, it invades and compresses adjacent structures. Abdominal cancer, for example, often compresses the viscera and causes bowel obstruction. Cancer may obstruct lymph flow and penetrate serous cavities, causing pleural effusion and ascites. In its late stages, cancer often causes pain (see Chapter 48). In fact, pain is probably one of the most dreaded aspects of cancer. Pain management is one of the major treatment concerns for persons with incurable cancers.

Abnormalities in a person's energy, carbohydrate, lipid, and protein regulation are common manifestations during progressive tumor growth. Many cancers are associated with weight loss and wasting of body fat and lean protein, a condition called *cancer cachexia*. Although anorexia, reduced food intake, and abnormalities of taste are common in people with cancer and are often accentuated by treatment methods, the extent of weight loss and protein wasting cannot be explained in terms of diminished food intake alone. It has been suggested that a cytokine (hormonelike protein produced by inflammatory cells; see Chapter 13) called *tissue necrosis factor* (*TNF*) contributes to the tissue wasting that occurs in people with cancer.[19, 20] Tissue necrosis factor, also called *cachectin*, is produced by macrophages in response to tumor growth or tissue destruction; it has been credited with suppressing the enzymes needed for fat storage; hence, the loss of fat tissue. The actions of TNF range from eliciting fever and other inflammatory responses to mediating endotoxic shock secondary to trauma, burns, and sepsis. The role of TNF and its full impact on cancer cachexia are uncertain. It has been suggested by some that the hormone may be an endogenous antineoplastic agent.[20]

In addition to signs and symptoms at the sites of primary and metastatic disease, cancer can produce manifestations in sites that are not directly affected by the disease. Such manifestations are collectively referred to as *paraneoplastic syndromes*. Some of these manifestations are caused by the elaboration of hormones by cancer cells, and others are due to the production of circulating factors that produce nonmetastatic hematopoietic, neurologic, and dermatologic syndromes. For example, cancers may produce procoagulation factors that contribute to an increased risk of venous thrombosis. It is estimated that about 7% of people with cancer are affected by these syndromes.[21] The three most common endocrine syndromes associated with cancer are (1) the syndrome of inappropriate antidiuretic hormone (ADH) secretion (see Chapter 29), (2) Cushing's syndrome due to ectopic adrenocorticotropic hormone (ACTH) production (see Chapter 45), and (3) hypercalcemia (see Chapter 29). Hypercalcemia of malignancy does not appear to be related to parathyroid hormone but to some other circulating factor or factors. The paraneoplastic syndromes may be the earliest indication that a person has cancer; they may also signal early recurrence of the disease in previously treated people. In some people with cancer, a paraneoplastic syndrome such as hypercalcemia can be disabling and even life-threatening.

In summary, neoplasms may be either benign or malignant. Tumors are named by the addition of the suffix *-oma* to the name of the tissue type. The term *carcinoma* refers to a malignant tumor of epithelial cell origin, and the term *sarcoma* refers to a malignant tumor of mesenchymal cell origin. Benign and malignant tumors differ in terms of (1) cell characteristics, (2) manner of growth, (3) rate of growth, (4) potential for metastasis, (5) ability to produce generalized effects, (6) tendency to cause tissue destruction, and (7) capacity to cause death. The growth of a benign tumor is restricted to the site of origin, and the tumor will not usually cause death unless it interferes with vital functions. Cancer or malignant neoplasms, on the other hand, grow wildly and without organization, spread to distant parts of the body, and cause death unless checked.

There are two types of cancer—solid tumors and hematologic tumors. Solid tumors are initially confined to a specific organ or tissue, whereas hematologic cancers are disseminated from the onset. Cancer is a disorder of cell proliferation and differentiation. Cancer cells are often poorly differentiated in comparison to normal cells; they display abnormal membrane characteristics, have abnormal antigens, produce abnormal biochemical products, and have abnormal karyotypes. All cancers result from nonlethal genetic changes that transform a normal cell into a cancer cell. The spread of cancer occurs via three pathways: (1) direct invasion and extension, (2) seeding of cancer cells within body cavities, and (3) metastatic spread through the blood or lymph pathways. Only a small clone of cancer cells is capable of metastasis. In order to metastasize, a cancer cell must be able to break loose from the primary tumor, invade the surrounding extracellular matrix and gain access to a blood vessel, survive its passage in the bloodstream, emerge from the bloodstream at a favorable location, invade the surrounding tissue, and begin to grow.

■ CARCINOGENESIS AND CAUSES OF CANCER

Because cancer is not a single disease, it is reasonable to assume that it does not have a single cause. More likely, cancer occurs because of interactions between multiple risk factors or repeated exposure to a single carcinogenic (cancer-producing) agent. Among the risk factors that have been linked to cancer are heredity, chemical and environmental carcinogens, cancer-causing viruses, and immunologic defects. All cancers result from nonlethal genetic changes that transform a normal cells into cancer cells.

ONCOGENESIS

The term *oncogenesis* refers to a genetic mechanism whereby normal cells are transformed into cancer cells. Two kinds of genes control normal cell growth and replication: growth-promoting regulatory genes (proto-oncogenes) and growth-inhibiting regulatory genes (anti-oncogenes).[6,7] These genes have been implicated as principal targets of genetic damage that occurs during the development of a cancer cell. Such genetic damage may be acquired by the action of chemicals, radiation, or viruses, or it may be inherited in the germ line. Most cancers are probably multifactorial in origin, with several factors acting in concert or sequentially to produce the multiple genetic abnormalities that are characteristic of cancer cells.

Oncogenes are mutations of normal growth-regulating genes. The oncogene theory dates back to 1911 when Francis Peyton Rous discovered a virus that causes sarcomas in chickens. Over the years, various oncogenic viruses have been identified that can produce cancerous transformations in laboratory cell cultures and animals. As the research with virus-induced cell transformation progressed, it was discovered that normal cells contain DNA sequences similar to the viral genes that cause cancerous transformation of laboratory cells. These DNA sequences, called *proto-oncogenes*, have essential roles in regulating the growth and proliferation of normal cells. Proto-oncogene products may act as growth factors, as receptors for growth factors, or as second messengers that transmit growth factor signals. The involvement of these genes in the cancer process is due to a somatic mutation that takes place in a specific target tissue, converting its proto-oncogenes into oncogenes.

A more recent discovery identified a different class of genes, the *cancer suppressor* or *anti-oncogenic genes*. These tumor-suppressing genes seem to be involved in controlling cellular growth. When this type of gene is inactivated, a block to proliferation is removed and the cells begin a program of unregulated growth. The products of these genes may act at many of the same sites as the growth-promoting proto-oncogenes. It has been suggested that cells have companion growth-suppressing anti-oncogenes that are paired with the growth-promoting proto-oncogenes. Of particular interest is the p53 gene located on the short arm of chromosome 17.[8] This gene codes for a protein that is pivotal in growth regulation apparently functioning as a suppressor of tumor growth.

Normally, proto-oncogenes are specifically turned on for only a brief period in the cell cycle. When their oncogenes or their products are altered by mutation, they may operate continuously, causing unregulated cell growth. Significantly, it appears that the acquisition of a single oncogene is not sufficient to convert cells into full-blown tumor cells. Instead, cancerous transformation appears to require the activation of many independently mutated genes.

HEREDITY

Certain types of cancers seem to run in families. Breast cancer, for example, occurs more frequently in women whose grandmothers, mothers, aunts, and sisters also have had a cancerous disease. The genetic predisposition for development of cancer has been documented for a number of cancerous and precancerous lesions that follow mendelian inheritance patterns. Cancer is found in approximately 10% of people having one affected first-degree relative, in approximately 15% of people having two affected family members, and in 30% of people having three affected family members.[9]

Among the inherited forms of cancer are retinoblastoma and multiple polyposis of the colon. In about 40% of cases, retinoblastoma is inherited as an autosomal dominant trait; the remaining cases are nonhereditary. The penetrance of the genetic trait is high; in carriers of the dominant retinoblastoma gene, the penetrance for this gene is 95% for at least one tumor, and the affected person may be unilaterally or bilaterally affected.[10] Familial polyposis of the colon also follows an autosomal dominant inheritance pattern. People who inherit the gene develop polypoid adenomas of the colon, and almost all are fated to develop cancer by age 50.[3] Retinoblastoma and heritable forms of cancer are discussed further in the section of the chapter on childhood cancers.

CARCINOGENS

A carcinogen is an agent capable of causing cancer. The role of environmental agents in causation of cancer was first noted in 1775 by Sir Percivall Pott, who related the high incidence of scrotal cancer in chimneysweeps to their exposure to coal soot. In 1915, Yamagiwa and Ichikawa conducted the first experiments in which a chemical agent was used to produce cancer. These investigators found that a cancerous growth developed when they painted a rabbit's ear with coal tar. Coal tar has since been found to contain potent polycyclic aromatic hydrocarbons. Since then, many carcinogenic agents have been identified. In fact, it has been estimated that 80% to 85% of human cancers are associated with exposure to environmental or chemical agents (Chart 5-1).[11]

Chemical Carcinogens. Literally hundreds of chemical carcinogens exist; some have been found to cause cancers in animals and others are known to cause cancers in humans. These agents include both natural (*e.g.*, aflatoxin B_1) and artificial products (*e.g.*, vinyl chloride). The transformation of normal cells to cancer cells by carcinogenic agents is a multistep process that can be divided into two stages: initiation and promotion.[11] *Initiation* results from exposure of cells to an appropriate dose of a carcinogenic agent, rendering it likely to give rise to a tumor. It is not, however, sufficient for tumor formation. Initiation is rapid and irreversible and is thought to produce permanent changes in the DNA of a target cell. Because the effects of initiating agents are irreversible, multiple divided doses may achieve the same effect as comparable doses delivered at the same time. *Promotion* involves the induction of cancer in initiated cells. Cells that have been irreversibly initiated may be promoted even after long latency periods. The latency period varies with the type of agent, the dosage, and the characteristics of the target cells. Chemical carcinogens are called *complete carcinogens* because they can both initiate and promote neoplastic transformation.

Carcinogenic agents can be divided into two categories: (1) direct-reacting agents, which do not require activation in the body to become carcinogenic, and (2) indirect-reacting agents, called *procarcinogens*, which become active only after metabolic conversion.[3] The carcinogenicity of some chemicals is augmented by agents that by themselves have little or no cancer-causing ability. These agents are called *promoters*. It is believed that promoting agents exert their effect by changing the expression of genetic material within a cell, increasing DNA synthesis, enhancing gene amplification (number of gene copies that are made), and altering intercellular communication. Some hormones, for example, may alter the endocrine balance and thus act as promoters. Several carcinogenic agents may act together or with other types of carcinogenic influences such as viruses or radiation to produce cancer.[3]

Both direct- and indirect-acting agents form highly reactive species (electrophiles and free radicals) that bind with the nucleophilic residues on DNA, RNA, or cellular proteins. The action of these reactive species tends to cause cell mutation or alteration in synthesis of cell enzymes and structural proteins in a manner that alters cell replication and interferes with cell regulatory controls. Antioxidants such as vitamins A, C, and E inhibit the formation of free radicals and may thus inhibit the damaging effects of carcinogens on DNA.

The direct-acting agents are, in general, weak carcinogens and, depending on the dose and duration of exposure, may cause cancer.[3] Among these direct-acting agents are the alkylating drugs used in the treatment of cancer (to be discussed).

The indirect-acting procarcinogens require metabolic conversion to active carcinogens. Among the most potent of the procarcinogens are the polycyclic hydrocarbons. The polycyclic hydrocarbons are of particular interest because they are produced in the combustion of tobacco and are present in cigarette smoke. They are also produced from animal fat in the process of broiling meats and are present in smoked meats and fish. Another class of procarcinogens are the aromatic amines and azo dyes. The carcinogenicity of these agents is exerted mainly in the liver where the metabolic process that activates the procarcinogen occurs. An exception is beta-naphthylamine, which is broken down in the urine and causes bladder cancer. It has been responsible for a 50-fold increase in bladder cancer in workers exposed to aniline dye and rubber industries.[3] Some of the azo dyes have been developed into food colors, which are federally regulated in the United States. Aflatoxin B_1 is a naturally occurring carcinogen produced by some strains of *Aspergillus*, a mold that grows in improperly stored grains and nuts. It may be found in peanuts and peanut butter. There is a high correlation between dietary levels of this food contaminant and liver cancer in some parts of Africa and the Far East. Hepatitis B is also endemic in these areas, and it has been suggested it may contribute to carcinogenic effects of aflatoxin B_1.[3]

Many cancers are associated with lifestyle risk factors such as smoking, dietary factors, and alcohol consumption. Cigarette smoke contains both procarcinogens and promoters. It is directly associated with lung cancer and has been linked with cancers of the pancreas, kidney, and bladder. Chewing tobacco or tobacco products increases the risk of cancers of the oral cavity and esophagus.[12] It has been estimated that 30% of current cancer deaths in the United States are related to tobacco. Not only is the smoker at risk, but others sharing the smoker's environment may also be at risk.

There is strong evidence that certain elements in the diet contribute to cancer risk. For example, benzopyrene may be produced when meat and fish are charcoal broiled or smoked or when any food is fried in fat that has been reused repeatedly. Nitrosamines, which are powerful carcinogens, may be formed from nitrites derived from nitrates that have been ingested in vegetables and foods to which nitrates have been added as a preservative. Formation of these nitrosamines may be inhibited by the presence of antioxidants such as vitamin C in the stomach. Cancer of the colon has been associated with the type and amount of fat consumed in the diet. A high-fat diet leads to increased flow of primary bile acids. The primary bile acids are converted to secondary bile acids in the presence of anaerobic bacteria in the colon. The secondary bile acids, lithocholic acid and deoxycholic acid, are promoters.[11] Reducing the level of total fat in the diet reduces bile acid levels. The addition of fiber to the diet dilutes the concentration of bile acids and reduces the promoting potential.

Alcohol modifies the metabolism of carcinogens in the liver and esophagus.[11] It is also believed to influence the transport of carcinogens, increasing the contact between an externally induced carcinogen and the stem cells that line the upper oral cavity and esophagus. The carcinogenic effect of cigarette smoke can be enhanced by concomitant consumption of alcohol; people who both smoke and drink considerable amounts of alcohol are at increased risk for development of cancer of the oral cavity and esophagus.

The effects of carcinogenic agents are usually dose dependent—the larger the dose or the longer the duration of exposure, the greater the risk that cancer will develop. Some chemical carcinogens may act in concert with other carcinogenic influences such as viruses or radiation to induce neoplasia. There is usually a time delay ranging from 5 to 30 years from the time of chemical carcinogen exposure to the development of overt cancer. This is unfortunate, because many people may have been exposed to the agent and its carcinogenic effects before the association is recognized. This occurred, for example, with the use of diethylstilbestrol, which was widely used in the United States from the mid 1940s to 1970 to prevent miscarriages. But it was not until the late 1960s that many cases of vaginal adenosis and adenocarcinoma in young women were found to be a result of their exposure *in utero* to diethylstilbestrol.[13]

Radiation. Among the well-documented causes of cancer is radiation, including ultraviolet rays from sunlight, x-rays, radioactive chemicals, and other forms of radiation. As with other carcinogens, the effects of radiation are usually additive, and there is usually a long delay between the time of exposure and the time that cancer can be detected. This is true of skin cancer, which is caused by overexposure to the sun and is many years in the making. Skin cancer is an occupational hazard of farmers and sailors, particularly those who work in the southwest United States. Equally hazardous is the practice of sunbathing to achieve a suntan.

Another example of the ultimate consequences of radiation exposure was the therapeutic radiation of the head and neck—particularly in infants and small children to reduce the tonsils or thymus—in which there was a time lag as long as 35 years before thyroid cancer was detected.[14] Even more dramatic are the long-term effects of radiation on the survivors of the atomic blasts in Hiroshima and Nagasaki: between 1950 and 1970, the death rate from leukemia alone in the most heavily exposed population groups in Hiroshima was 147 per 100,000, or 30 times the expected rate.[15]

ONCOGENIC VIRUSES

An oncogenic virus is a virus that can induce cancer. Viruses, which are small particles containing genetic (DNA or RNA) material, enter a host cell and become incorporated into its chromosomal DNA or take control of the cell's machinery for the purpose of producing viral proteins. A large number of DNA and RNA (retroviruses) viruses have been shown to be oncogenic in animals. However, only a few viruses have been linked to cancer in humans.[3,11] Among the recognized oncogenic viruses in humans is the human T cell leukemia virus-1, human papilloma virus, Epstein-Barr virus, and hepatitis B virus. Herpes simplex II has been also been associated with cervical cancer, but the evidence supporting its role as a carcinogenic influence is less clear.

Although there are a number of retroviruses (RNA viruses) that cause cancer in animals, there is only one known human retrovirus that is associated with cancer: the *human T cell leukemia virus-1 (HTLV-1)*. HTLV-1 is associated with a form of T cell leukemia/lymphoma that is endemic in certain parts of Japan, some areas of the Caribbean, Africa, and is found sporadically elsewhere including the United States. Like the human immunodeficiency virus (HIV), HTLV-1 is attracted to the CD4+ T cells and hence this subset of T cells is the major target for cancerous transformation. The virus requires transmission of infected T cells by way of sexual intercourse, infected blood, or breast milk. Leukemia develops in about 1% of infected people and has a long latency period of 20 to 30 years.[3] A second type of HTLV virus, HTLV-2, has been isolated from the T-lymphocyte variety of hairy cell leukemia. However, this type of leukemia is mainly a disease of B-lymphocytes with relatively few cases of the T-lymphocyte type.

Three DNA viruses have been implicated in human cancers: the human papilloma virus, Epstein-Barr virus, and the hepatitis B virus. The transforming DNA viruses form stable associations with the human genome using genes that allow them to complete their replication cycle and be expressed in transformed cells. There is strong evidence to suggest that the DNA viruses act in concert with other factors to cause cancer.

There are over 50 genetically different types of *human papilloma viruses (HPV)*. Some types (types 1, 2, 4, 7) have been shown to cause benign squamous papillomas (warts). HPVs have also been implicated in squamous cell carcinoma of the cervix and anogenital region. HPV type 16 and 18 have been found in 75% to 100% of squamous cell carcinomas of the cervix and presumed precursors (severe cervical dysplasia and carcinoma in situ).

Epstein-Barr virus (EBV) has been implicated in the pathogenesis of two human cancers: Burkitt's lymphoma and nasopharyngeal cancer. Burkitt's lymphoma, a tumor of B-lymphocytes, is endemic in parts of Africa and sporadically elsewhere. In people with normal immune function, the EBV-driven B-cell proliferation is readily controlled and the person becomes asymptomatic or develops a self-limited episode of infectious mononucleosis (see Chapter 16). In regions of the world where Burkitt's lymphoma is endemic, concurrent malaria or other infections cause impaired immune function, allowing sustained B-lymphocyte proliferation. Nasopharyngeal cancer is endemic in southern China, and EBV virus is found in all tumors.

Although epidemiologic data support a relationship between the *hepatitis B virus (HBV)* and cancer of liver, the role of the tumor virus in tumor production is uncertain. The incidence of cancer of the liver is high in southeastern Africa and Asia where the incidence of HBV is endemic.

IMMUNOLOGIC DEFECTS

There is growing evidence for the immune system's participation in resistance against the progression and spread of cancer. The central concept, known as the *immune surveillance hypothesis* which was first proposed by Paul Ehrlich in 1909, postulates that the immune system plays a central role in resistance against the development of tumors.[16] In addition to cancer–host interactions as a mechanism of cancer development, immunologic mechanisms provide a means for the detection, classification, and prognostic evaluation of cancers, and as a potential method of treatment. *Immunotherapy* (discussed later in this chapter) is a cancer treatment modality designed to heighten the patient's general immune responses so as to increase tumor destruction.

It has been suggested that the development of cancer might be associated with impairment or decline in the surveillance capacity of the immune system. For example, increases in cancer incidence have been observed in people with immunodeficiency diseases and in people with organ transplants who are receiving immunosuppressant drugs. The incidence of cancer is also increased in the elderly, in whom there is a known decrease in immune activity. The association of Kaposi's sarcoma with AIDS further emphasizes the role of the immune system in preventing malignant cell proliferation.

It has been shown that most tumor cells have molecular configurations that can be specifically recognized by immune T cells or by antibodies and hence are termed *tumor antigens*.[17] The most relevant tumor antigens fall into two categories: (1) unique tumor-specific antigens found only on tumor cells and (2) tumor-associated antigens found on tumor cells and also on normal cells. Quantitative and qualitative differences permit the use of these tumor-associated antigens to distinguish cancer cells from normal cells.

Virtually all of the components of immune system have the potential for eradicating cancer cells, including T-lymphocytes, B-lymphocytes and antibodies, macrophages, and natural killer (NK) cells (see Chapter 13). The T-cell response is undoubtedly one of the most important host responses for control of growth of antigenic tumor cells; it is responsible for both direct killing of tumor cells and for activation of other components of the immune system. The T-cell immunity to cancer cells reflects the function of two subsets of T cells: the CD4 helper T cells and CD8 cytotoxic T cells. Figure 5-8 illustrates the function of T-cell immunity in the lysis of cancer cells. The finding of tumor-reactive antibodies in the serum of people with cancer supports the role of the B cell as a member of the immune surveillance team. Antibodies can destroy cancer cells through complement-mediated mechanisms or through antibody-dependent cellular cytotoxicity in which the antibody binds the cancer cell to another effector cell such as the NK cell that does the actual killing of the cancer cell. NK cells do not require antigen recognition and can lyse a wide variety of target cells. The cytotoxic activity of NK cells can be augmented by the lymphokines, interleukin 2 (IL-2), and interferon, and, thus, NK activity can be amplified by immune T-cell responses.[18] Macrophages are important in tumor immunity as antigen-presenting cells to initiate the immune response and as potential effector cells to participate in tumor cell lysis.

In summary, because cancer is not a single disease, it is reasonable to assume that it does not have a single cause. Multiple factors probably interact at the genetic level to transform normal cells into cancer cells. This transformation process is called oncogenesis. Two kinds of genes control normal cell growth and replication: growth-promoting regulatory genes (proto-oncogenes) and growth-inhibiting regulatory genes (anti-oncogenes). These genes are implicated as principal targets of genetic damage that occurs during the development of a cancer cell. Such genetic damage may be acquired by the action of chemicals (chemical carcinogens), radiation, or viruses or it may be inherited in the cell line.

■ DIAGNOSIS AND TREATMENT

DIAGNOSTIC METHODS

The methods used in the diagnosis and staging of cancer are determined largely by the location and type of cancer suspected. A number of diagnostic procedures are used in diagnosis of cancer, including x-ray studies; endoscopic examinations; urine and stool tests; blood tests for tumor markers; bone marrow aspirations; ultrasound imaging; magnetic resonance imaging (MRI); and computed tomography (CT scan). Three diagnostic methods are discussed in this chapter: the Pap smear, tissue biopsy, and tumor markers.

THE PAP SMEAR

The Pap smear is an example of the type of test called *exfoliative cytology*. It consists of microscopic examination of a properly prepared slide by a cytotechnologist or pathologist for the purpose of detecting the presence of abnormal cells. The usefulness of exfoliative cytology relies on the fact that the cancer cells lack the cohesive properties and intercellular junctions that are characteristic of normal tissue; without these characteristics, cancer cells tend to exfoliate and become mixed with secretions surrounding the tumor growth. The American Cancer Society recommends that the test be done annually to detect cervical cancer in women who are or have been sexually active and who have reached age 18. After three consecutive normal findings, the test may be performed less frequently at the discretion of the physician.[1] Exfoliative cytology can also be performed on other body secretions, including nipple drainage, pleural or peritoneal fluid, gastric washings, and others.

BIOPSY

A tissue biopsy is the removal of a tissue specimen for microscopic study. It can be obtained by needle aspiration (needle biopsy) or by endoscopic methods, such as bronchoscopy or cystoscopy, which involve the passage of a scope through an orifice and into the involved structure. In some instances a surgical incision is made. If the tumor is small, the entire tumor may be removed; if the tumor is too large to be removed, a specimen may be excised for examination. Tissue diagnosis is of critical importance in designing the treatment plan should cancer cells be found.

TUMOR MARKERS

Tumor markers are substances that are produced by tumor cells or substances released from normal cells in response to the presence of tumor. Some substances such as hormones and enzymes are produced normally by the tissue involved but become overexpressed as a result of cancer. Other tumor markers, such as oncofetal proteins, are produced during fetal development and are induced to reappear later in life as a result of benign and malignant neoplasms. Tumor markers are used for screening, for diagnosis, for establishing prognosis, for monitoring treatment, and for detecting relapse.

As diagnostic tools, tumor markers have limitations. The value of a marker depends on its sensitivity, specificity, proportionality, and feasibility.[22] Sensitivity implies that the marker is apparent early in the development of the tumor and has few false

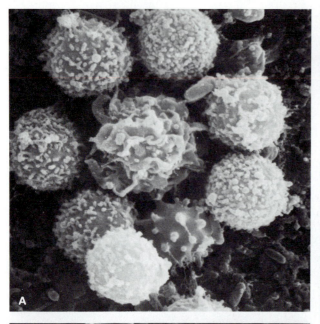

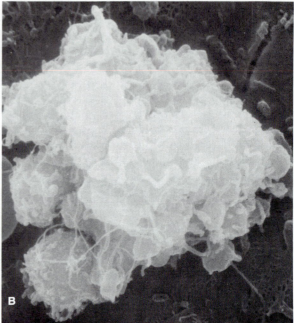

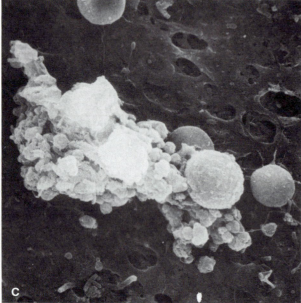

FIG. 5-8. A scanning electron micrograph showing the combination of a cancer cell and lymphocytes removed from the same patient and studied in the laboratory. (**A**) The lymphocytes surround the cancer cell (60 min). (**B**) Lymphocytes attack the cancer cell (150 min). (**C**) The integrity of the cancer cell has been destroyed (240 min). (Courtesy of Kenneth Siegesmund, Ph.D., and Burton A. Waisbren, Sr., M.D., Anatomy Department, The Medical College of Wisconsin)

negatives. Specificity indicates that the marker is specific for cancer and is not elevated in other disease conditions (*e.g.*, has few false positives). Proportionality means that the level of marker accurately reflects the growth of the tumor. Feasibility implies that the methods are readily available, easy to use, and that the cost is not prohibitive. Nearly all markers can be elevated in benign conditions, and most are not elevated in the early stages of malignancy. Hence, tumor markers have limited value as screening tests. Extremely elevated levels of a tumor marker can indicate a poor prognosis or need for more aggressive treatment. Perhaps the greatest value of tumor markers is in monitoring therapy in people with widespread cancer. Nearly all markers show an asso-

ciation with the clinical course of the disease. The levels of nearly all markers decline with successful treatment and increase with recurrence of the tumor. The markers that have been most useful in practice have been human chorionic gonadotropin (HCG), CA-125, prostate-specific antigen (PSA), prostatic acid phosphatase (PAP), α-fetoprotein (AFP), and carcinoembryonic antigen (CEA).

HCG is a hormone normally produced by the placenta. It is used as a marker for diagnosing, prescribing treatment, and following the disease course in people with high-risk gestational trophoblastic tumors. PSA and PAP are used as markers in prostatic cancer, and CA-125 is used as a marker in ovarian cancer.

Some cancers express fetal proteins. The two that have proven the most useful as tumor markers are AFP and CEA. AFP is synthesized by the fetal liver, yolk sac, and gastrointestinal tract and is the major serum protein in the fetus. Elevated levels are encountered in people with primary liver cancers and have also been observed in some testicular, ovarian, pancreatic, and stomach cancers. CEA is normally produced by embryonic tissue in the gut, pancreas, and liver and is elaborated by a number of different cancers. Dependent on the serum level adopted for significant elevation, CEA is elevated in approximately 60% to 90% of colorectal carcinomas, 50% to 80% of pancreatic cancers, and 25% to 50% of gastric and breast tumors.[3] As with most other tumor markers, elevated levels of both CEA and AFP are found in other noncancerous conditions, and elevated levels of both depend on tumor size so that neither is useful as an early test for cancer.

STAGING AND GRADING OF TUMORS

There are two basic methods for classifying cancers: (1) grading according to the histologic or cellular characteristics of the tumor and (2) staging according to the clinical spread of the disease. Both methods are used to prognosticate the course of the disease and to aid in selecting an appropriate treatment or management plan. Grading of tumors involves the microscopic examination of cancer cells to determine their level of differentiation and the number of mitoses. Cancers are classified as grades I, II, III, and IV with increasing anaplasia. Staging of cancers uses methods to determine the progress and spread of the disease. It may use surgery to determine tumor size and lymph node involvement.

The clinical staging of cancer is intended to provide a means by which information related to the progress of the disease, the methods and success of treatment modalities, and the prognosis can be communicated to others. The TNM system, which has evolved from the work of the International Union Against Cancer (IUAC) and the American Joint Committee on Cancer Staging and End Stage Reporting (AJCCS), is used by many cancer facilities. This system, which is briefly described in Chart 5-2, quantifies the disease into stages, using three tumor components: (1) *T* stands for the extent of the primary tumor, (2) *N* refers to the involvement of the regional lymph nodes, and (3) *M* describes the extent of the metastatic involvement. The time of staging is indicated as cTNM, clinical-diagnostic staging; pTNM, postsurgical resection–pathologic staging; sTNM, surgical-evaluative staging; rTNM, retreatment staging; and aTNM, autopsy staging.[23]

CHART 5-2: TNM CLASSIFICATION SYSTEM

T*Subclasses

Tx—tumor cannot be adequately assessed
T0—no evidence of primary tumor
TIS—carcinoma *in situ*
T1, T2, T3, T—progressive increase in tumor size or involvement

N† Subclasses

Nx—regional lymph nodes cannot be assessed clinically
N0—no evidence of regional node metastasis
N1, N2, N3—increasing involvement of regional lymph nodes

M‡ Subclasses

Mx—not assessed
M0—no distant metastasis
M1—distant metastasis present, specify site(s)

*T = Primary tumor.
†N = Regional lymph nodes.
‡M = Distant metastasis.
[Developed from Beahrs, O. H., & Myers, M. H. [eds.]. [1988]. *Manual for staging of cancer* [3rd ed., p. 7]. Philadelphia: J.B. Lippincott.]

CANCER TREATMENT

The goals of treatment methods fall into three categories: *curative*, *palliative*, and *adjunctive*. The most common modalities are surgery, radiation, chemotherapy, and endocrine therapy. Biotherapy has been added to the list of treatment modalities. Interferon and hyperthermia are being used on an experimental basis. A practice in the treatment of cancer is the use of a carefully planned program that combines the benefits of multiple treatment modalities and the expertise of a team of medical specialists such as a medical oncologist, surgical oncologist, and radiologist.

SURGERY

Surgery is used for diagnosis, the staging of cancer, the removal of the tumor, and palliation (relief of symptoms) when cure cannot be effected. The type of surgery to be used is determined by the extent of the disease and the structures involved. When the tumor is small, the entire lesion can often be removed; when the tumor is large or involves vital tissues, surgical removal may be impossible.

Surgical techniques have been expanded to include electrosurgery, cryosurgery, chemosurgery, and laser surgery. *Electrosurgery* uses the cutting and coagulating effects of high-frequency current applied by needle, blade, or electrodes. Once considered a palliative type of procedure, it is now being used as an alternative treatment for certain cancers of the skin, oral cavity, and rectum. *Cryosurgery* involves the instillation of liquid nitrogen into the tumor through a probe. It is used in treating cancers of the oral cavity, brain, and prostate. *Chemosurgery* is used in skin cancers. It involves the use of a corrosive paste in combination with multiple frozen sections to ensure complete removal of the tumor. *Laser surgery* uses a laser beam to resect a tumor. It has been used effectively in retinal and vocal cord surgery.

Cooperative efforts between cancer centers throughout the world have helped to standardize and improve surgical procedures, determine which cancers benefit from surgical intervention, and establish in what order surgical and other treatment modalities should be used. Increased emphasis has also been placed on the development of surgical techniques, such as limb salvage surgery, which is used in the treatment of osteogenic sarcoma to preserve functional abilities while permitting complete removal of the tumor.

RADIATION THERAPY

Over 50% of patients with cancer receive radiation therapy, either alone or in combination with other forms of treatment. Radiation can be used singly as the primary method of treatment, as presurgical or postsurgical therapy, with chemotherapy, or with chemotherapy and surgery. It can also be used as a palliative treatment to reduce symptoms in people with advanced cancers. Radiation is often chosen as the sole treatment modality with the curative intent in Hodgkin's disease, skin cancers, oral cancers of the larynx (permitting cure with loss of voice), prostate cancers, and cancers of the vagina and uterine cervix.

Ionizing radiation was discovered by Marie and Pierre Curie and Wilhelm Conrad Roentgen just before the turn of the century. Development of the first cathode ray tube followed, during the 1920s, along with quantitative methods for measuring radiation dosage. The first use of radium to treat cancer occurred 1 to 2 years after development of the cathode ray tube. During this same period, Claude Regaud (Foundation Curie in Paris) was able to show that fractionated—small, sublethal—doses of radiation could permanently halt spermatogenesis, whereas no single lethal dose could do so without causing severe damage to the surrounding tissues. This observation linked external radiation to the treatment of cancer. Another advance in radiation therapy followed the atomic bomb, with the development of radioactive cobalt. Since then, advances in technology have resulted in the development of sophisti-

cated equipment that produces high-voltage x-ray and electron beams capable of delivering a therapeutic dose of radiation to the tumor with limited morbidity to surrounding tissues.

Mechanisms of Action. Ionizing radiation affects cells by direct ionization of molecules. The most common effect of x-rays and gamma rays is indirect ionization, which is produced when the primary radiation interacts with free or loosely bonded electrons, which subsequently produce ionization or free radicals that interact with critical cell components (see Chapter 2). Radiation exerts its greatest effect during certain stages of the cell cycle, particularly during early DNA synthesis in the S or synthesis phase and in the M or mitotic phase of the cycle.[24] It can immediately kill cells, delay or halt cell cycle progression, or at dose levels commonly used in radiation therapy it can cause damage within the nucleus that results in cell death after replication. Cell damage may be sublethal, in which case the stand of DNA can repair itself if there is time before the next radiation insult.[25] Double-strand breaks in DNA are generally believed to be the primary damage that leads to radiation death in cells. The result of unrepaired DNA is that cells may continue to function until they undergo cell mitosis, at which time the genetic damage from the irradiation may result in death of the cell. The clinical significance being that the rapidly proliferating and poorly differentiated cells of a cancerous tumor are more likely to be injured by radiation therapy than are the slower proliferating cells of normal tissue. To some extent, however, radiation is injurious to all rapidly proliferating cells including those of the bone marrow and the mucosal lining of the gastrointestinal tract. In addition to its lethal effects, radiation also produces sublethal injury. Recovery from sublethal doses of radiation occurs in the interval between the first dose of radiation and subsequent doses. This is why large total doses of radiation can be tolerated when they are divided into multiple smaller fractionated doses. Normal tissue is usually able to recover from radiation damage more readily than cancerous tissue.

Radiation Sensitivity and Responsiveness. The term *radiosensitivity* describes the inherent properties of a tumor that determine its responsiveness to radiation. It varies widely among the different types of cancers. For example, lymphomas are highly radiosensitive, whereas rhabdomyosarcomas and melanomas are much less so. The radiation dose that is chosen for treatment of a particular cancer is determined by factors such as the radiosensitivity of the tumor type, size of the tumor, and, more importantly, the tolerance of the surrounding tissues. The ability to give graded, fractional doses of radiation and quantitate the number of cells surviving permits the development of a dose–response curve. With the use of fractionated doses, it is more likely that the cancer cells will be dividing and in the vulnerable period of the cell cycle. This dose also allows time for normal tissues to repair the radiation damage.

Studies are being conducted in hopes of finding ways to increase the radiosensitivity of tumors by altering their DNA in a manner that either makes it more sensitive to radiation or less able to repair radiation damage.

Radiation responsiveness describes the manner in which a radiosensitive tumor responds to irradiation. One of the major determinants of radiation responsiveness is tumor oxygenation. This is because oxygen is a rich source of free radicals that form and destroy essential cell components during irradiation. Many rapidly growing tumors outgrow their blood supply and become deprived of oxygen. The hypoxic cells of these tumors are more resistant to radiation than normal or well-oxygenated tumor cells. Therefore, methods of ensuring adequate oxygen delivery, such as adequate hemoglobin levels, are important. Agents that act as radiosensitizers are being investigated. These agents increase the production of free radicals during radiation in a manner similar to oxygen.

Administration. Ionizing radiation includes two distinct forms: electromagnetic waves and fast, high-energy moving particles. Electromagnetic radiation consists of x-rays and gamma rays. X-rays are produced by electrons hitting a target, and gamma rays are emitted from the spontaneous decay of radioactive isotopes such as cobalt and cesium. The electromagnetic radiation is energetic and extremely penetrating. Particulate radiation used in radiotherapy includes electrons, protons, pions, and heavy ions. These particles are accelerated by electrical magnetic fields in linear accelerators and cyclotrons.

A number of types of equipment and beams can be used for administering radiation therapy. Large radiotherapy centers have a selection suitable to the treatment of almost any malignancy in any part of the body.

Therapy can be delivered by either external beam radiation machines that have sources of radiation located some distance from the patient (sometimes called *teletherapy*) or by short-distance therapy (*brachytherapy*) in which a sealed radioactive source is placed close to or directly in the tumor site. Radioisotopes, with a short half-life, may be injected or given by mouth as a palliative or curative treatment for some forms of cancer.

External beam radiation machines deliver a penetrating radiation dose depending on the energy or voltage rating that is used. The higher the energy, the greater the depth of penetration. The early forms of radiation therapy used x-ray machines with energy from 100 to 250 kV. These machines delivered low-penetrance rays that exerted their maximum tumor dose within 1 to 2 cm of the skin surface. They are now used only in superficial skin lesions or tumors located near the skin surface. The newer megavoltage machines produce x-rays by allowing high-energy electrons to be accelerated by microwaves. These x-rays are much more penetrating and allow for treatment from a number of directions (cross firing). This allows for delivery of curative doses of radiation without causing extensive damage to skin or other tissues. The megavoltage rays also spare bone structures more than lower energy x-rays. Various beam-modifying wedges, rotational techniques, and other specific approaches are used to increase the radiation damage to the tumor site while sparing the normal surrounding tissues. Cobalt 60 machines deliver gamma rays that are comparable to megavolt x-rays. They were once the most common type of equipment used, but because the radiation source is a radioactive isotope it is undergoing decay and needs to be replaced every 5 to 6 years to avoid lengthy treatment times. As the name implies, linear accelerators produce megavoltage electromagnetic wave radiation by accelerating electrons in a straight line. Linear accelerators have distinct advantages, including the speed with which treatment can be given. This reduces the time the patient must spend in awkward and uncomfortable positions. Some linear accelerators are also equipped to produce particulate radiation. With particulate radiation, most of the energy is expended at a certain depth, sparing surrounding tissues.

Brachytherapy involves the insertion of sealed radioactive sources into a body cavity (intracavitary) or directly into body tissues (interstitial). Radiation sources are sealed within applicators of almost any size or shape. Most commonly they are packed into needles, beads, seeds, ribbons, or catheters, which are then implanted directly into the tumor. Removable devices make it possible to insert a radioactive material into a tumor area for a period of time (1 or 2 days to a week) and remove it. The radioactive sources used most commonly for this purpose are cesium-137, and iridium-192, and iodine-125. Cancer of the cervix and uterus is often treated with removable cesium insertions or iridium implants. Radioactive materials with a relatively short half-life, such as gold-198, radon, iodine-125, or palladium-103, are commonly encapsulated and used in permanent implants. This type of treatment is used for oral, bladder, and prostate cancers.

Unsealed internal radiation sources are either injected intravenously, administered by mouth, or instilled into a body cavity. Iodine-131, which is given by mouth, is used in the treatment of thyroid cancer. Gold-198 and phosphorus-32 are instilled directly into body cavities to control effusions (collections of fluid within a serous cavity).

Internal radiation sources are a source of radiation exposure as long as a sealed implant remains in the body or an unsealed implant or injected radioisotope emanates rays of radiant energy. It is essential that the type of ray that is being emitted and the half-life of the radioisotope be considered when care is provided for a person receiving internal radiation. Some radioisotopes, such as phosphorus-32, produce only beta rays, which do not create a radiation hazard because of the limited range of beta radiation. Others, such as cesium implants, pose a radiation hazard because they emit gamma rays. Institutions that practice nuclear medicine must be licensed by the Atomic Energy Commission and have a radiation safety officer, who has the responsibility of establishing policies and maintaining radiation safety within the institution.

Adverse Effects. Radiation cannot distinguish between malignant cells and the rapidly proliferating cells of normal tissue. During radiation treatment, injury to normal cells can produce adverse effects. Radiation effects are dose and fractionation dependent. Tissues that are most frequently affected are the skin, the mucosal lining of the gastrointestinal tract, and the bone marrow. Anorexia, nausea, emesis, and diarrhea are common depending on the site of treatment. These can usually be controlled by medication and dietary measures. Other systemic signs include fatigue, profuse perspiration, and even chills. These effects are temporary and reversible.

Radiation also causes bone marrow depression and affects the blood count and predisposes to infection and bleeding. The first cells to decrease are the leukocytes, then the thrombocytes (platelets), and finally the red blood cells. Frequent blood counts are used during radiation therapy to monitor bone marrow function.

External beam radiation must first penetrate the skin; depending on the total dose and type of radiation used, reactions of the skin may develop. With moderate doses of radiation to the skin, the hair falls out either spontaneously or when being combed, after the 10th to the 14th day; with larger doses, erythema develops (much like a sunburn) and may turn brown; and, at higher doses, there are patches of dry or moist desquamation. Fortunately, epithelialization takes place after the treatments have been stopped. Mucosities, desquamation of the oral and pharyngeal mucous membranes, which may sometimes be severe, may occur as a predictable side effect

in people receiving head and neck irradiation. The most severe effect is dry mouth due to the fact that the parotid gland is within the treatment field.

PHARMACOLOGIC THERAPY

Pharmacologic therapy is aimed at curing existing cancers, preventing local recurrence and metastatic spread, or reducing or controlling tumor size for palliative purposes. Pharmacologic methods include cancer chemotherapy cytotoxic agents, hormonal agents, and biotherapy. The discussion in this chapter is intended as an overview, and readers are referred to other references for a more complete discussion of these agents.

Chemotherapy. In the past four decades, cancer chemotherapy has evolved as a major treatment modality. Over 30 different chemotherapeutic drugs are used alone or in various combinations. Administering higher doses of multiple drugs may be used as a strategy to achieve cure or optimal palliation; however, the adverse drug interactions and side effects can be unpredictable and intensified. Chemotherapeutic drugs may be the chief form of treatment, or they may be used as adjuncts to other treatments. Chemotherapy is the primary treatment for most hematologic and some solid tumors, including choriocarcinoma, acute and chronic leukemia, Burkitt's lymphoma, and multiple myeloma.

Cancer chemotherapeutic drugs exert their effects through several mechanisms. At the cellular level, they exert their lethal action by creating adverse conditions that prevent cell growth and replication. These mechanisms include disrupting production of essential enzymes; inhibiting DNA, RNA, and protein synthesis; and preventing cell mitosis.

For most chemotherapy drugs, the relationship between tumor cell survival and drug dose is exponential, with the number of cells surviving being proportional to drug dose and the number of cells at risk for exposure being proportional to destructive action of the drug.[26] They are most effective in treating tumors that have a high growth fraction because of their ability to kill rapidly dividing cells. Exponential killing implies that a proportion or percentage of tumor cells (*e.g.*, 90%) are killed, rather than an absolute number (*e.g.*, 1 million); thus, multiple courses of treatment are needed if the tumor is to be eradicated.

The anticancer drugs may be classified as either cell-cycle specific or cell-cycle nonspecific. Drugs are cell-cycle specific if they exert their action during a specific phase of the cell cycle. For example, methotrexate, an antimetabolite, acts by interfering with DNA synthesis and thereby interrupts the S phase of the cell cycle. Drugs that are cell-cycle nonspecific affect cancer cells through all the phases of the cell cycle. The alkylating agents, which are cell-cycle nonspecific, act by disrupting DNA when the cells are in the resting state as well as when they are dividing. Figure 5-9 illustrates the site of action of various cancer drugs. Chemotherapeutic drugs that have similar structures and effects on cell function are generally grouped together, and these drugs usually have similar toxic effects and side effects. Because they differ in their mechanisms of action, combinations of cell-cycle–specific and cell-cycle–nonspecific agents are often used to treat cancer.

Combination chemotherapy has been found to be more effective than treatment with a single drug. With this method, several drugs with different mechanisms of action, metabolic pathways, times of onset of action and recovery, side effects, and onsets of side effects are used. The regimens for combination therapy are often referred to by acronyms. Two well-known combinations are MOPP (mechlorethamine, Oncovin (vincristine), procarbazine, and prednisone), used in the treatment of Hodgkin's disease, and CMF (cyclophosphamide, methotrexate, and

5-fluorouracil), used in the treatment of breast cancer. The maximum possible drug doses are usually used to ensure the maximum cell-kill. Routes of administration and dosage schedules are carefully designed to ensure optimal delivery of the active forms of the drugs to a tumor during the sensitive phase of the cell cycle.

Many of these drugs are administered intravenously. Venous access devices are often used for people with poor venous access and those who require frequent or continuous intravenous therapy. It can be used for home administration of chemotherapy drugs, blood sampling, and administration of blood components.[27] These systems use an implanted venous catheter with vascular access ports. In some cases, the drugs are administered by continuous infusion using a special ambulatory infusion pump that allows the people to remain at home and maintain their activities.

Adverse Effects. Because cancer cells derive from normal cells, they retain many of the latter's properties; thus, chemotherapeutic drugs affect both the neoplastic cells and the rapidly proliferating cells

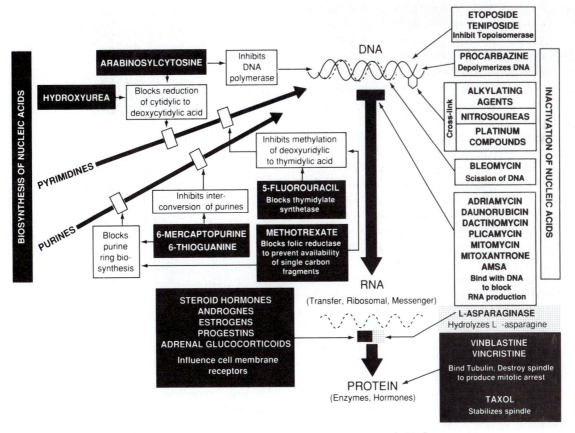

FIG. 5-9. Mechanism of action of chemotherapeutic agents. (Krakow, I. H. [1991]. Cancer chemotherapeutic and biologic agents. *CA—A Cancer Journal for Clinicians, 41,* 268)

of normal tissue. The *nadir* (lowest point) is the point of maximal toxicity for a given adverse effect of a drug and is stated in the time it takes to reach that point. The nadir for leukopenia with thiotepa occurs at 14 days after initiation of treatment. Because many toxic effects of chemotherapeutic drugs persist for some time after the drug is discontinued, the nadir times and recovery rates are useful guides in evaluating the effects of cancer therapy.

Anorexia, nausea, vomiting, and diarrhea are common problems associated with cancer chemotherapy. They occur within minutes or hours of drug administration and are thought to be due to stimulation of the chemoreceptor trigger zone (vomiting center) in the medulla or the autonomic nervous system. The symptoms usually subside within 24 to 48 hours and often can be relieved by antiemetics.[28] Some drugs cause stomatitis and damage to the rapidly proliferating cells of the gastrointestinal tract mucosal lining. Most chemotherapeutic drugs suppress bone marrow function and formation of blood cells, leading to anemia, leukopenia, and thrombocytopenia. With severe granulocytopenia, there is risk of developing serious infections. Hair loss results from impaired proliferation of the hair follicles and is a side effect of a number of cancer drugs; it is usually temporary, and the hair tends to regrow when treatment is stopped. The rapidly proliferating structures of the reproductive system are particularly sensitive to the action of the cancer drugs. Women may experience changes in menstrual flow or amenorrhea. Men may develop decreased sperm count (oligospermia) or absence of sperm (azoospermia). Many of these agents may also have teratogenic or mutagenic effects leading to fetal abnormalities.

Because cancer drugs are mutagenic, special care is required when handling or administering the drugs. Drugs, drug containers, and administration equipment require special disposal as hazardous waste. The Occupational Safety and Health Administration (OSHA) has developed special guidelines for the safe handling and disposal of antineoplastic drugs as well for accidental spills and exposure.[29]

Epidemiologic studies have shown an increased risk of second malignancies such as acute nonlymphocytic leukemia after long-term use of alkylating agents[30, 31] and semustine[32] for treatment of various forms of cancer. These second malignancies are thought to result from direct cellular changes produced by the drug or from suppression of the immune response.

Hormone Therapy. Hormone therapy consists of administration of hormones or hormone blocking drugs. It is used for cancers that are responsive to or dependent on hormones for growth. The actions of hormones depends on the presence of specific receptors in the tumor. Among the tumors known to be responsive to hormonal manipulations are those of the breast, prostate, adrenal gland, and uterine endometrium. Hormones commonly used for cancer treatment include estrogens (diethylstilbestrol, estradiol), androgens (testosterone), and progestins (hydroxyprogesterone). Hormone therapy also involves use of the adrenal corticosteroid hormones. These compounds inhibit mitosis and are cytotoxic to cells of lymphocytic origin. Hormones are cell-cycle nonspecific and are thought to alter the synthesis of RNA and proteins by binding to receptor sites. Hormone blocking drugs include the antiestrogen drugs tamoxifen and leuprolide (a gonadotropin-releasing hormone analog that blocks both estrogens and androgens) and the antiadrenal drug aminoglutethimide. The side effects of hormonal treatment are directly related to the normal action of the hormones. Because dosages of these drugs are usually higher than those that normally occur in the body, the normal actions of the hormone are accentuated.

Biotherapy. Biotherapy involves the use of biologic response modifiers that change the person's own biologic response to cancer. Although biotherapy relies heavily on immune mechanisms, it is not limited to them.[33] Three major mechanisms by which biotherapy exerts its effects are: (1) modification of host responses, (2) direct destruction of cancer cells, and (3) modification of tumor cell biology. Some agents, such as interferons, may use more than one mechanism. Immunotherapy remains largely investigational and is often used in conjunction with other forms of treatment. Four types of biologic response modifiers are being used or investigated: active immunotherapy, interferon therapy, adoptive therapy, and monoclonal antibodies. *Active immunotherapy* focuses on stimulating immune response. One such agent is BCG (bacille Calmette-Guérin), an attenuated strain of the bacterium that causes bovine tuberculosis. BCG acts as a nonspecific stimulant of the immune system. A second method involves the use of vaccines made from the patient's own tumor (autologous) or from pooled tumor-associated antigens (allogeneic) that have been obtained from a number of tumors. Active immunotherapy has been studied as treatment for melanoma, renal-cell carcinoma, and leukemia.

Interferons (*IFN*) are a group of cytokines (see Chapter 13) that are synthesized by a number of cells in response to a variety of stimuli including viral infections. There are three broad groups of interferons: alpha (α), beta (β), and gamma (γ), each group differing in terms of their cell surface receptors.[34] The exact physiologic roles of each of the interferons remain unclear. They appear to inhibit viral replication and may also be involved in inhibiting tumor protein synthesis and in prolonging the cell cycle and increasing the percentage of cells in the G_0 phase.[14] In addition, interferons stimulate NK cells and T-lymphocyte killer cells.

α-Interferon, the most widely studied, has been shown to have antitumor and antiviral effects against various tumor and tumor-related viruses. Until recently, the availability of interferon was limited because it could only be obtained from white blood cells and fibroblasts. Large amounts can now be produced using techniques of recombinant DNA synthesis. It has been approved by the Federal Drug Administration for use with hairy cell leukemia, AIDS-related Kaposi's sarcoma, and condylomata acuminata (genital warts).[34] Its use with other cancers, including renal-cell carcinoma, colorectal cancer, cutaneous T-cell lymphoma, and multiple myeloma, is being investigated. Research is focusing on combining interferons with other forms of cancer therapy and establishing optimal doses and treatment protocols.

Adoptive immunotherapy uses lymphokine-activated NK cells or tumor-specific T-cell immunity as a means of eradicating cancer cells. Originally, only *lymphokine-activated killer* (*LAK*) cells were used.[17] These NK cells are grown in culture supported by the lymphokine, interleukin-2. Because NK cells are nonspecific in their function, LAK cells attack both normal and tumor cells. The technique of adoptive therapy has been expanded to the production of tumor-specific T cells. These cells are derived from a person's own *tumor-infiltrating lymphocytes* (*TIL* cells) that have been expanded in the laboratory so that a large amount of cells are available for reinfusion. Because the TIL cells are tumor-specific, they do not attack normal host cells.

In summary, the methods used in diagnosis of cancer vary with the type of cancer that is present and its location. Because many cancers are curable if diagnosed early, health care practices designed to promote early detection are important. These practices include breast self-examination in the female, testicular self-examination in the male, and consulting of a physician when any of the early warning signals of cancer are present. Pap smear and tissue biopsy are used to detect the presence of cancer cells and in diagnosis. There are two basic methods of classifying tumors: (1) grading according to the histologic or tissue characteristics and (2) clinical staging according to spread of the disease. Histologic studies are done in the laboratory using cells or tissue specimens. The TNM system for clinical staging of cancer uses tumor size, lymph node involvement, and presence of metastasis.

Treatment plans that use more than one type of therapy, often in combination, are providing cures for a number of cancers that a few decades ago had a poor prognosis and are increasing the life expectancy in other types of cancer. Surgical procedures are more precise as a result of improved diagnostic equipment and new techniques such as laser surgery. Radiation equipment and radioactive sources permit greater and more controlled destruction of cancer cells while causing less damage to normal tissues. Combination chemotherapy regimens have provided cures for cancers that were previously viewed as uncurable. Successes with use of immunotherapy and interferon offer hope that the body's own defenses can be used in fighting cancer.

■ CHILDHOOD CANCERS

In the United States, cancer is the leading cause of death due to disease in children 1 to 15 years of age. There were an estimated 7800 new cases of childhood cancer in 1992.[1] The spectrum of cancers that affect children differs markedly from those that affect adults. Although most adult cancers are of epithelial cell origin (*e.g.*, lung cancer, breast cancer, and colorectal cancers), childhood cancers usually involve the hematopoietic system, nervous system, or connective tissue. Chart 5-3 lists the most common forms of solid childhood cancers. The discussion in this chapter focuses on three forms of solid childhood cancers: neuroblastoma, Wilms' tumor, and retinoblastoma. Leukemia, lymphoma, and Hodgkin's disease are discussed in Chapter 16, and Ewing's sarcoma and osteogenic sarcoma are discussed in Chapter 57.

As with adult cancers, there is probably no one cause of childhood cancer. However, many forms of childhood cancer repeat within families and may result from polygenic or single-gene inheritance, chromosomal aberrations (*e.g.*, translocations, deletions, insertions, inversions, duplications), exposure to mutagenic environmental agents, or a combination of these factors (see Chapter 4). If one child develops cancer, the risk of cancer in siblings is approximately twice that of the general population, and, if two children develop the disease, the risk is even greater.

Heritable forms of cancer tend to have an earlier age of onset, a higher frequency of multifocal lesions within a single organ, and bilateral involvement of paired organs or multiple primary tumors. The two-

---

CHART 5-3: COMMON SOLID TUMORS OF CHILDHOOD

Brain and nervous system tumors
  Medulloblastoma
  Glioma
Neuroblastoma
Wilms' tumor
Rhabdomyosarcoma and embryonal sarcoma
Retinoblastoma
Osteosarcoma
Ewing's sarcoma

hit hypothesis has been used as one explanation of heritable cancers.[36] The first hit (mutation) occurs prezygotically (in germ cells before conception) and is present in the genetic material of all somatic cells. Cancer subsequently develops in one or several somatic cell lines that undergo a second mutation.

It has also been shown that children with heritable disorders are at increased risk for developing certain forms of cancer. For example, Down's syndrome is associated with increased risk of leukemia; primary immunodeficiency disorders (see Chapter 15) are associated with lymphoma, leukemia, and brain cancer; and xeroderma pigmentosum is associated with basal and squamous cell carcinoma, and melanoma.

DIAGNOSIS AND TREATMENT

The early diagnosis of childhood cancers is often overlooked because of the signs and symptoms are often similar to those of common childhood diseases and cancer occurs less frequently in children than in adults. Symptoms of prolonged fever, unexplained weight loss, and growing masses (especially in association with weight loss) should be viewed as warning signs of cancer in children.

Diagnosis of childhood cancers involves many of the same methods that are used in adults. Accurate disease staging is especially beneficial in childhood cancers, in which the potential benefits of treatment must be carefully weighed against potential long-term effects (to be discussed).

The treatment of childhood cancers is complex, intensive, prolonged, and continuously evolving. Improved therapy and supportive care have led to progressive increases in survival. Among white children, the 5-year survival rate for all cancer sites is 67%; bone cancer, 56%; neuroblastoma, 55%; brain and central nervous system (CNS), 84%; Wilms' tumor, 87%; and Hodgkin's disease, 87%.[1]

NEUROBLASTOMA

Neuroblastoma originates in the embryonic neural-crest tissue of the sympathetic nervous system that normally develops into the adrenal glands and sympathetic ganglia. It is the most common malignancy in infants, accounting for 50% of all neonatal and 30% of infant malignancies. Congenital and even fetal neuroblastoma have been reported. Neuroblastoma represents 7% of all childhood cancers, yet results in 15% of all cancer-related deaths.

The most common presenting symptoms of neuroblastoma are pain, abdominal mass (caused by the tumor or its extension to the liver), lesions other than in the abdomen, and malaise. The abdominal distention may be asymptomatic but is often associated with anorexia, malaise, vague abdominal pain, and diarrhea. Most children have involved regional lymph nodes and metastasis at the time of diagnosis. Tumors that arise within the paravertebral ganglia tend to grow through the intervertebral foramen, causing spinal cord compression. This is a medical emergency. Tumors arising in the mediastinum can cause airway compression; those that affect the sympathetic ganglia can produce Horner's syndrome (*e.g.,* constricted pupil, drooping eyelid, and lack of sweating on the affected side). There may also be excess production and excretion of the catecholamines that cause unexplained episodes of flushing and sweating. However, hypertension is rare despite the alterations in catecholamine release.

Newer diagnostic methods include body scanning with ^{131}I-meta-iodo-benzyl-guanidine (MIBG), an agent that is taken up by the neuroblasts.[37] The treatment is based on age and extent of disease. Localized tumors are usually removed surgically. The tumor is sensitive to certain chemotherapeutic drugs, and combination chemotherapy has contributed to the successful treatment of the neuroblastoma.

WILMS' TUMOR

Wilms' tumor, or nephroblastoma, is a malignant embryonic tumor of the kidney. It is one of the most common malignant tumors in children, occurring most commonly in children between 1 and 5 years of age.[36] It occurs in both heritable and sporadic forms. In children with the heritable form, the neoplasm develops earlier and is more likely to be bilateral. Familial cases are inherited as an autosomal dominant disorder. About 30% of the offspring of people with bilateral or known Wilms' familial disease will develop Wilms' tumor.[36] According to the two-hit hypothesis, the first hit is inherited and the second hit is acquired. In the sporadic form, both hits are acquired. About 15% of children with Wilms' tumor, especially those with bilateral disease, have other congenital anomalies including other genitourinary anomalies (5%), unilateral hypertrophy of some part of the body (hemihypertrophy, 2%), absence of the iris (aniridia, 1%).

The most common presenting sign of Wilms' tumor is a large abdominal or flank mass first noted by the parents. Abdominal pain occurs in about 40% of children and may be severe enough to suggest an acute abdominal pathology. Hypertension, usually mild, is found in 60% to 90% of children. Fever may occur, sometimes in relation to an associated urinary tract infection.

Treatment involves surgery, chemotherapy, and radiotherapy (the tumor is radiosensitive). The overall cure rate is over 80%.[36]

RETINOBLASTOMA

Retinoblastoma is a malignant tumor of the nuclear layer of the retina. It is relatively rare (200 new cases/year) and usually occurs in children under 2 years of age. The disorder has been traced to a single gene located on the long arm of chromosome 13. Retinoblastoma serves as a model for childhood cancers that involve gene inactivation. In this rare type of cancer, a mutation in both members of a single gene pair that is located on the long arm of chromosome 13 is needed to block the expression of the retinoblastoma suppressor gene and induce neoplasia. Children with a familial form of the disease apparently inherit one defective gene in a germ cell and acquire the second in a somatic cell of the developing retina. In children with sporadic forms of the disorder, both alleles are mutated in retinal cells.

The condition typically presents as the cat's eye reflex (whitish appearance of the pupil) and strabismus (crossed eyes). The parents are usually the first to notice the eye disorder. Red and painful eyes are a late sign of the disorder. Limited vision or loss of vision is also a late sign. Bilateral involvement occurs in about 30% of cases and is associated with the heritable form of the disease.[37]

Diagnostic methods include ophthalmoscopic examination usually under general anesthesia. Staging procedures include CT scan of the head. Cerebral spinal fluid examination, chest x-ray, skeletal studies, and bone marrow examination may be done if advanced disease is suspected.

Treatment includes irradiation, photocoagulation, and cryotherapy with a focus on preserving sight. The eye may need to be removed (enucleated) in advanced disease, in which case chemotherapy and radiation may be used to control spread of the disease.

ADULT SURVIVORS OF CHILDHOOD CANCER

With improvement in treatment methods, the number of children who survive childhood cancer is continuing to increase.[38, 39] Unfortunately, therapy may produce late sequelae, such as impaired growth, neurologic dysfunction, hormonal dysfunction, cardiomyopathy, pulmonary fibrosis, and risk of second malignancies. Although cures for large numbers of children have only been possible since the 1970s, much is already known about the potential for delayed effects.

Children reaching adulthood after cancer therapy may have reduced physical stature because of the therapy they received—particularly radiation, which retards the growth of normal tissues along with cancer tissue. The younger the age and the higher the radiation, the greater the deviation from normal growth. There is also concern that CNS radiation as a prophylactic measure in childhood leukemia has an effect on cognition and learning. Children less than 6 years old at the time of radiation and those receiving the highest radiation doses are most likely to have subsequent cognitive difficulties.

Delayed sexual maturation in both boys and girls can result from irradiation of the gonads. Delayed sexual maturation is also related to treatment of children with alkylating agents. Cranial irradiation may result in premature menarche in girls, with subsequent early closure of the epiphysis and a reduction in final growth achieved. Data related to fertility and health of the offspring of childhood cancer survivors are just becoming available.

Vital organs such as the heart and lungs may be affected by cancer treatment. Children who received anthracyclines (doxorubicin or daunorubicin) may be at risk for developing cardiomyopathy and congestive heart failure. Pulmonary irradiation may cause lung dysfunction and restrictive lung disease. Drugs such as bleomycin, methotrexate, and bisulfan can also cause lung pathology.

For survivors of childhood cancers, the risk of second cancers is reported to range from 3% to 12%. There is a special risk of second cancers in children with the retinoblastoma gene. Because of this risk, children who have been treated for cancer should be followed routinely.

In summary, although most adult cancers are of epithelial cell origin, most childhood cancers usually involve the hematopoietic system, nervous system, or connective tissue. Heritable forms of cancer tend to have an earlier age of onset, a higher frequency of multifocal lesions within a single organ, and bilateral involvement of paired organs or multiple primary tumors. Three common types of childhood cancer are neuroblastoma, Wilms' tumor, and retinoblastoma. Neuroblastoma originates in the embryonic neural-crest tissue of the sympathetic nervous system that normally develop into the adrenal glands and sympathetic ganglia; Wilms' tumor, or nephroblastoma, is a malignant embryonic tumor of the kidney; and retinoblastoma is a malignant tumor of the nuclear layer of the retina. The early diagnosis of childhood cancers is often overlooked because the signs and symptoms are often similar to those of other childhood diseases. With improvement in treatment methods, the number of children who survive childhood cancer is continuing to increase. As these children approach adulthood, there is continued concern that the therapy that saved their lives may produce late sequelae, such as impaired growth, neurologic dysfunction, hormonal dysfunction, cardiomyopathy, pulmonary fibrosis, and risk of second malignancies.

■ REFERENCES

1. *Cancer facts 1992.* (1992). New York: American Cancer Society.
2. Prescott, D.M., & Flexer, A.S. (1986). *Cancer: The misguided cell* (p. 61). Sunderland, MA: Sinauer.
3. Kumar, V., Cotran, R.S., & Robbins, S.L. (1992). *Basics of pathology* (5th ed., pp. 171–215). Philadelphia: W.B. Saunders.
4. Zetter, B.R. (1990). The cellular basis of site specific tumor metastasis. *New England Journal of Medicine, 322,* 605–612.
5. Liotta, L.A. (1992). Cancer cell invasion and metastasis. *Scientific American, 266*(2), 54–63.
6. Weinberger, R.A. (1991). A short guide to oncogenes and tumor-suppressing genes. *Journal of National Institutes of Health Research, 3*(1), 45–47.
7. Yarbro, J.W. (1992). Oncogenes and cancer suppressor genes. *Seminars in Clinical Oncology, 8*(1), 30–39.
8. Levine, A.J. (1992). The p53 tumor-suppressor gene. *New England Journal of Medicine, 326,* 1350–1352.
9. Lynch, H.T. (1976). Familial risk and cancer control. *Journal of the American Medical Association, 236*(6), 585.
10. Knudson, A.G. (1974). Heredity and human cancer. *American Journal of Pathology, 77*(1), 77.
11. McMillan, S. (1992). Carcinogenesis. *Seminars in Oncology Nursing, 8*(1), 10–19.
12. Weisburger, J.H., & Horn, C.L. (1991). The causes of cancer. In A.I. Holleb, D.J. Fink, & G.P. Murphy. *American Cancer Society textbook of clinical oncology* (pp. 80–98). Atlanta: American Cancer Society.
13. Poskanzer, D.C., & Herbst, A. (1977). Epidemiology of vaginal adenosis and adenocarcinoma associated with exposure to stilbestrol in utero. *Cancer, 39*(4), 1792.
14. Favus, M.J., Schneider, A.B., Stachura, M.E., et al. (1976). Thyroid cancer occurring as a late consequence of head and neck irradiation: Evaluation of 1056 patients. *New England Journal of Medicine, 294,* 1019.
15. Jablon, S., & Kato, H. (1972). Studies of the mortality of A-bomb survivors: 5. Radiation dose and mortality, 1950–1970. *Radiation Research, 50,* 649.
16. Burnett, F.M. (1967). Immunologic aspects of malignant disease. *Lancet, 1,* 1171.
17. Haberman, R.B. (1991). Principles of tumor immunology. In A.I. Holleb, D.J. Fink, & G.P. Murphy. *American Cancer Society textbook of clinical oncology* (pp. 69–79). Atlanta: American Cancer Society.
18. Stites, D.P., & Terr, A.I. (1991). *Basic and clinical immunology* (7th ed.). San Mateo, CA: Appleton & Lange.
19. Beutler, B., & Cerami, A. (1990, February 15). The tumor necrosis factors: Cachectin and lymphotoxin. *Hospital Practice, 25*(2A), 45–56.
20. Rothstein, J.L., et al. (1986). Tumor necrosis factor: A potent effector molecule for tumor cell killing by activated macrophages. *Proceedings of the National Academy of Sciences of the United States of America, 83,* 8318.
21. Ihde, D.C. (1987, August 15). Paraneoplastic syndromes. *Hospital Practice, 22,* 105.
22. Collins, M.C. (1990). Tumor markers and screening tools in cancer detection. *Nursing Clinics of North America, 25,* 283–290.
23. Beahrs, O.H., & Myers, M.H. (Eds.). (1983). *Manual for staging of cancer* (2nd ed., p. 6). Philadelphia: J.B. Lippincott.
24. Fu, K.K., & Phillips, T.L. (1991). Radiation therapy: Basic principles and clinical applications. In L.W. Way (Ed.). *Current surgical diagnosis & treatment* (9th ed., pp. 79–94). San Mateo, CA: Appleton & Lange.
25. Hendrickson, F.R., & Withers, H.R. (1991). Principles of radiation oncology. In A.I. Holleb, D.J. Fink, & G.P. Murphy. *American Cancer Society textbook of clinical oncology* (pp. 35–46). Atlanta: American Cancer Society.
26. Cooper, M.R., & Cooper, M.R. (1991). Principles of medical oncology. In A.I. Holleb, D.J. Fink, & G.P. Murphy. *American Cancer Society textbook of clinical oncology* (pp. 47–68). Atlanta: American Cancer Society.
27. Groenwald, S.L., Frogge, M.H., Goodman, M., & Yarbo, C.H. (1990). *Cancer nursing: Principles and practice* (pp. 251–255). Columbia, MO: Jones Bartlett.
28. Gralla, R.J. (1992). Antiemetic drugs for chemotherapeutic support. *Cancer* (Suppl), *70*(4), 1003–1006.
29. U.S. Department of Labor. Office of Occupational Medicine, Occupational Safety and Health Administration (OSHA). (1986). *Work practice guidelines for personnel dealing with cytotoxic (antineoplastic) drugs,* Publ. no. 8-1.1. Washington, DC: U.S. Department of Labor.
30. Pederson-Bjergaard, J., & Larsen, S.O. (1982). Incidence of acute nonlymphocytic leukemia, preleukemia and acute myeloproliferative syndrome up to 10 years after treatment of Hodgkin's disease. *New England Journal of Medicine, 307,* 964.
31. Coltman, C.A., Jr., & Dixon, D.O. (1982). Second malignancies complicating Hodgkin's disease: A Southwest Oncology Group 10 year followup. *Cancer Treatment Reports, 66,* 1023.
32. Boise, J.D., Greene, M.H., Killen, J.Y., et al. (1983). Leukemia and preleukemia after adjuvant treatment of gastrointestinal cancer with semustine. *New England Journal of Medicine, 309,* 1079.
33. Mayer, D.K. (1990). Biotherapy: Recent advances and nursing implications. *Nursing Clinics of North America, 25,* 291–308.
34. Itri, L.M. (1992). The interferons. *Cancer* (Suppl), *70*(4), 940–944.
35. Goldstein, D., & Laszio, J. (1988). The role of interferon in cancer therapy: A current perspective. *CA: A Cancer Journal for Clinicians, 38*(5), 258.
36. Pui, C-H., & Crist, W.M. (1991). Pediatric solid tumors. In A.I. Holleb, D.J. Fink, & G.P. Murphy. *American Cancer Society textbook of clinical oncology* (pp. 453–480). Atlanta: American Cancer Society.
37. Crist, W.M., & Kun, L.E. (1991). Common solid tumors in childhood. *New England Journal of Medicine, 324,* 461–471.
38. Meadows, A.T. (1991, February). Follow-up and care of childhood cancer survivors. *Hospital Practice, 15,* 99–108.
39. Carter, M., Thompson, E.I. &, Simone, J.V. (1991). The survivors of childhood cancer. *Nursing Clinics of North America, 38,* 505–526.

■ BIBLIOGRAPHY

Appelbaum, J.W. (1992). The role of the immune system in the pathogenesis of cancer. *Seminars in Oncology Nursing, 8*(1), 51–62.

Bates, S.E. (1991). Clinical application of serum tumor markers. *Annals of Internal Medicine, 115*(8), 623–638.

Bingham, B. (1985). Hazards to health care workers from antineoplastic drugs. *New England Journal of Medicine, 313,* 1220–1221.

Bishop, J.M. (1987). The molecular genetics of cancer. *Science, 235*, 305.

Buckley, I. (1988). Oncogenes and the nature of malignancy. *Advances in Cancer Research, 50*, 71.

Cawley, M.M. (1990). Recent advances in chemotherapy: Administration and nursing implications. *Nursing Clinics of North America, 25*(2), 377–391.

Cole, J.S., & Grube, J. (1992). Progress and prospects for human cancer vaccines. *Journal of the National Cancer Institute, 24*(1), 18–21.

DeLast, C.A., & Lampkin, B.C. (1992). Long-term survivors of childhood cancer: Evaluation and identification of sequelae of treatment. *CA: A Cancer Journal for Clinicians, 42*(5), 263–282.

Dudjak, L.A. (1992). Cancer metastasis. *Seminars in Oncology Nursing, 8*(1), 40–50.

Galassi, A. (1992). The next generation: New chemotherapy agents for the 1990s. *Seminars in Oncology Nursing, 8*(2), 83–94.

Glickman, A.S. (1987). Radiologic basis of brachytherapy. *Seminars in Oncology Nursing, 3*(1), 3–6.

Greenberg, P.D., & Riddel, S.R. (1992). Tumor specific T-cell immunity: Ready for prime time? *Journal of the National Cancer Institute, 14*, 105961.

Helman, L.J., & Thiele, C.J. (1991). New insights into the causes of cancer. *Pediatric Clinics of North America, 38*, 201–221.

Lind, J. (1991). Tumor cell growth and cell kinetics. *Seminars in Oncology Nursing, 8*(1), 3–9.

Maddock, P.G. (1987). Brachytherapy sources and applicators. *Seminars in Oncology Nursing, 3*(1), 15–22.

McGuire, P., & Moore, K. (1990). Recent advances in childhood cancer. *Nursing Clinics of North America, 25*(2), 447–460.

Mundy, G.R. (1987). Ectopic hormonal syndromes in neoplastic disease. *Hospital Practice, 22*(4), 179.

Old, L.J. (1988). Tumor necrosis factor. *Scientific American, 258*(5), 59.

Schiffman, M.H. (1992). Recent progress in defining the epidemiology of human papillomavirus infection and cervical neoplasia. *Journal of the National Cancer Institute, 84*(6), 394–398.

DEVELOPMENTAL ASPECTS OF ALTERED HEALTH

CHAPTER 6

CONCEPTS OF ALTERED HEALTH IN CHILDREN

MARIANNE SIGDA
JUDY WRIGHT LOTT

■ OBJECTIVES

After you have studied this chapter, you should be able meet the following objectives:

■ Describe the major events that occur during prenatal development from fertilization to birth.

■ Describe the major physical differences of infancy, early childhood, early to late school years, and adolescence.

■ Identify reasons for abnormal uterine growth.

■ State the major causes of illness and death in children of all ages.

■ Describe assessment methods for determination of gestational age.

■ Differentiate between organic and nonorganic failure to thrive syndrome.

■ Discuss the common health problems of early school years.

■ Explain how the common health care needs of the premature infant differ from the health care needs of the full-term newborn or infant.

■ Discuss common health problems of the child in early to late school age.

■ Discuss how the physical changes that occur during adolescence can influence the health care needs of the adolescent.

Carol Mattson Porth: PATHOPHYSIOLOGY: CONCEPTS OF
ALTERED HEALTH STATES, 4th ed. © 1994, 1990, 1986, 1982
J.B. Lippincott Company

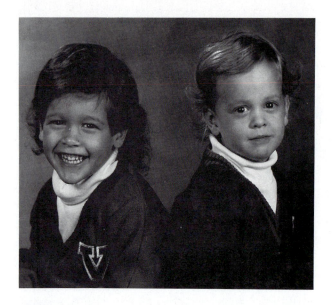

Children are not merely small adults. Their level of maturity in terms of physical and psychological development strongly influences the type of illnesses they experience and their responses to these illnesses. Although many signs and symptoms are the same in people of all ages, some diseases and complications are more likely to occur in the child. This chapter provides an overview of the developmental stages of childhood and their relationship to the health care needs of children. Specific diseases are presented throughout other sections of the book.

At the beginning of the 20th century, a child's chances of obtaining adulthood in the United States were limited. The infant mortality rate was 200 infant deaths per 1000 live births. Infectious diseases were rampant, and children were especially vulnerable. With the introduction of antibiotics, infectious disease control, and nutritional and technologic advances, infant mortality decreased dramatically. In 1989, infant mortality for the United States, 9.8 deaths per 1000 live births, was the lowest ever recorded. However, when this infant mortality rate is compared with the rates of other developed countries, the United States is ranked number 21 out of 25 countries.[1] Also of great concern is the difference in mortality rates for white and African-American infants. In 1989, the mortality rates for white and African-American infants were 8.2 and 17.7 deaths per 1000 live births, respectively, with the leading cause of death in African-American infants being prematurity and low birth weight (LBW). For white infants, the leading cause of death is congenital anomalies.[1-3]

Although the efforts to improve these rates are aimed at improving access to prenatal care, the underlying etiologies of two major causes of neonatal (infants less than 28 days of age) mortality, congenital anomalies and preterm delivery, are still poorly understood, despite continuing research. Many of the major causes of postneonatal (infants from 28 days to 11 months) deaths from infectious diseases (pneumonia and influenza), accidents, and adverse effects are preventable through health promotion such as well-baby care, immunizations, and teaching of parenting skills.

■ GROWTH AND DEVELOPMENT

The term *growth and development* describes a process whereby a fertilized ovum becomes an adult person.[4] Physical growth describes changes in the body as a whole or in its individual parts. Development, on the other hand, embraces other aspects of differentiation such as changes in body function and psychosocial behaviors.

Physical growth occurs in a caphalocaudal direction. Relative body proportions change over the lifespan. In early fetal development, the head is the largest part of the body, but this changes as the individual grows. Figure 6-1 shows the changes in body proportions from the second fetal month until age 25.

The average newborn weighs approximately 3000 to 4000 g and is 50 to 53 cm in length. The 1st year is a period of rapid growth demonstrated by lengthening of the trunk and accumulation of subcutaneous fat. After the 1st year and entering into puberty, the legs grow more rapidly than any other part.

The onset of puberty is marked by a significant alteration in body proportions, secondary to the effects of the pubertal growth spurt. The feet and hands are the first to increase. Because the trunk grows faster than the legs, at adolescence a large portion of the increase in height is a result of trunk growth. The brain is another organ that undergoes a period of rapid growth. At birth, the brain is 25% of adult size; at 1 year, it is 50% of adult size; and at 5 years, it is 90% of adult size. The size of the head reflects brain growth.[1,2]

Linear growth is a result of skeletal growth. Once maturation of the skeleton is complete, linear growth is complete. By 2 years of age, length will be 50% of adult height. Beginning with the 3rd year, the growth rate will be 5 to 6 cm for the next 9 years. During the adolescent period there is a growth spurt. Males may add approximately 20 cm and females 16 cm to their height during time. Terminal height is reached by 16.5 years in females and 17.75 years in males. Weight is rapidly increased after birth. By 6 months

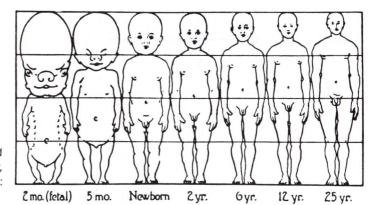

FIG. 6-1. Changes in body proportions from the 2nd fetal month to adulthood. (From Robbins, W.J., Brody, S., Hogan, A.G., et al. [1928]. *Growth.* New Haven: Yale University Press. By permission of publisher)

2 mo.(fetal)   5 mo.   Newborn   2 yr.   6 yr.   12 yr.   25 yr.

the birth weight is doubled, and by 1 year it is tripled. The average weight increase is 2 to 2.75 kg per year until the adolescent growth spurt begins.[1,2]

Growth and development encompass a complex interaction between genetic and environmental influences. The experience of each child is unique, and the patterns of growth and development may be profoundly different for individual children within the context of what is termed "normal." Because of the wide variability, these norms can often be expressed only in statistical terms.

Evaluation of growth and development requires comparison of an individual's growth and development to a standard of growth and development. Statistics are calculations derived from measurements that are used to describe the sample measured and/or to make (infer) predictions about the rest of the population that the sample represented. Since all individuals grow and develop at different rates, the standard for growth and development must somehow take this individual variation in account. The standard is typically derived from measurements made on a sample of individuals deemed representative of the total population. When multiple measurements of biologic variables such as height, weight, head circumference, and blood pressure are made, the majority of the values fall around the center or middle of all the values. Plotting the data on a graph yields a "bell-shaped" curve, which depicts the normal distribution of these continuously variable values (Figure 6-2).

The mean and stanadard deviation are common statistics used in describing the characteristics of a population. The *mean* represents the average of the measurements. It is simply the sum of the values divided by the number of values. A normal bell-shaped curve is symmetric, with the mean falling in the center of the curve and with one-half of the values falling on either side of the mean. The *standard deviation (SD)* determines how far a value varies or deviates from the mean. The points one standard devia-

tion above and below the mean include 68% of all values, two standard deviations 95% of all values, and three standard deviations 99.7 values. Thus, if a child's height is within one standard deviation of the mean, he or she is as tall as 68% of children in the population. If a child's height is greater than three standard deviations, he or she is taller than 99.7% of children in the population.[5]

The bell-shaped curve can also be marked by percentiles, which are useful for comparison of an individual's values to other values. When quantitative data are arranged in ascending and descending order, a middle value called the *median* can be described with half (50%) of the values falling on either side. The values can be further divided into percentiles. A percentile is a number that indicates the percentage of values for the population that are equal to or below the number. Percentiles are most often used to compare an individual's value with a set of norms. They are used extensively to develop and interpret physical growth charts and measurements of ability and intelligence.

PRENATAL GROWTH AND DEVELOPMENT

Human development is considered to begin with fertilization, the union of sperm and ovum resulting in a zygote. The process begins with the intermingling of a haploid number of paternal (23 X or Y) and maternal (23 XX) chromosomes in the ampulla of the oviduct that fuse to form a zygote. Within 24 hours, the unicellular organism becomes a 2-cell organism and, within 72 hours, a 16-cell organism, called a *morula*. This series of mitotic divisions is called *cleavage*. During cleavage, the rapidly developing cell mass travels down the oviduct to the uterus by a series of peristaltic movements. The morula enters the uterus about 3 days after fertilization. On the 4th day, the morula is separated into two parts by fluid from the uterus. The outer layer gives rise to the

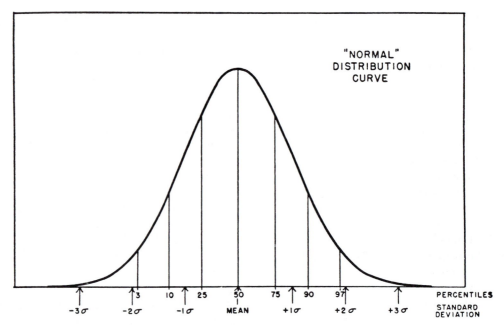

FIG. 6-2. "Normal" (gaussian) distribution curve. This curve represents the theoretical distribution of values for many biologic measurements. The percentiles indicate certain positions within this distribution, as do the standard deviations from the mean. (From Nelson, W.E. [Ed.]: [1959]. *Textbook of pediatrics* [7th ed., p. 18]. Philadelphia; W.B. Saunders)

placenta (trophoblast), and the inner layer gives rise to the embryo (embryoblast). The structure is now called a *blastocyte*. By the 6th day, the blastocyte attaches to the endometrium epithelium. This is the beginning of implantation, and it is completed during the 2nd week of development.[6]

Prenatal development is divided into two main periods. The first period, or *embryonic*, period, begins during the 2nd week and continues through the 8th week after fertilization. During the embryonic period, the main organ systems are developed and many function at a minimal level. The second, or *fetal*, period begins during the 9th week. During the fetal period, the growth and differentiation of the body and organ systems occur.

EMBRYONIC DEVELOPMENT

With the onset of embryonic development, which begins during the 2nd week of gestation, the trophoblast continues its rapid proliferation and differentiation, whereas the embryoblast evolves into a bilaminar embryonic disk. This flattened, circular plate of cells gives rise to all three germ layers of the embryo (ectoderm, mesoderm, endoderm).

The 3rd week is a period of rapid development noted for the conversion of the bilaminar embryonic disk into a trilaminar embryonic disk through a process called *gastrulation*.[6] The ectoderm differentiates

into the epidermis and nervous system, and the endoderm gives rise to the epithelial linings of the respiratory passages, digestive tract, and glandular cells of organs such as the liver and pancreas. The mesoderm becomes smooth muscle tissue, connective tissue, blood vessels, blood cells, bone marrow, skeletal tissue, striated muscle tissue, and reproductive and excretory organs. The notochord, which is the primitive axis about which the axial skeleton forms, is also formed during the 3rd week (see Chapter 47). The neurologic system begins its development during this period. *Neurulation*, a process that involves formation of the neural plate, neural folds, and their closure, is completed by the 4th week. Disturbances during this period can result in brain and spinal defects such as spina bifida. The cardiovascular system is the first functional organ system to develop. The primitive heart, which beats and circulates blood, develops during this period (see Chapter 23).

By the 4th week, the neural tube is formed.[6] The embryo begins to curve and fold into a characteristic C-shaped structure. The limb buds are visible as well as the otic pits (primordia of the internal ears) and the lens placodes (primordia of the lens of the eyes). The 5th week is notable for the rapid growth of the head secondary to brain growth.

During the 6th week, the upper limbs are formed by fusion of the swellings around the branchial groove. In the 7th week, there is the beginning of the digits, and the intestines enter the umbilical cord (umbilical herniation).[6] By the 8th week, the embryo is "human-like" in appearance; eyes are open, eyelids and ear auricles are easily identified.

FETAL DEVELOPMENT

During the 9th to 12th weeks, fetal head growth slows, whereas body length growth is greatly accelerated. By the 11th week, the intestines in the proximal portion of the cord have returned to the abdomen. The primary ossification centers are present in the skull and long bones, and maturation of the fetal external genitalia is established by the 12th week. During the fetal period, the liver is the major site of red blood cell formation (erythropoiesis); at 12 weeks, this activity has decreased and erythropoiesis begins in the spleen. Also, urine begins to form during the 9th to 12th week and is excreted into the amniotic fluid.[6]

The 13th through 16th weeks are notable for ossification of the skeleton, scalp hair patterning, and differentiation of the ovaries. By the 17th through 20th week, growth has slowed. The fetal skin is covered with a fine hair called *lanugo* and a white cheese-like material called *vernix caseosa*. Eyebrows and head hair are visible. In male fetuses, the testes begin to descend, and, in female fetuses, the uterus is formed. Brown fat also forms during this period. Brown fat is a specialized type of adipose tissue that produces heat by oxidizing fatty acids. It is similar to white fat but has larger and more numerous mitochondria, which provide its brown color. Brown fat is found near the heart and blood vessels that supply the brain and kidneys and is thought to play a role in maintaining the temperature of these organs during exposure to environmental changes that occur after birth.

During the 25th through 26th weeks, there is a significant fetal weight gain. The type II alveolar cells of the lung begin to secrete surfactant (see Chapter 26). The pulmonary system becomes more mature and able to support respiration during the 26th through 29th weeks (see Chapter 27). Breathing movements are present secondary to central nervous system (CNS) maturation. There is also an increasing amount of subcutaneous fat, with white fat making up 3.3% of body weight.

The 30th through 34th weeks are significant for an increasing amount of white fat (8% of body weight), which gives the fetal limbs an almost chubby appearance.[6] During the 35th week, grasp and the pupillary light reflex are present.

Expected time of birth is 264 days or 38 weeks after fertilization or 40 weeks after the last menstrual period (LMP).[6] At this time, the neurologic, cardiovascular, and pulmonary systems are developed enough for the baby to make the transition to extra-uterine life. The survival of the newborn depends on this adaptation once the placenta is removed.

Fetal Growth and Weight Gain. Normal growth progresses through three phases. During the first stage (embryonic and early fetal life), there is growth through cell multiplication or hyperplasia. During this phase, new cells are formed through mitosis, which is the basis for organ and tissue development and growth.[7–9]

During the second stage of growth (middle of gestation), hyperplasia continues, although at a slower rate, and growth is through enlargement of existing cells by addition of cytoplasm or hypertrophy.

The last phase of growth (end of gestation) is primarily hypertrophy (cell enlargement) although some hyperplasia is ongoing. As cells enlarge, cellular differentiation is occurring and hyperplasia is decreasing. This occurs after a few weeks of rapid hyperplasia. The process of growth is ongoing, and hypertrophy and hyperplasia continue after birth.

Fetal weight gain is linear beginning at 20 weeks gestation. until 38 weeks gestation. In the last half of pregnancy, the fetus gains 85% of birth weight. After 38 weeks of gestation, the rate of growth declines, probably related to the constraint of uterine size and decreased placental function. After birth, weight gain reaches intrauterine rates.

Birth weight can be affected by a variety of factors including maternal nutrition, genetic factors, maternal chronic diseases, placental abnormalities, sex, socioeconomic factors, multiple births, chromosomal abnormalities, and infectious diseases.

BIRTH WEIGHT AND GESTATIONAL AGE

At birth, the average weight of the full-term newborn is 3000 to 4000 g. In the past, infant weighing less than 2500 g were classified as premature. In 1961, infants weighing less than 2500 g were classified as low birth weight (LBW). Lubchenco and Battagila established standards for birth weight, gestational age, and intrauterine growth in the United States in the 1960s (Fig. 6-3).[10,11] With these standards, gestational age can be assessed and normal and abnormal growth can be identified. The *Colorado Growth Curve* places newborns into percentiles.[10] The 10th through 90th percentiles of intrauterine growth encompass 80% of births.[14] Growth is considered abnormal when a newborn falls above or below the 90th and 10th percentiles, respectively.

An infant is considered term when born between the beginning of the 38th week and completion of the

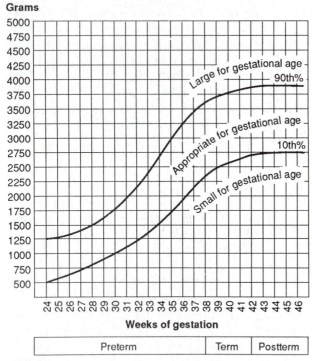

Grams

FIG. 6-3. Classification of newborns by birth weight and gestational age. (Redrawn from Battaglia, F.C., & Lubchenco, L.O. [1967]. A practical classification of newborn infants by weight and gestational age. *Journal of Pediatrics, 71*, 159)

41st week. An infant is considered premature when born before the end of the 37th week and postmature when born at the onset of the 42nd week. The lowest rates of mortality occurs among newborns with weight between 3000 and 4000 g with gestational ages 38 to 42 weeks.[7-9]

ABNORMAL INTRAUTERINE GROWTH

Growth of the fetus in the uterus depends on a multitude of factors, both intrinsic and extrinsic. Optimal fetal growth depends on efficient placental function, adequate provision of energy and growth substrates, appropriate hormonal environment, and adequate room in the uterus. Birth weight variability in a population is primarily determined by maternal heredity, intrinsic fetal growth potential, and environmental factors. Abnormal growth, which can occur at any time during fetal development, can have immediate as well as long-term consequences for the infant.

Small for Gestational Age. Small for gestational age (SGA) is a term that denotes fetal undergrowth. SGA is defined as birth weight less than two standard deviations below the mean for gestational age or be-

low the 10th percentile. It is often used interchangeably with intrauterine growth retardation (IUGR). Worldwide, between 30% and 40% of infants born at weights less than 2500 g are SGA. Mortality of severely affected SGA infants is five to six times that of a normally grown infant of comparable gestation age. Fetal growth retardation can occur anytime during fetal development. Depending on the time of insult, the infant can have symmetric or proportional growth retardation or asymmetric or disproportional growth retardation. Impaired growth that occurs early in pregnancy during the hyperplastic phase of growth results in a symmetric growth retardation. Because mitosis is affected, organ and tissues are smaller because of decreased cell number. Head circumference, length, and weight usually are represented within similar percentile grids, although the head may be smaller, as in microcephaly.[12] This is irreversible postnatally. Causes of proportional IUGR include chromosomal abnormalities, congenital infections, and exposure to environmental toxins.

Impaired growth that occurs later in pregnancy during the hypertrophic phase of growth results in asymmetric growth retardation.[7-9] Infants with IUGR due to intrauterine malnutrition often have weight reduction out of proportion to length or head circumference and exhibit sparing of impaired head and brain growth.[15] Tissues and organs are small because of decreased cell size, not decreased cell numbers. Postnatally, the impairment may be partially corrected with good nutrition.

Maternal, placental, and environmental factors affect fetal growth. Because of the effects on the placenta (it is also undergrown), the risk for perinatal complications is higher. These include birth asphyxia, hyperglycemia, polycythemia, meconium (the dark green mucilaginous newborn stool) aspiration, and hypothermia. The long-term effects of growth retardation depend on the timing and severity of the insult. Many of these infants have been found to have developmental disabilities on follow-up examination, especially if the growth retardation was symmetric. They may remain small, especially if the insult occurs early. If the insult occurs later because of placental insufficiency or uterine restraint, with good nutrition catch-up growth can occur and the infant may attain appropriate growth.

Large for Gestational Age. Large for gestational age (LGA) is a term that denotes fetal overgrowth. The definition of LGA is birth weight greater than two standard deviations above the mean for gestation or above the 90th percentile. The excessive growth may be due to a genetic predisposition or stimulated by abnormal conditions in utero. Infants of diabetic mothers may be LGA, especially if the diabetes was poorly controlled during pregnancy. Maternal hyperglycemia exposes the fetus to increased levels of glucose, which stimulates fetal secretion of insulin. Insulin increases fat disposition, and the result is a macrosomic infant. Babies with macrosomia have enlarged viscera and are large and plump due to an increase in body fat. Complications when an infant is LGA include birth asphyxia and trauma due to mechanical difficulties during the birth process, hypoglycemia, and polycythemia.[7–9]

ASSESSMENT METHODS

The methods of assessing gestation can be divided into two categories: prenatal assessment and postnatal assessment.

Prenatal assessment of gestational age most commonly includes careful menstrual history, physical milestones during pregnancy (uterine size, detection of fetal heart rate and movements), and prenatal tests for maturity (ultrasound, amniotic fluid studies). Nägele's rule uses the first day of the last menstrual period (LMP) to calculate the day of labor by adding 7 days to the LMP and counting back 3 months.[7] This method can often be inaccurate if the mother is not a good historian or has a history of irregular menses, which interferes with identification of a normal cycle.

Postnatal assessment of gestational age is most commonly done by examination of physical external and neuromuscular characteristics either alone or in combination. The most common methods used in nurseries today were developed by Dubowitz (1970) or Ballard. The Dubowitz method is comprehensive and includes 21 criteria using both external physical (11) and neuromuscular (10) signs (Fig. 6-4).[13] The estimate of gestational age is best done within 48 hours of birth and is accurate within 2 weeks. The method is less accurate for infants born at gestational age less than 30 weeks. The Ballard method is an abbreviated Dubowitz method that includes 12 criteria using 6 external physical and 6 neuromuscular signs.[14] This method is accurate for gestational ages 26 to 44 weeks.

In summary, growth and development begin with union of ovum and sperm and is ongoing throughout a child's life to adulthood. Abnormalities during this process can have profound effects on the person. Perinatal development is composed of two periods—the embryonic period and the fetal period. During these periods, the zygote becomes the newborn with the organ maturity to make the adjustments necessary for extrauterine life. Infants born before this process is completed are called premature and can have major problems with extrauterine adjustments. Postnatal growth is rapid and ongoing and proceeds in an orderly and predictable manner.

■ INFANCY

Infancy is defined as that time from birth to about 18 months of age. This is a period of rapid physical growth and maturation. The infant begins life as a relatively helpless organism and, through a process of progressive development, gains the skills to interact and cope with the environment. The infant begins life with a number of primitive reflexes and little body control. By 18 months, a child is able to run, grasp, and manipulate objects, feed self, play with toys, and communicate with others.

GROWTH AND DEVELOPMENT

Physical growth is rapid during infancy. After birth, there is a period of relative starvation as the infant adjusts to enteral feeding. Infants lose about 5% to 10% of their birth weight, but, within days, they begin to gain weight and by 2 weeks are back to birth weight. Average birth weight for a term newborn is 3000 to 4000 g, and this weight is doubled by 6 months and tripled by about 1 year after birth.

The median height at birth is 49.9 cm for girls and 50.5 cm for boys. During the first 6 months, height increases by 2.5 cm per month. By 1 year, the increase in length is 50% of the birth length. This increase is primarily in trunk growth. Median head circumference at birth is 34.5 cm for girls and 34.8 cm for boys. There is rapid increase in head circumference the first year, which is a good indicator of brain growth. Head circumference increases by 1.5 cm per month the first 6 months and 0.5 cm per month the second 6 months. Chest circumference at birth is smaller than head circumference. By 1 year, the head and chest are approximately equal in circumference. After 1 year, chest circumference exceeds head circumference.[2]

After birth, the majority of organ systems continue to grow and mature in an orderly fashion. Variations in growth and development are responsible for the differences in body proportions. For example, during the fetal period, the head is the predominant part due to the rapidly growing brain, whereas, during infancy, the trunk predominates and, in childhood, the legs predominate. The patterns of growth are cephalocaudal, proximodistal, and mass to specific.

Organ systems must continue to grow and mature after delivery. Many are at a minimal level of functioning at birth. This often places them at risk for health problems. One example is the nervous system. Neurologic development and maturation continue after birth. At birth, the average brain weighs about 325 g. By 1 year, the weight has tripled and the

A

NEURO-LOGICAL SIGN	SCORE					
	0	1	2	3	4	5
POSTURE						
SQUARE WINDOW (WRIST)	90°	60°	45°	30°	0°	
ANKLE DORSI-FLEXION	90°	75°	45°	20°	0°	
ARM RECOIL	180°	90-180°	<90°			
LEG RECOIL	180°	90-180°	<90°			
POPLITEAL ANGLE	180°	160°	130°	110°	90°	<90°
HEEL TO EAR						
SCARF SIGN						
HEAD LAG						
VENTRAL SUSPENSION						

B

EXTERNAL SIGN	SCORE				
	0	1	2	3	4
OEDEMA	Obvious oedema hands and feet, pitting over tibia	No obvious oedema hands and feet, pitting over tibia	No oedema		
SKIN TEXTURE	Very thin, gelatinous	Thin and smooth	Smooth, medium thickness Rash or superficial peeling	Slight thickening Superficial cracking and peeling esp hands and feet	Thick and parchment-like, superficial or deep cracking
SKIN COLOUR (Infant not crying)	Dark red	Uniformly pink	Pale pink variable over body	Pale Only pink over ears, lips, palms or soles	
SKIN OPACITY (trunk)	Numerous veins and venules clearly seen, especially over abdomen	Veins and tributaries seen	A few large vessels clearly seen over abdomen	A few large vessels seen indistinctly over abdomen	No blood vessels seen
LANUGO (over back)	No lanugo	Abundant, long and thick over whole back	Hair thinning especially over lower back	Small amount of lanugo and bald areas	At least half of back devoid of lanugo
PLANTAR CREASES	No skin creases	Faint red marks over anterior half of sole	Definite red marks over more than anterior half, indentations over less than anterior third	Indentations over more than anterior third	Definite deep indentations over more than anterior third
NIPPLE FORMATION	Nipple barely visible, no areola	Nipple well defined, areola smooth and flat diameter <0.75 cm.	Areola stippled, edge not raised diameter <0.75 cm.	Areola stippled, edge raised diameter >0.75 cm.	
BREAST SIZE	No breast tissue palpable	Breast tissue on one or both sides 0.5 cm diameter	Breast tissue both sides, one or both 0.5 cm	Breast tissue both sides, one or both 1 cm	
EAR FORM	Pinna flat and shapeless, little or no incurving of edge	Incurving of part of edge of pinna	Partial incurving whole of upper pinna	Well-defined incurving whole of upper pinna	
EAR FIRMNESS	Pinna soft, easily folded, no recoil	Pinna soft, easily folded, slow recoil	Cartilage to edge of pinna, but soft in places, ready recoil	Pinna firm, cartilage to edge, instant recoil	
GENITALIA MALE	Neither testis in scrotum	At least one testis high in scrotum	At least one testis right down		
FEMALES (With hips half abducted)	Labia majora widely separated, labia minora protruding	Labia majora almost cover labia minora	Labia majora completely cover labia minora		

FIG. 6-4. (**A**) Neurologic characteristics of the Dubowitz examination. Neurologic criteria are recorded and added to a final score as performed for the physical assessment. (**B**) External characteristics of the Dubowitz examination. Physical criteria are recorded and a final score is obtained following the addition of each category's score. (Dubowitz, L., & Dubowitz, V. [1977]. *Gestational age of the newborn*. Reading, MA: Addison-Wesley)

brain weighs about 1000 g. The maturation process includes an increase in neuron size, in size and number of glial cells, in myelinization, and in interneural connections and branching of axons and dendrites. As this maturation progresses, the level of functioning of the infant increases from simple to complex, from primitive reflexes to purposeful movement. The development of fine and gross motor skills follows the principles of cephalocaudal and proximodistal maturation.[1, 15]

The respiratory system must make the transition from an intrauterine to an extrauterine existence. On-set of respiration must begin at birth for survival. The first breaths expand the alveoli and initiate gas exchange. The infant's respiratory rate is initially rapid and primarily abdominal, but, with maturation, it gradually slows. Maturation of the respiratory system includes increases in the number of alveoli and the growth of the airways. Infants are obligatory nose breathers until 3 to 4 months of age; any upper airway obstruction may cause respiratory distress.[1, 15] The trachea is small and close to the bronchi and its branching structures enabling infectious agents to be easily transmitted throughout the lungs. The softness of the supporting cartilage in the trachea, along with its small diameter, places the infant at risk for airway obstruction. The eustachian tube is short and straight and closely communicates with the ear, putting the infant at risk for middle ear infections.

Birth initiates major changes in the cardiovascular system. The fetal shunts, the foramen ovale and ductus arteriosus, begin to close, and the circulation of blood changes from a series to a parallel circuit (see Chapter 23). At birth, the heart lies in the thoracic cavity, and its size is large in relation to the chest cavity. The size and weight of the heart double the first year. Initially, the right ventricle is more muscular than the left ventricle, but this reverses in infancy. The heart rate gradually slows, and systolic blood pressure rises.

The gastrointestinal system is immature, and the majority of digestive processes are poorly functioning until approximately 3 months of age. Solid food may pass incompletely digested and be evident in the stool. At birth, sucking may be poor and require several days to become effective. The tongue thrust reflex is present and aids in sucking, but it disappears around 6 months of age. Stomach capacity increases rapidly the first months, but, due to the limited capacity and rapid emptying, infants require frequent feeding.[1,15]

The infant's genitourinary system is functionally immature at birth. There is difficulty in concentrating urine, and the ability to adjust to a restricted fluid intake is limited. The small bladder capacity causes frequent voiding.

By 24 weeks gestation age, all the nerve cells are present and growth is primarily due to an increase in cytoplasm. The most rapid period of brain growth is between 15 to 20 weeks of postnatal age, at which time there is a significant increase in neurons. Another period of significant growth is between 30 weeks and 1 year of age. Neurologic growth and maturation continue into adolescence. The best indicator of brain growth is head circumference. Head circumference increases six times during the first year of life. At birth, the cerebral cortex is one half adult thickness. The brain surface is initially smooth, but, with the advancing development that continues throughout childhood, the sulci deepen. Brain maturation includes increased interconnections between neurons and myelination of nerves. In a cephalocaudal and proximodistal sequence, myelination begins at the spinal cord and cranial nerves followed by myelination of the brain stem and corticospinal tracts.[1,2,6]

The first year of life is also filled with psychosocial developmental milestones for the infant. Basic needs must be met before the infant can accomplish these developmental tasks. Erikson described the development of a sense of trust as the task of the first stage.[16] If trust is not acquired, the infant develops mistrust of others and frustration with its inability to control the surrounding environment.

COMMON HEALTH PROBLEMS

The birth process is a critical event. Prenatal influences, birth trauma, and prematurity have an immediate impact on survival and health. The common health problems in this section have been divided into three sections: (1) health problems of the newborn, (2) special needs of the premature infant, and (3) health problems of the infant.

HEALTH PROBLEMS OF THE NEWBORN

Apgar Score. The Apgar score, devised by Dr. Virginia Apgar, is a scoring system that evaluates infant well-being at birth.[17] The system is composed of five categories (heart rate, respiratory effort, muscle tone, reflex irritability, color) with a total score ranging from 0 to 10 depending on the degree to which these qualities are presented. Evaluations are performed at 1 minute and 5 minutes after delivery. A score of 0 to 3 is indicative of severe distress; 4 to 6 of moderate distress; and 7 to 10 of mild to no distress. The majority of infants score from 6 to 7 at 1 minute and 8 to 9 at 5 minutes. If the score is 7 or less, the evaluation should be repeated every 5 minutes until a score of 7 or greater is obtained. An abnormal score at 5 minutes is more predictive of survival and neurologic outcome than at 1 minute.[7,15]

Birth Injuries. Injuries sustained during the birth process are responsible for a significant amount of neonatal mortality and morbidity. In 1988, birth injuries ranked as the eighth cause of death in the United States. Predisposing factors for birth injuries include macrosomia, prematurity, cephalopelvic disproportion, and dystocia (abnormal labor or childbirth).[7,18,19]

Caput succedaneum is a localized area of scalp edema caused by sustained pressure of the presenting part against the cervix. There is an accumulation of serum or blood above the periosteum from the high pressure caused from the obstruction. The caput succedaneum may extend across suture lines and have overlying petechiae, purpura, or ecchymosis. No treatment is needed, and it usually resolves over the first week of life.[7,19]

Cephalohematoma is a subperiosteal collection of blood from ruptured blood vessels. The margins are sharply delineated and do not cross suture lines. It is usually unilateral, but it may be bilateral and it usually occurs over the parietal area. The swelling may not be apparent for 24 to 48 hours because subperiosteal bleeding is slow. The overlying skin is not discolored. An underlying skull fracture may be present. Treatment is not needed unless the cephalohematoma is large and results in severe blood loss or significant hyperbilirubinemia. Skull fracture and intracranial hemorrhage are associated complications. An uncomplicated cephalohematoma usually resolves within 2 weeks to 3 months.[7, 19]

Skull fractures are uncommon because the infant's compressible skull is able to mold to fit the contours of the birth canal. But fractures can occur and usually follow a forceps delivery or severe contraction of the pelvis associated with prolonged, difficult labor. Skull fractures may be linear or depressed. Uncomplicated linear fractures are often asymptomatic and do not require treatment. Depressed skull fractures are observable by the palpable indentation of the infant's head. They require surgical intervention if there is compression of underlying brain tissue. A simple linear fracture usually heals within several months.[7, 19]

The *clavicle* is the most frequently fractured bone during the birth process. It is more common in LGA infants and occurs when delivery of the shoulders is difficult in vertex (head) or breech presentations. The infant may or may not demonstrate restricted motion of the upper extremity, but passive motion elicits pain. There may be discoloration or deformity, and, on palpation, crepitus (crackling sound from bones rubbing together) and irregularity may be found. Treatment consists of immobilizing the affected arm and shoulder and providing pain relief.[7, 19]

The *brachial plexuses* are situated above the clavicles in the anterolateral bases of the neck. They are composed of the spinal roots of the fifth cervical nerves through the first thoracic nerves. During vertex deliveries, excessive lateral traction of the head and neck away from the shoulders causes a stretch injury to the brachial plexus on that side. In a breech presentation, excessive lateral traction on the trunk before delivery of the head may tear the lower roots of the cervical cord. Also, if the breech presentation includes delivery with the arms overhead, an injury to the fifth and sixth cervical roots may result. When injury to the brachial plexus occurs, it causes paralysis of the upper extremity. The paralysis is often incomplete. Brachial plexus injuries include three types: (1) Erb-Duchenne paralysis (upper arm); (2) Klumpke's paralysis (lower arm); and (3) paralysis of the entire arm. Risk factors include difficult, traumatic delivery and LGA infants while trying to deliver the shoulders. Erb-Duchenne paralysis occurs with injury to the fifth and sixth cervical roots. It is the most common type of brachial plexus injury and

presents with variable degrees of paralysis of the shoulder and arm. The position of the affected arm is adducted and internally rotated, with extension at the elbow, pronation of the forearm, and flexion of the wrist. When the infant is lifted, the affected extremity is limp. The Moro reflex is impaired or absent. Grasp reflex is present.[7, 19]

Klumpke's paralysis results from injury to the eighth cervical and first thoracic roots. It is rare and presents with paralysis of the hand. The infant has wrist drop, the fingers are relaxed, and the grasp reflex is absent. The Moro reflex is impaired with the upper extremity extending and abducting normally while the wrist and fingers remain flaccid.

Treatment of brachial plexus injuries includes immobilization, appropriate positioning, and an exercise program. Most infants recover in 3 to 6 months. Recovery from lower arm paralysis is less successful, and the infant may develop a claw deformity.[7, 19]

Congenital Malformations. Congenital malformations are anatomic or structural abnormalities present at birth (see Chapter 4). They are a major cause of morbidity and mortality in children. In the perinatal period, 20% of deaths are attributed to congenital malformations. The malformations may be minor or major, detectable at birth or not detectable for years. Some stages of embryonic development are more at risk than others for development of congenital malformations after teratogen exposure. The causes of congenital malformations may be divided into genetic, environmental, or multifactorial.[5]

SPECIAL NEEDS OF THE PREMATURE INFANT

Infants born before 37 weeks gestation are considered premature. They often fall into the LBW category. The health of the LBW infant is directly related to its gestational age. Mortality and morbidity are increased in the premature population and are inversely proportional to the length of gestation. Therefore, the shorter the time of gestation, the more risk of death or disability. This is secondary to the immaturity of the organ systems, which interferes with the successful transition to an extrauterine life. Immaturity predisposes this population to the complications of prematurity. Also within this group are those premature infants who have grown abnormally during their shortened gestation, being either LGA or SGA. Abnormal growth places an added stress on their transition to extrauterine life.

Despite the advances in obstetric management in the past 30 years, the rate of premature delivery has not significantly changed. In the United States, over 9% of infants are born before 37 weeks gestation.

LBW and prematurity often go hand in hand. The majority of infants less than 2500 g and almost all less than 1500 g are premature. In the United States, LBW is responsible for two thirds of the neonatal deaths despite an increase in survival of the LBW infant. The birth rate of LBW infants was approximately 6.8% in 1985, and LBW accounted for 20% of all postnatal deaths. Contributing risk factors for prematurity are also associated with LBW. Risk factors associated with prematurity and LBW include maternal age (younger than 16, older than 35), race (African-American more than white), socioeconomic status, marital status (single more than married), smoking, substance abuse, malnutrition, poor or no prenatal care, medical risks predating pregnancy, and medical risks in current pregnancy.[7, 9]

The premature infant is poorly equipped to withstand the rigors of extrauterine transition. The organ systems are immature and may not be able to sustain life. The respiratory system may not be able to support gas exchange; the skin may be thin and gelatinous and easily damaged; the immune system is compromised and may not effectively fight infection; and the lack of subcutaneous fat puts the infant at risk for temperature instability. Complications of prematurity include respiratory distress syndrome (RDS), pulmonary hemorrhage, transient tachypnea, congenital pneumonia, pulmonary air leaks, bronchopulmonary dysplasia, recurrent apnea, glucose instability, hypocalcemia, hyperbilirubinemia, anemia, intraventricular hemorrhage, necrotizing enterocolitis (NEC), circulatory instability, hypothermia, bacterial or viral infection, retinopathy of prematurity, and disseminated intravascular coagulopathies.

Respiratory Problems. Respiratory distress syndrome (RDS), frequently referred to as hyaline membrane disease (HMD), is the most common complication of prematurity. In the United States, approximately 10% to 15% of infants less than 2500 g and 60% of infants at 29 weeks gestation develop RDS. The incidence of RDS is lower in African-American infants than in white infants and lower in female infants than in male infants. The primary problem is the lack of surfactant in the lungs. Surfactant is produced by type II alveolar cells in the lungs. It is a combination of several phospholipids that lowers the alveolar surface tension and facilitates lung expansion (see Chapters 26 and 27). At 24 weeks gestation, there are small amounts of surfactant as well as few terminal air sacs (primitive alveoli) with underdeveloped pulmonary vascularity. If an infant is born at this time, there is little chance of survival. By 26 to 28 weeks, there is usually sufficient surfactant and lung development to permit survival. The availability of exogenous surfactant replacement therapy has im-

proved the outcome of RDS and has been recognized as the main factor responsible for the 6.2% fall in the 1989/1990 infant mortality rate in the United States. However, because the survival of the sickest infants has improved and because their management is more complex, the incidence of complications has increased. These include air leak syndromes, bronchopulmonary dysplasia, and intracranial hemorrhage.[7, 20]

Apnea and periodic breathing are common problems in premature infants. The respiratory center in the medulla oblongata is underdeveloped in the premature infant; therefore, the ability for sustained ventilatory drive is often impaired. *Apnea* is defined as cessation of breathing; it is characterized by failure to breath for 20 seconds or more and is often accompanied by bradycardia or cyanosis. In infants less than 1.5 kg, 50% require intervention for significant apnea spells. Apnea may be due to an underlying disease process such as infection. This is not apnea of prematurity and should not be treated as such. *Periodic breathing* commonly occurs in those infants less than 1.8 kg. It is intermittent failure to breathe in durations less than 10 seconds to 15 seconds. Management of apnea and periodic breathing includes use of medications or ventilatory support until the CNS is developed and able to sustain adequate ventilatory drive.[7, 20]

Intraventricular Hemorrhage. Intraventricular hemorrhage (IVH) is a common problem almost exclusive to premature infants. It is a common problem, second only to RDS as the major cause of death in the premature infant. In infants less than 35 weeks gestation or 1400 g birth weight, the incidence is 40% to 50% with the most immature at the highest risk of IVH. The hemorrhage often occurs in a subependymal germinal matrix layer. This is a periventricular structure located between the caudate nucleus and the thalamus at the level of or slightly posterior to the foramen of Monro. The germinal matrix is an early developmental structure that contains a fragile vascular area that is poorly supported by connective tissue. By term, this structure is gone.

Risk factors for IVH include pneumothorax, hypotension, acidosis, coagulopathy, transport, volume expansion, and bicarbonate infusion. Mechanisms for cause of IVH include an hypoxic-ischemic insult resulting in cerebral hyperperfusion in their germinal matrix area causing vessel rupture. Another proposed mechanism is disruption of vascular integrity in the germinal matrix caused by hypotension, and, if followed by an increase in arterial pressure, rupture of damaged capillaries results. Four grades of hemorrhage have been identified.[7, 21] The majority of hemorrhages resolve, but the more severe hemorrhages may lead to an obstruction to the flow of cerebrospinal fluid causing a progressive hydrocephalus.

Necrotizing Enterocolitis. Necrotizing enterocolitis (NEC) is an acquired gastrointestinal disease process that is a major problem in preterm infants. The incidence is 1% to 5% of admissions to the neonatal intensive care unit (NICU). Although, approximately 90% of infants affected are preterm infants less than 1500 g, 10% of infants affected are term infants. Mortality varies from 20% to 40%. The exact etiology of NEC is unknown but is thought to be multifactorial. Risk factors for NEC include birth asphyxia, umbilical artery catheterization, patent ductus arteriosus, polycythemia, enteral feeding, and medications such as indomethacin, vitamin E, and xanthines.[22] There is agreement that the process begins with diminished perfusion of the intestinal wall, which results in ischemia and hypoxia that leads to necrosis and gangrene. Although bacterial infection plays a role in the disease, it is not thought to be the initiating event. Milk feeding has been implicated. Approximately 93% of infants who develop NEC have been fed enterally.[12] Human milk and commercial formulas serve as substrates for bacterial growth in the gut.

The ileum is most commonly affected, followed by the ascending colon, cecum, transverse colon, and rectosigmoid. The necrosis of the intestine may be superficial, affecting only the mucosa or submucosa, or may extend through the entire intestinal wall. Perforation can occur and lead to peritonitis.

The manifestations of NEC are variable, but the usual presentation includes abdominal distention, gastric aspirates, bilious stools, lethargy, apnea, and hypoperfusion. The infant often appears septic. Laboratory examination may reveal leukocytosis or leukopenia, neutropenia, thrombocytopenia, glucose instability, electrolyte imbalance, metabolic acidosis, hypoxia, hypercapnia, and disseminated intravascular coagulation (DIC). Blood cultures are positive only about 30% of the time. Microorganisms reported in NEC include *Escherichia coli*, *Klebsiella*, enterobacter, *Pseudomonas*, *Salmonella*, *Clostridium difficile*, and *Clostridium perfringens*.[22]

Clinical diagnosis is primarily radiographic. The radiographic hallmark of NEC is pneumatosis intestinalis or intramural air. Pneumoperitoneum is indicative of intestinal perforation. A large stationary distended loop of intestine on repeated x-rays may indicate gangrene, whereas a gasless abdomen may indicate peritonitis.[22]

Treatment includes cessation of feedings, stomach decompression, broad-spectrum antibiotic coverage, and supportive treatment. Intestinal perforation requires surgical intervention. Intestinal resection of dead intestine with diverting ostomy is the procedure of choice.[21, 22]

HEALTH PROBLEMS OF THE INFANT

Infants are prone to numerous health problems during the first year of life. They may become serious if not recognized and treated appropriately. A significant amount may be precipitated by the relative immaturity of the organ systems. Infants are prone to have nutritional disturbances, feeding difficulties, problems with food allergies, gastroesophageal reflux, and colic. Injuries, the major cause of death during infancy, are due to events such as aspiration of foreign objects, suffocation, motor vehicle accidents, falls, poisoning, burns, and drowning. Childhood diseases may be a problem if the infant is not adequately immunized.

Nutrition. Good nutrition is important during infancy because of the rapid growth that occurs. Human milk or commercial infant formulas form the basis for the early nutritional needs of the newborn and young infant. The American Academy of Pediatrics recommends breast-feeding for the first 12 months of life. Human milk from a well-nourished mother is easily digested and typically provides sufficient nutrients and calories for normal growth and development. Human milk also has the added benefit of offering some immune protection to the infant in most cases. Fluoride is added from birth, and iron is added at approximately 6 months of age when the fetal iron stores are depleted.

Mothers who do not choose to breast-feed their child or who are unable to breast-feed may choose a commercial formula. Several companies produce infant formulas that contain the essential nutrients for infants. Although there are some minor differences, most infant formulas are similar, regardless of which company produced the formula.

Some infants may experience difficulties in consuming mother's milk or infant formulas that are based on cow's milk, due to lactase deficiency. Lastase is an enzyme that breaks down lactose, the carbohydrate found in human milk and cow's milk. There are infant formulas available that contain carbohydrates other than lactose. These formulas are made from soy beans. Other feeding intolerances may also occur. Treatment of any milk or formula intolerance depends on identification of the specific offender and elimination of it from the diet. Newborns and infants frequently exhibit ''spitting up'' or regurgitation of formula, despite the absence of a formula intolerance. Generally, cow's milk-based formulas are preferable to soy-based formulas, and changing to a soy-based formula should only be undertaken when there is a proven case of intolerance. Thus, it is important that all claims of formula intolerance be thoroughly investigated before an infant is changed to a soy-based formula. Education of the parents about the signs and symptoms of intolerance, as well as reassurance that "spitting up" of formulas is normal, may be all that is required. An infant who is gaining weight, appears alert and well-nourished, has adequate stools, and demonstrates normal hunger is unlikely to have a formula intolerance.

One area of infant nutrition that is still subject to much variation is the introduction of solid foods. There is a great deal of variation regarding when to start solid foods and what solid foods to introduce. Generally, human milk or iron-fortified infant formulas should supply the majority of infant nutrition during the first year of life. However, solid foods are usually introduced beginning at 6 months. When solid foods are being introduced, they should be considered as supplemental to the total nutrition and not as the main component of nutrition. Solid foods should be introduced only by spoon feeding. The addition of cereal to formula in bottle or in "infant feeders" is not recommended. It has never been shown that early introduction of solid foods causes the infant to sleep longer at night. Bland infant cereals, such as rice cereal, are usually introduced first. Slow progression to the addition of individual vegetables, fruits, and, finally, meats occurs as the infant learns to chew and swallow food. Infants also become able to drink from a cup rather than a bottle during this time. The addition of desserts is not recommended because these add calories without adding substantial nutrition. Sometime between 9 months and 12 months, the infant's intake of solid foods and formula increases and infant can be weaned from the breast or bottle. Much anxiety can accompany weaning, so it should be done gradually. Mothers may need reassurance that their infant is progressing normally at that time.

Irritable Infant Syndrome or Colic. Colic is generally defined as paroxysmal abdominal pain or cramping in an infant and is usually manifested by loud crying, drawing up of the legs to the abdomen, and extreme irritability. Episodes of colic may last from several minutes to several hours a day. During this time, most efforts to soothe the infant or relieve the distress are not successful. Colic is most common in infants under 3 months of age but can persist for up to 9 months. Caring for an infant with colic can be frustrating. There is no one single etiologic factor that causes colic; therefore, the treatment of colic is not precise. Many nonmedical techniques as well as pharmacologic preparations such antispasmodics, sedatives, and antiflatulents have been tried. Non-

pharmacologic interventions should be attempted before administration of drugs. Support of the parents is probably the single most important factor in treatment of colic. Many times the mother (or primary care provider) may be afraid to state just how frustrated she is with her inability to console the infant. An open discussion of this frustration can help the mothers or care providers recognize that their feelings of frustration are normal; frequently, this gives them the added support needed to deal with their infant.

Failure to Thrive. Failure to thrive is a term that refers to inadequate growth of the child from the inability to obtain or use essential nutrients. Failure to thrive may be organic or nonorganic (see Chapter 45). Organic failure to thrive is the result of a physiologic cause that prevents the infant from obtaining or using nutrients appropriately. An example of organic failure to thrive is inadequate growth of an infant with deficient energy reserve due to a congenital defect that makes sucking and feeding difficult. Inorganic failure to thrive is the result of psychological factors that prevent adequate intake of nutrition. An example of nonorganic failure to thrive is inadequate weight gain caused by inadequate intake of nutrients due to parental neglect.

Diagnosis as to the type of failure to thrive depends on careful examination and history of the infant and serial follow-up and evaluation. An individual infant's growth can be compared to the standards for normal growth and development. Cases of organic failure to thrive are usually easier to diagnose than cases of nonorganic failure to thrive. Diagnosis of nonorganic failure to thrive requires extensive investigation of history, family situation, relationship of the care provider to the infant, and evaluation of feeding practices. The nonorganic basis should be considered early in every case of failure to thrive.

Therapy for failure to thrive depends on the etiology. Because long-term nutritional deficiencies can result in impaired physical and intellectual growth, provision of optimal nutrition is essential. Methods to increase nutritional intake by adjusting caloric density of the formula or by parenteral nutrition may be required in cases of organic failure to thrive.

Sudden Infant Death Syndrome. Sudden infant death syndrome (SIDS) or crib death refers to sudden unexplained death of an infant under 1 year of age, after autopsy, investigation of the death scene, and review of the history. SIDS is the leading cause of death in infants between 1 month and 1 year of age. Approximately 7000 infants succumb to SIDS each year.[24, 25]

The exact cause of SIDS is unknown. Theories of

etiology center on brain stem abnormality, which prevents effective control of cardiorespiratory control. Features of SIDS included prolonged sleep apnea, increased frequency of brief inspiratory pauses, excessive periodic breathing, and impaired response to increased carbon dioxide or decreased oxygen. A diagnosis of SIDS can only be made if an autopsy is performed to rule out other causes of death. Differentiation of child abuse from SIDS is an important consideration, and each case of SIDS must be subjected to careful examination.

Support of the family of an infant with SIDS is crucial. Parents frequently feel guilty or inadequate as parents. The fact that there must be close scrutiny to differentiate a SIDS death from a death by child abuse adds to the guilt and disappointment felt by the family. It is important that once a diagnosis of SIDS is made, that the parents and other family members receive information about SIDS. Health care providers need to be fully aware of resources available to families with a SIDS death. The siblings of the child who died should not be overlooked. Children also need information and support to get through the grief process. Children may blame themselves for the death or fear that they, too, will die of SIDS. Yet, many times, they are not given information because the adults are trying to protect them.

Injuries. Injuries are the major cause of death in infants between 6 months and 12 months of age. Aspiration of foreign objects, suffocation, falls, poisonings, drowning, burns, and other bodily damage may occur because of the infant's increasing ability to investigate the environment. Childproofing the environment can be an important precaution to prevent injuries. No home or environment can be completely childproofed, however; close supervision of the child by a competent care provider is essential to prevent injury.

Motor vehicle accidents are responsible for a significant number of infant deaths. After 1 year of age, motor vehicle accidents become the number one cause of accidental death. Most states require that infants be placed in an approved infant safety restraint while riding in a vehicle. The middle of the back seat is considered the safest place for the infant to ride. Many hospitals do not discharge a baby unless there is a safety restraint system in the car. If a family cannot afford a restraint system, programs are available that donate or loan the family a restraint. Health care providers must be involved in educating the public about the dangers of carrying infants in vehicles without taking proper precautions to protect them.

Immunizations. One of the most dramatic improvements in infant health has been related to wide-spread immunization of infants and children to the major childhood communicable diseases including diphtheria, pertussis, tetanus, polio, measles, mumps, rubella, hepatitis, and *Hemophilus influenzae* (type B). Immunizations to these infectious diseases have greatly reduced morbidity and mortality of infants and young children. These immunizations are given at standard times as part of health promotion in infants and children. However, these immunization programs have not completely eradicated these diseases but have only lowered their prevalence. Immunization programs are only effective if all children receive the immunizations. Although most immunizations can be received through local health departments at no or low cost, many infants or young children do not routinely receive immunizations or do not receive the full regimen of immunizations. Methods to improve compliance and access to immunizations continue to be needed.

In summary, infancy is defined as that period of time from birth to 18 months. During this time, growth and development are ongoing. The relative immaturity of many of the organ systems places the infant at risk for a variety of illnesses. Birth initiates many changes in the organ systems as a means of adjusting to postnatal life. The birth process is a critical event, and maladjustments and injuries during the birth process are a major cause of death or disability. Premature delivery is a significant health problem in the United States. The premature infant is at risk for numerous health problems secondary to the interruption of intrauterine growth and immaturity of organ systems.

■ EARLY CHILDHOOD

Early childhood is considered the period of 18 months through 5 years. During this time, the child passes through the stages of toddler (18 months to 3 years) and preschooler (3 years through 5 years). There are many changes as the child moves from infancy through the toddler and preschool years. The major achievements are the development and refinement of locomotion and language, which take place as children progress from dependence to independence.[7, 20]

GROWTH AND DEVELOPMENT

Early childhood is a period of continued physical growth and maturation. Compared with infancy, physical growth is not as dramatic. Weight gain during the toddler stage is 1.8 to 2.7 kg per year (an average of 2.3 kg per year). At 2 years, the average weight is 12 kg, and by 2½ years the birth weight has quadrupled. By the preschool years, growth slows considerably. The average weight gain is still approximately 2.3 kg per year, and almost all organ systems have reached full maturity. At 3 years, the average weight is 14.5 kg, and by 6 years it has increased to 21 kg. During early childhood, height increases an average 7.5 cm per year and is primarily through increase in leg length. At 2 years of age, the average height is 86.6 cm, and by 6 years it has reached 116 cm. In the first 2 years of life, head circumference increases by 2.5 cm per year. After 2 years of age, head circumference growth slows, and, by 5 years, the average increase in head circumference is 1.25 cm per year.[1,15]

The maturation of organ systems is ongoing during early childhood. The respiratory system continues its growth and maturation, but, because of the relative immaturity of the airway structures, otitis media and respiratory infections are common. The barrel-shaped chest that is characteristic of infancy has begun to change to a more adult shape. The respiratory rate of infancy has slowed and averages 20 to 30 beats/min. Respirations remain abdominal until 7 years of age.[1,15]

Neural growth remains rapid during early childhood. All brain cells are present by 12 months of age. Growth is primarily hypertrophic. The brain is 90% of adult size by 2 years of age. The cephalocaudal, proximodistal principle is followed as myelinization of the cortex, brain stem, and spinal cord is completed. The spinal cord is completely myelinated by 2 years of age. At that time, the control of anal and urethral sphincter and the motor skills of locomotion can be achieved and mastered. The continuing maturation of the neuromuscular system is increasingly evident as complex gross and fine motor skills are acquired throughout early childhood.

Growth and maturation in the musculoskeletal system continue with ossification of the skeletal system, growth of the legs, and changes in muscle and fat proportions. Legs grow faster than the trunk in early childhood; after the first year of life, 66% of the increase in height is leg growth. Muscle growth is balanced by a corresponding decrease in adipose tissue accumulation.[19,20]

During early childhood, many important psychosocial tasks are mastered by the child. Independence begins to develop, and the child is on the way to becoming a social being in control of the environment. Development and refinement of gross and fine motor abilities allow involvement with an infinite amount of tasks and activities. Learning is ongoing and progressive and includes interactions with others, appropriate social behavior, and sex role functions. Erikson described the tasks that must be accomplished in early childhood.[16] The toddler must acquire a sense of autonomy while overcoming a sense of doubt and shame. The preschooler must acquire a sense of initiative and develop a conscience.[1,15]

COMMON HEALTH PROBLEMS

Early childhood years can pose significant health risks to the growing and maturing child. Injuries are the leading cause of death in children ages 1 to 4 years. Only adolescents have more. Locomotion together with a lack of awareness of danger places toddlers and preschoolers at special risk for injuries. Motor vehicle accidents are responsible for almost 50% of all accidental deaths in this group. Many of the injuries and deaths can be prevented by appropriate restraints in car seats and seatbelts. Other major causes of injuries include drowning, burns, poisoning, falls, aspiration and suffocation, and bodily damage.[1,15]

Infectious diseases can be a problem for children during early childhood because of their susceptibility. This may also be the time when children first enter day care, which increases their exposure to other children as well as infectious diseases. The major disorders include the communicable childhood diseases (chickenpox, measles, roseola, mumps, pertussis, rubella, scarlet fever), conjunctivitis, and intestinal parasitic infections.[1,15]

Child maltreatment is an increasing problem in the United States. In 1985, over 1.9 million cases of abuse were reported to child protective services. Child maltreatment includes neglect (physical and emotional), physical abuse, and sexual abuse. Neglect is the most common type of maltreatment and can take the form of deprivation of basic necessities or failure to meet the child's emotional needs. It is often attributed to poor parenting skills. Physical abuse is the deliberate infliction of injury. The cause is probably multifactorial with predisposing factors that include the parent, child, and environment. Sexual abuse is on the rise and includes a spectrum of types. The typical abuser is male. Children often do not report the abuse because they are afraid of not being believed.[1,15]

In summary, early childhood is defined as that period of time from 18 months to 5 years of age—the toddler and preschool years. Growth and development continue but are not as dramatic as during the prenatal and infancy periods. Early childhood is a time when the majority of organ systems reach maturity and the child becomes an independent, mobile being. There continues to be significant health risks during this period, especially in regards to infectious diseases and injuries. Injuries are the leading cause of death during this period. Child abuse is rapidly increasing as a major health problem during this period of development.

■ EARLY SCHOOL YEARS TO LATE CHILDHOOD

In this text, early school years or late childhood is defined as the period in which a child begins school through the beginning of adolescence. These 6 years involve a great deal of change, but when one recollects "childhood," these are the years most often remembered. The experiences of this period have a profound effect on the physical, cognitive, and psychosocial development of the child, which, in turn, influence the adult that the child will become.

GROWTH AND DEVELOPMENT

Although physical growth is steady throughout the early school years, it is slower than the previous periods and the adolescent period to follow. During late childhood, children typically gain approximately 2 to 3 kg and grow an average of 5 cm per year. The average 6-year-old child is 116 cm tall and weighs about 21 kg. By age 12, the same child may weigh 40 kg and be 150 cm tall. There is only a slight difference in the body sizes of males and females during this period, with boys being just a little taller and heavier than girls.[1, 15]

During late childhood, a child's legs grow longer, posture improves, and their center of gravity descends to a lower point. These changes make children more graceful and help them be successful at climbing, bike riding, roller skating, and other physical activities. Body fat distribution decreases and, in combination with the lengthening skeleton, gives the child a thinner appearance. As the body fat decreases, lean muscle mass increases. By age 12, both boys and girls have doubled their body strength and physical capabilities. Although muscular strength increases, the muscles are still relatively immature and injury from overstrenuous activities, such as difficult sports, can occur. With the gains in length, the head circumference decreases in relation to the height, waist circumference decreases in relation to height, and leg length increases in relation to height.[1, 15]

Facial proportions change as the face grows faster in relation to the rest of the cranium. The brain and skull grow very little during late childhood. Primary teeth are lost and replaced by permanent teeth. When the permanent teeth first appear, they may appear to be too big for the mouth and face. This is a temporary imbalance that is alleviated as the face grows.[1, 15]

Caloric requirements usually are lower when compared to previous periods and to the adolescent period to follow. Cardiac growth is slow. Heart rate and respiratory rates continue to decrease, and blood pressure gradually rises. Growth of the eye continues, and the normal farsightedness of the preschool child is gradually converted to 20/20 vision by about 11 to 12 years. Frequent vision assessment is recommended during late childhood as part of normal routine health screenings.[1, 15]

Bone ossification continues, but mineralization is not completed. Bones cannot resist muscle pressure and pull as well as mature bones. Precautions should be taken to prevent alterations in bone structure, such as providing properly fitting shoes and adequate desks to prevent poor posture. Children should be routinely checked for scoliosis (see Chapter 57) often during this period.

Toward the end of late childhood, the physical differences between the two sexes become apparent. Females usually enter pubescence about 2 years before males, resulting in noticeable differences in height, weight, and development of secondary sex characteristics. There is also a lot of individual variation among children of the same sex. These differences can be extremely difficult for children to cope with.

Entry into the school setting has a major impact on the psychosocial development of the child at this age. The child begins to form relationships with other children, forming groups. Peers become more important as the child moves out of the security of the family and into the bigger world. Usually during this period children begin to form closer bonds with individual "best friends." However, the best friend relationships may frequently change. The personality of the person begins to appear. Although the personality is still developing, the basic temperament and approach to life become apparent. Although changes in personality occur with maturity, the basic elements may not change. The major task of this stage, as identified by Erikson, is the development of industry or accomplishment.[16] Failure to meet this task results in a sense of inferiority or incompetence, which can impede further progress.

COMMON HEALTH PROBLEMS

Because of the high level of immune system competence in late childhood, children have an immunologic advantage over earlier years. Respiratory infections are the leading cause of illness at this time, followed by gastrointestinal disorders. The chief cause of mortality is accidents, primarily motor vehicle accidents. Immunization against the major communicable diseases of childhood has greatly improved the health of children in their early childhood years.

Health promotion includes appropriate dental care. The incidence of dental caries has decreased since the addition of fluoride to most water systems in the United States. However, there is still a high incidence of dental caries during late childhood that is related to inadequate dental care and a high amount of sugar in their diet. Children at the early part of this stage may not be as effective in brushing their teeth and may require adult assistance, but they may be reluctant to allow parental help. Infections with bacterial and fungal agents are a common problem in childhood. These infections commonly occur as respiratory, gastrointestinal, or skin diseases. Infections of the skin occur more frequently in this age group than in any other age group, probably related to increased exposure to skin lesions.

Other acute or chronic health problems may surface for the first time. Asthma, caused by allergic reactions, frequently manifests for the first time during the early school years. Epilepsy may also first be diagnosed during this period. Many childhood cancers also may appear. Developmental disabilities or specific learning disabilities may initially become apparent as the child enters school.

In summary, early school years to late childhood are defined as that period of time from beginning school through adolescence. During these 6 years, growth is steady but much slower than in the previous periods. Entry into school begins the formation of relationships with peers and has a major impact on psychological development. This is a wonderful period of relatively good health secondary to an immunologic advantage, but respiratory disease poses a leading cause of illness and motor vehicles accidents are the major cause of death. Several chronic health problems such as asthma, epilepsy, and childhood cancers may surface during this time.

■ ADOLESCENCE

Adolescence is a transitional period between childhood and adulthood. During adolescence, there are significant physical, social, psychological, and cognitive changes. The changes of adolescence do not occur on a strict timeline; instead, the changes occur at different times according to a unique internal calendar known only to the person. For definition's sake, adolescence is considered to begin with the development of secondary sex characteristics around 11 or 12 years of age, and to end with the completion of somatic growth from about 18 to 20 years of age. Females generally begin and end adolescence earlier than males. The adolescent period is conveniently referred to as the "teen-aged years" from age 13 years through 19 years.

GROWTH AND DEVELOPMENT

Adolescence is influenced by hormonal activity influenced by the CNS. Physical growth occurs simultaneously with sexual maturation.

Adolescents typically experience gains of 20% to 25% in linear growth. An adolescent "growth spurt," which lasts approximately 24 to 36 months, accounts for the majority of this somatic growth. The age at onset, the duration, and the extent of the growth vary between males and females and among individuals. In females, the growth spurt usually begins around 10 to 14 years of age. It begins earlier in females than in males and ends earlier with less dramatic changes in weight and height. Females generally gain about 5 to 20 cm in height and from 7 to 25 kg in weight. Most females have completed their growth spurt by age 16 or 17 years. Males begin their growth spurt later, but it is usually more pronounced with an increase in height of from 10 to 30 cm and an increase in weight from 7 to 30 kg. Males may continue to gain in height until age 18 to 20 years. Increases in height are possible until about 25 years of age.[26]

The changes in physical body size are not random but have a characteristic pattern. Growth in arms, legs, hands, feet, and neck appear first, then increases in hip and chest sizes occur, followed in several months by increases in shoulder width and depth and increases in trunk length. These changes may be difficult for the adolescent and parents. Adolescents may change shoe sizes several times over several months. Although brain size is not significantly increased during adolescence, the size and shape of the skull and facial bones change. The features of the face may appear to be out of proportion until full adult growth is attained.[1,26]

Muscle mass and strength also increase during adolescence. Sometimes there may be a discrepancy between the growth of bone and muscle mass, creating a temporary dysfunction with slower or less smooth movements resulting from the mismatch of bone and muscle. Body proportions undergo typical changes during adolescence. In males, the thorax becomes broader, and the pelvis remains narrow. In females, the opposite occurs: the thorax remains narrow and the pelvis widens.

Organ systems also undergo changes in function, and some actually have changes in structure. The heart increases in size as the result of increased muscle cell size. Heart rate decreases to normal adult rates, whereas blood pressure increases rapidly to adult rates. Circulating blood volume and hemoglobin concentration increase. Males demonstrate greater changes in blood volume and higher hemoglobin concentrations, due to the influence of testosterone and the relatively higher muscle mass.

With adolescence, skin become thicker and additional hair growth occurs in both sexes. Sebaceous and sweat gland activity increases. Plugged sebaceous glands frequently result in acne (see Chapter 11). Increased sweat gland activity results in perspiration and body odor. The eyes undergo changes that may contribute to increased myopia. Auditory acuity actually peaks in adolescence and begins to decline after about age 13. Voice changes are of significant importance during adolescence for both sexes; however, the change is more pronounced in males. The voice change results from the growth of the larynx. There is more growth of the larynx of males than females. The paranasal sinuses reach adult proportion, which increases the resonance of the voice, adding to the adult sound of the voice.[1, 26]

Changes in the endocrine system are of great importance in the initiation and continuation of the adolescent growth spurt. The hormones involved include growth hormone (GH), thyroid hormones, adrenal hormones, insulin, and the gonadotropic hormones. GH regulates growth in childhood but is essentially replaced by sex hormones as the primary impetus for growth during adolescence. The exact role of GH in the adolescent growth spurt is unclear. Thyroid hormone, a significant hormone in the regulation of metabolism during childhood, continues to be important during adolescence. Again, the relationship of thyroid hormone to the other hormones and its role in the adolescent growth spurt is unclear. The thyroid gland become larger during adolescence, and it is believed that production of thyroid hormones is increased during this period. Insulin is necessary for appropriate growth at all stages, including adolescence. Insulin must be present for GH to be effective. The pancreatic islets of Langerhans increase in size during adolescence.[1, 15, 26]

The anterior pituitary gland produces the gonadotropic hormones, follicle-stimulating hormone (FSH), and luteinizing hormone (LH). These hormones influence target organs to secrete sex hormones. The ovaries respond by secreting estrogens and progesterone, and the testes by producing androgens, resulting in the maturation of the primary sex characteristics and the appearance of secondary sex characteristics. Primary sex characteristics are those involved in reproductive function (internal and external genitalia). The secondary sex characteristics are the physical signs that signal the presence of sexual maturity but are not directly involved in reproduction (pubic and axillary hair). Androgens initiate the beginning of the growth spurt. Sex hormones, including androgens, also conclude height growth by causing bone age maturity, epiphyseal closure of bones, and discontinuation of skeletal growth.

The dramatic and extensive physical changes that occur during the transition from child to adult are matched only by the psychosocial changes that occur during the adolescent period. It is not possible to develop one "guide" that adequately describes and explains the tremendous changes that occur during adolescence because the experience is unique for each adolescent. There are, fortunately, some commonalities within the process, which can be used to facilitate understanding of the changes. The transition from child to adult is not a smooth, continuous, or uniform process. There are frequent periods of rapid change, followed by brief plateaus. These periods can change with little or no warning, which makes living with an adolescent difficult at times.

One fact that people who deal with adolescents must remember is that, no matter how rocky the transition from child to adult, adolescence is not a permanent disability! Eighty percent of adolescents go through adolescence with little or no lasting difficulties. Health care professionals who care for adolescents may need to offer support to worried parents that the difficulties their adolescent is experiencing, and that the entire family is experiencing as a result, may be normal. The adolescent may also need reassurance that his or her feelings are not abnormal.[1, 15, 26]

Common concerns identified by adolescents include conflicts with parents, conflicts with siblings, concerns about school, and concerns about peers and peer relationships. Personal identity is an overwhelming concern expressed by adolescents. Common health problems experienced by adolescents are headache, stomach ache, and insomnia. These disorders may be psychosomatic in origin. Adolescents also may exhibit situational anxiety and mild depression. The health care worker may need to refer adolescents for specialized counseling or medical care if any of the health care concerns are exaggerated.

Parents of adolescents may also have concerns about their child during the adolescent period. Common concerns related to the adolescent's behavior include: rebelliousness, wasting time, risk-taking behaviors, mood swings, drug experimentation, school problems, psychosomatic complaints, and sexual activity.[19, 20, 32] Several "tasks" that adolescents need to fulfill have been identified. These tasks include: (1) achieving independence from parents, (2) adopting peer codes and making personal lifestyle choices, (3) forming or revising individual body image and coming to terms with one's body image if it is not "perfect," and (4) establishing sexual, ego, vocational, and moral identities.[26] The period of adolescence is one of transition from childhood to adulthood. It is filled with conflicts as the adolescent attempts to "take on" an adult role. Communication with the adolescent and family can help make the transition less stressful.

COMMON HEALTH PROBLEMS

Adolescence is considered to be a relatively healthy period; however, significant morbidity and mortality do occur. Health promotion is of extreme importance during the adolescent period. There are fewer actual physical health problems during this period, but there is a greater risk of morbidity and mortality from other causes, such as accidents, homicide, or suicide. Several factors contribute to the risk for injury during adolescence. The adolescent is unable to predict potentially dangerous situations, possibly due to a discrepancy between physical maturity and cognitive and emotional development. Certain behavioral and developmental characteristics of the adolescent exaggerate this problem. Adolescents may feel the need to challenge parental or other authority. They also have a strong desire to "fit in" with the peer group. Adolescents exhibit a type of magical thinking and have a need to experiment with potentially dangerous situations or behaviors.

Over 80% of deaths during adolescence are attributed to injuries. Leading causes of nonintentional injuries are automobile accidents (#1), motorcycle accidents, and drowning (#2). Other accidental injuries include falls, striking objects, firearm mishaps (#3), and sports. Accidental injuries kill more adolescents every year than all other causes of death combined, with males accounting for four out of five injury victims. Automobile accidents account for 50% of all deaths of adolescents from ages 16 through 19.[1, 15, 26] Drowning, which is more common in males than females, decreases in prevalence after age 18. Most drownings occur on weekends, from May through August, are associated with alcohol use, and occur in fresh water rather than in the ocean. Firearm injuries are the third leading cause of nonintentional mortality in adolescents. Firearm accidents occur much more frequently to males between the ages of 15 to 24 than to males of any other age.[1] Many of these accidents occur in the adolescent's home while cleaning or playing with the gun.

Other nonintentional causes of death include poisoning, skateboard injuries, all-terrain vehicle (ATV) accidents, and participation in sports. However, the majority of sports injuries are not fatal. Approximately one-third to one-half of all injuries occur in the school. Falls are the most common cause of injury in high schools, with contusions, abrasions, swelling, sprains, strains, and dislocations being the most common injuries.[1, 26] Cancer is the fourth leading cause of death in adolescents, but it is the leading cause of death from nonviolent sources. There is an increased incidence of certain types of cancer during adolescence, including lymphomas, Hodgkin's disease, and bone and genital tumors. Leukemia is the leading cause of cancer mortality in people aged 15 to 24 years.[26]

Adolescents also are subject to intentional injuries, such as homicide and suicide. Suicide rates have risen dramatically in adolescents since the 1950s, to approximately 13 to 14 per 100,000. Most of the increase can be attributed to the greater number of suicides committed by white males. It is also thought that the actual rate of adolescent suicide may be higher than what is reported, due to underreporting on death certificates.[26] Almost 60% of suicides involved firearms.

The increasing prevalence of sexual activity among adolescents has created unique health problems. These include adolescent pregnancy, sexually transmitted diseases, and human immunodeficiency virus (HIV) transmission. Associated problems include substance abuse, such as alcohol, tobacco, inhalants, and other illicit drugs. Health care providers must not neglect discussing sexual activity with the adolescent. Nonjudgmental, open, factual communication is essential for dealing with an adolescent's sexual practices. Discussion of sexual activity is frequently difficult for the adolescent and the adolescent's family. If a relationship exists between the adolescent and the health care provider, this may provide a valuable forum for the adolescent to get accurate information about safe sex, including contraception and avoidance of high-risk behaviors for acquiring sexually transmitted diseases or acquired immunodeficiency syndrome (AIDS).[26]

Substance abuse among adolescents increased rapidly in the 1960s and 1970s but has declined since that time. However, substance abuse is still prevalent in the adolescent age group. Health care workers must be knowledgeable about the symptoms of drug abuse, the consequences of drug abuse, and the appropriate management of adolescents with substance abuse problems. Substance abuse among adolescents includes tobacco products, both cigarettes and "smokeless" tobacco (e.g., snuff and chewing tobacco). Other substances include alcohol, marijuana, stimulants, inhalants, cocaine, hallucinogens, tranquilizers, and sedatives. Adolescents are at high risk for succumbing to the peer pressure to participate in substance abuse. They have a strong desire to "fit in" and be accepted by their peer group. It is difficult for them to "just say no." Adolescents also are "magical thinkers." They just don't believe that they will get "hooked" or that the bad consequences will happen to them. Additionally, adolescents, as well as the rest of society, are constantly bombarded with the glamorous side of substance use. Television shows, movies, and magazine advertisements, just to name a few examples, are filled with beautiful, healthy, successful, happy, and popular people who are smoking cigarettes or drinking beer or other alcoholic beverages. Adolescents are trying to achieve that lifestyle depicted in those ads—it takes tremendous willpower to resist that temptation. It is important that adolescents be provided with "the rest of the story" through education and constant communication.[1, 26]

Pregnancy has become a major problem of the teen years. Statistics from the Guttmacher Institute (1990) reveal that approximately 1 million of the 9 million adolescents in the United States become pregnant annually.[33] Four out of every 10 teenage females become pregnant before reaching age 20. One fifth of all pregnancies occur within the first month after beginning sexual activity; one half occur within the first 6 months of sexual activity. Of the slightly over 1 million adolescent pregnancies, 47% delivered, 40% had therapeutic abortions, and 13% had spontaneous abortions. Adolescent pregnancy carries significant risks to the mother and to the fetus or newborn. The topic of adolescent pregnancy involves issues related to physical and biologic maturity of the adolescent, growth requirements of the adolescent and fetus, and unique prenatal care requirements of the pregnant adolescent. Additionally, emotional and psychological issues regarding relationships of the adolescent within her family and with the father of the baby, as well as how the pregnancy will affect the future of the adolescent, must be considered.[32]

In summary, adolescence is a transitional period between childhood and adulthood. It begins with development of secondary sex characteristics (11 to 12 years) and ends with cessation of somatic growth (18 to 20 years). This is a period of major growth spurt, which is more pronounced in males. The endocrine system is of great importance with its numerous hormonal changes and their initiation and continuation of the growth spurt. Psychosocial changes are just as major as the physical changes during this period and often place tremendous pressure on relationships between adults and the adolescent.

Adolescence is a relatively healthy period, but significant morbidity and mortality exist from accidents, homicide, and suicide. The increasing prevalence of sexual activity and substance abuse places the adolescent at risk for HIV infection, alcohol, tobacco, and other drug abuse, as well as adolescent pregnancy.

■ REFERENCES

1. Wong, D.L., & Rollins, J.H. (1993). *Essentials of pediatric nursing* (pp. 3–4, 105–156, 343–365, 423–444, 446–466). St. Louis: Mosby–Year book.
2. Whaley, L.F. & Wong, D.L. (1991). *Nursing care of infants and children* (pp. 4–28, 78–100, 268–309). St. Louis: Mosby–Year Book.
3. Infant Mortality—United States, 1989. *Morbidity and Mortality Weekly Report, 42*(5).
4. Behrman, R.E. (Ed.). (1992). *Nelson textbook of pediatrics* (14th ed., pp. 13–43). Philadelphia: W.B. Saunders.
5. Hermanson, M. (1990). *Biostatistics: Some basic concepts.* Patterson, NY: Caduceus Medical Publishers.
6. Moore, K.L. (1988). *The developing human* (4th ed.). Philadelphia: W.B. Saunders.
7. Korones, S.B. (1986). Significance of the relationship of birth weight to gestational age. In S.B. Korones (Ed.). *High risk newborn infants: The basis for intensive nursing care* (pp. 38–85, 205–287, 364–392, 111–150). St. Louis: C.V. Mosby.
8. Kliegman, R.M. (1992). Intrauterine growth retardation: Determinants of aberrant fetal growth. In A.A. Fanaroff & R.J. Martin (Eds.). *Neonatal–perinatal medicine: Diseases of the fetus and infant* (pp. 149–185). St. Louis: Mosby–Year Book.
9. Charlton, V. (1991). Fetal growth, nutritional issues. In W.H. Tauesch, R.A. Ballard, & M.E. Avery (Eds.). *Diseases of the Newborn* (pp. 58–65). Philadelphia: W.B. Saunders.
10. Luchenco, L.O., Hansman, C., Dressler, M., et al. (1963). Intrauterine growth as estimated from liveborn birthweight data at 24 to 42 weeks of gestation. *Pediatrics, 32,* 793–800.
11. Battaglia, F.C., & Luchenco, L.O. (1967). A practical classification of newborn infants by weight and gestational age. *Journal of Pediatrics, 71,* 159.
12. Oski, F.A., DeAngelis, C.D., Feign, R.D., & Warshaw, J.B. (1990). *Principles and practice of pediatrics* (pp. 304–305, 390–397). Philadelphia: J.B. Lippincott.
13. Dubowitz, L.M., Dubowitz, V., & Goldberg, C. (1970). Clinical assessment of gestational age in the newborn infant. *Journal of Pediatrics, 77,* 1.
14. Ballard, J.L., Novak, K., & Driver, M. (1979). A simplified score on assessment of fetal maturation in newly born infants. *Journal of Pediatrics, 95*(5), 769.
15. Mott, S.R., Fazekas, N.F., & James, S.R. (1985). *Nursing care of children and families: A holistic approach.* Reading, MA: Addison-Wesley.
16. Erikson, E. (1963). *Childhood and society.* New York: W.W. Norton.
17. Apgar, V. (1953). A proposal for a new method of evaluation of the newborn infant. *Current Research in Anesthesia and Analgesia, 32,* 260.
18. Kehrberg, D.D. (1986). Immediate care. In N.S. Streeter (Ed.). *High-risk neonatal care* (pp. 25–37). Rockville, MD: Aspen.
19. Mangurten, H.H. (1992). Birth injuries. In A.A. Fanaroff & R.J. Martin (Eds.). *Neonatal–perinatal medicine: Diseases of the fetus and infant* (pp. 346–371). St. Louis: Mosby–Year Book.
20. Fanaroff, A.A., & Martin, R.J. (1992). The respiratory distress syndrome and its management. In A.A. Fanaroff & R.J. Martin (Eds.). *Neonatal–perinatal medicine: Diseases of the fetus and infant* (pp. 810–819). St. Louis: Mosby–Year Book.
21. Papile, L. (1992). Periventricular–intraventricular hemorrhage. In A.A. Fanaroff & R.J. Martin (Eds.). *Neonatal–perinatal medicine: Diseases of the fetus and infant* (pp. 719–728). St. Louis: Mosby–Year Book.
22. Byrne, W.J. (1991). Disorders of the intestines and pancreas. In W.H. Tauesch, R.A. Ballard, & M.E. Avery (Eds.). *Diseases of the newborn* (pp. 681–693). Philadelphia: W.B. Saunders.
23. Crissinger, K.D., Ryckman, F.C., Flake, A.W., & Ballstreri, W.F. (1992). Necrotizing enterocolitis. In A.A. Fanaroff & R.J. Martin (Eds.). *Neonatal–perinatal medicine: Diseases of the fetus and infant* (pp. 1068–1072). St. Louis: Mosby–Year Book.
24. Valdes-Dopena, M. (1992). The sudden infant death syndrome: Pathologic findings. *Clinical Perinatology, 19,* 701–716.
25. Hoffman, H.J., & Hellman, L.S. (1992). Epidemiology

of the sudden death infant syndrome: Maternal, neonatal, and postnatal risk factors. *Clinical Perinatology, 19,* 717–738.

26. Neinstein, L.S., & Kaufman, F.R. (1991). *Adolescent health care: A practical guide* (pp. 3–37, 561–575). Baltimore: Urban & Schwarzenberg.

■ BIBLIOGRAPHY

Brouillette, R.T., Weese-Mayer, D.E., & Hunt, C.E. (1990). Breathing control disorders in infants and children. *Hospital Practice, 25*(8A), 82–103.

Castiglia, P.T. (1992). Alcohol use by children. *Journal of Pediatric Health Care, 6*(5), 271.

Castiglia, P.T. (1990). Suicide in adolescents. *Journal of Pediatric Health Care, 4*(3), 149.

Crawford, T.O. (1992). Clinical evaluation of the floppy infant. *Pediatric Annals, 21*(6), 348–354.

D'Apolito, K. (1991). What is an organized infant? *Neonatal Network, 10*(1), 23–29.

Dine, M.S., Gartside, P.S., Glueck, C.J., et al. (1981). Relationship of head circumference to length in the first 400 days of life: A mnemonic. *Pediatrics, 67,* 506–507.

Havens, D.M., & Bodenhorn, K. (1992). Standards for pediatric immunization practices. *Journal of Pediatric Health Care, 6*(5), 275.

Hein, K. (1989). Commentary on adolescent acquired immunodeficiency syndrome: The next wave of human immunodeficiency virus epidemic? *Adolescent AIDS, 114*(1), 114.

Lobo, M.L., Barnard, K.E., & Coombs, J.B. (1992). Failure to thrive: A parent–infant interaction. *Journal of Pediatric Nursing, 7*(4), 251.

Manley, L.K. (1987). Pediatric trauma: Initial assessment and management. *Journal of Emergency Nursing, 13*(2), 77–87.

Marchal, F., Bairam, A., & Vert, P. (1987). Neonatal apnea and apneic syndromes. *Clinical Perinatology, 14,* 509–529.

Mathew, O.P., Thoppil, C.K., & Belan, M. (1991). Motor activity and apnea in preterm infants. *American Review of Respiratory Disease, 144,* 842–844.

Miller, H.C., & Jekel, J.F. (1985). Diagnosing intrauterine growth retardation in newborn infants. *Perinatology and Neonatology, 9,* 35.

Phelps, W.M. (1990). Cerebral birth injuries: Their orthopedic classification and subsequent treatment. *Clinical Orthopaedics and Related Research, 253,* 4.

Roberts, P.M. (1990). NEC: Etiology, treatment, prevention, and nursing care. *Critical Care Nursing, 10*(4), 38–54.

Stahlman, M.T. (1989). Medical complications of premature infants. *New England Journal of Medicine, 320,* 1551–1553.

CHAPTER 7

CONCEPTS OF ALTERED HEALTH IN OLDER ADULTS

JANICE KUIPER PIKNA

◼ OBJECTIVES

After you have studied this chapter, you should be able to meet the following objectives:

◼ State a philosophy of aging that incorporates the positive aspects of the aging process.

◼ Compare the focus of programmed change and stochastic theories of aging.

◼ Describe common skin changes that occur with aging.

◼ Explain how muscle changes that occur with aging affect high-speed performance and endurance.

◼ Describe the process of bone loss that occurs with aging.

◼ State the common changes in blood pressure regulation that occur with aging.

◼ List the changes in respiratory function that occur with aging.

◼ Relate aging changes in neural function to the overall function of the body.

◼ Briefly discuss the effects of aging on vision and hearing.

◼ Define the term xerostomia and cite two factors that predispose the older population to this condition.

◼ State the significance of decreased lean body mass on interpretation of the GFR using serum creatinine levels.

◼ Compare information obtained from functional assessment versus that obtained by doing a physical examination used to arrive at a medical diagnosis.

◼ Cite the difference between chronic and transient urinary incontinence.

◼ State four risk factors for falls in older individuals.

◼ List five symptoms of depression in older adults.

◼ Define the term "talking therapy."

◼ Name a tool that can be used for assessing cognitive function.

◼ State the difference between delirium and dementia.

◼ List five factors that contribute to adverse drug reactions in the elderly.

Carol Mattson Porth: PATHOPHYSIOLOGY: CONCEPTS OF
ALTERED HEALTH STATES, 4th ed. © 1994, 1990, 1986, 1982
J.B. Lippincott Company

"For age is opportunity no less than youth, itself, though in another dress. And as the evening twilight fades away the sky is filled with stars, invisible by day."
                                        HENRY WADSWORTH LONGFELLOW

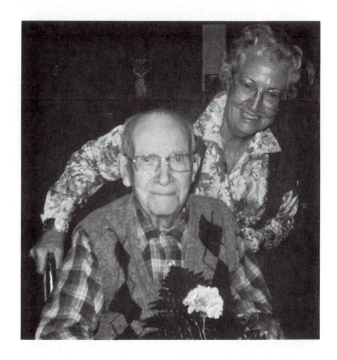

Aging is a natural, lifelong process that brings with it unique biopsychosocial changes. These changes create special health care needs for the older adult population that merit consideration. Because the prediction for the future is a continuous rise in the older adult population, there is a need to focus on the special health care needs of this group.

Gerontology is the discipline that studies aging and the aged from biological, psychological, and sociological perspectives. It explores the dynamic processes of complex physical changes, adjustments in psychological functioning, and alterations in social identities. Through a holistic approach, health care providers specializing in gerontology seek to assist the older adult in maximizing functional abilities while attempting to prevent and minimize illness and disability.

An important first distinction is that aging and disease are not synonymous. Unfortunately, a common assumption is that growing older is inevitably accompanied by illness, disability, and overall decline in function. The fact is that the aging body can accomplish most, if not all, of the functions of its youth; the difference is that it may take longer, require greater motivation, and be less precise. But as in youth, maintenance of physiologic function occurs through continued use.

■ WHO ARE THE ELDERLY?

The older adult population is typically defined in chronologic terms and generally includes individuals 65 years of age and older. This age was chosen somewhat arbitrarily, and historically it is linked to the Social Security Act of 1935. With this Act, the first national pension system in the United States, which designated 65 years as the pensionable age, was developed. Since then, the expression "old age" has been understood to apply to anyone over 65 years. Because there is considerable heterogeneity among this group, older adults are often subgrouped into young-old (ages 65–74 years), middle-old (75–84 years), and old-old (85+ years) to more accurately reflect changes in function that occur. Age parameters, however, are somewhat irrelevant, as chronologic age is a poor predictor of biologic function. However, chronologic age does help to quantify the number of individuals in a group and allows predictions to be made for the future.

In 1989, 12.5% of the total United States popula-

tion (approximately 31 million) was 65 years of age or older, and the proportion has increased yearly. This figure represents a 21% increase in the number of older Americans since 1980, compared with an increase of only 8 percent for the under-65 population. The older adult population is expected to grow to 65.6 million over age 65 by the year 2030 (Fig. 7-1). Furthermore, the older adult population is itself getting older. Average life expectancy has increased as a re-

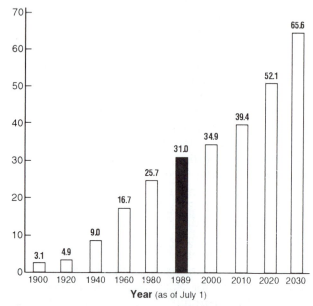

Note: Increments in years on horizontal scale are uneven

FIG. 7-1. Number of persons aged 65 years and older, 1990 to 2030 (in millions). (American Association of Retired Persons. [1990]. *A profile of older Americans.* Washington, DC: AARP)

sult of overall advances in health care technology, improved nutrition, and improved sanitation. Women who are now 65 years of age can expect to live an additional 18.6 years (83.6 years old), and men an additional 14.8 years (79.8 years old).[1]

Aging can be thought of somewhat as a women's issue since women tend to outlive men. In 1989, there was a sex ratio of 145 women for every 100 men over 65 years in the United States. This ratio increases in the old-old age group, with a high of 258 women for every 100 men for individuals 85 years of age or older.[1] Marital status also changes with advancing age. In 1989, half of all older women living in the community were widows, and there were five times as many widows (8.3 million) as there were widowers (1.7 million).

Although 3.4 million older adults were in the work force in 1989 (either working or actively seeking work), the vast majority were retired. Retirement presents a significant role change for older adults. Attitudes and adjustment to retirement are influenced by preretirement lifestyles and values. Individuals with leisure pursuits during their work life seem to adjust better to retirement than those whose lives were dominated by work. For many of today's cohort of older adults, the work ethic of the Great Depression remains profoundly ingrained as the central purpose in life. Thus when work is gone, a significant loss is felt and something must be substituted in its place. Because leisure has not always been a highly valued activity, older adults may have difficulty learning to engage in meaningful leisure pursuits.[2]

Loss of productive work is just one of many losses that can accompany the aging process. Loss of a spouse is a highly significant life event that commonly has negative implications for the survivor. Experts cite an increased mortality among recently bereaved older adults (especially men), an increased incidence of depression, psychological distress and loneliness, and higher rates of chronic illness. Loss of physical health and loss of independence are other changes that can affect the psychosocial aspects of aging, as can relocation, loss of friends and relatives, and changes in the family structure.

Poverty is common among the elderly population. In 1989, about 3.4 million (11.4%) of persons 65 years of age and older lived below the poverty line, with a median income of $13,107 for men and $7,655 for women. The income for African-American elderly was even lower. Social Security was the primary source of income (39%) for older adults, followed by asset income (25%), earnings (17%), public and private pensions (17%), and all other sources (2%).[1*]

*Data reported for noninstitutionalized elderly only.

Contrary to popular belief, the vast majority of older adults live in community settings. Most live in some type of family setting, whether with a spouse, their children or other relatives, whereas about 30% live alone.[1] Only 5.6 percent of all individuals 65 years of age and older reside in long-term care facilities or nursing homes. However, this number increases to 22 percent for persons 85 years of age or older.[1]

Older adults are the largest consumers of health care. In 1987, health care costs for persons over age 65 amounted to $162 billion dollars, or 36% of the nation's total personal health care expenditures. Of this, hospital expenses accounted for the largest share (42%), followed by costs for physicians (21%) and nursing home care (20%). Benefits from government programs, including Medicare and Medicaid, covered about two-thirds of these health care expenditures.[1]

■ THEORIES OF AGING

The lifestyle changes that occur with aging have been described in various developmental theories, probably the most widely known being Erikson's eight stages of development (1963). According to his theory, the first seven developmental stages span the period from childbirth through middle adulthood. The eighth stage focuses on "ego integrity versus despair" of older adulthood. Ego integrity is the acceptance of one's life in relation to humanity and one's place in history. Lack of ego integrity leads to despair, signified by a nonacceptance of one's lifestyle and a fear of death. Despair may be manifested as apathy, depression, or decreased life satisfaction.[3,4]

The stages of physical change that occur as part of the aging process are less well articulated. A number of theories attempt to explain aging through a variety of scientific observations at the molecular, cellular, systemic, and organic levels. Currently, no one theory explains all of the aging processes, but each holds some clues. In reality, it is reasonable to suppose that there are multiple influences that affect the aging process.

The various theories of aging can be categorized into two types: (1) programmed change theories and (2) stochastic theories. *Programmed change* theories propose that the changes that occur with aging are genetically programmed; *stochastic* theories maintain that the changes result from an accumulation of random events or damage due to environmental hazards.

One programmed change theory involves the immune system. It postulates that the involution of the thymus gland, a process that begins during adolescence, affects the integrity of the immune system. Specifically, it is the T cell–dependent immune functions that become progressively impaired, and this may, in part, explain how aging occurs.[5] Also in the area of programmed change theory, Moorhead and Hayflick observed more than 25 years ago that cultured human fibroblasts have a limited ability to replicate (about 50 population doublings) and then die.[6, 7] The inability to replace cells may also contribute to the aging process.

More recently, it was reported that the administration of the human growth hormone to healthy elderly men who had low levels of the growth hormone and insulin-like growth factor reversed changes in lean body mass and adipose tissue. The magnitude of the changes was equivalent to those incurred during 10 to 20 years of aging. This, too, may partly answer the aging question.[8]

The free radical theory is a stochastic idea in which aging is thought to be partially due to the effects of free radical damage. When paired electrons are transiently separated, they produce free radicals that may cause cellular damage (see Chapter 2). Over time, the cumulative effects of free radical damage are theorized to cause cellular dysfunction and, in turn, may result in aging.[9]

Another damage theory, the wear and tear theory, proposes that accumulated damage to vital parts of the cell leads to aging and death. Cellular DNA is cited as an example. If repair to damaged DNA is incomplete or defective, as is thought to occur with aging, declines in cellular function might occur.[10, 11]

The above theories help to explain the phenomenon of aging. Scientists continue to study these processes in pursuit of a better understanding of the aging process.

In summary, aging is a natural, lifelong process that brings with it unique biopsychosocial changes. Aging is not synonymous with disease or ill health. The aging body can accomplish most if not all of the functions of its youth; the difference is that it may take longer, require greater motivation, and be less precise.

The older adult population is typically defined in chronologic terms as individuals 65 years of age and older and can be further defined as (1) young-old (ages 65–74 years), (2) middle-old (75–84 years), and (3) old-old (85 + years). The number of older people has increased and is expected to continue to grow in the future, with an anticipated 65.6 million Americans over age 65 by the year 2030.

There are two main types of theories used to explain the changes that occur with aging: programmed change theories, which propose that aging changes are genetically programmed, and stochastic theories, which maintain that aging changes result from an accumulation of random events or damage due to environmental hazards.

■ PHYSICAL CHANGES WITH AGING

Overall, there is a general decline in the structure and function of the body with advancing age. The decline results in a decreased reserve capacity of the various organ systems that consequently produces reduced homeostatic capabilities, making the older adult more vulnerable to stressors such as illness, trauma, surgery, medications, and environmental changes.

Research to identify true age-related changes as opposed to disease states is difficult. Studies using cross-sectional methodologies are the easiest to perform; however, mortality can confound the results. Although longitudinal studies tend to be more precise, they require years to perform and may not be able to account for numerous variables that enter into the aging equation, such as environment, occupation, and diet.[12] However, it is important to distinguish, as much as possible, those changes that occur in the body as a result of aging from those that occur from disease. This distinction allows for more accurate diagnosis and treatment of disease conditions and helps to avoid inappropriate labeling of aging changes.

SKIN

Changes in the skin more obviously reflect the aging process than do changes in other organ systems (see Chapter 11). Aging can impinge upon the primary functions of the skin: protection from the environment, temperature regulation, maintenance of fluid and electrolyte balance, sensory regulation, and excretion of metabolic wastes. Sun and harsh weather accelerate aging of the skin.

Overall, with aging the skin becomes wrinkled and dry, with uneven pigmentation. There is a decrease of approximately 20% in the thickness of the dermis, or middle layer of skin, which gives the skin an overall thin and transparent quality. This is especially true for areas exposed to sunlight. Dermal collagen fibers rearrange and degenerate, resulting in decreased skin strength and elasticity. Cellularity and vascularity of the dermis decrease with advancing age and can cause vascular fragility, leading to senile purpura (skin hemorrhages) and slow skin healing. Delayed wound healing may also be influenced by other factors such as poor nutrition and circulation and changes in immune function.[13, 14]

The function of the sebaceous (oil) glands diminishes with age and leads to a decrease in sebum secretion. The decrease in size, number, and function of the eccrine sweat glands causes a decrease in their capacity to produce sweat. Fingernails and toenails become dull, brittle, and thick, mostly as a result of decreased vascularity of the nailbeds. Age-related changes in hair occur as well. Owing to a decline in melanin production by the hair follicle, about half of the population over 50 years of age has at least 50 percent gray hair, irrespective of sex or hair color. Changes in hair growth and distribution are also seen.[13, 14] Hairs on the scalp, axillae, and pubis become fewer, and the hairs of the ears and nostril coarsen.

Skin disorders are very common among the older adult population and can include skin cancers, keratoses (warty lesions), xerosis (excessive dryness), dermatitis, and pruritus (generalized itching).

MUSCULOSKELETAL FUNCTION

Current debates about changes in the musculoskeletal system attempt to differentiate normal aging from disuse changes that occur with a sedentary lifestyle. Much of what was previously considered aging is now regarded as functional disuse.[15] With aging there is a reduction in muscle size and strength that is related to a loss of muscle fibers as well as a reduction in the size of the existing fibers. Although the decline in strength that occurs with aging cannot be halted, its progress can be slowed with exercise.[16] Aging, however, does not appear to affect endurance. In fact, when corrected for strength and cardiopulmonary changes, endurance may be enhanced in the elderly because type I muscle fibers, which affect endurance, are thought to remain consistent with age. There does tend to be a decline in high-speed performance and reaction time due to a decrease in type II muscle fibers, although this is still under debate.[17] Impairments in the nervous system can also cause movements to slow.

Numerous studies have reported a loss of bone mass with aging, regardless of gender, race, or body size. With aging the process of bone formation (renewal) is slowed in relation to bone resorption (breakdown), resulting in a loss of bone mass and weakened bone structure. This is especially true for postmenopausal women. By age 65, most women have lost two-thirds of their skeletal mass, probably owing to a decrease in estrogen production.[17] Skeletal bone loss is not a uniform process. Beginning around age 30, bone loss begins predominantly in the trabecular bone (the fine network of bony struts and braces in the medullary cavity) of the heads of the femora and radii and in the vertebral bodies.[15, 17] By age 80, women will have lost nearly 43% of their trabecular bone, and men 27%. This process becomes pathologic (i.e., osteoporosis) when it significantly in-

creases the predisposition to fracture and associated complications (see Chapter 57).

Changes in stature also occur with aging. There is a progressive decline in height, especially among older women, which is mainly attributed to compression of the spinal column. Body composition changes as well. The amount of fat increases, and lean body mass along with total body water decreases with advancing age.[18]

CARDIOVASCULAR FUNCTION

Cardiovascular disease remains the leading cause of morbidity and mortality in older adults. Thus, it is often difficult to separate true age-related changes in the cardiovascular system from disease processes. In spite of aging changes and cardiovascular disease, overall cardiovascular function at rest in most healthy elderly persons is considered adequate to meet the body's needs.

The aorta and arteries tend to become stiffer and less distensible with age. Although approximately 50% of older adults suffer from hypertension, the disorder is not considered a normal age-related process.[19] The elevation in blood pressure is more pronounced for systolic blood pressure than for diastolic blood pressure, probably as a result of increased aortic stiffness. In the elderly, compensatory cardiovascular mechanisms are often delayed or insufficient, so that a drop in blood pressure due to position change or consumption of a meal is common.[20] Orthostatic hypotension, or a significant drop in systolic blood pressure upon assumption of the upright position, is more common among the elderly (see Chapter 21). Even in the absence of orthostatic hypotension, the elderly respond to postural stress with diminished changes in heart rate and diastolic pressure. The alteration in orthostatic response to aging is usually due to changes in autonomic function, circulatory inadequacy, or both.[21]

Senescent cardiac muscle typically displays a decreased response to beta-adrenergic stimulation and circulating catecholamines, and there is increased diastolic stiffness that impedes diastolic filling, probably due to a slower rate of diastolic relaxation. Although early diastolic filling decreases by approximately 50% between ages 20 and 80 years, filling volumes are maintained, most likely as a result of an enhanced atrial contraction and its contribution to ventricular filling.[22] The afterload (opposition to left ventricular ejection) rises steadily with age as the ascending aorta becomes more rigid and the resistance in peripheral arterial vessels increases. Although the overall size of the heart does not increase, the thickness of the left ventricular wall may increase with age, due in part to the increased afterload that develops because of blood vessel changes.[22, 23] The resting heart rate remains unchanged or decreases only slightly with age; however, the maximum heart rate than can be achieved during maximal exercise is decreased.

Earlier studies suggested that cardiac output at rest declines with age.[24] However, more recent data in which subjects were highly screened to exclude cardiovascular disease showed that resting cardiac output is unaffected by age.[25] Interestingly, cardiac output is maintained in healthy older adults during exercise in spite of the decreased heart rate response. This appears to be due to a greater stroke volume resulting from increased end-diastolic volume (Frank-Starling mechanism) during exercise.[23, 26]

RESPIRATORY FUNCTION

As lung function declines with age, it is often difficult to differentiate the effects of age from environmental and disease factors. A progressive loss of recoil within the lung is due to changes in the elastin and in the composition of the collagen. Calcification of the soft tissues of the chest wall causes increased stiffness and thus increases the workload of the respiratory muscles. There is a loss of alveolar structure that decreases the surface area of gas exchange. Although the total lung capacity remains constant, the consequences of these changes result in an increased residual lung volume, a decreased functional reserve capacity, and a decline in vital capacity. There is a linear fall in arterial oxygen tension (PO_2) of about 20 mmHg from ages 20 years to 70 years. This is thought to be primarily due to the ventilation-perfusion mismatching of the aging lung.[27]

Maximal oxygen consumption (VO_2max), a measure used to determine overall cardiopulmonary function, declines with age. Numerous studies have indicated that VO_2max can improve significantly with exercise and that the VO_2max of older adult master athletes can meet and exceed that of their younger counterparts.

NEUROLOGIC FUNCTION

Changes in neurologic function occur with normal aging, but overall they do not interfere with day-to-day routines unless specific neurologic diseases come into play. The weight of the brain decreases with age, and there is a loss of neurons in the brain and spinal cord. Neuron loss is most pronounced in the cerebral cortex, especially in the superior temporal area. Additional changes take place within the neurons and supporting cells. Atrophy of the neuronal dendrites results in impaired synaptic connections, diminished electrochemical reactions, and neural dysfunction. Synaptic transmissions are also affected by changes in the chemical neurotransmitters dopamine, acetylcholine, and serotonin. As a result, there is a slowing of many neural processes. Lipofuscin deposits (yellow, insoluble intracellular material) are found in greater amounts in the aged brain.[28, 29]

Sensorimotor changes show a decline in motor strength, slowed reaction time, diminished reflexes (especially in the ankles), and proprioception changes. These changes can cause the balance problems and slow, more deliberate movements that are frequently seen in older individuals.[28, 29]

Even though changes in the brain are associated with aging, overall cognitive abilities remain intact. Although language skills and attention are not altered with advanced age, performance and constructional task abilities can decline, as can short-term memory and immediate recall. A change in personality is considered unusual with normal aging. If personality changes occur, then evaluation is in order. Dementia and/or depression can frequently be the cause.[28, 30]

SPECIAL SENSES

Sensory changes with aging can greatly affect the older adult's level of functioning and quality of life. Vision and hearing impairments due to disease states, for example, can interfere with written and verbal communication and may lead to social isolation and depression.

Vision. There is a general decline in visual acuity with age, and nearly all individuals over 55 years of age require eyeglasses for either reading or distance. The decline occurs as a result of a smaller pupil diameter, loss of refractive power of the lens, and an increase in the scattering of light.[31] The most common visual problem among older adults is presbyopia, or difficulty focusing on near objects. It is due mainly to a decreased elasticity of the lens and atrophy of the ciliary muscle (see Chapter 52).[32]

Glare and abrupt changes in light pose particular problems for older adults. Both are reasons why the elderly frequently give up night driving; they also increase their risk for falls and injury.[31] Color discrimination changes also take place with aging. In particular, older adults have more difficulty identifying blues and greens. This is thought to be related to problems associated with filtering short wavelengths of light (violet, blue, green) through a yellowed, opaque lens.[33] Corneal sensitivity may also diminish with age, so that older adults may be less aware of injury or infection.

Ophthalmologic diseases and disorders are common in the elderly. Cataracts, glaucoma, and macular degeneration are seen frequently and can greatly impair vision and function. Low-vision aids, such as special magnifiers and high-intensity lighting that mimics sunlight, can assist in optimizing vision in otherwise uncorrectable ophthalmologic problems.

Hearing. Hearing loss is very common among older adults, and some degree of impairment is almost inevitable with advancing age. It has been reported that 24% of independent individuals 65 to 74 years of age and 39% of those 75 years of age and older have a hearing impairment,[34] whereas as many as 70% of institutionalized older adults have difficulty hearing.[35]

Presbycusis, or the hearing loss of old age, is characterized by a gradual, progressive onset of bilateral and symmetric sensorineural hearing loss of high-frequency tones (see Chapter 53). Speech discrimination, or the ability to understand the spoken word, is often impaired. Specific consonant sounds that are commonly problematic include s, z, sh, ch, and dg, as in u*s*, *z*ebra, ben*ch*, and nu*dg*e.[36] Accelerated speech and shouting can also increase distortion and further compound the problem. When speaking to hearing-impaired older adults, it is helpful to face them directly so they can observe lip movements and facial expressions. Speech should be slow and direct. Loudness can be irritating. Rephrasing misunderstood messages can also improve understanding of the spoken word. Hearing aids can be effective for various levels of hearing loss and may greatly improve the ability to hear and communicate.

Cerumen (ear wax) impaction in the external auditory canal is also commonly seen in older adults and can impair hearing. The cerumen glands, which are modified apocrine sweat glands, atrophy and produce drier cerumen. This may be partially responsible for more frequent cerumen impactions in the older adult population.[37]

Taste and Smell. The evidence regarding taste sensitivity changes is inconclusive. Recent studies have indicated that decrements in the ability to discriminate tastes are not as great as previously thought. The sense of smell declines after the fifth decade, perhaps as the result of observed generalized atrophy of the olfactory bulbs and a moderate loss of olfactory neurons. Because both taste and smell are necessary for the enjoyment of food flavor, older adults may not enjoy eating as much as in their youth. Drugs and disease also may affect taste. Alterations in taste and smell, along with other factors

such as eating alone, decreased ability to prepare and purchase food, and the high cost of some foods, may account for poor nutritional intake in some older adults.

IMMUNE FUNCTION

It appears that there is an overall decline in immune system capabilities with aging that can pose an increased risk for some infections. Most notably, involution of the thymus gland is complete by about age 45 to 50, and although the total number of T cells remains unchanged, there are changes in the function of helper T cells that alter the cellular immune response of older adults. There is also evidence of an increase in various autoantibodies (*e.g.*, rheumatoid factor) as a person ages, increasing the risk of autoimmune disorders. Clinically, older adults are more susceptible to urinary tract infections, respiratory tract infections, wound infections, and nosocomial infections. An increased mortality rate from influenza and bronchopneumonia is also seen in the older adult population.[38–40] Local organ factors and coincident diseases probably play a bigger role in the acquisition of these infections than age-related changes in immunity.

GASTROINTESTINAL FUNCTION

The gastrointestinal tract, on the whole, shows less age-associated change in function than many other organ systems. Although tooth loss is common and about 40% of the current older adult population is edentulous, it is not considered part of the normal aging process. Poor dental hygiene with associated caries and periodontal disease are the main reasons for the loss. Toothlessness can lead to dietary changes and can be associated with malnutrition. Use of dentures can enhance mastication; however, taste sensation is inhibited. Because of improved dental technology as well as the fluoridated water supply, more people will be able to keep their teeth into their late years. Xerostomia (dry mouth) is also common, but it is not universal among older adults and typically occurs as a result of decreased salivary secretions. Other causes of dry mouth can include medications, such as anticholinergics and tranquilizers, radiation therapy, and obstructive nasal diseases that induce mouth breathing.[12]

Esophageal function is essentially preserved with aging. Soergel and his colleagues (1964) coined the term "presbyesophagus" to denote esophageal changes among older adults, such as decreased esophageal motility and inadequate relaxation of the lower esophageal sphincter.[41] There is current debate as to whether these changes are truly age-related or related to or caused by disorders such as diabetes mellitus or neuropathies.

Atrophy of the gastric mucosa and a decrease in gastric secretions can be seen in older adults. Achlorhydria (a decrease in hydrochloric acid secretion) occurs, probably as a result of a loss of parietal cells. Although not universal, achlorhydria is more prevalent among older adults and can cause impaired gastric absorption of substances requiring an acid environment.[42]

The small intestine shows some age-related morphological changes, such as mucosal atrophy; however, absorption of nutrients and other functions appears to remain intact. Diverticuli of the colon are common among older adults: more than 50% of individuals over age 80 have diverticular disease. The high incidence appears to be mainly due to a low-fiber diet.[43] Constipation, or infrequent passage of hard stool, is another frequently occurring phenomenon. It is often attributed to immobility and decreased physical activity, a low-fiber diet, decreased fluid intake, and medications; malignancies and other disease states can also be responsible. Complications of constipation can include fecal impaction or obstruction, megacolon, rectal prolapse, hemorrhoids, and laxative abuse.[12]

RENAL FUNCTION

Although age-related anatomic and physiologic changes occur, the aging kidney remains capable of maintaining fluid and electrolyte balance remarkably well. Aging changes result in a decreased reserve capacity, which may alter the kidney's ability to maintain homeostasis in the face of illnesses or stressors.

Overall, there is a general decline in kidney mass with aging, predominantly in the renal cortex. The number of functional glomeruli decreases by 30% to 50%, with an increased percentage of sclerotic and/or abnormal glomeruli.[44, 45]

Numerous cross-sectional and longitudinal studies have documented a steady, age-related decline in total renal blood flow of about 10% per decade after age 20, so that the renal blood flow of an 80-year-old averages approximately 300 mL/minute compared with 600 mL/minute in a younger adult. The major decline in blood flow occurs in the cortical area of the kidney, causing a progressive age-related decrease in the *glomerular filtration rate* (*GFR*). Serum creatinine, a by-product of muscle metabolism, is often used as a measure of GFR. It is important to note that the decline in GFR that occurs with aging is not accompanied by an equivalent increase in serum creatinine

levels because the production of creatinine is reduced as muscle mass declines with age. Serum creatinine levels are often used as an index of kidney function when prescribing and calculating drug doses for medications that are eliminated through the kidneys; this has important implications for older adults. If not carefully addressed, improper drug dosing can lead to an excess accumulation of circulating drugs and result in toxicity. A formula that adjusts for age-related changes in serum creatinine for individuals 40 through 80 years is available (see Chapter 33).

Renal tubular function declines with advancing age, and the ability to concentrate and dilute urine in response to fluid and electrolyte impairments is diminished. The aging kidney's ability to conserve sodium in response to sodium depletion is impaired and can result in hyponatremia. A decreased ability to concentrate urine, an age-related decrease in responsiveness to antidiuretic hormone, and an impaired thirst mechanism may account for the older adult's easier predisposition to dehydration during periods of stress and illness.[46, 47] Older adults are also more prone to hyperkalemia and hypokalemia when stressed than are younger individuals. An elevated serum potassium may result from a decreased GFR, lower renin and aldosterone levels, and changes in tubular function. Low potassium levels, on the other hand, are more commonly caused by gastrointestinal disorders or diuretic use.[45, 47] Both are not the result of aging.

GENITOURINARY FUNCTION

Changes in the bladder occur with the aging process. Overall, the smooth muscle and supportive elastic tissue are replaced with fibrous connective tissue. This can cause incomplete bladder emptying and a diminished force of urine stream. Bladder capacity also decreases with age, whereas the frequency of urination increases. As elastic tissue and muscles weaken, stress incontinence becomes more prevalent. In aging women, atrophy of perineal structures can cause the urethral meatus to recede along the vaginal wall. Atrophy of other pelvic organs occurs in the aging woman as well, owing to diminished estrogen production after menopause—vaginal secretions diminish; the vaginal lining is thinner, drier, less elastic and more easily traumatized; and normal flora are altered. These changes can result in vaginal infections, pruritus, and painful intercourse.[48, 49]

In aging men, benign prostatic hyperplasia is very common (see Chapter 36). Incidence progressively increases to about 90% of men who are 80 years old. Although the condition is often asymptomatic, it can cause obstructive symptoms such as urinary hesitancy, diminished force of stream, retention, and postvoid dribbling; it can also cause irritative symptoms such as frequency, nocturia, urgency, and even urge incontinence. The development of benign prostatic hyperplasia is thought to be hormonally mediated, and approximately 50% of men require prostatectomy for symptom relief.[48, 50] Medical therapies for benign prostatic hyperplasia are being actively investigated.

Although penile erections take longer to develop owing to changes in neural innervation and vascular supply, sexual activity remains possible into late life for men as well as for women. Causes of impotence in men can be multifactorial and can include cardiovascular disease such as angina with exertion, arthritis with functional immobility, medication use, and psychological changes. Impotence should not be considered normal aging, and complaints about sexual dysfunction warrant investigation.

In summary, there is a general decline in the structure and function of the body with advancing age, resulting in a decreased reserve capacity of the various organ systems, including the skin and the musculoskeletal, cardiorespiratory, nervous and sensory, immune, gastrointestinal, and genitourinary systems. This results in a reduction of homeostatic capabilities, making the older adult more vulnerable to stressors such as illness, trauma, surgery, medication administration, and environmental changes.

■ FUNCTIONAL PROBLEMS OF AGING

Although aging is not synonymous with disease, the aging process does lend itself to an increased incidence of illness. This is especially true for chronic diseases. It has been estimated that 86% of older adults have at least one chronic condition, and most actually suffer from more than one. The extent of these problems is described in Table 7-1. Older adults are more apt to experience a decline in overall health and function due to the increases in incidence of chronic illness with advancing age. Because aging also brings with it a decreased ability to maintain homeostasis, illnesses often present in an atypical manner.

In addition to chronic illnesses, older adults suffer disproportionately from functional disabilities, or the inability to perform a necessary activity of daily living. It is most likely that the decrements in health that can accompany the aging process are responsible for functional disabilities. Among the more common functional problems of the older adult are urinary incontinence, falls, depression, dementia, and delirium.

TABLE 7-1. COMMON HEALTH PROBLEMS IN THE ELDERLY

HEALTH PROBLEMS	% WITH PROBLEM
Arthritis	49
Hypertension	37
Hearing impairments	32
Heart disease	30
Cataracts	17
Sinusitis	17
Orthopedic impairments	16
Visual impairments	9
Diabetes	9
Tinnitus	8
Varicose veins	8

(Data from American Association of Retired Persons. [1990]. *A profile of older Americans.* Washington, DC: AARP)

FUNCTIONAL ASSESSMENT

The evaluation of the older adult's functional abilities is a key component in gerontologic health care. Medical diagnoses alone are incomplete without an assessment of function–for example, two older adults with similar medical diagnoses of arthritis, hypertension, and osteoporosis can be at opposite ends of the spectrum of functional abilities.

Assessing functional status can be done in many different ways using a variety of methods. Measures of function should attempt to systematically and objectively evaluate the level at which an individual is functioning in a variety of areas, including biological, psychological, and social health.

Selection of a screening tool to measure function depends on the purpose of data collection, the individual or target population to be assessed, availability and applicability of the instruments, reliability and validity of the screening tools, and the setting or environment.[51] An issue that arises when assessing function is the question of capability versus performance. For example, an older adult might be able to bathe without supervision; however, the long-term care facility where the person resides may discourage it for safety reasons. Among the more commonly used assessment tools are those that measure (1) the ability to perform activities of daily living and (2) cognitive function.

Activities of Daily Living. When evaluating levels of function, determination of the older adult's ability to perform *activities of daily living* (*ADL*) and *instrumental activities of daily living* (*IADL*) should be included. Activities of daily living are basic self-care tasks, such as bathing, dressing, grooming, ambulating, transferring (*e.g.*, from a chair to bed), feeding, and communicating. Instrumental activities of daily living are more complex tasks that are necessary to function in society, such as writing, reading, cooking, cleaning, shopping, laundering, climbing stairs, using the telephone, managing money, managing medications, and using transportation. The IADL tasks indirectly examine cognitive abilities as well in that they require a certain level of cognitive skills to complete.

A number of tools are available for measuring functional status. One commonly used measure is the Index of Activities of Daily Living. Developed by Katz in 1963 and revised in 1970, it summarizes performance in six functions: bathing, dressing, toileting, transferring, continence, and feeding. It is used as an assessment tool to determine the need for care and the appropriateness of treatment and as a teaching aid in rehabilitation settings. Through questioning and observation, the rater forms a mental picture of the older adult's functional status as it existed during a 2-week period preceding the evaluation, using the most dependent degree of performance.[52–54] Numerous studies using the Katz Index tool show significant validity and reliability. The advantage of the tool is that it is easy to administer and provides a "snapshot" of the older adult's level of physical functioning. The disadvantage is that it does not include IADL categories that are of equal importance, especially for older adults living in the community.

URINARY INCONTINENCE

Urinary incontinence, or involuntary loss of urine, plagues approximately 30% of community-living individuals over age 60, 50% of hospitalized older adults, and 60% of residents in long-term care facilities.[54–56] These estimates may be low because individuals often fail to report symptoms of urinary incontinence, perhaps owing to the attached social stigma. Health care professionals often neglect to elicit such information as well.

Incontinence is an expensive problem. A conservative estimate of cost for direct care of adults with incontinence is over $10 billion annually.[57] Urinary incontinence can have deleterious consequences, such as social isolation and embarrassment, depression and dependency, skin rashes and pressure sores, urinary tract infections, and financial hardship. Although urinary incontinence is a common disorder, it is not considered a normal aspect of aging. Studies reveal that 60% to 70% of community-dwelling older adults with urinary incontinence can be successfully treated and even cured.

Changes in the micturition cycle that accompany the aging process make the older adult prone to urinary incontinence. A decrease in bladder capacity, in bladder and sphincter tone, and in the ability to inhibit detrusor (bladder muscle) contractions, combined with the nervous system's increased variability to interpret bladder signals, can cause incontinence (see Chapter 34). Impaired mobility and a slower reaction time can also aggravate incontinence problems.

The causes of incontinence can be divided into two categories: transient and chronic. Of particular importance is the role of pharmaceuticals as a cause of transient urinary incontinence. Numerous medications, such as long-acting sedatives and hypnotics, psychotropics, and diuretics, can induce incontinence. Treatment of transient urinary incontinence is aimed at ameliorating or relieving the cause in the assumption that the incontinence will resolve.

Chronic, or established, urinary incontinence occurs as a result of detrusor overactivity with inappropriate bladder contractions; detrusor underactivity, or failure of the bladder to contract causing overflow leakage; urethral incompetence, in that the bladder pressure overcomes the resistance of the urethra; or outlet obstruction with resulting overflow incontinence, as with prostatic enlargement or urethral stricture. Chronic urinary incontinence can also be classified according to the type of problem that occurs. *Stress incontinence* describes an involuntary loss of urine with an increase in intraabdominal pressure, as with coughing or laughing. *Urge incontinence* is leakage of urine because of an inability to delay voiding after the sensation of bladder fullness is perceived. *Overflow incontinence* is leakage of urine resulting from an overdistended bladder. *Functional incontinence*, or urine leakage due to toileting problems, occurs because cognitive, physical, or environmental barriers impair appropriate use of the toilet.[48, 54, 58]

TREATMENT

Once a specific diagnosis of urinary incontinence is established, treatment is aimed at correcting or ameliorating the problem. Probably the most effective interventions for older adults with incontinence are behavioral techniques. These strategies involve educating the individual and providing reinforcement for effort and progress. Techniques include bladder training and retraining, timed voiding or habit training, prompted voiding, pelvic floor muscle (Kegel) exercises, and dietary and fluid intake modifications. Biofeedback, which may be appropriate for some older adults, uses electrical or mechanical instruments to relay information to individuals about their physiologic functions and can be helpful when used in conjunction with other behavioral treatment techniques.[48, 54] Use of pads or other absorbent products should be seen as a temporary help measure and not as a cure. Numerous types of products are available to meet many different consumer needs. The ideal absorbent product should contain the urine completely and prevent leakage onto clothing and furniture, be comfortable and easy to wear, disguise or contain odor, be inconspicuous under clothing, be easy to dispose of or clean, and be reasonably priced and readily available.[48]

Pharmacologic intervention may be helpful for some individuals. Estrogen replacement therapy in postmenopausal women, for example, may help to relieve stress incontinence. Drugs with anticholinergic and bladder smooth muscle relaxant properties (*e.g.*, oxybutynin) may help with urge incontinence. These medications are not without side effects, however, and these must be carefully weighed against the possible benefits.

Surgical intervention may help to relieve urinary incontinence symptoms in appropriate patients. Bladder neck suspension may assist with stress incontinence unrelieved by other interventions, and prostatectomy for men with overflow incontinence is appropriate. Older adults may have medical conditions that preclude surgery. Other treatments include intermittent self-catheterization for some types of overflow incontinence.[54, 58]

FALLS

Falls are a common source of concern for the older adult population. The literature reveals that 30% of community-dwelling individuals over 65 years of age and 50% of nursing home residents fall each year.[59] Most falls do not result in serious injury, but the potential for serious complications and even death is real. Accidents are the sixth leading cause of death among older adults, with falls ranking first in this category.[60] Hip fractures are one the most feared complication from a fall. More than 200,000 individuals fracture a hip each year, the vast majority being elderly women.[61] Significant morbidity occurs as a result of a hip fracture. The literature varies, but up to 50% of older adults who sustain a hip fracture are reported to require nursing home care for at least 1 year and up to 20% die in the year following a hip fracture. Other bones frequently fractured by older adults who fall are the humerus, wrist, and pelvis. These bones bear the brunt of osteoporotic changes and, as a result, are more vulnerable to injury. Soft tissue injuries such as sprains and strains can also result from falls.

Restrictions on an individual's activity may occur due to a fear, on the part of the individual or caregiver, of possible falling. These anxieties may lead to unnecessary restrictions in independence and mobility and are commonly mentioned as a reason for institutionalization.[62, 63]

Although some falls have a single, obvious cause, such as a slip on a wet or icy surface, most are the result of several factors. Risk factors that predispose to falling include a combination of age-related biopsychosocial changes, chronic illnesses, and situational and environmental hazards. Gait and stability require the integration of information from the special senses, the nervous system, and the musculoskeletal system. As a result, both age-related and disease-related changes in neural function can affect ambulation. Changes in gait and posture that occur in healthy aged individuals serve to contribute to the problem of falls: the older person's stride shortens; the elbows, trunk, and knees become more flexed; toe and heel lift decreases while walking; and sway while standing increases. In addition, muscle strength and postural control of balance decrease, proprioception input diminishes, and righting reflexes slow. All these factors predispose the older adult to the possibility of falling.[58, 64]

Because the central nervous system integrates sensory input and sends signals to the effector components of the musculoskeletal system, any alteration in neural function can predispose to falls. For this reason, falls have been associated with strokes, Parkinson's disease, and normal pressure hydrocephalus. Similarly, diseases or disabilities that affect the musculoskeletal system, such as arthritis, muscle weakness, or foot deformities, are associated with an increase in the incidence of falls. Age- and disease-related alterations in vision and hearing impair sensory input and can contribute to falls. Vestibular system alterations, such as benign positional vertigo or Ménière's disease, cause balance problems that can result in falls. Cognitive impairments such as dementia have been associated with an increased risk of falling, most likely because of impaired judgment and problem-solving abilities. Input from the cardiovascular and respiratory systems influences both function and ambulation. Cardiovascular diseases, especially postural hypotension, can cause recurrent falls, either solely or in association with the previously mentioned factors. The dramatic drop in blood pressure upon rising that is seen in postural hypotension can cause falls due to syncope and dizziness. Table 7-2 summarizes the possible causes of falls.

Medications are an important and potentially correctable cause of instability and falls. Centrally-acting medications, such as sedatives and hypnotics, have been associated with an increase in the risk of falling and injury. Diuretics can cause volume deple-

TABLE 7-2. CAUSES OF FALLS

Accidents
  True accidents (trips, slips, etc.)
  Interactions between environmental hazards and factors increasing susceptibility
Syncope (sudden loss of consciousness)
Drop attacks (sudden leg weaknesses, without loss of consciousness)
Dizziness and/or vertigo
  Vestibular disease
  CNS disease
Orthostatic hypotension
  Hypovolemia or low cardiac output
  Autonomic dysfunction
  Impaired venous return
  Prolonged bed rest
  Drug-induced hypotension
Drug-related causes
  Diuretics
  Antihypertensives
  Tricyclic antidepressants
  Sedatives
  Antipsychotics
  Hypoglycemics
  Alcohol
Specific disease processes
  Acute illness of any kind ("premonitory fall")
  Cardiovascular
    Arrhythmias
    Valvular heart disease (aortic stenosis)
    Carotid sinus syncope
Neurologic causes
  Transient ischemic attack (TIA)
  Stroke (acute)
  Seizure disorder
  Parkinson's disease
  Cervical or lumbar spondylosis (with spinal cord or nerve root compression)
  Cerebellar disease
  Normal-pressure hydrocephalus (gait disorder)
  CNS lesions (*e.g.*, tumor, subdural hematoma)
Idiopathic (no specific cause identifiable)

(Kane, R.L., Ouslander, J.G., & Abrass, I.B. [1989]. *Essentials of geriatrics* [2nd ed.]. New York: McGraw-Hill)

tion, electrolyte disturbances, and fatigue, predisposing to falls. Antihypertensives can cause fatigue and postural hypotension or impair mental alertness and result in falls as well.[58, 63]

Environmental hazards play a significant role in falling. More than 70% of falls occur in the home and often involve objects that are tripped over, such as cords, scatter rugs, and small items left on the floor. Poor lighting, ill-fitting shoes, surfaces with glare, and improper use of ambulatory devices such as canes or walkers also contribute to the problem.[62]

PREVENTION OF FALLS

Preventing falls is the key to controlling the potential complications that can result. Because falling is generally multifactorial, the aim of the clinical evaluation is to identify risk factors that can be modified. Assessment of sensory, neurologic, and musculoskeletal systems; direct observation of gait and balance; and a careful medication inventory can help identify possible causes. Treatment can include a variety of interventions, such as surgery for cataracts or cerumen removal for hearing impairment related to excessive ear wax accumulation. Other interventions may include podiatric care, discontinuation or alteration of the medication regimen, exercise programs, physical therapy, and appropriate adaptive devices. The home should also be assessed by an appropriate health care professional (*e.g.*, occupational therapist) and recommendations made regarding modifications to promote safety. Simple changes such as removing scatter rugs, improving the lighting, and installing grab bars in the bathtub can help prevent falling. These interventions can maximize the older adult's independence and prevent the morbidity and mortality that can occur as a result of a fall.[62]

DEPRESSION

Depression is a significant health problem that affects the older adult population. Estimates of depression in the elderly vary widely; however, there is a consensus that the size of the problem is underestimated owing to misdiagnosis and mistreatment. Approximately 15% of community-dwelling older adults are thought to have depressive symptoms. The estimate drops to about 3% when diagnosis is restricted to major depression. Depressive symptoms are seen in about 15% to 25% of nursing home residents.[65]

The term depression is used to describe either a symptom, syndrome, or disease. As listed in the 1987 American Psychiatric Association Diagnostic and Statistical Manual (DSM-IIIR), the criteria for the diagnosis and treatment of a major depression include at least five of the following: (1) appetite and weight changes; (2) sleep disturbance; (3) motor agitation or retardation; (4) fatigue and loss of energy; (5) depressed or irritable mood; (6) loss of interest or pleasure in usual activities; (7) feelings of worthlessness, self-reproach, or excessive guilt; (8) suicidal thinking or attempts; and (9) difficulty with thinking or concentration.[66]

Depressive symptomatology can be incorrectly attributed to the aging process, making recognition and diagnosis difficult. Depressed mood, the signature symptom of depression, may be less prominent in the older adult and more somatic complaints reported, confusing the diagnosis. Physical illnesses can complicate the diagnosis as well. Depression can be a symptom of a medical condition, such as pancreatic cancer, hypo/hyperthyroidism, pneumonia and other infections, congestive heart failure, dementia, and stroke, to name a few. Medications such as sedatives, hypnotics, steroids, antihypertensives, and analgesics can also induce a depressive state. In addition, numerous confounding social problems such as bereavement, loss of job or income, and loss of social support can often obscure or complicate the diagnosis.[66,67]

The course of depression in older adults is similar to that in younger people. Recurrence occurs in up to 40% of people. Suicide rates are the highest in the elderly. There is a linear increase in suicide with age, most notably among white men over the age of 60. Although the exact reasons are unclear, it may be due to the emotional alienation that can accompany the aging process, combined with complex biopsychosocial losses.[66-69]

DIAGNOSIS AND TREATMENT

Because diagnosis of depression can be difficult, use of a screening tool may help to objectively measure affective functioning. The Geriatric Depression Scale, an instrument of known reliability and validity, was developed to measure depression specifically in the noninstitutionalized older adult population.[70] The 30-item dichotomous scale elicits information on topics relevant to symptoms of depression among older adults, such as memory loss and anxiety. Many other screening tools, each with its own advantages and disadvantages, exist to evaluate the older adult's level of psychological functioning, either in its entirety or as specific, separate components of function.[70]

Treatment goals for older adults with depression are to decrease the symptoms of depression, improve the quality of life, reduce the risk of recurrences, improve health status, decrease health care costs, and decrease mortality.[65] Pharmacotherapy (*i.e.,* use of antidepressants) is thought to be effective in the older adult population. Because of the common anticholinergic and cardiovascular side effects, however, these medications warrant cautious use. Initially they should be given in low doses and titrated according to response and side-effect profile. Significant antidepressant response in older adults generally requires at least 6 to 12 weeks of therapy.[66,67]

Electroconvulsive therapy (ECT) may be the treatment of choice for older adults with severe, pharmacologically resistant major depressive episodes. Studies indicate that individuals over the age of 60 are the largest group of patients who receive ECT. Despite the negative publicity that has been associated

with ECT, the evidence for its short-term efficacy in the treatment of depression is strong. Unfortunately, relapse after ECT is frequent, and alternative treatment strategies, including maintenance ECT or maintenance antidepressants post-ECT, are being researched.[67-69]

"Talking therapy," such as supportive counseling or psychotherapy, is considered to be an important part of the treatment regimen, either alone or in combination with pharmacotherapy or ECT. Alterations in life roles, lack of social support, and chronic medical illnesses are just a few examples of life event changes that may require psychosocial support and new coping skills. Counseling in the older adult population requires special considerations. Individuals with significant vision, hearing, or cognitive impairments may require special approaches. Additionally, many elderly do not see themselves as depressed and reject referrals to mental health professionals. Special efforts are needed to engage these individuals in treatment. Family therapy can be beneficial as a way to help the family understand more about depression and its complexities and as an important source of support for the older adult.[65] Although depression can impose great risks for older adults, it is thought to be the most treatable psychiatric disorder in late life and therefore warrants aggressive case-finding and intervention.

DEMENTIA

Dementia is a very complex and devastating problem that is a major cause of disability in the older adult population. Although the actual prevalence of dementia is unknown, estimates range from 2.5% to 24.6% of those over 65, with the number increasing with advanced age. In fact, a community-based study in East Boston by Evans and colleagues (1989) indicated that 47.2% of those over 85 years of age had dementia.[71] In long-term care facilities, up to 50% of residents have cognitive impairments.[30]

Although there is often decline in intellectual function with aging, dementia, or "senility," is not a normal aging process. Dementia is a syndrome of acquired, persistent impairment in several domains of intellectual function, including memory, language, visuospatial ability, and cognition (abstraction, calculation, judgment, and problem solving). Mood disturbances and changes in personality and behavior often accompany the intellectual deterioration. (Chart 54-1, Chapter 54) describes the diagnostic criteria for dementia as presented in the DSM-IIIR.

Dementia can result from a wide variety of conditions, including degenerative, vascular, neoplastic, demyelinating, infectious, inflammatory, toxic, metabolic, and psychiatric disorders. Up to 70% of older adults with dementia (4 million Americans) are thought to have Alzheimer's disease, a chronic, progressive neurologic disorder of unknown cause. Multi-infarct dementia is the second most common disorder, with up to 30% of dementias attributed to this vascular disorder in which multiple emboli disseminate throughout the brain, causing infarctions.[30, 72]

DIAGNOSIS AND TREATMENT

Much work is being done in the diagnosis and treatment of dementia, in particular of Alzheimer's disease. Currently there are no specific diagnostic tests to determine the presence of Alzheimer's disease, so the diagnosis is essentially made by excluding other possible causes of the dementia symptoms. Experimental medications to halt further cognitive decline from dementia are being evaluated.

A commonly used measure of cognitive function is the Mini Mental State Examination (MMSE) developed by Folstein and colleagues in 1975. This tool provides a brief, objective measure of cognitive functioning and has been widely used. The MMSE, which can be administered in 5 to 10 minutes, consists of a variety of questions that cover memory, orientation, attention, and constructional abilities.[73] The test has been studied and found to fulfill its original goal of providing a brief screening tool that quantifies cognitive impairments and documents cognitive changes over time.[74] However, it has been cautioned that this examination should not be used by itself as a diagnostic tool to identify dementia.

Management of older adults with Alzheimer's disease and other dementias generally involves assuming increasing responsibility for and supplying increasing care to individuals as the illness renders them incapable. Impaired judgment and cognition can prevent the older adult from making reasonable decisions and choices and eventually threatens their overall well-being. Family members often assume the monumental task of caring for older adults with dementia until the burden becomes too great, at which time many older adults are relocated to long-term care facilities.

Some specific behavioral problems are commonly seen in older adults with dementia, including agitation, depression, hallucinations, aggressiveness, and wandering. There may be a need to utilize low doses of pharmacologic agents such as neuroleptics, antidepressants, and antipsychotics. Nonpharmacologic interventions can help control behavioral problems and might preclude the need for medications. Ensuring that the individual's physical needs, such as hygiene, bowel and bladder elimination, safety, and nutrition are met will help prevent catastrophic reactions. Providing a consistent routine in familiar surroundings will also help to alleviate stress. Matching the cognitive needs of the older adult by avoiding both understimulation and overstimulation will assist in preventing behavior problems.[75]

The work of Hall (1987) shows promising results in the care of older adults with Alzheimer's disease. Hall's conceptual model, progressively lowered stress threshold (PLST), proposes that the demented individual's ability to tolerate any type of stress progressively declines as the disease advances. Interventions for the older adult with dementia, therefore, center on eliminating and avoiding stressors as a way to prevent dysfunctional behaviors. These stressors include fatigue, change of routine, excessive demands, overwhelming stimuli, and physical stressors. Hall's work with the PLST model, currently under way using a longitudinal experimental design, is demonstrating encouraging results. Individuals are noted to awaken less at night, use less sedatives and hypnotics, eat better, socialize more, function at a higher level, and experience fewer episodes of anxiety, agitation, and other dysfunctional behaviors.[76, 77]

DELIRIUM

It is important to distinguish dementia from *delirium*, also referred to as acute confusional state. The demented older adult is far more likely to become delirious. The onset of delirium in the demented individual may be mistaken as an exacerbation of the dementia and consequently not treated.[78, 79]

Delirium is an acute disorder developing over a period of hours to days and is frequently seen in hospitalized elderly patients. Prevalence rates range from 30% to 70% of hospitalized individuals over 70 years of age and up to 90% of older adults admitted to psychiatric hospitals.[78] Delirium is defined by the DSM-IIIR (1987) as an organic mental syndrome featuring a global cognitive impairment, disturbances of attention, reduced level of consciousness, increased or decreased psychomotor activity, and a disorganized sleep-wake cycle. The severity of the symptoms tends to fluctuate unpredictably but is often more pronounced at night.[66]

Delirium can be a presenting feature of a physical illness and may be seen with disorders such as myocardial infarction, pneumonia and other infections, cancer, and hypothyroidism. Patients suffering from drug toxicities may also present with delirium.

The exact reason that delirium occurs is unclear. It is speculated that the decreased central nervous system capacity in older adults may precipitate delirium. Other possible contributing factors include vision and hearing impairments, psychological stress, and diseases of other organ systems.[78] Delirium has a high mortality rate, ranging between 20% and 40%. In addition, agitation, disorientation, and fearfulness—the key symptoms of delirium—place the individual at high risk for injuries such as a fracture due to a fall.

DIAGNOSIS AND TREATMENT

Diagnosis of delirium involves recognition of the syndrome and identification of its causes. Management involves treatment of the underlying disease condition and symptomatic relief through supportive therapy (good nutrition and hydration, rest, comfort measures, and emotional support). Prevention of delirium is the overall goal; avoidance of the devastating and life-threatening acute confusional state is the key to successful management and treatment.

In summary, health care for older adults requires unique considerations, taking into account both age-related physiologic changes and specific disease states common in this population. Although aging is not synonymous with disease, the aging process does lend itself to an increased incidence of illness. The overall goal is to assist the older adult in maximizing independence and functional capabilities and minimizing disabilities that can result from various acute and chronic illnesses.

The evaluation of the older adult's functional abilities is a key component in gerontological health care. Medical diagnoses alone are incomplete without an assessment of function. When evaluating levels of function, determination of the older adult's ability to perform activities of daily living (ADL) and instrumental activities of daily living (IADL) should be included.

Among the functional disorders that are common in the older population are urinary incontinence, falls, depression, delirium, and dementia. The older adult is especially prone to urinary incontinence due to changes in the micturition cycle that accompany the aging process. Behavioral techniques can be an effective way to treat incontinence problems in the older adult population. Falls are a common source of concern for the older adult population; although most falls do not result in serious injury, the potential for serious complications and even death is real. Most falls are the result of several risk factors, including age-related biopsychosocial changes, chronic illness, and situational and environmental hazards. Depression is a significant but treatable health problem that is often misdiagnosed and mistreated in the older adult population. Delirium is an acute confusional disorder developing over a period of hours to days and is often seen as a presenting feature of a physical illness or drug toxicity. Dementia is a syndrome of acquired, persistent impairment in several domains of intellectual function, including memory, language, visuospatial ability, and cognition (abstraction, calculation, judgment, and problem solving). Although there is often a slight decline in intellectual function with aging, dementia is not a normal aging process.

■ DRUG THERAPY IN THE OLDER ADULT

Drug therapy in the older adult population is a complex phenomenon influenced by numerous biopsychosocial factors. The elderly are the largest group of consumers of both prescription and over-the-counter (OTC) drugs, spending about $10 billion annually. The average older adult uses 4.5 prescription and 2.1 OTC medications and fills between 12 to 17 prescriptions yearly.[80, 81] The incidence of adverse drug reactions in the elderly is two to three times that found in young adults. This is considered to be a conservative estimate because drug reactions are less well recognized in older adults and because reactions can often mimic symptoms of specific disease states.

Errors in the administration of medications and in compliance are high in the older adult population, estimated by several authors to be between 25% and 50% for community-dwelling elderly. Reasons for this high volume of errors are numerous. Poor manual dexterity, failing eyesight, lack of understanding about the treatment regimen, attitudes and beliefs about medication use, mistrust of health care providers, and forgetfulness or confusion are but a few factors that can affect the adherence to medication regimens. The role of the health care provider can also contribute to improper medication use. There can be a tendency to treat symptoms with drugs rather than fully investigate the etiology of those symptoms. To compound matters, accurate diagnosis of specific disease states can be difficult, as older adults tend to underreport symptoms and because presenting symptoms are often atypical.

Age-related physiologic changes also account for adverse effects of medications. Generally speaking, the absorption of drugs remains essentially unchanged with age, even though the gastric pH is known to elevate and gastric emptying time can be delayed. Changes in drug distribution, however, are clinically significant. Because lean body mass and total body water decreases with advancing age, water-soluble drugs such as digoxin and propranolol tend to have a smaller volume of distribution, resulting in higher plasma concentrations for a given dose and increased likelihood of a toxic reaction. Conversely, fat-soluble drugs such as diazapam are more widely distributed and accumulate in fatty tissue owing to an increase in adipose tissue with aging. This can cause a delay in elimination and accumulation of the drug over time (prolonged half-life) with multiple doses of the same drug. Drug metabolism through the liver is thought to be altered owing to the decrease in hepatic blood flow seen in the older adult. Renal excretion controls the elimination of drugs from the body, and because kidney function declines with age, the rate of drug excretion decreases. This can result in an increased half-life of drugs and is why estimates of creatinine clearance are recommended to determine drug dosing.[82, 83]

Drug use for older adults warrants a cautious approach. "Start low and go slow" is the adage governing drug prescribing in geriatric pharmacology. Very often older adults can achieve therapeutic results on small doses of medications. If necessary, dosing can then be titrated slowly according to response.

Further complicating matters is the issue of polypharmacy in older adults, since they often have multiple disorders that may require multiple drug therapies. Polypharmacy increases the risk of drug interactions and adverse drug reactions and decreases compliance. Drugs and disease states can also interact, causing adverse effects. For example, psychotropic drugs administered to older adults with dementia may cause a worsening of confusion; beta-blocking agents administered to an individual with chronic obstructive pulmonary disease may induce bronchoconstriction; and nonsteroidal anti-inflammatory medications given to an older adult with hypertension can raise blood pressure further.

The use of certain types of medications carries a high risk for older adults and should be avoided if possible. Generally speaking, long-acting drugs or drugs with prolonged half-lives can be problematic. Many sedatives and hypnotics fit into this category, and drugs such as diazepam and flurazepam should be avoided. If these types of agents are indicated, smaller doses of shorter-acting drugs such as orazepam should be considered. Other classes of drugs, such as antidepressants and anxiolytics, may provide the necessary symptomatic relief and may be more appropriate for older adults. Use of these agents warrants caution, however, with consideration for the unique pharmacokinetic changes that accompany aging. Unfortunately, the short-acting agents are not without side effects either. Drugs that possess anticholinergic properties should be used with caution. Anticholinergics are used for a variety of conditions; however, side effects such as dry mouth and eyes, blurred vision, and constipation are common. These drugs can also cause more serious side effects, such as confusion, urinary retention, and orthostatic hypotension. Agents that enter the central nervous system, including narcotics and alcohol, can cause a variety of problems, most notably delirium. These problems most likely occur as a result of a decreased central nervous system reserve capacity.[80, 84]

Because of the serious implications of medication use in the elderly, strategies need to be used to enhance therapeutic effects and prevent harm. Careful evaluation of the need for the medication by the health care provider is the first step. Once decided, analysis of the individual's current medication regimen and disease states is necessary to prevent drug interactions, drug–disease interactions, and adverse responses. Dosing should be at the low end, and frequency of drug administration should be kept to a minimum to simplify the routine and enhance compliance. Timing the dose to a specific activity of daily living (*e.g.*, "Take with breakfast") can also improve compliance, as can special packaging devices such as pill boxes and blister packs. The cost of medications is another important factor to older adults on reduced, fixed incomes. Choosing less expensive products of equal efficacy can increase compliance. Finally, the importance of educating the individual about the medication cannot be overemphasized. Health care professionals need to provide both oral and written information on the principles of medication use and on the specific medications being utilized. This will facilitate active, involved participation by the older adult and enhance the individual's ability to make informed decisions.[83, 84]

In summary, drug therapy in the older adult population is a complex phenomenon influenced by numerous biopsychosocial factors, and errors in administration of medications are frequent in the older adult population. Poor manual dexterity, failing eyesight, lack of understanding of the treatment regimen, attitudes and beliefs about medication use, mistrust of health care providers, and forgetfulness or confusion are but a few factors that can affect the adherence to medication regimens.

■ REFERENCES

1. American Association of Retired Persons. (1990). *A profile of older Americans*. Washington DC: AARP.
2. Glick, R. (1982). Assessing the quality of life. *Perspectives on Aging*, 11(3), 11–16.
3. Erikson, E. (1963). *Childhood and society*. New York: W.W. Norton.
4. Erikson, E.H., Erikson, J.M., & Kivirck, H.Q. (1986). *Vital involvement in old age*. New York: W.W. Norton.
5. Rowe, J.W., & Schneider, E.L. (1990). Aging processes. In Abrams, W.B., & Berkow, R. (Eds.). *The Merck manual of geriatrics* (pp. 303–308). Rahway NJ: Merck Sharp & Dohme Research Laboratories.
6. Hayflick, L. (1985). Theories of biological aging. *Experimental Gerontology*, 10, 145–159.
7. Hayflick, L. (1979). Cell biology of aging. *Federation Proceedings*, 38, 1847–1850.
8. Rudman, D., Feller, A.G., Hoskote, N.S., et al. (1990). Effects of human growth hormone in men over 60 years old. *New England Journal of Medicine*, 323, 1–6.
9. Harmon, D. (1983). Free radicals and the orientation, evolution, and present status of free radical theory of aging. In Armstrong, D., et al. (Eds.). *Aging, Vol. 27. Free radicals in molecular biology* (pp. 1–12). New York: Raven Press.
10. Blass, J.P., Cherniack, E.P., & Weksler, M.E. (1992).

Theories of aging. In Calkins, E., Ford, A.B., & Kratz, P.R. (Eds.). *Practice of geriatrics* (2nd ed., pp. 10–18). Philadelphia: W.B. Saunders.

11. Holliday, R. (1990). The limited proliferation of cultured human diploid cells: Regulation and senescence. *Journal of Gerontology, 45*, B36–B41.

12. Duthie, E.H., Jr. (1990). Geriatric medicine. In Kochar, M.S., & Kutty, K. (Eds.). *Concise textbook of medicine* (2nd ed., pp. 359–380). New York: Elsevier.

13. Phillips, T.J., & Gilchrest, B.A. (1990). Skin changes and disorders. In Abrams, W.B., & Berkow, R. (Eds.). *The Merck manual of geriatrics* (pp. 1025–1054). Rahway NJ: Merck Sharp & Dohme Research Laboratories.

14. Macmillan, A.L. (1989). Aging and the skin. In Brocklehurst, J.C. (Ed.). *Textbook of geriatric medicine and gerontology* (3rd ed., pp. 899–914). Edinburgh: Churchill Livingstone.

15. Wilmore, J.H. (1991). The aging of bone and muscle. *Clinics in Sports Medicine, 10*, 231–244.

16. Spirduso, W.W. (1982). Physical fitness in relation to motor aging. In Mortimer, J.A., Pirozzolo, F.J., & Maletta, G.J. (Eds.). *The aging motor system: Advances in neurogerontology, Vol. 3* (pp. 120–151). New York: Praeger Publishers.

17. Scileppi, K.P. (1985). Aging of the musculoskeletal system. In Sculco, T.P. (Ed.). *Orthopedic care of the geriatric patient* (pp. 3–11). St. Louis: C.V. Mosby.

18. Fulop, T., Worum, I., Csongor, J., et al. (1985). Body composition in elderly people. *Gerontology, 31*, 150–157.

19. U.S. Department of Health and Human Services. (1980). *Statement on hypertension in the elderly* (pp. 1–7). Bethesda MD: National Institutes of Health.

20. Wei, J.Y. (1992). Age and the cardiovascular system. *New England Journal of Medicine, 327*, 1735–1739.

21. Smith, J.J., & Porth, C.J.M. (1990). Age and the response to orthostatic stress. In Smith, J.J. (Ed.). *Circulatory response to the upright position* (p. 136). Boca Raton, FL: CRC Press.

22. Lakatta, E.G. (1990). Changes in cardiovascular function with aging. *European Heart Journal, 11*(Suppl C), 22–29.

23. Morley, J.E., & Reese, S.S. (1989). Clinical implications of the aging heart. *American Journal of Medicine, 86*, 77–86.

24. Branfronbrener, M., Landowne, M., & Shock, N.W. (1955). Changes in cardiac output with age. *Circulation, 12*, 557–566.

25. Rodeheffer, R.J., Gerstenblith, G., Becker, L.C., et al. (1984). Exercise cardiac output is maintained with advancing age in healthy human subjects: Cardiac dilatation and increased stroke volume compensate for diminished heart rate. *Circulation, 69*, 203–213.

26. VanTosh, A., LaKatta, E.G., Fleg, J.L., et al. (1980). Ventricular changes during submaximal exercise: Effect of aging in normal man. *Circulation, 62*(4, PtII), 111–129.

27. Levitzsky, M.G. (1984). Effects of aging on the respiratory system. *Physiologist, 27*, 102.

28. Morris, J.C., & McManus, D.Q. (1991). The neurology of aging: Normal and pathological change. *Geriatrics, 46*(8), 47–54.

29. Paulson, G.W. (1983), Disorders of the central nervous system in the aged. *Medical Clinics of North America, 67*, 345–359.

30. Cummings, J.L., & Benson, D.F. (1992). *Dementia: A clinical approach* (2nd ed.). Boston: Butterworth-Heinemann.

31. Werner, J.S., Peterzell, D.H., & Scheetz, A.J. (1990). Light, vision, and aging. *Optometry and Vision Science, 67*, 214–229.

32. Langsten, R.H.S. (1990). The aging eye. In Schrier, R.W. (Ed.). *Geriatric medicine* (pp. 119–128). Philadelphia: W.B. Saunders.

33. Corso, J.F. (1971). Sensory changes and age effects in normal adults. *Journal of Gerontology, 26*, 90–105.

34. Rees, T.S., & Duckert, L.G. (1990). Auditory and vestibular dysfunction in aging. In Hazzard, W.R., Andres, R., Bierman, E.L., & Blass, J.P. (Eds.). *Principles of geriatric medicine and gerontology* (pp. 432–444). New York: McGraw-Hill.

35. Schrow, R., & Nerbonne, M. (1980). Hearing level in nursing home residents. *Journal of Speech and Hearing Disabilities, 45*, 124.

36. Blair, K.A. (1990). Aging: Physiological aspects and clinical implications. *Nurse Practitioner, 15*(2), 14–28.

37. Meyerhoff, W., & Patt, B.S. (1992). Otologic disorders. In Calkins, E., Ford, A.B., & Katz, P.R. (Eds.). *Practice of geriatrics* (pp. 247–255). Philadelphia: W.B. Saunders.

38. Schneider, E.L. (1983). Infectious diseases in the elderly. *Annals of Internal Medicine, 98*, 395–400.

39. Haddy, R.I. (1988). Aging, infections and the immune system. *Journal of Family Practice, 27*, 409–413.

40. Kay, M.M.B. (1990). Immunologic problems. In Schrier, R.W. (Ed.). *Geriatric medicine* (pp. 376–398). Philadelphia: W.B. Saunders.

41. Soergel, K.H., Zboralske, F.E., & Amberg, J.R. (1964). Presbyesophagus: Esophageal motility in nonagenarians. *Journal of Clinical Investigation, 43*, 1472.

42. Nelson, J.B., & Castell, D.O. (1990). Aging of the gastrointestinal system. In Hazzard, W.R., Andres, R., Bierman, E.L., et al. (Eds.). *Principles of geriatric medicine and gerontology* (2nd ed., pp. 593–608). New York: McGraw-Hill.

43. Parks, T.G. (1975). Natural history of diverticular disease. *Clinical Gastroenterology, 4*, 53.

44. Epstein, M. (1979). Effects of aging in the kidney. *Federation Proceedings, 38*, 168.

45. Samiy, A.H. (1983). Renal disease in the elderly. *Medical Clinics of North America, 67*, 463–480.

46. Levi, M., & Schrier, R.W. (1990). Renal disease. In Schrier, R.W. (Ed.). *Geriatric medicine* (pp. 189–206). Philadelphia: W.B. Saunders.

47. Beck, L.H., & Burkart, J.M. (1990). Aging changes in renal function. In Hazzard, W,R,, Andres, R., Bierman, E.L., et al. (Eds.). *Principles of geriatric medicine and gerontology* (2nd ed., pp. 555–564). New York: McGraw-Hill.

48. Jeter, K., Fuller, N., & Norton, C. (1990). *Nursing for continence*. Philadelphia: W.B. Saunders.

49. McGuire, E.J., DeLancey, J.O.L., & Elkins, T. (1990). Female genitourinary disorders. In Abrams, W.B., & Berkow, R. (Eds.). *Merck manual of geriatrics* (pp. 624–631). Rahway, NJ: Merck, Sharp & Dohme Research Laboratories.

50. Freed, S.Z. (1986). Genitourinary disease in the elderly. In Rossman, I. (Ed.). *Clinical geriatrics* (3rd ed., pp. 352–363). Philadelphia: J.B. Lippincott.

51. Kane, R.A., & Kane, R.L. (1981). *Assessing the elderly: A practical guide to measurement*. Lexington, MA: Lexington Books.

52. Katz, S., Ford, A.B., Moskowitz, R.W., et al. (1963). Studies of illness in the aged: The Index of ADL. *Journal of the American Medical Association, 185*, 914–919.

53. Katz, S., Downs, T.D., Cash, H.R., et al. (1970). Progress in development of the Index of ADL. *Gerontologist, 10*, 20–30.

54. Aging for Health Care Policy and Research. (1992). *Urinary incontinence in adults: Guideline report* (AHCPR Publication No. 92-0039). Rockville, MD: AHCPR.

55. Ouslander, J., & Uman, G. (1985). Urinary incontinence: Opportunities for research, education, and improvement in medical care in the nursing home setting. In Schreider, E. (Ed.). *The teaching nursing home* (pp. 73–196). New York: Raven Press.

56. Diokno, A.C., Brock, B.M., Braun, M.B., et al. (1986). Prevalence of urinary incontinence and other urological symptoms in the noninstitutionalized elderly. *Journal of Urology, 136*, 1022–1025.

57. Hu, T.W. (1990). Impact of urinary incontinence on health-care costs. *Journal of the American Geriatric Society, 38*, 292–295.

58. Kane, R.L., Ouslander, J.G., & Abrass, J.B. (1989). *Essentials of clinical geriatrics* (2nd ed.). New York: McGraw-Hill.

59. Rubenstein, L.Z., Robbins, A.L., Schulman, B.L., et al. (1988). Falls and instability in the elderly. *Journal of the American Geriatric Society, 36*, 266–278.

60. Baker, S.P., & Harvey, A.H. (1985). Fall injuries in the elderly. *Clinics in Geriatric Medicine, 1*, 501–508.

61. National Center for Health Statistics. (1986). 1985 summary, National Hospital Discharge Survey: Advanced data from Vital and Health Statistics, 127, DHHS(PHS) 86–1250. Hyattsville, MD: Department of Health and Human Services.

62. Tinetti, M. (1990). Falls. In Hazzard, W.R., Andres, R., Bierman, E.L., & Blass, L.E. (Eds.). *Principles of geriatric medicine and gerontology* (2nd ed., pp. 1192–1199). New York: McGraw-Hill.

63. Smallegan, M. (1983). How families decide on nursing home admission. *Geriatric Consultant, 2*, 21.

64. Surdarsky, L. (1990). Geriatrics: Gait disorders in the elderly. *New England Journal of Medicine, 322*, 1441–1446.

65. *Diagnosis and treatment of depression in late life.* (1991). Reprinted from NIH Consensus Development Conference Consensus Statement, November 4–6.

66. American Psychiatric Association. (1987). *Diagnostic and statistical manual of mental disorders* (3rd ed., rev.). Washington, DC: American Psychiatric Association.

67. Blazer, D. (1990). Depression. In Hazzard, W.R., Andres, B., Bierman, E.L., & Blass, J.P. (Eds.). *Principles of geriatric medicine and gerontology* (2nd ed., pp. 1010–1018). New York: McGraw-Hill.

68. Blazer, D.G., Bachar, J.R., & Manton, K.G. (1986). Suicide in late life: Review and commentary. *Journal of the American Geriatric Society, 34*, 519–525.

69. Hay, D.P. (1990). Electroconvulsive therapy, mental health and aging. *International Journal of Technology and Aging, 3*(1), 39–45.

70. Yesavage, J.A., Brink, T.L., Rose, T.L., et al. (1983). Development and validation of a geriatric depression scale: A preliminary report. *Journal of Psychiatric Research, 17*, 37–49.

71. Evans, D.A., Funkenstein, H., Albert, M.S., et al. (1989). Prevalence of Alzheimer's disease in a community population of older persons: Higher than previously reported. *Journal of the American Medical Association, 262*, 2551–2556.

72. Folstein, M.R., & Folstein, S.E. (1990). Syndromes of altered mental state. In Hazzard, W.R., Andres, R., Bierman, E.L., & Blass, J.P. (Eds.). *Principles of geriatric medicine and gerontology* (2nd ed., pp, 1089–1101). New York: McGraw-Hill.

73. Folstein, M.F., Folstein, B.E., & McHugh, P.R. (1975). "Mini-Mental State": A practical method for grading the cognitive state of patients for the clinician. *Journal of Psychiatric Research, 12*, 189–198.

74. Tombough, T.N., & McIntyre, N.J. (1992). The "Mini-Mental State examination": A comprehensive review. *Journal of the American Geriatric Society, 40*, 922–935.

75. Richards, B.S. (1990). Alzheimer's disease: A disabling neurophysiological disorder with complex nursing implications. *Archives of Psychiatric Nursing, 4*(1), 39–42.

76. Hall, G.R., & Buckwalter, K.C. (1987). Progressively lowered stress threshold: A conceptual model for care of adults with Alzheimer's disease. *Archives of Psychiatric Nursing, 1*, 399–406.

77. Hall, G., Kirschling, M.V., & Todd, S. (1986). Sheltered freedom—an Alzheimer's unit in an ICF. *Geriatric Nursing, 7*, 232–236.

78. Foley, J.M. (1982). Delirium. In Calkins, E., Ford, A.B., & Katz, P.R. (Eds.). *Practice of geriatrics* (2nd ed., pp. 305–308). Philadelphia: W.B. Saunders.

79. Lipowski, Z.J. (1990). Delirium in older patients. *Journal of the American Medical Association, 40*, 829–838.

80. Baum, C., Kennedy, D.L., Forbes, M.B., et al. (1985). Drug use and expenditures in 1982. *Journal of the American Medical Association, 253*, 382–386.

81. Ostran, J.R., Hammarlund, E.R., Christensen, D.B., et al. (1985). Medication usage in an elderly population. *Medical Care, 23*, 157–164.

82. Montamort, S.C., Cusack, B.J., & Vestal, R.E. (1989). Management of drug therapy in the elderly. *New England Journal of Medicine, 321*, 303–309.

83. Beers, M.H. (1992). Medication use in the elderly. In Calkins, E., Ford, A.B., & Katz, P.R. (Eds.). *Practice of geriatrics* (2nd ed., pp. 33–49). Philadelphia: W.B. Saunders.

84. Kuiper Pikna, J., & Porth, C.M. (1990). The medication-taking behaviors reported by community-dwelling individuals 65 years of age and older. (Unpublished.)

ALTERATIONS IN INTEGRATED BODY FUNCTIONS

C H A P T E R   8

STRESS AND ADAPTATION

Stress
Stressors
The Stress Response
Manifestations of the Stress
Response

Adaptation
Constancy of the Internal
Environment
Homeostasis
Control Systems

System Efficiency
Feedback Systems
**Factors Affecting Adaptation
to Stress**

■ OBJECTIVES

After you have studied this chapter, you should be able to meet the following objectives:

■ State Selye's definition of stress.
■ Define *stressor*.
■ Cite two factors that influence the nature of the stress response.
■ Compare specific and nonspecific stress responses.
■ Explain the interactions of the nervous system in mediating the stress response.
■ Describe the stress responses of the autonomic nervous system, the endocrine system, the immune system, and the musculoskeletal system.
■ Explain the purpose of adaptation.

■ Describe the components of a simple control system.
■ Describe the function of a negative feedback system.
■ Cite Cannon's four features of homeostasis.
■ List at least six factors that influence a person's adaptive capacity.
■ Relate experience and previous learning to the process of adaptation.
■ Contrast anatomic and physiologic reserve.
■ Propose a way by which social support may serve to buffer stress.

Health is a dynamic state in which energy must be expended continuously to adapt to life stresses. Much of this energy is used to recruit physiologic and psychological behaviors that oppose or compensate for perceived threats to the integrity of the internal environment. In this respect, the human body is truly an amazing structure—able to withstand exposure to environmental stresses while maintaining its internal environment within the confines of what is termed *normal*. From astronauts who have traveled to the moon and from explorers of the ocean's depths, we have learned that vital physiologic functions such as heart rate, blood *p*H, and body temperature remain remarkably similar to those observed under normal environmental conditions. Even in advanced disease states, the body retains much of its adaptive capacity and is able to maintain the internal environment within relatively normal limits.

Carol Mattson Porth: PATHOPHYSIOLOGY: CONCEPTS OF ALTERED HEALTH STATES, 4th ed. © 1994, 1990, 1986, 1982 J.B. Lippincott Company

■ STRESS

Interest in the roles that stress and altered adaptive processes play in the development of disease has increased. Hypertension, heart disease, and peptic ulcer are but a few of the diseases associated with stress. Stress may contribute directly to the production of disease, or it may contribute to the development of behaviors such as smoking, overeating, and drug abuse, which increase the risk of disease.

Stress has been defined in many ways. To the physicist, the term refers to a force, strain, or pressure applied to a system. To the lay person, stress frequently implies exposure to excessive demands or environmental conditions that cause emotional upset and tension. To the psychologist, stress can be anything that alters the psychological homeostatic processes.[1] To the anthropologist, stress is adversity: coercion between people or between the environment and humans, or between history and humankind.[2] Hans Selye, the world-renowned endocrinologist and pioneer in the field of stress research, has described stress as the nonspecific response of the body to any demand made on it.[3]

STRESSORS

The events or environmental agents responsible for initiating the stress response are called *stressors*. According to Selye, stressors may be endogenous, arising from within the body, or exogenous, arising from outside the body.[3] Stressors can be physical, psychological, or sociologic. They include mental and physical effort, extremes of temperature, hunger, thirst, and fatigue, and other everyday experiences. Mason has suggested that emotional reactions to the stressor serve as the final common pathway for the stress response, emphasizing the need to consider the impact that learning and emotion have on the response.[4]

Of particular interest are the differences in the body's response to stressors that threaten the integrity of the body's physiologic environment and those that threaten the integrity of the person's psychosocial environment. Many of the body's responses to physiologic stressors are controlled on a moment-by-moment basis by feedback mechanisms that limit their utilization and duration of action. For example, the baroreflex-mediated rise in heart rate that occurs when one moves from the recumbent to the standing position is almost instantaneous and subsides within seconds. Furthermore, the response to physiologic stressors that threaten the integrity of the internal environment is specific to the stress—the body does not usually raise the body temperature when a rise in heart rate is needed. In contrast, the response to

psychological stressors is not regulated with the same degree of specificity and feedback control—instead, the effect may be inappropriate and sustained.

THE STRESS RESPONSE

In explaining the stress response, Selye proposed that two factors determine the nature of the stress response: (1) the properties of the stressor and (2) the conditioning of the person being stressed.[3] Most stressors produce both specific and nonspecific responses. For example, the joy of becoming a new parent and the sorrow of losing a parent are completely different experiences, yet their stressor effect—the nonspecific demand for adjustment to a new situation—can be similar. The specific stress responses alert a person to the presence of the stressor, whereas the nonspecific effects, which involve neuroendocrine responses such as increased autonomic nervous system activity, are designed to maintain or reestablish normality and are independent of specific responses. The ability of the same stressor to produce different responses and disorders in different people indicates the adaptive capacity of the person, or what Selye termed *conditioning factors*. These conditioning factors may be internal (genetic predisposition, age, sex, or others) or external (exposure to environmental agents, treatment with certain drugs, or dietary factors).[3]

MANIFESTATIONS OF THE STRESS RESPONSE

The manifestations of the stress response—a pounding headache, cold moist hands, a stiff neck, and increased incidence of infections—reflect, for the most part, the nonspecific aspects of the stress response. They include responses of the autonomic nervous system, the endocrine system, the musculoskeletal system, and the immune system. The integration of these responses, which occurs at the level of the central nervous system (CNS), is elusive and complex. It relies on communication between the cerebral cortex, the limbic system, the thalamus, the hypothalamus, and the reticular formation and reticular activating system (Fig. 8-1). The thalamus functions as a relay center and is important in sorting out and distributing sensory input. The reticular formation modulates mental alertness, autonomic nervous system activity, and skeletal muscle tone; but it does this using input and output from other neural structures. Likewise, the hypothalamus modulates the functioning of both the endocrine and the autonomic nervous system. The limbic system is involved with the emotional components (fear, excitement, rage,

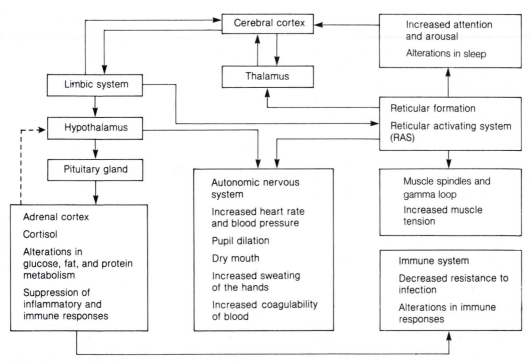

FIG. 8-1. Stress pathways. The *broken line* represents negative feedback.

anger) of the stress response, and the cerebral cortex is involved with vigilance, cognition, and focused attention.

Musculoskeletal Responses. The musculoskeletal tension that occurs during the stress response reflects the increased activity of the reticular formation and its influence on the muscle spindles and the gamma loop (descending neural pathways, gamma motor neurons, spindle muscle fibers, afferent neurons, and alpha motor neurons), which control muscle tone. Muscle tension can remain as a prolonged manifestation of the stress response and can cause stiffness of the neck, backache, headaches, and other complaints.

Autonomic Nervous System Responses. The sympathetic division of the autonomic nervous system confers an adaptive advantage during a stress situation. The sympathetic nervous system manifestation of the stress reaction has been termed the *fight-or-flight response.* This is the most rapid of the stress responses and represents the basic survival response of our primitive ancestors when confronted with the perils of the wilderness and its inhabitants. In the presence of danger, the alternatives were clear—run away or stand up and fight. The heart and respiratory rates increase, the hands and feet become moist, the pupils dilate, the mouth becomes dry, and the activity of the gastrointestinal (GI) tract decreases. The autonomic nervous system is also in-

volved in less-threatening situations. For example, the autonomic nervous system controls the circulatory responses to activities of daily living such as moving from the seated or lying, to the standing position.

Endocrine Responses. A wide variety of hormones are highly responsive to stressful situations. The most widely studied hormonal mechanisms have been those associated with the hypothalamic–pituitary–adrenal axis that regulates body levels of adrenocortical hormones (mainly cortisol). The production of cortisol by the adrenal gland is controlled by the adrenocorticotropic hormone (ACTH) from the anterior pituitary. ACTH, in turn, is controlled by the corticotropin-releasing hormone (CRH) from the hypothalamus. The influence of emotion and stress on cortisol production is largely through the CNS by way of the hypothalamus. Cortisol is involved in maintaining blood glucose levels, facilitating fat metabolism, supporting vascular responsiveness, and modulating CNS function. In addition, cortisol affects mineral turnover in bone, hematopoiesis, gastric acid secretion, protein and collagen synthesis, immune responses, and renal function.

Other hormones, such as growth hormone, thyroid hormone, vasopressin, the sex hormones, and others, are also involved in the stress response. Stress is associated with inhibition of thyroid hormone, the purpose of which may be to conserve energy during stress. Likewise, both the reproductive hormones and growth hormone are inhibited by various components of the hypothalamic–pituitary–adrenal axis.[5]

As a young medical student, Selye noted that patients suffering from diverse disease conditions had many signs and symptoms in common. He noted that "whether a man suffers from a loss of blood, an infectious disease, or advanced cancer, he loses his appetite, his muscular strength, and his ambition to accomplish anything; usually the patient also loses weight and even his facial expression betrays that he is ill."[3] Selye referred to this as the "syndrome of just being sick." To Selye, the response to stress was a process that enabled the body to resist the stressor in the best possible way by enhancing the function of the system best able to respond to it. He termed this response the *general adaptation syndrome (GAS)*. The GAS involves three stages: (1) the alarm stage, (2) the stage of resistance, and (3) the stage of exhaustion. The hypothalamic–pituitary–adrenal axis assumes a pivotal role in stress homeostasis during the alarm stage. Selye observed a triad of adrenal enlargement, thymus atrophy, and gastric ulcers in the rats used in his original studies. During the alarm stage, no one organ system is predominantly active. The most appropriate channels of defense are recruited during the stage of resistance. During this second stage, the increased cortisol levels that were present during the first stage drop, because they are no longer needed. During the third stage—the stage of exhaustion—the reaction spreads because of wear and tear on the most appropriate channel of adaptation.[6]

Selye contended that many ailments, such as various emotional disturbances, mildly annoying headaches, insomnia, upset stomach, gastric and duodenal ulcers, and certain types of rheumatic disorders, as well as cardiovascular and kidney diseases, appear to be initiated or encouraged by the "body itself because of its faulty adaptive reactions to potentially injurious agents."[3]

Immunologic Responses. There is increasing interest in the effect that stress has on the immunologic responses. The occurrence of the oral disease acute necrotizing gingivitis, in which the normal bacterial flora of the mouth becomes invasive, is well known by dentists to be associated with acute stress, such as final exams.[7] Similarly, herpes simplex I (cold sores) often develops during periods of inadequate rest, fever, ultraviolet radiation, and emotional upset. In this case, the resident herpes virus is kept in check by body defenses, most likely by T-lymphocytes, until a stressful event occurs and causes suppression of the immune system. It was shown that psychological stress was associated in a dose–response manner with an increased risk of developing the common

cold, and this risk was attributable to increased rates of infection rather than frequency of symptoms after infection.[8]

The exact mechanism by which stress produces its effect on the immune response is unknown and probably varies from person to person, depending on genetic endowment and environmental factors. It is known, however, that the stress response induces changes in a number of hormonal factors that affect the immune response. The hallmark of the stress response, as first described by Selye, is the presence of conditions (increased corticosteroid production and atrophy of the thymus) known to suppress the immune response. This process can be used clinically, as in the administration of pharmacologic preparations of the corticosteroid hormones to suppress the inflammatory and immune response. The existence of a feedback loop between the immune system and the hypothalamic–pituitary–adrenal system suggests the intriguing possibility that there may be interaction between the two systems in decreasing resistance to infection and in the surveillance function of the immune system in preventing cancer (see Chapter 5). The receptors for a number of CNS-controlled hormones and neuromediators reportedly have been found on lymphocytes. Among these are receptors for glucocorticoids, insulin, testosterone, catecholamines, estrogens, histamine, acetylcholine, and growth hormone.[9] The presence of a hormone receptor on a cell suggests that the cell's function is influenced by the hormone.

Much of the literature regarding stress and the immune response focuses on the causal role of stress in immune-related diseases. It has been suggested that the reverse may occur; emotional and psychological stress may be a manifestation of alterations in the CNS resulting from the immune response. In the case of cancer, this could mean that the subjective feelings of helplessness and hopelessness that have been repeatedly related to the onset and progression of cancers may arise secondary to the central nervous system effects of products released by immune cells during the early stage of the disease.[10]

In summary, stress is defined in many ways. Hans Selye, the world-renowned endocrinologist and pioneer in the field of stress research, defined stress as the nonspecific response of the body to any demands made on it. The event or environmental agent that produces the stress is called a stressor. Stressors may be physical, psychological, or social. They include mental and physical effort, extremes of temperature, hunger, thirst, fatigue, and other everyday experiences. Most stressors produce both specific and nonspecific responses. The specific responses alert the person to the nature of the stressor and assist in establishing definitive measures to deal with it. The nonspecific responses are designed to maintain or reestablish normality.

■ ADAPTATION

The ability to adapt to a wide range of environments and stressors is not peculiar to humans. According to René Dubos (a microbiologist noted for his study of human response to the total environment), "adaptability is found throughout life and is perhaps the one attribute that distinguishes most clearly the world of life from the world of inanimate matter."[11] Living organisms, no matter how primitive, do not submit passively to the impact of environmental forces. They attempt to respond adaptively, each in its own unique and most suitable manner. The higher the organism on the evolutionary scale, the larger its repertoire of adaptive mechanisms and its ability to select and limit aspects of the environment to which it responds. The most fully evolved mechanisms are the social responses through which individuals or groups modify their environments, their habits, or both, to achieve a way of life that is suited to their needs.[11]

Human beings, because of their highly developed nervous system and intellect, usually have alternative mechanisms for adapting and have the ability to control many aspects of their environment. Air conditioning and central heating limit the need to adapt to extreme changes in environmental temperature. The control of microbial growth, immunization, and the availability of antibiotics eliminate the need to respond to common infectious agents. On the other hand, modern technology creates new challenges for adaptation and provides new sources of stress, such as increased noise, air pollution, exposure to chemicals that reduce the microbial agents in the environment and increase the shelf life of the foods we eat, and changes in the biologic rhythms imposed by shift work and transcontinental flights.

CONSTANCY OF THE INTERNAL ENVIRONMENT

The environment in which body cells live is not the external environment that surrounds the organism, but a local fluid environment that surrounds each cell. It is from this internal environment that body cells receive their nourishment, and it is into this fluid that they secrete their wastes. Even the contents of the GI tract and lungs do not become part of the internal environment until they have been absorbed into the extracellular fluid. A multicellular organism is able to survive only as long as the composition of the internal environment is compatible with the survival needs of the individual cells. Even a small change in the *p*H of the body fluids can disrupt the metabolic processes of individual cells. Claude Bernard, a nineteenth-century physiologist, was the first to describe clearly the central importance of a stable internal environment (*milieu interne*). Bernard recognized that body fluids that surround the cells and the various organ systems provide the means for exchange between the external and the internal environments.

HOMEOSTASIS

The concept of a stable internal environment was supported by Walter B. Cannon, who emphasized that this kind of stability, which he termed *homeostasis*, was achieved through a system of carefully coordinated physiologic processes that oppose change. He pointed out that these processes were largely automatic.

Cannon emphasized that homeostasis involves not only resistance to external disturbances, but also resistance to disturbances from within. In his book *Wisdom of the Body*, published in 1939, Cannon presented four tentative propositions to describe the general features of homeostasis:

1. Constancy in an open system, such as our bodies represent, requires mechanisms that act to maintain this constancy. Cannon based this proposition on insights into the ways by which steady states such as glucose concentrations, body temperature, and acid–base balance were regulated.

2. Steady-state conditions require that any tendency toward change be automatically met with factors that resist change. An increase in blood sugar results in thirst as the body attempts to dilute the concentration of sugar in the extracellular fluid.

3. The regulating system that determines the homeostatic state consists of a number of cooperating mechanisms acting simultaneously or successively. Blood sugar is regulated by insulin, glucagon, and other hormones that control its release from the liver or its uptake by the tissues.

4. Homeostasis does not occur by chance, but is the result of organized self-government. With this postulate, Cannon emphasized that, when a factor is known to shift homeostasis in one direction, it is reasonable to expect the existence of mechanisms that have the opposite effect. In the homeostatic regulation of blood sugar, one would expect to find mechanisms that both raise and lower blood sugar.[12]

CONTROL SYSTEMS

The ability of the body to function under conditions of change in the internal and external environment depends on the thousands of control systems that serve to regulate body function. The body's control systems regulate cellular function, control the life processes, and integrate the interrelated functions of the different organ systems.

The most intricate of these control systems is the genetic control system that regulates cellular function, including cell structure and replication. Other control systems regulate function within organs and systems, whereas still others operate throughout the body to integrate the functions of the different organ systems. The concentration of carbon dioxide in the extracellular spaces is regulated by the respiratory and nervous systems, and the blood sugar concentration is controlled mainly by the liver and pancreas.

A homeostatic control system is a collection of interconnected components that function to keep a physical or chemical parameter of the body relatively constant. At least three essential components exist in a control system: (1) a *sensor*, which detects changes in product or function, (2) a *comparator*, which compares the sensed value with an acceptable range, and (3) an *effector system*, which returns the function or product to the acceptable range (Fig. 8-2).

SYSTEM EFFICIENCY

The effectiveness of a system is determined by the amount of change (amplification or gain) that occurs within the system in response to changes in external chemical or physical parameters. In his textbook of physiology, Guyton uses the example of a 1-degree Fahrenheit change in body temperature (from 98°F to 99°F) that occurs when the ambient temperature is increased from 60°F to 110°F.[13] As body temperature

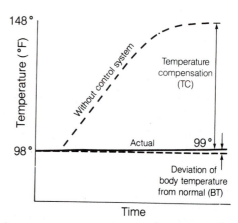

FIG. 8-3. Effects on body temperature of suddenly increasing the air temperature 50°F, showing the hypothetical effect without a control system and the actual effect with a normal control system. (Guyton, A. [1986]. *Textbook of medical physiology* [7th ed.]. Philadelphia: W.B. Saunders)

rises because of the change in external temperature, sensors in the system detect the error, and sufficient compensation, in terms of radiation and evaporative heat losses from the skin, returns the temperature to within 1 degree Fahrenheit of the set point of the system. Were it not for the efficiency of the control system, the body temperature would have risen 50 degrees Fahrenheit instead of 1 degree Fahrenheit (Fig. 8-3).

FEEDBACK SYSTEMS

Most control systems in the body operate by *negative feedback mechanisms*, which function in a manner similar to the thermostat on a heating system. When the monitored function decreases below the set point of the system, the feedback mechanism causes the function to increase, and when the function is increased above the set point, the feedback mechanism causes it to decrease (Fig. 8-4). For example, in the negative feedback mechanism that controls blood glucose levels, an increase in blood glucose stimulates an increase in insulin, which enhances the removal of glucose from the blood. When sufficient glucose has left the bloodstream to cause blood glucose levels to fall, the release of glucose from the liver and the recruitment of other counterregulatory mechanisms cause the blood glucose to return to normal.

The reader is likely to ask why most physiologic control systems function under negative rather than *positive feedback mechanisms*. The answer is that a positive feedback mechanism interjects instability rather than stability into a system. It produces a vicious circle in which the initiating stimulus produces more of the same. In a positive feedback system, exposure to an increase in environmental temperature would

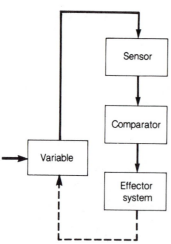

FIG. 8-2. A simple control system consisting of a sensor that monitors a physiologic variable, a comparator that compares the actual value of the monitored variable with the setpoint of the system, and an effector system that functions to correct the disturbance (*solid line*). The *broken line* represents feedback control.

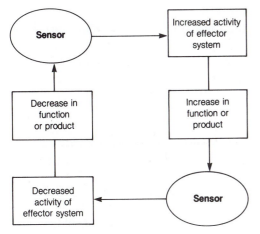

FIG. 8-4. Negative feedback control of a body function, hormone level, or biochemical product.

invoke compensatory mechanisms designed to increase rather than decrease body temperature.

■ FACTORS AFFECTING ADAPTATION TO STRESS

Adaptation and homeostasis are idealized concepts. In practice, the body has available to it a wide variety and range of responses for adjusting to the external and internal environments, and conditions do not always return to their original state.

Generally speaking, adaptation affects the whole person. When adapting to stress, the body uses those behaviors that are most efficient and effective—it does not use long-term mechanisms when short-term adaptation mechanisms are sufficient. The increase in heart rate that accompanies a febrile illness is a temporary response designed to deliver additional oxygen to the tissues during the short period when the elevated temperature increases the metabolic needs of the tissues (the increase in heart rate also expedites delivery of heat-carrying blood to the skin surface, where the heat can be lost to the external environment). On the other hand, adaptive responses such as hypertrophy of the left ventricle in people with systemic hypertension are long-term responses.

Adaptation is affected by a number of factors, including previous experience and learning, physiologic reserve, time, genetic endowment and age, health status, nutrition, sleep–wake cycles, and psychosocial factors (Fig. 8-5).

Previous Experience and Learning. Dubos cites the case of an old Chinese fisherman (the type depicted on the scrolls of the Sung era) as an example of the effect that experience and learning have on adaptation.[11]

The fisherman appears fully at ease and relaxed in his primitive boat, floating on a misty lake, or even a polluted and crowded harbor. He has probably experienced many tribulations in the course of his years of struggle and poverty, but has survived by becoming almost totally identified with his environment. In fact he is so well adapted to it that he will probably live for many more years, without modern comfort, sanitation, or medical care, just by letting his existence be ruled by what he considers to be the unalterable laws of the seasons and nature. In the course of his life, he developed different protective mechanisms that increased his immunologic, physiologic, and psychic resistance to the physicochemical hardships, the parasites, and the social conflicts which threatened him every day. Finally, he has elected to spend the rest of his life in the environment in which he has evolved and to which he has become adapted. Robust though he appears and really is, he probably would soon become sick if he moved into an area where the parasites, physiologic stresses, and social customs differ from the ones among which he has spent his early life.

Physiologic Reserve. The trained athlete is able to increase cardiac output six- to sevenfold during exercise. The safety margin for adaptation of most body systems is considerably greater than that needed for normal activities. The red blood cells carry more oxygen than the tissues can use, the liver and fat cells store excess nutrients, and bone tissue has a storage of calcium in excess of that needed for normal neuromuscular function. The ability of body systems to increase their function given the need to adapt is

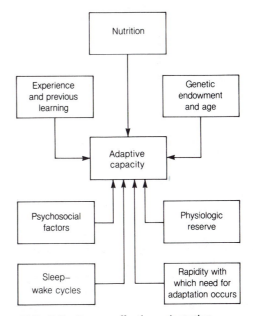

FIG. 8-5. Factors affecting adaptation.

known as the *physiologic reserve*. Many of the body organs, such as the lungs, kidneys, and adrenal glands, are paired to provide not only a physiologic but an *anatomic reserve* as well. Both organs are not needed to ensure the continued existence and maintenance of the internal environment. Many people function normally with only one lung or one kidney. In kidney disease, for example, signs of renal failure do not occur until about 90% of the functioning nephrons have been destroyed.

Time. Adaptation is most efficient when changes occur gradually rather than suddenly. It is possible, for instance, to lose a liter or more of blood through chronic GI bleeding over a period of a week without developing signs of shock. However, a sudden hemorrhage that causes loss of an equal amount of blood is apt to cause hypotension and shock.

Genetic Endowment. Adaptation is further affected by the availability of adaptive responses and flexibility in selecting the most appropriate and economical response. The greater the number of available responses, the more effective the capacity to adapt.

Genetic endowment can ensure that the systems that are essential to adaptation function adequately. Even a gene that has deleterious effects may prove adaptive in some environments. In Africa, the gene for sickle cell anemia persists in some populations because it provides some resistance to the parasite that causes malaria.

Age. The capacity to adapt is decreased at the extremes of age. The ability to adapt is impaired by the immaturity of an infant much as it is by the decline in functional reserve that occurs with age. For example, the infant has difficulty concentrating urine because of immature renal structures and is therefore less able than an adult to cope with decreased water intake or exaggerated water losses. A similar situation exists in the elderly due to age-related changes in renal function.

Health Status. Health status, both physical and mental, determines physiologic and psychological reserves and is a strong determinant of the ability to adapt. For example, people with heart disease are less able to adjust to stresses that require the recruitment of cardiovascular responses. Likewise, severe emotional stress often produces disruption of physiologic function and limits the ability to make appropriate choices related to long-term adaptive needs. Those who have worked with acutely ill people know that the will to live often has a profound influence on survival during life-threatening illnesses.

Nutrition. There are 50 to 60 essential nutrients, including minerals, lipids, certain fatty acids, vitamins, and specific amino acids. Deficiencies or excesses of any of these nutrients can alter one's health status and impair the ability to adapt. The importance of nutrition to enzyme function, immune response, and wound healing is well known. On a worldwide basis, malnutrition may be one of the most common causes of immunodeficiency. Among the problems associated with dietary excess are obesity and alcohol abuse. Obesity is a common problem. It predisposes to a number of health problems, including atherosclerosis and hypertension. Alcohol is a well-known nutrient that is often used in excess. It acutely affects the brain function and, with long-term use, can seriously impair the function of the liver, brain, and other vital structures.

Sleep–Wake Cycles. Sleep is considered to be a restorative function in which energy is restored and tissues are regenerated.[14] Sleep occurs in a cyclic manner, alternating with periods of wakefulness and energy utilization. In the past 20 to 30 years, it has become increasingly evident that biologic rhythms play an important role in adaptation to stress, the development of illness, and response to medical treatment. Many rhythms such as sleep, rest and activity, work and leisure, and eating and drinking oscillate with a frequency similar to that of the 24-hour light–dark solar day. The term *circadian*, from the Latin *circa* (about) and *dies* (day), is used to describe these 24-hour diurnal rhythms. The stress of sleep disorders and alterations in the sleep–wake cycle has been shown to alter immune function,[15] the normal pattern of normal circadian pattern of hormone secretion, immune function, and both physical and psychological functioning.

The two most common manifestations of an alteration in the sleep–wake cycle are insomnia and sleep deprivation or increased somnolence. In some people, stress may produce sleep disorders, and, in others, sleep disorders may lead to stress. Acute stress and environmental disturbances, loss of a loved one, recovery from surgery, and pain are common causes of transient and short-term insomnia. Air travel and jet lag are another cause of altered sleep–wake cycles as is shift work. In people with chronic insomnia, the bed often acquires many unpleasant secondary associations and becomes a place of stress and worry rather than a place of rest.[16]

Psychosocial Factors. A number of studies relate social factors and life events to illness. Scientific interest in the social environment as a cause of stress has gradually broadened to include the social environment as a resource that modulates the relationship between stress and health. Presumably, people who can mobilize strong supportive resources from within their social relationships are better able to withstand the negative effects of stress on their health. Studies suggest that social support has both direct and indirect positive effects on health status and serves as a buffer or modifier of the physical and psychosocial effects of stress.[17]

Social networks contribute in a number of ways to a person's psychosocial and physical integrity. The configuration of significant others that constitutes this network functions to mobilize the resources of the person; these people share the person's tasks and provide monetary support, materials and tools, and guidance in improving problem-solving capabilities.[18] People with ample social networks are not as likely to experience many types of stress such as being homeless or being lonely.[19] There is also evidence that people who have social supports or social assets may live longer and have a lower incidence of somatic illness.[20, 21]

Social support has been viewed in terms of both the number of relationships a person has and the person's perception of these relationships. Thus, close relations with others can involve not only positive effects but also the potential for conflict and may, in some situations, leave the person less able to cope with life stressors. There is also the belief that social supports are likely to be protective only in the presence of stressful circumstances.[22]

Holmes and Rahe defined *social stressors* as any set of circumstances the advent of which signifies or requires changes in a person's ongoing life pattern.[23] According to this definition, exposure to social stresses does not cause disease but may alter the person's susceptibility at a particular time and may therefore serve as a precipitating factor. A Schedule of Recent Experiences, developed by Holmes and Rahe, is an instrument used to measure recent life experiences. The scale lists 43 life changes (*e.g.*, promotion, divorce, being fired) to which subjects respond by indicating how many times in the preceding year each event has occurred. Each event is rated with a score, and the sum of these scores is used to determine the amount of stress associated with recent life change events.

In summary, physiologic adaptation involves the ability to maintain the constancy of the internal environment in the face of a wide range of changes in the internal and external environments. It involves control systems that regulate cellular function, control life's processes, and integrate the function of the different body systems. Adaptation is affected by a number of factors, including experience and previous learning, the rapidity with which the need to adapt occurs, genetic endowment and age, health status, nutrition, sleep–wake cycles, and psychosocial factors.

■ REFERENCES

1. Burchfield, S.R. (1979). The stress response: A new perspective. *Psychosomatic Medicine, 41*, 661.
2. Hartmann, F. (1982). An anthropological consideration of the stress response. *Contributions to Nephrology, 30, 7.*
3. Selye, H. (1973). The evolution of the stress concept. *American Scientist, 61*, 692.
4. Mason, J.W. (1971). The re-evaluation of the concept of nonspecificity in stress theory. *Journal of Psychiatric Research, 7*, 323.
5. Chrousos, G.P., & Gold, P.W. (1992). The concepts of stress and stress system disorders. *Journal of the American Medical Association, 267*, 1244–1252.
6. Selye, H. (1974). *Stress without distress* (p. 6). New York: New American Library.
7. Dworkin, S.F. (1969). Psychosomatic concepts and dentistry: Some perspectives. *Journal of Peridontology, 40*, 647.
8. Cohen, S., Tyrrell, D.A.J., & Smith, A.P. (1991). Psychological stress and susceptibility to the common cold. *New England Journal of Medicine, 325*, 606–612.
9. Solomon, G.F., & Amkraut, G.F. (1981). Psychoneuroendocrinological effects on the immune response. *Annual Review of Microbiology, 35*, 155–184.
10. Dantzer, R., & Kelley, K.W. (1989). Stress and immunity: An integrated view of relationships between the brain and immune system. *Life Sciences, 44*, 1995–2008.
11. Dubos, R. (1965). *Man adapting* (pp. 256, 258, 261, 264). New Haven: Yale University Press.
12. Cannon, W.B. (1932). *The wisdom of the body* (pp. 299–300). New York: W.W. Norton.
13. Guyton, A.C. (1986). *Textbook of medical physiology* (7th ed., p. 8). Philadelphia: WB Saunders.
14. Adams, K., & Oswold, I. (1983). Protein synthesis, bodily renewal and sleep wake cycle. *Clinical Science, 65*, 561–567.
15. Gillin, J.C., & Byerley, W.F. (1990). The diagnosis and management of insomnia. *New England Journal of Medicine, 322*, 239–248.
16. Moldofsky, H., Lue, F.A., Davidson, J.R., et al. (1989). Effects of sleep deprivation on human immune functions. *FASEB Journal, 3*, 1972–1977.
17. Broadhead, W.E., Kaplan, B.H., James, S.A., et al. (1983). The epidemiologic evidence for a relationship between social support and health. *American Journal of Epidemiology, 117*, 521–537.
18. Greenblatt, M., Becerra, R.M., & Serafetinides, E.A. (1982). Social networks and mental health: An overview. *American Journal of Psychiatry 139*(8), 977.
19. House, J.S., Robbins, C., & Metzner, H.L. (1982). The association of social relationships and activities with mortality: Prospective evidence from the Tecumseh Community Health Study. *American Journal of Epidemiology, 116*, 123.
20. Berkman, L.F., & Syme, S. (1979). Social networks, host resistance, and mortality: A nine-year follow-up study of Alameda County residents. *American Journal of Epidemiology, 109*, 186.
21. Tilden, V.P., & Weinert, C. (1987). Social support and the chronically ill individual. *Nursing Clinics of North America, 33*, 613–620.
22. Kaplan, B.H., Cassel, J., & Gore, S. (1977). Social support and health. *Medical Care, 15*(5, Suppl), 48.
23. Holmes, T.H., & Rahe, R.H. (1967). The social readjustment rate scale. *Journal of Psychosomatic Research, 11*, 213.

CHAPTER 9

ALTERATIONS IN ACTIVITY TOLERANCE

MARY KAY JIRICKA

■ OBJECTIVES

After you have studied this chapter, you should be able to meet the following objectives:

- Describe the body's physiologic response to exercise and work.
- Identify one physical method and two paper and pencil tools to assess work performance.
- Differentiate between acute and chronic fatigue.
- Define *chronic fatigue syndrome*.
- Describe physical assessment findings, presenting symptomatology, and laboratory values associated with chronic fatigue syndrome.
- Describe the effects of gravity on the body.
- Describe the effects of immobility and prolonged bedrest on the cardiovascular, pulmonary, renal, musculoskeletal, metabolic, and gastrointestinal body systems.

- Discuss changes in fluid and electrolyte balance associated with immobility and prolonged bedrest.
- Identify alterations in serum electrolyte and hematologic values that are related to immobility and prolonged bedrest.
- Discuss changes in sensory perception that are consequences of immobility and prolonged bedrest.
- Identify alterations in physical assessment findings that are related to the effects of immobility and prolonged bedrest.
- Describe treatment interventions that counteract the negative effects of immobility and prolonged bedrest.

Carol Mattson Porth: PATHOPHYSIOLOGY: CONCEPTS OF
ALTERED HEALTH STATES, 4th ed. © 1994, 1990, 1986, 1982
J.B. Lippincott Company

Health includes both physical and psychological components; it involves the ability to work, exercise, participate in leisure activities, and perform activities of daily living. To be able to perform these activities requires that the body have sufficient physiologic and psychological energy and stamina. When the body can no longer meet these energy demands, fatigue occurs. Fatigue may be acute, as in that resulting from increased physical activity, or it may be chronic in nature. Lack of health, or disease, also affects a person's activity reserve and imposes certain restrictions such as bedrest and immobility on the ability to perform work and perform other activities. The content in this chapter focuses on: (1) activity tolerance, the ability to do work, and the body's response to exercise; (2) activity intolerance and fatigue; and (3) activity intolerance as it relates to the physiologic and psychosocial responses to immobility and bedrest.

■ ACTIVITY TOLERANCE AND WORK PERFORMANCE

Activity is defined as the process of exerting energy for the purpose of accomplishing an effect. Human beings interact with their environment in a pattern of activity cycles. These cycles include periods of rest and periods of activity and have both physical and psychological elements. Rest is characterized by inactivity and requires minimal energy expenditure. In contrast to rest, activity denotes the process of movement and requires the expenditure of energy. One form of activity is exercise. Like activity, exercise is characterized by movement and energy expenditure. However, exercise differs from activity in that it results in an overall conditioning of the body when performed on a regular basis, whereas activity does not condition the body. This section of the chapter focuses on the physiologic and psychosocial responses to activity, specifically the effects of exercise and increased workload on the body.

PHYSIOLOGIC RESPONSES

Physical activity or exercise involves four major components: (1) muscle strength, flexibility, and endurance; (2) cardiopulmonary fitness; (3) availability of energy substrates to meet the increased energy demands imposed by increased physical activity; and (4) motivation and mental endurance.

CARDIOPULMONARY RESPONSES

The cardiopulmonary responses, which include the circulatory functions of the heart and blood vessels and the gas exchange functions of the respiratory system, work to supply oxygen and energy substrates to the working muscle groups and exchange oxygen and carbon dioxide with the atmosphere. Aerobic or cardiopulmonary exercise involves repetitive and rhythmic movements; it uses large muscle groups and results in the body's ability to perform vigorous exercise for an extended period of time.[1]

As the cardiovascular system responds to increased activity and exercise, the heart rate, the amount of blood that the heart pumps with each beat (stroke volume), and arterial blood pressure increase. The increase in heart rate is mediated by way of the autonomic nervous system and intrinsic cardiovascular mechanisms. In anticipation of exercise, the limbic system and the hypothalamus stimulate cardiovascular centers in the medulla that inhibit parasympathetic slowing of heart rate and stimulate release of the sympathetic neurotransmitters, norepinephrine and epinephrine, that increase heart rate and cardiac contractility. At the start of exercise, heart rate rises immediately and continues to increase until a plateau is reached. This plateau, or steady-state heart rate, is maintained until the exercise, or activity, is terminated. Also contributing to the increased heart rate are intrinsic mechanisms in the heart. During exercise, increased blood return to the heart stimulates right atrial stretch receptors that serve to increase the heart rate. Release of epinephrine and norepinephrine from the adrenal glands helps to sustain the increased heart rate.[3]

During exercise, the cardiac output may increase from a resting level of 4 to 8 L/min to as high as 15 L/min for women and to as high as 22 L/min for men. The increase in cardiac output is due to an increase in heart rate and stroke volume. One factor that is thought to contribute to the cardiac output is the stimulation of the heart muscle by epinephrine and norepinephrine. These neurotransmitters cause the heart to beat faster and more forcefully. Another factor that contributes to the increased cardiac output is the stretching of the myocardial fibers by the increased blood return. The increased stretch of the myocardial fibers results in a more forceful contraction and a more complete emptying of the ventricles with each beat, a response called the *Frank-Starling mechanisms* (see Chapter 22).[2,3]

With the onset of exercise, the systolic blood pressure increases. This is due to the increase in cardiac output and is reflected by the increased volume of blood being ejected from the heart. The diastolic blood pressure changes little during exercise. This is believed to be related to the peripheral vasodilatation that occurs from the metabolic waste products that accumulate during exercise. The increased systolic pressure and the fact that the diastolic blood pressure does not change results in an increase of mean arterial pressure. The increase in mean arterial pressure is necessary so that organ systems of high priority can continue to be perfused.[2,3]

The respiratory system has the role of exchanging oxygen and carbon dioxide. During exercise, the respiratory system must increase the rate of gas exchange. This takes place through a series of physiologic responses. With the increase in cardiac output, a greater volume of blood under slightly increased pressure is delivered to the pulmonary vessels in the lungs. This results in opening of more pulmonary capillary beds so there is better alveolar perfusion and a more efficient exchange of oxygen and carbon dioxide.[2]

In addition to pulmonary perfusion being enhanced during exercise, pulmonary ventilation is also increased. The respiratory rate and tidal volume increase, resulting in an increase in minute ventilation. This response is controlled by chemoreceptors, located in the medulla and aorta and carotid arteries, that monitor blood gases and pH. During exercise, decreases in blood oxygen and pH along with increases in carbon dioxide stimulate an increase in the rate and depth of respiration.[2,3]

NEUROMUSCULAR RESPONSES

The integration of the neurologic and musculoskeletal systems is essential for the body to have movement and participate in activity. To initiate and sustain increased activity, muscle strength, flexibility, and endurance are needed. *Muscle strength* is defined as the ability of muscle groups to produce force against resistance. Flexibility involves the range of movement of joint(s), whereas muscle endurance refers to the ability of the body (or muscle groups) to perform increased activity for an extended period of time.[1]

Skeletal muscles are adapted by heredity and activity for the type of work they predominately perform. Skeletal muscle consists of two types of muscle fibers. There are slow twitch (type I) and fast twitch (type II) muscle fibers. Major muscle groups are classified according to how fast a muscle contraction is produced in response to an electrical stimulus. Each muscle group is characterized as either type I or type II muscle.

Slow twitch fibers, which are smaller than fast twitch fibers, tend to produce less overall force. But although they are smaller, slow twitch fibers are more energy efficient than fast twitch fibers. Slow twitch fibers predominate in the large muscle groups such as the leg muscles and, therefore, play a major role in sustaining activity during prolonged exercise or endurance activities. During periods of sustained inactivity, such as prolonged immobility or bedrest, it is the slow twitch fibers that are primarily affected and quickly decondition.[3]

In contrast to slow twitch fibers, fast twitch fibers are larger and fatigue more easily. Fast twitch muscle fibers are most common in smaller muscle groups such as those found in the arms and eye. Fast twitch fibers predominate during activities where short bursts of intense energy are required, such as sprinting or weight-lifting activities. Anabolic steroids enhance fast twitch fiber activity.[2]

During aerobic activity, working muscles use oxygen 10 to 20 times faster than nonworking muscles. This increased oxygen demand is met by both an increase in cardiac output and an increase in blood flow through the working muscles. The increase in blood flow does not begin at the onset of exercise but occurs gradually as the workload increases. It is achieved by way of two mechanisms: (1) dilation of blood vessels in the working muscles and (2) constriction of blood vessels in the organs of low priority.[2,3]

Dilation of blood vessels in the working muscles is a result of increased blood flow to the muscles and increased venous return from the working muscles. Increased blood flow to working muscles is achieved by relaxation of the arterioles and the precapillary sphincters. In addition, chemical changes such as decreased oxygen and pH and increased levels of potassium, adenosine, carbon dioxide, and phosphate contribute to the local control of muscle blood flow during prolonged exercise and during recovery from exercise.[2] Increased venous return is facilitated by the alternate contraction and relaxation of working muscles.

The second mechanism that increases blood flow to working muscles is the diversion of blood from visceral organs to the working muscles. The amount of blood diverted from visceral organs is proportional, so as exercise is increased more blood is diverted to working muscles. The exact mechanism for this response is uncertain.[2]

METABOLIC AND THERMAL RESPONSES

To perform physical activities, the body requires energy sources. Energy is obtained from creatine phosphate (a stored form of muscle energy), glucose, glycogen, and fatty acids. As the activity begins, especially aerobic activity, the body uses its energy sources in a characteristic pattern. The first sources for energy are stored adenosine triphosphate (ATP), creatine phosphate, and muscle glycogen. These energy sources are used for short intense periods of activity of 1 to 2 minutes. The process of using these fuels for energy is by way of anaerobic metabolism. If the activity is to be performed for a longer period of 3 to 40 minutes, muscle glycogen and creatine phosphate are used to meet the energy requirements by way of both anaerobic and aerobic metabolism. For intense prolonged periods of activity that last over 40 minutes, aerobic metabolism is essential. Muscle glycogen, glucose, and fatty acids are used for energy sources during prolonged activity.[2]

For increased activity, the person must consume a balanced diet that is high in carbohydrate. General recommendations for a balanced diet include: (1) 60% carbohydrate sources (80% complex carbohydrates and 20% sugar), (2) 30% fat sources (mainly polyunsaturated fats), and (3) 10% protein.[2] Although proteins are not used as energy sources during increased activity, they have an essential role in the building and rebuilding of tissues and organs. During increased activity and exercise, it is essential that the person maintain adequate hydration. Increased activity can result in loss of fluids from the vascular compartment. If allowed to progress, the person may experience severe dehydration that may lead to vascular collapse. Before and during vigorous activity, a person should replenish body fluids with water.[2]

Under normal resting conditions, the body is able to maintain its temperature within a set range. It does this by way of two mechanisms. The first mechanism used by the body to regulate temperature is to change blood flow to the skin. When the blood vessels of the skin dilate, warm blood is shunted from the core of the body to the skin surface where heat is more easily lost to the surrounding environment. The second mechanism by which the body loses heat is sweat secretion. The evaporation of sweat from the skin surface contributes to the loss of heat from the body. However, with vigorous exercise and depending on environmental conditions, the body may be unable to regulate its temperature.

With sufficient training, the body adapts and is able to regulate its temperature efficiently under conditions of strenuous exercise. The body adapts by increasing the rate of sweat production. The trained body begins to sweat sooner, often within 1 to 2 minutes of the start of exercise. Sweat production begins even before the core temperature rises, thus a cooling effect is initiated soon after the start of exercise. In the trained or conditioned person, the sweat produced is more dilute than sweat produced by a nontrained person. Sweat normally contains large amounts of sodium chloride; production of a dilute sweat allows for evaporative cooling to take place while sodium chloride is conserved. Also, there occurs a shift of plasma proteins so that there is an increase in the amount of proteins in the blood. These proteins exert an osmotic gradient effect that draws fluid from the interstitial space into the vascular compartment. This contributes to an increase in the vascular volume that can be delivered to the working muscles and contribute to more efficient heat dissipation.[2]

PSYCHOLOGICAL RESPONSES

There is a mental component to the performance of increased activity and exercise. The mental aspect entails the motivation to initiate an activity, or exercise program, and the dedication to incorporate the regimen into one's lifestyle. Positive effects of regularly performed exercise include increased energy and motivation, positive self-image and self-esteem, decreased anxiety, better management of one's life stresses, and increased perceived locus of control.[1]

ASSESSMENT OF ACTIVITY TOLERANCE

The assessment of a person's ability to tolerate exercise and perform work can be conducted in several ways. One method is to administer a paper and pencil test. There are several tests that can be administered that enable people to describe their normal activities, their perceived level of activity tolerance, or their level of fatigue. One example of a paper and pencil test is the Human Activity Profile (HAP).[4] The HAP was originally developed to assess the quality of life for people participating in a rehabilitation program for chronic obstructive pulmonary disease (COPD). After investigating numerous physiologic and psychological measures, it was noted that the most important aspect of quality of life was the amount of daily activity the person is able to perform. The HAP consists of 94 items that represent common activities that require known amounts of average energy expenditure. The person marks each item on the tool based on whether he or she is still able to perform the activity or has stopped performing the activity.

A second example of a paper and pencil test is the Fatigue Severity Scale (Chart 9-1).[5] This tool consists of nine statements that describe symptoms of fatigue. People are instructed to choose a number from 1 to 7 that best indicates their agreement with each statement. The tool is brief, easy to administer, and easily interpreted. Paper and pencil tests provide an objective way to assess a person's activity tolerance.

Another method to use to assess activity tolerance is ergometry. Ergometry is a procedure for determining physical performance capacity. The ergometer is a specific tool that imposes a constant level of work. A specified workload (expressed in terms of watts or joules per second) is imposed while the person performs the task. During the performance of the work, the person's physiologic status is monitored, as well as his or her subjective assessment of the work.[3]

Two examples of ergometers include the bicycle ergometer and the treadmill ergometer. A bicycle

CHART 9-1: FATIGUE SEVERITY SCALE*

1. My motivation is lower when I am fatigued.
2. Exercise brings on my fatigue.
3. I am easily fatigued.
4. Fatigue interferes with my physical functioning.
5. Fatigue causes frequent problems for me.
6. My fatigue prevents sustained physical functioning.
7. Fatigue interferes with carrying out certain duties and responsibilities.
8. Fatigue is among my three disabling symptoms.
9. Fatigue interferes with my work, family, or social life.

   * Patients are instructed to choose a number from 1 to 7 that indicates their degree of agreement with each statement where 1 indicates strongly disagree and 7 indicates strongly agree.
   (Krupp, L. B., LaRocca, N. G., Muir-Nash, J., & Steinberg, A. D. [1989]. The fatigue severity scale: Application to patients with multiple sclerosis and systemic lupus erythematosus. *Archives of Neurology, 46,* 1122)

ergometer is a stationary bicycle that has a friction belt attached. The front wheel of the bicycle is rotated, and the braking force of the belt can be adjusted to alter the workload.

A treadmill ergometer is more frequently used to assess workload performance, especially cardiac function. During treadmill testing, the person walks or runs on a moving belt. The workload can be altered by changing the speed and incline of the treadmill. This change is usually done in predetermined stages. During treadmill testing, the electrocardiogram (ECG) is monitored continuously; the blood pressure is checked intermittently. Usually the person being tested continues to exercise, completing successive stages of the test, until exhaustion or a predetermined heart rate, or maximal heart rate, is reached.[6]

Maximal heart rate is estimated by age. Tables of maximal heart rate by age are available, but, as a general rule, the predicted maximal heart rate can be estimated by subtracting age from 220 (*e.g.*, the target heart rate for a 40 year old would be 180 beats/min). The person may continue to exercise until the predicted maximal heart rate is achieved, or until a percentage (*i.e.*, 85% to 90%) of the predicted maximal rate is reached.[6]

Metabolic equivalents (METs) are commonly used to express workload at various stages of work. One MET is equivalent to the energy expended in a resting position. METs are multiples of the basal metabolic rate, and, as the type of activity performed (*i.e.*, walking, running) is changed, the MET requirement also changes. For example, walking at 4 miles per hour (mph), cycling at 11 mph, playing tennis (singles), or doing carpentry requires 5 to 6 METs. Running 6 mph requires 10 METs, and running 10

mph requires 17 METs. Physically trained people are able to achieve workloads beyond 16 METs. Healthy sedentary people are seldom able to exercise beyond 10 or 11 METs. In people with coronary artery disease, workloads of 8 METs often produce angina.[6]

During exercise stress testing, people often are asked to rate their subjective feelings of the exercise experience. A commonly used tool to measure the person's feelings of the amount of work being performed is the Borg Rating of Perceived Exertion (RPE) Scale.[7] The RPE Scale is based on research that correlates heart rate to feelings of perceived exertion. The scale values range from 6 through 20. As the person is performing the exercise, he or she is asked to select a number that best corresponds to his or her feelings of exertion for the work being performed. The numbers and expressions describing perceived levels of exertion are often posted on the wall where the exercise is being performed. Number 7 represents "very, very light" exertion; number 9, "very light" exertion; number 11, "fairly light" exertion; number 13, "somewhat hard" exertion; number 15, "hard" exertion; number 17, "very hard" exertion; and number 19, "very, very hard" exertion.[7] The numeric values on the RPE Scale increase linearly with workload, and the total scale reflects a tenfold increase in heart rate. Therefore, as the person begins to exercise, he or she is asked to rate the intensity of the work being performed. The person selects a number from the RPE Scale, and this number should approximate the heart rate when that number is multiplied by ten (*e.g.*, if the person rates the exercise experience as a 7, the heart rate should be 70 beats/minute).

A newer category scale with ratio properties has also been developed. The numbers on this scale range from 0 to 10, with 0 representing "nothing at all"; 0.5, "very, very weak"; and 10, "very, very strong." With this method, the expressions and the numbers they represent are placed in the correct position for a ratio scale. For example, since 1 represents "very weak," 0.5 represents "very, very weak" or half that intensity.[7b]

In summary, the response of the body to increased activity and exercise assumes that a healthy, normal person is performing the increased activity. In disease states, especially diseases of the cardiovascular, pulmonary, or musculoskeletal systems, the body's response to increased activity is compromised. The normal physiologic responses cannot be elicited. When a person experiences disease, activities of daily living, as well as an exercise regimen, must be adapted to their physiologic limitations.

The body reacts to the increased activity of exercise by a series of physiologic responses that increase its level of performance. Heart rate, cardiac output, and stroke volume increase to deliver more blood to working muscles. Minute ventilation and diffusion of oxygen and carbon dioxide increase to provide oxygen more efficiently to meet the rising metabolic demands. Local changes in the arterioles and capillaries contribute to enhanced perfusion of the working muscles. Lastly, over time, and with training, temperature regulation is altered so the body is able to perform activity without increasing its core temperature. Activity tolerance is assessed by use of paper and pencil tests or bicycle or treadmill ergometry. People are required to perform a prescribed amount of work. While performing this work, people are monitored for their cardiovascular response and their subjective feelings of exertion for the specified amount of work being performed.

■ ACTIVITY INTOLERANCE AND FATIGUE

Activity intolerance can be defined as "a state in which a person has insufficient physical or psychological energy to endure or complete required or desired daily activity."[8] How frequently, intensely, and long people are able to carry out their activities depends on a balance between available energy (needed oxygen and nutrients) and the energy that is required to complete the desired task. Factors that influence this balance of energy include: (1) overall physical condition (*e.g.*, level of fatigue, deconditioning, disease, and pain), (2) psychosocial factors (*e.g.*, depression and anxiety), and (3) lifestyle factors (*e.g.*, obesity, smoking, lack of regular exercise).[9] This section focuses on fatigue, specifically acute fatigue and the chronic fatigue syndrome.

MECHANISMS OF FATIGUE

Fatigue is a state that is experienced by everyone at some time in their life. Fatigue can be physical, as in the case of extreme exercise in healthy people, or it can be a normal symptom that is experienced by people with limited exercise reserve such as people with impaired cardiorespiratory function, anemia, malnutrition, or those on certain types of drug therapy. Fatigue may also be related to lack of sleep or mental stress. Like dyspnea and pain, fatigue is a subjective symptom. Fatigue is often described as a subjective feeling of tiredness that varies in terms of pleasantness, intensity, and duration and is often influenced by the time of day and a person's biorhythms.[11] It is different from the normal tiredness that people experience at the end of the day. Tiredness is relieved by a good night's sleep, whereas fatigue persists despite sufficient or adequate sleep. Fatigue is one of the most common symptoms reported to physicians, yet it is one of the least understood health care problems.

According to Piper,[10,11] fatigue may be related

to two major types of stressors—situational and developmental. Situational stressors are situation specific and can be associated with five factors: (1) the environment (*e.g.*, excessive noise, temperature extremes, changes in weather), (2) drug-related incidents (*e.g.*, use of tranquilizers, alcohol, toxic chemical exposure), (3) treatment-related therapies (*e.g.*, chemotherapy, radiation therapy, surgery, anesthesia, diagnostic testing), (4) physical exertion (*e.g.*, exercise), and (5) nonphysical exertion (*e.g.*, monotony). Developmental stressors are associated with two main factors, physical factors due to a disease process and emotional factors.

The factors contributing to fatigue are numerous and interrelated, making assessment complex and identification difficult. So too is the physiologic explanation of fatigue. When fatigue is related to mental factors or emotional stress, the physiologic explanation of fatigue is associated with the function of the reticular activating system (RAS). The RAS, which is located in the reticular formation of the pons and midbrain, is responsible for maintaining wakefulness. A feedback system between the RAS and the cerebral cortex exists. Stimulation of this system results in wakefulness; conversely, inhibition results in fatigue.[10]

ACUTE PHYSICAL FATIGUE

Acute fatigue has a rapid onset, is perceived to be a normal response to the activity being performed, has a short duration in which the fatigue is relieved when the activity ceases, and serves as a protective mechanism. Although acute physical fatigue can develop when insufficient oxygen or nutrients are delivered to the muscle, for the purpose of this chapter, acute fatigue is defined as muscle fatigue associated with increased activity or exercise that is carried out to the point of exhaustion.

Physical conditioning can influence the onset of acute fatigue. People who engage in regular exercise are able to perform an activity for longer periods of time before acute fatigue develops than sedentary people. They are probably able to do so because their muscles use oxygen and nutrients more efficiently and because their circulatory and respiratory systems are better able to deliver oxygen and nutrients to the exercising muscles.[2]

Acute physical fatigue occurs more rapidly in deconditioned muscle. For example, acute fatigue is often seen in people who have been on bedrest because of a surgical procedure, or in people who have had their activity curtailed because of chronic illnesses such as heart and respiratory diseases. In this example, the acute fatigue is often out of proportion to the activity that is being performed (*e.g.*, dangling at the bedside, sitting in a chair for the first time). When resuming activity for the first time after a prolonged period of bedrest or inactivity, the person may experience tachycardia and hypotension that is greater than was expected because of the period of inactivity. A possible explanation for this phenomenon is the deconditioning of type I (slow twitch) muscle fibers. Unless these parameters are changed by medications such as β-adrenergic blocking drugs, heart rate and blood pressure become particularly sensitive indicators of activity tolerance or intolerance.

Another example of people who experience acute physical fatigue are those people who require the use of assistive devices. This is true of people in wheelchairs and those using assistive devices after losing a limb. The upper arm muscles are less well adapted to prolonged exercise than the leg muscles. This is because arm muscles are primarily composed of type II muscle fibers. Type II muscle fibers, which are used when the body requires short bursts of energy, fatigue quickly. As a result, people who use wheelchairs or a pair of crutches may quickly experience fatigue until their arms become conditioned to the increased activity.

CHRONIC FATIGUE

A second type of activity intolerance is chronic fatigue. Chronic fatigue differs from acute fatigue in terms of onset, intensity, perception, duration, and relief. In contrast to acute fatigue, chronic fatigue has a more gradual insidious onset, is typically perceived as being unusually intense for the amount of activity performed, lasts longer than 1 month, and is not relieved by cessation of activity. Although acute fatigue often serves a protective function, chronic fatigue is not protective. Chronic fatigue may even lead to aversion of activity and be further accompanied by a desire to escape certain activities. Many diseases and chronic health conditions cause people to experience chronic fatigue. When associated with a specific disease, there often exists a physiologic basis for the fatigue. When the physiologic problem is corrected, the fatigue may be relieved.[10, 11]

Chronic fatigue is one of the more common problems experienced by people with chronic health problems (Table 9-1). It limits the amount of activity that a person can perform and may interfere with employment, the performance of activities of daily living, and the quality of life in general. Although fatigue is often viewed as a symptom of anxiety and depression, it is important to recognize that these psychological manifestations may be a symptom of the fatigue. For example, people with persistent fatigue due to a chronic illness may have to curtail their work schedules, decrease social activities, and limit their usual family responsibilities. These lifestyle changes may be the reasons for the depression rather than the depression being a cause of the fatigue.

Chronic fatigue is a common problem in people with cancer, particularly people who are undergoing cancer treatment (chemotherapy or radiation therapy). Studies involving patients receiving chemotherapy for a variety of different types of cancers report incidences of fatigue ranging from 59% to 82%.[12] In all of these studies, fatigue was the most common and distressing side effect of the treatment. In people receiving radiation therapy, the incidence of fatigue ranged from 65% to 100% and was rated as the most severe effect of the treatment, especially during the last week of the treatment.[12] A possible explanation for the fatigue that occurs in people with cancer involves a chemical mediator called tumor necrosis factor (TNF). TNF is a chemical mediator secreted by activated macrophages, some tumor cells, and some T lymphocytes (see Chapter 13). It causes depletion of the protein stores of skeletal muscle. As a result, muscle wasting occurs, and people have to expend more energy to perform simple activities such as sitting and standing.[13]

CHRONIC FATIGUE SYNDROME

Chronic fatigue syndrome (CFS) is an illness that can affect the entire body. It is described as disabling fatigue of at least 6 months duration that is often preceded by flulike symptoms. CFS is the chief complaint of 10% to 20% of patients seen in primary care clinics.[14, 15] Reports of CFS have emerged from the United States, Canada, Australia, and Europe.

In the United States, CFS first came to prominence in 1985 at Lake Tahoe, Nevada. At the Incline Village resort, approximately 200 residents (1% of the population) reported a "mono" flulike illness to their primary care physicians. The physicians examining these patients were aware of the medical literature that described the possible association of the Epstein-Barr virus (EBV) with chronic mononucleosis. Because such a large number of the population reported the same symptoms, the Centers for Disease Control (CDC) was asked to investigate this "epidemic." The CDC declared this reported epidemic resulted from the attitude or activity of the physician in the area and discounted the link between EBV and the chronic fatigue syndrome. This incident brought national prominence to CFS and caused other people with similar complaints to organize and request that this syndrome be further investigated.[17]

TABLE 9-1. CHRONIC ILLNESSES AND CAUSES OF CHRONIC FATIGUE

CHRONIC ILLNESS	CAUSES OF CHRONIC FATIGUE
AIDS	Impaired immune function, anorexia, muscle wasting, psychosocial factors associated with the disease
Anemia	Decreased oxygen-carrying capacity of the blood
Cancer	Presence of chemical products and catabolic processes associated with tumor growth; anorexia and difficulty eating; effects of chemotherapy and radiation therapy; psychosocial factors (depression, grieving, hopelessness, and fear)
Cardiac disease	Poor tissue perfusion
Chronic lung disease	Impaired gas exchange and increased breathing effort
Neurologic disorders	
Multiple sclerosis	Muscle weakness associated with impaired nerve transmission
Myasthenia gravis	Muscle weakness associated with decreased acetylcholine receptors at the myoneural junction
Renal failure	Accumulation of metabolic wastes; electrolyte imbalances; decreased oxygen-carrying capacity due to impaired erythropoietin production
Metabolic disorders	
Hypothyroidism	Decreased metabolic rate
Diabetes mellitus	Impaired glucose utilization and associated fluid and electrolyte disorders
Obesity	Imbalance between nutritional intake and energy expenditure; increased weight increases the workload of the body
Steroid myopathy	Muscle wasting due to impaired protein and glycogen synthesis

Definition. CFS may be described in several ways. Common descriptions include: (1) a state of abnormal exhaustion that follows normal activities; (2) a decrease in energy for tasks that require sustained attention; and (3) a global disturbance in the ability to act.[14] In 1988, a working case definition for CFS was developed by the CDC. This definition describes CFS as a complex syndrome that includes: (1) the major criteria of (a) debilitating fatigue that has been present for at least 6 months and (b) that cannot be explained in terms of other conditions that produce similar symptoms of fatigue; (2) is accompanied by complaints (symptom criteria) that include (a) mild fever, (b) sore throat, (c) painful cervical or axillary lymph nodes, (d) unexplained general muscle weakness, (e) prolonged generalized fatigue after levels of exercise that would have previously been well tolerated, (f) generalized headaches that are different from those that the person normally experiences, (g) migratory arthralgia, (h) neuropsychological complaints (photophobia, transient scotoma, forgetfulness, excessive irritability, confusion, difficulty thinking), (i) inability to concentrate, depression, (j) sleep disturbances (hypersomnia or insom-

nia, and (k) description of the main symptom complex developing over a few hours or days; and (3) physician-documented findings of (a) low-grade fever, (b) nonexudative pharyngitis, and (c) palpable or tender cervical or axillary lymph nodes. For a case definition of CFS to be made, criteria 1 (both a and b) must be present, along with 6 or more of the 11 symptom criteria and 2 or more of the physician-documented findings, or 8 or more of the 11 symptom criteria. All symptoms must be present for at least 6 months.[17, 18]

Pathophysiology. Despite much research and the development of several theories, the pathophysiology of CFS is unknown. It is known that the fatigue experienced in CFS is similar to the fatigue associated with therapeutic doses of α-interferon, suggesting a possible link to an underlying viral infection. Most theories have identified infectious agents such as EBV, human herpesvirus 6, enterovirus, human retrovirus, *Mycobacterium tuberculosis*, *Borrelia burgdorferi*, *Brucella*, and *Candida* to be associated with the syndrome. Yet none of these agents has conclusively been associated with the development of CFS. Also associated with CFS are neuropsychiatric factors as well as a primary immunodysregulatory phenomenon. Other theories that have postulated causes of CFS identify a genetic predisposition, dysfunction in the hypothalamus–pituitary–adrenal axis, and an as yet unidentified infectious organism.[18, 19]

The association of psychiatric disorders to CFS is difficult to evaluate. There is much overlap between psychiatric disorders and the reactive depression of CFS. It is known that people with CFS have an increased occurrence and lifetime prevalence of depression that is greater than the depression associated with other chronic diseases. In as much as 40% to 50% of the cases of CFS, depression preceded the development of CFS.[19]

The role of the immune system in CFS demonstrates both qualitative and quantitative abnormalities. It is hypothesized that the immune system may overreact to an environmental agent (most likely an infectious agent) or internal stimuli and be unable to self-regulate after the infectious insult is over. One suggestion is that a viral infection may produce continued suppression of the immune system. Mononuclear cells from people with CFS have a decreased response to antigenic stimulation and proliferate at half the normal rate. A deficiency in natural killer cells has been proposed to explain many of these abnormalities. These lymphocytes participate in transfer of delayed hyersensitivity and production of interleukin-2 and τ-interferon.[19, 20]

Manifestations. One of the most important assessment finding is the person's subjective complaint of fatigue. The person reports feeling well one day and experiencing an insidious onset of overwhelming fatigue the next day. Often the symptom of fatigue is preceded by a cold or flulike illness. Frequently, the person describes the illness as reoccurring. With each subsequent episode of the illness, the fatigue increases.

Physical assessment findings include low-grade fever. The fever is intermittent and occurs only when the illness reoccurs. Other assessment findings include nonexudative pharyngitis, palpable and tender cervical lymph nodes, a mildly enlarged thyroid gland, wheezing, splenomegaly, myalgias, arthralgias, and heme-positive stool with subsequent negative sigmoidoscopies.

Psychological problems include impaired cognition that the person describes as an inability to concentrate and to perform previously mundane tasks. Also reported are mood and sleep disturbances, balance problems, visual disturbances, and varying degrees of anxiety and depression. The presence of depression in approximately 50% of the cases of CFS has generated much discussion regarding

whether depression is a cause of CFS or a comorbid condition.[16, 19, 20]

Before making the diagnosis of CFS, laboratory values to monitor include complete blood count, serum electrolytes, glucose, calcium, phosphorus, total protein, Lyme titers, and renal, liver, and thyroid function tests, along with a urinalysis and stool guaiac. Laboratory and other diagnostic test results demonstrate minor abnormalities, but not of sufficient magnitude to be reflective of the degree of fatigue present. Common laboratory abnormalities include atypical lymphocytosis, mild anemia, elevation of the sedimentation rate, decreased serum phosphorus, iron deficiency, and elevated liver function tests. Chest x-rays are normal.

The diagnosis of CFS is made by the physician integrating the entire clinical picture of patient symptomatology, physical assessment findings, laboratory results, and any other diagnostic tests that have been conducted. The patient symptoms must be present for at least 6 months. In some cases, the symptoms have been present for as long as 1 to 2 years before the diagnosis of CFS is made. CFS is often a diagnosis of exclusion. The physician must first rule out any infectious processes and any psychological diagnoses.

Treatment. The treatment of CFS tends to be nonspecific. It centers on patient education, emotional support, treatment of symptoms, and overall management of general health. During the diagnostic work-up, people need to be supported and reassured that their symptoms are real and not all in their head. Local and national support groups are available for people who experience CFS.

Symptom treatment consists of developing an exercise program that helps the person regain strength. People with CFS have a decreased aerobic capacity. An activity program that gradually increases in intensity is recommended. Initially, the activity program should be short—3 to 5 minutes in length—and gradually increase in intensity by 20% every 2 to 3 weeks.[20] Along with a structured activity program, people should be encouraged to be as active as possible as they resume their activities of daily living.

Nutritional support is important. A low-fat, low-to-moderate protein, high–complex-carbohydrate diet is recommended along with a multivitamin, multimineral supplement. For overweight people, weight loss is recommended. Alcohol should be avoided because it exacerbates the symptoms of CFS.[21]

Analgesics and antiinflammatory nonsteroidal medications are beneficial in treating the symptoms of myalgia and arthralgia. Antidepressants may be used to treat symptoms of depression, however the medication(s) should not be used in isolation and appropriate supportive treatment and counseling also must be provided to the person.

A holistic approach to the treatment of CFS is essential. With proper treatment and support, 40% to 50% of the people with CFS demonstrate improvement at 1 year follow-up.[22] Relapses can occur. Therefore, it is imperative that people diagnosed with CFS continue to receive follow-up care and treatment on a regular basis.

In summary, fatigue is a nonspecific, self-recognized state of physical and psychological exhaustion. It results in the person not being able to perform routine activities and is not relieved with sleep or rest. Acute fatigue results from excessive use of the body or a specific muscle group and is often related to depletion of energy sources. Chronic fatigue is often associated with a specific disease or chronic illness and may be relieved when the effects of the disease are corrected. Chronic fatigue syndrome is a complex illness that has physiologic and psychological manifestations. It is characterized by debilitating fatigue. Diagnosis is often made by a process of elimination, and treatment requires a holistic approach.

■ BEDREST AND IMMOBILITY

Immobility and bedrest are two common forms of inactivity. Immobility may be dictated by injury that requires stabilization to facilitate the healing process, or it may result from conditions that limit physical reserve. The effects of immobility can be restricted to a single extremity that is encased in a plaster cast, involve both legs as in a person confined to a wheel-chair, or involve the entire body as in a person confined to bedrest. Bedrest and immobility are associated with various complications that include generalized weakness, orthostatic intolerance, atelectasis, pneumonia, pulmonary emboli, thrombophlebitis, muscle atrophy, osteoporosis, urinary retention, constipation, and impairment in sensory perception (Table 9-2). This section of the chapter describes the physiologic changes that occur with bedrest and immobility and treatment interventions to counteract their effects.

Bedrest is one of the oldest and most commonly used methods of treatment for various medical conditions and diagnoses. Historically, before the 1940s, bedrest was prescribed for 2 weeks after childbirth, 3 weeks after herniorrhaphy, and 4 to 6 weeks after myocardial infarction. It was believed that the complex biochemical and physical demands of physical activity diverted energy from the restorative and reparative processes of healing. Rest in bed was regarded as tantamount to optimal rest of the heart and entire body.

During World War II, the shortage of hospital beds and medical personnel forced early mobilization of many patients. As often happens with this kind of action, it was soon discovered that early mobilization lessened complications and improved patient outcome. The National Aeronautics and Space Administration (NASA) conducted research that described the damaging effects of prolonged inactivity and weightlessness. These studies indicate that weightlessness and the antigravity effects of bedrest produce similar responses.

TABLE 9-2. COMPLICATIONS OF BEDREST AND IMMOBILITY

SYSTEM	COMPLICATION
Cardiovascular	Decreased cardiac output, contributing to decreased aerobic capacity; orthostatic intolerance; venous thrombophlebitis
Pulmonary	Atelectasis; relative hypoxemia; pneumonia
Musculoskeletal	Muscle atrophy and loss of strength; decreased muscle oxidative capacity contributing to decreased aerobic capacity; osteoporosis (bone loss); contractures; osteoarthritis
Gastrointestinal	Constipation
Genitourinary	Incontinence; renal calculi
Skin	Pressure ulcers
Functional	Impaired ambulation and activity tolerance
Psychological	Sensory deprivation; altered sensory perception

(Harper, C. M. & Lyles, Y. M. [1988]. Physiology and complications of bed rest. *Journal of the American Geriatric Society, 36*[11], 1048)

ANTIGRAVITY EFFECTS OF BEDREST

The supine position that often accompanies immobility and bedrest interferes with the effects of gravity. The force of gravity exerts beneficial effects on the body. As the body maintains a supine position, the absence of the force of gravity leads to many of the deconditioning effects associated with immobility and bedrest.

While upright, the body interferes with the force of gravity in a variety of ways. The skeletal muscles contract and exert pressure against veins and lymph vessels. This contraction counteracts the force of gravity that would cause blood and fluid to pool in the lower extremities. Thus blood is kept moving through the circulatory system. Bones remain stronger because longitudinal weight bearing keeps essential minerals, such as calcium, inside the structure of the bone.

During bedrest, the forces of gravity and hydrostatic pressure are removed from the cardiovascular system. In the standing position, approximately 500 to 700 mL (10%) of the body's blood volume becomes sequestered in the lower extremities. This results in a temporary decrease in venous return to the heart, which, in turn, decreases the cardiac output. Under normal conditions, cardiovascular reflexes respond by increasing heart rate and systemic vascular resistance to maintain blood pressure. With prolonged bedrest, these hemodynamic changes are maintained, except for heart rate, which increases approximately 0.5 beat/min each day.[23]

PHYSIOLOGIC RESPONSES

CARDIOVASCULAR RESPONSES

After a period of bedrest, the cardiovascular system becomes deconditioned resulting in an exaggeration of the hemodynamic changes normally seen with standing after brief bedrest. This deconditioning is manifest in three major alterations: (1) postural hypotension, (2) increased cardiac workload, and (3) venous stasis and potential for deep venous thrombosis. Bedrest also causes a negative fluid balance.

One of the most striking responses to assumption of the supine position during bedrest is the alteration of blood flow. There is a shift of fluid from the lower to the upper part of the body. In the supine position, approximately 500 mL of blood is redistributed from the lower extremities to the central circulation. Most of this blood is diverted to the lungs; a small portion is diverted to the arms and head. The increase in central circulation results in an increase in stroke volume, which results in an increase in cardiac output. In the supine position, the normal cardiac output is 7 to 8 L/min compared with a cardiac output of 5 to 6 L/min for a person in the standing position. The increase in stroke volume and cardiac output is accompanied by a slight decrease in heart rate and systemic vascular resistance and the maintenance in blood pressure. With increased fluid shifted to the head and thoracic cavity, the person may experience headache, swelling of the nasal sinuses, nasal congestion, and puffiness of the eyelids.[28]

The increase in plasma volume in the central cavity stimulates baroreceptors. The stimulation of the baroreceptors results in an inhibition of antidiuretic hormone (ADH) and aldosterone with a resultant water and sodium (natriuresis) diuresis. In the supine position, diuresis begins on the first day with the shift of blood from the lower extremities to the thoracic cavity. Accompanying the loss of water and sodium is an increase in hematocrit, hemoglobin, and red cell mass, probably attributed to the loss of plasma volume. Also seen at this time are the isotonic losses of chloride, potassium, protein, albumin, creatinine, and glucose.

After about 4 days of bedrest, fluid losses reach an equilibrium. A possible explanation for this centers on the theory that fluid is lost from the vascular compartment with a subsequent iso-osmotic shift of fluids from the extravascular space. Extravascular hydration is sacrificed to maintain adequate isotonic vascular volume. With a decrease in the extravascular volume and the reestablishment of intravascular volume, the osmolar receptors inhibit diuresis and natriuresis. Despite the reestablishment of intravascular volume, the extravascular spaces remain dehydrated.[24]

Postural Blood Pressure. During bedrest, the forces of gravity and hydrostatic pressure are removed from the cardiovascular system. After 3 to 4 days of bedrest, the resumption of the upright position results in postural intolerance. Standing after prolonged bedrest results in a decrease in central blood volume as blood is displaced to the lower extremities and dependent parts of the body. Decreases in stroke volume and cardiac output occur along with increases in heart rate and systemic vascular resistance. The signs and symptoms of postural intolerance include tachycardia, nausea, diaphoresis, and sometimes syncope. This response is believed to be due to β-adrenergic and sympathetic vagal stimulation. The reason for this is not completely understood because catecholamine levels and adrenergic receptor sensitivity do not change significantly with bedrest.

Cardiac Workload and Exercise Tolerance. The major cardiovascular manifestation of deconditioning associated with bedrest is an increased workload on the heart. Initially, when a person assumes the supine position, venous return to the heart increases along with an increase in stroke volume and cardiac output, which, in turn, is accompanied by a slight decrease in heart rate. Over time, cardiac output and stroke volume stabilize, whereas heart rate increases. During periods of tachycardia, the time the heart spends in diastole is decreased. With decreased time spent in diastole, the heart does not have sufficient time to fill with blood. Thus the heart has to work harder (expend more energy and use more oxygen) to perfuse vital organs and meet the metabolic demands of the body. This response is exaggerated when a person has to assume the upright position and begin activity after a prolonged period of bedrest. Research has demonstrated that when people begin submaximal exercise after prolonged bedrest, heart rate increases while stroke volume and cardiac output decrease. Furthermore, 5 to 10 weeks of reconditioning exercise were required for return of heart rate, stroke volume, and cardiac output parameters to prebedrest levels.[26, 27]

Venous Stasis. Venous stasis in the legs results from lack of skeletal muscle pump function that promotes venous return to the heart. The skeletal muscle pump function is removed after assumption of the supine position; additionally, there is mechanical compression of veins due to the position of the lower extremities against the bed. This increased pressure damages the intima of the vessel and causes platelets to adhere easily to the damaged vessel. Over time, this may be the basis for clot formation. The development of deep vein thrombosis (DVT) is the third major complication of bedrest. It is believed that three possible factors of immobility combine to predispose a person to thrombus formation: (1) venous stasis, (2) application of external pressure from the mattress against the veins, and (3) hypercoagulability of the blood. However, most people who develop DVT have additional risk factors in place in addition to bedrest.[23] The development of DVT also predisposes to the development of pulmonary emboli. As people begin to resume activity patterns, the risk that large thrombi may dislodge and work their way through the circulatory system and lodge in a pulmonary blood vessel increases.

Blood Coagulability. Various theories exist that describe the possible causes of hypercoagulability and clot formation. One theory cites the development of dehydration, which often occurs with bedrest, as responsible. Dehydration leads to an increased number of formed elements in the blood and contributes to increased blood viscosity. Increased viscosity contributes to clotting. Another theory cites the role of calcium. During bedrest, demineralization of bone occurs, and calcium and other minerals are released into the bloodstream. Calcium activates the conversion of prothrombin to thrombin, and thrombin becomes the activating enzyme that converts fibrinogen to fibrin. Fibrin initiates the process for clot formation.[29, 30]

PULMONARY RESPONSES

Bedrest and assumption of the supine position produce changes in lung volumes and the mechanics of breathing. When a person is supine, the diaphragm moves toward the head and causes a decrease in the size of the thoracic compartment. Also, chest expansion is limited due to the resistance of the bed. These limitations to the thoracic cavity hinder normal lung expansion. As a result, a decrease in both lung compliance and in elastic recoil of the lungs occurs. In the supine position, normal tidal volume breathing is a function of the abdominal muscles; this is in contrast to breathing in the upright position, in which normal breathing is primarily a function of rib cage movement. Tidal volume and functional residual capacity are decreased, and the efficiency and effectiveness of ventilation are hindered. People must work harder to breathe and, thus, take fewer deep breaths. Alveoli tend to collapse, resulting in areas of atelectasis and a decrease in the surface for gas exchange. These changes in function contribute to respiratory complications associated with bedrest: atelectasis, accumulation of secretions, hypoxemia, and pulmonary emboli.

Atelectasis is characterized by localized area(s) of lung collapse (see Chapter 27). It is caused by impaired mucociliary clearance of the airway resulting in pooling of secretions. Also, poor fluid intake and dehydration may cause secretions to become thick and tenacious. Stasis of secretions provides an ideal medium for bacterial growth, especially pneumococcic, staphylococcic, and streptococcic organisms. To prevent the complication of pneumonia from developing, people must perform coughing and deep breathing exercises. However, with the combined need of overcoming resistance to chest and lung expansion and obstructed airways, more energy is required to breathe. More oxygen is used, and more carbon dioxide is produced causing the person to expend more energy to get less air.

URINARY TRACT RESPONSES

The kidneys are designed to function optimally with the body in the erect position. The anatomy of the kidney is such that urine flows from the kidney pelvis by gravity, whereas the action of peristalsis moves urine through the ureters to the bladder. Prolonged bedrest affects the renal system by altering the composition of body fluids and predisposing to the development of kidney stones. In the supine position, urine is not readily drained from the renal pelvis. Bedrest may also predispose to urinary tract infections and urinary incontinence because of positional changes and difficulty emptying the bladder.

A major complication of prolonged bedrest is the increased risk of developing kidney stones. Prolonged bedrest causes muscle atrophy, protein breakdown, decalcification of bone, hypercalcemia and hyperphosphatemia, and increased risk of developing calcium-containing kidney stones.[31] The urine becomes saturated with calcium salts (calcium oxalate and calcium phosphate) as a result of the hypercalcemia and hyperphosphatemia; stasis of urine resulting from the supine position favors crystallization of the stone-forming calcium salts. Moreover, urine levels of citrate, a prominent inhibitor of calcium stone formation, do not increase during bedrest.[30, 31] Dehydration further increases urine concentration of stone-forming elements and risk of kidney stone formation. The pathogenesis and manifestations of kidney stones are discussed in Chapter 32.

Urinary tract infections and incontinence may also occur. The cause of incontinence is inadequate emptying of the bladder while the person is in the supine position. This position contributes to stagnation of urine in the bladder and may predispose the person to bladder and urinary tract infections.

MUSCULOSKELETAL RESPONSES

Muscles are only as strong as they need to be to perform the work at hand. Disuse atrophy leads to loss of about one eighth of the muscle's strength with each week of disuse.[32] Weight loss occurs when normally healthy people are subjected to periods of prolonged bedrest. The weight loss occurs when people are placed on controlled diets, as well as when people are allowed to eat ad libitum.[33] The reduction in weight is associated with the loss of lean muscle mass and loss of fat content. The larger the muscle, and the better trained the muscle, the faster the loss of muscle strength and the quicker the deconditioning occurs. This is best illustrated by the example that leg muscles lose strength and mass more quickly than muscles of the arms when people are placed on prolonged bedrest.

In addition to loss of strength, muscles atrophy, change shape and appearance, and shorten when immobilized. There is also a decrease in the oxidative capacity of the muscle mitochondria. These changes affect both individual muscle fibers and total muscle mass.[23] Atrophy of muscles is reflected as an increase in urinary nitrogen excretion and a decrease in muscle weight. Because of the decreased oxidative capacity of the mitochondria, muscles fatigue more easily.

Muscle atrophy not only contributes to wasting and weakening of muscle tissue, it also plays a role in the development of contractures. A contracture is the abnormal shortening of muscle tissue rendering the muscle highly resistant to stretch. As previously described, muscles weaken and shorten with disuse. Contractures occur when muscles do not have the necessary strength to maintain their integrity (their proper function and full range of motion). Contractures mainly develop over joints when there is an imbalance in the muscle strength of the antagonistic muscle groups. If allowed to progress, the contracture eventually involves not only the muscle groups, but the tendons, ligaments, and joint capsule. The joint becomes limited in its full use and range of motion. Proper body alignment decreases the risk for the development of contractures.[30]

Another consequence of prolonged immobility and bedrest on the musculoskeletal system is the development of osteoporosis. Bone is a dynamic tissue that undergoes continual deposition and replacement of minerals in response to the dual stimuli of weight bearing and muscle pull. With immobility and bedrest, calcium loss from the bone begins almost immediately.

Osteoblast cells function to form the osseous matrix of the bone, whereas the osteoclast cells work continually to destroy the bone matrix. Through their opposing forces, bone material is continually turned over and new bone is regenerated. Osteoblasts depend on the stress of mobility and weight bearing to perform their function. During immobility and bedrest, the process of building new bone stops, but the osteoclast cells continue to perform their function. This results in structural changes in the bone as the bone decalcifies. There is also an increase in the excretion of bone phosphorus and nitrogen. This demineralization of the bone is known as osteoporosis. Despite the calcium loss from the bone, serum calcium remains normal because the excess calcium is excreted in the urine and feces.

People who experience osteoporosis from prolonged immobility and bedrest develop soft spongy bones. The bones may easily compress and become deformed. Also, because of lack of structural firmness, the bones may easily fracture. People with osteoporosis encounter much pain when they begin weight-bearing activities. Despite the lack of calcium in the bone, a diet high in calcium does not enhance bone uptake of calcium. Unneeded calcium is added to the excess calcium that is already being excreted in the urine. Often this may precipitate the formation of calcium-containing renal stones. The best measure to prevent the occurrence of osteoporosis is to begin weight bearing as soon as possible.

SKIN

Except for the soles of the feet, the skin is not designed for weight bearing. However, during bedrest, the large surface area of the skin bears weight and is in constant contact with the surface of the bed. Constant pressure is transmitted to the skin, subcutaneous tissue, and muscle, especially to those tissues over bony prominences. This constant contact causes increased pressure and impairs normal capillary blood flow, which interferes with the exchange of nutrients and waste products. Tissue ischemia and necrosis may result and lead to the development of pressure ulcers. Also contributing to the development of pressure ulcers is moisture from the skin being in constant contact with bed linens, and the forces of friction and shear.

METABOLIC AND ENDOCRINE RESPONSES

When a person is placed on bedrest, the basal metabolic rate falls in response to the decreased energy requirements of the body. Anabolic processes are slowed, and catabolic processes become accelerated. As a result, protein breakdown occurs and leads to a protein deficiency and a negative nitrogen balance. People in a negative nitrogen balance experience nausea and anorexia. Insulin plays a role in regulating protein metabolism and glucose utilization. It does this primarily by inhibiting protein breakdown.

With bedrest, people experience an impaired glucose tolerance. During bedrest, it takes more insulin to maintain serum glucose. Research has demonstrated that after 10 days of bedrest there is a 100% increase in basal insulin concentration to maintain normal glucose control.[34] Thus, there appears to exist an induced insulin resistance that helps explain the negative nitrogen balance seen in patients who experience prolonged bedrest.

Possible reasons to explain glucose unresponsiveness to the hyperinsulinemia include: (1) a change in the action of insulin because of the release of a substance that acts as an insulin inhibitor (this substance is believed to act at cell membrane binding sites); (2) a change in some aspect of cellular membrane function; and (3) blockage of the function of a second factor that has insulinlike activity. Research has demonstrated that there is a factor, or factors, present that are activated with physical exercise. These factors respond to the quantity of energy expenditure and are necessary for insulin, and possibly

glucose, to function normally. Therefore, in the absence of activity, the action of these factors may be suppressed. A final explanation to describe glucose unresponsiveness to hyperinsulinemia is a combination of the above-mentioned causes.[33, 35]

Also seen with people who experience prolonged periods of bedrest is a change in the circadian release of various hormones. Normally, insulin and growth hormone peak twice a day. In subjects who experienced 30 days of bedrest, a single daily peak of these hormones occurred. Other hormonal changes include an afternoon peak of epinephrine rather than the normal early morning peak, and an early morning peak of aldosterone rather than the usual noonday peak that is seen in normally active people.[35]

GASTROINTESTINAL RESPONSES

Gastrointestinal responses to bedrest vary. Constipation and fecal impaction are frequent complications that occur when people experience prolonged periods of immobility and bedrest. With inactivity, there is slowed movement of feces through the colon. The act of defecation requires the integration of the abdominal muscles, the diaphragm, and the levator ani. Muscle atrophy and loss of tone occur in the immobilized person and interfere with the normal act of defecation. Lack of privacy and the supine position may compound normal defecation.

SENSORY RESPONSES

Immobility reduces the quality and quantity of sensory information available from kinesthetic, visual, auditory, and tactile sensation. It also reduces the ability of the person to interact with the environment. Decreased kinesthetic stimulation occurs from both immobilization and assumption of the supine or recumbent position. Responses to decreased kinesthetic stimulation include an impaired functioning of thought processes and decreased sensory perception. Prolonged immobility and bedrest have been associated with a number of impaired sensory responses. Common occurrences include both visual and auditory hallucinations, vivid dreams, inefficient thought processes, loss of contact with reality, and alteration in tactile stimulation.

In addition to sensory deprivation related to prolonged bedrest and immobility, people may experience a sensory monotony from the hospital environment. Repetitious and meaningless sounds from cardiac monitors, respirators, and hospital personnel, along with an environment that may be void of light and a day–night cycle also contribute to impaired sensory perception.

TIME COURSE OF PHYSIOLOGIC RESPONSES

The deconditioning responses to the inactivity of immobility and bedrest affect all body systems. One of the important factors to keep in mind is the rapidity with which the changes occur, and the length of time required to overcome these effects. The body responds in a characteristic pattern to the effects of the supine position and bedrest. During the first 3 days of bedrest, one of the first changes to occur is a massive diuresis. Accompanying the diuresis are increases in serum osmolality, hematocrit, venous compliance, and an increase of urinary sodium and chloride excretion. Fluid losses stabilize by about the 4th day.

By days 4 to 7, there are changes in the hemolytic system. Fibrinogen increases along with increases in fibrinolytic activity and prolonged clotting time. The cardiovascular system responds with a decrease in cardiac output and stroke volume. No change is seen in heart rate and blood pressure. The basal metabolic rate decreases and the person begins to develop an insulin intolerance and a negative nitrogen balance.

Days 8 to 14 are characterized by additional effects on the hemolytic system. Decreases are seen in the number of red blood cells, and the phagocytic ability of leukocytes. Also, people begin to experience a decrease in lean body mass.

After 15 days of bedrest, osteoporosis and hypercalcuria occur. Also occurring is a decrease in aerobic power, changes in the cyclic excretion of some hormones, and alterations in the person's thought pattern and sensory perception (Table 9-3).[36]

PSYCHOSOCIAL RESPONSES

Immobility often sets the stage for changes in a person's response to illness. People not only adapt to prolonged bedrest and immobility through a series of physiological responses, but changes in affect, perception, and cognition as well. Affective changes include increased anxiety, fear, depression, hostility, rapid mood changes, and alterations with normal sleep patterns. These changes in mood not only occur with hospitalized patients who are subjected to periods of prolonged bedrest and immobility, but

TABLE 9-3. PHYSIOLOGIC CHANGES DURING BEDREST

0–3 DAYS	4–7 DAYS	8–14 DAYS	OVER 15 DAYS
Increases in:	Increases in:	Increases in:	Increases in:
Urine volume	Urine creatinine, hydroxy-	Urine pyrophosphate	Peak hypercalciuria
Urine Na, Cl, Ca, and os-	proline, PO_4, N, and K	Sweating sensitivity	Sensitivity to thermal
mol excretion	excretion	Exercise hyperthermia	threshold
Plasma osmolality	Plasma globulin, phosphate	Exercise maximal heart rate	Auditory threshold (sec-
Hematocrit	and glucose levels		ondary)
Venous compliance	Blood fibrinogen		
	Fibrinolytic activity and		
	clotting time		
	Visual focal point		
	Hyperthermia of eye con-		
	junctiva, dilation of reti-		
	nal arteries and veins		
	Auditory threshold		
Decreases in:	Decreases in:	Decreases in:	Decreases in:
Total fluid intake	Near point of visual acuity	Red blood cell mass	Bone density
Extracellular and intracellu-	Orthostatic tolerance	Leukocyte phagocytosis	
lar fluid	Nitrogen balance	Tissue heat conductance	
Calf blood flow		Lean body mass	
Resting heart rate			
Secretion of gastric acid			
Glucose tolerance			

(Greenleaf, J. E. [1984]. Physiological responses to prolonged bedrest and fluid immersion in humans. *Journal of Applied Physiology: Respiratory, Environmental and Exercise Physiology, 57*[3], 619–633)

also occur in people in confinement, such as astronauts and prisoners.[23]

Research of immobilized or isolated people has demonstrated that the motivation to learn decreases with periods of prolonged immobility as does the ability to learn and retain new material and transfer newly learned material to a different situation. In addition, people are less able and less motivated to perform problem-solving activities; they are less able to concentrate and discriminate information.[29] These studies present major implications for the timing of patient education as well as the preparation of education materials.

Prolonged bedrest and immobility also contribute to the social isolation of the hospitalized person. Confined to a hospital bed, the person is not able to assume certain societal roles. The roles of spouse, parent, sibling, worker, friend are altered either temporarily or permanently while the person is hospitalized. People may respond to this isolation by exhibiting various effective and ineffective coping behaviors, which include increased anxiety, depression, restlessness, fear, and rapid mood changes.

INTERVENTIONS

A holistic approach should be initiated when caring for people who are immobile or require prolonged periods of bedrest. Interventions and treatment should include actions that address the person's physical and psychosocial needs. The goals of care for the immobilized person include structuring a safe environment in which the person is not at risk to incur any nosocomial complications, providing diversional activities to offset problems with sensory deprivation, and preventing complications of bedrest by implementing a multidisciplinary plan of care.

In summary, during the last 75 years, the use of bedrest has taken a complete reversal as a standard of treatment for a variety of medical conditions. Over time, research findings have described the deleterious consequences of inactivity. All body systems are affected by complications of immobility and prolonged bedrest.

The responses to bedrest and immobility affect all body systems. One of the important factors is the rapidity with which the changes occur, and the long time required to overcome the effects of prolonged bedrest and immobility. Adverse effects of prolonged immobility and bedrest include a decreased cardiac output, orthostatic intolerance, dehydration, potential for thrombophlebitis, pneumonia, formation of renal calculi, development of pressure ulcers, sensory deprivation, and impaired thought processes.

■ REFERENCES

1. Allan, J.D. (1992). Exercise program. In G.M. Bulechek & J.C. McCloskey (Eds.). *Nursing interventions: Essential nursing treatments* (2nd ed., pp. 406–424). Philadelphia: W.B. Saunders.
2. Lamb, D.R. (1984). *Physiology of exercise: Responses and adaptations.* New York: Macmillan.
3. Ulmer, H.V. (1983). Work physiology; Environmental physiology. In R.F. Schmidt & G. Thews (Eds.). *Human physiology* (pp. 548–564). New York: Springer-Verlag.
4. Daughton, D.M., & Fix, J.A. (1986). *Human activity profile manual.* Omaha, NE: Psychological Assessment Resources.
5. Krupp, L.B., LaRocca, N.G., Muir-Nash, J., et al. (1989). The Fatigue Severity Scale: Application to patients with multiple sclerosis and systemic lupus erythematosus. *Archives of Neurology, 46,* 1121–1123.
6. Cantwell, J.D. (1984). Exercise and coronary heart disease: Role of primary prevention. *Heart & Lung, 13,* 6–13.
7. Borg, G.A.V. (1973). Perceived exertion: A note on ''history'' and methods. *Medicine and Science in Sports, 5*(2), 90–93.
7b. Borg, G.A.V. (1982). Psychophysical bases of perceived exertion. *Medicine and Science in Sports and Exercise, 14*(5), 377–381.
8. Carroll-Johnson, R. (Ed.). (1989). *Classification of nursing diagnoses: Proceedings of the eighth conference.* Philadelphia: J.B. Lippincott.
9. MacLean, S. (1991). Activity intolerance. In M. Maas, K. Buckwalter, & M.A. Hardy (Eds.). *Nursing diagnoses and interventions for the elderly* (pp. 252–262). Redwood City, CA: Addison-Wesley Nursing.
10. Piper, B.F. (1986). Fatigue. In V.K. Carrieri, A.M. Lindsey, & C.W. West (Eds.). *Pathophysiological phenomena in nursing: Human responses to illness.* Philadelphia: W.B. Saunders.
11. Piper, B.F. (1989). Fatigue: Current bases for practice. In S.G. Funk, E.M. Tornquist, M.T. Champagne, L.A. Copp, & R.A. Wiese (Eds.). *Key aspects of comfort: Management of pain, fatigue, and nausea* (pp. 187–198). New York: Springer.
12. Nail, L.M., & King, K.B. (1987). Fatigue. *Seminars in Oncology Nursing, 3,* 257–261.
13. St. Pierre, B.A., Kasper, C.E., & Lindsey, A.M. (1992). Fatigue mechanisms in patients with cancer: Effects of tumor necrosis factor and exercise on skeletal muscle. *Oncology Nursing Forum, 19*(3), 419–425.
14. Matthews, D.A., Manu, P., & Lane, T.J. (1991). Evaluation and management of patients with chronic fatigue. *The American Journal of Medical Sciences, 302*(5), 269–277.
15. Shafran, S.D. (1991). The chronic fatigue syndrome. *American Journal of Medicine, 90*(6), 730–739.
16. Gorensek, M.J. (1991). Chronic fatigue and depression in the ambulatory patient. *Primary Care, 18*(2), 397–419.
17. Holmes, G.P., Kaplan, J.E., Gantz, N.M., et al. (1988). Chronic fatigue syndrome: A working case definition. *Annals of Internal Medicine, 108,* 387–389.
18. Holmes, G.P. (1991). Defining the chronic fatigue syndrome. *Reviews of Infectious Diseases, 13*(Suppl 1), S53–55.
19. Cho, W.K., & Stollerman, G.H. (1992). Chronic fatigue syndrome. *Hospital Practice, 27*(9), 221–245.
20. Calabrese, L., Danao, T., Camara, E., & Wilke, W. (1992). Chronic fatigue syndrome. *American Family Physician, 45*(3), 1205–1213.

21. Portwood, M.F. (1988). Chronic fatigue syndrome—A diagnosis for consideration. *Nurse Practitioner, 13*(2), 11–23.
22. Kroenke, K. (1991). Chronic fatigue syndrome: Is it real? *Postgraduate Medicine, 89*(2), 44–55.
23. Harper, C.M., & Lyles, Y.M. (1988). Physiology and complications of bed rest. *Journal of the American Geriatric Society, 36*(11), 1047–1054.
24. Rubin, M. (1988). The physiology of bed rest. *American Journal of Nursing, 88*(1), 50–58.
25. Hyatt, K.H., Kamenetsky, L.G., & Smith, W.M. (1969). Extravascular dehydration as an etiologic factor in postrecumbency orthostatism. *Aerospace Medicine, 40*(6), 644–650.
26. Taylor, H.L., Henschel, A., Brozek, J., et al. (1949). Effects of bed rest on cardiovascular function and work performance. *Journal of Applied Physiology, 2*(5), 223–239.
27. Saltin, B., Blomquist, G., Mitchell, J.H., et al. (1968). Responses to exercise after bed rest and after training: A longitudinal study of adaptive changes in oxygen transport and body composition. *Circulation, 38*(7S), 1–78.
28. Winslow, E.H. (1985). Cardiovascular consequences of bed rest. *Heart & Lung, 14*(3), 236–246.
29. Goldstrom, D.K. (1972). Cardiac rest: Bed or chair? *American Journal of Nursing, 72*(10), 1812–1816.
30. Olson, E.V., Thompson, L.F., McCarthy, J., et al. (1967). The hazards of immobility. *American Journal of Nursing 67*(4), 780–797.
31. Twang, T.S., Hill, D., Schneider, V., et al. (1988). Effect of bed rest on the propensity for renal stone formation. *Journal of Clinical Endocrinology and Metabolism, 66,* 109–112.
32. Corcoran, P.J. (1991). Use it or lose it: The hazards of bed rest and inactivity. *Western Journal of Medicine, 154*(5), 536–538.
33. Greenleaf, J.E., & Kozlowski, S. (1982). Physiological consequences of reduced physical activity during bed rest. In R.L. Terjung (Ed.). *Exercise and sports science review* (vol. 10, pp. 84–119). Syracuse, NY: American College of Sports Medicine.
34. Shangraw, R.E., Stuart, C.A., Prince, M.J., et al. (1988). Insulin responsiveness of protein metabolism in vivo following bedrest in humans. *American Journal of Physiology, 255,* E548–E558.
35. Dolkas, C.B., & Greenleaf, J.E. (1977). Insulin and glucose responses during bed rest with isotonic and isometric exercise. *Journal of Applied Physiology, 43*(6), 1033–1038.
36. Greenleaf, J.E. (1984). Physiological responses to prolonged bed rest and fluid immersion in humans. *Journal of Applied Physiology, 57*(3), 619–633.

ALTERATIONS IN BODY DEFENSES

CHAPTER 10

ALTERATIONS IN TEMPERATURE REGULATION

■ **OBJECTIVES**

After you have studied this chapter, you should be able to meet the following objectives:

■ Differentiate between body core temperature and skin temperature and relate the differences to methods used for measuring body temperature.

■ Describe the mechanisms of heat production in the body.

■ Define *conduction, radiation, convection*, and *evaporation* and relate them to the mechanisms for heat loss from the body.

■ Describe the four stages of fever.

■ Explain what is meant by intermittent, remittent, sustained, and relapsing fevers.

■ State the relationship between body temperature and heart rate.

■ Differentiate between the physiologic mechanisms involved in fever and hyperthermia.

■ List the possible mechanisms of drug-related fevers.

■ Compare the mechanisms of malignant hyperthermia and neuroleptic malignant syndrome.

■ Define *hypothermia*.

■ Compare the manifestations of mild, moderate, and severe hypothermia and relate to changes in physiologic functioning that occur with decreased body temperature.

Virtually all biochemical processes in the body are affected by changes in temperature. Metabolic processes speed up or slow down depending on whether body temperature is rising or falling. Body temperature is normally maintained within a range of 35.9°C to 37.4°C (96.6°F to 99.3°F). Within this range there are individual differences and diurnal variations; internal core temperatures reach their highest point in late afternoon and evening and their lowest point in the early morning hours (Fig. 10-1). This chapter is organized in three sections: regulation of body temperature, fever and hyperthermia, and hypothermia.

Carol Mattson Porth: PATHOPHYSIOLOGY: CONCEPTS OF
ALTERED HEALTH STATES, 4th ed. © 1994, 1990, 1986, 1982
J.B. Lippincott Company

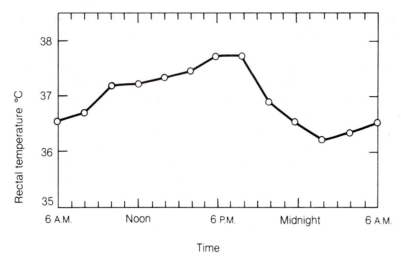

FIG. 10-1. Normal diurnal variations in body temperature.

■ BODY TEMPERATURE REGULATION

Body temperature reflects the difference between heat production and heat loss and varies with exercise and extremes of environmental temperature. Properly protected, the body can function in environmental conditions that range from −50°C (−58°F) to +50°C (122°F). Individual body cells, however, cannot tolerate such a wide range of temperatures—at −1°C (32°F) ice crystals form, and at +45°C (113°F) cell proteins coagulate.[1]

Most of the body's heat is produced by the deeper core tissues (muscles and viscera) of the body, which are insulated from the environment and protected against heat loss by the subcutaneous tissues and skin (Fig. 10-2). Adipose tissue is a particularly good insulator, conducting heat only one third as effectively as other tissues. Heat loss occurs when the heat from the body's inner core is transferred to the skin surface by the circulating blood. If no heat were lost by the body at rest, the temperature of the body would rise 1°C (1.8°F)/h; with light work, the temperature would rise 2°C/h.

Temperatures differ in various parts of the body, core temperatures being higher than those at the skin surface. Generally the rectal temperature is used as a measure of core temperature. Core temperatures may also be obtained from the esophagus using a flexible thermometer, from a pulmonary artery catheter that is used for thermodilution measurement of cardiac output, or from a urinary catheter with thermosensor that measures the temperature of urine in the bladder. Because of location, pulmonary artery and esophageal temperatures closely reflect the temperature of the heart and thoracic organs. The oral temperature, taken sublingually, is usually 0.2°C (0.36°F) to 0.51°C (0.9°F) lower than the rectal temperature. The axillary temperature can also be used

as an estimate of core temperature. However, the parts of the axillary fossa must be pressed closely together because this method requires considerable heat to accumulate before the final temperature is reached.

Tympanic membrane thermometry has been introduced as a method of measuring body temperature. The method uses infrared sensor to measure

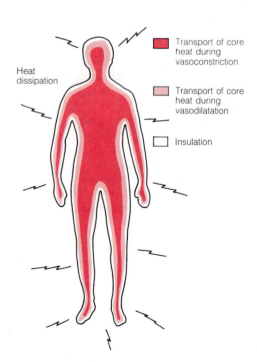

FIG. 10-2. Control of heat loss. Body heat is produced in the deeper core tissues of the body, which is insulated by the subcutaneous tissues and skin to protect against heat loss. During vasodilatation, circulating blood transports heat to the skin surface, where it dissipates into the surrounding environment. Vasoconstriction decreases the transport of core heat to the skin surface, and vasodilatation increases transport.

the flow of heat from the tympanic membrane and ear canal. Ear thermometry is easy to use and has been reported to correlate well with rectal temperatures. The method has become popular in the pediatric setting because of its ease and speed of measurement, acceptability to parents and children, and cost savings in personnel time required to take a child's temperature.[2]

Body temperature is regulated by the thermoregulatory center in the hypothalamus. This center integrates input from various thermal receptors located throughout the body with output responses that either conserve body heat or increase its dissipation. It is the temperature of the body core rather than surface temperature that is regulated. The thermostatic set point of the thermoregulatory center is set so that the temperature of the body is regulated within the previously mentioned normal range of 35.9°C to 37.4°C. When body temperature begins to rise above the normal range, heat-dissipating behaviors are initiated; when the temperature falls below the normal range, heat production is increased. Core temperatures above 41°C (105.8°F) or below 34°C (93.2°F) usually mean that the body's ability to thermoregulate is impaired (Fig. 10-3). Body responses that produce, conserve, and dissipate heat are described in Table 10-1. Spinal cord injuries that transect the cord at T6

or above can seriously impair temperature regulation. This is because the hypothalamus can no longer control skin blood flow or sweating.

Aside from the body's thermoregulatory mechanisms, people engage in other voluntary behaviors to help regulate body temperature. These behaviors include the selection of proper clothing and regulation of environmental temperature through heating systems and air conditioning. Body positions that hold the extremities close to the body prevent heat loss and are commonly assumed in cold weather.

MECHANISMS OF HEAT PRODUCTION

The body's main source of heat production is metabolism. There is a 0.56°C (1°F) increase in body temperature for every 7% increase in metabolism. The sympathetic neurotransmitters, epinephrine and norepinephrine, which are released when an increase in body temperature is needed, act at the cellular level to shift metabolism so energy production is reduced and heat production is increased. This may be one of the reasons fever tends to produce feelings of weakness and fatigue. Thyroid hormone increases cellular metabolism, but this response usually requires several weeks to reach maximal effectiveness.

Fine involuntary actions such as shivering and chattering of the teeth can produce a three- to fivefold increase in body temperature. Shivering is initiated by impulses from the hypothalamus. The first muscle change that occurs with shivering is a general increase in muscle tone followed by an oscillating rhythmic tremor involving the spinal-level reflex that controls muscle tone. Because no external work is performed, all the energy liberated by the metabolic processes from shivering is in the form of heat.

Physical exertion increases body temperature. With strenuous exercise, more than three quarters of the increased metabolism resulting from muscle activity appears as heat within the body and the remainder appears as external work.

MECHANISMS OF HEAT LOSS

Most of the body's heat losses occur at the skin surface as heat from the blood moves to the skin and from there into the surrounding environment. There are numerous arteriovenous (AV) shunts under the skin surface that allow blood to move directly from the arterial to the venous system. These AV shunts are much like the radiators in a heating system. When the shunts are open, body heat is freely dissipated to the skin and surrounding environment; when the shunts are closed, heat is retained in the body. The

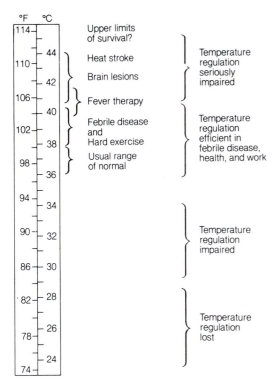

FIG. 10-3. *Body temperatures under different conditions.* (Dubois, E. F. [1948]. *Fever and the regulation of body temperature.* Springfield, IL: Charles C. Thomas)

TABLE 10-1. HEAT LOSS AND HEAT GAIN RESPONSES USED IN REGULATION OF BODY TEMPERATURE

HEAT GAIN		HEAT LOSS	
Body Response	Mechanism of Action	Body Response	Mechanism of Action
Vasoconstriction of the superficial blood vessels	Confines blood flow to the inner core of the body, with the skin and subcutaneous tissues acting as insulation to prevent loss of core heat	Dilatation of the superficial blood vessels	Delivers blood containing core heat to the periphery where it is dissipated through: Radiation Conduction Convection
Contraction of the pilomotor muscles that surround the hairs on the skin	Reduces the heat loss surface of the skin	Sweating	Increases heat loss through evaporation
Assumption of the huddle position with the extremities held close to the body	Reduces the area for heat loss		
Shivering	Increases heat production by the muscles		
Increased production of epinephrine	Increases the heat production associated with metabolism		
Increased production of thyroid hormone	Is a long-term mechanism that increases metabolism and heat production		

blood flow in the AV shunts is controlled almost exclusively by the sympathetic nervous system in response to changes in core temperature and environmental temperature. Contraction of the pilomotor muscles of the skin, which raises skin hairs and produces goose bumps, reduces the surface area available for heat loss.

Heat is lost from the body through radiation, conduction, and convection from the skin surface; through the evaporation of sweat and insensible perspiration; through the warming and humidifying of inspired air; and through urine and feces. Of these mechanisms, only heat losses that occur at the skin surface are directly under hypothalamic control.

CONDUCTION

Conduction is the direct transfer of heat from one molecule to another. Blood carries, or conducts, heat from the inner core of the body to the skin surface. Normally only a small amount of body heat is lost through conduction to a cooler surface. Cooling blankets or mattresses that are used for reducing fever rely on conduction of heat from the skin to the cool surface of the mattress. Heat can also be conducted in the opposite direction—from the external environ-

ment to the body surface. For instance, body temperature may rise slightly after a hot bath.

Water has a specific heat several times greater than air, so water absorbs far greater amounts of heat than air. Hence, the loss of body heat can be excessive and life-threatening in situations of cold water immersion or cold exposure in damp or wet clothing.

The conduction of heat to the body's surface is influenced by blood volume. In hot weather, the body compensates by increasing blood volume as a means of dissipating heat. People who are not acclimated to a hot environment can increase their total blood volume by 10% within 2 to 4 hours of heat exposure. A mild swelling of the ankles during hot weather provides evidence of blood volume expansion. Exposure to cold produces a cold diuresis and a reduction in blood volume as a means of controlling the transfer of heat to the body's surface.

RADIATION

Radiation is the transfer of heat through the air or a vacuum. Heat from the sun is carried by radiation. Heat loss by radiation varies with the temperature of the environment. Environmental temperature must be less than that of the body for heat loss to occur.

Normally about 60% to 70% of body heat is dissipated by radiation.

CONVECTION

Convection refers to heat transfer through the circulation of air currents. Normally a layer of warm air tends to remain near the body's surface; convection causes continual removal of the warm layer and replacement with air from the surrounding environment. The wind-chill factor that is often included in the weather report combines the effect of convection due to wind with the actual still-air temperature.

EVAPORATION

Evaporation involves the use of body heat to convert water on the skin to water vapor. Water that diffuses through the skin independent of sweating is called *insensible perspiration*. Insensible perspiration losses are greatest in a dry environment. Sweating occurs through the sweat glands and is controlled by the sympathetic nervous system. Unlike other sympathetically mediated functions, in which the catecholamines serve as neuromediators, sweating is mediated by acetylcholine. This means that anticholinergic drugs, such as atropine, can interfere with heat loss by interrupting sweating.

Evaporative heat losses involve both insensible perspiration and sweating, with 0.58 calories being lost for each gram of water that is evaporated.[3] As long as body temperature is greater than the atmospheric temperature, heat is lost through radiation. However, when the temperature of the surrounding environment becomes greater than skin temperature, evaporation is the only way the body can rid itself of heat. Any condition that prevents evaporative heat losses causes the body temperature to rise.

In summary, body temperature is normally maintained within a range of 35.9°C to 37.4°C (96.6°F to 99.3°F). Most of the body's heat is produced by metabolic processes that occur within deeper core structures (muscles and viscera) of the body. Heat loss occurs at the body's surface when heat from core structures is transported to the skin by the circulating blood. Heat is lost from the body through radiation, conduction, convection, and evaporation. The thermoregulatory center in the hypothalamus functions to modify heat production and heat losses as a means of regulating body temperature.

■ INCREASED BODY TEMPERATURE

Fever and hyperthermia describe an increase in body temperature that is outside the normal range. True fever is a disorder of thermoregulation in which there is upward displacement of the hypothalamic set point for temperature control. In hyperthermia the set point is unchanged, but the mechanisms that control body temperature are ineffective in meeting the challenge of maintaining body temperature during exposure to high ambient temperature or the excess heat production that occurs with strenuous exertion.

FEVER

The literature on fever dates back to the writings of Hippocrates, which contain many descriptions of the febrile-course diseases, such as typhoid fever.[4] However, it was not until the development of the thermometer that actual measurements of body temperature became possible. One of the first studies of body temperature was reported in 1868 by the German physician Carl Wunderlich, who, during a 20-year period, studied the body temperature of 25,000 patients with observations made twice daily with a foot-long thermometer held in the axilla for 20 minutes.[5] Wunderlich observed that the thermometer was a useful instrument for providing insight into the condition of the sick. Today, temperature is one of the most frequent physiologic responses to be monitored during illness.

MECHANISMS

Fever, or pyrexia, describes an elevation in body temperature that is caused by an upward displacement of the set point of the hypothalamic thermoregulatory center. When the fever has broken, the set point returns to its prefever setting. Fevers that are regulated by the hypothalamus usually do not rise above 41°C (105.8°F), suggesting a built-in thermostatic safety mechanism. Temperatures above that level are usually the result of superimposed activity, such as convulsions, hyperthermic states, or direct involvement of the temperature control center. The mechanisms for controlling temperature are not well developed in the infant. Hence, in infants under 3 months, a mild elevation in temperature (*i.e.*, rectal temperature of 38°C [100.4°F]) can indicate serious infection and requires immediate medical attention.[6] The presence of fever in elderly people is also more likely to indicate serious infection or disease.[7] This is because the elderly often have a lower baseline temperature and, although they increase their temperature during an infection, it may fail to reach a level that is equated with significant fever.[8]

Fever can be caused by a number of microorganisms and substances that are collectively called *exogenous pyrogens*. Exogenous pyrogens induce host cells to produce a fever-producing mediator called *endogenous pyrogen*. Research has identified at least three chemical substances that act as endogenous pyrogens: interleukin-1 (IL-1), interleukin-6 (IL-6), and tumor necrosis factor (TNF).[9] These chemical mediators, also known as *cytokines*, are synthesized by a number of body cell types, including endothelial cells, epithelial cells, lymphocytes, fibroblasts, and macrophages. The endogenous pyrogens produce fever by increasing the set point of the hypothalamic thermoregulatory center, probably through the action of prostaglandin E. In addition to their fever-producing actions, the endogenous pyrogens mediate a number of other responses. For example, IL-1 is an inflammatory mediator that produces other signs of inflammation such as leukocytosis, anorexia, and malaise (see Chapter 13).

Many noninfectious disorders, such as myocardial infarction, pulmonary emboli, and neoplasms, produce fever. In these conditions, the injured or abnormal cells incite the production of endogenous pyrogen. For example, trauma and surgery can be associated with up to 3 days of fever.[10, 11] Some malignant cells, such as those of leukemia and Hodgkin's disease, secrete endogenous pyrogen.

A fever that has its origin in the central nervous system (CNS) is sometimes referred to as a *neurogenic fever*. It is usually caused by CNS trauma, intracerebral bleeding, or an increase in intracranial pressure. Neurogenic fevers are characterized by a high temperature that is resistant to antipyretic therapy and is not associated with sweating.

PURPOSE

The purpose of fever is not completely understood. However, from a purely practical standpoint, fever is a valuable index to health status. For many people, fever signals the presence of an infection and may legitimize the need for medical treatment. In ancient times, fever was thought to "cook" the poisons that caused the illness. With the availability of antipyretic drugs in the late 19th century, the belief that fever was useful began to wane, probably because most antipyretic drugs also had analgesic effects. There is little research to support the belief that fever is harmful unless the temperature rises above 40°C (104°F). Animal studies have demonstrated a clear survival advantage in infected members with fever as compared with animals that were unable to develop a fever. It has been shown that small elevations in temperature like those that occur with fever enhance immune function. There is increased motility and activity of the white blood cells, stimulation of interferon production, and activation of T cells.[12, 13] Many of the microbial agents that cause infection grow best at normal body temperatures, and their growth is inhibited by temperatures within the fever range. For

example, the rhinoviruses responsible for the common cold are cultured best at 33°C (91.4°F), which is close to the temperature in the nasopharynx; temperature-sensitive mutants of virus that cannot grow at temperatures above 37.5°C (99.5°F) produce fewer signs and symptoms.[14]

PATTERNS

The patterns of temperature change in people with fever vary and may provide information about the nature of the causative agent.[15, 16] These patterns can be described as intermittent, remittent, sustained, or relapsing. An *intermittent* fever is one in which temperature returns to normal at least once every 24 hours. In a *remittent* fever, by contrast, the temperature does not return to normal and varies a few degrees in either direction. In a *sustained* or *continuous* fever the temperature remains above normal with minimal variations. A *recurrent* or *relapsing* fever is one in which there is one or more episodes of fever, each as long as several days, with one or more days of normal temperature between episodes.

Critical to the analysis of a fever pattern is the relationship of heart rate to the level of temperature elevation. Normally a 1°C rise in temperature produces a 15-beat/min increase in heart rate (1°F, 10 beats/min).[15] Most people respond to an increase in temperature with an appropriate increase in heart rate. The observation that a rise in temperature is not accompanied by the anticipated change in heart rate can provide useful information about the cause of the fever. For example, a heart rate that is slower than would be anticipated can occur with Legionnaires' disease and drug fever, and a heart rate that is more rapid than anticipated can be symptomatic of hyperthyroidism and pulmonary emboli.

MANIFESTATIONS

The physiologic behaviors that occur during the development of fever can be divided into four stages: (1) a prodrome, (2) a chill during which the temperature rises, (3) a flush, and (4) defervescence. During the first or prodromal period, there are nonspecific complaints such as mild headache and fatigue, general malaise, and fleeting aches and pains. Vasoconstriction and piloerection usually precede the onset of shivering. At this point the skin is pale and covered with goose flesh. There is a feeling of being cold and an urgency to put on more clothing or covering and to curl up in a position that conserves body heat. The prodromal stage is followed by the second stage—the onset of a generalized shaking chill; and even as the temperature rises, there is the uncomfortable sensation of being chilled. When the shivering has caused the body temperature to reach the new set point of the temperature control center, the shivering ceases and a sensation of warmth develops. At this point, the third stage begins, during which cutaneous vasodilation occurs and the skin becomes warm and flushed. The fourth, or defervescence, stage of the febrile response is marked by the initiation of sweating. Not all people proceed through the four stages of fever development. Sweating may be absent, and fever may develop gradually with no indication of a chill or shivering.

Common manifestations of fever are anorexia, myalgia, arthralgia, and fatigue. These discomforts are worse when the temperature rises rapidly or exceeds 39.5°C (103.1°F). Respiration is increased, and the heart rate is usually elevated. The occurrence of chills commonly coincides with the introduction of pyrogen into the circulation. Many of the manifestations of fever are related to the increases in the metabolic rate, increased need for oxygen, and use of body proteins as an energy source. Dehydration occurs because of sweating and the rapid respiratory rate that results in increased vapor losses. With prolonged fever, there is increased breakdown of endogenous fat stores. If fat catabolism is rapid, metabolic acidosis may result.

Headache is a common accompaniment of fever and is thought to result from the vasodilation of cerebral vessels occurring with fever. Delirium is possible when the temperature in fever exceeds 40°C (104°F). In the elderly, confusion and delirium may follow moderate elevations in temperature. Owing to increasingly poor oxygen uptake by the aging lung, pulmonary function may prove to be a limiting factor in the hypermetabolism that accompanies fever in older people. Confusion, incoordination, and agitation commonly reflect cerebral hypoxemia. Febrile convulsions can occur in some children. They usually occur with rapidly rising temperatures or at a threshold temperature that differs with each child.

Herpetic lesions, or fever blisters, that develop in some people during fever are due to a separate infection by the type I herpes simplex virus that established latency in the regional ganglia and that is reactivated by a rise in body temperature.

TREATMENT

The methods of fever treatment focus on (1) modification of the external environment as a means of increasing heat transfer from the internal to the external environment, (2) support of the hypermetabolic state that accompanies fever, (3) protection of vulnerable body organs and systems, and (4) treatment of the infection or condition causing the fever. Because fever is a disease symptom, its manifestation suggests the need for treatment of the primary cause.

Modification of the environment ensures that the environmental temperature facilitates heat transfer away from the body. Sponge baths (with cool water or an alcohol solution) can be used to increase evaporative heat losses. More profound cooling can be accomplished through the use of a cooling mattress, which facilitates the conduction of heat from the body into the coolant solution that circulates through the mattress. Care must be taken so that cooling methods do not produce vasoconstriction and shivering that decrease heat loss and increase heat production.

Adequate fluids and sufficient amounts of simple carbohydrates are needed to support the hypermetabolic state and to prevent the tissue breakdown that is characteristic of fever. Additional fluids are needed for sweating and to balance the insensible water losses from the lungs that accompany an increase in respiratory rate. Fluids are also needed to maintain an adequate vascular volume for heat transport to the skin surface.

Antipyretic drugs, such as aspirin and acetaminophen, are often used to alleviate the discomforts of fever and protect vulnerable organs, such as the brain, from extreme elevations in body temperature. These drugs act by resetting the hypothalamic temperature control center to a lower level.

HYPERTHERMIA

Hyperthermia describes an increase in body temperature that occurs without a change in the set point of the hypothalamic thermoregulatory center. It includes (in order of increasing severity), heat cramps, heat syncope, heat exhaustion, and heatstroke. Malignant hyperthermia describes a rare genetic disorder of anesthetic-related hyperthermia. Fever and hyperthermia may also occur as the result of a drug reaction.

A number of factors predispose to hyperthermia. If muscle exertion is continued for long periods in warm weather, as often happens with athletes, military recruits, and laborers, excessive heat loads are generated.[17] Adequate circulatory function is essential for heat dissipation. Elderly people and people with cardiovascular disease are at increased risk. Drugs that increase muscle tone and metabolism or reduce heat loss can impair thermoregulation. Infants and small children who are left in a closed car for even short periods of time in hot weather are potential victims of hyperthermia. Florence Nightingale in *Notes on Nursing* observed that an excess of blankets is the commonest cause of fever in the hospital.[18]

HEAT CRAMPS

Heat cramps are slow, painful, skeletal muscle cramps and spasms, usually in the muscles that are most heavily used, that last for 1 to 3 minutes. Cramping results from salt depletion that occurs when fluid losses due to heavy sweating are replaced by water alone. The muscles are tender, and the skin is usually moist. Body temperature may be normal or slightly elevated. There is almost always a history of vigorous activity preceding the onset of symptoms.

Treatment consists of drinking an oral saline solution and resting in a cool environment. Because absorption is slow and unpredictable, salt tablets are not recommended. Salt tablets can also cause gastric irritation, vomiting, and cerebral edema. Strenuous physical activity should be avoided for several days, while dietary sodium replacement is continued.

HEAT SYNCOPE

Heat syncope is characterized by a sudden episode of unconsciousness resulting from cutaneous vasodilation and subsequent hypotension. Usually the episode follows vigorous exercise. The systolic blood pressure is usually less than 100 mmHg, the pulse is weak, and the skin is cool and moist. The treatment consists of recumbency and rest in a cool place and administration of fluids by mouth or intravenously.

HEAT EXHAUSTION

Heat exhaustion is related to a gradual loss of salt and water, usually after prolonged and heavy exertion in a hot environment. The symptoms include thirst, fatigue, nausea, oliguria, giddiness, and finally delirium. Gastrointestinal flulike symptoms are common. Hyperventilation in association with heat exhaustion may contribute to heat cramps and tetany by causing respiratory alkalosis. The skin is moist, the rectal temperature is usually over 37.8°C (100°F), and the heart rate is elevated (usually more than half again the normal resting rate). Signs of heat syncope and heat cramps may accompany heat exhaustion.

Like heat cramps, heat exhaustion is treated by rest in a cool environment, the provision of adequate hydration, and salt replacement. Intravenous fluids are administered when adequate oral intake cannot be achieved.

HEATSTROKE

Heatstroke is a severe, life-threatening failure of thermoregulatory mechanisms resulting in an excessive rise in body temperature—a core temperature greater than 40°C (104°F), absence of sweating, and loss of consciousness. Evaporation serves as the major mechanism for heat dissipation in a warm environment, and conditions that interrupt this mechanism predispose to increased body temperature and heatstroke.

Heatstroke is seen most commonly in the elderly and disabled. Mortality may be as high as 80% in people over 65 years of age. In the United States, approximately 5000 deaths occur each year from heatstroke, two thirds of these in people over age 60 years.[19] In the elderly, the problem is often one of impaired heat loss and failure of homeostatic mechanisms, so body temperature rises with any increase in environmental temperature. Elderly people with decreased perception of environmental temperature changes and decreased mobility are at particular risk, because they may also be unable to take appropriate measures such as removing clothing, moving to a cooler environment, and increasing fluid intake. This is particularly true of elderly people who live alone in small and poorly ventilated housing units and who may be too confused or weak to complain or seek help at the onset of symptoms.

The symptoms of heatstroke include dizziness, weakness, emotional lability, nausea and vomiting, confusion, delirium, blurred vision, convulsions, collapse, and coma. The skin is hot and usually dry, and the pulse is typically strong initially. The blood pressure may be elevated at first, but hypotension develops as the condition progresses. As vascular collapse occurs, the skin becomes cool.

Associated abnormalities include electrocardiograph changes consistent with heart damage, blood coagulation disorders, potassium and sodium depletion, and signs of liver damage.

Treatment consists of rapidly reducing the core temperature. Care must be taken that the cooling methods used do not produce vasoconstriction or shivering and thereby decrease the cooling rate or induce heat production. Two general methods of cooling are used. One method involves submersion in cold water or application of ice packs, and the other, spraying the body with tepid water while a fan is used to enhance heat dissipation through convection. Whatever method is used, it is important that the temperature of vital structures, such as the brain, heart, and liver, be reduced rapidly because tissue damage ensues when core temperatures rise above 43°C (109.4°F). Selective brain cooling has been reported by fanning the face during hyperthermia.[20] Blood flows from the emissary venous pathways of the skin on the head through the bones of the skull to the brain. In hyperthermia, face fanning is thought to cool the venous blood that flows through these emissary veins and thereby produce brain cooling by enhancing heat exchange between the hot arterial blood and the surface-cooled venous blood within the intracranial venous spaces.

MALIGNANT HYPERTHERMIA

Malignant hyperthermia is an autosomal-dominant metabolic disorder in which heat generated by uncontrolled skeletal muscle contraction can produce severe and potentially fatal hyperthermia. The muscle contraction is caused by an abnormal release of intracellular calcium from the mitochondria and sarcoplasmic reticulum (see Chapter 1).

In affected people, an episode of malignant hyperthermia is triggered by exposure to certain stresses or general anesthetic agents. The incidence of malignant hyperthermia from anesthetic agents is 1 in 15,000 in children and 1 in 50,000 to 100,000 in adults.[21] The syndrome is most frequently associated with the halogenated anesthetic agents and the depolarizing muscle relaxant succinylcholine.[22] There are also various nonoperative precipitating factors, including trauma, exercise, environmental heat stress, and infection. The condition is particularly dangerous in a young person who has a large muscle mass to generate heat.

During malignant hyperthermia the body temperature can rise as high as 43°C (109.4°F) at a rate of 1°C every 5 minutes. An initial sign of the disorder, when the condition occurs during anesthesia, is skeletal-muscle rigidity. Cardiac arrhythmias and a hypermetabolic state follow in rapid sequence unless the triggering event is immediately discontinued. In addition to discontinuing the triggering agents, treatment includes measures to cool the body and the administration of dantrolene, a muscle relaxant drug. There is no accurate screening test for the condition. A family history of malignant hyperthermia should be considered when general anesthesia is needed, because there are anesthetic agents available that do not trigger the hyperthermic response.

DRUG FEVER AND NEUROLEPTIC MALIGNANT SYNDROME

Drug fever has been defined as fever coinciding with the administration of a drug and disappearing once the drug has been discontinued.[23–25] Drugs can induce fever by several mechanisms: they can interfere with heat dissipation; they can alter temperature regulation by the hypothalamic centers; they can act as direct pyrogens; they can injure tissues directly; or they can induce an immune response.[22] Peripheral heat dissipation can be impaired by atropine, antihistamines, and tricyclic antidepressants, which de-crease sweating, or by sympathomimetic drugs, which produce peripheral vasoconstriction. Thyroid hormone can increase heat production. Bleomycin (an anticancer drug), amphotericin B (an antifungal drug), and allergic extracts and vaccines that contain bacterial and viral products can all act to induce the release of pyrogens. Intravenously administered drugs can lead to infusion-related phlebitis with production of cellular pyrogens that produce fever. Treatment with anticancer drugs can cause the release of endogenous pyrogen from the cancer cells that are destroyed. Antipsychotic drugs have been shown to produce a life-threatening form of malignant hyperthermia.

Hypersensitivity Reactions. The most common cause of drug fever is a hypersensitivity reaction. Hypersensitivity drug fevers develop after several weeks of exposure to the drug, cannot be explained in terms of the drug's pharmacologic action, are not related to dose, disappear when the drug is stopped, and reappear when the drug is readministered. The fever pattern is typically spiking in nature and exhibits a normal diurnal rhythm.[26] In addition, people with drug fevers often experience other signs of hypersensitivity reactions, such as arthralgias, urticaria, myalgias, gastrointestinal discomfort, and rashes. The person may be unaware of the fever and appear to be well for the degree of fever that is present. Often a fever precedes other more serious effects of a drug reaction; for this reason, the early recognition of drug fever is important. In a study of 68 cases of drug fever, of which 31 were fatal, an early fever was present in 30% of the cases.[27] Some of the most commonly cited causes of drug fever are aminosalicylic acid (an antituberculosis drug), amphotericin B, antihistamines, barbiturates, cocaine derivatives, methyldopa (an antihypertensive drug), novobiocin (an antibiotic), penicillin, and quinidine sulfate (a cardiac dysrhythmic drug).[24] This list is not inclusive; many other drugs can induce drug fever. Drug fever should be suspected whenever the temperature elevation is unexpected and occurs despite improvement in the condition for which the drug was prescribed.

Neuroleptic Malignant Syndrome. Neuroleptic malignant syndrome, which is usually explosive in onset, consists of hyperthermia, muscle rigidity, alterations in consciousness, and autonomic nervous system dysfunction. The hyperthermia is accompanied by tachycardia (120 to 180 beats/min) and cardiac dysrhythmias, labile blood pressure (70/50 mmHg to 180/130 mmHg), postural instability, dyspnea, and tachypnea (18 to 40 breaths/min).[28] Permanent brain damage may result, and the mortality rate is nearly 30%.[29]

The disorder is associated with neuroleptic medications and may occur in up to 1% of people taking such drugs.[28] Some of the most commonly implicated drugs are haloperidol, chlorpromazine, thioridazine, and thiothixene. All of these drugs block dopamine receptors in the basal ganglia and hypothalamus. Hyperthermia is thought to result either from alterations in the function of the hypothalamic thermoregulatory center caused by decreased dopamine levels or from uncontrolled muscle contraction like that occurring with anesthetic-induced malignant hyperthermia. Many of the neuroleptic drugs increase muscle contraction, suggesting that this mechanism might contribute to the neuroleptic malignant syndrome.

Treatment for neuroleptic malignant syndrome includes the immediate discontinuance of the neuroleptic drug, measures to decrease body temperature, and treatment of dysrhythmias and other complications of the disorder. Bromocriptine (a dopamine agonist) and dantrolene (a muscle relaxant) may be used as part of the treatment regimen.

In summary, fever and hyperthermia refer to an increase in body temperature outside the normal range. True fever is a disorder of thermoregulation in which there is an upward displacement of the set point for temperature control. In hyperthermia, the set point is unchanged, but the challenge to temperature regulation exceeds the thermoregulatory center's ability to control body temperature. Fever can be caused by a number of factors, including microorganisms, trauma, and drugs or chemicals, all of which incite the release of interleukin (formerly called endogenous pyrogen). The reactions that occur during fever consist of four stages: (1) a prodrome, (2) a chill, (3) a flush, and (4) defervescence. A fever can follow an intermittent, remittent, sustained, or recurrent pattern. The manifestations of fever are largely related to dehydration and an increased metabolic rate. The treatment of fever focuses on (1) modifying the external environment as a means of increasing heat transfer to the external environment; (2) supporting the hypermetabolic state that accompanies fever; (3) protecting vulnerable body tissues; and (4) treating the infection or condition causing the fever. Hyperthermia includes heat syncope, heat cramps, heat exhaustion, and heatstroke. Among the factors that contribute to the development of hyperthermia are prolonged muscular exertion in a hot environment, disorders that compromise heat dissipation, and hypersensitivity drug reactions. Malignant hyperthermia is an autosomal dominant disorder that can produce a severe and potentially fatal increase in body temperature. The condition is commonly triggered by general anesthetic agents and muscle relaxants used during surgery. The neuroleptic malignant syndrome is associated with neuroleptic drug therapy and is thought to result from alterations in the function of the thermoregulatory center or from uncontrolled muscle contraction.

■ DECREASED BODY TEMPERATURE

HYPOTHERMIA

Hypothermia is defined as a core (rectal, esophageal, or tympanic) temperature less than 35°C.[30–32] Core body temperatures in the range of 34°C to 35°C (93.2°F to 95°F) are considered mildly hypothermic; 30°C to 34°C (86°F to 93.2°F), moderately hypothermic; and less than 30°C (86°F), severely hypothermic.[33, 34] Accidental hypothermia may be defined as a spontaneous decrease in core temperature, usually in a cold environment and associated with an acute problem but without primary pathology of the temperature-regulating center. The term *submersion hypothermia* is used when cooling follows acute asphyxia such as occurs in drowning.[35] In children, the rapid cooling process, in addition to the diving reflex, which triggers apnea and circulatory shunting to establish a heart–brain circulation (see Chapter 22), may account for the surprisingly high survival rate after submersion. The diving reflex is greatly diminished in adults. Children have been reported to survive 10 to 40 minutes of submersion asphyxia.[36, 37] Controlled hypothermia may be used during certain types of surgeries to decrease brain metabolism.

Oral temperatures are markedly inaccurate during hypothermia because of severe vasoconstriction and sluggish blood flow. Although esophageal temperatures or temperatures obtained from a pulmonary artery catheter provide the most exact estimate of core temperature (near the heart) during hypothermia, these methods are often impractical; therefore, rectal temperatures are usually used. Most clinical thermometers measure temperature only in the range of 35°C to 42°C (95°F to 107.6°F); a special thermometer that registers as low as 25°C (77°F) or an electrical thermistor probe is needed for monitoring temperatures in people with hypothermia.[34]

Systemic hypothermia may result from exposure to prolonged cold (atmospheric or submersion). The condition may develop in otherwise healthy people in the course of accidental exposure. Because water conducts heat more readily than air, body temperature drops rapidly when the body is submerged in cold water or when clothing becomes wet. In people with altered homeostasis due to debility or disease, hypothermia may follow exposure to relatively small decreases in atmospheric temperature. Elderly and inactive people living in inadequately heated quarters are particularly vulnerable to hypothermia. Acute alcoholism is a common predisposing factor. People with cardiovascular disease, cerebrovascular disease, malnutrition, and hypothyroidism are also predisposed to hypothermia. The use of sedatives and tranquilizing drugs may be a contributing factor.

MANIFESTATIONS

With mild hypothermia, intense shivering generates heat and sympathetic nervous system activity is raised to resist lowering of temperature. Vasoconstriction can be profound, heart rate is accelerated, and stroke volume is increased. Blood pressure increases slightly, and hyperventilation is common. Exposure to cold augments urinary flow (cold diuresis) before there is any fall in temperature. Dehydration and increased hematocrit may develop within a few hours of even mild hypothermia, augmented by an extracellular-to-intracellular water shift.

With moderate hypothermia, shivering gradually decreases and the muscles become rigid. Shivering usually ceases at 27°C (80.6°F). Consciousness is usually lost at 30°C (86°F). Heart rate and stroke volume are reduced, and blood pressure falls. The greatest effect of hypothermia is exerted through a decrease in the metabolic rate, which falls to 50% of normal at 28°C (82.4°F).[38] Associated with this decrease in metabolic rate is a decrease in oxygen consumption and carbon dioxide production. There is roughly a 6% decrease in oxygen consumption per degree Celsius decrease in temperature. A decrease in carbon dioxide production leads to a decrease in respiratory rate. Respirations decrease as temperatures drop below 32.2°C (90°F). Decreases in mentation, the cough reflex, and respiratory tract secretions may lead to difficulty in clearing secretions and aspiration.

In terms of cardiovascular function, a gradual decline in heart rate and cardiac output occurs as hypothermia progresses. Blood pressure initially rises and then gradually falls. There is increased risk of dysrhythmia developing, probably from myocardial hypoxia and autonomic nervous system imbalance. Ventricular fibrillation is a major cause of death in hypothermia.

Carbohydrate metabolism and insulin activity are decreased, resulting in a hyperglycemia that is proportional to the level of cooling. A cold-induced loss of cell membrane integrity allows intravascular fluids to move into the skin, giving the skin a puffy appearance. Acid–base disorders occur with increased frequency at temperatures below 25°C (77°F) unless adequate ventilation is maintained. Extracellular sodium and potassium concentrations decrease, and chloride levels increase. There is a temporary loss of plasma from the circulation along with sludging of red blood cells and increased blood viscosity as the result of trapping in the small vessels and skin.

The signs and symptoms of hypothermia include poor coordination, stumbling, slurred speech, irrationality and poor judgment, amnesia, hallucinations, blueness and puffiness of the skin, dilation of the pupils, decreased respiratory rate, weak and irregular pulse, and stupor.

TREATMENT

The treatment of hypothermia consists of rewarming, support of vital functions, and the prevention and treatment of complications. There are three methods of rewarming: passive rewarming, active total rewarming, and active core rewarming. Passive rewarming is done by removing the person from the cold environment, covering with a blanket, supplying warm fluids (oral or intravenous), and allowing rewarming to occur at the person's own pace. Active total rewarming involves immersing the person in warm water or placing heating pads or hot water bottles on the surface of the body, including the extremities. Active core rewarming places major emphasis on rewarming the trunk, leaving the extremities, containing the major metabolic mass, cold until the heart rewarms.[31] Active rewarming can be done by instilling warmed fluids into the gastrointestinal tract; peritoneal dialysis; extracorporeal blood warming, in which blood is removed from the body and passed through a heat exchanger and then returned to the body; or warming by inhalation of an oxygen mixture warmed to 42°C to 46°C (107.6°F to 114.8°F).

People with mild hypothermia usually respond well to passive rewarming in a warm bed. People with moderate or severe hypothermia do not have the thermoregulatory shivering mechanism and require active rewarming. During rewarming, the cold acidotic blood from the peripheral tissues is returned to the heart and central circulation. If this is done too rapidly or before cardiopulmonary function has been adequately reestablished, the hypothermic heart cannot respond to the increased metabolic demands of warm peripheral tissues.

In summary, hypothermia is a potentially life-threatening disorder in which the body's core temperature drops below 35°C (95°F). Accidental hypothermia can develop in otherwise healthy people in the course of accidental exposure and in elderly or disabled people with impaired perception or response to cold. Alcoholism, cardiovascular disease, malnutrition, and hypothyroidism contribute to the risk of hypothermia. The greatest effect of hypothermia is a decrease in the metabolic rate, leading to a decrease in carbon dioxide production and respiratory rate. The signs and symptoms of hypothermia include poor coordination, stumbling, slurred speech, irrationality, poor judgment, amnesia, hallucinations, blueness and puffiness of the skin, dilation of the pupils, decreased respiratory rate, weak and irregular pulse, stupor, and coma. The treatment for moderate and severe hypothermia includes active rewarming.

■ REFERENCES

1. Vick, R. (1984). *Contemporary medical physiology* (p. 886). Menlo Park, CA: Addison Wesley.
2. Beach, P.S., & McCormick, D.P. (1991). Clinical applications of ear thermometry (editorial comment). *Clinical Pediatrics*, (Suppl), 3–4.
3. Guyton, A. (1991). *Textbook of medical physiology* (8th ed., p. 799). Philadelphia: W.B. Saunders.
4. Atkins, L. (1984). Fever: The old and new. *Journal of Infectious Diseases, 149*, 339–348.
5. Stein, M.T. (1991). Historical perspectives in fever and thermometry. *Clinical Pediatrics* (Suppl), 5–7.
6. Kruse, J. (1988). Fever in children. *American Family Practice, 37*(2), 127–135.
7. Keating, H.J., Klimek, J.J., Levine, D.S., et al. (1984). Effect of age on the clinical significance of fever in ambulatory adult patients. *Journal of the American Geriatric Society, 32*, 282–287.
8. Castle, S.C., Norman, D.C., Yeh, M., et al. (1991). Fever response in elderly nursing home residents: Are the older truly colder? *Journal of the American Geriatric Society, 39*, 853–857.
9. Dinarellos, C.A. (1989). The endogenous pyrogens. *Hospital Practice, 24*(11A), 111–128.
10. Fraser, I., & Johnstone, M. (1981). Significance of early postoperative fever in children. *British Medical Journal, 282*, 1299.
11. Pien, F.D., Ho, P.W.L., & Fergusson, D.J.G. (1982). Fever and infection after cardiac operation. *Annals of Thoracic Surgery, 33*, 382–384.
12. Kluger, M.J. (1986). Fever: A hot topic. *News of Physiologic Science, 1*, 25–28.
13. Roberts, N.J. (1979). Temperature and host responses. *Microbiological Reviews, 43*, 241–259.
14. Rodbard, D. (1981). The role of regional temperature in the pathogenesis of disease. *New England Journal of Medicine, 305*, 808–814.
15. McGee, Z.A., & Gorby, G.L. (1987). The diagnostic value of fever patterns. *Hospital Practice, 22*(10), 103–110.
16. Cunha, B.A. (1984). Implications of fever in the critical care setting. *Heart & Lung, 13*, 460–465.
17. Danzl, D.F. (1988). Hyperthermic syndromes. *American Family Practice, 37*(6), 157.
18. Nightingale, F. (1970). *Notes on nursing* (p. 45). London: Brandon/Systems Press.
19. Halle, A., & Repasy, A. (1987). Classic heatstroke: A serious challenge for the elderly. *Hospital Practice, 22*(5), 26–35.
20. Brinnel, H., Nagasaka, T., & Cabanac, M. (1987). Enhanced brain protection during passive hyperthermia in humans. *European Journal of Applied Physiology, 56*, 540–545.
21. Britt, B.A., & Kalow, W. (1970). Malignant hyperthermia: A statistical review. *Canadian Anaesthetic Society Journal, 17*, 293–315.
22. Nelson, T.E., & Flewellen, E.H. (1983). The malignant hyperthermia syndrome. *New England Journal of Medicine, 309*, 416–418.
23. Tabor, P.A. (1986). Drug-induced fever. *Drug Intelligence and Clinical Pharmacy, 20*, 413–420.
24. Mackowiak, P.A., & LeMaistre, C.F. (1986). Drug fever: A critical appraisal of conventional concepts. *Annals of Internal Medicine, 106*, 728–733.
25. Hofland, S.L. (1985). Drug fever: Is your patient's fever drug-related. *Critical Care Nurse, 5*, 29–34.
26. Musher, D.M., Fainstein, V., Young, E.J., et al. (1979). Fever patterns: Their lack of clinical significance. *Archives of Internal Medicine, 139*, 1225.
27. Cluff, L.E., & Johnson, J.E. (1964). Drug fever. *Progress in Allergy, 8*, 149–194.
28. Parker, W.A. (1987). Neuroleptic malignant syndrome. *Critical Care Nurse, 7*, 40–46.
29. Goldwasser, H.D., & Hooper, J.F. (1988). Neuroleptic malignant syndrome. *American Family Practice, 38*(5), 211–216.
30. Reuler, J.B. (1978). Hypothermia: Pathophysiology, clinical settings, and management. *Annals of Internal Medicine, 89*, 519–527.
31. Fitzgerald, F.T., & Jessop, C. (1982). Accidental hypothermia: A report of 22 cases and review of the literature. *Annual Review of Medicine, 127*.
32. Celestina, F.S., Van Noord, G.R., & Miraglia, C.P. (1988). Accidental hypothermia in the elderly. *Journal of Family Practice, 26*, 259–267.
33. Lønning, P.E., Skulberg, A., & Abyholm, F. (1986). Accidental hypothermia. *Acta Anaesthesiologica Scandinavica, 30*, 601–613.
34. Division of Environmental Hazards and Health Effects. (1985). Hypothermia-associated death—United States, 1968–1980. *Morbidity and Mortality Weekly Report, 34*(48).
35. Conn, A.W. (1979). Near drowning and hypothermia. *Canadian Medical Association Journal, 120*, 397–400.
36. Siebke, H., Beivik, H., & Rod, T. (1975). Survival after 40 minutes submersion with cerebral sequelae. *Lancet, 1*, 1275–1277.
37. Moss, J.F. (1988). The management of accidental severe hypothermia. *New York Journal of Medicine, 88*, 411–413.
38. Wong, K.C. (1983). Physiology and pharmacology of hypothermia. *Western Journal of Medicine, 138*, 227–232.

■ BIBLIOGRAPHY

Alexander, D., & Kelly, B. (1991). Responses of children, parents, and nurses to tympanic thermometry in the pediatric office. *Clinical Pediatrics* (Suppl), 53–59.

Bruce, J.L., & Grove, S.K. (1992). Fever: Pathology and treatment. *Critical Care Nurse, 12*(1), 40–49.

Enright, T., & Hill, M.G. (1989). Treatment of fever. *Focus on Critical Care, 16*(2), 96-102.

Hanson, M.A. (1991). Drug fever. *Postgraduate Medicine, 89*(5), 167–173.

Kimmel, S., & Gemmill, D.W. (1988). The young child with fever. *American Family Practice, 37*, 196.

Newman, J. (1985). Evaluation of sponging to reduce body temperature in febrile children. *Canadian Medical Association Journal, 132*, 641.

Steele, R.W., Tanaka, P.T., & Lara, R.P. (1970). Evaluation of sponging and of oral antipyretic therapy to reduce fever. *Journal of Pediatrics, 77*, 824.

Stern, R.C. (1978). Pathophysiologic basis for symptomatic treatment of fever. *Pediatrics, 59*, 92.

Styrt, B., & Sugarman, B. (1990). Antipyresis and fever. *Archives of Internal Medicine, 150*, 1589–1597.

CHAPTER 11

ALTERATIONS IN SKIN FUNCTION AND INTEGRITY

GLADYS SIMANDL

Structure of the Skin
  Epidermis
  Basement Membrane Zone
  Dermis
  Subcutaneous Tissue
  Skin Appendages
Manifestations of Skin Disorders
  Lesions and Rashes
  Pruritus

Developmental Skin Problems
  Disorders of Infancy
  Disorders of Childhood
  Disorders of Adolescence and
    Young Adulthood
  Disorders of Aging
Primary Disorders of the Skin
  Mechanical Processes

Infectious Processes
Inflammatory Skin Disorders
Allergic Skin Responses
  Drug-induced Skin Eruptions
Scabies, Lice, and Ticks
Photosensitivity and Sunburn
Neoplasms
Black Skin

■ OBJECTIVES

After you have studied this chapter, you should be able to meet the following objectives:

■ List the layers of the skin and describe their function.
■ Describe the following skin rashes and lesions: macule, patch, papule, plaque, nodule, tumor, wheal, vesicle, bulla, pustule, erosion, crust, ulcer, scale, fissure, lichenification, petechiae, ecchymosis.
■ Cite two theories used to explain the physiology of pruritus.
■ Differentiate between a strawberry hemangioma and a port-wine stain hemangioma in terms of appearance and outcome.
■ Describe the distinguishing features of rashes associated with roseola infantum, rubeola, rubella, chickenpox, and scarlet fever.
■ Define *keratosis* and compare the seborrheic and actinic keratoses.
■ Relate the behavior of fungi to the production of superficial skin lesions associated with tinea or ringworm.
■ Explain the dermatomal distribution of herpes zoster lesions.
■ Compare acne vulgaris, acne conglobata, and acne rosacea in terms of appearance and location of lesions.

■ Describe the appearance of psoriasis lesions.
■ Differentiate between lesions seen in infantile and adult forms of eczema.
■ Relate the life cycle of the *Sarcoptes scabiei* to the skin lesions seen in scabies.
■ Use knowledge of the life cycles of *Pediculus humanus corporis* and *Pediculus humanus capitis* to explain the lesions associated with body and head lice.
■ List three drugs that produce photosensitivity.
■ State the relationship between sun exposure and skin cancer.
■ Compare the appearance of basal cell carcinoma, squamous cell carcinoma, and malignant melanoma.
■ Cite changes in a mole that are suggestive of cancerous transformation.
■ Compare the appearance of atopic dermatitis, pityriasis rosea, psoriasis, tinea versicolor, and lichen planus in white and black skin.

Carol Mattson Porth: PATHOPHYSIOLOGY: CONCEPTS OF
ALTERED HEALTH STATES, 4th ed. © 1994, 1990, 1986, 1982
J.B. Lippincott Company

The skin is primarily an organ of protection. It is the largest organ of the body and forms the major barrier between the internal organs and the external environment. The skin of an average-sized adult covers approximately 18 ft² and weighs 6 lb to 9 lb.[1, 2] As the body's first line of defense, the skin is continuously subjected to potentially harmful environmental agents, including solid matter, liquids, gases, sunlight, and microorganisms. Although the skin may become bruised, lacerated, burned, or infected, it has remarkable properties that allow for a continuous cycle of healing, shedding, and cell regeneration.

In addition to protection, the skin serves several other important functions. The skin is richly innervated with pain, temperature, and touch receptors. Skin receptors relay the numerous qualities of touch, such as pressure, sharpness, dullness, and pleasure to the central nervous system (CNS) for localization and fine discrimination. Further, the skin is important in regulating body temperature (see Chapter 10). The skin also plays an essential role in vitamin D synthesis and fluid and electrolyte balance. Finally, a less well-known property of the skin is its ability to store glycogen and contribute to glucose metabolism.[3]

Importantly, skin may demonstrate outwardly what occurs in the body systemically. A number of systemic diseases are manifested by skin disorders (*e.g.*, systemic lupus erythematosus, several forms of cancer, and Kaposi's sarcoma associated with acquired immunodeficiency syndrome [AIDS]). This means that, although skin eruptions frequently represent primary disease of the skin, they may also be a manifestation of systemic disease.

The skin also has an elusive quality of reflecting emotional states regardless of disease. It is through the skin that warmth and human affection are given and received. The skin conveys notions of health, beauty, integrity, and love. Society emphasizes the body and, in particular, the skin to the degree that even slight imperfections may evoke a wide variety of human responses. As more is learned about the skin through scientific investigations, the importance of considering mind–body connectedness when working with people who have skin disorders is becoming increasingly apparent.

■ STRUCTURE OF THE SKIN

Because of the great variations in structure in different parts of the body, normal skin is difficult to describe.[4] Variations are found in the properties of the skin, such as the thickness of skin layers, the distribution of sweat glands, and the number and size of hair follicles. For example, the skin is thicker on the palms and soles of the feet, hair follicles are densely distributed in the scalp, and apocrine sweat glands are confined to the axillae and the anogenital area. Nevertheless, certain structural properties are common to all skin in all areas of the body. The skin is composed of two layers: the epidermis (outer layer) and the dermis (inner layer). A basement membrane zone (BMZ) divides the two layers. The subcutaneous tissue, a layer of loose connective and fatty tissues, binds the dermis to the underlying tissues of the body (Fig. 11-1).

EPIDERMIS

The functions of the skin depend on the properties of its outermost layer, the epidermis. The epidermis not only covers the body, but is also specialized to form the various skin appendages: hair, nails, and glandular structures. Its cells produce a fibrous protein called *keratin*, which is essential to the protective function of skin, and a pigment called *melanin*, which protects against ultraviolet radiation. The epidermis contains openings for two types of glands: sweat glands, which produce watery secretions, and sebaceous glands, which produce an oily secretion called *sebum*.

The keratinocyte is the major cell of the epidermis. The epidermis is composed of stratified squamous keratinized epithelium, which when viewed under the microscope is seen to consist of five distinct layers, or strata, that represent a progressive differentiation of keratinocytes: (1) the stratum germinativum, or basal layer; (2) the stratum spinosum; (3) the stratum granulosum; (4) the stratum lucidum; and (5) the stratum corneum.

The stratum germinativum, or stratum basale, is the first and deepest layer of the epidermis. It consists of a single layer of basal cells that are attached to the basement membrane. The basal cells, which are columnar in shape, produce new keratinocytes that move toward the skin surface to replace cells lost during normal skin shedding. Unlike the other layers of the epidermis, the basal cells do not migrate toward the skin surface, but remain stationary in the stratum germinativum.

The second layer, the stratum spinosum, is formed as the progeny of the basal cell layer move upward. This layer is two to four layers thick, and its cells become differentiated as they migrate outward, toward the skin surface. The cells of this layer are commonly referred to as prickle cells because they develop a spiny appearance as their cell borders interact.

The third layer, the stratum corneum, consists of dead, keratinized cells. This layer contains the most cell layers and the largest cells of any zone of the

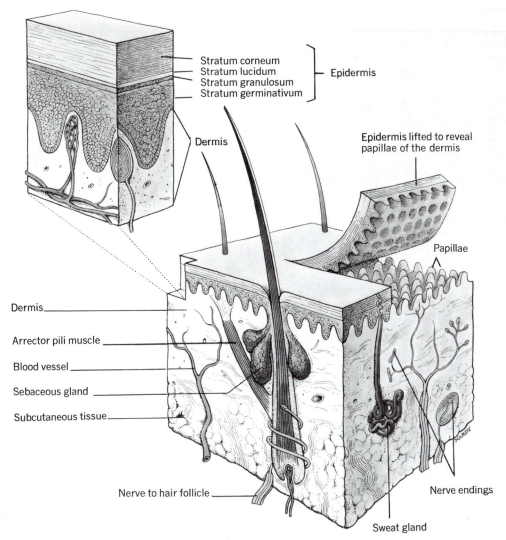

FIG. 11-1. *Three-dimensional view of the skin.* (Chaffee, E. E., & Lytle, I. M. [1980]. *Basic anatomy and physiology* [4th ed.]. Philadelphia: J.B. Lippincott)

epidermis. It ranges from 15 layers thick in areas such as the face to 25 layers or more on the arm. In specialized areas, such as the palms of the hands or soles of the feet, 100 or more layers are present.[5]

The stratum lucidum, or fourth layer, is thin and transparent. It consists of transitional cells that retain some of the functions of living skin cells from the layers below and resemble the cells of the stratum corneum. This layer can be seen on the palms of the hands and soles of the feet.

The stratum granulosum, the fifth layer of the epidermis, consists of granular cells that are the most differentiated cells of the living skin. The cells in this layer are unique in that two opposing functions are occurring simultaneously. While some cells are losing cytoplasm and DNA structures, others continue to synthesize keratin.

The keratinocyte that originates in the basal layer

changes morphologically as it is pushed toward the outer layer of the epidermis. For example, in the basal layer, the keratinocyte is round. As it is pushed into the stratum spinosum, the keratinocyte becomes multisided; it becomes flatter in the granular layer and is flattened and elongated in the stratum corneum (Fig. 11-2). Keratinocytes also change cytoplasmic structure and composition as they are pushed outward. This transformation from viable cells to the dead cells of the stratum corneum is called *keratinization.*

In addition to the keratinocytes, the epidermis has three other types of cells: melanocytes, Langerhans' cells, and Merkel's cells. These cells are also derived from the basal layer of the epidermis.

Melanocytes are pigment-synthesizing cells that are located at or in the basal layer. They function to produce pigment granules called melanosomes,

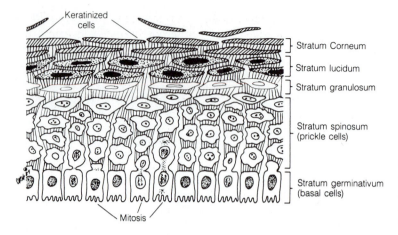

FIG. 11-2. Epidermal cells. The basal cells undergo mitosis and then change their size and shape as they move upward to produce new skin cells, which replace cells that are lost during normal cell shedding.

which contain melanin, the brown substance that gives skin its color. Although melanocytes remain in the basal layer, the melanosomes are transferred to the keratinocytes through a dendritic process. During this transfer, the normally round melanocytes become dendritic in shape. The dendrite tip of the melanocyte is engulfed by a nearby keratinocyte, and the melanosomes are transferred (Fig. 11-3). Each melanocyte is capable of supplying several keratinocytes with melanin. The amount of melanin in the keratinocytes determines a person's skin color. The

melanin pigment protects the skin from the ultraviolet sun rays, and exposure to ultraviolet rays increases the production of melanin. Black-skinned and white-skinned people have the same amount of melanocytes; however, the number of melanosomes produced differs greatly among individuals.

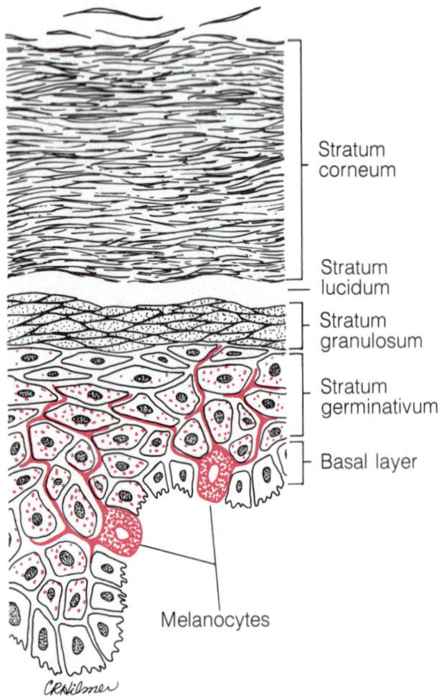

Langerhans' cells are located in the suprabasal layers of the epidermis and become established among the keratinocytes. They are few in number compared with the keratinocytes. They are derived from precursor cells originating in the bone marrow and continuously repopulate the epidermis.[6] Like melanocytes, they are dendritic in shape and have a clear cytoplasm. Microscopically, they resemble a tennis racquet and are therefore easy to differentiate from other skin cell types. The exact origin of these cells remains unknown, as does their function. Research has indicated that they may play a role in the cutaneous immune response and serve as a possible source of prostaglandins.[7,8]

Merkel's cells consist of free nerve endings attached to modified epidermal cells. Their origin remains unknown, and they are the least densely populated cell of the epidermis. Merkel's cells are found on the skin of the fingers, toes, lips, oral cavity, and outermost sheath of hair follicles (the touch areas). Merkel's cells function as mechanoreceptors, or touch receptors.[9]

The movement of the cells to the surface of the skin can best be described as random or nonsynchronized. Keratinocytes pass other keratinocytes, melanocytes, and Langerhans' cells as they migrate in a seemingly random fashion. However, the cells are connected with minute points of attachment called *desmosomes*. Desmosomes keep the cells from detaching and provide some structure to the skin while it is in perpetual motion. The basal layer, however, provides the underlying structure and stability for the epidermis.

FIG. 11-3. Melanocytes. The melanocytes, which are located in the basal layer of the skin, produce melanin pigment granules that give skin its color. The melanocytes have thread-like cytoplasmic-filled extensions that are used in passing the pigment granules to the keratinocytes.

BASEMENT MEMBRANE ZONE

The basement membrane zone (BMZ) is a layer of intercellular matrix that connects the epidermis to the dermis, both structures contributing to its formation. Characteristics of the BMZ have become more defined over the past few years. Essentially, the BMZ contains collagen fibers and glycoproteins and consists of four distinct layers, all contributing to the adhesion and elasticity of the skin. The collagen fibers provide the skin with tensile strength, anchorage, and elasticity. The glycoproteins are believed to be associated with cohesion. The function of the BMZ as a barrier remains debatable because many substances are able to penetrate it. Lymphocytes, neutrophils, and Langerhans' cells easily penetrate the BMZ; however, the BMZ has been found to bar larger molecules.

DERMIS

The dermis is the connective tissue layer that separates the epidermis from the subcutaneous fat layer. It supports the epidermis and serves as its primary source of nutrition. The two layers of the dermis, the papillary dermis and the reticular dermis, are composed of cells, fibers, and ground substances as well as nerves and blood vessels. The pilar (hair) structures and glandular structures are embedded in this layer and elaborated on in the epidermis.

The papillary dermis (pars papillaris) is a thin superficial layer that lies adjacent to the epidermis. It consists of collagen fibers and ground substance. The basal cells of the epidermis project into the papillary dermis, forming dermal papillae (see Fig. 11-1). Dermal papillae contain capillary venules, which serve to nourish the epidermal layers of the skin. This layer of the dermis is well vascularized. Lymph vessels and nerve tissue are also found in this layer.

The reticular dermis (pars reticularis) is the thicker area of the dermis and forms the bulk of the dermis. This is the layer from which the tough leather hides of animals are made. The reticular dermis is characterized by a mesh of three-dimensional collagen bundles interconnected with large elastic fibers and ground substance.

The ground substance is a viscid gel, rich in mucopolysaccharides. The collagen fibers are oriented parallel to the body's surface in any given area. These collagen bundles may be organized lengthwise, as on the abdomen, or in round blocks, as in the heel. The direction of surgical incisions is often determined by this organizational pattern. The epidermis extends deep into the reticular dermis and either terminates there or extends into the subcutaneous layer. Blood vessels, lymph vessels, and nerve fibers are found in this area. Extremely small nerve endings extend into the papillary dermis.

Cells found in the dermis include fibroblasts, macrophages, and mast cells. Limited numbers of lymphocytes are found around dermal blood vessels. Fibroblasts synthesize the connective tissue matrix. They also secrete enzymes needed to break down and thereby remodel the matrix. Macrophages are abundant in the dermis and serve to synthesize certain enzymes that enhance or suppress lymphocyte activity, certain prostaglandins, and interferon. Mast cells, which have a prominent role in IgE-mediated inflammation, are also present in the dermis. These cells are strategically located at body interfaces such as the skin and mucous membranes and are thought to interact with antigens that come in contact with the skin.

The microvasculature of the dermal papillae is linked to the larger vessels that exist between the dermal papillae. These vessels transport epidermal nutrients and waste products and also function in thermoregulation. The lymphatic system of the skin, which combats certain infectious skin invasions, is also limited to the dermis.

The innervation of the skin is complex. The skin, with its accessory structures, serves as an organ for receiving sensory information from the environment. Accordingly, it is well supplied with sensory nerves. In addition, it contains nerves that supply the blood vessels, sweat glands, and arrector pili muscles. The receptors for touch, pressure, heat, cold, and pain are widely distributed in the skin. Because of the variation in function among the different types of nerve endings, it is generally agreed that sensory modalities are not associated with a particular type of receptor. For example, the sensations of pain, touch, and pressure probably result from multiple stimuli. The final sensation may be the result of central summation in the CNS, which mediates patterned responses.

Most of the skin's blood vessels are under sympathetic nervous system control. The sweat glands are innervated by cholinergic fibers but controlled by the sympathetic nervous system. Likewise, the sympathetic nervous system controls the arrector pili (pilomotor) muscles that cause hairs on the skin to stand up. Contraction of these muscles tends to cause the skin to dimple, producing "goose pimples."

SUBCUTANEOUS TISSUE

The subcutaneous tissue layer consists primarily of fat and connective tissues that lend support to the vascular and neural structures supplying the outer layers of the skin. There is controversy about whether the subcutaneous tissue should be considered an actual layer of the skin. However, the eccrine glands and deep hair follicles extend to this layer, and several skin diseases involve the subcutaneous tissue.

SKIN APPENDAGES

The skin houses a variety of appendages including hair, nails, and sebaceous and sweat glands. The distribution as well as the function of the appendages varies.

Hair. Hair is a structure that originates from hair follicles in the dermis. Most hair follicles are associated with sebaceous glands, and these structures combine to form the pilosebaceous apparatus. The entire hair structure consists of the hair follicle, sebaceous gland, hair muscle (arrector pili), and, in some instances, the apocrine gland (see Fig. 11-1). Hair is a keratinized structure that is pushed upward from the hair follicle. Growth of the hair is centered in the bulb (base) of the hair follicle, and the hair undergoes changes as it is pushed outward. Hair has been found to go through cyclic phases identified as anagen (the growth phase), catagen (the atrophy phase), and telogen (the resting phase). A vascular network at the site of the follicular bulb nourishes and maintains the hair follicle. Melanocytes are found in the bulb and are responsible for the color of the hair. The arrector pili muscle, located under the sebaceous gland, provides a thermoregulation function by contracting and reducing the skin surface area that is available for the dissipation of body heat.

Sebaceous Glands. The sebaceous glands (see Fig. 11-1) secrete a fatty material called sebum, which lubricates hair and skin. Sebum prevents undue evaporation of moisture from the stratum corneum during cold weather and helps to conserve body heat. It is also thought to possess some bactericidal and fungicidal properties. The sebaceous glands are the structures that are most involved in the development of acne (discussed later in this chapter).

Sweat Glands. There are two types of sweat glands: eccrine and apocrine. Eccrine sweat glands are simple tubular structures that originate in the dermis and open directly to the skin surface. They vary in density and are located over the entire body surface. Their purpose is to transport sweat to the outer skin surface to regulate body temperature.

Apocrine sweat glands are fewer in number than eccrine sweat glands. They are larger and located deep in the dermal layer. They open through a hair follicle, even though a hair may not be present, and are found primarily in the axillae and groin. The major difference between these glands and the eccrine glands is that they secrete an oily substance. In animals, apocrine secretions give rise to distinctive odors that enable animals to recognize the presence of others. In humans, apocrine secretions are sterile until mixed with the bacteria on the skin surface; then they produce what is commonly known as body odor.

Nails. The nails are hardened keratinized plates that protect the fingers (fingernails) and toes (toenails) and enhance dexterity. The nails are the end-product of dead matrix cells that grow from the nail plate. Unlike hair, nails grow continuously unless permanently damaged or diseased.

In summary, the skin is primarily an organ of protection. It is the largest organ of the body and forms the major barrier between the internal organs and the external environment. In addition, the skin is richly innervated with pain, temperature, and touch receptors; it synthesizes vitamin D and plays an essential role in fluid and electrolyte balance. It contributes to glucose metabolism through its glycogen stores. The skin is composed of two layers, the epidermis and the dermis, separated by a basement membrane zone. A layer of subcutaneous tissue binds the dermis to the underlying organs and tissues of the body. The epidermis contains five layers, or strata, and is the outermost layer of the skin. The major cells of the epidermis are the keratinocytes, melanocytes, Langerhans' cells, and Merkel's cells. These cells, which remain in the stratum germinativum (or basal layer) of the epidermis, are the source of the cells in all five layers of the epidermis. The keratinocytes, which are the major cells of the epidermis, are transformed from viable keratinocytes to dead keratin as they move from the innermost layer of the epidermis (stratum germinativum) to the outermost layer (stratum corneum). The melanocytes are pigment-synthesizing cells that give skin its color. The dermis provides the epidermis with support and nutrition and is the source of blood vessels, nerves, and skin appendages (hair follicles and sebaceous glands, nails, and sweat glands).

■ MANIFESTATIONS OF SKIN DISORDERS

The skin is a unique organ in which numerous signs are immediately observable. These signs contribute to accurate diagnosis and treatment. In many cases, the skin may relay signs of other organic dysfunction. The most common manifestations of skin disorders are rashes, lesions, and pruritus.

LESIONS AND RASHES

Rashes are temporary eruptions of the skin, such as those associated with childhood diseases, heat rash, diaper rash, or drug-induced eruptions. The term *lesion* usually refers to a traumatic or pathologic loss of normal tissue continuity, structure, or function. Sometimes the components of a rash are referred to as lesions. Rashes and lesions may range in size from a fraction of a millimeter (as in petechiae) to many centimeters (as in a decubitus ulcer, or pressure sore). They may be blanched (white), reddened (erythematous), hemorrhagic or purpuric (containing blood), or pigmented. Skin lesions may occur as primary lesions arising in previously normal skin (Table 11-1); or they may develop as secondary lesions resulting from primary lesions.

PRURITUS

Pruritus, or itching, is a symptom common to many skin disorders. Pruritus may be present with dry skin and often accompanies major skin disorders. Itching may also be symptomatic of other organ disorders, such as diabetes mellitus or biliary disease, when no skin anomaly exists. Physiologically, two theories exist regarding itch. The first is that an anatomically distinct itch receptor exists, although none has been found to date, perhaps because of their scarcity and small size.[10] The second theory is that itching is the sensation experienced by a person when multiple nerve fibers in the skin are stimulated (*e.g.*, pain and touch). The CNS interprets these sensations as itch through central summation.

The latter theory, that itch and pain are transmitted through the same nerve pathways, is generally more accepted. However, the sensations are perceived as distinct from each other. Whether there are two receptors or one, the mediator of the itch response remains unknown. Several substances, such as histamine and morphine, are known to increase itching. Prostaglandins and warmth can also trigger the itch phenomenon.

The well-known response to an itch is scratching; this can cause skin excoriations. Excoriated skin is much more susceptible to infectious processes; therefore, measures to reduce pruritus and prevent scratching should be taken. People with pruritis should be instructed to keep their fingernails trimmed and use their entire hand to rub over large body surfaces.[11] Vasodilatation increases itching; therefore, a common method of reducing pruritus is the use of cold applications. Another treatment measure for self-limited or seasonal cases of pruritis includes moisturizing lotions and bath oils and the use of humidifiers. Application of topical corticosteroids may be helpful in some situations. Administration of systemic antihistamines, opiate antagonists, and cor-

---

TABLE 11-1. PRIMARY LESIONS (MAY ARISE FROM PREVIOUSLY NORMAL SKIN)

CIRCUMSCRIBED, FLAT, NONPALPABLE CHANGES IN SKIN COLOR	PALPABLE ELEVATED SOLID MASSES	CIRCUMSCRIBED SUPERFICIAL ELEVATIONS OF THE SKIN FORMED BY FREE FLUID IN A CAVITY WITHIN THE SKIN LAYERS
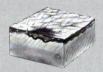		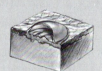
Macule—Small, up to 1 cm.* Example: freckle, petechia *Patch*—Larger than 1 cm. Example: vitiligo	*Papule*—Up to 0.5 cm. Example: an elevated nevus *Plaque*—A flat, elevated surface larger than 0.5 cm, often formed by the coalescence of papules *Nodule*—0.5 cm to 1–2 cm; often deeper and firmer than a papule *Tumor*—Larger than 1–2 cm *Wheal*—A somewhat irregular, relatively transient, superficial area of localized skin edema. Example: mosquito bite, hive	*Vesicle*—Up to 0.5 cm; filled with serous fluid. Example: herpes simplex *Bulla*—Greater than 0.5 cm; filled with serous fluid. Example: 2nd-degree burn *Pustule*—Filled with pus. Examples: acne, impetigo

*Authorities vary somewhat in their definitions of skin lesions by size. Dimensions given in this table should be considered approximate, not rigid.

(Bates, B. [1991] *A guide to physical examination and history taking* [5th ed.]. Philadelphia: J.B. Lippincott.)

ticosteroids may be indicated in people with severe pruritus.

In summary, skin lesions, rashes, and pruritus are common manifestations of skin disorders. Rashes are temporary skin eruptions. Lesions result from traumatic or pathologic loss of the normal continuity, structure, or function of the skin. Lesions may be vascular in origin; they may occur as primary lesions in previously normal skin; or they may develop as secondary lesions resulting from primary lesions. Pruritus, or itching, is a symptom common to many skin disorders. Scratching because of pruritus can lead to excoriation, infection, and other complications.

■ DEVELOPMENTAL SKIN PROBLEMS

Many skin problems occur more commonly in certain age groups. Because of aging changes, infants, adolescents, and elderly people tend to have different skin problems.

DISORDERS OF INFANCY

Infancy connotes the image of perfect, unblemished skin. For the most part, this is true; however, several congenital skin lesions, such as mongolian spots, hemangiomas, and nevi are associated with the early neonatal period. Table 11-2 summarizes common skin problems of the infant and small child.

Mongolian spots are caused by selective pigmentation. They usually occur on the buttocks or sacral area and are commonly seen in the yellow and black races. *Hemangiomas* are vascular disorders of the skin. Two types of hemangiomas are commonly seen in infants and small children: bright-red, raised strawberry hemangiomas and flat, reddish-purple port-wine stain hemangiomas. The strawberry hemangiomas begin as small red lesions that are noted shortly after birth. They may remain as small superficial lesions or extend to involve the subcutaneous tissue. Strawberry hemangiomas usually disappear before 5 to 7 years of age without leaving an appreciable scar. Port-wine stain hemangiomas are rare, usually occur on the face, and are disfiguring. They do not disappear with age, and there is no satisfactory treatment. Usually cover-up cosmetics are used in an attempt to conceal their disfiguring effects. The term *nevus*, discussed later in this chapter, is used to denote any congenital colored lesion.[12] Nevi may vary in shape or size, and they may be present at birth or develop later in life.

Because of its newness, infant skin is also sensitive to irritation, injury, and extremes of temperature. The contents of soiled diapers, if not changed

TABLE 11-2. COMMON SKIN LESIONS OF INFANTS AND SMALL CHILDREN

LESION	APPEARANCE
Congenital Dermatoses	
Hemangiomas	
Strawberry	Bright-red raised and rounded lesions; may enlarge with growth of infant and than regress; usually disappear by 5 to 7 years of age
Port-wine stain	Flat reddish-purple disfiguring lesion; usually found on the face; does not disappear with age
Mongolian spot	Light blue, gray-green to slate gray macule; commonly located in the lumbosacral area; usually disappears with age
Nevi (moles)	Vary in size, shape, and location; usually brown-black, flat or raised macules or papules; borders are usually well defined and rounded
Irritative and Inflammatory Dermatoses	
Cradle cap	Yellowish, greasy, and crusted collection of vernix and shedding skin on scalp
Prickly heat	Tiny vesicles usually located on the neck, back, chest, trunk, abdomen, and folds of skin; pruritus is common
Diaper rash	Erythematous macular rash; blister formation, excoriation, and infection may develop

frequently, can lead to contact dermatitis and bacterial infections. Prolonged exposure to a warm humid environment can lead to prickly heat, and too-frequent bathing can cause dryness and lead to skin problems. Baby lotions are helpful in maintaining skin moisture, whereas baby powder acts as a drying agent. Both are useful aids when used selectively and according to the nature of the skin problem (excessive moisture or dryness). Unnecessary bathing should be avoided, and clothing appropriate to the environment should be worn.

The appearance of *diaper rash* ranges from simple (widely distributed macules on the buttocks and anogenital areas) to severe (beefy, red, excoriated skin surfaces in the diaper area). It results from a combination of ammonia and other breakdown products of urine. The treatment includes frequent change of diapers with careful cleansing of the irritated area to remove the waste products. This is important particularly in hot weather. Exposing the irritated area to air is helpful. Use of plastic pants should be discouraged. Diapers washed in gentle detergent and thoroughly rinsed to remove all traces of waste products help to reduce the risk of diaper rash. Although disposable diapers may help in some cases, their plastic backing may further augment the problem unless they are changed frequently. For intractable, severe cases, the child should be seen by a physician for treatment of any secondary infections.

Prickly heat results from constant maceration of the skin because of prolonged exposure to a warm and humid environment; this leads to midepidermal obstruction and rupture of the sweat glands. Although commonly seen during infancy, prickly heat, or heat rash, may occur at any age. It most commonly occurs in hot, moist environments. The treatment includes the removal of excessive clothing, cooling the skin with warm water baths, drying the skin with powders, and avoiding hot, humid environments.

Cradle cap is a greasy crust or scale formation on the scalp. It is usually attributed to infrequent and inadequate washing of the scalp and is treated by mild shampooing and gentle combing to remove the scales. Application of oil is no longer recommended, because this can compound the problem. Selenium sulfate may be helpful in difficult cases. Caretakers should be advised about the need to agitate the scalp cells lightly so the build-up of keratinizing cells can be removed.

DISORDERS OF CHILDHOOD

As children become mobile and interact with the environment, they become susceptible to the myriad skin disorders affecting people of all ages. Children, because of their cognitive and physiologic development, are also more prone to accidents that may result in major skin trauma, such as lacerations and burns. Careful activity supervision consistent with the developmental needs of children is the prime factor in preventing these traumas. Besides interacting with the environment, children are frequently in close contact with other children. As a result, conditions such as head lice, tinea capitis, and impetigo are more frequently seen in children. Epidemiologically, the incidence of roseola, rubeola, rubella, and chickenpox is also highest in this age group; hence, these diseases have become known as the childhood diseases.

RASHES ASSOCIATED WITH CHILDHOOD DISEASES

Rubella. Rubella (3-day measles, German measles) is a childhood disease caused by the rubella virus. It is characterized by a diffuse, punctate, macular rash that begins on the trunk and spreads to the arms and legs. Mild febrile states occur; generally, the fever is less than 100°F. Postauricular, suboccipital, and cervical lymph node adenopathy is common. Coldlike symptoms usually accompany the disease in the form of cough, congestion, and coryza.

Rubella generally has no long-lasting sequelae; however, the transmission of the disease to pregnant women early in the gestation period may result in severe teratogenic effects in the unborn fetus. Among the teratogenic effects are cataracts, microcephaly, mental retardation, deafness, patent ductus arteriosus, glaucoma, purpura, and bone defects. Most states have laws requiring immunization to prevent the transmission of rubella to pregnant women. The incidence of rubella tripled between 1988 and 1991 in groups of unvaccinated adults, such as college students, work environments, and certain religious groups.[13] A concomitant increase in congenital rubella is expected. Immunization is accomplished by live-virus injection. A single injection after 15 months of age has produced a 98% to 99% immunity response in immunized children and is considered adequate in the prevention of rubella.[13] Many areas, however, require a second preschool or later dose of rubella vaccine to increase the immunity response of the vaccine. Cases of rubella in unimmunized children are rare provided the level of immunization in the general population remains high. As with rubeola, the treatment is symptomatic.

Roseola Infantum. Roseola infantum is a contagious viral disease of infants and small children, most frequently those between 6 and 18 months of age. It is caused by human herpesvirus-6 (HHV-6) and produces a characteristic maculopapular rash covering the trunk and spreading to the appendages. The rash is preceded by an abrupt onset of high fever (up to 105°F) and coldlike symptoms lasting 1 to 5 but usually 3 to 4 days. These symptoms improve at about the same time the rash appears. Unlike rubella, no cervical or postauricular lymph node adenopathy occurs. Roseola infantum is frequently mistaken for rubella. Rubella can usually be ruled out by the age of the child as well as the absence of lymph node adenopathy. Generally, children under 6 to 9 months do not develop rubella because they retain some maternal antibodies. Blood antibody titers may be taken to determine the actual diagnosis. In most cases, there are no long-term effects from this disease.

Treatment for roseola infantum is palliative; there is no vaccine for prevention. Antipyretic drugs such as acetaminophen and cooling baths are used to reduce the fever. Rest and fluids are recommended for recuperation and body rehydration. Pruritus may accompany the other symptoms, but this is rare.

Measles (Rubeola). *Measles* (rubeola, hard measles, 7-day measles) is an acute, highly communicable viral disease caused by morbillivirus. The characteristic rash is macular and blotchy; sometimes the macules become confluent. The rubeola rash usually begins on the face and spreads to the appendages. There are several accompanying symptoms: a fever of 100°F or greater, Koplik's spots (small, irregular red spots with a bluish white speck in the center) on the buccal mucosa, and mild to severe photosensitivity. Coldlike symptoms and general malaise and myalgia are often present. In severe cases, the macule may hemorrhage into the skin tissue or onto the outer body surface. This is called hemorrhagic measles. Measles is more severe in infants, adults, and malnourished children. There may be severe complications, including otitis media, pneumonia, and encephalitis. Antibody titers are drawn for a conclusive diagnosis of rubeola.

The treatment for measles is symptomatic. Children are isolated in a darkened room, antipyretic medications are given to reduce the fever, and rest and relaxation are encouraged. If marked dehydration exists or the symptoms are severe, a physician should be consulted.

Measles is a disease preventable by vaccine, and immunization is required by law in the United States. Immunization is accomplished by injection of a live-virus vaccine. A single injection after 15 months of age is usually sufficient to produce immunity. However, there has been a notable increase in the number of measles cases in the United States and other countries over the past few years. Measles outbreaks occur in unimmunized and underimmunized children: babies under 15 months of age, unimmunized inner-city preschool children, and previously vaccinated college-age students who received their immunizations before 15 months of age. A continuation of outbreaks of measles is expected. A second preschool dose of the vaccine results in a 95% seroconversion rate and is mandatory in most states. Revaccination of those entering educational and vocational institutions after high school is recommended.

Chickenpox (Varicella). Chickenpox (varicella) is a common communicable childhood disease. It is caused by the herpes zoster virus, which is also the agent in shingles (herpes zoster). The characteristic skin lesion occurs in three stages: macule, vesicle, and granular scab. The macular stage is characterized by rapid development (within hours) of macules over the trunk of the body, spreading to the limbs, buccal mucosa, scalp, axillae, upper respiratory tract, and conjunctiva. During the second stage, the macules vesiculate (become filled with water, or blister) and

may become depressed or umbilicated (raised blisters with depressed centers). The vesicles break open, and a scab forms during the third stage. Crops of lesions occur successively, so that all three forms of the lesion are usually visible by the third day of the illness. Mild to extreme pruritus accompanies these lesions and can be a complicating factor by leading to scratching and subsequent development of secondary bacterial infections. Chickenpox is also accompanied by coldlike symptoms, including cough, coryza, and sometimes photosensitivity. Mild febrile states usually occur. Side effects, such as pneumonia, septic complications, and encephalitis, are rare.

Live attenuated varicella vaccine has been demonstrated to be 100% effective in the prevention of chickenpox in healthy children and children who have leukemia.[14, 15] However, the cost of vaccinating children (and possibly the elderly) given the minimal side effects of the disease remains under debate. The drug, acyclovir, has been demonstrated to be effective in reducing the number of lesions and length of illness with healthy children when given within the first 24 hours of disease onset.[16] The treatment of chickenpox, however, remains primarily palliative. Antipyretic drugs such as acetaminophen are given to reduce fever; they may also relieve local discomfort. Pruritus is relieved with lukewarm baths and applications of topical antipruritics such as Caladryl lotion. Home remedies, such as baking soda or colloidal oatmeal baths, also relieve itching. The physician should be notified in cases of severe pruritus. Oral administration of diphenhydramine (Benadryl) or other antihistamines may be prescribed. Rest and fluids are important in recuperation and rehydration.

Scarlet Fever. Scarlet fever is a systemic reaction to the toxins produced by the group A beta-hemolytic streptococci. It occurs when the person is sensitized to the toxin-producing variants of streptococci. It frequently occurs in association with streptococcal sore throat (strep throat); but it may also be associated with a wound, skin infection, or puerperal infection. Scarlet fever is characterized by a pink punctate skin rash on the neck, chest, axillae, groin, and thighs. When palpated, the rash feels like fine sandpaper. There is flushing of the face with circumoral pallor. Other symptoms include high fever, nausea and vomiting, strawberry tongue, raspberry tongue, and skin desquamation. Complications of scarlet fever include otitis media, peritonsillar abscess, rheumatic fever, acute glomerulonephritis, and cholera. Penicillin is the drug of choice for treatment.

DISORDERS OF ADOLESCENCE AND YOUNG ADULTHOOD

The most common disorder of adolescence and young adulthood is acne vulgaris (discussed later in this chapter). The increased production of sex hormones and oils contributes to this problem. The problems associated with childhood diseases are less common in this age group; however, diseases such as pityriasis rosea are more commonly seen. Also, chronic skin diseases may exacerbate or change with the aging process.

DISORDERS OF OLD AGE*

An elderly person may experience a variety of skin disorders as well as exacerbation of earlier skin problems because of the aging process. Physiologically, in the skin of the elderly person, the dermal-epidermal junction is flattened; dermal and subcutaneous mass is lost; the capillary loops are shortened; and the number of melanocytes, Langerhans' cells, and Merkel's cells is reduced. This results in less padding, thinning of the skin, and changes in color and elasticity. The skin is much less resilient to environmental and mechanical trauma, and tissue repair takes longer. Similarly, there is less hair and nail growth, and the hair loses pigment.

Dry skin and pruritus associated with dry skin are common in the elderly. Reduced activity of the sebaceous glands and sweat glands contributes to this problem. For some elderly people, these changes may be a great help in clearing a lifelong struggle with acne.

The most common skin problems in the elderly are skin tags, keratoses, lentigines, and vascular lesions. Many of these problems reflect continued exposure to sun and weather over the years.

Skin tags are soft, pedunculated, brown or flesh-colored papules appearing on the front or side of the neck or in the axilla. Ranging in size from a pinhead to the size of a pea, the tags have the normal color and texture of the skin.

A *keratosis* is a horny growth or a condition characterized by an abnormal growth of the keratinizing cells of the epidermis. *Seborrheic keratoses* are sharply circumscribed, wartlike lesions that seem to rest on top of the skin. They usually begin as yellow-to-brown flat lesions of less than 1 cm and may become

* This section is reprinted from Porth, C., & Kapke, K. (1983). Aging and the skin. *Geriatric Nursing, 3,*160–161. Copyright American Journal of Nursing Company. Reprinted by permission.

larger, dark-brown to coal-black lesions with a greasy appearance.

Keratoses are usually found on the face or trunk, sometimes in the form of a solitary lesion and in other cases as literally hundreds of lesions. Although seborrheic keratoses are benign, they must be differentiated from nevi, or moles, which are formed from clusters of melanocytes, because a change in the color, texture, or size of a nevus may indicate malignant transformation to a melanoma.

Actinic (solar) keratoses are premalignant skin lesions that develop on sun-exposed areas. The lesions, ranging in size from 0.1 to 1 cm or larger, usually appear as dry, brown, and scaly areas, although some may have a shiny surface. A slight erythematous area often encircles the lesion. Actinic lesions are often multiple and more easily felt than seen. When scale is present, it is extremely adherent, and efforts at removal often cause capillary bleeding. The scale tends to recur when it is removed. Characteristic of actinic keratoses is the "weathered" appearance of the surrounding skin. Enlargement, induration, or ulceration of the lesions suggests malignant transformation.

Senile lentigines are the brown, so-called liver spots often seen on sun-exposed areas. Over-the-counter (OTC) creams and lotions containing hydroquinone (Eldoquin, Solaquin, and others) may be used to temporarily bleach these spots. This agent interferes with the synthesis of new pigment but does not destroy existing pigment.

In the concentration approved for over-the-counter (OTC) preparations, however, hydroquinone has limited usefulness. In the higher concentrations available in prescription preparations, hydroquinone may cause inflammation with burning, tingling, and stinging. Despite the limited usefulness of OTC preparations, their effects may make some people feel less self-conscious about skin discoloration. The success of treatment depends on avoiding sunlight completely or consistently applying a high-potency sunscreen.

Malignant lentigines, sometimes referred to as Hutchinson's melanotic freckles, begin as premalignant lesions arising from the melanocytes and are usually larger than the senile lentigines. They start as a small, light to dark-brown mottled area that is flat with the surface of the skin and grows laterally. Growth may continue at a variable rate over many years. As malignant changes occur, the area grows vertically and becomes elevated.

Vascular lesions consist of vascular tumors and chronically dilated blood vessels. *Senile angiomas* are small, ruby-red or purplish vascular tumors, usually compressible and found mainly on the trunk. *Senile ectasia* refers to a slightly raised erythematous papule that is composed of dilated capillaries. They are usually 2 to 5 mm in diameter and located on the trunk. *Telangiectases* are single dilated blood vessels (capillaries or terminal arteries) that appear most frequently on the cheeks and the nose—areas long exposed to excessive sunlight and harsh weather.

Venous lakes are usually seen on the exposed body parts, particularly the backs of the hands, ears, and lips. They consist of small, flat, bluish blood vessels that have a lakelike appearance. The color of the lesion can usually be blanched when sustained pressure is applied to one side. Senile angiomas and venous lakes can be removed by fulguration if a person desires.

In summary, many skin problems occur in specific age groups. Common in infants are diaper rash, prickly heat, and cradle cap. Rashes associated with such childhood diseases as roseola, rubeola, rubella, and chickenpox are seen in young children afflicted with these diseases. Acne vulgaris is a common disorder of adolescence and young adulthood. Skin changes that occur as a part of the aging process predispose the elderly to dry skin, keratosis, lentigines, and vascular skin lesions.

■ PRIMARY DISORDERS OF THE SKIN

Primary skin disorders are those originating in the skin. They include infectious processes, inflammatory conditions, allergic reactions, parasitic infestations, overexposure or hypersensitivity to sunlight, and neoplasms. Although most of these disorders are not life-threatening, they can affect the quality of life.

MECHANICAL PROCESSES

Areas of skin that are rubbed repeatedly may result in necrosis of the stratum spinosum. This can cause blisters, calluses, or corns.

A *blister* is a vesicle or fluid-filled papule. Blisters of mechanical origin form from the repeated friction caused by repeated rubbing on a single area of the skin. Histologically, there is degeneration of epidermal cells and a disruption of intercellular junctions that causes the layers of the skin to separate. As a result, fluid accumulates and a noticeable bleb forms on the skin surface. Blisters are best protected by adding layers of padding (such as adhesive bandages or gauze) to prevent further blister formation. Breaking the skin of a blister to remove the fluid is inadvisable because of the risk of secondary infections.

Prolonged repeated rubbing or pressure can pro-duce a *callus* or area of increased skin production (hyperkeratosis). Increased cohesion between cells results in both hyperkeratosis and decreased skin shedding.

Corns are small, well-circumscribed, conical keratinous thickenings of the skin. They usually appear on the toes from rubbing or ill-fitting shoes. The actual corn is a small, encapsulated body of hardened keratinous material. Pain often accompanies corns. Corns may be surgically removed, but they recur if the causative agent is not removed.

INFECTIOUS PROCESSES

The skin is subject to invasion by a number of microorganisms. Normally, the skin flora, sebum, immune responses, and other protective mechanisms guard the skin against infection. Depending on the virulence of the infecting agent and the competence of the host's resistance, infections may result.

FUNGAL INFECTIONS

Fungal (mycotic) infections of the skin are classified as superficial and deep types. The superficial infections are called *dermatophytoses*; they are commonly known as *tinea*, or *ringworm*. Different forms of tinea affect different body areas. Tinea can affect the body (tinea corporis), scalp (tinea capitis), hands (tinea manus), feet (tinea pedis), nails (tinea unguium), or groin and upper aspects of the thigh (tinea cruris or jock itch). Deep fungal infections involve the epidermis, dermis, and subcutis. Infections that are typically superficial may exhibit deep involvement in immunosuppressed individuals.

A fungus is a free-living saprophytic plantlike organism (see Chapter 12). Certain strains of fungi are considered normal flora. Fungi causing superficial skin infections live on the dead, keratinized cells of the epidermis. They emit an enzyme that enables them to digest keratin, which results in superficial skin scaling, nail disintegration, and hair structure breakage. An exception to this is the invading fungus of tinea versicolor, which does not produce a keratolytic enzyme. Individual species of three genera have been identified as the invading fungi in most forms of tinea: *Microsporum, Epidermophyton*, and *Trichophyton*.

Diagnosis of fungal infections is primarily done by microscopic examination of skin scrapings. Hyphae are threadlike filaments that grow from spores and are visible microscopically. Mycelia are macroscopic aggregations of hyphae. The fungal spores, the reproducing bodies of fungi, are rarely seen on skin scrapings. Potassium hydroxide (KOH) preparations are used to prepare slides of skin scrapings. The

KOH disintegrates human tissue and leaves behind the hyphae for examination. With another method of diagnosis, a Wood's light (ultraviolet light) is directed onto the affected area; under the light, many fungi fluoresce a green to yellow-green color.

Tinea Corporis. Tinea corporis (ringworm of the body) can be caused by any of the fungal agents. Usually, it is caused by *Microsporum canis* or *Microsporum audouini;* less frequently, it is caused by *T. rubrum* or *T. mentagrophytes.*

The lesions vary depending on the fungal agent. However, the most common types of lesions are round, oval, or circular patches (Fig. 11-4). There is central clearing of the patches with raised red borders consisting of vesicles, papules, or pustules. The lesion begins as a red papule and enlarges with central healing. The borders are sharply defined; lesions may coalesce. Pruritus, a mild burning sensation, and erythema frequently accompany the skin lesion.

Tinea corporis affects all ages. However, children seem most prone to infection. Transmission is most commonly from kittens, puppies, and other children who have infections. Less common forms are from foot and groin infections.

Treatment of mild cases is generally with OTC antifungal preparations containing tolnaftate or undecylenic acid. Tinactin contains a 1% tolnaftate base, whereas Desenex and other name brands contain undecylenic acid. Both of these topical agents are effective if used correctly. Griseofulvin, the prototype oral prescription antifungal agent, is warranted in severe cases. Newer synthetic antifungal agents, called azole compounds and allylamines, such as ketoconazole and fluconazole, have been used effectively in the treatment of tinea corporis and other ringworms. Although griseofulvin is a fungistatic agent, the synthetic agents are considered to be fun-

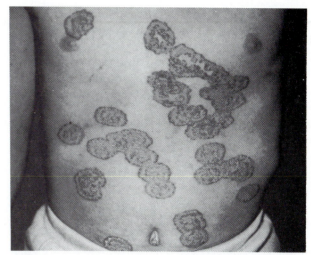

FIG. 11-4. Tinea corporis. (Sauer, G. C. [1980]. *Manual of skin diseases* [4th ed.]. Philadelphia: J.B. Lippincott)

gicidal and therefore more effective. However, the synthetic agents have more serious side effects, such as hepatic toxicity. Topical preparations of these synthetic fungicidals (*e.g.,* Lotrimin) are available and produce less severe side effects.

Tinea Capitis. Tinea capitis (ringworm of the scalp) is separated into two types: primary (non-inflammatory) and secondary (inflammatory). Primary lesions characteristically present as grayish, round, hairless patches, or balding spots, on the head. The lesion varies in size and is most commonly seen on the back of the head (Fig. 11-5). Mild erythema, crust, or scale may be present. The child is usually symptomless, although occasionally pruritus may exist. The primary form of tinea capitis is caused by *Microsporum audouini* and *Microsporum canis* transferred from kittens, puppies, and other humans. Epidemics have occurred from *T. tonsurans* and *Micro-*

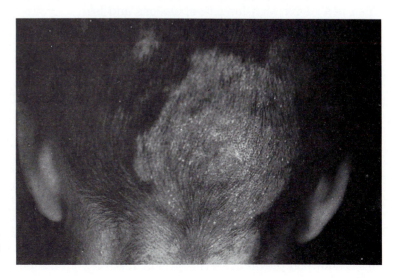

FIG. 11-5. Tinea capitis. (Sauer, G. C. [1980]. *Manual of skin diseases* [4th ed.]. Philadelphia: J.B. Lippincott)

sporum audouini and represent human-to-human transmission.

Children aged 3 to 8 are primarily affected. Tinea capitis seldom occurs in an adult; this has been partially attributed to the higher content of fatty acids in the sebum after puberty, a finding that has generated the development of several antifungal agents with fatty acid bases. These antifungal agents revolutionized treatment, replacing the old remedies in which children were often subjected to head shavings and use of harsh shampoos and salves.

The inflammatory type of tinea capitis is caused by a virulent strain of *T. mentagrophytes, T. verrucosum,* and *Microsporum gypseum.* The onset is acute, and lesions are usually localized to one area. The initial lesion consists of a pustular scaly round patch with broken hairs. A secondary bacterial infection is common and may lead to a painful circumscribed, boggy, and indurated lesion called a *kerion.* The highest incidence is in children and in farmers who work with infected animals.

The treatment for both forms of tinea capitis is primarily griseofulvin, an oral antifungal agent. The synthetic antifungals have been effective modalities as well. Topical ointments are sometimes indicated in addition to oral medications. Wet packs and medicated shampoos, along with antibiotics, may be prescribed for the secondary types of infection.

Tinea Pedis. Tinea pedis (athlete's foot, ringworm of the feet) is a common skin disorder primarily affecting the spaces between the toes, the soles of the feet, or the sides of the feet. It is caused by *T. mentagrophytes* and *T. rubrum.* The lesions vary from a mild scaling lesion to a painful exudative, erosive, inflamed lesion with fissuring. Lesions are often accompanied by pruritus and foul odor.

Evidence suggests that athlete's foot occurs in two forms, simple and complex. Simple forms of tinea pedis have high fungal populations and low bacterial growths. They are characterized by mild to moderate skin peeling and are largely asymptomatic. Complex tinea pedis has a higher bacterial count (*Proteus* and *Pseudomonas*) with a receding fungal count. Complex forms involve maceration of tissue, inflammation, and fissuring. Pruritus and pain are often present.[17]

Some people are prone to chronic tinea pedis. Mild forms are more common during dry environmental conditions. Exacerbations in the mild form occur as a result of hot weather, sweating, and exercise, or when the feet are exposed to moisture or occlusive shoes. Tinea pedis may occur alone or in combination with other infections such as tinea corporis or tinea cruris. Patches may occur on the hands; this is known as the intradermal, or dermatophytid, reaction.

Simple forms of tinea pedis are treated with topical application of antifungals such as tolnaftate. In the past, complex cases have been treated with oral griseofulvin and topical antifungal agents. Based on their study, Klingman and Leyden[17] suggest the combination of antibiotics (neomycin sulfate) and tolnaftate in the treatment of complex forms. Other treatment and preventive modalities include scrupulous cleansing and drying of affected areas, clean dry socks, and changing of socks daily. When bathed, the feet should be dried after other parts of the body to prevent spread of the disease.

Tinea Unguium. Tinea unguium, or ringworm of the nails (onychomycosis), is a chronic fungal infection of the nails of the hands or feet. Tinea of the toenails is common; tinea of the fingernails is less common. Toenail infection is common in people prone to chronic infections of tinea pedis. Often, the infection in the toenails becomes a ready source for future infections of the foot. It may begin from a crushing injury to a toenail or from the spread of tinea pedis. Usually tinea unguium is caused by *T. rubrum* or *T. mentagrophytes.* The infection usually begins at the tip of the nail, where the fungus digests the keratin of the nail. Initially, the nail appears opaque, white, or silvery. The nail then turns yellow or brown. This condition remains unchanged for years and may involve only one or two nails. Generally, there is no discomfort. Gradually, the nail thickens and becomes frail as the infection spreads to the entire nail and nail plate. The nail cracks and thickens, and the nail plate separates from the nail bed as the nail becomes permanently discolored and distorted. Spreading to other nails may occur. The synthetic antifungal agents have been effective to varying degrees with both forms of tinea. However, patients need to be monitored closely for the side effects of the drugs.

The prognosis for fungal infections of the toenail is poor. The treatment usually involves oral griseofulvin for up to 1 year. It rarely produces a cure, and some authorities recommend not using griseofulvin or only using the drug with removal of the infected toenails. Even with this therapy, recurrence is frequent. Fingernail infections are more easily treated. Oral griseofulvin therapy for 6 months to 1 year has been successful but depends on the persistence of both the therapist and the patient.

Tinea Manus. Tinea manus (ringworm of the hands) is rarely a primary infection. The primary site of infection is usually tinea pedis with tinea manus occurring as a secondary infection. A diagnostic differentiation among hand diseases is that tinea manus usually occurs only on one hand, whereas other infectious processes, such as contact dermatitis and psoriasis, affect both hands.

The same fungal agents responsible for tinea pedis are found active in tinea manus, *T. rubrum* and *T. mentagrophytes*. The characteristic lesion is a blister on the palm or finger surrounded by erythema. Chronic lesions are scaly and dry. Cracking and fissuring may occur. The lesions may spread to the plantar surfaces of the hand; if chronic, tinea manus may lead to tinea of the fingernails. The treatment of choice is oral griseofulvin therapy for approximately 3 months. The synthetic antifungal drugs have also been effective.

Tinea Versicolor. Tinea versicolor is a fungal infection involving the upper chest, the back, and sometimes the arms. The causative agent is *Malassezia furfur*. The infection occurs primarily in young adults in tropic and temperate regions; however, cases have been reported in the northern states.

The characteristic lesion is a yellow, pink, or brown sheet of scaling skin. The name *versicolor* is derived from the multicolored variations of the lesion. The patches are depigmented and do not tan when exposed to ultraviolet light, and the skin has an overall appearance of being "dirty." These cosmetic defects often bring the patient to the physician in the summer months. The theory is that the fungus filters the ultraviolet light, thus preventing tanning. In darker-skinned people, the depigmented areas are more apparent.

Selenium sulfide, found in several shampoo preparations, has been an effective fungistatic treatment measure. Boiling or steam-pressing clothes may help in the prevention of recurrence. Ketoconazole and fluconazole, because of its fungicidal properties, have become the drugs of choice. However, recurrences after drug therapy have occurred.

Dermatophytid Reaction. A secondary skin eruption may occur in people allergic to one of the dermatophytes, and this is called a dermatophytid, or intradermal (ID), reaction. It may occur during an acute episode of a fungal infection. The most common reaction occurs on the hands, in response to tinea pedis. The lesions are vesicles with erythema extending over the palms and fingers of the hand; extension to other areas may occur. Less commonly, there can be a more generalized reaction in which papules or vesicles erupt on the trunk or extremities. These eruptions may resemble tinea corporis and may become excoriated and infected with bacteria. Treatment is directed at the primary site of infection. The ID reaction resolves in most cases without intervention if the primary site is cleared.

Candidal (Monilial) Infections. Candidiasis (moniliasis) is a fungal infection caused by *Candida albicans*. This yeastlike fungus is a normal inhabitant of the gastrointestinal tract, mouth, and vagina (see genital *C. albicans*, Chapter 39). The skin problems that result are due to the release of irritating toxins on the skin surface. Some conditions predispose a person to candidal infections, such as diabetes mellitus, antibiotic therapy, pregnancy, use of birth control pills, poor nutrition, and immunosuppressed diseases. Oral candidiasis may be the first sign of HIV infection.

C. albicans thrives in warm, moist intertriginous areas of the body. The rash is red with well-defined borders. Patches erode the epidermis, and there is scaling. Mild to severe itching and burning often accompany the infection. Severe forms of infection may involve pustules or vesiculopustules. A differential diagnostic feature of candidal in comparison with tinea infection is the presence of satellite lesions. These satellite lesions are maculopapular and are found outside the clearly demarcated borders of the candidal infection. The appearance of candidal infections varies according to the site. Table 11-3 summarizes site characteristics.

Treatment measures vary according to the location. Preventive measures, such as wearing rubber gloves, are encouraged for people with infections of the hands. Intertriginous areas, caused by the macerating effect of heat and moisture, are often separated

TABLE 11-3. CANDIDAL INFECTIONS: LOCATION AND APPEARANCE OF LESIONS	
LOCATION	**APPEARANCE**
Breasts, groin, axillae, anus, umbilicus, toe or fingerwebs	Red lesions with well-defined borders and presence of satellite lesions; lesions may be dry or moist
Vagina	Red, oozing lesions with sharply defined borders and inflamed vagina; cervix may be covered with moist, white plaque, cheesy, foul-smelling discharge; presence of pruritus and burning
Glans penis (balanitis)	Red lesions with sharply defined borders; penis may be covered with white plaque; presence of pruritus and burning
Mouth (thrush)	Creamy white flakes on a red, inflamed mucous membrane; papillae on tongue may be enlarged
Nails	Red, painful swelling around nail bed; common in people who often have their hands in water

with clean cotton cloth. Nystatin (Mycostatin), an antibiotic available in tablets, powder, or vaginal suppositories, is effective in control of infection. Oral synthetic agents, such as ketoconazole and fluconazole, have also been effective.

BACTERIAL INFECTIONS

Bacteria are considered normal flora of the skin. Most bacteria are not pathogenic; however, when pathogenic bacteria invade the skin, superficial or systemic infections may develop. Bacterial infections are classified as primary, or superficial, and secondary, or deep. Impetigo is an example of a primary bacterial infection, and infected ulcers are an example of a secondary bacterial infection.

Bacterial infections are usually cultured for diagnosis. In addition to antibiotic therapy, the treatment of bacterial infections often includes hygiene education, general isolation procedures, and dietary management.

Impetigo. Impetigo is a common superficial bacterial infection caused by staphylococci or group A beta-hemolytic streptococci (GABHS). Historically, there has been a shift from a higher incidence of GABHS type impetigo to *Staphylococcus aureus* as the predominant causal agent. It is most common among young infants and children, although older children and adults occasionally contract the disease. It is highly communicable in the younger population.

GABHS impetigo initially appears as a small vesicle or pustule, or a large bulla. The primary lesion ruptures, leaving a denuded area that discharges a honey-colored serous liquid; the liquid hardens on the skin surface and deposits a honey-colored crust with a stuck-on appearance (Fig. 11-6). New vesicles erupt within hours. Pruritus often accompanies the disease, and the skin excoriations that result from scratching multiply the infection sites. A possible complication of untreated GABHS impetigo is poststreptococcal glomerulonephritis (see Chapter 32). Lesions are most often found on the face, but they can occur anywhere on the body.

Staphylococcus aureus impetigo first manifests as a vesicle. The vesicle becomes seropurulent with a surrounding erythematous base. The pustules rupture, favoring spread of the lesions. A less common form of *Staphylococcus aureus* infection, called Ritter's disease, manifests with a diffuse scarlatiniform erythema resembling its common description, "scalded skin syndrome." If untreated, both forms of impetigo can last for weeks and may continue to spread and become deeper bacterial infections requiring emergency medical attention.

The treatment of impetigo has changed consis-

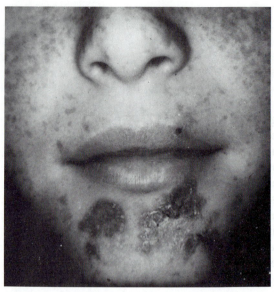

FIG. 11-6. The crusted lesions of impetigo. (Demis, D. J. [Ed.]. [1985]. *Clinical dermatology.* Philadelphia: Harper & Row)

tent with the causative agent. With the lessened incidence of GABHS impetigo, there has been a concomitant decrease in the administration of systemic doses of antibiotics for its treatment. For *Staphylococcus aureus*, topical mupirocin (Bactroban) has proved clinically effective with few side effects. Bullous or severe forms of impetigo should be treated individually by a physician.

Ecthyma is an ulcerative form of impetigo, usually secondary to minor trauma. It frequently occurs on the buttocks and thighs of children. The lesions are similar to those of GABHS impetigo. A vesicle or pustule ruptures, leaving a skin erosion or ulcer that weeps and dries to a crusted patch, often resulting in scar formation. With extensive ecthyma, there is a low-grade fever and extension of the infection to other organs. The treatment is the same as for GABHS impetigo (*i.e.,* removal of crusts by soaking and application of topical antibiotics). In severe cases, oral or intramuscular antibiotics are indicated.

VIRAL INFECTIONS

Viruses are intracellular pathogens. They have no organized cell structure but consist of a DNA or RNA core surrounded by a protein coat (see Chapter 12). Viruses rely completely on live cells for reproduction. The viruses seen in skin lesion disorders tend to be DNA-containing viruses. Viruses invade the keratinocyte, begin to reproduce, and cause cellular proliferation or cellular death. The rapid increase in viral skin diseases has been attributed to the use of birth control medication and corticosteroid drugs, which have immunosuppressive qualities, and the use of antibiotics, which alter the bacterial flora of the skin.[18] As the number of bacterial infections has decreased, there has been a proportional rise in viral skin diseases.

Verrucae. Verrucae, or warts, are common benign papillomas caused by DNA-containing papovaviruses. Although warts vary in gross appearance depending on their location, they all have a similar histologic appearance (Table 11-4). The wart is not a mass of uniform tumor cells but, like other skin diseases, is an exaggeration of the normal skin composition. There is an irregular thickening of the stratum spinosum and greatly increased thickening of the stratum corneum. Human papillomavirus (HPV) is the subgroup of the papovaviruses that cause human warts. There are over 60 types of HPVs found on the skin and mucous membranes of humans. A great amount of these are genital or sexually transmitted (see Chapter 39); the remainder account for warts that commonly appear on the hands and feet. The nongenital warts, types 1, 2, 3, and 4, are generally not precancerous. They are known as plantar warts, common warts, and flat warts. Wart transmission occurs usually through skin contact.

Warts resolve spontaneously when immunity to the virus develops. The immune response may be delayed for years; after 5 years, most warts that are left untreated have disappeared. In earlier years, treatment measures were directed at eradicating all wart tissue, primarily by excision. Because this fre-

quently left scars, treatment was directed at irritation of the wart with liquid nitrogen or acid chemicals. Cryotherapy and salicylic acid paint or plasters have been effective. More recently, laser therapy of various types has been successful in wart eradication. Interestingly, given the resolution rate of most warts, self-hypnosis with imagery has also been successful in the mitigation and elimination.[19]

Herpes Simplex (Cold Sore, Fever Blister). Herpes simplex virus (HSV) infections of the skin and mucous membrane are common (Fig. 11-7). Two types of herpesvirus infect humans, type I and type II. Both HSV I and HSV II cause genital herpes. However, most infections that occur above the waist are caused by HSV I. HSV I may be transmitted to other parts of the body through the occupational hazards that exist in athletics and some professions, such as dentistry and medicine. HSV I may also be transmitted by kissing or oral sex. Type II is responsible for most infections in the genital region (see Chapter 39).

Herpesvirus lesions usually begin with a burning or tingling sensation. Vesicles and erythema follow and progress to pustules, ulcers, and crusts before healing. The lesion is most common on the lips, face, and mouth. Pain is common, and healing takes place within 10 to 14 days.

HSV infections are of two types: primary and secondary. The primary infection usually consists of a high fever, sore throat, painful vesicles, and ulcers of the tongue, palate, gingiva, buccal mucosa, and lips. The primary infection results in the develop-

TABLE 11-4. TYPES AND CHARACTERISTICS OF VERRUCAE (WARTS)

TYPE	LOCATION	APPEARANCE
Verruca vulgaris (common warts)	Anywhere on the skin, usually on the hands	Ragged dome-shape with growth above the skin surface
Verruca filiformis	Eyelids, face, neck	Long finger-like projections
Verruca plana (flat wart)	Forehead, dorsum of hand	Small flat tumors, may be barely visible
Verruca plantaris (plantar wart)	Sole of foot	Flat to slightly raised growth extending deep into skin; painful; bleeding occurs with superficial trimming; coalesced plantar warts are referred to as mosaic warts
Condyloma acuminata	Mucous membrane of the penis, female genitalia, perianal areas, and rectum	Large moist projections with rough surfaces; usually pink or purple in color

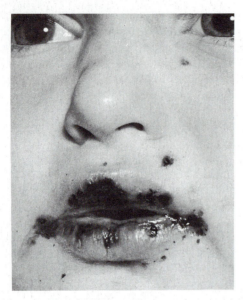

FIG. 11-7. Primary herpes simplex in a two-year-old child. (Sauer, G. C. [1980]. *Manual of skin diseases* [4th ed.]. Philadelphia: J.B. Lippincott)

ment of antibodies to the virus so that recurrences (secondary infections) are more localized and less severe. After an initial infection, the herpesvirus persists in the trigeminal and other ganglia in the latent state. Recurrent lesions are common in a small percentage of people; precipitating factors may be stress, sunlight exposure, menses, or injury.

There is no cure for herpes simplex; most treatment measures are palliative. Lidocaine (Xylocaine) or diphenhydramine (Benadryl) application and aspirin help relieve pain. Cold compresses help in the acute stages. Severe forms have been treated with idoxuridine (IDI, Stoxil), which prevents certain aspects of DNA synthesis and thereby inhibits viral reproduction without causing cell injury. To date, the most effective treatment has been the drug acyclovir. Acyclovir is an antimetabolite that inhibits herpesvirus replication. It is given orally or intravenously and is the prototype of all the antiviral drugs.

Herpes Zoster. Herpes zoster (shingles) is an acute localized inflammatory disease of a dermatome segment of the skin. It is caused by the same herpesvirus (varicella-zoster) that causes chickenpox. It is believed to be the result of reactivation of a latent varicella-zoster virus that has been present in the sensory dorsal ganglia since childhood infection. During an episode of shingles, the reactivated virus travels from the ganglia to the skin of the corresponding dermatome.

The clinical picture of herpes zoster is the eruption of vesicles with erythematous bases that are restricted to skin areas supplied by sensory neurons of a single or associated group of dorsal root ganglia. Eruptions are generally unilateral in the thoracic region, trunk, and face. In immunosuppressed people, the lesions may extend beyond the dermatome. New crops of vesicles erupt for 3 to 5 days along the nerve pathway. The lesions are deeper and more confluent than those of chickenpox. The vesicles dry, form crusts, and eventually fall off. The lesions usually clear in 2 to 3 weeks. Severe pain and paresthesia are common. In the elderly, herpes zoster is a particularly serious condition that may be long-lasting and eventually lead to death. Pain reports from elderly people indicate an increased severity and lengthy episodes of up to 1 year. The reason may be greater involvement of small nerve fibers due to loss of large nerve fibers associated with aging. Postherpetic neuralgia is the most important complication occurring in people over the age of 50. Eye involvement can result in permanent blindness and occurs in a large percentage of cases involving the ophthalmic division of the trigeminal nerve (Fig. 11-8). The occurrence of herpes zoster in all people warrants closer scrutiny and assessment. In people at risk for HIV infection, development of herpes zoster may be one sign that precedes marked depression of cellular immunity associated with AIDS.

The treatment of choice in herpes zoster is early oral or intravenous doses of acyclovir. Despite side effects, such as decreased renal function, nausea, vomiting, and abdominal pain, acyclovir remains the drug of choice for immunosuppressed people as

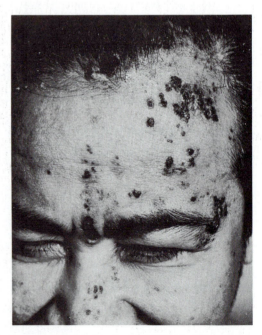

FIG. 11-8. Herpes zoster involving the ophthalmic branch of the trigeminal nerve. (Sauer, G. C. [1985]. *Manual of skin disease* [5th ed.]. Philadelphia: J.B. Lippincott)

well. Narcotic analgesics may be used to decrease the pain response. Also, nerve blocks may be used in the early management of herpetic pain. Systemic corticosteroids have been effective in some cases, but their use remains controversial. Local treatment measures include Burow's solution compresses, aqueous alcohol lotions, calamine lotion, and starch shake lotions.

INFLAMMATORY SKIN DISORDERS

The inflammatory skin diseases listed here are generally of unknown cause or etiology. They are usually localized to the skin and are rarely associated with a specific internal disease. They produce marked variations in normal skin, usually papulosquamous in nature. Inflammation and erythema are common. These disorders, which include acne, lichen planus, psoriasis, and pityriasis rosea, are among the most common skin disorders.

ACNE

Acne is commonly referred to as a disorder of the pilosebaceous (hair and sebaceous gland) unit. The sebaceous glands empty into the hair follicle, and the pilosebaceous unit opens to the skin surface by means of a widely dilated opening called a *pore* (see Fig. 11-4). The sebaceous glands are largest on the face, scalp, scrotum, but are present in all areas of the skin except for the soles of the feet and palms of the hands. The sebaceous cells are derived from the epidermal keratin cell and have a structure similar to epidermal cells except that they accumulate lipid droplets. The sebaceous glands produce a complex lipid mixture called *sebum*, from the Latin word meaning tallow or grease. Sebum consists of a mixture of free fatty acids, triglycerides, diglycerides, monoglycerides, sterol esters, wax esters, and squalene. Sebum production occurs as a holocrine process in which the sebaceous cells are completely broken down and their lipid contents are emptied through the sebaceous duct into the hair follicle. The amount of sebum produced depends on two factors: (1) the size of the sebaceous gland, and (2) the rate of cellular growth. Sebaceous cell proliferation and sebum production are uniquely responsive to direct hormonal stimulation by androgen. In men, testicular androgens are the main stimulus for sebaceous activity; in women, adrenal and ovarian androgens maintain sebaceous activity.

Acne lesions consist of comedones (whiteheads and blackheads), papules, pustules, and, in severe cases, cysts. Noninflammatory acne consists primarily of comedones, whereas inflammatory acne consists of

erythematous-based pustules and cysts. Blackheads are plugs of material that accumulate in sebaceous glands that open to the skin surface. The color of blackheads results from melanin that has moved into the sebaceous glands from adjoining epidermal cells. Whiteheads are pale, slightly elevated papules with no visible orifice. The inflammatory lesions are believed to develop from the escape of sebum into the dermis and the irritating effects of the fatty acids that are contained in the sebum.

There are several forms of acne. Three types of acne occur during different stages of the life cycle: acne vulgaris is the most common form among adolescents and young adults; acne conglobata develops later in life; and acne rosacea occurs in older adults. There are numerous other types of acne with varying etiologic agents and influences.

Acne Vulgaris. Acne vulgaris develops in about 80% to 90% of all people during adolescence or young adulthood and accounts for about 25% of all visits to the dermatologist. In women, acne may persist up to 30 years of age; however, the overall incidence is higher in men.[21]

Acne vulgaris lesions form primarily on the face and neck and, to a lesser extent, on the back, chest, and shoulders (Fig. 11-9). The lesions are thought to

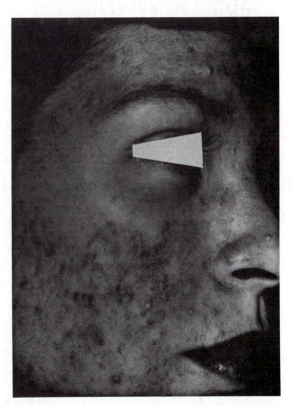

FIG. 11-9. Acne vulgaris. (Demis, D. J. [Ed.]. [1985]. *Clinical dermatology*. Philadelphia: Harper & Row)

result from increased activity of the sebaceous glands and plugging of the pilosebaceous ducts.

The cause of acne vulgaris remains unknown; it may be multifactorial. Several contributing factors have been examined: (1) the influence of androgens on sebaceous cell activity; (2) increased proliferation of the keratinizing epidermal cells that form the sebaceous cells; (3) increased sebum production in relation to the severity of the disease; (4) decreased amounts of linoleic acid in the sebum; and (5) presence of the *Propionibacterium acnes* organism. The *Propionibacterium acnes* organism contains lipases, and these enzymes can result in lipolysis and production of the free fatty acids that produce inflammation.[21]

Over the years, several factors have been studied empirically and debunked as causal or contributing agents. Included are: (1) diets high in fatty content, (2) certain foods, such as chocolate, (3) acne as an infectious process, and (4) makeup. However, many therapists continue to advise general hygienic and preventive measures as a child nears puberty. These include washing the involved areas, avoiding touching the face with the hands, shampooing hair and scalp regularly, keeping hair away from the face, avoiding the use of creams and moisturizers, and using water-based, rather than oil-based, makeup. Exposure to sunlight is often helpful, whereas squeezing, rubbing, or picking of comedones should be avoided. A balanced diet is recommended; stressful or fatigue-producing activities should be minimized. Hygienic and preventive measures are also used to treat acne. Mild forms of acne respond well to stringent hygiene measures in addition to the topical application of acne creams, ointments, and lotions. Numerous commercial products are available that contain peeling, drying, and antibiotic agents. Products with resorcinol, salicylic acid, or sulfur bases are helpful in drying and peeling the skin. Oil-based preparations should be avoided, because they may contribute to the problem.

Treatment of severe acne is based on four objectives supported by current knowledge of the condition: (1) correction of the defect in epidermal cell proliferation, (2) lessening of sebaceous gland activity, (3) reduction of the *Propionibacterium acnes* population, and (4) reduction of the inflammatory process. Many of the treatment modalities may be used alone or in combination with other treatments. An important treatment measure is sensitivity to the acne client's emotional needs.

Acne creams and lotions contain keratolytic agents such as sulfur, salicylic acid, and resorcinol that act as chemically abrasive agents to loosen comedones and exert a peeling effect on the skin. Tretinoin (Retin-A), an acid derivative of vitamin A, is a stronger keratolytic agent, but it is irritating. It helps remove comedones by increasing mitotic activity at the base of the follicle. Comedones are pushed out from below. Because tretinoin is applied topically, it remains chiefly on the epidermis with minimal absorption into the circulation.

Oral low-dose tetracycline has been used effectively for years. Tetracycline has no effect on sebum production, but it does decrease the amount of free fatty acids. Tetracycline requires a sufficient treatment period to establish effective blood levels. Side effects are minimal, which is why the drug has remained so useful. However, it does have teratogenic effects and should not be given to pregnant women. Erythromycin, another antibiotic, also has been effective in acne treatment. Of the antimicrobial drugs, dapsone has been effective in severe cystic acnes. However, the side effects are many, and the drug should be used with caution and close monitoring. Tetracycline, erythromycin, and clindamycin are available for topical application.

Estrogens decrease sebum production; however, because of the high dosages required, they are contraindicated in men. In women, estrogen therapy is administered in 2-week or 3-week treatment periods and regulated with the menstrual cycle. Side effects are those associated with any estrogen therapy, such as nausea, weight gain, spotting, breast tenderness, amenorrhea, thromboembolic disorders, and a possible increased risk of cancer.

Glucocorticoid therapy has been limited primarily to severe resistive cases. The therapy results in remarkable healing, yet acne usually returns after the therapy has been terminated.

Isotretinoin (Accutane), an orally administered synthetic retinoid or acid form of vitamin A, has revolutionized the treatment of recalcitrant cases of acne and cystic acnes. Its effects are thought to be related more to hormonal activity rather than the vitamin activity its origin would indicate.[22] In carefully planned dosages, oral isotretinoin has cleared major cases of acne and initiated long-term remissions of the disease. It is administered for 3-month to 4-month treatment periods. Although the exact mode of action is not known, it decreases sebaceous gland activity, reduces the *Propionibacterium acnes* count, and has an antiinflammatory effect. Because of its many side effects, it should only be used in people with severe acne. Side effects are dryness of the mouth and other mucous membranes, conjunctivitis, musculoskeletal system abnormalities, and elevated liver and serum lipid levels. Isotretinoin is also a major teratogen that causes brain, heart, and ear malformations. Women on isotretinoin should be strongly advised not to become pregnant; some physicians require written contracts from women to this end.

Other treatment measures for acne include surgery, ultraviolet irradiation, cryotherapy, and intralesional glucocorticosteroid injection. Acne surgery involves the aspiration of comedones with small-bore needles or devices designed to extract comedone contents. Scarring is a common sequela if done improperly. The use of ultraviolet irradiation, which involves exposure to either hot or cold quartz lights for specified periods, remains controversial, but continues to be used in treatment of some forms of acne. Cryotherapy (freezing with carbon dioxide slushes, liquid nitrogen, dry ice, or acetone) has been effective in promoting healing of lesions by removing the outer layers of skin. Intralesional injection of corticosteroids using a syringe or needleless injector is limited to severe nodulocystic forms of acne. It has been effective in promoting cyst healing, but usually has to be repeated frequently.

Acne Conglobata. Acne conglobata occurs later in life and is a chronic form of acne. Comedones, papules, pustules, nodules, abscesses, cysts, and scars occur on the back, buttocks, and chest, and, to a lesser extent, on the abdomen, shoulders, neck, face, upper arms, and thighs. The comedones have multiple openings, and their discharge is odoriferous, serous, and purulent or mucoid. Healing leaves deep keloidal lesions. Afflicted people have anemia and increased white blood cell counts, sedimentation rates, and neutrophil counts. The treatment is difficult and stringent. It often includes debridement, systemic corticosteroid therapy, oral retinoids, and systemic antibiotics.

Acne Rosacea. Acne rosacea is a chronic acne that occurs in middle-aged and older adults. The characteristic lesion is an erythema or telangiectasia with or without acneiform components (comedones, pustules, nodules). The cause is unknown, and the onset is insidious. It begins with redness over the nose and cheeks and may extend to the chin and forehead. After years of affliction, acne rosacea may develop into an irregular, bullous hyperplasia (thickening) of the nose, known as *rhinophyma*. The sebaceous follicles and openings enlarge, while the skin color changes to a purple red. Treatment measures are similar to those for acne vulgaris; there is no specific treatment. Patients are told to avoid vascular-stimulating agents such as heat, cold, sunlight, hot liquids, highly seasoned foods, and alcohol. Rhinophyma can be treated surgically.

Other Acnes. There are numerous other forms of acne. The symptoms vary depending on the source or age of onset. Treatment measures for these acnes vary depending on the precipitating agent and the extent of the lesions. Many of the previously discussed treatment measures have been used with varying degrees of success.

Acne fulminans is manifested by a sudden eruption of large, inflamed, tender lesions on the back and chest that ulcerate, heal, and scar. Teenage boys are most affected by this type of acne. *Steatocystoma multiplex* consists of an eruption of many cystic lesions of various sizes on the trunk of men and women of young adult age. *Neonatal acne* occurs on the newborn infant, typically on the nose and cheeks; it usually clears without treatment. *Drug acnes* occur as an untoward reaction to certain pharmacologic agents, most commonly steroids, iodides (in cough mixtures), and bromides (in sedatives).

Acne that results from the exposure to occupational compounds or chemicals is called *occupational acne*. Many of the precipitating agents are the same as those that may cause allergic responses, cutting oils being the most offensive. *Acne cosmetica* is believed to be caused by cosmetics. The exact etiologies are unknown because of the variety of cosmetic agents used by women. Even after cosmetic use has been discontinued, this acne usually persists and is difficult to heal. *Acne detergicans* is believed to be caused by compulsive washing of the face with soaps, whereas *acne mechanica* develops from repeated trauma to the skin. A common form of acne mechanica is seen on football players from the rubbing of their helmets. *Pomade acne* follows the hairline and is most commonly seen on African-American males. *Acne excoriée des jeunes filles* is a mild form of acne seen in adolescent girls. The lesions spread from scratching and picking that are believed to be of emotional origin.

LICHEN PLANUS

The term *lichen* is of Greek origin and means *tree-moss*. The term is applied to skin disorders characterized by small, firm, papular lesions that are set close together. Lichen planus is a relatively common chronic, pruritic disease involving inflammation and papular eruption of the skin and mucous membranes. Idiopathic lichen planus is of unknown etiology, but, like other diseases, it is associated with a variety of drugs and chemicals in susceptible people. Lichen planus may involve a cell-mediated immune response that occurs in the basal cells. There is basal cell degeneration with reduced cell mitosis. There are variations in the pattern of lesions (annular, linear) as well as differences in the sites (mucous membranes, genitalia, nails, scalp). The characteristic lesion is a shiny white-topped, purple, polygonal papule. These lesions appear on the wrist, ankles, and trunk of the body (Fig. 11-10).

In the majority of people, lichen planus is a self-limiting disease. Treatment measures include discon-

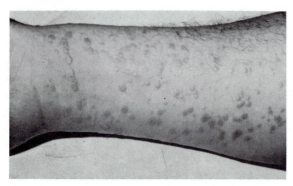

FIG. 11-10. Lichen planus. Note the discrete papules on the forearm. On the wrist, the papules have a linear configuration. (Demis, D. J. [Ed.]. [1985]. *Clinical dermatology.* Philadelphia: Harper & Row)

tinuation of all medications, followed by treatment with topical corticosteroids and occlusive dressings. Systemic corticosteroids may be indicated in severe cases. Intralesional injections of triamcinolone acetonid suspension (a corticosteroid preparation) has produced occasional cures. Antipruritic agents are helpful in reducing itch.

PSORIASIS

Psoriasis is a common, papulosquamous disease characterized by white, scaling patches of various sizes. Psoriasis occurs worldwide, although the incidence is lower in warmer, sunnier climates. In the United States, it affects 1% of the population. The average age of onset is in the third decade.

The disease, which can persist throughout life and exacerbate at unpredictable times, is classified as a chronic ailment. A few cases, though, have been known to clear and not recur. The cause of psoriasis is unknown. Approximately one third of the cases have a genetic history, indicating a hereditary factor. Skin trauma is a common precipitating factor in people predisposed to the disease (prepsoriasis). This reaction of the skin to the original trauma, which can be of any type, is called the Koebner reaction. There appears to be an association between psoriasis and arthritis. Psoriatic arthritis occurs in 5% to 7% of people with psoriasis. The association between alcohol consumption and psoriasis remains under investigation. Many people with psoriasis drink because of frustration with the disease process and available treatment modalities. Alcohol tends to worsen the disease. Alcohol as a risk factor in the development of the disease has also been reported.[23]

Histologically, the migration time of the keratinocyte from the basal cell layer of the stratum corneum decreases from the normal 14 days to approximately 4 to 7 days. This process is *hyperkeratosis*. In psoriasis, there is thinning of the suprapapillary plate and clubbing of the dermal papillae. Capillary beds show permanent damage even when the disease is in remission or has resolved.

There are various forms of psoriasis. A chronic stationary form called *psoriasis vulgaris* is the most common form. The lesions may occur anywhere on the skin, but most often involve the elbows, knees, and scalp (Fig. 11-11). The primary lesions are papules that vary in shape. The papules form into plaques with thick and silvery scales. A differential diagnostic finding is that the plaques bleed from minute points when removed, which is known as *Auspitz* sign. Secondary lesions are uncommon, but there may be excoriation, thickening, or oozing. In African Americans, the plaques may turn purple.

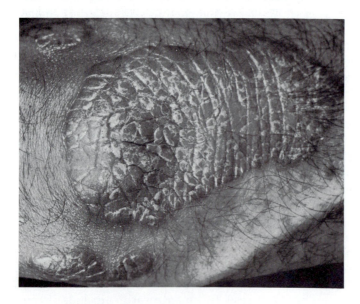

FIG. 11-11. Psoriasis on the elbow. (Sauer, G. C. [1985]. *Manual of skin diseases* [5th ed.]. Philadelphia: J.B. Lippincott)

Another form of psoriasis, called *eruptive* (*gut-tata*) psoriasis, is more common as an early onset form of the disease. Its lesions are smaller and usually limited to the upper trunk and extremities. Generalized pustular psoriasis is a distinct form of the disease that is distinguished by a fever that lasts for several days after eruptions of small pustules. The pustules occur over the trunk and extremities and may include nail beds, palms of the hands, and soles of the feet. Psoriatic erythroderma affects all body surfaces including the hands, feet, nails, trunk, and extremities. *Psoriasis annularis* is a rare form of the disease, and, as its name implies, the lesions are annular in shape.

There are a variety of treatment regimens for psoriasis. Anthralin applied topically has been effective in resolving lesions in approximately 2 weeks. A variation of the treatment, called the Ingram method, involves coal tar applications, ultraviolet-B (UVB) radiation, followed by anthralin paste application. Coal or wood tar (crude tar or wood extract) is one of the oldest and yet one of the most effective forms of treatment. The skin is covered with a film of coal tar for a period of up to several weeks. The exact mechanism of action of the tar products is unknown, but the side effects of the treatment are few. Coal tar preparations may contain other compounds. The Goeckerman regimen consists of combining the therapeutic effects of coal tar and ultraviolet light. Unfortunately, coal tar treatments are less accessible given the restrictions of third-party payers.

Topical, systemic, and intralesionally applied corticosteroids are useful in the treatment of psoriasis. Topical corticosteroids are most effective if they are potent and used under occlusive dressings. Severe cases or acute exacerbations of the disease may warrant the use of systemic corticosteroid therapy. The intralesional injection of the corticosteroid drug, triamcinolone, has proven effective in resistant lesions.

The preferred treatment modality is photochemotherapy using a light-activated form of the drug methotrexate—methoxsalen (8-MOP). Methoxsalen is a psoralen, a light-activated drug that exerts its actions when exposed to ultraviolet-A (UVA) rays in the 320-nm to 400-nm wavelength range. The combination treatment regimen of psoralen (P) and UVA is known by the acronym PUVA. Methotrexate, which is also used in cancer treatment, is an antimetabolite that inhibits DNA synthesis and thus prevents cell mitosis. Methotrexate has been effective in treating psoriasis when given without phototherapy, but the drug has many side effects, including nausea, malaise, leukopenia, thrombocytopenia, and liver function abnormalities. Because methoxsalen is inert until it is exposed to UVA light, its effects are limited to the skin cells that are exposed to both the drug and the UVA light. Methoxsalen is given orally before UVA exposure. Activated by UVA, methoxsalen inhibits DNA synthesis and thus prevents cell mitosis, thereby decreasing the hyperkeratosis that occurs with psoriasis. The treatment produces a remission, but not a cure. Even though there has been a high success rate with PUVA treatment, it must be used cautiously, because it can induce accelerated aging of exposed skin cancer, development of cataracts, and alterations in immune function. In addition, the skin remains sensitive to sunlight until the methoxsalen is excreted, so that people receiving PUVA treatment should be cautioned to avoid sun exposure for 8 hours after treatment.

Cyclosporine has been used in the treatment of psoriasis and other T cell mediated skin disorders. It is a potent immunosuppressive drug used to prevent rejection in organ transplantation. Its use is limited to severe psoriasis because of severe side effects, including renal dysfunction, hypertension, and increased risk of cancers. Intralesional cyclosporine has also been effective.

Retinoids are under investigation for the treatment of psoriasis. Climatotherapy (moving to a warm climate with saltwater baths for 4 to 6 weeks) has also been an effective treatment. All treatments are palliative, because a cure for psoriasis has not yet been developed.

PITYRIASIS ROSEA

Pityriasis rosea is a skin rash of unknown origin that primarily affects young adults. The incidence is highest in spring and fall. The belief is that it could be viral; the picornavirus is under investigation. Cases occur in clusters and among people who are in close contact with each other, indicating an infectious spread; however, there are no data to support communicability.

The characteristic lesion is a macule or papule with surrounding erythema. The lesion spreads with central clearing much like tinea corporis. This initial lesion is a solitary lesion called the herald patch and is usually on the trunk or neck. As the lesion enlarges and begins to fade away (2 to 10 days), successive crops of lesions appear on the trunk and neck. The extremities, face, and scalp may be involved, and mild to severe pruritus may occur. The disease is self-limiting and usually disappears within 6 to 8 weeks. Treatment measures are palliative and include topical steroids, antihistamines, and colloid baths. Systemic corticosteroids may be indicated in severe cases.

ALLERGIC SKIN RESPONSES

Allergic skin responses involve the body's immune system and are caused by hypersensitivity reactions (see Chapter 12). They include contact dermatitis, atopic and nummular eczema, and drug reactions.

CONTACT DERMATITIS

Contact dermatitis is a common inflammation of the skin. There are two types of contact dermatitis—irritant and allergic. Irritant contact dermatitis occurs in people who are in contact with a sufficient amount of the irritant to cause a reaction (Fig. 11-12). It can occur from mechanical means such as rubbing (wool, fiberglass), chemical irritants (those found in common household cleaning products), or environmental irritants (plants, urine). An example is the increased incidence of contact dermatitis from synthetic latex products, specifically, the increased use of rubber gloves and condoms due to the HIV epidemic. Allergic contact dermatitis is the cell-mediated allergy response brought about by sensitization to an allergen. It is a type IV sensitivity (see Chapter 14). This type depends on hapten migration into the skin to produce an immune reaction. Many contact allergens are capable of producing the inflammatory skin response (Table 11-5). The crude forms of many naturally occurring substances are rarely allergenic. Additives such as dyes and perfumes account for the major sources of known allergens. Additional examples are poison ivy, chemicals, and metal sources such as jewelry.

The initial contact dermatitis lesion ranges from a mild erythema with edema to vesicles or large bullae. Secondary lesions from bacterial infection

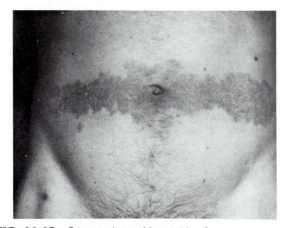

FIG. 11-12. Contact dermatitis resulting from a component of rubber. (Demis, D. J. [Ed.]. [1985]. *Clinical dermatology.* Philadelphia: Harper & Row)

TABLE 11-5. SOURCES OF CONTACT DERMATITIS ALLERGENS

SOURCES	POSSIBLE ALLERGENS
Clothing	Raw material such as wool, polyester, cotton, dyes and sizers in new fabrics and clothing; detergents used to wash clothing
Cosmetics	Dyes, perfumes, oils (*e.g.,* lanolin, coconut oil, olive oil, palm oil)
Cleaning products (soaps, detergents)	Fats, alkali, perfumes, dyes, formaldehyde, hydrochloric acid, sodium carbonate, ammonium hydroxide, and germicidal agents
Occupational exposure	Metals, metal salts, and alloys (nickel); resin, natural and synthetic; tung oil, linseed oil, turpentine; usually the allergens are from the processing of rubber rather than crude rubber (acids, alkalis, solvents, soaps, dust, heat) and are more common from rubber products (gloves, footwear, condoms)
Plants and woods	Ragweed; lichens; poison ivy, oak, and sumac; pine (more from resin and turpentine); caterpillars; and growth on trees and plants
Soap ingredients Fats	Coconut oil, olive oil, palm oil, rosin, and fish or whale oil
Alkali	Sodium hydroxide, potassium hydroxide, sodium carbonate, trisodium phosphate, sodium tripolyphosphate, pyrophosphate, sodium silicate
Perfumes	Seed oil, oil of bergamot, bitter almond oil, eucalyptus oil, geranium oil, lavender oil, peppermint oil, rosemary oil, musk
Coloring agents	D&C yellow No. 11, eosin, rhodamine, fuchsin, ultramarine green

may occur. Lesions can occur almost anywhere on the body. The typical poison ivy lesion consists of vesicles or bullae in a linear pattern. The vesicles and bullae break and weep, leaving an excoriated area.

Treatment measures are aimed at removing the source of the irritant. In some cases, this may mean that the person needs to modify his or her behavior in the home or workplace to avoid the irritant. The actual treatment regimen differs according to the type of irritant and the severity of the reaction. Minor cases are treated by washing the affected areas to remove further sources of irritation, applying antipruritic creams and lotions, and bandaging the exposed areas. More extreme cases are treated with wet dressings, systemic corticosteroids, and oral antihistamines.

ECZEMA

There are two forms of eczema, atopic and nummular. Atopic eczema (also called atopic dermatitis) is a common skin disorder that occurs in two clinical forms, infantile and adult. It is associated with a type I hypersensitivity reaction (see Chapter 14). There is usually a family history of asthma, hay fever, or atopic dermatitis. The infantile form is characterized by vesicle formation, oozing, and crusting with excoriations. It usually begins in the cheeks and may progress to involve the scalp, arms, trunk, and legs (Fig. 11-13). The infantile form usually becomes mil-

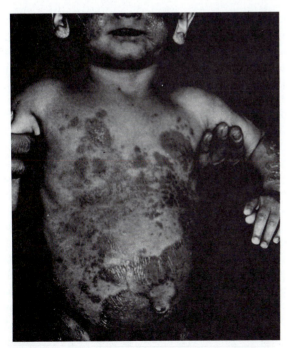

FIG. 11-13. Severe infantile atopic dermatitis. (Demis, D. J. [Ed.] [1985]. *Clinical dermatology.* Philadelphia: Harper & Row)

der and often disappears after the age of 3 or 4 years. Adolescents and adults generally have dry, leathery, and hyperpigmented or hypopigmented lesions located in the antecubital and popliteal areas that may spread to the neck, hands, feet, or eyelids, and behind the ears. Itching may be severe with both forms, and secondary infections are common.

The treatment measures for eczema are designed around the chronic nature of the disease. Exposure to environmental irritants and foods that cause exacerbation of the symptoms is avoided. Wool and lanolin (wool fat) often aggravate the condition. Dryness of the skin often causes the condition to become worse. For this reason, bathing and the use of soap and water should be reduced. Avoidance of temperature changes and stress helps to minimize abnormal and cutaneous vascular and sweat responses. Acute weeping lesions are treated with soothing lotions, soaps, baths, or wet dressings. Subacute or subsiding lesions may be treated with lotions containing mild antipruritic agents. Chronic dry lesions are treated with ointments and creams containing lubricating, keratolytic, and antipruritic agents as indicated. Topical or systemic corticosteroid therapy may be indicated for severe cases.

The exact etiology of nummular eczema is unknown. There is usually a history of asthma, hay fever, or atopic dermatitis. Lesions consist of coin-shaped (nummular) papulovesicular patches mainly involving the arms and legs. The disease is chronic and most often occurs in elderly men. Lichenification and secondary bacterial infections are common. Ingestion of iodides and bromides usually aggravates the condition. The treatment is palliative. Frequent bathing and foods rich in iodides and bromides should be avoided. Topical corticosteroids and antibiotics are prescribed as necessary.

DRUG-INDUCED SKIN ERUPTIONS

Without exception, any drug can cause a localized or generalized skin eruption. Generally, topical drugs are responsible for a localized contact dermatitis type of rash, whereas systemic drugs cause generalized skin lesions. Table 11-6 describes the characteristics of selected drug-induced skin eruptions.

The diagnosis of a drug sensitivity depends almost entirely on accurate reporting by the patient, because the lesions from drug sensitization differ greatly. Drug reactions mimic almost all other skin lesions described in this chapter. The treatment is aimed at eliminating the offending drug. Mild skin eruptions are treated symptomatically, whereas severe systemic drug eruptions often require systemic corticosteroid therapy and antihistamines.

TABLE 11-6. TYPES OF RASHES ASSOCIATED WITH DRUG-INDUCED SKIN ERUPTIONS

DRUGS	TYPE OF RASH
Barbiturates, arsenic, sulfonamides, quinine	Resembles measles
Barbiturates, arsenic, codeine, morphine	Resembles scarlet fever
Bismuth, gold, barbiturates	Resembles pityriasis rosea
Quinine, procaine, antihistamines	Eczematous
Isoniazid, para-aminosalicylic acid combinations	Resembles nummular eczema
Penicillin, salicylates, opium	Urticaria
Bromides, iodides, testosterone, ACTH	Pustular (acne)
Sulfonamides, penicillin, phenylbutazone	Vesicular, bullous
Quinacrine, arsenic, gold	Lichen planus
Contraceptive drugs, quinacrine	Pigment changes
Arsenic, mercury	Keratosis and epitheliomas

SCABIES, LICE, AND TICKS

The skin is susceptible to a variety of disorders as a result of an invasion or infestation by bugs, ticks, or parasites. The rash, or sometimes singular lesion, differs depending on the causative agent.

SCABIES

Scabies is caused by a mite (*Sarcoptes scabiei*) that burrows into the epidermis. After a female mite is impregnated, she burrows into the skin and lays two to three eggs each day for 4 or 5 weeks. Three to 5 days later, the eggs hatch and the larvae migrate to the skin surface. At this point, they burrow into the skin only for food or for protection. The larvae molt and become nymphs; they molt once more to become adults. Once they are impregnated, the cycle is repeated.

The characteristic lesion is a small burrow, approximately 2 mm long, that may be red to red-brown in color. Small vesicles may cover the burrows. The areas most commonly affected are the interdigital web of the finger, flexor surface of the wrist, inner surface of the elbow, axilla, female nipple, penis, belt line, and gluteal crease. Pruritus is common and may

result from the burrows, the fecal material of the mite, or both. Excoriations may develop from scratching, and secondary bacterial infections and severe skin lesions may occur if the condition is untreated.

Scabies affects all people in all socioeconomic classes. Usually more prevalent in times of war and famine, it reached pandemic proportions in the 1970s, perhaps as a result of poverty, sexual promiscuity, and worldwide travel.

Diagnosis is done by skin scrapings. Mineral oil is applied to the skin, and a scraping is obtained. A positive diagnosis relies on the presence of the mite or its feces. The treatment is simple and curative. Lindane lotion or cream (Kwell) is applied over the entire skin surface for 12 hours. Repeat applications may be recommended in certain cases, but one treatment is usually sufficient. Controversy exists over bathing before the treatment. Some physicians no longer recommend bathing before the treatment, perhaps to enhance full drug effectiveness.[20] Clothes and towels are disinfected with hot water and detergent. Treatment of outer clothing and furniture is unnecessary because the mite cannot live away from the body for more than a few hours. If symptoms persist after treatment, the patient should be advised not to retreat the condition without consulting the physician. A red-brown nodule, thought to be an allergic response from the mite parts left on the skin, may form after treatment.

PEDICULOSIS

Pediculosis is the term for infestation with lice (genus *Pediculus*). Lice are gray, gray-brown, or red-brown, oval, wingless insects that live off the blood of humans and animals. Lice are host-specific; lice that live on animals do not transfer to humans, and vice versa. Lice are also host-dependent; they cannot live apart from the host beyond a few hours. As with scabies, the incidence of pediculosis increased in the 1970s to pandemic levels, probably because of increases in poverty, sexual experiences, and worldwide travel.

Three types of lice affect humans: *Pediculus humanus corporis* (body lice), *Pediculus pubis* (pubic lice), and *Pediculus humanus capitis* (head lice). Although these three types differ biologically, they have similar life cycles. The life cycle of a louse consists of an unhatched egg or "nit," three molt stages, an adult reproductive stage, and death. Before adulthood, lice live off the host and are incapable of reproduction. After fertilization, the egg is laid by the female louse along a hair shaft. These nits appear pearl-gray to brown. Depending on the site, a female louse can lay anywhere between 150 and 300 nits in her life. The life span of a feeding louse is 30 to 50 days. Lice are equipped with stylets that pierce the skin. Their saliva contains an anticoagulant that prevents host blood from clotting while the louse is feeding. A louse takes up to 1 mg of blood during a feeding.

Pediculosis Corporis. Pediculosis corporis is infestation with *Pediculus humanus corporis*, or body lice, which are chiefly transferred through contact with infested clothing and bedding. The lice live in the clothes fibers, coming out only to feed. Unlike the pubic louse and the head louse, the body louse can survive 10 to 14 days without the host. The typical lesion is a macule at the site of the bite. Papules and wheals may develop. The infestation is pruritic and evokes scratching that brings about a characteristic linear excoriation. Eczematous patches are frequently found. Secondary lesions may become scaly and hyperpigmented and leave scars. Areas typically affected are the shoulders, trunk, and buttocks. The presence of nits in the seams of clothes confirms a diagnosis of body lice. Treatment measures consist of eradicating the louse and nits both on the body and on clothing. Washing clothes in hot water and steam pressing or dry-cleaning them are recommended. Special attention is given to the seams. Merely storing clothing in plastic bags for 2 weeks rids clothes of lice. Many physicians prefer not to treat the body unless nits are in evidence on hair shafts. If treatment is indicated, lindane shampoo or topical preparations containing gamma benzene hexachloride, pyrethrum, or malathion are recommended.

Pediculosis Pubis. Pediculosis pubis (the infestation known as crabs, or pubic lice) is a nuisance disease that is uncomfortable and embarrassing. The disease is spread by intimate contact with someone harboring *Phthirus pubis*. Lice and nits are located in the pubic area of males and females. Occasionally, they may be found in secondary sex sites such as the beard in males or the axilla in males and females. Symptoms include intense itching and irritation of the skin. Diagnosis is made on the basis of symptoms and microscopic examination. The treatment is the same as that used for head lice.

Pediculosis Capitis. Pediculosis capitis, or infestation with head lice, primarily affects white-skinned people; it is relatively unknown in darker-skinned people. In addition, the incidence is higher in female children, although hair length has not been indicated as a contributing factor. Infestations of head lice are usually confined to the nape of the neck and behind the ears. Less frequently, head lice are found on the beard, pubic areas, eyebrows, and body hairs.

Head lice are primarily transmitted by human-to-human contact. A positive diagnosis depends on the presence of firmly attached nits on hair shafts.

Crawling adults are rarely seen. Pruritus and scratching of the head are the primary indicators that head lice may be present. The scalp may appear red and excoriated from scratching. In severe cases, the hair becomes matted together in a crusty foul-smelling "cap." An occasional morbilliform rash, which may be misdiagnosed as rubella, may occur with lymphadenopathy.

Head lice are treated with lindane (Kwell). The medicated shampoo is applied to dry hair in sufficient quantity to wet the hair and skin. After the hair and head are massaged, small amounts of water are added to produce a lather. The head is scrubbed for 4 minutes, rinsed, and dried. The treatment may be repeated after 1 week to eliminate the hatching nits. Dead nits may be removed with a fine-toothed comb.

TICKS

Ticks are insects that live in woods and underbrush. They attach to human and animal hosts and burrow into the epidermis, where they feed on blood. The tick bite is not problematic; the dangers stem rather from the infectious bacteria or viruses that they carry to human hosts. There are many tickborne illnesses, including Central European encephalitis, Q fever, babesiasis, and relapsing fever. A common tickborne disease in the United States is Rocky Mountain spotted fever (RMSF), which is caused by a tick that carries *Rickettsia rickettsii*. RMSF used to be localized to the Rocky Mountain area, but by 1982 most states had reported a case of RMSF.

The initial tick bite appears as a papule or macule with or without a central punctum. The tick burrows in and enlarges as it feeds. The tick must be attached to the human host for 4 to 6 hours before the rickettsiae are activated by the blood. Rickettsiae are found in the tick feces and body parts. The rickettsiae enter the bloodstream and multiply in the body tissues. Within 4 to 8 days, the patient experiences fever, headache, muscle aches, nausea, and vomiting. A rash that starts on the wrist or ankle follows. The characteristic rash is a macular or maculopapular rash that spreads to the rest of the body. Other symptoms include generalized edema, conjunctivitis, petechial lesions, photophobia, lethargy, confusion, and cranial nerve deficits.

The treatment for RMSF requires hospitalization and antibiotic therapy. The most important measure is to prevent tick bites by using insect repellents while engaged in activities in the woods. Once a tick has attached itself, it is important to remove all the body parts to limit the possibility of infection. Ticks may be removed by slowly pulling them, dousing them with mineral oil or alcohol before removing them with a tweezers, or applying a hot match to the end of the tick. The latter method is not the most effective, because the tick may regurgitate into the open wound.

Lyme disease is the most common tickborne disease in the United States, characterized by a distinctive skin lesion, erythema chronicum migrans (ECM). It is a red macule or papule that extends in an annular fashion with a central clearing, which has been called the *bull's eye*. The disease is caused by a spirochete, *Borrelia burgdorferi*, and occurs in three stages: (1) appearance of the ECM, often accompanied by malaise, fatigue, fever, headache, and lymphadenopathy; (2) cardiac and neurologic manifestations that present weeks to months later; and (3) arthritis, which develops weeks to years later in about 60% of cases. The disease was first reported in Europe in the early 1900s and in the United States in 1976. It was named Lyme disease after the town in Connecticut where the disease was discovered due to the efforts of a mother who reported eight cases of juvenile arthritis. Incidence rates are highest in three geographic areas in the United States: (1) coastal northeastern (Massachusetts to Maryland), (2) midwest (Minnesota and Wisconsin), and western (California, Oregon, Utah, and Nevada). Differences exist in the symptoms between Europe and United States; for example, the arthritis symptoms occur more frequently in the United States. Research continues in an effort to standardize and improve the inaccuracies of serologic testing methods for diagnosis. Preventive measures include using tick repellents, wearing clothing that covers the body, and checking for and removing ticks every 3 to 4 hours. Transmission of the disease occurs only if the tick has fed for several hours on the host. Treatment consists of tetracycline and penicillin therapy and is most effective if initiated during the ECM stage. Longer courses of therapy are indicated in the presence of latent forms of the disease. Ceftriaxone, an antibiotic, is under investigation for its potential merit in the treatment of the arthritis symptoms.

PHOTOSENSITIVITY AND SUNBURN

Physical and mechanical stimuli such as fire, electromagnetic radiation, and ionizing radiation can cause skin burns. Many of these burns occur accidentally in the home or workplace. UVB radiation, or sunlight, also causes skin changes. The obvious and desired skin change is tanning; yet most forms of skin cancer are directly related to sun exposure. Besides cancerous lesions, several skin alterations, such as senile lentigines, have been linked to UVB exposure. Exposure to the sun, as well as harsh weather, has also been linked to early wrinkling and aging of the skin.

Some drugs are classified as photosensitive drugs because they produce an exaggerated response to ultraviolet light when the drug is taken in combination with sun exposure (Chart 11-1).

The skin, as an organ, is the protective shield against harmful UVB rays from the sun. Living epidermal cells are damaged when 280-nm to 310-nm wavelengths penetrate the skin.

The wavelength of sunlight in an area is determined by the ozone layer. Ozone absorbs wavelengths shorter than 320 nm; the shortest wavelength of sunlight reaching the earth is about 290 nm. The diminishing ozone layer surrounding the earth is believed to be a critical factor in increased ultraviolet light exposure and concomitant increased incidence of cancerous skin lesions over the past decade. Smoke and fog may play a part in reducing the intensity of ultraviolet radiation.[24]

With UVB exposure, human cells release vasoactive and injurious chemicals, resulting in vasodilation and sunburn. The melanin in the stratum corneum protects the skin by absorbing the ultraviolet rays, and the skin responds to sunlight exposure by increasing its melanin content as a means of preventing destruction of the lower skin layers.

Sunburn ranges from mild to severe. A mild sunburn consists of varying degrees of redness 2 to 12 hours after exposure to the sun. Varying degrees of inflammation, vesicle eruption, weakness, chills, fever, malaise, and pain accompany more severe forms of sunburn. Scaling and peeling follow any overexposure to sunlight. Black skin also burns and may appear grayish or gray-black.

The Food and Drug Administration (FDA) requires a rating on all commercial suntan preparations based on their ability to occlude UVB rays. The ratings are generally on a scale of 1 to 35, with 1 being least occlusive to sunlight. Total sun-blocking agents with ratings of 35 and higher are available on the market. Para-aminobenzoic acid (PABA) is the most effective blocking ingredient in many suntan creams. Suntan creams should be used diligently and according to the person's tendency to burn rather than

---

CHART 11-1: SOME DRUGS THAT INDUCE PHOTOSENSITIVITY

Sulfonamides
Thiazide diuretics
Furosemide
Sulfonylurea hypoglycemia agents
Tetracycline (particularly demeclocycline)
Phenothiazine, antipsychotic drugs
Nalidixic acid

tan. If the desired outcome of sun exposure is a good suntan, prevention of excessive exposure to harmful ultraviolet rays is the best policy. Early morning and late afternoon sun exposures are less harmful because the ultraviolet rays are longer. Although longer wavelength rays are less apt to cause severe sunburn, they, too, have been implicated in the development of skin cancers. Given the alarming increase in the rates of cancerous lesions in the adolescent and young adult populations, the popular slogan, "no tan is the best tan," may be the best policy. An estimated 78% decrease in skin cancers would occur if children under 18 used sunscreens with a blocking agent of at least 15.[25]

Another preventive measure includes knowing about sunlight and how to protect the skin. Shade does not necessarily protect people from the sun's rays, because ultraviolet rays are reflected from many surfaces. Sand is a good reflector of sunlight. Therefore, a person can get sunburned even while sitting under an umbrella on a sandy beach. Water absorbs ultraviolet light and does not reflect it, as is commonly thought.[24]

Severe sunburns are treated with boric acid soaks and topical creams to limit pain and maintain skin moisture. Extensive second- and third-degree burns require hospitalization and specialized burn care techniques.

NEOPLASMS

There are a number of premalignant and malignant skin lesions. Most of these are found on the skin surfaces exposed to sun and harsh weather. Nevi are common benign tumors of the skin. Cancer of the skin is the most common of all cancers. The American Cancer Society reports that there were an estimated 600,000 new cases of skin cancer in 1990. Most of them were highly curable basal or squamous cell carcinoma.[26]

NEVI

Nevi, or moles, are common congenital or acquired tumors of the skin. Almost all adults have nevi, some in greater numbers than others. Nevi can be pigmented or nonpigmented, flat or elevated, and hairy or nonhairy. Pigmented nevi are derived from neural crest-derived cells (nevocellular nevi) that include modified melanocytes of various shapes. Histologically, most nevi begin as aggregates of well-defined cells located within the lower epidermal layer that lies adjacent to the dermis. These nevi are called *junctional nevi*. Eventually, nevus cells begin to grow into the dermis. *Compound nevi* contain both epidermal

and dermal components. *Dermal nevi* are located within the dermis.

Generally, nevocellular nevi are tan to deep brown, uniformly pigmented, small papules with well-defined and rounded borders. Blue nevi have a blue-black color. Moles are important because of their capacity for transformation to malignant melanomas. The relationship between preexisting benign nevi and malignant melanoma is unclear. Although the average person has about 20 moles, only 4 people out of 100,000 develop a malignant melanoma. Two types of pigmented nevus are associated with malignant transformation; these are the congenital melanocytic nevi and the large atypical or dysplastic nevi (discussed later in this chapter). Because of the possibility of malignant transformation, any mole that undergoes a change in size, thickness, or color, causes itching, or bleeds, warrants immediate medical attention.

BASAL CELL CARCINOMA

Basal cell carcinoma is the most common form of skin cancer (Fig. 11-14). Like other skin cancers, basal cell carcinoma has increased in occurrence over the past two decades. Light-skinned people are more susceptible; black- and brown-skinned people are rarely affected. It is a nonmetastasizing tumor that extends wide and deep if left untreated. These tumors are

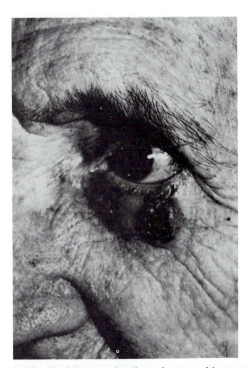

FIG. 11-14. Nodular basal cell carcinoma with central ulceration. (Demis, D. J. [Ed.]. [1985]. *Clinical dermatology.* Philadelphia: Harper & Row)

most frequently seen on the head and neck and, less commonly, on the skin surfaces unexposed to the sun. Basal cell carcinoma usually occurs in people who are exposed to great amounts of sun.

The most common type of basal cell carcinoma is the nodular (noduloulcerative) basal cell epithelioma. It begins as a small, flesh-colored smooth pink translucent nodule that enlarges over time. Telangiectatic vessels are frequently seen beneath the surface. Over the years, a central depression forms that progresses to an ulcer surrounded by the original shiny, waxy border.

The second most common basal cell carcinoma is the superficial form, which is most often seen on the chest or back. It begins as a flat, nonpalpable erythematous plaque. The red scaly areas slowly enlarge with nodular borders and telangiectatic bases. This type of skin cancer is difficult to diagnose because it mimics other dermatologic problems.

In both cases, tumors are biopsied for diagnosis. The treatment depends on the site and extent of the lesion. The most important treatment goal is complete elimination of the lesion. Also important is the maintenance of function and optimal cosmetic effect. Curettage with electrodesiccation, surgical excision, irradiation, and chemosurgery are effective in removing all cancerous cells. Patients should be checked at regular intervals for recurrence.

SQUAMOUS CELL CARCINOMA

Squamous cell carcinomas are malignant tumors of the outer epidermis. An increase in the incidence of squamous cell carcinomas has occurred consistent with increased UVB exposure. There are two types of squamous cell carcinoma: intraepidermal squamous cell carcinoma and invasive squamous cell carcinoma. Intraepidermal squamous cell carcinoma remains confined to the epidermis for a long time, but may at some unpredictable time penetrate the basement membrane to the dermis and metastasize to the regional lymph nodes. Invasive squamous cell carcinoma can develop from intraepidermal carcinoma or from a premalignant lesion. It may be slow or fast growing with metastasis.

Squamous cell carcinoma is a scaly, keratotic slightly elevated lesion with an irregular border, usually with a shallow chronic ulcer. Later lesions grow outward, show large ulcerations, and have persistent crusts and raised, erythematous borders. These lesions occur on sun-exposed areas of the skin, particularly the nose, forehead, helixes of the ears, lower lip, and back of the hands (Fig. 11-15).

The mechanisms of squamous cell carcinoma development are unclear. Sunlight seems to be implicated as a causative factor. Most squamous cell cancers occur in sun-exposed areas of the skin. Outdoor

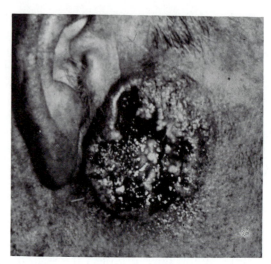

FIG. 11-15. *Squamous cell carcinoma.* (Demis, D. J. [Ed.]. [1985]. *Clinical dermatology.* Philadelphia: Harper & Row)

people are more affected, there is less incidence in dark-skinned people, and the incidence increases as the latitude decreases. Other suspected causes include exposure to arsenic, gamma radiation, tars, and oils.

Treatment measures are aimed at the removal of all cancerous tissue using methods such as electro-surgery, excision surgery, chemosurgery, or radiation therapy. After removal, the area is observed closely for signs of squamous cell carcinoma recurrence.

MALIGNANT MELANOMA

Malignant melanoma is a malignant tumor of the melanocytes. It is a rapidly progressing, metastatic form of cancer that accounts for 2.5% of all cancers.[27] It is the primary cause of death of all skin diseases. There has been a dramatic increase in the incidence of malignant melanoma over the past two decades with the incidence almost tripling over the past four decades. There is a concomitant 3% increase in mortality annually. The thinning of the ozone layer in the earth's stratosphere has been a central factor in this incidence rate.[28] Public health screening measures, early diagnosis, increased knowledge of precursor lesions, and greater public knowledge of the disease may also account for the increased incidence rates. These factors have also led to earlier intervention and increased survival rates of people who have malignant melanoma.

The incidence is highest in white, higher social class, professional indoor workers. Severe, blistering sunburns in early childhood and intermittent intense sun exposures (trips to sunny climates) contribute to increased susceptibility to melanoma in young and middle-aged adults. The rate of incidence is increased for people who immigrate to sunny locations. Incidence rates are higher in people who burn easily and tan minimally. The use of suntanning salons has also been implicated in the development of malignant melanoma. Malignant melanomas occur less in brown-skinned people and seldom in black-skinned people.[29, 30]

Malignant melanomas differ in size and shape (Fig. 11-16). Their exact etiology, specifically how and when a nevus converts to a melanoma, remains unknown. The vast majority seem to arise from pre-existing benign nevi or as new molelike growths.[27] Usually, they are slightly raised and black or brown. Borders are irregular, and surfaces are uneven. Periodically, melanomas ulcerate and bleed; there may be surrounding erythema, inflammation, and tenderness. Dark melanomas are often mottled with red, blue, and white shades. These three colors represent three concurrent processes: melanoma growth (blue), inflammation and the body's attempt to localize and destroy the tumor (red), and scar tissue formation (white). Malignant melanomas can appear anywhere on the body. They are frequently found on sun-exposed areas, but sun exposure alone does not account for the development of melanomas. In men, they are frequently found on the trunk, head, neck, and arms; in women, they are found on the legs, arms, trunk, head, and neck.

Four types of melanomas have been identified: superficial spreading melanoma, lentigo maligna melanoma, nodular melanoma, and acral-lentiginous melanoma.[29] Superficial spreading melanoma is characterized by a raised-edged nevus with lateral growth. It has a disorderly appearance in color and outline and tends to have a biphasic growth, horizontally and vertically. It typically ulcerates and bleeds with growth. This type of lesion accounts for 70% of all melanomas and is most prevalent in people who sunburn easily and have intermittent sun exposure. Lentigo maligna melanoma accounts for 4% to 10% of all melanoma. It is a slow-growing flat nevus and occurs primarily on sun-exposed areas of elderly people. This type is most closely associated with cumulative exposure to the sun. Nodular melanoma is raised and initially grows vertically, is of a uniform blue-black color, and is sharply delineated. These lesions tend to look like blood blisters. Acral-lentiginous melanoma occurs primarily in black- and brown-skinned people on the palms of the hands, soles of the feet, nail beds, and mucous membranes. It has the appearance of lentigo maligna.

Three precursor lesions have been identified in the development of melanoma: lentigo maligna, congenital melanocytic nevi, and dysplastic nevi. Recognition of these precursors is important to the early diagnosis and treatment of melanoma. Lentigo maligna is a flat lesion that looks like an irregular freckle. The lesion is tan-brown to black with irregular pigmentation and borders; it spreads and may look like a stain. Lentigo malignas frequently occur in elderly patients on sun-exposed areas. Congenital melanocytic nevi are large, brown to black hyperpigmented nevi that are present at birth. Generally, they are found on the hands, shoulders, buttocks, entire arm, or trunk of the body. Some involve large areas of the body in garmentlike fashion. These nevi darken with age, and hairs that are present in the lesion become coarser. Malignant changes often occur at an early age (generally by age 10).[12] Dysplastic nevi are flat to slightly raised lesions consisting of neural crest–derived cells (nevocellular nevi) and often have a diameter greater than 1 cm. A person may have hundreds of these lesions; typically, they occur on both sun-exposed and covered areas of the body. They vary in shade from brown and red to flesh tones with irregular borders. There is some familial tendency to develop dysplastic nevi.

The prognosis of malignant melanoma depends on the depth of the lesion and the extent of the disease process. Stage I patients have no evidence of tumor growth in regional lymph nodes, and the disease process is limited to the localized lesion area. Survival rates for these people, with surgical intervention, is uncertain but is longer than for either of the other two stages. Stage II melanomas have metastasized to the regional lymph nodes. Five- to 10-year survival rates have been reported for people in this stage of the disease process. Stage III malignant melanoma involves metastasis to distant organs in the body. The prognosis is poor, with survival ranging up to 16 months.[31]

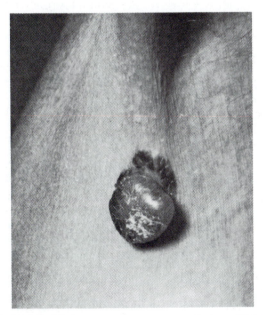

FIG. 11-16. Malignant melanoma on posterior axillary fold (K.C.G.H.). (Sauer, G. C. [1980]. *Manual of skin diseases* (4th ed.). Philadelphia: J.B. Lippincott)

The best treatment is early detection. An ABCD rule has been developed to aid in early diagnosis and timely treatment of malignant melanoma. It stands for asymmetry, border irregularity, color variegation, and diameter greater than 0.6 (pencil eraser size) cm. Patients should be taught to watch for these changes in existing nevi or the development of new nevi: color changes, variegation, irregular borders, bleeding, and growth of nevi. All people should use sun-blocking agents when exposed to the sun, but it is imperative with those whose skin burns easily. Treatment measures vary depending on the severity. Deep and wide excisions with skin grafts are used. Systemic immunotherapy, chemotherapy, and radiation therapy are indicated when the disease becomes systemic.

In summary, primary disorders of the skin include infectious processes, inflammatory conditions, allergic reactions, parasitic infestations, skin reactions to sunlight, and neoplasms. Superficial fungal infections are called dermatophytoses and are commonly known as tinea, or ringworm; they include tinea corporis, tinea capitis, tinea barbae, tinea manus, tinea pedis, tinea unguium, and tinea versicolor. Impetigo, which is caused by staphylococci or beta-hemolytic streptococci, is the most common superficial bacterial infection. Viruses are responsible for verrucae (warts), herpes simplex I lesions (cold sores or fever blisters), and herpes zoster (shingles). Noninfectious inflammatory skin conditions such as acne, lichen planus, psoriasis, and pityriasis rosea are generally of unknown etiology. They are usually localized to the skin and are rarely associated with specific internal disease. Allergic skin responses involve the body's immune system and are caused by hypersensitivity reactions to allergens, environmental agents, drugs, and other substances. The skin is sensitive to a number of disorders resulting from invasion or infestation by bugs, ticks, or parasites. The rash or bite from such invasion is usually singular and varies with the agent. Neoplasms of the skin include basal cell carcinoma, squamous cell carcinoma, and melanoma, with basal cell carcinoma being the most common form. Repeated exposure to the ultraviolet rays of the sun is the principal cause of skin cancer.

■ BLACK SKIN

There are several skin disorders common to African Americans that are not commonly found in whites. Similarly, many skin disorders that affect white-skinned people do not affect darker-skinned people, such as skin cancers. Literature related specifically to black skin disorders is rare; frequently, common occurrences in black skin are mistaken for anomalies.

The greater number of melanosomes produced and transferred to the keratinocyte is responsible for the darker pigmentation in African Americans. In other words, African Americans do not have more melanocytes than whites, but the production of pigment is increased. Skin pallor, cyanosis, and erythema are more difficult to see in African-Americans. Also,

normal variations in skin structure and skin tones make evaluation of black skin difficult (Table 11-7). Often, verbal histories must be relied on to indicate skin changes. Hypopigmentation refers to a loss of pigmentation, and hyperpigmentation refers to excessive melanin production. Often these signs accompany black skin disorders and are important to accurate diagnosis. The appearances of skin disorders listed in Table 11-8 are common to the African American who represents a blend of African Negro, European Caucasian, and Native American.

Vitiligo is a pigmentary problem of concern to darkly pigmented people of all races. It also affects whites, but not as often. The lesion is a macular depigmentation with definite borders on the face, axillae, neck, or extremities. The borders are smooth. The patches vary in size from small to large macules involving great skin surfaces. The large macular type is much more common. Depigmented areas, which burn in sunlight, appear white or flesh-colored or sometimes grayish-blue. Vitiligo appears at any age, in men and women alike, and usually occurs before the age of 21 years. It has been on the rise in India, Pakistan, and Far Eastern countries. Although the cause is unknown, inheritance and autoimmune fac-

TABLE 11-7. COMMON NORMAL VARIATIONS IN BLACK SKIN

VARIATION	APPEARANCE
Futcher (Voigt's) line	Demarcation between darkly pigmented and lightly pigmented skin in upper arm; follows spinal nerve distribution; common in black and Japanese populations
Midline hypopigmentation	Line or band of hypopigmentation over the sternum, dark or faint, lessens with age; common in Latin American and black populations
Nail pigmentation	Linear dark bands down nails or diffuse nail pigmentation, brown, blue or blue-black
Oral pigmentation	Blue to blue-gray pigmentation of oral mucosa; gingivae also affected
Palmar changes	Hyperpigmented creases, small hyperkeratotic papules, and tiny pits in creases
Plantar changes	Hyperpigmented macules, can be multiple with patchy distribution, irregular borders, and variance in color

(Developed from information in Rosen, T., & Martin, S. [1981]. *Atlas of black dermatology.* Boston: Little, Brown.)

TABLE 11-8. APPEARANCE OF COMMON DISORDERS OF BLACK SKIN

DISORDER	APPEARANCE
Hot-comb alopecia	Well-defined patches of scalp alopecia on crown; extends down; decreased number of follicular orifices, hair loss irreversible; due to use of hot comb with petroleum, more common with Afro hairstyles
Infantile acropustulosis	Crops of vesicopustules for 7 to 10 days, followed by a 2- to 3-week remission before recurrence; pruritus; affects palms and soles of feet in children 2 to 10 months of age; resolves by 3 years of age
Keloids	Firm, smooth, shiny hairless elevated scars, sometimes hyperpigmented; often with symptomatic pruritus, tenderness, or pain; extremely common even with simple wounds on ears, neck, jaw, cheeks, upper chest, shoulders, and back
Mongolian spot	Very common; ill-defined light blue to slate gray macule in lumbosacral area; usually disappears, but may persist through adulthood
Atopic dermatitis	Follicular lesion development that progresses to a lichenification stage; hyperpigmented lichenifications are interspersed with excoriated pink patches; common in blacks
Pityriasis rosea	Lesions are salmon-pink, dull-red, or dark-brown; profuse fine scales, not commonly seen in white skin; postinflammatory pigmentary changes are more common in blacks
Psoriasis	Does not commonly occur in blacks; distribution is similar, but the plaques are bright-red, violet, or blue-black; pigment changes may persist after treatment
Tinea versicolor	Common in blacks, increased incidence in tropical climates; hypopigmented or extremely hyperpigmented patches, gray to dark brown; occurs more often on the face in blacks than in whites
Lichen planus	Papules are deep purple from pigmentary leakage; oral lesions are uncommon; hypertrophic lesions are more common in blacks than in whites

(Developed from information in Rosen, T. & Martin S. [1981]. *Atlas of black dermatology*. Boston: Little, Brown.)

tors have been implicated. Vitiligo also seems to be implicated as a cutaneous expression of a systemic disorder, especially thyroid disease.[32] The areas affected enlarge over time.

Treatment regimens for vitiligo remain experimental. PUVA treatment has been successful in patients who have involvement of 40% or more of the skin surface. Cosmetics and sunscreens are used for camouflage.

In summary, black skin has an increased number of melanosomes. Thus, skin pallor, cyanosis, and erythema are more difficult to evaluate. Some skin disorders that are common in African Americans are not common in whites, and vice versa. The manifestations of common skin disorders are also different. Vitiligo, a condition of depigmentation, is a problem of concern to darkly pigmented people of all races.

■ REFERENCES

1. Arey, L.B. (1974). *Human histology* (p. 186). Philadelphia: W.B. Saunders.
2. Jacob, S.W., Fracone, C.A., & Lossow, W.J. (1978). *Structure and function in man* (4th ed., p. 75). Philadelphia: W.B. Saunders.
3. Arndt, K.A., & Jick, H. (1976). Rates of cutaneous reactions to drugs. *Journal of the American Medical Association, 235,* 918.
4. Pinkus, H., & Mehregan, A.H. (1981). *A guide to der-* *matohistopathology* (3rd ed., p. 5). New York: Appleton-Century-Crofts.
5. Holbrook, K.A., & Odland, G.F. (1974). Regional differences in the thickness (cell layers) of the human stratum corneum: An ultrastructural analysis. *Journal of Investigative Dermatology, 62,* 415.
6. Katz, S.I., Tamaki, K., & Sachs, D.H. (1979). Epidermal Langerhans cells are derived from cells originating in the bone marrow. *Nature, 282,* 324.
7. Silberberg-Sinakin, I., Baer, R.L., & Thorbekke, G. (1978). Langerhans cells: A review of their nature with emphasis on their immunologic functions. *Progress in Allergy, 24,* 268.
8. Tamaki, K., Stingl, G., & Katz, S.J. (1980). The origin of Langerhans cells. *Journal of Investigative Dermatology, 74,* 309.
9. Hartschuh, W., & Grube, D. (1979). The Merkel cell—a member of the APUD cell system: Fluorescence and electron microscopic contribution to the neurotransmitter function of the Merkel cell granules. *Archives of Dermatological Research, 265,* 115.
10. Herndon, J.H. (1982). Pruritus. In S.L. Moschella (Ed.). *Dermatology update* (pp. 185–196). New York: Elsevier Biomedical.
11. Greco, P.J., & Ende, J. (1992). An office-based approach to the patient with pruritis. *Hospital Practice, 27*(May 30), 121.
12. Robbins, S.L., Cotran, R.S., & Kumar, V. (1984). *Pathologic basis of disease* (3rd ed., pp. 1275, 1279, 1298). Philadelphia: W.B. Saunders.
13. Benenson, A.S. (Ed.). (1990). *Control of communicable diseases in man*. Washington, DC: American Public Health Association.
14. Arbeter, A., Starr, S.E., & Plotkin, S.A. (1986). Var-

icella vaccine studies in healthy children and adults. *Pediatrics, 78,* Suppl 748–756.

15. Hardy, I., Gershon, A.A., Steinberg, S.P., et al. (1991). Varicella Vaccine Collaborative Study Group: The incidence of zoster after immunization with live attenuated varicella vaccine: A study in children with leukemia. *New England Journal of Medicine, 325,* 1545–1550.

16. Dunkle, L.M., Arvin, A.M., Whitley, R.J., et al. (1991). A controlled trial of acyclovir for chickenpox in normal children. *New England Journal of Medicine, 325,* 1539–1554.

17. Klingman, A.M., & Leyden, J. (1981). The interaction of fungi and bacteria in the pathogenesis of athlete's foot. In H.I. Maibach & R. Aly (Eds.). *Skin microbiology: Relevance to clinical infection* (pp. 203–219). New York: Springer-Verlag.

18. Nasemann, T. (1977). *Viral diseases of the skin, mucous membrane and genitalia.* Philadelphia: W.B. Saunders.

19. Spanes, N.P., Williams, V., & Gwynn, M.I. (1990). Effects of hypnotic, placebo, and salicyclic acid treatments on wart regression. *Psychosomatic Medicine, 52,* 109.

20. Parish, L.C., Witkowski, J.A., & Cohen, H.B. (1983). Clinical picture of scabies. In L.C. Parish, W.B. Nutting, & R.M. Schwartzman (Eds.). *Cutaneous infestations of man and animal* (pp. 70–78. New York: Praeger.

21. Strauss, J.S. (1984). Biology of the sebaceous gland and the pathophysiology of acne vulgaris. In N.A. Soter & H.P. Baden (Eds.). *Pathophysiology of dermatologic diseases* (pp. 159–173).

22. Dicken, C.H. (1984). Retinoids: A review. *Journal of the American Academy of Dermatology, 11*(4), 541–552.

23. Poikolainen, K., Reunala, T., Karvonen, J., Lauharanta, J., & Karkkainin, P. (1990). Alcohol intake: A risk factor for psoriasis in young and middle aged men? *British Medical Journal, 300,* 780–783.

24. Pathak, M.A., Fitzpatrick, T.B., Greiter, F., & Kraus, E.W. (1987). Preventive treatment of sunburn, dermatoheliosis, and skin cancer with sun protective agents. In T.B. Fitzpatrick, A.Z. Eisen, K. Wolf, & K.F. Austen (Eds.). *Dermatology in medicine: Textbook and atlas* (pp. 1507–1522). New York: McGraw-Hill.

25. Stern, R.S., Weinstein, M.C., & Baker, S.G. (1986). Risk reduction for nonmelanoma skin cancer with childhood sunscreen use. *Archives of Dermatology, 122,* 537–545.

26. Friedman, R.J., Reigel, D.S., Berson, D.S., et al. (1991). Skin cancer: Basal cell and squamous cell carcinoma. In A.I. Holleb, D.J. Fink, G.P. Murphy (Eds.). *Clinical oncology* (7th ed., pp. 290–303). New York: American Cancer Society.

27. Sherman, C.D., McCune, C.S., & Rubin, P. (1983). Malignant melanoma. In P. Rubin (Ed.). *Clinical oncology* (6th ed., p. 190). New York: American Cancer Society.

28. Fitzpatrick, T.B. (1990). Trends in dermatology: Ozone depletion and the dermatologist: Need we prepare for the consequences of a UVB "holocaust" in the next decades? In A.J. Sober & T.B. Fitzpatrick (Eds.). *The year book of dermatology* (pp. xiii–xxii). St. Louis: C.V. Mosby.

29. Balch, C.M., Houghton, A.N., Milton, G.W., et al. (Eds.). (1992). *Cutaneous melanoma* (2nd ed.). Philadelphia: J.B. Lippincott.

30. Koh, H.K. (1991). Cutaneous melanoma. *New England Journal of Medicine, 325,* 171–182.

31. Sober, A.J., Rhodes, A.R., Day, C.L., Fitzpatrick, T.B., & Mihm, M.C. (1983). Primary melanoma of the skin: Recognition of precursor lesions and estimation of prognosis in Stage I. In T.B. Fitzpatrick, A.Z. Eisen, K. Wolff, I.M. Freedburg, & K.F. Austen (Eds.). *Update: Dermatology in general medicine.* New York: McGraw-Hill.

32. Mosher, D.B., Pathak, M.A., & Fitzpatrick, T.B. (1983). Vitiligo: Etiology, pathogenesis, diagnosis, and treatment. In T.B. Fitzpatrick, A.Z. Eisen, K. Wolff, I.M. Freedburg, & K.F. Austen (Eds.). *Update: Dermatology in general medicine.* New York: McGraw-Hill.

◼ BIBLIOGRAPHY

Abel, E. (Ed). (1992). *Photochemotherapy in dermatology.* New York: Igaku-Shoin.

Arnold, M.L., Odam, R.B., & James, W.D. (Eds.). (1990). *Andrew's diseases of the skin: Clinical dermatology* (8th ed.). Philadelphia: W.B. Saunders.

Banov, C.H., Epstein, & Grayson, L.D. (1992). When an itch persists. *Patient Care,* March 15, 75–88.

Benenson, A.S. (Ed.). (1990). *Control of communicable diseases in man.* Washington, DC: American Public Health Association.

Brunnel, P.A. (1991). Chickenpox—examining our options. *New England Journal of Medicine, 325,* 1577–1579.

Cohen, S. (1978). Skin rashes in infants and children. *American Journal of Nursing, 78,* 1.

Cunliffe, W.J. (1987). Evolution of a strategy for treatment of acne. *Journal of the American Academy of Dermatology, 16,* 591–599.

Epstein, J.H. (1990). Phototherapy and photochemistry. *New England Journal of Medicine, 322,* 1149–1151.

Koh, H.K. (1991). Cutaneous melanoma. *New England Journal of Medicine, 325,* 171–182.

Lowe, N.J. (1991). Systemic treatment of severe psoriasis. *New England Journal of Medicine, 324,* 33–34.

Malloy, B.M., & Perez-Wood, R.C. (1991). Neonatal skin care: Prevention of skin breakdown. *Pediatric Nursing, 17*(1), 41–48.

Marzulli, F.N., & Maibach, H.I. (Eds.). (1991). *Dermatotoxicology.* New York: Hemisphere.

NIH Consensus Conference. (1992). Diagnosis and treatment of early melanoma. *Journal of the American Medical Association, 268,* 1314.

Phillips, R.J., & Dover, J.S. (1992). Recent advances in dermatology. *New England Journal of Medicine, 326,* 167–178.

Rook, A., & Dawber, R. (Eds.). (1990). *Diseases of the hair and scalp.* Oxford: Blackwell.

Slaven, R.G., & Ducomb, D.F. (1989). Allergic contact dermatitis. *Hospital Practice, 24*(7), 39–51.

Sober, A.J., & Fitzpatrick, T.B. (Eds.). (1990). *The year book of dermatology.* St. Louis: C.V. Mosby.

CHAPTER 12

MECHANISMS OF INFECTIOUS DISEASE

W. MICHAEL DUNNE, JR.

Terminology
Agents of Infectious Disease
   Viruses
   Bacteria
     Spirochetes
     Mycoplasmas
   Rickettsiae and Chlamydiae
   Fungi

   Parasites
Mechanisms of Infection
   Epidemiology of Infectious
     Diseases
   Portal of Entry
   Source
   Symptomatology
   Disease Course

Site of Infection
Virulence Factors
Diagnosis of Infectious Diseases
Therapy of Infectious Diseases
   Antimicrobial Agents
   Immunotherapy
   Surgical Intervention

■ OBJECTIVES

After you have studied this chapter, you should be able to meet the following objectives:

- Define *host, infectious disease, colonization, microflora, commensalism, mutualism, parasitic relationship, virulence, pathogen,* and *saprophyte.*
- Describe the concept of host–microorganism interaction.
- Explain the mechanisms of reproduction for viruses, bacteria, rickettsiae, and chlamydiae, fungi, and parasites.
- Use the concepts of incidence, portal of entry, source of infection, symptomatology, disease course, site of infection, agent, and host characteristics to explain the mechanisms of infectious diseases.
- Differentiate between incidence and prevalence and among endemic, epidemic, and panepidemic.
- Describe the stages of an infectious disease after the point at which the potential pathogen enters the body.

- List the systemic manifestations of infectious disease.
- State the two criteria used in the diagnosis of an infectious disease.
- Explain the difference between culture, serology, and antigen or metabolite detection methods for diagnosis of infectious disease.
- Cite three general intervention methods that can be used in treatment of infectious illnesses.
- State four basic mechanisms whereby antibiotics exert their action.
- Differentiate between the terms *bactericidal* and *bacteriostatic.*
- Explain the actions of IGIV and cytokines in treatment of infectious illnesses.

Carol Mattson Porth: PATHOPHYSIOLOGY: CONCEPTS OF ALTERED HEALTH STATES, 4th ed. © 1994, 1990, 1986, 1982 J.B. Lippincott Company

All living creatures share two basic purposes in life—survival and reproduction. This tenet applies equally to humans and to members of the microbial world, including bacteria, viruses, fungi, and protozoa. To satisfy these goals, organisms must extract nutrients essential for growth and proliferation from the environment; for countless organisms, that environment is the human body. Normally, the contact between humans and microorganisms is incidental and in certain situations may actually benefit both organisms. Under extraordinary circumstances, however, the invasion of the human body by microorganisms can produce harmful and potentially lethal consequences. These consequences are collectively termed *infectious diseases*.

■ TERMINOLOGY

All scientific disciplines evolve with a distinct vocabulary, and the study of infectious diseases is no exception. Therefore, the most appropriate way to approach this subject is with a brief discussion of the terminology used to characterize interactions between humans and microbes.

Any organism capable of supporting the nutritional and physical growth requirements of another is called a *host*. Throughout this chapter, the term *host* most often refers to humans supporting the growth of microorganisms. The term *infection* describes the presence and multiplication of a living organism on or within the host. Occasionally, the terms infection and *colonization* are used interchangeably.

One common misconception should be dispelled early on; not all contacts between microorganisms and humans are injurious. The exposed surfaces of the human body (internal and external) are normally and harmlessly inhabited by a multitude of bacteria collectively referred to as the *normal microflora* (Table 12-1). Although the colonizing bacteria acquire nutritional needs and shelter, the host is not adversely affected by the relationship. An interaction such as this is called *commensalism*. The term *mutualism* is applied to an infection in which the microorganism and the host derive benefits from the interaction. For example, certain inhabitants of the human intestinal

TABLE 12-1. LOCATION AND VARIETY OF NONPATHOGENIC NORMAL HUMAN MICROFLORA

AREA	SITE(S)	BACTERIA	
		Gram-positive	Gram-negative
Upper respiratory tract	Mouth, nose	+ + +	+ + +
	Nasopharynx	(Aerobes and	(Aerobes and
	Throat	anaerobes)	anaerobes)
Lower respiratory tract	Larynx	0	0
	Trachea	0	0
	Lungs	0	0
External surfaces	Skin	+ + + +	+
	Outer ear	(Aerobes and	(Transient)
	Eyes	anaerobes)	0
Upper gastro-intestinal tract	Stomach	+	+
	Duodenum	(Transient)	(Transient)
	Esophagus	0	0
	Jejunum	0	0
Lower gastro-intestinal tract	Ileum	+ + +	+ + + +
	Colon	(Predominantly anaerobes)	(Predominantly anaerobes)
External genito-urinary tract	Vagina	+ +	+ +
	Anterior urethra	0	0
Internal genito-urinary tract	Cervix, ovaries	0	0
	Fallopian tubes	0	0
	Uterus, prostate	0	0
	Bladder, kidney	0	0
	Testes, epididymis	0	0
Body fluids	Blood, urine	0	0
	Spinal fluid	0	0
	Synovial fluid	0	0
	Peritoneal fluid	0	0

Key: 0 = none; + = rare; + + = few; + + + = moderate; + + + + = many.

tract extract nutrients from the host and, in turn, secrete essential vitamin by-products of metabolism (*e.g.*, vitamin K), which are absorbed and used by the host. A *parasitic relationship* is one in which only the infecting organism benefits from the relationship. If the host sustains injury or pathologic changes in response to a parasitic infection, the process is called an *infectious disease*.

The severity of an infectious disease can range from mild to life-threatening depending on many variables including the health of the host at the time of infection and the *virulence* (disease-producing potential) of the microorganism. A select group of microorganisms called *pathogens* are so virulent that they are rarely found in the absence of disease. Fortunately, there are few human pathogens among the microbial world. Most microorganisms are harmless *saprophytes*, (*i.e.*, free living organisms obtaining their growth from dead or decaying organic material from the environment). All microorganisms, even saprophytes and members of the normal flora, can be *opportunistic pathogens*, capable of producing an infectious disease when the health and immunity of the

host have been severely weakened by illness, famine, or medical therapy.

In summary, throughout life humans are continuously and harmlessly colonized by a multitude of microscopic organisms. This relationship is kept in check by the intact defense mechanisms of the host (mucosal and cutaneous barriers, normal immune function) and the innocuous nature of most environmental microorganisms. Those factors that either weaken the resistance of the host or increase the virulence of colonizing microorganisms can disturb the equilibrium of the relationship and cause disease. The degree to which the balance is shifted in favor of the microorganism determines the severity of illness.

■ AGENTS OF INFECTIOUS DISEASE

The agents of infectious disease include viruses, bacteria, rickettsiae, and chlamydiae, fungi, and parasites.

VIRUSES

Viruses are the smallest obligate intracellular pathogens. They are incapable of replication outside of a living cell. They have no organized cellular structures

MYCOBACTERIA	PARASITES	MYCOPLASMAS	FUNGI	CHLAMYDIA/ RICKETTSIA	SPIROCHETES
+	+	+	+	0	+
0	(Protozoans)	0	(Yeast)	0	0
0	0	0	0	0	0
0	0	0	0	0	0
0	0	0	0	0	0
+	0	0	+	0	0
0	0	0	(Yeast)	0	0
0	0	0	0	0	0
+	0	0	0	0	0
(Transient)					
0	0	0	0	0	0
0					
+	+	0	+	0	+
0	(Protozoans)	0	(Yeast)		0
0	0	+	+	0	+
0	0	0	(Yeast)	0	0
0	0	0	0	0	0
0	0	0	0	0	0
0	0	0	0	0	0
0	0	0	0	0	0
0	0	0	0	0	0
0	0	0	0	0	0
0	0	0	0	0	0
0	0	0	0	0	0
0	0	0	0	0	0

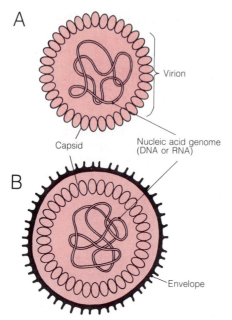

FIG. 12-1. The structure of viruses. The basic structure of a virus includes a protein coat surrounding an inner core of nucleic acid (either DNA or RNA). Some viruses may also be enclosed in a lipoprotein outer envelope.

but simply consist of a protein coat (capsid) surrounding a nucleic acid core (genome) of either RNA or DNA—never both (Fig. 12-1). Some viruses are enclosed within a lipoprotein envelope derived from the cytoplasmic membrane of the parasitized host cell. Certain viruses are continuously shed from the infected cell surface enveloped in buds pinched from the cytoplasmic membrane. Enveloped viruses include members of the herpesvirus group and paramyxoviruses such as influenza.

Viruses must penetrate a susceptible living cell and use the biosynthetic machinery of the cell to produce viral progeny. The process of viral replication is shown in Figure 12-2. Not all viral agents cause the lysis and death of the host cell during the course

of replication. Still other viruses enter the host cell and insert their genetic material (genome) into the host cell chromosome where the genome remains in a latent, nonreplicating state for long periods without causing disease. Under the appropriate stimulation, the virus undergoes active replication and produces symptoms of disease months to years later. Members of the herpesvirus group and adenovirus are the best examples of latent viruses. Herpesviruses include the viral agents of chickenpox and zoster (shingles), genital herpes, cytomegalovirus infections, infectious mononucleosis, and fever blisters. In each of these, the resumption of the latent viral replication may produce symptoms of primary disease (*e.g.,* genital herpes) or cause an entirely different symptomatology (*e.g.,* shingles instead of chickenpox).

Within the past decade, members of the retrovirus group have received considerable attention after identification of the human immunodeficiency viruses (HIV) as the causative agent of acquired immunodeficiency syndrome (AIDS). The retroviruses have a unique mechanism of replication; after entry into the host cell, the viral RNA genome is first translated into DNA by a viral enzyme called reverse transcriptase. The viral DNA copy is integrated into the host chromosome and exists in a latent state similar to the herpesviruses. Reactivation and replication require a reversal of the entire process. Some retroviruses lyse the host cell during the process of replication. In the case of HIV, the infected cells regulate the immunologic defense system of the host and their lysis leads to a permanent suppression of the immune response. In addition to causing infectious diseases, certain viruses also have the ability to transform normal host cells into malignant cells during the replication cycle. This group of viruses is referred to as *oncogenic* and includes certain retroviruses and DNA viruses such as the herpesviruses, adenoviruses, papovaviruses.

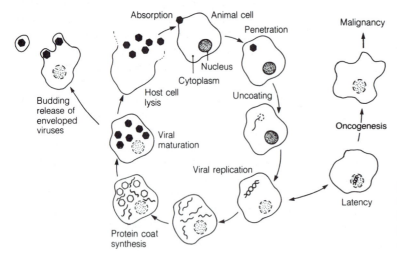

FIG. 12-2. Schematic representation of the many possible consequences of viral infection of host cells, including cell lysis (poliovirus), continuous release of budding viral particles or latency (herpesviruses) and oncogenesis (papovaviruses).

The viruses of humans and animals have been categorized somewhat arbitrarily according to various characteristics including the type of viral genome, the mechanism of replication (the retroviruses), the mode of transmission (anthropodborne viruses or enteroviruses), and the type of disease produced (hepatitis A and B viruses) just to name a few.

BACTERIA

Bacteria are autonomously replicating unicellular organisms known as *prokaryotes* because they lack an organized nucleus. Compared with nucleated eukaryotic cells (see Chapter 1), the structure of the bacterial cell is small and relatively primitive (Fig. 12-3). Bacteria approximate the size of the eukaryotic mitochondria (about 1 μm in diameter) and may, in fact, be the evolutionary ancestors of mitochondria.

Bacteria contain no organized intracellular organelles and only a single chromosome (genome) of DNA. Many bacteria transiently harbor smaller extrachromosomal pieces of circular DNA called plasmids. Occasionally, plasmids contain genetic information that increases the virulence of the organism. Similar to eukaryotic cells, but unlike viruses, bacteria contain both DNA and RNA.

The prokaryotic cell is organized into an internal compartment called the *cytoplasm*, which contains the reproductive and metabolic machinery of the cell. The cytoplasm is surrounded by a flexible lipid membrane (cytoplasmic membrane), which, in turn, is enclosed within a rigid cell wall. The structure and synthesis of the cell wall determine whether the microscopic shape of the bacterium is spherical (*cocci*), helical (*spirilla*), or elongate (*bacilli*). Most bacteria produce a cell wall composed of a distinctive polymer known as *peptidoglycan*. This polymer is only produced by prokaryotes—not eukaryotes—and, therefore, is an ideal target for antibacterial therapy. Several bacteria synthesize an extracellular capsule composed of protein or carbohydrate. The capsule protects the organism from environmental hazards such as the immunologic defenses of the host.

Certain bacteria are motile as the result of external whiplike appendages called *flagella*. The rotary action of the flagella transports the organism through a liquid environment like a propeller. Bacteria can also produce hairlike structures projecting from the cell surface called *pili* or *fimbriae*, which enable the organism to adhere to surfaces such as mucous membranes or other bacteria.

Most prokaryotes reproduce asexually by simple cellular division. The number of planes in which an organism divides can influence the microscopic morphology. For instance, when the cocci divide in chains, they are called *streptococci;* in pairs, *diplococci;* and in clusters, *staphylococci.* The growth rate of bacteria varies significantly among different species and depends to a great deal on physical growth conditions and the availability of nutrients. In the laboratory, a single bacterium placed in a suitable growth environment such as an agar plate reproduces to the extent that it forms a visible colony composed of millions of bacteria within a few hours.

The physical appearance of the colony can be distinctive for each type of bacteria. Some bacteria produce highly resistant *spores* when faced with an unfavorable environment. The spores exist in a quiescent state almost indefinitely until suitable growth conditions are encountered. The spores germinate, and the organism resumes normal metabolism and replication.

Bacteria are extremely adaptable life forms. They inhabit almost every environmental extreme on earth including humans. However, each individual bacterial species has a well-defined set of growth parameters including nutrition, temperature, light, humidity, and atmosphere. Bacteria with extremely strict growth requirements are called *fastidious*. For example, *Neisseria gonorrhoeae*, the bacterium that causes gonorrhea, cannot live for extended periods outside the human body. Some bacteria require oxygen for growth and metabolism and are called *aerobes;* others cannot survive in an oxygen-containing environment and are called *anaerobes*. An organism capable of adapting its metabolism to aerobic or anaerobic conditions is termed *facultatively anaerobic.*

In the laboratory, bacteria are generally classified according to the microscopic appearance and staining properties of the cell. Gram's stain, originally developed in 1884 by the Danish bacteriologist Christian Gram, is still the most widely used staining procedure. Bacteria are designated *gram-positive* if they are stained purple by a primary basic dye (usually crystal violet); organisms that are not stained by the crystal violet but are counterstained a red color by a second dye (safranin) are called *gram-negative*. Staining characteristics and microscopic morphology are used in combination to describe bacteria. For example, *Streptococcus pyogenes*, the agent of scarlet fever and rheumatic fever, is a gram-positive streptococcus that is spherical, grows in chains, and stains purple by Gram's stain. *Legionella pneumophila*, the bacterium responsible for legionnaire's disease, is a gram-negative rod. For purposes of identification and classification, each member of the bacterial kingdom is categorized into a small group of biochemically and genetically related organisms called the *genus* and further subdivided into distinct individuals within the genus called *species*. The genus and species as-

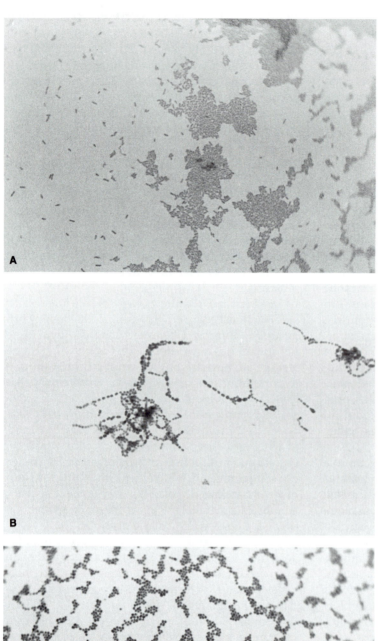

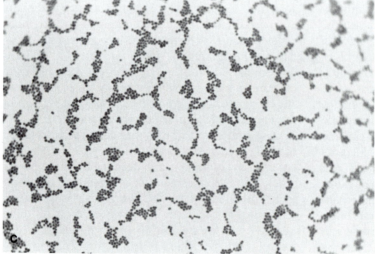

FIG. 12-3. A sampling of the microscopic morphology of bacteria demonstrating the variability of size and shape including bacilli (**A**), streptococci, (**B**), staphylococci (**C**), and diplococci (**D**). Also shown (**E**) is an electron micrograph of a cross-sectioned gram-negative bacterium showing the simple procaryotic cell structure including the cytoplasm (*c*), cytoplasmic membrane (*m*), and the bacterial cell wall (*w*).

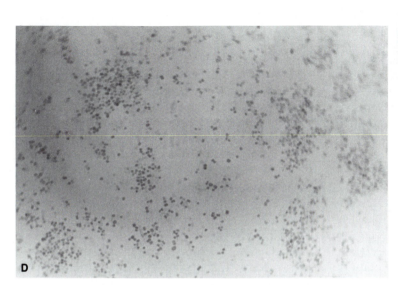

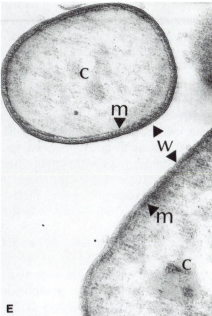

signment of the organism is reflected in its name (*e.g.*, *Staphylococcus* [genus] *aureus* [species]).

SPIROCHETES

The spirochetes are an eccentric category of bacteria that are mentioned separately because of their unusual cellular morphology and mechanism of motility. Technically, the spirochetes are gram-negative rods but are distinctive in that the cell is helical in shape and the length of the organism is many times its width. A series of filaments are wound about the cell wall and extend the entire length of the cell. These filaments propel the organism through an aqueous environment in a corkscrew motion. Spirochetes are anaerobic or facultatively anaerobic organisms and contain three genera: *Leptospira, Borrelia*, and *Treponema*. Each genus has both saprophytic and pathogenic strains. The pathogenic leptospires infect a wide variety of wild and domestic animals. Infected animals shed the organisms into the environment through the urinary tract. Transmission to humans occurs by contact with infected animals or urine-contaminated surroundings. Leptospires gain access to the host directly through mucous membranes or breaks in the skin. In contrast, the borreliae are transmitted from infected animals to humans through the bite of an arthropod vector such as lice or ticks. Included among the genus *Borrelia* are the agents of relapsing fever (*B. recurrentis*) and Lyme disease (*B. burgdorferi*). Pathogenic *Treponema* species require no intermediates and are spread from person to person by direct contact. The most important member of the genus is *Treponema pallidum*, the cause of syphilis.

MYCOPLASMAS

The mycoplasmas are unicellular prokaryotes capable of independent replication. These organisms are less than one third the size of bacteria and contain a small DNA genome approximately one half the size of the bacterial chromosome. The cell is composed of cytoplasm surrounded by a membrane, but, unlike bacteria, the mycoplasmas do not produce a rigid peptidoglycan cell wall. As a consequence, the microscopic appearance of the cell is highly variable, ranging from coccoid forms to filaments, and the mycoplasmas are resistant to cell wall inhibiting antibiotics (*e.g.*, penicillins and cephalosporins). The mycoplasmas of humans are divided into three genera: *Mycoplasma, Ureaplasma*, and *Acholeplasma*. The first two of these require cholesterol from the environment to produce the cell membrane; the *Acholeplasma* do not. In the human host, mycoplasmas are commensals. However, a number of species are capable of producing serious diseases including pneumonia (*Mycoplasma pneumoniae*), genital infections (*Mycoplasma hominis* and *U. urealyticum*), and maternally transmitted respiratory infections to low birth weight infants (*U. urealyticum*).

RICKETTSIAE AND CHLAMYDIAE

The rickettsiae and chlamydiae combine the characteristics of both viral and bacterial agents to produce disease in humans. Both are obligate intracellular pathogens like the viruses and yet both synthesize a rigid peptidoglycan cell wall, reproduce asexually by cellular division, and contain both RNA and DNA similar to the bacteria.

The rickettsiae depend on the host cell for essential vitamins and nutrients, whereas the chlamydiae appear to scavenge intermediates of energy metabolism such as adenosine triphosphate (ATP). The rickettsiae infect but do not produce disease in the cells of certain arthropods such as fleas, ticks, and lice. The organisms are accidentally transmitted to humans through the bite of the arthropod (vector) and produce a number of potentially lethal diseases including Rocky Mountain spotted fever and epidemic typhus.

The chlamydiae are slightly smaller than the rickettsiae but are structurally similar. Unlike the rickettsiae, chlamydiae are transmitted directly between susceptible vertebrates without an intermediate arthropod host. Transmission and replication of chlamydiae occur through a defined life cycle. The infectious form, called an *elementary body*, attaches to and enters the host cell where it transforms into a larger *reticulate body*. The latter undergoes active replication into multiple elementary bodies, which are shed into the extracellular environment to initiate another infectious cycle. Chlamydial diseases of humans include sexually transmitted genital infections (see Chapter 39), ocular infections, and pneumonia of the newborn (*Chlamydia trachomatis*), as well as respiratory disease acquired from infected birds (*Chlamydia psittaci*).

FUNGI

The fungi are free-living, eukaryotic saprophytes found in every habitat on earth. Some are members of the normal human microflora. Fortunately, few fungi are capable of causing diseases in humans, and most of these are incidental self-limited infections of skin and subcutaneous tissue. Serious fungal infections are rare and usually initiated through puncture wounds or inhalation. Despite their normally harmless nature, fungi can cause serious life-threatening opportunistic diseases when host defense capabilities have been disabled.

The fungi can be separated into two groups, yeasts and molds, based on rudimentary differences in their morphology (Fig. 12-4). The yeasts are single-celled organisms, approximately the size of a red blood cell, that reproduce by a budding process. The buds separate from the parent cell and mature into identical daughter cells. Molds, on the other hand, produce long, hollow, branching filaments called *hyphae*. Some molds produce cross walls, which segregate the hyphae into compartments—others do not.

A limited number of fungi are capable of growing as yeasts at one temperature and as molds at another. These organisms are called dimorphic fungi and include a number of human pathogens such as the agents of blastomycosis, histoplasmosis, and coccidioidomycosis (San Joaquin fever).

The visual appearance of a fungal colony tends to reflect its cellular composition. Colonies of yeast are generally smooth with a waxy or creamy texture. Molds tend to produce cottony or powdery colonies composed of mats of hyphae collectively called a *mycelium*. The mycelium can penetrate the growth surface or project above the colony like the roots and branches of a tree. Both yeasts and molds produce a rigid cell wall layer that is chemically unrelated to the peptidoglycan of bacteria, and, therefore, is not susceptible to the effects of penicillinlike antibiotics.

Most fungi are capable of either sexual or asexual reproduction. The former process involves the fusion of zygotes with the production of a recombinant zygospore. Asexual reproduction involves the formation of highly resistant spores called *conidia* or *sporangio spores*, which are borne by specialized structures that arise from the hyphae. Molds are identified in the laboratory by the characteristic microscopic appearance of the asexual fruiting structures and spores. Just like the bacterial pathogens of humans, fungi can only produce disease in the human host if they can grow at the temperature of the infected body site. For example, a number of fungal pathogens called the *dermatophytes* are incapable of growing at core body temperature (37°C) and the infection is limited to the cooler cutaneous surfaces. Diseases caused by these organisms (ringworm, athlete's foot, jock itch) are collectively called superficial mycoses. Systemic mycoses are serious fungal infections of deep tissues and, by definition, are caused by organisms capable of growth at 37°C. Yeasts such as *Candida albicans* are commensals of the skin, mucous membranes, and gastrointestinal tract and are capable of growth at a wider range of temperatures. Intact immune mechanisms and competition for nutrients provided by the bacterial flora normally keep colonizing fungi in check. Alterations in either of these components by disease states or antibiotic therapy can upset the balance, permitting fungal overgrowth and setting the stage for opportunistic infections.

PARASITES

In a strict sense, any organism that derives benefits from its biologic relationship with another organism is a parasite. In the study of microbiology, however, the term *parasite* has evolved to designate members of the animal kingdom that infect and cause disease in

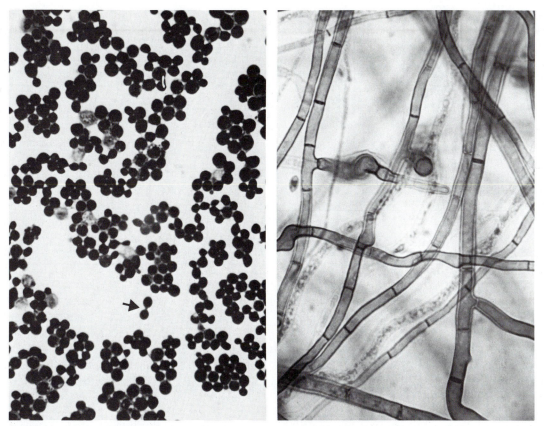

FIG. 12-4. The microscopic morphology of the fungal pathogens of humans. The yeasts (*left*) are single-celled organisms that reproduce by a budding process (*arrow*). The molds (*right*) produce long branched or unbranched filaments called *hyphae*. A number of fungal pathogens called *dimorphic fungi* can exist either as yeasts or molds depending on the temperature of the environment.

other animals and includes protozoa, helminths, and arthropods.

The protozoa are unicellular animals with a complete complement of eukaryotic cellular machinery including a well-defined nucleus and organelles. Reproduction may be sexual or asexual, and life cycles may be simple or complicated with several maturation stages requiring more than one host for completion. Most are saprophytes, but a few have adapted to the accommodations of the human environment and produce a variety of diseases including malaria, amebic dysentery, and giardiasis. Protozoan infections can be passed directly from host to host (*e.g.,* sexual contact), indirectly through contaminated water or food, or by way of an arthropod vector. Direct or indirect transmission results from the ingestion of highly resistant cysts or spores that are shed in the feces of an infected host. When the cysts reach the intestine, they mature into vegetative forms called trophozoites which, in turn, are capable of asexual reproduction or cyst formation. Most trophozoites are motile by means of flagella, cilia, or ameboid motion.

The helminths are a collection of wormlike parasites, which include the roundworms (nematodes), tapeworms (cestodes), and flukes (trematodes). The helminths reproduce sexually within the definitive host, and some require an intermediate host for the development and maturation of offspring. Humans can serve as the definitive or intermediate host and in certain diseases (*e.g.,* trichinosis) as both. Transmission of helminth diseases occurs primarily through the ingestion of fertilized eggs (ova) or the penetration of infectious larval stages through the skin—either directly or with the aid of an arthropod vector. Helminth infections can involve many organ systems and sites including the liver and lung, urinary and intestinal tracts, circulatory and central nervous systems, and muscle. Although most helminth diseases have been eradicated from the United States, they are still a major health concern of developing nations.

The parasitic arthropods of humans and animals include the vectors of infectious diseases (*i.e.,* ticks, mosquitoes, and biting flies) and the ectoparasites. The ectoparasites infest external body surfaces and cause localized tissue damage or inflammation secondary to the bite or burrowing action of the arthro-

TABLE 12-2. COMPARISON OF CHARACTERISTICS OF HUMAN MICROBIAL PATHOGENS

ORGANISM	DEFINED NUCLEUS	GENOMIC MATERIAL	SIZE*	INTRACELLULAR/ EXTRACELLULAR	MOTILITY
Virus	No	DNA or RNA	0.02–0.3	I	–
Bacteria	No	DNA	0.5–15	I/E	±
Mycoplasmas	No	DNA	0.2–0.3	E	–
Spirochetes	No	DNA	6–15	E	+
Rickettsias	No	DNA	0.2–2	I	–
Chlamydia	No	DNA	0.3–1	I	–
Yeasts	Yes	DNA	2–60	I/E	–
Molds	Yes	DNA	2–15 (hyphal width)	E	–
Protozoans	Yes	DNA	1–60	I/E	+
Helminths	Yes	DNA	2mm–>1 m	E	+

*Micrometers unless indicated.

pod. The most prominent human ectoparasites are mites (scabies), chiggers, lice (head, body, and pubic), and fleas. Transmission of ectoparasites occurs directly by contact with immature or mature forms of the arthropod or its eggs found on the infested host or the host's clothing, bedding, or grooming articles (*e.g.,* combs and brushes). Many of the ectoparasites are vectors of other infectious diseases including endemic typhus and bubonic plague (fleas) and epidemic typhus (lice). A summary of the salient characteristics of human microbial pathogens is presented in Table 12-2.

In summary, this section of the chapter underscores the extreme diversity of prokaryotic and eukaryotic microorganisms capable of causing infectious diseases in humans. With the advent of immunosuppressive medical therapy and immunosuppressive diseases such as AIDS, the number and type of potential microbic pathogens, the so-called opportunistic pathogens, have increased dramatically. However, the majority of infectious illnesses in humans continue to be caused by only a small fraction of the organisms that comprise the microscopic world.

■ MECHANISMS OF INFECTION

EPIDEMIOLOGY OF INFECTIOUS DISEASES

Epidemiology, in the context of this chapter, is the study of factors, events, and circumstances that influence the transmission of infectious diseases among humans. The ultimate goal of the epidemiologist is to devise strategies that interrupt or eliminate the spread of an infectious agent. To accomplish this, infectious diseases must be classified according to incidence, portal of entry, source, symptomatology,

disease course, site of infection, agent, and host characteristics so that potential outbreaks may be predicted and averted or appropriately treated. Each of these categories is discussed in detail with the exception of agents and host, which have already been reviewed.

Epidemiology is a science of rates. The expected frequency of any infectious disease must be calculated so that gradual or abrupt changes in frequency can be observed. The term *incidence* is used to describe the number of new cases of an infectious disease that occur within a defined population (*e.g.,* per 100,000 people) over an established period of time (monthly, quarterly, yearly). Disease prevalence indicates the number of active cases at any given time. A disease is considered endemic in a particular geographic region if the incidence and prevalence are expected and relatively stable. An epidemic describes an abrupt and unexpected increase in the incidence of disease over endemic rates. A pandemic refers to the spread of disease beyond continental boundaries. The advent of rapid, worldwide travel has increased the likelihood of pandemic transmission of pathogenic microorganisms.

PORTAL OF ENTRY

The portal of entry refers to the process by which a pathogen enters the body, gains access to susceptible tissues, and causes disease. Among the potential modes of transmission are penetration, direct contact, ingestion, and inhalation.

Penetration. Any disruption in the integrity of the body's surface barrier (*e.g.,* skin and mucous membranes) is a potential site for invasion of microorganisms. The break may be the result of an accidental injury (abrasions, burns, penetrating wounds), medical procedures such as surgery or catheterization, a primary infectious process that produces surface lesions like chickenpox or impetigo, or direct inoculation from intravenous drug use, animal or arthropod bites. The latter mode of transmission can be extremely dangerous because large numbers of organisms can be introduced directly into vital sites, bypassing the host's primary immune defense systems.

Direct Contact. Some pathogens are transmitted directly from infected tissue or secretions to exposed, intact mucous membranes without a prerequisite for damaged mucosal barriers. This is especially true of certain sexually transmitted diseases (STDs) such as gonorrhea, syphilis, chlamydia, and herpes where exposure of uninfected membranes to pathogens occurs during intimate contact.

The transmission of STDs is not limited to sexual contact. *Vertical transmission* of these agents (*i.e.*, from mother to child) can occur across the placenta or during birth when the mucous membranes of the child come in contact with infected vaginal secretions of the mother. When an infectious disease is transmitted from mother to child during gestation or birth, it is classified as a *congenital infection*. The most frequently observed congenital infections include the parasite *Toxoplasma gondii*, rubella, cytomegalovirus, herpes simplex viruses, and syphilis (the so-called *TORCH* infections), varicella-zoster (chickenpox), and paravirus B19. The severity of congenital defects associated with these infections depends greatly on the gestational age of the fetus when transmission occurs, but most of these agents can cause profound mental retardation and neurosensory deficits.

Ingestion. The entry of pathogenic microorganisms or their toxic products through the oral cavity and gastrointestinal tract represents one of the more efficient means of disease transmission in humans. Many bacterial, viral, and parasitic infections, including cholera, typhoid fever, dysentery (amoebic and bacillary), food poisoning, traveler's diarrhea, and hepatitis A are initiated through the ingestion of contaminated food and water. This mechanism of transmission necessitates that an infectious agent survives the low *p*H and enzyme activity of gastric secretions and the peristaltic action of the intestines in numbers sufficient to establish infection (infectious dose). Ingested pathogens also must compete successfully with the normal bacterial flora of the bowel for nutritional needs. People with reduced gastric acidity (achlorhydria) due to disease or medication are more susceptible to infection by this route because the number of ingested microorganisms sur-

viving the gastric environment is greater. Ingestion has also been postulated as a means of transmission of HIV infection from mother to child through breastfeeding.

Inhalation. The respiratory tract of healthy people is equipped with a multitiered defense system to prevent potential pathogens from entering the lungs. The surface of the respiratory tree is lined with a layer of mucus that is continuously swept up and away from the lungs and toward the mouth by the beating motion of ciliated epithelial cells. Humidification of inspired air increases the size of aerosolized particles, which are effectively filtered by the mucous membranes of the upper respiratory tract. Coughing also aids in the removal of particulate matter from the lower respiratory tract. Respiratory secretions contain antibodies and enzymes capable of inactivating infectious agents. Particulate matter and microorganisms that ultimately reach the lung are cleared by phagocytic cells. Despite this impressive array of protective mechanisms, a number of pathogens can invade the human body through the respiratory tract, including agents of bacterial pneumonia (*Streptococcus pneumoniae, Legionella pneumophila*), meningitis and sepsis (*N. meningitidis* and *Hemophilus influenzae*), tuberculosis, and the viruses responsible for measles, mumps, chickenpox, influenza, and the common cold. Defective pulmonary function or mucociliary clearance caused by noninfectious processes such as cystic fibrosis, emphysema, or smoking can increase the risk of inhalation-acquired diseases.

It is important to remember that the portal of entry does not dictate the site of infection. Ingested pathogens may penetrate the intestinal mucosa, disseminate through the circulatory system, and cause diseases in other organs such as the lung or liver. Whatever the mechanisms of entry, the transmission of infectious agents is directly related to the number of infectious agents absorbed by the host.

Source. The source of an infectious disease refers to the location, host, object, or substance from which the infectious agent was acquired: essentially the who, what, where, and when of disease transmission. The source may be endogenous (*i.e.*, acquired from the host's own microbial flora as would be the case in an opportunistic infection) or exogenous (*i.e.*, acquired from sources in the external environment such as the water, food, soil, or air). The infectious agent can originate from another human being, as from mother to child during gestation (congenital infections) or birth (perinatal infections). Zoonoses are a category of infectious diseases passed from other animal species to humans. Examples of zoonoses include cat-scratch disease, rabies, and visceral or cutaneous larval migrans. The spread of infectious diseases including Lyme disease, malaria, yellow fever, and trypanosomiasis through biting arthropods (vectors) has already been mentioned.

Source can denote a place. For instance, infections that develop in patients while they are hospitalized are termed *nosocomial*, and those that are acquired outside of health-care facilities are called *community acquired*.

The source may also pertain to the body substance that is the most likely vehicle for transmission, such as feces, blood, body fluids, respiratory secretions, and urine. Infections can be transmitted from person to person through shared inanimate objects (fomites) contaminated with infected body fluids. An example of this mechanism of transmission would include the spread of the HIV and hepatitis B virus through the use of shared syringes by intravenous drug users.

SYMPTOMATOLOGY

The term *symptomatology* refers to the collection of signs and symptoms expressed by the host during the disease course. This is also known as the *clinical picture* or disease presentation and can be characteristic of any given infectious agent. In terms of pathophysiology, symptoms are the outward expression of the struggle between invading organisms and the retaliatory inflammatory and immune responses of the host (see Chapter 13). The symptoms of an infectious disease may be specific and reflect the site of infection (*e.g.*, diarrhea, rash, convulsions, hemorrhage). Conversely, symptoms such as fever, myalgia, headache, and lethargy are relatively nonspecific and can be shared by a number of diverse infectious diseases. The symptoms of a diseased host

might be obvious, as in the cases of chickenpox or measles. Other covert symptoms, such as hepatitis or an increased white blood cell count, may require laboratory testing to detect. Accurate recognition and documentation of symptomatology can aid in the diagnosis of an infectious disease.

DISEASE COURSE

The course of any infectious disease can be divided into several distinguishable stages after the point of time in which the potential pathogen enters the host. These stages are: the incubation period, the prodromal stage, the acute stage, the convalescent stage, and the resolution stage (Fig. 12-5). These stages are based on the progression and intensity of the host's symptoms over time. The duration of each phase and the pattern of the overall illness can be specific for different pathogens, thereby aiding in the diagnosis of an infectious disease.

Incubation Period. The incubation period is the phase during which the pathogen begins active replication without producing recognizable symptoms in the host. The incubation period may be short, as in the case of salmonellosis (6 to 24 hours) or prolonged such as hepatitis B (50 to 180 days). The duration of the incubation period can be influenced by additional factors including the general health of the host, the portal of entry, and the infectious dose of the pathogen.

Prodromal Stage. The hallmark of the prodromal stage is the initial appearance of symptoms in the host, although the clinical presentation during this time may be only a vague sense of malaise. The host may experience mild fever, myalgia, headache, and

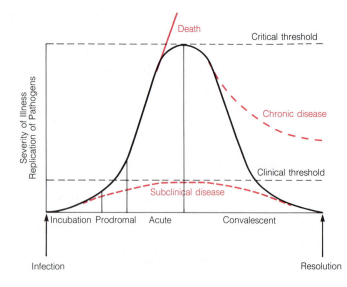

FIG. 12-5. *The stages of a primary infectious disease as they appear in relation to the severity of symptoms and the numbers of infectious agents. The clinical threshold corresponds with the initial expression of recognizable symptoms whereas the critical threshold represent the peak of disease intensity.*

fatigue. These are constitutional changes shared by a great number of disease processes. Once again, the duration of the prodromal stage can vary considerably from host to host.

Acute Stage. The acute stage is the period during which the host experiences the maximum impact of the infectious process corresponding to rapid proliferation and dissemination of the pathogen. During this phase, toxic by-products of microbial metabolism, cell lysis, and the immune response mounted by the host combine to produce tissue damage and inflammation. The symptoms of the host are pronounced and more specific than the prodromal stage, usually typifying the pathogen and site(s) of involvement.

Convalescent Stage. The convalescent period is characterized by the containment of infection, progressive elimination of the pathogen, repair of damaged tissue, and resolution of associated symptoms. Similar to the incubation period, the time required for complete convalescence may be days, weeks, or months depending on the type of pathogen and the voracity of the host's immune response.

Resolution. The resolution is the total elimination of a pathogen from the body without residual signs or symptoms of disease. Several notable exceptions of the classic presentations of an infectious process have been recognized. *Chronic* infectious diseases have a markedly protracted and sometimes irregular course. The host may experience symptoms of the infectious process continuously or sporadically for months or years without a convalescent phase. In contrast, *subclinical* or *subacute* illness progresses from infection to resolution without clinically apparent symptoms. A disease is termed *insidious* if the prodromal phase is protracted; a *fulminant* illness is characterized by abrupt onset of symptoms with little or no prodrome. Obviously, fatal infections are variants of the typical disease course.

SITE OF INFECTION

The anatomic location of an infectious process is usually designated by adding the suffix *-itis* to the name of the involved tissue (*e.g.*, bronchitis, infection of the bronchi and bronchioles; encephalitis, brain infection; carditis, infection of the heart). These are general terms, however, and they apply equally to inflammation due to infectious and noninfectious causes. The suffix *-emia* is used to designate the presence of a substance in the blood; hence, the terms *bacteremia*, *viremia*, and *fungemia* describe the presence of these infectious agents in the bloodstream. The term *sepsis*, or *septicemia*, refers to the presence of microbial toxins in the blood.

The site of an infectious disease is determined ultimately by the type of pathogen, the portal of entry, and competence of the host's immunologic defense system. Many pathogenic microorganisms are restricted in their capacity to invade the human body. *Mycoplasma pneumoniae*, influenza viruses, and *Legionella pneumophila* rarely cause disease outside the respiratory tract; infections caused by *N. gonorrhoeae* are generally confined to the genitourinary tract; and shigellosis and giardiasis seldom extend beyond the gastrointestinal tract. These are considered localized infectious diseases. The bacterium *Helicobacter pylori* is an extreme example of a site-specific pathogen. *Helicobacter pylori* is considered a probable agent of gastric ulcers and has not been implicated in disease processes elsewhere in the human body. Bacteria such as *Hemophilus influenzae* type b, a prominent pathogen of young children; *Salmonella typhi*, the cause of typhoid fever; and *B. burgdorferi*, the agent of Lyme disease, tend to disseminate from the primary site of infection to involve other locations and organ systems. These are examples of systemic pathogens. Most systemic infections disseminate throughout the body by way of the circulatory system.

An abscess is a localized pocket of infection composed of devitalized tissue, microorganisms, and the host's phagocytic white blood cells—in essence, a stalemate in the infectious process. The spread of the pathogen has been contained by the host, but white cell function within the toxic environment of the abscess is hampered, and the elimination of microorganisms is retarded. Abscesses, in general, must be surgically drained to effect a complete cure. Similarly, infections of biomedical implants such as catheters, artificial heart valves, and prosthetic bone implants are seldom cured by the host's immune response and antimicrobial therapy. The infecting organism colonizes the surface of the implant producing a dense matrix of cells, host proteins, and capsular material called a *biofilm*, necessitating the removal of the device.

VIRULENCE FACTORS

Virulence factors are substances or products generated by infectious agents that enhance their ability to cause disease. Although number and type of microbial products that fit this description are numerous, they can generally be grouped into four categories: (1) toxins, (2) adhesion factors, (3) evasive factors, and (4) invasive factors (Table 12-3).

TABLE 12-3. EXAMPLES OF VIRULENCE FACTORS PRODUCED BY PATHOGENIC MICROORGANISMS

FACTOR	CATEGORY	ORGANISM	EFFECT ON HOST
Cholera toxin	Exotoxin	*Vibrio cholerae* (bacterium)	Secretory diarrhea
Diphtheria toxin	Exotoxin	*Corynebacterium diphtheriae* (bacterium)	Inhibits protein synthesis
Lipopolysaccharide	Endotoxin	Many gram-negative bacteria	Fever, hypotension, shock
Toxic shock toxin	Enterotoxin	*Staphylococcus aureus* (bacterium)	Rash, diarrhea, vomiting, hepatitis
Hemagglutinin	Adherence	Influenzae virus	Establishment of infection
Pili	Adherence	*Neisseria gonorrhoeae* (bacterium)	Establishment of infection
Leukocidin	Evasive	*Staphylococcus aureus*	Kills phagocytes
IgA protease	Evasive	*Hemophilus influenzae* (bacterium)	Inactivates antibody
Capsule	Evasive	*Cryptococcus neoformans* (yeast)	Prevents phagocytosis
Collagenase	Invasive	*Pseudomonas aeruginosa* (bacterium)	Penetration of tissue
Protease	Invasive	*Aspergillus* (mold)	Penetration of tissue
Phospholipase	Invasive	*Clostridium perfringens* (bacterium)	Penetration of tissue

Toxins. Toxins are substances that alter or destroy the normal function of the host or host's cells. Toxin production is a trait chiefly monopolized by bacterial pathogens, although certain fungal and protozoan pathogens also elaborate substances toxic to humans. Bacterial toxins have a diverse spectrum of activity and exert their effects on a wide variety of host target cells. For classification purposes, however, the bacterial toxins can be divided into two main types: *exotoxins* and *endotoxins*.

Exotoxins are proteins released from the bacterial cell during growth. Bacterial exotoxins enzymatically inactivate or modify key cellular constituents leading to cell death or dysfunction. Diphtheria toxin, for example, inhibits cellular protein synthesis; botulism toxin decreases the release of neurotransmitter from cholinergic neurons, causing flaccid paralysis; tetanus toxin decreases the release of neurotransmitter from inhibitory neurons, producing spastic paralysis; and cholera toxin induces fluid secretion into the lumen of the intestine, causing diarrhea. Other examples of exotoxin-induced diseases include pertussis (whooping cough), anthrax, traveler's diarrhea, toxic shock syndrome, and a host of foodborne illnesses (food poisoning). Bacterial exotoxins that produce vomiting and diarrhea are sometimes referred to as *enterotoxins*. There has been a resurgent interest in streptococcal pyrogenic exotoxin A (SPEA), an exotoxin produced by certain strains of group A, beta-hemolytic streptococci (*Streptococcus pyogenes*) that causes a life-threatening toxic shock–like syndrome similar to the disease associated with tampon use produced by *Staphlococcus aureus*. The streptococcal form of intoxication is sometimes called *Henson's disease* because it was this infection that caused the death of the famous puppeteer Jim Henson.

By comparison, endotoxins do not contain protein, are not actively released from the bacterium during growth, and have no enzymatic activity. Rather, endotoxins are complex molecules composed of lipid and polysaccharides found in the cell wall of gram-negative bacteria. Studies of different endotoxins have indicated that the lipid portion of the endotoxin confers the toxic properties to the molecule. Endotoxins are potent activators of a number of regulatory systems in humans. A small amount of endotoxin in the circulatory system (endotoxemia) can induce clotting, bleeding, inflammation, hypotension, and fever. The sum of the physiologic reactions to endotoxins is sometimes called *endotoxic shock*.

Adhesion Factors. No interaction between microorganisms and humans can progress to infection or disease if the pathogen is unable to attach to and colonize the host. The process of microbial attachment may be site specific (mucous membranes or skin surfaces), cell specific (T-lymphocytes, respiratory epithelium), or nonspecific (moist or charged surfaces). In any of these cases, adhesion requires a positive interaction between the surfaces of host cells and the infectious agent. The site to which microorganisms adhere is called a *receptor*, and the reciprocal molecule or substance that binds to the receptor is called a *ligand* or *adhesin*. Receptors may be proteins, carbohydrates, lipids, or complex molecules composed of all three. Similarly, ligands may be simple or complex molecules, and in some cases, highly specific structures. Ligands that bind to specific carbohydrates are called *lectins*. Certain bacteria produce hairlike structures protruding from the cell surface called *pili* or *fimbriae*, which anchor the organism to receptors on host cell membranes to establish an infection. Many viral agents including influenza, mumps, measles, and adenovirus produce filamentous appendages or spikes called *hemagglutinins*, which recognize carbohydrate receptors on the surfaces of specific cells in the upper respiratory tract of the host. After initial attachment, a number of bacterial agents become embedded in a gelatinous matrix of polysaccharides called a slime or mucous layer. The slime layer serves two purposes: it anchors the agent firmly to host tissue surfaces, and it protects the agent from the immunologic defenses of the host.

Evasive Factors. A number of factors produced by microorganisms enhance virulence by evading various components of the host's immune system. Extracellular polysaccharides (capsules, slime, or mucous layers) discourage engulfment and killing of pathogens by the phagocytic white blood cells (neutrophils and macrophages) of the host. Certain bacterial, fungal, and parasitic pathogens avoid phagocytosis by excreting leukocidins—toxins that deplete the host of neutrophils and macrophages by causing specific and lethal damage to the cytoplasmic membrane of white blood cells. Other pathogens, such as the bacterial agents of listeriosis and legionnaires' disease are adapted to survive and reproduce within phagocytic white blood cells after ingestion, avoiding or neutralizing the usually lethal products contained within the lysosomes of the cell. Other unique strategies employed by pathogenic microbes to evade immunologic surveillance have evolved solely to avoid recognition by host antibodies. Strains of *Staphylococcus aureus* produce a surface protein (protein A), which immobilizes immunoglobulin G, holding the antigen-binding region harmlessly away from the organisms. This pathogen also secretes a unique enzyme called coagulase. Coagulase converts soluble human coagulation factors into a solid clot, which envelops and protects the organism from phagocytic host cells and antibody. *Hemophilus influenzae* and *N. gonorrhoeae* secrete enzymes that cleave and inactivate secretory immunoglobulin A, thus neutralizing the primary defense of the respiratory and genital tracts at the site of infection.

Borrelia species, including the agents of Lyme disease and relapsing fever, alter surface antigens during the disease course to avoid immunologic detection. So it appears that the ingenuity to devise strategic defense systems and stealth technologies is not limited to humans. Viruses such as HIV cause impaired function of immunoregulatory cells. Although this property certainly increases the virulence of these agents, it is not considered a virulence factor in the true sense of the definition.

Invasive Factors. Simply defined, invasive factors are products produced by infectious agents that facilitate the penetration of anatomic barriers and host tissue. In general, most invasive factors are enzymes capable of destroying cellular membranes (phospholipases), connective tissue (elastases, collagenases), intercellular matrices (hyaluronidase), and structural protein complexes (proteases). It is the combined effects of invasive factors, toxins, and antimicrobial and inflammatory substances released by host cells to counter infection that mediate the tissue damage and pathophysiology of infectious diseases.

DIAGNOSIS OF INFECTIOUS DISEASES

The diagnosis of an infectious disease requires two criteria: the recovery of a probable pathogen or evidence of its presence from the infected site(s) of a diseased host and accurate documentation of clinical signs and symptoms (symptomatology) compatible with an infectious process. In the laboratory, the diagnosis of an infectious agent is accomplished using three basic techniques: (1) culture, (2) serology, or (3) the detection of characteristic antigens or metabolites produced by the pathogen.

Culture refers to the propagation of a microorganism outside of the body usually on or in artificial growth media such as agar plates or broth (Fig. 12-6). The specimen from the diseased host is inoculated into broth or on to the surface of an agar plate, and the culture is placed in a controlled environment (incubator) until the growth of microorganisms becomes detectable. In the case of a bacterial pathogen, identification is based on microscopic appearance and Gram's stain reaction, shape, texture, and color (morphology) of the colonies, and by a panel of reactions that "fingerprint" salient biochemical characteristics of the organism. Certain bacteria such as *Mycobacterium leprae*, the agent of leprosy, and *Treponema pallidum*, the syphilis spirochete, do not grow on artificial media and require additional methods of identification. Fungi and mycoplasmas are cultured in much the same way as bacteria but with more reliance on microscopic and colonial morphology for identification. Chlamydia, rickettsia, and all human viruses are obligate intracellular pathogens. As a result, the propagation of these agents in the laboratory requires the inoculation of eukaryotic cells grown in culture (cell cultures). A cell culture consists of a flask containing a single layer, or monolayer, of eukaryotic cells covering the bottom and overlaid with broth containing essential nutrients and growth factors. When a virus infects and replicates within cultured eukaryotic cells, it produces pathologic changes in the appearance of the cell called cytopathic effect or CPE (Fig. 12-7). CPE can be detected microscopically, and the pattern and extent of cellular destruction is often characteristic of a particular virus. Although

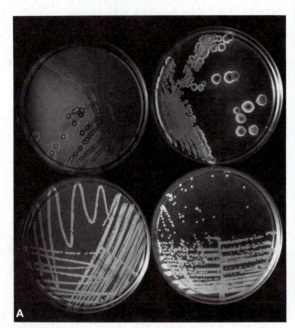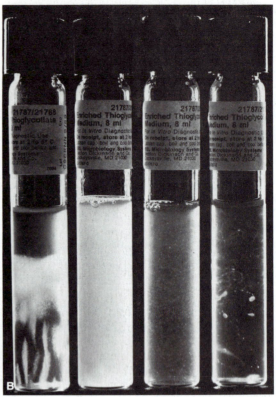

FIG. 12-6. Variability of the macroscopic appearance of bacterial cultured on solid, agar-containing medium (**A**) or liquid broth medium (**B**). On solid surfaces, bacteria form distinct colonies, which increase in size and cell density with time until nutrients are depleted. Bacteria cultured in broth form a variety of growth patterns ranging from particulate to homogenous, turbid suspensions. Anaerobic bacteria cultured in liquid medium tend to grow best at the bottom of the tube where the concentration of molecular oxygen is lowest.

culture media have been developed for the growth of certain human protozoa and helminths in the laboratory, the diagnosis of parasitic infectious diseases has traditionally relied on microscopic, or, in the case of worms, visible identification of organisms, cysts, or ova directly from infected patient specimens.

Serology, the study of serum, is an indirect means of identifying infectious agents by measuring serum antibodies in the diseased host. A tentative diagnosis can be made if the antibody level, also called *antibody titer*, against a specific pathogen rises during the acute phase of the disease and falls during convalescence. Serologic identification of an infectious agent is not as accurate as culture, but it may be a useful adjunct, especially for the diagnosis of diseases caused by pathogens that cannot be cultured (*e.g.*, hepatitis B virus). The measurement of antibody titers has another advantage in that specific antibody types such as IgM and IgG are produced by the host during different phases of an infectious process; IgM-specific antibodies generally rise and fall during the acute phase, whereas the synthesis of the IgG class of

antibodies increases during the acute phase and remains elevated until or beyond resolution. Measurements of class-specific antibodies are also useful in the diagnosis of congenital infections. IgM antibodies do not cross the placenta, whereas certain IgG antibodies are transferred passively from mother to child during the final trimester of gestation. Consequently, an elevation of pathogen-specific IgM antibodies found in the serum of a neonate must have originated from the child and, therefore, indicates congenital infection. A similarly increased IgG titer in the neonate does not distinguish congenital from maternal infection.

The technology of *direct antigen detection* has evolved rapidly over the past decade and in the process has revolutionized the diagnosis of infectious diseases. Antigen detection incorporates features of culture and serology but reduces by a fraction the time required for diagnosis. In principle, this method relies on purified antibodies to detect antigens of infectious agents in specimens obtained from the diseased host. The source of antibodies used for antigen detec-

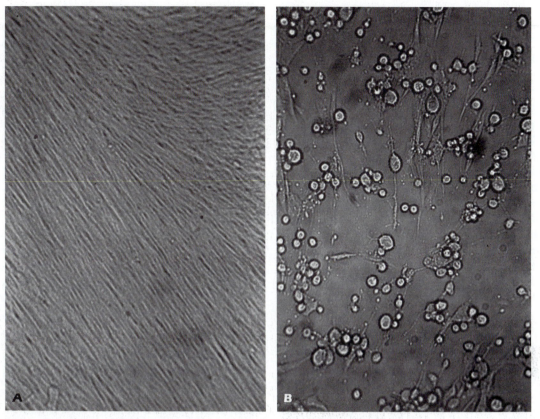

FIG. 12-7. The microscopic appearance of a monolayer of uninfected human fibroblasts grown in cell culture (**A**) and the same cells after infection with herpes simplex virus (**B**) demonstrating the cytopathic effect (CPE) caused by viral replication and concomitant cell lysis.

tion can be animals immunized against a particular pathogen or *hybridomas*. Hybridomas are created by fusing normal antibody-producing spleen cells from an immunized animal with malignant myeloma cells, which synthesize large quantities of antibody. The result is a cell that produces an antibody called a *monoclonal antibody*, which is highly specific for a single antigen and a single pathogen. Regardless of the source, the antibodies are labeled with a substance that allows microscopic or overt detection when bound to the pathogen or its products. Generally, the three types of labels used for this purpose are fluorescent dyes, enzymes, and particles such as latex beads. Fluorescent antibodies allow visualization of an infectious agent with the aid of a fluorescent microscope. Depending on the type of fluorescent dye used, the organism may appear a bright green or orange color against a black background, making detection extremely easy. Enzyme-labeled antibodies function in a similar manner. The enzyme is capable of converting a colorless compound into a colored substance, thereby permitting detection of antibody bound to an infectious agent without the use of a fluorescent microscope. Finally, particles coated with

antibodies clump together, or agglutinate, when the appropriate antigen is present in a specimen. Particle agglutination is especially useful when examining infected body fluids such as urine, serum, or spinal fluid.

The identification of infectious agents through the detection of sequences of DNA or RNA unique to a single agent has undergone rapid development and use over the past few years. Several techniques have been devised to accomplish this goal, each having different degrees of sensitivity regarding the number of organisms that need to be present in a specimen for detection. The first of these methods is called *DNA probe hybridization*. Small fragments of DNA are cut from the genome of a specific pathogen and labeled with compounds (*e.g.*, radioisotopes or photoemitting chemicals) that allow detection. The labeled DNA ''probes'' are added to specimens from an infected host. If the pathogen is present, the probe attaches to the complementary strand of DNA on the genome of the infectious agent permitting rapid diagnosis. The use of labeled probes have allowed visualization of particular agents within and around individual cells in histologic sections of tissue. The second and most sensitive method of DNA detection to be developed is called the polymerase chain reaction or PCR. This method incorporates two unique reagents: a specific pair of oligonucleotides (usually more than 25 nucleotides in length) called primers and a heat-stable DNA polymerase. To perform the assay, the primers are added to the specimen containing the suspect pathogen and the sample is heated to melt all the DNA present in the specimen and allowed to cool. The primers locate and bind only to the complementary target DNA of the pathogen in question. The heat-stable polymerase begins to replicate the DNA from the point at which the primers attached similar to two trains approaching one another on separate but converging tracks. After the initial cycle, DNA polymerization ceases at the point where the primers were located, producing a strand of DNA with a distinct size depending on the distance separating the two primers. The specimen is heated again, and the process starts anew. After many cycles of heating, cooling, and polymerization, a large number of uniformly sized DNA fragments are produced only if the specific pathogen (or its DNA) is present in the specimen. The polymerized DNA fragments are separated by electrophoresis and visualized with a dye. The size of the polymerized fragments are compared to positive controls containing the specific agent and a diagnosis is made. PCR is an extremely useful and powerful tool. In some circumstances, this method can detect as few as one virus or bacterium in a single specimen. This method also allows laboratorians to diagnose infections caused by microorganisms that are impossible or difficult to grow in culture. Many variations of *gene amplification* techniques similar to PCR are being developed with the promise of increased sensitivity and automated methods that would bring this technology out of research laboratories and into routine diagnostic laboratories.

THERAPY OF INFECTIOUS DISEASES

The goal of treatment for an infectious disease is complete removal of the pathogen from the host and the restoration of normal physiologic function to damaged tissues. Most infectious diseases of humans are self-limiting (*i.e.*, they require little or no medical therapy for a complete cure). When an infectious process gains the upper hand and therapeutic intervention is essential, the choice of treatment may be medicinal through the use of antimicrobial agents; immunologic with antibody preparations, vaccines, or substances that stimulate and improve the host's immune function; or surgical by removing infected tissues. The decision of which therapeutic modality

or combination of therapies is based on the extent, urgency, and location of the disease process, the pathogen, and the availability of effective antimicrobial agents.

ANTIMICROBIAL AGENTS

The use of chemicals, potions, and elixirs in the treatment of infectious diseases dates back to the earliest records of human medicine. Over 2000 years ago, Greek and Chinese physicians recognized that certain substances were useful for preventing or curing wound infections. Although the biologic activity of these compounds was not understood, some may have inadvertently contained by-products of molds that resemble modern antibiotics. From that time until the late 1800s when the relationship between infection and microorganisms was finally accepted, the evolution of antiinfective therapy was less than explosive. It was not until the advent of World War II, after the introduction of sulfonamides and penicillin, that the development of antimicrobial compounds matured into a science of great consequence. Today, the comprehensive list of effective antiinfective agents is burgeoning. Most antimicrobial compounds can be categorized roughly according to mechanism of antiinfective activity, chemical structure, and target pathogen (*e.g.*, antibacterial, antiviral, antifungal, or antiparasitic agents).

Antibacterial Agents. Antibacterial agents are generally called antibiotics. Most antibiotics are actually produced by other microorganisms—primarily bacteria and fungi—as by-products of metabolism and, in general, are only effective against other prokaryotic organisms. An antibiotic is considered *bactericidal* if it causes irreversible and lethal damage to the bacterial pathogen and *bacteriostatic* if its inhibitory effects on bacterial growth are reversed when the agent is eliminated. Antibiotics can be classified into families of compounds with related chemical structure and activity (Table 12-4).

Not all antibiotics are effective against all pathogenic bacteria. Some agents are only effective against gram-negative bacteria, others are specific for gram-positive organisms. The so-called broad-spectrum antibiotics, such as the newest class of cephalosporins, are active against a wide variety of gram-positive and gram-negative bacteria. Members of the *Mycobacterium* genus, including *Mycobacterium tuberculosis*, are extremely resistant to the effects of the major classes of antibiotics and require an entirely different spectrum of agents for therapy. The four basic mechanisms of the antibiotics are: (1) inhibition of bacterial peptidoglycan synthesis (penicillins, cephalosporins, glycopeptides); (2) inhibition of bacterial protein syn-

TABLE 12-4. CLASSIFICATION AND ACTIVITY OF THE ANTIBACTERIAL AGENTS (ANTIBIOTICS)			
FAMILY	**EXAMPLE**	**TARGET SITE**	**SIDE EFFECTS**
Penicillins	Ampicillin	Cell wall	Allergic reactions
Cephalosporins	Cephalexin	Cell wall	Allergic reactions
Monobactams	Aztreonam	Cell wall	Skin rash
Aminoglycosides	Tobramycin	Ribosomes (protein synthesis)	Hearing loss
			Nephrotoxicity
Tetracyclines	Doxycycline	Ribosomes (protein synthesis)	Gastrointestinal irritation
			Allergic reactions
			Teeth and bone dysplasia
Macrolides	Clindamycin	Ribosomes (protein synthesis)	Colitis
			Allergic reactions
Sulfonamides	Sulfadiazine	Folic acid synthesis	Allergic reactions
			Anemia
			Gastrointestinal irritation
Glycopeptides	Vancomycin	Ribosomes (protein synthesis)	Allergic reactions
			Hearing loss
			Nephrotoxicity
Quinolones	Ciprofloxacin	DNA synthesis	Gastrointestinal irritation
Miscellaneous	Chloramphenicol	Ribosomes (protein synthesis)	Anemia
			Hepatotoxicity
	Rifampin	Ribosomes (protein synthesis)	Allergic reactions
	Trimethoprim	Folic acid synthesis	Same as sulfonamides

thesis (aminoglycosides, macrolides, tetracyclines, chloramphenicol, and rifampin); (3) interruption of nucleic acid synthesis (fluoroquinolones, nalidixic acid); and (4) interference with normal metabolism (sulfonamides and trimethoprim).

Despite lack of antibiotic activity against eukaryotic cells, many cause unwanted or toxic side effects in humans including allergic responses (penicillins, cephalosporins, sulfonamides, and glycopeptides), hearing and kidney impairment (aminoglycosides), and liver or bone marrow toxicity (chloramphenicol). Of greater concern is the increasing prevalence of bacteria resistant to the effects of antibiotics. The ways in which bacteria acquire resistance to antibiotics are becoming as numerous as the number of antibiotics. Bacterial resistance mechanisms include the production of enzymes that inactivate antibiotics, genetic mutations that alter antibiotic binding sites, alternative metabolic pathways that bypass antibiotic activity, and changes in the filtration qualities of the bacterial cell wall that prevent access of antibiotics to the target site within the organism. It is the continuous search for a better mousetrap that makes antiinfective therapy such a fascinating aspect of infectious diseases.

Antiviral Agents. Unlike antibiotics, the list of effective antiviral agents, although increasing, is relatively small. The reason for this is host toxicity—viral replication requires the use of eukaryotic host cell enzymes and the drugs that effectively interrupt viral replication are likely to interfere with host cell reproduction as well. Almost all antiviral compounds are artificial, and, with few exceptions, the primary target of antiviral compounds is viral RNA or DNA synthesis. Agents such as acyclovir, ganciclovir, vidarabine, and ribavirin mimic the nucleoside building blocks of RNA and DNA. During active viral replication, the nucleoside counterfeits inhibit the host or viral enzymes required to duplicate the viral genome, thus preventing the spread of infectious viral progeny to other susceptible host cells. Similar to the specificity of antibiotics, antiviral agents may be active against RNA viruses only, DNA viruses only, or occasionally both. Antiviral agents such as zidovudine, ddI, and ddC, which are under evaluation in the treatment of AIDS, have targeted the HIV-specific enzyme, reverse transcriptase, for inhibition. This key enzyme is essential for viral replication and has no counterpart in the infected eukaryotic host cells. Experimental approaches to antiviral therapy include compounds that inhibit viral attachment to susceptible host cells and drugs that prevent uncoating of the viral genome once inside the host cell and agents such as foscarnet that directly inhibit viral DNA polymerase. Although the treatment of viral infections with antimicrobial agents is a relatively recent endeavor, reports of viral mutations resulting in resistant strains have already appeared in medical journals.

Antifungal Agents. The target site of the two most important families of antifungal agents is the cytoplasmic membranes of yeasts or molds. Fungal membranes differ from human cell membranes in that they contain the sterol ergosterol instead of cholesterol. The polyene family of antifungal compounds (amphotericin B, nystatin) preferentially bind to ergosterol and form holes in the cytoplasmic membrane causing leakage of the fungal cell contents and, eventually, lysis of the cell. The imidazole class of drugs (fluconazole, itraconazole, ketoconazole) inhibit the synthesis of ergosterol, thereby damaging the integrity of the fungal cytoplasmic membrane. Both types of drugs bind, to a certain extent, to the cholesterol component of host cell membranes and elicit a variety of toxic side effects in treated patients. The nucleoside analogue 5-fluorocytosine (5-FC) disrupts fungal RNA and DNA synthesis but without the toxicity associated with the polyene and imidazole drugs. Unfortunately, 5-FC demonstrates little or no antifungal activity against molds or dimorphic fungi and is primarily reserved for infections caused by yeasts.

Antiparasitic Agents. Because of the extreme diversity of human parasites and their growth cycles, a review of current antiparasitic therapies and agents would be highly impractical and lengthy. Similar to other infectious disease caused by eukaryotic microorganisms, treatment of parasitic illnesses is based on exploiting essential components of the parasite's metabolism or cellular anatomy that are not shared by the host. Any relatedness between the target site of the parasite and the cells of the host increases the likelihood of toxic reactions in the host. Continued development of improved antiparasitic agents suffers greatly from economic considerations as well. Parasitic diseases of humans are primarily the scourge of poor, underdeveloped, third-world nations. As a result, financial incentives to produce more effective therapies are nonexistent. Resistance among human parasites to standard, effective therapy is also a major concern. In Africa, Asia, and South America, the incidence of chloroquine-resistant malaria (*Plasmodium falciparum*) is on the rise. Resistant strains require more complicated, expensive, and potentially toxic therapy with a combination of agents.

IMMUNOTHERAPY

One of the most recent and exciting approaches to the treatment of infectious diseases is immunotherapy. This strategy involves supplementing or stimulating the host's immune response so that the spread of a pathogen is limited or reversed. Several products are available for this purpose including intravenous immune globulin (IVIG) and cytokines. IVIG is a pooled preparation of antibodies obtained from normal, healthy immune human donors that is infused as an intravenous solution. In theory, pathogen-specific antibodies present in the infusion facilitate neutralization, phagocytosis, and clearance of infectious agents above and beyond the capabilities of the diseased host. Hyperimmune immunoglobulin preparations, which are also commercially available, contain high titers of antibodies against specific pathogens including hepatitis B virus, cytomegalovirus, rabies, and varicella-zoster (chickenpox) virus. Cytokines are substances produced by human white blood cells that, in small quantities, stimulate white cell replication, phagocytosis, antibody production, and the induction of fever, inflammation, and tissue repair—all of which counteract infectious agents and hasten recovery. With the advent of genetic engineering and cloning, many cytokines, including interferon and interleukins, have been produced in the laboratory and are being evaluated experimentally as antiinfective agents. As we learn more about the action of cytokines, we are beginning to appreciate that some of the adverse reactions associated with infectious processes are due to our own inflammatory response. Intervention therapies designed to inactivate certain cytokines (*e.g.*, tumor necrosis factor) have proven to be helpful in animal models of infection. It is not unlikely that therapies based on the regulation of the inflammatory response will become widely used in human medicine over the next few years.

One of the most efficient (and often overlooked) means of preventing infectious diseases is immunization. Proper and timely adherence to recommended vaccination schedules in children and boosters in adults effectively reduces the senseless spread of vaccine-preventable illnesses such as measles, mumps, pertussis, and rubella, which still occur in the United States with alarming frequency.

SURGICAL INTERVENTION

Before the discovery of antimicrobial agents, surgical removal of infected tissues, organs, or limbs was occasionally the only option available to prevent the demise of the infected host. Today, medicinal therapy with antibiotics and other antiinfective agents is an effective solution for a great majority of infectious diseases. However, surgical intervention is still an important option for cases in which (1) the pathogen is resistant to available treatments, (2) containment of rapidly progressing infectious process is the only means of saving the patient (gas gangrene), or (3) access to an infected site by antimicrobial agents is limited and surgical drainage (abscesses), cleaning of the site (debridement), or removal of organs or necrotic tissue (*e.g.*, appendectomy) will hasten the recovery process. In certain situations, surgery may be the only means of effecting a complete cure, as in the case of endocarditis (infected heart valves) in which the diseased valve must be replaced with a mechanical or biologic valve to restore normal function.

In summary, the ultimate outcome of any interaction between microorganisms and the human host is decided by a complex and ever-changing set of variables that take into account the overall health and physiologic function of the host, and the virulence and infectious dose of the microbe. In many instances, disease is an inevitable consequence, but with continued advancement of science and technology, the vast number of cases can either be eliminated or rapidly cured with appropriate therapy. It is the intent of those who study infectious diseases to understand thoroughly the pathogen, the disease course, the mechanisms of transmission, and the host response to infection. This knowledge will lead to development of improved diagnostic techniques, revolutionary approaches to antiinfective therapy, and, hopefully, the eradication or control of those microscopic agents that cause frightening devastation and loss of life throughout the world.

■ BIBLIOGRAPHY

Beachey, E.H. (1981). Bacterial adherence: Adhesin-receptor interactions mediating the attachment of bacteria to mucosal surfaces. *Journal of Infectious Diseases, 143*, 325.

Blaser, M.J. (1992). *Helicobacter pylori*: Its role in disease. *Clinical Infectious Diseases, 15*, 386–391.

Brenner, D.J., et al. (1991). Proposal of *Afipia* gen. no., with *Afipia felis* sp. nov. (formerly the cat scratch bacillus), *Afipa cleve landensis* sp. nov. (formerly the Cleveland Clinic Foundation strain), *Afipia broomeae* sp. nov., and three unnamed genospecies. *Journal of Clinical Microbiology, 29*, 2450–2460.

Donowitz, G.R., & Mandell, G.L. (1988). Beta-lactam antibiotics (parts 1 and 2). *New England Journal of Medicine, 318*, 419, 490.

Flier, J. S., & Underhill, L. H. (1986). Medical consequences of persistent viral infections. *N Engl J Med, 314*(6), 359.

Guyer, R.L., & Koshland, D.E., Jr. (1989). The molecule of the year. *Science, 246*, 1543–1544.

Jones, J.E. (1988). Pinworms. *American Journal of Family Practice, 38*(3), 159.

Krogfelt, K.A. (1991). Bacterial adhesion: Genetics, biogenetics, and role in pathogenesis of fimbrial adhesions of *Eschereichia coli. Review of Infectious Disease, 13*, 721–735.

Lennette, E.H., Balows, A., Hausler, W.J., Jr., et al. (Eds.). (1985). *Manual of clinical microbiology*. Washington, DC: American Society for Microbiology.

Musher, D.M. (1988). The gram-positive cocci: I. Streptococci. *Hospital Practice, 23*(3), 63.

Musher, D.M. (1988). The gram-positive cocci: II. Staphylococci. *Hospital Practice, 23*(4), 179.

Musher, D.M. (1988). The gram-positive cocci: III. Resistance to antibiotics. *Hospital Practice, 23*(5), 105.

Petri, W.A. (1988). Tick-borne diseases. *American Family Practice, 37*(6), 95.

Sharp, A.H., & Fields, B.N. (1985). Pathogenesis of viral infections. *New England Journal of Medicine, 312*(8), 486.

Sheagren, J.N. (1984). *Staphlococcus aureus. New England Journal of Medicine, 3109*(21,22), 1437.

Stechenberg, B.W. (1988). Lyme disease: The latest great imitator. *Pediatric Infectious Disease, 7*, 402.

Treadwell, T.L. (1988). Gram-negative bacteremia. *Hospital Practice, 23*(7), 117.

Vacheron, F., Mandine, E., Lenaour, P., et al. (1992). Inhibition of production of tumor necrosis factor by monoclonal antibodies to lipopolysaccharides. *Journal of Infectious Diseases, 165*, 873–878.

Van de Perre, P., Lepage, P., Homsy, J., et al. (1992). Mother-to-infant transmission of human immunodeficiency virus by breast milk: Presumed innocent or presumed guilty? *Clinical Infectious Diseases, 15*, 502–507.

Wright, S.W., & Trott, A.T. (1988). North American tick-borne diseases. *Annals of Emergency Medicine, 17*(9), 964.

Zanetti, G., Glauser, M.P., & Baumgartner, J.D. (1991). Use of immunoglobulins in prevention and treatment of infection in critically ill patients: Review and critique. *Review of Infectious Diseases, 13*, 985–992.

C H A P T E R   1 3

INFLAMMATION AND IMMUNITY

MARK LAROCCO

■ OBJECTIVES

After you have studied this chapter, you should be able to meet the following objectives:

■ State the purpose of inflammation.

■ State the five cardinal signs of acute inflammation and describe the physiologic mechanisms involved in production of each of these signs.

■ Describe the hemodynamic and cellular phases of the inflammatory response.

■ Name and state the function of the granulocytes.

■ Contrast acute and chronic inflammation.

■ Name and describe the five types of inflammatory exudates.

■ Explain the significance of the major histocompatibility complex (MHC) and the human leukocyte antigen (HLA).

■ Differentiate between the central and peripheral lymphoid structures.

■ Trace the differentiation of the T-lymphocytes from bone marrow stem cells to mature regulatory and effector cells.

■ Trace the differentiation of a B-lymphocyte from a bone marrow stem cell to a mature plasma cell or memory cell.

■ State the function of the five classes of immunoglobulins.

■ Describe the function of the macrophage.

■ Describe the characteristics of an antigen.

■ Differentiate between passive and active immunity.

■ Contrast humoral and cell-mediated immunity.

■ Relate the complement system to the immune response.

■ Relate the actions of the cytokines to the immune response.

■ Characterize the changes in the immune response that occur in the elderly.

Carol Mattson Porth: PATHOPHYSIOLOGY: CONCEPTS OF
ALTERED HEALTH STATES, 4th ed. © 1994, 1990, 1986, 1982
J.B. Lippincott Company

Inflammation is the "reaction of vascularized living tissue to local injury."[1] Although the effects of inflammation are often viewed as undesirable because they are unpleasant and cause discomfort, the process is essentially a beneficial one that allows a person to live with the effects of everyday stress. Without the inflammatory response, wounds would not heal and minor infections would become overwhelming. On the other hand, inflammation also produces undesirable effects. The crippling effects of rheumatoid arthritis, for example, have their origin in the inflammatory response.

The *immune system* is a complex network of specialized organs and cells that protects the body from destruction by foreign agents and microbial pathogens, and degrades and removes damaged or dead cells. The immune system also exerts a surveillance function to prevent the development and growth of malignant cells. The immune system consists of the immune cells and the lymphoid organs and tissues. In many respects, the complexity of the immune system parallels that of the nervous system. It is able to distinguish self from nonself, remember previous experiences, and react accordingly.[2] Once a person has the mumps, the immune system remembers the experience and protects against getting the disease again. Not only is the immune system capable of memory, it is also able to respond with great diversity and specificity. It can recognize many millions of nonself molecules and produce specific molecules that match up with and counteract each of them.

■ THE INFLAMMATORY RESPONSE

The causes of inflammation are many and varied. Although it is common to equate inflammation with infection, it is important to recognize that almost all types of injury are capable of inciting the response and that only a small number of inflammatory responses are related to infections. The injurious agents that cause inflammation can arise from outside the body (*exogenous*) or from within the body (*endogenous*). Common causes of inflammation are trauma, surgery, infection, caustic chemicals, extremes of heat and cold, immune responses, and ischemic damage to body tissues.

Although the inflammatory response can be initiated by a wide variety of injurious agents, the sequence of physiologic events that follow is remarkably similar. An acute inflammatory response follows the same course, whether the injury is caused by a streptococcal infection or by tissue necrosis associated with myocardial infarction. The extent of the injury varies, and the site of inflammation is different, but the tissue response and systemic manifestations are similar. The body, however, uses only those behaviors in the sequence that are needed to minimize tissue damage. A small area of local swelling and redness may be sufficient to prevent injury from a mosquito bite, whereas other, more serious conditions, such as appendicitis, may incite leukocytosis, fever, and formation of an exudate.

Inflammation can be acute or chronic. Acute inflammation is the typical short-term response associated with all types of tissue injury. It involves hemodynamic changes, formation of an exudate, and the presence of granular leukocytes. Chronic inflammation follows a less uniform and more persistent pattern. It involves the presence of nongranular leukocytes and usually results in more extensive formation of scar tissue and deformities.

Inflammatory conditions are named by adding the suffix -*itis* to the affected organ or system. For instance, neuritis refers to inflammation of a nerve, pericarditis to inflammation of the pericardium, and appendicitis to inflammation of the appendix. A further description of the inflammatory process might indicate whether the process was acute or chronic and what type of exudate was formed (*e.g.*, acute fibrinous pericarditis).

ACUTE INFLAMMATION

The classic description of acute inflammation has been handed down through the ages. In the first century A.D., the Roman physician Celsus described the local reaction to injury in terms of what has come to be known as the cardinal signs of inflammation. These signs are *rubor* (redness), *tumor* (swelling), *calor* (heat), and *dolor* (pain). In the second century. A.D., the Greek physician Galen added a fifth cardinal sign, *functio laesa* or loss of function.

The manifestations of acute inflammation can be divided into two categories, *vascular* and *cellular blood cell responses*. At the biochemical level, many of the responses that occur during acute inflammation are associated with the release of chemical mediators. Both the hemodynamic responses and white blood cell responses contribute to the *inflammatory exudates* that characterize the acute inflammatory response. Each of these aspects of acute inflammation is discussed separately.

VASCULAR RESPONSE

The vascular, or hemodynamic, changes that occur with inflammation begin almost immediately after injury and are initiated by a momentary constriction of small vessels in the area. This momentary period of vasoconstriction is followed immediately by vasodilation of the arterioles and venules that supply the area. As a result, the area becomes congested, causing the *redness* and *warmth* characteristic of acute inflammation. Accompanying this hyperemic response is an increase in capillary permeability, which allows fluid to escape into the tissue and cause *swelling*. *Pain* and *impaired function* follow as the result of tissue swelling and release of chemical mediators.

The hemodynamic changes that occur during the early stages of inflammation are beneficial in that they aid in controlling the effects of the injurious agent. During this stage, the exudation of fluid out of the capillary into the tissue spaces helps dilute the toxic and irritating agents. As fluid moves out of the capillary, stagnation of flow and clotting of blood in the small capillaries that supply the inflamed area occur. This aids in localizing the effects of the injury.

Depending on the severity of injury, the hemodynamic changes that occur with the inflammatory reaction follow one of three patterns of response. The first is an immediate transient response, which occurs with minor injury. The second is an immediate sustained response, which occurs with more serious injury and continues for several days and results in actual damage to the vessels in the area. The third type of response is a delayed response—the increase in capillary permeability is delayed for a period of 4 to 24 hours. A delayed response often accompanies radiation types of injuries, such as a sunburn.

CELLULAR RESPONSE

The cellular stage of acute inflammation is marked by movement of white blood cells (leukocytes) into the area of injury. This stage includes (1) the margination or pavementing of white blood cells, (2) emigration of white blood cells, (3) chemotaxis, and (4) phagocytosis. A description of white blood cells precedes the discussion of cellular events that occur in acute inflammation.

The leukocytes, or white blood cells (WBCs), develop from the primordial stem cells located in the bone marrow. The leukocytes are larger and less numerous than the red blood cells. There are two types of white blood cells, granular and nongranular leukocytes (Fig. 13-1).

Granular Leukocytes. The granular leukocytes are identifiable because of their cytoplasmic granules and are commonly referred to as granulocytes. In addition to their cytoplasmic granules, these white blood cells have distinctive multilobar nuclei. The granulocytes are divided into three types (neutrophils, eosinophils, and basophils) according to the staining properties of the granules.

The *neutrophils*, which constitute 60% to 70% of

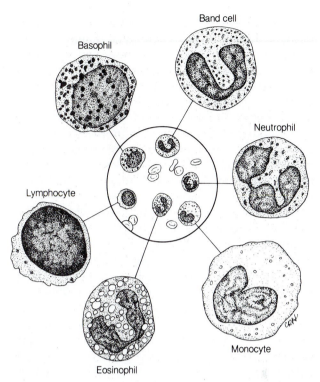

FIG. 13-1. *White blood cells involved in the inflammatory response.*

the total number of WBCs, have granules that are neutral and hence do not stain with either an acid or a basic dye. These granules contain enzymes that are used in destroying and degrading bacteria and correspond to lysosomes found in other cells (see Chapter 1). Because these WBCs have nuclei that are divided into three to five lobes, they are often called *polymorphonuclear (PMN) leukocytes*. The neutrophils are the first cells to arrive at the site of inflammation, usually appearing within 90 minutes of injury. The neutrophil count increases greatly during the inflammatory process. When this happens, immature forms of neutrophils are released from the bone marrow. These immature cells are often called *bands* or *stabs* because of the horseshoe shape of their nuclei. After being released from the bone marrow, circulating neutrophils have a life span of only about 10 hours and, therefore, must be constantly replaced if their numbers are to be adequate. This requires an increase in circulating WBCs, a condition called *leukocytosis*.

The cytoplasmic granules of the *eosinophils* stain red with the acid dye eosin. These leukocytes constitute 1% to 3% of the total number of white blood cells and increase during allergic reactions and parasitic infections. It is thought that they detoxify the agents or chemical mediators associated with allergic reactions and assist in terminating the response.

The granules of the *basophils* stain blue with a

basic dye. These cells constitute only about 0.3% to 0.5% of the white blood cells. The granules in the basophils contain heparin and histamine. The basophils are thought to be involved in allergic and stress responses.

Nongranular Leukocytes. There are two groups of nongranular leukocytes, the monocytes and the lymphocytes. The *monocytes* are the second order of cells to arrive at the inflammation site; their arrival usually requires 5 hours or more. Within 48 hours, however, the monocytes are usually the predominant cell type in the inflamed area. Monocytes are the largest of the white blood cells and constitute about 3% to 8% of the total leukocyte count. The circulating life span of the monocyte is three to four times longer than that of the granulocytes, and these cells survive for a longer period in the tissues. The monocytes, which are phagocytic cells, are often referred to as *macrophages*. The monocytes engulf larger and greater quantities of foreign material than the neutrophils. These leukocytes play an important role in chronic inflammation and are also involved in the immune response. When the monocyte leaves the vascular system and enters the tissue spaces, it becomes known as a *histiocyte*. Histiocytes function as macrophages in the inflamed area. They can also proliferate to form a capsule, enclosing foreign material that cannot be digested.

The *lymphocytes* constitute 20% to 30% of the WBCs count. There are two types of lymphocytes: B cells and T cells. The B cells differentiate to form antibody-producing plasma cells and are involved in humoral immunity. The T cells are concerned with cell-mediated immunity.

Margination and Pavementing. During the early stages of the inflammatory response, fluid leaves the capillaries of the microcirculation causing blood viscosity to increase. As this occurs, the leukocytes begin to *marginate*, or move to the periphery of the blood vessel. As the process continues, the marginated leukocytes begin to adhere to the vessel lining in preparation for emigration from the vessel. The cobblestone appearance of the vessel lining due to margination of leukocytes has led to the term *pavementing.*

Emigration of Leukocytes. *Emigration* is a mechanism whereby the leukocytes extend pseudopodia (false feet), pass through the capillary walls by ameboid movement, and migrate into the tissue spaces. The movement of white blood cells through the wall of the capillary occurs by means of a process called *diapedesis*. Along with the emigration of leukocytes, there is also an escape of red cells from the capillary.

The red cells may escape singly or in small jets at points where the capillaries have become distended.

Chemotaxis. The leukocytes, after emigrating through the vessel wall, wander through the tissue space guided by the presence of bacteria and cellular debris. The process by which leukocytes are attracted to bacteria and cellular debris is called *chemotaxis*. Chemotaxis can be positive or negative, meaning that it can act either to attract or to repel the leukocytes. Many substances are capable of acting as chemotaxic agents, including infectious organisms, complement (to be discussed), and tissue debris.

Phagocytosis. In the final stage of the cellular response, the neutrophils and monocytes engulf and degrade the bacteria and cellular debris in a process called *phagocytosis* (Fig. 13-2). The neutrophils are sometimes called *microphages* because they concentrate on the phagocytosis of bacteria and small particles. The monocytes, or macrophages, remove tissue debris and larger particles from the area of inflammation.

Phagocytosis involves four distinct but interrelated steps: (1) chemotaxis, (2) opsonization, (3) engulfment, and (4) intracellular killing. Neutrophil and macrophage chemotaxis can be stimulated by many factors including complement, chemotactic factors produced by leukocytes, and compounds elaborated by bacteria. Opsonization renders pathogens more susceptible to ingestion by phagocytic cells by providing binding sites for attachment of the phagocyte

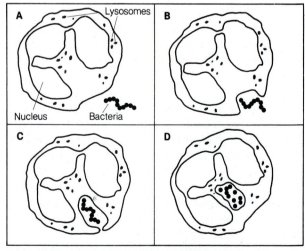

FIG. 13-2. Phagocytosis by a neutrophil. In **A**, a neutrophil has emigrated from the capillary; in **B**, it is attracted to the bacteria through chemotaxis; and in **C**, it engulfs the bacteria. **D** shows the final stages of phagocytosis: the bacteria are degraded by the enzymes and digestive materials contained in the cytoplasmic granules of the neutrophil.

to the pathogen. Two opsonins are immunoglobulin (IgG) and the C3b fragment of complement.

Engulfment occurs once the phagocyte recognizes the agent as foreign. Cytoplasm-filled extensions of the cell membrane surround and enclose the agent, forming a membrane-enclosed phagocytic vesicle or phagosome. Interiorization occurs as the phagosome breaks away from the cell membrane and moves inside the cell. Once inside the cell, the phagosome merges with a lysosome and lysosomal enzymes digest the agent (see Chapter 1).

Intracellular killing of pathogens is accomplished through a number of mechanisms associated with an acid pH environment, enzymes, and oxygen-dependent myeloperoxidases and peroxides. Neutrophils contain granules that participate in destruction of the agent. Neutrophils are generally concerned with phagocytosis of bacteria and organisms that rely on evading phagocytosis for survival.

INFLAMMATORY MEDIATORS

Although inflammation is precipitated by injury and cell death, its signs and symptoms are produced by chemical mediators. Mediators can be classified by function: (1) those with vasoactive and smooth muscle constricting properties such as histamine, prostaglandins, leukotrienes, platelet activating factor (PAF), and adenosine; (2) chemotactic factors such as complement fragments (high and low molecular weight polypeptides, which stimulate chemotaxis of neutrophils and eosinophils); (3) enzymes derived from mast cells, which can cleave complement and activate kallikrein; and (4) reactive molecules liberated from neutrophils and eosinophils, which when released into the extracellular environment can cause damage to the surrounding tissue.[3] Table 13-1 describes the prominent manifestations of inflammation and the chemical substances that mediate their occurrence.

Histamine. Histamine is widely distributed throughout the body. It can be found in platelets, basophils, and mast cells. Histamine causes dilatation of arterioles and enhanced permeability of capillaries and venules. It is the first mediator in the initial inflammatory response. Antihistamine drugs suppress this immediate transient response induced by mild injury.

Plasma Proteases. The plasma proteases consist of the kinins, complement and its fractional components, and clotting factors. One of the kinins, bradykinin, causes increased capillary permeability and pain. The complement system consists of a number of component proteins and their cleavage products.

TABLE 13-1. SIGNS OF INFLAMMATION AND CORRESPONDING CHEMICAL MEDIATORS

INFLAMMATORY RESPONSE	CHEMICAL MEDIATOR
Swelling, redness, and tissue warmth (vasodilation and capillary permeability)	Histamine Prostaglandins Leukotrienes Bradykinin Platelet-activating factor
Tissue damage	Lysosomal enzymes of neutrophils and macrophages
Chemotaxis	Complement fractions
Pain	Prostaglandins Bradykinin
Fever	Interleukin-1 Tumor necrosis factor
Leukocytosis	Interleukin-1, other cytokines

These substances interact with the antigen–antibody complexes and mediate immunologic injury and inflammation. The clotting system (see Chapter 17) contributes to the vascular phase of inflammation, mainly through fibrinopeptides that are formed during the final step of the clotting process.

Prostaglandins. The prostaglandins, so named because they were first identified in the prostate gland, are ubiquitous tissue proteins composed of lipid-soluble acids derived from arachidonic acid, which is stored in cell membrane phospholipids. The synthesis of prostaglandins occurs in two stages: (1) arachidonic acid is liberated from the phospholipids of the cell membrane and (2) converted to prostaglandins. This second stage requires the enzyme cyclo-oxygenase. Prostaglandins contribute to vasodilation, capillary permeability, and the pain and fever that accompany inflammation. There are a number of prostaglandins. The stable prostaglandins (PGE_1 and PGE_2) induce inflammation and potentiate the effects of histamine and other inflammatory mediators. The prostaglandin thromboxane A_2 promotes platelet aggregation and vasoconstriction. Prostacycline (PGI_2) has the opposite effect. It relaxes vascular smooth muscle and inhibits platelet aggregation. Drugs such as aspirin and indomethacin (a nonsteroidal antiinflammatory drug) inhibit prostaglandin synthesis by suppressing cyclo-oxygenase activity. The glucocorticoid hormones secreted from the adrenal cortex (or given as a drug) are known to curtail the availability of arachidonic acid for prostaglandin production.[4] The glucocorticoid drugs have come to be known as antiinflammatory drugs because of their ability to suppress the inflammatory response.

Leukotrienes. The leukotrienes are a group of chemical mediators capable of inciting the inflammatory response. Their name was chosen because they were discovered on the leukocyte and they have a chemical triene structure. One of the leukotrienes causes slow and sustained constriction of the bronchioles and is an important inflammatory mediator in bronchial asthma and immediate hypersensitivity reactions (see Chapter 27). The leukotrienes have also been reported to have an effect on: the permeability of the postcapillary venules; the adhesion properties of the endothelial cells; the extravasation of the white blood cells; and the chemotaxis of PMN cells, eosinophils, and monocytes.[5] Like the prostaglandins, the leukotrienes are formed from arachidonic acid but they use the lipoxygenase pathway, which involves the enzyme lipoxygenase. Thus, it appears that prostaglandins and leukotrienes are part of a larger biologic control system based on arachidonic acid. Depending on the active enzymes in the stimulated cell, arachidonic acid can be converted to several biologically active compounds, which regulate various cellular responses to injury.

Platelet Activating Factor Generated from a complex lipid stored in cell membranes, PAF affects a variety of cell types and induces platelet aggregation. It activates neutrophils and is a potent eosinophil chemoattractant. When injected in the skin, PAF causes a wheal-and-flare reaction and leukocyte infiltration. When inhaled, it causes bronchospasm, eosinophilic infiltrate, and nonspecific bronchial hyperreactivity.

CYTOKINES

Cytokines are hormonelike polypeptides that are produced during the initial response to a foreign agent or substance. They participate in a variety of cellular responses, particularly as modulators of the immune response (to be discussed). They are produced by many different cell types but principally by macrophages and activated lymphocytes. Cytokines are usually named for the cell that produced them (*e.g.*, lymphokines, monokines). Most cytokines have more than one biologic property and share a number of overlapping functions (Table 13-2). Cytokines play an important role in host resistance and have been identified as important mediators of inflammation. Interleukin-1 (formerly known as endogenous pyrogen), tumor necrosis factor α (cachectin), and α-interferon are cytokines involved in the induction of fever, leukocytosis, and secondary cytokine stimulation.[6]

INFLAMMATORY EXUDATES

Characteristically, the acute inflammatory response involves production of exudates. These exudates can vary in terms of fluid, plasma protein, and cell content. Acute inflammation can produce serous, fibrinous, membranous, purulent, and hemorrhagic exudates. Inflammatory exudates are often composed of a combination of these types.

Serous Exudate. The initial exudate that enters the inflammatory site is largely plasma. Serous drainage is a watery exudate low in protein content. A blister contains serous fluid. A catarrhal inflammation is one that affects the mucous membranes and is associated with an increase in watery secretions and desquamation of the epithelial cells. Hay fever is an example of a catarrhal inflammatory response.

Fibrinous Exudate. Fibrinous exudates contain large amounts of fibrinogen and form a thick and sticky meshwork, much like the fibers of a blood clot. Fibrinous exudates are frequently encountered in the serous cavities of the body. Acute rheumatic fever often causes development of a fibrinous pericarditis. A fibrinous exudate must be removed through fibrinolytic activity of enzymes before healing can take place. Failure to remove the exudate leads to ingrowth of fibroblasts and subsequent development of scar tissue and adhesions. A fibrinous exudate may be beneficial in that it tends to glue the inflamed structures together, thereby preventing the spread of infection. In appendicitis, for example, the initial formation of a fibrinous exudate serves to localize the organisms in the region of the appendix and thus prevents the generalized spread of the infection to the peritoneal cavity.

Membranous Exudate. Membranous or pseudomembranous exudates develop on mucous membrane surfaces. The development of a membranous exudate occurs as necrotic cells become enmeshed in a fibrinopurulent exudate that coats the mucosal surface. *Diphtheria* was known for its ability to produce a membranous exudate on the surface of the trachea and major bronchi. *Thrush* is a monilial infection of the oral cavity that produces patches of membranous inflammation. *Membranous enterocolitis* is a severe membranous inflammatory condition of the bowel mucosa related to a disturbance in the normal bowel flora due to treatment with a variety of broad-spectrum antibiotics.

TABLE 13-2. CHARACTERISTIC BIOLOGIC PROPERTIES OF HUMAN CYTOKINES

CYTOKINE	BIOLOGIC PROPERTIES
Interleukin-1 (alpha and beta)	Activates resting T cells; is cofactor for hematopoietic growth factor; induces fever, sleep, ACTH release, neutrophilia, and other systemic acute-phase responses; stimulates synthesis of lymphokines, collagen, and collagenases; activates endothelial and macrophagic cells; mediates inflammation, catabolic processes, and nonspecific resistance to infection
Interleukin-2	Growth factor for activated T cells; induces the synthesis of other lymphokines; activates cytotoxic lymphocytes
Interleukin-3	Supports the growth of pluripotent (multilineage) bone-marrow stem cells; is growth factor for mast cells
Interleukin-4	Growth factor for activated B cells, resting T cells, and mast cells; induces class I (DR) expression on B cells; enhances cytotoxic T cells; activates macrophages
Interleukin-5	B cell differentiating and growth factor; promotes differentiation of eosinophils; promotes antibody production (IgA)
Interleukin-6	Acts as cofactor for immunoglobulin production by B cells; growth factor for hybridomas, myelomas, and plasmacytomas; stimulates hepatocytes to produce acute phase proteins
Interleukin-7	Stimulates pre-B cells and thymocytes. Stimulates myeloid precursors and megakaryocytes
Interleukin-8	Chemoattracts neutrophils and T-lymphocytes; regulates lymphocyte homing and neutrophil infiltration
Gamma-interferon	Induces class I, class II (DR), and other surface antigens on a variety of cells, activates macrophages and endothelial cells; augments or inhibits other lymphokine activities; augments natural killer cell activity; exerts antiviral activity
Interferon (alpha and beta)	Exerts antiviral activity; induces class I antigen expression; augments natural killer cell activity; has fever-inducing and antiproliferative properties
Tumor necrosis factor (alpha and beta)	Direct cytotoxin for some tumor cells; induces fever, sleep, and other systemic acute-phase responses; stimulates the synthesis of other cytokines, collagen, and collagenases; activates endothelial and macrophagic cells; mediates inflammation, catabolic processes, and septic shock
Colony-stimulating factor (CSF)	
Granulocyte-macrophage CSF	Promotes neutrophilic, eosinophilic, and macrophagic bone marrow colonies, activates mature granulocytes
Granulocyte CSF	Promotes neutrophilic colonies
Macrophage CSF	Promotes macrophagic colonies
T-cell growth factor-β	Is chemotactic for fibroblasts; inhibits proliferation of endothelial cells, epithelial cells, and T- and B-lymphocytes; suppresses NK cell activity

Purulent Exudate. A purulent (suppurative) exudate contains pus, which is composed of the remains of white blood cells, proteins, and tissue debris. Purulent infections are caused by a number of pyogenic or pus-forming bacteria. An *abscess* is a localized collection of pus. Abscesses may occur at the site of injury, or they may develop as the result of metastatic spread of infectious organisms and tissue debris through the bloodstream. An abscess is encapsulated in a so-called pyogenic membrane, which consists of layers of fibrin, inflammatory cells, and granulation tissue. An abscess may need to be incised and the pus removed before healing can occur.

Cellulitis, or phlegmonous inflammation, is a subgroup of suppurative infections that involve massive necrosis of tissue along with production of purulent infiltrates. Instead of producing small localized collections of pus, certain pyogenic organisms (usually the streptococci) elaborate a large amount of spreading factor, the *hyaluronidases*, which break down the fibrin meshwork and other barriers designed to localize the infection.

Hemorrhagic Exudate. A hemorrhagic exudate occurs in situations in which severe tissue injury causes damage to blood vessels or when there is diapedesis of red blood cells from the capillaries. Often a hemorrhagic exudate accompanies other forms of exudate. A *serosanguineous* exudate describes a combination of serous and hemorrhagic exudates.

RESOLUTION OF ACUTE INFLAMMATION

Acute inflammation can be resolved in one of three ways: (1) it can undergo resolution, with the injured area returning to normal or near-normal appearance and function; (2) it can progress, and suppurative processes may develop; or (3) it can proceed to the chronic phase. In the process of responding to injury, the body uses only those behaviors in the inflammatory sequence that are necessary to prevent or halt the destruction of tissue.

THE ACUTE-PHASE RESPONSE

Infection, injury, and inflammatory processes produce a constellation of systemic effects that are often collectively referred to as the *acute-phase response*. The acute-phase response, which usually begins within hours or days of the onset of inflammation or infection, includes: leukocytosis, fever and increased metabolism (see Chapter 10), increased erythrocyte sedimentation rate (ESR), decreased plasma iron levels and anemia, skeletal muscle catabolism and negative nitrogen balance, anorexia, and increases in lassitude and sleep.[7–9]

The manifestations of the acute-phase response, which has the characteristics of a generalized host response irrespective of the localized or systemic nature of the inciting agent, are associated with the production of cytokines, particularly interleukin-1 (IL-1), tumor necrosis factor α (TNF-α), and α-interferon.[7,10] These cytokines affect the thermoregulatory center in the hypothalamus to produce fever, the most obvious sign of the acute-phase response. Interleukin-1 and other cytokines induce an increase in the number and immaturity of circulating neutrophils by stimulating their production in the bone marrow. Neutrophil activation is also up-regulated. Sleepiness, a common feature of the acute-phase response, results from the effects of IL-1 and TNF-α on the central nervous system.

During the acute-phase response, the liver dramatically increases the synthesis of acute-phase proteins such as fibrinogen and the C-reactive protein, which may serve several different nonspecific host-defense functions.[8] These acute-phase proteins contribute to the increased sedimentation rate of the erythrocytes. There is evidence that decreased levels of serum iron have an important protective role in combating various bacteria.[7] Sequestering of iron in the liver during the acute-phase response causes a rapid drop in serum iron levels, contributing to the development of anemia in some people. Other factors such as decreased red-cell survival also contribute to the anemia, but the role of interleukin in this process is unclear.

The metabolic changes that occur with the acute-phase response include skeletal muscle catabolism and liberation of amino acids that are used in the synthesis of lymphokines, immunoglobulins, fibroblasts, and collagen needed for repair of injured tissue. Fat metabolism decreases during the acute-phase response, whereas amino acids are used for glucose production and energy. A common manifestation of infection and inflammation is a decrease in food appetite that occurs at a time during which metabolism and the need for energy substrates are often markedly increased. This acute-phase anorexia can be a major factor in the negative nitrogen balance and body weight loss that occurs with injury and infection.

Disorders of interleukin production and its effects may contribute to the pathology of some chronic inflammatory conditions. Elevated levels have been reported in the serum of people with fever, sepsis, and Crohn's disease. Interleukin has also been detected in joint effusions of people with rheumatoid arthritis and other joint disease.

The numerous effects of interleukin in producing the acute-phase response can be used as a means for monitoring the inflammatory process. The measurement of fever, white blood cell count, and ESR are well-established procedures for monitoring many disease states. The ESR is a laboratory test that measures the speed at which erythrocytes settle when an anticoagulant is added to the blood. In this test, the blood to which the anticoagulant is added is placed in a long, narrow tube and the speed at which the cells settle is observed. Methods for measuring interleukin-1 have also been developed.[7] Although these methods are not standardized, it seems likely that they will be refined and used to monitor the inflammatory response.

CHRONIC INFLAMMATION

To this point, we have discussed acute inflammation associated with a self-limiting stimulus, such as a burn or infection, that is rapidly controlled by host defenses. Chronic inflammation, on the other hand, is self-perpetuating and may last for weeks, months, or even years. It may develop in the course of a recurrent or progressive acute inflammatory process or as the result of a low-grade smoldering response that fails to evoke an acute response. Characteristic of chronic inflammation is an infiltration by mononuclear cells (macrophages, lymphocytes, and plasma cells) rather than neutrophils, such as occurs in acute inflammation. Chronic inflammation also involves the proliferation of fibroblasts rather than exudates. As a result, the risk of scarring and deformity developing is usually considerably greater than in acute inflammation.

In contrast to agents that provoke sufficient initial tissue injury to evoke the acute inflammatory response, agents that evoke chronic inflammation are typically low-grade persistent irritants that are unable to penetrate deeply or spread rapidly. Among the causes of chronic inflammation are foreign bodies such as talc, silica, asbestos, and certain surgical suture materials. Many viruses provoke a chronic inflammatory response, as do certain bacteria, fungi, and larger parasites of moderate to low virulence. Examples are the tubercle bacillus, the treponema of syphilis, and the actinomyces. The presence of injured or altered tissue, such as that surrounding a tumor or healing fracture, may also incite chronic inflammation. In many cases of chronic inflammation, such as sarcoidosis, the inciting agent is unknown. Little is known about the mediators of the chronic inflammatory response. Immunologic mechanisms are thought to play an important role in chronic inflammation.

There are two patterns of chronic inflammation: (1) a nonspecific chronic inflammation and (2) granulomatous inflammation.

NONSPECIFIC CHRONIC INFLAMMATION

Nonspecific chronic inflammation involves a diffuse accumulation of macrophages and lymphocytes at the site of injury. Macrophages are accumulated from three sources: (1) continued recruitment of monocytes, the precursors of tissue macrophages, from the circulation in response to chemotaxic factors; (2) local proliferation of macrophages after they have left the bloodstream; (3) prolonged survival and immobilization of macrophages within the inflammatory site.[1] These mechanisms lead to fibroblast proliferation with subsequent scar formation that, in many cases, replaces the normal supporting connective tissue elements or the functional parenchymal tissue of the involved structure. For example, scar tissue resulting from chronic inflammation of the bowel causes narrowing of the bowel lumen, and in chronic glomerulonephritis there is a loss of functional nephrons.

GRANULOMATOUS INFLAMMATION

A granulomatous lesion is a form of chronic inflammation. A granuloma is typically a small, 1- to 2-mm lesion in which there is a massing of macrophages surrounded by lymphocytes. These modified macrophages resemble epithelial cells and are sometimes called *epithelioid cells*. Like other macrophages, the epithelioid cells that form a granuloma are derived from blood monocytes. Granulomatous inflammation is associated with foreign bodies such as splinters, sutures, silica, and talc particles, and with microorganisms such as those that cause tuberculosis, syphilis, sarcoidosis, deep fungal infections, and brucellosis. These types of agents have one thing in common—they are poorly digested and are usually not easily controlled by other inflammatory mechanisms.

The epithelioid cells in granulomatous inflammation may either clump in a mass (granuloma) or coalesce, forming a large multinucleated giant cell that attempts to surround the foreign agent. Some giant cells may contain as many as 200 nuclei. A giant cell is usually surrounded by granuloma cells, and a dense membrane of connective tissue eventually encapsulates the lesion and isolates it. A tubercle is a granulomatous inflammatory response to the tubercle bacillus. Peculiar to the tuberculosis granuloma is the presence of a caseous (cheesy) necrotic center. In the past, surgical gloves were dusted with talc so they could be slipped on easily, but particles of talc frequently ended up in the surgical field and caused granulomatous lesions to develop. Surgical gloves are now dusted with an absorbable starch that does not cause this problem.

In summary, inflammation describes a local response to tissue injury and can present as an acute or chronic condition. Acute inflammation is the local response of tissue to a nonspecific form of injury. The classic signs of inflammation are redness, swelling, local heat, pain, and loss of function. The inflammatory response is orchestrated by chemical mediators such as histamine, prostaglandins, PAF, adenosine, complement fragments, and reactive molecules that are liberated from the granulocytes. Acute inflammation involves a hemodynamic phase during which blood flow and capillary permeability are increased and a cellular phase during which phagocytic WBCs called *granulocytes* move into the area to engulf and degrade the inciting agent. Chemical mediators called *cytokines* participate in the cellular responses, particularly those involving the immune response. Acute inflammation involves the production of exudates containing serous fluid (serous exudate), red blood cells (hemorrhagic exudate), fibrinogen (fibrinous exudate), products of mucous membrane and fibrinogen breakdown products (membranous exudate), and tissue debris and WBC breakdown products (purulent exudate).

In contrast to the acute inflammatory process which is self-limiting, chronic inflammation is more prolonged and is usually caused by persistent irritants, most of which are insoluble and resistant to phagocytosis and other inflammatory mechanisms. Chronic inflammation involves the presence of mononuclear cells (lymphocytes, plasma cells, and macrophages) rather than granulocytes and proliferation of fibroblasts that cause scarring and deformity rather than formation of an exudate as in acute inflammation.

■ THE IMMUNE SYSTEM

The immune system consists of the immune cells and the central and peripheral lymphoid structures. The central immune organs, the bone marrow and the thymus, are the sites of immune cell production. The peripheral lymphoid structures consist of lymph nodes, spleen, tonsils, intestinal lymphoid tissue, and aggregates of lymphoid tissue occurring in non-lymphoid organs. The immune cells interact with antigens in the peripheral lymphoid structures. The lymphoid organs are connected by networks of lymph channels and blood vessels. The immune cells travel throughout the body and into and out of the lymphoid tissue. As they move throughout the body, the immune cells selectively seek out and destroy foreign antigens and materials, while recognizing and sparing the host cells that are identified as self.

Within the last several decades, major scientific advances have enhanced the understanding of the immune system. To a great extent, these advances have resulted from several new technologies including methods for developing monoclonal antibodies and advances in molecular biology used to determine the genetic basis for antigen recognition.

Monoclonal antibodies are produced in a laborious process that fuses an antibody-producing spleen cell from an animal (usually a mouse) with a malignant myeloma cell. The fusion of the two cells results in a single fused cell, or clone, capable of producing a highly specific antibody. The precision of the monoclonal antibody is such that it recognizes a single antigenic site, such as one of those located on the cell surface of hematopoietic or tumor cells.

The stages in the life history of an immune cell are marked by expression of a changing variety of membrane-bound antigen markers. These antigens are not present on bone marrow stem cells but develop as an expression of the differentiation process. For example, membrane-bound antigens differ among T cells according to their level of maturation and among subsets of mature T cells such as CD4+ and CD8+ cells. Thus, monoclonal antibodies can be used for distinguishing among cells of mononuclear phagocytic lineage, in delineating between B cells and T cells, and in differentiating subsets of T cells. It was through the use of monoclonal antibodies that the pathogenesis of acquired immunodeficiency syndrome (AIDS) was made possible.

SELF VERSUS NONSELF: THE ROLE OF THE MAJOR HISTOCOMPATIBILITY COMPLEX ANTIGENS

The ability of the immune system to distinguish self from nonself resides in cell surface antigens that are unique to each person. These antigens are coded by a large cluster of genes called the *major histocompatibility complex* (MHC) located on the short arm of the sixth chromosome. In humans, the histocompatibility antigens are called the *human leukocyte antigens* (HLA) because they were first detected on the leukocyte. The histocompatibility antigens are similar in many respects to the ABO antigens found on red blood cells, which are matched for transfusion purposes.

The histocompatibility antigens are inherited as part of the genetic makeup of a person. Seven closely linked gene loci—HLA-A, HLA-B, HLA-C, HLA-D, HLA-DR, HLA-DQ, and HLA-DP—have been identified. Each of the seven gene loci is occupied by multiple alleles, or alternate genes, that code for the development of each cell surface antigen. There are at least 24 possible gene products or antigens for the A loci and 50 antigens for the B loci. Each of the antigens is numbered, HLA-A1, HLA-A2, and so on. An international workshop meets every 2 to 3 years to update the nomenclature of the HLA complex.

A person's HLA type is inherited. Because of their close linkage, the combination of HLA genes at each locus is usually inherited as a unit. This unit is called a *haplotype*. Each person inherits a chromosome from each parent and, therefore, has two HLA haplotypes for each gene locus. By simple mendelian inheritance, there is a 25% chance that two siblings will share the same haplotype, a 50% chance that they will share one haplotype, and a 25% chance that they will share no haplotype. Unlike blood types, common HLA types are highly unlikely. When one considers that there are at least 24 gene products for the HLA-A locus and 50 gene products for the HLA-B gene locus, the diversity of HLA types among the general population becomes tremendous. With the exception of identical twins, the chances of two people having exactly the same HLA type are unlikely. The typing of histocompatibility antigens is important in tissue grafting and organ transplantation. The closer the matching of HLA types, the less the chance of rejection.

Based on their tissue distribution and structure, HLA antigens have been subdivided into three categories: classes I, II, and III.[3] Class I MHC antigens, referred to as the *classic histocompatibility antigens*, include the HLA-A, HLA-B, and HLA-C antigens. These antigens are glycoproteins found on the surface of virtually all nucleated cells. Class II MHC antigens include the HLA-D, HLA-DR, HLA, HLA-DQ, and HLA-DP antigen. These are surface glycoproteins found only on cells of the immune system, such a B-lymphocytes and macrophages. Class III molecules include components of complement. Class III molecules are soluble and do not act as transplantation antigens.

IMMUNE CELLS

The primary cells of the immune system are the small WBCs called *lymphocytes*. Lymphocytes represent 20% to 30% of the leukocytes (Fig. 13-3). Like other blood cells, they are derived from stem cells in the bone marrow that differentiate into lymphocytic precursor cells called *lymphoblasts* (Fig. 13-4). One class of lymphocytes, the B-lymphocytes (B cells), undergoes maturation in the bone marrow. The other class of lymphocytes, the T-lymphocytes (T cells), completes maturation in the thymus. About 60% to 70% of the lymphocytes are T cells, and 10% to 20% are B cells.[1] Most of the remaining lymphocytes are not identified as either T cells or B cells, but as a cell population called natural killer cells. Under the microscope, both T-lymphocytes and B-lymphocytes have similar appearances. However, both types of lymphocytes express different surface antigens and both have functional properties that distinguish them. Within both lymphocyte populations are subsets of cells with their own special properties. In addition to lymphocytes, cells of the mononuclear phagocytic system, monocytes and macrophages, serve as accessory cells for the immune system. The macrophages capture the antigen, process it, and present it to the lymphocytes.

Both B-lymphocytes and T-lymphocytes manifest immunologic specificity (*i.e.*, they are programmed to respond to a specific antigen). B-cell specificity is

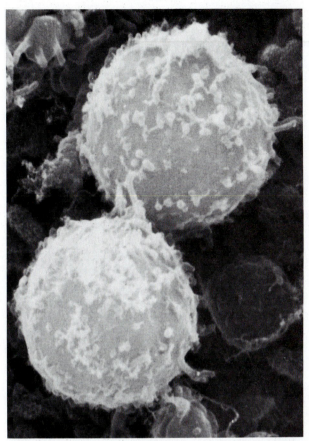

FIG. 13-3. A scanning micrograph of two lymphocytes. (Courtesy of Kenneth Siegesmund, Ph.D., Anatomy Department, Medical College of Wisconsin)

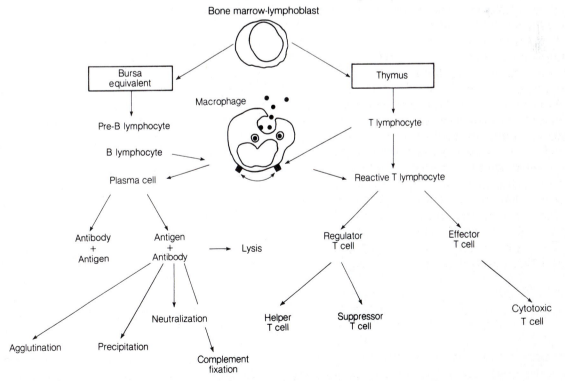

FIG. 13-4. The development of cellular and humoral immunity.

expressed as antibody receptor proteins, and T-cell specificity is expressed as cell surface receptors. Within the T-cell and B-cell populations are both effector cells and memory cells. Effector cells (activated T cells and antibody-producing plasma cells of the B-cell population) are instrumental in causing destruction of the antigen. Effector cell specificity is accomplished through an antigen-stimulated gene reshuffling process, resulting in a clone of cytotoxic T cells or plasma cells with receptors that exactly match those of the stimulating antigen. In the case of the plasma cells, the antigen receptors are expressed on the antibody (immunoglobulin) that is produced. Memory cells are formed after initial exposure to the antigen. They revert to an inactive state but are able to proliferate rapidly and increase the intensity of the immune response with subsequent exposure to the specific antigen of which they have a memory. There is considerable interaction among immune cells. Only certain antigens stimulate B cells. With most immune responses that elicit a humoral (antibody) response, T-lymphocytes interact with B-lymphocytes, facilitating their activation and regulating their differentiation. The functions of the macrophage are essential to both T-cell and B-cell function.

T-LYMPHOCYTES

The T-lymphocytes function in the activation of other T cells and B cells, in the control of viral infections, in the rejection of grafts of foreign tissues, and in delayed hypersensitivity reactions (see Chapter 14). Collectively, these immune responses are referred to as cell-mediated or cellular immunity. The T cells take the lead in the immune response when they recognize an antigen presented on the surface of macrophages. Activated in this way, T cells produce soluble factors that recruit other T cells and B cells. T-lymphocytes can only recognize an antigen when it is associated with MHC membrane-bound products. This dual recognition of both nonself antigen and the self MHC gene products is important for activation of both cytotoxic effector cells and immunoregulatory cells.[11]

The T-lymphocytes arise from precursors in the bone marrow and travel to the thymus where they are programmed to differentiate into T cells. T cells have a life span of years; they leave the hymus and circulate throughout the body in the bloodstream. Selected subpopulations of T cells transiently seed the lymph nodes, spleen, or other peripheral immune tissues and reenter the circulation in a lymphaticovenous communication system.

There are two populations of T cells: regulatory T cells and effector T cells. Both regulatory and effector T cells synthesize and release cytokines. The T-cell regulatory functions involve amplification of cell-mediated cytotoxicity by other T cells and immunoglobulin production by B cells. Regulatory T cells act by either enhancing or suppressing the action of the B-lymphocytes. These cells are called the helper and suppressor T cells. The helper T cells may be the switch to the immune system. B cells can recognize antigen independent of T-cell stimulation, but their proliferation and terminal differentiation require activation by helper T cells. The suppressor T cells seem to be equally important in regulating the immune response by providing negative feedback; they make the immune response self-limiting. The cytotoxic or killer T cells serve as effector cells. The cytotoxic T cell destroys by binding to cell surface antigens on the target cell and releasing lymphokines that destroy the cell membrane on the target cell. The close contact between the cytotoxic T cell and the target cell ensures that neighboring cells are not indiscriminately destroyed.

The mature T cells contain surface antigens called *clusters of differentiation* (CD). These antigens serve as markers to define functionally distinct T-cell subsets. About 70% of mature cells carry the CD4+ antigen and 30% carry the CD8+ antigen. The CD4+ cells act as helper and inducer T cells by recognizing processed antigen in association with class II MHC products.

The CD8+ cells are either suppressor or cytotoxic T cells; they recognize antigens in association with class I MHC gene products. All T cells recognize antigens by a membrane structure called the CD3+/T-cell antigen receptor complex.[12]

B-LYMPHOCYTES

The B-lymphocytes are responsible for humoral immunity. Humoral immunity provides for elimination of bacterial invaders, neutralization of bacterial toxins, prevention of viral reinfection, and immediate allergic responses (see Chapter 14).

The B-lymphocytes can be identified by the presence of B-cell antigens, immunoglobulin and complement receptors, and class II MHC antigens on their surface. They are called *B-lymphocytes* because, in fowl, B-cell precursors migrate from the bone marrow to a hindgut structure, the bursa of Fabricius, where they differentiate and mature. Because mammals do not have a bursa of Fabricius, the differentiation of B cells is thought to occur in the bone marrow.

During the maturation process, the premature or *pre-cells* rearrange their immunoglobulin genes and begin to express surface immunoglobins that have not as yet interacted with antigen. At this stage, the B cells leave the bone marrow; they enter the circulation and migrate to the spleen or other peripheral lymphoid structures. The migration of the B cells from the bone marrow to the spleen is an antigen-independent process. In the absence of antigen stimulation, the life of a B cell ends after this process. Most B cells reaching the spleen die within a few days.[13] B cells that encounter antigens complementary to their surface immunoglobulins and receive T-cell help undergo a series of changes that transform them into immunoglobulin (antibody)-secreting plasma cells and memory cells. The antigen molecules that bind to immunoglobulin receptors are taken into the B cell and are partially digested, and the antigen fragments are recycled to the B-cell surface and expressed in association with the class II MHC antigens. The combination of antigen fragments and the MHC molecules are recognized by helper T cells. In this way, B cells can present antigen to helper T cells and stimulate the production of T-cell lymphokines that stimulate the antigen-presenting B cell to divide and undergo terminal differentiation into mature plasma cells, which produce thousands of antibody molecules per second before their death a day or so later.[13] Memory cells that retain the antibody-producing information are also produced after primary exposure to antigen.

The immunoglobulins have been divided into five classes: IgG, IgA, IgM, IgD, and IgE (Table 13-3). Each of the immunoglobulins is composed of two heavy (H) chains and two light (L) chains (Fig. 13-5). The heavy chains in each of the classes of immunoglobulins are antigenically distinctive, and this distinction permits division of the immunoglobulins into classes through the use of immunoelectrophoresis. The amino acid sequence of each of the heavy chains and each of the light chains has a constant (C) region and a variable (V) region. An antigen reacts with the variable region. Each different type of immunoglobulin is produced by a separate clone of B cells and has a different amino acid sequence in the variable region, which provides it with the specificity needed to react with a single antigen. Clonal diversity is generated during the early stages of B-cell differentiation—a process that involves a series of immunoglobulin-gene rearrangements. As the immature B cell achieves a functional gene arrangement for immunoglobulin production, it begins to express membrane-bound IgM molecules. Over the next couple of days, most B cells also begin to produce IgD. Within each B-cell clone, some members switch from the expression of IgM and IgD to the expression of IgG, IgA, or IgE.[14]

IgG (gamma globulin) is the most abundant of the immunoglobulins. It circulates in body fluids and is the only immunoglobulin that crosses the placenta. In the past several years, it has been found that there are four subsets of IgG (IgG1, IgG2, IgG3, and IgG4).

TABLE 13-3. CLASSES OF IMMUNOGLOBULINS

CLASS	PERCENTAGE OF TOTAL	CHARACTERISTICS
IgG	75.0	Present in majority of B cells; contains antiviral, antitoxin, and antibacterial antibodies; only immunoglobulin that crosses the placenta; responsible for protection of newborn; activates complement and binds to macrophages
IgA	15.0	Predominant immunoglobulin in body secretions, such as saliva, nasal and respiratory secretions, breast milk; protects mucous membranes
IgM	10.0	Forms the natural antibodies such as those for ABO blood antigens; prominent in early immune responses; activates complement
IgD	0.2	Action is not known; may affect B-cell maturation
IgE	0.004	Binds to mast cells and basophils; involved in allergic and hypersensitivity reactions

IgG1 is the predominant subclass (58% to 71% of the total IgG), IgG2 (19% to 31%), IgG3 (5% to 8%), and IgG4 (1% to 5%).[15] IgG subclass restrictions have been reported for antibodies against many bacterial and viral antigens. For example, tetanus toxoid antibody is found predominantly with the IgG1 subclass and IgG2 appears to be specific for bacteria that are encapsulated with a polysaccharide covering such as pneumococcus, *Hemophilus influenzae*, and *Neisseria meningitides*.

IgA, the second most abundant of the immunoglobulins, is found in saliva, tears, and bronchial, gastrointestinal, prostatic, and vaginal secretions. It is a secretory immunoglobulin and is considered to be a primary defense against local infections. The difference in protection afforded by the IgG and the IgA immunoglobulins can be illustrated using the two types of polio vaccine—Salk and Sabin. With

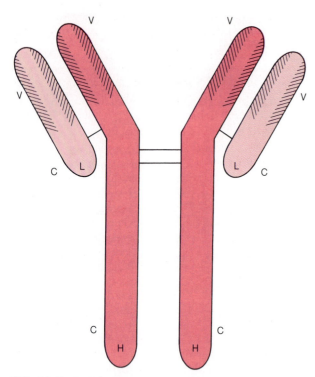

FIG. 13-5. Basic immunoglobulin structure formed from four polypeptide chains bound together. Light chains (L), heavy chains (H), constant amino acid region (C), and variable amino acid region (V). Antigens bind to the variable region of the immunoglobulin.

some viral infections, such as poliovirus, systemic infection follows an initial mucosal phase during which the virus replicates in the mucosa of the portal of entry. In these infections, circulating IgG antibodies are important in preventing systemic disease. The Salk polio vaccine (killed virus administered by injection) prompts the production of systemic IgG antibodies and protects against the systemic effects of the virus. However, the Salk vaccine does not stimulate production of IgA secretory antibodies, and there can be growth of the organisms in the gastrointestinal tract and establishment of a carrier state. With the oral Sabin polio vaccine, IgA secretory antibody production is induced and virus replication and subsequent mucosal penetration are prevented as is systemic dissemination of the virus and development of the carrier state.

IgE is involved in allergic and hypersensitivity reactions. It binds to mast cells and causes release of histamine and other mediators of allergic reactions.

MACROPHAGES

The monocytes and tissue macrophages are a part of the mononuclear phagocyte system, formerly called the *reticuloendothelial system*. All of the cells of the mononuclear phagocytic system arise from a com-

mon precursor in the bone marrow that gives rise to the blood monocytes, which migrate to the various tissues where they are transformed into macrophages.[16] The tissue macrophages are scattered in connective tissue or clustered in organs such as the lung (alveolar macrophages), liver (Kupffer's cells), spleen sinusoids, lymph nodes, peritoneum, central nervous system (microglial cells), and other areas. Langerhans' cells are macrophages that are located in the skin; they are involved in cell-mediated immune reactions of the skin such as delayed contact hypersensitivity and they play an important role in induction of allergic contact sensitivity (see Chapter 14).[17]

The cells of the mononuclear phagocyte system, also called *accessory cells*, are antigen-processing cells (APC). They participate in the immune response by capturing and breaking down microorganisms and antigen-containing substances and presenting the antigen to the lymphocytes in a form that increases its immunogenicity (Fig. 13-6). In the process of phagocytosis, the macrophage ingests the foreign substance, digests it, and moves the antigen fragments to the cell surface along with class II MHC gene products. The combined antigen fragments and class II MHC gene products are recognized by T cells. The interaction between the modified antigen particles on the macrophage receptors and the lymphocyte stimulates lymphocyte differentiation and proliferation. These receptor–site interactions also appear to pro-

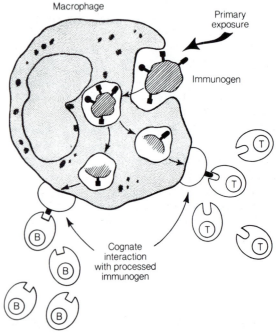

FIG. 13-6. The interaction between the immunogen (antigen), macrophage, and T-lymphocytes and B-lymphocytes.

vide the stage for T-cell and B-cell interactions; they facilitate the helper role of the T-lymphocytes in terms of B-cell function. The interaction between antigen-presenting macrophages and T cells appears to be limited to helper T cells that bear the CD4 protein on their membrane. Because the helper T cell cannot be triggered by free antigens, presentation of antigen by macrophages or other accessory cells is essential for induction of cell-mediated immunity.[18] Macrophages also produce interleukin, which is a mediator for the inflammatory process, and they can act under T-cell influence to destroy bacteria and tumor cells. Lymphokines produced by the effector T cells cause migration or activation of the macrophages.

Although macrophages can ingest microorganisms and other foreign antigens before the development of specific antibodies, the process is accelerated when antibodies are present. Frequently, soluble proteins that are injected in deaggregated form as vaccine antigens are not attracted to accessory cells and do not provoke antibody formation. For this reason, immunization vaccines are often developed by creating particulate immunogens (alum precipitation or formation of oily droplets), which incite antibody formation and carry the antigen to the accessory cell.[19] As soon as antibody is formed, any remaining soluble antigen is rapidly taken into accessory cells within hours.

NATURAL KILLER CELLS

Natural killer (NK) cells are lymphocytes that are functionally, genotypically, and phenotypically distinct from T cells, B cells, and monocyte-macrophages. The NK cell is defined as an effector cell that displays MHC-unrestricted cytotoxicity toward tumor cells and virus-infected cells.[20] Many NK cells appear as large granular lymphocytes noted for their indented nuclei and abundant pale cytoplasm containing azurophilic granules. The granules may be related to cytotoxicity. Augmentation of NK-cell activity in vitro occurs after exposure to IL-2; this phenomenon is called *lymphokine-activated killer (LAK) activity*. Natural killer cells also participate in antibody-dependent cellular cytotoxicity (ADCC), a mechanism whereby a cytotoxic effector cell can kill an antibody-coated target cell.[3] The role of NK cells is probably one of immune surveillance and host resistance to infection.

LYMPHOID ORGANS

THYMUS

The thymus is an elongated flat bilobed structure that is located in the neck below the thyroid gland and extends into the upper part of the thorax behind the top of the sternum. The thymus is a fully developed organ at birth and weighs about 15 to 20 g.[21] After birth, the thymus grows slowly, reaching a maximum size of about 40 g at puberty. It regresses in size, its lymphoid tissue being replaced by adipose tissue so that in the adult its substance is difficult to distinguish from the adipose tissue in which it is embedded. Nevertheless, some thymus tissue persists into old age.

The function of the thymus is central to the development of the immune system. During embryonic development, the thymus is the first organ to begin the manufacture of lymphocytes. There is evidence that precursor cells of some of the nonthymic lymphoid tissues (*e.g.*, lymph nodes and spleen) originate in the thymus and migrate at various times before and after birth to sites where they establish germinal centers for maintaining the body's immunologic defenses. Impaired thymus function has been associated with immunologic deficiency disorders. If the thymus is removed from certain animals at birth or it is congenitally absent, as it is in certain human conditions, there is a decrease of lymphocytes in the blood, a marked depletion or absence of T-lymphocytes, and an absence of thymus-dependent lymphocytes in the peripheral lymphoid tissues.[22]

Thymic epithelial cells produce soluble factors that influence the growth and maturation of T cells. Maturation of the lymphocytes in the thymus takes about 2 to 3 days, after which the mature lymphocytes migrate from the thymus gland into the bloodstream. From the bloodstream, they enter the inner cortex of the lymph nodes, the periarterial sheaths of the spleen, and other thymus-dependent regions of the peripheral lymphoid tissue.[22] In addition to lymphocytes that arise from resident cells within the thymus, certain hematopoietic cells from the bone marrow are capable of migrating to the thymus where they are somehow instructed to become mature lymphocytes. Before birth, the thymus is the major source of lymphocytes; in later life, the precursor cells migrate to the thymus.

LYMPH NODES

The lymph nodes serve two functions: (1) they remove foreign materials from lymph before it enters the bloodstream and (2) they are centers for proliferation of immune cells. They are located along the lymph ducts, which lead from the tissues to the thoracic duct. Each lymph node processes lymph from a discrete, adjacent anatomic site (see Fig. 16-2). Many lymph nodes are situated in the axillae, groin, and along the great vessels of the neck, thorax, and abdomen.[23] A lymph node consists of an outer cortex and inner medulla and is surrounded by a connective tissue capsule. Lymph enters the node through afferent channels that penetrate the capsule and leaves through the deep indentation in the hilus. Because of the lymph nodes' spongelike structure, the macrophages, lymphocytes, and granulocytes flow slowly through them. The reticular meshwork serves as a surface on which macrophages attach and phagocytose antigens. The T-lymphocytes are more abundant in the medullary portion of the node, and the B-lymphocytes are more abundant in the cortex. The T-lymphocytes proliferate on antigenic stimulation and create germinal centers in the medullary region after stimulation. These centers contain macrophages, growing T-lymphocytes, and smaller adult cells. The cortical germinal centers contain mainly B-lymphocytes and appear to be concerned with antibody production.

SPLEEN

The spleen, which is roughly the size of a clenched fist, is located in the abdomen at the level of the 9th, 10th, and 11th ribs. The spleen is composed of red and white pulp. The red pulp is well supplied with arteries and is the area where senescent and injured red blood cells are destroyed. The white pulp contains concentrated areas of lymphocytes called periarterial lymphoid sheaths, which surround the central arterioles. Although T-lymphocytes are found in the spleen, it is primarily a B-lymphocyte-containing organ.

OTHER LYMPHOID TISSUES

The tonsils have a structure similar to the lymph, thymus, and lymph nodes. Like the thymus, the tonsils are rather large during childhood and regress in size with age. Other important collections of lymphoid tissue exist in the appendix and in the Peyer's patches of the intestine.

In summary, the immune system is a complex network of organs and cells that serve to protect the body against invasion by foreign agents and proliferation of abnormal and malignant cells. The immune system is able to distinguish self from nonself through cell surface antigens coded by the MHC genes on the sixth chromosome. There are two classes of MHC antigens: Class I gene products found on most nucleated body cells and class II products found on selected immune cells.

The immune system includes the immune cells and the central and peripheral lymphoid organs. The central lymphoid structures consist of the bone marrow and thymus gland where blood cells are produced. The bone marrow is the source of the immune cells. The peripheral lymphoid structures consist of the lymph nodes, spleen, tonsils, intestinal lymphoid tissue, and aggregates of other lymphoid tissue. The interaction between antigens and immune cells occurs in the peripheral lymphoid structures.

The primary cells of the immune system are the B-lymphocytes, which are the source of antibodies, and the T-lymphocytes, which are the source of cell-mediated immunity. The proliferation and maturation of B-lymphocytes occur in the bone marrow. When fully differentiated, the B-lymphocyte becomes an antibody or immunoglobulin-producing plasma cell. There are five classes of immunoglobulins (IgA, IgD, IgE, IgG, and IgM), each produced by a separate clone of B cells. The T-lymphocytes travel from the bone marrow to the thymus where they are programmed to differentiate into mature and functional T cells. The helper T cells, a subset of T cells, act as a switch for the immune response. They are necessary for B-cell proliferation and differentiation. The macrophages, which are members of the mononuclear phagocytic system, are antigen-capturing cells. They capture, modify, and present antigen to the lymphocytes in a form that increases its antigenicity. NK cells are lymphocytes distinctly different from T cells. They serve as effector cells in destroying tumor cells and virus-infected cells.

■ IMMUNITY AND IMMUNE MECHANISMS

Immunity is a normal adaptive response designed to protect the body against potentially harmful foreign substances, infections, and other sources of nonself antigens. Immunity can be either natural or acquired. *Natural immunity* is species specific. It is the reason that humans do not contract certain animal diseases, such as feline distemper. *Innate immunity* is the immunity one is born with. It is genetically controlled and involves natural immunity, heredity, race, and sex. *Acquired immunity* is that protection which a person gains through active or passive means.

The *immune response* describes the interaction between an antigen (immunogen) and an antibody (immunoglobulin) or reactive T-lymphocyte. The process of acquiring the ability to respond to an antigen is known as immunization.

Active immunity is acquired through immunization or actually having a disease. It is long-lived immunity developed by the body's own immune system. Active immunity does not provide immediate protection after first exposure to an invading agent or vaccine. It takes a few days to weeks before the immune response is sufficiently developed to contribute to the destruction of the pathogen. However, the immune system is usually able to react within minutes to hours to subsequent exposure to the same agent.

Passive immunity is temporary immunity transmitted or borrowed from another source. An infant receives passive immunity from its mother in utero and from antibodies that it receives from its mother's breast milk. Passive immunity can also be transferred through injection of antiserum, which contains the antibodies for a specific disease, or through the use of pooled gamma globulin, which contains antibodies for a number of diseases. Both antiserum and gamma globulin are obtained from blood plasma.

ANTIGENS

An antigen is any substance recognized as foreign (nonself) by the immune system. An antigen can be a microorganism, such as a virus or a bacterium, or it can be a foreign protein or polysaccharide. Tissues or cells from another person, unless it is an identical twin, can also act as antigens. Antigens have specific *antigenic determinant sites*, or *epitopes*, which interact with immune cells to induce the immune response. All antigens carry different epitopes, allowing the immune system to recognize the antigen as nonself and as different from other antigens. The number of antigenic determinant sites on a molecule is roughly proportional to its molecular weight, with one site existing for each 10,000 or so units of molecular weight. A complete antigen has two or more sites. Large protein and polysaccharide molecules make good antigens because of their complex chemical structure and multiple antigenic determinant sites. Smaller molecules (those with a molecular weight of less than 10,000) usually make poor antigens.[3] Some substances cannot act as antigens by themselves, but have antigenic determinant sites and can combine with carrier substances and act as antigens. These substances, which usually have a low molecular weight, are called *haptens*. House dust, animal danders, and plant pollens are haptens.

The site of access to the body may influence the antigenic strength of a substance. For example, the digestive enzymes often hydrolyze and destroy the antigenic quality of otherwise fully antigenic materials. When these same substances are given parenterally (injected), greater amounts of the antigen are available for interacting with the antigen-processing cells. The oral polio vaccine is one exception; when taken into the gastrointestinal tract, it invades the lining of the intestine and reproduces itself.[21]

IMMUNE MECHANISMS

Immune mechanisms are of two types: specific and nonspecific. There are two types of specific immunologic responses, humoral and cell-mediated, that not only recognize self from nonself, but also distinguish among antigens. Nonspecific immunologic defense mechanisms such as the complement system, some cytokines, and phagocytosis can recognize self from nonself, but cannot distinguish between agents or pathogens.

HUMORAL IMMUNITY

Humoral immunity depends on B-lymphocytes and plasma cell production of immunoglobulins. Antigen–antibody reactions can take several forms. Combination of antigen with antibody can result in precipitation of antigen–antibody complexes, agglutination or clumping of cells, neutralization of bacterial toxins, lysis and destruction of pathogens or cells, adherence of antigen to immune cells, facilitation of phagocytosis through opsonization, and complement activation. Some of these reactions, such as opsonization, occur because of complement activation.

Two types of responses occur in the development of humoral immunity (Fig. 13-7). A primary immune response occurs when the antigen is first introduced into the body. During this primary response, there is a latent period before the antibody can be detected in the serum. This latent period involves the recognition of antigen by the APC and recognition by helper T cells. The antigen recognition receptor sites on helper T cells are similar to those expressed by the immunoglobulins. A T-cell receptor has a variable region that is modified to match the antigenic determinant in association with class II MHC molecules on the APC.[12] The activated helper T cell produces cytokines to further stimulate the immune system. In humoral immunity, activated helper T cells trigger B cells to proliferate and differentiate into a clone of plasma cells that will produce antibody. This period usually takes from 48 to 72 hours, after which the detectable antibody titer continues to rise for a period of 10 days to 2 weeks. Recovery from many infectious diseases occurs at about the time during the primary response when the antibody titer is reaching its peak. The secondary response occurs

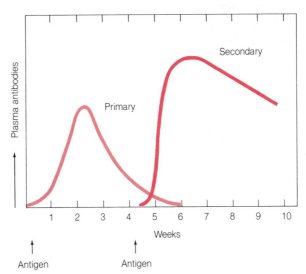

FIG. 13-7. *Primary and secondary phases of the humoral immune response to the same antigen.*

on second or subsequent exposures to the antigen. During the secondary response, the rise in antibody titer occurs sooner and reaches a higher level.

During the primary response, B cells are activated to proliferate and differentiate into antibody-secreting plasma cells. A fraction of activated B cells do not differentiate in plasma cells. Such B cells form a pool of memory cells. During the secondary response, the memory cells recognize the antigen and stimulate production of plasma cells, which produce the specific antibody. The booster immunization given for some infectious diseases, such as tetanus, makes use of the secondary response. For a person who has been previously immunized, administration of a booster shot causes an almost immediate rise in antibody titer to a level sufficient to prevent development of the disease.

CELL-MEDIATED IMMUNITY

In cell-mediated immunity, the action of the T-lymphocytes and the macrophages predominates. The most aggressive phagocyte, the activated macrophage, becomes so only after exposure to a T-cell lymphokine. Cell-mediated immunity provides protection against viruses and cancer cells. In addition to its protective effects, cell-mediated immunity is responsible for delayed hypersensitivity and transplant reactions.

The antigen recognition receptor sites on the T cell are similar to those expressed by the immunoglobulins. A T-cell receptor site has a variable region that is modified to match the particular antigen that a particular clone of T cells has been programmed to defend against. Activated T cells exert their effect through the synthesis of lymphokines. Once T cells have been activated by signals required for antigen-specific activation, they release lymphokines, which act in an antigen-nonspecific manner on other populations of inflammatory cells, irrespective of their antigen specificity.

As in humoral immunity, there is a central role played by the APC–antigen–helper T-cell complex. However, in cell-mediated immunity, activated helper T cells secrete cytokines, which trigger the proliferation of cytotoxic T cells and induce macrophages into an activated state. T-cell activation is antigen specific, but activated macrophage function is not.

THE COMPLEMENT SYSTEM

The complement system is the primary mediator of the humoral immune response that enables the body to produce inflammation and facilitate the localization of an infective agent. The complement system, like the blood coagulation system, consists of a group of proteins that are normally present in the circulation as functionally inactive precursor components of the system. These proteins constitute 10% to 15% of the plasma-protein fraction. For a complement reaction to occur, each of the complement components must be activated in the proper sequence. Uncontrolled activation of the complement system is prevented by the instability of the activated combining sites at each sequence of the process. In addition, several serum proteins have been identified that serve to modulate and limit activation of the complement system. There are two parallel but independent mechanisms for activation of the complement system: the classic and alternate pathways.

The classic complement pathway is activated when target cells are able to evoke a complement-fixing antigen–antibody response (Fig. 13-8). Only immune responses involving immunoglobulins IgG

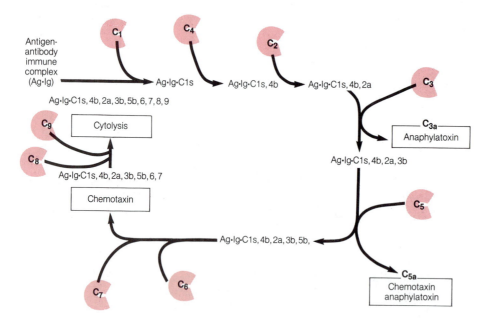

FIG. 13-8. Classic complement pathway and major biologic activities (in blocks).

(IgG1, IgG2, and IgG3) and IgM activate complement, and it is probable that complement is bound in all antigen–antibody reactions that involve these two classes of immunoglobulins. In addition, the classic complement pathway can be activated by a group of chemically diverse substances, including DNA, C-reactive protein, and certain cellular membranes and trypsinlike enzymes. Table 13-4 lists immune responses that occur as the result of complement fixation.

The alternate (properdin) pathway is activated by complex polysaccharides or enzymes. This system bypasses the first two steps of the classic complement pathway, but requires the presence of C3b.

After activation of the complement system, interactions ranging from lysis of a spectrum of different kinds of cells, bacteria, and viruses to direct mediation of the inflammatory process occur. First, complement has been shown to mediate the lytic destruction of many kinds of cells including red blood cells, platelets, bacteria, viruses, and lymphocytes. Either complement pathway may induce cytolysis. Second, a major biologic function of complement activation is opsonization—the coating of antigen–antibody complexes that facilitates clearance of these complexes by the fixed macrophage system. Third, chemotactic complement products can trigger

an influx of leukocytes that remain fixed in the area of complement activation through attachment to specific sites on C3b and C4b molecules. Fourth, production of anaphylatoxin and kinin products can lead to contraction of smooth muscle, increased vascular permeability, and edema. Fifth, complement-mediated phagocytosis facilitates the destruction of an infectious agent.

CYTOKINES AND THE IMMUNE RESPONSE

The last 10 years of immunologic research have produced an extraordinary amount of information on the role of cytokines as mediators of the immune response. Lymphokines (cytokines produced largely by T cells) act predominantly on lymphoid cells and are immunologically induced regulators of the immune response. These polypeptides function as intercellular signals that regulate local and, at times, systemic inflammatory responses. Cytokines modulate reactions of the host to foreign antigens or injurious agents by regulating the growth, mobility, and differentiation of leukocytes and other cells (see Table 13-2). A single purified cytokine can have multiple effects on cell growth and differentiation and display considerable overlap in their biologic activity on lymphoid, myeloid, and connective tissue target cells. In addition, biologically distinct cytokines may have similar effects by initiating the production of a cascade of identical cytokines or of one another.

Interleukin-1 (IL-1). The major function of IL-1 is as mediator of the inflammatory response in natural immunity. However, IL-1 also serves as a second signal in the activation of CD4+ T cells and the growth and differentiation of B cells. The major source of IL-1 is the mononuclear phagocyte, although it is produced by keratinocytes, dendritic cells, normal B cells, cultured T cells, fibroblasts, neutrophils, and smooth muscle cells.[24]

Interleukin-2. The presence of interleukin-2, formerly known as T-cell growth factor, is necessary for proliferation and function of helper, suppressor, and cytotoxic T-lymphocytes. Interleukin-2 interacts with T-lymphocytes by binding to specific membrane receptors that are present on activated T cells but not on resting T cells.[25] The expression of interleukin-2 receptors can be triggered by the binding of a specific antigen to the cell surface. Sustained T-cell proliferation relies on the presence of both interleukin-2 and interleukin-2 receptors—if either is missing, cell proliferation ceases and the cell dies.[26] Cyclosporin, a drug used to prevent rejection of heart, kidney, and liver transplants, functions primarily by inhibiting the synthesis of interleukin-2.

TABLE 13-4. COMPLEMENT-MEDIATED IMMUNE RESPONSES

RESPONSE	EFFECT
Cytolysis	Destruction of cell membrane of body cells or pathogens
Adherence of immune cells	Adhesion of antigens–antibody complexes to the inert surfaces of cells or tissues such as the reticuloendothelial cells that line the blood vessels and have the capacity for phagocytosis
Chemotaxis	Chemical attraction of phagocytic cells to foreign agents
Anaphylaxis	Degranulation of mast cells with release of histamine and other inflammatory mediators
Opsonization	Modification of the antigen so it can be easily digested by a phagocytic cell

Interferons. The interferons are a family of cytokines that protect neighboring cells from invasion by intracellular parasites. This includes viruses, rickettsia, malarial parasites, and other intracellular organisms. In addition, bacterial toxins, complex polysaccharides, and a number of other chemical substances are capable of inducing interferon production. Not all of these substances that induce interferon are antigenic. There are at least three types of interferon: α interferon (produced by leukocytes), β interferon (produced by fibroblasts), and γ interferon (produced by T cells). Interferon interacts at the gene level to inhibit translation of messenger RNAs, which regulate viral protein synthesis but not host protein synthesis. This antiviral activity can be transferred to neighboring cells without the continued presence of interferon. The actions of interferon are pathogen nonspecific (*i.e.*, they are effective against different types of viruses and intracellular parasites). They are, however, species specific. Animal interferons do not provide protection in humans. Interferon produced during immune reactions is primarily γ interferon. The immunodeficiency activities of γ interferon include activation of macrophages, generation of cytotoxic lymphocytes, and enhancement of NK cell activity.[6]

Tumor Necrosis Factor. Like IL-1, TNF is a cytokine with multiple immunologic and inflammatory effects. It was first described as an activity in serum that induced hemorrhagic necrosis in certain tumors and later independently discovered as *cachectin*, a circulating mediator of wasting during parasitic disease.[10] TNF is produced by activated macrophages and other cells such as activated T cells and activated NK cells. Besides functioning as a major chemical mediator in the inflammatory response, TNF may function as a costimulator for T-cell activation and slightly up-regulates antibody production by B cells. This cytokine is an especially potent stimulator of IL-1, Il-6, and IL-8. In the setting of bacterial sepsis, high serum levels of TNF may mediate endotoxic shock.[10]

Hematopoietic Colony Stimulating Factor. Colony stimulating factors (CSF) are cytokines that stimulate a limited number of pluripotent stem cells, present predominantly in the bone marrow, to produce large numbers of platelets, erythrocytes, neutrophils, monocytes, esosinophils, and basophils. The CSF were named according to the type of target cell they act on (see Table 13-2). The GM-CSF acts on the bipotential stem cells to produce monocytes and granulocytes; G-CSF primarily induces granulocyte proliferation; and M-CSF is a mononuclear phagocyte progenitor. Other cytokines, including IL-1, IL-2, IL-3, IL-4, IL-5, IL-6, and IL-7, may influence hematopoiesis, directly or indirectly, during the immune response.[6]

AGING AND THE IMMUNE RESPONSE

Aging is characterized by a declining ability to adapt to environmental stresses. One of the factors thought to contribute to this problem is a decline in immune responsiveness. This includes changes in both cell-mediated and antibody-mediated immune responses. Elderly people tend to be more susceptible to infections, they have more evidence of autoimmune and immune complex disorders than younger people, and they have a higher incidence of cancer. In addition, experimental evidence suggests that vaccination is less successful in inducing immunization in older people than younger adults.[27] However, the effects of altered immune function on the health of elderly people is clouded by the fact that age-related changes or disease may affect the immune response.

The alterations in immune function that occur with advanced age are not fully understood. There is a decrease in the size of the thymus gland, which is thought to affect T-cell function. The size of the gland begins to decline shortly after sexual maturity, and by age 50 it has usually diminished to 15% or less of its maximum size.[28] There are conflicting reports regarding age-related changes in the peripheral lymphocytes. Some researchers have reported a decrease in the absolute number of lymphocytes, and others have found little if any change. The most common finding is a slight decrease in the proportion of T cells to other lymphocytes and decrease in both CD4+ and CD8+ cells.

What is probably more evident is altered response of the immune cells to antigen stimulation, with increasing proportions of lymphocytes becoming unresponsive while the remainder continue to function relatively normally. Both T- and B-cell compartments show deficiencies in activation. In the T-cell compartment, the CD4+ subset is most severely affected. In addition, there is evidence that aged T cells have diminished synthesis of lymphokines that drive the proliferation of lymphocytes and diminished expression of the receptors that interact with those lymphokines. For example, it has been shown that IL-2 synthesis decreases markedly with aging.[29] Although B-cell function is compromised somewhat with age, the range of antibodies that can be recognized is not diminished. If anything, the repertoire is increased to the extent that B cells begin to recognize some self-antigens as foreign antigens. This may be the basis for the increased incidence of autoimmune disease in the elderly.

In summary, immunity is the resistance to a disease that is provided by the immune system. An immune response involves an antigen, an antibody, or an effector T cell. It can be acquired actively (through immunization or actually having a disease) or passively (by receiving antibodies or immune cells from another source). Antigens have antigenic determinant sites, which the immune system uses to recognize the antigen as nonself and to distinguish it from other antigens. Immune mechanisms can be classified into two types: specific and nonspecific. Specific immunity involves humoral and cellular mechanisms; it can recognize self from nonself and can distinguish between antigens. Nonspecific immune mechanisms can distinguish between self and nonself but cannot differentiate between antigens. It includes the complement system, lyphokines, and phagocytic functions of the neutrophils and macrophages. The lymphokines (cytokines produced largely by T cells) function as intercellular signals that regulate immune and inflammatory responses. The effectiveness of the immune response decreases with aging. Elderly people tend to be more susceptible to infections, they have more evidence of autoimmune and immune complex disorders than younger people, and they have a higher incidence of cancer.

■ REFERENCES

1. Cotran, R.S., Kumar, V., & Robbins, S.L. (1989). *Pathologic basis of disease* (4th ed., pp. 39, 64, 165–167). Philadelphia: W.B. Saunders.
2. National Institutes of Health. (1983). *Understanding the immune system*, No. 8429. Washington, DC: US Dept of Health and Human Services.
3. Stites, D.P., & Terr, A.I. (1991). *Basic and clinical immunology* (7th ed., pp. 46, 69–70, 101, 154). San Mateo, CA: Lange.
4. Claman, H.N. (1983). Glucocorticoids I: Anti-inflammatory mechanisms. *Hospital Practice, 18*(7), 123.
5. Samuelsson, B. (1981). Leukotrienes: Mediators of immediate hypersensitivity reactions and inflammation. *Science, 220*, 568.
6. Arai, K., Lee, F., Miyajima, A., et al. (1990). Cytokines, coordinators of immunity and inflammation. *Annual Review of Biochemistry, 59*, 783.
7. Dinarello, C.A. (1984). Interleukin and the pathogenesis of the acute-phase response. *New England Journal of Medicine, 311*, 1413.
8. Dinarello, C. (1986). Interleukins. *Annusl Review of Medicine, 37*, 173.
9. Duff, G. (1985). Many roles for interleukin. *Nature, 313*, 353.
10. Beutter, B., & Cerami, A. (1988). The biology of cachectin-TNF: A primary mediator of the host response. *Annual Review of Immunology, 7*, 625.
11. Royer, H.D., & Rienherz, E.L. (1987). T lymphocyte ontogeny, function, and relevance to clinical disorders. *New England Journal of Medicine, 317*, 1136.
12. Clevers, H., Alarcon, B., & Wileman, T. (1988). The T cell receptor/CD3 complex: A dynamic protein ensemble. *Annual Review of Immunology, 6*, 629.
13. Cooper, M.D. (1987). B lymphocytes. *New England Journal of Medicine, 317*, 1452.
14. Rosen, F.S., Cooper, M.D., & Wedgwood, R.J.P. (1984). The primary immunodeficiencies (first of two parts). *New England Journal of Medicine, 311*, 235.
15. Ochs, H.D., & Wedgwood, R.J. (1987). IgG subclass deficiencies. *Annual Reveiew of Medicine, 38*, 325.
16. Johnson, R.B. (1988). Monocytes and macrophages. *New England Journal of Medicine, 318*, 747.
17. Lasser, A. (1983). The mononuclear phagocytic system: A review. *Human Pathology, 14*, 108.
18. Unanue, E.R., & Allen, P.M. (1987). The immunoregulatory role of the macrophage. *Hospital Practice, 22*(4), 87.
19. Nossal, G.J.V. (1987). The basic components of the immune system. *New England Journal of Medicine, 316*, 1320.
20. Trinchieri, G. (1989). Biology of natural killer cells. *Advances in Immunology, 47*, 187.
21. Barrett, J.T. (1983). *Textbook of immunology* (4th ed., pp. 79, 215–216, 212). Philadelphia: W.B. Saunders.
22. Smith, L.H., & Their, S.O. (1981). *Pathophysiology* (p. 167). Philadelphia: W.B. Saunders.
23. Cormack, D.H. (1987). *Ham's histology* (9th ed., p. 249). Philadelphia: J.B. Lippincott.
24. Dinarello, C.A. (1988). Biology of interleukin-1. *FASEB Journal, 2*, 108.
25. Dinarello, C.A., & Mier, J.W. (1987). Lymphokines. *New England Journal of Medicine, 317*, 940.
26. Dinarello, C.A., & Mier, J.W. (1986). Interleukins. *Annual Review of Medicine, 37*, 173.
27. Powers, D.C. (1992). Immunologic principles and emerging strategies of vaccination for the elderly. *Journal of the American Geriatrics Society, 40*(1), 81–94.
28. Weksler, M.E. (1981). The senescence of the immune response. *Hospital Practice, 16*(10), 55.
29. Weigle, W.O. (1989, December 15). Effects of aging on the immune system. *Hospital Practice, 24*.

■ BIBLIOGRAPHY

Adams, D.O. (1989). Molecular interactions in macrophage activation. *Immunology Today, 10*, 33.

Baily, J.M. (1992). *Prostaglandins, leukotrienes, lipoxins, and PAF: Mechanisms of action, molecular biology and clinical application.* Proceedings of the Eleventh International Washington Spring Symposium, New York: Plenum Press.

Faltynok, C.R., & Kung, H.F. (1988). The biochemical mechanism and actions of interferons. *Biofactors, 1*, 277.

Kimball, E.S. (1991). *Cytokines and inflammation.* Boca Raton: CRC Press.

Lehrer, R.I. (1988). Neutrophils and host defense. *Annals of Internal Medicine, 109*, 127.

Miyajma, A. (1988). Coordinate regulation of immunologic and inflammatory responses by T cell dependent lymphokines. *FASEB Journal, 2*, 2462.

Mizel, S.B. (1987). Interleukin-1 and T cell activation. *Immunology Today, 8*, 330.

Nicola, N.A. (1989). Hematopoietic cell growth factors and their receptors. *Annual Review of Biochemistry, 58*, 45.

Romagnani, S., & Abbas, A.K. (1990). *Cytokines: Basic principles and clinical applications.* New York: Raven Press.

Schumaker, V.N. (1987). Activation of the first component of complement. *Annual Review of Immunology, 5,* 21.

Waldman, T.A., & Tsudd, M. (1987). Interleukin-2 receptors: Biology and therapeutic potential. *Hospital Practice, 22*(1), 77.

Warren, J.S. (1990). Interleukins and tumor necrosis factor in inflammation. *Critical Reviews in Clinical Laboratory Sciences, 28,* 37.

Whicher, J.T., & Evans, S.W. (1992). *Biochemistry of inflammation.* Boston: Kluwer Academic Publishers.

Young, J.D., & Cohn, Z.A. (1988). How killer cells kill. *Scientific American, 258*(1), 38.

CHAPTER 14

ALTERATIONS IN THE IMMUNE RESPONSE

W. MICHAEL DUNNE, JR.

Immunodeficiency Disease
  Humoral (B-cell)
    Immunodeficiencies
  Cellular (T-cell)
    Immunodeficiencies
  Combined T- and B-cell
    Immunodeficiencies
  Disorders of the Complement
    System

Disorders of Phagocytosis
Allergic and Hypersensitivity
  Disorders
  IgE-mediated Allergic and Atopic
    Disorders
  Immune Complex Allergic
    Diseases
  Cell-Mediated Hypersensitivity
    Disorders

Transplantation
  Immunopathology
  Host-Versus-Graft Disease
  Graft-Versus-Host Disease
Autoimmune Disease
  Probable Mechanisms
  Diagnosis of Autoimmune
    Disorders

■ OBJECTIVES

After you have studied this chapter, you should be able to meet the following objectives:

■ List the most important categories of immuno-deficiency disease and state one example of each category.

■ Relate the function of the complement system to the manifestations of hereditary angioneurotic edema.

■ State the proposed mechanisms of dysfunction and manifestations in primary disorders of phagocytosis.

■ Compare the immune mechanisms involved in type I, II, III, and IV hypersensitivity immune reactions.

■ List the goals for treatment of seasonal pollen allergy and allergic bronchitis.

■ Compare the hypersensitivity reactions associated with serum sickness and the Arthus reaction.

■ Discuss the rationale for matching of HLA and MHC types in organ transplantation.

■ Compare the immune mechanisms involved in transplant rejection and graft-versus-host disease.

■ Discuss the role of the suppressor and helper T cells in the regulation of self-tolerance.

■ Describe three or more postulated mechanisms underlying autoimmune disease.

The human immune network is a multifaceted defense system that has evolved to protect against invading microorganisms, prevent the proliferation of cancer cells, and mediate the healing of damaged tissue. Under normal conditions, the immune response deters or prevents disease. Occasionally, how-ever, the inadequate, inappropriate, or misdirected activation of the immune system can produce debilitating or life-threatening illnesses typified by immunodeficiency states, allergic or hypersensitivity reactions, transplantation pathophysiology, and autoimmune disorders. The variety of immunologic disorders that

Carol Mattson Porth: PATHOPHYSIOLOGY: CONCEPTS OF ALTERED HEALTH STATES, 4th ed. © 1994, 1990, 1986, 1982 J.B. Lippincott Company

directly or indirectly lead to pathologic conditions in humans are discussed in this chapter.

■ IMMUNODEFICIENCY DISEASE

Immunodeficiency can be defined as an abnormality in one or more branches of the immune system that renders a person susceptible to diseases normally prevented by an intact immune system. Four major categories of immune mechanisms defend the body against infectious or neoplastic disease: (1) humoral or antibody-mediated immunity (B-lymphocytes), (2) cell-mediated (T-lymphocytes and lymphokines) immunity, (3) the complement system, and (4) phagocytosis (neutrophils and macrophages). Although not usually included in a discussion of the immune system, disorders that breech the integrity of natural barriers such as skin, mucous membranes, and secretory antimicrobial enzymes (*e.g.*, lysozyme in tears and the hydrolytic enzymes in saliva) can also produce a state of immunodeficiency.

Abnormalities of the immune system can be classified as primary (*i.e.*, congenital or inherited) or secondary if the immunodeficiency is acquired later in life. Secondary immunodeficiency can be the result of infection (acquired immunodeficiency syndrome; AIDS), neoplastic disease (lymphoma), or immunosuppressive therapy (cyclosporin). Regardless of the cause, both primary and secondary deficiencies can produce the same spectrum of disease. The severity and symptomatology of the various immunodeficiencies depend on the disorder and extent of immune system involvement. The various categories of immunodeficiency are summarized in Chart 14-1. AIDS is discussed in Chapter 15.

HUMORAL (B-CELL) IMMUNODEFICIENCIES

Humoral immunodeficiency can range from a transient decrease in immunoglobulin levels during early infancy to inherited disorders that interrupt the production of one or all of the immunoglobulins. During the first few months of life, infants are protected from infection by IgG class antibodies that have been transferred from the maternal circulation during gestation. IgA, IgM, IgD, and IgE do not normally cross the placenta. The presence of elevated levels of IgA or IgM in the infant cord blood suggests premature antibody production due to an intrauterine infection. An infant's level of maternal IgG gradually declines (the approximate half-life of circulating antibody is 23 days) over a period of about 6 months. Concomitant with the loss of maternal antibody, the infant's immature humoral immune system begins to function,

and, between the ages of 1 and 2 years, the child's antibody production reaches adult levels.

Antibody production depends on the differentiation of B stem cells within the bone marrow to mature, immunoglobulin-producing plasma cells. This maturation cycle initially involves the production of surface IgM, migration from the marrow to the peripheral lymphoid tissue, and switching to the specialized production of IgG, IgA, IgD, IgE, or IgM antibodies after antigenic stimulation (Fig. 14-1).

Transient Hypogammaglobulinemia of Infancy. Any abnormality that blocks or prevents the maturation of B stem cells can produce a state of immunodeficiency. For example, certain infants may experience a delay in the maturation process of B cells that leads to a prolonged deficiency in IgG levels (IgM and IgA levels are normal) beyond 6 months of age. The total number and antigenic response of circulating B cells is normal, but the chemical communication between B and T cells that leads to clonal proliferation of antibody-producing plasma cells seems to be reduced. This condition is referred to as *transient hypogammaglobulinemia of infancy*. The result of this condition is usually limited to repeated bouts of upper respiratory and middle ear infections, and this usually resolves by the time the child is 2 to 4 years of age.

X-linked and Common Variable Hypogammaglobulinemia. At the opposite end of the spectrum of B-cell immunodeficiencies is a serious inherited X-linked disorder called *Bruton's hypogammaglobulinemia* that only affects males. As the name implies, children with this disorder have essentially undetectable levels of all serum immunoglobins. As a result, they are susceptible to meningitis and recurrent otitis media, sinus and pulmonary infections with encapsulated organisms such as *Streptococcus pneumoniae*, *Hemophilus influenzae* type b, or *Neisseria meningitidis*. Many children with this disorder have severe tooth decay. The central defect in this syndrome appears to prevent continued differentiation of pre-B cells. Subsequently, there is an absence of both mature circulating B cells and plasma cells. Symptoms of the disorder usually coincide with the loss of maternal antibodies. A clue to the presence of the disorder is failure of an infection to respond completely and promptly to antibiotic therapy. Diagnosis is based on demonstration of low or absent serum immunoglobulins. Therapy is based on monthly administration of intravenous immunoglobulin and prompt antimicrobial therapy for suspected infections. The prognosis of this condition depends on the prompt recognition and treatment of infections. Chronic pulmonary disease is an ever-present danger; pulmonary function is usually assessed annually in children over 10 years of age.

CHART 14-1: IMMUNODEFICIENCY STATES

Humoral (B-Cell) Immunodeficiency

Primary
  Transient hypogammaglobulinemia of infancy
  X-linked hypogammaglobulinemia
  Common variable immunodeficiency
  Selective deficiency of IgG, IgA, IgM
Secondary
  Increased loss of immunoglobulins (nephrotic syndrome)

Cellular (T-Cell) Immunodeficiency

Primary
  Congenital thymic aplasia (DiGeorge's syndrome)
  Abnormal T-cell production (Nezelof's syndrome)
Secondary
  Malignant disease (Hodgkin's disease and others)
  Transient suppression of T-cell production and function due to an acute viral infection such as measles
  AIDS
  Purine nucleoside phosphorylase (PNP) or adenosine deaminase (ADA) deficiency

Combined B-Cell and T-Cell Immunodeficiency

Primary
  Severe combined immunodeficiency (autosomal or sex-linked recessive)
  Wiskott-Aldrich syndrome (immunodeficiency, thrombocytopenia, and eczema)
  Ataxia and telangiectasia
Secondary
  Irradiation
  Immune suppressant and cytotoxic drugs
  Aging

Complement Disorders

Primary
  Angioneurotic edema (complement 1 inactivator deficiency)
  Selective deficiency in a complement component
Secondary
  Acquired disorders that involve complement utilization

Phagocytic Dysfunction

Primary
  Chronic granulomatous disease
  Glucose-phosphate dehydrogenase deficiency
  Job's syndrome
  Chédiak-Higashi syndrome
  CD11/CD18 deficiency
Secondary
  Drug induced (*e.g.*, corticosteroid and immunosuppressive therapy)
  Diabetes mellitus

  Examples are not inclusive.

Another disorder of B-cell maturation, which is similar to Bruton's hypogammoglobulinemia, is a condition called *common variable immunodeficiency* or *late onset hypogammaglobulinemia*. In this syndrome, however, the terminal differentiation of mature B cells to plasma cells is blocked. The result is markedly reduced serum immunoglobulin levels, normal numbers of circulating B-lymphocytes, and a complete absence of germinal centers and plasma cells in lymph nodes and the spleen. The symptomatology is similar to that of Bruton's hypogammaglobulinemia (*i.e.*, recurrent otitis media and sinus and pulmonary infections with encapsulated organisms), but the onset of symptoms occurs much later in life (between ages 15 and 35 years), and distribution of disease between males and females is equal. People with late onset hypogammaglobulinemia also have increased tendency to develop chronic lung disease, auto-

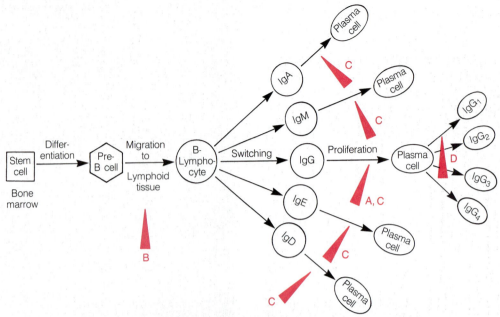

FIG. 14-1. Stem cells to mature immunoglobulin-secreting plasma cells. *Arrows* indicate the stage of the maturation process that is interrupted in: (*A*) transient hypoglobulinemia, (*B*) Bruton's hypogammaglobulinema, (*C*) common variable immunodeficiency, and (*D*) IgG subclass deficiency.

immune disorders, hepatitis, gastric carcinoma, and chronic diarrhea with associated malabsorption. Approximately one half of people with the disorder have evidence of abnormal T-cell immunity, suggesting that this syndrome is a complex immunodeficiency. Treatment methods are similar to those used for Bruton's hypogammaglobulinemia.

Selective Immunoglobulin Deficiencies. *Selective IgA deficiency* is the most common type of immunoglobulin deficiency affecting nearly 1 of every 500 people. The syndrome is characterized by moderate to marked reduction in levels of serum and secretory IgA. It is likely that the cause of this deficiency is a block in the pathway that promotes terminal differentiation of mature B cells to IgA secreting plasma cells. Approximately two thirds of people with selective IgA deficiency have no overt symptoms, presumably because IgG and IgM levels are normal and compensate for the defect. At least 50% of affected children overcome the deficiency by the age of 14 years. People with markedly reduced levels of IgA often experience repeated upper respiratory and gastrointestinal infections and have increased incidence of allergies such as asthma, autoimmune disorders, and malignancies. In addition, they can develop antibodies against IgA which, in turn, could lead to an anaphylactic response when given blood components containing IgA. There is no treatment available for selective IgA deficiency unless there is a concomitant reduction in IgG levels.

An *IgG subclass deficiency* is another type of selective immunoglobulin deficiency. Children who are prone to multiple upper respiratory and middle ear infections throughout the year are sometimes afflicted with an IgG subclass deficiency. This deficiency alters their ability to produce antibodies against polysaccharide antigens. As discussed in Chapter 13, IgG immunoglobulins can be divided into four subclasses (IgG1–4) based on structure and function. The majority of circulating IgG belongs to IgG1 (70%) and IgG2 (20%) subclasses. In general, antibodies directed against protein antigens belong to IgG1 and IgG3 subclasses, whereas antibodies directed against carbohydrate and polysaccharide antigens are primarily IgG2 subclass. As a result, people who are deficient in IgG2 subclass antibodies can be at greater risk to develop sinusitis, otitis media, and pneumonia caused by polysaccharide encapsulated microorganisms such as *Streptococcus pneumoniae*, *Hemophilus influenzae* type b, and *Neisseria meningitidis*. Children with mild forms of the deficiency can be treated with prophylactic antibiotics to prevent repeated infections. Intravenous immune globulin (IVIG) can be given to children with severe manifestations of this deficiency. The use of polysaccharide vaccines conjugated to protein carriers can alleviate some of the infections because protein conjugated to protein carriers stimulate an IgG1 response.

Secondary deficiencies in humoral immunity can develop as a consequence of selective loss of immunoglobulins through the gastrointestinal or genitourinary tracts. Such is the case in people with nephrotic syndrome who, because of abnormal glomerular filtration, lose serum IgA and IgG in their urine (see Chapter 32). Because of its larger molecular size, IgM is not filtered into the urine and serum levels remain normal.

CELLULAR (T-CELL) IMMUNODEFICIENCIES

Unlike the B-cell lineage where a well-defined series of differentiation steps ultimately leads to the production of immunoglobulins, mature T-lymphocytes are composed of distinct subpopulations whose immunologic assignments are diverse. T cells can be functionally divided into helper, suppressor, and cytotoxic subtypes as well as a population of T cells that promote delayed hypersensitivity reactions. Collectively, T-lymphocytes protect against fungal, protozoan, viral, and intracellular bacterial infections; control malignant cell proliferation; and are responsible for coordinating the overall immune response.

There are few primary forms of T-cell immunodeficiency, probably because such severe defects in this branch of the immune response are lethal mutations. One such abnormality, called *DiGeorge's syndrome*, stems from an embryonic developmental defect. The defect is thought to occur during the 12th week of gestation at the time when the thymus gland, parathyroid gland, and parts of the head,

neck, and heart are developing. The syndrome can be caused by intrinsic factors such as chromosomal abnormalities or by extrinsic factors such as maternal alcoholism or diabetes. Babies born with this defect have partial or complete failure to develop the thymus and parathyroid glands and have congenital defects of the head, neck, and heart.

The extent of immune and parathyroid abnormalities is highly variable, as are the other defects. Occasionally, a child has no heart defect. In some babies, the thymus is not absent but is in an abnormal location and is extremely small. These babies can have partial DiGeorge's syndrome in which hypertrophy of the thymus occurs with development of normal immune function. The facial disorders can include hypertelorism (increased distance between the eyes), micrognathia (fish mouth), low-set posterior angulated ears, split uvula, and high arched palate (Fig. 14-2). Urinary tract abnormalities are also common. The most frequent presenting sign is hypocalcemia that develops in the first 24 hours of life. It is caused by the absence of the parathyroid gland and is resistant to standard therapy.

Children who survive the immediate neonatal period may develop recurrent or chronic infections due to impaired T-cell immunity. Additionally, there can be an absence of immunoglobulin production caused by a lack of T helper cell function. For children who do require treatment, thymus transplantation can be performed to reconstitute T-cell immunity. Bone marrow transplantation has also been successfully used to restore normal T-cell populations. If

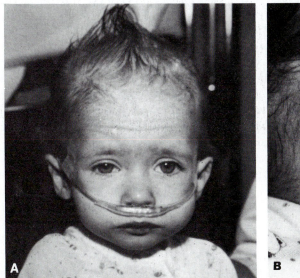 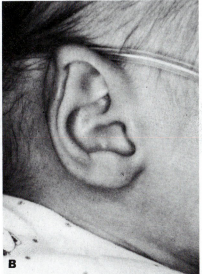

FIG. 14-2. Facial abnormalities in a child with DiGeorge's syndrome, as illustrated by hypertelorism, defective lowset ears, hypoplastic mandible, and bowing upward of the upper lip (**A**) and by closeup of the ears showing notched pinna and deficient helix formation (**B**). (Oski, F. A. [Ed.]. [1990]. *Principles and practice of pediatrics* [p. 193]. Philadelphia: J.B. Lippincott)

blood transfusions are needed, as during corrective heart surgery, special processing is required to prevent graft-versus-host disease (to be discussed).

A related disorder called *Nezelof's syndrome* is caused by a defect in thymus gland development with T-cell deficiency but without associated parathyroid dysfunction and other congenital deformities. The cause of the disorder is unknown. The syndrome occurs in both males and females.

Secondary deficiencies of T-cell function are more common and have been described in conjunction with acute viral infections (including measles and cytomegalovirus) and with certain malignancies such as Hodgkin's disease and other lymphomas. In the case of viruses, direct infection of specific T-lymphocyte subpopulations (*e.g.*, helper cells) by lymphotropic viruses such as HIV and human herpesvirus type 6 can lead to loss of cellular function and/or selective subtype depletion with a concomitant loss of immunologic responsibility associated with that subtype. On the other hand, people with neoplastic disorders can have impaired T-cell function based on unregulated multiplication or dysfunction of one particular subclone of T cells. The outward expression of this might be either an increased susceptibility to infections caused by normally harmless pathogens (called *opportunistic infections*) or failure to generate delayed-type hypersensitivity reactions (called *anergy*). People with anergy have a diminished or absent reaction to a battery of skin-test antigens, including *Candida* antigen and the tuberculin test even when infected with *Mycobacterium tuberculosis*.

A particularly severe secondary T-cell disorder stems from an inherited (autosomal recessive) deficiency in the enzyme *purine nucleoside phosphorylase* or *PNP*. Reduced levels of PNP lead to the accumulation of toxic intermediates of purine metabolism within T-lymphocytes causing cell death and/or loss of cell function. The B-cell immune response is usually normally. A related but distinct genetic defect leads to abnormally low levels of a lymphocytic cell enzyme called *adenosine deaminase* or *ADA*. Similar to PNP deficiency, this defect leads to accumulation of toxic metabolites within T-lymphocytes and causes cell death. Both of these conditions can be treated using enzyme replacement therapy.

COMBINED T- AND B-CELL IMMUNODEFICIENCIES

Disorders of the immune response that have elements of both B- and T-cell dysfunction fall under the broad classification of combined immunodeficiency syndrome (CIDS) and include a variety of inherited (autosomal recessive and X-linked) conditions. A single mutation in any one of the many genes that influence the lymphocytic response including lymphocyte receptors, cytokines, or major histocompatibility antigens (human leukocyte antigen; HLA) could lead to combined immunodeficiency. Regardless of the affected gene, the net result is a disruption in the normal communication system of B- and T-lymphocytes with deregulation of the immune response. The spectrum of disease resulting from CIDS ranges from mild to severe and ultimately fatal forms. The severe form is often referred to as severe combined immunodeficiency syndrome (SCIDS). Children with SCIDS have a disease course that resembles AIDS with chronic diarrhea and opportunistic infections that usually lead to death by the age of 2. Treatment consists of measures to prevent and control infections. Specific antibiotic treatment is used depending on the type of microorganism that is present. Gamma globulin (intramuscular or intravenous) may also be used. Immunizations with live attenuated viruses such as the polio virus should be avoided. SCIDS has been successfully treated with bone marrow transplantation. The successful transplants have come from HLA-matched siblings.

Ataxia-telangiectasia syndrome is also an inherited (autosomal recessive) disorder thought to be a mutation in a single gene located at chromosome 11q22-23. As the name implies, this syndrome is heralded by worsening cerebellar ataxia (poor muscle coordination) and the appearance of telangiectasias (lesions consisting of dilated capillaries and arterioles) on skin and conjunctival surfaces (Fig. 14-3). The ataxia usually goes unnoticed until the toddler begins to walk; the telangiectasias develop thereafter—especially on skin surfaces exposed to the sun. The ataxia progresses slowly and relentlessly to severe disability. Intellectual development is normal at first but seems to stop at the 10-year level in many of these children. In addition, children with this syndrome have associated deficiencies in both cellular and humoral components of the immune response including reduced levels of IgA, IgE, and IgG2, absolute lymphopenia, and a decrease in the T-helper:T-suppressor cell ratio. Subsequently, they are susceptible to recurrent upper and lower respiratory tract infections (particularly those caused by encapsulated bacteria) and have an increased risk for the development of malignancies. Death from malignant lymphoma is common.

Wiskott-Aldrich syndrome is an X-linked recessive disorder that becomes symptomatic during the first year of life. Infants with this syndrome are plagued by eczema, recurrent infections, and low platelet counts. Abnormalities of humoral immunity include decreased serum levels of IgM, and markedly elevated serum IgA and IgE concentrations. T-cell dys-

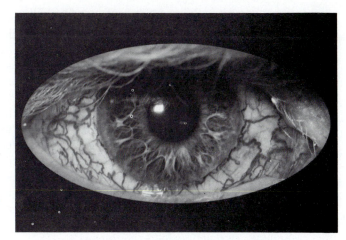

FIG. 14-3. Striking telangiectasis on the bulbar conjunctiva of a 22-year-old patient with ataxia-telangectasia. These dilated vessels typically appear between ages 2 and 5. (Oski, F. A. [Ed.]. [1990]. *Principles and practice of pediatrics.* [p. 189]. Philadelphia: J.B. Lippincott)

function is initially mild but progressively deteriorates, and patients become increasingly susceptible to develop malignancies of the mononuclear phagocytic system including Hodgkin's lymphoma and leukemia. Children with Wiskott-Aldrich syndrome typically are unable to produce antibody to polysaccharide antigens and therefore are susceptible to infections caused by encapsulated microorganisms. Bone marrow transplantation has been successful in children with Wiskott-Aldrich syndrome. Splenectomy may be used to control the thrombocytopenia in situations in which bone marrow transplantation cannot be done.

DISORDERS OF THE COMPLEMENT SYSTEM

The complement system is an integral part of the normal immune response. The activation of the complement network, either through the classic (antigen–antibody complexes) or alternative (binding of activated C3 to surfaces) pathways, promotes chemotaxis, opsonization, and phagocytosis of invasive pathogens, bacteriolysis, and anaphylactic reactions (see Chapter 25). It seems reasonable to predict that alterations in normal levels of complement or the absence of a particular complement component could create a state of immunodeficiency.

As with B- and T-cell deficiencies, complement disorders can be classified as primary if the deficiency is inherited or secondary if the condition develops due to another disease process. Most primary disorders of the complement system are transmitted as autosomal recessive traits and can involve one or more complement components. A C2 deficiency causes a susceptibility to multiple and potentially life-threatening infections caused by encapsulated bacteria, especially *Streptococcus pneumoniae*. People

with C2 deficiency are also at risk to develop autoimmune disorders that resemble lupus erythematosus. Similarly, people with *C3 deficiency* are predisposed to develop serious and recurrent infections caused by encapsulated bacteria and *Staphylococcus aureus* because of their inability to opsonize and lyse bacteria. Unlike people with C2 and C3 deficiencies, people with deficiencies in factors C1 (C1q,r, and s) and C4 are not necessarily at increased risk for recurrent infections because the alternative pathway can be activated normally through C3. However, many of them develop autoimmune diseases. Although people with deficiencies in the terminal components of complement (C5-C9) are susceptible to repeated episodes of meningitis and sepsis caused by *Neisseria meningitides* or systemic gonococcal disease, they are less likely to develop autoimmune disorders than people with other complement deficiencies.

Hereditary angioneurotic edema is a particularly interesting form of complement deficiency. People with this disorder do not produce a functional C1 inhibitor. Therefore, activation of the classic complement pathway is uncontrolled, leading to increased breakdown of C4 and C2 with concomitant release of C-kinin (a vasodilator). This, in turn, causes episodic attacks of localized edema involving the face, neck, joints, abdomen, and sites of trauma. If the trachea or larynx is involved, the episode can prove fatal. In most cases, the edema resolves within 2 to 3 days. The attacks associated with this inherited disease usually begin before the age of 2 and become progressively worse with age.

Secondary complement deficiencies can also occur in people with functionally normal complement systems due to rapid activation and turnover of complement components (as is seen in immune complex disease) or reduced synthesis of components as would be the case in chronic cirrhosis of the liver or malnutrition.

DISORDERS OF PHAGOCYTOSIS

The phagocytic system is composed primarily of mononuclear phagocytes and polymorphonuclear leukocytes. The former consists of circulating monocytes and tissue or fixed (splenic) macrophages whereas the latter includes neutrophils and eosinophils. The primary purpose of phagocytic cells is to migrate to the site of infection (chemotaxis), aggregate around the affected tissue (adherence), envelope invading microorganisms or foreign substances (phagocytosis), and generate microbactericidal substances (*e.g.*, enzymes or byproducts of metabolism) to kill the ingested pathogens. A defect in any of these functions or a reduction in the absolute number of available cells can essentially disrupt the phagocytic system. As with other alterations in immune function, defects in phagocytosis can be a primary or secondary disorder.

The most well-known disorder of phagocytosis is *chronic granulomatous disease* (*CGD*). In fact, CGD is a group of inherited disorders (X-linked or autosomal recessive) that greatly reduce or inactivate the ability of phagocytic cells to generate bactericidal byproducts of respiration (superoxide anion and hydrogen peroxide). People with CGD are subject to recurrent infections of the skin, liver, lung, and other soft tissues by organisms that produce the enzyme catalase (*e.g.*, *Staphylococcus aureus*). This enzyme catalyzes the reduction of hydrogen peroxide to oxygen and water. The end result is that polymorphonuclear leukocytes are unable to kill phagocytosed organisms through normal mechanisms. Organisms that do not produce this enzyme seldom cause infections in people with CGD. The disorder is diagnosed by examining the ability of a person's phagocytes to reduce a yellow dye (nitroblue tetrazolium; NBT) to a blue compound during active respiration. Treatment of the disorder is generally limited to the use of prophylactic antibiotics or white blood cell infusions.

Other disorders of phagocyte metabolism include myeloperoxidase deficiency, glucose-6-phosphate dehydrogenase deficiency, and glutathione peroxidase deficiency. Each of these metabolic disorders promotes an increased rate of infection in affected people but usually not with the frequency or severity seen in CGD.

Job's syndrome is a multisystem disorder that is inherited as an autosomal dominant trait. It is characterized by unregulated IgE synthesis, delayed or diminished polymorphonuclear neutrophil chemotaxis, recurrent infections of the skin and respiratory tract, and chronic eczema. The manifestations of the disorder become apparent early in infancy with the development of chronic mucocutaneous candidiasis and ''cold'' cutaneous abscesses (*i.e.*, without the usual symptoms of warmth, redness, and pain). Similar to CGD, the most common pathogen is *Staphylococcus aureus*, but children with the disorder are also susceptible to a multitude of bacterial and fungal infections. In addition to elevated IgE levels and poor chemotactic response, children with Job's syndrome frequently have coarse facial features, red hair, retarded growth, broad nasal bridge, eosinophilia, and osteoporosis.

By contrast, *Chédiak-Higashi syndrome* is an autosomal recessive disorder in which the central defect in phagocytic function is thought to be caused by abnormal cell membrane fluidity, poor cytoskeletal coordination, and poor fusion of neutrophilic granules with phagocytosed microorganisms. The end result is poor mobility of the phagocytes and delayed killing of ingested bacteria. As with other disorders of phagocytosis, children with Chédiak-Higashi syndrome are subject to repeated cutaneous and respiratory tract infections, usually caused by beta-hemolytic streptococci (*e.g.*, *Streptococcus pyogenes*) and *Staphylococcus aureus*. Other characteristics of the syndrome include partial albinism and bleeding disorders. Giant granules in the cytoplasm of neutrophils are pathognomonic of the condition.

An unusual but interesting disorder of phagocytic function is based on the absence or deficiency of glycoproteins that are normally present on the cell membrane of neutrophils and monocytes called the *CD11/CD18* complex. These glycoproteins are essential for just about all of the surveillance functions performed by phagocytes including adhesion, chemotaxis, phagocytosis, and the stimulation of oxidative metabolism that follows phagocytosis. The first indication of this deficiency in an infant is delayed umbilical separation followed by severe, recurrent infections caused by a wide variety of gram-positive and gram-negative bacteria. Children with complete lack of CD11/CD18 glycoproteins rarely survive beyond the first year of life, whereas those with a deficiency in CD11/CD18 production have a longer life span. Therapy for this deficiency includes prophylactic antibiotic therapy and/or bone marrow transplantation. In the future, this condition could be amenable to gene replacement therapy.

Secondary deficiencies of the phagocytic system can be caused by a number of circumstances (*e.g.*, opsonins [factors such as antibody and complement that coat the surface of a foreign substance and enhance phagocytosis] and chemotactic factors such as antibody and complement that coat the surface of microorganisms and promote increased migration of phagocytes to the site of infection and stimulate phagocytosis). Therefore, deficiencies of either of these opsonins reduce the overall effectiveness of phagocytes. Drugs that impair or prevent inflammation and T-cell function such as corticosteroids or cyclosporin A also alter phagocytic response through modulation of cytokines. People with diabetes mellitus also demonstrate poor phagocytic function, primarily due to altered chemotaxis. The reason for this dysfunction is not understood but is unrelated to the age or the severity of the metabolic disorder. Apparently, this is a separate genetic disorder that is coinherited at a higher frequency among people with diabetes and among family members. Finally, people with HIV infection and AIDS represent another form of acquired or secondary deficiency of phagocytic function. However, in this case, the deficiency is due to direct infection and destruction of helper T cells and monocytes/macrophages by the virus (see Chapter 15).

In summary, an immunodeficiency is defined as an absolute or partial loss of the normal immune response, which places a person in a state of compromise and increases the risk of developing infections or malignant complications. Immunodeficiency states can affect one or more of the four main components of the immune response: (1) antibody or humoral (B-cell) immunity; (2) cellular or T-cell immunity; (3) the complement system; and (4) the phagocytic system. The variety of defects known to involve the immune response can be classified as either primary (endogenous or inherited) or secondary (caused by exogenous factors such as drugs or infection). The extent to which any or all of these components are compromised dictates the severity of the immunodeficiency.

■ ALLERGIC AND HYPERSENSITIVITY DISORDERS

Allergic disorders can be defined as unfavorable physiologic consequences of antigen–antibody or antigen–lymphocyte interactions. In the vernacular, we refer to such disorders as allergies or allergic reactions focusing on the outward symptoms of rhinitis, sneezing, watery eyes, hives, and so forth, commonly associated with adverse immune reactions. However, allergic disorders also include normal yet unfavorable responses of the immune system that are not usually associated with allergies such as graft rejection or hemolytic anemia of the newborn.

The potential for developing an allergic disorder is programmed into everyone with a normal immune system, but those conditions most commonly termed as "allergies" (hay fever and asthma) only affect a small portion of the population and tend to follow family lines. Not all adverse reactions to environmental substances are true allergic disorders. For example, milk or lactose intolerance can be caused by an enzyme deficiency and, therefore, by definition, is not an allergic disorder.

Historically, allergic disorders have been categorized into two basic types: immediate and delayed-type hypersensitivity. The criteria for this classification involve the time between exposure to the inducing antigen or allergen, and the appearance of symptoms. Allergic responses can be further divided into four categories as defined by Gell, Combs, and Lachman (1975). These categories are referred to as type I, type II, type III, and type IV reactions.

Type I reactions are typified by allergic asthma and urticaria (hives), hay fever, angioedema, and anaphylactic shock. These conditions are triggered by the binding of an allergen to a specific IgE that is bound to the surface of a mast cell or basophil (Fig. 14-4). The resulting antigen–antibody complex promotes the release of histamine and other reactive mediators from the basophil/mast cell that produce the characteristic symptoms of asthma or hay fever. Type I reactions are predominantly of the immediate hypersensitivity type.

Type II reactions are the end result of direct interactions between IgG and IgM class antibodies and tissue or cell surface antigens with or without subse-

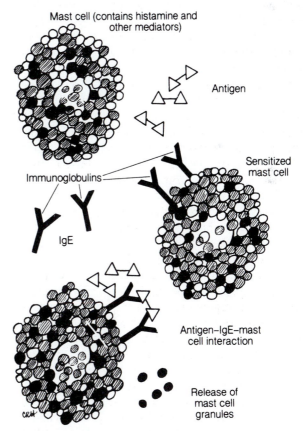

FIG. 14-4. Type I immune response that involves an allergen (antigen), immunoglobulin (IgE), and mast cell. Exposure to the allergen causes sensitization of the mast cell with subsequent binding of the allergen, which causes release of mast cell granules containing inflammatory mediators such as histamine and SRS-A.

quent activation of complement (Fig. 14-5). Examples of type II reactions include mismatched blood transfusion reactions, hemolytic disease of the newborn due to ABO or Rh incompatibility or certain drug reactions. In the latter, the binding of certain drugs to the surface of red or white blood cells elicits an antibody and complement response that lyses the drug-coated cell. Lytic drug reactions can produce transient anemia, leukopenia, or thrombocytopenia, which are corrected by the removal of the offending drug.

Type III reactions are caused by the formation of insoluble antigen–antibody complexes in the blood (Fig. 14-6). These complexes are eventually deposited within blood vessels or in the kidney; because immune complexes can activate complement, localized tissue damage can occur wherever these complexes are deposited. Type III reactions are responsible for the vasculitis seen in certain autoimmune diseases such as systemic lupus erythematosus (SLE) or the kidney damage seen with acute glomerulonephritis. Unlike type II reactions in which the damage is caused by direct and specific binding of antibody to tissue, the harmful effects of type III reactions are indirect (*i.e.*, secondary to the inflammatory response induced by activated complement).

Type IV reactions are synonymous with delayed-type hypersensitivity reactions and are caused by exposure of primed T-cell clones to the priming antigen. This contact leads to the synthesis and release of lymphokines and cytokines (Fig. 14-7), the recruitment of circulating and/or tissue macrophages to the

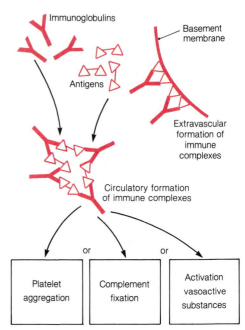

FIG. 14-6. Type III immune complex reactions that involve complement-activating IgG and IgM immunoglobulins with formation of bloodborne or extravascular immune complexes and their effects.

site of the interaction, proliferation of T cells, and localized inflammation. The end result is the typical induration reaction seen in a positive tuberculin test or contact dermatitis. Type IV reactions are also responsible for graft-versus-host and host-versus-graft disease after organ or bone marrow transplantation.

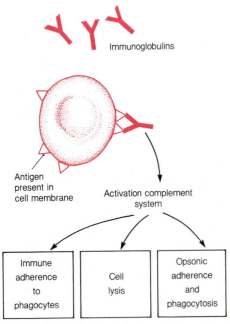

FIG. 14-5. Type II cytotoxic immune reactions that involve immunoglobulins (IgG and IgM) and cell-surface antigens with activation of the complement system.

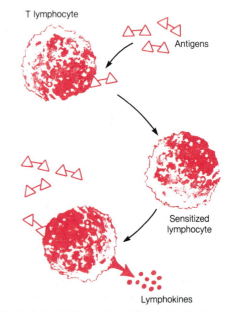

FIG. 14-7. Type IV immune response that involves an antigen, sensitized T-lymphocyte, and lymphokines. Exposure to the antigen causes sensitization of the lymphocyte with release of lymphokines on subsequent exposures.

IGE-MEDIATED ALLERGIC DISORDERS

There are two types of IgE-mediated allergic reactions—atopic disorders (allergic rhinitis, dermatitis, and gastroenteritis) and anaphylactic reactions (systemic anaphylaxis, urticaria, and angioedema).

ATOPIC DISORDERS

The term *atopic disorder* was coined to signify particular allergic disorders such as hay fever, asthma, or atopic dermatitis that tended to cluster along family lines (*i.e.*, there appeared to be a genetic predisposition to develop such disorders). At the root of most atopic allergies lies cell-associated IgE-class immunoglobulins—sometimes referred to as "skin-sensitizing antibody or reagins." It seems that people with atopic disorders respond to common environmental antigens (allergens) with an IgE response in the way that other people might elicit an IgM, IgG, or IgA immune response. People afflicted with atopic allergic conditions tend to have high serum levels of IgE and increased numbers of basophils and mast cells. Both basophils, which are blood cells, and mast cells, which are tissue cells, have granules that contain potent mediators of allergic reactions. These mediators are either preformed within the cell or activated through enzymatic processing. During priming stage, the allergen-specific or "sensitizing" IgE antibodies attach to receptors on the surface of these mast cells and basophils. After subsequent exposure, the sensitizing allergen binds to the cell-associated IgE and triggers a series of events that ultimately leads to degranulation of basophils and mast cells with concomitant activation and/or release of their allergy-producing mediators (see Fig. 14-4).

The most notable mediators of allergic reactions include histamine, complement, acetylcholine, slow-reacting substances, kinins, and eosinophil chemotactic factor. *Histamine* is a potent vasodilator that increases the permeability of capillaries and venules and causes smooth muscle contraction and bronchial constriction. Complement, when activated, leads to further release of histamine, stimulates the inflammatory response, and promotes leukocyte chemotaxis with secondary release of cytokines. Acetylcholine produces bronchial smooth muscle contraction and dilation of small blood vessels. The slow-reacting substances include both leukotrienes and prostaglandins. They produce responses similar to histamine and acetylcholine, although their effects are delayed and prolonged by comparison. The kinins, which are a group of potent inflammatory peptides, require activation through enzymatic modification. Once activated, these peptides produce vasodilata-

tion, smooth muscle contraction, leukocyte chemotaxis, and increased vascular permeability. Eosinophil chemotactic factor includes peptides released from mast cells and basophils after binding of surface IgE to allergen. These peptides prompt chemotaxis of eosinophils and leukocytes to the site of allergen contact. Additional mediators of atopic disorders include catecholamines, platelet activating factor, and 5-hydroxytryptamine (serotonin).

Although the IgE-triggered response is likely a key factor in the pathophysiology of atopic allergic disorders, it is certainly not the only factor and, in fact, may not be responsible for conditions such as atopic dermatitis and certain forms of asthma. In addition, many stimuli can induce conditions that are indistinguishable from atopic disorders yet bypass the immune response. It is possible, therefore, that people with atopic disorders are simply exquisitely responsive to the chemical mediators of allergic reactions rather than having hyperactive IgE immunity. The most notable examples of atopic allergic disorders are allergic rhinitis, atopic dermatitis, and food allergies. Bronchial asthma, sometimes classified as an atopic disorder, is discussed in Chapter 27.

Allergic Rhinitis. Allergic rhinitis can be divided into perennial and seasonal allergic rhinitis depending on the chronology of symptoms. People with the perennial type experience the characteristic symptoms of sneezing, itching, and watery discharge from the eyes and nose throughout the year whereas people with seasonal allergic rhinitis (also called hay fever) are plagued with intense symptoms in conjunction with periods of high pollen and mold counts. Typical allergens include pollens from ragweed, grasses, trees, and weeds; fungal spores; house dust mites; animal dander; and feathers. Either type of allergic rhinitis is predominantly the result of IgE-mediated histamine release and may affect one out of ten people in the general population. Diagnosis depends on a careful history and physical examination, microscopic identification of nasal eosinophilia, and skin testing to identify the offending allergen(s). Treatment is symptomatic in most cases and includes the use of oral antihistamines and decongestants. Nasal corticosteroids are often effective when used appropriately. Intranasal cromolyn may be useful, especially when administered before expected contact with an offending allergen. When possible, avoidance of the offending allergen is recommended. A program of desensitization may be used when symptoms are particularly bothersome. Desensitization involves frequent (usually weekly) injections of the offending antigen(s). The antigens, which are given in increasing doses, stimulate production of high levels of IgG, which acts as a blocking antibody by combining with the antigen before it can combine with the cell-bound IgE antibodies.

Atopic Dermatitis. Atopic dermatitis or eczema is another form of type I hypersensitivity that is highly associated with allergic rhinitis and asthma. The onset of atopic dermatitis typically begins in early childhood with 90% of all cases developing before the age of 5. During infancy, the characteristic skin lesions are erythematous papules or vesicles that alternately drain and crust over the surface. The forehead, cheeks, neck, and extensor surfaces are most often involved. At later ages, the lesions are generally dry and intensely pruritic and they develop on the anticubital and popliteal surfaces and the neck. Chronic scratching of the lesions occasionally leads to scarring and hypo- or hyperpigmentation. As with other atopic disorders, most people with atopic dermatitis have sensitizing antibodies to a variety of antigens, elevated IgE levels, eosinophilia, and a familial predisposition to develop atopic allergies. However, the pathophysiology associated with atopic dermatitis cannot be attributed to a hyperactive IgE immune response because the presence of sensitizing antibody is not a universal finding. Many environmental factors that circumvent the immune system can cause an exacerbation of the skin lesions. Possible defects in T-cell function have been identified in patients with this syndrome, indicating that, at the very least, this is a complex disorder. The course of atopic dermatitis is unpredictable, either diminishing with age or persisting for life. In some cases, the disease resolves spontaneously during the summer months. As with allergic rhinitis, treatment of atopic dermatitis is limited to symptomatic relief either with antihistamines or with topical or system corticosteroid therapy. Obviously, the best treatment is complete avoidance of the offending allergen. People who develop secondary bacterial infections are treated with the appropriate antibiotic therapy.

Food Allergies. Food allergies can occur at any age but, similar to atopic dermatitis and rhinitis, tend to manifest during childhood. Food allergies are usually considered type I allergic reactions and are often observed in conjunction with other atopic allergies. The allergic response is thought to occur after contact between specific food allergens and sensitizing IgE found in the intestinal mucosa causing local and systemic release of histamine and other mediators of the allergic response. In this disorder, allergens are usually food proteins and partially digested food products. Carbohydrates, lipids, or food additives, such as preservatives, colorings, or flavorings, are also potential allergens. Closely related food groups can contain common cross-reacting allergens. For example, some people are allergic to all legumes (beans,

peas, and peanuts). Some allergens are heat labile and are inactivated by cooking. Diagnosis of food allergies is usually based on careful food history, and treatment is based on avoidance.

NONATOPIC DISORDERS

The nonatopic allergic disorders are caused by IgE immunoglobulins but lack the genetic predisposition of atopic disorders. They include anaphylaxis (see Chapter 25) and urticaria. Angioedema, also categorized as a nonatopic disease, was discussed earlier.

Urticaria. *Urticaria* or hives is a common condition characterized by the appearance of raised, erythematous, pruritic skin lesions—the so-called wheal-and-flare reaction. These lesions appear to be the result of localized release (either IgE-mediated or nonimmune mechanisms) of histamine, although other activators of inflammation probably augment the condition. Episodes of urticaria are most often triggered by the ingestion of foods such as eggs or dairy products, certain fruits, chocolate, or wheat flour, to name a few. In addition, certain drugs (*e.g.,* penicillin and acetylsalicylic acid), insect bites, malignancies, autoimmune disorders, vaccines, and even exposure to extremes of temperature and light have been associated with hives. The best treatment is to avoid contact with the offending stimuli. After a reaction occurs, antihistamines or (in severe cases) epinephrine can be used to provide symptomatic relief. However, if the reaction occurs in subcutaneous or submucosal tissues (*e.g.,* airways), the condition (sometimes called angioedema) can be life threatening.

IMMUNE-COMPLEX ALLERGIC DISEASES

Immune-complex allergic disorders are mediated by the formation of insoluble antigen–antibody complexes that activate complement. Activation of complement by the immune complex generates chemotactic and vasoactive mediators that cause tissue damage by a variety of mechanisms including alterations in blood flow, vascular permeability, and the destructive action of inflammatory cells. Immune complex disorders can present with local manifestations as in the Arthus reaction or as a systemic reaction in serum sickness.

Arthus Reaction. The Arthus reaction is a term used by pathologists and immunologists to describe localized tissue necrosis (usually in the skin) caused by immune complexes. In the laboratory, an Arthus reaction can be produced by injecting an antigen preparation into the skin of an immune animal with high levels of circulating antibody. Within 4 to 10 hours, a red, raised lesion appears on the skin at the site of the injection. An ulcer often forms in the center of the lesion. Unlike type-I immune reactions, the Arthus reaction is not caused by IgE. It is thought that the injected antigen diffuses into local blood vessels, where it comes in contact with specific antibody (IgG) and precipitates a localized inflammatory response. Tissue sections of Arthus lesions show deposited immunoglobulin, complement, and fibrinolytic products within blood vessels. If the blood vessel bursts, hemorrhage into surrounding tissue is seen. If the blood vessel is occluded, the oxygen supply to surrounding tissue is interrupted (an ischemic event) causing cell death and tissue necrosis.

Serum Sickness. The term *serum sickness* was originally coined to describe a syndrome consisting of rash, lymphadenopathy, arthralgias, and occasionally neurologic disorders that appeared 7 or more days after injections of horse antisera. Although this therapy is rarely used today, the name remains. The most common contemporary causes of this allergic disorder include antibiotics (especially penicillin), various foods, drugs, and insect venoms.

Serum sickness can be classified as a type III immune complex reaction and is triggered by the deposition of insoluble antigen–antibody (IgM and IgG) complexes within blood vessels, joints, heart, and kidney tissue. The deposited complexes activate complement, increase vascular permeability, and recruit phagocytic cells, all of which tend to lead to focal tissue damage and edema. The signs and symptoms include urticaria, patchy or generalized rash, extensive edema (usually of the face, neck, and joints), and fever. In most cases, the damage is temporary and symptoms resolve within a few days. However, a prolonged and continuous exposure to the sensitizing antigen can lead to irreversible damage. In previously sensitized people, severe and even fatal forms of serum sickness may occur either immediately or within several days after the sensitizing drug or serum is administered. Treatment of serum sickness is generally directed toward removal of the sensitizing antigen and symptomatic relief. This may include aspirin for joint pain and antihistamines for pruritis. Epinephrine or systemic corticosteroids may be used for severe reactions.

CELL-MEDIATED HYPERSENSITIVITY DISORDERS

The effector T cells are responsible for certain forms of allergy, frequently referred to as delayed hypersensitivity. Delayed hypersensitivity reactions include allergic contact dermatitis and a much less frequent disease, hypersensitivity pneumonitis.

Allergic Contact Dermatitis. Allergic contact dermatitis denotes an inflammatory response confined to the skin that is initiated by reexposure to an allergen to which a person has previously become sensitized (*e.g.*, cosmetics, hair dyes, metals, and drugs applied to the skin). Contact dermatitis usually consists of erythematous macules, papules, and vesicles (blisters). The affected area often becomes swollen and warm, with exudation, crusting, and development of a secondary infection. The location of the lesions often provides a clue as to the nature of the antigen causing the disorder. The most common form of this condition is the dermatitis that follows an intimate encounter with poison ivy or oak antigens, although many other substances can trigger a reaction.

The mechanism of events that lead to prior sensitization to an antigen is not completely understood. It is likely that sensitization follows transdermal transport of an antigen with subsequent presentation to T-lymphocytes. Subpopulations of sensitized lymphocytes are distributed throughout the body so that subsequent cutaneous exposure to the offending antigen promotes a localized reaction regardless of the initial site of contact. The severity of the reaction associated with contact dermatitis ranges from mild to intense depending on the person and the allergen. Because this condition follows the mechanism of a delayed hypersensitivity response, the reaction does not become apparent for at least 12 hours and generally more than 24 hours after exposure. Depending on the antigen and the duration of exposure, the reaction may last from days to weeks and is typified by erythematous, vesicular, or papular lesions associated with intense pruritis and weeping. Diagnosis of contact dermatitis is made by noting the distribution of lesions on the skin surface and associating a particular pattern with exposure to possible allergens. If a particular allergen is suspected, a patch test can be used to confirm the suspicion. For this, the suspected allergen is applied to a gauze or patch that is taped to a hair-free surface for 48 hours. The patch is removed, and the surface is inspected daily for a response. Treatment is generally limited to the removal of the irritant, and topical application (*e.g.*, ointments and corticosteroid creams) to relieve symptomatic skin lesions and to prevent secondary bacterial infections. Severe reactions may require systemic corticosteroid therapy.

Hypersensitivity Pneumonitis. Hypersensitivity pneumonitis or allergic alveolitis is thought to be caused by the activation of pulmonary T cells, followed by the release of cytokine mediators of inflammation. The inflammatory response that ensues (generally several hours after exposure) produces labored breathing, dry cough, chills and fever, headache, and malaise. The symptoms usually subside within hours after the sensitizing antigen(s) are removed. A primary example of hypersensitivity pneumonitis is "farmers lung," a condition instigated by exposure to mold antigens while baling hay. Other sensitizing antigens include tree bark, sawdust, animal danders, and actinomycete bacteria that are occasionally found in humidifiers, hot tubs, and swimming pools. Treatment consists of identifying and avoiding the offending antigen(s). Severe forms of the disorder may be treated with systemic corticosteroid therapy.

Miscellaneous Nonatopic Disorders. Other conditions that can be classified as nonatopic allergic disorders include allergic bronchopulmonary aspergillosis, a syndrome similar to hypersensitivity pneumonitis resulting from chronic colonization of the respiratory tract by members of the fungal genus *Aspergillus* and the deposition of the organisms antigens within the lungs; Heiner's syndrome characterized by chronic upper respiratory symptoms in infants associated with antibodies to cow's milk antigens; and pulmonary eosinophilia, a condition characterized by the infiltration of the lung with eosinophils in conjunction with an elevated eosinophil count in the blood. Although the cause of this syndrome is not clear, it can be found in association with asthma, autoimmune disease, drug reactions, and parasitic infections.

In summary, hypersensitivity and allergic disorders are responses to environmental, food, or drug antigens that would not affect the majority of the population. There are four basic categories of hypersensitivity responses: (1) type I responses, which are mediated by the IgE-class immunoglobulins and include anaphylactic shock, hay fever, angioedema, and bronchial asthma; (2) type II cytotoxic reactions, which are characterized by hemolytic transfusion reactions and caused by immunoglobulin (IgG and IgM) activation of complement; (3) type III reactions, which result from the formation of insoluble antigen—antibody complexes that become deposited within blood vessels or in the kidney and cause localized tissue injury; and (4) type IV cell-mediated responses in which sensitized T-lymphocytes promote an inflammatory response when presented with the sensitizing antigen.

■ TRANSPLANTATION IMMUNOPATHOLOGY

Not long ago, transplantation of solid organs (*e.g.*, liver, kidney, heart) and bone marrow was considered experimental and reserved for people for whom alternative methods of therapy were exhausted and survival was unlikely. However, with a greater understanding of humoral and cellular immune regulation, the development of immunosuppressive drugs such as cyclosporin, and an appreciation of the role of the major histocompatibility complex (MHC) antigens, transplantation has become nearly routine and the subsequent success rate has been greatly enhanced.

In 1990, more than 4000 allogenic (see below) bone marrow transplantations were performed, and this procedure is a major therapeutic alternative for people with leukemia and lymphoma.

Regardless of the type of transplant, the cell surface antigens that determine whether transplanted tissue is recognized as foreign or native are the MHC, also called HLA in humans (see Chapter 13). Transplanted tissue can be categorized as allogenic if the donor and recipient are related or unrelated but share similar HLA types, syngeneic if the donor and recipient are identical twins, and autologous if donor and recipient are the same person. Donors of solid organ transplants can be living or dead (cadaver) and related or nonrelated (heterologous). When cells bearing foreign MHC antigens are transplanted, the recipient's immune system attempts to eliminate the donor cells, a process referred to as *host-versus-graft disease* (HVGD). Conversely, the cellular immunity of the transplanted tissue can attack unrelated recipient tissue causing a *graft-versus-host disease* (GVHD). Obviously, the likelihood of rejection varies indirectly with the degree of HLA (or MCH) relatedness between donor and recipient. With kidney transplants involving living-related donors, there is a 90% 1-year graft survival when the donor and recipient are identical twins as compared with 56% when donor and recipient do not share either HLA haplotype.

HOST-VERSUS-GRAFT DISEASE

Host-versus-graft rejection usually involves both cellular and humoral components and is a complex process. There are three basic patterns of transplant rejections: hyperacute, acute, and chronic. A hyperacute reaction occurs almost immediately after transplantation; in kidney transplants, it can often be seen at the time of surgery. As soon as blood flow from the recipient to the donor organ begins, it develops a cyanotic, mottled appearance. Sometimes the reaction takes hours to days to develop. The hyperacute response is produced by existing recipient antibodies to graft antigens that initiate an Arthus-type reaction in the blood vessels of the graft. These antibodies have usually developed in response to previous blood transfusions, pregnancies in which the mother develops antibodies to fetal antigens, or infections with bacteria or viruses possessing antigens that mimic MHC antigens.

Acute rejection generally occurs within the first few months after transplantation. In the patient with an organ transplant, acute rejection is evidenced by signs of organ failure. Acute rejection often involves both humoral and cell-mediated immune responses. Chronic host-versus-graft rejection occurs over a prolonged period of time and is largely heralded by a gradually rise in serum creatinine over a period of 4 to 6 months.

GRAFT-VERSUS-HOST DISEASE

In contrast to HVGD, three basic requirements are necessary for GVHD to develop: (1) the transplant must have a functional cellular immune component; (2) the recipient tissue must bear antigens foreign to the donor tissue, and (3) the recipient immunity must be compromised to the point that it cannot destroy the transplanted cells. We know that the primary agents of GVDH are T cells and that the antigens they recognize and attack are HLA. Once again, the greater the difference in tissue antigens between the donor and recipient, the greater the likelihood of GVHD. If the recipient has a normally functioning immune system, it quickly eradicates HLA-mismatched transplants making immunosuppression a necessity. Without appropriate therapy, most allogeneic (and even syngeneic or autologous) bone marrow transplant recipients develop some form of GVHD.

If GVHD occurs, the primary targets of the acute illness are the skin, liver, intestine, and cells of the immune system. Acute GVHD is characterized by a pruritic, maculopapular rash, which begins on the palms and soles and frequently extends over the entire body with subsequent desquamation. The epithelial layer is the primary site of injury. When the intestine is involved, symptoms include nausea, blood diarrhea, and abdominal pain. GVHD of the liver can lead to bleeding disorders and coma. GVHD is considered chronic if symptoms persist or begin 100 days or more after transplantation. Chronic GVHD is characterized by abnormal humoral and cellular immunity, severe skin disorders, and liver disease.

The pathogenesis of acute GVHD is initiated in three stages: (1) recognition and presentation by donor T cells of foreign recipient antigens; (2) activation of T cells through cytokines, and (3) multiplication of activated T cells. The actual tissue pathology observed with GVHD is produced directly by the action of cytotoxic T cells or indirectly through the release of inflammatory mediators such as tissue necrosis factor-alpha, interleukins, complement, and so forth. Conversely, chronic GVHD has all the markings of an autoimmune disorder in which activated T cells recognize minor MHC antigens common to all people (and, therefore, not foreign).

A third type of GVHD has been recognized that follows the transplantation of genetically identical tissue (*i.e.*, syngeneic or autologous). This variety of GVHC stems from the pretreatment conditioning regimen (*e.g.*, total body irradiation) or treatment with cytotoxic drugs. The conditioning therapy disrupts the normal immune surveillance system and allows "rogue" autoreactive T cells to proliferate and attack native tissue. Syngeneic GVHD is usually self-limited and not severe.

GVHD can be prevented by blocking any of the three steps of pathogenesis. For example, donor T-cells can be selectively removed from the transplanted tissue or destroyed using various treatments such as monoclonal antibodies with attached toxins equivalent to heat-seeking missiles). Alternatively, immunosuppressive or antiinflammatory drugs such as cyclosporin or glucocorticoids can be used to block T-cell activation and the action of cytokines.

In summary, organ and bone marrow transplantation has been enhanced by a greater understanding of humoral and cellular immune regulation, the development of immunosuppressive drugs such as cyclosporin, and an appreciation of the role of the MHC antigens. The likelihood of rejection varies indirectly with the degree of HLA (or MHC) relatedness between donor and recipient. A rejection can involve an attempt by the recipient's immune system to eliminate the donor cells (host-versus-graft disease) or an attack by the cellular immunity of the transplanted tissue on the unrelated recipient tissue (graft-versus-host disease).

■ AUTOIMMUNE DISEASE

To function properly, the immune system must be able to distinguish foreign antigens from native or "self" antigens. Normally, there is a high degree of immunologic tolerance to native antigens, which prevents the immune system from destroying the host. Autoimmune disorders result from the breakdown in the integrity of immune tolerance such that a humoral or cellular immune response can be mounted against host tissue or antigens leading to localized or systemic injury.

Autoimmune diseases can affect almost any cell or tissue in the body. There are known or suspected hematologic, rheumatologic, neurologic, and endocrine disorders associated with autoimmunity. Some autoimmune disorders, such as Hashimoto's thyroiditis, are tissue specific; whereas others, such as SLE, affect multiple organs and systems. Chart 14-2 lists some of the probable autoimmune diseases.

The ability of the immune system to distinguish foreign from native antigens is the responsibility of

---

CHART 14-2: PROBABLE AUTOIMMUNE DISEASES

Systemic

Mixed connective-tissue disease
Polymyositis-dermatomyositis
Rheumatoid arthritis
Scleroderma
Sjögren's syndrome
Systemic lupus erythematosus

Blood

Autoimmune hemolytic anemia
Autoimmune neutropenia and lymphopenia
Idiopathic thrombocytopenic purpura

Other Organs

Acute idiopathic polyneuritis
Atrophic gastritis and pernicious anemia
Autoimmune adrenalitis
Goodpasture's syndrome
Hashimoto's thyroiditis
Insulin-dependent diabetes mellitus
Myasthenia gravis
Premature gonadal (ovarian) failure
Primary biliary cirrhosis
Sympathetic ophthalmia
Temporal arteritis
Thyrotoxicosis (Graves' disease)
Ulcerative colitis

Examples are not inclusive.

HLA. HLA is encoded by MHC genes (see Chapter 13). Components of both humoral and cellular immunity can be detected in autoimmune disorders. One of the differences between the two components is that the B cell can respond to antigenic stimuli independent of the immune network like a loose cannon.

To elicit a T-cell response, the antigen must first be processed and presented on the surface of a phagocytic cell such as a macrophage that also displays MHC antigen. This dual recognition requirement acts like a security system and affects all T-cell subpopulations: cytotoxic T cells, which damage target cells directly, and the helper and suppressor T cells, which augment or restrict B- and T-cell function, respectively. Helper and suppressor T cells are the positive and negative feedback circuits of the immune system. Without these controls, an immune response would never accelerate to an effective level or would continue unabated causing undue destruction of the host.

Self-tolerance is the absence of an immune response directed against a person's own native tissue antigens. Because of the need for MHC recognition, a T-cell response directed against native antigens is rare. B cells, on the other hand, sometimes recognize native antigens complexed with smaller molecules or haptens as foreign and, without the control afforded by suppressor T cells, can ultimately mount an immune response. With a normally functioning cellular immune system, an abnormal B-cell response is held in check.

PROBABLE MECHANISMS

The event or events that trigger the development of an autoimmune response are not known. There may be the formation of antibodies directed against native tissue called *autoantibodies*, failure of the immune system to recognize native antigens as self, or the presence of abnormally potent antigens called *super antigens*.

There are multiple explanations for the formation of autoantibodies or failure to recognize native antigens as self. Proposed mechanisms include: (1) genetic abnormalities that predispose certain people to autoimmune processes, (2) interactions with chemical, physical, or biologic agents that trigger immunologic cross-reactions or recognition of native antigens, and (3) abnormalities in regulatory or surveillance systems that lead to an uncontrolled immune response. Because of the complexity of the immune system, it seems unlikely that autoimmune disorders arise from a single defect.

Genetic Predisposition. There is increasing evidence that genetic factors increase the incidence and severity of autoimmune diseases. This evidence is based on the familial clustering of several autoimmune diseases and the observation that certain inherited HLA types, which are inherited as part of the MHC, occur more frequently in people with a variety of immunologic and lymphoproliferative disorders. For example, 90% of people with ankylosing spondylitis carry the HLA-B27 antigen. By comparison, only 7% of a control group without the disease have the antigen. Other HLA-associated diseases are Reiter's syndrome and HLA-B27, rheumatoid arthritis and HLA-DR4, and SLE and HLA-DR3. The basis for these associations is not known. In the case of SLE, as many as six potentially abnormal gene loci could be involved in providing a veritable matrix of disease patterns. Because not all people with genetic predisposition develop autoimmunity, it would appear that other factors such as a "trigger event" interact to precipitate the altered immune state.

Interactions with Chemical and Microbial Agents. There are many ways in which chemical or microbial stimulants can evoke an altered immune response leading to an autoimmune disorder. Drugs and viruses can alter T-cell function so that maverick

B-cell responses against host cell antigens are not abated. It is possible that certain autoimmune disorders are due to "molecular mimicry" (*i.e.,* a foreign antigen so closely resembles a self antigen that antibodies produced against the former react with the latter). Also, a humoral or cellular response can be mounted against antigenically altered or injured tissue creating an immune process. In rheumatic fever and acute glomerulonephritis, for example, a protein in the cell wall of group A hemolytic streptococci has considerable homology with antigens in heart and kidney tissue, respectively. After infection, antibodies directed against the microorganism cause a classic case of mistaken identity, which leads to inflammation of the heart or kidney. Certain drugs, when bound to host proteins or glycoproteins, form a superantigen to which a humoral response is directed with substantial cross-reactivity to the original native protein. The antihypertensive agent methyldopa can bind to surface antigens on red cells to induce an antibody-mediated hemolytic anemia.

Disorders of Immune Regulatory or Surveillance Function. Because T cells regulate the immune response, an increasing T-helper : T-suppressor cell ratio can potentially lead to the development of autoimmune disorders. An example of this can be seen in people with multiple sclerosis where fluctuations in suppressor T-cell numbers parallel the intensity of the disease process.

Superantigens. A relatively new and exciting development in the understanding of certain immune disorders centers around the discovery of the so-called *superantigens*. Superantigens are a family of related substances including staphylococcal and streptococcal exotoxins that can short-circuit the normal sequence of events leading to activation of helper T cells. In essence, superantigens do not require processing and presentation by macrophages to induce a T-cell response. Normally, only a small percentage of the T-cell population is stimulated by the presence of processed antigens on the surface of macrophages. Superantigens, however, directly link the MHC-II complex molecules of antigen-presenting cells such as macrophages to T-cell receptors causing a massive release of T-cell inflammatory cytokines (primarily interleukin-2 and tumor necrosis factor) and an uncontrolled proliferation of T cells. The end result is either an acute and potentially life-threatening disease such as toxic shock syndrome or a chronic inflammatory process such as rheumatic fever. It is possible that, once we understand and control the effects of superantigen immune activation, we could eliminate a number of autoimmune disorders.

DIAGNOSIS OF AUTOIMMUNE DISORDERS

Criteria have been suggested for identifying autoimmune disease based on the following: (1) evidence of an autoimmune reaction, (2) determination that the immunologic findings are not secondary to another condition, and (3) the lack of other identified causes for the disorder. In the future, it is likely that autoimmune disorders will be diagnosed by directly identifying the gene(s) responsible for the condition as will soon be the case for cystic fibrosis. For now, however, the diagnosis of autoimmune disease is based primarily on clinical findings and serologic testing. The basis for most serologic assays is the demonstration of antibodies directed against tissue antigens or cellular components. For example, a child with chronic or acute history of fever, arthritis, and a macular rash along with high levels of antinuclear antibody carries a likely diagnosis of lupus erythematosus. The detection of autoantibodies in the laboratory is usually accomplished by one of three methods: indirect fluorescent antibody assays (IFA), enzyme-linked immunosorbent assay (ELISA), or particle agglutination of one kind or another. The rationale behind each of these methods is similar: the patient's serum is diluted and allowed to react with an antigen-coated surface (whole, fixed cells for the detection of antinuclear antibodies). In the case of IFA and ELISA, a second "labeled" antibody is added, which binds to the patient's antibody and forms a visible reaction. Particle agglutination assays are much simpler. The binding of the patient's antibody to antigen-coated particles causes a visible agglutination reaction. For most serologic assays, the patient's serum is serially diluted until it no longer produces a visible reaction (*e.g.,* 1 : 100 dilution). This is called a positive titer. Healthy people sometimes have low titers of antibody against cellular and tissue antigens, but the titers are usually far less than patients with autoimmune disease.

In summary, autoimmune diseases represent a disruption in self-tolerance that results in damage to body tissues by the immune system. Autoimmune diseases can affect almost any cell or tissue of the body. Normally self-tolerance is maintained by suppressor and helper T cells that recognize self-antigens and regulate and protect the body from inappropriate immune responses. Among the proposed mechanisms to explain the loss of self-tolerance and susceptibility to autoimmune disorders are: (1) genetic predisposition and influence of the HLA antigens in rejection of a person's own tissue, (2) interactions with chemical, physical, and biologic agents (*e.g.,* superantigens) that trigger an abnormal immune response, and (3) abnormalities in immune cells that lead to an inappropriate immune response directed against self-antigens. It is possible that, with a greater understanding of the events that trigger an abnormal immune response (*e.g.*, superantigens), we will be able to identify susceptible genotypes and prevent or delay the onset of autoimmune disorders.

■ BIBLIOGRAPHY

Anderson, K.C., & Weinstein, H.J. (1990). Transfusion-associated graft-versus-host disease. *New England Journal of Medicine, 323,* 315–321.

Behrman, R.E., Kliegman, R.M., Nelson, W., & Vaughn, V.C. (Eds.). (1992). *Nelson textbook of pediatrics* (14th ed., pp. 551–601). Philadelphia: W.B. Saunders.

Buckley, R.H., & Schiff, R.L. (1991). The use of intravenous immune globulin in immunodeficiency diseases (a review article). *New England Journal of Medicine, 325,* 109–117.

Cobern, G.T., & Main, E.K. (1991). Immunology of the maternal-placental interface in normal pregnancy. *Seminars in Perinatology, 15,* 196–205.

Cohen, I.R. (1988). The self, the world, and autoimmunity. *Scientific American, 258*(4), 52–60.

Colten, H.R. (1987). Hereditary angioneurotic edema, 1887 to 1987. *New England Journal of Medicine, 317,* 43–44.

Cotran, R.S., Kumar, V., & Robbins, S.L. (1989). *Robbins' pathologic basis of disease* (4th ed., pp. 172–224). Philadelphia: W.B. Saunders.

Dudley, D.J., & Wiedmeier, S. (1991). The ontogeny of the immune response: Perinatal perspectives. *Seminars in Perinatology, 15,* 184–195.

Fauci, A.S. (Moderator). (1983). Activation and regulation of human immune responses: Implications in normal and disease states (NIH Conference). *Annals of Internal Medicine, 99,* 61.

Ferrara, J.L.M., & Deeg, H.J. (1991). Mechanisms of disease: Graft-versus-host disease. *New England Journal of Medicine, 324,* 667–674.

Gell, R.G.H., Coombs, R.R.A., & Lachman, P.J. (Eds.). (1975). *Clinical aspects of immunology* (3rd ed.). Oxford: Blackwell Scientific.

Goroncy-Bermes, P., Dale, J.B., Beachey, E.H., et al. (1987). Monoclonal antibody to human renal glomeruli cross-reacts with streptococcal M protein. *Infection and Immunity, 55,* 2416–2419.

Herman, A., Kappler, J.W., Marrack, P., et al. (1991). Superantigens: Mechanisms of T-cell stimulation and role in immune disease. *Annual Review of Immunology, 9,* 745–772.

James, L.M., Ferrara, M.D., & Deeg, H.J. Graft-versus-host-disease (review article). *New England Journal of Medicine, 324,* 667–674.

Johnson, H.M., Russell, J.K., & Pontzer, C.H. (1992, April). Superantigens in human disease. *Scientific American, 266,* 92–101.

Kirkpatrick, C.H. (1987). Transplantation immunology. *Journal of the American Medical Association, 258,* 2993–3000.

Krensky, A.M., Crabtree, G., Davis, M.M., Parkman, P. (1990). T-lymphocyte–antigen interactions in transplant rejection. *New England Journal of Medicine, 322,* 510–518.

Pearlman, D.S., & Beirman, C.W. (1989). Allergic disorders. In E.R. Stiehm (Ed.). *Immunologic disorders in infants and children* (3rd ed., pp. 439–474). Philadelphia: W.B. Saunders.

Quie, P.G., & Abramson, J.S. (1989). Disorders of the polymorphonuclear phagocytic system. In E.R. Steihm (Ed.). *Immunologic disorders in infants and children* (3rd ed., pp. 343–363). Philadelphia: W.B. Saunders.

Schmalstieg, F.C. Leukocyte adherence defect. *Infectious Disease Journal, 7,* 867–872.

Shyur, S.D., & Hill, H.R. (1991). Immunodeficiency in the 1990s. *Pediatric Infectious Disease Journal, 10,* 595–611.

Stites, D.P., & Terr, A.L. (1991). *Basic and clinical immunology* (7th ed., pp. 319–362). Norwalk, CT: Appleton Lange.

Storb, R. (1991). Pathogenesis and recent therapeutic approaches to graft-versus-host disease. *Journal of Pediatrics, 118,* S10–S13.

Yu, D.T.Y., Choo, S.Y., & Schaack, T. (1989). Molecular mimicry in HLA-B27-related arthritis. *Annals of Internal Medicine, 111,* 581–591.

CHAPTER 15

ACQUIRED IMMUNODEFICIENCY SYNDROME (AIDS)

SUSAN E. DIETZ

■ OBJECTIVES

After you have studied this chapter, you should be able to meet the following objectives:

■ Briefly trace the history of the AIDS epidemic.

■ State the virus responsible for AIDS and explain how it differs from most other viruses.

■ Describe the mechanisms of HIV transmission and relate them to the need for public awareness and concern regarding the spread of AIDS.

■ Describe the universal precautions for HIV infection.

■ Discuss the CDC *Recommendations for Preventing the Transmission of HIV and HBV to Patients During Exposure-Prone Invasive Procedures.*

■ Describe diagnosis of AIDS using the CDC *AIDS Case Definition.*

■ Describe the alterations in immune function that occur in people with AIDS.

■ Relate the altered immune function in people with AIDs to the development of opportunistic infections, tuberulosis, and Kaposi's sarcoma.

■ Explain the possible significance of a positive antibody test for HIV infection.

■ Differentiate between the EIA (ELISA) and Western blot antibody detection tests for HIV infection.

■ List the four stages of AIDS and describe the symptoms, psychosocial issues, and management concerns for each stage.

■ Discuss the vertical transmission of HIV from mother to child and the impact of the AIDS epidemic on infants and children.

At the beginning of the AIDS epidemic, many Americans had little sympathy for people with AIDS. The feeling was that somehow people from certain groups deserved their illness. Let us put those feelings behind us. We are fighting a disease, not people. Those who are already afflicted are sick people and need our care as do all sick patients. The country must face this epidemic as a unified society. We must prevent the spread of AIDS while at the same time preserving humanity and intimacy.[1]

C. EVERETT KOOP, MD, ScD
Surgeon General (1981–1989)
U.S. Public Health Service

Carol Mattson Porth: PATHOPHYSIOLOGY: CONCEPTS OF
ALTERED HEALTH STATES, 4th ed. © 1994, 1990, 1986, 1982
J.B. Lippincott Company

Acquired immunodeficiency syndrome (AIDS) is caused by a retrovirus that selectively attacks and destroys the immune system. The Centers for Disease Control and Prevention (CDC) estimates that 1 million people in the United States are infected with human immunodeficiency virus (HIV).[2] The incidence and prevalence of HIV infection and AIDS in the United States have been highest in the East and West Coast regions and lowest in the northern Midwest and Mountain states. In addition, prevalence is greater in urban than in rural areas. Cases of HIV infection and AIDS have been concentrated among men between ages 20 to 39. The numbers of newly diagnosed AIDS cases and deaths continue to increase each year. Over 250,000 cases of AIDS have been diagnosed in the United States through December 1992.[3] Mortality increased from 31 deaths before 1981 to more than 170,000 through December 1992.[3] At least 40,000 new HIV infections occur each year in the United States. Some populations, such as African Americans and Hispanics, are disproportionately affected by this epidemic.

From 1988 through 1989, HIV infection increased from the 15th to the 11th leading cause of death in the United States. Of HIV-associated deaths in 1989, 63.9% were among white males; 24.8% among African-American males; 6.0% among African-American females; and 4.4% among white females. Most HIV-associated deaths occurred among people aged 25 to 44 years. For this age group, HIV infection was the second leading cause of death for men and the sixth leading cause of death for women.[4] In 1990, HIV infection/AIDS was the sixth leading cause of years of potential life lost (YPLL) before the age of 65 years. Although the YPLL before age 65 for most of the top 10 causes of death are stable or declining slightly, from 1989 to 1990 HIV showed the largest percentage increase (9.9%).[5] These trends reflect the youthfulness of those who have died of AIDS and the increasing number of deaths.

■ THE AIDS EPIDEMIC

The first recognized cases of AIDS occurred in the summer of 1981 when *Pneumocystis carinii* pneumonia (PCP) and Kaposi's sarcoma (KS) were reported in previously healthy people.[6] Both of these conditions previously occurred only in severely immunocompromised people. The condition became known in 1982 as the acquired immunodeficiency syndrome, although its causes and modes of transmission were not immediately obvious.[6]

An understanding of the virology of AIDS progressed with amazing efficiency; within 3 years after the first cases were recognized, the virus causing

AIDS was identified.[6] The virus was initially known by various names, including human T-lymphotropic, virus type 3, or human T-lymphadenopathy-associated virus (HTLV-III or LAV) and AIDS-associated retrovirus (ARV).[6] The internationally accepted term since 1986 has been human immunodeficiency virus (HIV).[7]

First described among homosexual men in June 1981, AIDS was recognized among injecting drug users the following year and among people with hemophilia, infants born to infected mothers, and as early as 1983 among heterosexual sex partners of people with AIDS.[8] Studies of these diverse groups led to the conclusion that AIDS is an infectious disease spread by blood, sexual contact, and perinatally from mother to child. The cumulative world total of AIDS cases was 11,965 through 1984.[9] Because HIV/AIDS occurs over a wide geographic area and affects an exceptionally high proportion of the population, it is often referred to as a pandemic. As of July 1, 1991, 371,802 cases of AIDS were reported officially from 163 countries to the World Health Organization. A more realistic estimate may be that over 1 million adults and 500,000 children worldwide have developed AIDS since it was first recognized.[10] Since reporting of cases is not uniform throughout the world, many countries may not be accurately represented in these figures.

The absence of a cure and preventive vaccine has led to broad and increasing public concern. Estimated inpatient hospital costs for a person with AIDS average $24,000, and outpatient costs average $8,000 for a total of $32,000 per year (in 1990 dollars).[11] Medical care costs for a person with HIV infection (not diagnosed with AIDS) are estimated at $5,150 per year (in 1990 dollars).[11] In addition, it is forecasted that the cost of treating all people with HIV infection and AIDS in the United States will increase 21% each year between 1991 and 1994.[11] These increases will lead to a total of $10.4 billion that will be spent on treating all people with HIV infection and AIDS in 1994.[11]

The development of AIDS appears to be directly related to the duration of HIV infection.[12] Cohort studies show that 51% of people who have seroconverted (developed antibodies as a result of infection with HIV) will develop HIV-related illness within 10 years. Some studies describe cases in which people are still free of clinical signs or symptoms more than 10 years after seroconversion.[13]

Infection with human immunodeficiency virus type 2 (HIV-2) is endemic in many countries in West Africa but generally much rarer in other parts of the world. Although data regarding HIV-2 transmission are limited, it appears to be transmitted in the same manner as HIV-1. HIV-2 can also cause immunodeficiency evidenced by a reduction in the number of lymphocytes. The spectrum of disease for HIV-2 is similar to that of HIV-1. Through 1991, 17 cases of HIV-2 were reported in the United States as compared to the estimated 40,000 new cases of HIV-1 infection each year. Because of the relatively rare occurrence of HIV-2 in the United States, there is little reason to believe it will have a major impact on morbidity and mortality over the short term. Long-term consequences will depend on its spread in the population.[14]

In summary, AIDS is an infectious disease of the immune system caused by the HIV. First described in June 1981, the disease is prevalent worldwide and is one of the leading causes of death among young adults in the United States. The severity of the clinical disease and the absence of a cure or preventive vaccine have increased public awareness and concern.

■ TRANSMISSION OF HIV INFECTION

HIV is transmitted from one person to another through sexual contact, by blood, or perinatally. HIV is not transmitted through casual contact. Several studies involving more than 1000 uninfected, non-sexual household contacts with people with HIV infection (including siblings, parents, and children) have shown no evidence of transmission.[15] HIV is not spread by mosquitoes or other insect vectors.[8] When infected blood, semen, or vaginal secretions from one person are deposited onto a mucous membrane or into the bloodstream of another person, transmission can occur.

Blood, semen, and vaginal/cervical secretions contain sufficient concentrations of HIV to transmit the infection.[8] Contact with semen occurs during sexual intercourse (vaginal and anal), oral sex (fellatio), and donor insemination. Exposure to vaginal/cervical secretions occurs during vaginal intercourse and oral sex (cunnilingus). In most cities in the United States, HIV is transmitted primarily through sexual contact. In the United States, 58% of AIDS cases are among men who have sex with men, and 6% of AIDS cases are related to infection through heterosexual contact.[4] In the developing world, heterosexual transmission is the major route of HIV infection.[8]

The sharing of injection needles, syringes, and other drug-injection paraphernalia contaminated with blood containing HIV is a direct route for transmission of HIV. Of the reported cases in the United States, 29% occurred among people who use injecting drugs, including 23% among people in whom injecting drug use is the only risk factor.[4] HIV-infected injecting drug users can pass the virus to

their needle-sharing and sex partners and, in the case of pregnant women, to their offspring.[8] Although alcohol, cocaine, and other noninjecting drugs do not directly transmit infection, their use alters perception of risk and reduces inhibitions about engaging in behaviors that pose a high risk of transmitting HIV infection.[12] The association between drug use and HIV infection is so high that they may be viewed as twin epidemics.

Transfusions of whole blood, plasma, platelets, or blood cells have resulted in transmission of HIV.[8] However, these routes of transmission account for only a small and declining percentage of AIDS in the United States (3% in adults and 13% in children).[4] All blood donations in the United States have been screened for HIV since mid-1985. There will continue to be cases of AIDS identified as being transmitted by transfusions for some time because of the long incubation period for AIDS.

The clotting factor used by people with hemophilia is derived from the pooled plasma of many donors. Before HIV testing was implemented in 1985, the virus was transmitted to people with hemophilia through infusions of clotting factor concentrates.[8] Although the clotting factor is heat-treated to kill HIV, 70% to 80% of people with hemophilia are already infected. Other blood products, such as gamma globulin or hepatitis B vaccine, have not been implicated in the transmission of HIV.[8]

HIV may be transmitted from infected women to their offspring by three routes: in utero through the maternal–placental circulation, by inoculation during labor and vaginal or cesarean delivery, and through infected breast milk after birth.[16] Transmission is predominantly in utero. Although studies of pregnancy outcomes have shown a wide range of infant infection rates, the rate of perinatal transmission is estimated from 25% to 35%.[16]

AIDS among health-care workers (HCWs) in the United States results primarily from infection that occurs outside the work setting. A small number of HCWs have been infected with HIV through occupational exposure.[3] The CDC recommends that Universal Blood and Body Fluid Precautions be used in encounters with all patients in the health-care setting (Chart 15-1).[17] Because HCWs may be caring for people whose HIV status is not known, adherence to the precautions is the most prudent way to prevent occupational exposure. Studies show that the occupational risk of acquiring HIV in the health-care setting is low. Occupational risk of infection for HCWs is most often associated with percutaneous inoculation (needlestick) of blood from a patient with HIV.[18] The risk of seroconversion after needlestick exposure to the blood of an HIV-infected patient is estimated to be less than 0.5%.[17]

CHART 15-1: GENERAL PRINCIPLES OF UNIVERSAL PRECAUTIONS*

1. Take care to prevent injuries when using needles, scalpels, and other sharp instruments or devices. Do not recap used needles by hand, and do not bend, break, or otherwise manipulate used needles by hand. Place used disposable syringes and needles, scalpel blades, and other sharp items in puncture-resistant containers for disposal. Locate the puncture-resistant containers as close to the treatment area as possible.
2. Use protective barriers (i.e., gloves, gowns, masks, protective eyewear) to prevent exposure to blood, body fluids containing visible blood, and other fluids to which universal precautions apply. The type of protective barrier(s) should be appropriate for the procedure being performed and the type of exposure anticipated.
3. Immediately and thoroughly wash hands and other skin surfaces that are contaminated with blood, body fluids containing visible blood, or other body fluids to which universal precautions apply.

* This list is abbreviated.
(Centers for Disease Control. [1988]. Update: Universal precautions for prevention of transmission of human immunodeficiency virus, hepatitis B virus, and other blood-borne pathogens in health-care settings. Morbidity and Mortality Weekly Report, 37, 377)

Evidence from CDC investigations suggests that the risk of transmission from infected HCWs to patients during invasive procedures is small. When recommended infection-control procedures are followed, the risk of transmitting hepatitis B virus (HBV) from an infected HCW to a patient is small, and the risk of transmitting HIV is likely to be even smaller. Although rare, the likelihood of patient exposure to an infected health-care worker's blood may vary depending on the procedure and on the skill and physical health of the infected worker (Chart 15-2).[19]

Evidence increasingly shows a relationship between other sexually transmitted diseases (STDs) and HIV infection. Research supports the hypothesis that the risk of HIV transmission is increased in the presence of genital ulcerative STDs (syphilis, herpes simplex virus [HSV], and chancroid) and nonulcerative STDs (gonorrhea, chlamydia, and trichomoniasis). Available data also suggest that HIV increases the duration and recurrence of lesions, treatment failures, and atypical presentation of genital ulcerative diseases. This "epidemiologic synergy" may be responsible for the explosive increase in HIV infection among some populations.[20]

The HIV-infected person is infectious even when no symptoms are present. The point at which antibodies to the virus can be detected in the blood of the infected person is called seroconversion. Seroconversion typically occurs within 1 to 3 but up to 6 months after exposure to HIV. An HIV-infected person can transmit the virus to others even before seroconversion. The time after infection and before seroconversion is known as the "window period."[20] Although infection rarely occurs from transfused blood that was screened for HIV antibody and found negative, the U.S. Food and Drug Administration (FDA) requires blood collection centers to screen potential donors through interviews designed to identify behaviors known to present risk for HIV infection. Also, because of the "window period," the decision on engaging in sexual or drug use behaviors that present a risk for transmission should not be based on the presence of a negative antibody test alone. More information regarding prevention of transmission is contained in the section entitled "Prevention of HIV Infection" later in this chapter.

In summary, HIV is transmitted from one person to another through sexual contact, blood exchange, or perinatally. Transmission occurs when the infected blood, semen, or vaginal secretions of one person are deposited onto a mucous membrane or into the bloodstream of another person. The primary route of transmission is through intimate sexual contact. Although blood transmission may occur with injecting drug use, blood transfusion, or occupational exposure in a health-care setting, only a small percentage of HIV transmission is attributable to blood transfusion or occupational infection. Infected women may transmit the virus to their offspring in utero, during labor and delivery, or through breast milk. HIV infection is not transmitted through casual contact or by insect vectors. There is growing evidence of an association between other STDs and HIV infection. Infected people can transmit the virus to others before their infections can be detected by antibody tests.

■ PATHOPHYSIOLOGY OF AIDS

Since the first description of AIDS, considerable strides have been taken in understanding the pathophysiology of the disease. The virus, its mechanism of action, HIV antibody screening tests, and some treatment methods were discovered within a few years after the recognition of the first cases.

HIV belongs to a class of viruses called retroviruses, which carry their genetic information in RNA rather than DNA (see Chapter 12). HIV infects a limited number of cell types in the body including a subset of lymphocytes called CD4+ T-cells (also known as helper or T4-lymphocytes)[8] and macrophages.[22] HIV has also been found in brain tissue. The CD4 receptor molecule enables HIV to establish infection. A surface protein on the viral envelope of HIV, gp120, binds to the CD4 receptor on the surface

CHART 15-2: RECOMMENDATIONS FOR PREVENTING THE TRANSMISSION OF HIV AND HBV TO PATIENTS DURING EXPOSURE-PRONE INVASIVE PROCEDURES

To minimize the risk of HIV or HBV transmission, the following measures are recommended:

▪ All health-care workers (HCWs) should adhere to universal precautions, including the appropriate use of handwashing, protective barriers, and care in the use and disposal of needles and other sharp instruments. HCWs who have exudative lesions or weeping dermatitis should refrain from all direct patient care and from handling patient-care equipment and devices used in performing invasive procedures until the condition resolves. HCWs should also comply with current guidelines for disinfection and sterilization of reusable devices used in invasive procedures.

▪ Currently available data provide no basis for recommendations to restrict the practice of HCWs infected with HIV or HBV who perform invasive procedures not identified as exposure-prone, provided the infected HCWs practice recommended surgical or dental technique and comply with universal precautions and current recommendations for sterilization/disinfection.

▪ Exposure-prone procedures should be identified by medical/surgical/dental organizations and institutions at which the procedures are performed.

▪ HCWs who perform exposure-prone procedures should know their HIV antibody status. HCWs who perform exposure-prone procedures and who do not have serologic evidence of immunity to HBV from vaccination or from previous infection should know their HBsAg status and, if that is positive, should also know their HBeAg status.

▪ HCWs who are infected with HIV or HBV (and are HBeAg positive) should not perform exposure-prone procedures unless they have sought counsel from an expert review panel and been advised under what circumstances, if any, they may continue to perform these procedures.* Such circumstances would include notifying prospective patients of the HCW's seropositivity before they undergo exposure-prone invasive procedures.

▪ Mandatory testing of HCWs for HIV antibody, HBsAg is not recommended. The current assessment of the risk that infected HCWs will transmit HIV or HBV to patients during exposure-prone procedures does not support the diversion of resources that would be required to implement mandatory testing programs. Compliance by HCWs with recommendations can be increased through education, training, and appropriate confidentiality safeguards.

* The review panel should include experts who represent a balanced perspective. Such experts might include all of the following: a) the HCWs personal physician(s), b) an infectious disease specialist with expertise in the epidemiology of HIV and HBV transmission, c) a health professional with expertise in the procedures performed by the HCW, and d) state or local public health official(s). If the HCW's practice is institutionally based, the expert review panel might also include a member of the infection-control committee, preferably a hospital epidemiologist. HCWs who perform exposure-prone procedures outside the hospital/institutional setting should seek advice from appropriate state and local public health officials regarding the review process. Panels must recognize the importance of confidentiality and the privacy rights of infected HCWs.
(Centers for Disease Control. [1991]. Recommendations for preventing transmission of human immunodeficiency virus and hepatitis B virus to patients during exposure-prone invasive procedures. *Morbidity and Mortality Weekly Report, 40,* 1–9)

of the lymphocyte. Although T-lymphocytes seem to have the highest density of CD4 receptors, the molecule is also present on other cells, such as monocytes and macrophages. After attaching to the CD4 receptor, the virus enters the lymphocyte and sheds its protein coat. Viral RNA is transcribed into DNA using a unique enzyme called reverse transcriptase. A second strand is produced to form a DNA duplex, called proviral DNA, the DNA that is integrated into the host cell DNA. The infection enters a latent phase that may last for several years. During this time, infected people remain asymptomatic although serologic tests can identify antibodies to HIV proteins. These antibodies are usually detectable as early as 1 to 3 months after infection. The presence of these antibodies does not convey any protection against the virus.[22]

The CD4 + T-cells are necessary for normal immune function (see Chapter 13). Among other functions, the CD4 + T-cell recognizes foreign antigens, infected cells, and helps activate the antibody-producing B-lymphocytes. The CD4 + T-cells also orchestrate cell-mediated immunity, in which cytotoxic CD8 + T-cells and natural killer cells directly destroy foreign antigens. Phagocytic monocytes and macrophages are also influenced by CD4+ T-cells. By infecting and selectively destroying CD4+ T-cells, which are pivotal cells in the immune response, HIV strips the person with AIDS of protection against common organisms and cancerous cells that might arise as mutations during cell division.

CLINICAL MANIFESTATIONS

Some people develop an acute mononucleosis–like syndrome soon after infection with HIV.[23] This acute phase may include fever, sweats, myalgia, arthralgias, malaise, sore throat, nausea, vomiting, and headache. Physical findings include generalized lymphadenopathy, hepatic and splenic enlargement, and transient macular erythematous rashes.[24]

The acute phase may be followed by a latent period of as many as 10 years before many other symptoms occur. Previously, people with symptoms who had not yet developed AIDS were referred to clinically as having AIDS-related complex (ARC). During this time, people with HIV infection present with lymphadenopathy. Persistent HIV-related lymphadenopathy is usually defined as lymph nodes that are chronically swollen for more than 3 months in at least two locations, not including the groin.[25] The lymph nodes may be sore or visible externally. Lymphadenopathy may be accompanied by fatigue, fever, weight loss, night sweats, and diarrhea.

The onset of severe illness is usually precipitated by an opportunistic infection. Opportunistic infections involve common organisms that normally do not produce infection unless there is impaired immune function. With immune system failure, these infections become progressively more severe and difficult to treat. The presence of an opportunistic infection or neoplasm is an essential feature in the diagnosis of AIDS (Chart 15-3). The complications of AIDS include opportunistic infections of the respiratory and gastrointestinal tract, central nervous system (CNS) involvement, KS, and the wasting syndrome.

RESPIRATORY MANIFESTATIONS

Pneumocystis carinii pneumonia is the most common opportunistic disease in people with AIDS. PCP is caused by a fungus that is common in soil, houses, and many other places in the environment. In people with healthy immune systems, the fungus does not cause infection or disease. In people with AIDS, *Pneumocystis carinii* can multiply quickly in the lungs and cause pneumonia.[26] These symptoms may be acute or gradually progressive. People may complain of chest pain or sputum production. Physical examination may demonstrate only fever and tachypnea; rales may be absent

and breath sounds may be normal. Chest x-ray may show interstitial infiltrates, but normal chest film does not rule out PCP. The specific diagnosis can be made in some people by examination of induced sputum, but most require bronchoalveolar lavage or lung biopsy.

Other organisms that cause pulmonary infections in people with AIDS include *Mycobacterium tuberculosis*, cytomegalovirus (CMV), *Mycobacterium avium*-complex (MAC), *Toxoplasma gondii*, and *Cryptococcus neoformans*.[25] Pneumonia may also occur because of more common pulmonary pathogens, including *Streptococcus pneumoniae*, *Hemophilus influenzae*, and *Legionella pneumophila*. Some people may be infected with multiple organisms.[26]

MYCOBACTERIUM TUBERCULOSIS

From 1985 to 1991, there was a 16% increase in the number of cases of tuberculosis reported annually in the United States—a marked change from the average annual decline of 6% during the preceding 30 years. A number of factors contributed to this increase; the most profound is the epidemic of HIV infection. People infected with *Mycobacterium tuberculosis* (*i.e.*, those with positive tuberculin skin tests) are more likely to develop tuberculosis if they are infected with HIV. Equally important, HIV-infected people exposed to tuberculosis are likely to have rapidly progressive primary disease instead of a subclinical tuberculosis infection. The clinical presentation of tuberculosis in people infected with HIV differs from that in people with normal cellular immunity. With HIV present, tuberculosis usually presents diffuse pulmonary infiltrates or thoracic lymphadenopathy and extrapulmonary involvement that extends to the CNS (tuberculosis meningitis).[27]

Over the last three decades, tuberculosis has responded well to therapy. However, from 1988 to 1991, there were at least six outbreaks of tuberculosis that were resistant to multiple drugs. The transmission of drug-resistant disease has occurred between patients, from patients to health-care workers or prison guards, and from patients to family members. About 90% of the cases of drug-resistant tuberculosis have occurred in HIV-infected people. Mortality rates from disease of this type range from 70% to 90%, with a median of 4 to 16 weeks from diagnosis to death.[27]

GASTROINTESTINAL MANIFESTATIONS

Esophageal candidiasis is another common opportunistic infection occurring among people with AIDS.[26] Other opportunistic organisms causing esophagitis include CMV and herpes simplex virus.[26] People experiencing these infections usually complain of painful swallowing or retrosternal pain. Endoscopy, with

CHART 15-3: AIDS CASE DEFINITION*

A case of AIDS can be diagnosed under the following conditions:

I. Without an HIV antibody test or one with inconclusive results, the absence of other causes of immunodeficiency and a definitive diagnosis of:
  ■ Candidiasis of the esophagus, trachea, bronchi, or lungs
  ■ Cryptococcosis, extrapulmonary
  ■ Cryptosporidiosis with diarrhea persisting over 1 month
  ■ Cytomegalovirus disease of an organ other than the liver, spleen, or lymph nodes in a patient over 1 month of age
  ■ Herpes simplex virus infection causing a mucocutaneous ulcer that persists longer than 1 month; or bronchitis, pneumonia, or esophagitis for any duration affecting a patient over 1 month of age
  ■ Kaposi's sarcoma affecting a patient under 60 years of age
  ■ Lymphoma of the brain (primary) affecting a patient under 60 years of age
  ■ Lymphoid interstitial pneumonia and/or pulmonary lymphoid hyperplasia affecting a child under 13 years of age
  ■ *Mycobacterium avium* complex or *M. kansasii* disease, disseminated (at other than or in addition to the lungs, skin, or cervical or hilar lymph nodes)
  ■ *Pneumocystis carinii* pneumonia
  ■ Progressive multifocal leukoencephalopathy
  ■ Toxoplasmosis of the brain affecting a patient over 1 month of age

II. With laboratory evidence of HIV infection and a definitive diagnosis of:
  ■ The combination of at least two bacterial infections within a 2-year period, multiple or recurrent, affecting a child under 13 years of age (septicemia, pneumonia, meningitis, bone or joint infection, or abscess of an internal organ or body cavity—excluding otitis media or superficial skin or mucosal abscesses, caused by *Hemophilus*, *Streptococcus*, or other pyogenic bacteria)
  ■ Coccidioidomycosis, disseminated
  ■ HIV encephalopathy (HIV infection or AIDS dementia)
  ■ Hystoplasmosis, disseminated
  ■ Isoporiasis with diarrhea persisting over 1 month
  ■ Kaposi's sarcoma
  ■ Lymphoma of the brain (primary)
  ■ Other non-Hodgkins lymphoma of B-cell or unknown immunogenic phenotype
  ■ Any mycobacterial disease caused by mycobacteria other than *M. tuberculosis*, disseminated
  ■ Disease caused by *M. tuberculosis*, extrapulmonary
  ■ HIV wasting syndrome (emaciation, "slim disease")

III. When laboratory test results are negative for HIV infection, and:
  ■ All other causes of immunodeficiency are excluded
  ■ The patient has had a definitively diagnosed case of any of the diseases in list II and a helper T-lymphocyte count under 400/mm.

* Subject to revision by CDC, which periodically proposes changes.
(Centers for Disease Control. [1987]. Revision of the CDC surveillance case definition for acquired immunodeficiency syndrome. *Morbidity and Mortality Weekly Report, 36*, 35)

esophageal brushings or biopsy, is required for definitive diagnosis.

Diarrhea or gastroenteritis also occurs commonly in people with AIDS. Symptoms may be the result of protozoal infection by *Cryptosporidium*.[26] This watery diarrhea may produce large volumes of stool per day and last for months. Such severe symptoms lead to weakness and death from fluid loss. The organism is identified by examining and culturing the stool specimen.

NERVOUS SYSTEM MANIFESTATIONS

Neurologic complications of HIV infections occur frequently and may affect either the peripheral or CNS. These complications arise from the direct effects of the retrovirus on the CNS and from opportunistic infections.[28] Neurologic symptoms may occur in HIV-infected people who are otherwise asymptomatic.[28] *Toxoplasma gondii* is a common opportunistic organism infecting the CNS in people with AIDS. The typical presentation includes fever, altered mental status, seizures, or motor deficits.[26] Computed tomography (CT scans) may show lesions, but brain biopsy is necessary in many cases for definitive diagnosis.

Primary CNS lymphoma and high-grade B-cell lymphoma have been diagnosed with increased frequency in people with AIDS. The latter tumors often present with extranodal involvement of the gastrointestinal tract, CNS, bone marrow, myocardium, or kidneys. The clinical course of these lymphomas is marked by rapid progression and death, despite treatment.[28]

A common neurologic syndrome attributed directly to HIV is called subacute encephalitis or AIDS dementia complex.[28] Although this neurologic syndrome occurs in more than 15% of people with AIDS, the prevalence in otherwise healthy seropositive people is not known. Marked by subtle cognitive or behavioral dysfunction occurring over weeks to months, people may initially develop memory loss, difficulty in concentrating, euphoria, social withdrawal, or lethargy. These early signs are easily confused with depression or drug abuse and may be ignored until they eventually progress to severe dementia with motor disturbances, ataxia, tremor, spasticity, and paraplegia. CT scans show a characteristic pattern of cerebral atrophy with prominent sulci and ventricles. Examination of the cerebrospinal fluid (CSF) typically shows a mild pleocytosis with an elevated protein or lowered glucose concentration.[28] AIDS dementia complex may initially occur without any other signs or symptoms of AIDS.

Cryptococcus neoformans is a fungus that typically causes meningitis with fever, stiff neck, and headache. Disseminated disease may be found in people with AIDS and may involve the lungs, kidneys, skin, and other organs.[25] Cryptococcal meningitis is diagnosed by laboratory testing of the CSF.

In addition to disorders of the CNS, HIV causes abnormalities of the peripheral nervous system in some people. A painful sensory neuropathy occurs in 30% to 50% of people with AIDS and in an unknown percentage of other HIV-infected people.[26] Painful dysesthesia, numbness, weakness, and those symptoms related to dysfunction of the autonomic nervous system may occur.

KAPOSI'S SARCOMA

Kaposi's sarcoma is a malignancy of endothothelial cells that line small blood vessels. An opportunistic cancer, KS occurs in immunosuppressed people (*e.g.*, transplant patients and people with AIDS). Before 1981, most cases of KS were found in North America among elderly men of Mediterranean or Eastern European Jewish descent and in Africa among young black adult males and prepubescent children. There is a great diversity in the clinical manifestations of KS. The disease usually begins as one or more macules, papules, or violet lesions that enlarge and become darker. They may coalesce to form raised plaques or tumors. These irregular-shaped tumors can be from one eighth of an inch to silver dollar size. Tumor nodules are frequently located on the trunk, neck, and head (especially the tip of the nose). They are usually painless in the early stages, but discomfort may develop as the tumor ages. Invasion of internal organs, including the lungs, gastrointestinal tract, and lymphatic system, occurs commonly. The tumors may obstruct organ function or rupture and cause internal bleeding. The progression of KS may be slow or rapid. Biopsy of suspicious lesions is needed to make a definitive diagnosis. Both chemotherapy and radiation therapy have been extensively used for palliative treatment of the tumors. Treatment of the malignancy alone is unlikely to improve survival because most patients die of opportunistic infections rather than tumor effects.[26]

WASTING SYNDROME

HIV wasting syndrome is formally considered in the case definition of AIDS.[25] The syndrome is common in people with HIV infection or AIDS. In Africa, AIDS has become known as "slim disease" because of this condition. With the wasting syndrome, there is profound involuntary weight loss (over 10% of baseline body weight), severe diarrhea, and chronic weakness with fever. This diagnosis is used when no other opportunistic infections or neoplasms can be identified as causing these symptoms.[25]

AIDS IN CHILDREN

Although AIDS cases among children who became infected through receiving blood products or blood transfusions before donor screening are still being identified, almost all of the current transmission of HIV infection to children in the United States occurs perinatally. Studies show that virtually 100% of infants born to seropositive mothers test antibody positive at birth, but one third or fewer of the infants are actually infected. Uninfected infants usually lose maternal antibody (IgG) between 6 and 12 months of age, but a small proportion may retain maternal antibody for up to 18 months. Although a positive antibody test alone does not diagnose HIV infection in the newborn, the test does identify a perinatally exposed infant who requires careful follow-up and management. Clinical evaluation and repeated testing over at least the first 2 years of life are the primary means of diagnosis in these infants. Infants who remain HIV-antibody positive beyond 15 to 18 months of age are considered infected.[29] Thus, seropositive children who die in the first year of life cannot easily be counted as infected or uninfected unless they have a clinical and immunologic picture characteristic of AIDS or direct evidence of the virus (*e.g.*, a positive HIV culture). Infected infants usually appear well for the first few months of life, although immune abnormalities can sometimes be detected. A number of children have remained well or with mild symptoms for more than 5 years.[16]

The case definitions for children and adults are similar except that two conditions, lymphoid interstitial pneumonitis and recurrent serious bacterial infections, are applicable to children only.[25] Worldwide, studies indicate that HIV transmission from an infected woman to her child ranges from 10% to 50%. Most of the larger studies with sufficient follow-up of infants in Europe and the United States indicate infection rates between 25% and 35%. It remains unclear when most of the maternal infant transmission takes place: early in pregnancy, later in pregnancy, or around delivery. Maternal cofactors (*e.g.*, maternal health status, drug use) are also poorly understood. Most evidence suggests that transmission is predominantly in utero. Breast-feeding is also a route of transmission.[16]

Among children reported to CDC in 1988 and 1989, 34% had PCP, 28% had lymphoid interstitial pneumonitis (LIP), 24% had recurrent serious bacterial infections, and 13% had *Candida* esophagitis. Wasting syndrome was reported in 16%, and HIV encephalopathy was reported in 13% of the children; various other conditions were reported in fewer than 10%. Clinical presentation and age at diagnosis are related to survival of children with AIDS. Overall, 57% of the children reported to CDC in 1988 and 1989 were alive 12 months after diagnosis. A major cause of early mortality for HIV-infected children is PCP. The 1-year survival rate was only 30% for children under 12 months with PCP compared with 55% for children under 12 months with other conditions. Survival rates for older children were 48% for those with PCP and 72% for those with other conditions.[16]

Infants clearly progress faster than adults in developing immunodeficiency and related illnesses. Modeling of the incubation period for infants suggests that 3 years is the median age at diagnosis. In adults, the median incubation period is probably nearer 10 years. Few adults develop AIDS in the first 3 years after infection. The relative immaturity of the immune system of infants may account for the more rapid progression as may many other factors such as route of infection and dose of virus. Infants born to infected mothers are significantly more likely to develop AIDS in the first year of life than those infants infected by blood transfusions.[16]

Therapeutic interventions for children, especially zidovudine, appear to delay the progression of HIV infection to AIDS. Even without antiviral medication, early diagnosis of infection and supportive therapy are likely to slow the course of the disease in children.[16] The American Academy of Pediatrics recommends that HIV testing should be offered to all pregnant women and women of childbearing age in the United States by informing them of the availability of counseling and testing. In addition, the Academy recommends that testing should be routinely recommended and encouraged for all pregnant women and women of childbearing age at increased risk because of high-risk behavior. The potential benefits of voluntary testing for mothers and newborns include reduced morbidity because of intensive treatment and supportive health care, the opportunity for early antiviral therapy, and information regarding the risk of transmission from breast milk.[30]

DIAGNOSIS

The most accurate and cost-effective method for identifying HIV is the utilization of antibody detection tests. The first commercial assays for HIV were introduced in 1985 to screen donated blood. Since then, use of antibody detection tests has been expanded to include evaluating people at increased risk for HIV infection and as a component of the case definition of AIDS. The enzyme immunoassay (EIA), also known as enzyme-linked immunosorbent assay (ELISA), and the Western blot (WB) assay are in widespread use.[25] In light of the psychosocial issues related to HIV and AIDS, sensitivity and confidentiality must be maintained whenever testing is implemented. If testing is conducted for the purpose of determining a person's HIV status, it must be carried out with pre- and post-test counseling and with the consent of the person being tested.

The EIA detects antibodies produced in response to HIV infection and is based on the light absorbance of antigen–antibody complexes in sample wells compared to control wells.[22] The test kit contains beads or microtiter wells coated with HIV antigens. When a serum sample is added, HIV antibodies in the serum bind to the antigen-coated surface. A second antibody linked to an enzyme is added to combine with the antigen–antibody complexes. These steps are separated by washings and incubations before a substrate for the enzyme is added. Color development, indicating the amount of bound HIV antibody, is measured with a spectrophotometer. The test is considered reactive if the measured light absorbance is greater than a cut-off value established from known positive and negative controls.[22] Samples that are repeatedly reactive are tested by a supplemental test such as the Western blot.[25]

The Western blot assay allows identification of antibodies to specific viral antigens. Before the test, HIV antigens prepared from a virus culture are separated by electrophoresis and transferred (blotted) to nitrocellulose paper, which is subsequently cut into strips.[22] The serum sample is added to a strip, allowing specific HIV antibodies to bind with specific viral antigen bands. The reaction is carried out similarly to the EIA. This technique permits the identification of antibodies to specific HIV proteins and glycoproteins.[22] When certain combinations of the antibody bands are identified, the test is considered positive. In public health practice, the Western blot is run only on those samples that are repeatedly reactive on the EIA.

Serologic tests for detecting HIV antibodies are sensitive and specific. When serum tests are strongly reactive or border line by EIA and also positive by Western blot, the person is considered to be infected with HIV.[25] Both tests are important because, in some situations, misinformation can be generated by EIA testing alone. The EIA test has a high predictive value when used in groups with a high prevalence of infection (e.g., sexually active homosexual men).[31] However, when the EIA test is used in groups of low prevalence of infection (e.g., blood donors), most of the positive results turn out to be false-positive.[31]

Polymerase chain reaction (PCR) is a technique for HIV detection, although availability of the test is limited. Because the amount of viral DNA in the HIV-infected cell is small compared with the amount of human DNA, direct detection of the virus' genetic material is difficult. PCR is a method for amplifying the viral DNA up to 1 million times or more to increase the probability of detection. PCR detects the presence of the virus rather than the antibody to the virus as in the EIA and WB tests. PCR may be useful in diagnosing HIV infection in infants born to infected mothers.[29]

TABLE 15-1. PHYSICAL EXAMINATION—CURRENT SIGNS, SYMPTOMS, AND COMPLAINTS

SYSTEM	SIGNS/SYMPTOMS/COMPLAINTS	ETIOLOGIES TO CONSIDER
General	Fatigue, weight loss	All HIV-related diseases
	Parotid swelling	HIV (in children)
Lymph nodes	Swelling of nodes, particularly posterior, cervical, axillary, epitrochlear	HIV, cytomegalovirus (CMV), syphilis, lymphoma, Kaposi's sarcoma (KS), TB
Dermatologic	Skin discoloration, rash, scaling, alopecia, eruptions (vesicles, macules, papules, nodules)	Seborrheic dermatitis, KS, varicella-zoster, herpes simplex molluscum contagiosum, psoriasis, cryptococcosis, condylomata acuminatum, other fungal infections
Oral	White lesions	Candidiasis, oral hairy leukoplakia
	Erythematous purplish lesion	KS
	Ulcers	Aphthous ulcers, herpes simplex, CMV
	Odynophagia, pharyngitis	Esophageal candidiasis, herpes simplex, CMV, KS
Visual	Visual field defects	CMV, HIV, toxoplasmosis
	Retinal hemorrhage, exudate	CMV, toxoplasmosis
Cardiopulmonary	Persistent dry cough, dyspnea, chest tightness, rales, rhonchi	*Pneumocystis carinii* pneumonia (PCP), bacterial infection, cryptococcosis, fungal infection, TB, *mycobacterium avium* complex (MAC), CMV, KS
Hematologic	Easy bruising	Idiopathic thrombocytopenic purpura (ITP)
Gastrointestinal	Diarrhea, anorexia, nausea, vomiting	Parasitic infestation, bacterial infection, CMV, HIV, anorexia nervosa
Abdominal	Hepatomegaly	Hepatitis, CMV, lymphoma, TB, MAC, toxoplasmosis
	Splenomegaly	ITP, HIV
Genitourinary	Rashes, lesions, ulcers, chancres	Herpes simplex, syphilis, chancroid, KS molluscum
	Dysuria, discharge	Gonorrhea, nongonococcal urethritis
	Abnormal Pap smear	Human papilloma virus (HPV), Herpes simplex, cervicitis, candidiasis, trichomoniasis, cervical cancer
Anorectal	Anal pain	Herpes simplex, condyloma, hemorrhoids, fissures/fistulas, CMV, lymphoma, KS
	Violaceous macules, nodules	KS, squamous cell carcinoma, HPV, syphilis
Neurologic	Headaches, weakness, seizures	Cryptococcosis, toxoplasmosis, lymphoma, progressive multifocal leukoencephalopathy (PML), encephalopathy, myopathy, neuropathy, radiculopathy, herpes simplex, HIV
	Loss of memory, loss of concentration, sadness, mood swings	HIV, other encephalopathy, depression, dementia, endocrine disturbance
	Numbness, dyskathesia	HIV, varicella zoster
	Motor/sensory deficits	Toxoplasmosis, lymphoma, PML, HIV

(American Medical Association. [1991]. *HIV early care/AMA physician guidelines* (p. 8). Chicago, American Medical Association.)

EARLY MANAGEMENT

Once HIV infection is confirmed, laboratory and other test results are combined with the results of the physical examination to determine the stage of the disease. A diagnostic schedule has been suggested by the American Medical Association for an initial work-up and ongoing evaluation of an HIV-infected person (Table 15-1). These recommendations are subject to change as medical knowledge of HIV clinical course increases and more interventions become available.

Absolute CD4+ T-cell counts are the most frequently used indicators of immune system function. A decrease in the absolute CD4+ T-cell count (below 500) is associated with the appearance of opportunistic infections and illnesses.[31] A careful physical examination and evaluation of recent complaints and symptoms are crucial components of the initial staging process. Table 15-1 summarizes important considerations for both the initial and subsequent examinations, as suggested by the American Medical Association.

TREATMENT ISSUES

There is no cure for AIDS. Opportunistic diseases are treated individually with standard and experimental protocols such as antibiotics, antifungals, and anticancer therapies. An increasing number of therapeutics are being approved by the Food and Drug Administration (FDA) for treatment of HIV. More than a dozen medicines are already approved, and almost 100 others are in development for treatment of AIDS and HIV-related conditions.[33]

Azidothymidine (AZT, Retrovir, or zidovudine), the first AIDS-specific drug to be approved, is a competitive inhibitor of reverse transcriptase and inhibits viral replication. Clinical trials showed that AZT increased survival of people with AIDS.[34] Didanosine (ddI or VIDEX) is the second drug to be approved as an antiviral. Didanosine is indicated in the treatment of adults and pediatric patients (over 6 months of age) who have an advanced HIV infection, are intolerant of zidovudine, or have demonstrated significant clinical or immunologic deterioration during therapy with zidovudine. Antiviral therapies are prescribed to improve the overall survival time of people with HIV infection as well as to slow the progression to AIDS. Other drugs have been approved and are commonly used for the treatment of opportunistic infections including PCP, toxoplasmosis, KS, cryptococcal meningitis, and cytomegalovirus retinitis.[33]

Theoretically, other infections might increase HIV-related disease progression through activation of the immune system.[35] Therefore, people with HIV should be advised to avoid infections as much as possible and seek evaluation promptly whenever they occur. Immunization is important because people infected with HIV are at risk of developing many infectious diseases. Some of these diseases can be avoided by vaccination while the immune system's responsiveness is relatively intact. Vaccines for the following infections are suggested: hepatitis B, pneumococcal, *Hemophilus influenzae* type b, and influenza.[36] Bacille Calmette Guérin (BCG), oral typhoid vaccine, or live-virus vaccines should not be given to people with HIV infection or AIDS.[36] People with asymptomatic HIV infection should be vaccinated against measles, mumps, and rubella.[36] People with HIV infection should be encouraged to avoid alcohol, nonprescription drugs, and smoking. A balanced diet, moderate exercise, and stress management are all positive factors in maintaining a healthy lifestyle.[32] Once a diagnosis of AIDS has been made, the survival rate is approximately 50% at 1 year and 15% at 5 years.[37]

PSYCHOSOCIAL ISSUES

The psychological effects of HIV infection or AIDS may be just as significant as the physical effects. The dramatic impact of this catastrophic illness is compounded by complex reactions from members of the health-care team, the person with HIV/AIDS, his or her partner, friends, and family.[38] These reactions may be influenced by inadequate information, fear of contagion, shame, prejudices, and condemnation of risk behaviors. In addition to the fear and grief associated with death, the person with HIV/AIDS may also experience guilt, anger, and uncertainty. Questioning and self-examination are common as the person attempts to understand what is happening. Preexisting psychiatric conditions may be present, particularly alcohol and drug abuse. Appropriate treatment should be made available when alcohol or other drug dependence is noted.

The person with HIV infection or AIDS may feel helpless, hopeless, stigmatized, and out of control.[38] HIV/AIDS affects all spheres of life. Isolated from peers and with a weakened sense of identity, the person may be anxious, depressed, and miserable. Acknowledging a diagnosis of AIDS may be the first indication to family and colleagues of otherwise hidden lifestyles (*i.e.,* homosexuality or drug use). This increases the strain on relationships with important support people. Diagnosis and treatment of cognitive and affective disorders are essential parts of ongoing care for the HIV-infected person. The emotional stress, feelings of isolation, and sadness experienced by the person with HIV/AIDS can be overwhelming. People with the disease must have as much information and control over activities as possible.[38] They should be encouraged to direct their energies in a positive manner and continue with their social and group activities as long as such activities can be tolerated. All appropriate social support systems (*e.g.*, AIDS service organizations, community groups, religious organizations) should be used whenever possible.

To deal with these complex issues, the healthcare team must recognize and accept their fears, prejudices, and emotions concerning those with HIV/AIDS. Personal feelings must not prevent caregivers from acknowledging the intrinsic human worth of all people and their right to be treated with dignity and respect.[38] Members of the health-care team should have adequate support for their own emotional needs generated from working with people with AIDS. Grief, anxiety, and concern over stigmatization are normal feelings. They should be acknowledged and dealt with through peer support or professional counseling to reduce burnout and emotional strain.

In summary, HIV, a retrovirus, infects the body's CD4+ T-cells and macrophages. HIV genetic material becomes integrated into the host cell DNA. Manifestations of infection, such as acute mononucleosislike symptoms, may occur shortly after infection or appear after a latent phase that may last many years. The end of the latent period is marked by the onset of severe opportunistic infections and cancers. The complications of these infections, manifested throughout the respiratory, gastrointestinal, and nervous systems, include pneumonia, esophagitis, diarrhea, gastroenteritis, tumor, wasting syndrome, altered mental status, seizures, and motor deficits. HIV is diagnosed by the enzyme immunoassay and the Western blot assay—antibody detection tests, which are sensitive, specific, and reliable. The emotional stress, feelings of isolation, and sadness experienced by the person with HIV/AIDS can be overwhelming. Diagnosis and treatment of cognitive and affective disorders are an essential part of ongoing care for the HIV-infected person. Appropriate treatment should be made available when alcohol or other drug dependence is noted.

■ PREVENTION OF HIV INFECTION

Because there is no cure for HIV/AIDS, adopting risk-free or low-risk behavior is the best protection against the disease. Abstinence or long-term, mutually monogamous sexual relationships between two uninfected partners are ways to avoid HIV infection and other sexually transmitted diseases. Proper use of latex condoms may provide protection from the disease by not allowing contact with semen or vaginal secretions during intercourse.[39] "Natural" or "lambskin" condoms do not provide the same protection

from HIV as latex because of the larger pores in the material.[39] Only water-based lubricants should be used with condoms; petroleum (oil-based) products weaken the structure of the latex.[39]

The use of injecting drugs provides another opportunity for HIV transmission. Avoiding recreational drug use and particularly the practice of sharing needles are important to AIDS prevention. Substances that alter inhibitions can lead to risky sexual behavior. For example, smoking cocaine (known as "crack") heightens the perception of sexual arousal, and this can influence the user to practice unsafe sexual behavior.[12] In addition, the addictive nature of many recreational drugs can lead to an increase in the frequency of unsafe sexual behavior and the number of partners as the user engages in sex exchanged for money or drugs.[12] People concerned about their risk should be encouraged to get information and counseling about their infection status.

Public health programs for HIV prevention rely on principles developed in other control efforts, such as STD prevention, and are creating new systems specific to the epidemic. In fact, HIV has had a profound impact on the public health system in the United States. Although standard methods for disease intervention and statistical analysis are applied to HIV, public health programs have become more responsive to community concerns, confidentiality, and long-term follow-up of clients as a direct result of the HIV epidemic. Testing for HIV antibodies and counseling have become widely available in the United States.

Education continues to be the mainstay of HIV prevention programs. Individual education regarding HIV transmission, personal risk, and possible prevention techniques/skills is delivered to people in clinical settings as well as to those at high risk of infection in community settings. Community-wide education is provided in schools, in the workplace, and in the media. Training for professionals can have an impact on HIV and is an important element of prevention. The constant addition of new information on HIV makes prevention education ever changing and challenging.

UNIVERSAL PRECAUTIONS

Universal precautions are intended to prevent parenteral, mucous membrane, and nonintact skin exposures of health-care workers to bloodborne pathogens. These precautions apply to all body fluids that might contain HIV (*i.e.*, blood, semen, vaginal/cervical secretions).[17] Blood is the single most important source of HIV pathogens in the occupational setting. Universal precautions also apply to semen and vaginal/cervical secretions. Although semen and vaginal/

cervical secretions have been implicated in sexual transmission of HIV, they have not been implicated in occupational transmission from patient to health-care worker. Because the associated risk of transmission is unknown, universal precautions should also be used with tissues and fluids that ordinarily would be handled with aseptic technique such as cerebrospinal, pleural, peritoneal, pericardial, and amniotic fluids.[17] Universal precautions do not apply to the following fluids, unless they contain visible blood, because the risk of transmission is extremely low or nonexistent: feces, nasal secretions, sputum, sweat, tears, urine, saliva, and vomitus. Epidemiologic studies have not shown HIV to be transmitted by any of these fluids in health-care or community settings.[17] General infection control practices include the use of gloves for digital examinations of mucous membranes and endotracheal suctioning and hand-washing after contact with body fluids. The general principles of universal precautions are listed in Chart 15-1. The U.S. Occupational Safety and Health Administration (OSHA) has enacted regulations that mandate hospitals and other health-care employers to provide personal protective equipment to employees who may come in contact with blood or other potentially infectious materials.[40] Personal protective equipment includes gloves, gowns, laboratory coats, face shields or masks, eye protection, mouth pieces, resuscitation bags, and pocket masks or other ventilation devices.[40]

Study results indicate that HIV is sensitive to chemical disinfectants. Commonly used germicides at the manufacturer recommended concentrations inactivate HIV within 2 to 10 minutes. Sodium hypochlorite (household bleach) in a water dilution from 1:10 to 1:100 and 70% alcohol (ethyl, isopropyl) inactivated the virus within 1 minute of contact.[41] The results of these studies do not necessitate any changes in recommended procedures for sterilization or disinfection in public, private, or health-care facilities.[42]

In summary, risk-free or low-risk behavior is the best protection against HIV infection because there is no cure for AIDS. Abstinence or long-term mutually monogamous sexual relationships between two uninfected partners, use of condoms, avoiding drug use and the sharing of needles, and the practice of universal precautions by health-care workers are essential to stopping the spread of HIV.

■ REFERENCES

1. Koop, C.E. (1986). *The Surgeon General's report on acquired immune deficiency syndrome* (p. 6). Washington, DC: US Department of Health and Human Services.
2. Centers for Disease Control. (1990). Estimates of HIV prevalence and projected AIDS cases: Summary of a workshop, October 31–November 1, 1989. *Morbidity and Mortality Weekly Report, 39,* 110–119.
3. Centers for Disease Control. (1993, February). *HIV/AIDS Surveillance Report,* pp. 1–23
4. Centers for Disease Control. (1992). Mortality patterns—United States, 1989. *Morbidity and Mortality Weekly Report, 41,* 121–125.
5. Centers for Disease Control. (1992). Years of potential life lost before ages 65 and 85—United States, 1989–1990. *Morbidity and Mortality Weekly Report, 41,* 313–315.
6. Curran, J.W., Morgan, W.M., Hardy, A.M., et al. (1985). The epidemiology of AIDS: Current status and future prospects. *Science, 229,* 1352.
7. Montagnier, L., & Alizon, M. (1986). The human immune deficiency virus (HIV): An update. In J.C. Gluckman & E. Vilmer (Eds.). *Proceedings of the Second International Conference on AIDS* (p. 13). Paris: Elsevier.
8. Friedland, G.H., & Klein, R.S. (1987). Transmission of the human immunodeficiency virus. *New England Journal of Medicine, 317,* 1125.
9. Centers for Disease Control. (1988). Update: Acquired immune deficiency syndrome (AIDS)—worldwide. *Morbidity and Mortality Weekly Report, 37,* 224.
10. Mann, J.M. (1992). AIDS—The second decade: A global perspective. *Journal of Infectious Diseases, 165,* 245–250.
11. Hellinger, F.J. (1991). Forecasting the medical care costs of the HIV epidemic: 1991–1994. *Inquiry, 28,* 213–225.
12. National Research Council. (1989). AIDS—sexual behavior and intravenous drug use. Washington, DC: National Academy Press.
13. Rutherford, G.W., Lifson, A.R., Hessol, N.A., et al. (1990). Course of HIV-1 infection in a cohort of homosexual and bisexual men: An 11-year follow-up study. *British Medical Journal, 301,* 1183–1188.
14. O'Brien, T.R., George, J.R., & Holmberg, S.D. (1992). Human immunodeficiency virus type-2 infection in the United States—epidemiology, diagnosis, and public health implications. *Journal of the American Medical Association, 267,* 2775—2779.
15. Gershon, R.R.M., Vlahov, D., & Nelson, K.E. (1990). The risk of transmission of HIV-1 through non-percutaneous, non-sexual modes—a review. *AIDS, 4,* 645–650.
16. Oxtoby, M.J. (1990). Perinatally acquired human immunodeficiency virus infection. *Pediatric Infectious Disease Journal, 9,* 609–619.
17. Centers for Disease Control. (1988). Update: Universal precautions for prevention of transmission of human immunodeficiency virus, hepatitis B virus, and other blood-borne pathogens in health-care settings. *Morbidity and Mortality Weekly Report, 37,* 377.
18. Centers for Disease Control. (1988). Update: Acquired immunodeficiency syndrome and human immunodeficiency virus infection among health-care workers. *Morbidity and Mortality Weekly Report, 37,* 229.
19. Centers for Disease Control. (1991). Recommendations for preventing transmission of human immunodeficiency virus and hepatitis B virus to patients during exposure-prone invasive procedures. *Morbidity and Mortality Weekly Report, 40,* 1–9.
20. Wasserheit, J.N. (1992, March/April). Epidemiological synergy—interrelationships between human immunodeficiency virus infection and other sexually transmitted diseases. *Sexually Transmitted Diseases,* pp. 61-77.
21. Horsburgh, C.R., Jason, J., Longini, I.M., et al. (1989, September). Duration of human immunodeficiency vi-

rus infection before detection of antibody. *Lancet, 16,* 637–639.

22. Levy, J.A. (1988). The human immunodeficiency virus (HIV) and its pathogenic properties. In R.F. Schinaz & A.J. Nahmias (Eds.). *AIDS in children, adolescents and heterosexual adults* (pp. 117–125). New York: Elsevier.

23. Ho, D.D., Sarngadharan, M.G., Resnick, L., et al. (1985). Primary human T-lymphotropic virus type III infection. *Annals of Internal Medicine, 103,* 880.

24. Lemp, G.A., Hessol, N.A., Rutherford, G.W., et al. (1988). Projections of AIDS morbidity/mortality in San Francisco using epidemic models. In *Proceedings of the IV International Conference on AIDS* (p. 4682). Stockholm, Sweden.

25. Centers for Disease Control. (1987). Revision of the CDC surveillance case definition for acquired immunodeficiency syndrome. *Morbidity and Mortality Weekly Report, 36,* 3S.

26. Sherertz, R.A. (1985). Acquired immune deficiency syndrome. *Medical Clinics of North America, 69,* 637.

27. Snider, D.E., & Roper, W.L. (1992). The new tuberculosis. *New England Journal of Medicine, 326,* 703–705.

28. Price, R.W., Brew, B., Sidtis, J., et al: (1988). The brain in AIDS: Central nervous system HIV-1 infection and AIDS dementia complex. *Science, 239,* 586.

29. Rogers, M.F., Ou, C.Y., Kilbourne, B., & Schochetman, G. (1991). Advances and problems in the diagnosis of human immunodeficiency virus infection in infants. *Pediatric Infectious Disease Journal, 10,* 523–531.

30. American Academy of Pediatrics. (1992). Perinatal human immunodeficiency virus (HIV) testing. *Pediatrics, 89,* 791–793.

31. Francis, D.P., & Chin, J. (1987). The prevention of acquired immunodeficiency syndrome in the United States. *Journal of the American Medical Association, 257,* 1357.

32. American Medical Association. (1991). *HIV early care/ AMA physician guidelines* (p. 8). American Medical Association.

33. The Pharmaceutical Manufacturers Association. (1992, April). 1991 survey report on AIDS medicines in development. *AIDS Patient Care,* pp. 86–92.

34. Fischl, M.A., Richman, D., Grieco, M., et al. (1987). The efficacy of azidothymidine (AZT) in the treatment of patients with AIDS and AIDS-related complex. A double-blind, placebo controlled trial. *New England Journal of Medicine, 317*(4), 185.

35. Quinn, T.C., Piot, P., & McCormick, J.B., et al. (1987). Serologic and immunologic studies in patients with AIDS in North America and Africa. The potential role of infectious agents as cofactors in human immunodeficiency virus infection. *Journal of the American Medical Association, 257,* 2617.

36. Centers for Disease Control. (1991). Update on adult immunization—recommendations of the Immunization Practices Advisory Committee (ACIP). *Morbidity and Mortality Weekly Report, 40,* 13.

37. Rothenberg, R., Woelfel, M., Stoneburner, R., et al. (1987). Survival with the acquired immunodeficiency syndrome. *New England Journal of Medicine, 317,* 1297.

38. O'Brien, A.M., Oerlemans-Bunn, M., & Blachfield, J.C. (1987). Nursing the AIDS patient at home. *AIDS Patient Care, 1,* 21.

39. Centers for Disease Control. (1988). Condoms for the prevention of sexually transmitted diseases. *Morbidity and Mortality Weekly Report, 37,* 133–137.

40. Department of Labor, Occupational Safety and Health Administration. (1991, December 6). Occupational exposure to bloodborne pathogens: Final rule (29 CFR 1910.1030). *Federal Register,* pp. 64004–64182.

41. Resnick, L., Veren, K., Salhuddin, S.K., et al. (1986). Stability and inactivation of HTLV-III/LAV under clinical and laboratory environments. *Journal of the American Medical Association, 255,* 1887.

42. Martin, L.S., McDougal, J.S., & Loskoske, S.L. (1985). Disinfection and inactivation of the human T-lymphotropic virus type III/lymphadenopathy-associated virus. *Journal of Infectious Diseases, 152,* 400.

■ BIBLIOGRAPHY

Blendon, R.J., Donelan, K., & Knox, R.A. (1992). Public opinion and AIDS—lessons for the second decade. *Journal of the American Medical Association, 267,* 981–986.

Burroughs, M.H., & Edelson, P.J. (1991). Medical care of the HIV-infected child. *Pediatric Clinics of North America, 38,* 45–67.

Caldwell, M.B., & Rogers, M.F. (1991). Epidemiology of pediatric HIV infection. *Pediatric Clinics of North America, 38,* 1–16.

Centers for Disease Control. (1992). Recommendations for prophylaxis against *Pneumocystis carinii* pneumonia for adults and adolescents infected with human immunodeficiency virus. *Morbidity and Mortality Weekly Report, 41*(RR-4), 1–11.

Darrow, W.W. (1991). AIDS: socioepidemiologic responses to an epidemic. In R. Ulack & W.F. Skinner (Eds.). *AIDS and the social sciences: Common threads* (pp. 82–99). Lexington: The University Press of Kentucky.

Farizo, K.M., Buehler, J.W., Chamberland, M.E., et al. (1992). Spectrum of disease in persons with human immunodeficiency virus infection in the United States. *Journal of the American Medical Association, 267,* 1798–1805.

Flaskerud, J.H., & Ungvarski, P.J. (1992). *HIV/AIDS: A guide to nursing care.* Philadelphia: W.B. Saunders.

Gold, J.W. (1992). HIV-1 infection/diagnosis and management. *Medical Clinics of North American, 76,* 1–18.

Graham, N., Zeger, S.L., Park, L.P., et al. (1992). The effects on survival of early treatment of human immunodeficiency virus infection. *New England Journal of Medicine, 326,* 1037–1042.

Hinman, A.R. (1991). Strategies to prevent HIV infection in the United States. *American Journal of Public Health, 81,* 1557–1559.

Hoyt, M.J., & Staats, A. (1991). Wasting and malnutrition in patients with HIV/AIDS. *Journal of the Association of Nurses in AIDS Care, 2,* 16–26.

Kassler, W.J., & Wu, A.W. (1992). Addressing HIV infection in office practice. *Primary Care, 19,* 19–33.

Phillips, T.J., & Dover, J.S. (1992). Human immunodeficiency virus infection. *New England Journal of Medicine, 326,* 172–178.

Prober, C.G., & Gershon, A.A. (1991). Medical management of newborns and infants born to human immunodeficiency virus seropositive mothers. *Pediatric Infectious Disease Journal, 10,* 684–695.

CHAPTER 16

DISORDERS OF WHITE BLOOD CELLS AND LYMPHOID TISSUES

■ OBJECTIVES

After you have studied this chapter, you should be able to meet the following objectives:

■ List the cells and tissues of the hematopoietic system.

■ Trace the development of the different blood cells from their origin in the pluripotent bone marrow stem cell to their circulation in the bloodstream.

■ Define the terms *leukopenia, neutropenia, granulocytopenia,* and *aplastic anemia.*

■ Cite two general causes of neutropenia.

■ Describe the mechanism of symptom production in neutropenia.

■ List the signs and symptoms of infectious mononucleosis.

■ Describe the pathogenesis of infectious mononucleosis.

■ Use the predominant cell type and classification as acute or chronic to describe the four general types of leukemia.

■ State the warning signs of acute leukemia.

■ Explain the manifestations of leukemia in terms of altered cell differentiation.

■ Describe the following complications of acute leukemia and its treatment: leukostasis, tumor lysis syndrome, hyperuricemia, and blast crisis.

■ State the difference between syngeneic, allogeneic, and autologous bone marrow transplantation.

■ Compare the lymphoproliferative disorders associated with Hodgkin's disease and non-Hodgkin's lymphoma.

■ Contrast and compare the signs and symptoms of Hodgkin's disease and non-Hodgkin's lymphoma.

■ Describe the lymphoproliferative disorder that occurs with multiple myeloma.

■ Explain the origin of the Bence Jones protein that appears in the urine in multiple myeloma.

The white blood cells protect the body against invasion by foreign agents. They include both phagocytic cells (granulocytes and monocytes) and the immune cells (B lymphocytes, or B cells, and T lymphocytes, or T cells). Disorders of white blood cells fall into two broad categories: deficiency disorders and proliferative disorders. This chapter focuses on disorders of white blood cell deficiency, infectious mononucleosis, the leukemias, and the lymphomas. Disorders of the thrombocytes and hemostasis are discussed in

Carol Mattson Porth: PATHOPHYSIOLOGY: CONCEPTS OF ALTERED HEALTH STATES, 4th ed. © 1994, 1990, 1986, 1982 J.B. Lippincott Company

Chapter 17 and those of red blood cells are discussed in Chapter 18. The functions of white blood cells in inflammation and immunity are discussed in Chapter 13.

■ HEMATOPOIETIC AND LYMPHOID TISSUE

The hematopoietic system encompasses all the blood cells, their precursors, and their derivatives (red blood cells, thrombocytes or platelets, and white blood cells). It includes the *myeloid*, or bone marrow, tissue in which the white blood cells are formed, and the *lymphoid tissues* of the lymph nodes, thymus, and spleen, in which blood cells circulate and mature.

WHITE BLOOD CELLS

The white blood cells include granulocytes (neutrophils, eosinophils, and basophils), monocytes (macrophages), and lymphocytes. Granulocytes and monocytes originate in bone marrow and circulate in the blood. T cells and B cells originate in bone marrow, mature in lymphoid tissue (thymus gland and bursa equivalent), and migrate between blood and lymph.

BONE MARROW

The entire hematopoietic system, in all its complexity, arises from a small number of stem cells that not only differentiate to form blood cells but also replenish bone marrow by a process of self-renewal. All the hematopoietic precursors, including the erythroid (red cell), myelocyte (granulocyte and monocyte), lymphocyte (T cell and B cell), and megakaryocyte (platelet) series, are derived from a small population of cells called the *pluripotent stem cells* (Fig. 16-1). These cells are capable of providing progenitor cells (parent cells) for both lymphopoiesis and hematopoiesis (processes by which myeloid and lymphoid blood cells are made). Several levels of differentiation lead to the development of committed unipotential cells, which are the progenitors for each of the blood cell types. The progenitor cells lose their capacity for self-renewal but retain the potential to differentiate into erythrocytes, monocytes, megakaryocytes, or lymphocytes. The term *colony-forming unit* is used to designate the myeloid and lymphoid progenitor cells; the term *burst-forming unit* is used to designate the precursors of the red blood cells.[1]

Under normal conditions, the number of each type of circulating blood cell and their total body mass remain constant. This regulation of blood cells is thought to be at least partially controlled by hormone-like messengers, called *cytokines*, that regulate the function of other cells, in this case the blood cell

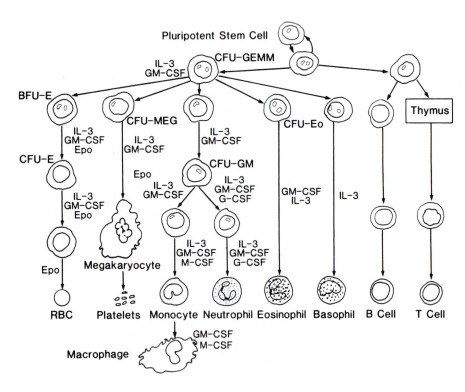

FIG. 16-1. *Stem cell maturation. BFU, burst-forming unit; CFU, colony-forming unit; CSF, colony-stimulating factor; GM, granulocyte-macrophage; GEMM, granulocyte-erythrocyte-macrophage-megakaryocyte; Epo, erythropoietin; IL-3, interleukin-3. (Developed by Dr. David H. Johnson.) (Hays, K. [1990]. Physiology of normal bone marrow. Seminars in Oncology Nursing, 6[1], 3–8)*

precursors. Many types of cytokines exist, including interleukins, interferons, and colony-stimulating factors (CSFs). The CSFs are a family of glycoproteins that support hematopoietic colony formation. There are three lineage-specific CSFs: erythropoietin, granulocyte colony-stimulating factor, and monocyte–macrophage colony-stimulating factor. There are also nonspecific CSFs that support the proliferation of the earlier hematopoietic precursors. Although the CSFs act at different points in the proliferation and differentiation pathway, there is overlap in their functions. In addition, other cytokines, such as interleukin-1, interleukin-4, interleukin-6, and interferon, act synergistically to support the functions of the CSFs (see Chapter 13).

The identification and characterization of the various cytokines and growth factors have led to their use in a wide range of clinical diseases. The diseases include bone marrow failure, hematopoietic neoplasms, infectious diseases, congenital and myeloproliferative disorders.[1] Many of these uses are investigational. Interferons are being used to treat some forms of leukemia.

Bone Marrow Aspiration and Biopsy. Samples of bone marrow may be obtained for diagnostic purposes by using bone marrow aspiration or bone marrow biopsy.

With bone marrow aspiration, a special bone marrow needle is inserted into the marrow cavity of the bone and a sample of marrow is withdrawn. The preferred site for this procedure in patients over the age of 12 to 18 months is the posterior iliac crest. Other sites include the anterior iliac crest, sternum, and spinous processes T10 through L4. The sternum is not commonly used in children because the cavity is too shallow and there is danger of mediastinal and cardiac perforation.[2] Aspiration disturbs the marrow architecture. Hence this technique is used primarily to determine the types of cells present and their relative numbers. Stained smears of bone marrow aspirates usually are subjected to the following studies: (1) determination of the erythroid-to-myeloid cell count (normal ratio 1:3), (2) differential cell count, (3) search for abnormal cells, (4) evaluation of iron stores in reticulum cells, and (5) special stains and immunochemical studies.[3]

Bone marrow biopsy requires a special needle. The most common site is the posterior iliac crest. In this procedure, a sample of bone marrow tissue is removed and its architecture is studied. Bone marrow biopsy is used to determine the marrow-fat ratio and to detect the presence of fibrosis, vasculitis, plasma cells, granulomas, and cancer cells.

The major hazard of these procedures is the slight risk of hemorrhage. This risk is increased in patients whose platelet count is low.

LYMPHOID TISSUES

The body's lymphatic system, which consists of the lymphatic vessels, lymph nodes, spleen, and thymus, is made up of lymphoid tissue. Lymph is body fluid that originates as excess fluid from the capillaries. It is returned to the vascular compartment and the right side of the heart through lymphatic vessels.

The lymph nodes, which are situated along the lymphatic channels, filter the lymph before it is returned to the circulation (Fig. 16-2). Lymph enters a lymph node through afferent lymphatic channels, percolates through a labyrinthine system of minute channels lined with endothelial and phagocytic cells, and then emerges through efferent lymphatic vessels. A number of efferent vessels join to form collecting trunks. Each collecting trunk drains a definite area of the body. By filtering bacteria and other particulate matter, the lymph nodes serve as a secondary line of defense even when clinical disease is not present. In the event of malignant neoplasm development, cancer cells are filtered and retained by the lymph nodes for a period of time before being disseminated to other parts of the body. Because of their contribution to the development of the immune system, lymph nodes are relatively large at birth and atrophy throughout life.

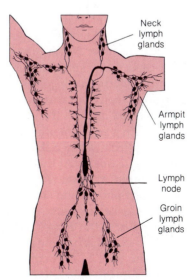

Neck
lymph
glands

Armpit
lymph
glands

Lymph
node

Groin
lymph
glands

FIG. 16-2. Location of some of the lymph nodes in the human body. (*What you need to know about Hodgkin's disease.* [1981]. Washington, DC: Department of Health and Human Services)

■ DISORDERS OF WHITE BLOOD CELL DEFICIENCY

The number of leukocytes, or white blood cells, in the peripheral circulation normally ranges from 5,000 to 10,000/μL of blood. About 50% to 70% of the leukocytes are granulocytes (50% to 70% neutrophils, 1% to 4% eosinophils, and 0.4% basophils), 20% to 30% are lymphocytes, and 2% to 8% are monocytes. The term *leukopenia* describes an absolute decrease in white blood cell numbers. The disorder may affect any of the specific types of white blood cells, but most often it affects the neutrophils, which are the predominant type of granulocyte.

Neutrophils, the predominant leukocyte in the circulation, have a brief existence between their formation in bone marrow and their phagocytic and microbial activity in the tissue sites of inflammation. They are primarily responsible for maintaining normal host defenses against invading microorganisms. The mature neutrophil has a segmented, multilobe nucleus and its cytoplasm contains fine granules. Enzymes associated with these granules are capable of degrading various natural and synthetic substances, including complex polysaccharides, proteins, and lipids. These enzymes are important in maintaining normal host defenses and in mediating inflammation.

Neutrophils originate in the myeloblasts that are found in bone marrow. Myeloblasts do not normally appear in the peripheral circulation. Their presence suggests a disorder of blood cell proliferation and differentiation. Myeloblasts differentiate into promyelocytes and then myelocytes. A cell is not called a myelocyte until it has at least 12 granules.[4] Myelocytes mature to become metamyelocytes (from the Greek word *meta*, meaning beyond), at which point they lose their capacity for mitosis. Subsequent development of the neutrophil involves reduction in size, with transformation from an indented to an oval to a horseshoe-shaped nucleus (band cell) and then to a mature cell with a segmented nucleus. Neutrophil development (from stem cell to mature neutrophil) takes about 2 weeks. At this point, the neutrophil enters the bloodstream. After their release from marrow, neutrophils spend only a short time (1 to 2 days) in the circulation before moving into the tissues. Their survival in the tissues is short (about 5 days). They die either in discharging their function or of senescence. The pool of circulating neutrophils (those that appear in the blood count) are in rapid equilibrium with a similar-sized pool of cells marginating along the walls of small blood vessels.[5] Epinephrine, exercise, and corticosteroid drug therapy can cause rapid increases in the circulating neutrophil count by shifting cells from the marginating pool to the circulating pool. Endotoxins have the opposite effect, producing a transient decrease in the number of neutrophils.

NEUTROPENIA

Neutropenia (also called *granulocytopenia*) refers specifically to a decrease in neutrophils. It commonly is defined as a circulating neutrophil count of less than 1500 cells/μL. Agranulocytosis, which denotes a severe granulocytopenia, is characterized by a circulating neutrophil count of less than 500 cells/μL.[3]

CAUSES

Neutropenia can occur because (1) neutrophil production fails to keep pace with granulocyte turnover or (2) the removal of neutrophils from circulating blood is accelerated. The causes of neutropenia are summarized in Table 16-1.

Impairment of Granulopoiesis. Impairment of granulopoiesis occurs as a complication of certain procedures, such as chemotherapy and irradiation, and conditions, such as aplastic anemia, which interfere with the formation of all blood cells. Overgrowth of neoplastic cells in nonmyelocytic leukemia and lymphoma may suppress the function of neutrophil precursors. Because of the neutrophil's short life span (about 1 day in the peripheral blood), neutropenia occurs rapidly when granulopoiesis is impaired. Under these conditions, neutropenia usually is accompanied by thrombocytopenia (platelet deficiency). In *aplastic anemia*, all of the myeloid stem cells are affected, resulting in anemia, thrombocytopenia, and agranulocytosis.

Periodic or cyclic neutropenia is a genetic disorder (autosomal dominant with various expression) that begins in infancy and persists for decades.[3] It is characterized by periodic neutropenia that develops every 21 to 30 days and lasts about 3 to 6 days. Although the cause is undetermined, it is thought to result from impaired feedback regulation of granulocyte production and release.

Transient neutropenia occurs in neonates whose mothers have hypertension. It usually lasts from 1 to 60 hours but can persist for 3 to 30 days. This type of neutropenia, which is associated with increased risk of nosocomial infection, is thought to result from transiently reduced neutrophil production.[6]

Accelerated Removal of Granulocytes. The removal of neutrophils from the circulation may be accelerated in a number of conditions. Infections may drain neutrophils from the blood faster than they can be replaced. Autoimmune disorders or idiosyncratic

CAUSE	MECHANISM
Accelerated removal (*e.g.*, inflammation and infection)	Removal of neutrophils from the circulation exceeds production
Drug-induced granulocytopenia	
Defective production	
Cytotoxic drugs used in cancer therapy	Predictable damage to percursor cells, usually dose dependent
Phenothiazine, thiouracil, chloramphenicol, phenylbutazone, and others	Idiosyncratic depression of bone marrow function
Hydantoinates, primidone, others	Intramedullary destruction of granulocytes
Immune destruction	Immunologic mechanisms with cytolysis or leukoagglutination
Aminopyrine, others	
Periodic or cyclic neutropenia (occurs during infancy and later)	Unknown
Neoplasms involving bone marrow (*e.g.*, leukemias and lymphomas)	Overgrowth of neoplastic cells, which crowd out granulopoietic precursors
Idiopathic neutropenia that occurs in the absence of other disease or provoking influence	Autoimmune reaction
Felty's syndrome	Intrasplenic destruction of neutrophils

drug reactions may cause increased and premature destruction of neutrophils. In splenomegaly, neutrophils may be trapped in the spleen along with other blood cells. In Felty's syndrome (a variant of rheumatoid arthritis), there is increased destruction of neutrophils in the spleen.

Most cases of neutropenia are drug-related. Chemotherapeutic drugs used in the treatment of cancer (*e.g.*, alkylating agents and antimetabolites) cause predictable dose-dependent suppression of bone marrow function. The term *idiosyncratic* is used to describe drug reactions that are different from the effects obtained in most people and that cannot be explained in terms of allergy. A number of drugs, such as chloramphenicol (an antibiotic), phenothiazine tranquilizers, sulfonamides, propylthiouracil (used in treatment of hyperthyroidism), and phenylbutazone (used in the treatment of arthritis), may cause idiosyncratic depression of bone marrow function. Some drugs, such as hydantoin derivatives and primidone (used in the treatment of seizure disorders), can cause intramedullary destruction of granulocytes and thereby impair production. In addition, many idiosyncratic cases of drug-induced neutropenia are thought to be caused by immunologic mechanisms, with the drug or its metabolites acting as antigens (or haptens) to incite the production of antibodies reactive against the neutrophils. Neutrophils possess not only HLA antigens but also other antigens specific to a given leukocyte line. Anti-

bodies to these specific antigens have been identified in some cases of drug-induced neutropenia.

MANIFESTATION AND TREATMENT

Because the neutrophil is essential to the cellular phase of inflammation, infections are common in persons with neutropenia, and extreme caution is needed to protect them from exposure to infectious organisms. Infections that might go unnoticed in a person with a normal neutrophil count may prove fatal in a person with neutropenia.

The clinical features of neutropenia usually stem from severe infections that are characteristic of the disorder. These infections commonly are caused by organisms that colonize the skin and the gastrointestinal tract. Signs and symptoms initially include malaise, chills, and fever, followed by extreme weakness and fatigability. The white blood cell count often is reduced to $1000/\mu L$ and, in certain cases, may fall to 200 to $300/\mu L$. Ulcerative necrotizing lesions of the mouth are common in neutropenia. Ulcerations of the skin, vagina, and gastrointestinal tract may also occur.

Antibiotics are used to treat infections in those situations in which neutrophil destruction can be controlled or the neutropoietic function of the bone marrow can be recovered. Corticosteroid therapy and neutrophil transfusions are also used. The prognosis is variable and depends on the cause.

In summary, neutropenia, a marked reduction in the number of circulating neutrophils, is one of the major disorders of the white blood cells. It can result from defective neutrophil production or the accelerated removal of neutrophils from the circulation. Severe neutropenia can occur as a complication of lymphoproliferative diseases, in which neoplastic cells crowd out neutrophil precursor cells, or of radiation therapy or treatment with cytotoxic drugs, which destroy neutrophil precursor cells. Neutropenia may also be encountered as an idiosyncratic reaction to various drugs. Because the neutrophil is essential to the cellular stage of inflammation, severe and often life-threatening infections are common in persons with neutropenia.

■ INFECTIOUS MONONUCLEOSIS

Infectious mononucleosis is a self-limiting lymphoproliferative disorder caused by the Epstein-Barr virus (EBV). One of the herpesviruses, EBV is ubiquitous in all human populations. Infectious mononucleosis is most prevalent in adolescents and young adults in the upper socioeconomic classes in developed countries. This is probably because the disease, which is relatively asymptomatic when it occurs during childhood, confers complete immunity to the virus. In upper socioeconomic families, exposure to the virus may be delayed until late adolescence or early adulthood. In such people, the mode of infection, size of the viral pool, and physiologic and immunologic condition of the host may determine whether or not the infection occurs.

Infectious mononucleosis has been called the ''kissing disease,'' and evidence suggests that exposure to EBV-contaminated saliva is one of the main modes of transfer. The virus undergoes a replicative cycle in the oropharyngeal epithelium and then invades the blood by selectively infecting B cells, a cell population that has specific surface receptors for the virus. It is shed from the oropharynx for up to 18 months after primary infection; thereafter, it may be spread intermittently by people who are EBV-seropositive despite the absence of clinical disease.[7] Immunosuppressed people shed the virus more frequently. Asymptomatic shedding of EBV by healthy people accounts for most of the spread of infectious mononucleosis, despite the fact that it is not a highly contagious disease.

PATHOGENESIS

Infectious mononucleosis is characterized by fever, generalized lymphadenopathy, sore throat (pharyngitis), and the appearance in the blood of atypical lymphocytes. In the course of infection, EBV invades the B cells of oropharyngeal lymphoid tissues. Replication of the virus ensues, with the subsequent death of the B cells and release of the virus into the blood,

causing the febrile reaction and specific immunologic responses. Concurrent with the febrile reaction, antiviral antibodies (immunoglobulin M and immunoglobulin G) appear and the virus disappears from the blood. Other viral-determined antibodies also develop, including the well-known *heterophil* (also known as the *Paul-Bunnel* antibody) that is used in the diagnosis of infectious mononucleosis.

Although infectious B cells and free virions disappear from the blood, some EBV-transformed B cells remain in the circulation with the genome of the virus integrated into their genetic structure. These B cells display virus-directed membrane antigens. These B cell antigens stimulate production of both cytotoxic (CD4) and suppressor (CD8) T cells. Together, the suppressor–cytotoxic (CD8) T cells are the atypical lymphocytes seen in the blood of patients with infectious mononucleosis. The proliferation of atypical lymphocytes throughout the body is responsible for the lymphadenopathy and hepatosplenomegaly. The progressive increase in the number of EBV-specific antibodies and cytotoxic (CD8) T cells eventually brings the disease under control and eliminates the latently infected B cells.[7]

MANIFESTATIONS

The onset of infectious mononucleosis usually is insidious. During the prodromal period, which lasts for 1 to 2 weeks, there is fever, pharyngitis, fatigue, general malaise, and anorexia. Occasionally, the disorder comes on abruptly with a high fever. Severe pharyngitis is the symptom that most frequently prompts people to seek medical attention. It usually is maximal for 5 to 7 days and persists for 7 to 14 days. Severe toxic pharyngotonsillitis may cause airway obstruction.

Lymphadenopathy is present in 90% of cases, with symmetrically enlarged and often tender lymph nodes. Its duration is variable but seldom exceeds 3 weeks.

Hepatitis and splenomegaly are common manifestations of infectious mononucleosis and, as explained earlier, are thought to be immune-mediated. Hepatitis is characterized by hepatomegaly, nausea, anorexia, and jaundice. Although discomforting, it usually is a benign condition that resolves without causing permanent liver damage. The spleen may be enlarged two to three times its normal size, and rupture of the spleen is an infrequent complication.

A rash that resembles rubella develops in 10% to 15% of cases.[7] Treatment with amoxacillin or ampicillin frequently produces skin eruptions.[8] The reason for this is unknown.

Fewer than 1% of cases, mostly in the adult age group, develop complications referable to the central nervous system (CNS). These complications include cranial nerve palsies, encephalitis, meningitis, transverse myelitis, and Guillain-Barré syndrome.

The peripheral blood usually shows an increase in the number of leukocytes, with a white blood cell count between 12,000 and 18,000/μL, 95% of which are lymphocytes. The rise in white blood cells begins during the 1st week, rises even higher during the 2nd week of the infection, and then returns to normal around the 4th week. Although leukocytosis is common, leukopenia may be seen in some people during the first 3 days of the illness. Atypical lymphocytes are frequent, constituting more than 20% of the total lymphocyte count. Heterophil antibodies usually appear during the 2nd or 3rd week and decline after the acute illness has subsided. They may, however, be detectable for up to 9 months after onset of the disease.

Most persons with infectious mononucleosis recover without incident. The acute phase of the illness usually lasts for 2 to 3 weeks, after which recovery occurs rapidly. Some degree of debility and lethargy may persist for 2 to 3 months.

DIAGNOSIS AND TREATMENT

Diagnosis is based on the clinical features (fever, pharyngitis, and lymphadenopathy) coupled with the presence of atypical lymphocytes and heterophil antibodies. EBV-specific antibody studies may facilitate diagnosis in heterophil-negative cases.

Treatment usually is symptomatic and supportive. It includes bed rest and analgesics, such as aspirin, to relieve the fever, headache, and sore throat. In cases of severe pharyngotonsillitis, corticosteroids are given to reduce inflammation.

In summary, infectious mononucleosis is a self-limited lymphoproliferative disorder caused by the B lymphocytotropic EBV, a member of herpesvirus family. The highest incidence of infectious mononucleosis is found in adolescents and young adults and is seen more frequently in the upper socioeconomic classes of developed countries. The disease is characterized by fever, generalized lymphadenopathy, sore throat (pharyngitis), and the appearance in the blood of atypical lymphocytes and several antibodies, including the well-known heterophil antibodies that are used in the diagnosis of infectious mononucleosis.

■ NEOPLASTIC DISORDERS OF HEMATOPOIETIC ORIGIN

Neoplastic disorders of hematopoietic origin include the leukemias, multiple myeloma, and the lymphomas. The process of cell proliferation and differentiation, neoplasia, and methods of cancer treatment are discussed in Chapter 5.

LEUKEMIAS

The leukemias are malignant neoplasms of the hematopoietic stem cells. They are characterized by diffuse replacement of bone marrow with immature neoplastic cells. In most cases, the leukemic cells spill out into the blood, where they are seen in large numbers. The term *leukemia* (*white blood*) was first used by Virchow to describe a reversal of the usual ratio of red blood cells to white blood cells. Leukemia is thought to arise after the malignant transformation of a single hematopoietic cell line. The leukemic cells proliferate mainly in the bone marrow, circulate in the blood, and infiltrate the spleen, lymph nodes, and other tissues.

Leukemia strikes about 28,000 persons in the United States each year. In 1992, about 27,200 new cases were diagnosed and 18,200 persons died of this disease.[9] More children are stricken with leukemia than with any other form of cancer, and it is the leading cause of death in children aged 3 to 14. Although leukemia commonly is thought of as a childhood disease, it strikes more adults than children (27,700 adults per year compared with 2,500 children).

Recent advances in molecular biology have contributed greatly to an understanding of leukemic cell types, including the early stages of cell differentiation and gene function. This information has greatly influenced the diagnosis, treatment, and prognosis of patients with leukemia.

CLASSIFICATION

The leukemias commonly are classified according to their predominant cell type (lymphocytic or myelocytic) and whether the condition is acute or chronic. Thus, a rudimentary classification system divides leukemia into four types: acute lymphocytic (lymphoblastic) leukemia (ALL), chronic lymphocytic leukemia (CLL), acute myelocytic (myeloblastic) leukemia (AML), and chronic myelocytic leukemia (CML). The lymphocytic leukemias involve the lymphoid precursors that originate in the bone marrow but infiltrate the spleen, lymph nodes, CNS, and other tissues. The myelocytic leukemias, which involve the pluripotent myeloid stem cells in bone marrow, interfere with the maturation of all blood cells, including the granulocytes, erythrocytes, and thrombocytes.

ALL is the most common leukemia in childhood with a peak incidence between ages 2 and 4. CLL affects older people; fewer than 10% of those who develop the disease are younger than age 50. AML is seen most often between the ages of 13 and 39 years and chronic myelocytic leukemia between ages 30 and 50 years.

CAUSES

The causes of leukemia are unknown. The incidence of leukemia among people who have been exposed to high levels of radiation is unusually high. The number of cases of leukemia reported in the most heavily exposed survivors of the atomic blasts at Hiroshima and Nagasaki during the 20-year period from 1950 to 1970 was nearly 30 times the expected rate.[10] An increased incidence of leukemia also is associated with exposure to benzene as well as the use of antitumor drugs and chloramphenicol. Leukemia may occur as a second cancer after aggressive chemotherapy for other cancers, such as Hodgkin's disease,[11] gastrointestinal cancers,[12] ovarian cancer,[13] and ALL.[13–15] AML is the most common type of secondary cancer.

A significant number of cases of leukemia have been reported in identical twins. An identical twin of a person with acute leukemia has a 25% chance of developing the disease, whereas a fraternal twin has little excess risk.[3] Leukemia occurs relatively frequently in association with congenital chromosomal abnormalities such as Down's syndrome, Klinefelter's syndrome, and Turner's syndrome.

Advances in cytogenetic studies have made it increasingly evident that many forms of leukemia are associated with nonrandom chromosomal changes (usually translocations). For example, the Philadelphia chromosome (translocation from chromosome 22 to chromosome 9) is present in about 90% of people with CML.[16] In many cases, these chromosomal aberrations, which are present at diagnosis, disappear with treatment and remission and reappear with relapse. The underlying cause of these chromosomal changes is unknown. It is now possible, however, to try to correlate the chromosomes that are affected with the genes involved. This may lead to increased understanding of the pathogenesis of leukemia and to the discovery of new methods of diagnosis and treatment.

CLINICAL MANIFESTATIONS

A leukemic cell is an immature and mobile type of white blood cell. As explained in Chapter 5, differentiation of a cell line determines its structure, function, and life span. Because leukemic cells are immature and poorly differentiated, they are capable of an increased rate of proliferation and have a prolonged life span. They also cannot perform the functions of mature leukocytes; that is, they are ineffective as phagocytes or immune cells. Because they proliferate rapidly, leukemic cells interfere with the maturation of normal bone marrow cells, including the erythroblasts (red blood cells) and the megakaryoblasts (platelets). Being mobile, they can travel throughout the circulatory system, cross the blood–brain barrier, and infiltrate many body organs.

ACUTE LEUKEMIAS

Acute leukemia is a cancer of the hematopoietic stem cells. It usually has a sudden and stormy onset of signs and symptoms related to depressed bone marrow function (Table 16-2). Most patients present within 3 months of the onset of symptoms. They may have mild pancytopenia (anemia, thrombocytopenia, and neutropenia), normal leukocyte count and absence of blast cells, or leukocytosis and circulating blast cells. Generalized lymphadenopathy, splenomegaly, and hepatomegaly caused by infiltration of leukemic cells occur in all acute leukemias but are more common in ALL.[17]

A definitive diagnosis of acute leukemia is based on blood and bone marrow studies; it requires the demonstration of leukemic cells in the peripheral blood, bone marrow, or extramedullary tissue. Laboratory findings reveal the presence of immature (blast) white blood cells in the circulation and bone marrow, where they may constitute 60% to 100% of the cells.[17] These cells suppress the normal hematopoietic stem cells in the marrow. Consequently, there is a loss of mature myeloid cells, such as erythrocytes, granulocytes, and platelets. Anemia is almost always present, and the platelet count is decreased.

According to the American Cancer Society, the warning signs and symptoms of acute leukemia are fatigue, pallor, weight loss, repeated infections, easy bruising, and nosebleeds and other types of hemorrhage.[9] These features may appear suddenly in children. Both ALL and AML are characterized by fatigue resulting from anemia; bleeding secondary to decreased platelet count; and bone marrow involvement, including subperiosteal infiltration, marrow expansion, and bone resorption, which causes bone tenderness and pain. Infection results from neutropenia, with the risk of infection becoming high as the neutrophil count falls below 500/μL.

Signs and symptoms of CNS involvement occur in both ALL and AML and include headache, nausea, vomiting, cranial nerve palsies, and, sometimes, seizures and coma. The latter two are more common in children than in adults and in ALL than in AML. *Leukostasis*, a condition in which the circulating blast count is markedly elevated (usually more than 100,000 μL), leading to impaired circulation, presents as headache, confusion, and dyspnea. A medical emergency, it requires leukapheresis (removal of white blood cells) and chemotherapy.[18]

Hyperuricemia occurs as the result of increased

TABLE 16-2. CLINICAL MANIFESTATIONS OF LEUKEMIA AND THEIR PATHOLOGIC BASIS*

CLINICAL MANIFESTATIONS	PATHOLOGIC BASIS
Bone marrow depression	
Malaise, easy fatigability	Anemia
Fever	Infection or increased metabolism by neoplastic cells
Bleeding	Decreased thrombocytes
Petechiae	
Ecchymosis	
Gingival bleeding	
Epistaxis	
Bone pain and tenderness in palpation	Subperiosteal bone infiltration, bone marrow expansion, and bone resorption
Headache, nausea, vomiting, papilledema, cranial nerve palsies, seizures, coma	Leukemic infiltration of central nervous system
Abdominal discomfort	Generalized lymphadenopathy, hepatomegaly, splenomegaly due to leukemic cell infiltration
Increased vulnerability to infections	Immaturity of the white cells and ineffective phagocytic and immune function
Hematologic abnormalities	
Anemia	Physical and metabolic encroachment of leukemic cells on red blood cell and thrombocyte precursors
Thrombocytopenia	
Hyperuricemia and other metabolic disorders	Abnormal proliferation and metabolism of leukemic cells

* Manifestations vary with the type of leukemia.

proliferation and metabolic alterations of the leukemic cells. It may increase before and during treatment and may require therapy with allopurinol to prevent renal complications secondary to uric acid crystallization in the urine.

Both chemotherapy and selective irradiation (*e.g.*, CNS irradiation) are used in the treatment of acute leukemia. Chemotherapy includes induction therapy designed to effect a remission, intensification therapy to further reduce the leukemic cell population, and maintenance therapy to maintain remissions. Remission is defined as eradication of leukemic cells as detectable by conventional technology. Massive necrosis of malignant cells can occur during the initial phase of treatment. This phenomenon, known as *tumor lysis syndrome*, can lead to life-threatening metabolic disorders, including hyperkalemia, hyperphosphatemia, hyperuricemia, hypomagnesemia, hypocalcemia, and acidosis. Prophylactic hydration with alkaline solutions is given to counteract these effects.[19]

Bone marrow transplantation from an identical twin (syngeneic transplantation) or an HLA-matched sibling or other major HLA-matched donor (allogeneic transplantation) has proved effective in both ALL and AML. The objective is to first treat the recipient of the transplant with high doses of chemotherapy alone or with irradiation to eliminate all the leukemic cells and then rescue the person from the effects of severe bone marrow suppression with normal transplanted bone marrow from a donor. Allogeneic transplantation is associated with substantial transplant-related risk, including graft-versus-host disease (see Chapter 14) and opportunistic infections. Autologous (self) transplantation has also been used in the treatment of acute leukemia. In this approach, the leukemic patient's own bone marrow is collected during remission, cryopreserved, and then reinfused after treatment to destroy all the leukemic cells. One of the problems with autologous bone marrow transplantation is the probable contamination of the remission bone marrow with leukemic cells. Various chemotherapeutic and immunologic agents have been used to eradicate residual tumor cells. One method under investigation involves purging the marrow with monoclonal antibodies that specifically bind and destroy the leukemic cells.

Acute Lymphocytic Leukemia. Acute lymphocytic leukemia primarily strikes children and young adults, accounting for 80% of childhood acute leukemias. The peak incidence occurs at about age 4. ALL can be classified according to the origin of the lymphocytes: early pre–B cell precursor, pre–B cell, mature B cell, and immature T cell. The vast majority of ALLs are of B-cell origin, mainly of the early B precursor type.

ALL is treated with combination chemotherapy. Systemic chemotherapeutic agents cannot cross the blood–brain barrier and eradicate leukemic cells that have entered the CNS. Cranial irradiation combined with intrathecal chemotherapy often is used as a prophylactic measure to prevent CNS recurrence. Concern over the potential adverse effects of intracranial therapy, however, has prompted reappraisal of the treatment strategies. CNS irradiation usually is reserved for children with initial CNS leukemia or who are at high risk for CNS relapse.[17] The long-term effects of treatment on childhood cancer survivors is discussed in Chapter 5. Although CNS involvement is a major problem in children, the incidence in adults at the time of diagnosis is less than 10%.

Acute lymphocytic leukemia is one of the outstanding examples of a once fatal disease that is now treatable and potentially curable with combination chemotherapy. More than 90% of children with ALL have complete remission, and about 60% are alive 5 years later. The prognosis in adults in more variable.

Acute Myelocytic Leukemia Acute myelocytic leukemia, also called acute nonlymphocytic leukemia, is chiefly an adult disease with a median age of about 50 years.[19] However, it is also seen in children and young adults.

Of all the leukemias, AML has the strongest linkage with toxins and underlying congenital and hematologic disorders. It is the type of leukemia associated with Down's syndrome and the most frequent second cancer seen in people who have been treated for other types of cancer.[19]

The AMLs are an extremely heterogeneous group of disorders. Some arise from the multipotent stem cells in which myeloblasts predominate, and others arise from the monocyte–granulocyte precursor, giving rise to myelomonocytic leukemia. Based on the line of differentiation and the maturity of the cells, AMLs have been divided into seven subtypes in the widely used French-American-British classification system (Table 16-3). In addition to the common manifestations of acute leukemia (fatigue, weight loss, fever, easy bruising), certain presentations are distinctive for the subtypes. Infiltration of the skin, gums, and other soft tissue is particularly common in the monocytic form (M5) of leukemia, whereas disseminated intravascular coagulation poses a serious complication of promyelocytic leukemia (M3).

AML is treated with intensive chemotherapy to effect aplasia of the bone marrow. During this period, supportive transfusion and antibiotic therapy often are needed. If remission is achieved, some type of continuing chemotherapy is used. In some cases, bone marrow transplantation may be performed.

Chemotherapy induces complete remission in 70% of all people with AML, about one fourth of whom achieve long-term disease-free survival or cure.[19]

CHRONIC LEUKEMIAS

Chronic leukemias have a more insidious onset than acute leukemias and may be discovered during a routine medical examination with blood count. CML

TABLE 16-3. FAB CLASSIFICATION FOR AML*		
CLASS		**PERCENTAGE OF AML**
M1	AML without differentiation	20
M2	AML with differentiation	29–30
M3	Promyelocytic leukemia	5–7
M4	Acute myelomonocytic leukemia	22–30
M5	Acute monocytic leukemia	10–19
M6	Acute erythroleukemia	1–5
M7	Acute megakaryoblastic leukemia	2–5

* FAB, French-American-British; AML, acute myelocytic leukemia.
Developed from information in Kumar, V.K., Cotran, R.S., & Robbins, S.L. (1992). *Basic pathology* (5th ed., pp. 365–372). Philadelphia: W.B. Saunders; Champlin, R., & Gold, D.W. (1991). The leukemias. In J.D. Wilson, E. Braunwald, K.J. Isselbacher (Eds.). *Harrison's principles of internal medicine* (12th ed.). New York: McGraw-Hill.

is predominantly a disorder of adults, but it can affect children as well. CLL is a disorder of older adults.

Chronic Myelocytic Leukemia. A myeloproliferative disorder, CML involves expansion of all bone marrow elements. The bone marrow cells of the CML line have the Philadelphia chromosome, suggesting a mutation in the multipotential stem cell as the initiating event. CML is divided into three stages: (1) chronic or stable, (2) accelerated, and (3) acute or blast crisis. Early in the course, the clinical features are mild and nonspecific.

The finding of abnormal blood counts on routine testing frequently leads to the diagnosis of CML. The most characteristic laboratory finding at presentation is leukocytosis with immature cell types in the peripheral blood. Anemia and, eventually, thrombocytopenia develop. Anemia causes weakness, easy fatigability, and exertional dyspnea. Splenomegaly is present in 50% of cases at the time of diagnosis; hepatomegaly is less common, and lymphadenopathy is relatively uncommon. Splenomegaly often causes a feeling of abdominal fullness and discomfort. Bleeding and easy bruising may arise from dysfunctional platelets. Within an average of 3 to 4 years, most cases undergo transformation to the blast phase, which is heralded by the accelerated phase. During the accelerated phase, constitutional symptoms such as low-grade fever, night sweats, and weight loss develop due to rapid proliferation and hypermetabolism of the leukemic cells. Erratic fluctuations in white blood cell and platelet counts may accompany the accelerated phase. The blast crisis represents evolution to acute leukemia, either myeloid or lymphoid. Constitutional symptoms become more pronounced during this period, and splenomegaly may increase significantly. Isolated infiltrates of leukemic cells can involve the skin, lymph nodes, bones, and CNS. If very high blast counts (more than 100,000/μL) are present, symptoms of leukostasis may occur. The prognosis for patients who are in the blast crisis stage is very poor.

The treatment of chronic leukemia varies with the type of leukemic cell that is present, the stage of the disease, other health problems, and the person's age. Often the treatment is palliative. The median survival is 3 to 4 years, with less than 30% of people living 5 years after diagnosis. Curative treatment for CML consists of high-dose chemotherapy and, possibly, bone marrow transplantation. α-Interferon has recently been evaluated in the treatment of CML. This biologic response modifier induces hematologic remission in up to 80% of cases, and in 56% of these, the number of Philadelphia chromosomes that reactively divide is reduced.[19]

Chronic Lymphocytic Leukemia. Mainly a disease of older people, CLL typically follows a slow, chronic course. For these people, reassurance that they can live a normal life for many years is important. Complications such as autoimmune thrombocytopenia and hemolytic anemia may be managed with corticosteroid treatment, or a splenectomy may be necessary.

CLL is a disorder of immunologically incompetent lymphocytes. The finding of abnormal, small lymphocytes of the CLL lineage in peripheral blood and bone marrow is a prerequisite for the diagnosis of CLL, except when complete remission has occurred. The person with CLL is predisposed to infection and the development of autoimmune phenomenon because of the immunologic incompetence of the expanding lymphocyte population. Generalized lymphadenopathy with palpable lymph nodes in the cervical, axillary, inguinal, and femoral regions is common. The spleen and liver may be enlarged. Anemia, thrombocytopenia, and neutropenia may result from bone marrow infiltration.

The treatment of CLL is variable. Most early cases require no specific treatment. Indications for chemotherapy include progressive fatigue, troublesome lymphadenopathy, anemia, and thrombocytopenia.

Hairy cell leukemia, a rare but malignant variant of CLL, is characterized by the presence of leukemic cells that have fine, hair-like cytoplasmic projections. It occurs mainly in older men. The most common physical finding is splenomegaly, which commonly is massive and may be the only presenting sign. Pancytopenia resulting from bone marrow failure and splenic sequestration is seen in more than 50% of cases. The course of the disease is chronic, and the median survival has been about 6 years. In the past, the treatment of choice was splenectomy. This procedure raises the blood count and relieves symptoms in many people. α-Interferon has recently produced responses in a high number of cases and has led to the disappearance of the disease for some time. Also, two experimental drugs, deoxycoformycin and 2-chlorodeoxyadenosine, have proved promising.[18]

LYMPHOMAS

The lymphomas—Hodgkin's disease and non-Hodgkin's lymphomas—represent malignant neoplasms of cells native to lymphoid tissue (lymphocytes and histiocytes) and their precursors or derivatives.[20] The seventh most common cancer in the United States,[21] the lymphomas are among the most studied human tumors and among the most curable.

HODGKIN'S DISEASE

Hodgkin's disease is a malignant neoplasm of the lymphatic structures. An English physician, Thomas Hodgkin, first described the disease in 1832. About 7400 new cases of Hodgkin's disease were reported in 1992, of which 1500 resulted in death.[9] Distribution of the disease is bimodal; the incidence rises sharply after age 10, peaks in the late 20s, and then declines until age 45. After age 45, the incidence again increases steadily with age.[21] In 60% to 90% of people with localized Hodgkin's disease, the possibility of a definitive "cure" (normal life expectancy for the patient's age for 10 or more years after treatment) exists.

The cause of Hodgkin's disease is unknown. There is a long-standing suspicion that the disease may begin as an inflammatory reaction to an infectious agent. This belief is supported by epidemiologic data that include the clustering of the disease among family members and among students who have attended the same school. There also seems to be an association between the presence of the disease and a deficient immune state. As with other forms of cancer, it is likely that no single agent is responsible for the development of Hodgkin's disease.

Hodgkin's disease is characterized by painless and progressive enlargement of a single node or group of nodes. It is believed to originate within one area of the lymphatic system and, if unchecked, will spread throughout the lymphatic network. The initial lymph node involvement typically is above the level of the diaphragm, and the cervical chain or supraclavicular nodes most commonly are affected. An exception is in elderly people, in whom the subdiaphragmatic lymph nodes may be the first to be involved. Involvement of the retroperitoneal lymph nodes, liver, spleen, and bone marrow occurs after the disease becomes generalized.

The malignant proliferating cells may invade almost any area of the body and may produce a wide variety of signs and symptoms. Low-grade fever, night sweats, unexplained weight loss, fatigue, pruritus, and anemia are indicative of disease spread. In the advanced stages of Hodgkin's disease, the liver, lungs, digestive tract, and, occasionally, CNS may be affected.

As the disease progresses, the rapid proliferation of abnormal lymphocytes leads to an immunologic defect, particularly in cell-mediated responses, rendering the person more susceptible to bacterial, viral, fungal, and protozoal infections. Neutrophilic leukocytosis and mild normocytic normochromic anemia are common. Eosinophilia may also occur. Leukopenia usually is a late manifestation. Hypergammaglobulinemia is common during the early stages of the disease, whereas hypogammaglobulinemia may develop in advanced disease.

The staging of Hodgkin's disease is of great clinical importance because the choice of treatment and the prognosis are ultimately related to the distribution of the disease. Staging is determined by the number of lymph nodes that are involved, whether the lymph nodes are on one or both sides of the diaphragm, and whether there is disseminated disease involving the bone marrow and liver. In addition, patients are designated stage A if they lack constitution symptoms and stage B if they experience significant weight loss, fever, and night sweats.

A definitive diagnosis of Hodgkin's disease requires that the Reed-Sternberg cell be present in a biopsy specimen of lymph node tissue. Although the question of neoplastic lineage remains unclear, evidence suggests that the Reed-Sternberg cell, a distinctive giant tumor cell, is derived from the macrophage–monocyte line. This cell may also be found in other disorders, such as infectious mononucleosis. Computed tomographic scans of the abdomen commonly are used in screening for involvement of abdominal and pelvic lymph nodes. Radiologic visualization of the abdominal and pelvic lymph structures can be achieved through the use of bipedal lymphangiography. In this diagnostic test, radiopaque dye is injected into the lymphatic channels of the lower leg, enabling visualization of the iliac and para-aortic nodes. Nuclear studies, such as a gallium scan (in which the tumor takes up the radionuclide), or a staging laparotomy, to detect abdominal nodes and inspect the liver, also may be done.

Both radiation and chemotherapy are used in treating the disease. Most patients with localized disease are treated with radiation therapy. Disseminated Hodgkin's disease usually is treated with combination therapy.

NON-HODGKIN'S LYMPHOMAS

The non-Hodgkin's lymphomas are a group of neoplastic disorders of the lymphoid tissue, usually the lymph nodes. Unlike Hodgkin's disease, which is initially localized to a single group of lymph nodes, the non-Hodgkin's lymphomas typically are multicentric in origin and spread early to various tissues throughout the body, especially the liver, spleen, and bone marrow. In 1992, about 41,000 new cases were reported in the United States and about 19,400 deaths were related to these disorders.[9]

A viral etiology is suspected in at least some of the lymphomas. Cell cultures and immunologic studies of one type of lymphoma, Burkitt's lymphoma, which is found in some parts of Africa, have implicated EBV without proving a causal relation. Serologic studies have also demonstrated an association between the HTLV-I retrovirus and T-cell leukemia/lymphoma. Non-Hodgkin's lymphomas are also seen with increased frequency in people with acquired immunodeficiency syndrome and in those who have received chronic immunosuppressive therapy after kidney or liver transplantation.

As tumors of the immune system, non-Hodgkin's lymphomas may originate from B cells, T cells, or histiocytes (macrophage–monocytes). The vast majority of these lymphomas are of B-cell origin; most of the remaining are of T-cell origin. Histiocytic forms of lymphoma are rare. Non-Hodgkin's lymphomas commonly are divided into three groups, depending on the grade of the tumor: (1) low-grade lymphomas, which are predominantly B-cell tumors; (2) intermediate-grade lymphomas, which include B-cell and some T-cell lymphomas; (3) high-grade, which are largely immunoblastic (B-cell), lymphoblastic (T-cell), Burkitt's, and non-Burkitt's lymphomas.

The signs and symptoms of non-Hodgkin's lymphomas are similar to those of Hodgkin's disease, except for the early involvement of the oropharyngeal lymphoid tissue, skin, gastrointestinal tract, and bone marrow. Leukemic transformation with high peripheral lymphocyte counts occurs in about 13% of persons with non-Hodgkin's lymphomas. There is increased susceptibility to bacterial, viral, and fungal infections associated with hypogammaglobulinemia and poor humoral antibody response, rather than impaired cellular immunity, as seen in Hodgkin's disease.

As with Hodgkin's disease, a lymph node biopsy is used to confirm the diagnosis. Bone marrow biopsy, blood studies, abdominal computed tomographic scans, and nuclear medicine studies often are used to determine the stage of the disease. Treatment depends on the stage of the disease and includes chemotherapy and radiation therapy.

MULTIPLE MYELOMA

Multiple myeloma is a plasma cell cancer of the osseous tissue. In the course of its dissemination, it also may involve nonosseous sites. It is characterized by the uncontrolled proliferation of an abnormal clone of plasma cells, usually of the immunoglobulin G or immunoglobulin A type. In 1992, about 12,500 new cases of multiple myeloma and 9,200 deaths caused by the disease were reported in the United States.[9] Less than 2% of cases occur before age 40, after

which the incidence increases continuously through age 80.[22]

In multiple myeloma, plasma cells that are seldom found in healthy bone marrow proliferate and erode into the hard bone, predisposing to pathologic fractures and hypercalcemia caused by bone dissolution. Paraproteins secreted by the plasma cells may cause a hyperviscosity of body fluids and may break down into amyloid, a proteinaceous substance deposited between cells, causing heart failure and neuropathy. In some forms of multiple myeloma, the plasma cells produce only *Bence Jones proteins*, abnormal proteins that consist of the light chains of the immunoglobulin molecule. Because of their low molecular weight, Bence Jones proteins are excreted in the urine. Many of these abnormal proteins are directly toxic to renal tubular structures, which may lead to tubular destruction and, eventually, renal failure. The malignant plasma cells can also form tumors (plasmacytomas) that have a tendency to cause spinal cord compression.

Bone pain, concentrated in the back, typically is one of the first symptoms present in this form of cancer. Bone destruction also impairs the production of erythrocytes and leukocytes and predisposes to anemia and recurrent infections. Many patients experience weight loss and weakness. Neurologic manifestations caused by neuropathy or spinal cord compression and signs of renal failure also may be present. Treatment is largely palliative and consists mainly of chemotherapy. The combination of α-interferon and chemotherapy has produced remission.[23] Bone marrow transplantation has been used on younger patients. Although the initial response is promising, this approach remains experimental.[24]

In summary, lymphoproliferative disorders affect the cells of the lymphoreticular system, including the lymphocytes and plasma cells. Malignant lymphoproliferative disorders include the leukemias, Hodgkin's disease, non-Hodgkin's lymphomas, and multiple myeloma. Leukemias are classified according to cell type (lymphocytic or myelocytic) and whether the disease is acute or chronic. The lymphocytic leukemias, most common in children, involve the lymphoid precursors that originate in bone marrow but infiltrate the spleen, lymph nodes, CNS, and other tissues. The myelocytic leukemias, which are seen more often in adults, involve the pluripotent myeloid stem cells in bone marrow and interfere with the maturation of all blood cells, including granulocytes, erythrocytes, and thrombocytes. The warning signs and symptoms of acute leukemia are fatigue, paleness, weight loss, repeated infections, easy bruising, and nosebleeds and other hemorrhages. In children, these symptoms may appear suddenly.

The lymphomas—Hodgkin's disease and non-Hodgkin's lymphomas—represent malignant neoplasms of cells native to lymphoid tissue (lymphocytes and histiocytes) and their precursors or derivatives. They are among the most studied human tumors and among the most curable. Hodgkin's disease is characterized by painless and progressive enlargement of a single node or group of nodes. It is believed to originate within one area of the lymphatic system and, if unchecked, will spread throughout the lymphatic network. Non-Hodgkin's lymphomas are a group of neoplastic disorders of the lymphoid tissue, usually the lymph nodes. Unlike Hodgkin's disease, which is initially localized to a single group of lymph nodes, most non-Hodgkin's lymphomas are multicentric in origin and spread early to various tissues throughout the body, especially the liver, spleen, and bone marrow. Multiple myeloma results in the uncontrolled proliferation of plasma cells, usually a single clone of immunoglobulin G– or immunoglobulin A–producing cells.

■ REFERENCES

1. Hays, K. (1990). Physiology of normal bone marrow. *Seminars in Oncology Nursing, 6*(1), 3–8.
2. Fishbach, F. (1992). *A manual of laboratory and diagnostic tests* (4th ed., pp. 20–24). Philadelphia: J.B. Lippincott.
3. Beck, W.S. (Ed.). (1991). *Hematology* (5th ed., pp. 16–20, 371–388). Cambridge, MA: MIT Press.
4. Cormack, D.H. (1987). *Ham's histology* (9th ed, pp. 226–228). Philadelphia: J.B. Lippincott.
5. Smith, L.H., & Their, S.O. (1981). *Pathophysiology* (p. 421). Philadelphia: W.B. Saunders.
6. Koenig, J.M., & Christensen, R.D. (1989). Incidence, neutrophil kinetics, and natural history of neonatal neutropenia associated with maternal hypertension. *New England Journal of Medicine, 321,* 557–562.
7. Schooley, R.T. (1991). Epstein-Barr virus infections including infectious mononucleosis. In J.D. Wilson, E. Braunwald, K.J. Isselbacher, et al. (Eds.). *Harrison's principles of internal medicine* (pp. 689–692). New York: McGraw-Hill.
8. Cotran, R.S., Kumar, V., & Robbins, S.L. (1989). *Pathologic basis of disease* (4th ed., pp. 323–325, 704–705). Philadelphia: W.B. Saunders.
9. American Cancer Society. (1987). *Cancer facts and figures 1987.* Atlanta: American Cancer Society.
10. Jablon, S., & Kato, H. (1972). Studies of the mortality of A-bomb survivors. *Radiation Research, 50,* 658.
11. Pederson-Bjergaard, J., & Larsen, S.O. (1982). Incidence of acute nonlymphocytic leukemia, preleukemia and acute myeloproliferative syndrome up to 10 years after treatment for Hodgkin's disease. *New England Journal of Medicine, 307,* 964.
12. Boise, J.D., Greene, M.H., Killen, J.Y., et al. (1983). Leukemia and preleukemia after adjuvant treatment of gastrointestinal cancer with semustine. *New England Journal of Medicine, 309,* 107.
13. Collman, C.A., & Dahlberg, S. (1990). Treatment-related leukemia. *New England Journal of Medicine, 322,* 52–53.
14. Pui, C., Behm, F.G., & Raimondi, S. (1989). Secondary acute myeloid leukemia in children treated for acute lymphoid leukemia. *New England Journal of Medicine, 321,* 136–142.
15. Negalia, J.P., Meadows, A.T., & Robison, L.L. (1991). Secondary neoplasms after acute lymphoblastic leukemia in children. *New England Journal of Medicine, 325,* 1330–1336.
16. Kurzrock, R., Gulterman, J.U., & Talpaz, M. (1988). The molecular genetics of Philadelphia chromosome–positive leukemia. *New England Journal of Medicine, 319,* 990–998.
17. Pui, C., & Rivera, G.K. (1991). Childhood leukemia. In A.I. Hollieb, D.J. Fink, & G. Murphy (Eds.). *American Cancer Society textbook of clinical oncology* (pp. 433–452). Atlanta: American Cancer Society.
18. Linker, C. (1992). Blood. In S.A. Schroeder, L.M. Tierney, S.J. McPhee, et al. (Eds.). *Current medical diagnosis and treatment* (pp. 408–425). E. Norwalk, CT: Appleton & Lange.
19. Mitus, A.J., & Rosenthal, D.S. (1991). Adult leukemias. In A.I. Hollieb, D.J. Fink, & G. Murphy (Eds.). *American Cancer Society textbook of clinical oncology* (pp. 410–432). Atlanta: American Cancer Society.
20. Kumar, V.K., Cotran, R.S., & Robbins, S.L. (1992). *Basic pathology* (5th ed., pp. 365–372). Philadelphia: W.B. Saunders.
21. Eyre, H.J., & Farver, M.L. (1991). Hodgkin's disease and nonmalignant lymphoma. In A.I. Hollieb, D.J. Fink, & G.P. Murphy (Eds.). *American Cancer Society textbook of clinical pharmacology* (pp. 377–396). Atlanta: American Cancer Society.
22. Bubley, G.J., & Schnipper, L.E. (1991). Multiple myeloma. In A.I. Hollieb, D.J. Fink, & G.P. Murphy (Eds.). *American Cancer Society textbook of clinical pharmacology* (pp. 397–409). Atlanta: American Cancer Society.
23. Oken, M.M. (1992). New agents for the treatment of multiple myeloma and non-Hodgkin's lymphoma. *Cancer, 70*(Suppl. 4), 946–948.
24. Gahrton, G., Tura, S., & Ljungman, P. (1991). Allogeneic bone marrow transplantation in multiple myeloma. *New England Journal of Medicine, 325,* 1267–1273.

■ BIBLIOGRAPHY

Alkire, K., & Collingwood, J. (1990). Physiology of blood and bone marrow. *Seminars in Oncology Nursing, 6*(2), 99–108.

Buchsbaum, R.J., & Schwartz, R.S. (1990). Cellular origins of hematologic neoplasms. *New England Journal of Medicine, 322,* 694–696.

Canello, G.P., & Portlock, C.S. (1992, March 15). Hodgkin's today: It's curable. *Patient Care,* pp. 174–192.

Cheson, B.D., & Lacerna, L. (1989). Autologous bone marrow transplantation: Current status and future directions. *Annals of Internal Medicine, 110,* 51–65.

Chetham, M.M. (1991). Infectious mononucleosis in adolescents. *Pediatric Annals, 20,* 206–212.

Desforges, J.F. (1986). Blast crisis—reversing the direction. *New England Journal of Medicine, 315,* 1478.

Ferrara, J.L.M., & Deeg, H.J. (1991). Graft-versus-host disease. *New England Journal of Medicine, 324,* 667–674.

Freireich, E.J. (1986). Hematologic malignances: Adult acute leukemia. *Hospital Practice, 21*(6), 91.

Lehrer, R.I. (Moderator). (1988). UCLA Conference: Neutrophils and host defense. *Annals of Internal Medicine, 109*(2), 127.

Sullivan, J.L. (1988). Epstein-Barr virus and lymphoproliferative disorders. *Seminars in Hematology, 25,* 269–279.

CHAPTER 17

ALTERATIONS IN HEMOSTASIS

KATHRYN J. GASPARD

Mechanisms of Hemostasis
Vessel Spasm
Formation of the Platelet Plug
Blood Coagulation
Clot Retraction
Clot Dissolution (Fibrinolysis)

Hypercoagulability States
Increased Platelet Function
Increased Clotting Activity
Bleeding Disorders
Platelet Defects

Coagulation DefectsVascular
Disorders
Effects of Drugs on Hemostasis
Anticoagulant Drugs
Thrombolytic Drugs

■ OBJECTIVES

After you have studied this chapter, you should be able to meet the following objectives:

■ State the five stages of hemostasis.
■ Describe the formation of the platelet plug.
■ State the purpose of coagulation.
■ State the function of clot retraction.
■ Trace the process of fibrinolysis.
■ Compare normal and abnormal clotting.
■ State the causes and effects of increased platelet function.
■ State two conditions that contribute to increased clotting activity.
■ State the mechanisms of drug-induced thrombocytopenia and idiopathic thrombocytopenia and the differing features in terms of onset and resolution of the disorders.

■ Describe the manifestations of thrombocytopenia.
■ Describe the role of vitamin K in coagulation.
■ State three common defects of coagulation factors and the causes of each.
■ Differentiate between the mechanisms of bleeding in hemophilia A and von Willebrand's disease.
■ Describe the physiologic basis of acute disseminated intravascular clotting.
■ Describe the effect of vascular disorders on hemostasis.
■ State the mechanism by which aspirin, warfarin, and heparin alter blood clotting.
■ State the mechanism and use of thrombolytic drugs.

The term *hemostasis* refers to the stoppage of blood flow. The normal process of hemostasis is regulated by a complex array of activators and inhibitors that maintain blood fluidity and prevent blood loss from vessels. Hemostasis is normal when it seals a blood vessel, thereby preventing blood loss and hemorrhage. It is abnormal when it causes inappropriate blood clotting or when clotting is insufficient to stop the flow of blood from the vascular compartment. Disorders of hemostasis fall into two main categories:

Carol Mattson Porth: PATHOPHYSIOLOGY: CONCEPTS OF
ALTERED HEALTH STATES, 4th ed. © 1994, 1990, 1986, 1982
J.B. Lippincott Company

(1) the inappropriate formation of clots within the vascular system (thrombosis) and (2) the failure of blood to clot in response to an appropriate stimulus (bleeding).

■ MECHANISMS OF HEMOSTASIS

Hemostasis is divided into five stages: (1) vessel spasm, (2) formation of the platelet plug, (3) blood coagulation or development of an insoluble fibrin clot, (4) clot retraction, and (5) clot dissolution. These steps are summarized in Chart 17-1.

VESSEL SPASM

Vessel spasm is initiated by endothelial injury and caused by local and humoral mechanisms. A spasm constricts the vessel and reduces blood flow. It is a transient event that usually lasts less than 1 minute. Thromboxane A_2, released from the platelets, contributes to vasoconstriction.[1]

FORMATION OF THE PLATELET PLUG

The platelet plug, the second line of defense, is initiated as platelets come in contact with the vessel wall. Platelets, or thrombocytes, are large fragments from the cytoplasm of bone marrow stem cells called the megakaryocytes. They are enclosed in a membrane but have no nucleus. Their life span is only 8 to 9 days. Platelet production presumably is controlled by a substance called thrombopoietin. The source of thrombopoietin is unknown, but it appears that its production and release are regulated by the number of platelets in the circulation. The newly formed platelets that are released from the bone marrow spend up to 8 hours in the spleen before they are released into the blood. Formation of the platelet plug also involves a small protein molecule called *von Wil-*

lebrand's factor. This factor is produced by the endothelial cells of blood vessels and circulates in the blood attached to coagulation factor VIII.

Formation of a platelet plug involves both adhesion and aggregation of platelets (Fig. 17-1A). Platelets are attracted to a damaged vessel wall, become activated, and change from smooth disks to spiny spheres, exposing receptors on their surfaces. Adhesion to the vessel subendothelial layer occurs when the platelet receptor binds to von Willebrand's factor at the injury site, bridging the platelet to exposed collagen. Platelet aggregation occurs as platelets become attached to one another, forming a meshwork. Adenosine diphosphate, thrombin, and thromboxane A_2 (a prostaglandin), released by the platelets, induce the aggregation process.

The coagulation factors become activated on the platelet surface to finally convert fibrinogen to fibrin, thereby stabilizing the platelet plug (Fig. 17-1B). De-

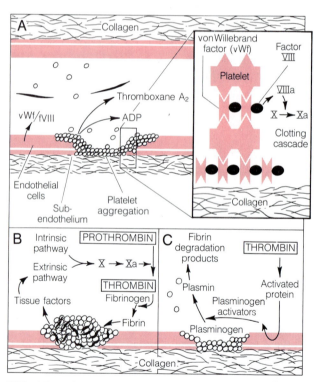

FIG. 17-1. (**A**) The platelet plug occurs seconds after vessel injury. Von Willebrand's factor, released from the endothelial cells, binds to platelet receptors and thus causes *adhesion* of platelets to the exposed collagen. Platelet *aggregation* is induced by release of thromboxane A_2 and adenosine diphosphate. (**B**) Coagulation factors, activated on the platelet surface, lead to the formation of thrombin and fibrin, which stabilize the platelet plug. (**C**) Control of the coagulation process and clot dissolution are governed by thrombin and plasminogen activators. Thrombin activates protein C, which stimulates the release of plasminogen activators. The plasminogen activators in turn promote the formation of plasmin, which digests the fibrin strands.

CHART 17-1: STEPS IN HEMOSTASIS

Vessel spasm
Formation of the platelet plug
Platelet adherence to the vessel wall
Platelet aggregation to form the platelet plug
Blood coagulation
Activation of the intrinsic or extrinsic coagulation
    pathway
Conversion of fibrinogen to fibrin
Clot retraction
Clot dissolution (fibrinolysis)

fective platelet plug formation causes bleeding in people who are deficient in receptor sites or von Willebrand's factor. In addition to sealing vascular breaks, platelets play an almost continuous role in maintaining normal vascular integrity. People with platelet deficiency have increased capillary permeability and develop small skin hemorrhages from the slightest trauma or change in blood pressure.

BLOOD COAGULATION

Blood coagulation is the process by which fibrin strands create a meshwork that cements blood components together (Fig. 17-2). It results from activation of either the intrinsic or the extrinsic coagulation pathways (Fig. 17-3). The intrinsic pathway, which is a relatively slow process, occurs in the vascular system; the extrinsic pathway, which is a much faster process, occurs in the tissues. The terminal steps in both pathways are the same: the activation of factor X and thrombin-induced formation of fibrin, the material that stabilizes a clot. Both pathways are needed for normal hemostasis, and many interrelations exist

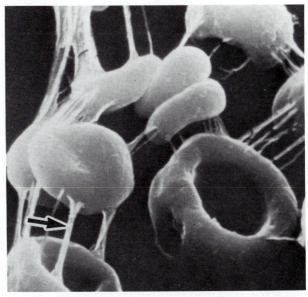

FIG. 17-2. Scanning electron micrograph of a blood clot (×5000). The fibrous bridges (indicated by the *arrow*) that form a meshwork between red blood cells are fibrin fibers. (Chaffee, E. E., & Lytle, I. M. [1980]. *Basic physiology and anatomy* [4th ed.]. Philadelphia: J.B. Lippincott)

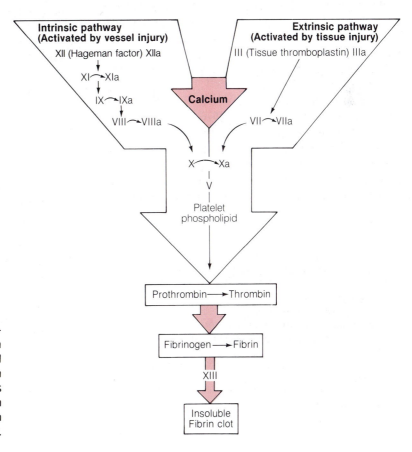

FIG. 17-3. Intrinsic and extrinsic coagulation pathways. The terminal steps in both pathways are the same. Calcium, factors X and V, and platelet phospholipids combine to form prothrombin activator, which then converts prothrombin to thrombin. This interaction causes conversion of fibrinogen into the fibrin strands that create the insoluble blood clot.

between them.[2] Bleeding, when it occurs because of defects in the extrinsic system, usually is not as severe as that which results from defects in the intrinsic pathway. Both systems are activated when blood passes out of the vascular system. The intrinsic system is activated as blood comes in contact with the injured vessel wall; the extrinsic system is activated when blood is exposed to tissue extracts.

The purpose of the coagulation process is to form an insoluble fibrin clot. This process is controlled by many substances that either promote clotting (procoagulation factors) or inhibit it (anticoagulation factors). Each of the procoagulation factors, identified by Roman numerals, performs a specific step in the coagulation process. The action of one coagulation factor is designed to activate the next factor in the sequence (cascade effect). Because most of the inactive procoagulation factors are present in the blood at all times, the multistep process ensures that a massive episode of intravascular clotting does not occur by chance. It also means that abnormalities of the clotting process occur when one or more of the factors are deficient or when conditions lead to inappropriate activation of any of the steps. Calcium (factor IV) is required in all but the first two steps of the clotting process. The body usually has sufficient amounts of calcium for these reactions. Inactivation of the calcium ion is used to prevent blood that has been removed from the body from clotting. The addition of citrate to blood stored for transfusion purposes prevents clotting by combining with the calcium ions. Both oxalate and citrate often are added to blood samples used for analysis in the clinical laboratory.

Coagulation is also regulated by several natural anticoagulants. Antithrombin III inactivates coagulation factors and neutralizes thrombin. When complexed with naturally occurring heparin, its action is accelerated and provides protection against uncontrolled thrombus formation on the endothelial surface. Protein C, on combining with its receptor, thrombomodulin, inhibits thrombin and several coagulation factors. Protein S accelerates the action of protein C. Deficiencies of antithrombin III, protein C, or protein S result in hypercoagulable states and increased risk for thromboembolism.[3]

CLOT RETRACTION

After the clot has formed, clot retraction, which requires large numbers of platelets, contributes to hemostasis by joining the edges of the broken vessel.

CLOT DISSOLUTION (FIBRINOLYSIS)

The dissolution of a blood clot begins shortly after its formation; this allows blood flow to be reestablished

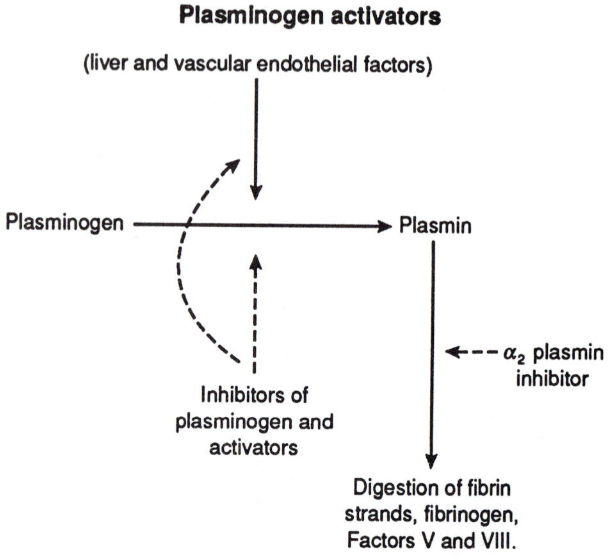

FIG. 17-4. Fibrinolytic system and its modifiers. The *solid lines* indicate activation, and the *broken lines* indicate inactivation.

and permanent tissue repair to take place (see Figure 17-1C). The process by which a blood clot dissolves is called fibrinolysis. As with clot formation, clot dissolution requires a sequence of steps controlled by activators and inhibitors (Fig. 17-4). *Plasminogen*, the proenzyme for the fibrinolytic process, normally is present in the blood in its inactive form. It is converted to its active form, *plasmin*, by plasminogen activators formed in the vascular endothelium, liver, and kidneys. The plasmin formed from plasminogen digests the fibrin strands of the clot as well as certain clotting factors, such as fibrinogen, factor V, and factor VIII. Circulating plasmin is rapidly inactivated by α_2-plasmin inhibitor, which limits fibrinolysis to the local clot and prevents it from occurring in the entire circulation.

There are two naturally occurring plasminogen activators: tissue-type plasminogen activator (t-PA) and urokinase-type plasminogen activator.[1] The liver, plasma, and vascular endothelium are the major sources of physiologic activators. These activators are released in response to a number of stimuli, including vasoactive drugs, venous occlusion, elevated body temperature, and exercise. The activators are unstable and rapidly inactivated by inhibitors synthesized by the endothelium and the liver. For this reason, chronic liver disease may cause altered fibrinolytic activity. A major inhibitor, PAI-1, in high concentrations has been associated with deep vein thrombosis and myocardial infarction.[4]

In summary, hemostasis is designed to maintain the integrity of the vascular compartment. The process is divided into five phases: (1) vessel spasm, which constricts the size of the vessel and reduces blood flow; (2) platelet adherence and formation of the platelet plug; (3) formation of the fibrin clot, which cements the platelet plug together; (4) clot retraction, which pulls the edges of the injured vessel together; and (5) clot dissolution, which involves the action of plasmin that dissolves the clot and allows blood flow to be reestablished and tissue healing to take place. Blood coagulation requires the stepwise activation of coagulation factors, carefully controlled by activators and inhibitors.

■ HYPERCOAGULABILITY STATES

There are two general forms of hypercoagulability states or thrombosis: (1) conditions that create increased platelet function and (2) conditions that cause accelerated activity of the coagulation system. Arterial thrombi are composed of platelet aggregates, and venous thrombi are fibrin complexes that result from excess coagulation.[5] Chart 17-2 summarizes conditions commonly associated with hypercoagulability states. (Thrombosis is discussed more fully in Chapter 20.)

INCREASED PLATELET FUNCTION

The causes of increased platelet function are (1) disturbances in flow and endothelial damage and (2) increased sensitivity of platelets to factors that cause adhesiveness and aggregation. Atherosclerotic plaques disturb flow, cause endothelial damage, and promote platelet adherence. Platelets that adhere to the vessel wall release growth factors that cause proliferation of smooth muscle and thereby contribute to the development of atherosclerosis. Smoking, elevated levels of blood lipids and cholesterol, hemodynamic stress, diabetes mellitus, and immune mechanisms may cause vessel damage, platelet adherence, and, eventually, thrombosis. Cancer, inflammation, and myeloproliferative disease often are associated with an elevated platelet count and a tendency toward thrombosis.[6]

INCREASED CLOTTING ACTIVITY

Factors that increase the activation of the coagulation system are (1) stasis of blood flow and (2) alterations in the coagulation components of the blood (either an increase in procoagulation factors or a decrease in anticoagulation factors). Stasis causes the accumulation of activated clotting factors and platelets and prevents their interactions with inhibitors. Slow and disturbed flow is a common cause of venous thrombosis in the immobilized or postsurgical patient. Heart failure also contributes to venous congestion and thrombosis. Elevated levels of estrogen increase coagulation factors. The incidence of stroke, thromboemboli, and myocardial infarction is greater in women who use oral contraceptives, particularly after age 35, and in heavy smokers.[7] Clotting factors are also increased during normal pregnancy; these changes, along with limited activity during the puerperium (immediate post-birth period), predispose to venous thrombosis. Hypercoagulability is common in cancer and sepsis. Many tumor cells are thought to release tissue factor molecules, which, along with the increased immobility and sepsis seen in patients with malignant disease, contribute to thrombosis in these patients.

A reduction in anticoagulants such as antithrombin III, protein C, and protein S predisposes to venous thrombosis.[3] Deficiencies of these inhibitor proteins are uncommon, inherited defects.

In summary, hypercoagulability causes excessive clotting and contributes to thrombus formation. It results from (1) conditions that create increased platelet function or (2) conditions that cause accelerated activity of the coagulation system. Increased platelet function usually results from disorders such as atherosclerosis that damage the vessel endothelium and disturb blood flow or from conditions such as smoking that cause increased sensitivity of platelets to factors that promote adhesiveness and aggregation. Factors that cause accelerated activity of the coagulation system include the stasis of blood flow, resulting in an accumulation of coagulation factors, and alterations in the components of the coagulation system (either an increase in procoagulation factors or a decrease in anticoagulation factors).

CHART 17-2: CONDITIONS ASSOCIATED WITH HYPERCOAGULABILITY STATES

Increased Platelet Function

Atherosclerosis
Diabetes mellitus
Smoking
Elevated blood lipid and cholesterol levels
Increased platelet levels

Accelerated Activity of the Clotting System

Pregnancy and the puerperium
Use of oral contraceptives
Postsurgical state
Immobility
Congestive heart failure
Malignant diseases

■ BLEEDING DISORDERS

Bleeding disorders or impairment of blood coagulation can result from defects in any of the factors that contribute to hemostasis. Defects are associated with latelets, coagulation factors, and vascular integrity.

PLATELET DEFECTS

Bleeding can occur as a result of either a decrease in the number of circulating platelets (thrombocytopenia) or impaired platelet function (thrombocytopathia).

The depletion of platelets must be relatively severe (10,000 to 20,000/μL compared with the normal values of 150,000 to 400,000/μL) before hemorrhagic tendencies become evident. Bleeding that results from platelet deficiency is characterized by petechiae (pinpoint purplish red spots) and purpura (purple areas of bruising) on the arms and thighs. Bleeding from mucous membranes of the nose, mouth, gastrointestinal tract, and vagina is characteristic.[8] Bleeding of the intracranial vessels is a rare danger with severe platelet depletion.

THROMBOCYTOPENIA

Platelets are produced by cells in the bone marrow and then stored in the spleen before being released into the circulation. Consequently, a decrease in the number of circulating platelets, a condition called *thrombocytopenia*, can result from a decrease in platelet production by the bone marrow, an increased pooling of platelets in the spleen, or decreased platelet survival.

Loss of bone marrow function in aplastic anemia (discussed in Chapter 18) or replacement of bone marrow by malignant cells, such as occurs in leukemia, results in decreased production of platelets. Radiation therapy and drugs such as those used in the treatment of cancer may depress bone marrow function and reduce platelet production. On the other hand, there may be normal production of platelets but excessive pooling of platelets in the spleen. The spleen normally sequesters about 30% to 40% of the platelets. When the spleen is enlarged (splenomegaly), however, as many as 80% of the platelets can be sequestered in the spleen. In acute disseminated intravascular clotting (DIC), excessive platelet consumption leads to a deficiency. Premature destruction of platelets occurs by a variety of immune mechanisms (*i.e.*, antibodies produced against the platelet).

Drug-Induced Thrombocytopenia. Some drugs, such as quinine, quinidine, and certain antibiotics, induce thrombocytopenia. These drugs act as a hapten (see Chapter 13) and induce antigen–antibody response and formation of immune complexes that cause platelet destruction. In people with drug-associated thrombocytopenia, there is a rapid fall in platelet count within 2 to 3 days of resuming a drug that the person has previously taken for 7 or more days (the time needed to develop an immune response) after starting a drug for the first time. The platelet count rises rapidly once the drug is discontinued. The anticoagulant drug heparin has been increasingly implicated in thrombocytopenia.[9]

Idiopathic Thrombocytopenic Purpura. *Idiopathic thrombocytopenic purpura*, an autoimmune disorder of unknown mechanisms, results in platelet antibody formation and excess destruction of platelets. Although the antibody may bind to platelets in the circulation, the platelets are destroyed in the spleen. In children, acute idiopathic thrombocytopenic purpura commonly follows a viral infection and is a self-limited disorder. In contrast, the adult form seldom follows an infection and usually is chronic. It is a disease of young people, with a peak incidence between ages 20 and 50, and is seen twice as often in females as in males. The condition typically presents precipitously with signs of bleeding, often into the skin (purpura and petechiae) or oral mucosa. Other common types of bleeding are epistaxis (nosebleeds) and abnormal menstrual bleeding. Because the spleen is the site of platelet destruction, splenic enlargement is common. Diagnosis usually is based on severe thrombocytopenia (platelet counts less than 10,000/μL) and splenomegaly. Tests for the platelet antibody are available but lack specificity (*e.g.*, they react with platelet antibodies from other sources). Treatment includes the use of corticosteroid drugs, splenectomy, and, in cases of severe bleeding, high-dose intravenous immunoglobulin.

THROMBOCYTOPATHIA

Impaired platelet function may result from inherited disorders of adhesion (*e.g.*, von Willebrand's disease, discussed later) or acquired defects caused by drugs, disease, or extracorporeal circulation.

Aspirin, which inhibits the production of thromboxane A_2 required for platelet aggregation, is one of the most common causes of platelet impairment. The effect of aspirin on platelet aggregation lasts for the life of the platelet—usually about 7 to 8 days. Nonsteroidal antiinflammatory drugs have a similar effect that is reversible in about 6 hours.[10] Aspirin commonly is used to prevent formation of arterial thrombi. A 1989 report indicated a 44% reduction in risk of myocardial infarction in people over age 50 who had taken low doses of aspirin.[11] Chart 17-3 lists other drugs that impair platelet function. Defective platelet function is also common in uremia, presumably because of unexcreted waste products. Cardiopulmonary bypass also causes platelet defects and destruction.

CHART 17-3: DRUGS THAT MAY PREDISPOSE TO BLEEDING

Interference with Platelet Production or Function

Acetazolamide
Alcohol
Antimetabolite and anticancer drugs
Antibiotics such as penicillin and the cephalosporins
Aspirin and salicylates
Carbamazepine
Clofibrate
Colchicine
Dextran
Dipyridamole
Thiazide diuretics
Gold salts
Heparin
Nonsteroidal anti-inflammatory drugs
Quinine derivatives (quinidine and hydroxychloroquine)
Sulfinpyrazone
Sulfonamides

Interference with Coagulation Factors

Amiodarone
Anabolic steroids
Coumadin
Heparin

Decrease in Vitamin K Levels

Antibiotics
Clofibrate

COAGULATION DEFECTS

Impairment of blood coagulation can result from deficiencies of one or more of the known clotting factors. Deficiencies can arise because of defective synthesis, inherited disease, or increased consumption of the clotting factors.

IMPAIRED SYNTHESIS

Coagulation factors V, VII, IX, X, XI, and XII; prothrombin; and fibrinogen are synthesized in the liver. In liver disease, synthesis of these clotting factors is reduced and bleeding may result. Of the coagulation factors synthesized in the liver, factors VII, IX, and X and prothrombin require the presence of vitamin K for normal activity. In vitamin K deficiency, the liver produces the clotting factor but in an inactive form. Vitamin K is a fat-soluble vitamin that is continuously being synthesized by intestinal bacteria. This means that a deficiency in vitamin K is not likely to occur unless intestinal synthesis is interrupted or absorption of the vitamin is impaired. Vitamin K deficiency can occur in the newborn infant prior to the establishment of the intestinal flora; it can

also occur as a result of treatment with broad-spectrum antibiotics that destroy intestinal flora. Because vitamin K is a fat-soluble vitamin, its absorption requires bile salts. A vitamin K deficiency, therefore, may result from impaired fat absorption caused by liver or gallbladder disease.

HEREDITARY DISORDERS

Hereditary defects have been reported for each of the clotting factors; most, however, are rare diseases. The most common are factor VIII deficiencies. Hemophilia A affects 1 in 10,000 males, and von Willebrand's disease occurs in 1 in 10,000 persons.[12] Factor IX deficiency (hemophilia B) occurs in about 1 in 50,000 persons and is genetically and clinically similar to hemophilia A.

Hemophilia. Circulating factor VIII is a complex molecule of three subunits. The first, factor VIII coagulant protein is the functional portion produced by the liver and endothelial cells. The second, von Willebrand's factor, synthesized by the endothelium and megakaryocytes, binds and stabilizes factor VIII in the circulation and is required for platelet adhesion. The third subunit, factor VIII–related antigen, has no known function in coagulation.

Hemophilia is a sex-linked recessive disorder that primarily affects males. Although it is a hereditary disorder, there is no family history of the disorder in about one third of newly diagnosed cases, suggesting that it has arisen as a new mutation.[12] About 90% of persons with hemophilia produce insufficient quantities of the factor and 10% produce a defective form. The percentage of normal factor VIII activity in the circulation varies with the severity of hemophilia (*i.e.*, 5% to 20% in mild hemophilia, 1% to 5% in moderate hemophilia, and 1% or less in severe forms of hemophilia). In mild or moderate forms of the disease, bleeding usually does not occur unless there is a local lesion or trauma. The mild disorder may not be detected in childhood. On the other hand, in severe hemophilia, bleeding usually is present in childhood (it may be noted at the time of circumcision) and is both spontaneous and severe. Bleeding occurs in soft tissues, the gastrointestinal tract, and the hip, knee, and ankle joints. Joint bleeding is followed by fibrosis and contractures and is a major cause of disability. Minimizing injury and preventing bleeding are primary concerns.

When bleeding occurs, factor VIII replacement therapy is initiated. *Cryoprecipitate*, prepared from fresh frozen plasma, contains factor VIII. Highly purified factor VIII and factor IX concentrates are also available for people with severe hemophilia. Before blood was tested for infectious diseases, these products were prepared from multiple donor samples and carried a high risk of exposure to viruses for hepatitis and acquired immunodeficiency syndrome. Pasteurized or antibody-purified concentrates have reduced the transmission of hepatitis viruses and human immunodeficiency virus. In addition, the lyophilized concentrates make self-administration convenient. Factor VIII produced by recombinant DNA technology promises to eliminate the risk of disease transmission and will soon be available for patient use.[2]

Von Willebrand's Disease. Von Willebrand's disease, which typically is diagnosed in adulthood, is the most common hereditary bleeding disorder. Transmitted as an autosomal trait, it is caused by a deficiency of von Willebrand's factor. This deficiency results in reduced platelet adhesion (discussed previously). Because von Willebrand's factor carries factor VIII, its deficiency may also be accompanied by reduced levels of factor VIII and results in defective clot formation. Symptoms include bruising, excessive menstrual flow, and bleeding from the nose, mouth, and gastrointestinal tract. Many people with the disorder are diagnosed when surgery or dental extraction results in prolonged bleeding.[13] In severe cases, cryoprecipitate is infused to replace von Willebrand's factor and factor VIII. Many people can now be treated with desmopressin acetate (DDAVP), a synthetic analogue of the hormone vasopressin, which stimulates the endothelial cells to release von Willebrand's factor and factor VIII. DDAVP can also be used to treat mild hemophilia A and platelet dysfunction caused by uremia, heart bypass, and the effects of aspirin.[14]

ABNORMAL CONSUMPTION

Disseminated intravascular coagulation (DIC) is a paradox in the hemostatic sequence in which blood coagulation, clot dissolution, and bleeding all take place at the same time. The condition begins with massive activation of the coagulation sequence that overwhelms the normal control mechanisms. Clot formation consumes all available coagulation proteins and platelets, and severe hemorrhage results. The fibrinolytic system is activated, releasing products of fibrin degradation, which act as natural anticoagulants and contribute to further bleeding.

DIC is not a primary disorder; it occurs as a complication in various disease conditions. The coagulation process can be initiated by activation of either the extrinsic pathway, through liberation of tissue factors, or the intrinsic pathway, through extensive endothelial damage caused by viruses, infections, and immune mechanisms or stasis of blood. Obstetric disorders that involve necrotic placental or fetal tissue commonly are associated with DIC. Other

inciting clinical conditions include massive trauma, burns, sepsis, shock, meningococcemia, and malignant disease. Chart 17-4 summarizes the conditions associated with DIC.

Although the coagulation and formation of microemboli initiate the events that occur in DIC, its acute manifestations usually are more directly related to the bleeding problems that occur. The bleeding may be present as petechiae, purpura, oozing from puncture sites, or severe hemorrhage. Uncontrolled postpartum bleeding may indicate DIC. Microemboli may obstruct blood vessels and cause tissue hypoxia and necrotic damage to organ structures, such as the kidneys, heart, lungs, and brain. A form of hemolytic anemia may develop as red cells are damaged as they pass through vessels partially blocked by thrombus.

The treatment of DIC is directed toward managing the primary disease, replacing clotting components, and preventing further activation of clotting mechanisms. Transfusions of fresh frozen plasma, platelets, or fibrinogen-containing cryoprecipitate may correct the clotting factor deficiency. Heparin may be given to decrease blood coagulation, thereby

---

CHART 17-4: CONDITIONS THAT HAVE BEEN ASSOCIATED WITH DIC

Obstetric Conditions

Abruptio placenta
Dead fetus syndrome
Preeclampsia and eclampsia
Amniotic fluid embolism

Cancers

Metastatic cancer
Leukemia

Infections

Acute bacterial infections (*e.g.,* meningococcal meningitis)
Acute viral infections
Rickettsial infections (*e.g.,* Rocky Mountain spotted fever)
Parasitic infection (*e.g.,* malaria)

Shock

Septic shock
Severe hypovolemic shock

Trauma or Surgery

Burns
Massive trauma
Surgery involving extracorporeal circulation
Snake bite
Heatstroke

Hematologic Conditions

Blood transfusion reactions

interrupting the clotting process. Heparin therapy is controversial, however, and the risk of hemorrhage may limit its use to severe cases. It typically is given as a continuous intravenous infusion that can be interrupted promptly if bleeding is accentuated.

VASCULAR DISORDERS

Vascular disorders may cause bleeding from small blood vessels. These disorders occur because of structurally weak vessels or vessels that have been damaged by inflammation or immune responses. Among the vascular disorders that cause bleeding are hemorrhagic telangiectasia, an uncommon autosomal dominant trait in which there are dilatations of capillaries and arterioles; vitamin C deficiency (scurvy), in which the vessel walls become extremely fragile because of failure of the endothelial cells to be cemented together properly and failure to form the collagen fibers that normally are present in the vessel walls; Cushing's disease, in which excess corticosteroid hormone causes protein wasting and loss of vessel tissue support; and senile purpura (bruising in elderly people). Vascular defects also occur in the course of DIC as a result of the presence of the microthrombi and corticosteroid therapy.

Vascular disorders are characterized by easy bruising and the spontaneous appearance of petechiae and purpura of the skin and mucous membranes. In people with bleeding disorders caused by vascular defects, the platelet count and other tests for coagulation factors are normal.

In summary, bleeding disorders or impairment of blood coagulation can result from defects in any of the factors that contribute to hemostasis: platelets, coagulation factors, or vascular integrity. The number of circulating platelets can be decreased (thrombocytopenia) or platelet function can be impaired (thrombocytopathia). Impairment of blood coagulation can result from deficiencies of one or more of the known clotting factors. Deficiencies can arise because of defective synthesis (liver disease or vitamin K deficiency), inherited diseases (hemophilia or von Willebrand's disease), or increased consumption of the clotting factors (DIC). Bleeding may also occur from structurally weak vessels that result from impaired synthesis of vessel wall components (vitamin C deficiency, excessive cortisol levels as in Cushing's disease, or the aging process) or that have been damaged by genetic mechanisms (hemorrhagic telangiectasis) or the presence of microthrombi.

■ EFFECTS OF DRUGS ON HEMOSTASIS

A number of drugs serve to either enhance or impair hemostasis. Oral contraceptives and corticosteroids are associated with an increase in coagulation factors. Drugs that impair platelet production and function

and those that interfere with coagulation are summarized in Chart 17-3.

ANTICOAGULANT DRUGS

Therapeutic agents commonly are used to prevent thrombus formation. Antiplatelet drugs, particularly aspirin, are used to prevent arterial thrombi. In low doses, aspirin increases survival after myocardial infarction, decreases the incidence of stroke, and assists in maintaining the patency of bypass grafts.[14]

The anticoagulant drugs warfarin and heparin are used to prevent venous thrombi and thromboembolic disease, such as deep vein thrombosis and pulmonary embolism. Warfarin acts by decreasing prothrombin and other procoagulation factors. It blocks the regeneration of vitamin K and, therefore, reduces its availability to participate in synthesis of the vitamin K–dependent coagulation factors in the liver. Warfarin's maximum effect takes 36 to 72 hours because of preformed clotting factors that remain in the circulation. It is given orally and interacts with many drugs. The major adverse effect is bleeding, which can be reversed with vitamin K.

Heparin is naturally formed in large quantities in mast cells and in the basophilic cells of the blood. Pharmacologic preparations of heparin are extracted from animal tissues. Heparin must be injected because it is not absorbed in the gastrointestinal tract. It binds to antithrombin III, forming a complex that inactivates some clotting factors and inhibits the action of thrombin. The effect of heparin is immediate and is reversed with protamine sulfate.

THROMBOLYTIC DRUGS

Thrombolytic drugs convert plasminogen to plasmin and, therefore, cause lysis of an existing clot. They are used to treat acute coronary occlusion, deep vein thrombosis, and pulmonary embolism. Streptokinase, a protein elaborated by certain β-hemolytic streptococci, is inexpensive and widely used but may cause hypersensitivity reactions in people previously infected with streptococcus. Urokinase, prepared from human kidney cells, is also effective but costly. An alternative fibrinolytic drug, t-PA, is produced by DNA recombinant techniques and identical to the natural tissue plasminogen activator. t-PA is localized to the clot, binding more avidly to the fibrin than streptokinase. It is used early in acute myocardial infarction to limit damage and preserve left ventricular function.[15] Anisoylated plasminogen streptokinase activator complex (antistreplase; APSAC) is a conjugate of streptokinase that is inactive until the anisolyl group is activated, which gradually occurs after it is injected. The drug is concentrated at the site of the thrombus and is activated locally. It can be injected as a bolus and provide continuing thrombolytic activity.

In summary, a number of drugs serve to either enhance or impair hemostasis. Oral contraceptives and corticosteroids are associated with an increase in coagulation factors. Therapeutic agents commonly are used to prevent thrombus formation. Antiplatelet drugs, particularly aspirin, are used to prevent arterial thrombi. The anticoagulant drugs warfarin and heparin are used to prevent venous thrombi (e.g., deep vein thrombosis) and emboli. Thrombolytic drugs convert plasminogen to plasmin and, therefore, cause lysis of an existing clot. They frequently are used to treat acute coronary occlusion.

▪ REFERENCES

1. Jaffe, E.A. (1990). Vascular function in hemostasis. In W.J. Williams, E. Beutler, A.J. Erslev, & M.A. Lichtman (Eds.). *Hematology* (4th ed., p. 1327). New York: McGraw-Hill.
2. Roberts, H.R., & Lozier, J.N. (1992). New perspectives on the coagulation cascade. *Hospital Practice, 27,* 97.
3. Moake, J.L. (1991). Hypercoagulable states: New knowledge about old problems. *Hospital Practice, 26,* 31.
4. Rosenberg, R.D. (1991). Hemorrhagic disorders: 1. Protein interactions in the clotting mechanism. In W.S. Beck (Ed.). *Hematology* (5th ed., p. 540). Cambridge, MA: MIT Press.
5. Clark, W.G., Brater, D.C., & Johnson, A.R. (1992). *Goth's medical pharmacology* (13th ed., p. 452). St. Louis: Mosby-Year Book.
6. Rifkind, R.A., Bank, A., Marks, P.A., Kaplan, K.L., Ellison, R.R., & Lindenbaum, J. (1986). *Fundamentals of hematology* (3rd ed., p. 183). Chicago: Year Book Medical Publishers.
7. Goldfien, A. (1989). The gonadal hormones and inhibitors. In B.G. Katzung (Ed.). *Basic and clinical pharmacology* (4th ed., p. 505). E. Norwalk, CT: Appleton & Lange.
8. Babior, B.M., & Stossel, T.P. (1990). *Hematology: A pathophysiological approach* (2nd ed., p. 213). New York: Churchill Livingstone.
9. Harrington, L., & Hufnagel, J.M. (1990). Heparin-induced thrombocytopenia and thrombosis: A case study. *Heart and Lung, 19,* 93–99.
10. Kuter, D.J. (1991). Hemorrhagic disorders: 2. Platelets. In W.S. Beck (Ed.). *Hematology* (5th ed., p. 571). Cambridge, MA: MIT Press.
11. Steering Committee Physicians' Health Study Research Group. (1989). Final report on the aspirin content of the ongoing physicians' health study. *New England Journal of Medicine, 321,* 129.
12. Kuter, D.J., & Rosenberg, R.D. (1991). Hemorrhagic disorders: 2. Disorders of hemostasis. In W.S. Beck (Ed.). *Hematology* (5th ed., p. 588). Cambridge, MA: MIT Press.
13. Rapaport, S.I. (1987). *Introduction to hematology* (2nd ed., pp. 510, 528). Philadelphia: J.B. Lippincott.
14. Aledort, L.M. (1989). New approaches to management of bleeding disorders. *Hospital Practice, 24,* 207.
15. Schreiber, T.L. (1989). Aspirin and thrombolytic therapy for acute myocardial infarction: Should the combination now be routine therapy? *Drugs, 38,* 180.
16. Simoons, M.L. (1989). Thrombolytic therapy in acute myocardial infarction. *Annual Review of Medicine, 40,* 181.

▪ BIBLIOGRAPHY

Andrew, M., Paes, B., Milner, R., et al. (1987). Development of the human coagulation system in the full-term infant. *Blood, 70,* 165.

Beller, F.K., & Ebert, C. (1985). Effects of oral contraceptives on blood coagulation. A review. *Obstetrical and Gynecological Survey, 40,* 425.

Benedict, C.R., Mueller, S., Anderson, H.V., & Willerson, J.T. (1992). Thrombolytic therapy: A state of the art review. *Hospital Practice, 27,* 61.

Bennett, J.S. (1992). Mechanisms of platelet adhesion and aggregation: An update. *Hospital Practice, 27,* 124.

Berkman, S.A. (1992). Current concepts in anticoagulation. *Hospital Practice, 27(2),* 187.

Bloom, A.L. (1991). Von Willebrand factor: Clinical features of inherited and acquired disorders. *Mayo Clinic Proceedings, 66,* 743.

Brettler, D.B., & Levine P.H. (1989). Factor concentrates for treatment of hemophilia: Which one to choose? *Blood, 73,* 2067.

Broze, G.J. (1992). Why do hemophiliacs bleed? *Hospital Practice, 27,* 71.

Carr, M.E. (1987). Disseminated intravascular coagulation: Pathogenesis, diagnosis, and therapy. *Journal of Emergency Medicine, 5,* 311.

Gerrard, J.M. (1988). Platelet aggregation: Cellular regulation and physiologic role. *Hospital Practice, 23,* 89.

Hirsh, J. (1991). Heparin. *New England Journal of Medicine, 324,* 1565.

Kurachi, K., Yao, S., Furukawa, M., et al. (1992). Deficiencies in factors IX and VIII: What is now known. *Hospital Practice, 27(2),* 41.

Lucas, F.V., & Miller, M.L. (1988). The fibrinolytic system. *Cleveland Clinic Journal of Medicine, 55,* 531.

Mannucci, P.M., Schimpf, K., Abe, T., et al. (1992). Low risk of viral infection after administration of vapor-heated factor VIII concentrate. *Transfusion, 32,* 134.

Patrono, C. (1989). Aspirin and human platelets: From clinical trials to acetylation of cyclooxygenase and back. *TIPS, 10,* 453.

Robertson, G.L., & Harris, A. (1989). Clinical use of vasopressin analogues. *Hospital Practice, 24,* 114.

Salzman, E.W., Weinstein, M.J., & Weintraub, R.M. (1986). Treatment with desmopressin acetate to reduce blood loss after cardiac surgery. *New England Journal of Medicine, 314,* 1402.

Scharfstein, J., & Loscalzo, J. (1992). Molecular approaches to antithrombotic therapy. *Hospital Practice, 27,* 77.

Sherry, S., & Marder, V.J. (1991). Thrombosis, fibrinolysis, and thrombolytic therapy: A perspective. *Progress in Cardiovascular Diseases, 34(2),* 89.

Weintraub, P.S. (1987). Hemophilia A: Virus transmission and immunity in factor VIII therapy. *Laboratory Manual, 25,* 53.

Wu, K.K. (1992). Endothelial cells in hemostasis: Thrombosis and inflammation. *Hospital Practice, 27(4),* 145.

ALTERATIONS IN OXYGENATION OF TISSUES

CHAPTER 18

THE RED BLOOD CELL AND ALTERATIONS IN OXYGEN TRANSPORT

KATHRYN J. GASPARD

◼ OBJECTIVES

After you have studied this chapter, you should be able to meet the following objectives:

◼ Trace the development of a red blood cell from erythroblast to erythrocyte.

◼ Describe the formation, transport, and elimination of bilirubin.

◼ Explain the function of the enzyme glucose-6-phosphate dehydrogenase in the red blood cell.

◼ State the meaning of the red blood cell count, percentage of reticulocytes, hemoglobin, hematocrit, mean corpuscular volume, and mean corpuscular hemoglobin concentration as it relates to the diagnosis of anemia.

◼ Describe the manifestations of anemia and their mechanisms.

◼ Explain the difference between intravascular and extravascular hemolysis.

◼ Compare the hemoglobinopathies associated with sickle cell anemia and thalassemia.

◼ Explain the cause of sickling in sickle cell anemia.

◼ Cite common causes of iron-deficiency anemia in infancy, adolescence, and adulthood.

◼ Describe the relation between vitamin B_{12} deficiency and megaloblastic anemia.

◼ List three causes of aplastic anemia.

◼ Compare characteristics of the red blood cells in acute blood loss, hereditary spherocytosis, sickle cell anemia, iron-deficiency anemia, and aplastic anemia.

◼ Compare polycythemia vera and secondary polycythemia.

◼ Differentiate between red cell antigens and antibodies in people with type A, B, AB, or O blood.

◼ Explain the determination of the Rh factor.

◼ List the signs and symptoms of a blood transfusion reaction.

◼ Cite the function of hemoglobin F in the neonate and describe the red blood cell changes that occur during the early neonatal period.

◼ Cite the factors that predispose to hyperbilirubinemia in the infant.

◼ Describe the pathogenesis of hemolytic disease of the newborn.

Carol Mattson Porth: PATHOPHYSIOLOGY: CONCEPTS OF ALTERED HEALTH STATES, 4th ed. © 1994, 1990, 1986, 1982 J.B. Lippincott Company

■ Compare conjugated and unconjugated bilirubin in terms of production of encephalopathy in the neonate.

■ Explain the action of phototherapy in the treatment of hyperbilirubinemia in the neonate.

■ State the changes in the red blood cells that occur with aging.

Although the lungs provide the means for gas exchange between the external and internal environment, it is the hemoglobin in the red blood cells that transports oxygen to the tissues. The red blood cells also function as carriers of carbon dioxide and participate in acid–base balance. The function of the red blood cells, in terms of oxygen transport, is discussed in Chapter 26, and acid–base balance is covered in Chapter 30. This chapter focuses on the red blood cell, anemia, and polycythemia.

■ THE RED BLOOD CELL

The mature red blood cell (erythrocyte) is a non-nucleated concave, spherical disk (Fig. 18-1). This shape serves to increase the surface area available for diffusion of oxygen and allows the cell to change in volume and shape without rupturing its membrane. The biconcave form presents the plasma with a surface 20 to 30 times greater than if the red blood cell were an absolute sphere. The erythrocytes, 500 to 1000 times more numerous than other blood cells, are the most common type of blood cell.

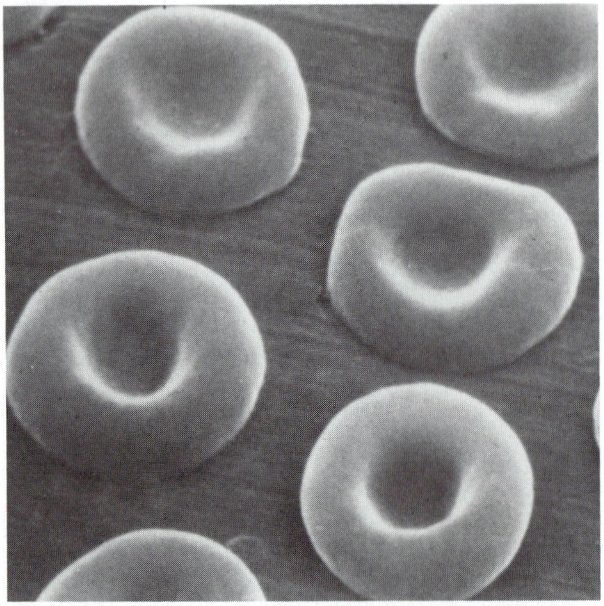

The function of the red blood cell, facilitated by the hemoglobin molecule, is to transport oxygen to the tissues. In addition, hemoglobin binds some carbon dioxide and carries it from the tissues to the lungs. The hemoglobin molecule is composed of two pairs of structurally different polypeptide chains (Fig. 18-2). Each of the four polypeptide chains is attached to a heme unit, which in turn surrounds an atom of iron that binds oxygen. The rate at which hemoglobin is synthesized depends on the availability of iron for heme synthesis. The lack of iron results in relatively small amounts of hemoglobin in the red blood cells.

There are two types of normal hemoglobin: adult hemoglobin (HbA) and fetal hemoglobin (HbF). *HbA* consists of a pair of α *chains* and a pair of β *chains*. *HbF* is the predominant hemoglobin in the fetus from the 3rd through the 9th month of gestation. It has a pair of γ *chains* substituted for the β chains. Because of this chain substitution, HbF has a high affinity for oxygen. This facilitates the transfer of oxygen across the placenta. HbF is replaced within 6 months of birth with HbA.

FIG. 18-1. Scanning micrograph of normal red blood cells (×5000). The normal concave appearance of these cells is apparent. (Courtesy STEM Laboratories and Fischer Scientific Company)

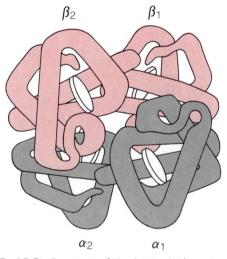

FIG. 18-2. Structure of the hemoglobin molecule.

RED CELL PRODUCTION AND REGULATION

Erythropoiesis is the production of red blood cells. After birth, red cells are produced in the red bone marrow. Until age 5, almost all bones produce red cells to meet growth needs. After this period, bone marrow activity gradually declines; after age 20, red cell production takes place mainly in the membranous bones of the vertebrae, sternum, ribs, and pelvis.[1] With this reduction in activity, the red bone marrow is replaced with fatty yellow bone marrow.

The red cells derive from the erythroblasts, which are continuously being formed from the primordial stem cells in the bone marrow (Fig. 18-3). In developing into a mature red cell, the primordial stem cell moves through a series of divisions, each producing a smaller cell. Hemoglobin synthesis begins at the erythroblast stage and continues until the cell becomes an erythrocyte. During its transformation from normoblast to reticulocyte, the red blood cell loses its nucleus. The period from stem cell to emergence of the reticulocyte in the circulation normally takes about 1 week. Maturation of reticulocyte to erythrocyte takes about 24 to 48 hours. During this process, the red cell loses its mitochondria and ribosomes along with its ability to produce hemoglobin and engage in oxidative metabolism. Most maturing red cells enter the blood as reticulocytes. About 1% of red blood cells are generated from bone marrow each

day; therefore, the reticulocyte count serves as an index of the erythropoietic activity of the bone marrow.

The red blood cell relies on glucose and the glycolytic pathway for its metabolic needs. The enzyme-mediated anaerobic metabolism of glucose generates adenosine triphosphate (ATP), needed for normal membrane function and ion transport. The depletion of glucose or the functional deficiency of one of the glycolytic enzymes leads to the premature death of the red blood cell. An offshoot of the glycolytic pathway provides a large amount of 2,3-diphosphoglycerate (2,3-DPG), which reduces the affinity of hemoglobin for oxygen. This facilitates the release of oxygen at the tissue level, particularly in hypoxia and anemia.[2]

Two additional pathways prevent the oxidation of hemoglobin by environmental oxidants. The methemoglobin reductase pathway prevents the oxidation of hemoglobin to methemoglobin, a nonfunctional molecule with reduced oxygen-carrying capacity. The pentose phosphate pathway depends on the enzyme glucose-6-phosphate dehydrogenase (G6PD). In the presence of environmental oxidants, G6PD activity prevents oxidative denaturation of hemoglobin, with resultant red cell injury and lysis.[3]

Erythropoiesis is governed, for the most part, by tissue oxygen needs. *Hypoxia* is the main *stimulus* for red cell production but does not act directly on the bone marrow. Instead, oxygen is sensed by the kidneys, which then produce the hormone *erythro-*

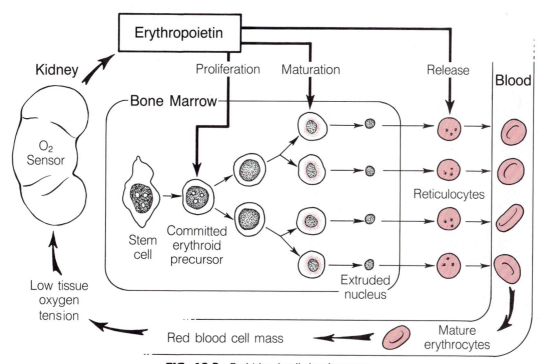

FIG. 18-3. Red blood cell development.

poietin. Erythropoietin, a glycoprotein with a molecular weight of about 38,000, is produced primarily by the interstitial and endothelial cells that line the peritubular capillaries.[4] About 5% to 10% of erythropoietin is released by the liver and other tissues.

Erythropoietin takes several days to effect this release of red blood cells from the bone marrow, and only after 5 or more days does red blood cell production reach maximum. Erythropoietin probably binds to a specific bone marrow receptor and stimulates committed stem cells to differentiate into erythroblasts.[5] Because red blood cells are released into the blood as reticulocytes, the percentage of these cells is higher when there is a marked increase in red blood cell production. In some severe anemias, for example, the reticulocytes may account for as much as 30% of the total red cell count. In some situations, red cell production is so accelerated that numerous normoblasts appear in the blood. Human erythropoietin (EPO) is now produced by deoxyribonucleic acid (DNA)-recombinant technology. It has revolutionized the management of anemia in chronic renal failure; other potential uses include controlling blood loss during surgery.[6]

RED CELL DESTRUCTION

Mature red blood cells have a life span of about 4 months, or 120 days. As the red blood cell ages, a number of changes occur. The metabolic activities within the cell decrease, enzyme activity falls off, and ATP, potassium, and membrane lipids decrease. The rate of red cell destruction (1% per day) normally is equal to red cell production, but in some conditions, such as hemolytic anemia, the cell's life span may be shorter.

The destruction of red blood cells is accomplished by a group of large phagocytic cells found in the spleen, liver, bone marrow, and lymph nodes. These phagocytic cells recognize old and defective red cells and ingest and destroy them in a series of enzymatic reactions. During these reactions, the amino acids from the globulin chains and iron from the heme units are salvaged and reused. The bulk of the heme unit is converted to bilirubin (the pigment of bile), which is insoluble in plasma and attaches to the plasma proteins for transport. Bilirubin is removed from the blood by the liver and conjugated with glucuronide to render it water-soluble so that it can be excreted in the bile. The plasma-insoluble form of bilirubin is referred to as unconjugated bilirubin; the water-soluble form is referred to as conjugated bilirubin. Serum levels of conjugated and unconjugated bilirubin can be measured in the laboratory and are reported as direct and indirect, respectively.

If red cell destruction and consequent bilirubin production are excessive, unconjugated bilirubin accumulates in the blood. This results in a yellow discoloration of the skin—*jaundice* (discussed in Chapter 42).

When red blood cell destruction takes place in the circulation, as in hemolytic anemia, the hemoglobin remains in the plasma. The plasma contains a hemoglobin-binding protein called haptoglobin. Other plasma proteins, such as albumin, may also bind hemoglobin. With extensive intravascular destruction of red blood cells, hemoglobin levels may exceed the hemoglobin-binding capacity of haptoglobin. When this happens, free hemoglobin appears in the blood (hemoglobinemia) and is excreted in the urine (hemoglobinuria). Because excessive red blood cell destruction can occur in hemolytic transfusion reactions, urine samples are tested for free hemoglobin after a transfusion reaction.

LABORATORY TESTS

Red blood cells can be studied by means of a sample of blood (Table 18-1). In the laboratory, automated blood cell counters rapidly provide accurate measurements of red cell content and cell indices. The *red blood cell count* measures the *total number* of red blood cells in a cubic millimeter of blood. The *percentage of reticulocytes* (normally about 1%) provides an index of the rate of red cell production. The *hemoglobin* (grams per 100 mL of blood) measures the *hemoglobin content* of the blood. The major components of blood are the red cell mass and plasma volume. The *hematocrit* measures the volume of red cell mass in 100 mL of plasma volume. To determine the hematocrit, a sample of blood is placed in a glass tube, which is then centrifuged to separate the cells and the plasma. The hematocrit may be deceptive because it varies with the quantity of extracellular fluid present, rising with dehydration and falling with overexpansion of extracellular fluid volume.

Red cell indices are used to distinguish types of anemias by size or color of red cells. The *mean corpuscular volume (MCV)* reflects the *volume* or *size* of the red cells. The MCV falls in microcytic (small cell) anemia and rises in macrocytic (large cell) anemia. Some anemias are normocytic (*i.e.*, cells are of normal size or MCV. The *mean corpuscular hemoglobin concentration (MCHC)* is the *concentration of hemoglobin* in each cell. Anemias are described as normochromic (normal color or MCHC) or hypochromic (decreased color or MCHC). Mean cell hemoglobin (MCH) refers to the mass of the red cell and is less useful in classifying anemias.

A stained blood smear provides information

TABLE 18-1. STANDARD LABORATORY VALUES FOR RED BLOOD CELLS

TEST	NORMAL VALUES	SIGNIFICANCE
Red blood cell count (RBC)		
Men	4.2–5.4 million/µL)	Number of red cells in the blood
Women	3.6–5 million/µL	
Reticulocytes	1.0%–1.5% of total RBC	Rate of red cell production
Hemoglobin		
Men	14–16.5 g/dL	Hemoglobin content of the blood
Women	12–15 g/dL	
Hematocrit		
Men	40%–50%	Volume of cells in 100 mL of blood
Women	37%–47%	
Mean corpuscular volume	85–100 fL/red cell	Size of the red cell
Mean corpuscular hemoglobin concentration	31–35 g/dL	Concentration of hemoglobin in the red cell
Mean cell hemoglobin	27–34 pg/cell	Red cell mass

about the size, color, and shape of red cells as well as the presence of immature or abnormal cells. If blood smears are abnormal, examination of the bone marrow may be important. Marrow commonly is aspirated with a special needle from the posterior iliac crest or the sternum. The aspirate is stained and observed for number and maturity of cells and abnormal types.[7]

In summary, the red blood cell provides the means for transporting oxygen from the lungs to the tissues. Red cells develop from stem cells in the bone marrow and are released into the blood as reticulocytes, where they become mature erythrocytes. The life span of a red blood cell is about 120 days. Red cell destruction normally occurs in the spleen, liver, bone marrow, and lymph nodes. In the process of destruction, the heme portion of the hemoglobin molecule is converted to bilirubin. Bilirubin, which is insoluble in plasma, attaches to plasma proteins for transport in the blood. It is removed from the blood by the liver and conjugated to a water-soluble form so that it can be excreted in the bile.

■ ANEMIA

In anemia, the number of circulating red blood cells or the hemoglobin level, or both, may be abnormally low, resulting in diminished oxygen-carrying capacity. There may be (1) excessive loss (bleeding) or destruction (hemolysis) of red blood cells or (2) deficient red blood cell production because of a lack of nutritional elements or bone marrow failure.

MANIFESTATIONS

Anemia is not a disease but rather an indication of some disease process or alteration in body function. The manifestations of anemia can be grouped into three categories: (1) impaired oxygen transport, (2) alterations in red cell structure, and (3) signs and symptoms associated with the pathologic process that is causing the anemia. The manifestations of anemia also depend on its severity, the rapidity of its development, and the patient's age and health status. With rapid blood loss, circulatory shock and circulatory collapse may occur. On the other hand, the body adapts to slowly developing anemia, and the loss of red cell mass may reach 50% without the occurrence of signs and symptoms.[4]

In anemia, the oxygen-carrying capacity of hemoglobin is reduced, causing tissue hypoxia. Tissue hypoxia can give rise to angina, night cramps, fatigue, weakness, and dyspnea. The redistribution of the blood from cutaneous tissues or a lack of hemoglobin causes pallor of the skin, mucous membranes, conjunctiva, and nail beds. Tachycardia and palpitations may occur as the body tries to compensate with an increase in cardiac output. A flow-type systolic murmur, resulting from changes in blood viscosity, may occur. Ventricular hypertrophy and high-output heart failure may develop in severe anemia or in elderly people even at hemoglobin levels of 10 g/dL.[8] Erythropoietin activity is accelerated and may be recognized by diffuse bone pain and sternal tenderness. The production of 2,3-DPG is a compensatory mechanism that reduces the hemoglobin affinity for oxygen, as evidenced by a shift to the right in the oxygen–hemoglobin saturation curve; this causes more oxygen to be released to the tissues rather than remaining bound to hemoglobin. In addition to the common anemic manifestations, hemolytic anemias are accompanied by jaundice, caused by increased blood levels of bilirubin. In aplastic anemia, petechiae and purpura (red spots caused by small-vessel bleeding) are the result of reduced platelet function.

BLOOD LOSS ANEMIA

With anemia caused by bleeding, iron and other components of the erythrocyte are lost from the body. Blood loss may be acute or chronic. In the acute form, there is a risk of hypovolemia and shock rather than anemia (see Chapter 25). The red cells are normal in size and color. A fall in the red blood cell count, hematocrit, and hemoglobin results from hemodilution caused by movement of fluid into the vascular compartment. The hypoxia that results from blood loss stimulates red cell production by the bone marrow. If the bleeding is controlled and sufficient iron stores are available, the red cell concentration returns to normal within 3 to 4 weeks. Chronic blood loss does not affect blood volume but instead leads to iron-deficiency anemia. The red cells that are produced have too little hemoglobin, giving rise to microcytic hypochromic anemia.

HEMOLYTIC ANEMIAS

Hemolytic anemia is characterized by the premature destruction of red cells with retention in the body of iron and the other products of red cell destruction. Almost all types of hemolytic anemia are distinguished by the presence of normocytic and normochromic red cells. Because of the red blood cell's shortened life span, the bone marrow usually is hyperactive, resulting in an increase in the number of reticulocytes in the circulating blood. As with other types of anemias, there is easy fatigability, dyspnea, and other signs and symptoms of impaired oxygen transport. In addition, mild jaundice often is present. In hemolytic anemia, red cell breakdown can occur within the vascular compartment, or it can result from phagocytosis by the reticuloendothelial system. Intravascular hemolysis is manifested by hemoglobinemia and hemoglobinuria.

The cause of hemolytic anemia can be either intrinsic or extrinsic to the red blood cell. Intrinsic causes include defects of the red cell membrane, the various hemoglobinopathies, and inherited enzyme defects. Acquired forms of hemolytic anemia are caused by agents extrinsic to the red blood cell, such as drugs, bacterial and other toxins, antibodies, and trauma. Although all these factors can cause premature and accelerated destruction of red cells, they cannot all be treated in the same way. Some respond to splenectomy, others respond to treatment with adrenocorticosteroid hormones, and still others do not resolve until the primary disorder is corrected.

INHERITED DISORDERS OF THE RED CELL MEMBRANE

Hereditary spherocytosis, transmitted as an autosomal dominant trait, is the most common inherited disorder of the red cell membrane. The disorder leads to gradual loss of the membrane surface during the life span of the red blood cell, resulting in a tight sphere instead of a concave disk. Although the spherical cell retains its ability to transport oxygen, its shape renders it susceptible to destruction as it passes through the venous sinuses of the splenic circulation. A life-threatening aplastic crisis may occur when a sudden disruption of red cell production (in most cases caused by a viral infection) causes a rapid drop in hematocrit and the hemoglobin level. The disorder usually is treated with splenectomy to reduce red cell destruction.

HEMOGLOBINOPATHIES

Abnormalities in hemoglobin structure can lead to accelerated red cell destruction. Two main types of hemoglobinopathies can cause red cell hemolysis: (1) the abnormal substitution of an amino acid in the hemoglobin molecule, as in sickle cell anemia, and (2) defective synthesis of one of the polypeptide chains that form the globin portion of hemoglobin, as in the thalassemias.

Sickle Cell Anemia. Sickle cell disease affects about 50,000 (0.1% to 0.2%) black Americans. About 9% of black Americans carry the trait.[9] In sickle cell anemia, there is a defect in the β chain of the hemoglobin molecule, with an abnormal substitution of a single amino acid. Sickle hemoglobin (HbS) is transmitted by recessive inheritance and can be present as either sickle cell trait (heterozygote) or sickle cell disease (homozygote). In the heterozygote, only about 40% of the hemoglobin is HbS, whereas in the homozygote, almost all the hemoglobin is HbS.

In the homozygote, the HbS becomes sickled when deoxygenated. Sickling occurs when one HbS molecule interacts with another, causing a semisolid polymer that changes the shape and deformability of the cell (Fig. 18-4). These deformed red cells obstruct blood flow in the microcirculation, causing tissue hypoxia. The person with sickle cell trait who has less HbS has little tendency to sickle except in hypoxia. HbF does not interact with HbS; therefore, most children with sickle cell anemia do not begin to experience the effects of the sickling until sometime after 4 to 6 months of age, when the HbF has been replaced by HbS.

The factors associated with sickling include exer-

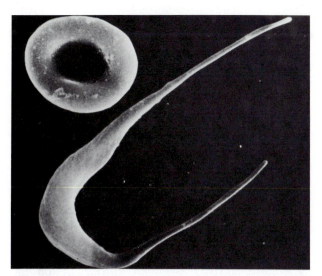

FIG. 18-4. Photograph of a sickled cell and a normal red blood cell taken under the auspices of the Comprehensive Sickle Cell Center, University of Miami. (Photo by Dr. Bruce R. Cameron) (Smeltzer, S. C., & Bare, B. G. [1992]. *Brunner and Suddarth's textbook of medical-surgical nursing* [7th ed., p. 795]. Philadelphia: J.B. Lippincott)

tion, infection, other illnesses, hypoxia, acidosis, dehydration, or even such trivial incidents as reduced oxygen tension induced by sleep. Hardly an organ is spared in sickle cell anemia. Affected people develop severe anemia, painful crises, organ damage, and chronic hyperbilirubinemia. A painful crisis results from vessel occlusion and can occur suddenly in almost any part of the body. Common sites are the abdomen, chest, and joints. Infarctions caused by sluggish blood flow may cause chronic damage to the liver, spleen, heart, kidneys, and other organs. The hyperbilirubinemia that results from the breakdown products of hemoglobin often leads to the production of pigment stones in the gallbladder. Children experience growth retardation and reduced spleen function with frequent infections.

There is no known cure or therapeutic regimen that prevents the problems associated with sickle cell anemia, and treatment is largely supportive. The patient is advised to avoid situations that precipitate sickling episodes, such as infections, cold exposure, severe physical exertion, acidosis, and dehydration. Infections are aggressively treated, and blood transfusions may be warranted in a crisis. A promising experimental treatment using hydroxyurea allows synthesis of more HbF and less HbS, thereby decreasing sickling.[10]

Thalassemias. In contrast to sickle cell anemia, the thalassemias result from absent or defective synthesis of either the α or the β chains of hemoglobin.

The β-thalassemias represent a defect in β-chain synthesis, and the α-thalassemias represent a defect in α-chain synthesis. The defect is inherited as a mendelian trait, and a person may be heterozygous for the trait and have a mild form of the disease or be homozygous and have the full-blown disease. Like sickle cell anemia, the thalassemias occur with high degree of frequency in certain populations. The β-thalassemias, sometimes called *Cooley's anemia* or *Mediterranean anemia*, are most common in Mediterranean populations (southern Italy and Greece), and the α-thalassemias are most common among Asians. Both α- and β-thalassemias are common in Africans and black Americans.

Two factors contribute to the anemia that occurs in thalassemia: reduced hemoglobin synthesis and an imbalance in globin chain production. In both α- and β-thalassemia, defective globin chain production leads to deficient hemoglobin production and the development of a hypochromic microcytic anemia. The unaffected type of chain continues to be synthesized, accumulates in the red cell, and contributes to red cell destruction and anemia. In β-thalassemia, the excess α chains are denatured to form precipitates (Heinz bodies) within the bone marrow red cell precursors. These Heinz bodies impair DNA synthesis and cause damage to the red cell membrane. Severely affected red cell precursors are destroyed in the bone marrow, and those that escape intramedullary death are at increased risk of destruction in the spleen.

The clinical manifestations of β-thalassemias are based on the severity of the anemia. The presence of one normal gene in heterozygous people usually results in sufficient normal hemoglobin synthesis to prevent severe anemia. People who are homozygous for the trait have severe transfusion-dependent anemia. Severe growth retardation is present in children with the disorder. An increased hematopoiesis causes bone marrow expansion and increases iron absorption, and splenomegaly and hepatomegaly result from increased red cell destruction. Bone marrow expansion leads to thinning of the cortical bone, with new bone formation evident on the maxilla and frontal bones of the face (chipmunk facies). The long bones, ribs, and vertebrae may become vulnerable to fracture. Frequent transfusions prevent most of these complications and enable the patient to survive to the second or third decade.[11] Excess iron stores, which accumulate secondary to increased dietary absorption and repeated transfusions, are deposited in the myocardium, liver, and pancreas and induce organ injury and congestive heart failure.

Synthesis of the α-globin chains of hemoglobin is controlled by two pairs of genes; hence, α-thalassemia shows great variations in severity. Silent carriers have deletion of a single α-globin gene and are asymptomatic. The severest form of α-thalassemia occurs in infants in whom all four α-globin genes are deleted. Such a defect results in a hemoglobin molecule (Hb Bart's) that is formed exclusively from the chains of HbF. Hb Bart's, which has an extremely high oxygen affinity, cannot release oxygen in the tissues. Affected infants suffer from severe hypoxia and either are stillborn or die shortly after birth. Deletion of three of the four α-chain genes leads to unstable aggregates of β chains called *hemoglobin H* (HbH). The β chains are more soluble than the α chains; therefore, their accumulation is less toxic to the red cells, so that senescent, rather than precursor, red cells are affected. Most people with HbH have only mild to moderate hemolytic anemia, and manifestations of ineffective erythropoiesis (bone marrow expansion and iron overload) are absent.

INHERITED ENZYME DEFECTS

The most common inherited enzyme defect that results in hemolytic anemia is a deficiency of G6PD. The gene that determines this enzyme is located on the X chromosome, and the defect is expressed only in males and homozygous females. There are many genetic variants of this disorder. The African variant has been found in 10% of black Americans.[9] The disorder makes red cells more vulnerable to oxidants and causes direct oxidation of hemoglobin to methemoglobin as well as the denaturing of the hemoglobin molecule to form *Heinz* bodies. Hemolysis usually occurs as the damaged red blood cells move through the narrow vessels of the spleen, causing hemoglobinemia, hemoglobinuria, and jaundice. In blacks, the defect is mildly expressed and is not associated with chronic hemolytic anemia unless triggered by oxidant drugs or infection. The antimalarial drugs primaquine and quinacrine, the sulfonamides, nitrofurantoin, aspirin, phenacetin, and other drugs cause hemolysis. Free radicals generated by phagocytes during infections are possible triggers also.[12] A severer deficiency of G6PD is found in people of Mediterranean descent (eg, Sardinians, Sephardic Jews, and Arabs). In some of these people, chronic hemolysis occurs in the absence of exposure to oxidants. The disorder can be diagnosed through the use of a G6PD assay or screening test.

ACQUIRED HEMOLYTIC ANEMIAS

A number of acquired factors, exogenous to the red blood cell, produce hemolysis by direct membrane destruction or by antibody-mediated lysis. Various drugs, chemicals, toxins, venoms, and infections such as malaria destroy red cell membranes. Hemo-

lysis may also be caused by mechanical factors such as prosthetic heart valves, vasculitis and severe burns. Some hemolytic anemias are immune-mediated (*i.e.*, caused by antibodies that destroy the red cell). Autoantibodies may be produced by a person in response to drugs and disease. Alloantibodies come from an exogenous source and are responsible for transfusion reactions and hemolytic disease of the newborn.

The antibodies that cause red cell destruction fall into two categories: warm-reacting antibodies of the immunoglobulin G (IgG) type, which are maximally active at 37° C, and cold-reacting antibodies of the immunoglobulin M (IgM) type, which are optimally active at or near 4° C.

The warm-reacting antibodies cause no morphologic or metabolic alteration in the red cell. Instead, they react with antigens on the red cell membrane, causing destructive changes that lead to spherocytosis, with subsequent phagocytic destruction in the spleen or reticuloendothelial system. They lack specificity for the ABO antigens but may react with the Rh antigens. The hemolytic reactions associated with the warm-reacting antibodies have varied causes; about 60% are idiopathic, 25% to 30% are drug-induced, and most of the remainder are related to cancers of the lymphoproliferative system (chronic lymphocytic leukemia and lymphoma) or collagen diseases (systemic lupus erythematosus).[13] The antihypertensive drug α-methyldopa produces almost 70% of drug-induced hemolysis, and penicillin accounts for about 23%.[14]

The cold-reacting antibodies activate complement. Chronic hemolytic anemia caused by cold-reacting antibodies occurs with lymphoproliferative disorders and as an idiopathic disorder of unknown cause. The hemolytic process occurs in distal body parts, where the temperature may fall below 30° C. Vascular obstruction by red cells results in pallor, cyanosis of the body parts exposed to cold temperatures, and Raynaud's phenomenon (see Chapter 20). Hemolytic anemia caused by cold-reacting antibodies develops in only a few people.

The Coombs' test, or antiglobulin test, is used to diagnose hemolytic anemia. It detects the presence of antibody or complement on the surface of the red cell. The direct antiglobulin test (DAT) detects the antibody on red blood cells. In this test, red cells that have been washed free of serum are mixed with anti-human globulin reagent. The red cells agglutinate if the reagent binds to and bridges the antibody or complement on adjacent red cells. The DAT is positive in autoimmune hemolytic anemia, erythroblastosis fetalis (Rh disease of the newborn), transfusion reactions, and drug-induced hemolysis. The indirect antiglobulin test (IAT) detects the presence of antibody in the serum and is positive in the presence of specific antibodies. It is used for antibody detection and crossmatching before transfusion.

ANEMIAS OF DEFICIENT RED CELL PRODUCTION

Anemia may result from the decreased production of erythrocytes by the bone marrow. A deficiency of nutrients for hemoglobin synthesis (iron) or DNA synthesis (cobalamin or folic acid) may reduce red cell production by the bone marrow. A deficiency of red cells also results when the marrow itself fails or is replaced by nonfunctional tissue.

IRON-DEFICIENCY ANEMIA

Iron is an integral constituent of the heme in the hemoglobin molecule, and its deficiency leads to a decrease in hemoglobin synthesis with a decrease in serum iron. The red cells are decreased in number and are microcytic, hypochromic, and often malformed (poikilocytosis). The laboratory values indicate reduced MCHC and MCV. Membrane changes may predispose to hemolysis, causing further loss of red cells.

Body iron is repeatedly reused. When red cells become senescent and are broken down, their iron is released and reused in the production of new red cells. The normal diet contains about 12 to 15 mg of iron of which about 1 mg is absorbed daily.[15] In iron deficiency, absorption increases. Less than 1 mg of iron normally is lost from the body daily. About 30% of body iron is stored in the bone marrow, spleen, muscle, and other organs; the remainder is present in the form of hemoglobin.

In the adult, chronic blood loss is the usual reason for iron deficiency. In men and postmenopausal women, blood loss may be due to gastrointestinal bleeding, such as occurs with peptic ulcer, intestinal polyps, hemorrhoids, or cancer. Excessive aspirin intake may cause undetected gastrointestinal bleeding. In women, blood lost during menstruation may contain from 0.7 to 2.0 mg of iron, causing deficiency.[15] Although cessation of menstruation spares iron loss in the pregnant woman, iron requirements increase at this time. The expansion of the mother's blood volume requires about 480 mg of additional iron and the growing fetus requires about 390 mg, averaging about 3.6 mg of iron daily.

A child's growth places extra demands on the body: blood volume increases, with a greater need for iron. Iron requirements are proportionally higher in infancy (3 to 24 months) than at any other age,

although they are also increased in childhood and adolescence.

In infancy, the two main causes of iron-deficiency anemia are low iron levels at birth (because of maternal deficiency) and a diet consisting mainly of cow's milk, which is low in absorbable iron. Thirty percent of infants in low-income populations are reported to be anemic.[16]

The signs and symptoms of iron-deficiency anemia are related to impaired oxygen transport and lack of hemoglobin. Depending on the severity of the anemia, fatigability, palpitations, dyspnea, angina, and tachycardia may occur. Epithelial atrophy is common and results in waxy pallor, brittle hair and nails, smooth tongue, sores in the corners of the mouth, and, sometimes, dysphagia and decreased acid secretion. A poorly understood symptom that sometimes is seen is pica, the bizarre compulsive eating of ice or dirt.

The treatment of iron-deficiency anemia is directed toward controlling chronic blood loss, increasing dietary intake of iron, and administering supplemental iron. Ferrous sulfate, which is the usual oral replacement therapy, replenishes iron stores in 3 to 6 months.[17] Parenteral iron may be given if oral forms are not tolerated. Special care is required when administering an iron preparation (such as Imferon) intramuscularly; it must be injected deeply by pulling the skin to one side before inserting the needle (Z-track) to prevent leakage into the tissues with skin discoloration.

MEGALOBLASTIC ANEMIAS

Megaloblastic anemias are caused by abnormal nucleic acid synthesis that results in enlarged red cells (MCV greater than 100) and deficient nuclear maturation. Cobalamin (vitamin B_{12}) and folic acid deficiencies result in megaloblastic anemia. (One form of megalo blastic anemia, unresponsive to either vitamin B_{12} or folic acid therapy, is not discussed here.) Because megaloblastic anemias develop slowly, there are often few symptoms until the anemia is far advanced.

Cobalamin (Vitamin B_{12})–Deficiency Anemia. Vitamin B_{12} is essential for the synthesis of DNA. When it is deficient, nuclear maturation and cell division, especially of the rapidly proliferating red cells, fail to occur. Moreover, when vitamin B_{12} is deficient, the red cells that are produced are abnormally large, have flimsy membranes, and are oval rather than biconcave. These oddly shaped cells have a short life span that can be measured in weeks rather than months. The MCV is elevated and the MCHC is normal. The most common form of anemia caused by vitamin B_{12} deficiency is pernicious anemia, resulting from diminished intestinal absorption of B_{12}. The absorption of vitamin B_{12} in the intestine requires the presence of *intrinsic factor*, which is produced by the gastric mucosa. Intrinsic factor binds to vitamin B_{12} in food, protects it from the enzymatic actions of the gut, and facilitates its absorption. As discussed in Chapter 41, chronic atrophic gastritis is an autoimmune disorder that destroys the gastric mucosa and produces antibodies that interfere with the action of intrinsic factor, which leads to pernicious anemia.

Neurologic changes accompany the disorder. Degeneration of the dorsal and lateral columns of the spinal cord causes symmetric paresthesias of the feet and fingers, which eventually progress to spastic ataxia. Lifelong treatment consisting of intramuscular injections of vitamin B_{12} reverse the anemia and improve the neurologic changes.

Folic Acid–Deficiency Anemia. Folic acid is also required for red cell maturation, and its deficiency produces the same type of red cell changes that occur in vitamin B_{12}–deficiency anemia (*i.e.*, increased MCV and normal MCHC). Symptoms are also similar, but the neurologic manifestations are not present.

Folic acid is readily absorbed from the intestine. It is found in vegetables (particularly the green leafy types), fruits, cereals, and meats. Much of the vitamin, however, is lost in cooking. The most common cause of folic acid deficiency is malnutrition, especially in association with alcoholism, and malabsorption syndromes such as sprue. Because pregnancy increases the need for folic acid 5- to 10-fold, a deficiency can occur at this time. Poor dietary habits, anorexia, and nausea are other reasons for folic acid deficiency during pregnancy. In neoplastic disease, tumor cells compete for folate, and deficiency is common.[18] Some drugs used to treat seizure disorders (*e.g.*, primidone, phenytoin, and phenobarbital) and triamterene (a diuretic) predispose to a deficiency by interfering with folic acid absorption. Methotrexate (a folic acid analogue used in the treatment of cancer) impairs the action of folic acid by blocking its conversion to the active form.

BONE MARROW DEPRESSION (APLASTIC ANEMIA)

Aplastic anemia describes a primary condition of bone marrow stem cells that results in a reduction of all three hematopoietic cell lines (red cells, white cells, and platelets) with fatty replacement of bone marrow. True red cell aplasia (in which only the red cells are affected) can occur but is rare.

Anemia results from the failure of the marrow to replace senescent red cells that are destroyed and leave the circulation, although the cells that remain are of normal size and color. At the same time, because the leukocytes, particularly the neutrophils, and the thrombocytes have a short life span, a deficiency of these cells usually is apparent before the anemia becomes severe.

The onset of aplastic anemia may be insidious, or it may strike with suddenness and great severity. It can occur at any age. The initial presenting symptoms include weakness, fatigability, and pallor caused by anemia. Petechiae (small punctate skin hemorrhages) and ecchymoses (bruises) often are present on the skin, and there may be bleeding from the nose, gums, vagina, or gastrointestinal tract because of decreased platelet levels. The decrease in the number of neutrophils increases susceptibility to infection.

Among the causes of aplastic anemia are exposure to high doses of radiation and chemical agents that are toxic to bone marrow. The best-documented of the identified toxic agents are benzene, the antibiotic chloramphenicol, and the alkylating agents and antimetabolites used in the treatment of cancer (see Chapter 5). Aplastic anemia caused by exposure to a chemical agent may be an idiosyncratic reaction; that is, it affects only certain susceptible people. Such reactions often are severe and sometimes irreversible and fatal. Aplastic anemia can develop in the course of many infections and has been reported most often as a complication of viral hepatitis, mononucleosis, and other viral illnesses, including acquired immunodeficiency syndrome. In two thirds of cases, the cause is unknown, and these are termed *idiopathic aplastic anemia*.

Therapy for aplastic anemia in the young and severely affected includes bone marrow transplantation. Histocompatible donors supply stem cells to replace the patient's destroyed marrow cells. Graft-versus-host disease and infections are major risks of the procedure, yet up to 70% survival is reported.[19] Immunosuppressive therapy with lymphocyte immune globulin (antithymocyte globulin) prevents suppression of proliferating stem cells, producing remission in 50% of patients.[19] Patients with aplastic anemia should avoid the offending agents and be treated with antibiotics for infection. Red cell transfusions to correct the anemia and platelets and corticosteroid therapy to minimize bleeding may also be required.

Bone marrow depression often occurs secondary to cancer treatment. Chemotherapy and irradiation commonly cause anemia and deficiency of platelets and leukocytes as a result of bone marrow depression.

CHRONIC DISEASE ANEMIAS

Chronic renal failure almost always results in a normocytic, normochromic anemia, primarily because of a deficiency of erythropoietin. Uremic toxins also interfere with the actions of erythropoietin and red cell production. In addition, they cause hemolysis and bleeding tendencies, which contribute to the anemia. Until recently, dialysis and red cell transfusions were the only therapy. Recombinant erythropoietin injected several times a week for 12 or more weeks dramatically elevates the hemoglobin level and hematocrit and eliminates the need for transfusions.[19]

Anemia often occurs as a complication of chronic infections, inflammation, and cancer. Many other underlying causes shorten the life span of red cells and reduce iron availability. Mild to moderate anemia usually is not treated.

In summary, anemia describes a condition in which the red cell mass is decreased. It is not a disease but a manifestation of some disease process or alteration in body function. Anemia typically is caused by the excessive loss of red cells (blood loss or destruction) or by impaired production. The manifestations of anemia include those associated with (1) impaired oxygen transport, (2) alterations in red blood cell structure, and (3) the signs and symptoms of the underlying process causing the anemia.

■ TRANSFUSION THERAPY

Anemias of various causes are treated with transfusions of whole blood or red blood cells only when oxygen delivery to the tissues is compromised, as evidenced by measures of oxygen transport and use as well as hemoglobin and hematocrit.[20] Acute massive blood loss usually is replaced with whole blood transfusion. Most anemias, however, are treated with transfusions of red cell concentrates, which supply only the blood component that is deficient. Since the 1960s, devices that mechanically separate a unit of blood into its constituents provide not only red cell components but also platelets, fresh frozen plasma, cryoprecipitate, and clotting factor concentrates. In this way, a unit of blood can be used efficiently for several recipients to correct specific deficiencies.

Several red cell components that are used for transfusion are prepared and stored under specific conditions and have unique uses, as described in Table 18-2. These red cell components are derived principally from voluntary blood donors.

The use of *autologous* donation and transfusion has recently been advocated. Autologous transfusion refers to the procedure of receiving one's own blood—usually to replenish a surgical loss—thereby eliminating the risk of blood-borne disease or transfusion reaction. Up to 10% of red cell transfusions could be provided by the recipient.[21] Autologous blood can be provided by several means: predeposit, hemodilution, and intraoperative salvage. A patient who is anticipating elective surgery (plastic or orthopedic) may predeposit blood (*i.e.*, have his blood collected up to 6 weeks in advance and stored) for later transfusion during the surgery. Hemodilution involves phlebotomy before surgery with transfusion of the patient's blood at the completion of surgery. The procedure requires the use of fluid infusions to maintain blood volume and is limited to open heart surgery. Intraoperative blood salvage is the collection of blood shed from the operative site for reinfusion into the patient. Semiautomated devices are used to collect, anticoagulate, wash, and resuspend red cells for reinfusion during many procedures, including vascular, cardiac, and orthopedic surgery.[20]

Before red cells or whole blood from a volunteer donor source is transfused, a series of procedures are required to ensure a successful transfusion. Donor and recipient samples are typed to determine ABO and Rh groups and screened for unexpected red cell antibodies. Donor samples are also tested for blood-borne diseases, such as hepatitis B and hepatitis C, and for human immunodeficiency virus types 1 and 2. The crossmatch is performed by incubating the donor cells with the recipient's serum and observing for agglutination. If none appears, the donor and recipient blood types are compatible.

ABO BLOOD GROUPS

ABO compatibility is essential for effective transfusion therapy and requires knowledge of ABO antigens and antibodies. There are four major ABO blood groups as determined by the presence or absence of two red cell antigens (A and B). People who have neither A nor B antigens are classified as having type O blood; those with A antigens are classified as having type A blood; those with B antigens, as having type B blood; and those with both A and B antigens, as having type AB blood (Table 18-3). The ABO blood groups are genetically determined. The type O gene is apparently functionless in production of a red cell antigen. Each of the other genes is expressed by the presence of a strong antigen on the surface of the red cell. Six genotypes, or gene combinations, result in four phenotypes, or blood type expressions.

ABO antibodies predictably develop in the serum of people whose red cells lack the corresponding antigen. Thus, people with type A antigens on their

TABLE 18-2. RED BLOOD CELL COMPONENTS USED IN TRANSFUSION THERAPY

COMPONENT	PREPARATION	USE	LIMITATIONS
Whole blood	Drawn from donor Anticoagulant-preservative solutions added, usually citrate-phosphate-dextrose (CPDA-1) adenine. Stored at 1°–6°C until expiration up to 35 days.	Replacement of blood volume and oxygen-carrying capacity lost in massive bleeding.	Contains few viable platelets or granulocytes and is deficient in coagulation factors V and VIII. May cause hypervolemia, febrile and allergic reactions and infectious disease (i.e., hepatitis and AIDS).
Red blood cells	Removal of two thirds of plasma by centrifugation. Additive solution contains adenine and dextrose to extend shelf life up to 42 days and maintain ATP levels.	Standard transfusion to increase oxygen-carrying capacity in chronic anemia and slow hemorrhage. Reduce danger of hypervolemia.	Contains no viable platelets or granulocytes. Risk of reactions and infectious disease.
Leukocyte-poor red blood cells	Removal of 70%–90% of leukocytes, platelets, and debris by centrifugation or filtration.	Reduces risk of nonhemolytic febrile reactions in susceptible people.	Preparation may reduce red cell mass to 70%; 24-hr outdate and infectious disease risk.
Washed red blood cells	Red cells are washed in normal saline solution and centrifuged several times to remove plasma and constituents.	Reduces risk of febrile and allergic reactions.	Loss of red cell mass, 24-hr outdate, costly preparation, and infectious disease risk.
Frozen red blood cells	Red cells are mixed with glycerol to prevent ice crystals from forming and rupturing the cell membrane. Cells must be thawed, deglycerolized, and washed before transfusing.	Reduces risk of severe febrile reactions. Preserves rare and autologous (self-donated) units for transfusion up to 10 years.	Costly and lengthy preparation. Loss of red cell mass, 24-hr outdate, and infectious disease risk.

ATP, adenosine triphosphate.
(Data from Reynolds, A., & Steckler, D. [1986]. *Practical aspects of blood administration* [pp. 43–93]. Arlington, VA: American Association of Blood Banks; and Widmann, F.K. [Ed.] [1985]. *Technical manual* [9th ed., pp. 35–58]. Arlington, VA: American Association of Blood Banks)

red cells develop type B antibodies; people with type B antigens develop type A antibodies in their serum; people with type O blood develop both type A and type B antibodies; and people with type AB blood develop neither A nor B antibodies. The ABO antibodies usually are not present at birth but begin to develop at ages 3 to 6 months and reach maximum levels between ages 5 and 10 years.[22]

RH TYPES

The D antigen of the Rh system is also important in transfusion compatibility and is routinely tested. The Rh type is coded by three gene pairs: C, c, D, d, and E, e. Each allele, with the exception of d, codes for a specific antigen. The D antigen is the most immunogenic. People who express the D antigen are termed Rh positive, whereas those who do not express the D antigen are Rh negative. Unlike serum antibodies for the ABO blood types, which develop spontaneously after birth, Rh antibodies develop after exposure to one or more of the Rh antigens. About 50% to 75% of Rh-negative people develop the antibody to D antigen if they are exposed to Rh-positive blood.[14] Because it takes several weeks to produce antibodies, a reaction may be delayed and usually is mild. If subsequent transfusions of Rh-positive blood are given to a person who has become sensitized, the person may have a severe immediate reaction.

TABLE 18-3. ABO SYSTEM FOR BLOOD TYPING

GENOTYPE	RED CELL ANTIGENS	BLOOD TYPE	SERUM ANTIBODIES
OO	None	O	AB
AO	A	A	B
AA	A	A	B
BO	B	B	A
BB	B	B	A
AB	AB	AB	None

BLOOD TRANSFUSION REACTIONS

The seriousness of blood transfusion reactions prompts the need for extreme caution when blood is administered. Because most transfusion reactions are due to clerical errors or misidentification, care should be taken to correctly identify the recipient and the transfusion source.[20] The recipient's vital signs should be monitored before and during the transfusion, and careful observation for signs of transfusion reaction is imperative.

The most feared and lethal transfusion reaction is the destruction of donor red cells by the reaction with antibody in the recipient's serum. This immediate hemolytic reaction usually is caused by ABO incompatibility. The signs and symptoms of such a reaction include sensation of heat along the vein where the blood is being infused, flushing of the face, urticaria, headache, pain in the lumbar area, chills, fever, constricting pain in the chest, cramping pain in the abdomen, nausea, vomiting, tachycardia, hypotension, and dyspnea. If any of these adverse effects occur, the transfusion should be stopped immediately. Access to a vein should be maintained because it may be necessary to administer intravenous medications and take blood samples. The blood must be saved for studies to determine the cause of the reaction. Hemoglobin that is released from the hemolyzed donor cells is filtered in the glomeruli of the kidneys. Two possible complications of a blood transfusion reaction are oliguria and renal shutdown because of the adverse effects of the filtered hemoglobin on renal tubular flow. Therefore, the urine should be examined for the presence of hemoglobin, urobilinogen, and red blood cells.

A febrile reaction, the most common transfusion reaction, occurs in about 2% of transfusions.[20] Recipient antibodies directed against the donor's white cells cause chills and fever. Antipyretics are used to treat this reaction. Future febrile reactions may be avoided by the use of leukocyte-poor blood.

Allergic reactions are due to patient antibodies against donor proteins, particularly immunoglobulin A. Urticaria and itching occur and can be relieved with antihistamines. Susceptible people may be transfused with washed red cells to prevent reactions.

Delayed hemolytic reactions may occur more than 10 days after transfusion and are due to undetected antibodies in the recipient's serum. The reaction is accompanied by a fall in hematocrit, but most recipients are asymptomatic.

In summary, transfusion therapy provides the means for replacement of red blood cells and other blood components. Red blood cells contain surface antigens, and reciprocal antibodies are found in the serum. Four major ABO blood types are determined by the presence or absence of two red cell antigens: A and B. The presence of the D antigen determines the Rh-positive type; absence of the D antigen determines the Rh-negative type. ABO and Rh types must be determined in recipient and donor blood before transfusion to ensure compatibility.

■ POLYCYTHEMIA

In contrast to anemia, polycythemia is an abnormally high total red blood cell mass. It is categorized as relative, primary, or secondary. In *relative polycythemia*, the hematocrit rises because of a loss of plasma volume without a corresponding decrease in red cells. *Primary polycythemia* (*polycythemia vera*) is a proliferative disease of the bone marrow characterized by an absolute increase in total red blood cell mass accompanied by elevated white cell and platelet counts. It most commonly is seen in men aged 40 to 60. *Secondary polycythemia* results from an increase in the level of erythropoietin. This elevation is related to living at high altitudes, chronic heart and lung disease, and smoking (all causes of hypoxia).

In polycythemia vera, the signs and symptoms are related to increased blood viscosity, hypermetabolism, and an increase in the red cell count, hemoglobin level, and hematocrit. The increased blood volume gives rise to hypertension. The patient may complain of headache, inability to concentrate, and some difficulty in hearing because of decreased cerebral blood flow. There is a plethoric appearance, or dusky redness—even cyanosis—particularly of the lips, fingernails, and mucous membranes. Because of the concentration of blood cells, the person may experience itching and pain in the fingers or toes, and the hypermetabolism may induce night sweats and weight loss. With the increased blood viscosity and stagnation of blood flow, thrombosis and hemorrhage are possible.

Relative polycythemia is corrected by increasing the vascular fluid volume. Treatment of secondary polycythemia focuses on relieving hypoxia. For example, continuous low-flow oxygen therapy can be used to correct the severe hypoxia that occurs in some people with chronic obstructive lung disease. This form of treatment is thought to relieve the pulmonary hypertension and polycythemia and to delay the onset of cor pulmonale. The goal of treatment in primary polycythemia is to reduce blood viscosity. This can be done by withdrawing blood by means of phlebotomy or by suppressing bone marrow function by using chemotherapy or radiation therapy.

In summary, polycythemia describes a condition in which the red blood cell mass is increased. It may be relative in type, with the red cell mass increased because of a loss of vascular fluid; primary, with proliferative changes in the bone marrow; or secondary, with elevated erythropoietin levels caused by hypoxia.

■ AGE-RELATED CHANGES IN RED BLOOD CELLS

RED CELL CHANGES IN THE NEONATE

At birth, changes in the red blood cell indices reflect the transition to extrauterine life and the need to transport oxygen from the lungs (Table 18-4). Hemoglobin concentrations at birth are high, reflecting the high synthetic activity *in utero* to provide adequate oxygen delivery.[23] Toward the end of the first postnatal week, hemoglobin concentration begins to decline, gradually falling to a minimum value at about age 2 months. Red cell count, hematocrit, and MCV likewise fall. The factors responsible for the decline include reduced red cell production and plasma dilution caused by increased blood volume with growth. Neonatal red cells also have a shorter life span of 50 to 70 days and are thought to be more fragile.

During the early neonatal period, there is also a switch from HbF to HbA. The amount of HbF in term infants varies from 53% to 95% and decreases by about 3% per week after birth.[24] At age 6 months, HbF usually accounts for less than 2% of total hemoglobin. The switch to HbA provides greater unloading of oxygen to the tissues, since HbA has a lower affinity for oxygen compared with HbF. Infants who are small for gestational age or born to diabetic or smoking mothers or who experienced hypoxia *in utero* have higher total hemoglobin levels, higher HbF levels, and a delayed switch to HbA.

A *physiologic anemia of the newborn* develops at about age 2 months. It seldom is symptomatic and cannot be altered by nutritional supplements. *Anemia of prematurity*, an exaggerated physiologic response

TABLE 18-4. RED CELL VALUES FOR TERM INFANTS

AGE	RBC × 10⁶/μL MEAN ± SD	Hb, g/dL MEAN ± SD	Hct, % MEAN ± SD	MCV, fl MEAN ± SD
Days				
1	5.14 ± 0.7	19.3 ± 2.2	61 ± 7.4	119 ± 9.4
4	5.00 ± 0.6	18.6 ± 2.1	57 ± 8.1	114 ± 7.5
7	4.86 ± 0.6	17.9 ± 2.5	56 ± 9.4	118 ± 11.2
Weeks				
1–2	4.80 ± 0.8	17.3 ± 2.3	54 ± 8.3	112 ± 19.0
3–4	4.00 ± 0.6	14.2 ± 2.1	43 ± 5.7	105 ± 7.5
8–9	3.40 ± 0.5	10.7 ± 0.9	31 ± 2.5	93 ± 12.0
11–12	3.70 ± 0.3	11.3 ± 0.9	33 ± 3.3	88 ± 7.9

Hb, hemoglobin; Hct, hematocrit; MCV, mean corpuscular volume. (Adapted from Matoth, Y., Zaizor, R., & Varsano, I. [1971]. Postnatal changes in some red cell parameters. *Acta Paediatrica Scandinavica, 60,* 317)

in low-birthweight infants, is thought to be due to poor erythropoietin response. The hemoglobin level rapidly declines after birth to a low of 7 to 10 g/dL at about age 6 weeks. Signs and symptoms include apnea, poor weight gain, pallor, decreased activity, and tachycardia. In infants born before 33 weeks' gestation or those with hematocrits below 33%, the clinical features are more evident. A recent study suggests that the protein content of breast milk may not be sufficient for hematopoiesis in the premature infant. Protein supplementation significantly elevates the hemoglobin concentrations at ages 4 to 10 weeks.[23]

Anemia at birth, characterized by pallor, congestive heart failure, or shock, usually is caused by hemolytic disease of the newborn. Bleeding from the umbilical cord, internal hemorrhage, congenital hemolytic disease, or frequent blood sampling are other possible causes of anemia. The severity of symptoms and presence of coexisting disease may warrant red cell transfusion.

HYPERBILIRUBINEMIA IN THE NEONATE

Hyperbilirubinemia, an increased level of serum bilirubin, is a common cause of jaundice in the neonate. A benign self-limited condition, it most often is related to the developmental state of the neonate. Fewer cases of hyperbilirubinemia are pathologic and may lead to kernicterus and serious brain damage.

In the 1st week of life, about 60% of term and 80% of preterm neonates are jaundiced.[25] This *physiologic jaundice* appears in term infants on the 2nd or 3rd day of life, and bilirubin levels peak at less than 12 mg/dL. This complication probably is related to the increased fetal red cell breakdown and the inability of the immature liver to conjugate bilirubin. Premature infants exhibit a similar rise in serum bilirubin level, perhaps because of poor hepatic uptake and reduced albumin binding of bilirubin. The rise is slower, appearing at day 3 or 4, and peak levels of bilirubin are higher (greater than 15 mg/dL). Most neonatal jaundice resolves within 1 week and is untreated.

When jaundice appears at atypical times (*i.e.*, at birth or after 1 week), the cause is sought to prevent exaggerated hyperbilirubinemia and its toxic consequences. Many factors cause elevated bilirubin levels in the neonate: breastfeeding, hemolytic disease of the newborn, hypoxia, infections, acidosis, and albumin-binding drugs (*e.g.*, furosemide, hydrocortisone, gentamicin, and digoxin).[26] Bowel or biliary obstruction and liver disease are less common causes. Associated risk factors include prematurity, Asian ancestry, and maternal diabetes.

Breast milk jaundice occurs in about 1 in 200 breastfed babies.[25] These neonates develop significant levels of unconjugated bilirubin 4 to 7 days after birth and reach maximum levels in the 3rd week of life. This type of jaundice disappears if breastfeeding is discontinued. Nursing can be resumed in 3 to 4 days without any hyperbilirubinemia ensuing. It is thought that the breast milk contains fatty acids that inhibit bilirubin conjugation in the neonatal liver. A factor in milk is also thought to increase the absorption of bilirubin in the duodenum.

Hyperbilirubinemia places the neonate at risk of developing a neurologic syndrome called *kernicterus*. This condition is caused by the accumulation of unconjugated bilirubin in brain cells. Unconjugated bilirubin is lipid-soluble, crosses the permeable blood–brain barrier of the neonate, and is deposited in cells of the basal ganglia to cause brain damage. Symptoms may appear 2 to 7 days after birth or later in the neonatal period. Lethargy, poor feeding, and short-term behavioral changes may be evident in mildly affected infants. Severe manifestations include rigidity, tremors, ataxia, and hearing loss. Fatal cases are followed by seizures and death. Most survivors are seriously damaged and by age 3 exhibit involuntary muscle spasm, seizures, mental retardation, and deafness.

The potential for developing kernicterus is related to the level of unconjugated bilirubin in the serum, regardless of cause, and predisposing factors such as gestational age and weight. Signs and symptoms of kernicterus in term infants occur at indirect bilirubin levels of 25 to 30 mg/dL; less mature or ill infants are susceptible at lower levels.[27] Infants at risk for developing kernicterus are those with (1) clinically apparent jaundice in the first 24 hours; (2) an increase in total serum bilirubin of more than 5 mg/dL/d; (3) total bilirubin concentration higher than 12 mg/dL in full-term or 14 mg/dL in preterm infants; (4) direct serum bilirubin levels higher than 1 mg/dL); and (5) visible jaundice lasting for more than 1 week in full-term infants or 2 weeks in premature infants.[25]

Hyperbilirubinemia in the neonate is treated with phototherapy or exchange transfusion. Phototherapy is more commonly used to treat jaundiced infants and reduce the risk of kernicterus. Exposure to fluorescent light in the blue range of the visible spectrum (420- to 470-nm wave length) reduces bilirubin levels. Bilirubin in the skin absorbs the light energy and is converted to a structural isomer that is more water-soluble and can be excreted in the stool and urine. Effective treatment depends on the area of skin exposed and the infant's ability to metabolize and excrete bilirubin. Frequent monitoring of bilirubin levels, body temperature, and hydration is critical to the infant's care. Exchange transfusion is considered when signs of kernicterus are evident or hyperbilirubinemia is sustained or rising and unresponsive to phototherapy.

HEMOLYTIC DISEASE OF THE NEWBORN

Erythroblastosis fetalis, or hemolytic disease of the newborn, occurs in Rh-positive infants of Rh-negative mothers who have been sensitized. The mother can produce anti-Rh antibodies from pregnancies in which the infants are Rh positive or by blood transfusions of Rh-positive blood. The Rh-negative mother usually becomes sensitized during the first few days after delivery when fetal Rh-positive red cells from the placental site are released into the maternal circulation. Because the antibodies take several weeks to develop, the first Rh-positive infant of an Rh-negative mother usually is not affected. Infants with Rh-negative blood have no antigens on their red cells to react with the maternal antibodies and are also not affected.

Once an Rh-negative mother has been sensitized, the Rh antibodies from her blood are transferred to subsequent babies through the placental circulation. These antibodies react with the red cell antigens of the Rh-positive infant, causing agglutination and hemolysis. This leads to severe anemia with compensatory hyperplasia and enlargement of the blood-forming organs, including the spleen and liver, in the fetus. Liver function may be impaired, with decreased production of albumin causing massive edema called *hydrops fetalis*. If blood levels of unconjugated bilirubin are abnormally high because of red cell hemolysis, there is danger of the infant's developing kernicterus. Only 10% of infants so affected survive.[28]

Three recent advances have served to decrease the threat to infants born to Rh-negative mothers: (1) prevention of sensitization, (2) intrauterine transfusion to the affected fetus, and (3) exchange transfusion. The injection of *Rh immune globulin* (gamma globulin containing Rh antibody) prevents sensitization in Rh-negative mothers who have given birth to Rh-positive infants if administered within 72 hours of delivery, abortion, genetic amniocentesis, or fetal–maternal bleed. Once sensitization has developed, the immune globulin is of no value.

Since 1968, the year Rh immune globulin was introduced, the incidence of sensitization of Rh-negative women has dropped by more than 80%.[29] Early prenatal care and screening of maternal blood continue to be important in reducing immunization. Efforts to improve therapy are aimed at production of monoclonal anti-D, the Rh antibody.

In the past, about 20% of erythroblastotic fetuses died *in utero*. It is now possible to increase the chance of survival of such infants by studying the amniotic fluid to determine the bilirubin concentration, which reflects the severity of the disease. If the fetus is erythroblastotic, intrauterine transfusions of red cells are given into the fetus's peritoneal cavity or by the more difficult direct intravascular technique.[28] Exchange transfusions are administered after birth. In this technique, 10 to 20 mL of the infant's blood is removed and replaced with an equal amount of type O Rh-negative blood. This procedure is repeated until twice the blood volume of the infant has been exchanged. The exchange transfusion removes 85% to 90% of the hemolyzed red cells and about 25% of the total bilirubin, thus treating the anemia and hyperbilirubinemia.[28]

RED CELL CHANGES WITH AGING

Aging is also associated with red cell changes. Bone marrow cellularity declines with age from about 50% cellularity at age 65 to about 30% at age 75. The decline may be due to osteoporosis.[30]

Hemoglobin levels decline after middle age. In studies of men over age 60, mean hemoglobin levels ranged from 15.3 to 12.4 g/dL with the lowest levels found in the oldest people. The decline is less in women, with mean levels ranging from 13.8 to 11.7 mg/dL.[24] In most asymptomatic elderly people, lower hemoglobin levels are due to iron deficiency. Orally administered iron is poorly utilized in older adults, despite normal iron absorption. Underlying neoplasms may contribute to anemia in this population, apart from the effects of aging.

■ REFERENCES

1. Guyton, A. (1990). *Textbook of medical physiology* (8th ed., p. 356). Philadelphia: W.B. Saunders.
2. Babior, B.M., & Stossel, T.P. (1990). *Hematology: A pathophysiological approach* (2nd ed., pp. 29–31). New York: Churchill Livingstone.
3. Rifkind, R.A., Bank, A., Marks, P.A., Kaplan, K.L., Ellison, R.R., & Lindenbaum, J. (1986). *Fundamentals of hematology* (3rd ed., p. 73). Chicago: Year Book Medical Publishers.
4. Beck, W.S. (1991). Erythropoiesis and introduction to the anemias. In W.S. Beck (Ed.). *Hematology* (5th ed., pp. 27, 29). Cambridge, MA: MIT Press.
5. Erslev, A.J. (1990). Production of erythrocytes. In W.J. Williams, E. Beutler, A.J. Erslev, & M.A. Lichtman (Eds.). *Hematology* (4th ed., pp. 394–395). New York: McGraw-Hill.
6. Eschbach, J.W., Egrie, J.C., Downing, M.R., Browne, J.K., & Adamson, J.W. (1987). Correction of the anemia of end-stage renal disease with recombinant human erythropoietin. *New England Journal of Medicine, 316,* 73.
7. Beck, W.S. (1991). Hematopoiesis. In W.S. Beck (Ed.). *Hematology* (5th ed., p. 17). Cambridge, MA: MIT Press.
8. Hillman, R.S., & Finch, C.A. (1985). *Red cell manual* (5th ed., p. 33). Philadelphia: F.A. Davis.

9. Chandrasoma, P., & Taylor, C.R. (1991). *Concise pathology* (p. 394). E. Norwalk, CT: Appleton & Lange.
10. Rodgers, G.P. (1991). Recent approaches to the treatment of sickle cell anemia. *Journal of the American Medical Association, 265*(16), 2097.
11. Nathan, D.G. (1991). The thalassemias. In W.S. Beck (Ed.). *Hematology* (5th ed., p. 213). Cambridge, MA: MIT Press.
12. Beck, W.S., & Tepper, R.I. (1991). Hemolytic anemias IV. Metabolic disorders. In W.S. Beck (Ed.). *Hematology* (5th ed., p. 293). Cambridge, MA: MIT Press.
13. Churchill, W.H., Jr., & Jandl, J.H. (1991). Hemolytic anemias II. Immunohemolytic anemias. In W.S. Beck (Ed.). *Hematology* (5th ed., p. 246). Cambridge, MA: MIT Press.
14. Committee on Technical Manual. Widmann, F.K. (Ed.). (1985). *Technical manual* (9th ed., pp. 260, 128). Arlington, VA: American Association of Blood Banks.
15. Beck, W.S. (1991). Hypochromic anemias I. Iron deficiency and excess. In W.S. Beck (Ed.). *Hematology* (5th ed., p. 135). Cambridge, MA: MIT Press.
16. Lane, M., & Johnson, C.L. (1981). Prevalence of iron deficiency. In F.A. Oski & H.A. Pearson (Eds.). *Iron nutrition revisited—infancy, childhood, adolescence: Report of the Eighty-Second Ross Conference on Pediatric Research* (pp. 31–46). Columbus, OH: Ross Laboratories.
17. Ries, C.A., & Santi, D.V. (1989). Agents used in anemias. In B.G. Katzung (Ed.). *Basic and clinical pharmacology* (4th ed., p. 397). E. Norwalk, CT: Appleton & Lange.
18. Beck, W.S. (1991). Megaloblastic anemias II. Folic acid deficiency. In W.S. Beck (Ed.). *Hematology* (5th ed., p. 126). Cambridge, MA: MIT Press.
19. Beck, W.S. (1991). Normocytic anemias. In W.S. Beck (Ed.). *Hematology* (5th ed., pp. 72, 78). Cambridge, MA: MIT Press.
20. Huestis, D.W., Bove, J.R., & Case, J. (1988). *Practical blood transfusion* (4th ed., pp. 211, 226, 254, 259). Boston: Little, Brown.
21. Toy, P.T.C.Y., Strauss, R.G., Stehling, L., et al. (1987). Predeposited autologous blood for elective surgery. *New England Journal of Medicine, 316*, 517.
22. Pittiglio, D.H. (Ed.). (1983). *Modern blood banking and transfusion practices* (pp. 91–92). Philadelphia: F.A. Davis.
23. Brown, M.S. (1988). Physiologic anemia of infancy: Nutritional factors and abnormal states. In J.A. Stockman & C. Pochedly (Eds.). *Developmental and neonatal hematology* (pp. 252, 274). New York: Raven Press.
24. Segel, G.B., & Oski, F.A. (1990). Hematology of the newborn. In W.J. Williams, E. Beutler, A.J. Erslev, & M.A. Lichtman (Eds.). *Hematology* (4th ed., p. 100). New York: McGraw-Hill.
25. Behrman, R.E., Kliegman, R.M., Nelson, W.E., & Vaughan, V.C. (Eds.). (1992). *Nelson textbook of pediatrics* (14th ed., pp. 476–479). Philadelphia: W.B. Saunders.
26. Hazinski, M.F. (1992). *Nursing care of the critically ill child* (2nd ed., p. 739). St. Louis: Mosby-Year Book.
27. Cashore, W.J. (1990). Neonatal hyperbilirubinemia. In F.A. Oski, C.D. DeAngelis, R.D. Feigin, & J.B. Warshaw (Eds.). *Principles and practice of pediatrics* (p. 402). Philadelphia: J.B. Lippincott.
28. Bowman, J.M. (1988). Alloimmune hemolytic disease of the neonate. In J.A. Stockman & C. Pochedly (Eds.). *Developmental and neonatal hematology* (pp. 226, 232, 233). New York: Raven Press.
29. Bowman, J.M. (1988). The prevention of Rh immunization. *Transfusion Medicine Reviews, 2*, 129.
30. Williams, W.J. (1990). Hematology in the aged. In W.J. Williams, E. Beutler, A.J. Erslev, & M.A. Lichtman (Eds.). *Hematology* (4th ed., pp. 112–113). New York: McGraw-Hill.

▪ BIBLIOGRAPHY

Beutler, E. (1989). Glucose-6-phosphate dehydrogenase: New perspectives. *Blood, 73*, 1397.

Conley, C.L. (1990). Polycythemia vera. *Journal of the American Medical Association, 263*, 2481.

Fetus and Newborn Committee, Canadian Paediatric Society. (1986). Use of phototherapy for neonatal hyperbilirubinemia. *Canadian Medical Association Journal, 134*, 1237.

Goldberg, M.A., Brugnara, C., Dover, G.J., et al. (1990). Treatment of sickle cell anemia with hydroxyurea and erythropoietin. *New England Journal of Medicine, 323*, 366–372.

Golde, D.W., & Gasson, J.C. (1988). Hormones that stimulate the growth of blood cells. *Scientific American, 259*, 62.

Graf, H., Watzinger, U., et al. (1990). Recombinant human erythropoietin as adjuvant treatment for autologous blood donation. *British Medical Journal (Clinical Research Ed.), 300*, 1627.

Jaffe, E.R. (1991) Chronic nonspherocytic hemolytic anemia and G6PD deficiency. *Hospital Practice, 26*, 57–70.

Kodish, E., Lantos, J., Stocking, C., et al. (1991). Bone marrow transplantation for sickle cell disease. *New England Journal of Medicine, 325*, 1349.

Lee, D., & Napier, J.A. (1990). ABC of transfusion. Autologous transfusion. *British Medical Journal (Clinical Research Ed.), 300*, 737.

Lucarelli, G., Galimberti, M., et al. (1990). Bone marrow transplantation in patients with thalassemia. *New England Journal of Medicine, 322*, 417.

Maisels, M., Gifford, K., Antle, C., et al. (1988). Jaundice in the healthy newborn infant: A new approach to an old problem. *Pediatrics, 81*, 505.

McDonagh, K.T., Dover, G.J., et al. (1990). Manipulation of HbF production with hematopoietic growth factors. *Progress in Clinical and Biological Research, 316B*, 307.

Menitove, J.E. (1990). Current risk of transfusion-associated human immunodeficiency virus infection. *Archives of Pathology and Laboratory Medicine, 114*, 330.

Miller, C.B., Jones, R.J., et al. (1990). Decreased erythropoietin response in patients with the anemia of cancer. *New England Journal of Medicine, 322*, 1689.

Perutz, M.F. (1990). Mechanisms regulating the reactions of human hemoglobin with oxygen and carbon monoxide. *Annual Review of Physiology, 52*, 1.

Platt, O.S., Thorington, B.D., Brambilla, D.J., et al. (1991). Pain in sickle cell disease—rates and risk factors. *New England Journal of Medicine, 325*, 11.

Ranney, H.M. (1992). The spectrum of sickle cell. *Hospital Practice, 27*, 133–163.

Spivak, J.L. (1989). Erythropoietin: A brief review. *Nephron, 52*, 289.

THE CIRCULATORY SYSTEM AND CONTROL OF BLOOD FLOW

■ OBJECTIVES

After you have studied this chapter, you should be able to meet the following objectives:

■ Describe the organization of the circulatory system.

■ Compare the distribution of blood flow and blood pressure in the systemic and pulmonary circulations.

■ Explain how vessel radius, vessel length, blood viscosity, and blood pressure affect blood flow.

■ Relate the cross-sectional area to pressure and the velocity of flow in a blood vessel.

■ Use Laplace's law to explain the effect of radius size on the pressure and wall tension in a vessel.

■ Compare laminar and streamlined flow in terms of the development of turbulent flow in the vascular system.

■ Describe the origin of the pressure pulse.

■ Define *mean arterial blood pressure* and state the rationale for its use.

■ Compare the structure of arteries, arterioles, veins, and capillaries.

■ Relate the effects of gravity to mechanisms of venous flow.

■ Define *microcirculation*.

■ Relate the function of capillaries in various organ systems to the size of the capillary pores.

■ Describe the organization and function of the lymphatic circulation.

■ Explain how the endothelium is thought to interact with various blood-borne substances in producing blood vessel dilatation or constriction.

■ Describe the regulation of blood flow in terms of local, neural, and humoral components.

The circulatory system, which consists of the heart and blood vessels, has one main function—transport. It delivers oxygen and nutrients needed for metabolic processes to the tissues, carries waste products from cellular metabolism to the kidneys and other excretory organs for elimination, and circulates electrolytes and hormones needed to regulate body function. Temperature regulation relies on the circulatory system for transport of core heat to the periphery, where it can be dissipated into the external environment. In addition, the circulatory system plays a vital role in the transport of various immune sub-

Carol Mattson Porth: PATHOPHYSIOLOGY: CONCEPTS OF ALTERED HEALTH STATES, 4th ed. © 1994, 1990, 1986, 1982 J.B. Lippincott Company

stances that contribute to the body's defense mechanisms. Amazingly, the blood flow to each tissue of the body is controlled in relation to tissue need. The purpose of this chapter is to discuss the organization of the circulatory system, the principles of blood flow, the structure and function of blood vessels, and the control of blood flow. Control of blood pressure is discussed further in Chapter 21, and control of cardiac function is discussed in Chapter 22.

■ ORGANIZATION OF THE CIRCULATORY SYSTEM

SYSTEMIC AND PULMONARY CIRCULATIONS

The circulatory system can be divided into two parts: the larger systemic circulation and the smaller pulmonary circulation (Fig. 19-1). The systemic, or *peripheral,* circulation supplies all the body's tissues with the exception of the lungs, which are supplied by the pulmonary circulation. Because the systemic circulation must transport blood to distant parts of the body, often against gravity, it functions as a high-pressure system (mean arterial blood pressure is

about 90 to 100 mmHg). The pulmonary circulation links the gas exchange function of the lungs with the transport function of the circulatory system. Because the lungs are located in the chest and in proximity to the heart, the pulmonary circulation functions as a low-pressure system (mean arterial blood pressure is about 12 mmHg). The low pressure of the pulmonary circulation allows blood to move more slowly, which is important for gas exchange. The pulmonary circulation along with the blood that is in the heart is also called the *central circulation.*

Each division of the circulation has a pump, an arterial system, capillaries, and a venous system. The systemic circulation consists of the aorta and its branches, the arterioles, the systemic capillaries, the systemic veins, and vena cavae. The pulmonary circulation consists of the pulmonary artery and its branches, the pulmonary capillaries, and the pulmonary veins. The heart is a four-chambered pump that propels blood through both divisions. It is divided into a right heart, which pumps blood to the pulmonary circulation, and a left heart, which pumps blood to the systemic circulation. Each side of the heart is further divided into two chambers, an atrium and a ventricle. The atria act as collection chambers for blood returning to the heart and as axillary pumps that assist in filling the ventricles. The ventricles are the main pumping chambers of the heart. The right ventricle pumps blood through the pulmonary artery to the lungs, and the left ventricle pumps blood through the aorta to the rest of the body.

In both the pulmonary and the systemic circulation, the blood vessels function in distribution, exchange, and collection of blood. The arteries and arterioles function as a distribution system to move blood to the tissues. The capillaries serve as an exchange system where the transfer of gases, nutrients, and waste products takes place. The venules and veins collect the blood and return it to the heart. Veins are equally important as reservoirs for blood storage.

The effective function of the circulatory system requires that the flow of blood is unidirectional and that the outputs of the right and left hearts are equal. Unidirectional flow through the heart is ensured by the heart valves. The distribution of pressure and volume throughout the circulatory system requires that both sides of the heart pump equal amounts of blood. If the output of the left heart were to fall below that of the right heart, blood would accumulate in the pulmonary circulation. If the right side of the heart pumped less than the left, blood would accumulate in the systemic circulation.

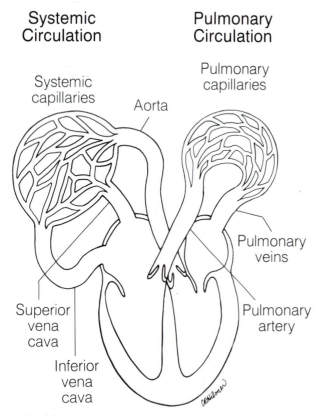

Systemic Circulation
Pulmonary Circulation

Systemic capillaries
Pulmonary capillaries
Aorta
Pulmonary veins
Pulmonary artery
Superior vena cava
Inferior vena cava

FIG. 19-1. Systemic and pulmonary circulations. The right side of the heart pumps blood to the lungs, and the left side of the heart pumps blood to the systemic circulation.

In summary, the circulatory system is designed to deliver nutrients to and remove waste products from body tissues. The heart pumps blood throughout the system. The blood vessels serve as tubes through which blood flows; the arterial system carries fluids from the heart to the tissues, and the veins carry them back to the heart. The circulatory system can be divided into two parts: the systemic and the pulmonary circulation. The systemic circulation, which is served by the left heart, supplies all the tissues except the lungs, which are served by the right heart and the pulmonary circulation. Blood moves throughout the circulation along a pressure gradient, moving from the high-pressure arterial system to the low-pressure venous system.

■ PRINCIPLES OF BLOOD FLOW

The function of the circulatory system is complex. The heart is an intermittent pump, and as a result, blood flow in the arterial circulation is pulsatile. The blood vessels are branched, distensible tubes of varying dimensions. The blood is a suspension of blood cells, platelets, lipid globules, and plasma proteins. Despite this complexity, the function of the circulatory system can be explained by the principles of basic fluid mechanics that apply to nonbiologic systems, such as household plumbing systems.

VOLUME, PRESSURE, AND FLOW

The most important characteristics of the circulation are *volume*, *pressure*, and *flow*. Blood volume is measured in milliliters (mL), blood pressure in millime-

ters of mercury (mmHg), and blood flow in mL/unit time. Blood flow in the circulatory system depends on a blood volume that is sufficient to fill the blood vessels and a pressure that provides the force to move blood through the circulatory system.

The total blood volume is a function of age and body weight, ranging from 85 to 90 mL/kg in the neonate to 70 to 75 mL/kg in the adult. As shown in Figure 19-2, about 4% of the blood is in the left heart, 16% is in the arteries and arterioles, 4% is in the capillaries, 64% is in the venules and veins, and 4% is in the right heart.[1]

Because the pulmonary and systemic circulations are connected and function as a closed system, blood can be shifted from one circulation to the other. In the pulmonary circulation, the blood volume (about 450 mL in the adult) can vary from as low as 50% of normal to as high as 200% of normal. Increases in intrathoracic pressure, which impede venous return to the right heart, can produce a transient shift from the central to the systemic circulation of as much as 250 mL of blood. Body position also affects the distribution of blood volume. In the recumbent position, about 25% to 30% of the total blood volume is in the central circulation.[1] On standing, about 26% to 30% of the central blood volume is rapidly displaced to the lower part of the body because of the forces of gravity.[1] Because the volume of the systemic circulation is about seven times that of the pulmonary circulation, a shift of blood from one

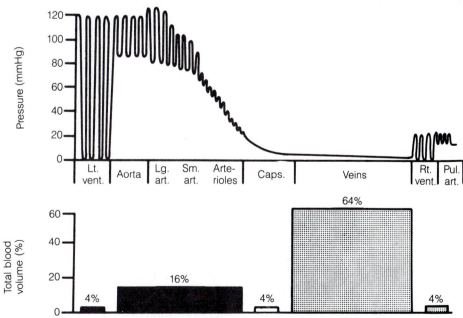

FIG. 19-2. Pressure and volume distribution in the systemic circulation. The graphs show the inverse relation between internal pressure and volume in different portions of the circulatory system. (Smith, J. J., & Kampine, J. P. [1984]. *Circulatory physiology: The essentials* [2nd ed.]. Baltimore: Williams & Wilkins)

system to the other has a much greater effect in the pulmonary than in the systemic circulation.

Blood moves from the arterial to the venous side of the circulation along a pressure gradient, going from an area of higher pressure to one of lower pressure. As shown in Figure 19-2, the pressure distribution in the different parts of the circulation is almost an inverse of the volume distribution. The pressure in the arterial side of the circulation, which contains only about one sixth of the blood volume, is much greater than the pressure on the venous side of the circulation, which contains about two thirds of the blood. This difference in pressure between the arterial and venous sides of the circulation (about 84 mmHg) provides the driving force for flow of blood in the systemic circulation. The pulmonary circulation has similar arterial–venous pressure differences, albeit of a lesser magnitude, that facilitate blood flow.

PRESSURE, RESISTANCE, AND FLOW

Blood flow is determined by two factors—a pressure difference between the two ends of a vessel or group of vessels and the resistance that blood must overcome as it moves through the vessel or vessels (Fig. 19-3). Vascular resistance cannot be measured directly. Instead, it is estimated, using cardiac output as a measure of flow and the pressure difference between two points in the circulation.

Vascular resistance = pressure difference/flow

The *systemic vascular resistance (SVR)*, or *total peripheral resistance (TPR)*, refers to the total resistance

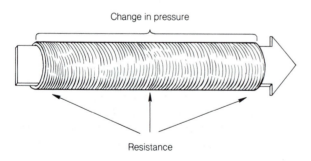

$$\text{Flow } Q = \frac{\text{Change in pressure} \times \pi \text{ radius}^4}{8 \times \text{length} \times \text{viscosity}}$$

FIG. 19-3. Factors that affect blood flow (Poiseuille's law). Increasing the pressure difference between the two ends of the vessel or enlarging the radius of the vessel causes flow to increase. Increasing the length of the vessel or the viscosity of the blood causes flow to decrease. Flow diminishes as resistance increases. Resistance is directly proportional to blood viscosity and the length of the vessel and inversely proportional to the fourth power of the radius.

the blood encounters as it flows through the systemic circulation. It considers the entire systemic circulation as a single tube that begins in the aorta and ends in the right atrium. The pressure difference between these two points is the mean arterial blood pressure (about 100 mmHg) minus the right atrial pressure (about 0 mmHg). The flow or cardiac output (CO) is about 100 mL/sec at rest. Thus, the SVR is 100/100, or 1 peripheral resistance unit (PRU). The total resistance in the pulmonary circulation is only about 0.12 PRU.[2] In this case, the blood flow is the same as in the systemic circulation, but the pressure difference between the pulmonary artery and the left atrium (16 mmHg minus 4 mmHg) is much less.

In the vascular system, resistance is affected by the vessel radius and the viscosity of the blood (see Fig. 19-3). Although the laws of physics state that flow is also affected by the length of a tube, the length of most blood vessels in the body is relatively fixed. A more important consideration is the radius of a blood vessel, which does change. Resistance to flow is related inversely to the fourth power of the radius. The larger the radius of a vessel, the less the resistance and the greater the flow. For example, the rate of flow is 16 times greater in a vessel with a radius of 2 mm than in a vessel with a radius of 1 mm. Thus, even small changes in a vessel's diameter can produce marked changes in blood flow. The reader is asked to consider the consequences of a 25%, 50%, and 75% narrowing of a coronary artery in terms of blood flow to the myocardium.

Viscosity is the resistance to flow caused by the friction of molecules in a fluid. Unlike water that flows through plumbing pipes, blood is a nonhomogeneous liquid. It contains blood cells, platelets, fat globules, and plasma proteins that increase its viscosity. The viscosity of a fluid is largely related to its thickness. The more particles that are present in a solution, the greater the frictional forces that develop between the molecules. The red blood cells, which constitute 40% to 45% of the formed elements of the blood, largely determine the viscosity of the blood. When measured in relation to water, the relative viscosity of plasma is 1.5, and at a normal hematocrit of 42 to 45, that of whole blood is 3.0.[2] Under special conditions, temperature may affect viscosity. There is a 2% rise in viscosity for each 1°C decrease in body temperature, a fact that helps explain the sluggish blood flow that is seen in people with hypothermia.

Because pressure is needed to overcome the resistance that blood encounters as it moves through the circulatory system, blood pressure is influenced greatly by the vascular resistance. Accordingly, arterial blood pressure (BP) can be estimated by multiplying the CO by the TPR (BP = CO × TPR).

VELOCITY, LAMINAR FLOW, AND TURBULENCE

Velocity is a distance measurement; it refers to the speed or linear movement with time (cm/sec) with which blood flows through a vessel. *Flow* is a volume measurement (mL/sec); it is determined by both the cross-sectional area of a vessel and the velocity of flow (Fig. 19-4). When the flow through a given segment of the circulatory system is constant—as it must be for continuous flow—the velocity is inversely proportional to the cross-sectional area (*e.g.*, the smaller the cross-sectional area of a vessel, the greater the velocity of flow). It is like cars moving from a two-lane to a single-lane section of a highway. To keep traffic moving at its original pace, cars would have to double their speed in the single-lane section of the highway.

The linear velocity of blood flow in the circulatory system varies widely from 30 to 35 cm/sec in the aorta to 0.2 to 0.3 mm/sec in the capillaries.[1] This is because the total cross-sectional area of all the systemic capillaries greatly exceeds the cross-sectional area of other parts of the circulation. As a result of this large surface area, the slower movement of blood allows ample time for exchange of nutrients, gases, and metabolites between the tissues and the blood.

Blood flow normally is laminar with the blood components arranged in layers so that the plasma is adjacent to the smooth, slippery endothelial surface of the blood vessel and the blood cells, including the platelets, are in the center or axis of the bloodstream (Fig. 19-5). This arrangement reduces friction by allowing the blood layers to slide smoothly over one another with the axial layer having the most rapid rate of flow. Under certain conditions, however, particularly at high velocities, flow becomes turbulent rather than laminar.

Turbulent flow is flow in which blood moves crosswise as well as lengthwise along a vessel in a manner similar to the eddy currents seen in a rapidly

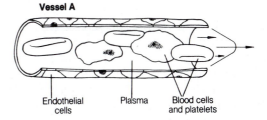

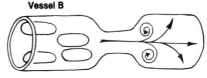

FIG. 19-5. Laminar and turbulent flow in blood vessels. Vessel *A* shows streamlined or laminar flow in which the plasma layer is adjacent to the vessel endothelial layer and blood cells are in the center of the bloodstream. Vessel *B* shows the presence of turbulent flow. The axial location of the platelets and other blood cells is disturbed.

flowing river at a point of obstruction (see Fig. 19-5). The tendency for turbulence to occur increases in direct proportion to the velocity of flow. Again, imagine the chaos as cars from a two- or three-lane highway converge on a single-lane section of the highway. The same type of thing happens in blood vessels that have been narrowed by disease processes, such as atherosclerosis. Turbulent flow predisposes to clot formation as platelets and other coagulation factors come in contact with the endothelial lining of the vessel. Turbulent flow often can be heard through a stethoscope. An audible murmur in a blood vessel is referred to as a *bruit*.

WALL TENSION, RADIUS, AND PRESSURE

In a blood vessel, wall tension is the force per unit length tangential to the vessel wall that opposes the distending pressure.[3] The relation between wall tension, pressure, and the radius of a vessel or sphere was described more than 200 years ago by the French astronomer and mathematician Pierre de Laplace.[3] This relation, which is expressed by the formula

Pressure (P) = 2 × tension (T)/radius (R)

has come to be known as *Laplace's law* (Fig. 19-6). Laplace's law states that the tension in the wall of a sphere is equal to the product of its radius and its transmural pressure (inside minus outside pressure). Laplace's law was later expanded to include wall thickness (T = P × R/wall thickness). Wall tension is inversely related to wall thickness such that the thicker the vessel wall, the less the tension and

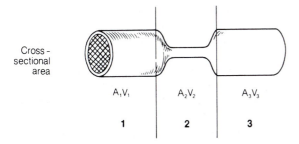

Cross-sectional area

A_1V_1 A_2V_2 A_3V_3

1   2   3

FIG. 19-4. Effect of cross-sectional area on velocity of flow. In section 1, velocity is low because of an increase in cross-sectional area. In section 2, velocity is increased because of a decrease in cross-sectional area. In section 3, velocity is again reduced because of an increase in cross-sectional area.

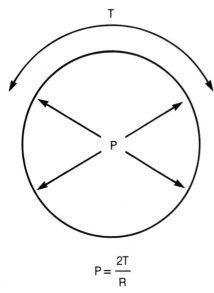

$$P = \frac{2T}{R}$$

FIG. 19-6. Law of Laplace (for a sphere $P = 2T/R$, and for a tube $P = T/R$), where P = the pressure needed to distend an elastic sphere or tube, T = the tension in the wall of the sphere or tube, and R = the radius of the sphere or tube.

vice versa. As discussed in Chapter 20, the principles related to wall thickness, wall tension, radius, and intraluminal pressure contribute to the progress and often the eventual rupture of arterial aneurysms. In hypertension, arterial vessel walls hypertrophy and become thicker, thereby minimizing wall stress.

Laplace's law can also be applied to the pressure required to maintain the patency of small blood vessels. Providing that the thickness of a vessel wall and its tension remain constant, it takes more pressure to overcome wall tension and keep a vessel open as its radius decreases in size. The *critical closing pressure* refers to point at which vessels collapse so that blood can no longer flow through them. In circulatory shock, for example, there is a decrease in both blood volume (and vessel radii) and blood pressure. As a result, many of the small vessels collapse as blood pressure drops to the point where it can no longer overcome the wall tension. The collapse of peripheral veins often makes it difficult to insert venous lines that are needed for fluid and blood replacement.

In summary, blood flow is controlled by many of the same mechanisms that control fluid flow in nonbiologic systems. It is influenced by vessel length, pressures differences, vessel radius, blood viscosity, cross-sectional area, and wall tension. The rate of flow is directly related to the pressure difference between the two ends of the vessel and the vessel radius and inversely related to vessel length and blood viscosity. The cross-sectional area of a vessel influences the velocity of flow; as the cross-sectional area decreases, the velocity is increased, and vice versa. Laminar blood flow is flow in which there is layering of blood components in the center of the bloodstream. This re-

duces frictional forces and prevents clotting factors from coming in contact with the vessel wall. In contrast to laminar flow, turbulent flow is disordered, in which the blood moves crosswise as well as lengthwise in blood vessels. At high velocities, flow often becomes turbulent rather than laminar. The relation between wall tension, transmural pressure, and radius is described by Laplace's law, which states that wall tension becomes greater as the radius decreases.

■ THE VASCULAR SYSTEM

BLOOD VESSEL STRUCTURE

Blood vessels are distensible tubes. All the blood vessels, except the capillaries, have walls composed of three layers or coats called tunicae (Fig. 19-7). The *tunica externa*, or *tunica adventitia*, is the outermost covering of the vessel. This layer is composed of fibrous and connective tissue that serves to support the vessel. The *tunica media*, or *middle layer*, is largely a smooth muscle layer that constricts to regulate and control the diameter of the vessel. The *tunica intima*, or *inner layer*, has an elastic layer that joins the media and a thin layer of endothelial cells that lie adjacent to the blood. The endothelial layer provides a smooth and slippery inner surface for the vessel. This smooth inner lining, as long as it remains intact, prevents platelet adherence and blood clotting. The layers of the different types of blood vessels vary with vessel function. The walls of the arterioles, which control blood pressure, have large amounts of smooth muscle. Veins are thin-walled, distensible, and collapsible vessels. Capillaries are single cell–thick vessels designed for the exchange of gases, nutrients, and waste materials.

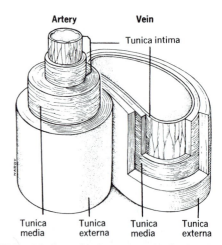

FIG. 19-7. Medium-sized artery and vein showing the relative thickness of the three layers. (Chaffee, E. E., & Lytle, I. M. [1980]. *Basic physiology and anatomy* [4th ed.]. Philadelphia: J.B. Lippincott)

VASCULAR SMOOTH MUSCLE

Smooth muscle contracts slowly and generates high forces for long periods with low energy requirements; it uses only $1/10$ to $1/300$ the energy of skeletal muscle. These characteristics are important in structures, such as blood vessels, that must maintain their tone day in and day out.

Although smooth muscle contains both actin and myosin filaments, these contractile filaments are not arranged in striations as they are in skeletal and cardiac muscle. Rather, smooth muscle fibers are linked together in a strong cable-like system that generates a circular pull as it contracts. Smooth muscle also lacks the fast sodium channels that function in the depolarization of striated skeletal and cardiac muscle (see Chapter 1). Instead, depolarization of smooth muscle occurs through calcium channels that are controlled by changes in the membrane potential or by receptor-mediated mechanisms. When smooth muscle is directly depolarized, a change in membrane potential causes calcium channels to open, allowing extracellular calcium ions to enter and initiate contraction. Receptor-activated channels involve the use of a second messenger, such as cyclic adenosine monophosphate (cAMP), and can be either excitatory or inhibitory. Sympathetic nervous system control of vascular smooth muscle occurs by way of receptor-activated channels. In general, α-adrenergic receptors are excitatory and produce vasoconstriction, and β-adrenergic receptors are inhibitory and produce vasodilation. Calcium-channel blocking drugs cause vasodilation by blocking calcium entry through the calcium channels.

VASCULAR ENDOTHELIUM

The endothelium, which lies between the blood and the vascular smooth muscle, serves as a physical barrier for vasoactive substances that circulate in the blood. Once thought to be nothing more than a single layer of cells that line blood vessels, it is now known that the endothelium plays an active role in controlling vascular function.

In capillaries, which are composed of a single layer of endothelial cells, the endothelium is active in transporting cell nutrients and wastes. In addition to its function in capillary transport, the endothelium removes vasoactive agents such as norepinephrine from the blood; it produces enzymes that convert precursors to active products (*e.g.*, angiotensin I to angiotensin II in lung vessels); and it secretes vasoactive substances such as prostacyclin, which inhibits platelet aggregation and produces vasodilation.

Of particular importance was the discovery, first reported in 1980, that the intact endothelium was able to produce a factor that caused relaxation of vascular smooth muscle. This factor was named *endothelial-derived relaxing factor (EDRF)*.[4,5] The discovery was an outcome of laboratory observations in which strips of vascular smooth muscle were exposed to agents known to produce relaxation. It was found that relaxation occurred only in vessel strips with an intact endothelium. Although the original discovery was made using acetylcholine, a number of other agents have since been shown to produce vascular relaxation in the same way. Thrombin was one of the first blood constituents shown to trigger EDRF. Aggregating platelets and the products they release also evoke endothelium-dependent vessel relaxation. This probably contributes to the protective role the endothelium plays in controlling platelet aggregation and thrombus formation. It also raises the question as to what happens in atherosclerotic vessels in which the endothelium has been injured or lost. In these vessels, the absence or dysfunction of the endothelium may favor the occurrence of abnormal vasoconstriction.

Recent evidence suggests the presence of an endothelial-derived contracting factor (EDCF). A reported stimulus for EDCF is hypoxia. In the pulmonary circulation, the production of EDCF could help to explain the vasoconstriction and pulmonary hypertension that occurs with hypoxia.

ARTERIAL SYSTEM

The arterial system consists of the large and medium-sized arteries and the arterioles. Arteries are thick-walled vessels with large amounts of elastic fibers. The elasticity of these vessels allows them to stretch during cardiac systole, when the heart contracts and blood enters the circulation, and to recoil during diastole, when the heart relaxes. The arterioles, which are predominantly smooth muscle, serve as resistance vessels for the circulatory system. They act as control valves through which blood is released as it moves into the capillaries. Sympathetic vasoconstrictor tone enables these vessels to constrict or to relax as needed to maintain blood pressure.

Arterial blood flow is pulsatile with fluctuating systolic and diastolic pressures; therefore, the average or *mean arterial pressure* often is used. Mean arterial pressure can be estimated by adding one third of the pulse pressure (difference between systolic and diastolic blood pressures) to the diastolic blood pressure. Blood encounters resistance as it travels through the arterial system, causing a progressive drop in pressure. The mean arterial pressure in the large arteries of the systemic circulation normally is about

90 to 100 mmHg; in the small arteries, it is 60 to 90 mmHg; and in the arterioles, it is 40 to 60 mmHg.

ARTERIAL PRESSURE PULSES

Blood enters the arterial circulation during ventricular systole. The intermittent pumping action of the ventricles produces a pressure pulse that serves as the driving force for the circulation. In the systemic circulation, the pressure pulse has its origin in the rapid ejection of blood from the left ventricle into the aorta at the onset of systole. This creates an impulse that is transmitted from molecule to molecule along the length of the vessel. In the aorta, this impulse, or pressure wave, is transmitted at a velocity of 4 to 6 m/sec, which is about 20 times faster than the actual flow of blood. These pressure waves are similar to those created by splashing water in a basin or tub. When taking a pulse, it is the pressure pulses that are felt, and it is the pressure pulses that produce the Korotkoff sounds heard during blood pressure measurement. The tip or maximum deflection of the pressure pulse coincides with the systolic blood pressure, and the minimum point of deflection coincides with the diastolic pressure.

As the pressure wave moves out through the aorta into the arteries, it is reflected backward and thus collides with the next advancing pressure wave (Fig. 19-8). Just as the waves created by splashing water in a tub increase in amplitude as they hit the edge of the tub and reverse their direction of movement, the pressure pulse increases as it moves to the peripheral arteries; therefore, the pulse pressure in the femoral artery, for example, usually is greater than that in the aorta. With peripheral arterial disease, resistance to transmission of the pressure wave increases and a delay occurs in the transmission of the reflected wave, so that the pulse decreases in amplitude.

After its initial amplification, the pressure pulse becomes smaller and smaller as it moves through the smaller arteries and arterioles, until it disappears entirely in the capillaries. This damping of the pressure pulse is caused by the resistance and distensibility characteristics of these vessels. The increased resistance of these small vessels impedes the transmission of the pressure waves. Their distensibility is great enough, however, that any small change in flow does not cause a pressure change. Although the pressure pulses usually are not transmitted to the capillaries, there are situations in which this does occur. For example, injury to a finger or other area of the body often results in a throbbing sensation. In this case, extreme dilatation of the small vessels in the injured area produces a reduction in the dampening of the pressure pulse. Capillary pulsations also occur in

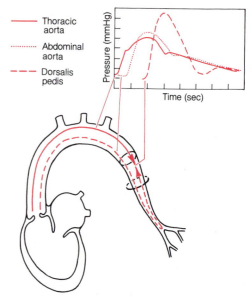

FIG. 19-8. *Amplification of the arterial pressure wave as it moves forward in the peripheral arteries. This amplification occurs as a forward-moving pressure wave merges with a backward-moving reflected pressure wave. The* inset *at upper right shows the increasing amplitude of the pressure pulse in the thoracic aorta, abdominal aorta, and dorsalis pedis.*

conditions that cause exaggeration of aortic pressure pulses, such as aortic regurgitation or patent ductus arteriosus (see Chapter 23).

VENOUS SYSTEM

The veins and venules are thin-walled, distensible, and collapsible vessels. The venules collect blood from the capillaries, and the veins transport blood back to the heart. The structure of the veins allows these vessels to act as a reservoir or blood storage system. Even though the veins are thin-walled, they are muscular. This allows them to contract or expand to accommodate varying amounts of blood.

The venous system is a low-pressure system that relies on changes in intraabdominal pressure and the action of muscle pumps to assist in the movement of blood back to the heart. Their pressure ranges from about 10 mmHg at the end of the venules to about 0 mmHg at the entrance of the vena cavae into the heart. The peripheral veins have valves that prevent the retrograde, or backward, flow of blood and aid in the return of blood to the heart.

Venous flow is designed to return the blood to the heart. The veins are capable of enlarging and storing large quantities of blood, which can be made available to the circulation as needed. Veins are innervated by the sympathetic nervous system. When blood is lost from the circulation, the veins constrict as a means of maintaining intravascular volume. The venous system is a low-pressure system, and when a person is in the upright position, blood flow in the venous system must oppose the effects of gravity. Valves in the veins of extremities prevent the retrograde flow, and with the help of skeletal muscles that surround and intermittently compress the veins in a milking manner, blood is moved forward to the heart. There are no valves in the abdominal or thoracic veins, and blood flow in these veins is heavily influenced by the pressure in the surrounding cavities.

As explained earlier in the chapter, flow in the circulatory system occurs along a pressure gradient, moving from the high-pressure arterial system to the low-pressure venous system. As blood enters the right atrium from the central veins, the pressure in the circulation normally drops to about 0 mmHg; it is this low atrial pressure that maintains the movement of blood into the right heart. Right atrial pressure is regulated by a balance between the ability of the heart to move blood out of the right atrium and through the left heart into the systemic circulation and the tendency of blood to flow from the peripheral veins into the right heart (called venous return). The difference between venous and right atrial pressure is called the *atrial filling pressure*. Blood moves from areas of higher to areas of lower pressure. When the heart pumps strongly, right atrial pressure decreases and atrial filling is enhanced. When atrial pressure rises, venous flow backs up.

Breathing and respiratory maneuvers also affect blood flow in the central veins and right atrium. The negative pressure generated within the thorax during inspiration is transmitted to the right atrium; this produces a decrease in right atrial pressure with a resultant increase in right atrial filling pressure and blood flow into the right heart. During expiration, when intrathoracic pressures are increased, blood flow is decreased.

MICROCIRCULATION

The metarterioles (capillary arterioles), capillaries, and venules of the circulatory system are collectively referred to as the *microcirculation*. It is here that the exchange of gases, nutrients, metabolites, and heat occurs. The lymphatic system represents an accessory system that removes excess fluid, proteins, and large particles from the interstitial spaces and returns it to the circulation. Because of their size, these proteins and large particles cannot be reabsorbed into the venous capillaries. The removal of proteins from the interstitial spaces is an essential function, without which death would occur in about 24 hours.[2]

CAPILLARIES

Capillaries are microscopic, single cell–thick vessels that connect the arterial and venous segments of the circulation. There are about 10 billion capillaries with a surface area of 500 to 700 m^2.[2]

The capillary wall is composed of a single layer of endothelial cells surrounded by a basement membrane (Fig. 19-9). Intracellular junctions join the capillary endothelial cells—these are called the *capillary pores*. Lipid-soluble materials diffuse directly through the capillary cell membrane. Water and water-soluble materials leave and enter the capillary through the capillary pores. The size of the capillary pores varies with capillary function. In the brain, the endothelial cells are joined by tight junctions that form the blood–brain barrier. This prevents substances that would alter neural excitability from leaving the capillary. In organs that process blood contents, such as the liver, capillaries have large pores so that substances can pass easily through the capillary wall. In the kidneys, the glomerular capillaries have small openings called *fenestrations*, which pass directly through the middle of the endothelial cells. Fenestrated capillary walls are consistent with the filtration function of the glomerulus.

The movement of fluids through the capillary pores occurs along a pressure gradient. At the arterial end, the intracapillary pressure (in the systemic circulation) is about 25 mmHg, dropping to about 10 mmHg at the venous end. Because of this pressure gradient, fluids are pushed out of the capillary at the arterial end and pulled back in at the venous end. Plasma proteins and other nondiffusible particles that remain in the capillary exert an osmotic force that contributes to pulling the fluid back into the venous end of the capillary. The mechanisms that control the distribution of fluids between the capillaries and the tissues are discussed in Chapter 29.

Blood enters the capillary through an arteriole and leaves by way of a small venule. The metarterioles serve as thoroughfare channels that link arterioles and capillaries (see Fig. 19-9). Precapillary sphincters control the flow of blood in the microcirculation. When the precapillary sphincters are open, blood flows through the capillary channels. Blood flow through capillary channels designed for exchange of nutrients and metabolites is called *nutritional flow*. In some parts of the microcirculation, blood flow bypasses the nutrient capillary bed, moving through a connection called an *arteriovenous (AV) shunt*, which directly connects an arteriole and a venule. This type of blood flow is called *nonnutrient flow* because it does not allow for nutrient exchange. Nonnutrient channels are important in terms of heat exchange. The AV shunts found in the microcirculation

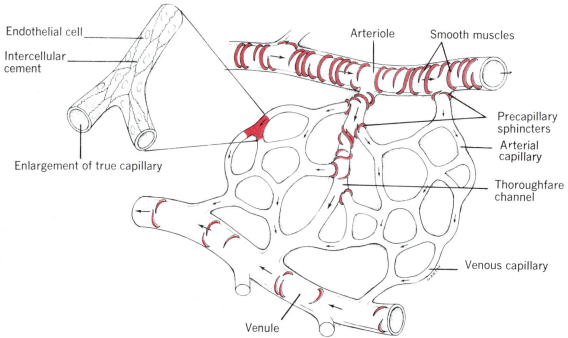

FIG. 19-9. Capillary bed. Precapillary sphincters are relaxed, thus permitting the flow of blood through the capillary network. A greatly magnified portion of capillary wall is shown in the inset (*upper left*). (Chaffee, E. E., & Lytle, I. M. [1980]. *Basic physiology and anatomy* [4th ed.]. Philadelphia: J.B. Lippincott)

of the skin are important in terms of temperature regulation.

The control of blood flow through the microcirculation performs two functions: (1) it provides for the tissue exchange of gases, nutrients, and metabolites and (2) it controls the peripheral vascular resistance of the circulatory tsystem. The total cardiac output travels through the microcirculation; therefore, the tone of these vessels, particularly the arterioles, determines the peripheral vascular resistance and the arterial blood pressure. If, for example, all the arterioles were to open fully, the peripheral vascular resistance, and thus the blood pressure, would fall catastrophically. These two somewhat conflicting functions require a degree of independent control over arteriole resistance and flow in the capillaries of the microcirculation. The nervous system controls the peripheral resistance by regulating the smooth muscle tone of the arterioles, and local factors control the precapillary sphincters, which regulate flow through the nutrient channels of the capillary bed.

LYMPHATIC SYSTEM

The lymphatic system, commonly called the *lymphatics*, serves almost all body tissues except cartilage, bone, epithelial tissue, and tissues of the central nervous system. Most of these tissues, however, have prelymphatic channels that eventually flow into areas supplied by the lymphatics. In addition to returning fluid and protein to the circulation, the lymph system filters the fluid at the lymph nodes and removes foreign particles such as bacteria.

The lymphatic system is made up of vessels similar to those of the circulatory system. These vessels commonly travel along with an arteriole or venule or with its companion artery and vein. The terminal lymphatic vessels are made up of a single layer of connective tissue with an endothelial lining and resemble blood capillaries. They lack tight junctions and are loosely anchored to the surrounding tissues by fine filaments. The loose junctions permit the entry of large particles, and the filaments hold the vessels open under conditions of edema, when the pressure of the surrounding tissues would otherwise cause them to collapse.[6] The lymph capillaries drain into larger lymph vessels that ultimately empty into the right and left thoracic ducts (Fig. 19-10). The thoracic ducts empty into the circulation at the junctions of the subclavian and internal jugular veins. About 120 mL of lymph flows into the circulation each hour through these channels.

Although not as distinct as in the circulatory system, the larger lymph vessels show evidence of having intimal, medial, and adventitial layers similar to blood vessels. The intima of these channels contain elastic tissue and an endothelial layer, and the

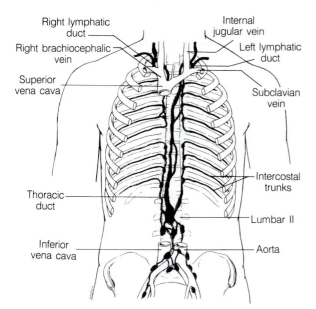

FIG. 19-10. Diagram showing course of thoracic duct and right lymphatic duct. Deep lymphatic vessels and nodes are also shown. (Chaffee, E. E., & Lytle, I. M. [1980]. *Basic physiology and anatomy* [4th ed.]. Philadelphia: J.B. Lippincott)

larger collecting lymph channels contain smooth muscle in their medial layer. Contraction of this smooth muscle assists in propelling lymph fluid toward the thorax. External compression of the lymph channels by pulsating blood vessels in the vicinity and active and passive movements of body parts also aid in forward propulsion of lymph fluid.

In summary, the walls of all blood vessels, except the capillaries, are composed of three layers: the tunica externa, tunica media, and tunica intima. The layers of the vessel vary with its function. Arteries are thick-walled vessels with large amounts of elastic fibers. The walls of the arterioles, which control blood pressure, have large amounts of smooth muscle. Veins are thin-walled, distensible, and collapsible vessels. Capillaries are single cell–thick vessels designed for the exchange of gases, nutrients, and waste materials.

Arterial flow is pulsatile; it reflects the intermittent contraction and relaxation of the heart. The pressure pulses that result from the pumping action of the heart are transmitted throughout the arterial system and reflect the energy that is imparted to the blood during systole. Venous flow is designed to return blood to the heart. It is a low-pressure system and relies on venous valves and the action of muscle pumps to offset the effects of gravity.

The capillaries, venules, and metarterioles of the circulatory system are collectively referred to as the *microcirculation*. It is here that the exchange of gases, nutrients, metabolites, and heat occurs. The control of blood flow through the microcirculation performs two functions: (1) it provides for the tissue exchange of gases, nutrients, and metabolites and (2) it controls the TPR of the circulatory system.

The lymphatic system represents an accessory system that

removes excess fluid, proteins, and large particles from the interstitial spaces and returns it to the circulation. Because of their size, these proteins and large particles cannot be reabsorbed into the venous capillaries.

■ CONTROL OF BLOOD FLOW

The function of the circulatory system is to supply the tissues with oxygen and nutrients and to remove metabolic wastes. To accomplish this function, blood flow must be regulated in relation to the local needs of the tissues and to provide the necessary cardiac output and arterial pressure to propel the blood forward. The local control of blood flow is regulated on a minute-to-minute basis in relation to tissue needs and on a more long-term basis through the development of collateral circulation. Neural mechanisms regulate the cardiac output and blood pressure needed to support these local mechanisms.

LOCAL CONTROL OF BLOOD FLOW

Local control is governed largely by the nutritional needs of the tissue. For example, blood flow to organs such as the heart, brain, and kidneys remains relatively constant, although blood pressure may vary over a range of 60 to 180 mmHg (Fig. 19-11). The ability of the tissues to regulate their own blood flow is called *autoregulation*. Autoregulation of blood flow is controlled by blood vessel distention or by local tissue factors, such as lack of oxygen or accumulation of tissue metabolites (*e.g.*, potassium, lactic acid, or adenosine, which is a breakdown product of ATP). It involves the selective opening and closing of capillary channels. Local control is particularly important

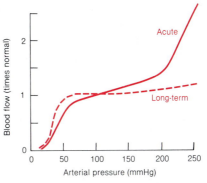

FIG. 19-11. Effect on blood flow through a muscle of increasing arterial pressure. The *solid curve* shows the effect if pressure is raised over a period of a few minutes. The *dashed curve* shows the effect if the arterial pressure is raised slowly over a period of many weeks. (Guyton, A. [1986]. *Medical physiology* [7th ed.]. Philadelphia: W.B. Saunders)

in tissues such as skeletal muscle, which has varying blood flow requirements according to the level of activity.

An increase in local blood flow is called *hyperemia*. When the blood supply to an area has been occluded and then restored, local blood flow through the tissues increases within seconds to restore the metabolic equilibrium of the tissues. This increased flow is called *reactive hyperemia*. The transient redness seen after leaning an arm on a hard surface is an example of reactive hyperemia. The ability of tissues to increase blood flow in situations of increased activity, such as exercising, is called *functional hyperemia*. Local control mechanisms rely on a continuous flow from the main arteries; therefore, hyperemia cannot occur when the arteries that supply the capillary beds are narrowed. For example, if a major coronary artery becomes occluded, the opening of channels supplied by that vessel cannot restore blood flow.

Vasodilator substances, formed in tissues in response to a need for increased blood flow, also aid in the local control of blood flow. The most important of these are histamine, serotonin (5-hydroxytryptamine), the kinins, and the prostaglandins. *Histamine* increases blood flow. Most blood vessels contain histamine in mast cells and nonmast cell stores; when these tissues are injured, histamine is released. In certain tissues, such as skeletal muscle, the activity of the mast cells is mediated by the sympathetic nervous system; that is, when sympathetic control is withdrawn, the mast cells release histamine. This mechanism is augmented with withdrawal of vasoconstrictor activity. *Serotonin* is liberated from aggregating platelets during the clotting process; it causes vasoconstriction and plays a major role in control of bleeding. Serotonin is found in brain and lung tissues, and there is some speculation that it may be involved in the vascular spasm associated with some allergic pulmonary reactions and migraine headaches. The *kinins* (*kallidins* and *bradykinin*) are liberated from the globulin kininogen, which is present in body fluids. The kinins cause relaxation of arteriole smooth muscle, increase capillary permeability, and constrict the venules. In exocrine glands, the formation of kinins contributes to the vasodilation needed for glandular secretion. *Prostaglandins* are synthesized from constituents (the long-chain fatty acid arachidonic acid) of the cell membrane. Tissue injury incites the release of arachidonic acid from the cell membrane, which initiates prostaglandin synthesis. There are several prostaglandins (*e.g.*, E_2, F_2, and D_2), which are subgrouped according to their solubility; some produce vasoconstriction and some produce vasodilation. As a general rule of thumb, those in the E group are vasodilators and those in the F group are vasoconstrictors. The adrenal glucocorticoid hormones can produce an antiinflammatory response by blocking the release of arachidonic acid, thus preventing prostaglandin synthesis.

COLLATERAL CIRCULATION

Collateral circulation is a mechanism for the long-term regulation of local blood flow. In the heart and other vital structures, anastomotic channels exist between some of the smaller arteries. These channels permit perfusion of an area by more than one artery. When one artery becomes occluded, these anastomotic channels increase in size, allowing blood from a patent artery to perfuse the area supplied by the occluded vessel. For example, people with extensive obstruction of a coronary blood vessel may rely on collateral circulation to meet the oxygen needs of the myocardial tissue normally supplied by that vessel. As with other long-term compensatory mechanisms, the recruitment of collateral circulation is most efficient when obstruction to flow is gradual rather than sudden.

NEURAL CONTROL OF BLOOD FLOW

The neural control centers for regulation of cardiovascular function are located in the reticular formation of the lower pons and medulla of the brain. The area of the reticular formation in the brain that controls vasomotor function is called the *vasomotor center*. The sympathetic nervous system serves as the final common pathway for controlling the smooth muscle tone of the blood vessels. Most of the sympathetic preganglionic fibers that control vessel function travel in the intermediolateral column of the spinal cord and exit with the ventral nerves; they then synapse with postganglionic fibers in the paravertebral ganglia. The sympathetic neurons that supply the blood vessels maintain them in a state of tonic activity, so that even under resting conditions, the blood vessels are partially constricted. Vessel constriction and relaxation are accomplished by altering this basal input. Increasing sympathetic activity causes constriction of some vessels, such as those of the skin, the gastrointestinal tract, and the kidneys. Some blood vessels are supplied by both vasoconstrictor and vasodilator fibers. Skeletal muscle, for example, is innervated by both types of fibers; activation of sympathetic vasodilator fibers provides the muscles with increased blood flow during exercise. Although the parasympathetic nervous system contributes to the regulation of heart function, it has little, if any, control over blood vessels.

In summary, the mechanisms that control blood flow are designed to ensure delivery of blood to the capillaries in the microcirculation, where the exchange of cellular nutrients and wastes occurs. Local control is governed largely by the needs of the tissues and is regulated by local tissue factors such as lack of oxygen and the accumulation of metabolites. Hyperemia is a local increase in blood flow that occurs after a temporary occlusion of blood flow. It is a compensatory mechanism that serves to decrease the oxygen debt of the deprived tissues. Collateral circulation is a mechanism for long-term regulation of local blood flow that involves the development of collateral vessels. The vasomotor center of the reticular formation of the lower pons and medulla provides for neural control of blood flow by the sympathetic nervous system.

■   REFERENCES

1. Smith, J.J., & Kampine, J.P. (1989). *Circulatory physiology* (3rd ed., pp. 8, 24). Baltimore: Williams & Wilkins.
2. Guyton, A. (1991). *Medical physiology* (8th ed., pp. 89, 155, 157, 170, 180). Philadelphia: W.B. Saunders.
3. Johansen, K. (1982). Aneurysms. *Scientific American, 247*(1), 110.
4. Furchgott, R.F., & Zawadzki, J.V. (1980). The obligatory role of endothelial cells in relaxation of arterial smooth muscle by acetylcholine. *Nature, 288*, 373.
5. Vanhoutte, P.M. (1987). Endothelium and the control of vascular tissue. *News in Physiological Sciences, 2*(2), 21.
6. McCormack, D.H. (1987). *Ham's histology* (9th ed., p. 448). Philadelphia: J.B. Lippincott.

CHAPTER 20

ALTERATIONS IN BLOOD FLOW

**Mechanisms of Vessel
  Obstruction**
Alterations in Arterial Flow
  Atherosclerosis
    Risk Factors
    Cholesterol and Hyperlipidemia
  Aneurysms

Acute Arterial Occlusion
Peripheral Arterial Disease
  Raynaud's Syndrome
  Thromboangiitis Obliterans
    (Buerger's Disease)
  Atherosclerotic Occlusive Disease
Alterations in Venous Flow

Varicose Veins
Venous Thrombosis
**Alterations in External Forces
  That Impair Blood Flow**
Compartment Syndrome
Pressure Ulcers

■ OBJECTIVES

After you have studied this chapter, you should be able to meet the following objectives:

■ List five mechanisms of blood vessel obstruction.
■ Describe vessel changes that occur in atherosclerosis.
■ Cite two current theories used to explain the pathogenesis of atherosclerosis.
■ List three established risk factors in atherosclerosis.
■ List the five types of lipoproteins and state their function in terms of lipid transport.
■ State beneficial effects of controlling the fat and cholesterol content of the diet.
■ Distinguish among berry aneurysms, aortic aneurysms, and dissecting aneurysms.
■ List the signs and symptoms associated with thoracic and abdominal aneurysms.
■ State the signs and symptoms of acute arterial occlusion.
■ State a method for describing gradations in pulse volume.

■ Differentiate between the mechanisms of ischemia in Raynaud's syndrome and thromboangiitis obliterans (Buerger's disease).
■ State the signs and symptoms of chronic peripheral vascular disease.
■ Describe the effect of gravity on the venous system.
■ State the signs and symptoms of venous insufficiency.
■ Describe the pathology involved in venous thrombosis.
■ State five possible causes of compartment syndrome.
■ Explain why pulses and capillary refill time are not good assessment measures for compartment syndrome.
■ Cite two causes of pressure ulcers.
■ Explain how shearing forces contribute to ischemic skin damage.
■ List four measures that contribute to the prevention of pressure ulcers.

Carol Mattson Porth: PATHOPHYSIOLOGY: CONCEPTS OF
ALTERED HEALTH STATES, 4th ed. © 1994, 1990, 1986, 1982
J.B. Lippincott Company

Blood flow in both the arterial and the venous system depends on patent vessels and adequate perfusion pressure. Interruption of arterial flow impairs the delivery of oxygenated blood to the tissues. Alterations in venous flow obstruct the return of blood to the heart, causing congestion and edema. This chapter is organized into four sections: (1) mechanisms of vessel obstruction, (2) disorders of the arterial circulation, (3) alterations of the venous circulation, and (4) alterations in blood flow caused by external forces.

■ MECHANISMS OF VESSEL OBSTRUCTION

Blood flow is impeded by conditions that occlude blood vessels. As described in Chapter 19, the flow of blood through a vessel is directly related to the fourth power of the radius. Thus, decreasing the radius from 2 to 1 mm produces a 16-fold decrease in flow. A decrease in vessel radius and complete or partial occlusion of flow within a vessel can result from (1) vessel compression, (2) vasospasm, or (3) structural defects in the vessel wall (Fig. 20-1). Thrombi and emboli can also obstruct flow.

External forces can exert sufficient pressure to *compress* blood vessels and impair blood flow. Tumors may encroach on blood vessels as they grow. Although not intended, casts and circular dressings predispose to vessel compression, particularly when swelling occurs after these devices have been applied.

Vasospasm is a local or neurally mediated contraction of vascular smooth muscle that produces blood vessel narrowing (vasoconstriction). Exposure to cold causes severe vasoconstriction in many of the superficial blood vessels. Fortunately, local control mechanisms produce brief periods of vasodilation designed to maintain tissue oxygen needs. Those who have spent time on the ski slopes or elsewhere in the cold may have noticed the intermittent redness of their companions' noses during these periods of vasodilation. In certain disease states, vasospasm from exposure to cold or other stimuli is excessive and may lead to ischemia and tissue injury.

Structural changes in blood vessels can take many forms. Atherosclerosis causes rigidity and narrowing of large and medium-sized arteries. Defects in venous valves may impair blood flow in the venous system, causing varicose veins.

A *thrombus* is a blood clot. With formation of a thrombus, there is narrowing of the vessel lumen and obstruction of flow. Blood clotting is a homeostatic mechanism intended to seal off blood vessels, prevent bleeding, and maintain the continuity of the vascular system. Although thrombi can develop in either the arterial or the venous system, they are more common in the venous system. This is because the low-pressure characteristics of the venous system favor stasis of flow and aggregation of platelets and clotting factors. Alterations in hemostasis are discussed in Chapter 17.

An *embolus* is a foreign mass transported in the bloodstream. Although an embolus moves freely in the larger blood vessels, it becomes lodged and obstructs flow once it reaches a smaller vessel. An embolus can be a dislodged thrombus or can consist of air, fat, tumor cells, or other materials. About 95% of venous thrombi that become emboli have their origin in the deep veins of the legs. These emboli move through the venous system, into the right heart, and then into the pulmonary circulation where they can become lodged and obstruct blood flow. Arterial emboli commonly have their origin in the heart itself and can travel to the brain, spleen, kidneys, or vessels of the lower extremities before they become lodged and obstruct flow.

In summary, interruption of flow in either the arterial or the venous system interferes with the flow of oxygen and nutrients to the tissues. Occlusion of flow can result from (1) the presence of a thrombus, (2) emboli, (3) vessel compression, (4) vasospasm, or (5) structural changes within the vessel.

■ ALTERATIONS IN ARTERIAL FLOW

The arterial system distributes blood to all the various tissues in the body; pathology of the arterial system affects body function through impaired blood flow. The effect that impaired blood flow has on the

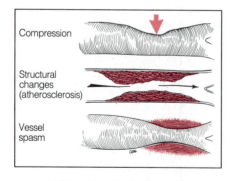
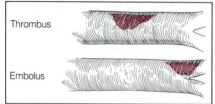

FIG. 20-1. Mechanisms of blood vessel occlusion.

body depends on the structures involved and the extent of altered flow. The term *ischemia* means the holding back of blood and refers to a reduction in arterial flow to a level that is insufficient to match the oxygen demands of the tissues. The discussion in this section focuses on arteriosclerosis, aneurysms, acute arterial occlusion, peripheral vascular diseases (Raynaud's syndrome and Buerger's disease), and assessment of arterial flow.

ATHEROSCLEROSIS

Atherosclerosis is a type of arteriosclerosis or hardening of the arteries. The term *atherosclerosis*, which comes from the Greek word *atheros* (meaning gruel or paste) and *sclerosis* (meaning hardness), is characterized by the formation of fibrofatty lesions in the intimal lining of the large and medium-sized arteries such as the aorta and its branches, the coronaries, and the large vessels that supply the brain.

As the leading cause of death in the United States, atherosclerosis contributed to 645,320 deaths from heart attack and stroke in 1989.[1] In 1988, the estimated cost of coronary heart disease and stroke was $48.7 billion in health care expenditures and lost productivity. The bright side of this grim picture is the recent decline in death rates from coronary heart disease. In 1978 alone, there were 114,000 fewer deaths among people aged 35 to 74 than would have been expected had the rate not declined from its high level in the 1960s.[2] This decline probably reflects new and improved methods of medical treatment as well as improved health care practices resulting from an increased public awareness of the factors that predispose to the development of this disorder.

Atherosclerosis begins as an insidious process, and clinical manifestations of the disease typically do not become evident for 20 to 40 years or longer. Fibrous plaques commonly begin to appear in the arteries of Americans in their 20s. Among 300 American soldiers (average age 22) killed during the Korean war, 77% had gross evidence of atherosclerosis.[3]

Atherosclerotic lesions are characterized by (1)

the accumulation of intracellular and extracellular lipids, (2) proliferation of vascular smooth muscle cells, and (3) formation of large amounts of scar tissue and connective tissue proteins.[4] The lesions begin as a gray to pearly white elevated thickening of the vessel intima with a core of extracellular lipid (mainly cholesterol, which usually is complexed to proteins) covered by a fibrous cap of connective tissue and smooth muscle. Later lesions contain hemorrhage, ulceration, and scar tissue deposits. As the lesions increase in size, they encroach on the lumen of the artery and eventually may either occlude the vessel or predispose to thrombus formation, causing a reduction of blood flow. Because blood flow is related to the fourth power of the radius, reduction in blood flow becomes more severe as the disease progresses.

RISK FACTORS

To date, the cause or causes of atherosclerosis have not been determined with certainty. Epidemiologic studies have, however, identified predisposing risk factors, which are listed in Table 20-1. Some of these risk factors can be changed and others cannot.

Risk factors such as heredity, male sex, and increasing age cannot be changed. It appears that the tendency to develop atherosclerosis runs in families. A number of genetically determined alterations in lipoprotein and cholesterol metabolism have been identified, and it seems likely that others will be identified in the future. The incidence of atherosclerosis increases with age. Men are at greater risk for developing coronary heart disease than are women; even though the death rate of women increases after menopause, it never reaches that of men. Race is also an inherited risk factor. More black Americans have hypertension than do whites, and consequently, their risk of developing atherosclerosis and coronary heart disease is increased.[1]

The major risk factors that can be changed include cigarette smoking, high blood pressure (see Chapter 21), and high blood cholesterol levels. Cigarette smoking is closely linked with coronary heart

TABLE 20-1. RISK FACTORS OF ATHEROSCLEROSIS

MAJOR RISK FACTORS THAT CANNOT BE CHANGED	MAJOR RISK FACTORS THAT CAN BE CHANGED	CONTRIBUTING FACTORS
Heredity	Cigarette smoking	Diabetes
Male sex	High blood pressure	Obesity
Increasing age	Blood cholesterol levels	Physical inactivity
		Stress

(*Heart facts 1992.* [1992]. Dallas: American Heart Association)

disease and sudden death. The risk of death from coronary heart disease is 70 to 200 times greater for men who smoke one or more packs of cigarettes per day than for those who do not.[5] The greatest effects of smoking are noted in young men and women, particularly those under age 55. The effects are directly related to the number of cigarettes smoked (packs/day/year). Risk factors such as high blood pressure and high blood cholesterol levels often can be controlled with the aid of a physician and other health professionals. The responsibility for changing other risk factors, such as smoking, rests largely with the person.

The association between coronary heart disease and contributing or "soft" factors is not as convincing as for the established risk factors. These "soft" risk factors commonly are linked with the established and other contributing risk factors. For example, obesity and physical inactivity often are observed in the same person. Furthermore, both of these conditions are reported to bring about elevations in blood lipid levels. Likewise, major risk factors such as cigarette smoking are closely associated with stress and personality patterns. Diabetes mellitus (type II) typically develops in middle-aged people and those who are overweight. Diabetes elevates blood lipid levels and otherwise increases the risk of atherosclerosis (see Chapter 46). Therefore, controlling other risk factors is particularly important in people with diabetes.

MECHANISMS OF DEVELOPMENT

Although the risk factors associated with atherosclerosis have been identified through epidemiologic studies, there are many unanswered questions regarding the mechanisms by which these risk factors contribute to the development of atherosclerosis. Research suggests that atherosclerosis results from endothelial injury, lipid (low-density lipoprotein [LDL] and cholesterol) infiltration, and smooth muscle proliferation.

The vascular endothelial layer acts as a selective barrier that protects the subendothelial layers from interacting with blood cells and blood components. The endothelial cells determine the nature of lipoproteins and other plasma constituents that reach the subendothelial space and vascular smooth muscle. They bind LDLs and modify them so that the LDLs can be ingested by macrophages; they produce vasoactive agents, growth factors, and growth inhibitors. The vascular endothelial cells are arranged in a single layer with cell-to-cell attachments. With repeated injury, the cell-to-cell attachments may be weakened and there may be impaired ability of the endothelium to regenerate. A number of factors are regarded as possible injurious agents, including products associated with smoking, immune mechanisms, and mechanical stress such as that associated with hypertension. If the injury is a single event, the lesion usually is reversible. If the original mechanism that led to vessel injury persists, there is less time for healing to occur and the lesion may become chronic.

Interactions between the endothelial layer and the white blood cells, particularly the monocytes (macrophages), normally occur throughout life; these interactions increase when blood cholesterol levels are elevated. One of the earliest responses to elevated cholesterol levels is the attachment of clusters of monocytes throughout the arterial tree.[6] The monocytes have been observed to move through the cell-to-cell attachments of the endothelial cells into the subendothelial spaces, where they contribute to the formation of fatty streaks. With continued enlargement of the fatty streaks, the cell-to-cell attachments are broken, the endothelial cells are pulled apart, and the underlying connective tissue is exposed. This provides the environment for platelet adherence, aggregation, and thrombosis.

Proliferation of vascular smooth muscle is also a feature in atherosclerotic plaque formation. One hypothesis of plaque formation is that endothelial injury is an initiating factor that permits platelets, cholesterol, and other blood components to come in contact with and stimulate abnormal proliferation of smooth muscle cells and connective tissue within the vessel wall (Fig. 20-2). Platelets contain a potent smooth muscle mitogenic actor that induces cell mitosis and proliferation. This factor is released from platelets when they aggregate over a denuded area on the vessel wall. Evidence suggests that LDLs act as cofactors that are necessary for growth and proliferation of vascular smooth muscle cells, but they are not able to stimulate the process by themselves.[7]

CHOLESTEROL AND HYPERLIPIDEMIA

Cholesterol is a waxy, fat-like substance that is essential to the growth and viability of body cells. It is an important component of cell membranes and is used in the synthesis of steroid hormones (eg, estrogens, testosterone, and cortisol). Although most cholesterol is found in cells, a small amount (about 7%) circulates in the blood serum.[5] It is the serum cholesterol that contributes to the formation of atherosclerotic plaques in arteries throughout the body.

According to the guidelines developed by the National Cholesterol Education Program's Expert Panel on Detection, Evaluation, and Treatment of High Blood Cholesterol in Adults, a cholesterol level of less than 200 mg/dL is considered desirable; levels between 200 and 239 mg/dL are borderline high; and

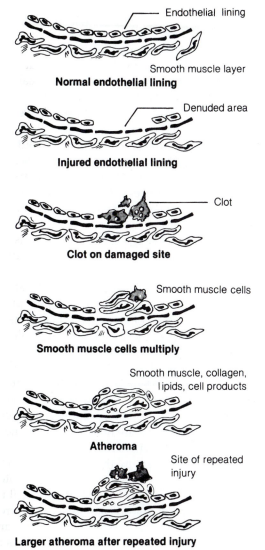

Normal endothelial lining

Injured endothelial lining

Clot on damaged site

Smooth muscle cells multiply

Atheroma

Larger atheroma after repeated injury

FIG. 20-2. Theory for evolution of atheroma. (Report of the 1977 Working Group to Review the Report by the National Heart and Lung Institute Task Force on Arteriosclerosis. [1977]. *Arteriosclerosis.* DHEW Publication No. NIH 81034)

levels equal to or greater than 240 mg/dL are high.[8] The Framingham Heart Study indicated that in men and women aged 35 to 44, serum cholesterol levels of 265 mg/dL or higher are associated with a five times greater risk of developing coronary heart disease than levels below 220 mg/dL.[9]

Lipoproteins. Because cholesterol and triglycerides are insoluble in plasma, they are encapsulated by special fat-carrying proteins—the lipoproteins—for transport in the blood. There are five classes of lipoproteins: (1) chylomicrons, (2) very low density lipoprotein (VLDL), (3) intermediate-density lipoprotein (IDL), (4) LDL, and (5) high-density lipoprotein (HDL). The naming of these lipoproteins is based on ultracentrifugation, by which the lipoproteins are

separated according to their density. Triglycerides have a lower density than cholesterol. Accordingly, VLDL carries large amounts of triglycerides compared with LDL. The lipoproteins can also be separated by electrophoresis, a technique that uses an electrical field to separate proteins. VLDL falls into the pre-beta band, LDL into the beta band, and HDL into the alpha band. β-VLDL, a cholesterol-enriched form of VLDL, migrates with the β-lipoproteins on electrophoresis. It is elevated in people who have an inherited form of hyperlipoproteinemia called *familial dysbetalipoproteinemia.*

Each type of lipoprotein consists of a large molecular complex of lipids and proteins called *apoproteins.*[10, 11] The major lipid constituents are cholesterol esters, triglycerides, nonesterified cholesterol, and phospholipids. The insoluble cholesterol esters and triglycerides are located in the hydrophobic core of the lipoprotein macromolecule, surrounded by phospholipids, nonesterified cholesterol, and apoproteins (Fig. 20-3). Both the nonesterified cholesterol and the triglycerides provide a negative electric charge that allows the lipoprotein to be soluble in plasma. There are four major classes of apoproteins, the major types being A (A-I, A-II, A-III, and A-IV), B-48, B-100, C (CI, CII, CIII), and E. The apoproteins control the interactions and ultimate metabolic fate of the lipoproteins. Some of the apoproteins activate the lipolytic enzymes that facilitate the removal of lipids from the lipoproteins; others serve as a reactive site that cellular receptors can recognize and use in endocytosis and the metabolism of the lipoproteins. The major apoprotein in LDL is B-100. Research findings suggest that genetic defects in apoproteins may be involved in hyperlipidemia and accelerated atherosclerosis.[12, 13]

The lipoproteins are synthesized in the small intestine and the liver. The chylomicrons, which are the largest lipoprotein molecules, are synthesized in the wall of the small intestine and carry large

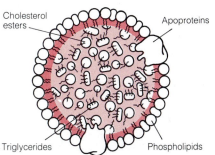

Cholesterol esters

Apoproteins

Triglycerides

Phospholipids

FIG. 20-3. *General structure of a lipoprotein. The cholesterol esters and triglycerides are located in the hydrophobic core of the macromolecule, surrounded by phospholipids and aproproteins.*

amounts of triglycerides (80% to 95% of their lipid content).[5] They are involved in the transport of exogenous triglycerides and cholesterol that have been absorbed from the gastrointestinal tract. Chylomicrons travel to the capillaries of adipose and skeletal muscle tissue; there they transfer their triglycerides to fat and muscle cells. The remaining cholesterol-containing chylomicron remnant particles are taken up by the liver. In this way, the chylomicrons transport dietary triglycerides to the tissues and cholesterol to the liver. The exogenous and endogenous pathways for cholesterol and triglyceride transport are shown in Figure 20-4.

The liver synthesizes and secretes VLDL and HDL. The VLDL contain about 75% triglycerides and 25% cholesterol.[5] They provide the primary pathway for transport of the endogenous triglycerides produced in the liver, as opposed to those obtained from the diet. Like chylomicrons, VLDLs carry their triglycerides to tissue capillaries for entry into fat and muscle cells. When the triglycerides have been removed from the VLDLs, the remaining remnants, which now contain about 45% cholesterol, are the IDLs. The IDLs are either taken up and broken down by the liver or converted to LDL by an intravascular process that removes much of the remaining triglycerides, leaving about 70% cholesterol.

LDL, sometimes called the "bad cholesterol," is the main carrier of cholesterol. LDL is removed from the circulation by both receptor-dependent and non–receptor-dependent mechanisms. Receptor-mediated transport of LDL involves binding to cell surface receptors followed by endocytosis, a phagocytic process in which LDL is engulfed and moved into the cell in the form of a membrane-covered endocytic vesicle. Within the cell, the endocytic vesicles fuse with lysosomes, and the LDL molecule is enzymatically degraded, causing free cholesterol to be released into the cytoplasm. Although most of the LDL receptors are located in the liver, other nonhepatic tissues (adrenal glands, smooth muscle cells, endothelial cells, and lymphoid cells) use the receptor-dependent pathway to obtain cholesterol needed for membrane and hormone synthesis. These tissues can control their cholesterol intake by adding or removing LDL receptors.

About two thirds of the LDL is removed by way of the receptor-dependent pathway. The remaining one third of LDL is removed by non–receptor-dependent mechanisms, including ingestion by phagocytic macrophages. In addition, nonreceptor uptake occurs in various other cells, particularly in the presence of high LDL levels. Macrophage uptake of LDL within the arterial wall can result in the accumulation of insoluble cholesterol ester, the formation of foam cells, and the development of atherosclerosis. When there is a decrease in LDL receptors or when LDL levels exceed receptor availability, the amount of LDL that must be removed by the non–receptor-dependent mechanisms is increased.

HDL is synthesized in the liver and often is referred to as the "good cholesterol." HDL participates in the reverse transport of cholesterol. Epidemiologic studies show an inverse relation between

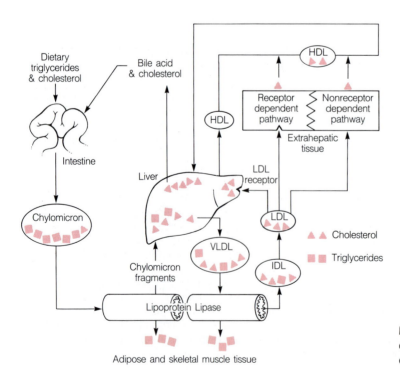

FIG. 20-4. Schematic representation of the exogenous and endogenous lipoprotein triglyceride and cholesterol transport.

HDL levels and the development of atherosclerosis. Although several explanations for the protective actions of HDL have been proposed, none has been proved. Probably HDL, which is low in cholesterol and rich in surface phospholipids, facilitates the clearance of cholesterol from atheromatous plaques and transports it to the liver where it may be excreted rather than reused in the formation of LDL. HDL is also believed to inhibit cellular uptake of LDL. It has been observed that regular exercise and moderate alcohol consumption increase HDL levels. Smoking and diabetes, which are in themselves risk factors for atherosclerosis, are associated with decreased levels of HDL. There are two subfractions of HDL, HDL_3 and its derivative HDL_2. Research suggests that both subfractions contribute to a decreased risk of atherosclerosis and myocardial infarction.[14]

Hyperlipidemia. Serum cholesterol levels may be elevated as a result of an increase in any of the lipoproteins: the chylomicrons, VLDL, IDL, LDL, or HDL. The commonly used classification system for hyperlipidemias is based on the type of lipoprotein involved (Table 20-2). Three factors—nutrition, genetics, and metabolic diseases—can raise blood lipid levels. Most cases of elevated levels of cholesterol are probably multifactorial. Some people may have increased sensitivity to dietary cholesterol; others, a lack of LDL receptors; and still others, an altered synthesis of the apoproteins, including oversynthesis of apoprotein B-100, the major apoprotein in LDL.

Causes of secondary hyperlipoproteinemia include obesity with high-caloric intake and diabetes mellitus. High-calorie diets increase the production of VLDL, with triglyceride elevation and high conversion of VLDL to LDL. Excess ingestion of cholesterol may reduce the formation of LDL receptors, and thereby decrease LDL removal. Diets that are high in triglycerides and saturated fats increase cholesterol synthesis and suppress LDL receptor activity. In diabetes mellitus, metabolic derangements cause an elevation of lipoproteins.

Many types of primary hypercholesterolemia have a genetic basis. There may be a defective synthesis of the apoproteins, a lack of receptors, defective receptors, or defects in the handling of cholesterol within the cell that are genetically determined. For example, the normal LDL receptor is deficient or defective in the genetic disorder known as *familial hypercholesterolemia* (type IIA). This autosomal dominant type of hyperlipoproteinemia results from a mutation in the gene specifying the receptor for LDL. Because most of the circulating cholesterol is removed by receptor-dependent mechanisms, blood cholesterol levels are markedly elevated in people with this disorder. The disorder is probably one of the most common of all mendelian disorders; the frequency of heterozygotes is 1 in 500 in the general population.[5] Heterozygotes have a two- to three-fold elevation of plasma cholesterol levels; in homozygotes, the elevation may be five-fold or greater. Although heterozygotes commonly have an elevated cholesterol level from birth, they do not develop symptoms until adult life, when they develop xanthomas (cholesterol deposits) along the tendons and atherosclerosis. Myocardial infarction before age 40 is common. Homozygotes are much more severely affected; they develop cutaneous xanthomas in child-

TABLE 20-2. CLASSIFICATION OF HYPERLIPOPROTEINEMIAS

TYPE	FAMILIAR NAME	LIPOPROTEIN ABNORMALITY	CAUSE
Type I	Exogenous dietary hyper-triglyceridemia	Elevated chylomicrons; triglycerides. Normal cholesterol	Dietary fat not cleared from the plasma
Type IIA	Hypercholesterolemia (familial)	Elevated LDL, cholesterol. Normal triglycerides	Hereditary metabolic defect
Type IIB	Combined hyperlipidemia	Elevated LDL, VLDL, cholesterol, triglycerides	Possible long-term dietary excess; hereditary component
Type III	Remnant hyperlipidemia	Increased beta-VLDL, cholesterol, triglycerides	Hereditary metabolic defect (familial dysbetalipoproteinemia)
Type IV	Endogenous hypertriglyceridemia	Elevated VLDL, triglycerides. Cholesterol normal or elevated	Excessive carbohydrate intake
Type V	Mixed hypertriglyceridemia	Elevated chylomicrons, VLDL, cholesterol. Triglycerides greatly increased	Possible metabolic defect

(From information in Robbins, S.L., & Kumar, V. [1987]. *Basic pathology* [4th ed., p. 289]. Philadelphia: W.B. Saunders; and Gotto, A.M. [1988]. Lipoprotein metabolism and etiology of hyperlipidemia. *Hospital Practice, 23* [Suppl 1], 4)

hood and many die of myocardial infarction by age 20.[14]

Diagnosis and Treatment. The National Institutes of Health Consensus Development Conference on Lowering Blood Cholesterol to Prevent Heart Disease recommended that (1) all Americans attempt to reduce their cholesterol intake; (2) people at moderate risk for coronary heart disease (cholesterol levels above the 75th percentile for Americans) and those at high risk (levels above the 90th percentile) be treated aggressively with diet; and (3) drugs be added to the regimen, particularly for high-risk people, if diet modification alone fails to lower cholesterol.[15]

It is recommended that all adults 20 years of age and older have their blood cholesterol level measured at least once every 5 years.[16] In most adults, a fasting serum cholesterol level using a venous blood sample is indicated. It is particularly important that people at high risk, such as those with a strong family history of coronary heart disease, be tested. This applies to children as well as adult family members. In people with cholesterol levels above 200 mg/dL, repeat measurements of serum cholesterol along with lipoprotein analysis may be indicated. LDL-cholesterol can be estimated using this approach. Capillary blood cholesterol testing methods provide a means for mass screening for hypercholesterolemia. The reliability of these methods, the education of the participants, and proper referral and follow-up in public screening programs all need special attention.[16]

The treatment of hypercholesterolemia focuses on dietary and life-style modifications; when these are unsuccessful, pharmacologic treatment is necessary. Three elements that affect dietary cholesterol and its lipoprotein fractions are (1) excess calorie intake, (2) saturated fats, and (3) cholesterol.[17] Excess calories consistently lower HDL and less consistently elevate LDL. Saturated fats in the diet can strongly influence cholesterol levels. Each 1% of saturated fat relative to caloric intake increases the cholesterol level an average of 2.8 mg/dL. Depending on individual differences, it raises both the VLDL and the LDL. Dietary cholesterol tends to increase LDL cholesterol. On an average, each 100 mg/dL of ingested cholesterol raises the serum cholesterol 8 to 10 mg/dL.[17]

Soluble fiber in the diet (pectin, bran, and guar) is another dietary intervention that has been shown to have moderate LDL- lowering effects. Most studies that have reported beneficial effects have used large amounts of fiber, which often produce adverse gastrointestinal effects; tolerance improves with prolonged usage.

Lipid-lowering drugs ultimately work by affecting cholesterol production, increasing intravascular breakdown, or removing cholesterol from the bloodstream. Drugs that act directly to decrease cholesterol levels also have the beneficial effect of further lowering cholesterol levels by stimulating the production of additional LDL receptors. This is how it occurs: When serum levels fall and cells need more cholesterol, the amount of messenger ribonucleic acid for LDL receptor biosynthesis rises and more receptors are found on the cell surface.

Five types of medications are available for treating hypercholesterolemia: (1) niacin and its congeners, (2) fibric acid agents, (3) bile acid–binding resins, (4) HMG-CoA reductase inhibitors, and (5) probucol. *Nicotinic acid* (a niacin congener) blocks the synthesis and release of VLDL by the liver, thereby lowering not only VLDL levels but IDL and LDL levels as well. The *fibric acid derivatives* (cholestyramine and colestipol) decrease the synthesis of VLDL from chylomicron fragments and enhance the intravascular lipolysis of VLDL and IDL. The *bile acid–binding resins* (clofibrate and gemfibrozil) bind and sequester cholesterol-containing bile acids in the intestine and prevent the reabsorption of cholesterol by way of the chylomicrons. *Inhibitors of HMG-CoA reductase* (lovastatin), a key enzyme in the cholesterol biosynthetic pathway, can reduce or block the hepatic synthesis of cholesterol. *Probucol* removes LDL from the circulation independently of LDL receptor activity. Because many of these drugs have significant adverse effects, they usually are used only in people with significant hyperlipidemia that cannot be controlled by other means, such as diet.

ANEURYSMS

An aneurysm is an abnormal localized vessel dilatation caused by weakness of the arterial wall. Aneurysms can assume several forms and may be classified according to their cause, location, and anatomic features (Fig. 20-5). A *berry aneurysm* consists of a small, spherical dilatation of the vessel and seldom is larger than 1.5 cm in diameter.[5] This type of aneurysm usually is found in the circle of Willis in the cerebral circulation. A *fusiform aneurysm* involves the entire circumference of the vessel and is characterized by a gradual and progressive dilatation of the vessel. These aneurysms, which vary in diameter (up to 20 cm) and length, may involve the entire ascending and transverse portions of the thoracic aorta or may extend over large segments of the abdominal aorta. A *saccular aneurysm* extends over part of the circumference of the vessel and appears saclike. They can vary in size up to 20 cm but typically are about 5 to 10 cm in diameter.[5] In a *dissecting aneurysm*, vessel dilatation occurs because of the accumulation of blood within the layers of the vessel wall. This occurs

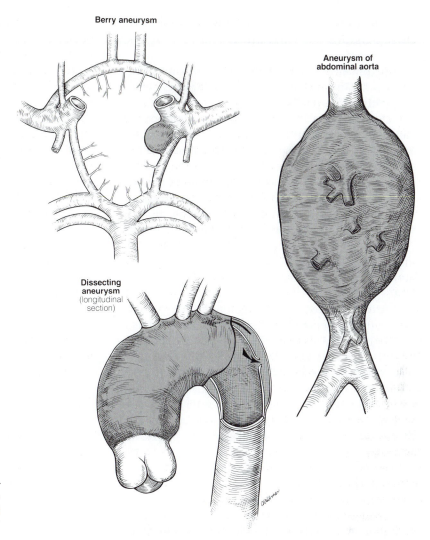

FIG. 20-5. Three forms of aneurysms—berry aneurysm in the circle of Willis, fusiform-type aneurysm of the abdominal aorta, and a dissecting aortic aneurysm.

when blood enters the wall of the artery, dissecting its layers to create a blood-filled cavity.

The weakness that leads to aneurysm formation may be due to several factors, including congenital defects, trauma, infections, and arteriosclerosis. Once initiated, the aneurysm grows larger as the tension on the vessel wall increases. If untreated, the aneurysm may burst because of internal pressure. Even an unruptured aneurysm can cause damage by exerting pressure on adjacent structures and interrupting blood flow.

AORTIC ANEURYSMS

Aortic aneurysms may involve any part of the aorta: the ascending aorta, aortic arch, descending aorta, or thoracicoabdominal aorta. Multiple aneurysms may be present. Aortic aneurysms were, until recently, largely caused by tertiary syphilis. Now, with better control of syphilis, atherosclerosis has become the leading cause of aneurysmal development. Athero-

sclerotic aneurysms are most common in men over age 50.

The signs and symptoms of an aortic aneurysm depend on its size and location. With aneurysms of the thoracic aorta, substernal, back, and neck pain may occur. There may also be dyspnea, stridor, or a brassy cough caused by pressure on the trachea. Hoarseness may result from pressure on the recurrent laryngeal nerve, and there may be difficulty swallowing because of pressure on the esophagus. The aneurysm can compress the superior vena cava, causing distention of neck veins and edema of the face and neck. It may also cause enlargement of the aorta in the areas of the aortic valve to the point of preventing complete valve closure and causing aortic regurgitation. An aortic aneurysm may also be asymptomatic, with the first evidence of its presence being associated with vessel rupture.

Most aneurysms of the abdominal aorta are below the level of the renal artery and involve the bifurcation of the aorta and proximal end of the common iliac arteries. Because an aneurysm is of arterial origin, a pulsating mass may provide the first evidence of the disorder. The mass may be discovered during a routine physical examination, or the affected person may complain of its presence. Calcification, which frequently exists on the wall of the aneurysm, may be detected during abdominal radiologic examination. Pain may be present and varies from mild midabdominal or lumbar discomfort to severe abdominal and back pain. The aneurysm may extend to and impinge on the renal, iliac, or mesenteric arteries. Stasis of blood favors thrombus formation along the wall of the vessel, and peripheral emboli may develop, causing symptomatic arterial insufficiency. With both thoracic and abdominal aneurysms, the most dreaded complication is rupture—the likelihood of rupture correlates with increasing aneurysm size.

Arteriography, using a radiopaque dye to render the aneurysm visible on x-ray film, may be used in diagnosis. Several noninvasive diagnostic techniques have recently come into use: ultrasonography, magnetic resonance imaging (MRI), and computed tomography (CT scan). Surgical repair, in which the involved section of the aorta is replaced with a synthetic graft of woven Dacron, frequently is the treatment of choice. Hypertension, if present, should be controlled.

DISSECTING ANEURYSMS

A dissecting aneurysm is an acute life-threatening condition. It involves hemorrhage into the vessel wall with longitudinal tearing (dissection) of the vessel wall to form a blood-filled channel. Unlike atherosclerotic aneurysms, dissecting aneurysms often occur without evidence of previous vessel dilatation. They can originate anywhere along the length of the aorta. The most common site in the ascending aorta is within a few centimeters of the aortic valve. The second most common site is the thoracic aorta just distal to the origin of the subclavian artery.[18, 19]

Dissecting aneurysms are caused by conditions that weaken or cause degenerative changes in the elastic and smooth muscle of the layers of the aorta. They are most common in the 40-to-60 age group and more prevalent in men than in women.[5] There is a history of hypertension in 94% of cases.[5] Dissecting aneurysms are also associated with connective tissue diseases, such as Marfan's syndrome. Aortic dissection may also occur during pregnancy because of histochemical changes in the aorta that occur during this time. Other factors that predispose to aortic dissection are congenital defects of the aortic valve (bicuspid or unicuspid valve structures) and aortic coarctation. Aortic dissection is a potential complication of cardiac surgery or catheterization. Surgically related dissection may occur at the points where the aorta has been incised or cross-clamped; it has also been reported at the site where the saphenous vein was sutured to the aorta during coronary artery bypass surgery.

Dissection usually is bidirectional, moving proximally toward the heart and distally into the descending aorta. When the ascending aorta is involved, expansion of the vessel wall may impair closure of the aortic valve. Although the length of dissection varies, it is possible for the abdominal aorta to be involved with progression into the renal, iliac, or femoral arteries. Partial or complete occlusion of the arteries that arise from the aortic arch or the intercostal or lumbar arteries may lead to stroke, ischemic peripheral neuropathy, or impaired blood flow to the spinal cord.

A major symptom of a dissecting aneurysm is the abrupt presence of excruciating pain described as tearing or ripping. The location of the pain may point to the site of dissection. Pain associated with dissection of the ascending aorta frequently is located in the anterior chest, whereas pain associated with dissection of the descending aorta often is located in the back. In the early stages, blood pressure typically is moderately or markedly elevated. Later, both the blood pressure and the pulse rate become unobtainable in one or both arms as the dissection disrupts arterial flow to the arms. Syncope, hemiplegia, or paralysis of the lower extremities may occur because of occlusion of blood vessels that supply the brain or spinal cord. Heart failure may develop when the aortic valve is involved.

Mortality caused by dissecting aneurysm is high. Within the first 48 hours, 50% of all untreated patients die, and 90% die within 6 weeks.[20] Aortic angiography, echocardiography, CT scans, and MRI studies aid in the diagnosis of dissecting aneurysm.

The treatment of dissecting aortic aneurysm may be medical or surgical. Aortic dissection is a life-threatening emergency situation; people with a probable diagnosis are stabilized medically even before the diagnosis is confirmed. Two important factors that participate in propagating the dissection are blood pressure and the steepness of the pulse wave. Without intervention, these forces continue to propagate the dissection. Therefore, medical treatment focuses on control of hypertension and the use of drugs that lessen the force of systolic blood ejection from the heart. Two commonly used drugs are intravenous sodium nitroprusside and a β-adrenergic blocking drug, given in combination. Surgical treatment consists of resection of the involved segment of the aorta and replacement with a prosthetic graft.

ACUTE ARTERIAL OCCLUSION

Acute arterial occlusion usually results from a thrombus or from emboli that originate in the heart. It usually is a complication of heart disease—ischemic heart disease with or without infarction, atrial fibrillation, or rheumatic heart disease. Trauma or arterial spasm caused by arterial cannulation is another cause.

The signs and symptoms of acute arterial occlusion depend on the artery involved and the adequacy of the collateral circulation. Emboli tend to lodge in bifurcations of the major arteries, including the aorta and iliac and the femoral and popliteal arteries. Occlusion in an extremity causes sudden onset of acute pain with numbness, tingling, weakness, pallor, and coldness. These changes are rapidly followed by cyanosis, mottling, and loss of sensory, reflex, and motor function. Pulses are absent below the level of the occlusion.

Treatment of acute arterial occlusion is aimed at restoring blood flow. Thrombolytic therapy (streptokinase or tissue plasminogen activator) may be used in an attempt to dissolve the clot. Anticoagulant therapy (heparin) usually is given to prevent extension of the embolus. An embolectomy—surgical removal of the embolus—may be indicated. It is important that application of heat and cold be avoided and that the extremity be protected from hard surfaces and overlying bedclothes.

PERIPHERAL ARTERIAL DISEASE

The peripheral arterial circulation usually is described as arterial circulation outside the heart. For our purposes, we will consider the peripheral circulation as that outside the pulmonary and cerebral circulation. Arteriosclerosis, discussed earlier, is a major cause of peripheral arterial disorders, often referred to as *peripheral vascular disease*. Two other conditions, Raynaud's phenomenon and thromboangiitis obliterans (Buerger's disease), are prototypes of peripheral arterial disease.

RAYNAUD'S SYNDROME

Raynaud's syndrome is a functional disorder caused by intense vasospasm of the arteries and arterioles in the fingers and, less often, the toes. Raynaud's syndrome is divided into two types: primary Raynaud's phenomenon, which occurs without demonstrable cause, and secondary Raynaud's phenomenon, which occurs secondary to some other disease condition. Primary Raynaud's phenomenon is seen in otherwise healthy young women, and it often is precipi-

tated by exposure to cold or by strong emotions. The cause of vasospasm in primary Raynaud's phenomenon is unknown. Hyperreactivity of the sympathetic nervous system has been suggested as a contributing cause.[22] Secondary Raynaud's phenomenon is associated with previous vessel injury, such as frostbite, occupational trauma associated with the use of heavy vibrating tools, collagen diseases, neurologic disorders, and chronic arterial occlusive disorders. Another occupation-related cause is the exposure to alternating hot and cold temperatures such as that experienced by butchers and food preparers.[21] Raynaud's phenomenon often is the first symptom of collagen diseases. In 70% of people with scleroderma, it is the first symptom; in lupus erythematosus, it is the presenting problem in 8% to 16% of cases.[23]

In Raynaud's disease or phenomenon, ischemia due to vasospasm causes changes in skin color that progress from pallor to cyanosis, a sensation of cold, and changes in sensory perception, such as numbness and tingling. The color changes usually are first noted in the tips of the fingers, later moving into one or more of the distal phalanges. After the ischemic episode, there is a period of hyperemia with intense redness, throbbing, and paresthesias. The period of hyperemia is followed by a return to normal color. If Raynaud's disease begins asymmetrically (does not affect both hands in the same manner), it usually becomes symmetrical within 4 to 6 months.[22] During the attack, there may be slight swelling. With repeated episodes of ischemia, the nails may become brittle, and the skin over the tips of the affected fingers may thicken. Nutritional impairment of these structures may give rise to arthritis. Ulceration and superficial gangrene of the fingers, although infrequent, may occur.

Treatment measures are directed toward eliminating factors that cause vasospasm and protecting the digits from trauma during an ischemic episode. Abstinence from smoking and protection from cold are priorities. Avoidance of emotional stress is another important factor in controlling the disorder because anxiety and stress may precipitate a vascular spasm in predisposed people. Vasoconstrictor medications, such as the decongestants contained in allergy and cold preparations, should be avoided. Treatment with vasodilator drugs may be indicated, particularly if episodes are frequent, because frequency encourages the potential for development of thrombosis and gangrene. The calcium-channel blocking drugs (diltiazem, nifedipine, and nicardipine) decrease the severity and frequency of attacks. Prazosin, a α-adrenergic receptor–blocking drug, may also be used. Intravenous infusion of prostaglandin E often is beneficial during an acute attack of vasospasm, and its effects may last for several weeks. Biofeedback training may be helpful in people with primary Raynaud's phenomenon but does not seem to be as effective in those with secondary Raynaud's phenomenon.[24] In the past, surgical interruption of sympathetic nerve pathways (sympathectomy) was an accepted form of therapy for people with severe symptomatology. The results were poor, however, and the procedure seldom is done today.

THROMBOANGIITIS OBLITERANS (BUERGER'S DISEASE)

Thromboangiitis obliterans is an inflammatory arterial disorder that causes thrombus formation. The disorder affects the medium-sized arteries, usually the plantar and digital vessels in the foot and lower leg. Arteries in the arm and hand may also be affected. Although primarily an arterial disorder, the inflammatory process often extends to involve adjacent veins and nerves. The cause of Buerger's disease is unknown. It is a disease of men between ages 25 and 40 who are heavy cigarette smokers.

Pain is the predominant symptom. During the early stages of the disease, there is intermittent claudication (pain, tension, weakness) of the calf muscles and the arch of the foot. In severe cases, pain is present even when the person is at rest. The impaired circulation increases sensitivity to cold. The peripheral pulses are diminished or absent, and there are changes in the color of the extremity. In moderately advanced cases, the extremity becomes cyanotic when the person assumes a dependent position, and the digits may turn reddish blue even when in a nondependent position. With lack of blood flow, the skin assumes a thin, shiny look and hair growth and skin nutrition suffer. Chronic ischemia causes thick, malformed nails. If the disease continues to progress, tissues eventually ulcerate and gangrenous changes arise that may necessitate amputation.

As part of the treatment program for thromboangiitis obliterans, it is mandatory that the person stop smoking cigarettes. Other treatment measures are of secondary importance and focus on methods for producing vasodilation and preventing tissue injury. Sympathectomy may be done to alleviate the vasospastic manifestations of the disease. Buerger's exercises take advantage of the gravitational effects of position change to improve blood flow to the affected part. The exercises consist of a cycle of positional changes that lasts about 2 minutes: legs horizontal, then elevated 45 degrees, then in a dependent position, and then horizontal again. The exercises usually are repeated five times and done three times a day.

Most patients are instructed to wiggle their toes while performing the exercises.

ATHEROSCLEROTIC OCCLUSIVE DISEASE

Atherosclerosis is an important cause of peripheral-vessel vascular disease. The superficial femoral and popliteal arteries are the most frequent sites for development of atherosclerotic occlusive disease. When it occurs in the lower leg and foot, the tibial, common peroneal, or pedal vessels are the arteries most commonly affected. As with atherosclerosis in other locations, the signs of vessel occlusion are gradual. The signs include intermittent claudication, atrophic changes and thinning of the skin and subcutaneous tissues of the lower leg, and diminution in the size of the leg muscles. The foot often is cool, and the popliteal and pedal pulses are weak or absent. Limb color blanches with elevation and becomes deep red when the leg is in the dependent position. Walking (slowly) to the point of claudication usually is encouraged because it increases the collateral circulation. Surgery (femoropopliteal bypass grafting using a section of saphenous vein) may be indicated in severe cases. Thromboendarterectomy with removal of the occluding core of atherosclerotic tissue may be done if the section of diseased vessel is short. Percutaneous transluminal angioplasty, in which a balloon catheter is inserted into the area of stenosis and the balloon inflated to increase vessel diameter, is another form of treatment.

ASSESSMENT OF ARTERIAL FLOW

There are a number of methods for assessing arterial blood flow and detecting arterial disease. These include monitoring of capillary refill time and peripheral pulses. Angiography, Doppler ultrasonic flow studies, and magnetic resonance imaging (MRI) may be used for a more definitive diagnosis.

Capillary refill time is an indicator of the efficiency of the microcirculation. It is measured by depressing the nail bed of a finger or toe until the underlying skin blanches. The refill time is normal if the capillary vessels refill within 3 seconds after pressure is released.[25]

The volume of the peripheral pulses and capillary refill time are useful indirect methods for assessing peripheral perfusion. Peripheral pulses can be palpated over vessels in the head, neck (carotid), and extremities. In situations associated with potential vessel spasm or thrombosis, it may be necessary only to check for the presence of pulses. In many situations, however, the pulse volume (weak and thready to strong and bounding) provides useful information about vascular volume and the condition of the arterial circulation. Arterial auscultation is used to listen to the flow of blood with a stethoscope. The term *bruit* is used to describe an audible murmur heard over a peripheral artery. It is caused by turbulent blood flow and is suggestive of obstructive arterial disease.

Doppler ultrasound flow studies use reflected ultrasound waves, which are transmitted back to the skin surface from a blood vessel to determine the direction and velocity of blood flow. Doppler studies can be used to establish the patency of a given blood vessel. It is useful in studying blood flow in the carotid arteries, abdominal vessels, fetal blood vessels, and peripheral blood vessels.

MRI is a noninvasive technique that can be used to study blood flow. The method uses a magnetic field to align the charges on blood components as they move through blood vessels. The aligned charges emit measurable radiofrequency signals, which can be detected electronically and recorded.

In summary, the arterial system distributes blood to all the various tissues of the body, and pathology of the arterial system exerts its effects through ischemia or impaired blood flow. There are two types of arterial disorders: (1) diseases such as atherosclerosis and peripheral arterial diseases that obstruct blood flow and (2) disorders such as aneurysms that weaken the vessel wall. Atherosclerosis, a leading cause of death in the United States, affects large and medium-sized arteries, such as the coronary and cerebral arteries. It has an insidious onset, and its lesions usually are far advanced before symptoms appear. Although the mechanisms of atherosclerosis are uncertain, risk factors associated with its development have been identified. These include (1) factors such as heredity, sex, and age, which cannot be controlled; (2) factors such as smoking, high blood pressure, high serum cholesterol levels, and diabetes, which can be controlled; and (3) other contributing factors such as obesity, lack of exercise, and stress. Cholesterol relies on lipoproteins (LDLs and HDLs) for transport in the blood. The LDLs, which are atherogenic, carry cholesterol to the peripheral tissues. The HDLs, which are protective, remove cholesterol from the tissues and carry it back to the liver for disposal. LDL receptors play a major role in removing cholesterol from the blood; people with reduced numbers of receptors are at particularly high risk for development of atherosclerosis.

Aneurysms are localized areas of vessel dilation caused by weakness of the arterial wall. A berry aneurysm, most often found in the circle of Willis in the brain circulation, consists of a small spherical vessel dilation. Fusiform and saccular aneurysms, most often found in the thoracic and abdominal aorta, are characterized by gradual and progressive enlargement of the aorta. They can involve part of the vessel circumference (saccular) or extend to involve the entire circumference of the vessel (fusiform). A dissecting aneurysm is an acute life-threatening condition. It involves hemorrhage into the vessel wall with longitudinal tearing (dissection) of the vessel wall to form a blood-filled channel. The most serious effect of aneurysms is rupture.

Peripheral arterial diseases affect blood vessels outside the heart and thorax. They include Raynaud's phenomenon, caused by vessel spasm; thromboangiitis obliterans (Buerger's disease), characterized by an inflammatory process that involves medium-sized arteries and adjacent veins and nerves of the lower extremities; and atherosclerotic occlusive disease. Peripheral vascular diseases evert their effect by producing ischemia of the tissues that the involved vessels supply.

■ ALTERATIONS IN VENOUS FLOW

Veins are low-pressure, thin-walled vessels that rely on the ancillary action of skeletal muscle pumps and changes in abdominal and intrathoracic pressure to return blood to the heart. Unlike the arterial system, the venous system is equipped with valves that prevent retrograde flow of blood. Although its structure enables the venous system to serve as a storage area for blood, it also renders the system susceptible to problems related to stasis and venous insufficiency. This section focuses on two common problems of the venous system: varicose veins and venous thrombosis. Pulmonary embolism, a complication of deep vein thrombosis, is discussed in Chapter 27.

VARICOSE VEINS

Varicose, or dilated, tortuous veins of the lower extremities are common and often lead to secondary problems of venous insufficiency. About 20% of the general population and as many as 50% of people over age 50 are affected by varicose veins. In people over age 30, four times as many women are affected as men, probably because of venous stasis caused by pregnancy.[5] Varicose veins are described as being primary or secondary. Primary varicosities originate in the superficial saphenous veins, and secondary varicose veins result from impaired flow in the deep venous channels.

A brief review of the anatomy of the venous system of the legs explains why varicosities may develop. The venous system in the legs might well be described as being composed of two venous channels: the superficial (saphenous and its tributaries) veins and the deep venous channels (Fig. 20-6). Perforating or communicating veins connect these two systems. Blood from the skin and subcutaneous tissues in the leg collects in the superficial veins and is then transported across the communicating veins into the deeper venous channels for return to the heart. When a person walks, the action of the muscle

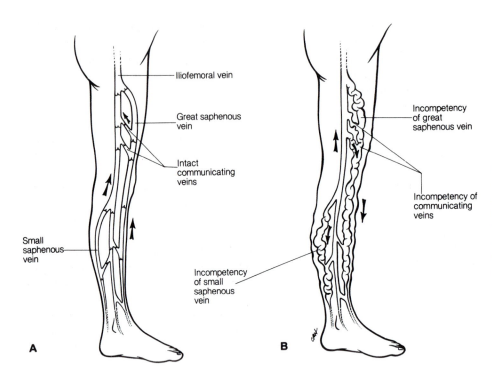

FIG. 20-6. Superficial and deep venous channels of the leg. View **A** shows normal venous structures and flow patterns. View **B** shows varicosities in the superficial venous system that are the result of incompetent valves in the communicating veins. The *arrows* in both views indicate the direction of blood flow. (Modified from Abramson, D. I. [1974]. *Vascular disorders of the extremities* [2nd ed.]. New York: Harper & Row)

pumps produces an increase in flow in the deep channels and facilitates movement of blood from the superficial to the deep veins.

Venous valves prevent the retrograde flow of blood and play an important role in the function of the venous system. Although these valves are irregularly located along the length of the veins, they are almost always found at junctions where the communicating veins merge with the larger deep veins and where two veins meet. The number of venous valves differs somewhat from one person to another, as does the structural competence, factors that may help to explain the familial predisposition to development of varicose veins.

MECHANISMS OF DEVELOPMENT

Varicose veins result from prolonged dilatation and stretching of the vessel wall as a result of increased venous pressure. One of the most important factors in the elevation of venous pressure is the hydrostatic effect associated with the standing position. When a person is in the erect position, the full weight of the venous columns of blood is transmitted to the leg veins. The effects of gravity are compounded in people who stand for long periods without using their leg muscles to assist in pumping blood back to the heart. Because there are no valves in the inferior vena cava or common iliac veins, blood in the abdominal veins must be supported by the valves located in the external iliac or femoral veins. When intraabdominal pressure increases, as it does during pregnancy, or when the valves in these two veins are absent or

defective, the stress on the saphenofemoral junction is increased. The high incidence of varicose veins in women who have been pregnant also suggests a hormonal effect on venous smooth muscle leading to venous dilatation and valvular incompetence.

Prolonged exposure to increases in pressure causes the venous valves to become incompetent so they no longer close properly. When this happens, blood regurgitates into the superficial veins. Furthermore, once varicose veins have developed, the venous structures become deformed, promoting further dilatation.

Another consideration is that the superficial veins have only subcutaneous fat and superficial fascia for support, whereas the deep venous channels are supported by muscle, bone, and connective tissue. Therefore, obesity increases the risk for varicose veins.

About 80% to 90% of venous blood from the lower extremities is transported through the deep channels. The development of secondary varicose veins becomes inevitable when flow in these deep channels is impaired or blocked. Among the causes of secondary varicose veins are thrombophlebitis, congenital or acquired arteriovenous fistulas, congenital venous malformations, and pressure on the abdominal veins caused by pregnancy or a tumor.

VENOUS INSUFFICIENCY

Signs and symptoms associated with varicose veins vary. Most women complain of their unsightly appearance. In addition to their cosmetic effects, varicose veins impair venous emptying, giving rise to a condition known as venous insufficiency. This condition often causes a sensation of progressive heaviness and, with prolonged standing, aching legs. In contrast to the ischemia caused by arterial insufficiency, venous insufficiency leads to tissue congestion, edema, and eventual impairment of tissue nutrition. The edema is exacerbated by long periods of standing. In its advanced form, impairment of tissue nutrition causes stasis dermatitis and the development of stasis or varicose ulcers. Stasis dermatitis is characterized by the presence of thin, shiny, bluish brown, irregularly pigmented desquamative skin that lacks the support of the underlying subcutaneous tissues. Minor injury leads to relatively painless ulcerations that are difficult to heal. The lower part of the leg is particularly prone to develop stasis dermatitis and varicose ulcers.

DIAGNOSIS AND TREATMENT

Several procedures are used to assess the extent of venous involvement associated with varicose veins. In one of these, the Trendelenburg's test, a tourniquet is applied to the affected leg while it is elevated and the veins are empty. The person then assumes the standing position, and the tourniquet is removed. If the superficial veins are involved, the veins distend quickly. To assess the deep channels, the tourniquet is applied while the person is standing and the veins are filled. The person then lies down and the affected leg is elevated. Emptying of the superficial veins indicates that the deep channels are patent. The Doppler ultrasonic flow probe may also be used to assess the flow in the large vessels. Angiographic studies using a radiopaque contrast medium are also used to assess venous function.

Once the venous channels have been repeatedly stretched and the valves rendered incompetent, little can be done to restore normal venous tone and function. Ideally, measures should be taken to prevent the development and progression of varicose veins. These measures center on avoiding any activities that involve prolonged elevation of venous pressure.

Treatment measures for varicose veins focus on improving venous flow and preventing tissue injury, such as avoiding prolonged standing and providing for frequent leg elevation. When correctly fitted, elastic support stockings compress the superficial veins, and thus prevent distention. These stockings should be applied before the standing position is assumed at a time when the leg veins are empty. Surgical treatment consists of removing the varicosities and the incompetent perforating veins, but it is limited to people with patent deep venous channels. Sclerotherapy, which usually is done on small residual varicosities, is another treatment measure; it involves the injection of a sclerosing agent into the collapsed superficial veins to produce fibrosis of the vessel lumen.

VENOUS THROMBOSIS

The presence of thrombus within a vein and the accompanying inflammatory response in the vessel wall are termed venous thrombosis, or thrombophlebitis. Thrombi can develop in either the superficial or the deep veins (deep vein thrombosis [DVT]). DVT most commonly occurs in the lower extremities, although the incidence of upper extremity venous thrombosis is increasing because of the greater utilization of subclavian vein catheters. The most important consequence of DVT is pulmonary embolism and the syndrome of chronic venous insufficiency. Superficial vein thrombosis, usually involving the greater or lesser saphenous veins or their tributaries, does not result in pulmonary emboli or chronic venous sufficiency. It is associated with intravenous catheters and infusions and varicose veins and may develop in association with DVT.[26]

In 1846, Virchow described the triad that has come to be associated with venous thrombosis: (1) stasis of blood, (2) increased blood coagulability, and (3) vessel wall injury.[27] Two of the three factors must be present for thrombi to form. A number of factors may be present that promote venous thrombosis (Chart 20-1). Bed rest and immobilization are associated with decreased blood flow and venous pooling in the lower extremities and with increased risk of DVT. People who are immobilized by a hip fracture, joint replacement, or spinal cord injury are particularly vulnerable to DVT. The risk of DVT is increased in situations of impaired cardiac function. This may account for the relatively high incidence in people with acute myocardial infarction and congestive heart failure. Elderly people are more susceptible than younger people, probably because disorders that produce venous stasis occur more frequently in older people. Hypercoagulability is a homeostatic mechanism designed to increase clot formation, and conditions that increase the concentration or activation of clotting factors predispose to DVT. Thrombosis can also be caused by deficiencies in certain plasma proteins that normally inhibit thrombus formation, such as antithrombin III, protein C, and protein S. The postpartum state is associated with increased levels of fibrinogen, prothrombin, and other coagulation factors. The use of oral contraceptives appears to increase coagulability and predispose to venous thrombosis. Certain cancers are associated with increased clotting tendencies, and although the reason for this is largely unknown, sub-

CHART 20-1: RISK FACTORS ASSOCIATED WITH VENOUS THROMBOSIS*

Venous Stasis

Bed rest
Immobility
Spinal cord injury
Acute myocardial infarction
Congestive heart failure
Shock
Venous obstruction

Hyperreactivity of Blood Coagulation

Stress and trauma
Pregnancy
Childbirth
Oral contraceptive use
Dehydration
Cancer

Vascular Trauma

Indwelling venous catheters
Surgery
Massive trauma or infection
Fractured hip
Orthopedic surgery

* Many of these disorders involve more than one mechanism.

stances that promote blood coagulation may be released from the tissues because of the cancerous growth. Also, when body fluid is lost because of injury or disease, the resulting hemoconcentration causes the clotting factors to become more concentrated.

MANIFESTATIONS

The most common signs and symptoms of thrombophlebitis are those related to the inflammatory process: pain, swelling, and deep muscle tenderness. Fever, general malaise, and an elevated white blood cell count and sedimentation rate are accompanying indications of inflammation. There may be tenderness and pain along the vein. Swelling may vary from minimal to maximal. Objective measurements of swelling can be obtained by measuring the circumference of the affected and unaffected extremities and comparing the difference.

The site of thrombus formation determines the location of the physical findings.[28] The most common site is in the venous sinuses in the soleus muscle and posterior tibial and peroneal veins. Swelling in these cases involves the foot and ankle, although it may be slight or absent. Calf pain and tenderness are common. Femoral vein thrombosis with calf thrombosis produces pain and tenderness in the distal thigh and popliteal area. Thrombi in ileofemoral veins produce the most profound manifestations with swelling, pain, and tenderness of the entire extremity. With DVT in the calf veins, active dorsiflexion produces calf pain (Homans' sign). The common sites of venous thrombosis are shown in Figure 20-7.

DIAGNOSIS AND TREATMENT

The risk of pulmonary embolism emphasizes the need for early detection and treatment of DVT. Several tests are useful for this purpose: ascending venography (done with the patient in the standing position but not bearing weight on the affected extremity), contrast DVT scans, Doppler ultrasonic flowmeter studies, and impedance plethysmography. The DVT scan involves the intravenous injection of radioactive fibrinogen (^{125}I), which becomes incorporated into any developing thrombus. The thrombus is then detected by a scintillation counter, which records the radioactivity at selected points in the extremity.

These methods assess venous flow or fibrinogen accumulation and are useful in monitoring people at risk for developing venous thrombosis. Whenever possible, venous thrombosis should be prevented, in preference to being treated. Early ambulation after childbirth and surgery is one measure that decreases the risk of thrombus formation. Exercising the legs and wearing support stockings improve venous flow. A further precautionary measure is to avoid assuming body positions that favor venous pooling. For example, in the hospitalized patient, if both the head and the knees of the hospital bed are raised, blood pools in the pelvic veins. Long, unbroken auto and plane trips also promote venous pooling and thrombus formation.

The objectives of treatment of venous thrombosis are to prevent formation of additional thrombi, prevent extension and embolization of existing thrombi, and minimize venous valve damage. Bed rest with elevation of the affected extremity is prescribed. In one study, contrast medium remained in the soleus veins, on average, for 10 minutes in supine patients whose legs were in the horizontal position.[29] This may explain why postoperative thrombi frequently originate in the soleus vein. A 15- to 20-degree elevation of the legs prevents stasis.[30] It is important that the entire lower extremity or extremities be carefully extended to avoid acute flexion of the knee or hip. Heat often is applied to the leg to relieve venospasm and to aid in the resolution of the inflammatory process. Bed rest usually is maintained until local tenderness and swelling have subsided. Gradual ambulation with elastic support is then permitted. Standing and sitting increase venous pressure

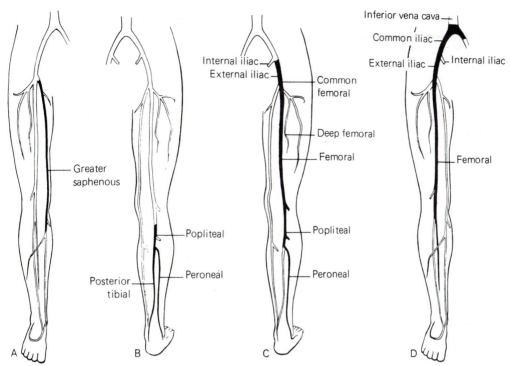

FIG. 20-7. Common pathways of venous thrombosis. (**A**) Superficial thrombophebitis. (**B**) Most common form of deep thrombophebitis. (**C** and **D**) Deep thrombophlebitis from the calf to iliac veins. (Haller, J. A., Jr. [1967]. *Deep thrombophlebitis: Pathophysiology and treatment.* Philadelphia: W.B. Saunders)

and are to be avoided. Elastic support is needed for 3 to 6 months to permit recanalization and collateralization and to prevent venous insufficiency.

Two anticoagulants, warfarin and heparin, are used both to treat and to prevent thrombophlebitis. *Treatment* typically is initiated with either continuous or periodic intravenous heparin infusions. This is followed by *prophylactic* therapy with either subcutaneous minidose heparin injections or oral warfarin sodium to prevent further thrombus formation. The mechanisms of action of the anticoagulant drugs are discussed in Chapter 17. Thrombolytic therapy (streptokinase or tissue plasminogen activator) may be used in an attempt to dissolve the clot.

In summary, the storage function of the venous system renders it susceptible to venous insufficiency, stasis, and thrombus formation. Varicose veins occur with prolonged distention and stretching of the superficial veins owing to venous insufficiency. Varicosities can arise because of defects in the superficial veins (primary varicose veins) or because of impaired blood flow in the deep venous channels (secondary varicose veins). Thrombophlebitis is an inflammation of a vein with thrombus formation. It is associated with vessel injury, stasis of venous flow, and hypercoagulability states. Thrombi can develop in either the superficial or the deep veins (DVT). Thrombus formation in deep veins is a precursor to venous insufficiency and embolus formation.

■ ALTERATIONS IN EXTERNAL FORCES THAT IMPAIR BLOOD FLOW

Blood flow in the circulatory system is brought about by pressure differences between the individual vascular regions, so that blood flows from regions of higher pressure to regions of lower pressure. The transmural pressure is pressure between the inside and the outside of a blood vessel. It is the pressure that holds blood vessels open and allows flow to occur. The external pressure normally is low enough that the transmural pressure is effectively the same as the intravascular pressure, and blood is able to move freely along an intravascular pressure gradient. Under certain conditions, the transmural pressure and blood flow can be considerably changed by local increases in external pressure. Two conditions that compromise blood flow because of increased external pressure are compartment syndrome and pressure ulcers.

COMPARTMENT SYNDROME

The muscles and nerves of an extremity are enclosed in a tough and inelastic fascial envelope called a *muscle compartment* (Fig. 20-8). Compartment syndrome

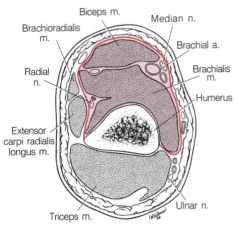

FIG. 20-8. Distal anterior arm muscle compartment showing the location of fascia, muscles, nerves, and blood vessels.

CHART 20-2: CAUSES OF COMPARTMENT SYNDROME

Decreased Compartment Size

Constrictive dressings and casts
Infiltration of intravenous fluids
Thermal injury and frostbite
Surgical closure of fascial defects

Increased Compartment Volume

Fractures and orthopedic surgery
Trauma and bleeding
Postischemic injury
Severe exercise
Prolonged immobilization with limb compression (*e.g.*, drug overdose)
Thermal injury and frostbite
Intravenous infiltration

describes a condition of increased pressure within a limited anatomic space (usually a muscle compartment) that impairs circulation and produces ischemic tissue injury. If the pressure in the compartment is sufficiently high, tissue circulation is compromised, causing death of nerve and muscle cells. Permanent loss of function and limb contracture may occur. The amount of pressure required to produce a compartmental syndrome depends on many factors, including the duration of the pressure elevation, the metabolic rate of the tissues, vascular tone, and local blood pressure. Less tissue pressure is required to stop circulation when hypotension or vasoconstriction is present. Intracompartmental pressures of 30 to 40 mmHg (normal is about 6 mmHg) are considered sufficient to impair capillary blood flow.[31] Nerve dysfunction (paresthesia and hypoesthesia) develops within 30 minutes of ischemia; muscle dysfunction, within 2 to 4 hours; and irreversible loss of function (contractures, sensory aberrations, and muscle weakness) begins after 12 to 24 hours of total ischemia.[32] Therefore, prompt diagnosis and decompression are essential to reinstate capillary pressure and prevent permanent disability.

Compartment syndrome can result from either a decrease in compartment size or an increase in the volume of its contents (Chart 20-2). The most common causes are crushing injuries, fractures, contusions, snake bites, postischemic swelling after arterial injury or thrombosis, severe exercise, limb compression owing to drug or alcohol overdose, and venous occlusion.

Decreased Compartment Size. Among the causes of decreased compartment size are constrictive dressings and casts, closure of fascial defects, and thermal injuries or frostbite. Splitting a cast or releasing the dressing usually is sufficient to relieve

most of the pressure. The appearance of a muscle hernia or fascial defect may be the result of increased compartmental pressure. This commonly is seen in people with chronic exercise-related compartment syndrome. Surgical closure of the hernia decreases compartmental size and may result in an acute compartment syndrome. In people with circumferential third-degree burns, the inelastic and constricting eschar produces a decrease in the size of the underlying compartments. Burns are also associated with the formation of massive edema and an increase in compartment volume. The combination of the two problems may lead to necrosis of the underlying neuromuscular tissues. Frostbite produces neuromuscular injury for similar reasons.

Increased Compartment Volume. Increased compartment volume can be caused by postischemic swelling, trauma, vascular injury and bleeding, infiltration of intravenous infusions, and venous obstruction. One of the most important causes of compartment syndrome is bleeding and edema caused by fractures and osteotomies (see Chapter 56). Contusions and soft tissue injury are also common causes of compartment syndrome. Bleeding can occur as a complication of arterial punctures, particularly in people with bleeding disorders or those who are receiving anticoagulant drugs. Infiltration of intravenous fluids can also restrict compartment size and cause compartment ischemia and postischemic swelling. Increased compartment volume may follow ischemic events, such as arterial occlusion, that are of sufficient duration to produce capillary damage, increased capillary permeability, and edema. During unattended coma caused by drug overdose or carbon monoxide poisoning, high compartment pressures are produced when an extremity is compressed by the weight of the overlying head or torso. Exercise may produce either acute or chronic elevations in compartment pressure. This condition commonly is referred to as *shin splints*.

DIAGNOSIS AND TREATMENT

It is important that a person at risk for development of compartment syndrome be identified and that proper assessment methods be instituted. Assessment should include pain assessment, examination of sensory (light touch and two-point discrimination) and motor function (movement and muscle strength), test of passive stretch, and palpation of the muscle compartments.

The most important symptom of compartment syndrome is unrelenting pain, usually described as a deep, throbbing sensation, that is greater than that expected for the primary problem, such as fracture or contusion. Pain with passive stretch is a common finding. Tenseness and tenderness of the involved compartment are specific symptoms of compartment syndrome. The skin over the compartment may become taut, shiny, warm, and red. Paresthesias progressing to anesthesia occur secondary to nerve involvement. Muscle weakness occurs owing to muscle ischemia. Although peripheral pulses and capillary refill time are parts of a complete assessment, they frequently are normal in the presence of compartment syndrome because the major arteries are located outside the muscle compartments. Although edema may make it difficult to palpate the pulse, the increased compartment pressure seldom is sufficient to occlude flow in a major artery. Doppler methods usually confirm the existence of a pulse.

Direct measurements of tissue pressure can be obtained using a needle or wick catheter inserted into the muscle compartment. This method is particularly useful in people who are unresponsive and in those with nerve deficits. Compartment decompression is recommended when pressures rise to 30 mmHg.

Treatment consists of reducing compartmental pressures. This entails cast splitting or removal of restrictive dressings. These procedures may be sufficient to relieve most of the underlying pressure and symptoms. Limb elevation is not recommended when compartment syndrome is suspected. Although elevation is widely used to promote venous drainage of an injured extremity, it may be detrimental in compartment syndrome. Because venous pressure must exceed tissue pressure, elevation of an extremity cannot augment venous drainage once intracompartment pressures are elevated. Furthermore, when an extremity is elevated, its arterial pressure falls because of the effects of gravity. Blood flow to an

extremity can be arrested because of diminution of arterial pressure in the elevated extremity. When compartment syndrome cannot be relieved by the measures described, a fasciotomy may become necessary. During this procedure, the fascia is incised longitudinally and separated so that the compartment volume can expand and blood flow can be reestablished. Because of potential problems with wound infection and closure, this procedure is performed as a last resort.

PRESSURE ULCERS

Pressure ulcers are ischemic lesions of the skin and underlying structures caused by external pressure that impairs the flow of blood and lymph. Pressure ulcers often are referred to as decubitus ulcers or bedsores. The word *decubitus* comes from the Latin term meaning lying down. A pressure ulcer, however, may result from pressure exerted in the seated as well as the supine position. Pressure ulcers are most likely to develop over a bony prominence, but they may occur on any part of the body that is subjected to external pressure, friction, or shearing forces.

The reported incidence and prevalence of pressure ulcers in hospital settings has ranged from 2.7% to 29.5%[33–35] and in skilled care and nursing home settings from 2.4% to 23%.[35,36] Several subpopulations are at particular risk, including people with quadriplegia, elderly people with restricted activity and hip fractures, and people in the critical care setting.

MECHANISMS OF DEVELOPMENT

Two factors contribute to the development of pressure ulcers: (1) external pressure that compress blood vessels and (2) friction and shearing forces that tear and injure vessels.

External Pressure. External pressure that exceeds capillary pressure (about 25 mmHg) interrupts the blood flow in the capillary beds. When this pressure is greater than the pressure in the arterioles, it also interrupts the flow in these vessels. A pressure exceeding 50 mmHg applied to the skin over a bony prominence is sufficient to interrupt the blood flow and cause ischemia.[37] If this pressure is applied constantly for 2 hours, oxygen deprivation coupled with an accumulation of metabolic end products leads to irreversible tissue damage. The same amount of pressure causes more damage when it is distributed over a small area than when it is distributed over a larger area. If a person weighing 70 kg with a total surface area of 1.8 m^2 were in the supine position, with pressure evenly distributed, the pressure at any given point would be 5.7 mmHg.[38] About 7 lb of pressure per square inch of tissue surface is sufficient to obstruct blood flow.[38]

Whether a person is sitting or lying down, the weight of the body is borne by tissues covering the bony prominences. Ninety-six percent of pressure ulcers are located on the lower part of the body, most often over the sacrum, the coccygeal areas, the ischial tuberosities, and the greater trochanter.[39] Pressure over a bony area is transmitted from the surface to the underlying dense bone; all the underlying tissue is compressed, with the greatest pressure at the surface of the bone and dissipating in a cone-like manner toward the surface of the skin (Fig. 20-9). Extensive underlying tissue damage can be present when a small superficial skin lesion is first noted. The skin lesion often is just the "tip of the iceberg."

Altering the distribution of pressure from one skin area to another prevents tissue injury. People unconsciously shift their weight to redistribute pressure on the skin and underlying tissues. During the night, for example, they turn in their sleep, preventing ischemic injury of tissues that overlie the bony prominences that support the weight of the body; the same is true for sitting for any length of time. The movements needed to shift the body weight are made unconsciously, and only when movement is restricted do they become aware of discomfort. Pressure ulcers most commonly occur with conditions in which normal sensation and movement to effect redistribution of body weight are impaired, such as spinal cord injury.

Friction and Shearing Forces. Shearing forces are caused by the sliding of one tissue layer over another with stretching and angulation of blood vessels causing injury and thrombosis. Clinically, injury caused by shearing forces commonly occurs when the head of the bed is elevated, causing the torso to slide down toward the foot of the bed. When this happens, friction and perspiration cause the skin and superficial fascia to remain fixed against the bed linens while the deep fascia and skeleton slide downward. The same thing can happen when people sitting up in a chair slide downward.

Another source of shearing forces is pulling rather than lifting a patient up in bed. In this case, the skin remains fixed to the sheet while the fascia and muscles are pulled upward.

PREDICTION AND PREVENTION

The prevention of pressure ulcers is preferable to treatment. In 1992, a special panel of the Agency for Health Care Policy and Research, the Panel for the Prediction and Prevention of Pressure Ulcers in Adults, released the Clinical Practice Guidelines for Pressure Ulcers in Adults.[40] The recommendations developed by the panel target four overall goals: (1) identifying at-risk people who need prevention and the specific factors placing them at risk, (2) maintaining and improving tissue tolerance to pressure to prevent injury; (3) protecting against the adverse effects of external mechanical forces (pressure, friction, and shear), and (4) reducing the incidence of pressure ulcers through educational programs.[40]

Risk Factor Assessment. Risk factors identified as contributing to the development of pressure ulcers were those related to sensory perception (ability to respond meaningfully to pressure-related discomfort), level of skin moisture, urine and fecal continence, nutrition and hydration status, mobility, circulatory status, and presence of shear and friction forces. Elderly people are particularly prone to develop pressure ulcers; in one institution, 76% of the pressure ulcers that occurred during two 6-month periods were in people over age 70.[41]

Numerous risk assessment tools exist; however,

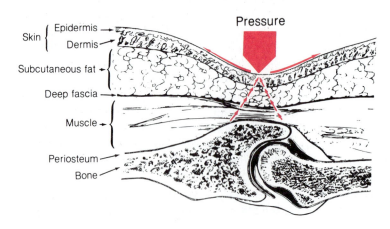

FIG. 20-9. Pressure over a bony prominence compresses all intervening soft tissue, with a resulting wide, three-dimensional pressure gradient that causes varying degrees of ischemia and damage. (Shea, J. D. [1975]. Pressure sores: Classification and management. *Clinical Orthopaedics and Related Research, 112,* 90)

only the Braden Scale and the Norton Scale have been extensively tested. The Norton Scale ranks risk owing to physical condition, mental condition, activity, mobility, and incontinence,[42] whereas the Braden Scale ranks sensory perception, moisture, activity, nutrition, and friction and shear.[43] Identifying patients who are at risk for development of pressure ulcers allows health care facilities to focus prevention measures on this group, which has been shown to reduce the incidence of pressure ulcers.

Skin Care and Early Treatment. Methods for preventing pressure ulcers include frequent position change, meticulous skin care, and frequent and careful observation to detect early signs of skin breakdown. All people at risk for pressure ulcers should have systematic skin inspection done at least once a day, with particular attention to bony prominences.[40] The bed linens should be kept clean, dry, and wrinkle free. The skin should be cleansed at the time of urine and fecal soiling with a mild cleansing agent that minimizes irritation and skin dryness. When soiling of the skin cannot be controlled, it is recommended that absorbent underpads or briefs be used to present a quick-drying surface for the skin. Topical agents that act as moisture barriers can also be used.

Adequate hydration of the stratum corneum appears to protect the skin against mechanical insult.[40] The skin should be kept clean and protected from environmental factors that cause drying. The level of skin hydration decreases with decreasing ambient air temperature, particularly when the relative humidity of the ambient air is low.[40] Dry skin should be treated with moisturizers. The prevention of dehydration also improves the circulation. It also decreases the concentration of urine, thereby minimizing skin irritation in people who are incontinent, and it reduces urinary problems that contribute to incontinence. Maintenance of adequate nutrition is important. Anemia and malnutrition contribute to tissue breakdown and delay healing once tissue injury has occurred.

The panel also recommended that the age-old practice of massaging over the bony prominences be avoided. Research suggests that using massage to stimulate blood and lymph flow may in fact decrease skin blood flow and increase the risk of deep tissue injury.[44, 45]

Protecting Against Mechanical Forces. Frequent change of position prevents tissue injury owing to pressure. People who are in bed and at risk for development of pressure ulcers should be repositioned at least every 2 hours if this is consistent with the overall treatment goals. It is recommended that people who are in a chair or wheelchair be repositioned every hour or put back to bed. People who are able to shift their weight should be advised to do so every 15 minutes.

Special pads and mattresses that distribute weight more evenly may be used. Silicone-filled pads, egg-crate cushions, turning frames, flotation pads, and other devices minimize contact pressure. Adequate exposure of the skin to air is necessary to avoid the buildup of heat and perspiration. Care should be taken to maintain the person at a position of 30 to 40 degrees to minimize slipping and shearing forces from sliding against the sheets. It is also important that the person be lifted and not dragged across the sheet. A lifting sheet works well for this purpose. Elevation of the ankles and heels off the sheets with foam pads can reduce skin breakdown in these areas of the body. The use of air cushions (donuts) is not recommended.

Casts, braces, and splints can exert extreme pressure on underlying tissues, and people with these devices require special attention to avoid skin breakdown.

STAGING AND TREATMENT

Pressure ulcers can be staged according to the following four categories recommended by the Panel for Prediction and Prevention of Pressure Sores in Adults[40] and the National Pressure Ulcer Advisory Panel.[46]

Stage I: Nonblanchable erythema of intact skin; the heralding of skin ulceration. Note: Reactive hyperemia normally can be expected to be present for one half to three fourths as long as the pressure occluded blood flow to the area; it should not be confused with a stage I pressure ulcer.

Stage II: Partial-thickness skin loss involving epidermis or dermis, or both. The ulcer is superficial and presents clinically as an abrasion, a blister, or a shallow crater.

Stage III: Full-thickness skin loss involving damage and necrosis of subcutaneous tissue that may extend down to but not through underlying fascia. The ulcer presents clinically as a deep crater with or without undermining of adjacent tissue.

Stage IV: Full-thickness skin loss with extensive destruction, skin necrosis, or damage to muscle, bone, or supporting structures (for example, tendon or joint capsule). Note: Undermining and sinus tracts may also be associated with stage IV pressure ulcers.

It was recognized that the staging criteria have the following limitations: (1) identification of stage I pressure ulcers may be difficult in people with darkly pigmented skin; and (2) when eschar is present, accurate staging of the pressure may be difficult until the eschar has sloughed or the wound has been debrided.

Once skin breakdown has occurred, special treatment measures are needed to prevent further ischemic damage, reduce bacterial contamination and infection, and promote healing. The treatment measures depend on the stage of the ulcer.[47] Stage I ulcers usually are treated with frequent turning and measures to remove pressure. Stage II ulcers are treated with saline or occlusive dressings to maintain a moist healing environment. Occlusive dressings (Bioclusive, Duoderm, Op-site, or Tegaderm) seal in the body's own defenses against invasion—leukocytes, plasma, and fibrin. They promote natural healing without the usual formation of a dry crust over the wound. Although these dressings are nonporous and prevent the escape of fluid, they are permeable to air and water vapor and prevent the growth of anaerobic bacteria. Stage III ulcers require debridement (removal of necrotic tissue and eschar). This can be done surgically, with wet-to-dry dressings, or through the use of proteolytic enzymes (Elase, Travase). Stage IV wounds are covered with nonadherent dressings, changed every 8 to 12 hours, depending on severity, degree of infection, and amount of exudate. Stage IV ulcers may require surgical interventions, such as skin grafts or myocutaneous flaps.

In summary, blood flow in the circulatory system is brought about by pressure differences between the arterial and venous systems and a transmural pressure (internal minus external) that holds the vessel open. Under certain conditions, such as compartment syndrome and pressure ulcers, increases in external pressures can exceed intravascular pressure and interrupt blood flow. Compartment syndrome is a condition of increased pressure within a muscle compartment that compromises blood flow and affords the potential for death of nerve and muscle tissue. It can result from either a decrease in compartment size (constrictive dressings, closure of fascial defects, thermal injury, or frostbite) or an increase in compartment volume (postischemic swelling, fractures, contusion and soft tissue trauma, bleeding caused by vascular injury, or venous congestion). Pressure ulcers are caused by ischemia of the skin and underlying tissues. They are caused by external pressure, which disrupts blood flow, or by shearing forces, which cause stretching and injury to blood vessels. Pressure ulcers are divided into four stages, according to the depth of tissue involvement. The prevention of pressure ulcers is preferable to treatment. The goals of prevention should include (1) identifying at-risk people who need prevention and the specific factors placing them at risk, (2) maintaining and improving tissue tolerance to pressure to prevent injury; (3) protecting against the adverse effects of external mechanical forces (pressure, friction, and shear), and (4) reducing the incidence of pressure ulcers through educational programs.

■ REFERENCES

1. *1992 Heart Facts*. (1992). Dallas: American Heart Association.
2. National Institutes of Health. (1981). *Report of the 1981 working group to review the report by the National Heart and Lung Institute task force on arteriosclerosis* (DHEW Publication No. NIH 81034, p. 37). Washington, DC: U.S. Government Printing Office.
3. Enos, W.F., Beyer, J.C., & Holmes, R.F. (1955). Pathogenesis of coronary artery disease in American soldiers killed in Korea. *Journal of the American Medical Association, 158*, 912.
4. Campbell, G.R., & Chambley-Campbell, J.H. (1981). Invited review: The cellular pathobiology of atherosclerosis. *Pathology, 13*, 424.
5. Cotran, R.S., Kumar, V., & Robbins, S.L. (1989). *Pathologic basis of disease* (4th ed., pp. 140, 141, 560, 561, 579, 582, 585). Philadelphi: W. B. Saunders.
6. Ross, R. (1986). The pathogenesis of atherosclerosis—an update. *New England Journal of Medicine, 314*(8), 488.
7. Smith, L.H., & Thier, S.O. (1981). *Pathophysiology* (p. 1163). Philadelphia: W.B. Saunders.
8. Report of the National Cholesterol Education Program's Expert Panel on Detection, Evaluation, and Treatment of High Blood Cholesterol in Adults. (1988). *Archives of Internal Medicine, 148*, 36–69.
9. Kannel, W.B., et al. (1976). A general cardiovascular risk profile: The Framingham Study. *American Journal of Cardiology, 38*, 46.
10. Gotto, A.M. (1988). Lipoprotein metabolism and the etiology of hyperlipidemia. *Hospital Practice, 23*(Suppl 1), 4.
11. Gwynne, J.T. (1988). Lipoprotein structure and metabolism. *Consultant, 28*(6), 6.
12. Mahley, R.W. (1988). Apolipoprotein E. Cholesterol transport protein with expanding role in cell biology. *Science, 240*, 622.
13. Editorial. (1988). Apolipoprotein B and atherogenesis. *Lancet, 1*, 1141.
14. Stamfer, M.J., Sacks, F.M., Salvini, S., et al. (1991). A prospective study of cholesterol, apoproteins and risk of myocardial infarction. *New England Journal of Medicine, 325*, 373–381.
15. Consensus Conference. (1984). Treatment of hypertriglyceridemia. *Journal of the American Medical Association, 251*, 1196.
16. U.S. Department of Health and Human Services. (1990). *A report of the expert panel on population strategies for blood cholesterol reduction*. NIH Publication No. 90: 30–47.
17. Goldberg, R.B. (1988). Dietary modification of cholesterol levels. *Consultant, 28*(Suppl 6), 35.
18. Knopp, R.H. (1988). New approaches to cholesterol lowering: Efficacy and safety. *Hospital Practice, 23* (Suppl 1), 22.
19. DeSanchis, R.W., Doroghazi, R.M., Austen, W.G., et al. (1987). Aortic dissection. *New England Journal of Medicine, 317*, 1060.
20. Webb, R.W., & Bunswick, R.A. (1980). Management of acute dissection of the aorta. *Heart and Lung, 9*, 284.

21. Lennihan, R., Porter, J.M., Summer, D.S., et al. (1988). Raynaud's phenomenon: A wrap-up. *Patient Care, 22*(3), 94.
22. Wigley, F.M. (1991). The differential diagnosis of Raynaud's phenomenon. *Hospital Practice, 26*(7A), 63–84.
23. Lipsmeyer, E.A. (1982). Raynaud's syndrome. *Journal of the Arkansas Medical Society, 79*, 63.
24. Gordon, R.S. From National Institutes of Health. (1979). Biofeedback for patients with Raynaud's vasospasm. *Journal of the American Medical Association, 242*, 509.
25. Miller, K.M. (1978). Assessing peripheral perfusion. *American Journal of Nursing, 78*, 1673.
26. Creager, M.A., & Dzaw, V.J. (1991). Vascular diseases of the extremities. In J.D. Wilson, E. Braunwald, K.J. Isselbacher, et al. (Eds.). *Harrison's principles of internal medicine* (12th ed., pp. 1024–1025). New York: McGraw-Hill.
27. Goldstone, J. (1991). Veins and lymphatics. In L.W. Way (Ed.). *Current surgical diagnosis and treatment* (9th ed., pp. 772–779). San Mateo, CA: Appleton & Lange.
28. Virchow, R. (1846). Weinere untersuchungen uber dic verstropfung der lungenrarterie und ihre folgen. *Beitrage zur Experimentelle Pathologie und Physiologie, 2*, 21.
29. Nicolaides, A.N., Kakkar, V.V., & Renney, J.T.G. (1971). Soleal sinuses and stasis. *British Journal of Surgery, 58*, 307.
30. Nicolaides, A.N., & Gordon-Smith, I. (1977). The prevention of deep venous thrombosis. In J.T. Hobbs (Ed.). *The treatment of venous disorders, a comprehensive review of current practice in the management of varicose veins and postthrombotic syndrome*. Philadelphia: J.B. Lippincott.
31. Matsen, F. (1975). Compartment syndrome: A unified concept. *Clinical Orthopaedics and Related Research, 113*, 8–13.
32. Ashton, H. (1962). Critical closing pressure in human peripheral vascular beds. *Clinical Science, 22*, 79.
33. Clark, M., & Kadhom, H.M. (1988). The nursing prevention of pressure sores in hospital and community patients. *Journal of Advanced Nursing, 13*, 365–373.
34. Meehan, M. (1990). Multisite pressure sore prevalence survey. *Decubitus, 3*, 14–17.
35. Langemo, D.K., Olson, B., Hunter, S., et al. (1989). Incidence and prediction of pressure ulcers in five patient care settings, extended care, home health, and hospice in one locale. *Decubitus, 2*(2), 42.
36. Young, L. (1989). Pressure ulcer prevalence and associated patient characteristics in one long-term facility. *Decubitus, 2*(2), 52.
37. Terry, C., & Silverstein, P. (Eds.). (1981). *Management of dermal ulcers*. Deerfield, IL: Travenol Laboratories.
38. Beland, I., & Passos, J.Y. (1981). *Clinical nursing* (4th ed., p. 1112). New York: Macmillan.
39. Reuler, J.B., & Cooney, T.G. (1981). The pressure sore: Pathophysiology and principles of management. *Annals of Internal Medicine, 94*, 661.
40. Panel for the Prediction and Prevention of Pressure Ulcers in Adults. (1992). *Pressure ulcers in adults: Prediction and prevention (clinical practice guidelines)* (DHHS, AHCPR Publication No. 92-0047). Washington, DC: U.S. Government Printing Office.
41. Anderson, K.E., & Korning, S.A. (1982). Medical aspects of decubitus ulcer. *International Journal of Dermatology, 5*, 265.
42. Braden, B.J. (1989). Clinical utility of the Braden Scale for predicting pressure ulcer risk. *Decubitus, 2*(3), 44–46, 50–51.
43. Norton, D. (1989). Calculating the risk: Reflections on the Norton Scale. *Decubitus, 2*(3), 24–31.
44. Ek, A.C., Gustafson, G., & Lewis, D.H. (1985). The local skin blood flow in areas at risk for pressure sores treated with massage. *Scandinavian Journal of Rehabilitation Medicine, 17*(2), 81–86.
45. Dyson, R. (1978). Bed sores—the injuries hospital staff inflict on patients. *Nursing Mirror, 146*(24), 30–32.
46. National Pressure Ulcer Advisory Panel. (1989). Pressure ulcers, incidence, economics, and risk assessment. Consensus Development Conference Statement. *Decubitus, 2*(2), 24–28.
47. Braun, J.L., Silvette, A.N., & Xakellis, G.G. (1992). What really works for pressure sores? *Patient Care, 30*, 63–83.

■ BIBLIOGRAPHY

American Journal of Nursing. (1992). How to predict and prevent pressure ulcers. *American Journal of Nursing, 92*(7), 52–60.

Bergstrom, N., & Braden, B. (1992). A prospective study of pressure sore risk among institutionalized elderly. *Journal of the American Geriatrics Society, 40*, 747–758.

Cooper, G.R., Myers, G.L., Smith, S.J., et al. (1992). Blood lipid measurements: Variations and practical utility. *Journal of the American Medical Association, 267*, 1652–1660.

Guaralnik, J.M., et al. (1988). Occurrence and predictors of pressure sores in the National Health and Nutrition Examination Survey followup. *Journal of the American Geriatrics Society, 36*, 7–12.

Johansen, K. (1982). Aneurysms. *Scientific American, 247*(1), 101.

Olin, J.W., & Graor, R.A. (1988). Thrombolytic therapy in treatment of peripheral arterial occlusions. *Annals of Emergency Medicine, 17*, 1210.

Resch, C.S., Kerner, E., Robson, M.C., et al. (1988). Pressure sore volume measurement. *Journal of the American Geriatrics Society, 36*, 444.

Ripsin, C.M., Keenan, J.M., Jacobs, D.R., et al. (1992). Oat products and lipid lowering: A meta-analysis. *Journal of the American Medical Association, 267*, 3317–3325.

Stump, D.C., & Mann, D.C. (1988). Mechanisms of thrombus formation and lysis. *Annals of Emergency Medicine, 17*, 1138.

Weingarten, J., & Teirney, L.M., Jr. (1987). Aortic dissection. *Western Journal of Medicine, 144*, 728.

ALTERATIONS IN BLOOD PRESSURE: HYPERTENSION AND ORTHOSTATIC HYPOTENSION

■ OBJECTIVES

After you have studied this chapter, you should be able to meet the following objectives:

- Define *arterial blood pressure, systolic blood pressure, diastolic blood pressure, pulse pressure*, and *mean arterial blood pressure*.
- Explain how cardiac output and peripheral vascular resistance interact in determining systolic and diastolic blood pressure.
- Explain the interaction of the autonomic nervous system, the baroreceptors and chemoreceptors, and the renin–angiotensin–aldosterone system on short-term regulation of blood pressure.
- Describe the effects of salt and water intake and mechanisms of renal elimination on the long-term regulation of blood pressure.
- Cite the definition of *hypertension* put forth by the Joint National Committee (JNC) on Detection, Evaluation, and Treatment of Hypertension.
- Differentiate among essential, secondary, and malignant forms of hypertension.
- Describe the possible influence of age, race, obesity, salt and other cation (potassium, calcium, and magnesium) intake, alcohol consumption, stress, and oral contraceptive medications on development of essential hypertension.

- Explain the changes in blood pressure that accompany normal pregnancy.
- Describe the four types of hypertension that can occur during pregnancy.
- Cite the criteria for the diagnosis of high blood pressure in children.
- Define *systolic hypertension* and relate the circulatory changes that occur with aging to the development of systolic hypertension.
- List two behavior modification strategies used in treatment of hypertension and explain their benefits in reducing blood pressure.
- List the three categories of drugs used to treat hypertension and state their action in control of high blood pressure.
- Define *orthostatic hypotension*.
- Explain how fluid deficit, medications, aging, disorders of the autonomic nervous system, and bedrest contribute to the development of orthostatic hypotension.

Carol Mattson Porth: PATHOPHYSIOLOGY: CONCEPTS OF
ALTERED HEALTH STATES, 4th ed. © 1994, 1990, 1986, 1982
J.B. Lippincott Company

The importance of measuring blood pressure and treating high blood pressure has been recognized for over 50 years. A speaker at the 1938 meeting of the Chicago Society of Internal Medicine stated:[1]

> . . . while it [measurement of blood pressure] does not carry an immediate purport in cases of acute illness as do the temperature and pulse; yet for long-term evaluation of health of the average person it is far more significant. No other commonly used test gives such quick and reasonably exact information regarding life expectancy.

The discussion in this chapter focuses on control of blood pressure and conditions of altered arterial pressure—hypertension and orthostatic hypotension.

■ CONTROL OF BLOOD PRESSURE

The arterial blood pressure is the driving force for blood flow in the circulatory system. Although blood pressure varies from moment to moment, it is perhaps the most controlled variable in the circulatory system.

THE PRESSURE PULSE

The arterial pressure reflects the intermittent ejection of blood from the left ventricle into the aorta. It rises during systole as the left ventricle contracts, and falls as the heart relaxes during diastole, giving rise to what is called a *pressure wave*. This pressure wave is responsible for the Korotkoff sounds heard when blood pressure is measured using a blood pressure cuff. The ejection of blood from the right ventricle into the pulmonary artery also produces pressure pulses, albeit of lesser magnitude than those of the systemic arterial pressure.

The contour of the arterial pressure tracing shown in Figure 21-1 is typical of the pressure changes that occur in the large arteries of the systemic circulation. There is a rapid rise in the pulse contour during left ventricular contraction, followed by a slower rise to peak pressure. About 70% of the blood that leaves the left ventricle is ejected during the first one third of systole (called the *rapid ejection period*); this accounts for the rapid rise in the pulse contour. The end of systole is marked by a brief downward deflection and formation of the *dicrotic notch*, which occurs when ventricular pressure falls below that in the aorta. The sudden closure of the aortic valve and the rebound energy it produces cause a brief rise in pressure immediately following the notch. As the ventricles relax and blood flows into the peripheral vessels during diastole, the arterial pressure falls rapidly at first and then declines slowly as the driving force decreases.

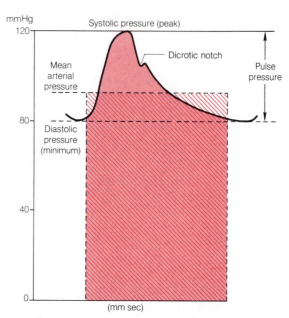

FIG. 21-1. Intraarterial pressure tracing made from the brachial artery. Pulse pressure is the difference between systolic and diastolic pressures. The *cross-hatched area* represents the mean arterial pressure, which can be calculated by using the formula mean arterial pressure = diastolic pressure + pulse pressure/3.

In healthy adults, the pressure at the height of the pressure pulse, called the *systolic pressure*, normally is about 120 mmHg, and the lowest pressure, called the *diastolic pressure*, is about 80 mmHg. The difference between the systolic and diastolic pressure (about 40 mmHg) is called the *pulse pressure*. It reflects the magnitude or height of the pressure pulse. The *mean arterial pressure* represents the average pressure in the arterial system during both ventricular contraction and relaxation (about 90 to 100 mmHg) and is depicted by the cross-hatched areas under the pressure tracing in Figure 21-1.

DETERMINANTS OF BLOOD PRESSURE

Arterial blood pressure is determined by the cardiac output (amount of blood that the heart pumps each minute [stroke volume × heart rate]) and the resistance that the blood encounters as it is being pumped through the peripheral circulation (called the *total peripheral resistance*); therefore, blood pressure can be expressed as the product of the two.

Blood pressure
= cardiac output × total peripheral resistance

The total peripheral vascular resistance reflects the tone of the resistance vessels and the viscosity of the blood; it is increased when resistance vessels constrict and when blood viscosity is increased. The term *total total peripheral resistance* (also called *peripheral or systemic vascular resistance*) is used to describe the sum of all the resistive forces that impede flow in the peripheral circulation. The body maintains its blood pressure by adjusting the cardiac output to compensate for changes in total peripheral resistance, and it changes the total peripheral resistance to compensate for changes in cardiac output.

In hypertension and disease conditions that affect blood pressure, changes in blood pressure are often described in terms of systolic, diastolic, pulse pressure, and mean arterial blood pressures. Each of these pressures contributes individually and collectively to blood flow in the various tissue beds of the body. The level to which each of these pressures rises and falls is influenced by the stroke volume, elastic properties of the aorta, and the total peripheral resistance.

SYSTOLIC BLOOD PRESSURE

The systolic pressure reflects the intermittent ejection of blood into the aorta (Fig. 21-2). As blood is ejected into the aorta, it stretches the vessel wall and produces a rise in aortic pressure. The extent to which the systolic pressure rises or falls is determined by the amount of blood ejected into the aorta (stroke volume), the velocity of ejection, and the elastic properties of the aorta. Systolic pressure increases when there is a rapid ejection of a large stroke volume or when the stroke volume is ejected into a rigid aorta. Only about one third of the ejected blood leaves the aorta during ventricular systole and normally the elastic walls of the aorta stretch to accommodate the blood that remains in the aorta; this prevents the pressure from rising excessively during systole and serves to maintain pressure during diastole. In some elderly people, the elastic fibers of the aorta lose some of their resiliency and the aorta becomes more rigid as a result of the aging process. When this occurs, the aorta is less able to stretch and buffer the pressure that is generated as blood is ejected into the aorta. This results in an elevated systolic pressure.

DIASTOLIC BLOOD PRESSURE

The diastolic pressure is maintained by the pressure that has been stored in the elastic walls of the aorta during systole (see Fig. 21-2). The level at which the diastolic pressure is maintained depends on (1) the condition of the arteries and their ability to stretch and store energy, (2) competency of the aortic valve, and (3) the resistance of the arterioles. The arteries are located between the outlet of the left heart (aortic valve) and the arterioles, which control the total pe-

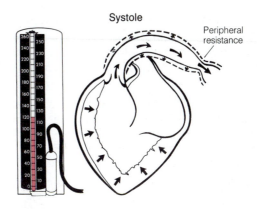

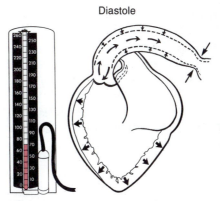

FIG. 21-2. *Diagram of the left side of the heart. Systolic blood pressure (**top**) represents the ejection of blood into the aorta during ventricular systole; it reflects the stroke volume, the distensibility of the aorta, and the velocity with which blood is ejected from the heart. Diastolic blood pressure (**bottom**) represents the pressure in the arterial system during diastole; it is largely determined by the peripheral vascular resistance.*

ripheral resistance and runoff of blood from the arterial circulation. When there is an increase in total peripheral resistance, as with sympathetic stimulation, diastolic blood pressure rises. With atherosclerosis, the smaller arteries may become rigid and unable to accept the runoff of blood from the aorta without producing an increase in diastolic pressure.

Closure of the aortic valve at the onset of diastole is essential to the maintenance of the diastolic pressure. When there is incomplete closure of the aortic valve, as in aortic regurgitation (see Chapter 23), the diastolic pressure drops as blood flows backward into the left ventricle.

PULSE PRESSURE

The pulse pressure reflects the pulsatile nature of the arterial blood flow and is an important component of blood pressure. During the rapid ejection period of ventricular systole, the volume of blood that is introduced into the arterial system exceeds the volume that exits. The pulse pressure reflects this difference. The pulse pressure rises when additional amounts of blood are ejected into the arterial circulation and it falls when the resistance to outflow is decreased. In hypovolemic shock, the pulse pressure declines due to a decrease in stroke volume and systolic pressure. This occurs despite an increase in peripheral resistance, which serves to maintain the diastolic pressure.

MEAN ARTERIAL BLOOD PRESSURE

The mean arterial blood pressure represents the average blood pressure in the systemic circulation. The mean arterial pressure determines tissue blood flow. Mean arterial pressure can be estimated by adding one third of the pulse pressure to the diastolic pressure (diastolic blood pressure + pulse pressure/3). Hemodynamic monitoring equipment in intensive and coronary care units usually computes mean arterial pressure automatically. Because it is a good indicator of tissue perfusion, the mean arterial pressure is often monitored, along with systolic and diastolic blood pressures, in critically ill patients.

BLOOD PRESSURE MEASUREMENT

Arterial blood pressure measurements are usually obtained by the indirect method using a sphygmomanometer and the auscultatory method. In the measurement of blood pressure, a cuff, which contains a rubber bladder, is placed around the upper arm. The bladder of the cuff is inflated to a point at which its pressure exceeds that of the artery, thus occluding the blood flow. The cuff is then slowly deflated until the pressure in the vessel once again exceeds the pressure in the cuff. At this time, a small amount of blood is forced through the partially obstructed artery; by placing a stethoscope over the brachial artery distal to the cuff, one can audibly monitor the tapping sounds that are produced. The auscultatory sounds, or tapping sounds, heard during blood pressure measurement are often referred to as Korotkoff sounds after the Russian physician who first described them (Table 21-1).

Blood pressure is recorded in terms of both systolic and diastolic pressures (*e.g.*, 120/70 mmHg). The initial tapping sound heard as blood is forced through the artery is the systolic pressure. Diastolic pressure reflects the point at which the sounds become muffled or are no longer heard; it represents the point at which arterial pressure is sufficient to prevent vessel compression by the cuff. It is recommended that the disappearance of sound (phase V) should be used for the diastolic reading.[2]

TABLE 21-1. KOROTKOFF SOUNDS	
Phase I	Period marked by the first tapping sounds, which gradually increase in intensity
Phase II	Period during which a murmur or swishing sound is heard
Phase III	Period during which sounds are crisper and greater in intensity
Phase IV	Period marked by distinct, abrupt muffling or by a soft blowing sound
Phase V	Point at which sounds disappear

Blood pressure can also be measured in the legs using a thigh cuff, or it can be measured in the forearm rather than the upper arm. When blood pressure is measured in the forearm, an appropriate sized cuff is placed below the elbow and the Korotkoff sounds are monitored over the radial artery. Forearm blood pressures are particularly useful in obese people, particularly when an appropriate sized cuff is not available for the upper arm. Automated or semiautomated methods of blood pressure measurement use a microphone, pulse sensor, or Doppler methods for detecting the equivalent of the Korotkoff sounds.

Intraarterial methods provide for direct measurement of blood pressure. Intraarterial measurement requires the insertion of a catheter into a peripheral artery. The arterial catheter is connected to a pressure transducer, which converts pressure into a digital signal that can be measured, displayed, and recorded.

MECHANISMS OF BLOOD PRESSURE CONTROL

Under ordinary conditions there are moment-by-moment variations in blood pressure related to activities of daily living such as moving from the supine to standing position, exercise, and emotional stress. Normally, blood pressure is regulated at levels sufficient to ensure adequate tissue perfusion. Blood pressure regulation requires the use of both short-term and long-term mechanisms.

SHORT-TERM REGULATION

Both neural and hormonal mechanisms function in the short-term regulation of blood pressure. The short-term adjustments (those occurring over seconds, minutes, or hours) are intended to correct temporary imbalances that occur during the performance of everyday activities such as physical exercise and changes in posture. These mechanisms are also responsible for maintenance of blood pressure at survival levels during life-threatening situations.

The neural mechanisms of blood pressure control, which are largely vested in the autonomic nervous system (ANS), include intrinsic circulatory reflexes, extrinsic reflexes, and higher neural control centers. The intrinsic reflexes, including the baroreflex and chemoreceptor-mediated reflex, are located within the circulatory system and are essential for rapid and short-term regulation of blood pressure. The extrinsic reflexes are found outside the circulation. They include blood pressure responses associated with such factors as pain, cold, and isometric handgrip exercise. The neural pathways for these reactions are largely unknown, and their responses are less consistent than those of the intrinsic reflexes. Among higher center responses are the central nervous system (CNS) ischemic response and those due to changes in mood and emotion. A number of hormones and humoral mechanisms contribute to blood pressure regulation, including the renin–angiotensin–aldosterone mechanism and vasopressin.

Baroreceptors. Baroreceptors are pressure-sensitive receptors located in the walls of blood vessels and the heart. The carotid and aortic baroreceptors are located in strategic positions between the heart and the brain (Fig. 21-3). The baroreceptors respond to a change in the stretch of the vessel wall by sending impulses to cardiovascular centers in the brain to effect appropriate changes in heart action and vascular smooth muscle tone. For example, a fall in blood pressure on moving from the lying to the standing position produces a decrease in the stretch of the aortic and carotid baroreceptors with a resultant increase in heart rate and vasoconstriction. The rapidity with which the baroreflex response occurs is such that a change in heart rate can often be observed within one or two heartbeats. The vasoconstrictor response may take several seconds to occur.

The carotid and aortic baroreceptors are often referred to as the high-pressure baroreceptors because they are located in the arterial side of the circulation. There are also low-pressure baroreceptors, which are located in the right atria and pulmonary artery (the low-pressure side of the circulation). As with other neural receptors, the baroreceptors adapt to prolonged changes in blood pressure and are probably of little importance in the long-term regulation of blood pressure.

Chemoreceptors. The chemoreceptors are sensitive to changes in the oxygen, the carbon dioxide, and the hydrogen ion content of the blood. The arterial chemoreceptors are located in the carotid bodies, which lie in the bifurcation of the two common carotids, and in the aortic bodies of the aorta (see Fig.

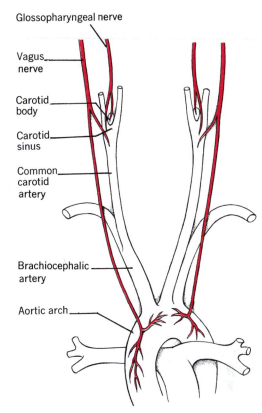

FIG. 21-3. Location and innervation of the aortic arch and carotid sinus baroreceptors and the carotid body chemoreceptors. (Chaffee, E. E. & Lytle, I. M. [1980]. *Basic physiology and anatomy* [4th ed.]. Philadelphia: J.B. Lippincott)

21-3). Because of their location, these chemoreceptors are always in close contact with the arterial blood. Although the main function of the chemoreceptors is to regulate ventilation, they also communicate with the vasomotor center and can induce widespread vasoconstriction. Whenever the arterial pressure drops below a critical level, the chemoreceptors are stimulated because of a diminished oxygen supply and a buildup of carbon dioxide and hydrogen ions. As discussed in Chapter 27, people with hypoxemia due to chronic lung disease may develop both systemic and pulmonary hypertension.

The Autonomic Nervous System. The neural control centers for the regulation of blood pressure are located in the reticular formation of the lower pons and medulla of the brain stem where the integration and modulation of ANS responses occur. The area of the reticular formation that controls blood vessel tone is called the *vasomotor center*. These brain stem centers receive information from many areas of the nervous system including the hypothalamus.

The ANS contributes to blood pressure control through both cardiac (heart rate and cardiac contractility) and vascular (peripheral vascular resistance) mechanisms. The heart is innervated by both the parasympathetic and sympathetic nervous systems. Parasympathetic innervation of the heart is by means of the vagus nerve. The effect of vagal stimulation on heart function is largely limited to heart rate, with increased vagal activity producing a slowing of the pulse. Stimulation of the sympathetic nervous system produces an increase in both heart rate and cardiac contractility. The sympathetic nervous system controls blood vessel tone. Even under resting or basal conditions the resistance vessels of the arterial system are partially constricted. The peripheral vascular resistance, a determinant of blood pressure, is controlled by altering this basal tone. The parasympathetic nervous system exerts little, if any, control over blood vessel function.

The actions of the ANS are mediated by chemical neurotransmitters. Acetylcholine is the postganglionic neurotransmitter for parasympathetic neurons, and norepinephrine is the main neurotransmitter for postganglionic sympathetic neurons. Sympathetic neurons also respond to epinephrine, which is released into the bloodstream by the adrenal medulla. The neurotransmitter dopamine can also act as a neuromediator for some sympathetic neurons.

The neuromediators exert their effect through membrane proteins called *receptors*. The neuromediators and receptors interact in a lock and key fashion, which ensures specificity of action. Receptors that interact with acetylcholine are called *cholinergic* receptors, and those that interact with the sympathetic neuromediators are called *adrenergic* receptors. There are two types of adrenergic receptors: alpha (α) and beta (β) receptors. In vascular smooth muscle, stimulation of α receptors produces vasoconstriction; stimulation of β receptors causes vasodilatation. Alpha receptors have been further subdivided into α_1 and α_2 receptors. α_1 receptors are found primarily at postsynaptic effector sites such as vascular smooth muscle. α_2 receptors are abundant in the CNS and act at presynaptic sites to produce feedback inhibition of sympathetic outflow. β_1 receptors are found primarily in the heart, and β_2 receptors are found in the bronchioles and in other sites that have β-mediated functions. In many tissues, the response that occurs is determined by the presence of a particular receptor type, which can vary from tissue to tissue. For example, in vascular smooth muscle that has α_1 receptors, sympathetic stimulation produces vasoconstriction; similar stimulation produces vasodilatation in other vessels that have β_2 receptors. The actions of the ANS are further discussed in Chapter 48.

The role of the ANS in control of blood pressure is only beginning to be understood. For example, central α_2-adrenergic receptors are known to inhibit sympathetic outflow from the brain. Several anti-hypertensive medications exert their effect at this level. α- and β-adrenergic receptors respond to endogenous or exogenous catecholamines (*e.g.*, drugs). Drugs that can selectively activate or block specific types of adrenergic receptors have been developed to treat high blood pressure.

The Central Nervous System Responses. It is not surprising that the CNS, which plays an essential role in regulating vasomotor tone and blood pressure, would have a mechanism for controlling the blood flow to the cardiovascular centers that control circulatory function. When the blood flow to the brain has been sufficiently interrupted to cause ischemia of the vasomotor center, these vasomotor neurons become strongly excited, causing massive vasoconstriction as a means of raising the blood pressure to levels as high as the heart can pump against. This response is called the CNS ischemic response, and it can raise the blood pressure to levels as high as 270 mmHg for as long as 10 minutes.[3] The CNS ischemic response is a last-ditch stand to preserve the blood flow to vital brain centers; it does not become activated until blood pressure has fallen to at least 60 mmHg, and it is most effective in the range of 15 to 20 mmHg. If the cerebral circulation is not reestablished within 3 to 10 minutes, the neurons of the vasomotor center cease to function, so that the tonic impulses to the blood vessels stop and the blood pressure falls precipitously.

The Cushing reflex is a special type of CNS reflex resulting from an increase in intracranial pressure. When the intracranial pressure rises to levels that equal intraarterial pressure, blood vessels to the vasomotor center become compressed, initiating the CNS ischemic response. The purpose of this reflex is to produce a rise in arterial pressure to levels above intracranial pressure so that the blood flow to the vasomotor center can be reestablished.

Renin–Angiotensin–Aldosterone Mechanism. The renin–angiotensin–aldosterone system plays a central role in blood pressure regulation. Renin is an enzyme that is synthesized and released from the kidneys when blood pressure drops to low. Factors that control renin release include renal blood flow and renal artery pressure. Renin levels increase as renal blood flow and renal artery pressure fall. Renin is also released in response to sympathetic stimulation.

Renin is an enzyme, not a vasoactive substance itself. It combines enzymatically with a plasma protein (*angiotensinogen*) that is present in the bloodstream to form angiotensin I (Fig. 21-4). Angiotensin I enters the circulation and travels to the small blood vessels of the lung, where it is converted to angioten-

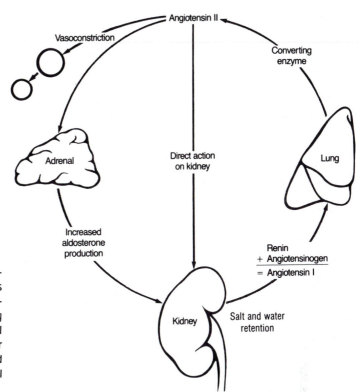

FIG. 21-4. Control of blood pressure by the renin–angiotensin–aldosterone system. Renin combines with the plasma protein angiotensinogen to form angiotensin I; angiotensin-converting enzyme in the lung converts angiotensin I to angiotensin II; angiotensin II produces vasoconstriction and increases salt and water retention through direct action on the kidney and through increased aldosterone secretion by the adrenal cortex.

sin II by the angiotensin-converting enzyme. There are several potential pathways whereby angiotensin II, the active component of the renin–angiotensin–aldosterone mechanism, could influence short- and long-term regulation of blood pressure: through vasoconstriction of blood vessels; through activation of the sympathetic nervous system or by potentiation of its effects; or through influence of fluid volume by thirst, direct renal mechanisms, or aldosterone.[4] Although angiotensin II has a short half-life of minutes, it is one of the most potent vasoconstrictors known. Angiotensin II exerts a direct effect on the kidneys to decrease the elimination of salt and water. It acts in a feedback manner to decrease renin release, and it stimulates the production and release of aldosterone from the adrenal cortex. Aldosterone provides more long-term regulation of blood pressure through salt and water retention.

Among people with hypertension, there is a subgroup that has high renin levels and another subgroup that has low renin levels with normal angiotensin and aldosterone levels. It has been proposed that the elevation of blood pressure in people in the high renin group is due to vasoconstriction, and in the low renin group it is due to volume expansion. Angiotensin-converting enzyme (ACE) inhibitors are used in the treatment of some people with hypertension, particularly those with high renin levels.[5] The ACE inhibitors not only reduce blood pressure, but they increase renal blood flow and the glomerular filtra-

tion, which is advantageous in certain types of hypertension.

Vasopressin. Vasopressin, or antidiuretic hormone (ADH), is released from the posterior pituitary gland in response to decreases in blood volume and blood pressure. Its release is mediated by the osmolality of body fluids and other stimuli. The antidiuretic actions of vasopressin are discussed in Chapter 29. Vasopressin has a direct vasoconstrictor effect on blood vessels, particularly those of the splanchnic circulation. However, long-term increases in vasopressin cannot maintain volume expansion or hypertension, and it does not enhance hypertension produced by sodium-retaining hormones or other vasoconstricting substances. Rather, it has been suggested that vasopressin plays a permissive role in hypertension by its fluid-retaining properties or that it acts as a neurotransmitter that serves to modify ANS function.[6]

LONG-TERM REGULATION

Both neural and hormonal regulation of blood pressure are short-term mechanisms that act rapidly to restore blood pressure. They are, however, ineffective in the long-term regulation of blood pressure; the day-by-day, week-by-week, and month-by-month regulation of blood pressure is vested in what

Guyton terms the "renal–body fluid pressure control system."[3]

The renal–body fluid system controls blood pressure by regulating extracellular fluid. When the body contains too much extracellular fluid, the arterial pressure increases; when too little fluid is present, it decreases. For example, an increase in arterial pressure greatly increases the rate at which both water (pressure diuresis) and sodium (pressure natriuresis) are excreted by the kidney. Figure 21-5 illustrates the control of blood pressure by renal output mechanisms. The only point on the graph at which the intake and output are balanced is at point A. At point B, where intake has increased almost fourfold, the blood pressure has increased to only 106 mmHg, demonstrating that the kidney adjusts the output of urine to balance the input. The function of the kidney in regulating body fluids is discussed in Chapter 31.

The only way to change the long-term regulation of blood pressure using the concept of the renal–body fluid control system is to change either the pressure range of the renal output curve or the net rate of intake. For example, kidney disease, which impairs salt and water excretion, results in a shift of the pressure range of the curve to the right so that points A and B occur at a higher arterial pressure. It is important to consider that the renal mechanisms control the blood volume at a level required to attain the blood pressure needed to balance the intake and output. In some situations such as hot weather, which produces vasodilatation, more volume is required to attain this balance.

The overall mechanism whereby increased extracellular volume elevates blood pressure is through an increase in blood volume, which in turn produces an increase in cardiac output. There are two different ways in which cardiac output increases blood pressure. One is through a direct effect on blood pressure; the other is through an indirect effect resulting from local autoregulation of blood flow. When excess blood flows through a tissue, local blood vessels constrict and return the flow to normal. When cardiac output is increased, all of the tissues are exposed to increased blood flow and autoregulation constricts blood vessels throughout the body; this, in turn, increases the total peripheral resistance, producing a further increase in blood pressure.[3]

In summary, the alternating contraction and relaxation of the heart produce a pressure pulse that moves the blood through the circulatory system. The elastic walls of the aorta stretch during systole and relax during diastole to maintain the diastolic pressure. The pressure pulse is responsible for the Korotkoff sounds heard when blood pressure is measured using a blood pressure cuff, and it is this impulse that is felt when the pulse is taken. Systolic pressure denotes the highest point of the pulse pressure, and diastolic denotes the lowest point. The pulse pressure is the difference between these two pressures. The mean arterial pressure reflects the average pressure throughout the cardiac cycle. It can be estimated by adding one third of the pulse pressure to the diastolic pressure. Systolic pressure is determined primarily by the characteristics of the stroke volume, whereas diastolic pressure is determined largely by the conditions of the arteries and arterioles and their abilities to accept the runoff of blood from the aorta. Blood pressure is determined by the cardiac output and total peripheral resistance.

Blood pressure can be measured either directly or indirectly. Direct measurement requires the insertion of a catheter into an artery. Clinical measurement of blood pressure is usually done by the indirect method using a blood pressure cuff and either the auscultatory or Doppler method.

Short-term and long-term mechanisms for blood pressure control normally maintain the mean arterial blood pressure within a range that is adequate for tissue perfusion. Short-term regulation of blood pressure involves neural and hormonal mechanisms; it occurs over minutes and hours and is intended to correct temporary imbalances in blood pressure, such as those caused by postural changes, exercise, or hemorrhage. Long-term mechanisms control the day-by-day, week-by-week, and month-by-month regulation of blood pressure and involve a change in the excretion of salt and water by the kidneys (the renal–body fluid pressure control system).

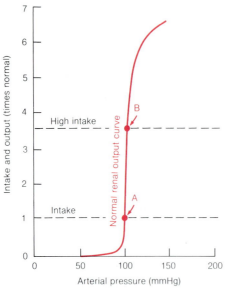

FIG. 21-5. Graphic representation of long-term regulation of blood pressure based on the renal–body fluid mechanism for pressure control. The steep part of the curve is the normal urinary output curve and indicates a 3.5 times normal intake 106 mmHg. (Guyton, A. [1981]. *Medical physiology* [6th ed.]. Philadelphia: W.B. Saunders)

■ HYPERTENSION

Hypertension, or high blood pressure, is probably the most common of all cardiovascular disorders. Almost 60 million people in the United States have an elevated blood pressure (140/90 mmHg or greater) or have reported being told by a physician that they have high blood pressure. The prevalence of hypertension increases with age, and the rate among African-Americans is higher than among white Americans. It occurs in all geographic areas of the country and affects people from low-, middle-, and upper-income groups. Hypertension is credited with causing 30,700 deaths annually; it takes its toll mainly through vascular complications that lead to stroke, coronary heart disease, and chronic renal failure.[13]

Hypertension is commonly divided into the categories of primary and secondary hypertension. In primary hypertension, often called essential hypertension, the chronic elevation in blood pressure occurs without evidence of other disease. In secondary hypertension, the elevation of blood pressure accompanies some other disorder, such as kidney disease. Malignant hypertension, as the name implies, is an accelerated form of hypertension. The discussion that follows focuses on these forms of hypertension, hypertension in children and the elderly, and the complications and treatment of hypertension.

ESSENTIAL HYPERTENSION

The fifth (1993) report of the Joint National Committee (JNC V) on Detection, Evaluation, and Treatment of High Blood Pressure of the National Institutes of Health has recommended criteria for the diagnosis of high blood pressure in individuals aged 18 years and older.[2] The diagnosis of hypertension is made if the systolic blood pressure is 140 mmHg or higher and diastolic blood pressure is 90 mmHg or higher when at least two blood pressure measurements are averaged on two or more subsequent visits (unless the systolic pressure is 210 mmHg or greater and/or diastolic pressure is 120 mmHg or greater). The 1993 report of the JNC includes a category of high normal blood pressure (systolic pressure of 130–139 mmHg and diastolic pressure of 85–89 mmHg) and categorizes high blood pressure into four stages based on systolic and diastolic blood pressures (Table 21-2). A consistently elevated systolic pressure of 160 mmHg or higher with a diastolic pressure of less than 90 mmHg represents isolated systolic hypertension.

The report emphasizes that obtaining one elevated blood pressure reading should not constitute the diagnosis of hypertension. Blood pressure measurements should be taken when the person is relaxed and has rested for at least 5 minutes and has not smoked or ingested caffeine within 30 minutes. A mercury manometer with the appropriately sized cuff or an aneroid manometer that is accurately calibrated should be used for blood pressure measurements. At least two measurements should be made at each visit in the same arm while the person is seated. The diastolic pressure is recorded at the disappearance of sound, or phase V of the Korotkoff sounds.[2]

RISK FACTORS

A number of factors interact in producing long-term elevations in blood pressure; these factors include hemodynamic, neural, humoral, and renal mecha-

TABLE 21-2. CLASSIFICATION OF BLOOD PRESSURE FOR ADULTS AGE 18 YEARS OR OLDER*		
CATEGORY	**SYSTOLIC (mmHg)**	**DIASTOLIC (mmHg)**
Normal	<130	<85
High normal	130–139	85–89
Hypertension†		
Stage 1 (Mild)	140–159	90–99
Stage 2 (Moderate)	160–179	100–109
Stage 3 (Severe)	180–209	110–119
Stage 4 (Very severe)	≥210	≥120

  * Not taking antihypertensive drugs and not acutely ill. When systolic and diastolic pressures fall into different categories, the higher category should be selected to classify the individual's blood pressure status. For instance, 160/92 mmHg should be classified as Stage 2, and 180/120 mmHg should be classified as Stage 4. Isolated systolic hypertension (ISH) is defined as SBP ≥140 mmHg and DBP <90 mmHg and staged appropriately (e.g., 170/85 mmHg is defined as Stage 2 ISH).

  † Based on the average of two or more readings taken at each of two or more visits following an initial screening.

  (Adapted from the National Heart, Lung, and Blood Institute. [1993]. *The fifth report of the National Committee on Detection, Evaluation, and Treatment of High Blood Pressure* [p. 4]. Bethesda, MD: NIH Publication No. 93-1088)

nisms. As with other disease conditions, it is improbable that there is a single cause responsible for the development of essential hypertension or, for that matter, that the condition is a single disease.

Because arterial blood pressure is the product of cardiac output and total peripheral resistance, all forms of hypertension involve hemodynamic mechanisms—either an increase in cardiac output or total peripheral resistance or a combination of the two. Many other factors such as the ANS, the kidneys, the electrolyte composition of the intracellular and extracellular fluids, cell membrane transport mechanisms, and humoral influences (*e.g.*, renin–angiotensin–aldosterone mechanism) play either an active or permissive role in regulating the hemodynamic mechanisms that control blood pressure.

Although the cause or causes of essential hypertension are largely unknown, several risk factors have been implicated as contributing to its development. These risk factors include family history, advancing age, race, and high salt intake. Other lifestyle factors can contribute to the development of hypertension by interacting with the risk factors. These lifestyle factors include obesity; excess alcohol consumption; intake of potassium, calcium, and magnesium; stress; and use of oral contraceptive drugs.

Family History. The inclusion of heredity as a contributing factor in the development of hypertension is supported by the fact that hypertension is seen most frequently among people with a family history of hypertension. Studies suggest that in people with a positive family history, the risk for developing essential hypertension is approximately twice that of people with a negative family history. The inherited predisposition does not seem to rely on other risk factors, but when they are present, the risk is apparently additive. This is particularly true of obesity. When obesity and a genetic predisposition are both present, the risk of developing hypertension becomes three to four times higher.[7] The pattern of heredity is unclear (*i.e.*, it is not known whether a single gene or multiple genes are involved). Whatever the explanation, the high incidence of hypertension among close family members seems significant enough to be presented as a case for recommending that people from so-called high-risk families be encouraged to participate in hypertensive screening programs.

Advancing Age. Maturation and growth are known to cause predictable increases in blood pressure. For example, in the newborn, arterial blood pressure is normally only about 50 mmHg systolic and 40 mmHg diastolic. Sequentially, blood pressure increases with physical growth from a value of 78 mmHg systolic at 10 days of age to 120 mmHg at the end of adolescence. Blood pressure usually continues to undergo a slow rate of increase during the adult years. The relationship between the aging process and hypertension is commonly accepted. The author can recall many older people describing the normal range of blood pressure as being "100 plus your age." Although this definition is not entirely correct, it is possible that the cardiovascular and ANS changes that are part of the normal aging process do, in fact, contribute to the increased blood pressures observed in older people. It must be remembered that people tend to age differently; this factor undoubtedly accounts for some of the great variations in blood pressure among elderly people. However, the finding of isolated systolic hypertension is common in the elderly population and is discussed later in this chapter.

Race. Hypertension is not only more prevalent in African-Americans than whites, it is also more severe. The National Health and Nutrition Examination Survey II, 1976–1980, reported that diastolic blood pressures were significantly greater for African-American than white men and women in age groups 35 years and above and that systolic pressures of African-American women at every age were greater than those of white women.[8] Furthermore, it has been reported that hypertension in African-Americans tends to appear earlier than in whites, and it is often not treated early enough or aggressively enough.[9] The result is a higher incidence of more severe hypertension in African-Americans.

The reasons for the increased incidence of hypertension in African-Americans is unknown. Studies have shown that African-American people with hypertension have lower renin levels than white people with hypertension.[9] It has been suggested that environmental stresses associated with poverty, low education, low occupational status, socioeconomic stress, and eating habits that include foods high in salt and fat and other nutritionally contraindicated foods may contribute to the risk of hypertension in African-Americans.[10] Because of their low-renin profile, African-Americans are reported to respond better to drugs, such as diuretics and calcium-channel blocking drugs, that do not exert their primary actions through renin mechanisms.[11]

High Salt Intake. Increased salt intake has long been suspected as an etiologic factor in the development of hypertension. The relationship between body levels of sodium and hypertension is based, at least partially, on the finding of a decreased incidence of hypertension among primitive, unacculturated people from widely differing parts of the world.

For example, among the Yanomamo Indians of northern Brazil, who excrete only about 1 mEq of sodium per day, the average blood pressure in men 40 to 49 years of age was 107/67 mmHg and 98/62 mmHg in women of the same age.[12] From childhood through adult life, acculturated societies consume 10 to 20 g of salt daily. Drinking water may be another source of increased sodium intake; in some cities there is considerable sodium in the water supply.

Just how increased salt intake contributes to the development of hypertension is still unclear. Evidence to support individual and group susceptibility to the hypertensive effects of sodium comes from observations made from the development of a strain of spontaneously hypertensive rats. These rats develop hypertension earlier than other strains, and their hypertension is more severe when extra salt is added to their diet. It may be that salt causes an elevation in blood volume, increases the sensitivity of cardiovascular or renal mechanisms to adrenergic influences, or exerts its effects through some other mechanism such as the renin–angiotensin–aldosterone mechanism. Interestingly, it has been observed that excessive salt intake does not cause hypertension in all people, nor does the reduction in salt intake reduce blood pressure in all hypertensives. This probably means that some people are more susceptible than others to the effects of increased sodium intake. The impact of long-term nationwide restriction of sodium consumption is not known; it could, for example, create problems in people who respond poorly to volume-depleting stresses in the absence of readily available salt in their diet.[13] Identification of people at risk who would specifically benefit from salt reduction would facilitate hypertension management.

Obesity. Excessive weight is commonly observed in association with hypertension. In a large nationwide screening program of more than a million people, it was found that the frequency of hypertension in overweight people 20 to 39 years of age was double that of people of normal weight and triple that of underweight people.[14] It has been suggested that fat distribution might be a more critical indicator of hypertension risk than actual overweight. The waist-to-hip ratio is commonly used to distinguish between waist (fat cell deposits in the abdomen) and hip or gluteal gynecoid obesity (fat cell deposits in the buttocks and legs). Studies have shown that there is a relationship between hypertension and increased waist-to-hip ratio even when body-mass index and skinfold thickness are taken into account.[15, 16] The exact mechanism by which obesity contributes to the development of hypertension is largely unknown, although it may be that mechanisms responsible for elevating blood pressure in the overweight person are related to the metabolic needs of the excess adipose tissue, along with the increased demands on the cardiovascular system to provide adequate blood flow through the enlarged tissue mass. It is also possible that the dietary habits of the overweight person include the ingestion of excessive amounts of salt along with increased caloric intake. Hyperinsulinemia (excess insulin in the blood), which reduces sodium excretion and causes neuroendocrine disturbances such as abnormalities of the sympathetic nervous system, may also contribute to the development of hypertension in obese people.[17] Whatever the cause, it is known that weight loss is effective in reducing blood pressure in a significant number of obese hypertensive people. In one study, it was shown that weight loss or sodium restriction in hypertensives controlled for 5 years more than doubled the success of withdrawal of drug therapy.[18]

Excess Alcohol Consumption. Studies have shown a significant relationship between alcohol consumption and hypertension;[19] it has been suggested that as much as 10% of hypertension cases can be related to alcohol consumption.[20] One of the first reports of a link between alcohol consumption and hypertension came from the Oakland–San Francisco Kaiser-Permanente Medical Care Program study of 84,000 people that correlated known drinking patterns and blood pressure levels.[21] This study revealed that the regular consumption of three or more drinks per day increased the risk of hypertension. Systolic pressures were more markedly affected than diastolic pressures. Blood pressure may improve or return to normal when alcohol consumption is decreased or eliminated.

Intake of Potassium, Calcium, and Magnesium. It has been proposed that it is the ratio of sodium to potassium in the diet, rather than increased sodium intake alone, that influences blood pressure.[22, 23] In terms of food intake, a diet high in sodium is generally low in potassium; conversely, a diet high in potassium is generally low in sodium. One of the major benefits of increased potassium intake is increased elimination of sodium. Other effects include a dampening of vasoconstrictor responses that are induced by norepinephrine and other vasoactive agents. A high-potassium diet does not appear to alter blood pressure in normotensive people, nor is there evidence to suggest a significant effect from giving potassium to hypertensives with normal potassium levels. The use of potassium supplements is expensive and possibly even hazardous for some people. Instead, it is recommended that high-potassium, low-sodium foods be substituted for high-sodium, low-potassium foods in the diet.[5]

The interrelationship of high blood pressure, calcium, and magnesium levels has been investigated.[24] Although there have been reports of high blood pressure in people with low calcium intake or lowering of blood pressure with increased calcium intake, the link between low calcium intake and hypertension is inconclusive.[25] Magnesium, which has been described as "nature's physiologic calcium blocker," is credited with blocking calcium entry into vascular smooth muscle cells, thereby decreasing vascular reactivity.[26] As with calcium, however, the benefits of supplementing magnesium intake in people with hypertension are controversial.

Stress. Physical and emotional stress undoubtedly contribute to transient alterations in blood pressure. Studies in which arterial blood pressure was continually monitored on a 24-hour basis as people performed their normal activities showed marked fluctuations in pressure associated with normal life stresses—increasing during periods of physical discomfort and family crisis and declining during rest and sleep.[27, 28] As with other risk factors, the role of stress-related episodes of transient hypertension in producing the chronically elevated pressures seen in essential hypertension is still speculative. It may be that vascular smooth muscle hypertrophies with increased activity in a manner similar to that of skeletal muscle or that the central integrative pathways in the brain become adapted to the frequent stress-related input.

Psychological techniques involving biofeedback, relaxation, and transcendental meditation have emerged as methods to control alterations in blood pressure. It is still too early to tell whether these techniques offer information about the role of stress in the production of hypertension or will prove useful in its treatment.

Use of Oral Contraceptive Drugs. Oral contraceptives cause a mild increase in blood pressure in many women and overt hypertension in about 5%.[29] Why this occurs is largely unknown, although it has been suggested that estrogen and progesterone are responsible for the effect. The fact that various contraceptive drugs contain different amounts and combinations of estrogen and progestational agents may contribute to the incidence of hypertension among different women. Fortunately, the hypertension associated with oral contraceptives usually disappears once the drug has been discontinued, although it may take as long as 6 months for this to happen. However, in some women the blood pressure may not return to normal; they may be among populations at risk for developing hypertension. The risk of hypertension-associated cardiovascular complications is found primarily in women over 35 years of age and in those who smoke.[29]

SIGNS AND SYMPTOMS

Essential hypertension is typically asymptomatic, and diagnosis is often made by chance during screening procedures or when a person seeks medical care for other purposes. Although headache is often considered to be an early symptom of hypertension, it is present only in a small number of hypertensives at the time of diagnosis. When present, the headache associated with hypertension is believed to be due to intense vasodilatation. It occurs most frequently on awakening and is usually felt in the back of the head or neck.

A common early symptom of long-term hypertension is nocturia, which indicates that the kidneys are losing their ability to concentrate urine. Other commonly associated signs and symptoms are probably related to the complications of hypertension—the long-term effects of blood pressure elevation on other organ systems in the body, such as the kidneys, eyes, heart, and blood vessels.

Aside from elevated blood pressure measurements, few diagnostic tests are useful in detecting and diagnosing essential hypertension. In this respect, the increased availability of hypertensive screening clinics provides a means for early detection. Laboratory tests, x-ray films, and other diagnostic tests are usually done to rule out secondary hypertension or associated complications.

EFFECTS

The complications and mortality associated with primary and secondary hypertension can be explained as the increased wear and tear on the heart and blood vessels. The 1993 report of the JNC uses the term target-organ disease to describe the cardiac, cerebrovascular, peripheral vascular, renal, and retinopathy complications associated with hypertension.[2]

The increase in the workload of the left ventricle as it pumps against the elevated pressures in the systemic circulation is directly related to the degree and duration of the hypertension. This increased work is the stimulus for ventricular muscle hypertrophy, and it increases the heart's need for oxygen. If the increased work demands exceed the heart's compensatory efforts, heart failure occurs because the heart can no longer pump effectively. (Heart failure is discussed in Chapter 24.) The person who develops coronary artery disease along with hypertension is at especially high risk because the heart's oxygen transport facilities are impaired in the presence of increased oxygen needs.

Arteries and arterioles throughout the body experience the effects of the mechanical stress associated with hypertension. Again, the severity and duration of the increase largely determine the extent of vascular changes. In general, hypertension has been implicated in accelerating the development of atherosclerosis, which causes a narrowing of the vessel lumen, and in weakening the vessels. Also, there is greater risk of aortic aneurysm, coronary heart disease, renal complications, retinopathy, and cerebral vascular disease.

The JNC V report emphasizes the need for early identification of target-organ disease and states that people with target-organ disease may require immediate treatment.

HIGH BLOOD PRESSURE IN PREGNANCY

About 10% of all pregnancies are accompanied by hypertension. The National High Blood Pressure Education Program's Working Group Report on High Blood Pressure in Pregnancy recommends four diagnostic categories for hypertension that occurs during pregnancy: (1) chronic hypertension, (2) preeclampsia-eclampsia, (3) chronic hypertension with superimposed preeclampsia-eclampsia, and (4) transient hypertension.[30] The report emphasizes a need to differentiate hypertension that precedes pregnancy from that developing during pregnancy.

The criteria for diagnosing hypertension in pregnancy are systolic pressure increases of 30 mmHg or greater and diastolic pressure increases of 15 mmHg or greater compared with the average values before 20 weeks' gestation. When previous blood pressures are not known, values of 140/90 mmHg or above are considered abnormal.

Preeclampsia, sometimes called *pregnancy-induced hypertension*, is characterized by the triad of hypertension of pregnancy as previously defined, proteinuria (300 mg/L in 24 hours), and edema (weight gain in excess of 2 lb/wk) developing after the 20th week of pregnancy. Eclampsia is an exaggerated form of preeclampsia that has progressed to include convulsions and finally coma. Preeclampsia usually presents after the 20th week of gestation but may occur earlier in pregnancy. The condition occurs primarily during first pregnancies and during subsequent pregnancies in women with chronic hypertension, multiple fetuses, diabetes mellitus, or coexisting renal disease. It is associated with a condition called a *hydatidiform mole* (abnormal pregnancy caused by a pathologic ovum, resulting in a mass of cysts). Of interest is the reversal of the diurnal pattern of blood pressure in preeclamptic hypertension—it is often highest during the night.

Chronic hypertension is considered as hypertension that is unrelated to the pregnancy. It is defined as (1) history of high blood pressure before pregnancy, (2) identification of hypertension before 20 weeks of pregnancy, and (3) hypertension that persists after pregnancy. In women with chronic hypertension, blood pressure often decreases in early pregnancy and increases during the last trimester (3 months) of pregnancy, resembling preeclampsia. Consequently, women with undiagnosed chronic hypertension who do not present for medical care until the later months of pregnancy may be incorrectly diagnosed as having preeclampsia. Furthermore, women with chronic hypertension are at increased risk for developing preeclampsia. Transient hypertension is a condition of high blood pressure that occurs during the last trimester or early post-delivery period, but resolves to normotensive levels within 10 days after delivery.

Defining the causes of hypertension in pregnancy is difficult because of the normal circulatory changes that occur.[31] Blood pressure normally decreases during the first trimester, reaches its lowest point during the second trimester, and gradually rises during the third trimester. The fact that there is a 40% to 60% increase in cardiac output during early pregnancy means the fall in blood pressure that occurs during the first part of pregnancy must be due to a decrease in peripheral vascular resistance. Because the cardiac output remains high throughout pregnancy, the gradual rise in blood pressure that begins during the second trimester probably represents a return of the peripheral vascular resistance to normal. Also, pregnancy is normally accompanied by increased levels of renin, angiotensin I and II, estrogen, progesterone, prolactin, and aldosterone, all of which may alter vascular reactivity. A major feature of preeclampsia is a marked increase in peripheral vascular resistance that is thought to result from exaggerated responsiveness to circulating angiotensin II and catecholamines. It has been suggested that preeclampsia may be associated with inappropriately increased production of prostaglandins with vasoconstrictor properties, or with either increased inactivation or diminished sythesis or release of another prostaglandin with vasodilator properties, or a combination of these events.

It is recommended that all pregnant women, including those with hypertension, refrain from alcohol and tobacco use. The role of calcium supplementation and low-dose aspirin therapy in preventing preeclampsia and chronic and transient hypertension is being investigated. Low-dose aspirin decreases thromboxane (a prostaglandin with vasoconstrictor properties) synthesis while sparing prostacyclin (a prostaglandin with vasodilator properties). Pregnant women with hypertension tend to have lower plasma volumes than do normotensive pregnant women. There is some indication that the severity of hypertension may reflect the degree of volume contraction. Therefore, salt restriction is usually not recommended during pregnancy.

HIGH BLOOD PRESSURE IN CHILDREN

Blood pressure is known to rise from infancy to late adolescence. During childhood, blood pressure is influenced by growth and maturation; therefore, blood pressure norms have been established using age (and height), race, and sex-specific percentiles to identify children for further follow-up and treatment.

The National Heart, Lung, and Blood Institute (NHLBI) convened its second task force in 1985 to (1) identify proper techniques for measuring blood pressure in infants (birth to 2 years), children (2 to 12 years), and adolescents (13 to 18 years); (2) characterize the existing base on blood pressure distribution throughout childhood and prepare distribution curves of blood pressure by height and weight information; (3) recommend blood pressure ranges for children denoting normal, high normal, and hypertensive; (4) present guidelines for detecting children with hypertension and, at the same time, guard against inappropriate labeling of children as hypertensive who are not hypertensive; (5) identify the appropriate diagnostic steps to be taken in the evaluation of children with hypertension; and (6) delineate nonpharmacologic and pharmacologic treatment strategies for management of children with hypertension.[32]

The task force classified blood pressure into three ranges: normal (systolic and diastolic pressures less than the 90th percentile for age and sex); high normal (systolic and/or diastolic blood pressures between the 90th and 95th percentile for age and sex); and high blood pressures or hypertension (average systolic and diastolic blood pressures equal to or greater than the 95th percentile for age and sex on at least three occasions). High blood pressure was further defined as significant hypertension (blood pressure between the 95th and 99th percentile for age and sex) and severe hypertension (blood pressure above the 99th percentile for age and sex). Table 21-3 presents classification of significant and severe blood pressure by age; the source of age-specific percentiles for blood pressure measurements in children appears in the references. The task force recommended further that children 3 years of age through adolescence should have their blood pressure taken once a year. It is recommended that phase IV Korotkoff sounds are used for diastolic pressure in infants and children 3 to 12 years of age. The phase V Korotkoff sound is used

TABLE 21-3. CLASSIFICATION OF HYPERTENSION IN THE YOUNG, BY AGE GROUP

AGE GROUP	95TH PERCENTILE (mmHg)	99TH PERCENTILE (mmHg)
Newborns— 7 days	SBP ≥ 96	SBP ≥ 106
Newborns (8–30 days)	SBP ≥ 104	SBP ≥ 110
Infants (<2 years)	SBP ≥ 112 DBP ≥ 74	SBP ≥ 118 DBP ≥ 82
Children (3–5 years)	SBP ≥ 116 DBP ≥ 76	SBP ≥ 124 DBP ≥ 84
Children (6–9 years)	SBP ≥ 122 DBP ≥ 78	SBP ≥ 130 DBP ≥ 86
Children (10–12 years)	SBP ≥ 126 DBP ≥ 82	SBP ≥ 134 DBP ≥ 90
Adolescents (13–15 years)	SBP ≥ 136 DBP ≥ 86	SBP ≥ 144 DBP ≥ 92
Adolescents (16–18 years)	SBP ≥ 142 DBP ≥ 92	SBP ≥ 150 DBP ≥ 98

Report of the Second Task Force on Blood Pressure Control in Children—1987. [1987]. *Pediatrics, 79,* 1.

with adolescents 13 to 18 years. As with adults, blood pressure should be obtained using the proper sized cuff and a well-functioning manometer. Repeated measurements over time, rather than a single isolated determination, are required to establish consistent and significant observations. Accurate blood pressure measurements are often difficult to obtain in infants and children who are restless; errors are easily generated in Korotkoff sounds if heavy pressure is exerted on the stethoscope. Doppler and oscillometric techniques can be used in infants and children to provide accurate systolic measurements; however, diastolic measurements are more difficult to obtain.

Children with high blood pressure, significant high blood pressure, or severe high blood pressure should be referred for medical evaluation and treatment as indicated. Treatment includes nonpharmacologic methods and, if necessary, pharmacologic therapy. The task force suggested use of the stepped-care approach for drug treatment of children who require antihypertensive medications.

HIGH BLOOD PRESSURE IN THE ELDERLY

Isolated systolic hypertension (systolic pressure greater than 160 mmHg and/or diastolic pressure less than 95 mmHg) is considered an abnormal clinical finding in old age.[33, 34] The prevalence of hypertension (both systolic and diastolic) in the elderly population of the United States ranges from 44% to 63% for whites and 60% to 76% for African-Americans, depending on the criteria used (*e.g.*, 160 mmHg or 140 mmHg systolic and 95 mmHg or 90 mmHg diastolic pressure). For years, systolic hypertension was considered innocuous and was not treated. The results of the Framingham study have shown, however, that there is approximately a two- to fivefold increase in death from cardiovascular disease associated with isolated systolic hypertension.[35]

Data from the Framingham study also indicate that hypertension, whether systolic or diastolic, is a risk factor for cardiovascular morbidity and mortality in older as well as younger people. Stroke is two to three times more common in elderly hypertensives than in age-matched normotensive subjects.[36]

The aging processes that tend to increase blood pressure are stiffening of the arteries, decreased baroreceptor sensitivity, increased peripheral vascular resistance, and decreased renal blood flow. Normally, other aging processes such as an increased volume capacity of the aorta, decrease in blood volume, and a decrease in cardiac output tend to counteract the rise in pressure. The disproportionate rise in systolic pressure observed in some elderly people is explained in terms of the increased rigidity of the aorta and peripheral arteries that accompanies the aging process; this is caused by a loss of elastic fibers in the media, an increase in the amount of collagen, calcium deposition in the media, and atheroma formation in the intima. Normally, the elastic properties of the aorta allow it to stretch during systole as a means of buffering the rise in pressure that occurs as blood is ejected from the heart. During diastole, the recoil of the elastin fibers serves to transmit the stored pressure to the peripheral arterioles as a means of maintaining the diastolic blood pressure. As the aorta loses its elasticity and becomes more rigid as a result of the aging process, the pressure generated during ventricular systole is transmitted to the peripheral arteries practically unchanged.

The Working Group on Hypertension in the Elderly, which met in 1985, recommended that blood pressure values in the elderly should be similar to those for the rest of the population.[34] For elderly people with elevations in both systolic and diastolic pressures, recommendations for detection and confirmation are the same as for younger people. For people with a systolic blood pressure greater than 160 mmHg and normal diastolic pressure on two separate visits, referral to a physician for further evaluation is recommended.

Blood pressure measurement methods require special considerations in the elderly. The indirect measurement of blood pressure (using a blood pressure cuff and the Korotkoff sounds), when compared with the direct intraarterial method, has been reported to give falsely elevated readings, especially of diastolic pressure, by as high as 15 to 30 mmHg.[37] This is because excessive cuff pressure is needed to compress the sclerotic arteries of some older people. A simple procedure called *Osler's maneuver* has been reported to differentiate people with true hypertension from those whose blood pressure is spuriously elevated because of excessive sclerosis of the large arteries.[38] This procedure involves inflating the blood pressure cuff above systolic pressure and carefully palpating the radial or brachial artery. Whenever either of these arteries remains clearly palpable (despite being pulseless), the person is said to be Osler-positive; when the artery is collapsed and not palpable, the person is said to be Osler-negative. On the other hand, in elderly people with hypertension, a silent interval—called the auscultatory gap—may occur between the end of the first and beginning of the third phases of the Korotkoff sounds, providing the potential for underestimating the systolic pressure, sometimes by as high as 50 mmHg.[39] Because the gap occurs only with auscultation, it is recommended that a preliminary determination of systolic blood pressure be made by palpation and the cuff be inflated above this value for auscultatory measurement of blood pressure. It is also recommended that the cuff be deflated slowly to avoid missing the first Korotkoff sounds.

There is often a transient fall in blood pressure during the first 2 to 3 minutes of standing, after which reflex-mediated increases in heart rate and total peripheral resistance (vascular constriction) usually return blood pressure to normal values. Because these reflexes are often less responsive in the elderly and may be impaired by hypertensive medications, it has been recommended that blood pressure be recorded 2 to 5 minutes after assumption of the standing position, as well as in the seated position.[2] This should be done not only during pretreatment examinations but during follow-up examinations once treatment has been instituted. This is done to detect the complication of postural hypotension, which can occur with some medications.

SECONDARY HYPERTENSION

Only 5% to 10% of hypertensive cases are classified as secondary hypertension (*i.e.*, hypertension due to another disease condition). In secondary hypertension, as with other alterations in physiologic function, the presence of an elevation in blood pressure may be a homeostatic response that is recruited in an effort to maintain body function at least partially. Or the elevated pressure may be due to an actual alteration in body structures that most frequently give rise to secondary hypertension: (1) renal disease, (2) vascular disorders, (3) alterations in endocrine function and hormone levels, and (4) acute brain lesions. To avoid duplication in descriptions, the mechanisms associated with elevations of blood pressure in these disorders are discussed briefly, and a more detailed discussion of specific disease disorders is reserved for other sections of this book.

KIDNEY DISEASE

With the dominant role that the kidney assumes in blood pressure regulation, it is not surprising that the largest single cause of secondary hypertension is renal disease. By controlling salt and water levels, the kidney is probably involved in virtually all types of hypertension. In renal disease, salt and water retention undoubtedly play a major role in elevated blood pressure. Also implicated in the development of renal hypertension is an imbalance between the vasoconstrictor and vasodepressor substances produced by the kidney.

Renovascular hypertension is a common cause of secondary hypertension; its prevalence has been estimated as 1% to 6% of all hypertensives.[40] This condition involves renal artery stenosis due to fibrous, fibromuscular, or atherosclerotic disease. In contrast to atherosclerosis, which most commonly occurs in older people, fibrous or fibromuscular renal artery disease is more common in women and tends to occur in younger age groups (30 and 40 year olds).

Diagnosis of renovascular disease often involves the use of angiographic studies. Angioplasty repair has been shown to be an effective long-term treatment for the disorder. Medical treatment includes the use of angiotensin-converting enzyme (ACE) inhibitors.

VASCULAR DISORDERS

Arteriosclerosis. As mentioned earlier in this chapter, hypertension predisposes to vascular disorders, and vascular pathology tends to produce or perpetuate hypertension. The effects of arteriosclerosis on blood pressure are generally interpreted as changes in total peripheral resistance. In arteriosclerosis of the aorta and large arteries, the rigid vessel walls resist the runoff of blood ejected from the heart during systole, so the blood pressure rises and remains elevated during diastole. When renal blood vessels are affected, additional renal mechanisms contribute to the blood pressure elevation. The exaggerated vascular changes seen in malignant hypertension are discussed later in this chapter.

Coarctation of the Aorta. An unusual form of hypertension occurs in coarctation of the aorta (adult form) in which there is a narrowing of that vessel as it exits from the heart, most commonly beyond the subclavian arteries (see Chapter 23). In the infantile form, the narrowing occurs proximal to the ductus arteriosus, in which case heart failure and other problems are present. As a result, many affected babies die within their first year of life. In the adult form of coarctation, there is often an increase in cardiac output that results from renal compensatory mechanisms. The ejection of a large stroke volume into a narrowed aorta with limited ability to accept the runoff results in an increase in systolic blood pressure and blood flow to the upper part of the body. Blood pressure in the lower extremities may be normal, although it is frequently low. For this reason, blood pressures in the legs may be assessed as a screening method for this disorder. The pulse pressure in the legs is almost always narrowed, and the femoral pulses are weak. Because the aortic capacity is diminished, there is usually a marked increase in pressure (measured in the arms) during exercise when both stroke volume and heart rate are exaggerated.

ALTERATIONS IN ENDOCRINE FUNCTION

Secondary hypertension due to endocrine disorders is rare; when it does occur, it is usually of adrenal origin and involves either the adrenal medullary or cortical tissue.

Pheochromocytoma. A *pheochromocytoma* is a tumor of chromaffin tissue usually found in the adrenal medulla; but it may also arise in other sites where there is chromaffin tissue, such as the sympathetic ganglia.[41] Like adrenal medullary cells, the tumor cells of a pheochromocytoma produce and secrete the catecholamines epinephrine and norepinephrine. Thus, the hypertension results from the massive release of these catecholamines. Often their release is paroxysmal rather than continuous, causing periodic episodes of hypertension, tachycardia, sweating, anxiety, and other signs of excessive sympathetic activity. Several tests are available to differentiate this type of hypertension from other types. The most commonly used diagnostic measure is the determination of urinary catecholamines and their metabolites, including vanillylmandelic acid (VMA).

Elevated Levels of Adrenocorticosteroid Hormones. Increased levels of *adrenocorticosteroid hormones* can also give rise to hypertension. Both primary hyperaldosteronism (excess production of aldosterone by the adrenal cortex) and excess levels of glucocorticoids (Cushing's disease or syndrome) tend to raise the blood pressure (see Chapter 45). These hormones facilitate salt and water retention by the kidney; the hypertension that accompanies excessive levels of either hormone is probably related to this factor. It has been observed that in primary hyperaldosteronism a salt-restricted diet often brings the blood pressure down. Because aldosterone acts on the distal renal tubule to promote sodium exchange for the potassium lost in the urine, people with hyperaldosteronism usually have decreased potassium levels. The drug spironolactone is an aldosterone antagonist and is therefore used in the medical management of patients with an excess of this hormone. The drug increases sodium excretion and potassium retention.

BRAIN LESIONS

The hypertension associated with brain lesions is usually of short duration and should be considered a protective homeostatic mechanism. It is mentioned here because it tells a lot about intracranial pressure and cerebral blood flow. The brain and other cerebral structures are located within the rigid confines of the skull with no room for expansion, and any increase in intracranial pressure tends to compress the blood vessels that supply the brain. Because adequate blood flow is essential to life, it is not surprising that brain lesions that increase intracranial pressure and impede cerebral blood flow trigger a vasoconstrictor response (Cushing's phenomenon) designed to elevate blood pressure as a way to restore blood flow to the brain. This flow is reestablished when the arterial pressure increases to a level higher than the increase in the intracranial pressure that caused the compression of the vessels. Should the intracranial pressure rise to the point that the blood supply to the vasomotor center becomes inadequate, vasoconstrictor tone is lost, and the blood pressure begins to fall.

MALIGNANT HYPERTENSION

A small number of people with secondary hypertension develop an accelerated and potentially fatal form of the disease—malignant hypertension. This is usually a disease of younger people, particularly young African-American men, women with toxemia of pregnancy, and people with renal and collagen diseases.

Malignant hypertension is characterized by marked elevations in blood pressure with diastolic values above 120 mmHg, renal disorders, vascular changes, and retinopathy. There may be intense arterial spasm of the cerebral arteries with hypertensive encephalopathy. Cerebral vasoconstriction is probably an exaggerated homeostatic response designed to protect the brain from excesses of blood pressure and flow. The regulatory mechanisms are often insufficient to protect the capillaries, and cerebral edema frequently develops. As it advances, papilledema (swelling of the optic nerve at its point of entrance into the eye) ensues, giving evidence of the effects of pressure on the optic nerve and retinal vessels. There may be headache, restlessness, confusion, stupor, motor and sensory deficits, and visual disturbances. In severe cases, convulsions and coma follow.

Prolonged and severe exposure to exaggerated levels of blood pressure in malignant hypertension injures the walls of the arterioles, and intravascular coagulation and fragmentation of red blood cells may occur. The renal blood vessels are particularly vulnerable to hypertensive damage. In fact, renal damage due to vascular changes is probably the most important prognostic determinant in malignant hypertension. Elevated levels of blood urea nitrogen and serum creatinine, metabolic acidosis, hypocalcemia, and proteinuria provide evidence of renal impairment.

The complications associated with a hypertensive crisis demand immediate and rigorous medical treatment. With proper therapy, the death rate from this cause can be markedly reduced, as can further episodes. Two drugs to treat hypertensive emergencies are mentioned here, although others also may be required to bring the blood pressure down to a safe level. These two drugs—diazoxide, which causes arteriolar dilatation, and sodium nitroprusside, a vasodilator that also affects the venous system—are administered intravenously.

TREATMENT OF HYPERTENSION

The main objective for treatment of essential hypertension is to achieve and maintain arterial blood pressure below 140/90 mmHg, with the goal of preventing morbidity and mortality. For persons with secondary hypertension, efforts are made to correct or control the disease condition that is causing the hypertension. Antihypertensive medications and other measures supplement the treatment for the underlying disease. The JNC V report on Detection, Evaluation, and Treatment of High Blood Pressure has developed a treatment algorithm for hypertension that includes both lifestyle modification and, when necessary, the use of pharmacologic agents to achieve and maintain systolic pressure below 140 mmHg and diastolic pressure below 90 mmHg (Fig. 21-6).[2]

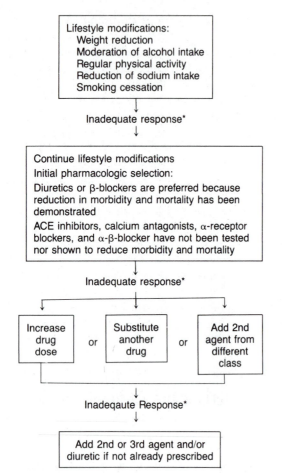

FIG. 21-6. Treatment algorithm. *Asterisk* indicates that response means the patient achieved goal blood pressure or is making considerable progress toward this goal. ACE, angiotensin-converting enzyme. (National Heart, Lung, and Blood Institute. [1993]. *The fifth report of the National Committee on Detection, Evaluation, and Treatment of High Blood Pressure.* [p. 16]. Bethesda, MD: NIH Publication No. 93-1088)

LIFESTYLE MODIFICATION

Lifestyle modification, previously referred to as non-pharmacologic therapy, includes weight reduction, reduction of sodium intake, regular physical activity, modification of alcohol intake, and smoking cessation. Other lifestyle modification strategies, such as increased intake of potassium, calcium, and magnesium or the use of relaxation and biofeedback, were not included in the JNC V report because of a lack of convincing data to justify recommendation.[2] In persons with stage 1 hypertension, an attempt to control blood pressure with weight loss and other lifestyle modifications should be tried for at least 3 to 6 months before initiating pharmacologic treatment.

Recognizing obesity as a major risk factor in essential hypertension, the committee recommended that all obese hypertensive adults be encouraged to participate in weight reduction programs with the goal of achieving a body weight within 15% of their desirable weight.

A high-salt diet may play a critical role in maintaining blood pressure elevation, and it may limit the effectiveness of some antihypertensive drugs. It was recommended that people with hypertension limit their salt intake to 70 to 100 mEq per day (*i.e.*, 1.5 to 2.5 g sodium or 4 to 6 g of salt). Because many prepared foods are high in sodium, merely refraining from use of the salt shaker is usually not sufficient. Instead, it was recommended that people consult package labels for the sodium content of canned foods, frozen foods, soft drinks, and other foods and beverages to reduce sodium intake adequately. Studies have suggested that in addition to excess salt intake, a reduction in potassium intake may contribute to elevated blood pressure levels. Therefore, an increased potassium intake is recommended for people with normal renal function. Although inadequate intake of calcium and magnesium has been reported to influence blood pressure, there is insufficient evidence in terms of the benefits and risks associated with increased intake of these two cations to suggest their supplementation.

A sedentary lifestyle has been cited as a risk factor in cardiovascular disease. Accordingly, a regular program of physical exercise (walking, biking, swimming) is protective, especially for those at increased risk for cardiovascular disease because of hypertension. Exercise may have further indirect benefits, such as weight loss or motivation for changing other risk factors. People with hypertension should be evaluated before beginning an exercise program of appropriate types of exercise. Weight lifting and other forms of isometric exercise can raise blood pressure acutely and should be done with caution.

Because of alcohol's association with high blood pressure, the JNC recommended restriction of alcohol consumption to no more than 1 oz per day (equal to 2 oz of 100-proof whiskey, approximately 8 oz of wine, or 24 oz of beer). Significant hypertension may develop during withdrawal from heavy alcohol consumption, but the pressor effects of alcohol withdrawal usually subside within a few days after alcohol consumption is reduced.

Although nicotine has not been associated with long-term elevations in blood pressure as in essential hypertension, it has been shown to increase the risk of heart disease. The fact that both smoking and hypertension are major cardiovascular risk factors should be reason enough to encourage the hypertensive smoker to quit. In addition, studies have also reported an interaction between smoking and the antihypertensive drug propranolol, in which smokers required larger doses of the drug to achieve similar reductions in blood pressure as compared to non-smokers.

There is conflicting evidence as to the direct effects of dietary fats on blood pressure. As with smoking, however, the interactive effects of saturated fats and high blood pressure as cardiovascular risk factors would seem to warrant dietary modification to reduce the intake of foods high in cholesterol and saturated fats.

Although biofeedback and relaxation methods have shown benefits for selective groups of people with hypertension, these methods have not been subjected to rigorous clinical investigation. Therefore, they may be suggested as adjunctive therapy rather than the sole treatment for hypertension.

PHARMACOLOGIC TREATMENT

The decision to initiate pharmacologic treatment is based on the severity of the hypertension, the presence of target-organ disease, and the existence of other conditions and risk factors. Drug selection is based on the stage of hypertension. Among the drugs used in the treatment of hypertension are diuretics, adrenergic inhibitors, vasodilators, angiotensin-converting enzyme inhibitors, and calcium-channel blocking drugs.

Diuretics, such as the thiazides, loop-diuretics, and the aldosterone antagonist (potassium-sparing) diuretics, produce a reduction in vascular volume and subsequent decrease in cardiac output and peripheral vascular resistance (see Chapter 31).

The *adrenergic inhibitors* exert their effects at various levels of the sympathetic nervous system. Some of the main actions of the β-adrenergic blockers are on β receptors in the heart and on renin release by the kidneys. The centrally acting inhibitors block sympathetic outflow from the CNS. Peripherally acting inhibitors depress the function of postganglionic neurons. α_1-Adrenergic blockers reduce the effect of the sympathetic nervous system on the vascular smooth muscle tone of the blood vessels that regulate the total peripheral vascular resistance. Inhibition of sympathetic activity often affects functions other than those related to blood pressure. The two divisions of the ANS have opposing and antagonistic actions. When the sympathetic nervous system is inhibited, the restraining effects on the parasympathetic nervous system are removed and manifestations of enhanced parasympathetic function such as increased gastrointestinal motility may occur. Accordingly, many of the side effects of adrenergic-inhibiting drugs are related to the altered autonomic responses—either decreased sympathetic function or increased parasympathetic function—they induce.

Vasodilator drugs promote a decrease in total peripheral vascular resistance by directly producing relaxation of vascular smooth muscle, particularly of the arterioles. These drugs often produce initial stimulation of the sympathetic nervous system and tachycardia and salt and water retention as a result of the decreased filling of the vascular compartment.

The *angiotensin-converting enzyme (ACE) inhibitors* act by decreasing angiotensin II levels and reducing its effect on vasoconstriction, aldosterone levels, intrarenal blood flow, and the glomerular filtration rate.

The *calcium-channel blockers* inhibit the movement of calcium into cardiac and vascular smooth muscle. Each of the different agents in this group acts in a slightly different way. They probably reduce blood pressure by several mechanisms, including a reduction of smooth muscle tone in the venous and arterial systems. Some calcium blockers have a direct myocardial effect that reduces the cardiac output through a decrease in cardiac contractility and a fall in heart rate. Other drugs influence venous tone and reduce the cardiac output through a decrease in venous return. Still others influence arterial vascular smooth muscle by either inhibiting calcium transport across the cell membrane channels or inhibiting the vascular response to norepinephrine or angiotensin.

The pharmacologic treatment of stage 1 and 2 hypertension is usually initiated when blood pressure remains elevated after a 3- to 6-month period of vigorous encouragement of lifestyle modification. Drug therapy is usually initiated using a single drug, usually a diuretic or β-blocker. The alternative drugs—calcium antagonists, angiotensin-converting enzyme inhibitors, α_1-receptor blockers and α-β-blockers—are considered to be equally effective and may be used. If the response to the initial drug is not adequate after 1 to 3 months, one of three approaches is used: (1) the dose can be increased if the initial dose was below the maximum recommended, (2) an agent from another class can be added, or (3) the initial drug can be discontinued and another drug substituted. Combining antihypertensive drugs with different modes of action will often allow smaller doses of drugs to be used to achieve blood pressure control, thereby minimizing the possibility of dose-dependent side effects from any one drug. With stage 3 and 4 hypertension, it is often necessary to add a second or third drug after a short interval if the treatment goal is not achieved.

Factors considered when hypertensive drugs are prescribed are the person's (1) lifestyle (people with a busy schedule may have problems with medications that must be taken three times a day), (2) demographics (some drugs are more effective in elderly or African-American people), (3) motivation for adhering to the drug regimen (some drugs can produce undesirable and even life-threatening consequences if discontinued abruptly), (4) other disease conditions and therapies, and (5) potential for side effects (*e.g.*, some drugs may impair sexual functioning or mental acuity; others have not been proved safe for women of childbearing age). The reader is referred to a pharmacology text for additional information on the side effects of the different antihypertensive drugs.

Another factor to be considered is the cost of the drug in relation to financial resources. There is a wide variation in the price of the different antihypertensive medications that should be considered when medications are prescribed. This is particularly important for low-income people with moderate to severe hypertension, because keeping costs at an affordable level may be the key to compliance. Studies by a nationwide Gallup survey revealed that 25% of people reported that paying for medication to treat their high blood pressure is "very much" or "somewhat" of a problem.[42]

For people with mild hypertension who have satisfactorily controlled their blood pressure through treatment for at least 1 year, reduction of medication using a reverse stepwise approach may be used, particularly if there has been successful adherence to nonpharmacologic methods of treatment.

In summary, hypertension is probably one of the most common cardiovascular disorders. It may occur as a primary disorder (essential hypertension) or as a symptom of some other disease (secondary hypertension). Hypertension can affect people of all age groups including children, pregnant women, and elderly people. The incidence of hypertension increases with age, is seen more frequently among African-Americans, and is linked to a family history of high blood pressure, obesity, and increased salt intake. Uncontrolled hypertension increases the risk of heart disease, renal complications, retinopathy, and stroke. Because hypertension occurs as a silent disorder, screening programs provide an effective means of early detection. The importance of screening lies in the fact that hypertension can usually be controlled and its complications can be prevented or minimized with appropriate treatment measures.

■ ORTHOSTATIC HYPOTENSION

After the assumption of the upright posture from the supine position, approximately 500 to 700 mL of blood are momentarily shifted to the lower part of the body, with an accompanying fall in central blood volume and arterial pressure.[43] Normally, this fall in blood pressure is transient, lasting through several cardiac cycles. This is because the baroreceptors located in the thorax and carotid sinus area sense the fall in blood pressure and initiate reflex constriction of the veins and arterioles as well as an increase in heart rate, which brings blood pressure back to normal. Within a few minutes of standing, blood levels of

ADH and sympathetic neuromediators increase as a secondary means of ensuring maintenance of normal blood pressure in the standing position. Muscle movement in the lower extremities also aids venous return to the heart by pumping blood out of the legs.

In people with healthy blood vessels and normal autonomic function, cerebral blood flow is usually not reduced in the upright position unless arterial pressure falls below 70 mmHg. The strategic location of the arterial baroreceptors between the heart and brain is designed to ensure that the arterial pressure is maintained within a range sufficient to prevent a reduction in cerebral blood flow.

Orthostatic or postural hypotension is an abnormal drop in blood pressure on assumption of the standing position. In the absence of normal circulatory reflexes or blood volume, blood pools in the lower part of the body when the standing position is assumed, cardiac output falls, and blood flow to the brain is inadequate. Dizziness, syncope (fainting), or both may occur. Although there is no firm agreement on the definition of orthostatic hypotension, many authorities use a drop in systolic of 20 mmHg or more or a drop in diastolic blood pressure of 10 mmHg or more as being diagnostic of the condition.[44] Some authorities regard the presence of orthostatic symptoms (*e.g.*, dizziness and syncope) as being more relevant than the numerical fall in blood pressure.[44] Kochar has developed a functional classification of orthostatic hypotension that uses both the drop in blood pressure and orthostatic symptoms (Chart 21-1).[45]

CAUSES

Orthostatic hypotension can present as an acute or chronic condition. The most common cause of acute orthostatic hypotension is a reduction in circulating

---

CHART 21-1: FUNCTIONAL CLASSIFICATION OF ORTHOSTATIC HYPOTENSION

Class 1   Asymptomatic postural hypotension (fall in either systolic or diastolic BP ≥ 20 mmHg)

Class 2   Lightheadedness (dizziness, giddiness) associated with postural hypotension but no history of syncope

Class 3   History of syncope (fainting) accompanied with postural hypotension

Class 4   Incapacitated because of severe dizziness or frequent syncope due to documented postural hypotension

(Kochar, M. S. [1990]. Orthostatic hypotension. In J. J. Smith [Ed.]. *Circulatory response to the upright posture* [p. 171]. Boca Raton, FL: CRC Press)

blood volume as a result of fluid depletion or blood loss. Chronic orthostatic hypotension is associated with medication use (antihypertensive or psychotropic drugs), aging, disorders of the ANS, and bedrest.

Fluid Deficit. Orthostatic hypotension is often an early sign of fluid deficit. When blood volume is decreased, the vascular compartment is only partially filled; although cardiac output may be adequate when a person is in the recumbent position, it often decreases to the point of causing weakness and fainting when the person assumes the standing position. Common causes of orthostatic hypotension related to hypovolemia are (1) excessive use of diuretics, (2) excessive diaphoresis, (3) loss of gastrointestinal fluids through vomiting and diarrhea, and (4) loss of fluid volume associated with prolonged bedrest.

Medication. Antihypertensive drugs and psychotropic drugs are the most common cause of chronic orthostatic hypotension. Table 21-4 lists some drugs that have the potential for causing orthostatic hypotension. In most cases, the orthostatic hypotension is well tolerated. If postural hypotension is of class 2 or more, it is recommended that the dosage of the drug be reduced or a different drug be used.[45]

Aging. Weakness and dizziness on standing are common complaints of elderly people. It has been estimated that 20% of medical outpatients over age 65 and 30% of those over age 75 experience orthostatic hypotension.[46, 47] Hypertension, which is more common among the elderly, predisposes to orthostatic hypotension. Because cerebral blood flow is primarily dependent on systolic pressure, patients with impaired cerebral circulation may experience symptoms of weakness, ataxia, dizziness, and syncope when their arterial pressure falls even slightly. This may happen in older people who are immobilized for brief periods of time or whose blood volume is decreased owing to inadequate fluid intake or overzealous use of diuretics.

Postprandial blood pressure falls in both fit and

TABLE 21-4. DRUGS KNOWN TO CAUSE ORTHOSTATIC HYPOTENSION*

DRUG GROUPS	SPECIFIC DRUGS	MECHANISM OF ACTION
Antihypertensive drugs	Pentolinium (Ansolysen) Trimetaphan (Arfonad)	Blocks transmission of sympathetic impulses at the autonomic ganglia
	Guanethidine (Ismelin)	Blocks sympathetic impulses at the post-ganglionic sites
	Methyldopa (Aldomet) Clonidin (Catapres)	Decreases sympathetic outflow from the central nervous system
	Hydralazine (Apresoline) Prazosin (Minipres) Minoxidil (Loniten)	Direct vasodilator action
Antiparkinsonian drugs	Levodopa preparation Amantadine (Symmetrel)	Vasodilatation due to β-adrenergic stimulation or α blockade of the peripheral vascular system
Antipsychotic drugs	Chlorpromazine (Thorazine) Thiethylperazine (Torecan) Thioridazine (Mellaril)	Loss of reflex vasoconstriction due to blocking of α-receptors; these drugs also impair sympathetic outflow from the brain
Calcium-channel blockers	Diltiazem (Cardizem) Nifedipine (Procardia) Verapamil (Calan, Isoptin)	Direct vasodilator action
Tricyclic and related antidepressant drugs	Amitriptyline (Elavil, Endep, Amitid, Amtril, others) Amoxapine (Asendin) Desipramine (Norepramine, Pertofrane) Doxepin (Adapin, Sinequan) Imipramine (Tofranil, Imavate, others) Nortriptyline (Aventyl, Pamelor) Maprotiline (Ludiomil) Traxodone (Desyrel)	Blocks norepinephrine uptake in central adrenergic neurons, with a resultant increase in stimulation of central α-adrenergic receptors, causing a decrease in peripheral sympathetic nervous system activity
Vasodilator drugs	Nitrates (nitroglycerin and long-acting nitrates)	Direct vasodilator action

* This list is not intended to be inclusive; it encompasses some of the widely prescribed drugs.

frail elderly people.[48, 49] The greatest postprandial changes occur after a high carbohydrate meal.[50] Although the mechanism responsible for these changes is not fully understood, it is thought to result from glucose-mediated impairment of baroreflex sensitivity and increased splanchnic blood flow mediated by insulin and vasoactive gastrointestinal hormones.

Disorders of Autonomic Nervous System Function. The sympathetic nervous system plays an essential role in adjustment to the upright position. Sympathetic stimulation increases heart rate and cardiac contractility and causes constriction of peripheral veins and arterioles. Orthostatic hypotension caused by altered autonomic function is common in peripheral neuropathies associated with diabetes mellitus, after injury or disease of the spinal cord, or as the result of a cerebral vascular accident in which sympathetic outflow from the brain stem is disrupted.

Bedrest. With prolonged bedrest there is a reduction in plasma volume, a decrease in venous tone, failure of peripheral vasoconstriction, and weakness of the skeletal muscles that support the veins and assist in returning blood to the heart (see Chapter 9). Physical deconditioning follows even short periods of bedrest. After 3 to 4 days, the blood volume is decreased. Loss of vascular and skeletal muscle tone is less predictable but probably becomes maximal after about 2 weeks of bedrest. Orthostatic intolerance is a recognized problem of space flight—a potential risk after reentry into the earth's gravitational field.

IDIOPATHIC ORTHOSTATIC HYPOTENSION

Idiopathic orthostatic hypotension is unrelated to drug therapy or pathologic conditions. It may be of two types: (1) idiopathic orthostatic hypotension not accompanied by other signs of neurologic deficits and (2) idiopathic hypotension accompanied by multiple neurologic deficits (Shy-Drager syndrome). The Shy-Drager syndrome is characterized by upper motor neuron damage with uncoordinated movements, urinary incontinence, constipation, and other signs of neurologic pathology. Disorders of ANS function are discussed further in Chapter 48.

DIAGNOSIS AND TREATMENT

Orthostatic hypotension can be assessed with the blood pressure cuff. A reading should be made when the patient is supine, immediately after assumption of the seated or upright position, and at 2- to 3-min-ute intervals for a period of 10 to 15 minutes. It takes about 10 minutes for the blood pressure to stabilize after lying down; therefore, it is recommended that people be supine for this period of time before standing. It is strongly recommended that a second person be available when blood pressure is measured in the standing position to prevent injury should the patient become faint. A tilt table can also be used for this purpose. With a tilt table, the recumbent patient can be moved to a head-up position without voluntary movement when the table is tilted.

People with a drop in blood pressure to orthostatic levels should be evaluated to determine the cause and seriousness of the condition. A history should be done to elicit information about symptoms, particularly dizziness and history of syncope and falls; medical conditions, particularly those such as diabetes mellitus that predispose to orthostatic hypotension; use of both prescription and over-the-counter drugs; and symptoms of ANS dysfunction such as impotence or bladder dysfunction. A physical examination should document blood pressure and heart rate in the supine, sitting, and standing positions in both arms and should note the occurrence of symptoms.

Treatment of orthostatic hypotension is usually directed toward alleviating the cause or, if this is not possible, toward helping the person learn ways to cope with the disorder and prevent falls and injuries. Correcting the fluid deficit and trying a different antihypertensive medication are examples of measures designed to correct the cause. Measures designed to help people prevent symptomatic orthostatic drops in blood pressure include: (1) gradual ambulation (i.e., sitting on the edge of the bed for several minutes and moving the legs to initiate skeletal muscle pump function before standing) to allow the circulatory system to adjust, (2) avoidance of situations that encourage excessive vasodilatation (such as drinking alcohol or exercising vigorously in a warm environment), and (3) avoidance of excess diuresis (use of diuretics), diaphoresis, or loss of body fluids. Tight-fitting elastic support hose or an abdominal support garment may help prevent pooling of blood in the lower extremities and abdomen.

In summary, orthostatic hypotension refers to an abnormal fall in both systolic and diastolic blood pressures that occurs on assumption of the upright position. An important consideration in orthostatic hypotension is the occurrence of dizziness and syncope. Among the factors that contribute to its occurrence are (1) decreased fluid volume, (2) medications, (3) aging, (4) defective function of the ANS, and (5) the effects of immobility. Diagnosis of orthostatic hypotension includes blood pressure measurement in both the supine and upright positions, a history of symptomatology, medication use, and disease conditions that contribute to a postural drop in blood pressure. Treatment includes correcting the reversible causes and assisting the person to compensate for the disorder and prevent falls and injuries.

■ REFERENCES

1. Robinson, S.C., & Brucer, M. (1939). Range of normal blood pressure: A statistical study of 11,383 people. *Archives of Internal Medicine, 64*(3):409.
2. The Fifth Report of the Joint National Committee on Detection, Evaluation, and Treatment of High Blood Pressure. NIH Publication No. 93–1088, January 1993.
3. Guyton, A. (1986). *Textbook of medical physiology* (7th ed., pp. 251, 257, 259). Philadelphia: W.B. Saunders.
4. Hall, J.H., Mizette, L., & Woods, L.L. (1986). The renin–angiotensin system and long-term regulation of arterial hypertension. *Journal of Hypertension, 4,* 387.
5. Weinberger, M.H. (1987). Angiotensin-converting enzyme inhibitors. *Medical Clinics of North America, 71*(5), 979.
6. Cowley, A.W., & Liard, J.F. (1988). Vasopressin and arterial pressure regulation. *Hypertension, 11*(Suppl I), 15.
7. Stamler, J., Stamler, R., Riedinger, W.F., et al. (1976). Hypertension screening in 1 million Americans. *Journal of the American Medical Association, 235*(21), 2299.
8. US Department of Health and Human Services. (1986). Blood pressure levels in people 18–74 years of age in 1976–80, and trends in blood pressure from 1960–80 in the United States. *Vital Health Statistics, 11*(234), 6–7.
9. Saunders, E. (1987). Hypertension in blacks. *Medical Clinics of North America, 71*(5), 1013.
10. Saunders, E. (1985). Special techniques in management of blacks. In W.D. Hall, E. Saunders, & N.B. Shulman (Eds.). *Hypertension in blacks, pathophysiology and treatment.* Chicago: Year Book Medical.
11. Saunders, E. (1986). Stepped care and profiled care in the treatment of hypertension: Considerations for black Americans. *American Journal of Medicine, 81*(Suppl 6C), 39.
12. Oliver, W.J., Cohen, E.L., & Neel, J.V. (1975). Blood pressure, sodium intake, and sodium related hormones in the Yanomamo Indians, a "no-salt" culture. *Circulation, 52*(1):146.
13. Laragh, J.H., & Pecker, M.S. (1983). Dietary sodium and essential hypertension: Some myths, hopes, and truths. *Annals of Internal Medicine, 98*(part 2), 735.
14. Stamler, R., Stamler, J., & Riedlinger, W.R. (1978). Weight and blood pressure. *Journal of the American Medical Association, 240,* 1607.
15. Lapidus, L., Bengstsson, C., Larsson, B., et al. (1984). Distribution of adipose tissue and risk of cardiovascular disease and death: A 12 year follow-up study in the population of Gothenburg, Sweden. *British Medical Journal, 289,* 1257.
16. Larrson, B., Svardsudd, K., Welin, L., et al. (1984). Abdominal adipose tissue distribution, obesity, and risk of cardiovascular disease: 13-year follow-up of participants in the study of men born in 1913. *British Medical Journal, 288,* 1401.
17. Dustan, H.P. (1983). Mechanisms of hypertension associated with obesity. *Annals of Internal Medicine, 98*(Part 2), 860.
18. Langford, H.G., Blaufox, D., Oberman, A., et al. (1985). Dietary therapy slows the return of hypertension after stopping prolonged medication. *Journal of the American Medical Association, 253*(5), 657.
19. Gruchow, H.W., Sobocinski, K.A., & Barboriak, J.J. (1985). Alcohol, nutrient intake, and hypertension in US adults. *Journal of the American Medical Association, 253*(11), 1567.
20. Kaplan, N.M. (1986). *Clinical hypertension* (4th ed., pp. 112, 113, 156, 294). Baltimore: Williams & Wilkins.
21. Klatsky, A.L., Freidman, G.D., & Siegelaub, A.B. (1977). Alcohol consumption and blood pressure. *New England Journal of Medicine, 296*(21), 1194.
22. Fregly, M.J. (1983). Estimates of sodium and potassium intake. *Annals of Internal Medicine, 98*(Part 2), 792.
23. Lanford, G.H. (1983). Dietary potassium and hypertension: Epidemiologic data. *Annals of Internal Medicine, 98*(Part 2), 770.
24. McCarron, D.A. (1983). Calcium and magnesium in human hypertension. *Annals of Internal Medicine, 98*(Part 2), 800.
25. Kaplan, N.M., & Meese, R.S. (1986). The calcium deficiency hypothesis of hypertension: A critique. *Annals of Internal Medicine, 105,* 947.
26. Iseri, L.T., & French, J.H. (1984). Magnesium: Nature's physiologic calcium blocker. *American Heart Journal, 108*(1), 188.
27. Bevan, A.T., Hanour, A.J., & Stott, F.H. (1969). Direct arterial pressure recording in unrestricted man. *Clinical Science and Molecular Medicine, 36,* 329.
28. Pickering, T., Harshfield, G.A., Kleinert, H.D., et al. (1982). Blood pressure during normal daily activities, sleep, and exercise. *Journal of the American Medical Association, 247*(7), 992.
29. Woods, J.W. (1988). Oral contraceptives and hypertension. *Hypertension, 11*(Suppl II), II1.
30. National High Blood Pressure Education Program Working Group Report on High Blood Pressure in Pregnancy. (1990). *American Journal of Obstetrics and Gynecology, 63* (5, Part I), 1689–1712.
31. Lindheimer, M.D., & Katz, A.I. (1985). Hypertension in pregnancy. *New England Journal of Medicine, 313*(11), 675.
32. National Heart, Lung and Blood Institute. (1987). Report of the Second Task Force on Blood Pressure Control in Children. *Pediatrics, 79*(1), 1.
33. Emerau, J.P., DeCamps, A., Manciet, A., et al. (1988). Hypertension in the elderly. *American Journal of Medicine, 84*(Suppl 1B), 92.
34. Working Group on Hypertension in the Elderly. (1986). Statement on hypertension in the elderly. *Journal of the American Medical Association, 256*(1), 70.
35. Kannel, W.B., Dawber, T.R., & McGee, D.L. (1980). Perspectives in systolic hypertension: The Framingham Study. *Circulation, 61,* 1179.
36. Shellke, R.B., Ostfeld, A.M., Klawans, H., et al. (1974). Hypertension and risk of stroke in an elderly population. *Stroke, 5,* 71.
37. Spence, J.D., Sibbald, W.J., & Cape, R.D. (1978). Pseudohypertension in the elderly. *Clinical Science and Molecular Medicine, 55,* 399s.
38. Messerli, F.H., Ventura, H.O., & Amodeo, C. (1985). Osler's maneuver and pseudohypertension. *New England Journal of Medicine, 312*(24), 1548.
39. Niarchos, A.P., & Laragh, J.H. (1980). Hypertension in the elderly: Diagnosis and treatment. *Modern Concepts in Cardiovascular Disease, 69,* 49.
40. Re, R.N. (1987). The renin–angiotensin system. *Medical Clinics of North America, 71*(5), 880.
41. Bravo, E.L., & Gifford, R.W. (1984). Pheochromocytoma:

Diagnosis, localization, and management. *New England Journal of Medicine, 311*(20), 1298.

42. Pauley, M.V., & Stason, W.B. (1986). Contemporary considerations in the treatment of hypertension. *American Journal of Medicine, 81*(Suppl 6C), 1.

43. Smith, J.J. & Porth, C.J.M. (1990). Age and the response to orthostatic stress. In J.J. Smith (Ed.). *Circulatory response to the upright posture* (pp. 121–138). Boca Raton, FL: CRC Press.

44. Lipsitz, L.A. (1989). Orthostatic hypotension in the elderly. *New England Journal of Medicine, 321*, 952–957.

45. Kochar, M.S. (1990). Orthostatic hypotension. In J.J. Smith (Ed.). *Circulatory response to the upright posture* (p. 170–179). Boca Raton, FL: CRC Press.

46. MacLennan, W.J., Hall, M.R., & Timothy, J.I. (1980). Postural hypotension in old age: Is it a disorder of the nervous system or blood vessels? *Age and Ageing, 12*, 25–32.

47. Caird, F.I., Andrews, G.R., & Kennedy, R.K. (1973). Effect of posture on blood pressure in the elderly. *British Heart Journal, 35*, 527–530.

48. Lipsitz, L.A., Lyquist, R.P., Wei, J.Y., et al. (1983). Postprandial reduction in blood pressure in the elderly. *New England Journal of Medicine, 309*, 81–86.

49. Westened, M., Lenders, J.W.M., & Thein, T.H. (1985). The course of blood pressure after a meal; A difference between young and elderly subjects. *Journal of Hypertension, 3*(Suppl 3), s417.

50. Potter, J.F., Heseltine, D., Matthews, J., et al. (1989). Effects of meal composition on the postprandial blood pressure, catecholamine and insulin changes in elderly subjects. *Clinical Science, 77*, 226.

▪ BIBLIOGRAPHY

Anastos, K., Charney, P., Charon, R. A., et al. (1991). Hypertension in women: What is really known. *Annals of Internal Medicine, 115*, 287–293.

Applegate, W.B. (1991). Systolic hypertension in older people. *Advances in Internal Medicine, 37*, 37–54.

Brunner, H.R. (1990). The renin–angiotensin system in hypertension: An update. *Hospital Practice, 25*(8A), 71–81.

Cunha, U.V. (1987). Management of orthostatic hypotension in the elderly. *Geriatrics, 42*(9), 61.

Cunningham, F.G., & Lindheimer, M.D. (1992). Hypertension in pregnancy. *New England Journal of Medicine, 326*, 92732.

Daniels, S.R. (1992). Primary hypertension in childhood and adolescence. *Pediatric Annals, 21*, 226–234.

Fletcher, A.E., & Bulpitt, C.J. (1992). How far should blood pressure be lowered? *New England Journal of Medicine, 326*, 251–253.

Francis, C.K. (1991). Hypertension, cardiac disease and compliance in minority patients. *American Journal of Medicine, 91*(Suppl A), IA-29S-36S.

Frohlich, E.D., Chobanian, A.V., Devereux, R.B., et al. (1992). The heart in hypertension. *New England Journal of Medicine, 327*, 998–1008.

Gistrap, L.C., & Gant, N.F. (1990). Pathophysiology of preeclampsia. *Seminars in Perinatology, 14*, 147–151.

Hoeldtke, R.D., & Carabello, B. (1987). Hemodynamic changes during food ingestion in a patient with postprandial hypotension. *Journal of the American Geriatric Society, 35*, 354.

Hollister, A.S. (1992). Orthostatic hypotension: Causes, evaluation, and management. *Western Journal of Medicine, 157*, 652–657.

Kaplan, N.M. (1992). Treatment of hypertensive emergencies and urgencies. *Heart Disease and Stroke, 1*, 373–378.

Laragh, J.H. (1992). The modern evaluation and treatment of hypertension: The causal role of the kidneys. *Journal of Urology, 147*, 1469–1477.

Lipsitz, L.A. (1989). Hypertension in the elderly. *Hospital Practice, 24*, 119–142.

Mann, S.J. (1992). Detection of renovascular hypertension—state of the art: 1992. *Annals of Internal Medicine, 117*, 845–853.

Memmer, M.K. (1988). Acute orthostatic hypotension. *Heart & Lung, 17*, 134.

Psaty, B.M., Furberg, C.D., Kuller, L.H., et al. (1992). Isolated systolic hypertension and subclinical cardiovascular disease in the elderly. *Journal of the American Medical Association, 268*, 1287–1291.

Rousseau, P.C. (1988). Postural hypotension in the elderly. *Hospital Practice, 23*(Oct 30), 74.

Schneider, R.E., & Messerli, F.H. (1987). Obesity hypertension. *Medical Clinics of North America, 71*, 991.

Shea, S., Misra, D., Ehrlich, M.H., et al. (1992). Predisposing factors for severe, uncontrolled hypertension in an inner-city minority population. *New England Journal of Medicine, 327*, 776–781.

Smith, J.J., & Porth, C.J.M. (1990). Age and the response to orthostatic stress. In J.J. Smith (Ed.). *Circulatory response to the upright posture* (pp. 121–138). Boca Raton, FL: CRC Press.

Walczak, M. (1991). Prevalence of orthostatic hypotension. *Journal of Gerontological Nursing, 17*(11), 26–29.

CHAPTER 22

CONTROL OF CARDIAC FUNCTION

■ OBJECTIVES

After you have studied this chapter, you should be able to meet the following objectives:

■ Describe how the ventricular wall thickness and the pressure generated by the right and left ventricles are related.

■ State the function of the pericardium.

■ Cite the function of the valvular structures of the heart.

■ State the function of the intercalated disks in cardiac muscle.

■ Trace an impulse that is generated in the sinoatrial node through the conduction system of the heart.

■ Relate systolic and diastolic changes in the left ventricular pressure and volume to changes in the electrocardiogram and phonocardiogram.

■ Define the terms *preload* and *afterload*.

■ Explain the effects that increased and decreased venous return to the heart have on cardiac output using Starling's law of the heart.

■ Describe the permeability of cells in the ventricular conduction system to sodium, potassium, and calcium ions during the five phases of an action potential.

■ Explain the importance of the plateau and length of the refractory period in cardiac muscle.

■ State the formula for calculating the cardiac output.

■ Define *cardiac reserve*.

■ Explain the function of the vessel endothelium in controlling blood vessel relaxation and contraction.

■ Cite the distribution of sympathetic and parasympathetic nervous system innervation and the effects on heart rate and cardiac contractility.

■ Describe the determinants of oxygen consumption by the myocardium.

The heart is a four-chambered muscular pump about the size of a man's fist that beats an average of 70 times a minute, 24 hours a day, 365 days a year for a lifetime. In 1 day, this pump moves more than 1800 gallons of blood throughout the body, and the work performed by the heart over a lifetime would lift 30 tons to a height of 30,000 ft. This chapter is divided into five parts: (1) the functional anatomy of the heart, (2) the cardiac conduction system and the electrical activity of the heart, (3) the cardiac cycle, (4) regulation of cardiac performance, and (5) the coronary circulation.

■ FUNCTIONAL ANATOMY OF THE HEART

The heart is located between the lungs in the mediastinal space of the intrathoracic cavity within a loose-fitting sac called the pericardium. It is suspended by the great vessels, with its broader side (base) facing upward and its tip (apex) pointing downward, forward, and to the left. The heart is positioned obliquely, so that the right side of the heart is almost fully in front of the left side of the heart with only a small portion of the lateral left ventricle on the frontal plane of the heart (Fig. 22-1). The impact of the heart's contraction is felt against the chest wall at a point between the fifth and sixth ribs, a little below the nipple and about 3 inches to the left of the midline. This is called the point of maximum impulse.

The heart is divided longitudinally into a right and a left pump, each composed of two muscular chambers: a thin-walled atrium, which serves as a reservoir for blood coming into the heart, and a thick-walled ventricle, which pumps blood out of the heart. The two halves of the heart are separated by the interatrial and interventricular septa.

The right side of the heart delivers blood to the lungs, where the blood is oxygenated and carbon dioxide is removed. Because of the proximity of the lungs to the heart and the low resistance to flow in the pulmonary circulation, the right side of the heart operates as a low-pressure pump (pulmonary artery pressure is about 22/8 mmHg).

In contrast to the right side of the heart, the left side of the heart must pump blood throughout the entire systemic circulation. Because of the distance the blood must travel and the resistance to blood flow, the left heart must operate as a high-pressure pump (systemic arterial blood pressure is about 120/70 mmHg). The increased thickness of the left ventricular wall results from the additional work this ventricle is required to perform.

Although the right and left sides of the heart function under different pressure requirements, both must pump the same amount of blood over a period of time. This concept has a particular meaning in relation to both right-sided and left-sided heart failure (see Chapter 24).

STRUCTURES OF THE HEART

The wall of the heart is composed of an outer epicardium, which lines the pericardial cavity; a fibrous skeleton; the myocardium or muscle layer; and the smooth endocardium, which lines the chambers of the heart.

PERICARDIUM

The pericardium forms a fibrous covering around the heart, holding it in a fixed position in the thorax. It provides both physical protection and a barrier to infection. The pericardium consists of a tough outer fibrous layer and an inner serous layer. The outer fibrous layer is attached to the great vessels that enter and leave the heart, the sternum, and the diaphragm. The fibrous pericardium is highly resistive to distention; it prevents acute dilatation of the heart chambers and exerts a restraining effect on the left ventricle. The inner serous layer consists of a visceral layer and a parietal layer. The visceral layer, also known as the epicardium, covers the entire heart and great vessels and then folds over to form the parietal layer that lines the fibrous pericardium (Fig. 22-2). Between the visceral and parietal layers is the pericardial cavity, a potential space that contains 30 to 50 mL of serous fluid. This fluid acts as a lubricant to minimize friction as the heart contracts and relaxes.

FIBROUS SKELETON

An important structural feature of the heart is its fibrous skeleton, which consists of four interconnecting valve rings and surrounding connective tissue. It separates the atria and ventricles and forms a rigid support for attachment of the valves and insertion of the cardiac muscle (Fig. 22-3). The tops of the valve rings are attached to the muscle masses of the atria, pulmonary trunks, and aorta. The bottoms are attached to the ventricular walls.

MYOCARDIUM

The myocardium, or muscular portion of the heart, includes the atrial and ventricular muscle fibers (which contract in a manner similar to that of skeletal muscle) and the specialized muscle fibers of the conduction system (which contract only slightly). Cardiac muscle cells have properties somewhere be-

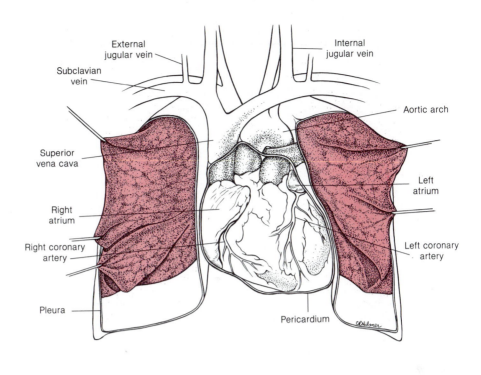

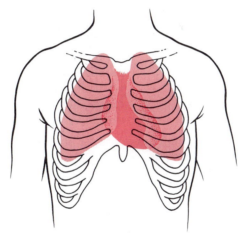

FIG. 22-1. (**Top**) Anterior view of the heart and great vessels. (**Bottom**) Position of the heart in relation to the skeletal structures of the chest cage.

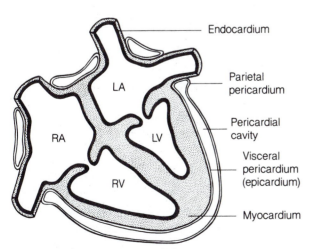

FIG. 22-2. Layers of the heart showing the visceral pericardium, the pericardial cavity, and the parietal pericardium.

tween those of skeletal and smooth muscle. They are small striated and branched cells with interconnecting fibers (Fig. 22-4). The cell membranes of the interconnecting fibers fuse to form tight junctions, or intercalated disks, which are low-resistance pathways for the passage of ions and electrical impulses from one cardiac cell to another. The myocardium, therefore, behaves as a single unit, or syncytium, rather than as a group of isolated units, as does skeletal muscle. When one myocardial cell becomes excited, the impulse travels rapidly to all the other cells.

ENDOCARDIUM

The endocardium is a thin, three-layered membrane that lines the heart. The innermost layer consists of smooth endothelial cells supported by a thin layer of

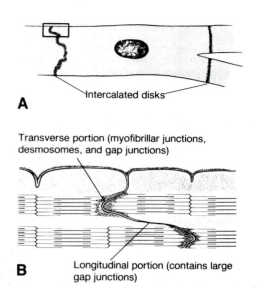

Intercalated disks

Transverse portion (myofibrillar junctions, desmosomes, and gap junctions)

B

Longitudinal portion (contains large gap junctions)

FIG. 22-4. (**A**) Cardiac muscle with intercalated disk at each end. (**B**) Area indicated in **A**, showing where cell junctions lie in the intercalated disks. (Cormack, D. H. [1992]. *Essential histology* [p. 225]. Philadelphia: J.B. Lippincott)

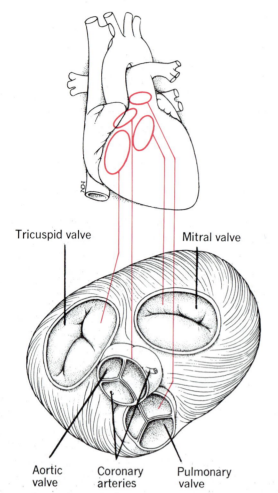

Tricuspid valve   Mitral valve

Aortic valve   Coronary arteries   Pulmonary valve

FIG. 22-3. Fibrous skeleton of the heart, which forms the four interconnecting valve rings and support for attachment of the valves and insertion of cardiac muscle. (Chaffee, E. E., & Lytle, I. M. [1980]. *Basic physiology and anatomy* [4th ed.]. Philadelphia: J.B. Lippincott)

connective tissue. The endothelial lining of the endocardium is continuous with the lining of the blood vessels that enter and leave the heart. The middle layer consists of dense connective tissue with elastic fibers. The outer layer, composed of irregularly arranged connective tissue cells, contains blood vessels and branches of the conduction system and is continuous with the myocardium.

HEART VALVES

For the heart to function effectively, blood must move forward through its chambers. This directional control is provided by the heart's two atrioventricular (AV; tricuspid and mitral) and two semilunar (aortic and pulmonic) valves (Fig. 22-5).

The AV valves control the flow of blood between the atria and the ventricles. The thin edges of the AV

valves form cusps, two on the left side of the heart (the bicuspid valve) and three on the right side (the tricuspid valve). The bicuspid valve is also known as the mitral valve. The AV valves are supported by the papillary muscles, which project from the wall of the ventricles, and the chordae tendineae, which attach to the valve. Contraction of the papillary muscles at the onset of systole ensures closure by producing

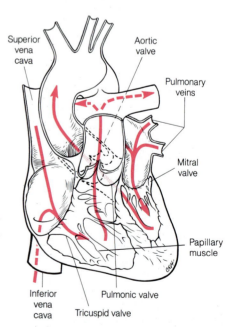

Superior vena cava

Aortic valve

Pulmonary veins

Mitral valve

Papillary muscle

Inferior vena cava

Pulmonic valve

Tricuspid valve

FIG. 22-5. Valvular structures of the heart. The atrioventricular valves are in an open position, and the semilunar valves are closed. There are no valves to control the flow of blood at the inflow channels (vena cava and pulmonary veins) to the heart.

tension on the leaflets of the AV valves before the full force of ventricular contraction pushes against them. The chordae tendineae are cord-like structures that support the AV valves and prevent them from everting into the atria during systole.

The aortic valve controls the flow of blood into the aorta; the pulmonic valve (also known as the pulmonary valve) controls blood flow into the pulmonary artery. The aortic and pulmonic valves often are referred to as the semilunar valves because their flaps are shaped like half-moons. Both the pulmonic and the aortic valve have three little teacup-shaped leaflets. These cup-like structures collect the retrograde, or backward, flow of blood that occurs toward the end of systole, enhancing closure. For the development of a perfect seal along the free edges of the semilunar valves, each valve cusp must have a triangular shape when it is closed, which is caused by a nodular thickening at the apex of each leaflet (Fig. 22-6). The openings for the coronary arteries are located in the aorta just above the aortic valve. There are no valves at the atrial sites (venae cavae and pulmonary veins) where blood enters the heart. This means that excess blood is pushed back into the veins when the atria become distended. For example, the jugular veins typically become prominent in severe right-sided heart failure when they normally should be flat or collapsed. Likewise, the pulmonary venous system becomes congested when outflow from the left atrium is impeded.

Heart Sounds. Closure of the heart valves produces vibrations of the surrounding heart tissues and blood that can be detected as the audible "lub-dup" sounds heard with a stethoscope during cardiac auscultation. There are four heart sounds. The first and second sounds are heard in all healthy people. The third and fourth heart sounds usually are not heard and may or may not indicate pathology.

The first and second heart sounds represent closure of the AV and semilunar valves, respectively. The first heart sound (lub), which has a lower pitch and lasts longer (about 0.14 second) than the second sound, marks the onset of systole and the closure of the AV valves. The second heart sound (dup) occurs with the closure of the semilunar valves; it is shorter (0.10 second) and has a higher pitch than the first heart sound. The second heart sound is a composite sound resulting from the closure of both the aortic and the pulmonic valve. The aortic valve normally closes slightly before the pulmonic valve, causing a separation of the two components of the second heart sound. During expiration, aortic valve closure precedes pulmonic valve closure by 0.02 to 0.04 second; during inspiration, this difference is increased to 0.04 to 0.06 second because there is an increase in venous return to the right heart, and as a result, it takes longer for the right ventricle to empty and the pulmonic valve to close. At the same time, less blood is returning to the left ventricle, causing the aortic valve to close slightly earlier. An audible widening of the second heart sound that occurs with inspiration is a normal finding. It often is referred to as a physiologic splitting and can be heard only in the left second intercostal space.

The third heart sound is low-pitched and occurs during rapid filling of the ventricles early in diastole, about 0.12 second after the second heart sound. It

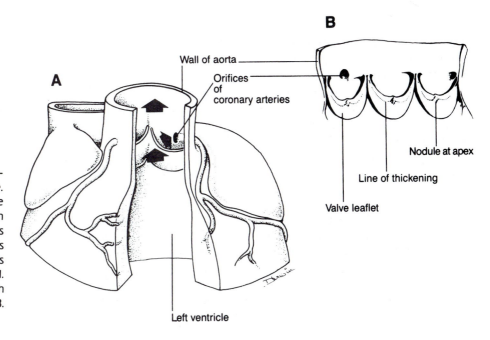

FIG. 22-6. Diagrammatic representation of the aortic valve. Its position at the base of the ascending aorta is indicated in **A**, and the appearance of its three leaflets when the aorta is cut open and spread out flat is depicted in **B**. (Cormack, D. H. [1987]. *Ham's histology* [9th ed., p. 432]. Philadelphia: J.B. Lippincott)

usually is heard only in young people or in people with heart failure. The fourth heart sound is produced by atrial contraction during the last third of diastole; it is audible only in conditions in which resistance to ventricular filling occurs during late diastole. The heart sounds and their relation to the cardiac cycle are shown in Figure 22-12.

The loudness of the first and second heart sounds depends on the rate of change in pressure across the valve. At high heart rates, intraventricular pressures rise rapidly, whereas atrial pressures remain relatively low. As a result, the first heart sound is intensified. The same principle occurs during exercise when the force of ventricular contraction is increased. Conversely, the intensity of the first heart sound is decreased when ventricular contractions are sluggish as a result of a weakened heart muscle. The loudness of the second heart sound is related to the rate of decrease in ventricular pressure at the end of systole. In people with hypertension, the second heart sound is accentuated because ventricular pressure is high at the time the aortic valve closes, and therefore, the rate at which ventricular pressure falls is accelerated.

Heart murmurs are caused by abnormal vibrations produced by turbulent blood flow. In the heart, turbulence occurs when the velocity of blood flow is increased, the valve diameter is decreased, or the viscosity of the blood is decreased. For example, very high velocities of flow may be reached when blood is ejected through a narrowed, or stenotic, heart valve. Severe anemia may reduce blood viscosity to the point at which turbulence occurs.

Auscultation to detect murmurs or abnormalities of the heart sounds is a valuable diagnostic procedure. Although auscultation of the heart does not involve the use of expensive equipment, it does require a trained ear and a thorough understanding of the physiologic events associated with valvular function and the cardiac cycle.

In summary, the heart is a four-chambered muscular pump that lies in the pericardial sac within the mediastinal space of the intrathoracic cavity. The wall of the heart is composed of an outer epicardium, which lines the pericardial cavity; a fibrous skeleton; the myocardium, or muscle layer; and the smooth endocardium, which lines the chambers of the heart. The right side of the heart pumps blood to the pulmonary circulation and the left side of the heart pumps blood to the systemic circulation. The four heart valves control the direction of blood flow as it moves through the heart. The AV valves control the flow of blood between the atria and the ventricles; the pulmonic valve controls the flow of blood from the right ventricle into the pulmonary artery; and the aortic valve controls the flow of blood from the left ventricle into the aorta. There are no valves at the atrial sites (venae cavae and pulmonary veins) where blood enters the heart; blood flows into the heart along a pressure gradient.

CONDUCTION SYSTEM AND ELECTRICAL ACTIVITY OF THE HEART

Heart muscle differs from skeletal muscle in its ability to generate and rapidly conduct its own action potentials (electrical impulses). This unique rhythmic property allows the heart to continue beating independently of the nervous system.

CARDIAC CONDUCTION SYSTEM

In certain areas of the heart, the myocardium has been modified to form the specialized cells of the conduction system. Although most myocardial cells are capable of initiating and conducting impulses, it is the heart's conduction system that maintains its pumping efficiency. Specialized pacemaker cells *generate* impulses at a faster rate than other types of heart tissue, and the conduction tissue *transmits* impulses at a faster rate than other types of heart tissue. Because of these properties, the conduction system can control the rhythm of the heart.

Each cardiac contraction is initiated by an impulse that originates in the sinoatrial (SA) node located in the posterior wall of the right atrium near the entrance to the superior vena cava. The SA node is called the *pacemaker* of the heart because it has the fastest inherent firing rate in the conduction system. Impulses from the SA node travel through the atria to the AV node (Fig. 22-7). There are at least four intraatrial pathways, including Bachmann's bundle, that connect the SA and AV nodes.[1]

The heart essentially has two conduction systems: one controls atrial activity and the other controls ventricular activity. These two systems are connected by the AV node. Within the AV node, atrial fibers connect with the very small junctional fibers of the node itself. The velocity of conduction through these fibers is very slow (about $1/25$ that of normal cardiac muscle), which greatly delays transmission of the impulse into the AV node.[2] A further delay occurs as the impulse travels through the AV node into the transitional fibers and finally into the bundle of His (also called the AV bundle). The delay in transmission of impulses through the AV node is important in that it allows the atria to empty before the ventricle contracts. Because the AV node provides the only connection between the two conduction systems, the atria and the ventricles beat independently of each other if the transmission of impulses through the AV node is blocked.

The Purkinje system, which supplies the ventricles, has large fibers that allow for rapid conduction and almost simultaneous excitation of the entire right

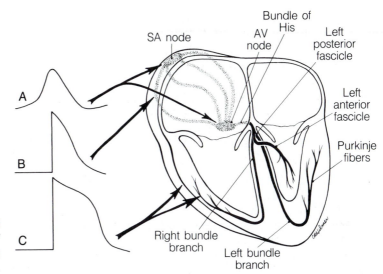

FIG. 22-7. Conduction system of the heart and action potentials. (**A**) Action potential of SA and AV nodes; (**B**) atrial muscle action potential; (**C**) action potential of ventricular muscle and Purkinje fibers.

and left ventricles. This rapid rate of conduction throughout the Purkinje system is necessary for the rapid and efficient ejection of blood from the heart. The Purkinje fibers originate in the AV node and then form the bundle of His, which extends through the fibrous tissue between the valves of the heart and into the ventricular system. The bundle of His divides almost immediately into right and left bundle branches as it reaches the interventricular septum. The bundle branches move through the subendocardial tissues toward the papillary muscles and then subdivide into the Purkinje fibers, which branch out and supply the outer walls of the ventricle. The left bundle branch fans out as it enters the septal area and divides further into two segments: the left posterior and left anterior fascicles.

ELECTROCARDIOGRAPHY

The electrocardiogram (ECG) is a recording of the electrical activity of the heart. The electric currents generated by the heart spread through the body to the skin, where they can be sensed by appropriately placed electrodes, amplified, and then recorded on an oscilloscope or chart recorder.

The deflection points of an ECG are designated by the letters P, Q, R, S, and T. Figure 22-8 shows the electrical activity of the conduction system on an ECG tracing. The P wave represents the SA node and atrial depolarization; the QRS complex (beginning of the Q wave to the end of the S wave) represents ventricular depolarization; and the T wave represents ventricular repolarization. The isoelectric line between the P wave and the Q wave represents depolarization of the AV node, bundle branches, and Purkinje system. Atrial repolarization occurs during ventricular depolarization and is hidden in the QRS complex. The ECG is discussed further in Chapter 23.

CARDIAC MUSCLE CONTRACTION

Cardiac muscle, like skeletal muscle, is composed of sarcomeres that contain myosin and actin filaments (see Chapter 1, Fig. 1-20).

Calcium ions are of particular importance in the regulation of cardiac muscle contraction. During an action potential, calcium is released from the sarcoplasmic reticulum and the transverse (T) tubules; these ions diffuse into the area of the actin and myosin filaments where they participate in the contractile process. Muscle relaxation results from (1) cessation of the calcium influx, (2) its removal from the actin–myosin sites, and (3) its energy-dependent reuptake from the cytoplasm into the sarcoplasmic reticulum and other storage sites. Compared with skeletal muscle cells, cardiac muscle cells are smaller, have less well defined sarcoplasmic reticulum, and have a shorter distance from the cell membrane to the myofibrils. Because of these differences, cardiac muscle relies more heavily than skeletal muscle on extracellular calcium ions for participation in the contractile process. The entry of extracellular calcium into myocardial cells is facilitated by two important mechanisms. Calcium enters the cell through the cell membrane, particularly during the plateau of the action potential. Calcium for cardiac muscle contraction also enters by means of the non–energy-dependent sodium–calcium exchange, in which two internal calcium ions are exchanged for one external sodium ion. Because of the normally low concentration of sodium within the cell, this mechanism usually is not an important source of calcium for cardiac contraction, but it may become important in conditions such as heart failure. Drugs such as digitalis, which block the sodium pump, increase the contractile properties of cardiac muscle by making more calcium available through this exchange system.

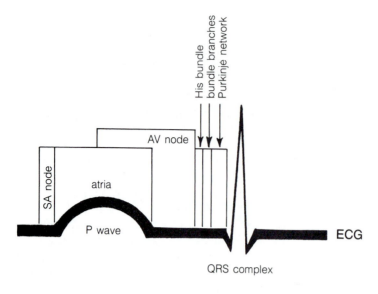

FIG. 22-8. Tissues depolarized by a wave of activation commencing in the SA node are shown in a series of blocks superimposed on the deflections of the electrocardiogram. (Katz, A.M. [1992]. *Physiology of the heart* [p. 483]. New York: Raven Press)

ACTION POTENTIALS

The action potential of a cardiac muscle is divided into five phases: (1) phase 0 is depolarization, which is characterized by the rapid upstroke of the action potential; (2) phase 1 is the brief period of repolarization; (3) phase 2 is the plateau, which lasts for 0.1 to 0.2 second; (4) phase 3 is the period of repolarization; and (5) phase 4 is the resting membrane potential. The plateau, or phase 2, of the action potential contributes to the unique electrical properties of cardiac muscle. It causes the action potential of cardiac muscle to last 20 to 50 times longer than that of skeletal muscle and causes a corresponding increased period of contraction.[1] Figure 22-9 shows the relation between the ECG and the phases of a cardiac muscle action potential.

The electrical activity of the myocardial cell depends on changes in the permeability of the cell membrane to cations, primarily sodium, potassium, and calcium. There are two types of membrane channels through which ions flow during the depolarization phase of the action potential: the fast channels and the slow channels. During phase 0, membrane permeability to sodium increases rapidly, resulting in the fast inward movement of current through the fast channels. Phase 1 occurs at the peak of the action potential and is characterized by an abrupt decrease in sodium permeability. If potassium permeability increased to its resting level at this time, as it does in nerve fibers or skeletal muscle, the cell would repolarize rapidly. Instead, potassium permeability is low, allowing for the membrane to remain depolarized throughout the phase 2 plateau of the action potential. Also contributing to the plateau is a slow inward current that develops during phase 0 when the membrane was partially depolarized and con-

tinues throughout the plateau. The slow channels, which are much more permeable to calcium than to sodium, also are called the calcium channels. During the phase 3 repolarization period, the slow inward current ceases and there is a sharp rise in potassium permeability. The rapid outward movement of the potassium ions during this phase facilitates the reestablishment of the resting membrane potential.

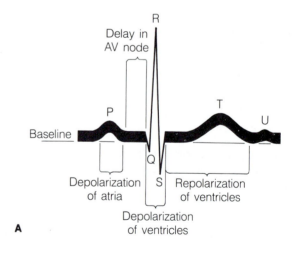

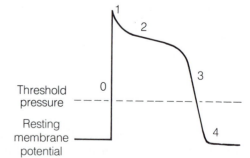

FIG. 22-9. Relation between electrocardiogram (**A**) and ventricular action potential (**B**).

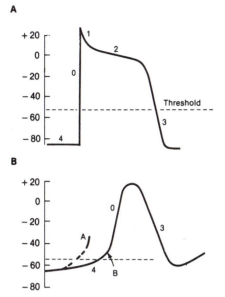

FIG. 22-10. Action potential of cardiac muscle and pacemaker cells. (**A**) Fast response that occurs in myocardial cells of atrial and ventricular muscle. The phases are identified by numbers: phase 4, resting membrane potential; phase 0, depolarization; phase 1, brief period of repolarization; phase 2, plateau; and phase 3, repolarization. (**B**) Slow response, SA and AV nodes. The slow response is characterized by a slow, spontaneous rise in the phase 4 membrane potential to threshold levels; it has a lesser amplitude and shorter duration than the fast response. Increased automaticity (A) occurs when the rate of phase 4 depolarization is increased.

Phase 4 corresponds to diastole; it is the period during which the membrane is impermeable to sodium. The calcium that enters the myocardial cells during an action potential is also involved in excitation–contraction coupling. Various factors may influence the slow inward current. The current is increased by catecholamines such as epinephrine and norepinephrine. This is probably the main mechanism whereby the catecholamines enhance cardiac contractility. Conversely, calcium-channel blocking drugs reduce the slow inward current and diminish the strength of cardiac contraction.

Action potentials from the contracting cells of the atria and the ventricles, the specialized intracardiac conduction system, and the distal portion of the AV node depend on both the fast and the slow channels. There are two main types of action potentials in the heart (Fig. 22-10). One type, the so-called fast response, occurs in the normal myocardial cells of the atria and the ventricles and in the Purkinje fibers (see Fig. 22-7B,C). The amplitude and the rate rise of phase 1 are important to the conduction velocity of the fast response. The other type, the so-called slow response, is found in the SA node, which is the natural pacemaker of the heart, and the conduction fibers of the AV node (see Fig. 22-7A). The hallmark

of these pacemaker cells is a spontaneous phase 4 depolarization. The membrane permeability of these cells allows a slow inward leak of current to occur through the slow channels during phase 4; this leak continues until the threshold for firing is reached, at which point the cell spontaneously depolarizes. The rate of pacemaker cell discharge varies with the resting membrane potential and the slope of phase 4 depolarization. The catecholamines (epinephrine and norepinephrine) increase the heart rate by increasing the slope or rate of phase 4. Acetylcholine, which is released during vagal stimulation of the heart, decreases the slope of phase 4.

The fast response of atrial and ventricular muscle can be converted to a slow pacemaker response under certain conditions. For example, such conversions may occur spontaneously in people with severe coronary artery disease, in areas of the heart where blood supply has been severely curtailed. Impulses generated by these cells can lead to ectopic beats and serious arrhythmias.

Refractory Period. The pumping action of the heart requires alternating contraction and relaxation. After an action potential, there is a refractory period during which the membrane is resistant to a second stimulus (Fig. 22-11). During the absolute refractory period, the membrane is insensitive to stimulation. The absolute refractory period is followed by the relative refractory period, during which a more intense stimulus is needed to initiate an action potential. This is followed by a supernormal excitatory period during which a weak stimulus can evoke a response. It is during this period that cardiac dysrhythmias develop (see Chapter 23). In skeletal muscle, the refractory

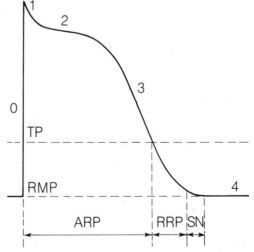

FIG. 22-11. Diagram of action potential of a ventricular muscle cell showing the RMP (resting membrane potential), ARP (absolute refractory period), RRP (relative refractory period), and SN (supernormal period).

period is very short compared with the duration of contraction, so that a second contraction can be initiated before the first is over, resulting in a summated tetanized contraction. In cardiac muscle, the absolute refractory period is almost as long as the contraction, and a second contraction cannot be stimulated until the first is over. The longer length of the absolute refractory period of cardiac muscle is important in maintaining the alternating contraction and relaxation that is essential to the pumping action of the heart and for the prevention of fatal arrhythmias.

In summary, the rhythmic contraction and relaxation of the heart rely on the specialized cells of the heart's conduction system. Specialized cells in the SA node have the fastest inherent rate of impulse generation and act as the pacemaker of the heart. Impulses from the SA node travel through the atria to the AV node and then to the AV bundle and the ventricular Purkinje system. The AV node provides the only connection between the atrial and ventricular conduction systems. The atria and the ventricles are independent of each other when AV node conduction is blocked.

The action potential of cardiac muscle is divided into five phases: phase 0 represents depolarization and is characterized by the rapid upstroke of the action potential; phase 1 is characterized by a brief period of repolarization; phase 2 consists of a plateau, which prolongs the duration of the action potential; phase 3 represents repolarization; and phase 4 is the resting membrane potential. Following an action potential, there is a refractory period during which the membrane is resistant to a second stimulus. During the absolute refractory period, the membrane is insensitive to stimulation. This period is followed by the relative refractory period, during which a more intense stimulus is needed to initiate an action potential. This is followed by a supernormal excitatory period, during which a weak stimulus can evoke a response.

■ CARDIAC CYCLE

The cardiac cycle can be divided into two parts: systole, the period during which the ventricles are contracting and blood is being ejected from the heart, and diastole, the period during which the ventricles are relaxed and the heart is filling with blood.

During diastole, the ventricles increase their volume to about 120 mL (called the end-diastolic volume), and at the end of systole, about 50 mL of blood remains in the ventricles (end-systolic volume). The difference between the end-diastolic volume and the end-systolic volume (about 70 mL) is the stroke volume. The portion of blood ejected during systole (stroke volume) divided by the end-diastolic volume is called the ejection fraction. There are simultaneous changes in left atrial pressure, left ventricular pressure, aortic pressure, ventricular volume, the ECG, and phonocardiogram during the cardiac cycle (Fig. 22-12).

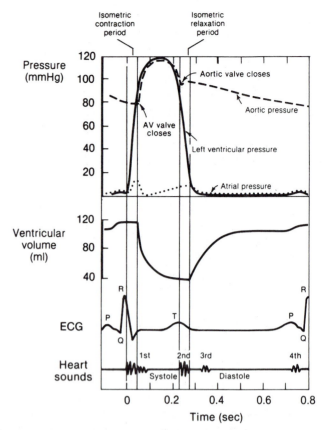

FIG. 22-12. Events in the cardiac cycle, showing changes in aortic pressure, left ventricular pressure, atrial pressure, left ventricular volume, the electrocardiogram, and heart sounds.

VENTRICULAR SYSTOLE AND DIASTOLE

During ventricular systole, the ventricles are contracting and blood is leaving the heart. The electrical activity, recorded on the ECG, precedes the mechanical events of the cardiac cycle. As the wave of depolarization (the QRS complex on the ECG) passes through the ventricles, it triggers a contraction. As the ventricles begin to contract, the AV valves close, giving rise to the first heart sound. After the AV valves close, there is an additional 0.02 to 0.03 second during which contraction is occurring in the ventricles, but the volume remains the same because both sets of valves are closed and no blood is leaving the heart. This period of the cardiac cycle, during which the heart muscle is undergoing isometric contraction, is called the *isovolumetric period*. The ventricular pressures rise abruptly during isometric contraction until left ventricular pressure is slightly higher than aortic pressure (and right ventricular pressure is about the same as pulmonary artery pressure). At this point, the semilunar valves open and blood is ejected from the heart. About 60% of the stroke volume is ejected during the first quarter of systole, and the remaining 40% is ejected during the next two quarters of systole.

Little blood is ejected from the heart during the last quarter of systole, although the ventricle remains contracted. At the end of systole, there is a precipitous fall in intraventricular pressures because of the relaxation of the ventricles. As this occurs, blood from the large arteries flows back toward the ventricles, causing the aortic and pulmonic valves to snap shut—an event that is marked by the second heart sound. The T wave on the ECG occurs during the last half of systole and represents repolarization of the ventricles.

The movement of blood into the aorta at the onset of systole causes the elastic fibers in the walls of the vessel to stretch and the pressure to rise. During the last quarter of systole, the aortic pressure begins to fall as blood flows out of the aorta into the peripheral vessels. At the end of ejection, the left ventricle begins to relax and its pressure falls below that in the aorta, at which point the aortic valve closes. The incisura, or notch, in the aortic pressure tracing represents closure of the aortic valve. Recoil of the elastic fibers in the aorta that were stretched during systole serve to maintain arterial blood pressure during the diastolic phase of the cardiac cycle.

After the semilunar valves close, the ventricles continue to relax for another 0.03 to 0.06 second (the *isometric relaxation* or *isovolumetric period*); during this time, the volume remains the same but the ventricular pressure drops until it becomes less than atrial pressure. At this time, the AV valves open and the blood that has been accumulating in the atria during systole flows into the ventricles. Most of ventricular filling occurs during the first third of diastole, which is called the *rapid filling period*. During the middle third of diastole, inflow into the ventricles is almost at a standstill. The last third of diastole is marked by atrial contraction, which gives an additional thrust to ventricular filling. When audible, the third heart sound is heard during the rapid filling period of diastole as blood flows into a distended or noncompliant ventricle. The fourth heart sound occurs during the last third of diastole.

ATRIAL SYSTOLE AND DIASTOLE

Atrial contraction occurs during the last third of diastole. It is preceded by the P wave on the ECG, which represents depolarization of the atria. There are three main atrial pressure waves that occur during the cardiac cycle. The *a* wave is caused by atrial contraction. The *c* wave occurs as the ventricles begin to contract, and their increased pressure causes the AV valves to bulge into the atria. The *v* wave results from a slow buildup of blood in the atria toward the end of systole when the AV valves are still closed. The atrial pressure waves are transmitted to the internal jugular veins as pulsations. These pulsations can

be observed visually and may be used to assess cardiac function. For example, exaggerated *a* waves occur when the right atrium has difficulty emptying into the right ventricle.

Although the main function of the atria is to store blood as it enters the heart, these chambers also act as primer pumps that aid in ventricular filling. This function becomes more important during periods of increased activity when the diastolic filling time is decreased or when heart disease impairs ventricular filling. In these two situations, the cardiac output would fall drastically were it not for the action of the atria. It has been estimated that atrial contraction can contribute as much as 30% to cardiac reserve during periods of stress, while having little or no effect on cardiac output during rest.

In summary, the cardiac cycle is divided into two parts: systole, during which the ventricles contract and blood is ejected from the heart, and diastole, during which the ventricles are relaxed and blood is filling the heart. The stroke volume (about 70 mL) represents the difference between the end-diastolic volume (about 120 mL) and the end-systolic volume (about 50 mL). The electrical activity of the heart, as represented on the ECG, precedes the mechanical events of the cardiac cycle. The heart sounds signal the closing of the heart valves during the cardiac cycle. Atrial contraction occurs during the last third of diastole. Although the main function of the atria is to store blood as it enters the heart, atrial contractions act to increase cardiac output during periods of increased activity when the filling time is reduced or in disease conditions in which ventricular filling is impaired.

■ REGULATION OF CARDIAC PERFORMANCE

The efficiency of the heart as a pump often is measured in terms of cardiac output. Cardiac output is the product of the stroke volume and the heart rate: cardiac output = stroke volume × heart rate. The cardiac output varies with body size and the metabolic needs of the tissues. It increases with physical activity and decreases during rest and sleep. The normal average cardiac output in normal adults ranges from 3.5 to 8.0 L/min. In the trained athlete, this value can increase to levels as high as 32 L/min during exercise. The *cardiac reserve* refers to the maximum percentage of increase in cardiac output that can be achieved above the normal resting level. The normal young adult has a cardiac reserve of about 300% to 400%.[2]

FACTORS THAT AFFECT CARDIAC OUTPUT

The heart's ability to increase its output according to body needs is mainly dependent on four factors: (1) the preload, or ventricular filling; (2) the afterload, or resistance to ejection of blood from the heart; (3) cardiac contractility; and (4) the heart rate.

PRELOAD

The volume achieved during diastolic filling of the ventricles is referred to as the preload because it is work imposed on the heart before the contraction begins. The preload varies with venous return to the heart, which in turn is determined by the right atrial pressure and mean systemic pressure. Preload contributes to the force of ventricular contraction by means of the Frank-Starling mechanism.

Right Atrial and Systemic Filling Pressures. During diastole, the ventricles fill with venous blood that has been returned to the atria. Venous return to the right atrium is determined by the right atrial and mean systemic filling pressures. The mean systemic filling pressure refers to the degree of filling of the systemic circulation and is the force that moves blood back to the heart. Venous return is greatest when the right atrial pressure is low and the mean systemic filling pressure is high. Because the heart is in the thoracic cavity, the right atrial pressure reflects the intrathoracic pressure. Therefore, venous return is increased during inspiration when the intrathoracic and right atrial pressures become more negative, and it is decreased during expiration when the intrathoracic and right atrial pressures become more positive.

Starling's Law of the Heart. The anatomic arrangement of the actin and myosin filaments in the myocardial muscle fibers is such that the tension or force of contraction is greatest when the muscle fibers are stretched just before the heart begins to contract. The maximum force of contraction is achieved when venous return produces an increase in ventricular filling (preload) such that the muscle fibers are stretched about two and one half times their normal resting length. When the muscle fibers are stretched to this degree, the actin and myosin filaments are in an optimal position for maximum contraction. The increased force of contraction that accompanies an increase in ventricular end-diastolic volume is referred to as the *Frank-Starling mechanism* or *Starling's law of the heart*. The Frank-Starling mechanism allows the heart to adjust its pumping ability to accommodate various levels of venous return. Cardiac output is less when decreased filling causes excessive overlap of the actin and myosin filaments or when the filaments are pulled too far apart because of excessive filling (Fig. 22-13).

AFTERLOAD

The afterload is the force, or resistance, against which the heart must pump to eject blood. It is the

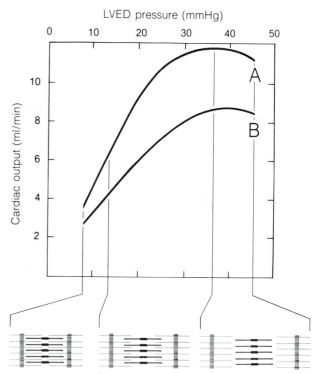

FIG. 22-13. (Top) Starling ventricular function curve. An increase in left ventricular end-diastolic (LVED) pressure produces an increase in cardiac output (*curve A*) by means of the Frank-Starling mechanism. The maximum force of contraction and increased stroke volume are achieved when diastolic filling causes the muscle fibers to be stretched about two and one half times their resting length. In *curve B*, an increase in cardiac contractility produces an increase in cardiac output without a change in LVED volume and pressure. **(Bottom)** Stretching of the actin and myosin filaments at the different LVED filling pressures.

work that is presented to the heart after the contraction has commenced. The arterial blood pressure is the main source of afterload strain on the heart. The afterload of the left ventricle is increased with narrowing (stenosis) of the aortic valve. In the late stages of aortic stenosis, the left ventricle may need to generate systolic pressures up to 300 mmHg to move blood through the diseased valve.[4]

CARDIAC CONTRACTILITY

Cardiac contractility refers to the ability of the heart to change its force of contraction without changing its resting (diastolic) length. The contractile state of the myocardial muscle is determined by biochemical and biophysical properties that govern the actin and myosin interactions within the myocardial cells. An *inotropic* influence is one that modifies the contractile state of the myocardium independent of the Frank-Starling mechanism. For instance, hypoxia exerts a negative inotropic effect by decreasing cardiac contractility, whereas sympathetic stimulation produces a positive inotropic effect by increasing it.

HEART RATE

The heart rate increases the frequency with which blood is ejected from the heart. As the heart rate increases, the time spent in diastole is reduced, and there is less time for the filling of the ventricles before the onset of systole. At a heart rate of 75 beats per minute, one cardiac cycle lasts 0.8 second, of which about 0.3 second is spent in systole and about 0.5 second in diastole. As the heart rate increases, the time spent in systole remains about the same, whereas that spent in diastole decreases. This leads to a decrease in stroke volume; at high heart rates, it may cause a decrease in cardiac output. In fact, one of the dangers of ventricular tachycardia is a reduction in cardiac output because the heart does not have time to fill adequately.

AUTONOMIC CONTROL OF CARDIAC FUNCTION

The autonomic nervous system modifies the activity of the conduction system and the contractile properties of the heart. The autonomic control of cardiac function is mediated by a number of sensors located throughout the circulatory system. For example, the baroreceptors, located in the aortic arch and carotid sinus, monitor blood pressure and effect changes in heart rate through the autonomic nervous system (see Chapter 19). There are also atrial and ventricular receptors that respond to distention and other stimuli.

PARASYMPATHETIC CONTROL OF CARDIAC FUNCTION

The parasympathetic outflow to the heart originates from the vagal nucleus in the medulla. The axons of these neurons pass to the heart in the cardiac branches of the vagus nerve. The parasympathetic nervous system has two effects on heart action: it slows the rate of impulse generation in the SA node and slows transmission of impulses through the AV node. As a consequence, there is a slowing of heart rate. The parasympathetic nervous system normally is tonically active and has a restraining effect on heart rate. Strong vagal stimulation can briefly stop impulse formation in the SA node or block transmission in the AV node. When this happens, there is a delay of about 10 to 15 seconds after which a ventricular pacemaker takes over, causing the ventricles to begin beating at a rate of 15 to 40 beats per minute. The neurotransmitter for the parasympathetic control of the heart is acetylcholine (cholinergic). The drug at-

ropine, which has an anticholinergic action, blocks vagal stimulation to the heart and causes the heart rate to increase.

SYMPATHETIC CONTROL OF CARDIAC FUNCTION

Sympathetic outflow to the heart and blood vessels arises from neurons located in the reticular formation of the brain stem. The axons of these neurons descend in the intermediolateral columns of the spinal cord; they exit from the upper thoracic segments of the spinal cord and synapse in the paravertebral ganglia with the postganglionic neurons that innervate the heart (see Chapter 48). Cardiac sympathetic fibers are widely distributed to the SA and AV nodes as well as the myocardium. Increased sympathetic activity produces an increase in both the heart rate and the velocity and force of cardiac contraction. The sympathetic control of cardiac function is mediated by the catecholamines. The actions of the sympathetic nervous system are mediated by β_1-adrenergic receptors. These receptors respond to norepinephrine released from the sympathetic neurons that innervate the heart and to catecholamines (epinephrine and norepinephrine) from the adrenal gland that circulate in the bloodstream. β-adrenergic blocking drugs are used to inhibit the effects of sympathetic stimulation on the heart.

AUTONOMIC RESPONSE TO CIRCULATORY STRESSES

The response of the cardiovascular system to the stresses of everyday living is mediated largely through the autonomic nervous system. These stresses include postural stress, Valsalva's maneuver, and face immersion.

Postural Stress. During movement from the supine to the standing position, about 20% of the blood in the heart and lungs is displaced into the legs.[4] The venous filling of the heart is decreased, the stroke volume falls, and blood pressure decreases. As the blood pressure drops, the baroreceptors are stimulated and produce a reflex-mediated increase in heart rate and peripheral vascular resistance. These responses prevent the blood pressure from falling excessively when the standing position is assumed. With prolonged standing, an increase in plasma volume and the action of the skeletal muscle pumps aid in the return of blood to the heart. Decreased tolerance of the upright position causes orthostatic hypotension, which is discussed in Chapter 21.

Valsalva's Maneuver. Valsalva's maneuver, which involves forced expiration against a closed glottis, incites a sequence of rapid changes in preload and afterload stresses along with autonomically mediated changes in the heart rate and total peripheral resistance.[5] Valsalva's maneuver is a normal accompaniment of many everyday activities. It is used in coughing, lifting, pushing, vomiting, and straining at stool. The pushing that occurs during the final stages of childbirth makes extensive use of the maneuver. The rise in intrathoracic pressure (often to levels of 40 mmHg or greater) during the strain of Valsalva's maneuver causes a decrease in venous return to the heart, with a resultant decrease in stroke volume output from the heart, a decrease in systolic and pulse pressures, and a baroreflex-mediated increase in the heart rate and the total peripheral resistance. Following the release of the strain, venous return is suddenly reestablished; both stroke volume and arterial blood pressure undergo marked but transient elevations. The sudden rise in arterial pressure that occurs at a time when reflex vasoconstriction is still present causes a vagal slowing of the heart rate that normally lasts for several beats. Valsalva's maneuver may be used as a method of testing circulatory reflexes because the increase in heart rate and total peripheral resistance that occur during Valsalva's strain, as well as the bradycardia that follows its release, are mediated through the baroreceptors and the autonomic nervous system.

Face Immersion (Diving Reflex). The diving reflex is a potent protective mechanism against asphyxia in birds and submerged vertebrates; it allows for gross redistribution of the circulation to ensure the oxygenation of the brain and heart. The diving response has three main features: (1) apnea, (2) an intense vagal slowing of heart rate, and (3) a powerful peripheral vasoconstriction. Except for the coronary and cerebral blood vessels, there is massive vasoconstriction to the extent that the circulation becomes in effect a heart–brain circuit.[6] Because of the severe vasoconstriction, arterial pressure remains relatively unchanged. The reflex enables the duck to remain submerged for 15 minutes, the sea lion for 30 minutes, and the whale for 2 hours.[6]

In humans, application of cold water to the face produces a similar reduction in the heart rate and in the skin and muscle blood flow. The slowing of the heart rate is greater with ice water than with cool water and greater with cool water than with cool air. Because of the powerful vagal effects, pathologic arrhythmias such as premature ventricular contractions can occur after only 30 seconds of diving.[6] Immersion of the face in ice water may be used clinically to terminate supraventricular paroxysmal tachycardia. Because the reflex is potent in the neonate, it may protect against asphyxia during the birth process. It has also been credited with increasing the chance of

survival of children who have accidentally fallen into cold water and remained submerged for longer periods than are associated with survival.

In summary, the efficiency of the heart as a pump often is measured in terms of cardiac output (the product of stroke volume and heart rate). The heart's ability to increase its output according to body needs depends on (1) the preload, or filling of the ventricles (end-diastolic volume); (2) the afterload, or resistance to ejection of blood from the heart; (3) cardiac contractility, which is determined by the interaction of the actin and myosin filaments of cardiac muscle fibers; and (4) the heart rate, which determines the frequency with which blood is ejected from the heart. The maximum force of cardiac contraction occurs when an increase in preload stretches muscle fibers of the heart to about two and one half times their resting length (Frank-Starling mechanism). The autonomic nervous system contributes to the regulation of cardiac output by altering the heart rate, cardiac contractility, preload, and afterload. Activation of the parasympathetic nervous system slows the heart rate. The sympathetic nervous system innervates the conduction system of the heart, the arterioles, and the veins; its stimulation produces an increase in heart rate and cardiac contractility, in preload (venous constriction), and in afterload (vasoconstriction). The autonomic nervous system plays a major role in regulating circulatory responses to everyday activities such as postural stress, Valsalva's maneuver, and exposure to cold.

■ CORONARY CIRCULATION

The blood supply for the heart is provided by the coronary arteries, which arise in the aorta just distal to the aortic valve (see Fig. 22-6). There are two coronary arteries: the right coronary artery, which mainly supplies the right ventricle and right atrium, and the left coronary artery, which divides near its origin to form the left circumflex artery and the anterior descending artery. The left coronary artery mainly supplies the left ventricle and left atrium. After passage through the arteries and capillary beds, most of the venous blood from the myocardium returns to the right atrium through the coronary sinus; some blood returns to the right atrium by way of the anterior coronary veins. There are also vascular channels that communicate directly between the vessels of the myocardium and the chambers of the heart; these are the arteriosinusoidal, arterioluminal, and thebesian vessels.

REGULATION OF CORONARY BLOOD FLOW

Blood flow in the coronary arteries is regulated by the metabolic and oxygen needs of the heart muscle. The exact means by which increased oxygen need causes coronary dilatation has not been determined. It is speculated that a decrease in the oxygen concentration of the coronary blood resulting from increased oxygen need or decreased oxygen delivery causes vasodilator substances to be released from cardiac muscle cells, and these cause the arterioles to dilate.[2] One of the vasodilator substances that has been implicated in the control of coronary blood flow is adenosine. With a decline in oxygen concentration, adenosine triphosphate (ATP) breaks down to form adenosine monophosphate, and small portions of this are further degraded to adenosine. After adenosine causes vasodilatation, much of it is reabsorbed back into cardiac cells and reused.

The autonomic nervous system exerts both direct and indirect effects on coronary blood flow. The direct effects result from the actions of the neurotransmitters of the autonomic nervous system. The indirect effects arise because of increased metabolic activity that occurs with autonomically mediated changes in heart rate and contractility. Both α-adrenergic receptors, which cause vessel constriction, and β-adrenergic receptors, which produce vessel dilatation, exist in the coronary vessels.

It has recently been shown that the intact endothelium of blood vessels produces vasodilator and vasoconstrictor substances, called *endothelium-derived relaxing factor* (EDRF) and *endothelium-derived contracting factor* (EDCF).[7] These substances, which are discussed in Chapter 19, interact with substances in the blood to produce local relaxation or constriction of blood vessels.

Coronary blood flow is also affected by the squeezing effect of the contracting myocardium on the blood vessels that course through it. During systole, the contraction of myocardial muscle compresses the coronary arteries and causes a reduction in blood flow. Because of the high pressure that the left ventricle must generate, the decrease in flow is greatest in the arteries that supply this chamber. About 70% of blood flow through the coronary arteries occurs during diastole. This is particularly significant in tachycardia when the increase in heart rate causes an increase in oxygen consumption, whereas the time spent in diastole is markedly reduced. An increase in heart rate probably has little effect on oxygen delivery in the normal heart because autoregulation causes the coronary arteries to dilate. On the other hand, rigid atherosclerotic vessels probably have a limited capacity for dilatation, in which case an increase in heart rate may impair oxygen delivery to the myocardium.

METABOLIC NEEDS OF THE MYOCARDIUM

The energy expended for myocardial contraction requires constant utilization of oxygen and other nutrients (fatty acids, glucose, and ketones). Although muscles can store limited supplies of nutrients, they cannot store oxygen. Oxygen must be supplied continuously for metabolic processes to continue. The oxygen supply for the heart is derived from the blood that flows through the coronary arteries. Under normal conditions, the heart extracts and uses about 60% to 80% of the oxygen from the blood flowing through the coronary arteries, compared with the 25% to 30% that is extracted by skeletal muscles. Because there is little oxygen reserve in the blood, the coronary arteries must increase their flow to meet the metabolic needs of the myocardium during periods of increased activity. The normal resting blood flow through the coronary arteries averages about 225 mL/min.[2] During strenuous exercise, coronary blood flow must increase four- to five-fold to meet the energy requirements of the heart.

The heart uses fats as a fuel source; about 70% of the heart's energy supply is derived from fatty acids, which must be metabolized by aerobic mechanisms. Under conditions of oxygen deprivation, the heart must convert to the anaerobic metabolism of glucose, with subsequent production of lactic acid, to meet its energy needs. Lactic acid is thought to be the source of pain stimulation during myocardial ischemia.

DETERMINANTS OF OXYGEN CONSUMPTION

The oxygen needs of the heart are determined by the tension that the heart must generate to pump blood, the stroke volume that is ejected, the contractile state of the heart, and the heart rate.

Oxygen consumption and the need for oxygen delivery by the coronary arteries are determined largely by the tension that the heart muscle must generate during contraction to eject blood into the aorta (left ventricle) and pulmonary artery (right ventricle) and the length of time that this tension must be maintained (tension × time). When the heart is dilated at the onset of systole, it must use additional energy just to overcome the wall tension and decrease its size before it can generate the pressure needed to eject blood. When some cardiac muscle fibers are damaged, others must take up the load. They do this by increasing their length; this causes the heart to dilate and produces an increase in wall tension (see Chapter 19, Laplace's law). The oxygen consumption is, therefore, greater for the same work load.

The stroke work is the effort the heart expends to pump blood. Work is defined as force multiplied by distance. For example, the work required to carry a heavy box up a flight of stairs is equal to the weight of the box multiplied by the height of the stairs. The main (external) work of the heart is determined by the amount of blood (like the weight of the box) that is pumped with each beat and the pressure (like the height of the stairs) that the ventricle must develop to move the blood into the aorta or pulmonary artery.

Stroke work = stroke volume
× mean arterial blood pressure

The stroke work of the left ventricle pumping against a mean systemic pressure of 85 mmHg is greater than the stroke work of the right ventricle pumping against a mean pulmonary artery pressure of 15 mmHg. Stroke work is increased in the presence of hypertension and in valvular disorders that reduce the size of the valve opening through which blood must be pumped.

The contractile state of the heart refers to its ability to change its force of contraction without a change in end-diastolic volume, heart rate, or arterial pressure. Oxygen consumed during the contractile state is used to produce and maintain the interactions between the actin and myosin filaments of the myocardial fibers. The cardiac glycosides (digitalis drugs) increase the myocardial contractility, allowing the heart to increase its stroke volume without an increase in metabolic demands. The catecholamines increase cardiac contractility, but they also increase the metabolic requirements of the myocardium.

The heart rate increases the myocardial oxygen requirements by increasing the frequency with which the heart goes through the processes that require oxygen consumption.

In summary, the blood supply for the heart is provided by the coronary arteries, which arise in the aorta just distal to the aortic valve. Coronary blood flow is regulated by the metabolic and oxygen needs of the heart muscle. The contraction of myocardial muscle fibers compresses the coronary arteries so that blood flow is greatest during diastole. Under normal conditions, the heart extracts 60% to 80% of the oxygen from the blood flowing through the coronary arteries, compared with the 25% to 30% that is extracted by skeletal muscle. Because the blood that flows through the coronary arteries contains little reserve oxygen, the coronary arteries must increase their flow during periods of increased activity. The oxygen needs of the heart are determined by the tension that the heart must generate to pump blood, the stroke volume that is ejected, and the heart rate.

■ REFERENCES

1. Berne, R.M., & Levy, M.N. (1988). *Physiology* (2nd ed., pp. 398–430). St. Louis: C. V. Mosby.
2. Guyton, A. (1991). *Textbook of medical physiology* (9th ed., pp. 221–244). Philadelphia: W.B. Saunders.
3. Katz, A.M. (1992). *Physiology of the heart*. New York: Raven Press.
4. Shepard, J.T., & Vanhoutte, P.M. (1979). *The human cardiovascular system* (p. 158). New York: Raven Press.
5. Porth, C.J.M., Bamrah, V.S., Tristani, F.E., et al. (1984). The Valsalva: Mechanisms and clinical implications. *Heart and Lung, 13*(5), 507.
6. Smith, J.J., & Kampine, J.P. (1990). *Circulatory physiology* (3rd ed.). Baltimore: Williams & Wilkins.
7. Vanhoutte, P. (1987). The endothelium and control of vascular tissue. *News in Physiological Sciences, 2*(1), 18.

CHAPTER 23

ALTERATIONS IN CARDIAC FUNCTION

LAURA BURKE
CAROL MATTSON PORTH

■ OBJECTIVES

After you have studied this chapter, you should be able to meet the following objectives:

■ Compare the manifestations of acute pericarditis with those of chronic pericarditis with effusion and constrictive pericarditis.

■ Relate the cardiac compression that occurs with cardiac tamponade to the clinical manifestations of the disorder, including pulsus paradoxus.

■ State the physiologic cause of myocardial ischemia.

■ Distinguish among classic angina, variant angina, unstable angina, silent myocardial ischemia, and myocardial infarction in terms of pathophysiology and symptomatology.

■ Compare the treatment goals for angina and silent myocardial ischemia with those for myocardial infarction.

■ Compare the procedures used in percutaneous transluminal coronary angioplasty and coronary bypass surgery.

■ Explain the mechanisms, criteria for use, and benefits of thrombolytic therapy in patients with myocardial infarction.

Carol Mattson Porth: PATHOPHYSIOLOGY: CONCEPTS OF
ALTERED HEALTH STATES, 4th ed. © 1994, 1990, 1986, 1982
J.B. Lippincott Company

■ Cite the benefits of an exercise program in patients with coronary heart disease.

■ Relate the activity of the cardiac conduction system to the mechanical functioning of the heart.

■ Cite the types of cardiac conditions that can be diagnosed using the ECG.

■ Describe methods used in the diagnosis of cardiac dysrhythmias.

■ Compare sinus dysrhythmia with atrial dysrhythmia.

■ Compare the effects of atrial flutter and atrial fibrillation on rhythm.

■ Describe the characteristics of first-, second-, and third- degree heart block.

■ Compare the effects of premature ventricular contractions, ventricular tachycardia, and ventricular fibrillation on cardiac function.

■ Explain the mechanisms, criteria for use, and benefits of electrolyte maintenance therapy, antidysrhythmic drugs, and internal cardioverter defibrillator therapy in people with recurrent, symptomatic dysrhythmias.

■ Compare the heart changes that occur with dilated, hypertrophic, and constrictive cardiomyopathies.

■ Distinguish between the role of infectious organisms and the immune system in myocarditis, rheumatic fever, Kawasaki's disease, and infective endocarditis.

■ Compare the effects of myocarditis, rheumatic fever, bacterial endocarditis, and Kawasaki's disease on cardiac structures and the function.

■ Compare the effects of stenotic and regurgitant mitral and aortic valvular heart disease on cardiovascular function.

■ Compare the methods of and diagnostic information obtained from cardiac auscultation, phonocardiography, and echocardiography as they relate to valvular heart disease.

■ Trace the flow of blood in the fetal circulation, and state the function of the foramen ovale and ductus arteriosus.

■ State the changes in circulatory function that occur at birth.

■ Compare the effects of left-to-right and right-to-left shunts on the pulmonary circulation and production of cyanosis.

■ Describe the anatomic defects and altered patterns of blood flow in children with atrial septal defects, ventricular septal defects, endocardial cushion defects, pulmonary stenosis, tetralogy of Fallot, patent ductus arteriosus, transposition of the great vessels, and coarctation of the aorta.

The latest estimates indicate that more than 42 million people in the United States have some form of cardiovascular disease. About 44% of all deaths—944,688 in 1989—result from cardiovascular disease.[1] Heart attack is the nation's number one killer; it is responsible for more than one third of all deaths and is the predominant cause of early disability in the American labor force. Each year, about 30,000 children are born with congenital heart defects and 1,131,000 children and adults are affected with rheumatic fever. In 1991, it was estimated that heart and blood vessel disease cost the nation an average of $108.9 billion. In an attempt to focus on common heart problems that affect people in all age groups, this chapter is organized into seven sections: (1) disorders of the pericardium, (2) coronary artery disease, (3) disorders of cardiac rhythm and conduction, (4) cardiomyopathies, (5) infectious and immunologic disorders, (6) valvular heart disease, and (7) congenital heart disease.

■ DISORDERS OF THE PERICARDIUM

The pericardium isolates the heart from other thoracic structures, maintains its position in the thorax, and prevents it from overfilling. The two layers of the pericardium are separated by a thin layer of serous fluid, which serves to prevent frictional forces from developing as the inner visceral layer, or epicardium, comes in contact with the outer parietal layer of the fibrous pericardium. The mechanisms that control the movement of fluid between the capillaries and the pericardial space are the same as those that control fluid movement between the capillaries and the interstitial spaces of other body tissues (see Chapter 29). The pericardial sac normally contains 30 to 50 mL of clear, straw-colored fluid.[2] Conditions that produce edema in other structures of the body, such as kidney disease and heart failure, may also produce an accumulation of fluid in the pericardial sac. This is called *pericardial effusion*. When the effusion is caused by serous transudate with a low specific gravity, it often is referred to as *hydropericardium*. Although 1 L or more of transudate may accumulate, volumes of more than 500 mL are uncommon.

The pericardium is subject to many of the same pathologic processes (*e.g.*, inflammation, neoplastic disease, and congenital disorders) that affect other structures of the body. Pericardial disorders usually are associated with or occur secondary to another disease, either within the heart or in the surrounding structures (Chart 23-1). The discussion in this chapter focuses on the pathologic processes associated

CHART 23-1: CLASSIFICATION OF DISORDERS OF THE PERICARDIUM

Inflammation

Acute inflammatory pericarditis
1. Infectious
    Viral (echo, coxsackie and others)
    Bacterial (tuberculosis, staphylococcus, strepto-
      coccus, and so forth)
    Fungal
2. Immune and collagen disorders
    Rheumatic fever
    Rheumatoid arthritis
    Systemic lupus erythematosus
3. Metabolic disorders
    Uremia and dialysis
    Myxedema
4. Ischemia and tissue injury
    Myocardial infarction
    Cardiac surgery
    Chest trauma
5. Physical and chemical agents
    Radiation therapy
    Untoward reactions to drugs, such as hydralazine,
      procainamide, and anticoagulants
Chronic inflammatory pericarditis
    Can be associated with most of the agents causing
      an acute inflammatory response

Neoplastic Disease

1. Primary
2. Secondary (carcinoma of the lung or breast, lym-
    phoma, and so forth)

Congenital Disorders

1. Complete or partial absence of the pericardium
2. Congenital pericardial cysts

with acute inflammation of the pericardium (pericarditis), pericardial effusion, and constrictive pericarditis.

TYPES OF PERICARDIAL DISORDERS

ACUTE PERICARDITIS

Acute pericarditis represents an acute inflammatory process and is characterized by chest pain, pericardial friction rub, and serial electrocardiographic (ECG) abnormalities.[3] It can result from a number of diverse causes. In many cases the condition is self-limited, resolving in 2 to 6 weeks; in other cases the same cause may persist over time and produce a recurrent subacute or chronic disease.

Acute pericarditis can be classified according to cause (infections, trauma, or rheumatic fever) or the nature of the exudate (fibrinous, purulent, hemorrhagic). Like other inflammatory conditions, acute pericarditis often is associated with increased capillary permeability. The capillaries that supply the serous pericardium become permeable, allowing plasma proteins, including fibrinogen, to leave the capillaries and enter the pericardial space. This results in an exudate that varies in type and amount, depending on the causative agent. It most commonly is fibrinous or serofibrinous (serous fluid mixed with fibrinous exudate) but may be hemorrhagic (contain red cells) or purulent (contain pus cells). Acute pericarditis frequently is associated with a fibrous exudate, which either heals by resolution or progresses to deposition of scar tissue and formation of adhesions between the layers of the serous pericardium.

Viral infections are the most common cause of acute pericarditis and are probably responsible for many cases classified as idiopathic pericarditis. Acute viral pericarditis is seen more frequently in men than in women and often is preceded by a prodromal phase during which fever, malaise, and other flulike symptoms are present. The condition usually lasts for several weeks, during which precordial pain, friction rub, and ECG changes are present. Although the acute symptoms may subside shortly, easy fatigability often continues for several months. Other causes of acute pericarditis are rheumatic fever, the postpericardiotomy syndrome, posttraumatic pericarditis, metabolic disorders (*e.g.*, uremia and myxedema), and pericarditis associated with connective tissue diseases (*e.g.*, systemic lupus erythematosus and rheumatoid arthritis). With the increased use of open heart surgery in the treatment of various heart disorders, the postpericardiotomy syndrome has become a commonly recognized form of pericarditis. Pericarditis with effusion is a common complication in people with renal failure, both in those with untreated uremia and in those being treated with hemodialysis.

Manifestations. The manifestations of acute pericarditis include a triad of chest pain, friction rub, and ECG changes. Acute pericarditis may also cause dyspnea. The clinical findings and other manifestations may vary according to the causative agent. Leukocytosis and an elevation in the erythrocyte sedimentation rate are common.

Nearly all people with acute pericarditis have chest pain. The pain usually is abrupt in onset, occurs in the precordial area, and is described as sharp. It may radiate to the neck, back, abdomen, or side. It typically is worse with deep breathing, coughing, swallowing, and positional changes. Many patients seek relief by sitting up and leaning forward. Only a small portion of the pericardium, the outer layer of the lower parietal pericardium below the fifth and sixth intercostal spaces, is sensitive to pain. This means that pericardial pain probably results from inflammation of the surrounding structures, particularly the pleura. Pain is more common when considerable effusion of fluid is present in the pericardial sac, probably because of the increased stretching of the lower parietal pericardium.

A pericardial friction rub, which is heard when a stethoscope is placed on the chest, results from rubbing and friction between the inflamed pericardial surfaces. The sound associated with a friction rub has been described as leathery or close to the ear. It is heard best when the patient is leaning forward in the seated position and the diaphragm of the stethoscope is placed firmly along the left sternal border over the xiphoid process or near the lower border of the sternum. The friction rub associated with acute pericarditis usually lasts from 7 to 10 days.[4]

Four stages of ECG changes occur during acute pericarditis: in stage 1, there is an acute elevation of the ST segment; in stage 2, the ST segment becomes isoelectric; in stage 3, the T wave becomes inverted; and in stage 4, the ECG returns to normal.[5] The ST-segment changes begin within hours to days after the onset of acute pericarditis. Serial ECGs are useful in differentiating between myocardial infarction, in which the ST segment does not return to the isoelectric line before the T-wave inversion occurs, and acute pericarditis, in which T-wave inversion occurs after the ST segment has returned to normal.

PERICARDIAL EFFUSION

Pericardial effusion refers to the presence of exudate in the pericardial cavity. Its major threat is compression of the heart chambers. The amount of exudate, the rapidity with which it accumulates, and the elasticity of the pericardium determine the effect the effusion has on cardiac function. Small pericardial effusions may produce no symptoms or abnormal clinical findings. Even a large effusion that develops slowly may cause few, if any, symptoms, providing the pericardium is able to stretch and avoid compressing the heart. On the other hand, a sudden accumulation of 200 mL may raise intracardiac pressure to levels that seriously limit the venous return to the heart. Symptoms of cardiac compression may also occur with relatively small accumulations of fluid when the pericardium has become thickened by scar tissue or neoplastic infiltrations.

Cardiac Tamponade. Cardiac tamponade is cardiac compression caused by excess fluid or blood in the pericardial sac. It can occur as the result of trauma, effusion, cardiac rupture, or dissecting aneurysm. The seriousness of the condition results from restriction in ventricular filling with a subsequent critical reduction in stroke volume and depends on the amount of fluid present and the rate at

which it accumulates. A rapid accumulation of fluid results in an increase in central venous pressure, a decrease in venous return to the heart, distention of the jugular veins, a decrease in cardiac output despite an increase in heart rate, a decrease in systolic blood pressure, and signs of circulatory shock.

Pulsus paradoxus refers to an exaggeration of the normal inspiratory decrease in systolic blood pressure and is a clinical indicator of cardiac tamponade.[6] The decreased intrathoracic pressure that occurs during inspiration normally accelerates venous flow, increasing right atrial and ventricular filling. This causes the interventricular septum to bulge to the left, producing internal compression of the left ventricle. In cardiac tamponade, the left ventricle is compressed from within by movement of the interventricular septum and from without by fluid in the pericardium (Fig. 23-1). With pulsus paradoxus, left ventricular output can decrease within a beat of the beginning of inspiration. Pulsus paradoxus can be determined by palpation or cuff sphygmomanometry. When pulsus paradoxus is present, the arterial

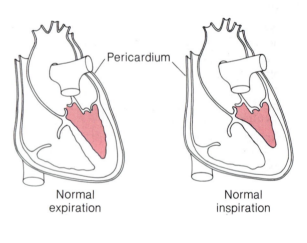

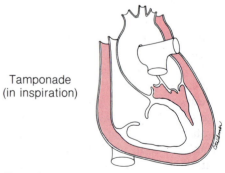

FIG. 23-1. *Effect of respiration and cardiac tamponade on ventricular filling and cardiac output. During inspiration venous flow into the right heart increases, causing the interventricular septum to bulge into the left ventricle. This produces a decrease in left ventricular volume, with a subsequent decrease in stroke volume output. In cardiac tamponade, the fluid in the pericardial sac produces further compression of the left ventricle, causing an exaggeration of the normal inspiratory decrease in stroke volume and systolic blood pressure.*

pulse (as palpated at the carotid or femoral artery) is reduced or absent during inspiration. Palpation provides only a gross estimate of the degree of paradoxus. Pulsus paradoxus is more sensitively estimated when the blood pressure cuff is inflated to a value above the systolic pressure and then deflated slowly at a rate of 2 mmHg per second until the first Korotkoff sound is detected with expiration. After the notation of this pressure, the cuff is deflated until the Korotkoff sounds can be heard throughout the respiratory cycle. A difference greater than 10 mmHg between inspiration and expiration is indicative of pulsus paradoxus. In cardiac tamponade, this implies a large reduction in ventricular volume.

Chronic Pericarditis With Effusion. Chronic pericarditis with effusion is characterized by an increase in inflammatory exudate that continues beyond the anticipated period. In some cases, the exudate persists for several years. In most cases of chronic pericarditis, no specific pathogen can be identified. The process commonly is associated with other forms of heart disease, such as rheumatic fever, congenital heart lesions, or hypertensive heart disease. Systemic diseases, such as lupus erythematosus, rheumatoid arthritis, scleroderma, and myxedema, are also causes of chronic pericarditis, as are metabolic disturbances associated with acute and chronic renal failure. Unlike those of acute pericarditis, the signs and symptoms of chronic pericarditis often are minimal; many times the disease is detected for the first time on routine chest film. As the condition progresses, the fluid may accumulate and compress the adjacent cardiac structures and impair cardiac filling.

CONSTRICTIVE PERICARDITIS

In constrictive pericarditis, scar tissue develops between the visceral and parietal layers of the serous pericardium. In time, the scar tissue contracts and interferes with cardiac filling, at which point cardiac output and cardiac reserve become fixed. Ascites is a prominent early finding and may be accompanied by pedal edema, dyspnea on exertion, and fatigue. The jugular veins are also distended. *Kussmaul's sign* is an inspiratory distention of the jugular veins caused by the inability of the right atrium, encased in its rigid pericardium, to accommodate the increase in venous return that occurs with inspiration.

DIAGNOSIS AND TREATMENT

Various diagnostic tests are used to confirm the presence of pericardial disease. These measures include auscultation, chest radiology, ECG, echocardiogra-

phy, radiation-scanning procedures, and computed tomography. The echocardiogram is the most definitive of these studies. Aspiration and laboratory analysis of the pericardial fluid may be used to identify the causative agent.

Treatment depends on the cause. When infection is present, antibiotics specific for the causative agent usually are prescribed. Antiinflammatory drugs may be given to minimize the inflammatory response and the accompanying undesirable effects. Pericardiocentesis, the removal of fluid from the pericardial sac, may be a life-saving measure in severe cardiac tamponade. Surgical treatment may be required in traumatic lesions of the heart or in constrictive pericarditis in which cardiac filling is severely impaired.

In summary, disorders of the pericardium include acute pericarditis, pericardial effusion, cardiac tamponade, and constrictive pericarditis. Acute pericarditis is characterized by chest pain, ECG changes, and a friction rub. Among its causes are infections, uremia, rheumatic fever, connective tissue diseases, and myocardial infarction. Pericardial effusion refers to the presence of an exudate in the pericardial cavity and can be either acute or chronic. It can increase intracardiac pressure, compress the heart, and interfere with venous return to the heart. The amount of exudate, the rapidity with which it accumulates, and the elasticity of the pericardium determine the effect the effusion has on cardiac function. Cardiac tamponade is a life-threatening cardiac compression resulting from excess fluid in the pericardial sac. In constrictive pericarditis, scar tissue develops between the visceral and parietal layers of the serous pericardium. In time, the scar tissue contracts and interferes with cardiac filling.

■ CORONARY ARTERY DISEASE

The term *coronary artery disease* describes heart disease caused by impaired coronary blood flow. Disease of the coronary vessels can cause angina, myocardial infarction, cardiac dysrhythmias, conduction defects, heart failure, and sudden death. Almost half of all cardiovascular deaths are due to coronary artery disease. In 1989, coronary artery disease caused 497,850 deaths; 6,160,000 persons have a history of angina, heart attack, or both.[1]

In most cases, coronary artery disease is caused by atherosclerosis (see Chapter 20). Atherosclerotic plaque fissures have been theorized to be the connecting link to various clinical syndromes associated with coronary artery disease. Coronary artery disease often is a silent disorder; most men and women over age 50 have moderately advanced coronary atherosclerosis, although the majority of these people have no symptoms of heart disease.[6]

Coronary artery disease can affect one or all of the coronary arteries (one-, two-, or three-vessel disease) and can be diffuse or localized to one area of a single vessel. At least 75% of the vessel lumen must be occluded before there is a significant reduction in blood flow.

CORONARY ARTERIES AND DISTRIBUTION OF BLOOD FLOW

There are two main coronary arteries, the left and the right, which arise from the coronary sinus just above the aortic valve (Fig. 23-2).

The left coronary artery extends for about 3.5 cm as the *left main coronary artery* and then divides into the anterior descending and circumflex branches. The *left anterior descending artery* passes down through the groove between the two ventricles, giving off *diagonal branches*, which supply the left ventricle, and *perforating branches*, which supply the anterior portion of the interventricular septum and the anterior papillary muscle of the left ventricle. The *circumflex* branch of the left coronary artery passes to the left and moves posteriorly in the groove that separates the left atrium and ventricle, giving off branches that supply the left lateral wall of the left ventricle.

The *right coronary artery* lies in the right atrioventricular groove, and its branches supply the right ventricle. The right coronary artery usually moves to the back of the heart where it forms the *posterior descending artery*, which supplies the posterior portion of the heart (the interventricular septum, atrioventricular node, and posterior papillary muscle).

The sinoatrial node usually is supplied by the right coronary artery. In about 10% of people, the left circumflex rather than the right coronary artery moves posteriorly to form the posterior descending artery.

Many factors interact in the control of coronary blood flow, including vessel diameter, aortic pressure, extravascular compression, presence of collateral channels, and vasodilator responses. Because the openings for the coronary arteries originate in the root of the aorta just outside the aortic valve, the primary factor responsible for perfusion of the coronary arteries is the aortic pressure, which is generated by the heart itself. Changes in aortic pressure produce parallel changes in coronary blood flow.

In addition to providing the aortic pressure that moves blood through the coronary vessels, the heart muscle influences blood supply by the squeezing effect that the contracting myocardium has on its intramyocardial and subendocardial blood vessels. The large epicardial coronary arteries lie on the surface of the heart, with smaller intramyocardial branches coming off and penetrating the myocardium and traveling to a network or plexus of subendocardial vessels.

During cardiac contraction the cardiac muscle squeezes toward the center of the heart, compressing both the intramyocardial blood vessels (Fig. 23-3) and the blood in the ventricles. As a result, the subendocardial vessels receive less blood than the outer epicardial vessels. The subendocardial vessels are more extensive than the vessels that supply the outer

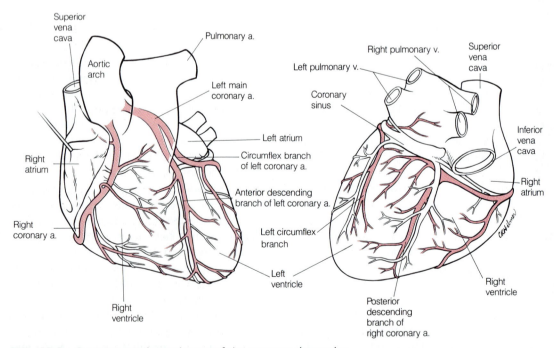

FIG. 23-2. Coronary arteries and some of the coronary sinus veins.

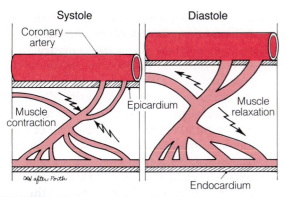

FIG. 23-3. The compressing effect of the contracting myocardium on intramyocardial blood vessels and subendocardial blood flow during systole and diastole.

layers of the heart, and they fill during diastole to compensate for the decreased flow that occurs during systole. Because subendocardial blood flow occurs during diastole, there is risk of myocardial ischemia and infarction when diastolic pressure is low and there is an elevation in diastolic intraventricular pressure sufficient to compress the vessels in the subendocardial plexus.[7] Intramyocardial blood flow is also affected by heart rate because at rapid heart rates, the time spent in diastole is greatly reduced.

Although there are no connections between the large coronary arteries, there are anastomotic channels that join the small arteries (Fig. 23-4). With gradual occlusion of the larger vessels, the smaller collat-

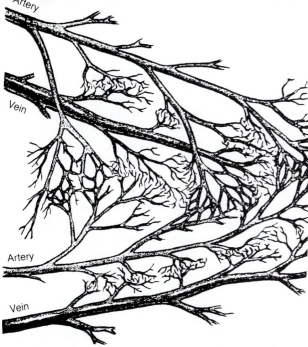

FIG. 23-4. Anastomoses of the smaller coronary arterial vessels. (Guyton, A. C. [1981]. *Textbook of medical physiology* [6th ed.]. Philadelphia: W.B. Saunders)

eral vessels increase in size and provide alternative channels for blood flow.[8] One of the reasons coronary artery disease does not produce symptoms until it is far advanced is that the collateral channels develop at the same time the atherosclerotic changes are occurring.

One of the characteristics of the coronary circulation is the ability of its vessels to dilate in the presence of increased metabolic activity. Although the mechanism for vasodilatation remains unsettled, numerous mediators, such as oxygen (hypoxia), carbon dioxide, lactic acid, potassium, and adenosine, have been suggested.[9]

Research has shown that the endothelial cells that line the arterial walls normally synthesize and release chemical mediators that produce vasodilatation (endothelium-derived relaxing factor [EDRF]) and vasoconstriction (endothelium-derived constricting factor [EDCF]).[9] EDRF maintains circulation of the blood by relaxing smooth muscle and promoting antiaggregation of platelets in arteries with intact endothelial cells. Some of the reported stimuli for release of EDRF in coronary blood vessels are acetylcholine, thrombin, norepinephrine, and vessel distention or shear stress of blood flow. For example, the endothelial cells of coronary arteries possess α_2-adrenergic receptors, which, when activated, cause release of EDRF. In laboratory experiments in which the endothelium has been removed, aggregating platelets produce massive vasoconstriction. This vasoconstriction does not occur when an intact endothelium is present, suggesting that aggregating platelets release substances that can trigger potent EDRF responses. One of the reported stimuli for EDCF is hypoxia. From these research observations, it has been proposed that the intact endothelium contributes to the regulation of blood flow by both (1) releasing factors that produce relaxation or constriction of vascular smooth muscle and (2) preventing aggregation and release of platelet factors that promote thrombus formation.

MYOCARDIAL ISCHEMIA

The term *ischemia* means to suppress or withhold blood flow. Myocardial ischemia occurs when the ability of the coronary arteries to supply blood is inadequate to meet the metabolic demands of the heart. Myocardial ischemia due to an inadequate blood supply may be caused by atherosclerotic lesions, vasospasm, thrombosis, or a combination of the three conditions. Metabolic demands of the heart are increased with everyday activities such as mental stress, exercise, and exposure to cold. In certain disease states, such as thyrotoxicosis, the metabolic demands may be so excessive that blood supply is inadequate despite normal coronary arteries. In other situations, such as aortic stenosis, the coronary arteries may not be diseased, but the perfusion pressure may be insufficient to provide adequate blood flow. Both symptomatic myocardial ischemia (angina pectoris) and silent (painless) myocardial ischemia are important functional indicators of active coronary artery disease and increased risk of myocardial infarction or sudden death.

ANGINA PECTORIS

The term *angina* (Latin) means to choke. Angina pectoris is a symptomatic paroxysmal pain or pressure sensation associated with transient myocardial ischemia. The pain typically is described as constricting, squeezing, or suffocating. It usually is steady, increasing in intensity only at the onset and end of the attack. The pain of angina commonly is located in the precordial or substernal area of the chest; it is similar to myocardial infarction in that it may radiate to the left shoulder, jaw, arm, or other areas of the chest (Fig. 23-5). In some people, the arm or shoulder pain may be confused with arthritis; in others, epigastric pain is confused with indigestion. The duration of angina is brief—seldom does it last for more than 5 minutes. There are three types of angina: classic angina, variant angina, and unstable angina.

Classic Angina. Classic angina, sometimes called exertional angina, is associated with atherosclerotic disease of the coronary arteries. It occurs when the metabolic needs of the myocardium exceed

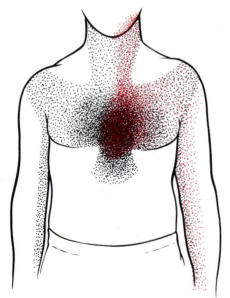

FIG. 23-5. Areas of pain due to angina. (Adapted from American Heart Association [1984]. *Heart facts 1984*)

the ability of the occluded coronary arteries to deliver adequate blood flow. Pain usually is precipitated by situations that increase the work demands of the heart, such as physical exertion, exposure to cold, and emotional stress. Despite the fact that the overwhelming majority of people with angina have atherosclerotic heart disease, angina does not develop in a considerable number of people with advanced coronary atherosclerosis. This is probably because of their sedentary life-style, the development of adequate collateral circulation, or the inability of these people to perceive pain. In many instances, myocardial infarction occurs without a history of angina.

Variant Angina. The syndrome of variant or Prinzmetal's angina was first described by Prinzmetal and associates in 1959.[10] Subsequent evidence suggests that variant angina is caused by spasms of the coronary arteries; thus, the condition is also called vasospastic angina. In most instances, the spasms occur in the presence of coronary artery stenosis; however, variant angina has occurred in the absence of visible disease. Unlike the classic form of angina, which occurs with exertion or stress, variant angina usually occurs during rest or with minimal exercise and frequently is nocturnal. It may be associated with rapid-eye-movement sleep. It commonly follows a cyclic or regular pattern of occurrence (*e.g.,* it happens at the same time each day). Dysrhythmias often are present when the pain is severe, and most people are aware of their presence during an attack. ECG changes are significant if recorded during an attack. The ST segment typically is elevated on the same lead during each attack, suggesting the involvement of a single vessel.

The mechanism of coronary vasospasm is uncertain. It has been suggested that it may result from hyperactive sympathetic nervous system responses, from a defect in the handling of calcium in vascular smooth muscle, or from a reduced production of prostaglandin I_2. The calcium-channel blocking drugs are effective in treating variant angina.

Unstable Angina. In unstable angina, an accelerated form of angina, the pain is characterized by a changing pattern. It begins to appear more frequently, is more severe, lasts longer, and may occur at rest. Sometimes unstable angina is called preinfarction angina because of its propensity for accelerating to myocardial infarction.

Unstable angina usually is triggered by a subtle or minor injury to a coronary atherosclerotic plaque. Although plaque disruption may occur with or without thrombosis, it increases the degree of coronary artery obstruction. When the original injury is mild, intermittent thrombotic occlusions may occur and cause episodes of anginal pain at rest. Additionally, vasoconstricting factors (thromboxane, serotonin, and platelet-derived growth factor) are released from platelets that aggregate at the site of injury. These platelet factors contribute, even at rest, to episodes of reduced coronary blood flow and either silent or symptomatic myocardial ischemia. Thrombus formation can progress until the coronary artery becomes occluded, leading to myocardial infarction. Ischemic episodes may also be precipitated by factors that increase the blood flow needs of the myocardium.[11]

SILENT MYOCARDIAL ISCHEMIA

Silent myocardial ischemia occurs in the absence of anginal pain. The factors that cause silent myocardial ischemia appear to be the same as those responsible for angina—impaired blood flow due to the effects of coronary atherosclerosis or vasospasm. Silent myocardial ischemia affects three populations: (1) people who are asymptomatic without other evidence of coronary heart disease, (2) people who have had a myocardial infarct and continue to have episodes of silent ischemia, and (3) people with angina who also have episodes of silent ischemia.

DIAGNOSTIC METHODS

The diagnosis of myocardial ischemia is based on history, ECG, response to the administration of nitroglycerin, and the results of exercise stress testing. Nuclear imaging or cardiac catheterization may be used to describe the location and extent of the disease.

Exercise Stress Testing. Exercise stress testing is a means of observing cardiac function under stress. Three types of tests are used: the step test, the bicycle ergometer, and the treadmill (discussed in Chapter 9). The presence of chest pain, severe shortness of breath, dysrhythmias, ST-segment changes on the ECG, or a decrease in blood pressure is suggestive of coronary heart disease, and if one or more of these signs or symptoms are present, the test usually is terminated.

Nuclear Imaging. Nuclear cardiology techniques involve the use of radionuclides (radioactive substances) and essentially are noninvasive. Three types of nuclear cardiology tests commonly are used: infarct imaging, myocardial perfusion imaging, and ventriculography. With all three types of tests, a scintillation camera is used to record the radiation emitted from the radionuclide.

Acute infarct imaging uses a radionuclide (*e.g.*, technetium pyrophosphate) that is taken up by the cells in the infarcted zone. With this method, the radionuclide becomes concentrated in the damaged myocardium, allowing its visualization as a "hot spot," or positive area, of increased uptake of the radionuclide.

Myocardial perfusion imaging uses radionuclides that are extracted from the blood and taken up by functioning myocardial cells. Thallium-201, an analogue of potassium, typically is used for this purpose. Thallium-201 is distributed to the myocardium in proportion to the magnitude of blood flow. After injection, an external detection device describes the distribution of the radioactive material. An ischemic area appears as a "cold spot" that lacks radioactive uptake. Thallium-201 can be used to assess myocardial blood flow during both rest and exercise.

Radionuclide ventriculography provides actual visualization of ventricular structures during systole and diastole and provides a means for evaluating ventricular function during rest and exercise. A radioisotope such as technetium-labeled albumin, which does not leave the capillaries but remains in the blood and is not bound to the myocardium, is used for this type of imaging. This type of nuclear imaging can be used to determine right and left ventricular volumes, ejection fractions, regional wall motion, and cardiac contractility. This method is also useful in the diagnosis of intracardiac shunts.

Radionuclide ventriculography can be performed using first-pass techniques in which the initial transit of the radioactive material is used in evaluating cardiovascular function. With this technique, the radionuclide bolus can be localized as it passes through the cardiac chambers, making it possible to visualize one side of the heart at a time. A second technique, called multigated acquisition (MUGA), produces computerized composite images of the heart that have been accumulated over hundreds of cardiac cycles. The distribution of these images is regulated by a gating signal from the ECG that controls the scintillation camera so that repeated images are taken during a designated portion of the cardiac cycle. This allows for calculation of left ventricular end-diastolic volumes, left ventricular end-systolic volumes, and left ventricular ejection fractions.

Cardiac Catheterization. Cardiac catheterization involves the passage of flexible catheters into the great vessels and chambers of the heart. In right heart catheterization, the catheters are inserted into a peripheral vein (usually the basilic or femoral) and then advanced into the right heart. The left heart catheter is inserted retrograde through a peripheral artery (usually the brachial or femoral) into the aorta and left heart. The cardiac catheterization laboratory, where the procedure is done, is equipped for viewing and recording fluoroscopic images of the heart and vessels in the chest and for measuring pressures within the heart and great vessels. There is also equipment for cardiac output studies and for obtaining samples of blood for blood gas analysis. Angiographic studies are made by injecting a contrast medium into the heart, so that an outline of the moving structures can be visualized and filmed. Coronary arteriography involves the injection of a contrast medium into the coronary arteries; this permits visualization of lesions within these vessels.

TREATMENT MEASURES

Measures for the treatment of myocardial ischemia usually are directed toward reducing the work demands of the heart or vessel constriction when coronary spasm or thrombosis is present. Treatment measures include nonpharmacologic and pharmacologic methods directed at reducing the preload and afterload work of the heart and measures such as percutaneous transluminal coronary angioplasty (PTCA) and coronary artery bypass surgery, which are used to improve blood flow to the myocardium.

Nonpharmacologic Methods. Nonpharmacologic treatment methods include the selective pacing of physical activities, stress reduction, avoidance of cold or other stresses that produce vasoconstriction, and weight reduction if obesity is present. Immediate cessation of activity often is sufficient to abort an anginal attack. Sitting down or standing quietly may be preferable to lying down because these positions decrease preload by producing pooling of blood in the lower extremities. Sudden exposure to cold increases vasoconstriction and afterload stress; thus, people with myocardial ischemia are cautioned against rapidly drinking large amounts of cold liquids (greater than 240 mL) and breathing extremely cold air. Anxiety often precipitates angina and silent myocardial ischemia because it causes an increase in both heart rate and blood pressure.

Pharmacologic Methods. Pharmacologic methods include the selective use of a combination of nitroglycerin and long-acting nitrates, β-adrenergic blocking drugs, and antiplatelet or anticoagulant drugs. Combination therapy decreases the incidence of symptoms and ischemia over single-drug therapy but has not conclusively reduced the incidence of myocardial infarction or death.[12]

Nitroglycerin (glycerol trinitrate) and long-acting nitrates such as isosorbide dinitrate and pentaerythritol tetranitrate promptly relieve anginal pain and silent myocardial ischemia. They are vasodilating drugs that relax both venous and arterial vessels.

Venous dilatation decreases venous return to the heart (preload), thereby reducing ventricular volume and compression of the subendocardial vessels, and returns the end-diastolic length of the ventricular muscle fibers to a more favorable position on the Starling curve. They also decrease the tension in the wall of the ventricle, so that less pressure is needed to pump blood, and reduce the amount of blood that needs to be pumped. Relaxation of the arteries reduces the pressure against which the heart must pump (afterload).

The extensive use of nitrates has led to the development of several delivery options. Nitroglycerin is absorbed into the portal circulation and destroyed by the liver when it is taken orally; therefore, it is administered by methods such as the sublingual (pill or spray) or topical (ointment or patch) route that bypass the portal circulation. Sublingual absorption is rapid, and pain relief usually begins in 30 seconds. Topical ointments have a duration of action of 4 to 6 hours. The adhesive patches have a longer duration of action (24 hours). Although they are costlier than the ointment, they increase compliance in many people. Topical forms of nitroglycerin are used prophylactically because of their prolonged action.

The β-*adrenergic blocking drugs* act as antagonists that block β-receptor–mediated functions of the sympathetic nervous system. There are two types of β-receptors: β₁- and β₂-receptors. β₁-receptors are found in the heart, and β₂-receptors are found in other parts of the body. Blockade of β₁-receptors in the heart reduces the heart rate, cardiac contractility, and myocardial oxygen consumption. Eight β-blocking drugs have been approved by the Food and Drug Administration (FDA): propranolol, nadolol, timolol, pindolol, acebutolol, labetalol, atenolol, and metoprolol. Of these drugs, atenolol and metoprolol are cardioselective in low doses (preferentially block β₁-receptors), whereas the other six drugs block both β₁- and β₂-receptors and are nonselective in their actions.

The *calcium-channel blocking drugs* sometimes are called calcium antagonists. Free intracellular calcium serves to link many membrane-initiated events with cellular responses, such as action potential generation and muscle contraction. Vascular smooth muscle lacks the sarcoplasmic reticulum and other structures necessary for intracellular storage of calcium; instead, it relies on the influx of calcium from the extracellular fluid into the cell to initiate and sustain contraction. In cardiac muscle, the slow inward calcium current contributes to the plateau of the action potential and to cardiac contractility. The slow calcium current is particularly important in the pacemaker activity of the sinoatrial (SA) node and the conduction properties of the atrioventricular (AV) node.

Several calcium-channel blocking drugs have

been approved by the FDA (diltiazem, nifedipine, verapamil, nicardipine, nitrendipine, bepredil, isradipine, and felodipine) for treatment of angina pectoris and cardiac dysrhythmias, cardiomyopathy, and hypertension. Although these eight drugs have different chemical structures and electrophysiologic effects, they are all effective in blocking a number of calcium-dependent functions; that is, they block the function of the calcium channels or enter the cell and substitute for calcium at intracellular receptor sites. Nicardipine, nitrendipine, and felodipine are considered vasoselective; they selectively dilate the vertebral, carotid, and coronary vessels, while having lesser vasodilatory effects on the mesenteric, femoral, and renal vessels, which significantly reduces the hypotensive effects often associated with the use of calcium-channel blocking drugs.

The therapeutic effect of the calcium antagonists results from coronary and peripheral artery dilatation and decreased myocardial metabolism associated with the decrease in myocardial contractility. The calcium-channel blockers also effectively reduce vasospasm in three quarters of patients with variant angina.[13] In clinical doses, verapamil and diltiazem depress the sinoatrial (SA) and atrioventricular (AV) nodes. The extent of slowing depends on the dose, route of administration, and concomitant use of other drugs. Verapamil may be administered intravenously for the termination of paroxysmal supraventricular tachycardia. Nifedipine, nicardipine, nitrendipine, and felodipine in the usual clinical doses have no direct effect on AV node conduction.

Percutaneous Transluminal Coronary Angioplasty and Coronary Artery Bypass Surgery. Percutaneous transluminal coronary angioplasty (PTCA) or coronary artery bypass surgery may be done to relieve coronary artery obstruction caused by atherosclerotic lesions. These procedures are indicated only when angiographic tests demonstrate that spasm occurs around an area of fixed obstruction but not in other coronary vessels or distal to the site of obstruction. They are not indicated for primary vasospastic angina because spontaneous remission of variant angina has been noted to occur 6 to 12 months after the acute phase, primarily in people with normal coronaries or with less than 70% diameter obstruction.[14, 15]

PTCA involves the dilatation of a stenotic coronary vessel. The procedure is similar to cardiac catheterization for coronary angiography. With PTCA, a double-lumen balloon dilatation catheter is introduced percutaneously into the femoral or brachial artery and then advanced under fluoroscopic view to the coronary ostium. It is then directed into the affected coronary artery and advanced until the balloon segment is within the stenotic area of the vessel.

Once in place, the balloon is inflated for 3 to 5 seconds using a pressure-controlled pump. Research suggests that the major mechanism of PTCA is "breaking," "cracking," "splitting," or "fracturing" of atherosclerotic plaque and stretching the plaque free wall segments of eccentric atherosclerotic lesions.[16]

PTCA is used to treat single-, double-, and triple-vessel disease with some or all stenoses amenable to dilation, acute coronary artery occlusion during a myocardial infarction, left main coronary artery disease, and stenosis of vein grafts from previous bypass surgery.[17, 18, 19] Although PTCA has about a 90% primary success rate, reclosure of dilated vessels occurs abruptly or restenoses within 6 months in about 20% to 40% of cases. Abrupt closure is more likely caused by arterial spasm or intimal dissection.

Because restenosis is common after PTCA, adjunctive therapies such as stents, lasers, and atherectomy are being tested. Studies on placement of a stent (hollow tube within the vessel) after PTCA show that the self-expanding stainless steel endoprosthesis has a dilating as well as a stenting role.[20, 21] The high incidence (7% to 48%) of subacute thrombosis and restenosis associated with stent usage is focusing subsequent research on new materials for stent construction and the timing for stent placement.[20] Although laser and thermal techniques have been useful additions to balloon dilation in peripheral vessels, additional research is needed to determine their effectiveness on coronary artery obstruction.[22] To date, laser and thermal techniques have been limited by inadequate delivery systems that create small recanalized channels and a high frequency of vessel perforation and thrombosis.[16] Atherectomy (cutting of the atherosclerotic plaque with a high-speed circular blade from within the vessel) is also being tested as a mechanical technique to treat restenosis lesions after PTCA.[16] Effectiveness studies have demonstrated comparable restenosis rates with atherectomy as compared with PTCA.[23]

The surgical treatment of coronary artery disease—*coronary artery bypass surgery*—remains popular for patients who have significant coronary artery disease uncontrolled by angioplasty or pharmacologic therapy. In this surgical procedure, revascularization of the myocardium is effected by placing a saphenous vein graft between the aorta and the affected coronary artery distal to the site of occlusion or by using the internal mammary artery as a means of revascularizing the left anterior descending artery or its branches. Figure 23-6 shows the placement of a saphenous vein graft and a mammary artery graft. Although it cannot be documented that this surgery significantly alters the progress of the disease, it does relieve pain, so that patients may have a more productive life. In three classic studies that examined the effect of bypass surgery on morbidity and mortality

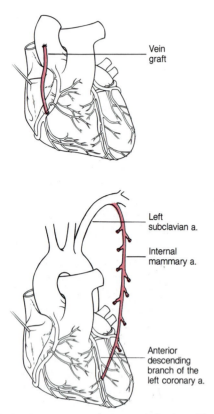

FIG. 23-6. Coronary artery revascularization. (**Top**) Saphenous vein bypass graft. The vein segment is sutured to the ascending aorta and the right coronary artery at a point distal to the occluding lesion. (**Bottom**) Mammary artery bypass. The mammary artery is anastomosed to the anterior descending left coronary artery, bypassing the obstructing lesion.

in people with mild to moderate angina, it was found that there was a significant reduction in angina, an improvement in exercise tolerance, and an improved quality of life. However, there was no significant decrease in myocardial infarction incidence.[24–27] Another study reported a 6-year chance of survival in 89% of bypass surgery patients who had a diagnosis of severe angina, two-vessel disease with at least one significant proximal lesion, and poor left ventricular function; this compared with a 76% chance of a 6-year survival in patients with similar pathology who underwent medical treatment.[28]

MYOCARDIAL INFARCTION

Myocardial infarction refers to the ischemic death of myocardial tissue associated with impaired blood flow sufficient to produce lethal cell injury. Obstructed blood flow can be caused by thrombosis, ulceration and hemorrhage in an atherosclerotic plaque, or prolonged vasospasm. It is also possible that a sudden increase in oxygen demand by the myocardium may contribute to the ischemic event.

Research has shown that 80% to 90% of transmural infarctions are caused by thrombosis of a coronary artery.[29] As discussed under unstable angina, it is possible that the event responsible for the infarct—vessel spasm or excessive myocardial oxygen demand—may also predispose to thrombus formation. Even though thrombosis may not be the initiating event in myocardial infarction, almost all patients dying of myocardial infarction have been found to have severe coronary atherosclerosis.[2]

An infarct may involve the endocardium, myocardium, epicardium, or a combination of these. An intramural infarct is one that is contained within the myocardium, whereas a transmural infarct involves all three layers of the heart. Most infarcts are transmural, involving the free wall of the left ventricle and the interventricular septum. The increased vulnerability of the left ventricle is probably related to its increased work demands. About 30% to 40% of infarcts affect the right coronary artery, 40% to 50% affect the left anterior descending artery, and the remaining 15% to 20% affect the left circumflex artery.[2] This distribution is depicted in Figure 23-7.

Although gross tissue changes are not apparent for hours after myocardial infarction (Table 23-1), it has been reported that the ischemic area ceases to function within a matter of minutes and that irreversible damage to cells occurs in about 40 minutes.

MANIFESTATIONS

The manifestations of myocardial infarction can be categorized into four groups: (1) pain and autonomic responses associated with the ischemic event; (2) weakness and signs related to impaired myocardial function; (3) dysrhythmias and ECG changes associated with changes in electrical conduction secondary to ischemia and death of myocardial cells; and (4) symptoms of inflammation and elevated serum enzyme levels indicative of tissue death.

The onset of myocardial infarction usually is abrupt, with pain as the significant symptom. The pain typically is severe and crushing, often described as being constricting, suffocating, or like "someone sitting on my chest." The pain usually is substernal, radiating to the left arm, neck, or jaw, although it may be experienced in other areas of the chest. Unlike that of angina, the pain associated with myocardial infarction is more prolonged and not relieved by rest or nitroglycerin, and narcotics frequently are required.

Gastrointestinal complaints are common. There may be a sensation of epigastric distress; nausea and vomiting may occur. These symptoms are thought to be related to the severity of the pain and vagal stimulation. The epigastric distress may be mistaken for

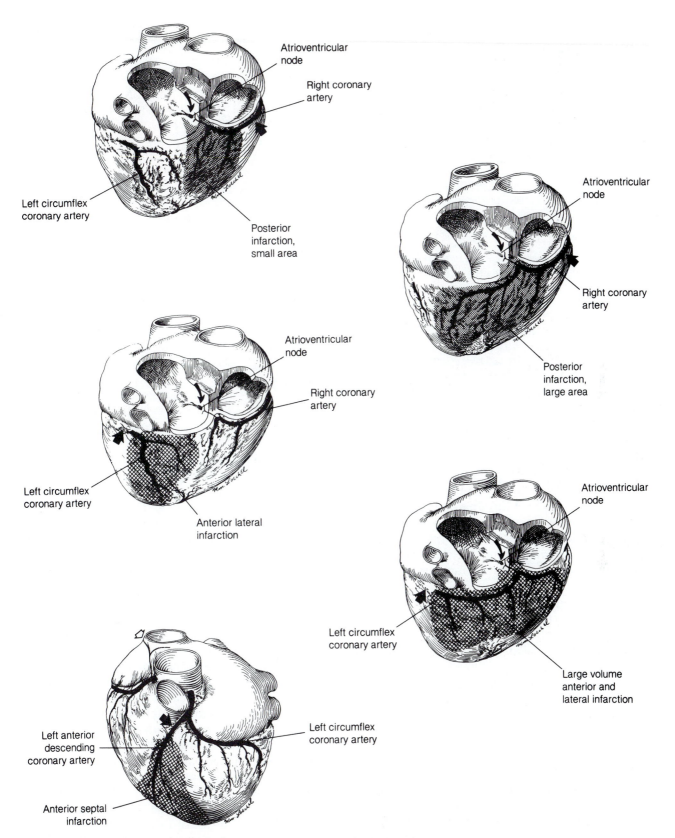

FIG. 23-7. Anatomy and distribution of the coronary arteries and the topography of infarction. *Shaded areas* represent extent of infarction. *Arrows* point to affected arteries. Percentages relate to persons with described involvement of right, left circumflex, or left anterior descending coronary artery. (James, T. N. [1962]. Arrhythmias and conduction disturbances in acute myocardial infarction. *American Heart Journal, 64* [3], 416)

TABLE 23-1. TISSUE CHANGES FOLLOWING MYOCARDIAL INFARCTION

TIME AFTER ONSET	GROSS TISSUE CHANGES
6–12 hours	No gross changes
18–24 hours	Pale to gray-brown Slight pallor of area
2–4 days	Necrosis of area is apparent. Area is yellow-brown in center and hyperemic around the edges
4–10 days	Area becomes soft; fatty changes in the center are well developed Hemorrhagic areas are present in the infarcted area. Rupture of the heart, when it occurs, happens during this period
10 days or more	Fibrotic (scar) tissue replacement and revascularization commences
6 weeks	Scar tissue replacement of necrotic tissue usually is complete; depends on size of infarct

(Developed from data in Robbins, S.L., Cotran, R., & Kumar, V. [1984]. *Pathologic basis of disease* [3rd ed., pp. 559–560]. Philadelphia: W.B. Saunders)

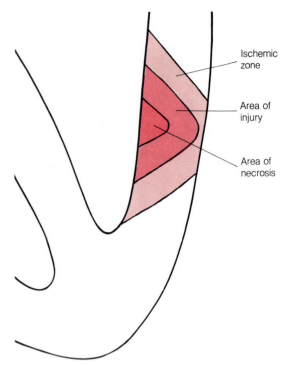

FIG. 23-8. Areas of tissue damage after myocardial infarction.

indigestion, and the patient may seek relief with antacids or other home remedies, which only delays getting medical attention. Complaints of fatigue and weakness, especially of the arms and legs, are common. Pain and sympathetic stimulation combine to give rise to tachycardia, anxiety, restlessness, and feelings of impending doom. The skin often is pale, cool, and moist. The impaired myocardial function may lead to hypotension and shock.

ECG changes may not be present immediately after the onset of symptoms, except as dysrhythmias. Premature ventricular contractions (PVCs) are common dysrhythmias after myocardial infarction. The occurrence of other dysrhythmias and conduction defects depends on the areas of the heart and conduction pathways that are included in the necrotic myocardium.

After a myocardial infarction, there usually are three zones of tissue damage: (1) a zone of myocardial tissue that becomes necrotic because of an absolute lack of blood flow; (2) a surrounding zone of injured cells, some of which will recover; and (3) an outer zone in which cells are ischemic and can be salvaged if blood flow can be reestablished (Fig. 23-8). The boundaries of these zones may change with time post infarct and with success of treatment measures to reestablish flow.

During the period of impaired blood flow, injured and ischemic cells revert to anaerobic metabolism with a resultant increase in lactic acid production, much of which is released into the local extracellular fluid. In addition, the necrotic cells become electrically inactive and their membranes become disrupted so that their intracellular contents, including potassium, are released into the surrounding extracellular fluid. This causes local areas of hyperkalemia, which can affect the membrane potentials of functioning myocardial cells. As a result of membrane injury and local changes in extracellular potassium and pH, some parts of the infarcted heart are unable to conduct or generate impulses, other areas are more difficult to excite, and still others are overly excitable. These different levels of membrane excitability in the necrotic, injured, and ischemic zones of the infarcted area set the stage for the development of dysrhythmias and conduction defects after myocardial infarction. Furthermore, each of these zones in the infarcted area conducts impulses differently. These changes in impulse conduction can be detected on the ECG and are the basis for determining whether an infarct has occurred and the area of the heart in which it is located. Typical ECG changes associated with death of myocardial tissue include prolongation of the Q wave, elevation of the ST segment, and inversion of the T wave. (The ECG changes are variable and complex, and interested readers and those intending to work in the coronary care unit are referred to specialty texts.)

In the infarcted area, cell death causes inflammation and the release of intracellular proteins and enzymes into the extracellular fluid. Fever and leukocytosis usually develop within about 24 hours and continue for 3 to 7 days. The erythrocyte sedimentation rate rises on the 2nd and 3rd days and remains elevated for 1 to 3 weeks. The level of myoglobin, an oxygen-carrying protein that normally is present in cardiac and skeletal muscle, elevates within 1 hour after myocardial cell death, with peak levels reached within 4 to 6 hours. Enzymes released include creatine phosphokinase (CPK), lactic dehydrogenase (LDH), and glutamic-oxaloacetic transaminase (GOT). As indicated in Figure 23-9, these proteins and enzymes become elevated at different times after infarction and provide useful diagnostic information. The protein myoglobin used in combination with the enzyme CPK (MB band) is reported to be a more reliable indicator for early detection of myocardial infarction than the ECG.[30]

COMPLICATIONS

The stages of recovery are closely related to the size of the infarct and the changes that have taken place within the infarcted area. Fibrous scar tissue lacks the contractile, elastic, and conductive properties of normal myocardial cells; hence, the residual effects as well as the complications are determined essentially by the extent and location of the injury. Among the complications of myocardial infarction are sudden death, heart failure and cardiogenic shock, pericarditis and Dressler's syndrome, thromboemboli, rupture of the heart, and ventricular aneurysms.

Sudden death due to coronary artery disease is death that occurs within 1 hour of the onset of symptoms. It usually is attributed to fatal dysrhythmias, which may occur without evidence of infarction. About 30% to 50% of people with acute myocardial infarction die of ventricular fibrillation within the first few hours after symptoms begin. Early hospitalization after onset of symptoms greatly improves chances of survival from sudden death. This is because the appropriate resuscitation facilities are immediately available when the fatal ventricular dysrhythmia occurs.

Depending on its severity, myocardial infarction has the potential for compromising the pumping action of the heart. Both heart failure (Chapter 24) and cardiogenic shock (Chapter 25) are dreaded complications of myocardial infarction.

Pericarditis may complicate the course of acute myocardial infarction. It usually appears on the 2nd or 3rd day after infarction. At this time, the patient experiences a new type of pain that is sharp and stabbing and aggravated with deep inspiration and positional changes. A pericardial rub may or may not be heard in all patients who have postinfarction pericarditis, and it often is transitory, usually resolving uneventfully. Dressler's syndrome describes signs and symptoms associated with pericarditis, pleurisy, and pneumonitis: fever, chest pain, dyspnea, and abnormal laboratory (elevated white blood cell count and sedimentation rate) and ECG findings. The symptoms may arise between 1 day and several weeks after infarction and are thought to represent a hypersensitivity response to tissue necrosis. Antiinflammatory agents or corticosteroid drugs may be used to reduce the inflammatory response.

Thromboemboli are a potential complication, arising either as venous thrombi or, occasionally, as a clot from the wall of the ventricle. Immobility and impaired cardiac function contribute to stasis of blood in the venous system. Elastic stockings, along with active and passive leg exercises, usually are included in the postinfarction treatment plan as a means of preventing thrombus formation. If a clot is detected on the wall of the ventricle (usually by echocardiography), treatment with anticoagulants is indicated.

The acute postmyocardial infarction period can

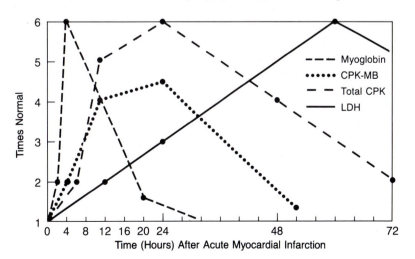

FIG. 23-9. Pattern of myoglobin and serum enzyme elevation (times normal) following acute myocardial infarction.

be complicated by rupture of the myocardium, the interventricular septum, or a papillary muscle. Myocardial rupture, occurring on the 7th to 10th day when the injured ventricular tissue is soft and weak, often is fatal. Necrosis of the septal wall or papillary muscle may also lead to the rupture of either of these structures with a worsening of ventricular performance. Surgical repair usually is indicated, but whenever possible it is delayed until the heart has had time to recover from the initial infarction. Vasodilator therapy and the aortic balloon counterpulsation pump may provide supportive assistance during this period.

An *aneurysm* is an outpouching of the ventricular wall. Scar tissue does not have the characteristics of normal myocardial tissue; when a large section of ventricular muscle is replaced by scar tissue, an aneurysm may develop (Fig. 23-10). This section of the myocardium does not contract with the rest of the ventricle during systole. Instead, it diminishes the pumping efficiency of the heart and increases the work of the left ventricle, thereby predisposing to heart failure. Ischemia in the surrounding area predisposes to the development of dysrhythmias, and stasis of blood within the aneurysm can lead to thrombus formation. Surgical resection often is corrective.

DIAGNOSIS AND TREATMENT

The diagnosis of myocardial infarction is based on the presence of prolonged chest pain and other signs of distress, changes in heart rate and blood pressure,

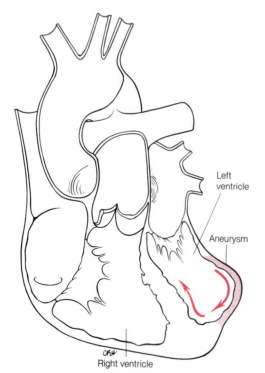

FIG. 23-10. Paradoxical movement of a ventricular aneurysm during systole.

ECG changes, and elevated serum myoglobin and cardiac enzyme levels. Nuclear imaging, specifically acute infarction imaging using technetium pyrophosphate, may be used to confirm the diagnosis.

The treatment methods for acute myocardial infarction are directed at (1) rapid recanalization of the occluded coronary artery; (2) pain relief, managing life-threatening complications; and (3) rehabilitation to maximize physical and psychological well-being during and after recovery. Controlled clinical trials have demonstrated that intravenously administered thrombolytic agents recanalize coronary arteries, reduce the size of the infarct, preserve left ventricular function, and reduce mortality.

The administration of oxygen augments the oxygen content of inspired air and increases the oxygen saturation of hemoglobin. Arterial oxygen levels may fall precipitously after myocardial infarction, and oxygen administration helps to maintain the oxygen content of the blood perfusing the coronary circulation.

The severe pain of myocardial infarction gives rise to anxiety and recruitment of autonomic nervous system responses, both of which increase the work demands of the heart. Morphine and meperidine (Demerol) often are given intravenously for pain relief because they have a rapid onset of action and the intravenous route does not elevate enzyme levels. Also, the intravenous route bypasses the variable rate of absorption of subcutaneous or intramuscular sites, which often are underperfused because of a decrease in cardiac output that occurs after infarction. Vasodilating drugs commonly are given because they decrease venous return (reduce preload) and arterial blood pressure (reduce afterload) and, thereby, reduce oxygen consumption. Morphine has vasodilator properties and often is used as the narcotic of choice in treatment of acute myocardial infarction. Intravenous nitroglycerin, another vasodilator, is also given to limit infarction size and is most effective if given with 4 hours of symptom onset.

Because sympathetic activity increases the metabolic activity of the myocardium and, consequently, myocardial oxygen consumption, β-adrenergic blocking drugs may be used to reduce sympathetic stimulation of the heart after myocardial infarction. These drugs decrease myocardial contractility (and cardiac work load), alter resting myocardial membrane potentials (and decrease dysrhythmia frequency), and may also redistribute coronary artery blood flow and improve myocardial blood supply.

Thrombolytic Agents. Thrombolytic drugs are used to dissolve blood and platelet clots; they react with plasminogen to create plasmin, which lyses fibrin clots and digests clotting factors V and VIII, prothrombin, and fibrinogen.[31] Several thrombolytic agents are approved by the FDA, including non–

fibrin-selective agents such as streptokinase, anisoylated plasminogen-streptokinase activator complex (APSAC), and urokinase and fibrin-selective agents such as recombinant tissue plasminogen activator (r-TPA) and prourokinase.

Intravenous or intracoronary artery infusion of thrombolytic agents is used as a treatment for people in whom myocardial infarctions are caused by intracoronary thrombi. These therapies act directly to improve myocardial blood supply. The treatment usually requires 20 to 40 minutes to reestablish blood flow; to be effective, the treatment must be done within 3 to 12 hours after the onset of the acute myocardial infarction period at a time when the heart tissue that is supplied by the affected vessel can still be salvaged. The patient must be a low-risk candidate for complications caused by bleeding.[32] When the drug is administered by intracoronary infusion, the procedure is carried out during cardiac catheterization using coronary arteriographic studies. Studies that have compared the three thrombolytic agents—streptokinase, APSAC, and r-TPA—found no significant differences between them in relation to mortality, morbidity, and left ventricular function. The optimal dose and the combination of thrombolytic agents with each other and with mechanical therapies are still under investigation.

PTCA and Bypass Surgery. PTCA and then, if needed, coronary artery bypass surgery may be used when the administration of a thrombolytic agent is contraindicated or ineffective.

It is now possible to open or dilate total and partial occlusions of coronary arteries with an inflatable balloon-tipped PTCA catheter. PTCA must be done within a few hours after the onset of infarction for maximal effectiveness. It more commonly is used after thrombolytic therapy to "salvage" or "rescue" the 20% to 25% of patients with persistently occluded arteries. Restenosis remains a problem, occurring in 20% to 40% of all patients who have been dilated.[18, 33] Further research is being done to test the effectiveness of additional therapies used in combination with PTCA, including stents, lasers, and atherectomy.[16] Studies have suggested that patients who present within the first 12 hours of symptom onset may benefit from elective rather than emergency PTCA after successful thrombolysis.[31, 32] Further studies on the progress of PTCA and thrombolytic therapy are in progress.

Although thrombolytic therapy and PTCA are the therapies of choice for acute myocardial infarction, emergency coronary bypass surgery is the next therapy of choice if the first two fail. Coronary artery bypass surgery is used to improve directly circulation to the myocardium, as described earlier in the chapter. Lower postoperative and long-term mortality rates have been reported for people with acute myocardial infarction who had coronary bypass surgery performed within 6 hours of symptom onset.[34]

Cardiac Rehabilitation Programs. Rehabilitation programs for people with myocardial infarction incorporate rest, exercise, and risk factor modification. Protecting the oxygen supply of the heart and decreasing the myocardial oxygen consumption as much as possible are concerns during the early treatment of myocardial infarction. Most people with myocardial infarction are maintained on bed rest for at least 24 hours, although the use of a bedside commode for elimination purposes may be allowed. This 24-hour period is followed by a gradual increase in activity, depending on the severity of the infarction and the presence of complications. Modifying the diet to include foods that are low in salt and cholesterol and easy to digest is another treatment measure used to decrease cardiac work. Stool softeners may be prescribed to prevent constipation and avoid straining with defecation.

An exercise program is an integral part of a cardiac rehabilitation program. It includes such activities as walking, swimming, and bicycling. These exercises involve changes in muscle length and rhythmic contractions of muscle groups. Most exercise programs are individually designed to meet each person's physical and psychological needs. The goal of the exercise program is to increase the maximal oxygen consumption by the muscle tissues, so that these people are able to perform more work at a lower heart rate and blood pressure. In addition to exercise, cardiac risk factor modification incorporates strategies for smoking cessation, weight loss, stress reduction, and control of hypertension and diabetes.

In summary, coronary artery disease usually is caused by atherosclerosis. It frequently is a silent disorder, and symptoms do not occur until the disease is far advanced. Myocardial ischemia occurs when there is a disparity between the metabolic needs of the myocardium and the amount of blood that the coronary arteries can deliver, and it may manifest itself as angina. There are three types of angina. Classic angina is associated with atherosclerosis of the coronary arteries, in which pain is precipitated by increased work demands on the heart and relieved by rest; variant angina is due to spasms of the coronary arteries; and unstable angina is an accelerated form of angina in which the pain occurs more frequently, is more severe, and lasts longer. Silent myocardial ischemia occurs without symptoms. Myocardial infarction refers to the ischemic death of myocardial tissue associated with obstructed blood flow in the coronary arteries owing to atherosclerosis or thrombosis. The infarct can involve the endocardium, myocardium, epicardium, or a combination of all three layers as well as the pericardium. The complications of myocardial infarction include potentially fatal dysrhythmias, heart failure, cardiogenic shock, pericarditis, thromboemboli, rupture of cardiac structures, and ventricular aneurysms.

■ DISORDERS OF CARDIAC RHYTHM AND CONDUCTION

The specialized cells in the conduction system manifest four inherent properties: (1) automaticity, (2) excitability, (3) conductivity, and (4) refractoriness (see Chapter 22). The term *dysrhythmia* refers to an alteration in cardiac rhythm. An alteration in any of these properties may produce dysrhythmias or conduction defects. There are many causes of altered cardiac rhythms, including congenital defects of the conduction system, degenerative changes, ischemia and myocardial infarction, fluid and electrolyte imbalances, and the effects of drug ingestion. Dysrhythmias are not necessarily pathologic; they can occur in the healthy as well as the diseased heart. Disturbances in cardiac rhythms exert their harmful effects by interfering with the heart's pumping ability. Rapid heart rates reduce the diastolic filling time, causing a subsequent decrease in the stroke volume output and in coronary perfusion while increasing the myocardial oxygen needs. Abnormally slow heart rates may impair the blood flow to vital organs such as the brain.

ELECTROCARDIOGRAPHY

ECG provides a practical, relatively inexpensive, and noninvasive method of viewing the electrical activity of the heart. No other area of cardiac function is so readily and easily monitored on a moment-by-moment basis. A description of the ECG is presented in this section of the chapter to help the reader understand disorders of cardiac rhythm and conduction.

The ECG is a recording of the electrical activity of the heart. The electric currents generated by the heart spread through the body to the skin, where they can be sensed by appropriately placed electrodes, amplified, and then recorded on an oscilloscope or chart recorder. The horizontal axis of the ECG measures time (seconds), and the vertical axis measures the amplitude of the impulse (millivolts). Each heavy vertical black line represents 0.2 second and each thin black line, 0.04 second (Fig. 23-11). On the horizontal axis, each heavy horizontal line represents 0.05 mV. The connections of the ECG are such that an upright deflection indicates a positive potential and a downward deflection indicates a negative potential.

The deflection points of an ECG are designated by the letters P, Q, R, S, and T. The P wave represents the SA node and atrial depolarization; the QRS complex (beginning of the Q wave to the end of the S wave) represents ventricular depolarization; and the T wave represents ventricular repolarization (see Chapter 22, Fig. 22-8). Atrial repolarization occurs during ventricular depolarization and is hidden in the QRS complex.

The process of impulse generation in the heart and other excitable tissue involves the movement or

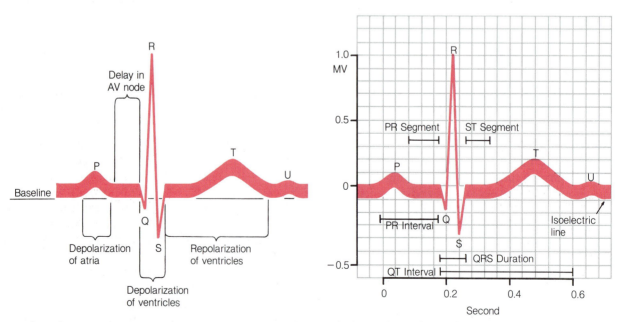

FIG. 23-11. Diagram of the electrocardiogram (lead II) and representative depolarization and repolarization of the atria and ventricle. The P wave represents atrial depolarization, the QRS complex ventricular depolarization, and the T wave ventricular repolarization. Atrial repolarization occurs during ventricular depolarization and is hidden under the QRS complex.

flow of electrically charged ions at the level of the cell membrane. The ECG represents the sum of all these impulses as they are conducted through the body fluids to the skin surface. The ECG records three types of electrical events: the resting membrane potential, depolarization, and repolarization. During the resting state, the membrane is impermeable to the flow of charge and charges of opposite polarity (positive on the outside and negative on the inside) become aligned along the membrane (Fig. 23-12). Depolarization occurs when the cell membrane becomes selectively permeable to a current-carrying ion such as sodium. During the process of repolarization, electrical charges move inward across the cell membrane and the membrane potential becomes reversed so that the inside becomes positive in relation to the outside. Repolarization involves the reestablishment of the resting membrane potential. During repolarization, membrane conductance or permeability for potassium becomes greatly increased, allowing the positively charged potassium ions to move outward across the membrane; this removes positive charges from inside the membrane, and the cell membrane again becomes negative on the inside and positive on the outside. The sodium–potassium membrane pump also assists in repolarization by pumping positively charged sodium ions out across the cell membrane.

The ECG records the potential difference in charge (in millivolts) that occurs between two electrodes as the depolarization and repolarization waves move through the heart and are conducted to the skin surface. The shape of the recorder tracing is determined by the direction in which the impulse spreads through the heart muscle in relation to electrode placement. A depolarization wave that moves toward the recording electrode registers as a positive, or upward, deflection. Conversely, if the impulse moves away from the recording electrode, the deflection is downward, or negative. When there is no flow of charge between electrodes, the potential is zero, and a straight line is recorded at the baseline of the chart. The ECG recorder is much like a camera in that it can record different views of the electrical activity of the heart, depending where the recording electrode is placed.

Conventionally, 12 leads are recorded for a diagnostic ECG, each viewing the electrical forces of the heart from a different position on the body's surface. Six limb leads view the electrical forces as they pass through the heart on the frontal plane of the body, and six chest leads view the electrical forces on the horizontal plane. The electrodes are attached to the four extremities or representative areas on the body (near the shoulders and lower chest or abdomen). The electrical potential recorded from any one extremity should be the same no matter where the electrode is placed on the extremity. Chest electrodes are moved to different positions on the chest. The right limb lead is used as a ground electrode. Additional electrodes may be applied to other areas of the body, such as the back, when indicated.

MECHANISMS OF DYSRHYTHMIAS AND CONDUCTION DISORDERS

Automaticity is the ability of certain cells of the conduction system to initiate spontaneously an impulse or action potential. The SA node has an inherent discharge rate of 60 to 100 times a minute; it normally acts as the pacemaker of the heart because it reaches the threshold for excitation before other parts of the conduction system have recovered sufficiently to be depolarized. If the sinus node fires more slowly or the SA node conduction is blocked, another site that is capable of automaticity takes over as pacemaker. Other regions that are capable of automaticity include the atrial fibers that have plateau-type action potentials, the AV node, the bundle of His, and the bundle-branch Purkinje fibers. These pacemakers have a slower rate of discharge. The AV node has an inherent firing rate of 40 to 60 times per minute and the Purkinje system, 30 to 40 times per minute. Even though the SA node is functioning properly, other cardiac cells can assume accelerated properties of automaticity and begin to initiate impulses when they are injured, oxygen-deprived, or exposed to certain chemicals or drugs.

An *ectopic pacemaker* is an excitable focus outside the normally functioning SA node. These pacemakers can reside in other parts of the conduction system or in muscle cells of the atria or ventricles. A premature contraction occurs when an ectopic pacemaker initiates a beat. Premature contractions do not follow the normal conduction pathways, they are not coupled with normal mechanical events, and they

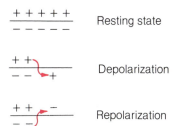

FIG. 23-12. The flow of charge during impulse generation in excitable tissue. During the resting state, opposite charges are separated by the cell membrane. Depolarization represents the flow of charge across the membrane, and repolarization the return of the membrane potential to its resting state.

often render the heart refractory or incapable of responding to the next normal impulse arising in the SA node. They occur without incident in people with healthy hearts in response to sympathetic stimulation or to stimulants such as caffeine. In the diseased heart, the premature contraction may lead to more serious dysrhythmias.

Excitability describes the ability of a cell to respond to an impulse and generate an action potential. Myocardial cells that have been injured or replaced by scar tissue do not possess normal excitability. For example, cells within the ischemic zone become depolarized during the acute phase of myocardial ischemia. These ischemic cells remain electrically coupled to the adjacent nonischemic area; thus, current from the ischemic zone can induce reexcitation of cells in the nonischemic zone.

Conductivity is the ability to conduct impulses, and *refractoriness* is the inability to respond to an incoming stimulus. The refractory period of cardiac muscle is the interval in the repolarization period during which an excitable cell has not recovered sufficiently to be reexcited (see Chapter 22, Fig. 22-10). Disturbances in either conductivity or refractoriness predispose to dysrhythmias.

An important condition in the development of dysrhythmias is the phenomenon of reentry. Reentry occurs when an impulse reexcites an area through which it previously traveled, disrupting the normal conduction sequence. For reentry to occur, there must be a unidirectional, or one-way, block in one limb of a conduction pathway (Fig. 23-13). When this occurs, the impulse is conducted through the unaffected limb of the pathway and then reenters the affected limb from the reverse direction, traveling through damaged or scarred myocardial tissue and creating the so-called *late potentials* that can be detected with a specially filtered signal-averaged ECG. If sufficient time has elapsed for the refractory period in the reentered area to have ended, a self-perpetuating circuitous-type movement can be initiated. The functional components of a reentry circuit can be large and include an entire specialized conduction system, or it can be microscopic; it can include myocardial tissue, AV nodal cells, or junctional cells.

TYPES OF DYSRHYTHMIAS

SINUS NODE DYSRHYTHMIAS

The normal rhythm of the heart with the sinus node in command is regular and ranges from 60 to 100 beats per minute. On the ECG, a P wave may be observed to precede every QRS complex.

Alterations in the function of the SA node lead to a change in the rate and regularity of the heartbeat.

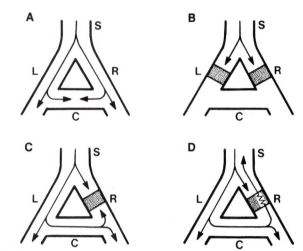

FIG. 23-13. The role of unidirectional block on reentry. (**A**) An excitation wave traveling down a single bundle (S) of fibers continues down the left (L) and right (R) branches. The depolarization wave enters the connecting branch (C) from both ends and is extinguished at the zone of collision. (**B**) The wave is blocked in the L and R branches. (**C**) Bidirectional block exists in branch R. (**D**) Unidirectional block exists in branch R. The antegrade impulse is blocked, but the retrograde impulse is conducted through and reenters bundle S. (Berne, R. M., & Levy, M. N. [1988]. *Physiology* [2nd ed.]. St. Louis: C.V. Mosby)

Sinus bradycardia describes a slow heart rate (less than 60 beats per minute). In sinus bradycardia, a P wave precedes each QRS; this confirms that the impulse is originating in the SA node rather than in a part of the conduction system that has a slower heart rate. Vagal stimulation decreases the firing rate of the SA node and conduction through the AV node to cause a decrease in the heart rate. A slow resting rate of 50 to 60 beats per minute may be normal in a well-trained athlete who maintains a large stroke volume. *Sinus tachycardia* refers to a rapid heart rate (100 to 160 beats per minute) that has its origin in the SA node (a P wave precedes every QRS complex). Sympathetic stimulation or withdrawal of vagal tone incites an increase in heart rate. Sinus tachycardia is normal during fever and exercise and in situations that incite sympathetic stimulation. *Sinus dysrhythmia* is a condition in which the heart rate speeds up and then slows down in an irregular but cyclic pattern; it often is associated with respiration and alterations in autonomic control. It is common and normal in young people. *Sinus arrest* refers to failure of the SA node to discharge and results in an irregular pulse. An escape rhythm develops as another pacemaker takes over. Sinus arrest may result in prolonged periods of asystole and often predisposes to other dysrhythmias. The causes of sinus arrest include disease of the SA node, digitalis toxicity, and excess vagal tone. The *sick sinus syndrome* is a term that describes a condition of periods of bradycardia alternating with tachycardia. The bradycardia is caused by disease of the sinus node (or other intraatrial conduction pathways) and the tachycardia, by paroxysmal atrial or junctional dysrhythmias.

DYSRHYTHMIAS THAT ORIGINATE IN THE ATRIA

The impulse from the SA node passes through the conductive pathways in the atria to the AV node. *Premature atrial contraction* can originate in the atrial conduction pathways or in atrial muscle cells. This contraction is transmitted to the ventricle as well as back to the SA node. The retrograde transmission to the SA node often interrupts the timing of the next sinus beat so that a pause occurs between the two normally conducted beats. *Atrial flutter* describes an atrial rate of 160 to 350 beats per minute. There is a delay in conduction through the AV node, and the ventricles respond to every second, third, or fourth beat (*e.g.*, when conduction from the atria to the ventricles is 3 : 1, an atrial flutter rate of 225 results in a ventricular rate of only 75). *Atrial fibrillation* describes an atrial rate in excess of 350, usually 450 to 600 beats per minute. Here, conduction through the AV node is totally disorganized, the peripheral pulse is grossly irregular, and a pulse deficit can be observed. The pulse deficit is the difference between the apical and peripheral pulses. In atrial fibrillation, the rate may be such that there is not sufficient stroke output with some beats to be felt at the wrist, causing a difference between the apical heartbeat and the peripheral pulses. Atrial fibrillation can occur as the result of left atrial distention caused by mitral stenosis. This is the most common atrial dysrhythmia in elderly people. Atrial fibrillation predisposes to thrombus formation in the atria, with subsequent risk of formation of systemic emboli. Figure 23-14 shows the ECG changes that occur with atrial dysrhythmias.

During rest and moderate activity, ventricular filling is not dependent on atrial contraction. Atrial contraction contributes only about 25% to 30% of cardiac reserve; therefore, atrial dysrhythmias may go unnoticed unless they are transmitted to the ventricle. In people with marginal cardiac output, the loss of atrial function may result in a sufficient decrease in cardiac output to produce symptoms.

DISORDERS OF AV CONDUCTION

The AV node provides the only connection for transmission of impulses between the atrial and ventricular conduction systems. Junctional fibers in the AV node have high resistance characteristics, which cause a delay in the transmission of impulses from the atria to the ventricles; this allows for filling of the

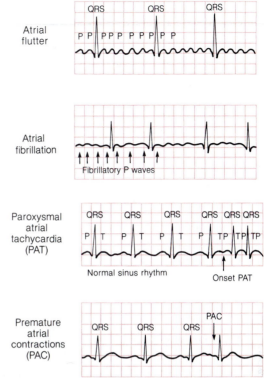

FIG. 23-14. Electrocardiographic (ECG) tracings of atrial dysrhythmias. Atrial flutter (*first tracing*) is characterized by the presence of atrial flutter (P) waves occurring at a rate of 160 to 350 beats per minute. The ventricular rate remains regular because of the conduction of every sixth atrial contraction. In atrial fibrillation (*second tracing*) there is an atrial rate in excess of 350 beats per minute; the P waves are no longer distinct and the ventricular rate becomes irregular. The *third tracing* illustrates paroxysmal atrial tachycardia (PAT), preceded by a normal sinus rhythm. The *fourth tracing* illustrates a premature atrial contraction (PAC).

ventricles and protects them from abnormally rapid rates that arise in the atria. Conduction defects most commonly are due to fibrosis or scar tissue in fibers of the conduction system. Conduction defects of the AV node can also occur as the result of digitalis toxicity.

Heart block occurs when conduction through the AV node is delayed or interrupted. It may occur in the AV nodal fibers or in the AV bundle (bundle of His), which is continuous with the Purkinje conduction system that supplies the ventricles. The PR interval on the ECG corresponds with the time that it takes for the cardiac impulse to travel from the SA node to the ventricular pathways; the normal range is 0.12 to 0.20 second.

A *first-degree heart block* occurs when conduction through the AV pathway is delayed and the PR interval is longer than 0.20 second (Fig. 23-15). In *second-degree block*, one or more of the atrial impulses are blocked. There are two types of second-degree block: the *Mobitz type I*, or *Wenckebach phenomenon*, describes

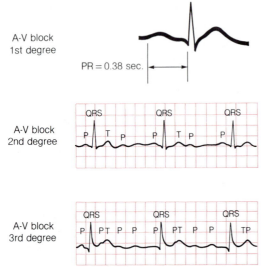

FIG. 23-15. Electrocardiographic (ECG) changes that occur with alterations in AV node conduction. The *top tracing* shows the prolongation of the PR interval, which is characteristic of first-degree AV block. The *middle tracing* illustrates Mobitz type II second-degree AV block, in which the conduction of one or more P waves is blocked. In third-degree AV block (*bottom tracing*), complete block in conduction of impulses through the AV node occurs, and the atria and ventricles each develop their own rate of impulse generation.

a progressive increase in the PR interval until the point at which one P wave is blocked; the *Mobitz type II block* (see Fig. 23-15) describes the situation in which there is a sudden block in one or more atrial impulses without an antecedent prolongation of the PR interval. In a Mobitz type II block, the ventricular rate is regular and reflects the degree of block; this type of block is significant because it often precedes complete heart block.

Third-degree, or *complete*, heart block occurs when the conduction link between the atria and the ventricles is lost (see Fig. 23-15); the atria continue to beat at a normal rate and the ventricles develop their own rate, which normally is slow (30 to 40 beats per minute). Complete heart block causes a decrease in cardiac output with possible periods of syncope (called a Stokes-Adams attack). Most persons with complete heart block require a pacemaker.

JUNCTIONAL DYSRHYTHMIAS

The AV node can act as a pacemaker in the event the SA node fails to initiate an impulse. Junctional fibers in the AV node or bundle can also serve as ectopic pacemakers, producing *premature junctional contractions*.

DISORDERS OF VENTRICULAR RHYTHM AND CONDUCTION

The junctional fibers in the AV node join with the bundle of His, which divides to form the right and left bundle branches; they then branch to form the Purkinje fibers, which supply the walls of the ventricles (see Chapter 22, Fig. 22-7). On leaving the junctional fibers, the cardiac impulse travels through the AV bundle, moves down the right and left bundle branches that lie beneath the endocardium on either side of the septum, and then spreads out through the walls of the ventricles. Interruption of impulse conduction through the bundle branches, called a *bundle-branch block*, usually does not cause alterations in the rhythm of the heartbeat; this is because the impulse typically is conducted along an alternate or detour pathway. It does, however, take longer for the impulse to be transmitted through the Purkinje system when there is a conduction defect; this produces changes in the QRS complex of the ECG and causes the QRS complex to be wider than the normal 0.08 to 0.12 second. The left bundle branch is divided into two parts called fascicles. A *hemiblock* refers to interruption of impulse conduction of one of the fascicles of the left bundle branch.

Dysrhythmias that arise in the ventricles commonly are considered more serious than those that arise in the atria because they afford the potential for interfering with the pumping action of the heart. A *premature ventricular contraction (PVC)* is caused by a ventricular ectopic pacemaker. After a PVC, the ventricle usually is not able to repolarize sufficiently to respond to the next impulse that arises in the SA node; this causes the compensatory pause, which occurs while the ventricle waits to reestablish its previous rhythm (Fig. 23-16). With a PVC, the diastolic volume usually is insufficient for ejection of blood into the arterial system; this causes a skipped beat. In the absence of heart disease, PVCs typically are not of great clinical significance. They can also occur in digitalis toxicity and in myocardial ischemia and infarction. A special pattern of PVC called *ventricular bigeminy* occurs in such a way that each normal beat is followed by or paired with a PVC. This pattern often is an indication of digitalis toxicity or heart disease. The occurrence of frequent PVCs in the diseased heart predisposes to other, more serious dysrhythmias, including ventricular tachycardia and fibrillation. *Ventricular tachycardia* describes a ventricular rate of 160 to 250 beats per minute; it is dangerous because it causes a reduction in the diastolic filling time to the point at which the cardiac output is severely diminished or nonexistent (see Fig. 23-16). In *ventricular fibrillation*, the ventricle quivers but does

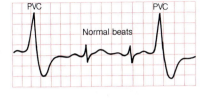

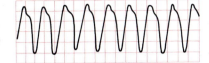

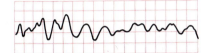

Premature ventricular contractions (PVC)

Normal beats

Ventricular tachycardia

Ventricular fibrillation

FIG. 23-16. Electrocardiographic (ECG) tracings of ventricular dysrhythmias. (*Top tracing*) Premature ventricular contractions (PVCs) originate from an ectopic focus in the ventricles, causing a distortion of the QRS complex. Because the ventricle usually cannot repolarize sufficiently to respond to the next impulse that arises in the SA node, a PVC is followed by a compensatory pause. (*Middle tracing*) Ventricular tachycardia is characterized by a rapid ventricular rate of 160 to 250 beats per minute and the absence of P waves. (*Bottom tracing*) In ventricular fibrillation there are no regular or effective ventricular contractions, and the ECG tracing is totally disorganized.

not contract; with the cessation of cardiac output, no pulse is palpable or audible.

DIAGNOSIS AND TREATMENT

The diagnosis of disorders of cardiac rhythm and conduction usually is made on the basis of the ECG. Further clarification of conduction defects and cardiac dysrhythmias can be done using electrophysiologic studies.

A resting ECG records the impulses of the heart as they occur during a limited period of time and during periods of inactivity. The resting ECG is the first approach to the clinical diagnosis of disorders of cardiac rhythm and conduction; it is limited, however, to events that occur during the period the ECG is being monitored.

Signal-averaged ECG is a special type of ECG that is used to detect late action potentials that are thought to originate from slow-conducting areas of the myocardium. Signal-averaging works by averaging together multiple QRS waveforms and creating a tracing that is an average of all the repetitive signals. The presence of late potentials indicates high risk for the development of sudden death.

Holter monitoring is one form of long-term mon-

itoring during which a person wears a 12-lead ECG recording device for 24 hours. During this time, the person also keeps a diary of his or her activities, which are later correlated with the ECG recording. Holter monitoring is useful for documenting rhythm and conduction abnormalities in people who have predictable symptoms.

Intermittent ECG recorders are also used in the diagnosis of dysrhythmias and conduction defects. With intermittent ECG recording, a monitoring lead ECG recording device, which either records or transmits by telephone the ECG to a recording machine, is worn. Some of these recorders have a patient-activated memory component to record the electrical events that precede the onset of symptoms. These types of ECG recordings are useful in people who have transient and unpredictable symptoms.

The exercise stress test (see Chapter 9) is useful in determining exercise-induced disorders of cardiac rhythm, particularly PVCs, because these dysrhythmias indicate a poorer prognosis in people with known coronary disease and recent myocardial infarction. Bicycle and treadmill exercise are equally effective in detecting exercise-induced PVCs.

An *electrophysiologic study* involves the passage of flexible catheters into the great vessels and chambers of the heart. Two or more multipolar catheters are inserted into the femoral, subclavian, or antecubital veins and positioned with fluoroscopy into the right atrium and right ventricle. Multipolar catheters can also be inserted into the left heart chambers by way of a peripheral artery. The catheter tips are positioned at several sites, and the endocardium is stimulated. Multiple atrial, AV junctional, and ventricular ECGs are recorded during the electrical stimulation. The catheters may also be used to pace the heart as part of the test. Overdrive pacing, cardioversion, or defibrillation may be necessary during the test to terminate tachycardia induced during the stimulation procedures. Electrophysiologic tests may be done to identify the location of additional electrical pathways between the ventricles and the atrial or ventricular tissue sites in which tachycardias originate. These tests may also be done repeatedly to test patient responses to drugs, devices such as implantable defibrillators, and surgical interventions used in the treatment of dysrhythmias.

The treatment of cardiac rhythm or conduction disorders is directed toward controlling the dysrhythmia, correcting the cause, and preventing more serious or fatal dysrhythmias. Correction may involve simply adjusting an electrolyte disturbance or withholding a medication such as digitalis. Preventing more serious dysrhythmias often involves drug therapy, electrical stimulation, or surgical intervention.

Antidysrhythmic drugs act by modifying disordered formation and conduction of impulses that induce cardiac muscle contraction. These drugs are classified into four groups: class I (IA, IB, IC), II, III, and IV. Class I drugs act by blocking the fast sodium channels. Class IA (quinidine, procainamide, disopyramide, moricizine) decrease automaticity by depressing phase 4 of the action potential, decrease conductivity by moderately prolonging phase 0, and prolong repolarization by extending phase 3 of the action potential (see Chapter 22 for a discussion of the phases of the cardiac action potential). Class IB drugs (lidocaine, phenytoin, tocainide, mexiletine, aprindine) decrease automaticity by depressing phase 4 of the action potential, have little effect on conductivity, decrease refractoriness by decreasing phase 2, and shorten repolarization by decreasing phase 3. Class IC drugs (flecainide, encainide, propafenone) decrease conductivity by markedly depressing phase 0 of the action potential but have little effect on refractoriness or repolarization. Class II drugs (propranolol, nadolol, atenolol, timolol, acebutolol, metoprolol, pindolol, esmolol) are β-adrenergic blocking drugs that act by blunting the effect of sympathetic nervous system stimulation on the heart. These drugs decrease automaticity by depressing phase 4 of the action potential; they also decrease heart rate and cardiac contractility. Class III drugs (amiodarone, bretyllium, sotalol) act by extending the action potential. They prolong repolarization by extending phase 3 of the action potential. Class IV drugs (verapamil, diltiazem, nifedipine, bepridil, nitrendipine, felodipine, isradipine, nicardipine) act by blocking the slow calcium channels, thereby depressing phase 4 and lengthening phases 1 and 2.

Two other types of antidysrhythmic drugs, the cardiac glycosides and adenosine, are not included in this classification schema. The cardiac glycosides (*e.g.*, digitalis drugs) slow the heart rate and are used in the management of dysrhythmias such as atrial tachycardia, atrial flutter, and atrial fibrillation. Adenosine, an endogenous nucleoside that is present in every human cell, is used for emergency intravenous treatment of paroxysmal supraventricular tachycardia involving the AV node. It interrupts AV node conduction and slows SA node firing.

The correction of conduction defects, bradycardias, and tachycardias can involve the use of an electronic pacemaker, cardioversion, or defibrillation. Electrical interventions can be used in both emergency and elective situations. A pacemaker is an electronic device that delivers an electrical stimulus to the heart. It is used to initiate heartbeats in situations when the normal pacemaker of the heart is defective or in complete heart block in which the rate of cardiac contraction and consequent cardiac output is inade-

quate to perfuse vital tissues. A pacemaker may be used as a temporary or a permanent measure. Internal temporary pacing involves the passage, under fluoroscopic or ECG direction, of a venous catheter with electrodes on its tip into the right atrium or ventricle, where it is wedged against the endocardium. External temporary pacing involves the placement of large patch electrodes on the chest wall. Permanent pacing requires the direct insertion of pacemaker electrodes into the epicardium or the transvenous insertion into the apex of the right ventricle, where the electrode comes in contact with the endocardium.

Defibrillation and synchronized cardioversion are two other reliable methods for treating ventricular fibrillation and are two of the effective methods of treating ventricular tachycardias as well. Defibrillation and synchronized cardioversion can be delivered externally through large patch electrodes on the chest or internally through small patch electrodes sewn into the epicardium or transvenous wires placed in the right ventricle. The electric current from the defibrillator or cardioverter interrupts the disorganized impulses, allowing the SA node to regain control of the heart. Electrical devices that combine antitachycardial pacing, cardioversion, defibrillation, and bradycardial pacing are under investigation.

Surgical interventions such as coronary artery bypass surgery, ventriculotomy, endocardial resection, radiofrequency ablation, and cryoablation may be used to improve myocardial oxygenation, remove dysrhythmogenic foci, or alter electrical conduction pathways. Coronary artery bypass surgery improves myocardial oxygenation. Ventriculotomy involves the removal of aneurysm tissue and the resuturing of the myocardial walls to eliminate the paradoxical ventricular movement and the foci of dysrhythmias. In endocardial resection, endocardial tissue that has been identified as dysrhythmogenic through the use of diagnostic tests is peeled away. Radiofrequency ablation uses radiofrequency energy waves to destroy defective or aberrant electrical conduction pathways. Cryoablation causes freezing and necrosis of defective or aberrant electrical conduction pathways. Both ablation techniques are used to treat recurrent, life-threatening supraventricular or ventricular tachycardias. Other surgical techniques, including transvenous electrocoagulation and laser ablation, are under investigation as potential treatment interventions for recurrent tachycardias.

In summary, disorders of cardiac rhythm arise as the result of disturbances in impulse generation or conduction of impulses in the heart. Cardiac dysrhythmias are not necessarily pathologic—they occur in healthy as well as diseased hearts. Sinus dysrhythmias have their origin in the SA node. They include sinus bradycardia (heart rate less than 60 beats per minute); sinus tachycardia (heart rate 100 to 160 beats per minute); sinus dysrhythmia, in which the heart rate speeds up and slows down; sinus arrest, in which there are prolonged periods of asystole; and the sick sinus syndrome, a condition characterized by periods of bradycardia alternating with tachycardia. Atrial dysrhythmias arise from alterations in impulse generation that occur within the conduction pathways or muscle of the atria. They include atrial premature contractions, atrial flutter (atrial depolarization rate of 160 to 350 beats per minute), and atrial fibrillation (atrial depolarization rate in excess of 350 beats per minute). Atrial dysrhythmias often go unnoticed unless they are transmitted to the ventricles. Alterations in the conduction of impulses through the AV node lead to disturbances in the transmission of impulses from the atria to the ventricles. There can be a delay in transmission (first-degree heart block), failure to conduct one or more impulses (second-degree heart block), or complete failure to conduct impulses between the atria and the ventricles (third-degree heart block). Conduction disorders of the bundle of His, called bundle-branch blocks, cause a widening of and changes in the configuration of the QRS complex of the ECG. Because of their potential for interfering with the pumping action of the heart, dysrhythmias that arise in the ventricles usually are considered more serious than those that arise in the atria. A PVC is caused by a ventricular ectopic pacemaker. Ventricular tachycardia is characterized by a ventricular rate of 160 to 250 beats per minute. Ventricular fibrillation (ventricular rate in excess of 350 beats per minute) is a fatal dysrhythmia unless it is successfully treated with defibrillation.

■ CARDIOMYOPATHIES

The cardiomyopathies are a group of disorders that affect the heart muscle. They can develop as either primary or secondary disorders. The primary cardiomyopathies, which are discussed in this chapter, are heart muscle diseases of unknown cause. Secondary cardiomyopathies are conditions in which the cardiac abnormality is due to another cardiovascular disease, such as myocardial infarction. In the United States, an estimated 1% of cardiac deaths can be attributed to primary cardiomyopathies. The onset of the primary cardiomyopathies often is silent, and the symptoms do not occur until the disease is well advanced. The diagnosis is suspected when a young, previously healthy normotensive person develops cardiomegaly and heart failure.

The International Society and Federation of Cardiology and the World Health Organization have categorized the primary cardiomyopathies into three groups: (1) dilated, (2) hypertrophic, and (3) restrictive (Fig. 23-17).[35]

DILATED CARDIOMYOPATHIES

The dilated, or congestive, cardiomyopathies are recognized by the dilatation of the heart chambers (often all four) and the impaired pumping function of

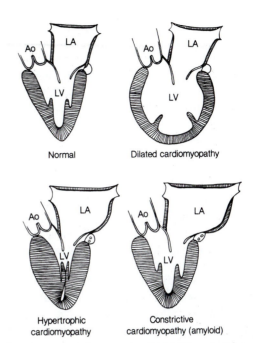

FIG. 23-17. The various types of cardiomyopathies compared with the normal heart. (Roberts, W. C., & Ferrans, V.J. [1975]. Pathologic anatomy of the cardiomyopathies. *Human Pathology, 6,* 289)

the ventricles, with increases in both end-systolic and end-diastolic volumes of the heart. There is a profound reduction in the left ventricular ejection fraction (the ratio of stroke volume to end-diastolic volume) to 40% or less, compared with a normal value of about 67%. Microscopically, there is evidence of scarring and atrophy of myocardial cells. The ventricular wall usually is thickened, and mural thrombi are common, most often in the left ventricle but also in the right ventricle or either atrium.

The cause of dilated cardiomyopathy is unknown. Infection and transient microvascular spasm of the precapillary arterioles leading to focal myocardial necrosis are proposed as two theories for the underlying cause of dilated cardiomyopathy.[36] The disease itself probably is the result of several factors acting in concert in a susceptible person, with infections, the puerperium, coexisting coronary artery disease, toxins such as alcohol, and other causes acting as risk factors.

There is considerable evidence that acute alcohol consumption reduces cardiac contractility and can produce dysrhythmias and conduction disorders. In the heart, the presence of alcohol or its metabolite, acetaldehyde, interferes with a number of cellular functions that involve the transport and binding of calcium. With chronic alcohol consumption, the toxic effects of alcohol on the myocardium can persist after the alcohol has been metabolized.

Although it is rare, congestive cardiomyopathy can also develop during the peripartum period. Most cases of peripartal cardiomyopathy have their onset within 5 weeks after giving birth, but a few women begin to develop symptoms during the last month of pregnancy.[37] The incidence of peripartal cardiomyopathy is significantly higher in black women over age 30, in a third or subsequent pregnancy, and in the presence of twins or toxemia.[37,38] The cause of the condition is unknown.

There are two possible outcomes of peripartal cardiomyopathy. In about half the cases, the heart returns to normal within 6 months and the chances for long-term survival are good. In these women, heart failure returns only during subsequent pregnancies. In the other half of the cases, the cardiomegaly persists, and the prognosis is poor and death is probable if another pregnancy occurs.

In dilated cardiomyopathy, heart failure occurs because the impairment of left ventricular ejection requires that the left ventricle dilate (Starling mechanism) to compensate for the fall in stroke volume that would otherwise occur. Dilation of the heart and pump failure may be present for years before symptoms are noted. Once symptoms have developed, the course of the disorder is distinguished by a propensity for development of heart failure, embolism, ventricular dysrhythmias, and poor prognosis. Three fourths of people die within 4 to 5 years of the time of diagnosis if dysrhythmias are left untreated. One fourth, however, do well for some unexplained reason. The most striking symptoms are right- and left-sided heart failure, dyspnea on exertion, paroxysmal nocturnal dyspnea, orthopnea, weakness, fatigue, ascites, and peripheral edema. On physical examination, an enlarged apical beat with the presence of a third and fourth heart sound, and a murmur associated with regurgitation of one or both AV valves frequently are found. The systolic pressure is either normal or low, and the peripheral pulses often are of low amplitude. Pulsus alternans, in which the pulse regularly alternates between weaker and stronger volume, may be present. Basilar rales frequently are present. Sinus tachycardia, atrial fibrillation, and complex ventricular dysrhythmias leading to sudden cardiac death are common.

The treatment of dilated cardiomyopathy is directed toward relieving the symptoms of heart failure, reducing the work load of the heart, or, in select cases, heart transplantation (see Chapter 24). Digoxin, diuretics, and afterload-reducing drugs are used to improve myocardial contractility and decrease left ventricular filling pressures. Avoiding myocardial depressants, including alcohol, and pacing rest with asymptomatic levels of exercise or activity are imperative. Proper electrolyte balance and internal cardioverter defibrillators are effective in controlling recurrent ventricular dysrhythmias associated with dilated cardiomyopathy.

HYPERTROPHIC CARDIOMYOPATHIES

Hypertrophic cardiomyopathy is characterized by a small left ventricular volume with hypertrophy of ventricular muscle mass. Although the hypertrophy may be symmetric, the involvement of the ventricular septum often is disproportionate, producing obstruction of the left ventricular outflow channel and dilated atria. Synonyms for this disorder include idiopathic hypertrophic subaortic stenosis and asymmetric septal hypertrophy.

A distinctive finding in hypertrophic cardiomyopathy is the microscopic presence of myofibril disarray. Instead of the normal parallel arrangement of myofibrils, the myofibrils branch off at random angles, sometimes at right angles to an adjacent fiber with which they may connect. Small bundles of fibers may course haphazardly through normally arranged muscle fibers.[2] It is thought that the presence of these disordered fibers may produce abnormal movements of the ventricles with uncoordinated contraction and impaired relaxation.[39]

Symptomatic hypertrophic cardiomyopathy commonly is a disease of young adulthood. The cause of the disorder is largely unknown. It often is of familial origin, the disorder being inherited as an autosomal dominant trait.

The manifestations of hypertrophic cardiomyopathy are variable; for reasons that are unclear, some people with the disorder remain stable for many years and gradually become more symptomatic as the disease progresses, whereas others experience sudden cardiac death as first evidence of the disease. Atrial fibrillation is a common precursor to sudden death in those who die of dysrhythmias. Dyspnea is the most common symptom associated with a gradual elevation in left ventricular diastolic pressure resulting from impaired ventricular filling and increased wall stiffness secondary to ventricular hypertrophy. Because of the obstruction to outflow from the left ventricle, the systolic pressure difference between the left ventricle and the aorta increases. Chest pain, fatigue, and syncope are also common and worsen during exertion.[40]

The treatment of hypertrophic cardiomyopathy includes medical and surgical management. The goal of medical management is to relieve the symptoms by lessening the pressure difference between the left ventricle and the aorta, thereby improving cardiac output. β-Adrenergic receptor–blocking drugs may be used in people with chest pain, dysrhythmias, or dyspnea. These drugs reduce the heart rate and myocardial contractility, allowing more time for ventricular filling and reduction of ventricular stiffness. The calcium-channel blocking drug verapamil has proved useful in relieving the symptoms of dyspnea, chest pain, and syncope.[41] Increased calcium uptake and increased intracellular calcium content are associated with an increased contractile state, a characteristic finding in patients with hypertrophic cardiomyopathy. Disopyramide and amiodarone are effective in controlling the supraventricular and complex ventricular tachydysrhythmias associated with hypertrophic cardiomyopathies. Both drugs may also reduce the subaortic gradient because of their negative inotropic effects.[41] Surgical treatment may be used if severe symptoms persist despite medical treatment. It involves incision of the septum (myotomy) with or without the removal of part of the tissue (myectomy) and is accompanied by all the risks of open heart surgery.

RESTRICTIVE CARDIOMYOPATHIES

Of the three categories of cardiomyopathies, the restrictive type is the least common in Western countries. With this form of cardiomyopathy, ventricular filling is restricted because of excessive rigidity of the ventricular walls, whereas the contractile properties of the heart remain relatively normal. The most common causes of restrictive cardiomyopathy are endocardial fibroelastosis and infiltrations, such as amyloidosis. Although the cause of fibroelastosis is unknown, about one third of cases are associated with congenital heart defects. The extent of the manifestations depends on the extent of the involvement. When there are only focal lesions, there may be few effects and normal longevity. On the other hand, when the lesions are diffuse, cardiac decompensation and death may result. The manifestations of restrictive cardiomyopathy resemble those of constrictive pericarditis.

In summary, the cardiomyopathies represent disorders of the heart muscle. Cardiomyopathies may present as primary or secondary disorders. Secondary cardiomyopathies are conditions in which damage to the cardiac muscle occurs as the result of another disease process, such as myocardial infarction. There are three main types of primary cardiomyopathies: (1) dilated, or congestive, cardiomyopathy, in which fibrosis and atrophy of myocardial cells with dilatation of all four heart chambers occur; (2) hypertrophic cardiomyopathy, characterized by a disproportionate involvement of the ventricular septum, causing obstruction of the left ventricular outflow channel, and a disarray in the organization of myocardial fibers and ventricular hypertrophy; and (3) restrictive cardiomyopathy, in which there is excessive rigidity of the ventricular wall. The cause of the primary cardiomyopathies is largely unknown. The disease is suspected when a young, previously healthy person develops cardiomegaly and heart failure.

■ INFECTIOUS AND IMMUNOLOGIC DISORDERS

MYOCARDITIS

Myocarditis is an acute inflammation of the myocardium. It can occur as a primary disease or as a secondary disorder, as in rheumatic fever. Viral myocarditis accounts for about 80% of cases and is the one that most often presents as a primary infection.[42] Bacterial myocarditis is relatively rare in relation to viral forms of the disease, the most common forms being associated with rheumatic fever and diphtheria toxins. Other causes of myocarditis are radiation therapy, hypersensitivity reactions, and any chemical or physical agent that induces acute myocardial necrosis and secondary inflammatory changes.[43]

ETIOLOGY AND MANIFESTATIONS

Viral myocarditis most often is caused by the coxsackie group of viruses, principally coxsackie B.[2] Viral infections, particularly of coxsackie group B origin, are also associated with dilated cardiomyopathies. The question has arisen as to whether such infections may initiate immunologic damage to the myocardium, possibly involving antimyocardial antibodies, that leads to changes later identified as cardiomyopathy.

Clinical manifestations of myocarditis vary from an absence of symptoms to profound heart failure or sudden death. When coxsackie myocarditis occurs in children or young adults, it often is symptomatic. It affects twice as many males as females.[2] Acute symptomatic myocarditis typically presents as malaise, dyspnea, low-grade fever, and a tachycardia that is more pronounced than would be expected with the level of fever that is present. There commonly is a history of an upper respiratory tract or gastrointestinal tract infection followed by a latent period of several days. In young adults, sudden death may be caused by viral myocarditis. Among adults, the disorder is more likely to be self-limited and benign. The ECG changes of acute myocarditis include ECG conduction disturbances such as ventricular dysrhythmias, AV junctional block, ST-segment elevation, T-wave inversion, and transient Q waves. Clinical symptoms include a flulike syndrome, fever, chest pain, leukocytosis, and elevations in serum levels of aspartate aminotransferase (formerly glutamic-oxaloacetic transaminase), alanine aminotransferase (formerly glutamic-pyruvic transaminase), and lactic dehydrogenase. Cardiac auscultation may reveal an S_3 ventricular gallop rhythm and a transient pericardial or pleurocardial rub. In most cases, myocarditis is transient, and symptoms subside within 1 to 2 months. With advanced disease, there is congestive heart failure that involves both ventricles.

DIAGNOSIS AND TREATMENT

The diagnosis of myocarditis involves viral antigen detection, serologic testing, and myocardial biopsy. Detection of the virus antigen or immunoglobulin M antibody response has been successful. Serologic testing allows determination of the stage of viral infection. Immunoglobulin G antibody titers peak after the 1st month of the disease. The presence of myofibril degeneration and increased interstitial lymphocytes confirm active inflammatory disease on myocardial biopsy.

Treatment focuses on symptom management and immunosuppressant therapy. Bed rest and activity restriction must be maintained until fever and cardiac symptoms subside to decrease the myocardial work load. Immunosuppressant therapy has been successful in resolving inflammation, as shown by repeated biopsies. People with chronic myocarditis show much greater improvement than those who have an acute form of the disease.

RHEUMATIC FEVER

Rheumatic fever is an acute, recurrent inflammatory disease that follows a throat infection with group A β-hemolytic streptococcus. The most serious aspect of rheumatic fever is chronic valvular heart disease that produces permanent cardiac dysfunction and, sometimes fatal, heart failure years later. The disease affects 2,150,000 adults and children in the United States. Considered a preventable form of heart disease, rheumatic fever caused 6000 deaths in 1989.[1] Although rheumatic fever is more prevalent in groups subjected to poor nutrition, crowded living conditions, and inadequate health care, there has been a recent resurgence of rheumatic fever in both underprivileged and middle- and upper-class families. The recent outbreaks are due to throat infections caused by a new strain of group A β-hemolytic streptococcus.

ETIOLOGY AND MANIFESTATIONS

Rheumatic fever is primarily a disease of schoolage children. The incidence of acute rheumatic fever peaks between ages 5 and 15.[2] The disease usually follows an inciting streptococcal throat infection by 1 to 4 weeks. It is of particular significance that rheumatic fever and its cardiac complications can be prevented by antibiotic treatment of the initial streptococcal throat infection.

The pathogenesis of the disease is unclear, and why only 3% of people with uncomplicated streptococcal infections develop rheumatic fever remains to be answered. The time frame for development of symptoms in relation to the sore throat as well as the presence of antibodies to the streptococcus organism strongly suggest an immunologic origin. Like other immunologic phenomena, rheumatic fever requires an initial sensitizing exposure to the offending (streptococcus) agent, and the risk of recurrence is high after each subsequent exposure. Rheumatic fever can present as an acute, recurrent, or chronic disorder.

The acute stage includes a history of an initiating streptococcal infection and subsequent involvement of the mesenchymal connective tissue of the heart, blood vessels, joints, and subcutaneous tissues. Common to all is the presence of a lesion called the *Aschoff body*. The Aschoff body is a localized area of tissue necrosis surrounded by immune cells. The recurrent phase usually involves extension of the cardiac effects of the disease. The chronic phase of rheumatic fever is characterized by permanent deformity of the heart valves and is a frequent cause of mitral valve stenosis. Chronic rheumatic heart disease usually does not appear until at least 10 years after the initial attack, sometimes decades later.[2]

Most children with rheumatic fever have a history of sore throat, headache, fever, abdominal pain, nausea, vomiting, swollen glands (usually at the angle of the jaw), and other signs and symptoms of a streptococcal infection. Other clinical features associated with an acute episode of rheumatic fever are related to the acute inflammatory process and the structures involved in the disease process. There are five major manifestations of rheumatic fever: (1) carditis, (2) polyarthritis, (3) chorea, (4) erythema marginatum, and (5) subcutaneous nodules. Minor manifestations can include arthralgia, fever, laboratory tests indicating elevated levels of acute-phase reactants, and prolonged R-R interval on the ECG.

Carditis. Rheumatic fever can affect any of the three layers of the heart: pericardium, myocardium, and endocardium. All three layers usually are involved. Rheumatic pericarditis causes the production of a fibrinous or serofibrinous exudate. For the most part, the myocarditis is reversible and produces minimal changes in cardiac function. The involvement of the endocardium and valvular structures produces the permanent and disabling effects of the disease. Although any of the four valves can be involved, the mitral and aortic valves most often are affected. During the acute inflammatory stage of the disease, the valvular structures become red and swollen; small vegetative lesions develop on the valve leaflets. The acute inflammatory changes gradually proceed to fibrous scar tissue development, which tends to contract and cause deformity of the valve leaflets and shortening of the chordae tendineae. In some cases, the edges or commissures of the valve leaflets fuse together as healing occurs.

The manifestations of rheumatic carditis include a heart murmur in a child without a previous history of rheumatic fever, change in the character of a murmur in a person with a previous history of the disease, cardiomegaly or enlargement of the heart, friction rub or other signs of pericarditis, and congestive heart failure in a child without discernible cause.[44]

Polyarthritis. Although not a cause of permanent disability, polyarthritis is the most common finding in rheumatic fever. The inflammatory process affects the synovial membrane of the joint, causing swelling, heat, redness, pain, tenderness, and limited motion. The arthritis is almost always migratory, affecting one joint and then moving to another. The joints most frequently affected are the larger ones, particularly the knees, ankles, elbows, and wrists. In untreated cases, the arthritis lasts about 4 weeks. A striking feature of rheumatic arthritis is the dramatic response (usually within 48 hours) to salicylates.[45]

Chorea. Chorea (Sydenham's chorea), sometimes called St. Vitus' dance, is the major central nervous system manifestation. It most frequently is seen in girls. There typically is an insidious onset of irritability and other behavior problems. The child often is fidgety, cries easily, begins to walk clumsily, and drops things. The choreic movements are spontaneous, rapid, purposeless, jerking movements that interfere with voluntary activities. Facial grimaces are common, and even speech may be affected. The chorea is self-limiting, usually running its course within a matter of weeks or months.

Erythema Marginatum. Erythema marginatum lesions are maplike macular areas most commonly seen on the trunk or inner aspects of the upper arm and thigh. Skin lesions are present only in about 10% of patients who have rheumatic fever; they are transitory and disappear during the course of the disease.

Subcutaneous Nodules. The subcutaneous nodules range in size from 1 to 4 cm; they are hard, painless, and freely movable and usually overlie the extensor muscles of the wrist, elbow, ankle, and knee joints. Subcutaneous nodules are rare, but when present, they most often occur in people with carditis.

Minor Manifestations. The minor manifestation provide evidence of an acute inflammatory process and cardiac manifestations. Elevated levels of acute-phase reactants are not specific for rheumatic fever but provide evidence of an acute inflammatory response. The erythrocyte sedimentation rate, C-reactive protein, and white blood cell count commonly are used; unless corticosteroids or salicylates have been used, the results of these tests are almost always elevated in people who present with polyarthritis, carditis, or chorea. These tests are also used to determine when the acute phase of the illness has subsided.

A prolonged P-R interval on the ECG is a nonspecific finding. It does not correlate with the ultimate development of chronic rheumatic heart disease.

DIAGNOSIS AND TREATMENT

The diagnosis of rheumatic fever is based on the Jones Criteria, which were initially proposed in 1955 and revised in 1984 and 1992 by a committee of the American Heart Association.[45] The criteria were developed because no single laboratory test, sign, or symptom is pathognomonic of the disease, although several combinations of them are diagnostic. The signs and symptoms of rheumatic fever are grouped into major and minor categories in the criteria. The presence of two major signs (carditis, polyarthritis, chorea, erythema marginatum, and subcutaneous nodules) or one major and two minor signs (arthralgia, fever, elevated levels of acute-phase reactants, or prolonged P-R interval) accompanied by evidence of a preceding group A streptococcal infection indicates a high probability of rheumatic fever.

Evidence of a streptococcal infection is established through the use of throat cultures, antigen tests, and antibodies to products liberated by the streptococcus. Throat cultures taken at the time of the acute infection usually are positive for group A streptococcus. It takes several days to obtain the results of a throat culture. The development of rapid tests for direct detection of group A streptococcal antigens have provided at least a partial solution for this problem. These tests use latex agglutination or an enzyme immunoassay and can be completed in a few minutes. Both types of tests are highly specific for group A streptococcus but are limited in terms of their sensitivity (*e.g.*, the person may have a negative test but have a streptococcal infection). Therefore, negative antigen tests should be confirmed with a throat culture when a streptococcal infection is suspected.

Group A streptococci elaborate a large number of extracellular products, including streptolysin O and deoxyribonuclease (DNase) B. The antibodies to these products are measured for retrospective confirmation of recent streptococcal infections in people thought to have acute rheumatic fever.[46]

Treatment is designed to control the acute inflammatory process and to prevent cardiac complications and recurrence of the disease. During the acute phase, prevention of residual cardiac effects is of primary concern; antibiotics, antiinflammatory drugs, and selective restriction of physical activities are prescribed. Recurrences of rheumatic fever are high, particularly in patients who have had carditis during their initial episode and in children. Penicillin (or another antibiotic in penicillin-sensitive patients) is used prophylactically for at least 5 years to prevent recurrence. Penicillin is also the antibiotic of choice for treating the acute illness. Salicylates and corticosteroids are also widely used.

Secondary prevention and compliance with a plan for prophylactic administration of penicillin require that the patient and the family understand the rationale for such measures as well as the measures themselves. Patients also need to be instructed to report possible streptococcal infections to their physicians. They should be instructed to inform their dentists about the disease so that they can be adequately protected during dental procedures that might traumatize the oral mucosa.

INFECTIVE ENDOCARDITIS

Infective, or bacterial, endocarditis is characterized by colonization or invasion of the endocardium by a microbiologic agent, leading to friable (easily crumbled) lesions laden with organisms—the so-called *infective vegetations*.[2] The disease commonly affects people with preexisting heart defects; the lesions of infective endocarditis usually attach to these defects. They most commonly involve a heart valve but may be attached to a septal lesion or the endocardial surface of the heart wall. In the preantibiotic era, infective endocarditis was almost always a fatal disease. Factors that determine the clinical presentation of infective endocarditis are (1) the nature of the infecting organism, (2) the presence of preexisting heart defects, and (3) the source of the infection, since endocarditis in drug users and infections acquired during heart surgery have special features.[47]

Almost any microorganism can cause endocarditis. The more virulent organisms, *Staphylococcus aureus* in particular, produce the more rapidly progressive and destructive infections. *Streptococcus viridans*, enterococci, and varieties of other gram-negative and gram-positive bacilli, yeasts, and fungi produce a more subacute process.[47]

Two predisposing factors contribute to the development of infective endocarditis: a damaged endocardial surface and a portal of entry by which the organism gains access to the bloodstream. The presence of valvular disease, rheumatic heart disease, or congenital heart defects provides an environment conducive to bacterial growth. In people with preexisting valvular or endocardial defects, simple gum massage or an innocuous oral lesion may afford the pathogenic bacteria access to the bloodstream. Also, transient bacteremia may emerge in the course of seemingly minor health problems, such as an upper respiratory tract infection, a skin lesion, or a dental procedure.

Although infective endocarditis frequently develops in an environment supported by a heart defect, this is not necessarily the case in intravenous drug abusers and hospital-acquired infections. Intravenous drug abuse is the major cause of infective endocarditis and the most common source of right-sided (tricuspid) lesions.[47] Although staphylococcal infections are frequent, these people may be infected with unusual organisms, such as gram-negative bacilli, yeasts, and fungi.

In hospital patients, infective endocarditis may arise as a complication of infected intravascular or urinary tract catheters. Infective endocarditis may also complicate prosthetic heart valve replacement. It can develop as an early infection that follows surgery or as a later infection that results from the long-term presence of the prosthesis. Infections of prosthetic valves account for 10% to 20% of cases of infectious endocarditis.

The vegetative lesion that is characteristic of infective endocarditis consists of a collection of pathogens and cellular debris enmeshed in the fibrin strands of clotted blood. These lesions may be singular or multiple, may grow to be as large as several centimeters, and usually are found loosely attached to the free edges of the valve surface. The loose organization of these lesions permits the organisms and fragments of the lesions to form emboli and travel in the bloodstream. The fragments may lodge in small blood vessels, causing small hemorrhages, abscesses, and infarction of tissue.

Infective endocarditis may occur in an acute or subacute form. *Acute infective endocarditis* is thought to primarily affect people with normal hearts, whereas *subacute infective endocarditis* most frequently is seen in patients with damaged hearts. The signs and symptoms include fever, change in the character of an existing heart murmur, and evidence of embolic distribution of the vegetative lesions. In the acute form, the fever usually is spiking and accompanied by chills. In the subacute form, the fever usually is low grade, of gradual onset, and frequently accompanied by other systemic signs of inflammation, such as anorexia, malaise, and lethargy. Cough, dyspnea, arthralgia or arthritis, diarrhea, and abdominal or flank pain may occur as the result of embolization.

Small petechial hemorrhages frequently result when emboli lodge in the small vessels of the skin, nail beds, and mucous membranes.

The clinical course of infective endocarditis is determined by the extent of heart damage, the type of organism involved, site of infection (right side of the heart versus left side of the heart), and whether embolization from the site of infection occurs. Destruction of infected heart valves is common with certain forms of organisms, such as *Staphylococcus aureus*. Peripheral embolization can establish metastatic infections and abscess formation; these are particularly serious when they affect organs such as the brain and kidneys. Right-sided endocarditis, which usually involves the tricuspid valve, leads to septic emboli traveling to the lung, causing infarction and lung abscesses.

DIAGNOSIS AND TREATMENT

The blood culture is the most significant diagnostic aid in infective endocarditis. A series of three to six cultures typically are obtained during a 36- to 48-hour period to ensure adequate sampling. The optimal time to obtain cultures is just before a temperature rise (*e.g.*, during the chill that precedes a fever).

Treatment focuses on identifying and destroying the causative organism, minimizing the residual cardiac effects, and treating the pathology induced by the emboli. The blood cultures usually identify the organism so that its sensitivity to antibiotics can be assessed. An appropriate antibiotic is prescribed to eradicate the pathogen. Surgery is indicated in the presence of moderate to severe heart failure, progressive renal failure, significant emboli, dysrhythmias, or left-sided endocarditis. Infected valves may need to be replaced.

Of great importance is the prevention of infective endocarditis in people with known risk. Prevention can be largely accomplished through prophylactic administration of an antibiotic before dental and other procedures that may cause bacteremia.[48, 49]

KAWASAKI'S DISEASE

Kawasaki's disease (also known as mucocutaneous lymph node syndrome) is an acute febrile disease of young children. First described in Japan in 1967 by Dr. Tomisaku Kawasaki, the disease affects the skin, brain, eyes, joints, liver, lymph nodes, and heart.[50–52] The disease can produce aneurysmal disease of the coronary arteries and is the most common cause of acquired heart disease in young children. More than 3000 children with Kawasaki's disease are diagnosed annually in the United States, and 0.5% to 1.0% of those die of complications of coronary artery involvement. Although first reported in Japanese children, the disease affects children of many races, occurs worldwide, and is increasing in frequency.

ETIOLOGY AND MANIFESTATIONS

The disease is characterized by a vasculitis (inflammation of the blood vessels) that begins in the small vessels (arterioles, venules, and capillaries) and progresses to involve some of the larger arteries, such as the coronaries. The cause of Kawasaki's disease is unknown, but it is thought to be of immunologic origin. Immunologic abnormalities that include increased activation of helper T cells and increased levels of immune mediators and antibodies that destroy endothelial cells have been detected during the acute phase of the disease. It has been hypothesized that some unknown antigen triggers the immune response. The nature of the antigen is unknown; it is speculated to be a common infectious agent (probably a virus) that triggers the response in a genetically predisposed child.

The course of the disease is triphasic and includes an *acute febrile phase* that lasts about 10 to 11 days; a *subacute phase* that follows the acute phase and lasts until days 21 through 25; and a *convalescent phase* that follows the subacute stage and continues until the signs of the acute-phase inflammatory response have subsided and the signs of the illness have disappeared.

The acute phase begins with an abrupt onset of fever followed by conjunctivitis, skin rash, involvement of the oral mucosa, redness and swelling of the hands and feet, and enlarged cervical lymph nodes. The fever typically is high, reaching 40°C (104°F) or more, has an erratic spiking pattern, is unresponsive to antibiotics, and persists for 5 or more days. The conjunctivitis, which is bilateral, begins shortly after the onset of fever, persists throughout the febrile course of the disease, and may last as long as 3 to 5 weeks. There is no exudate, discharge, or conjunctival ulceration, differentiating it from many other types of conjunctivitis. The rash usually is deeply erythematous and may take several forms, the most common being a nonpruritic urticarial rash with large erythematous plaques or a measles-type rash. Although the rash usually is generalized, it may be accentuated centrally or peripherally. Some children develop a perianal rash with a diaper-like distribution. Oropharyngeal manifestations include fissuring of the lips, diffuse erythema of the oropharynx, and hypertrophic papillae of the tongue, creating a strawberry appearance. The hands and feet become swollen and painful with reddened palms and soles. The rash, oropharyngeal manifestations, and changes in hands and feet appear within 1 to 3 days of fever onset and usually disappear as the fever subsides. Lymph node involvement is the least constant feature of the disease. It is cervical and unilateral with a single, firm, enlarged lymph node mass usually greater than 1.5 cm in diameter.

The subacute phase begins with the defervescence of fever and lasts until all signs of the disease have disappeared. During the subacute phase, desquamation (peeling) of the skin of the fingers and toetips begins and progresses to involve the entire surface of the palms and soles. Patchy peeling of skin areas other than the hands and feet may occur in some children.

The convalescent stage persists from the complete resolution of symptoms until all signs of inflammation have disappeared. This usually takes about 8 weeks.

In addition to the major manifestations that occur during the acute stage of the illness, there are a number of associated, less specific characteristics of the disease, including arthritis, urethritis and pyuria, gastrointestinal manifestations (diarrhea and abdominal pain), hepatitis, and hydrops of the gallbladder. Arthritis or arthralgia occurs in about 30% of children with the disease, characterized by symmetric joint swelling that involves both large and small joints. Central nervous system involvement occurs in almost all children and is characterized by pronounced irritability and lability of mood.

Cardiac involvement is the most important manifestation of Kawasaki's disease. Ten to 40% of children develop coronary vasculitis within the first 2 weeks of the illness, manifested by dilatation and aneurysm formation in the coronary arteries, as seen on two-dimensional echocardiography. The manifestations of coronary artery involvement include signs and symptoms of myocardial ischemia or, rarely, overt myocardial infarction or rupture of the aneurysm. Pericarditis, myocarditis, endocarditis, heart failure, and dysrhythmias may also develop.

DIAGNOSIS AND TREATMENT

As with rheumatic fever, the diagnosis of Kawasaki's disease is based on clinical findings, since no specific laboratory test for the disease exists.[53] In 1987, the CDC published diagnostic criteria that are used in establishing a diagnosis of Kawasaki's disease.[54] According to these criteria, a diagnosis of the disease is confirmed by the presence of a fever that lasts 5 or more days without another more reasonable explanation and the presence of at least four of the following acute-stage manifestations of the disease: (1) bilateral conjunctivitis, (2) oropharyngeal manifestations (injected or fissured lips, injected pharynx, or straw-berry tongue), (3) extremity changes (redness of the palms or soles, edema of the hands or feet, or generalized peeling of the skin of the hands or feet, usually beginning around the nails), (4) rash, and (5) cervical lymphadenopathy. Chest radiology, ECG, and two-dimensional echocardiography are used to detect coronary artery involvement and follow its progress. Coronary angiography may be used to determine the extent of coronary artery involvement.

Intravenous gamma globulin (IVGG) and aspirin are considered the best therapy for prevention of coronary artery abnormalities in children with Kawasaki's disease. It is recommended that all children diagnosed receive this treatment within the first 10 days of illness.[54] IVGG has been shown to be an effective treatment for Kawasaki's disease; it usually is given by daily infusion for 4 consecutive days. During the acute phase of the illness, aspirin usually is given in larger doses and for its antiinflammatory and antipyretic effects. After the fever is controlled, the aspirin dose is lowered and the drug is given for its anti–platelet-aggregating effects. Low-dose aspirin is administered during the period of greatest risk of cardiac thrombosis (days 14 through 35) and continued for 3 months to 1 year in children with evidence of coronary artery abnormalities.

Recommendations for cardiac follow-up evaluation (stress testing and, sometimes, coronary angiography) are based on the level of coronary artery changes. Anticoagulant therapy may be recommended for people with multiple or large coronary aneurysms. Some restrictions in activities such as competitive sports may be advised for children with significant coronary artery abnormalities.[53]

In summary, myocarditis is an acute inflammation of the myocardium, most often of viral origin. The manifestations of viral myocarditis range from absence of symptoms to sudden death. The disease usually is benign and self-limiting.

Rheumatic fever, which is associated with an antecedent group A streptococcal infection, is an important cause of heart disease. Its most serious and disabling effects result from involvement of the heart valves. Because there is no single laboratory test, sign, or symptom that is pathognomonic of acute rheumatic fever, the Jones Criteria are used to establish the diagnosis during the acute stage of the disease.

Infective endocarditis involves the invasion of the endocardium by pathogens that produce vegetative lesions on the endocardial surface. The loose organization of these lesions permits the organisms and fragments of the lesions to be disseminated throughout the systemic circulation. It can be caused by a number of organisms. Two predisposing factors contribute to the development of infective endocarditis: a damaged endocardium and a portal of entry through which the organisms gain access to the bloodstream.

Kawasaki's disease is an acute febrile disease of young children that affects the skin, brain, eyes, joints, liver, lymph nodes, and heart. The disease can produce aneurysmal disease

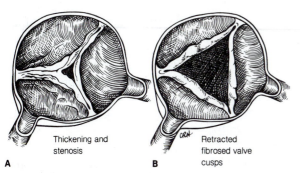

FIG. 23-18. Disease of the aortic valve as viewed from the aorta. **(A)** Stenosis of the valve opening. **(B)** An incompetent or regurgitant valve that is unable to close completely.

of the coronary arteries and is the most common cause of acquired heart disease in young children.

■ VALVULAR HEART DISEASE

Dysfunction of the heart valves can result from a number of disorders, including congenital defects, trauma, ischemic damage, degenerative changes, and inflammation. Rheumatic endocarditis is the most common cause. Its inflammatory changes cause scar tissue to form on the valve leaflets and the chordae tendineae with a subsequent shortening of the chordae and deformation of the valve structure. Two types of mechanical disruptions may occur in valvular disease: (1) narrowing or stenosis of the valve opening or (2) failure of a valve to close completely (Fig. 23-18). Although any of the four heart valves can become diseased, the most commonly affected are the mitral and aortic valves.

HEMODYNAMIC DERANGEMENTS

Valvular disease can be either stenotic (failure to open completely) or regurgitant (failure to close completely), but there often is a combination of stenotic and regurgitant effects. The influence of valvular disease on cardiac function is related to alterations in blood flow and increased work demands on the heart.

Stenosis causes a decrease in flow through the valve, with an increased work demand on the heart chamber in front of the diseased valve. In mitral stenosis, for example, the left atrium becomes distended and the work output required of this chamber is increased. As the condition advances, blood return from the lungs is impeded and the pulmonary circulation becomes congested. Blood flow through a normal valve can increase to five to seven times the resting value; consequently, valvular stenosis must

be severe before it causes life-threatening problems. The first evidence of symptoms usually is noted during situations of increased flow, such as exercise.

An *incompetent* (*regurgitant*) valve permits blood flow to continue while the valve is closed, flowing into the left ventricle during diastole when the aortic valve is affected and into the left atrium during systole when the mitral valve is diseased.

TYPES OF VALVULAR DISORDERS

AORTIC VALVE DEFECTS

The orifices of the coronary arteries are strategically located in the aorta, just distal to the aortic valve leaflets (Fig. 23-19). In aortic stenosis, the velocity of flow through the narrowed valve orifice is increased at the expense of the lateral pressure needed to perfuse the coronary arteries. In aortic regurgitation, failure of aortic valve closure during diastole causes diastolic pressure to fall; this decreases the pressure needed to perfuse the coronary arteries.

Aortic Valve Stenosis. Aortic stenosis causes resistance to ejection of blood into the aorta, so the work demands on the left ventricle are increased and the volume of blood ejected into the systemic circulation is decreased. The most common causes of aortic stenosis are rheumatic fever and congenital heart defects. In elderly people, it may be related to degenerative atherosclerotic changes of the valve leaflets.

Obstruction to aortic outflow causes a decrease in stroke volume, along with a reduction in systolic blood pressure and pulse pressure. Because of the narrowed opening, it takes longer for the heart to eject blood; the heart rate often is slow and the pulse is of low amplitude. Resistance to flow through the aortic valve gives rise to an auscultatory murmur in systole.

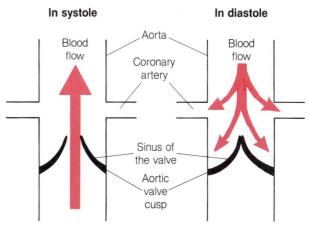

FIG. 23-19. Location of the orifices for the coronary arteries and the direction of blood flow during systole and diastole.

The onset of signs and symptoms of aortic stenosis depends, to a large extent, on the person's activity level. In people who lead sedentary lives, the disease may be far advanced before symptoms are noted. Exertional dyspnea is a common presenting symptom. It is characterized by vertigo and syncope when the stroke volume falls to levels insufficient for cerebral needs. Also, the combination of increased work demands on the hypertrophied left ventricle and decreased perfusion of the coronary vessels may cause angina.

Aortic Valve Regurgitation. An *incompetent aortic valve* allows blood to return to the left ventricle during diastole. This defect may result from conditions that cause scarring of the valve leaflets or from enlargement of the valve orifice to the extent that the valve leaflets no longer meet. Rheumatic fever ranks first on the list of causes of aortic regurgitation.

A widening of the pulse pressure, the result of an increased systolic pressure and decreased diastolic pressure, is characteristic of aortic regurgitation. Widening of the pulse pressure has two underlying mechanisms: first, there is an increase in the stroke volume (and systolic blood pressure) as the left ventricle ejects blood entering from the lungs as well as the blood that has leaked back across the aortic valve into the ventricle during diastole; second, because the aortic valve fails to close completely, diastolic pressure cannot be maintained. The left ventricle hypertrophies because of the increased volume load on this chamber. The turbulence of the flow across the aortic valve during diastole produces a high-pitched or blowing type of murmur.

The large stroke volume, wide pulse pressure, and rapid runoff of blood from the aorta produce characteristic changes in the peripheral pulses: prominent carotid pulsations in the neck, throbbing peripheral pulses, and a left ventricular impulse that causes the chest to move with each beat. The term *waterhammer* pulse often is used to describe the hyperkinetic peripheral pulse found in people with aortic regurgitation.

The symptoms of aortic regurgitation are those associated with heart failure: exertional dyspnea, dizziness, pulmonary edema, and orthopnea. Angina follows the impaired coronary perfusion owing to a low diastolic pressure and the increased work demands on the left ventricle. Patients with significant aortic regurgitation complain of throbbing of the chest caused by the hyperdynamic left ventricle.

MITRAL VALVE DEFECTS

The mitral valve controls the directional flow of blood between the left atrium and the left ventricle. The cusps of the AV valves are thinner than those of the semilunar valves; they are anchored to the papillary muscles by the chordae tendineae. During much of systole, the mitral valve is subjected to the high pressure generated by the left ventricle as it pumps blood into the systemic circulation, and the chordae tendineae prevent the eversion of the valve leaflets into the left atrium.

Mitral Valve Stenosis. Mitral valve stenosis is characterized by fibrous replacement of valvular tissue, along with stiffness and fusion of valve commissures. Involvement of the chordae tendineae causes shortening, which pulls the valvular structures more deeply into the ventricles. As the resistance to flow through the valve increases, the left atrial pressure rises and, eventually, dilatation of this heart chamber occurs. The increased left atrial pressure is transmitted to the pulmonary venous system, causing pulmonary congestion. The rate of flow across the valve depends on the size of the valve orifice, the driving pressure (atrial minus ventricular pressure), and the time available for flow during diastole. As the condition progresses, symptoms of decreased cardiac output occur during extreme exertion or other situations that cause tachycardia and, thereby, reduce diastolic filling time. In the late stages of the disease, pulmonary vascular resistance increases with the development of pulmonary hypertension; this increases the arterial pressure against which the right side of the heart must pump and, eventually, leads to failure of this side of the heart.

The signs and symptoms of mitral valve stenosis depend on the severity of the obstruction and are related to (1) elevation in left atrial pressure and pulmonary congestion, (2) decreased cardiac output owing to impaired left ventricular filling, and (3) left atrial enlargement with development of atrial arrhythmias and mural thrombi. The symptoms are those of pulmonary congestion, including nocturnal paroxysmal dyspnea and orthopnea. Premature atrial beats, paroxysmal atrial tachycardia, and atrial fibrillation may occur as a result of distention of the left atrium. Together, the fibrillation and distention predispose to mural thrombus formation, from which systemic emboli may form. Palpitations, chest pain, weakness, and fatigue are common complaints. The murmur of mitral valve stenosis is heard during diastole when blood is flowing through the constricted valve orifice; it is characteristically a low-pitched rumbling murmur, best heard at the apex of the heart. The first heart sound often is accentuated and somewhat delayed because of the increased left atrial pressure; an opening snap may precede the diastolic murmur as a result of the elevation in left atrial pressure.

Mitral Valve Regurgitation. Mitral valve regurgitation can result from many processes. Rheumatic heart disease is associated with a rigid and thickened valve that does not open or close completely. In addition to rheumatic disease, mitral regurgitation can result from rupture of the chordae tendineae or papillary muscles, papillary muscle dysfunction, or stretching of the valve structures due to dilatation of the left ventricle or valve orifice. Acute mitral valve regurgitation may occur abruptly, such as with papillary muscle dysfunction following myocardial infarction, valve perforation in infective endocarditis, or ruptured cordae tendinae in mitral valve prolapse.

With mitral valve insufficiency, blood from the left ventricle moves back into the left atrium during systole and is returned to the left ventricle during diastole. In acute regurgitation, left atrial pressure rises rapidly, leading to pulmonary edema if severe.

With chronic mitral regurgitation the left atrium enlarges gradually. Mitral regurgitation, like mitral stenosis, predisposes to atrial fibrillation. The degree of left ventricular enlargement reflects the severity of regurgitation. As the disorder progresses, left ventricular function becomes impaired and the left atrial pressure increases with the subsequent development of pulmonary hypertension. The increased volume work associated with mitral regurgitation is relatively well tolerated, and many people with the disorder remain asymptomatic for 10 to 20 years despite severe regurgitation. A characteristic feature of mitral valve regurgitation is an enlarged left ventricle and a pansystolic (throughout systole) murmur.

Mitral Valve Prolapse. Sometimes referred to as the floppy mitral valve syndrome, mitral valve prolapse has been reported to be present in 2.5% of males and 7.6% of females in the general population.[55] The disorder is seen three times more frequently in women than in men and may have a familial basis. Although the cause of the disorder is unknown, it has been associated with Marfan's syndrome, osteogenesis imperfecta, and other connective tissue disorders as well as cardiac, hematologic, neuroendocrine, metabolic, and psychological disorders.

Pathologic findings in mitral valve prolapse include a myxedematous (mucinous) degeneration of the spongiosum, which lies between the collagen and elastic tissue covering the atrial aspect of the valve and the thick layer of connective tissue that provides the main support for the valve, causing a redundancy of valve tissue and ballooning of the valve leaflets into the left atrium during systole when the ventricular pressure is high. It has also been suggested that certain forms of the disorder may arise from disorders of the myocardium that result in abnormal movement of the ventricular wall or papillary muscle; this places undue stress on the mitral valve. In epidemiologic survey studies, most people with the disorder were unaware that they had it. The most commonly encountered symptoms in the clinical setting are chest pain, weakness, dyspnea, fatigue, anxiety, palpitations, and light-headedness. The chest pain differs from that of angina in that it often is prolonged, ill-defined, and not associated with exercise or exertion. The pain has been attributed to ischemia resulting from traction of the prolapsing valve leaflets. It has recently been suggested that the anxiety, palpitations, and dysrhythmias that accompany the disorder may be due to an abnormal function of the autonomic nervous system that accompanies the disorder. Rare cases of sudden death have been reported in people with mitral valve prolapse, mainly in those with a family history of similar occurrences.

The disorder is characterized by a spectrum of auscultatory findings, ranging from a silent form to one or more midsystolic clicks followed by a late systolic murmur.[55] Various abnormal ECG changes can occur. Dysrhythmias may be brought out by exercise stress testing or 24-hour ECG monitoring. Echocardiographic studies have become a method for the diagnosis of mitral valve prolapse, and the availability of this technique has undoubtedly contributed to increased recognition of the problem, particularly in its asymptomatic form.

The treatment of mitral valve prolapse focuses on the relief of symptoms and the prevention of complications. The β-adrenergic blocking drugs have proved useful in treating the autonomic manifestations, chest discomfort, and dysrhythmias that occur in the symptomatic form of the disease. Infective endocarditis is an uncommon complication in patients with a murmur; antibiotic prophylaxis usually is recommended before dental treatments or surgery.

DIAGNOSTIC METHODS

Valvular defects usually are detected through cardiac auscultation. Diagnosis is aided by the use of cardiac auscultation (heart sounds), phonocardiography, echocardiography, and cardiac catheterization. Heart sounds are discussed in Chapter 22.

A permanent recording of the heart sounds can be made through the use of a recording called a *phonocardiogram*. This is obtained by placing a high-fidelity microphone on the chest wall over the heart while a recording is made. An ECG tracing usually is made simultaneously for timing purposes.

Echocardiography uses ultrasonography to record an image of heart structures. An ultrasound signal has a frequency greater than 20,000 Hz (cycles per second) and is inaudible to the human ear. Echocardiography uses ultrasound signals in the range of 2 million to 5 million Hz. The ultrasound signal is reflected (echoes) whenever tissue resistance to the transmission of the sound beam changes. It is possible to image the internal structures of the heart because the chest wall, blood, and different heart structures all reflect ultrasound differently.

The echocardiogram is useful for determining ventricular dimensions and valve movements, obtaining data on the movement of the left ventricular wall and septum, estimating diastolic and systolic volumes, and viewing the motion of individual segments of the left ventricular wall during systole and diastole. It can also be used for studying valvular disease and detecting pericardial effusion.

TREATMENT

The treatment of valvular defects consists of (1) medical management of heart failure and associated problems and (2) surgical intervention to either repair or replace the defective valve. Mitral commissurotomy is the surgical enlargement of a stenotic valve. It may be performed as either an open or a closed procedure. The open procedure requires extracorporeal circulation (cardiopulmonary bypass) but has the advantage of affording the surgeon direct visualization of the operative site. Valvular replacement, either with a prosthetic device or a homograft, usually is reserved for severe disease because the ideal substitute valve has not yet been invented. Percutaneous balloon valvuloplasty involves the opening of a stenotic valve by guiding an inflated balloon through the valve orifice. The procedure is done in the cardiac catheterization laboratory and involves the insertion of a balloon catheter into the heart by way of a peripheral blood vessel.

In summary, dysfunction of the heart valves can result from a number of disorders, including congenital defects, trauma, ischemic heart disease, degenerative changes, and inflammation. Rheumatic endocarditis is a common cause. Valvular heart disease produces its effects through disturbances in the blood flow. A stenotic valvular defect is one that causes a decrease in blood flow through a valve, resulting in impaired emptying and increased work demands on the heart chamber in front of the diseased valve. A regurgitant valvular defect permits the blood flow to continue when the valve is closed. Valvular heart disorders produce blood flow turbulence and often are detected through cardiac auscultation.

■ CONGENITAL HEART DEFECTS

About 8 out of every 1000 babies are born with a congenital heart defect. About 25% of these have a severe defect that would cause death within the 1st

year if it were not corrected. Premature infants have a higher incidence of congenital heart defects, most commonly patent ductus arteriosus and atrial septal defects. This section of the chapter provides an overview of congenital heart defects, including the embryonic development of the heart, fetal and postnatal circulation, hemodynamic manifestations of congenital heart defects, and a description of the more common defects. Depending on the type of defect present, children with congenital heart disease experience varying signs and symptoms associated with altered heart action, heart failure, pulmonary vascular disorders, and difficulty in supplying the peripheral tissues with oxygen and other nutrients.

EMBRYONIC DEVELOPMENT OF THE HEART

The heart is the first functioning organ in the embryo; its first pulsatile movements begin during the 3rd week after conception. This early development of the heart is essential to the rapidly growing embryo as a means of circulating nutrients and removing waste products. Most of the development of the heart and blood vessels occurs between the 3rd and 8th weeks of embryonic life.

The developing heart begins as two endothelial tubes that fuse into a single tubular structure.[56, 57] The early heart structures develop as the tubular heart elongates and forms alternate dilations and constrictions. A single atrium and ventricle along with the bulbus cordis develop first. This is followed by formation of the truncus arteriosus and the sinus venosus, a large venous sinus that receives blood from the embryo and developing placenta (Fig. 23-20). The early pulsatile-like movements of the heart begin in the sinus venosus and move blood out of the heart by way of the bulbus cordis, truncus arteriosus, and aortic arches.

A differential growth rate in the early cardiac structures, along with fixation of the heart at the venous and arterial ends, causes the tubular heart to bend over on itself. As the heart bends, the atrium and the sinus venosus come to lie behind the bulbus cordis, truncus arteriosus, and ventricle. This looping of the primitive heart results in the heart's alignment in the left side of the chest with the atrium located behind the ventricle. Malrotation during formation of the ventricular loop can cause various malpositions, such as dextroposition of the heart.

The embryonic heart undergoes further development as partitioning of the chambers occurs. Partitioning of the atrioventricular (AV) channel, atrium, and ventricle begins in the 4th week and essentially is complete by the 5th week. The separation of the heart begins as tissue bundles, called the *endocardial cushions*, form in the midportion of the dorsal and ventral

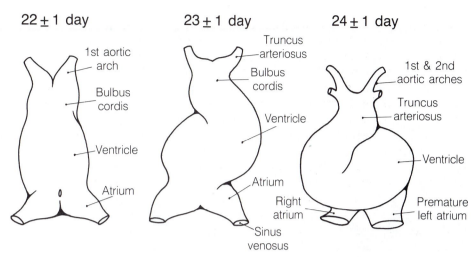

FIG. 23-20. Ventral view of the developing heart (20–25 days). (Adapted from Moore, K.L. [1977]. *The developing human* [2nd ed.]. Philadelphia: W.B. Saunders)

walls of the heart in the region of the AV canal and begin to grow inward. Until the separation begins, a single AV channel exists between the atria and the ventricles. As the endocardial cushions enlarge, they meet and fuse to form separate right and left AV channels (Fig. 23-21). The mitral and tricuspid valves develop in these channels. The endocardial cushions also contribute to formation of parts of the atrial and ventricular septum. Defects in endocardial cushion formation can result in atrial and ventricular septal defects, complete AV canal defect, and anomalies of the mitral and tricuspid valves.

Compartmentalization of the ventricles begins with the growth of the intraventricular septum from the floor of the ventricle moving upward toward the endocardial cushions. Fusion of the endocardial

cushions with the intraventricular septum usually is completed by the end of the 7th week.

Partitioning of the atrial septum is more complex and occurs in two stages, beginning with the formation of a thin crescent-shaped membrane called the *septum primum* that emerges from the anterior, superior portion of the heart and grows toward the endocardial cushions, leaving an opening called *ostium primum* between its lower edge and the endocardial cushions. A second membrane called *septum secundum* also begins to grow from the upper wall of the atrium on the right side of septum primum. As this membrane grows toward the endocardial cushions, it covers ostium secundum and forms an incomplete partition with an ovale opening called the *foramen ovale* (see Fig. 32-21). The upper part of the septum primum gradually disappears; the remaining part becomes the valve of the foramen ovale. The foramen ovale forms a communicating channel between the two upper chambers of the heart. This opening allows blood from the umbilical vein to pass directly into the left heart, bypassing the lungs. An ostium secundum defect, which is one type of atrial septal defect, is thought to arise from excessive absorption of septum primum.

To complete the transformation into a four-chambered heart, provision must be made for separating the blood pumped from the right side of the heart, which is to be diverted into the pulmonary circulation, from the blood pumped from the left side of the heart, which is to be pumped to the systemic circulation. This separation of blood flow is accomplished by developmental changes in the outlet channels of the tubular heart, the bulbus cordis, and the truncus arteriosus, which undergo spiral twisting and vertical partitioning (Fig. 23-22). As these vessels spiral and divide, the location of the aorta becomes posterior and to the right of the pulmonary artery. Impaired spiraling during this stage of development

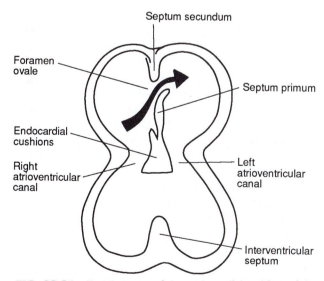

FIG. 23-21. Development of the endocardial cushions, right and left atrioventricular canals, interventricular septum, and septum primum and septum secundum of the foramen ovale. Note that blood from the left atrium flows through the foramen ovale to the left atrium.

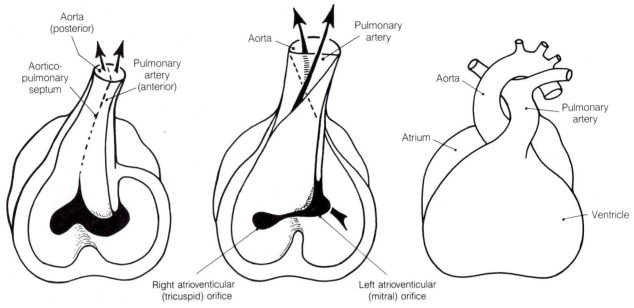

FIG. 23-22. Separation and twisting of the truncus arteriosus to form the pulmonary artery and aorta.

can lead to defects such as transposition of the great vessels.

In the process of forming a separate pulmonary trunk and aorta, a vessel called the *ductus arteriosus* develops. This vessel, which connects the pulmonary artery and the aorta, allows blood entering the pulmonary trunk to be shunted into the aorta as a means of bypassing the lungs. Like the foramen ovale, the ductus arteriosus usually closes shortly after birth.

FETAL AND PERINATAL CIRCULATION

The fetal circulation is different both anatomically and physiologically from the postnatal circulation. Before birth, oxygenation of blood occurs by way of the placenta, and after birth, it occurs by way of the lungs. The fetus is maintained in a low-oxygen state (Po_2 20 to 30 mmHg) and 60% to 70% saturation.[58, 59] To compensate, fetal cardiac output is higher than at any other time (400 to 500 mL/kg/min).

In the fetus, blood enters the circulation by way of the umbilical vein and returns to the placenta by way of the two umbilical arteries (Fig. 23-23). A vessel called the *ductus venosum* allows blood from the umbilical vein to bypass the hepatic circulation and pass directly into the inferior vena cava. From the inferior vena cava, blood flows into the right atrium and from there it is directed through the foramen ovale into the left atrium. Blood then passes into the left ventricle and is ejected into the ascending aorta to perfuse the

head and upper extremities. In this way, the best oxygenated blood from the placenta is used to perfuse the brain. At the same time, venous blood from the head and upper extremities returns to the right side of the heart by way of the superior vena cava, moves into the right ventricle, and is ejected into the pulmonary artery. The pulmonary vascular resistance is very high because the lungs are fluid-filled and the resultant alveolar hypoxia contributes to intense vasoconstriction. Because of the high pulmonary vascular resistance, the blood that is ejected into the pulmonary artery is diverted through the ductus arteriosus into the descending aorta. This blood perfuses the lower extremities and is returned to the placenta by way of the umbilical arteries.

At birth, the infant takes its first breath and switches from placental to pulmonary oxygenation of the blood. The most dramatic alterations in the circulation after birth are the elimination of the low-resistance placental vascular bed and the marked pulmonary vasodilation that is produced by initiation of ventilation. The pressure in the pulmonary circulation and the right side of the heart fall as fetal lung fluid is replaced by air and lung expansion decreases the pressure transmitted to the pulmonary blood vessels. Also with lung inflation, the alveolar oxygen tension increases, causing reversal of the hypoxemic-induced pulmonary vasoconstriction of the fetal circulation. Cord clamping and removal of the low-resistance placental circulation produce an increase in systemic vascular resistance and a resultant increase in left ventricular pressure. The resultant fall in right atrial pressure and rise in left atrial pressure

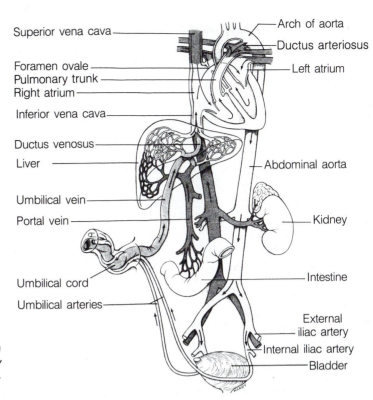

Superior vena cava — **Arch of aorta**

Ductus arteriosus

Foramen ovale — **Left atrium**
Pulmonary trunk
Right atrium

Inferior vena cava

Ductus venosus
Liver — **Abdominal aorta**

Umbilical vein

Portal vein — **Kidney**

Umbilical cord — **Intestine**
Umbilical arteries

External iliac artery
Internal iliac artery
Bladder

FIG. 23-23. Fetal circulation. (Redrawn from Chaffee, E.E., & Lytle, I.M. [1980]. *Basic physiology and anatomy* [4th ed., p. 353]. Philadelphia: J.B. Lippincott)

produce closure of the foramen ovale. Reversal of the fetal hypoxemic state also produces constriction of ductal smooth muscle, contributing to closures of the ductus arteriosus. Normally, both the foramen ovale and the ductus arteriosus normally close within the 1st day of life, effectively separating the pulmonary and systemic circulations.

After the initial precipitous fall in pulmonary vascular resistance, there is a more gradual decrease in pulmonary vascular resistance related to regression of the medial smooth muscle layer in the pulmonary arteries. During the first 2 to 9 weeks of life, there normally is a gradual thinning of the medial smooth muscle layer of pulmonary arteries that results in further decreases in pulmonary vascular resistance.[59] By the time a normal full-term infant is several weeks old, the pulmonary vascular resistance has fallen to adult levels.

Several factors, including prematurity, alveolar hypoxia, lung disease, and congenital heart defects, may affect postnatal vascular development.[59] If a baby is born prematurely, the smooth muscle layers of the pulmonary vasculature may develop incompletely or regress in a shorter period. Much of the development of the smooth muscle layer in the pulmonary arterioles occurs during the latter part of gestation; as a result, infants who are born prematurely have less medial smooth muscle. These infants follow the same pattern of smooth muscle regression, but because less muscle is present, their

muscle layer may regress in a shorter period. The pulmonary vascular smooth muscle in premature infants may also be less responsive to hypoxia. For these reasons, a premature infant may demonstrate a larger fall in pulmonary vascular resistance and a resultant shunting of blood from the aorta through the ductus arteriosus to the pulmonary artery within hours of birth.

The presence of hypoxia during the first days of life may delay or prevent the normal fall in pulmonary vascular resistance. During this period, the pulmonary arteries remain reactive and can constrict in response to hypoxia, acidosis, hyperinflation of the alveoli, and hypothermia. Alveolar hypoxia is one of the most potent stimuli for pulmonary vasoconstriction and of pulmonary hypertension in the neonate.

CAUSES OF CONGENITAL HEART DEFECTS

The major development of the fetal heart occurs between the 4th and 7th weeks of gestation; during this time, most congenital heart defects arise. The development of the heart may be altered as a result of environmental, genetic, and chromosomal influences.

Most cases of congenital heart defects are thought to be multifactorial in origin, meaning that they result from an interaction between a genetic predisposition to develop a heart defect and environmental influences. Infants born to parents with congenital heart defects or with siblings who have congenital heart defects are at higher risk. Some heart defects, such as coarctation of the aorta, atrial septal defect of the secundum type, and pulmonary valve stenosis, and certain ventricular septal defects have a stronger familial predisposition than others.

Chromosomal defects are thought to account for about 5% of congenital heart defects. Characteristic of these influences is the number of cardiac lesions observed in children born with Down's syndrome (trisomy of chromosome 21). A small number of cases (2% to 4%) are due to adverse maternal conditions and teratogenic influences, including maternal diabetes, congenital rubella, maternal alcohol ingestion, and treatment with anticonvulsant drugs.

HEMODYNAMIC DERANGEMENTS

Congenital heart defects produce their effects through abnormal shunting of blood and through alterations in pulmonary blood flow. They commonly are classified as congenital heart disease with cyanosis or congenital heart disease with little or no cyanosis.[60] Of the congenital defects discussed in this chapter, patent ductus arteriosus, atrial and ventricular septal defects, endocardial cushion defects, pulmonary valve stenosis, and coarctation of the aorta are considered defects with little or no cyanosis; both tetralogy of Fallot and transposition of the great vessels are considered defects with cyanosis.

SHUNTING OF BLOOD

Shunting of blood refers to the diverting of blood flow from one system to the other—from the arterial to the venous system (left-to-right shunt) or from the venous to the arterial system (right-to-left shunt). The shunting of blood in congenital heart defects is determined by the presence of an *abnormal opening* between the right and left circulations and the degree of resistance to flow through the opening.

The presence of a right-to-left shunt results in unoxygenated blood moving from the right side of the heart into the left side of the heart and then being ejected into the systemic circulation. Cyanosis develops when sufficient unoxygenated blood mixes with oxygenated blood in the left side of the heart. In left-to-right shunt, blood intended for ejection into the systemic circulation is recirculated through the right side of the heart and back through the lungs; this increased volume distends the right side of the heart and pulmonary circulation and increases the work load placed on the right ventricle. A child with a septal defect that causes left-to-right shunting usu-

ally has an enlarged right side of the heart and pulmonary blood vessels.

The vascular resistance of the systemic and pulmonary circulations may influence the direction of shunting. Because of the high pulmonary vascular resistance in the neonate, atrial and septal defects usually do not produce significant shunt or symptoms during the first weeks of life. As the pulmonary vascular smooth muscle regresses in the neonate, the resistance in the pulmonary circulation falls below that of the systemic circulation; in uncomplicated atrial or ventricular septal defects, blood shunts from the left side of the heart to the right. In more complicated ventricular septal defects, increased resistance to outflow may affect the pattern of shunting. For example, defects that increase resistance to aortic outflow (*e.g.*, aortic valve stenosis and coarctation of the aorta) increase left-to-right shunting, and defects that obstruct pulmonary outflow (*e.g.*, pulmonary valve stenosis or increased pulmonary vascular resistance) increase right-to-left shunting. Crying may increase right-to-left shunting in infants with septal defects by increasing pulmonary vascular resistance. This may be one of the reasons some infants with congenital heart defects become cyanotic during crying.

CHANGES IN PULMONARY VASCULAR RESISTANCE AND BLOOD FLOW

Many of the complications of congenital heart disorders result from their effect on the pulmonary circulation, which may be exposed to either an increase or a decrease in blood flow.

In contrast to the arterioles in the systemic circulation, the mature pulmonary arterioles are thin-walled vessels, so they can accommodate various levels of stroke volume from the right heart.

In a full-term infant who has a congenital heart defect that produces markedly increased pulmonary blood flow (such as a ventricular septal defect), the increased flow stimulates pulmonary vasoconstriction and prevents normal thinning of pulmonary vascular smooth muscle. These conditions delay or reduce the normal drop in pulmonary vascular resistance. As a result, symptoms related to increased pulmonary blood flow often are not apparent until the full-term infant is 4 to 12 weeks old.

Congenital heart defects that persistently increase pulmonary blood flow or pulmonary vascular resistance have the potential of causing pulmonary hypertension and producing pathologic changes in the pulmonary vasculature.

In situations in which the shunting of systemic blood flow into the pulmonary circulation threatens permanent injury to the pulmonary vessels, a surgical procedure may be done in an attempt to reduce the flow by increasing resistance to outflow from the right ventricle. This procedure, called *pulmonary banding*, consists of placing a constrictive band around the main pulmonary artery. The banding technique is used as a temporary measure to alleviate the symptoms and protect the pulmonary vessels in anticipation of later surgical repair of the defect. This procedure requires thoracotomy (opening the chest cavity) but does not necessitate cardiopulmonary bypass (use of the heart–lung machine).

Some congenital heart defects, such as pulmonary valve stenosis, decrease pulmonary blood flow, producing inadequate oxygenation of blood. The affected child may experience fatigue, exertional dyspnea, impaired growth, and even syncope.

SPECIFIC DEFECTS

Congenital heart defects can affect almost any of the cardiac structures or central blood vessels. Defects include communication between heart chambers, interrupted development of the heart chambers or valve structures, malposition of heart chambers and great vessels, and altered closure of fetal communication channels. The defect that is present reflects the embryo's stage of development at the time the defect occurred. Some congenital heart disorders, such as tetralogy of Fallot, involve several defects. The development of the heart is both simultaneous and sequential; a heart defect may reflect the multiple developmental events that were occurring simultaneously or sequentially. Table 23-2 summarizes the relative frequency of specific lesions.

PATENT DUCTUS ARTERIOSUS

Patent ductus arteriosus results from persistence of the fetal ductus beyond the prenatal period. In fetal life, the ductus arteriosus is the vital link by which blood from the right side of the heart bypasses the lungs and enters the systemic circulation (Fig. 23-24G). After birth, this passage is no longer needed, and it usually closes during the first 24 to 72 hours. The physiologic stimulus and mechanisms associated with permanent closure of the ductus are not entirely known, but the fact that infant hypoxia predisposes to a delayed closure suggests that the increase in arterial oxygen levels that occur immediately after birth play a role. Additional factors that contribute to closure are a fall in endogenous levels of prostaglandins and adenosine levels and the release of vasoactive substances. After constriction, the lumen of the ductus becomes permanently sealed with fibrous tissue within 2 to 3 weeks. Ductal closure may be de-

TABLE 23-2. RELATIVE FREQUENCY OF CONGENITAL HEART LESIONS*

LESIONS	PERCENTAGE OF ALL LESIONS
Ventricular septal defect	25–30
Atrial septal defect (secundum)	6–8
Patent ductus arteriosus	6–8
Coarctation of the aorta	5–7
Tetralogy of Fallot	5–7
Pulmonic valve stenosis	5–7
Aortic valve stenosis	4–7
Transposition of the great vessels	3–5
Hypoplastic left ventricle	1–3
Hypoplastic right ventricle	1–3
Truncus arteriosus	1–2
Total anomalous pulmonary venous return	1–2
Tricuspid atresia	1–2
Single ventricle	1–2
Double-outlet right ventricle	1–2
Others	5–10

* Excluding patent ductus arteriosus in preterm neonate, bicuspid aortic valve, peripheral pulmonary stenosis, and mitral valve prolapse. The endocardial cushion defects are included with specific defects (*e.g.*, ventricular septal and tricuspid atresia).
(From Behrman, R.E. [Ed.]. [1992]. *Nelson's textbook of pediatrics* [14th ed., pp. 1147–1191]. Philadelphia: W.B. Saunders)

layed or prevented in very premature infants probably as a result of a combination of factors, including decreased medial muscle in the ductus wall, decreased constrictive response to oxygen, and increased circulating levels of vasodilating prostaglandins. Hemodynamically significant patent ductus arteriosus is observed in about half of infants with a birthweight of less than 1000 g.[59] Ductal closure may also be delayed in infants with congenital heart defects that produce a decrease in oxygen tension.

As is true of other heart and circulatory defects, patency of the ductus arteriosus may be present in various forms; the opening may be small, medium-sized, or large. Once the infant's pulmonary vascular resistance falls, the patent ductus arteriosus provides for a continuous runoff of aortic blood into the pulmonary artery, causing a decrease in aortic diastolic (and mean arterial) pressure and a widening of the pulse pressure. With a large patent ductus, the runoff is continuous, resulting in increased pulmonary blood flow, pulmonary congestion, and increased resistance against which the right side of the heart must pump. Increased pulmonary venous return and increased work demands may lead to left ventricular failure.

Administration of indomethacin, an inhibitor of prostaglandin synthesis, is used as a treatment to

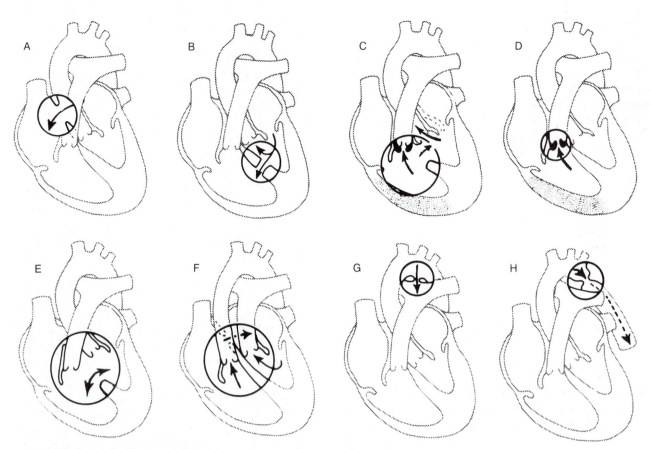

FIG. 23-24. Congenital heart defects. (**A**) Atrial septal defect. Blood is shunted from left to right. (**B**) Ventricular septal defect. Blood is usually shunted from left to right. (**C**) Tetralogy of Fallot. This involves a ventricular septal defect, dextroposition of the aorta, right ventricular outflow obstruction, and right ventricular hypertrophy. Blood is shunted from right to left. (**D**) Pulmonary stenosis, with decreased pulmonary blood flow and right ventricular hypertrophy. (**E**) Endocardial cushion defects. Blood flows between the chambers of the heart. (**F**) Transposition of the great vessels. The pulmonary artery is attached to the left side of the heart and the aorta to the right side. (**G**) Patent ductus arteriosus. The high pressure blood of the aorta is shunted back to the pulmonary artery. (**H**) Postductal coarctation of the aorta.

induce closure of a patent ductus arteriosus. If this method of treatment fails, surgical ligation may be needed.

The function of the ductus arteriosus in providing a right-to-left shunt in prenatal life has prompted the surgical creation of an aortic–pulmonary shunt as a means of improving pulmonary blood flow in children with severe pulmonary outflow disorders. Research has focused on the role of type E prostaglandins in maintaining the patency of the ductus; it has been found that by injecting prostaglandin E into the umbilical vein of infants who require a ductal shunt, closure has been delayed or prevented.

ATRIAL SEPTAL DEFECTS

In atrial septal defects, a hole in the atrial septum persists as a result of improper septal formation (see Fig. 23-24A). The two most common types of atrial septal defects are those that involve the ostium primum and ostium secundum, with those involving the latter being the most common. The defect is more common in females than in males. It may be single or multiple and vary in size from a small asymptomatic opening to a large symptomatic opening.

Most atrial septal defects are small, and the defect is discovered inadvertently during a routine physical examination. In the case of an isolated septal defect that is large enough to allow shunting, the flow of blood usually is from the left side to the right side of the heart because of the more compliant right ventricle and because the pulmonary vascular resistance is lower than the systemic vascular resistance. This produces right ventricular volume overload and increased pulmonary blood flow. The increased volume of blood that must be ejected from the right heart also prolongs closure of the pulmonary valve and produces a separation (fixed splitting) of the aortic and pulmonary components of the second heart sound.

Most children with atrial septal defects are asymptomatic. Older people (adolescents and young adults) may develop atrial fibrillation or atrial flutter and palpations because of atrial dilation. Because spontaneous closure occurs in some children, surgical treatment usually is delayed until the child is of school age. Transcatheter closure in the cardiac catheterization laboratory has proved effective. This procedure uses a double umbrella catheter with an umbrella placed on each side of the defect.[59] It often is used in children who have complex congenital heart defects that require multiple-stage surgical procedures. This can eliminate one surgical procedure. Surgical closure may be necessary when the defect does not close spontaneously or transcatheter closure is not deemed appropriate.

VENTRICULAR SEPTAL DEFECTS

A ventricular septal defect is an opening in the ventricular septum that results from a imperfect separation of the ventricles during early fetal development (see Fig. 23-24B). Ventricular septal defects are the most common form of congenital heart defect; they may be the only cardiac defect, or they may be one of multiple cardiac anomalies. In 20% of all people with congenital heart disease, a ventricular defect is the only abnormality. The ventricular septum originates from two sources: (1) the interventricular groove of the folded tubular heart that gives rise to the muscular part of the septum, and (2) the endocardial cushions that extend to form the membranous portion of the septum. The upper membranous portion of the septum is the last area to close, and it is here that most defects occur.

Depending on the size of the opening, the signs and symptoms of a ventricular septal defect may range from the presence of an asymptomatic murmur to congestive heart failure. If the defect is small, it allows a small shunt and small increases in pulmonary blood flow. These defects produce few symptoms, and about one third close spontaneously.[59] With medium-sized defects, a larger shunt occurs, producing a larger increase in pulmonary blood flow (twice as much blood may pass through the pulmonary circulation as through the systemic circulation). The increased pulmonary flow most often occurs under relatively low pressure. Most of the children with such defects are asymptomatic and have a low risk of developing pulmonary vascular disease.

Children with large defects have a large amount of pulmonary blood flow; because the defect is non-restrictive, the pressure in the left and right sides of the heart is equalized and blood is shunted from the left side of the heart into the pulmonary artery under high pressures that are sufficient to produce pulmonary hypertension. In these children, left-to-right shunting through the ventricular defect is lessened when pulmonary and systemic circulations offer equal resistance to flow. The child's symptoms improve during this time.[59] As the child's pulmonary vascular resistance increases further, a right-to-left shunt develops and the child demonstrates cyanosis. This reversal of the direction of shunt flow is called *Eisenmenger's syndrome.*

Most infants with a ventricular septal defect are asymptomatic during early infancy. This is because the higher pulmonary vascular resistance prevents shunting from occurring. Once an infant's pulmonary vascular resistance falls and a shunt develops, a characteristic systolic murmur develops. The infant with a large, uncomplicated ventricular septal defect usually is asymptomatic until pulmonary vascular resistance begins to fall at about 4 to 12 weeks. Once a large shunt develops, the mother reports that the infant breathes rapidly, feeds poorly, and is diaphoretic (signs of congestive heart failure). Right-to-left shunting produces cyanosis.

The treatment of a ventricular septal defect depends on the size of the defect and accompanying hemodynamic derangements. Children with small or medium-sized defects are followed closely in hopes that the defect will close spontaneously. Prophylactic antibiotic therapy is given during periods of increased risk of bacteremia. Cardiac catheterization may be performed in children with medium-sized or large defects who become symptomatic to document the location of the lesion, identify any associated heart defects, and determine the pulmonary vascular resistance. Congestive heart failure is treated medically. Surgical intervention is required for infants who do not respond to medical management. When possible, surgical closure of the defect is performed. Pulmonary artery banding may be done in cases of complex congenital defects with risk of pulmonary vascular involvement, in children with defects that are not amenable to medical or surgical treatment, or when the ventricular defect is only one of several defects present. The pulmonary band is removed when the ventricular defect is closed during open heart surgery at a later time.

ENDOCARDIAL CUSHION DEFECTS

The endocardial cushions form the AV canals, the upper part of the ventricular septum, and the lower part of the atrial septum. Endocardial cushion defects are responsible for about 5% of all congenital heart defects. Children with Down's syndrome have a high incidence of endocardial cushion defects, with estimates indicating that as many as 50% of such children have some form of endocardial cushion defect.

Because endocardial cushions contribute to multiple aspects of heart development, there a number of variations with this type of defect. The terms most commonly used to categorize endocardial cushion defects are partial and complete AV canal defects.[59] In partial AV canal defects, the two AV valve rings are complete and separate. The most common type of partial AV canal defect is an ostium primum defect with a cleft in the mitral valve. In complete canal defect, there is a common AV valve orifice along with defects in both the atrial and the ventricular septal tissue. Many variations of these two forms of endocardial cushion defect are possible (see Fig. 23-24E). Ebstein's anomaly is a defect in endocardial cushion development characterized by displacement of tricuspid valvular tissue into the ventricle. The displaced tricuspid leaflets are attached either directly to the right ventricular endocardial surface or to shortened or malformed chordae tendineae.

The direction and magnitude of shunt in children with endocardial cushion defects are determined by the combination of defects and the child's pulmonary and systemic vascular resistance. The hemodynamic effects of an isolated ostium primum defect are those of the previously described atrial septal defect. These children are largely asymptomatic during childhood. If a ventricular septal defect is present, pulmonary blood flow will be increased once pulmonary vascular resistance falls. Many children with ventricular septal defects have effort intolerance, easy fatigability, and recurrent infections, particularly when the shunt is large. The larger the defect, the greater the shunt and the higher the pressure in the pulmonary vascular system.

With complete AV canal defects, congestive heart failure and intercurrent pulmonary infections appear early in infancy. There is both left-to-right shunting and transatrial and transventricular mixing of blood. Pulmonary hypertension and increased pulmonary vascular resistance are common. Cyanosis develops with progressive shunting.

The treatment for endocardial cushion defects is determined by the severity of the defect. With an ostium primum defect, surgical repair usually is planned on an elective basis before the child enters school. Palliative or corrective surgery is required in infants with complete AV canal defects who develop congestive heart failure and do not respond to medical treatment. Total surgical repair of complete AV canal defects can now be accomplished with low operative risk.

PULMONARY STENOSIS

Pulmonary stenosis may occur as an isolated valvular lesion or in conjunction with more complex defects, such as tetralogy of Fallot. In isolated valvular defects, the pulmonary cusps may be absent or malformed, or they may remain fused at their commissural edges; all three abnormalities often are present.

Pulmonary valvular defects usually cause some impairment of pulmonary blood flow and increase the work load imposed on the right side of the heart (see Fig. 23-24D). Most children with pulmonic valve stenosis have mild to moderate stenosis that does not increase in severity. These children are largely asymptomatic. Severe defects are manifest by marked impairment of pulmonary blood flow that begins during infancy and is likely to become severer as the child grows. About one third of children under age 2 develop cyanosis.[59] The ductus arteriosus may provide the vital accessory route for perfusing the lungs in infants with severe stenosis. Also, when pulmonary stenosis is extreme, increased pressures in the right side of the heart may delay closure of the foramen ovale.

Treatment measures designed to maintain the patency of the ductus arteriosus may be used as a palliative measure to maintain or increase pulmonary blood flow in infants with severe pulmonary stenosis. Pulmonary valvotomy often is the treatment of choice. Transcatheter balloon valvuloplasty may be used in some infants with moderate degrees of obstruction. The procedure provides palliative improvement, although it is not known if the improvement is permanent.

TETRALOGY OF FALLOT

As the name implies, tetralogy of Fallot consists of four associated congenital heart defects: (1) ventricular septal defects that involve the membranous septum and the anterior portion of the muscular septum; (2) dextroposition or shifting to the right of the aorta, so that it overrides the right ventricle and is in communication with the septal defect; (3) obstruction or narrowing of the pulmonary outflow channel, including pulmonic valve stenosis, a decrease in the size of the pulmonary trunk, or both; and (4) hypertrophy of the right ventricle because of the increased work required to pump blood through the obstructed pulmonary channels (see Fig. 23-24C).

Most children with tetralogy of Fallot display varying degrees of cyanosis—hence the term *blue babies*. The cyanosis develops as the result of decreased pulmonary blood flow and because the right-to-left shunt causes mixing of unoxygenated blood with the oxygenated blood being ejected into the peripheral circulation. Hypercyanotic spells may occur during the first months of life. These spells typically occur in the morning during crying, feeding, or defecating. These activities increase the infant's oxygen requirements. In addition, crying and defecating may further increase pulmonary vascular resistance, thereby increasing right-to-left shunting and decreasing pulmonary blood flow. With the hypercyanotic spell, the infant becomes acutely cyanotic, hyperpneic, irritable, and diaphoretic. Later in the spell, the infant becomes limp and may lose consciousness. Placing the infant in the knee-chest position increases systemic vascular resistance and, as a result, increases pulmonary blood flow and decreases right-to-left shunting. During a hypercyanotic spell, toddlers and older children may spontaneously assume the squatting position; squatting functions like the knee-chest position to relieve the spell.[59]

Because of the hypoxemia that occurs in these children, palliative surgery designed to increase pulmonary blood flow often is needed during early infancy, with corrective surgery being done at a later age. Palliative surgery involves the creation of a surgical shunt to increase pulmonary blood flow. The most popular procedures use the subclavian artery or prosthetic material to create a shunt between the aorta and pulmonary artery.

TRANSPOSITION OF THE GREAT VESSELS

In complete transposition of the great vessels, the aorta originates in the right ventricle and the pulmonary artery originates in the left ventricle (see Fig. 23-24F). The defect is more common in infants whose mothers have diabetes and in male infants.[60] In infants born with this defect, survival depends on communication between the right and left sides of the heart, either in the form of a patent ductus arteriosus or septal defect. Prostaglandin E_1 may be administered in an effort to maintain the patency of the ductus arteriosus. Balloon atrial septostomy may be done to increase the blood flow between the two sides of the heart. In this procedure, a balloon-tipped catheter is inserted into the heart through the vena cava and then passed through the foramen ovale into the left atrium. The balloon is then inflated and brought back through the foramen ovale, enlarging the opening as it goes.

Corrective surgery is essential for long-term survival.[60] An arterial switch (Jantene) procedure may be done. This procedure, which corrects the relation of the systemic and pulmonary blood flows, is preferably performed in the first 2 weeks of life before postnatal reduction in pulmonary vascular resistance. An atrial switch procedure (Mustard, Senning) is performed on older children. Both of these procedures reverse the blood flow at the atrial level by the surgical formation of intraatrial baffles.

COARCTATION OF THE AORTA

Coarctation of the aorta is a localized narrowing of the aorta, either proximal (preductal or coarctation of infancy) or distal (postductal) to the ductus (see Fig. 23-24H). Most coarctations (about 98%) are of the postductal type. The anomaly occurs twice as often in males as in females. Coarctation of the aorta may be a feature of Turner's syndrome (see Chapter 4).

The classic sign of coarctation of the aorta is a disparity in pulsations and blood pressures in the arms and legs. The femoral, popliteal, and dorsalis pedis pulsations are weak or delayed in comparison with the bounding pulses of the arms and carotid vessels. The systolic blood pressure in the legs obtained by the cuff method normally is 10 to 20 mmHg higher than in the arms.[60] In coarctation, it is lower and may be difficult to obtain. The differential in blood pressure is common in children over age 1, about 90% of whom have hypertension in the upper extremities greater than the 95th percentile for age (see Chapter 21).[60]

Children with significant coarctation should be treated surgically, the optimal age for surgery being 2 to 4 years. If untreated, most people with coarctation of the aorta succumb between ages 20 and 40. The common serious complications are related to the hypertensive state.

In *preductal* or *infantile* coarctation, the ductus remains open and shunts blood from the pulmonary artery through the ductus arteriosus into the aorta. It frequently is seen with other cardiac anomalies and carries a high mortality. Because of the position of the defect, blood flow throughout the systemic circulation is reduced, and the affected infant develops heart failure at an early age because of the increased work load imposed on the left ventricle. Both medical and surgical methods are used to treat these infants.

MANIFESTATIONS AND TREATMENT

Congenital heart defects present with numerous signs and symptoms. Some defects, such as patent ductus arteriosus and small ventricular septal defects, close spontaneously, and in other, less severe defects, there are no signs and symptoms. The disorder typically is discovered during a routine health examination. Pulmonary congestion, cardiac failure, and decreased peripheral perfusion are the chief concerns in children with more severe defects. Such defects often cause problems shortly after birth or early in infancy. The child may exhibit cyanosis, respiratory difficulty, and fatigability and is likely to have difficulty with feeding and failure to thrive. A generalized cyanosis that persists longer than 3 hours after birth is suggestive of congenital heart disease.

One technique for evaluating the infant consists of administering 100% oxygen for 10 minutes. If the infant "pinks up," the cyanosis probably is due to respiratory problems. Because infant cyanosis may appear as a duskiness, it is important to assess the color of the mucous membranes, fingernails, toenails, tongue, and lips. Pulmonary congestion in the infant causes an increase in respiratory rate, orthopnea, grunting, wheezing, coughing, and rales. The baby whose peripheral perfusion is markedly decreased may appear to be in a shock-like state. The manifestations and treatment of heart failure in the infant and young child are similar to those in the adult (see Chapter 24), but the infant's small size and limited physical reserve make the manifestations more serious and treatment more difficult. The treatment plan usually includes supportive therapy designed to help the infant compensate for the limitations in cardiac reserve and to prevent complications. Surgical intervention often is required in severe defects; it may be done in the early weeks of life or, conditions permitting, delayed until the child is older. A discussion of congestive heart failure in children is presented in Chapter 24.

Most children with structural congenital heart disease and those who have had corrective surgery are at risk for development of infectious endocarditis. Because of this risk, these children should receive prophylactic antibiotic therapy during periods of increased risk of bacteremia.

In summary, the embryonic development of the heart occurs during weeks 3 through 8 after conception. During this time, development of the atrial and ventricular septa divides the embryonic tubular heart into a right side and a left side. The endocardial cushions develop to form separate right and left AV canals and the separation and spiraling of the bulbus cordis and truncus arteriosus separate the blood flow for the pulmonary and systemic circulations. At birth, the fetus takes its first breath and switches from placental to pulmonary oxygenation of blood; the foramen ovale and ductus arteriosus close, separating the pulmonary and systemic circulations; there is an almost immediate increase in systemic vascular resistance and left heart pressures and a decrease in pulmonary vascular resistance and right heart pressures. The smooth muscle layer in the pulmonary blood vessels undergoes gradual thinning during the first weeks of life, producing a further decrease in pulmonary vascular resistance.

Congenital heart defects affect about 8 out of every 1000 neonates and arise during the period of fetal heart development. The defect reflects the stage of development at the time the causative event occurred. A number of factors are thought to contribute to the development of congenital heart defects, including genetic and chromosomal influences, viruses, and environmental agents such as drugs and radiation. The cause of the defect often is unknown. The defect may produce no effects, or it may markedly affect cardiac function. Congenital heart defects commonly produce shunting of blood, either from the right to the left side of the heart or from the left to the right side of the heart. Left-to-right shunts typically increase the volume of the right side of the heart and pulmonary circulation, and right-to-left shunts transfer unoxygenated blood from the right side of the heart to the left side, diluting the oxygen content of blood that is being ejected into the systemic circulation and causing cyanosis. The direction and degree of shunt depend on the size of the defect that connects the two sides of the heart and the difference in resistance between the two sides of the circulation. Congenital heart defects commonly are classified into defects that produce cyanosis and those that produce little or no cyanosis. Depending on the severity of the defect, congenital heart defects may be treated medically or surgically. Both medical and surgical treatment often is indicated in children with severe defects.

■ REFERENCES

1. American Heart Association. (1992). *1992 Heart and stroke facts.* Dallas: American Heart Association.
2. Cotran, R.S., Kumar, V., & Robbins, S.L. (1989). *Pathologic basis of disease* (4th ed., pp. 597–656). Philadelphia: W.B. Saunders.
3. Braunwald, E. (1988). *Heart disease* (3rd ed., pp. 924, 944, 948, 1487–1491). Philadelphia: W.B. Saunders.
4. Spodick, D. (1971). Acoustic phenomena in pericardial disease. *American Heart Journal, 81,* 114–124.
5. Spodick, D. (1989). Pericarditis, pericardial effusion, cardiac tamponade, and constriction. *Critical Care Clinics, 5,* 455.
6. Sulzbach, L.M. (1989). Measurement of pulsus paradoxus. *Focus on Critical Care 16,* 142.
7. Guyton, A. (1991). *Medical physiology* (8th ed., pp. 238–239). Philadelphia: W. B. Saunders.
8. Gregg, D.E., & Patterson, R.E. (1980). Functional importance of coronary collaterals. *New England Journal of Medicine, 303*(24), 1404.
9. Berne, R.M., & Levy, L.M. (1992). *Cardiovascular physiology* (6th ed., pp. 266, 156–157). St. Louis: Mosby Year Book.
10. Prinzmetal, M., Kennamer, R., Merliss, R., et al. (1959). A variant form of angina pectoris. *American Journal of Medicine, 27,* 375–388.
11. Matriscians, L. (1992). Unstable angina: An overview. *Critical Care Nursing, 12,* 30.
12. Fluery, J. (1992). Long-term management of the patient with stable angina. *Nursing Clinics of North America, 27,* 205–230.
13. Pepine, C.J., El-Tamimi, H., & Lambert, C.R. (1992). Prinzmetal's angina (variant angina). *Heart Disease and Stroke, 1,* 281.
14. Freedman, S.B., Richmond, D.R., Alwyn, M., et al. (1987). Late follow-up (41 to 102 months) of medically treated patients with coronary artery spasm and minor atherosclerotic coronary obstructions. *American Journal of Cardiology, 57,* 1261.
15. Previtali, M., Panciroli, C., Ardissino, D. et al. (1987). Spontaneous remission of variant angina documented with Holter monitoring and ergonovine testing in pa-

tients treated with calcium antagonists. *American Journal of Cardiology, 59,* 235.

16. Waller, B.F. (1989). "Crackers, breakers, stretchers, drillers, scrapers, shavers, burners, welders and melters"—the future treatment of atherosclerotic coronary artery disease? A clinical-morphological assessment. *Journal of the American College of Cardiology, 13,* 969–987.

17. McKenna, M. (1992). Management of the patient undergoing myocardial revascularization: Percutaneous transluminal coronary angioplasty. *Nursing Clinics of North America, 27,* 231–256.

18. King, S.B., & Talley, J.D. (1989). Coronary arteriography and percutaneous transluminal coronary angioplasty: Changing patterns of use and results. *Circulation, 79*(Suppl. I), I-19.

19. Detre, K., Holubkov, R., Kelsy, S., et al. (1988). Percutaneous coronary angioplasty in 1985–1986 and 1977–1981. *New England Journal of Medicine, 318,* 265.

20. Bevens, M., & McLimore, E. (1992). Intracoronary stents: A new approach to coronary artery dilation. *Journal of Cardiovascular Nursing, 7,* 34–49.

21. Halfman-Franey, M., Tukan, T., Bergstrom, D., et al. (1991). Using stents in the coronary circulation: Nursing perspectives. *Focus on Critical Care 18,* 132.

22. Litvack, F., Grundfest, W.S., Segalowitz, J., et al. (1990). Interventional cardiovascular therapy by laser and thermal angioplasty. *Circulation, 81* (Suppl.), IV-109.

23. Speroni, R., Fiske, J., Frank, D., et al. (1992). Coronary atherectomy: Overview and implications for nursing. *Journal of Cardiovascular Nursing, 7,* 25.

24. CASS Principal Investigators and Associates. (1984). Myocardial infarction and mortality in the Coronary Artery Surgery Study (CASS) randomized trial. *New England Journal of Medicine, 310,* 750.

25. Varnaushas, E. (1985). The European Coronary Surgery Study Group: Survival, myocardial infarction, and employment status in a prospective randomized study of coronary artery bypass surgery. *Circulation, 72* (Suppl.), 90–101.

26. Detre, K.M., Taharo, T., Hultgren, H., et al. (1985). Long-term mortality and morbidity results of the Veterans Administration randomized trial of coronary artery bypass surgery. *Circulation, 72* (Suppl), 84–89.

27. CASS Principal Investigators and Associates. (1983). Coronary Artery Surgery Study (CASS): A randomized trial of coronary artery bypass surgery. Quality of life in patients randomly assigned to treatment groups. *Circulation, 68,* 951–960.

28. Mock, M.B., Fisher, L.D., Holmes, D.R., et al. (1988). Comparison of effects of medical and surgical survival in severe angina pectoris and two-vessel coronary artery disease with and without left ventricular dysfunction: A coronary artery surgery study. *American Journal of Cardiology, 61,* 1198.

29. DeWood, M.A., Spores, J., Notske, C., et al. (1980). Prevalence of total coronary occlusion during the early hours of transmural myocardial infarction. *New England Journal of Medicine, 303,* 897–902.

30. Gibler, W.B., Gibler, C.D., Weinshenker, E., et al. (1987). Myoglobin as an early indicator of acute myocardial infarction. *Annals of Emergency Medicine, 16,* 851–856.

31. Cole, P.L. (1991). Thrombolytic therapy: Then and now. *Heart and Lung, 10,* 542–551.

32. Daily, E.K. (1991). Clinical management of patients receiving thrombolytic therapy. *Heart and Lung, 20,* 552–563.

33. Yusup, S., Wittes, J., & Friedman, L. (1988). Overview of results of randomized clinical trials in heart disease. *Journal of the American Medical Association, 260,* 2088.

34. DeWood, M., & Berg, R. (1987). The role of surgical reperfusion in myocardial infarction. *Cardiology Clinics, 2,* 113.

35. Brandenburg, R.O., & Nishimura, R.A. (1985). Clinical differentiation of the cardiomyopathies. *Practical Cardiology, 11,* 149.

36. Casey, P.E. (1987). Pathophysiology of dilated cardiomyopathy: Nursing implications. *Journal of Cardiovascular Nursing 2,* 1.

37. Cragin, P. (1988). Peripartum cardiomyopathy. *Focus on Critical Care, 15,* 39.

38. Demakis, J.G., Shahbudin, H., Rahimtoola, M.B., et al. (1971). Natural course of peripartum cardiomyopathy. *Circulation, 44,* 1053–1061.

39. Bohachick, P., & Rongaus, A.M. (1984). Hypertrophic cardiomyopathy. *American Journal of Nursing, 84,* 320–326.

40. Courtney-Jenkins, A. (1987). The patient with hypertrophic cardiomyopathy. *Journal of Cardiovascular Nursing, 2,* 33.

41. Maron, B.J., Bonow, R.D., Cannon, R.D., et al. (1987). Hypertrophic cardiomyopathy, Part 2: Interrelations of clinical manifestations, pathophysiology, and therapy. *New England Journal of Medicine, 316,* 844–852.

42. Kawai, C., Matsumori, A., Fujiwara, H., et al. (1987). Myocarditis and cardiomyopathy. *Annual Review of Medicine, 38,* 227.

43. Peters, N.S., & Poole-Wilson, P.A. (1990). Myocarditis—continuing clinical and pathologic confusion. *American Heart Journal, 119,* 942–947.

44. Ad Hoc Committee to Revise Jones Criteria (modified) of the Council on Rheumatic Fever and Congenital Heart Disease of the American Heart Association. (1984). Jones Criteria (revised) for Guidance in the Diagnosis of Rheumatic Fever. *Circulation, 69,* 203A–208A.

45. Committee on Rheumatic Fever, Endocarditis, and Kawasaki Disease of the Council on Cardiovascular Disease in the Young of the American Heart Association. (1993). Guidelines for the diagnosis of rheumatic fever. *Journal of the American Medical Association, 268,* 2069–2073.

46. Bisno, A.L. (1991). Group A streptococcus infections and acute rheumatic fever. *New England Journal of Medicine, 325,* 783–794.

47. Massie, B.M., & Kokolow, M. (1993). Cardiovascular disease. In L.M. Tierney, S.J. McPhee, M.A. Papadakis, et al. (Eds.). *Current medical diagnosis and treatment* (pp. 284–288). Norwalk, CT: Appleton & Lange.

48. Committee on Rheumatic Fever, Endocarditis, and Kawasaki's Disease of the Council on Cardiovascular Disease in the Young, American Heart Association. (1990). Prevention of bacterial endocarditis. *Journal of the American Medical Association, 262,* 2919–2922.

49. Bisno, A.L. (1989). Antimicrobial prophylaxis for infective endocarditis. *Hospital Practice, 24*(3A), 209–225.

50. Barron, K.S., & Murphy, D.J. (1989). Kawasaki syndrome: Still a fascinating enigma. *Hospital Practice 24*(10A), 51–60.

51. Hicks, R.V., & Melish, M.E. (1986). Kawasaki syndrome. *Pediatric Clinics of North America, 33,* 1151–1175.

52. Rowley, A.H., Gonzalez-Crussi F., & Schulman, F. (1988). Kawasaki syndrome: A review article. *Review of Infectious Diseases, 10,* 1–15.

53. Schulman, S.T. (Ed.). (1989). Management of Kawa-

saki syndrome: A consensus statement prepared by North American participants of The Third International Kawasaki Disease Symposium, Tokyo, Japan, December, 1988. *Pediatric Infectious Disease Journal, 8,* 663–665.

54. Rauch, A.M. (1987). Kawasaki's syndrome: Review of new epidemiologic and laboratory evidence. *Pediatric Infectious Disease Journal, 6,* 1016–1021.

55. Levy, D., & Savage, D. (1987). Prevalence and clinical features of mitral valve prolapse. *American Heart Journal, 113,* 1281.

56. Moore, K.L. (1988). *The developing human* (4th ed., pp. 286–308). Philadelphia: W.B. Saunders.

57. Hazinski, M.F. (1983). Congenital heart disease in the neonate: Epidemiology, cardiac development, and fetal circulation. *Neonatal Network, 1*(2), 29–43.

58. Heyman, M.A., & Rudolph, A.M. (1972). Effects of congenital heart disease on fetal and neonatal circulations. *Progress in Cardiovascular Diseases, 14*(2), 115–143.

59. Hazinski, M.F. (1992). *Nursing care of the critically ill child* (2nd ed., pp. 12–131, 271–361). St. Louis: Mosby Year Book.

60. Behrman, R.E. (Ed.). (1992). *Nelsons textbook of pediatrics* (14th ed., pp. 1147–1191). Philadelphia: W.B. Saunders.

■ **BIBLIOGRAPHY**

Aktar, M., Avitall, B., Jazayeri, M., et al. (1992). Role of implantable cardioverter defibrillator therapy in the management of high-risk patients. *Circulation, 85* (Suppl. I), I-131.

Alyn, I.B., & Baker, L.K. (1992). Cardiovascular anatomy and physiology of the fetus, neonate, infant, child, and adolescent. *Journal of Cardiovascular Nursing, 6*(3), 1–11.

Antman, E.M., & Braunwald, E. (1990). Acute MI: Management in the 1990s. *Hospital Practice, 25*(7A), 65–82.

Borrow, K.M., & Karp, R. (1990). Atrial septal defect: Lessons from the past, directions for the future. *New England Journal of Medicine, 323,* 1698–1700.

Burge, D.J., & DeHoratius, R.J. (1992). Acute rheumatic fever. *Cardiovascular Clinics, 23,* 3–23.

Burke, L.J., & Norris, S.O. (1988). Nursing care of the patient with recurrent ventricular dysrhythmias. In L.S. Kern (Ed.). *Cardiac critical care nursing* (p. 143). Rockville, MD: Aspen.

Chapman, E.L., Strawn, R.M., & Stewart, B.P. (1992). Differentiating between ventricular tachycardia and supraventricular tachycardia in the clinical setting. *Focus on Critical Care, 19,* 87.

Cjuim, D., Ford, C.F., & Yursha-Johnson, M. (1991). Silent myocardial ischemia. *Focus on Critical Care, 18,* 295.

Cohn, P.F. (1992). Silent ischemia. *Heart Disease and Stroke, 1,* 295.

Deedwania, P.C., & Carbajal, E.V. (1991). Silent myocardial ischemia, a clinical perspective. *Archives of Internal Medicine, 151,* 2373.

Epstein, C.D. (1992). Changing interpretations of angina pectoris associated with transient myocardial ischemia. *Journal of Cardiovascular Nursing, 7,* 1.

Fowler, N.O. (1992). Pericardial disease. *Heart Disease and Stroke, 1,* 85.

Fuster, V., Badimon, L., Badimon, J.J., et al. (1992). The pathogenesis of coronary artery disease and the acute coronary syndromes (review articles, parts 1 and 2). *New England Journal of Medicine, 326,* 242–250, 310–318.

Givens, L., & Ricks, J. (1985). Assessment of clinical manifestations of cyanotic and acyanotic heart disease in infants and children. *Heart and Lung, 14,* 200.

Grady, K.L., & Costanzo-Nordin, M.R. (1989). Myocarditis: A review of a clinical enigma. *Heart and Lung, 18,* 347.

Grass, S., & Utz, S. (1986). Mitral valve prolapse: A review of the scientific and medical literature. *Heart and Lung, 15,* 507.

Katz, A.M. (1990). Cardiomyopathy of overload. *New England Journal of Medicine, 322,* 10010.

Manson, J.E., Tostenson, H., Satterfield, S., et al. (1992). The primary prevention of myocardial infarction (review article). *New England Journal of Medicine, 326,* 140616.

Mason, P., & McPherson, C. (1992). Implantable cardioverter defibrillator: A review. *Heart and Lung, 21,* 141.

Molavi, A. (1992). Endocarditis: Recognition, management, and prophylaxis. *Cardiovascular Clinics, 23,* 139.

Morody, F. (1990). Catheter ablation of accessory pathways. *Cardiology Clinic, 8,* 557.

Moss, A.J. (1992). Clues in diagnosing congenital heart defect. *Western Journal of Medicine, 156,* 392–398.

Owens-Jones, S.J., & Hopp, L. (1988). Viral myocarditis. *Focus on Critical Care, 15,* 25–37.

Page, G.G. (1986). Tetralogy of Fallot. *Heart and Lung, 15*(4), 390.

Pritchett, E.L.C. (1992). Management of atrial fibrillation (review article). *New England Journal of Medicine, 326,* 1264–1271.

Ross, A.M. (1990). Role of angioplasty in myocardial infarction management strategies: A review. *Heart and Lung, 19,* 604.

Ross, L., & Leary, E. (1992). Evaluating the patient with coronary artery disease. *Nursing Clinics of North America, 27,* 171.

Runge, M.S. (1992). The future of thrombolytic therapy. *Heart Disease and Stroke, 1,* 39.

Ruskin, J.N. (1987). Primary ventricular fibrillation. *New England Journal of Medicine, 317*(5), 307.

Selzer, A. (1987). Changing aspects of the natural history of valvular aortic stenosis. *New England Journal of Medicine, 317*(2), 91.

Speroni, R., Fishe, J., Frank, D., et al. (1992). Coronary atherectomy: Overview and implications for nursing. *Journal of Cardiovascular Nursing, 7,* 25.

Tamburro, P., & Wilber, D. (1992). Sudden death in idiopathic dilated cardiomyopathy. *American Heart Journal, 124,* 1035.

Vincent, R.N., & Collins, G.F. (1986). Cardiac embrylogy and fetal cardiovascular physiology. *Critical Care Quarterly, 9,* 1.

Wilson, W.R. (1992). Recognition and treatment of infective endocarditis. *Heart Disease and Stroke, 1,* 64.

Zaim, S., & Walter, P.F. (1992). Diagnosis and treatment of ventricular tachycardia. *Heart Disease and Stroke, 1,* 141.

C H A P T E R   2 4

HEART FAILURE

■ OBJECTIVES

After you have studied this chapter, you should be able to meet the following objectives:

- Explain the effect of cardiac reserve on symptom development in heart failure.
- Define the terms *preload*, *afterload*, and *cardiac contractility*.
- Explain how increased sympathetic activity, fluid retention, the Frank-Starling mechanism, and myocardial hypertrophy act as compensatory mechanisms in heart failure.
- Differentiate high-output versus low-output heart failure, systolic versus diastolic heart failure, and right-sided versus left-sided heart failure.
- Use the Starling curve to explain the development of dyspnea in heart failure.
- Explain the mechanisms involved in paroxysmal nocturnal dyspnea.
- Explain the cause of fluid retention and edema; nocturia; dyspnea and cough; fatigue, weakness, and confusion; hepatomegaly and liver dysfunction, ano-

rexia, and cardiac cachexia in persons with congestive heart failure.
- Relate the effect of left ventricular failure to the development of pulmonary edema.
- Describe the clinical picture of pulmonary edema.
- Describe the actions of digitalis and their effects on cardiac function.
- Explain the actions of diuretics, inotropic agents, and vasodilating drugs in the treatment of heart failure.
- Explain the rationale for placing a person with pulmonary edema in the seated position.
- Describe the manifestations of heart failure in infants and children.
- Cite how the aging process affects heart failure in the elderly.
- State how the signs and symptoms of heart failure may differ between younger and older adults.

Carol Mattson Porth: PATHOPHYSIOLOGY: CONCEPTS OF
ALTERED HEALTH STATES, 4th ed. © 1994, 1990, 1986, 1982
J.B. Lippincott Company

Heart failure represents the end result of the many conditions that impair the pumping ability of the heart. It has been estimated that 2.3 to 3 million persons in the United States are afflicted with heart failure.[1] Whereas the incidence of other cardiovascular disorders has decreased over the past several decades, heart failure has increased at a dramatic rate because more persons who normally would die of acute myocardial infarction are surviving, but with compromised ventricular function.[2] Despite advances in the understanding of heart failure and its treatment, about half of persons with mild to moderate heart failure die within 5 years.

Heart failure is not a specific disease but a condition that is characterized by the inability of the heart to pump blood commensurate with the metabolic needs of the body. It may result from a diseased heart that is unable to pump blood or from excessive demands placed on a normal heart. Congestive heart failure is accompanied by congestion of the body tissues. Heart failure may present as an acute condition (cardiogenic shock and acute pulmonary edema) or as a chronic condition (congestive heart failure). This chapter focuses on chronic heart failure and is divided into four sections: (1) physiology of heart failure, (2) congestive heart failure, (3) acute pulmonary edema, and (4) heart failure in children and the elderly. Acute heart failure, which occurs with cardiogenic shock, is discussed in Chapter 25.

■ PHYSIOLOGY OF HEART FAILURE

The heart has the amazing capacity to adjust its activity to meet the varying needs of the body—during sleep its output declines, and during exercise it increases markedly. The ability to increase cardiac output during increased activity is called the *cardiac reserve*. For example, competitive swimmers and long-distance runners have large cardiac reserves. During exercise the cardiac output of these athletes rapidly increases to as much as five to six times their resting level. In sharp contrast with the healthy athlete, persons with heart failure often use their cardiac reserve at rest. For them, just climbing a flight of stairs may cause shortness of breath because they have exceeded their cardiac reserve.

The physiology of heart failure involves an interplay between two factors: (1) the inability of the failing heart to maintain sufficient cardiac output to support body functions and (2) the recruitment of compensatory mechanisms designed to maintain the cardiac reserve.

CARDIAC OUTPUT

The cardiac output is the amount of blood that the heart pumps each minute. It reflects how often the heart beats each minute (heart rate) and how much blood the heart pumps with each beat (stroke volume) and can be expressed as the product of the heart rate and stroke volume (cardiac output = heart rate x stroke volume). Heart rate is regulated by the autonomic nervous system and by shifting the balance between sympathetic (adrenergic) activity, which accelerates heart rate, and parasympathetic (vagal) activity, which slows it down. Stroke volume is a function of preload, afterload, and cardiac contractility.

PRELOAD

The term *preload* is used to describe the tension that exists in the walls of the heart as a result of diastolic filling. It reflects venous return and the filling of the ventricles and is the work load that the heart encounters before it begins to contract. Both end-diastolic ventricular volume and end-diastolic ventricular pressure are measures of preload. In the clinical setting, pulmonary capillary wedge pressure (PCWP) and central venous pressure (CVP) are used to assess preload (discussed later). The heart may fail as a pump because the preload is excessively elevated, such as in valvular regurgitation, renal failure, or myocardial infarction.

AFTERLOAD

Afterload represents the force that the contracting heart must generate to eject blood from the filled heart. In the left heart, it represents all of the pre-ejection work that the left ventricle must do to generate sufficient pressure to open the aortic valve and eject blood into the aorta. The main components of afterload are ventricular wall tension and the systemic vascular resistance. There is an inverse relationship between afterload and ventricular emptying, such that elevated levels of afterload tend to impair emptying and increase ventricular work. Aortic stenosis and severe hypertension may excessively elevate afterload and contribute to the development of heart failure.

CARDIAC CONTRACTILITY

Cardiac contractility refers to the mechanical performance of the heart—the ability of the contractile elements of the heart muscle (actin and myosin filaments) to interact and shorten against a load. The ejection of blood from the heart during systole is dependent upon cardiac contractility. Sympathetic stimulation of the heart increases cardiac contractility, whereas hypoxia and ischemia decrease contractility. A decrease of cardiac contractility can result from loss of functional muscle tissue due to myocardial infarction or from conditions, such as cardiomyopathy, that diffusely affect the myocardium.

COMPENSATORY MECHANISMS

In heart failure, the cardiac reserve is largely maintained through four compensatory mechanisms: (1) sympathetic nervous system support mechanisms, (2) salt and water retention, (3) the Frank-Starling mechanism, and (4) myocardial hypertrophy. It is important to note that the healthy as well as the failing heart uses these same compensatory mechanisms. Hence in the failing heart, early decreases in cardiac function may go unnoticed because these compensatory mechanisms maintain the cardiac output. This is called *compensated heart failure.* Unfortunately, the mechanisms were not intended for long-term use; in severe and prolonged *decompensated heart failure* the compensatory mechanisms are no longer effective, and the compensatory mechanisms themselves worsen the failure. Figure 24-1 diagrams the mechanisms of compensated and decompensated heart failure.

SYMPATHETIC NERVOUS SYSTEM SUPPORT

Reflex stimulation of the sympathetic nervous system plays an important role in the compensatory response to a decrease in cardiac output and perhaps to the pathogenesis of heart failure.[3] Both afferent cardiac sympathetic tone and catecholamine levels are elevated during the late stages of most forms of heart failure. By direct stimulation of both heart rate and cardiac contractility as well as by regulation of vascular tone, the sympathetic nervous system helps to maintain perfusion of the various organs, particularly the heart and brain. In persons with more severe heart failure, blood from the skin, kidneys, and gastrointestinal tract is diverted to the more critical cerebral and coronary circulations. The negative aspects of these adaptations include an increase in vascular resistance and the afterload against which the heart must pump. There is also evidence that prolonged sympathetic stimulation may exhaust myocardial stores of norepinephrine and may lead to destruction of sympathetic nerve endings. Moreover, these effects are distributed unevenly across the myocardium and may have deleterious effects on cardiac structure and function over time. For example, they may adversely affect the balance between oxygen supply and demand in persons in whom this ratio is precariously balanced. The catecholamines may also contribute to the high rate of sudden death by promoting dysrhythmias.[3]

SODIUM AND WATER RETENTION

During heart failure, sodium and water retention increase vascular volume and venous return to the heart in a misdirected effort to increase the ventricular end-diastolic volume and cardiac output via the Frank-Starling mechanism. Although useful in cases of hypovolemia, this response serves to increase the volume load on an already overloaded heart in persons with heart failure.

One of the most important effects of lower cardiac output in heart failure is a reduction in renal blood flow and glomerular filtration rate, which leads to salt and water retention. Normally, the kidneys receive about 25% of the cardiac output, but this may be decreased to as low as 8% to 10% in persons with heart failure. With a decrease in renal blood flow there is a progressive increase in renin secretion by the kidneys along with parallel increases in circulating levels of angiotensin II. The increased concentration of angiotensin II contributes to a generalized and excessive vasoconstriction and provides a powerful stimulus for aldosterone production by the adrenal

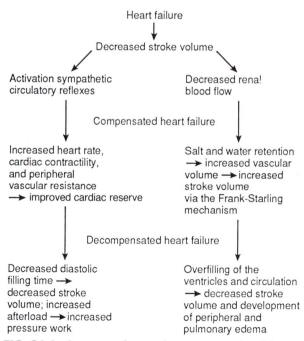

FIG. 24-1. *Sequence of events in compensated and decompensated heart failure.*

cortex. Aldosterone increases tubular reabsorption of sodium with an accompanying increase in water retention. Because aldosterone is metabolized in the liver, its levels are further increased when heart failure causes liver congestion. Angiotensin II also increases levels of antidiuretic hormone (ADH), which serves as a vasoconstrictor and inhibitor of water excretion (see Chapter 29). Currently, angiotensin-converting enzyme (ACE) inhibitor drugs, which block the conversion of angiotensin I to angiotensin II, are increasingly being used in the treatment of heart failure.[4]

A recently identified hormone called the *atrial natriuretic factor* (*ANF*), or *atriopeptin*, has been shown to affect fluid balance in heart failure.[5,6] ANF is a peptide hormone released from atrial cells in the heart in response to increased atrial pressure. The hormone produces rapid and transient natriuresis, diuresis, and moderate loss of potassium in the urine. Increased ANF has been found in adults with congestive heart failure, but the role of ANF in compensating for alterations in cardiac function that occur with heart failure is still unclear.

FRANK-STARLING MECHANISM

The Frank-Starling mechanism produces an increase in stroke volume by means of an increase in ventricular end-diastolic volume (preload). With increased diastolic filling, there is increased stretching of the myocardial fibers, more optimal approximation of the actin and myosin filaments, and a resultant increase in the force of the next contraction (see Chapter 22).

Cardiac output may be normal at rest in persons with heart failure due to increased ventricular end-diastolic volume and the Frank-Starling mechanism. This mechanism becomes ineffective, however, when the heart becomes overfilled and the muscle fibers are overstretched. With the deterioration of myocardial contractility, the ventricular function curve depicted in Figure 24-2 flattens out, so that with any given need for increased cardiac output, such as occurs with increased physical activity, there is a greater rise in left ventricular end-diastolic volume and pressure, with an elevation of pulmonary capillary pressure and development of dyspnea and pulmonary congestion.

The most important determinant of myocardial energy consumption is ventricular wall tension. Overfilling of the ventricle produces a decrease in wall thickness and an increase in wall tension. According to Laplace's law (explained in Chapter 19), wall tension is directly related to the product of intraventricular pressure and ventricle radius and inversely related to ventricular wall thickness ($T = [P \times R]/W$).

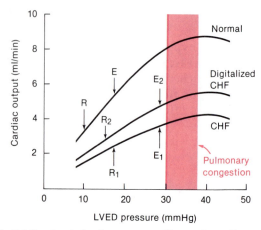

FIG. 24-2. Frank-Starling curves (*R* = resting; *E* = exercise; *LVED* = left ventricular end-diastolic; *CHF* = congestive heart failure). (Iseri, L. T., & Benvenuti, D. J. [1983]. Pathogenesis and management of congestive heart failure—revisited. *American Heart Journal, 105*(2), 346)

Because increased wall tension increases myocardial oxygen requirements, it can produce further impairment of cardiac function. The use of diuretics in persons with heart failure helps to reduce vascular volume and ventricular filling, thereby unloading the heart and reducing ventricular wall tension.

MYOCARDIAL HYPERTROPHY

Myocardial hypertrophy is a long-term compensatory mechanism. Cardiac muscle, like skeletal muscle, responds to an increase in work demands by undergoing hypertrophy. Hypertrophy increases the number of contractile elements (actin and myosin) in myocardial cells as a means of increasing their contractile performance.

Heart diseases that increase resistance to the ejection of blood from the ventricles are the greatest stimulus for hypertrophy. For example, the wall of the left ventricle may increase to six times its normal size in severe aortic stenosis. If portions of the heart muscle are damaged and replaced with scar tissue, the undamaged part of the myocardium often hypertrophies as a means of improving the pumping capacity of the ventricle. When the oxygen requirements of the increased muscle mass exceed the ability of the coronary vessels to bring blood to the area, myocardial hypertrophy is no longer beneficial. Also, some forms of hypertrophy may lead to abnormal remodeling of the ventricular wall with reduction in chamber size and impaired diastolic filling. In addition, abnormal growth of nonmyocardial tissue (*e.g.*, fibrous tissue) may produce stiffness of the ventricle and cause further impairment of ventricular function.

In summary, the physiology of heart failure reflects an interplay between a decrease in cardiac output that accompanies impaired function of the failing heart and the compensatory mechanisms designed to preserve the cardiac reserve. Four compensatory mechanisms contribute to the cardiac reserve: (1) increased activity of the sympathetic nervous system, (2) salt and water retention, (3) the Frank-Starling mechanism, and (4) myocardial hypertrophy. Hence, in the failing heart, early decreases in cardiac function may go unnoticed because these compensatory mechanisms maintain the cardiac output. This is called *compensated heart failure*. Unfortunately, the mechanisms were not intended for long-term use, and in severe and prolonged *decompensated heart failure*, the compensatory mechanisms are no longer effective and the mechanisms themselves further impair cardiac function.

■ CONGESTIVE HEART FAILURE

Congestive heart failure is heart failure that is accompanied by congestion of body tissues. It may occur as a primary condition caused by defective functioning of the heart itself or as a secondary disorder resulting from systemic diseases that place undue demands on the heart or influence its function. Primary disorders of the heart, such as coronary artery disease, valvular heart disease, and cardiomyopathies, account for most cases of heart failure. In persons with asymptomatic heart disease, heart failure may be precipitated by an unrelated illness or stress. Table 22-1 lists major causes of heart failure.

TYPES OF HEART FAILURE

Heart failure may be described as high-output or low-ouput failure, systolic or diastolic failure, and right-sided or left-sided failure.

HIGH-OUTPUT VERSUS LOW-OUTPUT FAILURE

An uncommon type of heart failure that is caused by an excessive need for cardiac output is often referred to as *high-output failure*. With high-output failure the function of the heart may be supranormal but inadequate owing to excessive metabolic needs. Causes of high-output failure include severe anemia, thyrotoxicosis, conditions that cause arteriovenous shunting, and Paget's disease. High-output failure tends to be specifically treatable. *Low-output failure* is caused by disorders that impair the pumping ability of the heart, such as ischemic heart disease and cardiomyopathy.

SYSTOLIC VERSUS DIASTOLIC FAILURE

Until recently, congestive heart failure viewed mainly in terms of backward and forward failure. *Backward failure* represents failure of one of the ventricles to discharge its content normally so that end-diastolic volume rises and the pressures and volumes in the atrium and venous system behind the ventricle become elevated. In contrast, *forward failure* is characterized by impaired output of blood into the arterial system emerging from the heart.

A more recent classification separates the pathophysiology of congestive failure into two new categories—systolic dysfunction and diastolic dysfunction.[7] With *systolic dysfunction* there is impaired ejection of blood from the heart during systole; with *diastolic dysfunction* there is impaired filling of the heart during diastole (Fig. 24-3). Many persons with heart disease fall into an intermediate category with elements of both systolic and diastolic dysfunction.[7,8]

TABLE 24-1. CAUSES OF HEART FAILURE

IMPAIRED CARDIAC FUNCTION	EXCESS WORK DEMANDS
Myocardial Disease	**Increased Pressure Work**
Cardiomyopathies	Systemic hypertension
Myocarditis	Pulmonary hypertension
Coronary insufficiency	Coarctation of the aorta
Myocardial infarction	
Valvular Heart Disease	**Increased Volume Work**
Stenotic valvular disease	Arteriovenous shunt
Regurgitant valvular disease	Excessive administration of intravenous fluids
Congenital Heart Defects	**Increased Perfusion Work**
	Thyrotoxicosis
	Anemia
Constrictive Pericarditis	

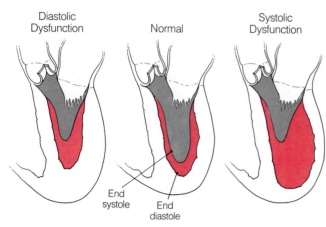

FIG. 24-3. Congestive heart failure due to systolic and diastolic dysfunction. Ejection fraction represents the difference between end diastolic function and end systolic volume. (**Middle**) Normal systolic and diastolic function with normal ejection fraction; (**left**) diastolic dysfunction with decreased ejection fraction due to decreased diastolic filling; (**right**) systolic dysfunction with decreased ejection fraction due to impaired systolic function.

Systolic Dysfunction. Systolic dysfunction involves a decrease in cardiac contractility and ejection fraction. It commonly results from conditions that impair the contractile performance of the heart (*e.g.,* ischemic heart disease and cardiomyopathy) or from hemodynamic conditions that produce a volume overload (*e.g.,* valvular insufficiency and anemia) or a pressure overload (*e.g.,* hypertension and valvular stenosis).

A normal ventricle ejects about two-thirds of the blood that is present in the ventricle at the end of diastole when it contracts. This is called the *ejection fraction*. In systolic heart failure, the ejection fraction declines progressively with increasing degrees of myocardial dysfunction. In very severe forms of heart failure, the ejection fraction may be as low as 15% to 20%. With a decrease in ejection fraction, there is a resultant increase in diastolic volume, ventricular dilation and ventricular wall tension, and a rise in ventricular end-diastolic pressure. The symptoms of persons with systolic dysfunction are mainly due to reductions in ejection fraction and cardiac output.

Diastolic Dysfunction. Diastolic dysfunction, which reportedly accounts for 25% to 40% of all cases of congestive heart failure, is characterized by smaller ventricular chamber size, ventricular hypertrophy, and poor ventricular compliance (ability to stretch during filling).[9,10] Because of impaired filling, congestive symptoms tend to predominate in diastolic dysfunction. Among the conditions that cause diastolic dysfunction are those that restrict diastolic filling (*e.g.,* mitral stenosis), those that increase ventricular wall thickness and reduce chamber size (*e.g.,* myocardial hypertrophy due to lung disease and hypertrophic cardiomyopathy), and those that delay diastolic relaxation (*e.g.,* aging and ischemic heart disease).

Aging is often accompanied by a delay in relaxation of the heart during diastole; as a result, diastolic filling begins while the ventricle is still stiff and resistant to stretching to accept an increase in volume. A similar delay occurs with myocardial ischemia, resulting from a lack of energy to break the rigor bonds that form between the actin and myosin filaments of the contracting cardiac muscle and to remove the calcium that activates muscle contraction.[11] Because tachycardia produces a decrease in diastolic filling time, persons with diastolic dysfunction often become symptomatic during activities and situations that increase heart rate.

RIGHT-SIDED VERSUS LEFT-SIDED HEART FAILURE

Congestive heart failure may also be classified according to the side of the heart (right or left) that is affected. An important feature of the circulatory system is that the right and left ventricles act as two pumps that are connected in series. To function effectively, both the right and left ventricles must maintain an equal output. Although the initial event that leads to heart failure may be primarily right-sided or left-sided in origin, long-term heart failure usually involves both sides. It is often easier, however, to understand the physiologic mechanisms associated with heart failure when right- and left-sided failure are considered separately.

Right-Sided Heart Failure. The right heart moves deoxygenated blood from the systemic circulation into the pulmonary circulation; consequently, when the right heart fails, there is accumulation or damming back of blood in the systemic venous system. This causes an increase in right atrial, right ventricular end-diastolic, and systemic venous pressures, with subsequent development of edema in the peripheral tissues and congestion of the abdominal organs. Because of the effects of gravity, the edema is most pronounced in the dependent parts of the body—in the lower extremities when the person is in the upright position and in the area over the sacrum when the person is supine. The accumulation of edema fluid is evidenced by a gain in weight. One pint of accumulated fluid results in a weight gain of 1 pound. Thus, daily measurement of weight can be used as a means of assessing fluid accumulation in congestive heart failure.

As venous distention progresses, blood backs

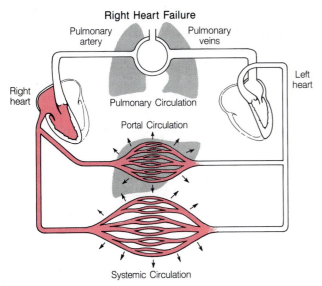

FIG. 24-4. Hemodynamic manifestations of right-sided heart failure.

up in the hepatic veins that drain into the inferior vena cava, and the liver becomes engorged. This may cause right upper quadrant pain. In severe and prolonged right-sided failure, liver function is impaired and hepatic cells may die. Congestion of the portal circulation may also lead to engorgement of the spleen and development of ascites. Congestion of the gastrointestinal tract may interfere with digestion and absorption of nutrients and cause anorexia and abdominal discomfort. The jugular veins, which are above the level of the heart, are normally collapsed in the standing position. In severe right-sided failure, the external jugular veins become distended and can be visualized when the person is standing. The hemodynamic manifestations of right-sided heart failure are depicted in Figure 24-4.

Left-Sided Heart Failure. The left side of the heart moves blood from the low-pressure pulmonary circulation into the high-pressure arterial side of the systemic circulation. With impairment of left heart function, there is a decrease in cardiac output, an increase in left atrial and left ventricular end-diastolic pressures, and congestion in the pulmonary circulation. An increase in pulmonary capillary pressure reflects the increased left atrial pressure and leads to pulmonary edema. In severe pulmonary edema, capillary fluid moves into the alveoli. The accumulated fluid in the alveoli and respiratory passages impairs the gas exchange function of the lung. With the decreased ability of the lungs to oxygenate the blood, the hemoglobin leaves the pulmonary circulation without being fully oxygenated. Cyanosis and shortness of breath result. The hemodynamic manifesta-

tions of left-sided heart failure are depicted in Figure 24-5.

MANIFESTATIONS

The signs and symptoms of congestive heart failure include edema, nocturia, shortness of breath, fatigue and limited exercise tolerance, signs of increased sympathetic activity, cyanosis, ascites, and cachexia. The severity and progression of symptoms depend on the extent and type of cardiac dysfunction that is present. Some persons with heart failure appear comfortable at rest. Others will become dyspneic during conversation or with minor activity.

Although a major compensatory mechanism in heart failure, the sympathetic nervous system is responsible for a number of physical signs and symptoms of heart failure. Peripheral vasoconstriction is manifested by pallor and coldness of the extremities and cyanosis of the nailbeds and digits. There may also be diaphoresis and tachycardia. Vasoconstriction may impede the loss of body heat and result in low-grade fever.

Fluid Retention and Edema. Many of the manifestations of congestive heart failure result from the increased capillary pressures that develop—in the peripheral circulation in right-sided heart failure and in the pulmonary circulation in left-sided heart failure. The increased capillary pressure reflects both an overfilling of the vascular system due to increased salt and water retention and venous congestion resulting from the impaired pumping ability of the heart.

Nocturia is a nightly increase in urine output that

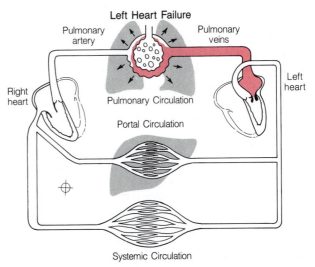

FIG. 24-5. Hemodynamic manifestations of left-sided heart failure.

occurs relatively early in the course of congestive heart failure. It results from the return to the circulation of edema fluids from the dependent parts of the body when the person assumes the supine position for the night. As a result, the cardiac output, renal blood flow, glomerular filtration, and urine output increase. When oliguria occurs, it is a late sign related to a severely reduced cardiac output.

Respiratory Manifestations. Shortness of breath due to congestion of the pulmonary circulation is one of the major manifestations of left-sided heart failure. Perceived shortness of breath (breathlessness) is called *dyspnea*. Dyspnea related to an increase in activity is called *exertional dyspnea*. *Orthopnea* is shortness of breath that occurs when a person is supine, or lying down. The gravitational forces that cause fluid to become sequestered in the lower legs and feet when the person is standing or sitting are removed when a person with congestive heart failure assumes the supine position; fluid from the legs and dependent parts of the body is mobilized and redistributed to an already distended pulmonary circulation. *Paroxysmal nocturnal dyspnea* is a sudden attack of dyspnea that occurs during sleep. It disrupts sleep, and the person awakens with a feeling of extreme suffocation that resolves when he or she sits up. Initially, the experience may be interpreted as awakening from a bad dream.

A subtle and often overlooked symptom of heart failure is a chronic dry, nonproductive cough, which becomes worse when the person is lying down. Bronchospasm due to congestion of the bronchial mucosa may be present, causing wheezing and difficulty in breathing. This condition is sometimes referred to as *cardiac asthma*.

Cheyne-Stokes respiration, also known as periodic breathing, is characterized by a slow waxing and waning of respiration. The person breathes deeply for a period of time when the Pco_2 is high and then slightly or not all when the Pco_2 falls. In persons with heart failure, the condition is thought to be caused by a prolongation of the heart-to-brain circulation, particularly in persons with hypertension and associated cerebral vascular disease.

Fatigue and Weakness. Fatigue and limb weakness often accompany diminished output from the left ventricle. Cardiac fatigue is different from emotional fatigue in that it is not present in the morning but appears and progresses as activity increases during the day. In acute or severe left-sided failure, cardiac output may fall to levels that are insufficient for providing the brain with adequate oxygen, and there are indications of mental confusion and disturbed behavior. Confusion, impairment of memory, anxiety, restlessness, and insomnia are common in elderly persons with advanced heart failure, particularly in those with cerebral atherosclerosis.

Cachexia and Malnutrition. Cardiac cachexia is a condition of malnutrition and tissue wasting that occurs in persons with end-stage heart failure. A number of factors probably contribute to its development, including fatigue and depression that interfere with food intake, congestion of the liver and gastrointestinal structures that impair digestion and absorption and produce feelings of fullness, and circulating toxins and mediators released from poorly perfused tissues that impair appetite and contribute to tissue wasting.

Cyanosis. Cyanosis is the bluish discoloration of the skin and mucous membranes due to the presence of excess desaturated hemoglobin in the blood; it is often a late sign of heart failure. Cyanosis may be central, due to arterial desaturation resulting from impaired pulmonary gas exchange, or peripheral, due to venous desaturation caused by extensive extraction of oxygen at the capillary level. *Central cyanosis* is caused by conditions that impair oxygenation of the arterial blood, such as pulmonary edema, left heart failure, or right-to-left shunting. *Peripheral cyanosis* is caused by conditions, such as low output failure, that cause delivery of poorly oxygenated blood to the peripheral tissues or by conditions, such as peripheral vasoconstriction, that cause excessive removal of oxygen from the blood. Central cyanosis is best monitored in the lips and mucous membranes since these areas are not subject to conditions such as cold that cause peripheral cyanosis.

DIAGNOSTIC METHODS

Diagnostic methods in heart failure are directed toward establishing the cause of the disorder and determining the extent of the dysfunction. Because heart failure represents the failure of the heart as a pump and can occur in the course of a number of heart diseases or other systemic pathologies, the diagnosis of heart failure is often based on signs and symptoms related to the failing heart itself, such as shortness of breath and fatigue, or to the compensatory mechanisms that represent excessive compensatory efforts, such as edema. The functional classification of the New York Heart Association is one guide to classifying the extent of dysfunction (Table 24-2).

Electrocardiographic findings may indicate underlying disorders of cardiac rhythm or conduction. Chest x-rays provide information about the size and

TABLE 24-2. NEW YORK HEART ASSOCIATION FUNCTIONAL CLASSIFICATION OF PATIENTS WITH HEART DISEASE

CLASSIFICATION	CHARACTERISTICS
Class I	Patients with cardiac disease but without the resulting limitations in physical activity. Ordinary activity does not cause undue fatigue, palpitation, dyspnea, or anginal pain.
Class II	Patients with heart disease resulting in slight limitations of physical activity. They are comfortable at rest. Ordinary physical activity results in fatigue, palpitation, dyspnea, or anginal pain.
Class III	Patients with cardiac disease resulting in marked limitation of physical activity. They are comfortable at rest. Less than ordinary physical activity causes fatigue, palpitation, dyspnea, or anginal pain.
Class IV	Patients with cardiac disease resulting in inability to carry on any physical activity without discomfort. The symptoms of cardiac insufficiency or of the anginal syndrome may be present even at rest. If any physical activity is undertaken, discomfort increases.

(Criteria Committee of the New York Heart Association. [1964]. *Diseases of the heart and blood vessels: Nomenclature and criteria for diagnosis* [6th ed., pp. 112–113]. Boston: Little, Brown)

shape of the heart and pulmonary vasculature. The cardiac silhouette can be used to detect cardiac hypertrophy and dilatation. Evidence of pulmonary venous hypertension and pulmonary congestion can also be detected on x-ray. Echocardiographic studies are used to reveal the size and function of cardiac valvular structures and the size and motion of both ventricles. It will also indicate pericardial effusion and determine the ventricular ejection fraction. Radionuclide angiography and cardiac catheterization are other diagnostic tests used to describe the underlying causes of heart failure.

Invasive hemodynamic monitoring is often used in the management of acute, life-threatening episodes of heart failure. These methods include the use of central venous pressure measurements, pulmonary capillary wedge pressures, thermodilution cardiac output measurements, and intraarterial measurements of blood pressure.

Central venous pressure (CVP) reflects the amount of blood returning to the heart. Measurements of central venous pressure are best obtained by means of a catheter inserted into the right atrium through a peripheral vein or by means of the right atrial port (opening) in a pulmonary artery catheter. This pressure is decreased in hypovolemia and increased in heart failure. The changes that occur in central venous pressure over time are usually more significant than the absolute numeric values obtained during a single reading.

Pulmonary capillary wedge pressure (PCWP) is obtained by means of a flow-directed, balloon-tipped pulmonary artery (Swan-Ganz) catheter. This catheter is introduced through a peripheral vein and is then advanced into the superior vena cava. The balloon is inflated with air once the catheter is in the right atrium; it then floats through the right heart and pulmonary artery until it becomes wedged in one of the small pulmonary arteries (Fig. 24-6). Once the catheter is in place, the balloon is inflated *only* when the PCWP is being measured. Continuous inflation of the balloon with its accompanying occlusion of a small pulmonary artery would cause necrosis of pulmonary tissue. With the balloon inflated, the catheter monitors pulmonary capillary pressures in direct communication with pressures from the left heart. The pulmonary capillary pressures provide a means of assessing the pumping ability of the left heart.

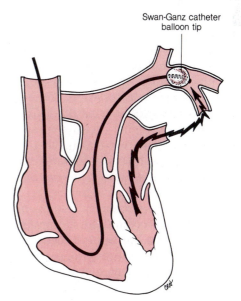

FIG. 24-6. Swan-Ganz balloon-tip catheter positioned in a pulmonary capillary. The pulmonary capillary wedge pressure, which reflects the left ventricular diastolic pressure, is measured with the balloon inflated.

One type of pulmonary artery catheter is equipped with a thermistor probe to obtain *thermodilution measurements of cardiac output*. In this method, a known amount of solution of a known temperature (iced or room temperature) is injected into the right atrium through an opening in the catheter, and the temperature of the blood is measured downstream in the pulmonary artery by means of a thermistor probe located at the end of that catheter. A microcomputer calculates blood flow (and cardiac output) using the difference between the temperatures recorded from the two sites.

Intraarterial blood pressure monitoring provides a means for continuous monitoring of blood pressure. It is used in persons with acute heart failure. Measurements are obtained through the use of a small catheter inserted into a peripheral artery, usually the radial artery. The catheter is connected to a pressure transducer, and beat-by-beat measurements of blood pressure are recorded. The monitoring system displays both the contour of the pressure waveform and a digital reading of the systolic, diastolic, and mean arterial pressures along with the electrocardiograph.

TREATMENT METHODS

Treatment of heart failure is directed toward the secondary consequences of circulatory failure as well as the primary source of the failure. Treatment measures include (1) correction of reversible causes such as anemia or thyrotoxicosis, (2) surgical repair of a ventricular defect or an improperly functioning valve, (3) pharmacologic and nonpharmacologic control of afterload stresses such as hypertension, (4) modification of activities and lifestyle to a level consistent with the functional limitations of a reduced cardiac reserve, and (5) use of medications to improve cardiac function and limit excessive compensatory mechanisms. Restriction of salt intake and diuretic therapy facilitate the excretion of edema fluid. Counseling, health teaching, and other assistive measures help persons with heart failure to manage their treatment regimen and cope with activity limitations and other manifestations of the disorder. In severe heart failure, restriction of activity, including bed rest if necessary, often facilitates temporary recompensation of cardiac function. However, there no convincing evidence that continued bed rest is of benefit or that it changes the course of the disease for persons who are able to maintain some degree of activity.

PHARMACOLOGIC TREATMENT

A number of medications are used in the treatment of heart failure, including inotropic agents, diuretics, and vasodilators.[12, 13] The choice of pharmacologic agents is determined by problems caused by the disorder (*e.g.,* systolic or diastolic dysfunction) and those brought about by activation of compensatory mechanisms (*e.g.,* excess fluid retention or inappropriate activation of sympathetic mechanism).

Diuretics. Diuretics are among the most frequently prescribed medications for heart failure. They promote the excretion of edema fluid and help to sustain cardiac output and tissue perfusion by reducing preload and allowing the heart to operate at a more optimal part of the Starling curve. Both thiazide and loop diuretics are used. In emergency situations, such as acute pulmonary edema, furosemide (Lasix) or bumetanide (Bumex) can be administered intravenously. When given intravenously, these drugs act quickly to reduce venous return through vasodilation so that right ventricular output and pulmonary vascular pressures are decreased. This response, which occurs when these drugs are administered intravenously, is extrarenal and precedes the onset of diuresis.

Inotropic Agents. Inotropic agents increase cardiac contractility irrespective of end-diastolic volume and pressure (preload). They include digitalis preparations, beta-adrenergic agonists, dopamine, and the newer nondigitalis noncatecholamine inotropic agents.

Digitalis has been a recognized treatment for congestive heart failure for the past 200 years. The various forms of digitalis are called *cardiac glycosides*. They improve cardiac function by increasing the force and strength of ventricular contraction. In addition, they slow the heart rate by decreasing SA node activity and decreasing conduction through the AV node, thus slowing heart rate and increasing diastolic filling time. Although not a diuretic, digitalis promotes urine output by improving cardiac output and renal blood flow. The digitalis drugs act by binding to sodium-potassium ATPase on the cell membrane and inhibiting the sodium pump. When intracellular sodium is increased because of inhibition of the sodium-potassium pump by digitalis, the exchange of intracellular calcium for extracellular sodium is inhibited; as a result, more calcium is available to activate the myocardial actin-myosin contractile apparatus.

The margin between therapeutic and toxic doses of digitalis is very narrow. The most serious side effect is digitalis-induced cardiac dysrhythmias. Such cardiac dysrhythmias can take many forms and can mimic most disturbances of cardiac rhythm. Anorexia, nausea, and vomiting are common gastrointestinal indications of toxicity. They may occur in patients receiving parenteral digitalis, which suggests that they are a result of disturbances in the central nervous system rather than of direct irritation of the gastrointestinal tract. Psychic and visual problems are signs of toxicity to the central nervous system. Confusion is a common sign of digitalis toxicity in the elderly. Low potassium, high calcium, and low magnesium blood levels predispose patients to digitalis toxicity, an important consideration in patients who are on digitalis because many of them are also taking diuretics, which promote potassium and magnesium losses. The elderly are at particular risk for developing digitalis toxicity.

A number of drugs have been shown to affect digitalis levels. Cholestyramine, some broad-spectrum antibiotics, antacids, and kaolin–pectin mixtures (*e.g.*, Kaopectate) may decrease absorption of the drug. Quinidine, verapamil, and amiodarone increase plasma levels of the drug by reducing both the volume of distribution and the excretion of the drug by the kidneys.

Laboratory methods allows the monitoring of serum digitalis levels. A digoxin antibody, digoxin immune fab (Digibind), that binds and inactivates digoxin is available and may be used in the treatment of life-threatening toxicities.

A new group of inotropic agents, the nondigitalis noncatecholamine phosphodiesterase inhibitors (amrinone, milrinone, enoximone, and piroximone), increase cardiac contractility without inhibiting the sodium-potassium membrane pump or activating adrenergic receptors.[14] These drugs inhibit the breakdown of cAMP with a subsequent increase in calcium influx similar to that caused by the beta-adrenergic agonists. Amrinone and milrinone also have a vasodilator effect, which may contribute to their usefulness in treating congestive heart failure. However, the value of these drugs for long-term use is still uncertain owing to the high incidence of adverse reactions.

Vasodilator Drugs. Vasodilator drugs produce relaxation of vascular smooth muscle. These drugs induce venous pooling of blood, relax the pulmonary arterial and venous vessels, and reduce the peripheral vascular resistance. With pooling of blood in the peripheral veins, less blood returns to the right heart for delivery to the pulmonary circulation. Relaxation of the pulmonary vessels diminishes the pressure in the pulmonary capillaries and allows fluid to be reabsorbed from the interstitium of the lung and from the alveoli. With a decrease in peripheral vascular resistance, there is less pressure against which the left heart must pump; thus the work of the left ventricle is decreased.

Among the vasodilators currently in use are the nitrates, hydralazine, prazosin, and the angiotensin-converting enzyme inhibitors. The nitrates produce relaxation of both arteriolar and venous smooth muscle. Sodium nitroprusside is a form of nitroglycerin given by continuous intravenous infusion in situations of acute heart failure. Oral and topical forms of nitroglycerin are used in the long-term management of ischemic heart disease. Hydralazine is a potent arteriolar dilator; it markedly reduces afterload and increases cardiac output. The combination of nitrates and oral hydralazine has proved effective in the management of persons with mild to moderate heart failure symptoms. The side effects of hydralazine (gastrointestinal upset, headaches, tachycardia, hypotension, and drug-induced lupus syndrome) limit its use in some persons. Prazosin, an oral alpha-adrenergic blocking drug that relaxes arterial smooth muscle, is being used selectively in the treatment of heart failure. However, its long-term benefits are not known.

In heart failure, renin activity is frequently elevated because of decreased renal blood flow. The net result is an increase in angiotensin II, which causes vasoconstriction and increased aldosterone production. Both of these mechanisms increase the workload of the heart. Angiotensin-converting enzyme (ACE) inhibitors (captopril, enalapril, and lisinopril), which prevent the conversion of angiotensin I to angiotensin II, have been effectively used in the treatment of heart failure. Some studies have shown that the ACE (ACE) inhibitors can relieve symptoms and increase survival in persons with symptomatic congestive heart failure.[4, 15]

MECHANICAL SUPPORT

In addition to pharmacologic methods, several types of mechanical support have been developed as a temporary measure to treat persons with acute myocardial pump failure. These methods include the aortic balloon pump (see Chapter 25) and ventricular assist devices.

Ventricular assist devices (VADs) are mechanical pumps that are used to support ventricular function.[16, 17] They are used to decrease the workload of the myocardium while maintaining cardiac output and systemic arterial pressure. This decreases the workload on the ventricle and allows it to rest and recover. The majority of VADs require an invasive open-chest procedure for implantation. They may be used in persons who fail or have difficulty weaning from cardiopulmonary bypass following cardiac surgery; those who develop cardiogenic shock following myocardial infarction; those with end-stage cardiomyopathy; and those who are awaiting cardiac transplantation. VADs can be used to support the function of the left ventricle, right ventricle, or both ventricles.

HEART TRANSPLANT

Heart transplant, once a scientific curiosity, has now become an established method of treatment for some persons with end-stage heart disease. Many of the successes of heart transplantation can be credited to improved methods of immunosuppressive therapy, which optimize survival and rehabilitation. In 1990, more than 2000 heart transplants were performed in the United States.[1] The 5-year survival rate for heart transplantations performed in high-volume transplant centers approaches 80%.[18] Despite the overall success of heart transplantation, donor availability and complications from infection, rejection, and immunosuppression drug therapy remain as problems.

Surgery is performed by placing the recipient on cardiopulmonary bypass and excising the diseased heart. An orthotopic cardiac approach is usually used to attach the donor heart (Fig. 24-7). Pacing wires are loosely attached to the right ventricle to assist with temporary pacing of the heartbeat in the event of bradycardia during the immediate postoperative phase. The heterotopic approach to heart transplantation is the surgical "piggy-backing" of a donor heart beside the recipient's own heart. The transplanted heart functions like a ventricular assist device. This procedure results in two beating hearts within a single chest cavity.[19]

Immediate postoperative care is directed toward maintaining hemodynamic stability, observing for bradyrhythmias and postoperative hemorrhage, and monitoring for transient renal failure. Subsequent postoperative management focuses on recognition and prevention of infection or rejection of the donor heart and monitoring of immunosuppressive therapy.

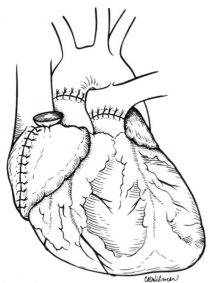

FIG. 24-7. Orthotopic heart transplantation and sites of donor heart attachment.

Cardiomyoplasty. An alternative to heart transplantation that is currently under investigation is a procedure called *cardiomyoplasty*.[20, 21] This procedure involves fashioning one of the patient's latissimus dorsi back muscles into a wrap that embraces the heart. A pacemaker, which is placed between the heart and the back muscle, stimulates the muscle to contract in synchrony with the left ventricle. Although the procedure is experimental, it provides an alternative to transplant for some persons, particularly when a donor heart is not available.

In summary, heart failure occurs when the heart fails to pump sufficient blood to meet the metabolic needs of body tissues. In congestive heart failure, there is a decrease in cardiac output along with fluid accumulation in body tissues. Heart failure may be described as high-output or low-output failure, systolic or diastolic failure, and right-sided or left-sided failure. With high-output failure the function of the heart may be supranormal but inadequate due to excessive metabolic needs, whereas low-output failure is caused by disorders that impair the pumping ability of the heart. With systolic dysfunction there is impaired ejection of blood from the heart during systole; with diastolic dysfunction there is impaired filling of the heart during diastole. Right-sided failure is characterized by congestion in the peripheral circulation, and left-sided failure by congestion in the pulmonary circulation.

The manifestations of congestive heart failure include edema, nocturia, fatigue and impaired exercise tolerance, cyanosis, signs of increased sympathetic nervous system activity, and impaired gastrointestinal function and malnutrition. In right-sided failure there is dependent edema of the lower parts of the body, engorgement of the liver, and ascites. In left-sided failure, shortness of breath and chronic nonproductive cough are common.

The diagnostic methods in heart failure are directed toward establishing the cause of the disorder and determining the extent of the dysfunction. Treatment is directed toward (1) correcting the cause whenever possible, (2) improving cardiac function, (3) maintaining the fluid volume within a compensatory level, and (4) developing an activity pattern consistent with individual limitations in cardiac reserve. Among the medications used in the treatment of heart failure are inotropic agents, diuretics, and vasodilator drugs. Heart transplant is becoming an established method of treatment for some persons with end-stage heart disease. The aortic balloon pump or ventricular assist devices may be used as temporary support measures for severe heart failure.

■ ACUTE PULMONARY EDEMA

Acute pulmonary edema is a life-threatening condition. It occurs as fluid accumulates in the interstitial spaces and alveoli of the lungs; this causes lung stiffness, makes lung expansion more difficult, and interferes with the gas exchange function of the lung. Although pulmonary edema is often associated with left heart failure, it can also result from increased permeability of the pulmonary capillary membrane, which in turn may be due to an infectious process, exposure to toxic gases, drug reactions, or other conditions. The following discussion centers on acute pulmonary edema due to heart failure.

With pulmonary edema due to heart failure, the contractile properties of the left ventricle are inadequate to eject all of the blood that enters from the lungs; this causes a sharp rise in left end-diastolic volume and pressure and a resultant increase in pulmonary venous and capillary pressures. Normally fluid does not leave the pulmonary capillaries and enter the intersititial lung tissue and alveolar spaces. This is because the pulmonary capillary pressure (normally about 10 mmHg) that serves to push fluid into the lung tissues is much lower than the capillary osmotic pressure (normally about 25 mmHg) that pulls fluid back into the capillary. Pulmonary edema develops when the pumping ability of the left ventricle is impaired to the extent that the pulmonary capillary pressure exceeds the capillary osmotic pressure.

MANIFESTATIONS

An episode of pulmonary edema usually occurs at night when the person has been reclining for a period of time. This is because the gravitational forces are removed from the circulatory system when a person lies down; as a result, edema fluid that had been sequestered in the lower extremities during the day is returned to the vascular compartment and redistributed to the pulmonary circulation. An acute episode of pulmonary edema may also occur as a complication of impaired cardiac pumping ability in myocardial infarction, or it may occur during rapid infusion of intravenous fluids or a blood transfusion in an elderly person or in a person with limited cardiac reserve.

A person with acute pulmonary edema is usually seen sitting and gasping for air. The apprehension is obvious. The pulse is rapid, the skin is moist and cool, and the lips and nailbeds are cyanotic. As the lung edema worsens and oxygen supply to the brain falls off, confusion and stupor appear. Dyspnea and air hunger are accompanied by a cough productive of frothy (resembling beaten egg whites) and often blood-tinged sputum—the effect of air mixing with serum albumin and red blood cells that have moved into the alveoli. The movement of air through the alveolar fluid produces fine crepitant sounds called *crackles*, which can be heard through a stethoscope placed on the chest. As fluid moves into the larger airways, the breathing becomes louder. The crackles heard earlier become louder and more coarse. In the terminal stage the breathing pattern is called the *death rattle*. In severe pulmonary edema, persons literally drown in their own secretions.

TREATMENT

Treatment of pulmonary edema is directed toward reducing the fluid volume in the pulmonary circulation. This can be accomplished by reducing the amount of blood that the right heart delivers to the lungs or by improving the work performance of the left heart.

A number of measures are available that decrease the blood volume in the pulmonary circulation; the seriousness of the pulmonary edema will determine which are to be used. One of the simplest measures to relieve orthopnea is assumption of the seated position. For many persons, sitting up or standing is almost instinctive and may be sufficient to relieve the symptoms associated with mild accumulation of fluid.

Measures to improve left heart performance focus on (1) decreasing the preload by reducing the filling pressure of the left ventricle and (2) reducing the afterload against which the left heart must pump. This can be accomplished through the use of vasodilator drugs, treatment of arrhythmias that impair cardiac function, and improvement of the contractile properties of the left ventricle with digitalis. Rapid digitalization may be accomplished with intravenous administration of the drug.

Oxygen therapy increases the oxygen content of the blood and helps relieve anxiety. Positive-pressure breathing increases the intraalveolar pressure, opposes the capillary filtration pressure in the pulmonary capillaries, and is sometimes used as a temporary measure to decrease the amount of fluid moving into the alveoli. Positive pressure breathing can be administered via a specially designed continuous positive airway pressure (CAPA) mask. In the most severe cases, however, endotracheal intubation and mechanical ventilation may be necessary.

Although its mechanisms of action are unclear, morphine sulfate is usually a drug of choice in acute pulmonary edema. Morphine relieves anxiety and depresses the pulmonary reflexes that cause spasm of the pulmonary vessels. It also increases venous pooling by vasodilation. Aminophylline is another drug, administered intravenously, that may be useful. It reduces bronchospasm, increases the glomerular filtration rate, and promotes urinary excretion of sodium and water.

In summary, acute pulmonary edema is a life-threatening condition. The accumulation of fluid in the interstitium of the lung and alveoli interferes with lung expansion and gas exchange. It is characterized by extreme breathlessness, rales, frothy sputum, cyanosis, and signs of hypoxemia. Measures to improve left heart performance focus on (1) decreasing the preload by reducing the filling pressure of the left ventricle and (2) reducing the afterload against which the left heart must pump. This can be accomplished through the use of vasodilator drugs, treatment of arrhythmias that impair cardiac function, and improvement of the contractile properties of the left ventricle with digitalis. Rapid digitalization may be accomplished with intravenous administration of the drug.

■ HEART FAILURE IN CHILDREN AND THE ELDERLY

The mechanisms of heart failure in children and the elderly are similar to that of adults. However, the etiologies and manifestations may differ because of age.

HEART FAILURE IN INFANTS AND CHILDREN

As in adults, heart failure in infants and children results from the inability of the heart to maintain the cardiac output required to sustain metabolic demands.[22–24] Congenital heart defects are the most common cause of congestive heart failure during childhood. Surgical correction of congenital heart defects may cause congestive heart failure as a result of intraoperative manipulation of the heart and resection of heart tissue, with subsequent alterations in pressure, flow, and resistance relationships.[22] Usually the heart failure that results is acute and resolves once the effects of the surgical intervention have subsided. Chronic congestive failure is occasionally observed in children with severe chronic anemia, inflammatory heart disease, end-stage congenital heart disease, or cardiomyopathy. Chart 24-1 lists some of the more common causes of heart failure in children. Inflammatory heart disorders (myocarditis, rheumatic fever, bacterial endocarditis, and Kawasaki disease), cardiomyopathy, and congenital heart disorders are discussed in Chapter 23.

MANIFESTATIONS

Many of the signs and symptoms of heart failure in infants and children are similar to those of adults. They include fatigue, effort intolerance, cough, anorexia, and abdominal pain. A subtle sign of cardiorespiratory distress in infants and children is a change in disposition or responsiveness, including irritability or lethargy. Sympathetic stimulation produces peripheral vasoconstriction and diaphoresis. Decreased renal blood flow often results in a urine output of less than 0.5 to 1.0 mL/kg/hr, despite adequate fluid intake.[22] When right ventricular function is impaired, systemic venous congestion develops. Hepatomegaly due to liver congestion is often one of the first signs of systemic venous congestion in in-

---

CHART 24-1: CAUSES OF HEART FAILURE IN CHILDREN

Newborn Period

Congenital heart defects
　Severe left ventricular outflow disorders
　　Hypoplastic left heart
　　Critical aortic stenosis or coarctation of the aorta
　Large arteriovenous shunts
　　Ventricular septal defects
　　Ductus arteriosus
　Transposition of the great vessels
Heart muscle dysfunction (secondary)
　Asphyxia
　Sepsis
　Hypoglycemia
Hematologic disorders (*e.g.*, anemia)

Infants 1 to 6 Months

Congenital heart disease
　Large arteriovenous shunts (ventricular septal defect)
Heart muscle dysfunction
　Myocarditis
　Cardiomyopathy
Pulmonary abnormalities
　Bronchopulmonary dysplasia
　Persistent pulmonary hypertension

Toddlers, Children, and Adolescents

Acquired heart disease
　Cardiomyopathy
　Viral myocarditis
　Rheumatic fever
　Endocarditis
　Systemic disease
　　Sepsis
　　Kawasaki's disease
　　Renal disease
　　Sickle cell disease
Congenital heart defects
　Nonsurgically treated disorders
　Surgically treated disorders

---

fants and children. However, dependent edema or ascites is rarely seen unless the central venous pressure is extremely high. Because of their short, fat necks, jugular venous distention is difficult to detect in infants, it is not a reliable sign until the child is of school age or older.

A third heart sound, or gallop rhythm, is a common finding in infants and children with heart failure. It results from rapid filling of a noncompliant ventricle. However, it is diffiuclt to distinguish at high heart rates.

Most commonly, children develop interstitial edema rather than alveolar pulmonary edema. This reduces lung compliance and increases the work of breathing, causing tachypnea and increased respiratory effort. Older children display use of accessory muscles (scapular and sternocleidomastoid). In infants head bobbing and nasal flaring may be noted.

Signs of respiratory distress are often the first and most noticeable signal of congestive heart failure in infants and young children. Pulmonary congestion may be mistaken for bronchiolitis or lower respiratory tract infections. The infant or young child with respiratory distress will often grunt with expiration. This grunting effort (essentially, exhaling against a closed glottis) is an instinctive effort to increase end-expiratory pressures and prevent collapse of small airways and atelectasis. Respiratory crackles (rales) are uncommon in infants and usually suggest respiratory tract infection. Wheezes may be heard, particularly if there is a large left-to-right shunt.

Infants with heart failure often have increased respiratory problems during feeding.[22, 24] The history is one of prolonged feeding with excessive respiratory effort and fatigue. Weight gain is slow owing to high energy requirements and low calorie intake. Other frequent manifestations of heart failure in infants are excessive sweating (due to increased sympathetic tone), particularly over the head and neck, and repeated lower respiratory tract infections. Peripheral perfusion is generally poor with cool extremities, tachycardia is common (resting >150/min), and respiratory rate is increased (resting rate >50/min).[22]

DIAGNOSIS AND TREATMENT

Diagnosis of congestive failure in infants and children is based on symptomatology, chest x-rays, electrocardiographic findings, echocardiographic techniques to assess cardiac structures and ventricular function (end-systolic and end-diastolic diameters), arterial blood gases to determine intracardiac shunting and ventilation/perfusion inequalities, and other laboratory studies to determine anemia and electrolyte imbalances.

Treatment of congestive failure in infants and children is similar to that in adults. It includes improvement of cardiac function and elimination of excess intravascular fluid. In addition, oxygen delivery must be supported and oxygen demands controlled or minimized. Whenever possible, the cause of the disorder is corrected (*e.g.*, medial treatment of sepsis and anemia and surgical correction of congenital heart defects). With congenital anomalies that are amenable to surgery, medical treatment is often needed for a time before surgery and is usually continued in the immediate postoperative period. For many children only medical management can be provided.

Medical management of heart failure in infants and children is similar to that in the adult, although it is tailored to the special developmental needs of the child. Inotropic agents such as digitalis are often used to increase cardiac contractility. Diuretics may be given to reduce preload and vasodilating drugs used to manipulate the afterload. Drug doses must be carefully tailored to control for the child's weight and conditions such as reduced renal function. Daily weighing and accurate measurement of intake and output is imperative during acute episodes of failure. Most children feel better in the semiupright position. An infant seat is useful for infants with chronic congestive heart failure. Activity restrictions are usually designed to allow children to be as active as possible within the limitations of their heart disease. Infants with congestive failure often have problems feeding. Small frequent feedings are usually more successful than larger, less frequent feedings. Severely ill infants may lack sufficient strength to suck and may need to be tube fed.

The treatment of heart failure in children should be designed to allow optimal physical and psychosocial development. It requires the full involvement of the parents, who are often the primary care providers; therefore parent education and support is essential.

HEART FAILURE IN THE ELDERLY

Congestive heart failure is one of the most common causes of disability is the elderly. The prevalence of heart failure increases with age—from 3% in persons aged 45 to 64 years, to 6% in persons aged 65 to 74 years, and to 10% for those aged 75 years and above.[25] Furthermore, congestive heart failure is associated with a high mortality rate in the elderly, particularly during the first year following diagnosis.[26] Repetitive readmissions to the hospital are also frequent, accounting for a substantial part of all inpatient Medicare expenditures.[27]

The causes of heart failure in the elderly are similar to those in younger persons. As in younger persons, hypertensive cardiovascular disease and ischemic heart disease are commonly present in elderly persons who develop heart failure. Valvular heart disease and cardiomyopathy, however, are the most frequent causes of heart failure in the elderly. Elderly persons also tend to develop cardiac failure when confronted with stresses that would not produce failure in younger persons. There is no evidence that the cardiovascular changes that occur with aging are sufficient to produce congestive heart failure. Moreover, the effects of heart failure in the elderly are often compounded by other disease conditions, such as hypertension and diabetes.

MANIFESTATIONS

The manifestations of congestive heart failure in the elderly are similar to those in younger individuals. However, the signs and symptoms are often masked by other disease conditions.[28] Lassitude is a common but nonspecific early symptom of cardiac failure. Nocturia is another early symptom but may be caused by prostatic hypertrophy. Dyspnea on exertion may result from lung disease, lack of exercise, and deconditioning. Lower extremity edema is commonly caused by venous insufficiency.

Among the acute manifestations of congestive heart failure in the elderly are increasing lethargy and confusion, probably the result of impaired cerebral perfusion. Activity intolerance is common. Instead of dyspnea, the prominent sign may be restlessness. Impaired perfusion of the gastrointestinal tract is a common cause of anorexia and profound loss of lean body mass. Loss of lean body mass may be masked by edema fluid.

The elderly also maintain a precarious balance between the managed symptom state and acute symptom exacerbation. During the managed symptom state they are relatively symptom free while adhering to their treatment regimen. Acute symptom exacerbation, often requiring emergency medical treatment, can be precipitated by seemingly minor conditions such as poor compliance with sodium restriction, infection, or stress. Failure to promptly seek medical care is a common cause of progressive acceleration of symptoms. The most common precipitating cause of acute symptom exacerbation in the hospital is the overzealous administration of intravenous fluids.[25]

DIAGNOSIS AND TREATMENT

The diagnosis of heart failure in the elderly is based on the history, physical examination, chest x-ray, and electrocardiograph findings. Often, however, the presenting symptoms of congestive heart failure are difficult to evaluate. Poor systemic perfusion may result in cerebrovascular accident, ischemia, confusional states, and symptoms of pulmonary embolism. These may so dominate the picture that underlying congestive failure is overlooked.

Treatment of congestive heart failure in the elderly involves many of the same methods as in younger persons. Activities are restricted to a level that is commensurate with the cardiac reserve. Seldom is bedrest recommended or advised. Bedrest causes rapid deconditioning of skeletal muscles and increases the risk of complications, such as orthostatic hypotension and thromboemboli. Instead, carefully prescribed exercise programs can help to maintain activity tolerance. Even walking around a room is usually preferable to continuous bedrest. Sodium restriction is usually indicated.

Age and disease-related changes increase the likelihood of adverse drug reactions and drug–drug interactions. Therefore, both drug dosage and the number of drugs that are prescribed should be kept to a minimum. Also, compliance with drug regimens is often difficult; the simpler the regimen, the more likely the older person will comply. In general, the treatment plan for elderly persons with congestive heart failure must be put in the context of the person's overall needs. Often an improvement in the quality of life may take precedence over increasing chances of survival.

In summary, the mechanisms of heart failure in children and the elderly are similar to those in adults. However, the etiologies and manifestations may differ because of age. In children congestive heart failure is most commonly seen during infancy and immediately after heart surgery. It can be caused by congenital and acquired heart defects and is characterized by fatigue, effort intolerance, cough, anorexia, abdominal pain, and impaired growth. Treatment of congestive heart failure in children includes correction of the underlying cause whenever possible. For congenital anomalies that are amenable to surgery, medical treatment is often needed for a time before surgery and is usually continued in the immediate postoperative period. For many children only medical management can be provided.

In the elderly, age-related changes in cardiovascular functioning contribute to congestive heart failure but are not in themselves sufficient to cause heart failure. The manifestations of congestive failure are often different and superimposed on other disease conditions; therefore, congestive heart failure is often more difficult to diagnose in the elderly than in younger persons. Because the elderly are more susceptible to adverse drug reactions and more problems with compliance, the number of drugs that are prescribed is kept to a minimum and the drug regimen is kept as simple as possible.

■ REFERENCES

1. American Heart Association. (1992). *1992 heart and stroke facts* (p. 35). Dallas: American Heart Association.
2. Packer, M. (1987). Prolonging life in patients with congestive heart failure: The new frontier. *Circulation, 75* (Suppl. IV), 1.
3. Daly, P.A., & Sole, M.J. (1990). Myocardial catecholamines and the pathophysiology of heart failure. *Circulation, 82* (Suppl. I), 35–43.
4. Kantner, T.R. (1992). ACE inhibitors in congestive heart failure. *Journal of Family Practice, 35,* 305–314.
5. Needleman, P., & Greenwald, J.E. (1986). Atriopeptin: A cardiac hormone intimately involved in fluid, electrolyte, and blood-pressure homeostasis. *New England Journal of Medicine, 314*(13), 828.
6. Raine, A.E.G., Pil, D., Erne, P. et al. (1986). Atrial natriuretic peptide and atrial pressure in patients with

congestive heart failure. *New England Journal of Medicine*, 315(9), 533.

7. Androli, T.E. (1991). Introduction: Modern aspects of congestive heart failure. *Hospital Practice*, April 15, 7–8.

8. Smith, T.W., & Kelly, R.A. (1991). Therapeutic strategies for CHF in the 1990s. *Hospital Practice*, 26(11A), 127–150.

9. Grossman, W. (1991). Diastolic dysfunction in congestive heart failure. *New England Journal of Medicine*, 325, 1557–1564.

10. Kessler, K.M. (1991). Diastolic heart failure. *Hospital Practice*, July 15, 137–164.

11. Katz, A.M. (1991). Energetics and the failing heart. *Hospital Practice*, August 15, 78–90.

12. Feldman, A.M. (1992). Can we alter survival in patients with congestive heart failure? *Journal of the American Medical Association*, 267, 1956–1961.

13. Arai, A.E., & Greenberg, B.H. (1990). Medical management of congestive heart failure. *Western Journal of Medicine*, 153, 406–414.

14. Dunbar, L.M. (1990). Emergency room management of congestive heart failure. *Hospital Practice*, 25 (Suppl. 1), 7–14.

15. The SOLVD Investigators. (1991). Effect of enalapril on survival in patients with reduced left ventricular ejection fractions and congestive heart failure. *New England Journal of Medicine*, 325, 293–302.

16. Elefteriades, J. (1988). Cardiac assist devices. *Cardiology Clinics*, 6, 449–459.

17. Vaska, P.L. (1991). Biventricular assist devices. *Critical Care Nursing*, 11(8), 52–60.

18. Futterman, L.G. (1988). Cardiac transplantation: A comprehensive nursing perspective, Part 1. *Heart and Lung*, 17, 499.

19. Rafalowski, M. (1991). The heterotropic heart transplant patient: Cardiac monitoring challenges. *Critical Care Nursing*, 11, 28–30.

20. Raymond, C. (1989). Cardiomyoplasty adds muscle to efforts to alleviated end-stage heart failure. *Journal of the American Medical Association*, 261, 503–504.

21. Anderson, D.R., Pchettino, A., & Hammond, R.L. (1991). Skeletal muscle as a myocardial substitute. *Proceedings of the Society for Experimental Biology and Medicine*, 197, 109–118.

22. Hazinski, F.H. (1992). *Nursing care of the critically ill child* (2nd ed., pp. 156–170). St. Louis: C.V. Mosby.

23. Ruggerie, D.P. (1990). Congestive heart failure. In Blumer, J.L. (Ed.). *A practical guide to pediatric intensive care* (3rd ed., pp. 104–119). St. Louis: Mosby-Year Book.

24. Behrman, R.E., Kliegman, R.M., Nelson, W.E., & Vaughan, V.C. (1992). *Nelson's texbook of pediatrics* (14th ed., pp. 1213–1216). Philadelphia: W.B. Saunders.

25. Luchi, R.J., Taffet, G.E., & Teasdale, T.A. (1991). Congestive heart failure in the elderly. *Journal of the American Geriatric Society*, 39, 810–825.

26. Taffet, G.E., Teasdale, T.A., Bleyer, A.J., et al. (1992). Survival of elderly men with congestiv heart failure. *Age and Ageing*, 21, 49–55.

27. Vinson, J.M., Rich, M.W., Sperry, J.C., et al. (1990). Early readmission of elderly patients with congestive heart failure. *Journal of the American Geriatric Society*, 38, 1290—1295.

28. Alpert, M.A. (1984). Cardiac failure in the elderly. *American Family Practice*, September, 123.

■ BIBLIOGRAPHY

Francis, G.S., & Cohn, J.N. (1990). Heart failure: Mechanisms of cardiac and vascular dysfunction and the rationale for pharmacologic intervention. *FASEB Journal*, 4, 3068–3075.

Gorlin, R. (1987). Treatment of congestive heart failure: Where are we going? *Circulation*, 75 (Suppl. IV), 108.

Hunt, S.A., & Schroeder, J.S. (1989). Managing patients after cardiactransplantation. *Hospital Practice*, 24(10A), 83–100.

Johnston, J. (1991). A new beginning: Current trends in pediatric heart transplantation. *Focus on Critical Care*, 18, 2328.

Katz, A.M. (1987). The physiologic approach to the treatment of heart failure. *Hospital Practice*, 22(2), 117.

Kitzman, D.W., & Edwards, W.D. (1990). Minireview: Age-related changes in the anatomy of the normal human heart. *Journal of Gerontology*, 45, M33–M39.

LaKatta, E.G. (1991). Excitation-contraction coupling in heart failure. *Hospital Practice*, 26(7A), 85–98.

Le Jemtel, T.H., Katz, S.D., & Sonneblick, E.H. (1991). Peripheral circulatory response in cardiac failure. *Hospital Practice*, 26(9A), 7582.

Leibovitch, E.R. (1991). Congestive heart failure: A current review. *Geriatrics*, 46, 43–52.

Marcus, F.I. (1992). Use and toxicity of digitalis. *Heart Disease and Stroke*, 1, 27–31.

CHAPTER 25

CIRCULATORY SHOCK

NANCIE URBAN

Types of Shock
  Hypovolemic Shock
  Cardiogenic Shock
  Obstructive Shock
  Distributive Shock
    Neurogenic Shock

Anaphylactic Shock
Septic Shock
Treatment Measures
Complications of Shock
  Shock Lung

Acute Renal Failure
Gastrointestinal Ulceration
Disseminated Intravascular
  Clotting
Multiple Organ Failure

■ OBJECTIVES

After you have studied this chapter, you should be able to meet the following objectives:

■ State a clinical definition of *shock*.
■ List the chief characteristics of hypovolemic shock, cardiogenic shock, obstructive shock, distributive shock, and septic shock.
■ List and describe the four stages of hypovolemic shock.
■ Trace the compensatory mechanisms that are activated in hypovolemic shock.
■ Characterize changes in cell metabolism that occur during shock.
■ Describe changes in thirst, skin blood flow, pulse rate, urine output, and sensorium that are indicative of shock.

■ State the basis of cardiogenic shock.
■ State the rationale for the use of the vasodilator drugs and the intraaortic balloon pump in cardiogenic shock.
■ State the common features of neurogenic shock, anaphylactic shock, and septic shock.
■ State the rationale for treatment measures to correct and reverse shock.
■ State a proposed mechanism for the development of septic shock.
■ Define multiorgan failure and cite its significance in shock.

The functions of the circulatory system are to perfuse body tissues and to supply them with oxygen. Circulatory shock can be described as a failure of the circulatory system with decreased peripheral perfusion or inadequate oxygenation of vital organs and cells of the body.[1] It is not a specific disease but can occur in the course of many life-threatening, traumatic, or disease states. Although circulatory shock produces hypotension, it should not be equated with a drop in blood pressure; in fact, hypotension often is a late sign and indicates a failure of compensatory mechanisms.[1]

Carol Mattson Porth: PATHOPHYSIOLOGY: CONCEPTS OF
ALTERED HEALTH STATES, 4th ed. © 1994, 1990, 1986, 1982
J.B. Lippincott Company

■ TYPES OF SHOCK

Adequate perfusion of body tissues depends on the pumping ability of the heart, a vascular system that transports blood to the cells and back to the heart, sufficient blood to fill the circulatory system, and tissues that are able to use and extract oxygen and nutrients from the blood. Shock can be classified into four major types: (1) hypovolemic, (2) cardiogenic, (3) obstructive, and (4) distributive. The four types of shock are summarized in Chart 25-1. Figure 25-1 diagrammatically compares normal circulation with the circulatory changes in each shock classification.

HYPOVOLEMIC SHOCK

Hypovolemic shock is characterized by a diminished blood volume such that there is inadequate filling of the vascular compartment (see Fig. 25-1). It occurs when there is an acute loss of 15% to 20% of the circulating blood volume. The decrease may be due to an external loss of whole blood (hemorrhage), plasma (severe burns), or extracellular fluid (gastrointestinal fluids lost in vomiting or diarrhea). Hypo-

---

CHART 25-1: CLASSIFICATION OF SHOCK

Hypovolemic

Loss of whole blood
Loss of plasma
Loss of extracellular fluid

Cardiogenic

Failure of the heart as a pump (myocardial damage or deterioration)
Severe alterations in rhythm (heart block or severe bradycardia, frequent or persistent tachycardia)
Mechanical defect (papillary muscle dysfunction or rupture, ventricular aneurysm, or ventricular septal defect)

Obstructive

Inability of the heart to fill properly (cardiac tamponade)
Obstruction to outflow from the heart (pulmonary embolus, cardiac myxoma, pneumothorax, or dissecting aneurysm)

Distributive

Loss of sympathetic vasomotor tone
Presence of vasodilating substances in the blood (anaphylactic, septic, or toxic shock syndrome)
Shunting of vascular fluid to the interstitial space (third spacing)
Arteriovenous shunting
Failure of body cells to use oxygen

---

volemic shock can also result from an internal hemorrhage or from third-space losses, when extracellular fluid is shifted from the vascular compartment to the interstitial space or compartment. Internal blood and fluid losses often are concealed. One source cites the case of an elderly man who suffered severe crushing injuries of both legs. The patient had no external evidence of bleeding yet required 8 L of blood over 7 hours for stabilization of vital signs.[2]

Of the four types of shock, hypovolemic shock has been the most widely studied and usually serves as a prototype in discussions of the manifestations of shock. Figure 25-2 shows the effect of removing blood from the circulatory system over a period of about 30 minutes.[3] About 10% can be removed without changing the cardiac output or arterial pressure. The reader is reminded that the average blood donor loses a pint of blood without suffering adverse effects. As increasing amounts of blood (10% to 25%) are removed, the cardiac output falls while the arterial pressure is maintained. This is because of sympathetic-mediated increases in heart rate and vasoconstriction. Because blood pressure is the product of cardiac output and systemic vascular resistance (BP = CO × SVR), an increase in systemic vascular resistance may maintain blood pressure in the presence of decreased blood volume and cardiac output. It is also apparent that cardiac output and tissue perfusion decrease before signs of hypotension occur. Both cardiac output and arterial pressure fall to zero when about 35% to 45% of the total blood volume has been removed.[3]

STAGES OF SHOCK

The progression of hypovolemic shock can be divided into four stages. During the *initial stage*, the circulatory blood volume is decreased but not enough to cause serious effects. The second stage is the *compensatory stage;* although the circulating blood volume is reduced, compensatory mechanisms are able to maintain blood pressure and tissue perfusion at a level sufficient to prevent cell damage. The third stage is the *progressive stage* or *stage of decompensated shock*. At this point, unfavorable signs begin to appear: the blood pressure begins to fall, blood flow to the heart and brain is impaired, capillary permeability is increased, fluid begins to leave the capillary, blood flow becomes sluggish, and the body cells and their enzyme systems are damaged. The fourth and final stage is the *irreversible stage*. In irreversible shock, even though the blood volume may be restored and vital signs stabilized, death ensues eventually. Although the factors that determine recovery from severe shock have not been clearly identified, it

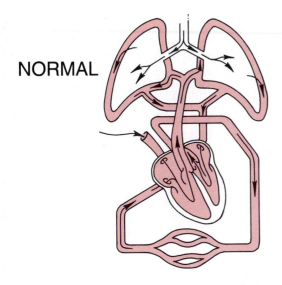

NORMAL

S H O C K

Hypovolemic   Cardiogenic   Obstructive   Distributive

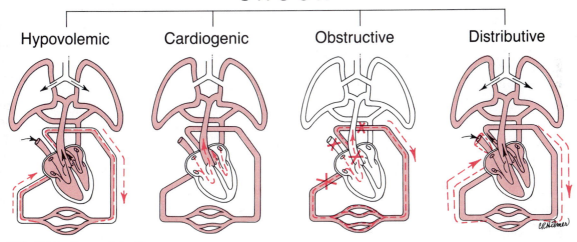

FIG. 25-1. Types of shock.

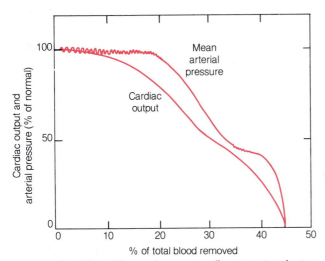

FIG. 25-2. Effect of hemorrhage on cardiac output and arterial pressure. (Guyton, A. C. [1986]. *Textbook of medical physiology* [7th ed.]. Philadelphia: W.B. Saunders)

appears that they are related to blood flow at the level of the microcirculation. The severity and clinical findings associated with hypovolemic shock are summarized in Table 25-1.

COMPENSATORY MECHANISMS

Without the compensatory mechanisms to maintain cardiac output and blood pressure, the loss of vascular volume would result in a rapid progression from the initial to the progressive and irreversible stages of shock. These compensatory mechanisms are directed at (1) maintaining cardiac output and blood pressure and (2) restoring blood volume.

The most immediate of the compensatory mechanisms are the sympathetic-mediated responses designed to maintain cardiac output and blood pressure. Within seconds after the onset of hemorrhage or the loss of blood volume, signs of sympathetic and

TABLE 25-1. CORRELATION OF CLINICAL FINDINGS AND THE MAGNITUDE OF VOLUME DEFICIT IN HEMORRHAGIC SHOCK

SEVERITY OF SHOCK	CLINICAL FINDINGS	PERCENTAGE OF REDUCTION IN BLOOD VOLUME* (mL)
None	None; normal blood donation	Up to 10 (500 mL)†
Mild	Minimal tachycardia	15–25 (750–1250)
	Slight decrease in blood pressure	
	Mild evidence of peripheral vaso-constriction with cool hands and feet	
Moderate	Tachycardia, 100–120 bpm	25–35 (1250–1750)
	Decrease in pulse pressure	
	Systolic pressure, 90–100 mmHg	
	Restlessness	
	Increased sweating	
	Pallor	
	Oliguria	
Severe	Tachycardia over 120 bpm	Up to 50 (2500)
	Blood pressure below 60 mmHg systolic and frequently unobtainable by cuff	
	Mental stupor	
	Extreme pallor, cold extremities	
	Anuria	

* Blood volume changes based on the clinical observations of Beecher et al.
† Based on blood volume of 7% in a 70-kg male of medium build.
(Weil, M., & Shubin, H. [1967]. *Diagnosis and treatment of shock.* [p. 118]. Baltimore: Williams & Wilkins)

adrenal medullary activity appear. These signs include tachycardia, increased cardiac contractility, and widespread vasoconstriction. The sympathetic vasoconstrictor response affects both the arterioles and the veins. Arteriolar constriction helps to maintain blood pressure by increasing the systemic vascular resistance, whereas venous constriction mobilizes blood that has been stored in the capacitance side of the circulation and increases venous return to the heart. There is considerable capacity for blood storage in the large veins of the abdomen and liver. About 350 mL of blood that can be mobilized in shock is stored in the liver. In the absence of sympathetic reflexes, only about 15% to 20% of the blood can be removed over a period of 30 minutes before death occurs, compared with the 30% to 40% that can be removed over a similar period with intact sympathetic innervation.[3] Sympathetic stimulation does not cause constriction of the cerebral and coronary vessels, and blood flow through the heart and brain is maintained at essentially normal levels as long as the mean arterial pressure remains above 70 mmHg.[3]

During the early stages of hypovolemic shock, vasoconstriction causes a reduction in the size of the vascular compartment and an increase in systemic vascular resistance. This response usually is all that is needed when the injury is slight, and blood loss is arrested at this point. As shock progresses, there are further increases in heart rate and cardiac contractility and vasoconstriction becomes more intense. There is vasoconstriction of the blood vessels that supply the skin, skeletal muscles, kidneys, and abdominal organs with a resultant decrease in blood flow. When acidosis becomes evident, the arterial chemoreceptors are activated and add an additional vasoconstrictor effect.

Compensatory mechanisms designed to restore blood volume include absorption of fluid from the interstitial spaces, conservation of salt and water by the kidneys, and thirst. Extracellular fluid is distributed between the interstitial spaces and the vascular compartment (Chapter 29). When there is a loss of vascular volume, capillary pressures decrease and water is drawn into the vascular compartment from the interstitial spaces. The maintenance of vascular volume is further enhanced by renal mechanisms that conserve fluid. The previously described decrease in renal blood flow, which results from sympathetic vasoconstriction, lowers the glomerular filtration rate and activates the renin-angiotensin mechanism

(Chapter 21). Activation of the renin-angiotensin mechanism results in the generation of angiotensin II, which is catalyzed by the converting enzyme that is present in the endothelium of the lung. Angiotensin II is a potent vasoconstrictor that acts directly on the kidneys to decrease excretion of both salt and water. It also increases aldosterone by the adrenal cortex, thus producing a further increase in sodium reabsorption by the kidney tubules. The decrease in blood volume also stimulates centers in the hypothalamus that regulate antidiuretic hormone (ADH) release and thirst. A decrease in blood volume of 10% is sufficient to stimulate both ADH release and thirst.[4] ADH, also known as *vasopressin*, constricts the peripheral arteries and veins and greatly increases water retention by the kidneys (Chapter 29).

The compensatory mechanisms that the body recruits in shock were not intended for long-term use. When injury is severe or its effects prolonged, the compensatory mechanisms begin to exert their own detrimental effects. The intense vasoconstriction causes a decrease in tissue perfusion, impaired cellular metabolism, release of vasoactive inflammatory mediators such as histamine, liberation of lactic acid, and cell death. Once circulatory function has been reestablished at the onset of shock, whether the shock will be irreversible or the patient will survive is determined largely at the cellular level.

FLOW IN THE MICROCIRCULATION

The delivery of oxygen and nutrients to body cells and the removal of metabolic waste products depend on adequate blood flow throughout the capillaries of the microcirculation. There are two types of capillary flow: *nutrient flow* and *nonnutrient flow*. Nutrient flow describes flow in the true capillary pathways that supply cells with oxygen and nutrients. In nonnutrient flow, blood is shunted directly from the arterial to the venous side of the circulation without passing through the true capillary pathways. Nonnutrient flow provides warmth, but not oxygen and nutrients, to the tissues. In septic shock, nonnutrient flow is increased and the skin is warm and flushed. On the other hand, both nutrient and nonnutrient flow are decreased in hypovolemic shock and the skin is cool and clammy.

In severe and prolonged shock, the vascular system fails. When this occurs, there is relaxation of the arterioles and venules, a fall in arterial pressure, and venous pooling of blood. At the capillary level, hypoxia and products of cell deterioration cause increased capillary permeability, stagnation of blood flow, the formation of small blood clots, and shifting of intravascular volume in the interstitium, a condition called *third spacing*.

CELLULAR CHANGES

At the cellular level, oxygen and nutrients supply the energy needed to maintain cellular function. Within the cell, oxygen and fuel substrates are converted to adenosine triphosphate (ATP), the cell's energy source. The cell uses ATP for a number of purposes, including operation of the sodium–potassium membrane pump that moves sodium out of the cell and potassium back into the cell.

The cell uses two pathways to convert nutrients to energy (see Chapter 1). The first is the *anaerobic* (nonoxygen) *glycolytic* pathway, which is located in the cytoplasm. Glycolysis converts glucose to ATP and pyruvate. The second pathway is the *aerobic* (oxygen-dependent pathway), called the *citric acid cycle* or *Krebs' cycle*, which is located in the mitochondria. When oxygen is available, pyruvate from the glycolytic pathway moves into the mitochondria and enters the citric acid cycle, where it is transformed into ATP and the metabolic by-products carbon dioxide and water. Fatty acids and proteins can also be metabolized in the mitochondrial pathway. When oxygen is lacking, pyruvate does not enter the citric acid cycle; instead, it is converted to lactic acid. In severe shock, cellular metabolic processes are essentially anaerobic, which means that excess amounts of lactic acid accumulate in both the cellular and the extracellular compartment.[5,6]

The anaerobic pathway, while allowing energy production to continue in the absence of oxygen, is relatively inefficient; it produces only 2 ATP units, whereas the citric acid cycle produces 36 ATP units. Without sufficient energy production, normal cell function cannot be maintained and the activity of the sodium–potassium membrane pump is impaired. As a result, sodium chloride accumulates within cells and potassium is lost from cells. The cells then swell, and their membranes become more permeable. In addition, mitochondrial activity becomes severely depressed and lysosomal membranes rupture, resulting in the release of enzymes that cause further intracellular destruction. This is followed by cell death and the release of intracellular contents into the extracellular spaces. Also, intracellular enzymes (*e.g.,* myocardial depressant factor [MDF] from pancreatic enzymes) and inflammatory mediators (*e.g.,* histamine, serotonin, and tissue necrosis factor) that produce changes in the microcirculation that adversely affect recovery from shock are released.

SIGNS AND SYMPTOMS

The signs and symptoms of hypovolemic shock are closely related to low peripheral blood flow and excessive sympathetic stimulation. For purposes of discussion, the manifestations of hypovolemic shock have been divided into the following categories: (1) thirst, (2) skin and body temperature changes, (3) arterial and venous pressure, (4) pulse rate, (5) urine output, and (6) changes in sensorium.

Thirst. An early symptom in hypovolemic shock, thirst is easily overlooked in situations in which concealed bleeding occurs. Explanations regarding the causes of thirst are many, although the underlying cause is probably related to decreased blood volume and increased serum osmolality (see Chapter 29). Many patients with trauma have a decreased renal blood flow because of an intense sympathetic nervous system stimulation, along with an increase in ADH levels, which causes water retention. Water should, therefore, be given cautiously because water intoxication can occur in a patient who continues to drink water in the face of altered renal function.

Skin and Body Temperature. In hypovolemic shock, sympathetic stimulation leads to intense vasoconstriction of the skin vessels with activation of the sweat glands. As a result, the skin is cool and moist. When shock is due to hemorrhage, the loss of red blood cells leaves the skin and mucous membranes looking pale.

The decrease in body temperature, often observed in shock, reflects a decrease in the body's metabolic rate. There is a reported correlation between the temperature in the great toe (great toe temperature minus environmental temperature) and the survival rate in shock, in that patients who had increases in toe temperature during dopamine treatment for shock had the highest survival rate. These differences were not accounted for by a simultaneous increase in rectal temperature and were, therefore, thought to reflect differences in peripheral blood flow to the distal extremities.[7]

Pulses and Pressures. An increase in heart rate often is an early sign of shock. Like vasoconstriction, the tachycardia of early shock is a sign of sympathetic nervous system response to injury. Tachycardia may also reflect emotional aspects surrounding injury or the pain associated with trauma. Blood volume and vessel tone are reflected in the quality of the pulse. A weak and thready pulse indicates vasoconstriction and a reduction in filling of the vascular compartment. In addition, decreased intravascular volume with poor cardiac output results in decreased venous return to the heart and a fall in central venous pressure (CVP).

Considerable controversy exists over the value of blood pressure measurements in the diagnosis and management of shock. This is because compensatory mechanisms tend to preserve blood pressure until shock is relatively far advanced. Furthermore, an adequate arterial pressure does not ensure adequate perfusion of vital organs such as the liver and kidneys. This is not to imply that blood pressure should not be measured in patients at risk for developing shock, but it does indicate the need for other assessment measures by which shock may be detected at an earlier stage.

In shock, blood pressure commonly is measured intraarterially because the sphygmomanometer may not always provide an accurate measurement. Systolic pressures measured by cuff methods typically are lower than those measured intraarterially. This is because in shock, increased vascular resistance in the upper extremities alters the hemodynamic events that produce the Korotkoff sounds. Thus, the first tapping sounds detectable with the stethoscope may be heard at a pressure that is considerably lower than that measured from the artery. The *Doppler method*, in which blood pressure is measured noninvasively by ultrasound, may provide a more accurate estimate of Korotkoff sounds when they are no longer audible through the stethoscope. In some instances, this method may be used as an alternative to continuous intraarterial monitoring.

Urine Output. Urine output decreases in the initial stages of shock. Compensatory mechanisms decrease renal blood flow as a means of diverting blood flow to the heart and brain. Oliguria of 20 mL/h or less is indicative of severe shock and inadequate renal perfusion. Continuous measurement of urine output is essential for assessing the circulatory status of the patient in shock.

Sensorium. Restlessness and apprehension are common behaviors in early shock. As the shock progresses and blood flow to the brain decreases, the restlessness of an earlier stage is replaced by apathy and stupor. During this later stage, there is no longer an expression of concern about outcome and complaints of pain and discomfort cease. If shock is unchecked, the apathy progresses to coma. Coma caused by blood loss alone and not related to head injury or other factors usually is an unfavorable sign.

CARDIOGENIC SHOCK

Cardiogenic shock implies failure of the heart to pump blood adequately (see Fig. 25-1). It differs from hemorrhagic shock in that cardiac output falls despite normal or elevated blood volume and cardiac pressures. Cardiogenic shock can occur because of the damage to the heart that occurs during myocardial infarction; ineffective pumping caused by cardiac dysrhythmias; mechanical defects that may occur as a complication of myocardial infarction, such as ventricular septal defect; ventricular aneurysm; acute disruption of valvular function; or problems associated with open heart surgery.

The most common cause of cardiogenic shock is myocardial infarction. It develops in 15% to 20% of people admitted to hospitals with a diagnosis of myocardial infarction, and its severity and progression appear to be related to the amount of myocardium involved.[8] Most patients who die of cardiogenic shock have lost at least 40% of the contracting muscle of the left ventricle because of a recent infarct or a combination of recent and old infarcts. Cardiomyopathy (discussed in Chapter 23) is another common cause of cardiogenic shock. The condition, which causes progressive deterioration of the heart muscle, eventually produces a decrease in cardiac output sufficient to induce shock and death.

Cardiogenic shock can follow other types of shock associated with inadequate coronary blood flow, or it can develop because substances released from ischemic tissues impair cardiac function. One such substance, MDF, is released into the circulation during severe shock. MDF produces reversible (although often severe) myocardial depression, ventricular dilation, decreased left ventricular ejection fraction, and left ventricular diastolic pressure.[9] It is a key factor in the high mortality associated with septic shock and the syndrome of multiple organ failure.[10]

In all cases of cardiogenic shock there is failure to eject blood from the heart, hypotension, and inadequate cardiac output. Increased systemic vascular resistance often is present and contributes to the deterioration of cardiac function by increasing afterload or the resistance to ventricular systole. The filling pressure, or preload of the heart, is also increased as blood returning to the heart is added to blood that was previously returned but not pumped forward, resulting in an increase in end-systolic ventricular volume. Increased resistance to ventricular systole (afterload) combined with the decreased myocardial contractility causes the increased end-systolic ventricular volume and increased preload, all of which further complicate cardiac status.

The signs and symptoms of cardiogenic shock are consistent with those of severe heart failure (Chapter 24). The lips, nail beds, and skin are cyanotic because of stagnation of blood flow and increased extraction of oxygen from the hemoglobin as it passes through the capillary bed. Both CVP and pulmonary capillary wedge pressure (PCWP) rise as a result of volume overload caused by the pumping failure of the heart.

Treatment of cardiogenic shock requires a pre-carious balance between improving cardiac output, reducing the work load and oxygen needs of the myocardium, and preserving coronary perfusion. Fluid volume must be regulated within a level that maintains the filling pressure (venous return) of the heart and maximum utilization of the Frank-Starling mechanism without causing pulmonary congestion. The use of the pulmonary artery balloon-tipped catheter, or *Swan-Ganz* catheter (named for the persons who developed the technique), has provided a means for monitoring the circulatory filling pressure by measuring PCWP (see Chapter 24). When the catheter is positioned correctly and the balloon is inflated, the catheter obstructs forward blood flow, allowing left heart pressures to be reflected through the catheter tip.

Catecholamines increase cardiac contractility but must be used with caution because they also produce vasoconstriction and increase cardiac work load by increasing the afterload. The aortic balloon pump provides a means of increasing aortic diastolic pressure and enhances coronary and peripheral blood flow without increasing systolic pressure and the afterload, against which the left ventricle must pump.

OBSTRUCTIVE SHOCK

The term *obstructive shock* is used to describe circulatory shock that results from mechanical obstruction of the flow of blood through the central circulation (great veins, heart, or lungs; see Fig. 25-1). Obstructive shock may be caused by a number of conditions, including dissecting aortic aneurysm, cardiac tamponade, pneumothorax, atrial myxoma, or evisceration of abdominal contents into the thoracic cavity owing to a ruptured hemidiaphragm. The most frequent cause of obstructive shock is pulmonary embolism.

The primary physiologic results of obstructive shock are elevated right heart pressure and impaired venous return to the heart. Treatment modalities focus on correcting the cause of the disorder, frequently with surgical interventions such as pulmonary embolectomy, pericardiocentesis (removal of fluid from the pericardial sac) for cardiac tamponade, or the insertion of a chest tube for correction of a tension pneumothorax. In select cases of pulmonary embolus, thrombolytic drugs may be used to dissolve the clots causing the obstruction.

DISTRIBUTIVE SHOCK

Distributive shock is characterized by loss of blood vessel tone, enlargement of the vascular compartment, and displacement of the vascular volume away from the heart and central circulation. With distributive shock, the capacity of the vascular compartment expands to the extent that a normal volume of blood does not fill the circulatory system (see Fig. 25-1). Loss of vessel tone has two main causes: (1) a decrease in the sympathetic control of vasomotor tone and (2) the presence of vasodilator substances in the blood. There is a decrease in venous return in distributive shock, which leads to a diminished cardiac output, but not a decrease in total blood volume; hence, this type of shock often is referred to as *normovolemic shock*. There are three shock states that share the basic circulatory pattern of distributive shock: neurogenic shock, anaphylactic shock, and septic shock.

NEUROGENIC SHOCK

Neurogenic shock describes shock caused by decreased sympathetic control of blood vessel tone; there may be a defect in vasomotor center function in the brain stem or the sympathetic outflow to the blood vessels. Output from the vasomotor center can be interrupted by brain injury, the depressant action of drugs, general anesthesia, hypoxia, or lack of glucose (*e.g.*, insulin reaction). Fainting owing to emotional causes is a transient form of neurogenic shock. Spinal anesthesia or spinal cord injury above the midthoracic region can interrupt the transmission of outflow from the vasomotor center. The term *spinal shock* is used to describe the neurogenic shock that occurs in people with spinal cord injury. In contrast to hypovolemic shock, the heart rate in neurogenic shock often is slower than normal and the skin is dry and warm. This type of distributive shock is rare and usually transitory.

ANAPHYLACTIC SHOCK

Anaphylactic shock is characterized by massive vasodilation, pooling of blood in the peripheral blood vessels, and increased capillary permeability. This type of shock, which is a manifestation of systemic anaphylaxis, is due to an immunologically mediated reaction in which vasodilator substances such as histamine are released into the blood (see Chapter 14). These substances cause dilatation of both arterioles and venules along with a marked increase in capillary permeability. The vascular response in anaphylactic shock is accompanied by bronchospasm, contraction of gastrointestinal and uterine smooth muscle, and urticaria or angioedema. Despite recent advances in the understanding of mechanisms and mediators of the response, anaphylaxis is estimated to occur in as many as 1 in every 3000 patients and accounts for more than 500 deaths annually.[11] Among the most frequent causes of anaphylactic shock are reactions to drugs, such as penicillin; foods, such as nuts and shellfish;

and animal sera, such as tetanus antitoxin. The most common cause is stings from insects of the order Hymenoptera (bees, wasps, and fire ants).

The onset of anaphylaxis varies, depending on the sensitivity of the person and the rate and quantity of antigen exposure. Anaphylactic shock often develops suddenly; death can occur within a matter of minutes unless appropriate medical intervention is promptly instituted. Signs and symptoms associated with impending anaphylactic shock include abdominal cramps, apprehension, burning and warm sensation of the skin, itching, urticaria (hives), coughing, choking, wheezing, chest tightness, and difficulty in breathing. Once blood begins to pool peripherally, there is a precipitous drop in blood pressure and the pulse becomes so weak that it is difficult to detect. Life-threatening airway obstruction may ensue as a result of laryngeal edema or bronchial spasm.

The prevention of anaphylactic shock is preferable to treatment. Once a person has been sensitized to an antigen, the risk of a fatal outcome always exists. All patients should be carefully questioned about earlier drug reactions and should be told what medications they are to receive before the medications are administered. People with known hypersensitivities should carry some form of medical identification to alert medical personnel if they become unconscious or unable to relate this information. Most pharmacies can provide information about such medical identification. Such people should also be informed about what procedures to follow in case they are inadvertently exposed to the antigen that causes the anaphylactic reaction (*e.g.*, bee sting). In some situations, the administration of agents known to cause anaphylaxis to people at risk becomes medically necessary. Protocols have been developed to prevent or decrease the severity of the reaction. These protocols involve pharmacologic pretreatment to block or blunt the reaction.[11]

Because it is not always possible to prevent anaphylactic shock, all health care personnel should be aware of the characteristic signs and symptoms so that appropriate care can be instituted promptly. Treatment includes prompt discontinuance of the inciting agent and measures to decrease absorption; close monitoring of cardiovascular and respiratory function; and maintenance of adequate respiratory gas exchange, cardiac output, and tissue perfusion. Epinephrine constricts the blood vessels and relaxes the smooth muscle in the bronchioles; it usually is the first drug to be given to a patient believed to be experiencing an anaphylactic reaction. Other treatment measures include the administration of oxygen, antihistaminic drugs, and corticosteroids. Resuscitation measures may be required. It may be helpful to institute measures to decrease absorption when the antigenic agent has been injected into the tissues. This can be accomplished by the application of ice, which constricts the blood vessels. Measures to reduce absorption should not replace other treatment measures, but they may be particularly helpful in situations in which medical treatment is not immediately available; for example, application of ice may delay the absorption of the antigen from a bee sting so that there is time to secure medical attention.

SEPTIC SHOCK

Septic shock is associated with a severe, overwhelming infection. It most frequently is associated with gram-negative bacteremia, although it can be caused by gram-positive bacilli and other microorganisms.[12] Unlike other types of shock, septic shock commonly is associated with pathologic complications, such as pulmonary insufficiency (shock lung), disseminated intravascular coagulation (DIC), and multiple organ failure. First recognized as a clinical entity in the 1950s,[13] septic shock has now become the most common type of distributive shock. It currently has a mortality rate of about 50%.

Two major predisposing factors are involved in the development of septic shock: (1) access to the vascular compartment by an infectious agent and (2) a susceptible host. Elderly people and those with extensive trauma and burns, neoplastic disease, and diabetes are particularly susceptible to infection and the development of septic shock. Another cause is the presence of an indwelling urinary or intravenous catheter. It has been proposed that the rising incidence of septic shock is related to (1) the widespread use of antibiotics, with development of a reservoir of virulent and resistant organisms; (2) concentration in hospitals of larger numbers of infections; (3) more extensive operations on elderly and high-risk patients; (4) an increase in the number of patients suffering from severe trauma; and (5) use of steroids and immunosuppressant and anticancer drugs.[14]

Septic shock typically presents with fever, vasodilation, and warm, flushed skin. Mild hyperventilation, respiratory alkalosis, and abrupt alterations in personality and inappropriate behavior (owing to reduction in cerebral blood flow) may be the earliest signs and symptoms of septic shock. These manifestations, which are thought to be a primary response to the bacteremia, commonly precede the usual signs and symptoms of sepsis by several hours or days.

Two basic hemodynamic patterns appear to be associated with septic shock, depending on the patient's vascular volume at the onset of shock.[2] The first pattern is a hyperdynamic circulatory response that occurs in patients with a normal blood volume at the onset of sepsis. These patients have a high cardiac output, normal or increased CVP, increased pulse pressure, and warm and flushed skin. Because of these manifestations, this pattern of septic shock is referred to as *warm shock*. Hyperdynamic warm shock most frequently is seen in young healthy people, for example, young women who have had a septic abortion. The second response pattern is seen in patients who have a decreased blood volume at the onset of sepsis. They present with a low cardiac output, low CVP, and cold, cyanotic extremities, hence being referred to as *cold shock*. Whether septic shock begins as hyperdynamic warm shock or hypodynamic cold shock, the outcome is decreased cardiac output, compromised peripheral perfusion, and damage to vital organs unless aggressive treatment is instituted.

The mechanisms of distributive shock in sepsis are unclear. Evidence suggests that sepsis causes a cellular defect that inhibits oxygen utilization and occurs before hemodynamic changes such as hypotension occur.[2] In this situation, a hyperdynamic circulatory response is probably a compensatory mechanism to increase the blood flow and oxygen supply to deficient cells. Considerable research has been generated regarding the relation between mortality from septic shock and oxygen delivery or the ability of cells to use oxygen effectively. Many cases of septic shock demonstrate high mixed venous oxygen saturation, indicating a cellular inability to use delivered oxygen. Because of this, oxygen delivery for these people may need to exceed normal levels to preserve cellular oxygenation.[15–17]

Another possibility is that toxins from the sepsis-producing organisms incite an immune reaction, which leads to changes in vascular tone and permeability. The resulting vasodilatation and third-spacing of extracellular fluids combine to magnify the hypotensive effects of septic shock and increase the mortality. In laboratory animals, shock may be induced by the injection of purified endotoxin, which has a protein lipopolysaccharide composition.[18] The polysaccharide component of the endotoxin produces a complement-consuming anaphylaxis-like reaction during which vasoactive substances such as histamine and serotonin are liberated. The resulting vasodilatation and third-spacing yield profound hypotension, decreases in oxygen delivery to cells, and, eventually, cell destruction.

It seems probable that various organisms may produce septic shock through different mechanisms; this would account for the different hemodynamic responses seen in hyperdynamic, or warm, septic shock and those seen in hypodynamic, or cold, septic shock.

The treatment of septic shock focuses on the causative agent and support of the circulation. The administration of antibiotics specific to the infectious agent is essential. In addition, the cardiovascular status of the patient must be supported to maintain oxygen delivery to the cells. Aggressive fluid administration is needed to compensate for third-spacing, and equally aggressive use of vasopressors, such as epinephrine, norepinephrine bitartrate (Levophed), and phenylephrine (Neo-Synephrine), is needed to prevent vasodilation caused by endotoxins.[19] Studies support the early and aggressive use of positive inotropic drugs, such as dobutamine, to increase cardiac contractility and maintain oxygen delivery.[20] Of particular interest has been the development of human monoclonal antibodies to the endotoxins produced by the gram-negative sepsis.[21] Septic shock from causes other than gram-negative bacteria do not respond to the mortality-reducing effects of monoclonal antibodies.[22]

Toxic Shock. *Toxic shock*, a unique manifestation of a septic shock pattern, is clearly a life-threatening event. It is characterized by extreme hypotension, high fever, headache, dizziness, myalgia, confusion, rash, conjunctivitis, sore throat, vomiting, and watery diarrhea. Desquamation (peeling) of the skin on the hands and feet frequently occurs during convalescence.

Although some cases of toxic shock syndrome have been reported in men and children, by far the greatest number of cases occur in menstruating women. In one study of 37 cases reported during a 5-year period in Wisconsin, 35 occurred in menstruating women, and at least 10 of these women had one recurrent episode during subsequent menstrual periods.[23] Most of these women were tampon users. *Staphylococcus aureus* was the organism most frequently cultured from the cervix and vagina.[24] The onset of menstrual toxic shock syndrome occurs 1 to 11 days after vaginal bleeding begins, the median interval being 2 days.[25] Nonmenstrual toxic shock syndrome has been associated with surgical infections, nonsurgical infections of the skin or the subcutaneous or osseous tissues, and childbirth or abortion.

In summary, circulatory shock is an acute emergency situation in which body tissues are either deprived of oxygen or cellular nutrients or unable to use these materials in their metabolic processes. Shock may develop because there is not enough blood in the circulatory system (hypovolemic shock), the heart fails as a pump (cardiogenic shock), blood flow or venous return is obstructed (obstructive shock), or the tissues are unable to utilize oxygen and nutrients (distributive).

The manifestations of hypovolemic shock are related to low peripheral blood flow and excessive sympathetic stimulation. The low peripheral blood flow produces (1) thirst, (2) changes in skin temperature, (3) a fall in blood pressure and an increase in heart rate, (4) changes in venous pressure, (5) decreased urine output, and (6) changes in the sensorium. Signs and symptoms, such as changes in skin temperature (increased in septic shock and decreased in hypovolemic and

other forms of shock), may differ with the type of shock. The intense vasoconstriction that serves to maintain blood flow to the heart and brain causes a decrease in tissue perfusion, impaired cellular metabolism, liberation of lactic acid, and, eventually, cell death. Once circulatory function has been re-established at the onset of shock, whether the shock will be irreversible or the patient will survive is determined largely by changes that occur at the cellular level.

In cardiogenic shock, there is failure to eject blood from the heart, hypotension, and inadequate cardiac output. Both CVP and PCWP rise as a result of volume overload caused by the pumping failure of the heart. Obstructive shock is caused by mechanical obstruction to the flow of blood through the central circulation (great veins, heart, or lungs). The manifestations of obstructive shock are related to elevated right heart pressure and impaired venous return to the heart.

Distributive shock is characterized by loss of blood vessel tone and expansion of the vascular compartment to the extent that it cannot be filled by a normal volume of blood. The loss of vascular tone can be either neural (decreased sympathetic control of vasomotor tone) or humoral (presence of vasodilator substances in the blood). There are three shock states that share the basic circulatory pattern of distributive shock: neurogenic shock, anaphylactic shock, and septic shock. Septic shock, which is the most common of these three types, is associated with a severe, overwhelming infection and has a mortality rate of about 50%.

■ TREATMENT MEASURES

The treatment of circulatory shock is directed toward correcting or controlling the underlying cause and improving tissue perfusion.

In hypovolemic shock, the goal of treatment is to restore vascular volume. This can be accomplished through intravenous administration of fluids and blood. Plasma expanders (*dextrans and colloidal albumin solutions*) have a high molecular weight, do not necessitate blood typing, and remain in the circulation for longer periods than the crystalloids, such as glucose and saline. The dextrans must be used with caution because they may induce serious or fatal reactions, including anaphylaxis. Fluids and blood are best administered based on volume indicators such as CVP and PCWP. This is particularly important in pediatric patients, whose fluid balance allows less variation from normal before compromise to tissue perfusion results.[26]

CIRCULATORY ASSISTANCE

In hypovolemic shock, a pneumatic compression suit called *military antishock trousers (MAST)* may be used.[27] The MAST suit, which encases the legs and abdomen and can be inflated separately or wholly, compresses the blood vessels of the legs or abdomen and increases venous return to the heart. This *autotransfu-*

sion effect is particularly life-saving when used by emergency personnel in the field to manage hemorrhagic shock or traumatic shock. The MAST suit is contraindicated in cardiogenic shock because the increased venous return further overloads the failing heart.

In cardiogenic shock, treatment measures are directed toward reducing the work of the heart while improving its pumping efficiency. An intraaortic balloon pump may be used to supplement cardiac pumping in situations of severe cardiogenic shock when positive inotropic and vasodilator drugs prove insufficient to unload and support the failing heart. The balloon pump is inserted retrograde into the thoracic aorta through the femoral artery. The balloon, filled with helium, is synchronized to inflate during diastole and deflate during systole. Diastolic inflation creates a diastolic pressure wave that results in increased perfusion to all organs, including the myocardium. The sudden release of pressure at the onset of systole lowers resistance to ejection of blood from the left ventricle, thereby increasing the heart's

pumping efficiency without increasing the afterload and myocardial oxygen consumption.

VASOACTIVE DRUGS

Vasoactive drugs are agents capable of either constricting or dilating blood vessels. Considerable controversy exists about the advantages or disadvantages related to the use of these drugs. The major vasoactive drugs used to treat shock are summarized in Table 25-2.

There are two types of receptors for the sympathetic nervous system: alpha and beta. β-Receptors are further subdivided into β_1 and β_2. In the cardiorespiratory system, stimulation of the α-receptors causes vasoconstriction; stimulation of β_1-receptors causes an increase in heart rate and the force of myocardial contraction; and stimulation of β_2-receptors produces vasodilation of the skeletal muscle beds and relaxation of the bronchioles. Dopamine is prescribed to treat shock because it induces a more favor-

TABLE 25-2. VASOACTIVE DRUGS USED IN TREATMENT OF SHOCK

DRUG	MECHANISM	ACTION*
Epinephrine (Adrenalin)	Alpha Beta$_1$ and $_2$	Vasoconstriction (specific for anaphylactic shock) Increase in heart rate and cardiac contractility Causes a decrease in renal and splanchnic blood flow while increasing skeletal muscle flow
Norepinephrine (Levophed)	Alpha Beta$_1$	Vasoconstriction Increase in heart rate and cardiac contractility
Phenylephrine (Neo-Synephrine)	Alpha	Vasoconstriction
Isoproterenol (Isuprel)	Beta$_1$ Beta$_2$	Increase in heart rate and cardiac contractility Vasodilatation and perfusion of cerebral and renal tissue
Metaraminol (Aramine)	Alpha Beta$_1$	Vasoconstriction Increase in heart rate and cardiac contractility
Dopamine (Intropin)	Alpha Beta$_1$ Dopaminergic	Vasoconstriction with large doses Increased heart rate and cardiac contractility Vasodilatation of splanchnic and renal vessels
Dobutamine	Beta$_1$	Increases cardiac contractility with minimal increase in heart rate (specific in cardiogenic shock)
Nitroprusside (Nipride)	Dilator of venous and arterial smooth muscle	Decreases venous return to the heart, causing a decrease in end-diastolic volume and pressure Decreases systemic vascular resistance with a resultant decrease in left ventricular stroke work (specific for cardiogenic shock)
Nitroglycerin (Tridil)	Dilator of venous smooth muscle at any dose Dilator of arterial smooth muscle at high doses	Same as nitroprusside

* This list is not intended to be inclusive; it encompasses the drug actions related only to treatment of shock.

able array of α- and β-receptor actions than many of the adrenergic drugs. Dopamine is thought to increase blood flow to the kidneys, liver, and other abdominal organs while maintaining vasoconstriction of less vital structures, such as the skin and skeletal muscles, when given in low doses (less than 20 μg/kg/min). In severe shock, higher doses may be needed to maintain blood pressure. Once dopamine administration exceeds this low-dose range, it has vasoconstrictive effects on blood flow to the kidneys and abdominal organs that is similar to that of epinephrine. The vasodilators nitroprusside (Nipride) and nitroglycerin are used to treat cardiogenic shock. Nitroprusside causes both arterial and venous dilatation, thus producing a decrease in venous return to the heart with a reduction in arterial resistance against which the left heart must pump. Nitroglycerin focuses its effects on the venous vascular beds until, at high doses, it begins to dilate the arterial beds as well. The arterial pressure is maintained by an increased ventricular stroke volume ejected against a lowered systemic vascular resistance; this allows blood to be redistributed from the pulmonary vascular bed to the systemic circulation.

In summary, the treatment of shock depends on the cause and the type of shock that is present. It focuses on correcting or controlling the cause and improving tissue perfusion. In hypovolemic shock, the goal of treatment is to restore vascular volume. In cardiogenic shock, treatment is directed toward reducing the work load of the heart while improving its pumping efficiency. Vasoactive drugs, capable of either constricting or dilating blood vessels, may be used.

■ COMPLICATIONS OF SHOCK

Wiggers, a noted circulatory physiologist, has aptly stated, "Shock not only stops the machine, but it wrecks the machinery."[28] Indeed, many body systems are wrecked by severe shock. Five major complications of severe shock are (1) shock lung, (2) acute renal failure, (3) gastrointestinal ulceration, (4) DIC, and (5) multiple organ failure. Thus, the complications of shock are serious and often fatal.

SHOCK LUNG

Shock lung, or adult respiratory distress syndrome (ARDS), is a potentially lethal form of respiratory failure that can follow severe shock (see Chapter 28). The term *shock lung* was introduced during the Vietnam war to describe the progressive pulmonary failure seen in soldiers who suffered major trauma. The symptoms usually do not develop until 24 to 48 hours after the initial trauma; in some instances, they occur later. ARDS is thought to result from increased permeability of the pulmonary capillaries to water and plasma proteins.[29] Protein-rich fluids leak into the alveolar and interstitial spaces, impairing gas exchange and making the lung stiffer and more difficult to inflate. Some patients develop a hyaline membrane syndrome similar to that seen in respiratory distress syndrome in the neonate. The respiratory rate and effort of breathing increase. Arterial blood gas analysis establishes the presence of profound hypoxemia with hypercapnia, resulting from impaired matching of ventilation and perfusion and from the greatly reduced diffusion of blood gases across the thickened alveolar membranes.

The exact cause of ARDS is unknown. It has been suggested that the problem results from (1) a decrease in lung perfusion and ischemia of the type II alveolar cells, which produce surfactant; (2) oxygen toxicity; (3) neurogenic factors that cause pulmonary venoconstriction and pulmonary edema owing to sympathetic nervous factors; (4) fluid overload with stretching and disruption of the pulmonary capillaries; (5) damage to the lungs by endotoxins and substances released as the result of sepsis; and (6) prolonged hypotension. One widely accepted cause of ARDS is DIC and the presence of thromboemboli in the pulmonary microcirculation. Another proposed cause of ARDS is the release of free radicals (see Chapter 2) that are associated with altering both pulmonary capillary permeability and surfactant production.[18] It is possible that multiple mechanisms operate to cause a similar pattern of injury or to trigger a common response (*e.g.,* intravascular clotting), which, in turn, produces the pulmonary damage.

ACUTE RENAL FAILURE

The renal tubules are particularly vulnerable to ischemia, and *acute renal failure* is one important late cause of death in severe shock. In fact, sepsis and trauma account for most cases of acute renal failure. The endotoxins implicated in septic shock are powerful vasoconstrictors that are capable of activating the sympathetic nervous system and causing intravascular clotting. They have been shown to trigger all the separate physiologic mechanisms that contribute to the onset of acute renal failure. The degree of renal damage is related to the severity and duration of shock. The normal kidney is able to tolerate severe ischemia for 15 to 20 minutes. The renal lesion most frequently seen after severe shock is *acute tubular necrosis*. Acute tubular necrosis usually is reversible, although return to normal renal function may require weeks or months (see Chapter 33). Continuous monitoring of urine output during shock provides a means of assessing renal blood flow. Frequent monitoring of serum creatinine and blood urea nitrogen levels also provides valuable information regarding renal status.

GASTROINTESTINAL ULCERATION

The gastrointestinal tract is particularly vulnerable to ischemia because of the changes in distribution of blood flow to its mucosal surface. In shock, there is widespread constriction of blood vessels that supply the gastrointestinal tract; this causes a redistribution of blood flow such that mucosal perfusion is severely diminished. In fact, there is growing evidence that the splanchnic and mesenteric vascular beds experience disproportionately greater vasoconstriction in response to circulating catecholamines and angiotensin II than do other vascular beds.[30] As a result, superficial mucosal lesions of the stomach and duodenum can develop within hours of severe trauma, sepsis, or burn. Bleeding is a common symptom of gastrointestinal ulceration caused by shock. Hemorrhage has its onset usually within 2 to 10 days after the original insult and often begins without warning. In addition, poor perfusion in the gastrointestinal tract has been credited with allowing intestinal bacteria to enter the bloodstream, thereby contributing to the development of sepsis and shock.[31]

Gastric pH can be monitored by way of a nasogastric tube.[32] With a tube in place, gastric contents can be aspirated and the pH determined; depending on the pH, antacids can be instilled directly into the tube. Frequent pH monitoring is time-consuming, and sometimes it is difficult to obtain sufficient aspirate for pH testing. Technologic advances, such as nasogastric tubes with pH sensors on their tips, make this procedure less time-consuming and more accurate. Nasogastric tubes, when attached to level suction, also help to diminish the accumulation of hydrogen ions in the stomach. Histamine$_2$ antagonists may be given prophylactically to prevent gastrointestinal ulcerations caused by shock.

DISSEMINATED INTRAVASCULAR COAGULATION

DIC, a complication of septic shock, is characterized by the formation of small clots in the microcirculation. Consumption and depletion of platelets, fibrinogen, and other clotting factors occur, leading to the disruption of the normal clotting process with abnormal bleeding or hemorrhage (see Chapter 17).

MULTIPLE ORGAN FAILURE

Multiple organ failure is a particularly life-threatening complication of shock, especially septic shock. Mortality rates vary from 30% to 100%, depending on the number of organs involved.[33] If they are required for long periods, many of the compensatory mechanisms stimulated by shock become the cause of multiple organ failure. Selectively severe vasospasm such as occurs in the hepatic and mesenteric circulations and the release of endorphins that potentiate the hypotensive effects of vasodilation are two of many mechanisms that contribute to failure of multiple organ systems.[32, 33, 34] Interventions for multiple organ failure are focused on support of the affected systems.

In summary, the complications of shock result from the deprivation of circulation to vital organs or systems, such as the lungs, kidneys, gastrointestinal tract, and blood coagulation system. Shock lung, or ARDS, produces lung changes that occur with shock. It is characterized by changes in the permeability of the alveolar–capillary membrane with the development of interstitial edema and severe hypoxia that does not respond to oxygen therapy. The renal tubules are particularly vulnerable to ischemia, and acute renal failure is an important complication of shock. Gastrointestinal ischemia may lead to gastrointestinal bleeding and increased permeability to the intestinal bacteria that cause further sepsis and shock. DIC is characterized by the formation of small clots in the circulation. It is thought to be caused by sluggish blood flow in the microcirculation or inappropriate activation of the coagulation cascade because of toxins or other products released as a result of the shock state. Multiple organ failure, perhaps the most ominous complication of shock, rapidly depletes the ability of the body to compensate and recover from a shock state.

■ REFERENCES

1. Smith, J.J., & Kampine, J. (1990). *Circulatory physiology—the essentials* (3rd ed., p. 311). Baltimore: Williams & Wilkins.
2. MacLean, F.L. (1981). Shock: Causes and management of circulatory shock. In D.C. Sabiston (Ed.). *Davis-Christopher's textbook of surgery* (12th ed., pp. 58, 59). Philadelphia: W.B. Saunders.
3. Guyton, A.C. (1991). *Textbook of medical physiology* (8th ed., pp. 264–265). Philadelphia: W.B. Saunders.
4. Whitman, G. (1988). Tissue perfusion. In M. McKinney, D. Packa, & S. Dunbar (Eds.). *AACN clinical reference for critical-care nursing* (2nd ed., p. 129). New York: McGraw-Hill.
5. Guchschmidt, J., Oblitas, D., & Fried, J. (1991). Oxygen consumption in sepsis and septic shock. *Critical Care Medicine, 19*, 664–671.
6. Vincent, J.L., & DuFaye, P. (1983). Serial lactate determination during circulatory shock. *Critical Care Medicine, 11*, 449.
7. Ruiz, C.E., Weil, M.H., & Carlson, R.W. (1979). Treatment of circulatory shock with dopamine. *Journal of the American Medical Association, 242*(2), 167.

8. Makabali, C., Weil, M., & Henning, R.J. (1982). An update on the therapy for shock: Current concepts in mechanisms and management of circulatory shock. *Cardiovascular Review Report, 3,* 899.

9. Bone, R.C. (1991). The pathogenesis of sepsis. *Annals of Internal Medicine, 115,* 457–469.

10. Bochner, B.S., & Lichtenstein, L.M. (1991). Anaphylaxis. *New England Journal of Medicine, 324,* 1785–1790.

11. Parrillo, J.E. (Moderator, NIH Conference). (1990). Septic shock in humans. *Annals of Internal Medicine, 113,* 227–242.

12. Parker, M.M., & Parillo, J.E. (1983). Septic shock: Hemodynamics and pathogenesis. *Journal of the American Medical Association, 250,* 3324.

13. Waisbren, B.A. (1978). A paradigm that explains gram-negative shock. *American Journal of Medicine, 65,* 403–404.

14. (1987). Septic shock: A threat to the threatened. *Emergency Medicine, 19*(18), 24.

15. Tuchschmidt, J., Fried, J., Swinney, R., & Sharma, O.F. (1989). Early hemodynamic correlates of survival in patients with septic shock. *Critical Care Medicine, 17,* 719–723.

16. Edwards, J.D., Brown, G.C., Nightengale, P., Slater, R.M., & Fragher, E.B. (1989). Use of survivor's cardiorespiratory values as therapeutic goals in septic shock. *Critical Care Medicine, 17,* 1098–1103.

17. Gutierrez, G. (1991). Cellular energy metabolism during hypoxia. *Critical Care Medicine, 19,* 619–626.

18. Weil, M. (1977). Current understanding of mechanisms and treatment of circulatory shock caused by bacterial infection. *Annals of Clinical Research, 9,* 181.

19. Neugebauer, E., Dietrich, A., Lechleuthner, A., et al. (1992). Pharmacotherapy in shock syndromes. *Circulatory Shock, 36,* 312–320.

20. Vincent, J.L., Roman, A., & Kahn, R.J. (1990). Dobutamine administration in septic shock: Addition to standard protocol. *Critical Care Medicine, 18,* 689–693.

21. Wolff, S.M. (1991). Monoclonal antibodies and the treatment of gram-negative bacteremia and septic shock. *New England Journal of Medicine, 324,* 486–487.

22. Ziegler, E.J., Fisher, C.J., Sprung, C.L., et al. (1991). Treatment of gram-negative bacteremia and septic shock with HA-IA human monoclonal antibody against endotoxin. *New England Journal of Medicine, 324,* 429–436.

23. Davis, J.P., Chesney, M.D., Wand, P.J., et al. (1980). Toxic-shock syndrome. *New England Journal of Medicine, 303,* 1429.

24. Tofte, R.W., & Williams, D.N. (1983). Toxic shock syndrome. *Postgraduate Medicine, 73*(1), 175.

25. Shands, K.N., Schmid, G.P., & Bruce, B.D. (1980). Association of tampon use and *Staphylococcus aureus* and clinical features in 52 cases. *New England Journal of Medicine, 303,* 1436.

26. Perkins, R.M., & Levin, D.L. (1982). Shock in the pediatric patient: Therapy. *Pediatrics, 101,* 319–332.

27. Alfaro, R. (1982). Pneumatic antishock suits: When and how to use them. *Dimensions in Critical Care Nursing, 1*(1), 9.

28. Smith, J.J., & Kampine, J.P. (1980). *Circulatory physiology* (p. 298). Baltimore: Williams & Wilkins.

29. Tuchschmidt, J., Oblitas, D., & Fried, J. (1991). Oxygen consumption in sepsis and septic shock. *Critical Care Medicine, 19,* 664–671.

30. Buckley, G.B., Oshima, A., & Bailey, R.W. (1986). Pathophysiology of hepatic ischemia in cardiogenic shock. *American Journal of Surgery, 151,* 87.

31. Fink, M. (1991). Gastrointestinal mucosal injury in experimental models of shock, trauma and sepsis. *Critical Care Medicine, 19,* 627–641.

32. Collins, A.S. (1990). Gastrointestinal complications in shock. *Critical Care Clinics of North America, 2*(2), 269–276.

32. Carrico, C.J., Meakins, J.L., Marshall, J.C., et al. (1986). Multiple organ failure syndrome. *Archives of Surgery, 121,* 196.

33. Napolitano, L., & Chernou, B. (1988). Endorphins in circulatory shock. *Critical Care Medicine, 16,* 566.

34. Ruokonen, E., Takala, J., Kari, A., et al. (1991). Septic shock and multiple organ failure. *Critical Care Medicine, 19,* 1146–1151.

■ BIBLIOGRAPHY

Ayers, S.M. (1988). The prevention and treatment of shock in acute myocardial infarction. *Chest, 93,* 175–215.

Barone, J.E., & Snyder, A.B. (1991). Treatment strategies in shock: Use of oxygen transport measurements. *Heart and Lung, 20,* 81–86.

Bone, R.C. (1991). Multiple system organ failure and the sepsis syndrome. *Hospital Practice,* 101–126.

Broscious, S.K. (1991). Toxic shock syndrome and its potential complications. *Critical Care Nursing, 11*(4), 28–35.

Brossack, M.A., & Raffin, T.A. (1987). Importance of venous return, venous resistance and mean circulatory pressure in the physiology and management of shock. *Chest, 5,* 906–912.

Cerra, F.B. (1990). The multiple organ failure system. *Hospital Practice,* 169–175.

Hotter, A.N. (1990). The pathophysiology of multi-system organ failure in the trauma patient. *AACN Clinical Issues in Critical Care Nursing, 1*(3), 465–478.

Houston, M.C. (1990). Pathophysiology of shock. *Critical Care Clinics of North America, 2*(2), 143–149.

Klein, G.D. (1990). Physiologic response to traumatic shock. *AACN Clinical Issues in Critical Care Nursing, 1*(3), 505–521.

Mostow, S.R. (1991). Management of gram-negative septic shock. *Hospital Practice, 26*(8A), 121–130.

Stroud, M., Swindell, B., & Bernard, G.R. (1990). Cellular and humoral mediators of sepsis syndrome. *Critical Care Nursing Clinics of North America, 2*(2), 151–160.

Wolff, S.M. (1991). Monoclonal antibodies and the treatment of gram-negative bacteremia and shock. *New England Journal of Medicine, 324,* 486–487.

CHAPTER 26

CONTROL OF RESPIRATORY FUNCTION

■ OBJECTIVES

After you have studied this chapter, you should be able to meet the following objectives:

■ State the difference between the conducting and the respiratory airways.

■ Trace the movement of air through the airways beginning in the nose and oropharynx and moving into the respiratory tissues of the lung.

■ Describe the function of the mucociliary blanket.

■ Define the term *water vapor pressure* and cite the source of water for humidification of air as it moves through the airways.

■ Compare the supporting structures of the large and small airways in terms of cartilaginous and smooth muscle support.

■ Compare the function of the bronchial and pulmonary circulations that supply the lungs.

■ State the function of the three types of alveolar cells.

■ Relate Boyle's law to inspiration and expiration.

■ State the definition of intrathoracic, intrapleural, and intraalveolar pressures, and state how each of these pressures changes in relation to atmospheric pressure during inspiration and expiration.

■ Define *inspiratory reserve, expiratory reserve, vital capacity*, and *residual volume*.

■ Describe the method for measuring FEV_1.

■ State a definition of lung compliance.

■ Use Laplace's law to explain the need for surfactant in maintaining the inflation of small alveoli.

■ State the major determinant of airway resistance.

■ Explain why increasing lung volume (taking deep breaths) reduces airway resistance.

■ Trace the exchange of gases in the alveoli.

■ Explain why ventilation and perfusion must be matched.

■ Cite the difference between dead air space and shunt.

■ List four factors that affect the diffusion of gases in the alveoli.

■ Explain the difference between Po_2 and hemoglobin-bound oxygen.

■ Describe the transport of oxygen by hemoglobin.

■ Explain the significance of *shift to the right* versus *shift to the left* in the oxygen-hemoglobin dissociation curve.

■ Describe the function of the chemoreceptors in regulation of ventilation.

Carol Mattson Porth: PATHOPHYSIOLOGY: CONCEPTS OF
ALTERED HEALTH STATES, 4th ed. © 1994, 1990, 1986, 1982
J.B. Lippincott Company

Respiration provides the body with a means of gas exchange. It is the process whereby oxygen from the air is transferred to the blood and carbon dioxide is eliminated from the body. Internal respiration provides for gas exchange at the cellular level. Respiration can be divided into four parts: (1) ventilation, or the movement of air between the atmosphere and the respiratory portion of the lungs; (2) perfusion, or the flow of blood through the lungs; (3) diffusion, or the transfer of gases between the air-filled spaces in the lungs and the blood; and (4) the regulation and control of breathing by respiratory muscles and the nervous system. The discussion in this chapter focuses on the structure and function of the respiratory system as it relates to these aspects of respiration. The function of the red blood cell in the transport of oxygen is discussed in Chapter 18.

■ STRUCTURAL ORGANIZATION OF THE RESPIRATORY SYSTEM

The respiratory system consists of the air passages and the lungs. Functionally, the respiratory system can be divided into two parts: (1) the conducting airways through which air moves as it passes between the atmosphere and the lungs and (2) the respiratory tissues of the lungs, where gas exchange takes place.

LUNGS

The lungs are the functional structures of the respiratory system. In addition to their gas exchange function, they inactivate vasoactive substances such as bradykinin; they convert angiotensin I to angiotensin II; and they serve as a reservoir for blood. Heparin-producing cells are particularly abundant in the capillaries of the lung where small clots are trapped.

The lungs are soft, spongy, cone-shaped organs located side by side in the chest cavity (Fig. 26-1). They are separated from each other by the mediastinum (the space between the lungs) and its contents—the heart, blood vessels, lymph nodes, nerve fibers, thymus gland, and esophagus. The upper part of the lung, which lies against the top of the thoracic cavity, is called the *apex*, and the lower part, which lies against the diaphragm, is called the *base*. The lungs are divided into lobes: three in the right lung and two in the left (Fig. 26-2).

CONDUCTING AIRWAYS

The conducting airways consist of the nasal passages, mouth and pharynx, larynx, trachea, bronchi, and bronchioles (see Fig. 26-1). The air we breathe is

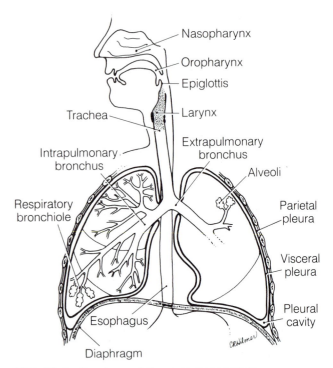

FIG. 26-1. Structures of the respiratory system.

warmed, filtered, and moistened as it moves through these structures. Body heat is transferred from the blood that flows through the walls of the air passages; the mucociliary blanket removes foreign materials; and water from the mucous membranes is used to moisten the air.

The conducting airways are lined with a *pseudostratified columnar epithelium* that contains mucus-secreting goblet cells and hair-like projections called *cilia*. The mucus produced by these cells forms a blanket-like layer, the *mucociliary blanket*, which protects the respiratory system and entraps dust and other foreign particles as they move through the conducting airways. The cilia, which constantly are in motion, move the mucociliary blanket with its entrapped particles escalator-fashion toward the oropharynx from where it is either expectorated or swallowed.

The function of the mucous escalator in clearing the lower airways and alveoli is optimal at normal oxygen levels and is impaired in situations of low and high oxygen levels. Clearance is stimulated by coughing. It is impaired by drying, for example, by heated but unhumidified indoor air during winter. Cigarette smoking also slows down or paralyzes the mucociliary escalator. This slowing allows the residue from tobacco smoke, dust, and other particles to accumulate in the lungs, decreasing the efficiency of this pulmonary defense system. There is also evidence that smoking causes hyperplasia of the goblet cells with a resultant increase in respiratory tract secretions and increased susceptibility to respiratory tract infections. As discussed in Chapter 27, these

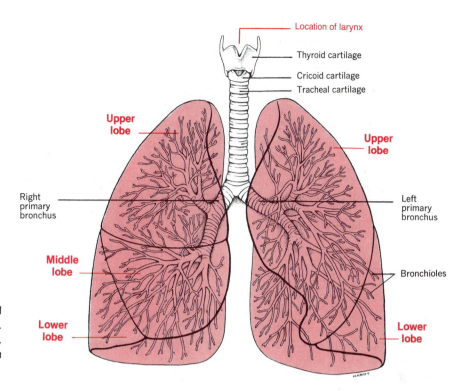

FIG. 26-2. Larynx, trachea, and bronchial tree (*anterior view*). (Chaffee, E. E., & Lytle, I. M. [1980]. *Basic physiology and anatomy* [4th ed.]. Philadelphia: J.B. Lippincott)

changes are thought to contribute to the development of chronic bronchitis and emphysema.

All the respiratory passages are kept moist by the mucus layer. Moisture is added to the air as it moves through the conducting airways. The capacity of the air to contain moisture or water vapor without condensation occurring increases as the temperature rises. Thus, the body-temperature air in the alveoli usually contains considerably more water vapor than the atmospheric-temperature air that we breathe. The difference between the water vapor contained in the air we breathe and that found in the alveoli is drawn from the moist surface of the mucous membranes that line the respiratory passages and is a source of insensible water loss (see Chapter 29). Under normal conditions, about 1 pint of water per day is lost in humidifying the air breathed. This amount is increased during fever caused by the temperature-associated increase in water vapor pressure within the lungs (to be explained). In addition, an increase in the respiratory rate usually accompanies fever, so that more air passes through the airways, withdrawing moisture from its mucosal surface. As a result, respiratory secretions thicken, preventing free movement of the cilia and impairing the protective function of the mucociliary defense system. This is particularly true in people whose water intake is inadequate.

Nasal Passages. The nose is the preferred route for the entrance of air into the respiratory tract during normal breathing. As air passes through the nasal passages, it is filtered, warmed, and humidified. The outer part of the nasal passages is lined with coarse hairs, which filter and trap dust and other large particles from the air. The upper portion of the nasal cavity is lined with mucous membrane that contains a rich network of small blood vessels; this portion of the nasal cavity supplies warmth and moisture to the air we breath.

Mouth and Pharynx. The mouth serves as an alternative airway when the nasal passages are plugged or when there is need for exchange of large amounts of air, such as occurs during exercise. The pharynx is the only opening between the nose and mouth and the lungs. Consequently, obstruction of the pharynx leads to immediate cessation of ventilation. Neural control of the tongue and pharyngeal muscles is impaired in coma and certain types of neurologic disease. In these conditions, the tongue falls back into the pharynx and obstructs the airway, particularly if the person is lying on the back. Swelling of the pharyngeal structures caused by injury or infection also predisposes a person to airway obstruction, as does the presence of a foreign body.

The epiglottis, also referred to as the *glottis*, is a thin, leaf-shaped structure that aids in covering the larynx during the act of swallowing to prevent food and fluids from entering the lungs. When the swallowing mechanism is partially or totally paralyzed, food and fluids can enter the trachea instead of the esophagus when a person attempts to swallow. These substances are not easily removed, and when they are pulled into the lungs, they can cause a serious inflammatory condition called *aspiration pneumonia*.

Larynx. The larynx connects the pharynx with the trachea. The walls of the larynx are supported by cartilaginous structures that prevent collapse during inspiration. The functions of the larynx can be divided into two categories: (1) those associated with speech and (2) those associated with protecting the lungs by preventing the entrance of substances other than air. The larynx is located in a strategic position between the upper airways and the lungs and sometimes is referred to as the *watchdog of the lungs.* When confronted with substances other than air, laryngeal muscles contract and close off the airway. At the same time, the cough reflex is initiated as a means of removing the foreign substance from the airway. Paralysis of the laryngeal muscles predisposes to aspiration of foreign materials into the lungs.

Tracheobronchial Tree. The tracheobronchial tree consists of the trachea, bronchi, and bronchioles and can be viewed as a system of branching tubes. It is similar to a tree whose branches become smaller and more numerous as they divide. There are about 23 levels of branching, beginning with the conducting airways and ending with the respiratory airways, where gas exchange takes place (Fig. 26-3).

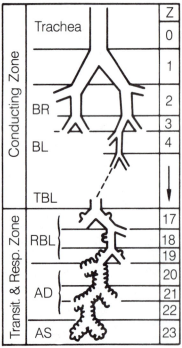

FIG. 26-3. *Idealization of the human airways according to Weibel (BR, bronchus; BL, bronchile; TBL, terminal bronchile; RBL, respiratory bronchiole; AD, alveolar duct; AS, alveolar sac). Note that the first 16 generations (Z) make up the conducting airways and that the last 7 make up the respiratory zone (or transitional and respiratory zone). (From Weibel, E. R. [1962]. Morphometry of the human lung [p. 111]. Berlin: Springer-Verlag)*

The trachea, or windpipe, is a continuous tube that connects the larynx and the major bronchi of the lungs (see Fig. 26-2). The walls of the trachea are supported by horseshoe-shaped cartilages, which prevent it from collapsing when the pressure in the thorax becomes negative.

The trachea divides to form the right and the left primary bronchus. Each bronchus enters the lung through a slit called the hilus. The point at which the trachea divides is called the *carina.* The carina is heavily innervated with sensory neurons, and coughing and bronchospasm result when this area is stimulated, as in tracheal suctioning. The right primary bronchus is shorter and wider and continues at a more vertical angle with the trachea than the left primary bronchus, which is longer and narrower and continues from the trachea at a more acute angle. For this reason, when an endotracheal tube is inserted to maintain a patent airway and facilitate ventilation, it is essential to secure the tube properly. If the tube should slip into the right main bronchus, it will prevent air from entering the left lung, causing it to collapse. Anatomic variations also make it easier for foreign bodies to enter the right main bronchus than to enter the left.

The right and left primary bronchi divide into secondary, or lobular, bronchi, which supply each of the lobes of the lungs. The right middle lobe bronchus is of relatively small caliber and length and sometimes bends sharply near its bifurcation. It is surrounded by a collar of lymph nodes that drain both the middle and the lower lobe and is particularly subject to obstruction. The secondary bronchi divide to form the segmental bronchi, which supply the bronchopulmonary segments of the lung. There are ten segments in the right lung and nine segments in the left lung (Fig. 26-4). These segments are identified according to their location in the lung (*e.g.,* the apical segment of the right upper lobe) and are the smallest named units in the lung. Lung lesions such as atelectasis and pneumonia often are localized to a particular bronchopulmonary segment.

The bronchi continue to branch, forming smaller bronchi, until they become the terminal bronchioles, the smallest of the conducting airways. The structure of the primary bronchi is similar to that of the trachea, in that these airways are supported by cartilaginous rings. As the bronchi move into the lungs, the horseshoe-shaped cartilage rings are replaced by irregular plates of cartilage. As these bronchi branch and become smaller, this cartilaginous support becomes thinner and finally disappears at the level of the bronchioles. Between the cartilaginous support and the mucosal surface are two crisscrossing layers of smooth muscle that wind in opposite directions (Fig. 26-5). Bronchospasm, or contraction, of these mus-

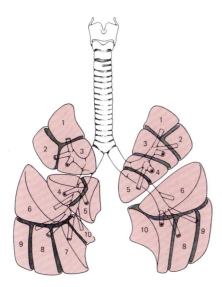

FIG. 26-4. Bronchopulmonary segments of the human lung. Left and right upper lobes: (1) apical, (2) posterior, (3) anterior, (4) superior, lingular, and (5) inferior lingular segments. Right middle lobe: (4) lateral and (5) medial segments. Lower lobes: (6) superior (apical), (7) medial-basal, (8) anterior-basal, (9) lateral-basal, and (1) posterior-basal segments. The medial-basal segment (7) is absent in the left lung. (From Fishman, A. P. [1980]. *Assessment of pulmonary function* [p. 19]. New York: McGraw-Hill)

cles causes narrowing of the bronchioles and impairs air flow.

LUNG CIRCULATION

The lungs are provided with a dual blood supply, the bronchial and the pulmonary circulation. The pulmonary circulation provides for the gas exchange function of the lungs, whereas the bronchial circulation supplies the cells of the lungs with blood to meet their nutritional needs. The bronchial arteries arise from the thoracic aorta and enter the lungs with the major bronchi, dividing and subdividing along with the bronchi as they move out into the lung and supplying them and other lung structures with oxygen. The capillaries of the bronchial circulation drain into the bronchial veins, the larger of which empties into the vena cava. The smaller of the bronchial veins empties into the pulmonary veins. This blood is unoxygenated because the bronchial circulation does not participate in gas exchange. As a result, this blood dilutes the oxygenated blood returning to the left side of the heart.

PLEURA

A thin, transparent, double-layered serous membrane, called the pleura, lines the thoracic cavity and encases the lungs. The outer parietal layer lies adja-

cent to the chest wall, and the inner, visceral layer adheres to the outer surface of the lung. The parietal pleura forms part of the mediastinum and lines the inner wall of the thoracic or chest cavity. A thin film of serous fluid separates the two pleural layers, and this allows the two layers to glide over each other and yet hold together, so there is no separation between the lungs and the chest wall. The pleural cavity is a potential space in which serous fluid or inflammatory exudate can accumulate. The term *pleural effusion* is used to describe an abnormal collection of fluid or exudate in the pleural cavity.

RESPIRATORY LOBULES

The gas exchange function of the lung takes place in the lobules of the lungs. Each lobule is supplied with structures that provide for gas exchange and the circulation of blood (see Fig. 26-5). Gas exchange takes place in the terminal respiratory bronchioles and the alveolar ducts and sacs. Blood enters the lobules through a pulmonary artery and then exits through a pulmonary vein. Lymphatic structures surround the lobule and aid in the removal of plasma proteins and other particles from the interstitial spaces.

The alveolar sacs are cup-shaped, thin-walled structures that are separated from each other by thin alveolar septa. Most of the septa are occupied by a single network of capillaries, so that blood is exposed to air on both sides. There are about 300 million alveoli in the human lung with a surface area of about

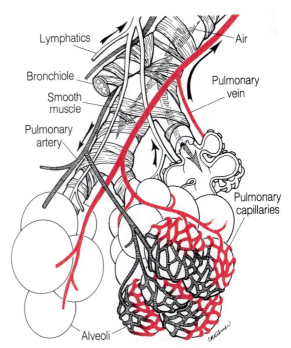

FIG. 26-5. Lobule of the lung showing the bronchial smooth muscle fibers, pulmonary blood vessels, and lymphatics.

50 to 100 m^2. Unlike the bronchioles, which are tubes with their own separate walls, the alveoli are interconnecting spaces that have no separate walls (Fig. 26-6). As a result of this arrangement, there is a continual mixing of air in the alveolar structures. Small holes in the alveolar walls, the pores of Kohn, probably contribute to the mixing of air under certain conditions.

The alveolar structures are composed of three types of cells: the alveolar macrophages, the type I alveolar cells, and the type II alveolar cells. The alveolar macrophages are responsible for the removal of offending substances from the alveolar epithelium. Available evidence suggests that smoking impairs the function of the macrophages. The type I alveolar cells are flat squamous epithelial cells across which gas exchange takes place. The type II alveolar cells produce surfactant, a lipoprotein substance that decreases the surface tension within the alveoli. This action allows for greater ease of lung inflation and helps to prevent the collapse of smaller airways.

In summary, the function of the respiratory system is to oxygenate and remove carbon dioxide from the blood. The lungs are the functional structures of the respiratory system. In addition to their gas exchange function, they inactivate vasoactive substances such as bradykinin; they convert angiotensin I to angiotensin II; and they serve as a reservoir for blood. The lungs are encased in a double-layered serous membrane called the pleura.

Functionally, the air passages of the respiratory system can be structurally divided into two parts: the conducting airways through which air moves as it passes into and out of the lungs and the respiratory tissues where gas exchange actually takes place. The conducting airways include the nasal passages, mouth and nasopharynx, larynx, and tracheobronchial tree. Air is warmed, filtered, and humidified as it passes through these structures. The function of the epiglottis and larynx is coordinated with the act of swallowing to prevent food and liquids from entering the trachea. The conducting airways are lined with pseudostratified columnar epithelium, which contains serous glands, goblet cells, and hair-like projections called cilia. The mucus produced by these cells forms the mucociliary blanket, which aids in removing dust and other foreign particles from the respiratory tract. Water is drawn from the mucociliary blanket to supplement the humidity of atmospheric air so that the air in the lungs can be saturated with water vapor. The lobules, which are the functional units of the lung, consist of the respiratory bronchioles, alveoli, and pulmonary capillaries. It is here that gas exchange takes place. Oxygen from the alveoli diffuses across the alveolar capillary membrane into the blood, and carbon dioxide from the blood diffuses into the alveoli.

■ EXCHANGE OF GASES BETWEEN THE ATMOSPHERE AND THE LUNGS

There is nothing mystical about ventilation in that it is purely a mechanical event that obeys the laws of physics as they relate to the behavior of gases. Some of these principles are summarized for the reader's review.

BASIC PROPERTIES OF GASES

The air we breathe is made up of a mixture of gases, mainly nitrogen and oxygen. These gases exert a combined pressure called the *atmospheric pressure*. At sea level (1 atmosphere), the atmospheric pressure is 760 mm of mercury (mmHg) or 14.7 lb per square inch. When measuring respiratory pressures, atmospheric pressure is assigned a value of 0. A respiratory pressure of +15 mmHg means that the pressure is 15 mmHg above atmospheric pressure, and a respiratory pressure of −15 mmHg is 15 mmHg less than atmospheric pressure. Respiratory pressures often are expressed in centimeters of water (cmH$_2$O). Multiplying by 1.35 (the specific gravity of mercury is 13.546) converts pressure expressed in millimeters of mercury to centimeters of water pressure.

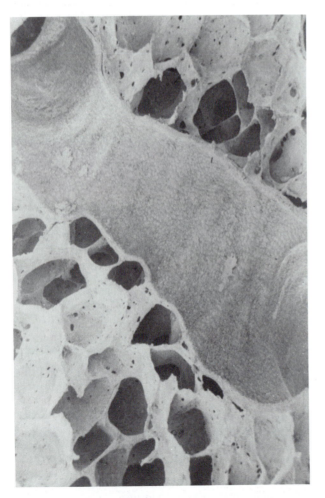

FIG. 26-6. Close-up of cross section of a small bronchus and surrounding alveoli. (Courtesy of Janice A. Nowell, of University of California, Santa Cruz)

The pressure exerted by a single gas in a mixture is called *the partial pressure*. The capital letter P followed by the subscript for the chemical name of the gas (P_{O_2}) is used to denote its partial pressure. The law of partial pressures states that the total pressure of a mixture of gases, as in the atmosphere, is equal to the sum of the partial pressures of the different gases in the mixture. If the concentration of oxygen at 760 mmHg is 20%, then its partial pressure is 152 mmHg (760 × 0.20).

Water vapor is different from other types of gases: its partial pressure is affected by temperature but not by atmospheric pressure. The relative humidity refers to the percentage of moisture in the air compared with the amount that the air can hold without causing condensation (100% saturation). Warm air holds more moisture than cold air. This is the reason that precipitation in the form of rain or snow commonly occurs when the relative humidity is high and there is a drop in atmospheric temperature. The air in the alveoli, which is 100% saturated and maintained at body temperature, is about 47 mmHg. The water vapor pressure must be included in the sum of the total pressure of the gases in the alveoli (*i.e.*, the total pressure of the other gases in the alveoli is 760 − 47 = 713 mmHg).

Air moves between the atmosphere and the lungs because of a pressure difference. According to Boyle's law, the pressure of a gas varies inversely with the volume of its container, provided the temperature remains constant. Thus, if equal amounts of a gas are placed in two different-sized containers, the pressure of the gas in the smaller container will be greater than the pressure in the larger container. The movement of gases is always from the container with the greater pressure to the one with the lesser pressure. The chest cavity can be viewed as a volume container. During inspiration, the size of the chest cavity increases and air moves into the lungs; during expiration, air moves out as the size of the chest cavity decreases.

MECHANICS OF BREATHING

Breathing is concerned with the movement of gases into and out of the lungs. It depends on a system of open airways and movement of the chest cage by the respiratory muscles.

CHEST CAGE AND RESPIRATORY MUSCLES

The lungs and major airways share the chest cavity with the heart, great vessels, and esophagus. The chest cavity is a closed compartment bounded on the top by the neck muscles and at the bottom by the diaphragm. The outer walls of the chest cavity are formed by 12 pairs of ribs, the sternum, the thoracic vertebrae, and the intercostal muscles that lie between the ribs. Mechanically, the act of breathing depends on the fact that the chest cavity is a closed compartment whose only opening to the exterior is the trachea.

During inspiration, the size of the chest cavity increases, the intrathoracic pressure becomes negative, and air is drawn into the lungs because intrathoracic pressure is less than atmospheric pressure. The diaphragm is the principal muscle of inspiration. When the diaphragm contracts, the abdominal contents are forced downward and the chest expands from top to bottom (Fig. 26-7). During normal levels of inspiration, the diaphragm moves about 1 cm, but this can be increased to 10 cm on forced inspiration. The diaphragm is innervated by the phrenic nerve roots, which arise from the cervical level of the spinal cord—mainly from C4 but also from C3 and C5. Paralysis of one side of the diaphragm causes the chest to move up rather than down during inspiration because of the negative pressure in the chest. This is called *paradoxical movement*.

The external intercostal muscles, which also aid in inspiration, connect to the adjacent ribs and slope downward and forward. When they contract, they raise the ribs and rotate them slightly so that the sternum is pushed forward; this enlarges the chest from side to side and from front to back. The intercostal muscles receive their innervation from the thoracic

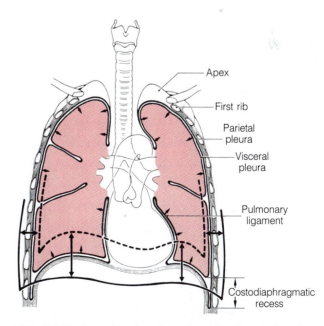

FIG. 26-7. Frontal section of the chest showing the location of the chest cage, lungs, mediastinum, and diaphragm. The *dotted lines* and *arrows* indicate the descent of the diaphragm during inspiration and the recoil during expiration. (From Fishman, A. P. [1980]. *Assessment of pulmonary function* [p. 19]. New York: McGraw-Hill)

level of the spinal cord. Paralysis of these muscles usually does not have a serious effect on respiration because of the effectiveness of the diaphragm.

The accessory muscles of inspiration include the scalene muscles and the sternocleidomastoid muscles. The scalene muscles elevate the first two ribs, and the sternocleidomastoid muscles raise the sternum to increase the size of the chest cavity (Fig. 26-8). These muscles contribute little to quiet breathing but contract vigorously during exercise. For the accessory muscles to assist in ventilation, they must be stabilized in some way. For example, people with bronchial asthma often brace their arms against a firm object during an attack as a means of immobilizing their shoulders so that the attached accessory muscles can exert their full effect on ventilation. The head commonly is bent backward as well, so that the scalene and sternocleidomastoid muscles can elevate the ribs more effectively. Other muscles that play a minor role in inspiration are the alae nasi, which produce flaring of the nostrils during obstructed breathing.

During expiration, the elastic components of the chest wall and lung structures that were stretched during inspiration recoil passively, causing lung volume to decrease so that the pressure within the lungs is greater than atmospheric pressure; therefore, air moves out of the lungs. When needed, the abdominal and the internal intercostal muscles can be used to increase expiratory effort (see Fig. 26-8). The increase in intraabdominal pressure that accompanies the forceful contraction of the abdominal muscles pushes the diaphragm upward and results in an increase in intrathoracic pressure. The internal intercostals move inward, pulling the chest downward, and are also used to increase expiratory effort.

RESPIRATORY PRESSURES

The pressure inside the airways and alveoli of the lungs is called the *intrapulmonary pressure* or *alveolar pressure*. The gases within this area of the lungs are in communication with atmospheric pressure (Fig. 26-9). When the glottis is open and air is not moving into or out of the lungs, as occurs just before inspiration or expiration, the intrapulmonary pressure is 0 or equal to atmospheric pressure.

The pressure in the pleural cavity is called the *intrapleural pressure*. It is always negative in relation to alveolar pressure (about −4 mmHg between breaths when the glottis is open and the alveolar spaces are open to the atmosphere). Both the lungs and the chest wall have elastic properties, each pulling in the opposite direction. If removed from the chest, the lungs would contract to a smaller size, and the chest wall, if freed from the lungs, would expand. The opposing forces of the chest wall and lungs create a pull against the visceral and parietal layers of the pleura, causing the pressure within the pleural cavity to become negative. During inspiration, the elastic recoil of the lungs increases, causing intrapleural pressure to become more negative than during expiration. Without the negative intrapleural pressure holding the lungs against the chest wall, their elastic recoil properties would cause them to collapse. Although intrapleural pressure is negative in relation to alveolar pressure, it may become positive in relation to atmospheric pressure (*e.g.,* during forced expiration and coughing).

The *intrathoracic* pressure is the pressure within the thoracic cavity. It is essentially equal to intrapleural pressure and is the pressure to which the heart and great vessels are exposed. Forced expiration

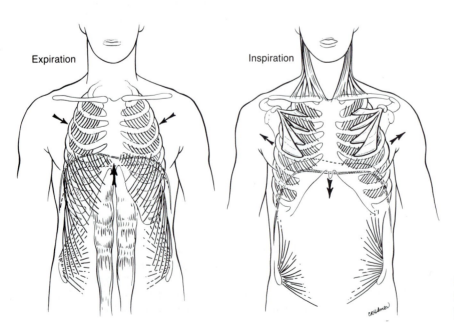

FIG. 26-8. Respiratory muscles during inspiration (*right*) and expiration (*left*).

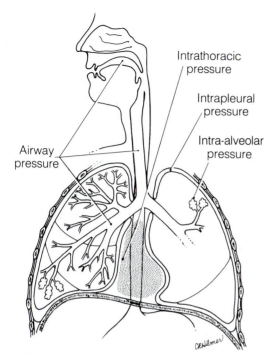

FIG. 26-9. Partitioning of respiratory pressures.

against a closed glottis compresses the air in the thoracic cavity and produces marked increases in intrathoracic pressure and intrapleural pressure.

LUNG COMPLIANCE

Lung compliance refers to the ease with which the lungs can be inflated. It can be compared to the ease of blowing up a new balloon versus one that is compliant from having been blown up before. Specifically, lung compliance describes the change in lung volume that can be accomplished with a given change in respiratory pressure.

$$\text{Compliance} = \frac{\text{change in volume}}{\text{change in pressure}}$$

The normal compliance of both lungs in the average adult is about 200 mL/cm water pressure. It would take more pressure to move the same amount of air into a noncompliant lung.

The elastic forces of the lung are determined by the elastic and collagen fibers. In the deflated lung, these fibers are partially contracted. When the lung is inflated, the elastic fibers are stretched out. Lung compliance is decreased in diseases such as interstitial lung disease and pulmonary fibrosis, which cause lung tissues to stiffen and lose their elasticity. Pulmonary congestion and edema produce a reversible decrease in pulmonary compliance. Pulmonary compliance is increased in elderly people and in those with emphysema, probably because lung tissues become permanently stretched owing to loss of elastic fibers.

Surface Tension. An important factor in lung compliance is the surface tension in the alveoli. The alveoli are lined with a thin layer of liquid, and it is at the liquid–air interface that surface tension develops. It arises because the forces that hold the liquid film together are stronger than those that hold the air molecules together. For example, it is surface tension that holds raindrops together. In the alveoli, excess surface tension causes the liquid film to contract, making lung inflation difficult.

The pressure in the alveoli (which are modeled as spheres with open airways projecting from them) can be predicted using Laplace's law (pressure = 2 × surface tension/radius). Thus, if the surface tension were equal throughout the lungs, the alveoli with the smallest radii would have the greatest pressure, and this would cause them to empty into the larger alveoli (Fig. 26-10). The reason this does not occur is because of special surface tension–lowering molecules, called *surfactant*, that line the inner surface of the alveoli.

Surfactant is a complex mixture of lipoproteins (largely phospholipids) and small amounts of carbohydrates that is synthesized within the type II alveolar cells. The surfactant molecule has two ends: a hydrophobic (water-insoluble) tail and a hydrophilic (water-soluble) group (Fig. 26-11). The hydrophilic group attaches to the fluid molecules and the hydrophobic tail attaches to the gas molecules, interrupting the intermolecular forces that are responsible for creating the surface tension. Surfactant exerts four important effects on lung inflation: (1) it lowers the surface tension; (2) it increases lung compliance, or ease of inflation; (3) it provides stability and more even inflation of the alveoli; and (4) it assists in preventing pulmonary edema by keeping the alveoli dry. Without surfactant, lung inflation would be extremely difficult, requiring intrapleural pressures of −20 to −30 mmHg compared with the −3 to −5 mmHg that normally is needed. Not only

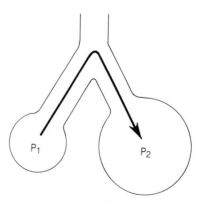

FIG. 26-10. Law of Laplace (P = 2T/R, p = pressure, T = tension, R = radius) depicting the effect of radius on the pressure and movement of gases in the alveolar structures. Air moves from P_1 with a small radius and higher pressure to P_2 with its larger radius and lower pressure.

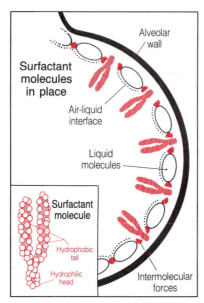

FIG. 26-11. Alveolar wall depicting the surface tension resulting from the intermolecular forces at the air–liquid interface; the surfactant molecule with its hydrophobic tail and hydrophilic head; and its function in reducing surface tension by disrupting the intermolecular forces.

does surfactant reduce the surface tension in the alveoli, but it does so more effectively in the small alveoli, which have the greatest tendency to empty into the larger alveoli and collapse. This is because the surfactant molecules are more densely packed in the small alveoli, and hence, the surface tension–reducing ability is greater than in larger alveoli, where the density of the molecules is less. Surfactant also helps to keep the alveoli dry and prevent pulmonary edema. As the surface tension created by the liquid film causes the alveoli to contract, water is pulled out of the pulmonary capillaries into the alveoli. By reducing these surface tension forces, surfactant helps to keep the alveoli dry.

The type II alveolar cells that produce surfactant do not begin to mature until the 26th to 28th week of gestation, and consequently, many premature babies have difficulty producing sufficient amounts of surfactant. This can lead to alveolar collapse and severe respiratory distress. This condition, called *respiratory distress syndrome*, is the single most common cause of respiratory disease in premature infants. There is also the potential for surfactant dysfunction in the adult. This usually occurs as the result of severe injury or infection and can contribute to the development of a condition called *adult respiratory distress syndrome* (see Chapter 28).

AIRWAY RESISTANCE

The volume of air that moves into and out of the air exchange portion of the lungs is directly related to the pressure difference between the lungs and the atmo-

sphere and inversely related to the resistance of the airways. Airway resistance normally is so small that only small changes in pressure are needed to move large volumes of air into the lungs. For example, the average pressure change that is needed to move a normal breath of 500 mL of air into the lungs is less than 1 mmHg. Because the resistance of the airways is inversely proportional to the fourth power of the radius, small changes in airway caliber, such as those caused by pulmonary secretions or bronchospasm, can produce a marked increase in airway resistance. For people with these conditions to maintain the same rate of air flow as before the onset of increased airway resistance, an increase in driving pressure (respiratory effort) is needed.

Airway resistance is greatly affected by lung volumes, being less during inspiration than during expiration. This is because elastic-type fibers connect the outside of the airways to the surrounding lung tissues. As a result, the airways are pulled open as the lungs expand during inspiration and they become narrower as the lungs deflate during expiration. This is one of the reasons people with conditions that increase airway resistance, such as bronchial asthma, usually have less difficulty during inspiration than during expiration.

Airway Resistance and Airflow. Air flows into and out of the lung along a pressure difference and against resistance. The pattern of airflow can be either laminar or turbulent, depending on the rate and pattern of flow. Laminar, or streamlined, airflow occurs at low flow rates in which the air stream is parallel with the sides of the airway. With laminar flow, the air at the periphery must overcome the resistance to flow, and as a result, the air in the center of the airway moves faster.

The French physician Poiseuille first described the pressure-flow characteristics of laminar flow in a straight circular tube, a relation that has become known as Poiseuille's law. According to Poiseuille's law, the resistance to flow is inversely related to the fourth power of the radius. Thus, if the radius is reduced by half, the resistance increases 16-fold.

In contrast to laminar flow, turbulent flow is disorganized flow in which the molecules of the gas move laterally, collide with one another, and change their velocities. Whether or not turbulence develops depends on the radius of the airways, the interaction of the gas molecules, and the velocity of airflow. It is most likely to occur when the radius of the airways is large and the velocity of flow is high. Turbulent flow occurs regularly in the trachea. Turbulence of airflow accounts for the respiratory sounds that are heard during chest auscultation (listening to the chest with a stethoscope).

In the bronchial tree with its many branches, laminar airflow probably occurs only in the very small airways where velocity of flow is low. Because the small airways contribute so little resistance, they constitute a silent zone. In small-airway disease (chronic obstructive pulmonary disease), it is probable that considerable abnormalities are present before the usual measurements of airway resistance can detect them.

Airway Compression. Airflow through the collapsible airways in the lungs depends on the distending airway (intrapulmonary) pressures that hold the airways open and the external (intrapleural or intrathoracic) pressures that surround and compress the airways. The difference between these two pressures (intrathoracic pressure − airway pressure) is called the *transpulmonary pressure*. For airflow to occur, the distending pressure inside the airways must be greater than the compressing pressure outside the airways.

During forced expiration, the transpulmonary pressure is decreased because of a disproportionate increase in the intrathoracic pressure compared with airway pressure. The resistance that air encounters as it moves out of the lungs causes a further drop in airway pressure (Fig. 26-12). If this drop in airway pressure is sufficiently great, the surrounding pressure compresses the collapsible airways (*i.e.,* those that lack cartilaginous support), causing airflow to be interrupted and air to be trapped in the alveoli. Although this type of airway compression is seen only during forced expiration in people with normal respiratory function, it may occur during normal breathing in people with lung diseases. For example, in conditions that increase airway resistance, such as emphysema, the pressure drop along the smaller airways is magnified and an increase in intrabronchial pressure is needed to maintain airway patency. Measures such as pursed-lip breathing increase airway pressure and improve expiratory flow rates in people with chronic obstructive lung disease. This is also the basis for using positive end-expiratory pressure in patients who are on mechanical ventilators. Infants who are having trouble breathing often grunt to increase their expiratory airway pressures and keep their airways open.

LUNG VOLUMES AND PULMONARY FUNCTION STUDIES

The amount of air that is inhaled or exhaled from various lung volumes can be measured with a spirometer (Fig. 26-13). With the type of spirometer shown in Figure 26-13, the bell, which is inverted over a water bath, moves down during inspiration and up during expiration, causing the pen to move up and down and mark the chart paper. Lung volumes and capacities are summarized in Table 26-1.

LUNG VOLUMES AND CAPACITIES

Lung volumes can be subdivided into four components: tidal volume, inspiratory reserve volume, expiratory reserve volume, and residual volume. The *tidal volume* (TV), usually about 500 mL, is the amount of air that moves into and out of the lungs during a normal breath. The maximum amount of air that can be inspired in excess of the normal TV is called the *inspiratory reserve volume* (IRV), and the maximum amount that can be exhaled in excess of the normal TV is the *expiratory reserve volume* (ERV). Some air—about 1200 mL—always remains in the lungs after forced expiration; this air is the *residual volume* (RV). The RV increases with age because there is more trapping of air in the lungs at the end of expiration.

Lung capacities include two or more lung volumes. The *vital capacity* equals the IRV plus the TV plus the ERV and is the amount of air that can be exhaled from the point of maximal inspiration. The *inspiratory capacity* equals the TV plus the IRV. It is the amount of air a person can breathe beginning at the normal expiratory level and distending the lungs to the maximal amount. The *functional residual capacity* is the sum of the RV and ERV; it is the volume of air that remains in the lungs at the end of normal expiration.

The *total lung capacity* is the sum of all the volumes in the lungs. The RV cannot be measured with the spirometer because this air cannot be expressed from the lungs. It is measured by indirect methods, such as the helium dilution methods, the nitrogen washout methods, or body plethysmography (see a respiratory physiology text for a description of these tests).

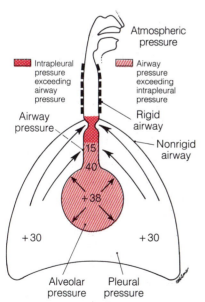

FIG. 26–12. *Mechanism that limits maximal expiratory flow rate. Forced expiration increases intrapleural pressure, causing airway compression of nonrigid airways where intrapleural pressure exceeds airway pressure.*

Within the figure:

Atmospheric pressure

Intrapleural pressure exceeding airway pressure

Airway pressure exceeding intrapleural pressure

Airway pressure

Rigid airway

Nonrigid airway

15

40

+38

+30

+30

Alveolar pressure

Pleural pressure

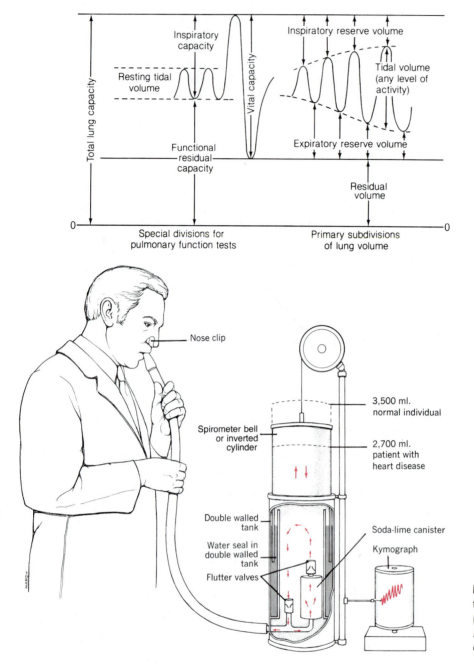

FIG. 26-13. Measurement of vital capacity using a spirometer. (Chaffee, E. E., & Lytle, I. M. [1980]. *Basic physiology and anatomy* [4th ed.]. Philadelphia: J.B. Lippincott)

PULMONARY FUNCTION STUDIES

The previously mentioned lung volumes and capacities are anatomic or static measures, determined by lung volumes, measured without relation to time. The spirometer is also used to measure dynamic lung function (ventilation with respect to time); these tests often are used in assessing pulmonary function. Pulmonary function is measured for various clinical purposes, including diagnosis of respiratory disease, preoperative surgical and anesthetic risk evaluation, and symptom and disability evaluation for legal or insurance purposes. The tests commonly are used in evaluating dyspnea, cough, wheezing, and abnormal radiologic or laboratory findings.

The *maximum voluntary ventilation* measures the volume of air that a person can move into and out of the lungs during maximum effort lasting for 12 to 15 seconds. This measurement usually is converted to liters per minute. The *forced expiratory vital capacity* (FVC) involves full inspiration to total lung capacity followed by forceful maximal expiration. Obstruction of airways produces a FVC that is lower than that observed with more slowly performed vital capacity measurements. The expired volume is plotted against time. The FEV_1 is the *forced expiratory volume* that can be exhaled in 1 second. The FEV_1 frequently is expressed as a percentage of the FVC. The FEV_1 and FVC are used in the diagnosis of obstructive lung disorders. The *forced inspiratory vital flow* (FIF) mea-

TABLE 26-1. LUNG VOLUMES AND CAPACITIES

VOLUME	SYMBOL	MEASUREMENT
Tidal volume (about 500 mL at rest)	TV	Amount of air that moves into and out of the lungs with each breath
Inspiratory reserve volume (about 3000 mL)	IRV	Maximum amount of air that can be inhaled from the point of maximal expiration
Expiratory reserve volume (about 1100 mL)	ERV	Maximum volume of air that can be exhaled from the resting end-expiratory level
Residual volume (about 1200 mL)	RV	Volume of air remaining in the lungs after maximal expiration. This volume cannot be measured with the spirometer; it is measured indirectly using methods such as the helium dilution method, the nitrogen washout technique, or body plethysmography
Functional residual capacity (about 2300 mL)	FRC	Volume of air remaining in the lungs at end-expiration (sum of RV and ERV)
Inspiratory capacity (about 3500 mL)	IC	Sum of IRV and TV
Vital capacity (about 4600 mL)	VC	Maximal amount of air that can be exhaled from the point of maximal inspiration
Total lung capacity (about 5800 mL)	TLC	Total amount of air that the lungs can hold; it is the sum of all the volume components after maximal inspiration. This value is about 20% to 25% less in females than in males.

sures the respiratory response during rapid maximal inspiration. Calculation of the airflow during the middle half of inspiration (FIF 25% to 75%) relative to the forced midexpiratory flow rate (FEF 25% to 75%) is used as a measure of respiratory muscle dysfunction, since inspiratory flow depends more on effort than does expiration. The pulmonary function tests are summarized in Table 26-2.

EFFICIENCY AND WORK OF BREATHING

The *minute volume* or total ventilation is the amount of air that is exchanged in 1 minute. It is determined by the metabolic needs of the body. The minute volume is equal to the TV multiplied by the respiratory rate, which is about 6000 mL (500 mL TV × respiratory

TABLE 26-2. PULMONARY FUNCTION TESTS*

TEST	SYMBOL	MEASUREMENT
Maximal voluntary ventilation	MVV	Maximum amount of air that can be breathed in a given time
Forced vital capacity	FVC	Maximum amount of air that can be rapidly and forcefully exhaled from the lungs after full inspiration. The expired volume is plotted against time.
Forced expiratory volume achieved in 1 sec	$FEV_{1.0}$	Volume of air expired in the first second of FVC
Percentage of forced vital capacity	$FEV_{1.0}$/FVC%	Volume of air expired in the first second, expressed as a percentage of FVC
Forced midexpiratory flow rate	FEF25%–75%	The forced midexpiratory flow rate determined by locating the points on the volume–time curve recording obtained during FVC corresponding to 25% and 75% of FVC and drawing a straight line through these points. The slope of this line represents the average midexpiratory flow rate.
Forced inspiratory flow rate	FIF25%–75%	FIF is volume inspired from RV at the point of measurement. FIF25%–75% is the slope of a line between the points on the volume pressure tracing corresponding to 25% and 75% of the inspired volume.

* By convention, all the lung volumes and rates of flow are expressed in terms of body temperature and pressure and saturated with water vapor (BTPS), which allows for a comparison of the pulmonary function data from laboratories with different ambient temperatures and altitudes.

rate of 12 breaths per minute) during normal activity. The efficiency of breathing is determined by matching the TV and respiratory rate in a manner that provides an optimal minute volume while minimizing the work of breathing.

The work of breathing is determined by the amount of effort required to move air through the conducting airways and by the ease of lung expansion (compliance). Expansion of the lungs is difficult for people with stiff and noncompliant lungs; these people usually find it easier to breathe if they keep their TV low and breathe at a more rapid rate (*i.e.,* 300 × 20 = 6000 mL) to achieve their minute volume and meet their oxygen needs. On the other hand, most people with obstructive airway disease find it less difficult to inflate their lungs but expend more energy in moving air through the airways. As a result, these people take deeper breaths and breathe at a slower rate (*i.e.,* 600 × 10 = 6000 mL) to achieve their oxygen needs.

In summary, the movement of air between the atmosphere and the lungs follows the laws of physics as they relate to gases. The air in the alveoli contains a mixture of gases, including nitrogen, oxygen, carbon dioxide, and water vapor pressure. With the exception of water vapor, each gas exerts a pressure that is determined by the atmospheric pressure and the concentration of the gas in the mixture. Water vapor pressure is affected by temperature but not atmospheric pressure. Air moves into the lungs along a pressure gradient. The pressure inside the airways and alveoli of the lungs is called *intrapulmonary,* or *alveolar, pressure;* the pressure in the pleural cavity, pleural pressure; and the pressure within the thoracic cavity, *intrathoracic pressure.*

Breathing is concerned with the movement of gases between the atmosphere and the lungs. It requires a system of open airways and pressure changes resulting from the action of the respiratory muscles in changing the volume of the chest cage. The diaphragm is the principal muscle of inspiration assisted by the external intercostal muscles. The accessory (scalene and sternocleidomastoid) muscles elevate the ribs and act as accessory muscles for inspiration. Expiration is largely passive, aided by the elastic recoil of the respiratory muscles that were stretched during inspiration. When needed, the abdominal and internal intercostal muscles can be used to increase expiratory effort. Lung volumes and lung capacities can be measured using a spirometer. Pulmonary function studies are used to assess ventilation with respect to time.

Lung compliance describes the ease with which the lungs can be inflated. It reflects the elasticity of the lung tissue and the surface tension in the alveoli. Surfactant molecules, produced by the type II alveolar cells, reduce the surface tension in the lungs and thereby increase lung compliance. Airway resistance refers to the impediment to flow that the air encounters as it moves through the airways. Minute volume is the amount of air that is exchanged in a minute (respiratory rate and tidal volume) and is determined by the metabolic needs of the body. The efficiency and work of breathing are determined by factors such as impaired lung compliance and airway diseases that increase the work involved to maintain the minute volume.

■ EXCHANGE AND TRANSPORT OF GASES IN THE BODY

The primary functions of the lungs are the oxygenation of the blood and the removal of carbon dioxide. Pulmonary gas exchange is conventionally divided into three processes: (1) ventilation or the flow of gases into the alveoli of the lungs, (2) perfusion of blood in the adjacent pulmonary capillaries, and (3) diffusion or transfer of gases between the alveoli and the pulmonary capillaries. The efficiency of gas exchange requires that there is alveolar ventilation adjacent to perfused pulmonary capillaries.

DISTRIBUTION OF VENTILATION

Ventilation refers to the exchange of gases in the respiratory system. There are two types of ventilation: pulmonary and alveolar. *Pulmonary ventilation* refers to the total exchange of gases between the atmosphere and the lungs; *alveolar ventilation* is the exchange of gases within the gas exchange portion of the lungs. The distribution of ventilation varies with lung volume and body position. It often is altered by bed rest and by disease conditions that affect the heart and the respiratory system.

Both lung volume and body position affect the regional distribution of ventilation in the top versus the bottom parts of the lungs. During full inspiration (high lung volumes) in the seated or standing position, the movement of the ribs causes a proportionately greater increase in lung volume at the bottom of the lungs. Also, the downward movement of the diaphragm expands the lower lobes of the lungs more than the upper lobes. As a result, more air moves into the lower lobes of the lungs. Because of the effects of gravity, this difference in distribution of ventilation is less pronounced at low lung volume. The difference in distribution of ventilation also disappears in the supine position, with the result that the top and the bottom of the lungs are equally ventilated. In that position, however, the ventilation of the lowermost (posterior) parts of the lungs exceeds that of the uppermost (anterior) parts of the lungs. In the lateral position (lying on the side), the dependent lung is best ventilated.

One of the reasons for the changes in regional distribution of ventilation that occur with a change in lung volume is related to differences in intrapleural pressure (less negative at the bottom of the lung compared with the top of the lung) that result from the effects of gravity and the weight of the lung as it moves downward in the chest cavity. At the end of maximal expiration at low lung volumes, the intrapleural pressure at the base of the lung exceeds airway pressure, causing airway collapse, so that air moves into the top part of the lungs. At larger lung volumes, there is greater chest expansion, which results in greater decreases in intrapleural pressure at the base of the lung so that the airways remain open and air preferentially moves into that portion of the lung.

Even at low lung volumes, some air remains in the alveoli of the lower portion of the lungs, preventing their collapse. According to the law of Laplace (discussed previously), the pressure needed to overcome the tension in the wall of a sphere or an elastic tube is inversely related to its radius; therefore, the small airways close first, trapping some gas in the alveoli. There may be increased trapping of air in the alveoli of the lower part of the lungs in older people and in those with lung disease (*e.g.*, emphysema). This is thought to be due to a loss in the elastic recoil properties of the lungs, so that the intrapleural pressure (created by the elastic recoil of the lung and chest wall) becomes less negative. In these people, airway closure occurs at the end of normal instead of low lung volumes, trapping larger amounts of air. The air trapping eventually causes an increase in the anteroposterior chest dimensions.

DISTRIBUTION OF BLOOD FLOW

The primary functions of the pulmonary circulation are to perfuse the gas exchange portion of the lung and to facilitate gas exchange. The pulmonary circulation serves several important functions in addition to gas exchange: it filters all the blood that moves from the right to the left side of the circulation; it removes most of the thromboemobi; and it serves as a reservoir of blood for the left side of the heart.

The gas exchange function of the lungs requires a continuous flow of blood through the respiratory portion of the lungs. Unoxygenated blood enters the lung through the pulmonary artery, which has its origin in the right side of the heart and enters the lung at the hilus, along with the primary bronchus. The pulmonary arteries branch in a manner similar to that of the airways. The small pulmonary arteries accompany the bronchi as they move down the lobules and branch to supply the capillary network that surrounds the alveoli (see Fig. 26-5).

The meshwork of capillaries in the respiratory portion of the lungs is so dense that the flow in these vessels often is described as being similar to a sheet of blood. The oxygenated capillary blood is collected in the small pulmonary veins of the lobules, and from there, it moves to the larger veins to be collected finally in the four large pulmonary veins that empty into the right atrium. The term *perfusion* is used to describe the flow of blood through the pulmonary capillary bed.

The pulmonary blood vessels are thinner, more compliant, and offer less resistance to flow than those in the systemic circulation, and the pressures in the pulmonary system are much lower (22/8 mmHg versus 120/70 mmHg). The low pressure and low resistance of this system accommodate the delivery of varying amounts of blood from the systemic circulation without producing signs and symptoms of congestion. The volume in the pulmonary circulation is about 500 mL, with about 100 mL of this volume being located in the pulmonary capillary bed. When the output of the right ventricle and input of the left ventricle are equal, pulmonary blood flow remains constant. Small differences between input and output can result in large changes in pulmonary volume if the differences continue for many heartbeats. The movement of blood through the pulmonary capillary bed requires that the mean pulmonary arterial pressure be greater than the mean pulmonary venous pressure. Pulmonary venous pressure increases in left-sided heart failure, allowing blood to accumulate in the pulmonary capillary bed and cause pulmonary edema. Acute pulmonary edema is discussed in Chapter 24.

As with ventilation, the distribution of pulmonary blood flow is affected by body position. In the upright position, the distance of the upper apices of the lung above the level of the heart may exceed the perfusion capabilities of the mean pulmonary arterial pressure (about 12 mmHg); therefore, blood flow in the upper part of the lungs is less than that in the base or bottom part of the lungs. In the supine position, the lungs and the heart are at the same level and blood flow to the apices and base of the lungs becomes more uniform. In this position, blood flow to the posterior or dependent portions (*e.g.*, bottom of the lung when lying on the side) exceeds flow in the anterior or nondependent portions of the lungs. In people with left-sided heart failure, congestion develops in the dependent portions of the lungs exposed to increased blood flow.

The blood vessels in the pulmonary circulation undergo marked vasoconstriction when they are exposed to hypoxia. The precise mechanism for this response is unclear. When alveolar oxygen levels drop below 70 mmHg, marked vasoconstriction may occur, and at very low oxygen levels, the local flow may be almost abolished. The vasoconstriction has the effect of directing blood flow away from the hypoxic regions of the lungs. These regions of low oxygen may result from bronchial obstruction. At high altitudes, generalized pulmonary vasoconstriction may occur, causing a marked increase in pulmonary arterial pressure. Other active responses of the pulmonary circulation have been described. A low blood *p*H causes vasoconstriction, especially when alveolar hypoxia is present (*e.g.*, during circulatory shock).

DIFFUSION

Gas exchange takes place in the alveoli. Here gases diffuse across the alveolar–capillary membrane, moving from an area of higher partial pressure to one of lower partial pressure. Oxygen moves from the alveoli into the capillaries, and carbon dioxide moves from the capillary network into the alveoli. There is rapid equilibration between the gases in the alveoli and those in the blood, such that the partial pressure of the blood gases at the venous end of the pulmonary capillary is about the same as in the alveoli.

Diseases that destroy lung tissue or increase the thickness of the alveolar–capillary membrane influence the diffusing capacity of the lungs. The removal of one lung, for example, reduces the diffusing capacity by one half. The thickness of the alveolar–capillary membrane and the distance for diffusion are increased in pulmonary edema and pneumonia. The administration of high concentrations of oxygen increases the difference in pressure between the two sides of the membrane and increases the diffusion of the gas. The characteristics of the gas and its molecular weight and solubility determine how rapidly it diffuses through the respiratory membranes. Carbon dioxide diffuses 20 times more rapidly than oxygen because of its greater solubility in the respiratory membranes. The factors that affect alveolar–capillary gas exchange are summarized in Table 26-3.

The diffusing capacity of the lung is a measure of the rate of transfer of gases through the alveolar–capillary membrane (measured in milliliters per minute). It is measured using a gas that readily diffuses across the membrane, is easily analyzed, and is af-fected by the same factors that influence oxygen diffusion. Carbon monoxide, which meets these criteria, commonly is used for this purpose. The test is done by having a person breathe a known concentration of carbon monoxide (usually for a 10-second breathhold). The volume of carbon monoxide that diffuses across the respiratory membranes is calculated from measurements of lung volume and changes in the carbon monoxide content of inspired and expired air. Because blood levels of carbon monoxide usually are zero, there is no back diffusion of the gas and the difference between the inspired and the expired carbon monoxide reflects the diffusion of the gas. The capacity for oxygen can be calculated using the diffusing capacity of carbon monoxide and known information about the solubility of the two gases. People who smoke or are exposed to carbon monoxide may have appreciable amounts of the gas in their lungs, invalidating the test results. The diffusing capacity of the lung is affected by conditions that alter the permeability of the alveolar–capillary membrane and the ability of the red blood cells to bind and transport the gas.

MATCHING OF VENTILATION AND PERFUSION

The gas exchange properties of the lung depend on the matching of ventilation and perfusion, so that equal amounts of air and blood are entering the respiratory portion of the lungs. Two factors may interfere with the matching of ventilation and perfusion: dead air space and shunt.

TABLE 26-3. FACTORS AFFECTING ALVEOLAR–CAPILLARY GAS EXCHANGE

FACTORS AFFECTING GAS EXCHANGE	EXAMPLES
Surface area available for diffusion	Removal of a lung or diseases such as emphysema and chronic bronchitis, which destroy lung tissue or cause mismatching of ventilation and perfusion
Thickness of the alveolar–capillary membrane	Conditions such as pneumonia, interstitial lung disease, and pulmonary edema, which increase membrane thickness
Partial pressure of alveolar gases	Ascent to high altitudes where the partial pressure of oxygen is reduced. In the opposite direction, increasing the partial pressure of a gas in the inspired air (e.g., oxygen therapy) increases the gradient for diffusion
Solubility and molecular weight of the gas	Carbon dioxide, which is more soluble in the cell membranes, diffuses across the alveolar–capillary membrane more rapidly than oxygen

Dead Air Space. Dead air space refers to the air that must be moved with each breath but does not participate in gas exchange. The movement of air through dead air space contributes to the work of breathing but not to gas exchange. There are two types of dead air space: that contained in the conducting airways (anatomic) and that contained in the respiratory portion of the lung (alveolar). The physiologic dead space includes the anatomic dead space plus the alveolar dead space. The volume of anatomic airway dead space is fixed and about 150 to 200 mL, depending on body size. It constitutes air contained in the nose, pharynx, trachea, and bronchi. The alveolar dead space is about 5 to 10 mL. In situations where alveoli are ventilated but deprived of blood flow, they do not contribute to gas exchange, and thus constitute alveolar dead space. The alveolar ventilation is equal to the minute ventilation minus the physiologic dead space ventilation. The creation of a tracheostomy decreases dead space ventilation and has the effect of decreasing the work of breathing.

Shunt. Shunt refers to blood that moves through the circulation without being oxygenated. There are two types of shunts: physiologic and anatomic. In a physiologic shunt, there is mismatching of ventilation and perfusion. As a result, there is not enough ventilation to provide the oxygen needed to oxygenate the blood flowing through the alveolar capillaries. In an anatomic shunt, blood moves from the venous to the arterial side of the circulation without moving through the lungs. Anatomic intracardiac shunting of blood because of congenital heart defects is discussed in Chapter 23. Physiologic shunting of

blood usually results from destructive lung disease, which impairs ventilation, or from heart failure, in which there is interference with movement of blood through sections of the lungs.

There are many causes of mismatched ventilation and perfusion, of which the most obvious are shown in Figure 26-14. This figure depicts three groups of alveoli with low, normal, and high ventilation-perfusion ratios. The ventilation-perfusion ratio in the center alveoli is normal, resulting in normal gas exchange and oxygen concentrations. Perfusion without ventilation (left) results in a low ventilation-perfusion ratio. This is the type of situation that occurs in atelectasis (see Chapter 27). Ventilation without perfusion (right) results in a high ventilation-perfusion ratio. An example of this type of situation is pulmonary embolism. The arterial blood leaving the pulmonary circulation reflects the mixing of the three alveolar–capillary units. Most of the situations in which ventilation and perfusion are mismatched are less obvious. In lung disease, for example, there may be altered ventilation in one area of the lung and altered perfusion in another area.

GAS TRANSPORT

The lungs enable inhaled air to come in proximity to blood flowing through the pulmonary capillaries so that exchange of gases between the external environment and the internal environment of the body can take place. Thus, the lungs restore the oxygen content of the arterial blood and remove carbon dioxide from the venous blood.

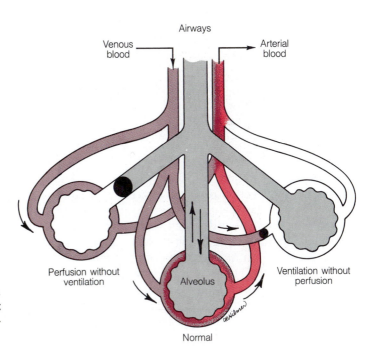

FIG. 26-14. Matching of ventilation and perfusion. (**Center**) Normal matching of ventilation and perfusion; (**left**) perfusion without ventilation (shunt); (**right**) ventilation without perfusion (dead air space).

The blood carries both oxygen and carbon dioxide in the dissolved state and in combination with hemoglobin. In addition, carbon dioxide is converted to bicarbonate and transported in that form.

The amount of a gas that will dissolve in plasma is determined by two factors: (1) the solubility of the gas in the plasma and (2) the partial pressure of the gas in the alveoli. Both oxygen and carbon dioxide dissolve in plasma. The presence of these dissolved gases is similar to the carbon dioxide that is dissolved in a capped bottle of a carbonated drink. In the case of the carbonated drink, the gas is dissolved under situations of increased pressure, which allows more gas to be dissolved. When the bottle cap is removed, the pressure is reduced; less gas remains in the dissolved state. Tiny bubbles form as the gas moves from the dissolved to the gaseous state.

In the clinical setting, blood gases are used to measure the level of dissolved oxygen (PO_2) and carbon dioxide (PCO_2). The letter P is used to indicate the partial pressure of the gas.

Arterial blood usually is used for measuring blood gases. Venous blood is not used because venous levels of oxygen and carbon dioxide reflect the metabolic demands of the tissues rather than the gas exchange function of the lungs. The PO_2 of arterial blood normally is above 80 mmHg, and PCO_2 is in the range of 35 to 45 mmHg.

OXYGEN TRANSPORT

Oxygen is transported in two forms: in chemical combination with hemoglobin and in the dissolved state. The hemoglobin in red blood cells serves as a transport vehicle for oxygen. It binds oxygen in the pulmonary capillaries and releases it in the tissue capillaries. As oxygen moves into or out of the red blood cells, it dissolves in the plasma. It is the dissolved form of oxygen that crosses the cell membrane and participates in cell metabolism. Only about 1% of the oxygen in the blood is carried in the dissolved state; the remainder is carried in combination with the hemoglobin.

Dissolved Oxygen. The partial pressure (PO_2) represents the level of dissolved oxygen in plasma. The amount of gas that can be dissolved in a liquid depends on the solubility of the gas and its pressure. The solubility of oxygen in plasma is fixed and very small. For every 1 mmHg of PO_2 present in the alveoli, 0.003 mL of oxygen becomes dissolved in 100 mL of plasma. This means that at a normal alveolar PO_2 of 100 mmHg, the blood carries only 0.3 mL of dissolved oxygen in each 100 mL of plasma. This amount is small compared with the amount that can be carried

in an equal amount of blood when oxygen is attached to hemoglobin.

Although the amount of oxygen carried in plasma under normal conditions is small, it can become a life-saving mode of transport in carbon monoxide poisoning when most of the hemoglobin sites are occupied by carbon monoxide and are unavailable for transport of oxygen. The use of a hyperbaric chamber, in which 100% oxygen can be administered at high atmospheric pressures, increases the amount of oxygen that can be carried in the dissolved state.

Hemoglobin Transport. Hemoglobin is a highly efficient carrier of oxygen, and about 98% to 99% of the oxygen used by body tissues is carried in this manner. Each gram of hemoglobin carries about 1.34 mL of oxygen when saturated. This means that a person with a hemoglobin of 14 g/100 mL of blood carries 18.8 mL of oxygen in each 100 mL of blood in the form of oxyhemoglobin.

In the lungs, oxygen moves across the alveolar–capillary membrane, through the plasma, and into the red blood cell where it forms a loose and reversible bond with the hemoglobin molecule. In normal lungs, this process is rapid, so that even with a fast heart rate, the hemoglobin is almost saturated with oxygen during the short time it spends in the pulmonary capillaries.

The oxygenated hemoglobin is transported in the arterial blood to the peripheral capillaries where the oxygen is released and made available to the tissues for use in cell metabolism. As the oxygen moves out of the capillaries in response to the needs of the tissues, the hemoglobin saturation, which was about 95% to 97% as the blood left the left side of the heart, drops to about 75% as the mixed venous blood returns to the right.

Oxygen–Hemoglobin Dissociation. Oxygen that remains bound to hemoglobin cannot participate in tissue metabolism. The efficiency of the oxygen dissociation transport system depends on the ability of the hemoglobin molecule to bind oxygen in the lungs and release it as it is needed in the tissues. The affinity of hemoglobin refers to its capacity to bind oxygen; thus, the hemoglobin binds oxygen more readily when affinity is increased and releases it more readily when affinity is decreased.

Hemoglobin's affinity for oxygen is influenced by pH, in that it binds oxygen more strongly under alkaline conditions and releases it more easily under acid conditions. Carbon dioxide moves out of the blood in the lungs, raising the pH and thereby increasing the oxygen affinity. In the tissues, a decrease in pH because of cellular release of carbon dioxide and metabolic acids lowers hemoglobin affinity for oxygen and thereby enhances its release.

The relation between the oxygen carried in combination with hemoglobin and the P_{O_2} of the blood is described by the *oxygen–hemoglobin dissociation* curve, which is shown in Figure 26-15. The curve is S-shaped, with the top flat portion representing the binding of oxygen by the hemoglobin in the lungs and the steep portion representing its release into the tissue capillaries. At about 100 mmHg P_{O_2}, a plateau occurs at which point the hemoglobin is about 98% saturated. Increasing the alveolar P_{O_2} above this level has no further effect on increasing hemoglobin saturation. Even at high altitudes, when the partial pressure of oxygen is considerably decreased, the hemoglobin remains relatively well saturated. At 60 mmHg P_{O_2}, the hemoglobin is still about 89% saturated.

The steep portion of the dissociation curve—between 60 and 40 mmHg—represents the removal of oxygen from the hemoglobin as it moves through the tissue capillaries. This portion of the curve is of great importance because it permits considerable transfer of oxygen from hemoglobin to the tissues with only a small drop in P_{O_2}. The tissues normally remove about 5 mL of oxygen per 100 mL of blood, and the hemoglobin of mixed venous blood as it returns to the right side of the heart is about 75%

saturated (P_{O_2}). In this portion of the dissociation curve, the rate at which oxygen is released from hemoglobin is largely determined by tissue utilization. During strenuous exercise, for example, the muscle cells may remove as much as 15 mL of oxygen per 100 mL of blood from hemoglobin.

Hemoglobin can be regarded as an oxygen buffer system that regulates oxygen pressure in the tissues. Thus, hemoglobin affinity for oxygen must change with the metabolic needs of the tissues. This change is represented by a shift to the right or left in the dissociation curve, as shown in Figure 26-15.

As the curve shifts to the right, the tissue P_{O_2} is greater for any given of level of hemoglobin saturation. A shift to the right represents reduced affinity of the hemoglobin for oxygen at any given P_{O_2}. It usually is caused by conditions such as fever or acidosis or by an increase in P_{CO_2}, which reflects increased tissue metabolism. High altitude and conditions such as pulmonary insufficiency, heart failure, and severe anemia also cause the oxygen dissociation curve to shift to the right.

A shift to the left in the oxygen dissociation curve represents enhanced affinity of hemoglobin for oxygen and occurs in situations associated with a decrease in tissue metabolism, such as alkalosis, decreased body temperature, and decreased carbon dioxide levels. The degree of shift can be determined by the P_{50}, or the partial pressure of oxygen that is needed to achieve a 50% saturation of hemoglobin. Returning to Figure 26-16, the reader will note that the dissociation curve on the left has a P_{50} of about 20 mmHg; the normal curve, a P_{50} of 26; and the curve on the right, a P_{50} of 35 mmHg.

CARBON DIOXIDE TRANSPORT

The transport of carbon dioxide, which is a by-product of tissue metabolism, is not nearly the problem of oxygen transport. Carbon dioxide is transported in the blood in three forms: as dissolved carbon dioxide, attached to hemoglobin, and as bicarbonate. As discussed in Chapter 30, acid–base balance is influenced by the amount of dissolved carbon dioxide and the bicarbonate level in the blood.

As carbon dioxide is formed during the metabolic process, it diffuses out of cells into the tissue spaces and then into the capillaries. On entering a capillary, carbon dioxide undergoes chemical and physical reactions that are essential for its transport. A small portion of the carbon dioxide is carried in the dissolved state (P_{CO_2}) to the lungs. The P_{CO_2} of arterial blood is about 40 mmHg, and the P_{CO_2} of venous blood is about 45 mmHg; the difference between the two values represents the amount of dissolved carbon dioxide carried in plasma. The amount of dis-

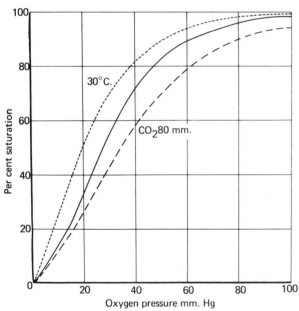

FIG. 26-15. *The oxygen–hemoglobin dissociation curve. Note that when the carbon dioxide is increased or when the blood pH is decreased, the curve is shifted to the right, and therefore, the hemoglobin binds less oxygen for any partial pressure of oxygen. When the curve is shifted to the left, as occurs when the carbon dioxide is decreased or the pH is increased, the opposite occurs. (Chaffee, E. E., & Lytle, I. M. [1980].* Basic physiology and anatomy *[4th ed.]. Philadelphia: J.B. Lippincott)*

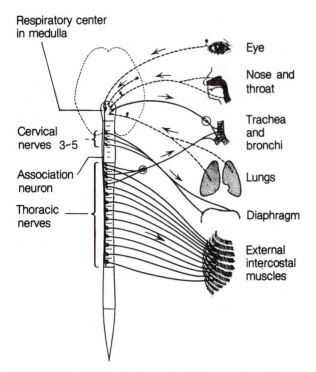

FIG. 26-16. Activity in the respiratory center. Impulses traveling over afferent neurons activate central neurons, which in turn activate the efferent neurons that supply the muscles of respiration. Thus, respiratory movements may be altered by a variety of stimuli. (Chaffee, E. E., & Greisheimer, E. M. [1974]. *Basic physiology and anatomy* [3rd ed.]. Philadelphia: J.B. Lippincott)

solved carbon dioxide that can be carried in plasma is determined by the partial pressure of the gas and its solubility coefficient (0.03 mL/100 mL/mmHg).

Dissolved carbon dioxide combines with water to form carbonic acid (H_2CO_3). This would be a slow reaction if it were not for an enzyme called *carbonic anhydrase*. Carbonic anhydrase, which increases the reaction between carbon dioxide and water about 5000-fold, is present in large quantities in red blood cells. Much of the carbon dioxide diffuses into red blood cells, where it reacts with water to form hydrogen and bicarbonate ions ($H_2CO_3 \leftrightarrows H^+ + HCO_3^-$) before it leaves the capillaries. In the red cell, the hydrogen ion that is generated from the carbonic anhydrase–mediated reaction combines with the hemoglobin, which is a powerful acid–base buffer. The bicarbonate ion that formed from the reaction diffuses into plasma, exchanged for a chloride ion in a bicarbonate–chloride shift. This is made possible by a special bicarbonate–chloride carrier protein in the red blood cell membrane. As a result of the bicarbonate–chloride shift, the chloride content of the red blood cell is greater in venous blood than in arterial blood. The reversible combination of carbon dioxide with water in the red blood cell accounts for 70% of all carbon dioxide transport.

In addition to the carbonic anhydrase–mediated reaction with water, carbon dioxide reacts directly with hemoglobin to form carbaminohemoglobin. The combination of carbon dioxide with hemoglobin is a reversible reaction that involves a loose bond, which allows for transport of carbon dioxide from tissues to the lungs, where it is released into the alveoli for exchange with the external environment. The release of oxygen from hemoglobin enhances the binding of carbon dioxide to hemoglobin in the peripheral capillaries; in the lungs, the combination of oxygen with hemoglobin displaces carbon dioxide. This is because the combination of oxygen with hemoglobin causes the hemoglobin to become a strong acid. In the lungs, the highly acidic hemoglobin has a lesser tendency to form carbaminohemoglobin, and carbon dioxide is released from hemoglobin into the alveoli. In the tissues, the release of oxygen from hemoglobin decreases the hemoglobin's acidity, thus increasing its ability to combine with carbon dioxide and form carbaminohemoglobin.

In summary, the primary function of the lungs is the oxygenation of the blood and the removal of carbon dioxide. Pulmonary gas exchange is conventionally divided into three processes: (1) ventilation or the flow of gases into the alveoli of the lungs, (2) perfusion of blood in the adjacent pulmonary capillaries, and (3) diffusion or transfer of gases between the alveoli and the pulmonary capillaries.

Ventilation refers to the movement of air between the atmosphere and the lungs. Pulmonary ventilation refers to the total exchange of gases between the atmosphere and the lungs, and alveolar ventilation refers to ventilation in the gas exchange portion of the lungs. The distribution of alveolar ventilation and pulmonary capillary blood flow varies with lung volume and body position. In the upright position and high lung volumes, ventilation is greatest in the lower parts of the lungs. The standing position also produces a decrease in blood flow to the upper parts of the lung, resulting from the distance above the level of the heart and the low mean arterial pressure in the pulmonary circulation.

The diffusion of gases in the lungs is influenced by four factors: (1) the surface area available for diffusion, (2) the thickness of the alveolar–capillary membrane through which the gases diffuse, (3) the differences in the partial pressure of the gas on either side of the membrane, and (4) the characteristics of the gas. The efficiency of gas exchange requires that there is matching of ventilation and perfusion, so that equal amounts of air and blood enter the respiratory portion of the lungs. Two factors—dead air space and shunt—interfere with matching of ventilation and perfusion and do not contribute to gas exchange. Dead air space occurs when areas of the lungs are ventilated but not perfused. Shunt is the condition under which areas of the lungs are perfused but not ventilated.

The blood transports oxygen to the cells and returns carbon dioxide to the lungs. Oxygen is transported in two forms: in chemical combination with hemoglobin and physically dissolved in plasma (Po_2). Hemoglobin is an efficient carrier of oxygen, and about 98% to 99% of oxygen is transported in this manner. Carbon dioxide is carried in three forms: as carbaminohemoglobin, as dissolved carbon dioxide, and as bicarbonate. Seventy to 80% of carbon dioxide in plasma is in the bicarbonate or dissolved form.

■ CONTROL OF BREATHING

Unlike the heart, which has inherent rhythmic properties and can beat independently of the nervous system, the muscles that control respiration require continuous input from the nervous system. Movement of the diaphragm, intercostal muscles, sternocleidomastoid, and other accessory muscles that control ventilation are integrated by neurons located in the pons and medulla. These neurons are collectively referred to as the *respiratory center*. The respiratory center consists of two dense bilateral aggregates of respiratory neurons involved in both initiating inspiration and expiration and incorporating afferent impulses into motor responses of the respiratory muscles. The first, or dorsal, group of neurons in the respiratory center is primarily concerned with inspiration. These neurons control the activity of the phrenic nerves and drive the second, or ventral, group of respiratory neurons. In addition, they probably integrate impulses from the lungs and airways into the ventilatory response. The second group of neurons, which contains both inspiratory and expiratory neurons, controls the spinal motor neurons of the intercostal and abdominal muscles. The pacemaker properties of the respiratory center result from the cycling of the two groups of respiratory neurons.

Axons from the neurons in the respiratory center cross in the midline and descend in the ventrolateral columns of the spinal cord. The tracts that control expiration and inspiration are spatially separated in the cord, as are the tracts that transmit specialized reflexes (*e.g.*, coughing and hiccoughing) and voluntary control of ventilation. Only at the level of the spinal cord are the respiratory impulses integrated to produce a reflex response. The neural control of ventilation is shown in Figure 26-16.

The control of breathing has both automatic and voluntary components. The automatic regulation of ventilation is controlled by input from two types of sensors or receptors: chemoreceptors, which monitor blood levels of oxygen, carbon dioxide, and *p*H and adjust ventilation to meet the changing metabolic needs of the body, and lung receptors, which monitor breathing patterns and lung function. Voluntary regulation of ventilation integrates breathing with voluntary acts such as speaking, blowing, and singing. These acts, initiated by the motor and premotor cortex, cause temporary suspension of automatic breathing. It has been suggested that alterations in the control of automatic and voluntary regulation of breathing may contribute to various forms of sleep apnea. This is discussed in Chapter 28.

The automatic and voluntary components of respiration are regulated by afferent impulses that come to the respiratory center from a number of sources. Afferent input from higher brain centers is evidenced by the fact that one can consciously alter the depth and rate of respiration. Fever, pain, and emotion exert their influence through lower brain centers. Vagal afferents from sensory receptors in the lungs and airways are integrated in the dorsal area of the respiratory center.

CHEMORECEPTORS

Tissue needs for oxygen and the removal of carbon dioxide are regulated by chemoreceptors that monitor blood levels of these gases. Input from these sensors is transmitted to the respiratory center, and ventilation is adjusted to maintain the arterial blood gases within a normal range.

There are two types of chemoreceptors: central and peripheral. The most important chemoreceptors for sensing changes in blood carbon dioxide content are the central chemoreceptors. These receptors are chemosensitive regions located in the medulla near the respiratory center and are bathed in cerebrospinal fluid. Although the central chemoreceptors monitor carbon dioxide levels, the actual stimulus for these receptors is provided by hydrogen ions that are present in the cerebrospinal fluid. This fluid is separated from the blood by the blood–brain barrier, which permits free diffusion of carbon dioxide but not bicarbonate or hydrogen ions. The carbon dioxide in turn combines rapidly with water to form carbonic acid, which dissociates into hydrogen ions. Thus, the carbon dioxide content in the blood regulates ventilation through its effect on the *p*H of the extracellular fluid of the brain. These chemoreceptors are extremely sensitive to short-term changes in carbon dioxide. The effect of an increase in plasma carbon dioxide levels on ventilation reaches its peak within a minute or so and then declines if the carbon dioxide level remains elevated. With long-term elevation in carbon dioxide, there occurs a compensatory increase in bicarbonate secretion into the cerebrospinal fluid, which acts as a buffer for the hydrogen ions. Thus, people with chronically elevated levels of carbon dioxide no longer respond to this stimulus for increased ventilation but rely on the stimulus provided by a decrease in blood oxygen levels.

Arterial oxygen levels are monitored by peripheral chemoreceptors located in the carotid and aortic bodies. Although these chemoreceptors also monitor carbon dioxide, they play a much more important role in monitoring arterial blood oxygen levels. These receptors exert little control over ventilation until the PO_2 has dropped below 60 mmHg. Hypoxia is the main stimulus for ventilation in people with chronic hypercapnia. If these people are given oxygen therapy at a level sufficient to increase the P_{O_2} above that needed to stimulate the peripheral chemoreceptors, their ventilation may be seriously depressed.

LUNG RECEPTORS

There are three types of lung receptors: stretch, irritant, and juxtacapillary (J). Stretch receptors are located in the smooth muscle layers of the conducting airways. They respond to changes in pressure within the walls of the airways. When the lungs are inflated, these receptors inhibit inspiration and promote expiration (Hering-Breuer reflex). They are important in establishing breathing patterns and in minimizing the work of breathing by adjusting respiratory rate and tidal volume to accommodate changes in lung compliance and airway resistance. Irritant receptors have a distribution similar to that of the stretch receptors. They can be mechanically stimulated by increases in airway pressure, changes in lung inflation, and changes in bronchial smooth muscle tone. Stimulation of the irritant receptors leads to airway constriction and a pattern of rapid, shallow breathing. This pattern of breathing probably protects respiratory tissues from the damaging effects of toxic inhalants. It is also thought that the mechanical stimulation of these receptors may ensure more uniform lung expansion by initiating periodic sighing and yawning. The function of the J receptors is uncertain; it is thought that they sense lung congestion. These receptors may be responsible for the rapid, shallow breathing that occurs with pulmonary edema, pulmonary embolism, and pneumonia.

COUGH REFLEX

Coughing is a neurally mediated reflex that protects the lungs from accumulation of secretions and from entry of irritating and destructive substances. It is one of the primary defense mechanisms of the respiratory tract.

The cough reflex is initiated by receptors located in the tracheobronchial wall; these receptors are extremely sensitive to irritating substances and to the presence of excess secretions. Afferent impulses from these receptors are transmitted through the vagus to the medullary center, which integrates the cough response.

Coughing itself requires the rapid inspiration of a large volume of air (usually about 2.5 L) followed by rapid closure of the glottis and forceful contraction of the abdominal and expiratory muscles. As these muscles contract, there is a marked elevation of intrathoracic pressures to levels of 100 mmHg or more.

The rapid opening of the glottis at this point leads to an explosive expulsion of air.

Many conditions can interfere with the cough reflex and its protective function. The reflex is impaired in people whose abdominal or respiratory muscles are weak. This problem can be caused by disease conditions that lead to muscle weakness or paralysis, by prolonged inactivity, or as an outcome of surgery involving these muscles. Bed rest interferes with expansion of the chest and limits the amount of air that can be taken into the lungs in preparation for coughing, so the cough is weak and ineffective. Disease conditions that prevent effective closure of the glottis and laryngeal muscles interfere with accomplishment of the marked increase in intrathoracic pressure that is needed for effective coughing. The presence of a nasogastric tube, for example, may prevent closure of the upper airway structures and may fatigue the receptors for the cough reflex that are located in the area. Last, the cough reflex is impaired when there is depressed function of the medullary centers in the brain that integrate the cough reflex. Interruption of the central integration aspect of the cough reflex can arise as the result of disease of this part of the brain or the action of drugs that depress the cough center.

Although the cough reflex is basically a protective mechanism, frequent and prolonged coughing can be exhausting and painful and can exert undesirable effects on the cardiovascular and respiratory systems and on the elastic tissues of the lungs. This is particularly true in young children and elderly people.

In summary, the respiratory system requires continuous input from the nervous system. Movement of the diaphragm, intercostal muscles, and other respiratory muscles are controlled by neurons of the respiratory center located in the pons and medulla. The control of breathing has both automatic and voluntary components. The automatic regulation of ventilation is controlled by two types of receptors: lung receptors, which protect respiratory structures, and chemoreceptors, which monitor the gas exchange function of the lungs by sensing changes in blood levels of carbon dioxide, oxygen, and pH. There are three types of lung receptors: stretch receptors, which monitor lung inflation; irritant receptors, which protect against the damaging effects of toxic inhalants; and J receptors, which are thought to sense lung congestion. There are two groups of chemoreceptors: central and peripheral. The central chemoreceptors are the most important in sensing changes in carbon dioxide levels and the peripheral chemoreceptors, in sensing arterial blood oxygen levels. Voluntary respiratory control is needed for integrating breathing and actions such as speaking, blowing, and singing. These acts, which are initiated by the motor and premotor cortex, cause temporary suspension of automatic breathing. The cough reflex protects the lungs from accumulation of secretions and from entry of irritating and destructive substances; it is one of the primary defense mechanisms of the respiratory tract.

▪ BIBLIOGRAPHY

Berne, R.M., & Levy, M.N. (1988). *Physiology* (2nd ed., pp. 575–635). St. Louis: C.V. Mosby.

Caminiti, S.P., & Young, S.L. (1991). The pulmonary surfactant system. *Hospital Practice, 26*(1A), 87–100.

Carpenter, K.D. (1989). Oxygen transport in the blood. *Critical Care Nurse, 11*(9), 2033.

Cormack, D.H. (1987). *Ham's histology* (9th ed., pp. 541–563). Philadelphia: J.B. Lippincott.

Davis, J.M., Venes-Meehan, K., Notter, R.H., et al. (1988). Changes in pulmonary mechanics after the administration of surfactant to infants with respiratory distress syndrome. *New England Journal of Medicine, 319,* 476.

Fishman, A.P. (1980). *Assessment of pulmonary function.* New York: McGraw-Hill.

Guyton, A. (1991). *Textbook of medical physiology* (8th ed., pp. 402–453, 501). Philadelphia: W.B. Saunders.

Reischman, R.R. (1988). Review of ventilation and perfusion physiology. *Critical Care Nurse, 8*(7), 24–28.

West, J.B. (1990). *Respiratory physiology* (4th ed.). Baltimore: Williams & Wilkins.

C H A P T E R   2 7

ALTERATIONS IN RESPIRATORY FUNCTION

■ OBJECTIVES

After you have studied this chapter, you should be able to meet the following objectives:

■ Describe the transmission of the common cold from one person to another.
■ State the reason that rest and drinking large amounts of liquids are helpful in treating influenza.
■ Differentiate between areas of the lung that are involved in lobar, bronchial, and viral pneumonias.
■ Differentiate between primary tuberculosis and reactivated tuberculosis on the basis of their pathophysiology.
■ State the mechanism for the transmission of fungal infections of the lung.
■ State the characteristics of pleural pain.
■ Explain why tension pneumothorax is a life-threatening emergency.
■ Relate the pathologic changes that occur with pleural effusion to the production of signs and symptoms.

■ Differentiate between primary and secondary atelectasis.
■ State the feature common to chronic obstructive pulmonary diseases.
■ Characterize the early and late phase response in the pathogenesis of bronchial asthma and relate to the current methods for treatment of the disorder.
■ Relate the pathologic changes that occur in bronchial asthma to the production of signs and symptoms.
■ Explain the distinction between chronic bronchitis and emphysema.
■ State the difference between chronic obstructive pulmonary diseases and interstitial lung diseases.
■ State the chief manifestations of bronchiectasis.
■ Describe the genetic abnormality responsible for cystic fibrosis and state its effect on lung function.

Carol Mattson Porth: PATHOPHYSIOLOGY: CONCEPTS OF
ALTERED HEALTH STATES, 4th ed. © 1994, 1990, 1986, 1982
J.B. Lippincott Company

523

- ■ Cite the characteristics of occupational dusts that determine their pathogenicity in terms of the production of pneumoconioses.
- ■ State the immediate effects of pulmonary embolism.
- ■ State three causes of pulmonary hypertension.
- ■ Describe the alterations in cardiovascular function that are characteristic of cor pulmonale.
- ■ List two symptoms of lung cancer that are related to the invasion of the mediastinum.
- ■ Cite three paraneoplastic manifestations of lung cancer.
- ■ Trace the development of the respiratory tract through the five stages of embryonic and fetal development.

- ■ Cite the function of surfactant in lung function in the neonate.
- ■ Cite the possible cause and manifestations of bronchopulmonary dysplasia.
- ■ Describe the physiologic basis for sternal and chest wall retractions and grunting, stridor, and wheezing as signs of respiratory distress in infants and small children.
- ■ Compare croup, epiglottitis, and bronchiolitis in terms of incidence by age, site of infection, and signs and symptoms.
- ■ List the signs of impending respiratory failure in small children.

Respiratory illnesses represent one of the more common reasons for visits to the physician, admission to the hospital, and forced inactivity among all age groups. Forty-seven million Americans—children and adults—suffer from one or more chronic respiratory diseases. For purposes of discussion, the content in this chapter has been organized under seven main headings: (1) respiratory tract infections, (2) disorders of lung inflation, (3) obstructive airway disease, (4) interstitial lung disease, (5) pulmonary vascular disease, (6) lung cancer, and (7) respiratory disorders in children. Alterations in ventilation and respiratory failure are discussed in Chapter 28.

■ RESPIRATORY TRACT INFECTIONS

Respiratory tract infections can involve the upper respiratory tract (nose, oropharynx, and larynx), the lower respiratory tract (lower airways and lungs), or both the upper and lower airways. The discussion in this section of the chapter focuses on the common cold, influenza, pneumonia, tuberculosis, and fungal infections of the lung. Acute respiratory infections in children are discussed in the last section of the chapter.

The respiratory tract is susceptible to infectious processes caused by many different types of microorganisms. For the most part, the signs and symptoms of respiratory tract infections depend on the function of the structure involved, the severity of the infectious process, and the person's age and general health.

Viruses are the most frequent cause of respiratory tract infections. They can range from a self-limiting cold to life-threatening pneumonia. Moreover, viral infections often lead to secondary bacterial in-

fections. Each viral species has its own pattern of respiratory tract involvement. The rhinoviruses remain strictly confined to the upper respiratory tract; the influenza viruses can infect both the upper and lower respiratory tracts; and measles and chickenpox viruses "pass through" the respiratory tract and do not cause respiratory symptoms until secondary viremic spread has occurred.[1] In addition to viruses, other microorganisms such as bacteria (*e.g.*, pneumococci, staphylococci), mycobacteria (*Mycobacterium tuberculosis*), fungi (histoplasmosis, coccidioidomycosis, and blastomycosis), and opportunistic organisms (*Pneumocystis carinii*) produce infections of the lung that cause significant morbidity and are among the major causes of death.

THE COMMON COLD

The common cold is a viral infection of the upper respiratory tract. It occurs more frequently than any other respiratory tract infection. Most adults have 2 to 4 colds per year; children may have up to 10 per year.[2] The condition usually begins with a feeling of dryness and stuffiness affecting mainly the nasopharynx; it is accompanied by excessive production of nasal secretions and lacrimation, or tearing of the eyes. Usually the secretions remain clear and watery. The mucous membranes of the upper respiratory tract become reddened, swollen, and bathed in secretions. Involvement of the pharynx and larynx causes sore throat and hoarseness. Headache and generalized malaise may be present. In severe cases there may be chills, fever, and exhaustion. The disease process is usually self-limiting, lasting about 7 days.

Although the condition can be caused by a number of viruses, the rhinovirus is the most common cause. The virus is rapidly spread from person to person. The first step in the spreading of the common cold is the shedding of viruses, the area of greatest potential being the nasal mucosa. Studies have shown that colds are spread most frequently in the home or school.[3,4] The fingers are the greatest source of spread, and the nasal mucosa and conjunctival surface of the eyes are the most important portals of entry of the virus. Cold viruses have been found to survive for 3.5 hours on the skin and hard surfaces, such as wood and plastic; survival is poor on facial tissue and porous cloth. The most highly contagious period is during the first 3 days after the onset of symptoms, and the incubation period is about 5 days. Studies suggest that the aerosol spread of colds through coughing and sneezing is much less important than the spread by fingers picking up the virus from contaminated surfaces and carrying it to the nasal membranes and eyes.[5,6] This suggests that careful attention to handwashing is one of the most important preventive measures for avoiding the common cold. Host defenses are also reported to influence the development of the common cold. Psychological stress, which is thought to influence immune function, is reported to increase the risk of developing a cold.[7]

A large number of over-the-counter (OTC) remedies are available for treating the common cold. Because the common cold is an acute and self-limiting illness in people who are otherwise healthy, treatment with antibiotics and other medications that are potentially harmful is contraindicated. Symptomatic treatment with rest and antipyretic drugs is all that is usually needed. There is some controversy about the use of vitamin C to reduce the incidence and severity of colds and influenza. Several studies have found an association between vitamin C intake and a reduced incidence,[8,9] whereas others have found that vitamin C had no effect on the number or severity of colds.[10] Antihistamines are popular OTC drugs because of their action in drying nasal secretions. However, they may dry up bronchial secretions and worsen the cough; in addition, they may cause dizziness, drowsiness, and impaired judgment. As with vitamin C, there is no evidence that they shorten the duration of the cold. Decongestant drugs (sympathomimetic agents) are available in OTC nasal sprays, drops, and oral cold medications. These drugs constrict the blood vessels in the swollen nasal mucosa and reduce nasal swelling. Rebound nasal swelling can occur with indiscriminate use of nasal drops and sprays. Oral preparations containing decongestants may cause systemic vasoconstriction and elevation of blood pressure when given in doses large enough to relieve nasal congestion; therefore, they should be avoided by people with hypertension, heart disease, hyperthyroidism, diabetes mellitus, and other health problems.

INFLUENZA

Influenza is a viral infection that can affect both the upper and lower respiratory tracts. It usually occurs in epidemics or pandemics. Until the advent of AIDS, it was the last uncontrolled pandemic killer of humans. More people died in the 1918/1919 influenza pandemic than in World War I. In the United States, 10,000 to 20,000 people die of influenza-related illness during nonpandemic years.[11] The majority of deaths are due to pneumonia or exacerbation of cardiopulmonary or other conditions; 80% to 90% of those who die are 65 years of age or older.[12] There are two antigenic types of the influenza virus (type A and type B). Both types of the virus cause similar manifestations.

The influenza virus causes three syndromes: an uncomplicated rhinotracheitis, a respiratory viral infection followed by a bacterial infection, and viral pneumonia. The incubation period for all three syndromes is 1 to 4 days. In the early stages, the symptoms of influenza are often indistinguishable from other viral infections. There is an abrupt onset of fever and chills, malaise, muscle aching, headache, profuse watery nasal discharge, nonproductive cough, and sore throat. One distinguishing feature of influenza viral infection is the rapid onset, sometimes in as little as 1 to 2 minutes, of profound malaise.[11] The infection causes necrosis and shedding of the serous and ciliated cells that line the respiratory tract, leaving gaping holes between the underlying basal cells, allowing extracellular fluid to escape. This is the reason for the "runny nose" that is characteristic of this phase of the infection. During recovery, the serous cells are replaced more rapidly than the ciliated cells. Mucus is produced, but the ciliated cells are unable to move it adequately; people recovering from influenza must continue to blow their nose to clear their sinuses and cough to clear their trachea.

The symptoms of uncomplicated rhinotracheitis usually peak by days 3 to 5 and disappear by days 7 to 10. People who develop secondary complications generally report that they were beginning to feel better when they experienced a return of symptoms. Frequent complications include sinusitis, otitis media, bronchitis, and bacterial pneumonia. Reye's syndrome (hepatic failure and encephalopathy) is a rare complication in young children.

The clinical course of influenza pneumonia progresses rapidly. It can cause hypoxemia and death within a few days of onset. The reason for the rapid onset is thought to relate to the mode of spread and the absence of an initial rhinotracheitis. If the virus is spread by fingers or large-droplet spray, as from sneezing or coughing, only the upper respiratory tract is involved. Infection of the upper respiratory tract is thought to give the immune system enough time to build the defenses needed to protect against viral pneumonia. When the virus is contained in small droplets, it can bypass the upper respiratory tract and travel directly into the lungs to establish infection.[11]

In influenza, the goals of treatment are designed to limit the infection to the upper respiratory tract. The symptomatic approach, which uses rest, keeping warm, and drinking large amounts of liquids, helps to accomplish this. Rest decreases the oxygen requirements of the body and reduces the respiratory rate and chance of spreading the virus from the upper to lower respiratory tract. Keeping warm helps maintain the respiratory epithelium at a core body temperature of 37°C (or higher if fever is present), thereby inhibiting viral replication, which is optimal at 35°C. This information also suggests that antipyretic drugs, such as acetaminophen, should not be given for low levels of fever but only for discomfort and high fever. Drinking large amounts of liquids ensures that the function of the epithelial lining of the respiratory tract is not further compromised by dehydration.[11]

Amantadine (an antiviral drug) is often effective in preventing symptomatic influenza A infections among high-risk groups during an outbreak.[13] It is only effective against influenza A and must be administered throughout the period of risk.

Influenza Immunization. Vaccines are available to protect against the influenzal infections. Immunization is recommended for high-risk groups who, because of their age or underlying health problems, are unable to cope well with the infection and often require medical attention, including hospitalization. For example, influenza outbreaks in nursing homes resulted in infection rates as high as 60%, with mortality rates of 30% or more.[14]

Several strains of the influenza virus are responsible for epidemics of the disease. These strains undergo small changes over time that affect their antigenicity and the host protection afforded by previous immunization. Influenza's impact is normally greatest when new strains appear against which the population lacks immunity. Therefore, the formulation of the influenza vaccine must be changed yearly in response to changes in the influenza virus. Each year the Public Health Advisory Committee on Immunization Practices updates its recommendations for the composition of the vaccine.

The Immunization Practices Advisory Committee recommends annual vaccination using inactivated influenza vaccine to prevent or minimize the effect of influenza infections in any person, 6 months of age or older, who is at high risk for complications of influenza.[13] Groups at highest risk for complications include: (1) people 65 years of age or older; (2) residents of nursing homes or other chronic-care facilities housing people of any age with chronic medical conditions; (3) adults or children with chronic disorders of the pulmonary or cardiovascular systems, including children with asthma; (4) adults and children who have required regular medical follow-up or hospitalization during the preceding year because of chronic metabolic diseases (*e.g.*, diabetes mellitus, renal dysfunction, sickle cell anemia, or immunosuppression); and (5) children or teenagers (6 months to 18 years) who are receiving long-term aspirin therapy (because of the risk of developing Reye's syndrome). Immunization is also recommended for groups (household members and health-care workers) that live with or care for people who at high risk for developing influenza complications. It is believed that the protection of people in the high-risk groups can be improved by reducing the chances of exposure to influenza from household contacts and health care providers.

PNEUMONIAS

Most of the agents that cause pneumonia and lower respiratory tract infections are inhaled into the lung in the air breathed. Normally, respiratory tract defense mechanisms would prevent these organisms from entering the lung. Loss of the cough reflex, damage to the ciliated endothelium that lines the respiratory tract, and lowered resistance to infection all increase susceptibility to pneumonia. Table 27-1 summarizes respiratory tract defense mechanisms along with factors that impair their effectiveness and thereby predispose to pneumonia.

The term *pneumonia* describes inflammation of parenchymal structures of the lung, such as the alveoli and the bronchioles. Etiologic agents include both infectious and noninfectious agents. For example, inhalation of irritating fumes or aspiration of gastric contents can result in severe pneumonia.

Although antibiotics have significantly reduced mortality due to pneumonias, these diseases remain an important immediate cause of death in the elderly and in people with debilitating diseases. Also, there have been subtle changes in the spectrum of microorganisms that cause infectious pneumonias, namely, a decrease in pneumonias caused by *Streptococcus pneumoniae* and an increase in pneumonias caused by other microorganisms such as *Pseudomonas, Candida* and other fungi, and nonspecific viruses. Many of these pneumonias occur in

**TABLE 27-1. RESPIRATORY DEFENSE MECHANISMS
AND CONDITIONS THAT IMPAIR THEIR EFFECTIVENESS**

DEFENSE MECHANISM	FUNCTION	FACTORS THAT IMPAIR EFFECTIVENESS
Nasopharyngeal defenses	Remove particles from the air; contact with surface lysosomes and immunoglobulins (IgA) protects against infection	IgA deficiency state, hay fever, common cold, trauma to the nose, others
Glottic and cough reflexes	Protect against aspiration into tracheobronchial tree	Loss of cough reflex due to stroke or neural lesion, neuromuscular disease, abdominal or chest surgery, depression of the cough reflex due to sedation or anesthesia, presence of a nasogastric tube (tends to cause adaptation of afferent receptors)
Mucociliary blanket	Removes secretions, microorganisms, and particles from the respiratory tract	Smoking, viral diseases, chilling, inhalation of irritating gases
Pulmonary macrophages	Remove microorganisms and foreign particles from the lung	Chilling, alcohol intoxication, smoking, anoxia

people with impaired immune defenses, including people who are on immunosuppressant drugs to prevent rejection of a bone marrow or organ transplant. *Pneumocystis carinii*, a virulent type of pneumonia, is associated with acquired immunodeficiency syndrome (AIDS).

Pneumonias are usually classified according to their etiologic agent and anatomic distribution. They are commonly classified as acute bacterial pneumonias and primary atypical pneumonias.

ACUTE BACTERIAL PNEUMONIAS

Bacterial pneumonias are typically associated with intraalveolar exudation resulting in consolidation of lung tissue. They tend to conform to one of two anatomic patterns: lobar pneumonia or bronchial pneumonia.

Lobar Pneumonia. Lobar pneumonia is an acute bacterial infection involving a large portion of an entire lobe of a lung (Fig. 27-1). Classically, lobar pneumonia occurs in otherwise healthy adults and is relatively uncommon in infants and the elderly. Approximately 90% to 95% of cases of lobar pneumonia are caused by pneumococcus (*Streptococcus pneumoniae*), types 1, 3, 7, and 2.[1] Type 3 causes a particularly virulent form of lobar pneumonia.

The tissue changes in lobar pneumonia are consistent with signs of acute inflammation. This acute inflammatory response can be divided into four stages: (1) congestion, (2) red hepatization, (3) gray hepatization, and (4) resolution. Often its progress is modified by antibiotic therapy. The *congestive stage* represents the initial inflammatory response and is characterized by vascular engorgement of the alveolar vessels and transudation of serous fluid into the alveoli. The period of congestion lasts about 24 hours and is followed by the stage of *red hepatization*. During this stage, there is extravasation of red blood cells and fibrin into the alveoli, and the lungs become firm and red with a liver-like appearance—hence the term red hepatization. The stage of *gray hepatization* is characterized by an accumulation of fibrin and the beginning disintegration of the inflammatory white and red cells. Sometimes the infection extends into the pleural cavity causing *empyema*—pus in the pleural cavity. In untreated pneumonia, the stage of *resolution* occurs in about 8 to 10 days and represents the enzymatic digestion and removal of the inflamma-

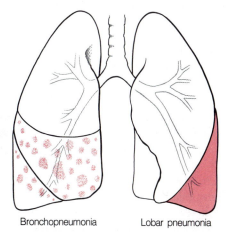

FIG. 27-1. Distribution of lung involvement in lobar and bronchial pneumonia.

Bronchopneumonia   Lobar pneumonia

tory exudate from the infected lung area. The exudate is either coughed up or removed from the lung by macrophages.

The signs and symptoms of lobar pneumonia coincide with the stage of the disease. The onset is usually sudden and is characterized by malaise, a severe shaking chill, and fever. The temperature may go as high as 106°F. During the congestive stage, coughing brings up a watery sputum and breath sounds are limited, with fine crackles. As the disease progresses, the character of the sputum changes; it may be blood-tinged (or rust-colored) to purulent. Pleuritic pain, a sharp pain that is more severe with respiratory movements, is common. With antibiotic therapy, fever usually subsides in about 48 to 72 hours and recovery is uneventful.[1]

Bronchopneumonia. In *bronchopneumonia*, there is a patchy consolidation with involvement of several lobules. The lesions tend to vary in size from 3 to 4 cm and, because of gravity, are more common in the lower and posterior portions of the lung (see Fig. 27-1). The disease frequently represents an extension of preexisting bronchitis or bronchiolitis. People with the disease often have a history of extended bedrest and immobility, malnutrition, serious health problems, and aspiration of gastric contents. Bronchopneumonia is considered to be a disease of the very young, the very old, and the debilitated—the very young because their immunologic reserve and respiratory defense mechanisms have not yet developed, and the very old because of a decline in immunity and because many have other diseases that predispose them to pneumonia.

In contrast to lobar pneumonia, which has a rapid onset, the early manifestations of bronchopneumonia are often insidious and in most cases include a low-grade fever (38°C to 39.5°C) along with a cough and expiratory crackles. Dyspnea may be present but is not common. Complications include formation of a lung abscess, empyema, and bacteremia.

Virtually any pathogenic organism can cause bronchopneumonia. The most common agents are staphylococci, *Hemophilus influenzae*, *Pseudomonas aeruginosa*, coliform bacteria, and the previously mentioned *Streptococcus pneumoniae*.[1] *Staphylococcus aureus* is an important cause of secondary bacterial pneumonia in children and healthy adults after viral respiratory tract infections. *Klebsiella pneumoniae* is the most common cause of gram-negative bacillary pneumonia, most frequently among debilitated and malnourished people. Hospitalized patients are susceptible to bacteria present in the environment. About two thirds of bronchopneumonias in hospitalized patients are pneumococcal pneumonias.[1] Proper handwashing by health care workers and de-

contamination of inhalation equipment are important in preventing these infections. Immunization to prevent pneumococcal pneumonia is recommended for high-risk groups.

Pneumococcal Immunization. A 23-valent pneumococcal vaccine, composed of antigens from 23 types of *Streptococcus pneumoniae* (pneumococcus), was licensed in the United States in 1983, replacing the 14-valent type licensed in 1977.

Vaccination with the pneumococcal vaccine is recommended for adults with chronic illnesses, particularly cardiovascular and pulmonary diseases, diabetes mellitus, alcoholism, who sustain increased morbidity with respiratory infections. Vaccination is also recommended for immunocompromised adults, those with other chronic illnesses associated with increased risk of pneumococcal infections, and for otherwise healthy older adults, especially those aged 65 and over. Children aged 2 years and older with chronic illnesses such as cardiovascular disease, sickle cell disease, splenectomy, Hodgkin's disease, nephrotic syndrome, cerebrospinal fluid leaks, or conditions associated with immunosuppression should also be immunized.

A single dose of pneumococcal vaccine usually confers lifetime immunity. There were early reports of adverse effects in people who had been revaccinated with pneumococcal vaccine. Subsequent reports have indicated few adverse effects occur when the interval between vaccination and revaccination is more than 5 years. However, revaccination should probably only be considered for those at highest risk for developing severe pneumococcal disease.[15]

Legionnaires' Disease. Legionnaires' disease is a form of bronchopneumonia caused by the hard-to-isolate gram-negative bacillus *Legionella pneumophila*, a member of the *Legionella* species. The organism is almost ubiquitous in water, particularly warm standing water. The disease was first recognized and received its name after an epidemic of severe and, for some, fatal pneumonia that developed among delegates to the 1976 American Legion convention held in a Philadelphia hotel. The spread of infection was traced to a water-cooled air-conditioning system. Although healthy people can develop the infection, the risk is greatest among people with chronic diseases or impaired cell-mediated immunity.

Symptoms of the disease typically begin about 2 to 10 days after infection with malaise, weakness, lethargy, fever, and dry cough. Depending on the severity of the disease, the initial manifestations are followed by recurring chills, dyspnea, weakness, confusion, pleuritic pain, and blood-stained sputum. Other manifestations include disturbances of central nervous system (CNS) function, gastrointestinal tract involvement, arthralgias, and elevation in body temperature, sometimes to over 104°F. The disease causes consolidation of lung tissues and impairs gas exchange. The mortality rate can be as high as 20% to 30% in previously healthy people and 80% in immunocompromised people.[16]

PRIMARY ATYPICAL PNEUMONIA

The term *primary atypical pneumonia* is used to describe acute respiratory infections that produce patchy inflammatory changes that are confined to the alveolar septum and the interstitium of the lung. The term *atypical* implies the lack of an alveolar exudate. The most common cause of primary atypical pneumonia is *Mycoplasma pneumoniae*. The mycoplasmas are the smallest free-living agents of disease, having characteristics of both viruses and bacteria. Less common offenders are *parainfluenza and respiratory syncytial viruses*. The influenza virus is the most common cause of viral pneumonia. A number of other viruses are sometimes implicated including measles and chickenpox.

***Mycoplasma* and Viral Pneumonias.** The clinical course among people with *Mycoplasma* and viral pneumonias varies widely from a mild infection (influenza A and B, adenovirus) that masquerades as chest cold to a more serious and even fatal outcome (chickenpox pneumonia). Often the symptoms are confined to fever, headache, and muscle aches and pains. Cough, when present, is characteristically dry, hacking, and nonproductive. Viruses impair the respiratory tract defenses and predispose to secondary bacterial infections with development of lobar or bronchopneumonia. Some viruses such as herpes simplex, varicella, and adenovirus may be associated with necrosis of the alveolar epithelium and acute inflammation.

PNEUMOCYSTIS PNEUMONIA

Pneumocystis carinii pneumonia is an opportunistic, often fatal form of lung infection seen in debilitated people and those with impaired immune function, particularly those with impaired cell-mediated immunity. *P. carinii* is a parasite of uncertain classification. Although the terminology applied to protozoa is used to describe the various stages of its life cycle, recent analysis suggests that it is a fungus or related to a fungus.[17] The organism can be found in the lungs of a variety of domesticated and wild animals and is distributed worldwide in humans. Nearly all children have acquired antibodies to *P. carinii* by their second birthday.[1] Only premature, malnourished, or debilitated infants develop symptomatic infections. In older children and adults, infections are usually only seen in the presence of immunosuppression or

immunodeficiency. It is seen in people treated with immunosuppressive or cytotoxic drugs or irradiation for management of organ transplantation or cancer. In the United States, *Pneumocystis* pneumonia develops in 75% to 80% of people with AIDS.[18, 19] Because it occurs so regularly in people with AIDS, it is used as a diagnostic criterion for the disease.

Although the mode of transmission is unknown, it is thought to be airborne. The onset of the disease is abrupt with high fever, tachypnea, shortness of breath, and a mild nonproductive cough, intercostal retractions, and cyanosis. In vulnerable hosts, the disease spreads rapidly throughout the lungs, producing involvement similar to that of adult respiratory distress syndrome (see Chapter 28). The infection produces an initial random and patchy involvement of the lungs. The *P. carinii* trophozoites attach and feed on alveolar epithelial cells but do not invade them. As they divide, some form cup- or boat-shaped cysts that can be detected microscopically. Microscopically, the walls of the involved alveoli become thickened and edematous and alveoli become filled with a foamy, protein-rich fluid. As the disease progresses, the gas-exchange function of the lungs becomes severely impaired.

The diagnosis of the disease depends on microscopic methods that use specific stains to identify the organism. Usually induced sputum specimens obtained after inhalation of hypertonic saline produced by a ultrasonic nebulizer are required for this purpose. Other methods for obtaining specimens include bronchoalveolar lavage and transbronchial lung biopsy.

Treatment includes the use of trimethoprim-sulfamethoxazole (TMP-SMZ) and pentamidine isethionate. Because of the risk of recurrence, the Centers for Disease Control recommend that prophylaxis (aerosolized pentamidine or TMP-SMZ) be provided for all HIV-infected adults who have had an episode of *Pneumocystis* or have T-helper lymphocytes less than 200/µL or less than 20% of total lymphocytes.[20]

TUBERCULOSIS

After decades of decline, the incidence of tuberculosis is increasing, particularly among people in the 25- to 44-year age group and among non-Hispanic blacks and Hispanics in all age groups. There were 25,701 new cases reported for 1990 (10.3 per 100,000), representing an annual increase of 9.4%.[21] In all age groups, reported cases increased among non-Hispanic blacks and Hispanics but decreased among non-Hispanic whites. In the 25- to 44-year age group, cases among non-Hispanic blacks increased by 22.6%, Hispanics by 34.5%, and non-Hispanic whites by 2.3%.[22] Tuberculosis is more common among the homeless, refugees from Asia and Central America, the elderly (particularly those in long-term care facilities), and people infected with the HIV virus. The HIV virus has emerged as the most important risk factor for the development of tuberculosis. In one state showing the highest number of AIDS cases, the seropositive rate was 46% in people with active or suspected tuberculosis.[23] Outbreaks of drug-resistant disease have occurred, complicating the selection of drugs and affecting the duration of treatment.

Tuberculosis is an infectious disease caused by *Mycobacterium tuberculosis*. *M. tuberculosis* (tubercle bacillus) are slender, rod-shaped, acid-fast organisms. They are similar to other bacterial organisms except for an outer waxy capsule that makes them more resistant to destruction (*e.g.*, the organism can persist in old necrotic and calcified lesions, still capable of initiating growth). Although tuberculosis can infect practically any organ of the body, the lungs are the most frequently involved. The tubercle bacilli are strict aerobes that thrive in PO_2 of 140 mmHg.[1] This explains their tendency to cause disease in the upper lobe or upper parts of the lower lobe of the lung where ventilation is greatest.

There are two forms of tuberculosis that pose a particular threat in humans—*M. tuberculosis hominis* (human tuberculosis) and *M. tuberculosis bovis* (bovine tuberculosis). Human tuberculosis is an airborne infection spread by minute, invisible particles, called *droplet nuclei*, that are harbored in the respiratory secretions of people with active tuberculosis.[24, 25] These droplet nuclei remain suspended in air and are circulated by air currents. They are so small that when inhaled they travel directly to the alveoli. Bovine tuberculosis is acquired by drinking milk from infected cows and initially affects the gastrointestinal tract. This form of tuberculosis has been virtually eradicated in North America and other developed countries as a result of rigorous controls on dairy herds and the pasteurization of milk. There has been a recent increase in the United States of atypical mycobacterial infections, including those caused by *M. kansasii* and *M. avium-intracellulare*. These atypical mycobacteria are predominantly opportunistic, causing infection in people with reduced immunity or preexisting lung disease. There is an increasing incidence of progressive systemic infection due to *M. avium-intracellulare* in people with AIDS.

PATHOGENESIS

The tubercle bacillus incites a distinctive chronic inflammatory response referred to as *granulomatous inflammation*. The destructiveness of the disease is due to the hypersensitivity response that the bacillus evokes rather than its inherent destructive capabilities. Cell-mediated immunity and hypersensitivity reactions contribute to the evolution of the disease.

Tuberculosis can occur as primary or reactivated infection. *Primary tuberculosis* occurs in a person lacking previous contact with the tubercle bacillus. It is typically initiated as a result of inhaling droplet nuclei that contain the tubercle bacillus. After inhalation, the droplet nuclei pass down the bronchial tree without settling on the epithelium and implant in a respiratory bronchiole or alveolus beyond the mucociliary system. Soon after entering the lung, the bacilli are surrounded and engulfed by macrophages. This is followed by the development of single graywhite circumscribed granulomatous lesion, called *Ghon's focus*, that contains the tubercle bacilli, modified macrophages, and other immune cells. Within 2 to 3 weeks, the central portion of Ghon's focus undergoes soft caseous (cheeselike) necrosis. This occurs at about the time that the tuberculin test becomes positive, suggesting that the necrosis is caused by the cell-mediated hypersensitivity immune response (see Chapter 14). During this same time, tubercle bacilli, either free or within macrophages, drain along the lymph channels to the tracheobronchial lymph nodes of the affected lung and there evoke caseous granulomas. The combination of the primary lung lesion and lymph node granulomas is called *Ghon's complex*.

The emergence of the hypersensitivity response plays a dominant role in limiting further replication of the bacilli. The immune response also provides protection against additional tubercle bacilli that may be inhaled at a later time. It has become apparent that infection with the HIV, because of its suppression of the immune response, predisposes to a much more severe form of tuberculosis.

When the number of organisms inhaled are small and the body's resistance is adequate, scar tissue forms and encapsulates the primary lesion. In time, most of these lesions become calcified and are visible on a chest x-ray film.

Occasionally, primary tuberculosis may progress, causing more extensive destruction of lung tissue. Often the granulomatous tissue erodes into a bronchus and the necrotic inflammatory tissue is discharged into it. An air-filled cavity forms, permitting bronchogenic spread of the disease. Tubercle bacilli also enter the sputum, allowing the person to infect others. In rare instances, tuberculosis may erode into a blood vessel, giving rise to hematogenic dissemination. *Miliary tuberculosis* describes minute lesions resulting from this type of dissemination and may involve almost any organ, particularly the brain, meninges, liver, kidney, and bone marrow.

Reactivated tuberculosis usually results from activation of a previously healed primary lesion. Less commonly it develops because of reinfection. It often occurs in situations of impaired body defense mechanisms. The partial immunity that follows initial exposure affords protection against reinfection and, to some extent, aids in localizing the disease should reactivation occur. The hypersensitivity reaction, on the other hand, is an aggravating factor in reactivation tuberculosis, as evidenced by the frequency of cavitation and bronchial dissemination. The cavities may coalesce to a size of up to 10 to 15 cm in diameter. Pleural effusion and tuberculous empyema are common as the disease progresses.

MANIFESTATIONS

Primary tuberculosis is usually asymptomatic, the only evidence of the disease being a positive tuberculin skin test and the presence of calcified lesions on the chest x-ray film. Uncommonly, the immune response is inadequate and progressive primary tuberculosis develops. The person with progressive primary or reactivation tuberculosis presents with symptoms of low-grade fevers, night sweats, easy fatigability, anorexia, and weight loss. There is development of a cough that is initially dry but later becomes productive of purulent and sometimes blood-tinged sputum. Dyspnea and orthopnea develop as the disease advances.

DIAGNOSIS

The most frequently used screening methods for tuberculosis are the tuberculin skin tests and chest x-ray studies. Bacteriologic studies (stain and cultures) of early morning sputum specimens are used to determine the presence of the organism. Often multiple specimens are necessary. Fiberoptic bronchoscopy may be used to obtain bronchial washings for bacteriologic studies. Drug sensitivity studies are done when there is a suspicion of a drug-resistant form of the disease.

The tuberculin skin test was introduced by Robert Koch in the late 19th century. The test measures delayed hypersensitivity (cell-mediated, type IV) that follows exposure to the tubercle bacillus. People who become tuberculin positive usually remain so for the rest of their lives. It is important to recognize that a positive reaction to the skin test does not mean that a person has active tuberculosis, only that there has been exposure to the bacillus and that cell-mediated immunity to the organism has developed.

The intracutaneous or Mantoux test is the standard skin test for suspected tuberculosis. It involves the intradermal injection of tuberculin (purified protein derivative standard [PPDS]). A positive reaction is evidenced by a discrete area of skin elevation of 10 mm or more.[24] People with HIV infection often have a reduced reaction to the tuberculin test because of impaired cellular immunity. A 5-mm or greater reaction is considered a positive test in people with or at high risk for HIV infections, close contacts of people with tuberculosis, and people with x-rays consistent with old healed tuberculosis. In people with tuberculosis, the area of elevation is often between 15 and 20 mm or more.[25] Both false-positive and false-negative reactions can occur. False-positive reactions are often due to cross-reactions with nontuberculosis mycobacteria (*e.g., M. kansasii* and *M. avium-intercellulare*). False-negative tests can occur because of immunodeficiency states that result from HIV infection, old age, corticosteroid treatment, concurrent infections, virus vaccinations, or improper testing techniques.

Multiple-puncture tests are available for screening purposes. This technique introduces tuberculin into the skin either by puncturing with an applicator with points that have been coated with dried tuberculin or by puncturing through a film of liquid tuberculin. A positive response is manifested by vesicle formation at the test site. The quantity of tuberculin introduced under the skin using the multiple puncture technique cannot be precisely controlled. For this reason, the multiple puncture methods are not intended as diagnostic tests but only for initial screening procedures in asymptomatic people who have not been exposed to someone with tuberculosis. Verification of the reaction to a multiple puncture test is recommended by use of the standard Mantoux test unless vesicle formation is present.

TREATMENT

Two groups of people meet the criteria established for the use of antimycobacterial therapy for tuberculosis: (1) people with active tuberculosis and (2) those who have contact with cases of active tuberculosis and who are at risk for developing an active form of the disease.

The primary drugs used in the treatment of tuberculosis are isoniazid (INH), rifampin, pyrazinamide, ethambutol, and streptomycin. Isoniazid is remarkably potent against the tubercle bacillus and is probably the most widely used drug for tuberculosis. Although its exact mechanism of action is unknown, it apparently combines with an enzyme that is needed by the INH-susceptible strains of the tubercle bacillus. Resistance to the drug develops rapidly, and combination with other effective drugs delays the development of resistance. Rifampin inhibits RNA synthesis in the bacillus. Although both ethambutol and pyrazinamide are known to inhibit the growth of the tubercle bacillus, their mechanisms of action are largely unknown. Streptomycin, the first drug found to be effective against tuberculosis, must be given by injection, which limits its usefulness, particularly in long-term therapy. It remains an important drug in tuberculosis therapy and is used primarily in people with severe, possibly life-threatening forms of tuberculosis.

Treatment of *active tuberculosis* requires the use of multiple drugs. Tuberculosis is an unusual disease in that chemotherapy is required for a long time. The tubercle bacillus is an aerobic organism that multiplies slowly and remains relatively dormant in oxygen-poor caseous material. It undergoes a high rate of mutation and tends to develop a resistance to any one drug. For this reason, multiple drug regimens are used for treating people with active tuberculosis.

Based on several recent trials, a marked change in chemotherapy for uncomplicated tuberculosis has developed. Short-course programs of therapy (usually for 6 to 9 months) have replaced the earlier 18- to 24-month multidrug regimens. Treatment may need to be prolonged in HIV-infected people and in people with drug-resistant strains of *M. tuberculosis.*

Prophylactic treatment is used for people who are infected with *M. tuberculosis* but without active disease.[25] This group includes people with a positive skin test who (1) have had close contact with active cases of tuberculosis; (2) have converted from a negative to positive skin test within 2 years; (3) have a history of untreated or inadequately treated tuberculosis; (4) have chest x-rays consistent with tuberculosis but no bacteriologic evidence of the active disease; (5) have special risk factors such as silicosis, diabetes mellitus, prolonged corticosteroid therapy, immunosuppression therapy, end-stage renal disease, chronic malnutrition due to any cause, hematologic or reticuloendothelial cancers, and those with positive HIV test or AIDS; and (6) are 35 years of age or under with a positive reaction of unknown duration. These people harbor a small number of microorganisms and are usually treated with isoniazid.

Recent outbreaks of multidrug-resistant (MDR) tuberculosis have posed a problem to the prophylactic treatment of exposed people, including health care workers. To date, most of the exposed people who have developed active MDR-tuberculosis were infected with the HIV virus; furthermore, the fatality rate among these people is high (72% to 89%). The Centers for Disease Control recommend that newly infected contacts who are at high risk for being infected with MDR strains of tuberculosis, particularly people with HIV infection, be treated with at least two drugs. When the strain of *M. tuberculosis* is resistant to isoniazid and rifampin, alternative drugs should be used. The suggested duration for alternative multidrug prevention therapy ranges from 6 to 12 months. Twelve months of therapy is recommended for people who have HIV infection or other immunosuppressive conditions.[26]

Success of chemotherapy for both prophylaxis and treatment of tuberculosis depends on strict adherence to a lengthy drug regimen. This is often a problem, particularly in asymptomatic people with tuberculosis infections and in poorly motivated groups such as intravenous drug abusers.

FUNGAL INFECTIONS

Although the spores of fungi are constantly present in the air we breathe, only a few reach the lung and cause disease. The most common of these are histoplasmosis, coccidioidomycosis, and blastomycosis. These infections are usually mild and self-limiting and are seldom noticed unless they produce local complications or progressive dissemination occurs. The signs and symptoms of these infections commonly resemble those of tuberculosis.

HISTOPLASMOSIS

Histoplasmosis, caused by the dimorphic fungus (see Chapter 12) *Histoplasma capsulatum*, is the most common fungal infection in the United States. Skin testing surveys suggest that 18% to 20% of people in the United States have been infected with the disease.[27] Most cases occur along the major river valleys of the Midwest—the Ohio, the Mississippi, and the Missouri. The organism grows in soil and other areas that have been enriched with bird excreta: old chicken houses, pigeon lofts, barns, and trees where birds roost. The infection is acquired by inhaling the fungal spores that are released when the dirt or dust from the infected areas is disturbed. The spores convert to the parasitic yeast phase when exposed to body temperature in the alveoli. The organisms are then carried to the regional lymphatics and from there are disseminated throughout the body in the bloodstream. They are removed from the circulation by fixed macrophages of the reticuloendothelial system. When delayed hypersensitivity develops (see Chapter 14), the macrophages are usually able to destroy the fungi.

The manifestations of histoplasmosis are strikingly similar to those of tuberculosis. Depending on the host's resistance and immunocompetence, the disease usually takes one of four forms: (1) latent asymptomatic disease, (2) self-limiting primary disease, (3) chronic pulmonary disease, or (4) disseminated infection. The average incubation period for the infection is about 14 days. Only 40% of infected people have symptoms, and only about 10% of these are ill enough to see a physician.[28] *Latent asymptomatic histoplasmosis* is characterized by evidence of healed lesions in the lungs or hilar lymph nodes accompanied by a positive histoplasmin skin test (analogous to the tuberculin test). *Primary pulmonary histoplasmosis* occurs in otherwise healthy people as a mild, self-limiting, febrile, respiratory infection. Its symptoms include muscle and joint pains and a nonproductive cough. Erythema nodosum (subcutaneous nodules) or erythema multiforme (hivelike lesions) sometimes appears. During this stage of the disease, chest x-rays usually show single or multiple infiltrates.

Chronic histoplasmosis resembles reactivation tuberculosis. Infiltration of the upper lobes of one or both lungs with cavitation occurs. This form of the disease is more common in middle-aged men who smoke and in people with chronic lung disease. The most common manifestations are productive cough, fever, night sweats, and weight loss. In many people, the disease is self-limiting. In others, there is progressive destruction of lung tissue and dissemination of the disease.

Disseminated histoplasmosis can follow either primary or chronic histoplasmosis but most often develops as an acute and fulminating infection in the very old or the very young or in people with compromised immune function. Although the macrophages of the reticuloendothelial system can remove the fungi from the bloodstream, they are unable to destroy them.[31] Characteristically, this form of the disease produces a high fever, generalized lymph node enlargement, hepatosplenomegaly, muscle wasting, anemia, leukopenia, and thrombocytopenia. There may be hoarseness, ulcerations of the mouth and tongue, nausea, vomiting, diarrhea, and abdominal pain. Often, meningitis becomes a dominant feature of the disease.

Absolute diagnosis of histoplasmosis requires identification of the organism on culture. The infection incites a delayed hypersensitivity immune response and the histoplasmin skin test is used to test for exposure to the organism. This test remains positive after the initial infection has occurred and does not indicate whether the disease is of recent or past origin. In addition to the delayed response, the humoral immune system responds to the acute infection by producing antibodies. Although these antibodies are not protective, they serve as markers of infection. These antibodies can be measured by means of the complement fixation (CF) test. An immunodiffusion (ID) test can also be used as a test for the antibodies. Both the CF and ID tests become positive 2 weeks after the onset of symptoms. The antifungal drugs amphotericin B and ketoconazole are used for people with disease severe enough to require treatment or those with compromised immune function who are at risk for developing disseminated disease. Amphotericin B is given intravenously and is usually the drug of choice in severe disease. The drug can impair kidney and liver function and produce anemia. Ketoconazole is given orally and takes up to 3 weeks to produce its effect.

COCCIDIOIDOMYCOSIS

Coccidioidomycosis is a common fungal infection caused by inhaling the spores of *Coccidioides immitis*. An estimated 100,000 new cases occur annually. It is most prevalent in the southwestern United States. About 80% of people in the San Joaquin Valley are coccidioidin-positive.[29] Because of its prevalence in this area, the disease is sometimes referred to as "San Joaquin fever" or "valley fever." The disease resembles tuberculosis, and its mechanisms of infection are similar to those of histoplasmosis.

The disease most commonly occurs as an acute, primary self-limiting pulmonary infection with or without systemic involvement, but in some cases it progresses to a disseminated disease. About 60% of exposed people only manifest a positive skin test (either coccidioidin skin test or spherulin skin test) and are unaware of the infection.[29] In the other 40%, the illness usually resembles influenza. There may be fever, a cough, and pleuritic pain, accompanied by erythema multiforme or erythema nodosum. The skin lesions are usually accompanied by arthralgias or arthritis without effusion, particularly of the ankles and knees. The terms "desert bumps" and "desert arthritis" are used to describe these manifestations. The presence of skin and joint manifestations indicates strong host defenses, because people who have had such manifestations seldom develop disseminated disease. Disseminated disease occurs in 1 out of 6000 infected people and in fewer than 0.5% of people with symptomatic disease. The commonly affected structures in disseminated disease are the lymph nodes, meninges, spleen, liver, kidney, skin, and adrenals. Meningitis is the most common cause of death.

Positive diagnosis of coccidioidomycosis can be made by direct visualization of spherules (multinucleated parasitic *C. immitis* cells) in the expectorated sputum after application of 10% potassium hydroxide. Although cultures can be used to identify the fungus, the results are positive in only about half of the cases. Furthermore, extreme caution is needed when handling this fungus because laboratory personnel can be easily infected. Two serologic tests, the tube-precipitin (TP) test and the complement-fixation (CF) test, are considered to be extremely useful in establishing a diagnosis of coccidioidomycosis. The CF test may be used in following the progress of the disease; an elevated CF titer is considered to indicate risk of disease dissemination. The skin tests with coccidioidin and spherulin do not indicate whether the disease is recent or has occurred in the past. Their main value is in epidemiologic studies and in confirming the diagnosis in people who convert from a negative to a positive test during an illness. As with histoplasmosis, the antifungal drugs amphotericin B and ketoconazole are used in the treatment of progressive or disseminated diseases.

BLASTOMYCOSIS

Blastomycosis is caused by the organism *Blastomyces dermatitidis*. It is characterized by local suppurative and granulomatous lesions of the lungs and skin. The disease is most commonly found in North America and is particularly prevalent in the southeastern and south central states.

The symptoms of acute infection are similar to those of acute histoplasmosis, including fever, cough, aching of the joints and muscles, and, uncommonly, pleuritic pain. In contrast to histoplasmosis, the cough in blastomycosis is often productive and the sputum is purulent. Acute pulmonary infections are usually self-limiting or progressive. Extrapulmonary spread most commonly involves the skin, bones, or prostate gland. These lesions may provide the first evidence of the disease.

The diagnosis of blastomycosis is more difficult than that of histoplasmosis. Visualization of the yeast in the sputum after application of 10% potassium hydroxide provides a presumptive diagnosis. When this fails, cultural isolation of the fungus is often attempted. The blastomycin skin test lacks specificity and is no longer available. The treatment of the progressive or disseminated form of the disease includes the use of amphotericin B or ketoconazole.

In summary, respiratory infections are the most common cause of respiratory illness. They include the common cold, influenza, pneumonias, tuberculosis, and fungal infections. The common cold occurs more frequently than any other respiratory infection. The fingers are the most incriminated source of transmission, and the most common portals of entry are the nasal mucosa and the conjunctiva of the eye. The influenza virus causes three syndromes: an uncomplicated rhinotracheitis, a respiratory viral infection followed by a bacterial infection, and viral pneumonia. Pneumonia describes an infection of the parenchymal tissues of the lung. Acute bacterial pneumonias are associated with intraalveolar exudation; they produce either lobar or bronchiogenic involvement of the lung. Lobar pneumonia involves a large portion or lobe of the lung and is usually caused by the *Streptococcus pneumoniae*. Bronchopneumonia is caused by a number of agents. It is characterized by patchy consolidation of several lobes of the lung and often affects people with other debilitating diseases. Legionnaires' disease is a form of bronchopneumonia caused by the gram-negative bacillus *Legionella pneumophila*. Viral or atypical pneumonia can occur as a primary infection, such as that caused by influenza virus, or as a complication of other viral infections, such as measles or chickenpox. Viral and atypical pneumonias involve the interstitium of the lung and often masquerade as chest colds. *Pneumocystis carinii* pneumonia is an opportunistic infection that occurs in debilitated people with impaired immune function, including people with AIDS.

Tuberculosis is a chronic respiratory infection caused by *Mycobacterium tuberculosis*. After decades of decline, the incidence of tuberculosis is increasing, particularly among people in the 25 to 44 year age group and among non-Hispanic blacks and Hispanics in all age groups. Tuberculosis is more common among the homeless, refugees from Asia and Central America, the elderly (particularly those in long-term care facilities), and people infected with the HIV virus. The HIV virus has emerged as the most important risk factor for the development of tuberculosis. In addition, the treatment of tuberculosis has been complicated by recent outbreaks of drug-resistant forms of the disease.

Infections caused by the fungi *Histoplasma capsulatum* (histoplasmosis), *Coccidioides immitis* (coccidioidomycosis), and *Blastomyces dermatitidis* (blastomycosis) resemble tuberculosis. These infections are common but seldom serious unless they produce progressive destruction of lung tissue or the infection disseminates outside the lungs.

■ DISORDERS OF LUNG INFLATION

Disorders of lung inflation are caused by conditions that produce lung compression or lung collapse. Air entering through the airways inflates the lung and the negative pressure in the pleural cavity keeps the lung from collapsing. There can be complete collapse of a entire lung as in pneumothorax or collapse of a segment of the lung as in atelectasis. Lung compression can result from fluid, blood, lymph, or air that has accumulated in the thoracic cavity.

DISORDERS OF THE PLEURA

The pleura is a thin double-layered membrane that encases the lungs. The inner visceral layer lies adjacent to the lung; the outer parietal layer lines the inner aspect of the chest wall, the superior aspect of the diaphragm, and the mediastinum. The visceral and parietal pleurae are separated by a thin layer of serous fluid, and the potential space between these two layers is called the *pleural cavity*. The right and left pleural cavities are separated by the mediastinum, which contains the heart and other thoracic structures. Both the chest wall and the lungs have elastic properties. Because of these elastic properties, there is a tendency for the chest wall to become larger and move outward and for the lungs to recoil or move inward and collapse (see Chapter 26). As a result of these two opposing forces, the pressure in the pleural cavity becomes negative in relation to alveolar pressure. It is the negative pressure within the pleural cavity that holds the lungs against the chest wall and keeps them from collapsing. Disorders of the pleura include pain, pneumothorax, and pleural effusion.

PLEURAL PAIN

Pain is one of the most frequent symptoms of conditions that cause inflammation of the pleura. Most commonly the pain is abrupt in onset: the person experiencing it can cite almost to the minute when the pain started. It is usually unilateral and tends to be localized to the lower and lateral part of the chest. Although the pain may radiate to the shoulder or abdomen, it seldom originates from the substernal, paravertebral, or any other central part of the chest. The pain is usually made worse by chest movements, such as deep breathing and coughing, that exaggerate pressure changes within the pleural cavity and increase movement of the inflamed or injured pleural surfaces. Because deep breathing is painful, tidal volumes are usually kept small and breathing becomes more rapid. Reflex splinting of the chest muscles may occur, causing a lesser respiratory excursion on the affected side.

It is important to differentiate pleural pain from pain produced by other conditions, such as musculoskeletal strain of chest muscles, bronchial irritation, and myocardial disease. Musculoskeletal pain may occur as the result of frequent forceful coughing. This type of pain is usually bilateral and located in the inferior portions of the rib cage where the abdominal muscles insert into the anterior rib cage. It is made worse by movements associated with contraction of the abdominal muscles. The pain associated with irritation of the bronchi is generally substernal and dull in character, rather than sharp. It is made worse with coughing but is not affected by deep breathing. Myocardial pain, which is discussed in Chapter 23, is usually located in the substernal area and is not affected by respiratory movements.

Although analgesic and narcotic drugs reduce awareness of pleural pain, these agents do not entirely relieve the discomfort associated with deep breathing and coughing. The nonsteroidal anti-inflammatory drug (NSAID) indomethacin has been used successfully to relieve pain and facilitate effective coughing.[30]

PNEUMOTHORAX

Normally the pleural cavity is free of air and contains only a thin layer of fluid. When air enters the pleural cavity, it is called *pneumothorax*. Pneumothorax causes partial or complete collapse of the affected lung. Pneumothorax can occur without obvious cause or injury (spontaneous pneumothorax) or as a result of direct injury to the chest or major airways (traumatic pneumothorax). Tension pneumothorax describes a life-threatening condition of excessive pressure within the pleural cavity.

Spontaneous Pneumothorax. Spontaneous pneumothorax occurs when an air-filled bleb, or blister, on the lung surface ruptures. Rupture of these blebs allows atmospheric air from the airways to enter the pleural cavity. Alveolar pressure is normally greater than pleural pressure; if communication develops between alveoli on the lung surface and the pleural space, air flows from the alveoli into the pleural space and the involved portion of the lung collapses as a result of its own recoil. Air continues to flow into the pleural space until a pressure gradient no longer exists or until the decline in lung size causes the leak to seal. Spontaneous pneumothoraces can be divided into primary and secondary pneumothoraces. *Primary spontaneous pneumothorax* occurs in otherwise healthy people. *Secondary spontaneous pneumothorax* occurs in people with underlying lung disease.

What causes the air-filled blebs responsible for spontaneous pneumothorax and the reasons why they rupture are largely unknown. In primary spontaneous pneumothorax, these blebs are usually located at the top of the lungs. The condition is seen most often in tall young men. It has been suggested that the difference in pleural pressure from the top to the bottom of the lung is greater in tall people and that this difference in pressure may contribute to the development of the blebs. Another factor that has been associated with primary spontaneous pneumothorax is smoking. Disease of the small airways related to smoking probably contributes to the condition.

Catamenial pneumothorax occurs in relation to the menstrual cycle and is usually recurrent.[30] Women with the condition usually develop symptoms within 24 to 48 hours of onset of menstrual flow. Although the cause of catamenial pneumothorax is unknown, it has been suggested that air may gain access to the peritoneal cavity during menstruation and then enter the pleural cavity through a diaphragmatic defect. Pleural and diaphragmatic endometriosis have also been implicated as causes of the condition.

Secondary spontaneous pneumothoraces are

usually more serious because they occur in people with lung disease. They are associated with many different types of lung conditions that cause trapping of gases and destruction of lung tissue, including asthma, tuberculosis, cystic fibrosis, sarcoidosis, bronchogenic carcinoma, and metastatic pleural diseases. The most common cause of secondary spontaneous pneumothorax is chronic obstructive pulmonary disease.

Traumatic Pneumothorax. Traumatic pneumothorax may be caused by penetrating or nonpenetrating injuries. Fractured or dislocated ribs that penetrate the pleura are the most common cause of pneumothorax due to nonpenetrating chest injuries. Hemothorax often accompanies these injuries. Pneumothorax may also accompany fracture of the trachea or major bronchus or rupture of the esophagus. People with pneumothorax due to chest trauma frequently have other complications and may require chest surgery. Medical procedures such as transthoracic needle aspirations, intubation, and positive pressure ventilation may occasionally cause pneumothorax. Pneumothorax may also occur as a complication of cardiopulmonary resuscitation.

Tension Pneumothorax. Tension pneumothorax is a life-threatening condition and occurs when injury to the chest or respiratory structures permits air to enter but not leave the pleural space (Fig. 27-2). This results in a rapid increase in pressure within the chest with compression atelectasis of the unaffected lung, a shift in the mediastinum to the opposite side of the chest, and compression of the vena cava with impairment of venous return to the heart.[30] Although tension pneumothorax can develop in people with spontaneous pneumothoraces, it is seen most often in people with traumatic pneumothoraces.

Manifestations. The manifestations of pneumothorax depend on its size and the integrity of the underlying lung. In spontaneous pneumothorax, manifestations of the disorder include development of pleuritic pain in an otherwise healthy person. There is an almost immediate increase in respiratory rate as a result of the activation of receptors that monitor lung volume; this may be accompanied by dyspnea. Heart rate is increased. An asymmetry of the chest may be present because of the air trapped in the pleural cavity on the affected side. This asymmetry may be evidenced during inspiration as a lag in the movement of the affected side (the affected side of the chest does not begin to move until the unaffected lung reaches the same degree of inspiration as the lung with the air trapped in the pleural space).

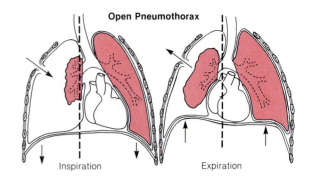

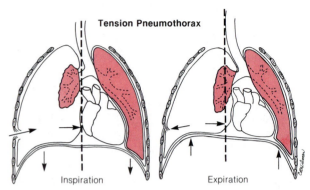

FIG. 27-2. Open or communicating pneumothorax (**top**) and tension pneumothorax (**bottom**). In an open pneumothorax, air enters the chest during inspiration and exits during expiration. There may be slight inflation of the affected lung due to a decrease in pressure as air moves out of the chest. In tension pneumothorax, air can enter but not leave the chest. As the pressure in the chest increases, the heart and great vessels are compressed and the mediastinal structures are shifted toward the opposite side of the chest. The trachea is pushed from its normal midline position toward the opposite side of the chest, and the unaffected lung is compressed.

Percussion of the chest produces a more hyperresonant sound, and breath sounds are decreased or absent over the area of the pneumothorax. With tension pneumothorax, the structures in the mediastinal space shift toward the opposite side of the chest (see Fig. 27-2). When this occurs, the position of the trachea, normally located in the midline of the neck, deviates with the mediastinum. The position of the trachea can be used as a means of assessing for a mediastinal shift. There may be distention of the neck veins and subcutaneous emphysema (movement of air into the subcutaneous tissues of the chest and neck) and clinical signs of shock.

Hypoxemia usually develops immediately after a large pneumothorax, followed by vasoconstriction of the blood vessels in the affected lung, causing the blood flow to shift to the unaffected lung. In people with spontaneous pneumothorax, this mechanism usually returns oxygen saturation to normal within about 24 hours. Hypoxemia is usually more serious in people with underlying lung disease who develop secondary spontaneous pneumothorax. In these people, the hypoxemia caused by the partial or total loss of the function of a lung can be life-threatening.

Diagnosis and Treatment. Diagnosis of pneumothorax can be confirmed by chest x-ray. Computed tomography (CT) scans may be used. Blood gas analysis may be done to determine the effect of the condition on blood oxygen levels.

The treatment varies with the cause and extent of the disorder. Even without treatment, air within the pleural space usually reabsorbs once the pleural leak seals. In small spontaneous pneumothoraces, the air usually reabsorbs spontaneously and only observation and follow-up chest x-rays are required. In larger pneumothoraces, the air is removed by needle aspiration or closed drainage system used with or without an aspiration pump. This type of drainage system allows the air to exit the pleural space through a one-way valve system to prevent the air from reentering the chest. This can be effected through a tube submerged in water or a drainage system with a one-way valve and no water. In secondary pneumothorax, surgical closure of the chest wall defect, ruptured airway, or perforated esophagus may be required.

Emergency treatment of tension pneumothorax involves the prompt insertion of a large-bore needle or chest tube into the affected side of the chest along with one-way valve drainage or continuous chest suction to aid in lung reexpansion. Sucking chest wounds, which allow air to pass in and out of the chest cavity, should be treated by promptly covering the area with an airtight covering (*e.g.*, Vaseline gauze or a firm piece of plastic). Chest tubes are inserted as soon as possible.

Because of the risk of recurrence, people with primary spontaneous pneumothorax should be advised against cigarette smoking, exposure to high altitudes, flying in nonpressurized aircraft, and scuba diving. Injection of a sclerosing agent (tetracycline) into the pleural space is sometimes used to prevent recurrence in these people.

PLEURAL EFFUSION

Normally only a thin layer (usually less than 10 to 20 mL) of serous fluid separates the visceral and parietal layers of the pleural cavity. *Pleural effusion* refers to a collection of fluid in the pleural cavity. The fluid may be a transudate, exudate, chyle, or blood.

Like edema developing elsewhere in the body, pleural effusion occurs when the rate of fluid formation exceeds the rate of its removal (see Chapter 29). Five mechanisms have been linked to the abnormal collection of fluid in the pleural cavity: (1) increased capillary pressure, as in congestive heart failure; (2) increased capillary permeability, which occurs with inflammatory conditions; (3) decreased colloidal osmotic pressure, such as the hypoalbuminemia occurring with liver disease and nephrosis; (4) increased negative intrapleural pressure, which develops with atelectasis; and (5) impaired lymphatic drainage of the pleural space, which is usually due to obstructive processes such as mediastinal carcinoma.[31]

Pleural effusion may involve the presence of a transudate or exudate, depending on the protein content of the fluid. A transudate has a protein content of less than 3.0 g/mL, and an exudate has a protein content greater than 3.0 g/mL. Additional characteristics that may be used to define a pleural exudate are (1) a pleural fluid-to-serum-protein ratio greater than 0.5, (2) a pleural fluid lactic acid dehydrogenase (LDH) level greater than two thirds the upper limit of normal, or (3) a pleural fluid-to-serum-LDH ratio exceeding 0.6.[32] LDH is an enzyme that is released from inflamed and injured pleural tissue; it is easily measured and is a useful marker for diagnosing exudative pleural disorders. Conditions that produce exudative pleural effusions are infections, pulmonary infarction, malignancies, rheumatoid arthritis, and lupus erythematosus.

Empyema refers to pus in the pleural cavity; it can be caused by direct spread from adjacent bacterial pneumonia, rupture of a lung abscess into the pleural space, invasion from a subdiaphragmatic infection, or infection associated with trauma.

Noninflammatory collections of serous fluid are called *hydrothorax*. The condition may be either unilateral or bilateral. The most common cause of hydrothorax is congestive heart failure. Other causes are renal failure, nephrosis, liver failure, malignancy, and myxedema.

Chylothorax refers to the presence of chyle in the thoracic cavity. Chyle, a milky fluid containing chylomicrons, is found in the lymph fluid originating in the gastrointestinal tract. The thoracic duct transports chyle to the central circulation. Chylothorax results from trauma, inflammation, or malignant infiltration obstructing chyle transport from the thoracic duct into the central circulation.

Hemothorax is the presence of blood in the thoracic cavity. Bleeding may arise from chest injury, a complication of chest surgery, malignancies, or rupture of a great vessel such as an aortic aneurysm. Hemothorax may be classified as minimal, moderate, or large.[33] A minimal hemothorax involves the presence of 300 to 500 mL of blood in the pleural space. Small amounts of blood are generally absorbed from the pleural space, and a minimal hemothorax generally clears in 10 to 14 days without complication. A moderate hemothorax (500 to 1000 mL blood) fills about one third of the pleural space and may produce signs of lung compression and loss of intravascular volume. It requires immediate drainage and replacement of intravascular fluids. A large hemothorax fills half or more of one side of the chest; it indicates the presence of 1000 mL or more of blood in the thorax and is usually caused by bleeding from a high-pressure vessel such as an intercostal or mammary artery. It requires immediate drainage and, if the bleeding continues, surgery to control the bleeding. One of the complications of untreated moderate or large hemothorax is fibrothorax—or the fusion of the pleural surfaces by fibrin, hyalin, and connective tissue—and in some cases calcification of the fibrous tissue, which causes restriction in lung expansion.

Manifestations. The manifestations of pleural effusion vary with the cause. Hemothorax may be accompanied by signs of blood loss, and empyema by fever and other signs of inflammation. Fluid in the pleural cavity acts as a space-occupying mass; it causes a decrease in lung volume on the affected side that is proportional to the amount of fluid collected. The effusion causes a mediastinal shift toward the contralateral side with a decrease in lung volume on that side as well. Characteristic signs of pleural effusion are dullness or flatness to percussion and diminished breath sounds. Pleuritic pain usually occurs only when inflammation is present, although a constant type of discomfort may be felt with large effusions. Usually 2000 mL or more of fluid must be present before dyspnea occurs. A minimum of 250 mL of unilateral fluid accumulation must be present before the condition can be detected on chest x-ray.

Diagnosis and Treatment. Thoracentesis is the aspiration of fluid from the pleural space. It is used to obtain a sample for both diagnostic and therapeutic purposes. The treatment of pleural effusion is directed at the cause of the disorder. With large effusions, thoracentesis may be used to allow reexpansion of the lung. A palliative method of treatment used when pleural effusion is due to a malignancy is the injection of a sclerosing agent into the pleural cavity; this causes obliteration of the pleural space and prevents the reaccumulation of fluid.

ATELECTASIS

Atelectasis means imperfect expansion; it refers to the incomplete expansion of a lung or portion of a lung. It can be caused by airway obstruction, lung compression such as occurs in pneumothorax or pleural effusion, or the increased recoil of the lung due to loss of pulmonary surfactant (discussed in Chapter 26). The disorder may be present at birth (primary atelectasis), or it may develop in the neonatal period or in later life (acquired or secondary atelectasis).

Primary atelectasis of the newborn implies that the lung has never been inflated. It is seen most frequently in premature and high-risk infants. A secondary form of atelectasis can occur in infants who established respiration and subsequently developed impairment of lung expansion. Among the causes of secondary atelectasis in the newborn are the respiratory distress syndrome associated with lack of surfactant and airway obstruction due to aspiration of amniotic fluid or blood. It results in a patchy form of atelectasis.

Acquired atelectasis occurs mainly in adults. It is most commonly caused by airway obstruction and lung compression (Fig. 27-3). Obstruction can be caused by a mucous plug within the airway or by external compression due to fluid, tumor mass, exudate, or other matter in the area surrounding the airway. A small segment of lung or an entire lung lobe may be involved in obstructive atelectasis. Complete obstruction of an airway is followed by the absorption of air from the dependent alveoli and collapse of that portion of the lung. Breathing high concentrations of oxygen, such as while on a ventilator, increases the rate at which gases are absorbed from the alveoli and predisposes to atelectasis.

Both chest expansion and breath sounds are decreased on the affected side. There may be intercostal retraction (pulling in of the intercostal spaces) over the involved area during inspiration. If the collapsed area is large, the mediastinum and trachea shift to the affected side. Signs of respiratory distress are proportional to the extent of lung collapse.

The danger of obstructive atelectasis increases after surgery. Anesthesia, pain, administration of

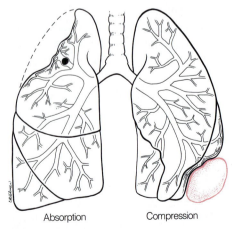

Absorption   Compression

FIG. 27-3. Atelectasis caused by airway obstruction and absorption of air from the involved lung area on the *left* and by compression of lung tissue on the *right*.

narcotics, and immobility tend to promote retention of viscid bronchial secretions and hence airway obstruction. Encouraging a patient to take deep breaths and cough, frequent changes of position, adequate hydration, and early ambulation decrease the likelihood of atelectasis developing.

Another cause of atelectasis is compression of lung tissue. It occurs when the pleural cavity is partially or completely filled with fluid, exudate, blood, a tumor mass, or air. It is most commonly observed in people with pleural effusion due to congestive heart failure or cancer. In compression atelectasis, the mediastinum shifts away from the affected lung.

Manifestations. The clinical manifestations of atelectasis include tachypnea, tachycardia, dyspnea, cyanosis, signs of hypoxemia, diminished chest expansion, absence of breath sounds, and intercostal retractions. Fever and other signs of infection may develop.

Diagnosis and Treatment. The diagnosis of atelectasis is based on signs and symptoms. Chest x-rays are used to confirm the diagnosis. CT scans may be used to designate the exact location of the obstruction.

Treatment depends on the cause and extent of lung involvement. It is directed at reducing the airway obstruction or lung compression and at reinflating the collapsed area of the lung. Ambulation and body positions that favor increased lung expansion are used when appropriate. Administration of oxygen may be needed to treat the hypoxemia. Bronchoscopy may be used as both a diagnostic and treatment method.

In summary, disorders of the pleura include pain, pneumothorax, and pleural effusion. Pain is commonly associated with conditions that produce inflammation of the pleura. Characteristically, it is unilateral, abrupt in onset, and exaggerated by respiratory movements. *Pneumothorax* refers to an accumulation of air in the pleural cavity with the partial or complete collapse of the lung. It can result from rupture of an air-filled bleb on the lung surface or from penetrating or nonpenetrating injuries. A tension pneumothorax is a life-threatening event in which air progressively accumulates within the thorax, causing not only the collapse of the lung on the injured side but also a progressive shift of the mediastinum to the opposite side of the thorax, producing severe cardiorespiratory impairment. *Pleural effusion* refers to the collection of fluid in the pleural cavity. The fluid may be a transudate (hydrothorax), exudate (empyema), blood (hemothorax), or chyle (chylothorax).

Atelectasis refers to an incomplete expansion of the lung. The disorder may be present at birth (primary atelectasis), or it may develop in the neonatal period or in later life (acquired or secondary atelectasis). Primary atelectasis occurs most often in premature and high-risk infants. Acquired atelectasis occurs mainly in adults and is most commonly caused by a mucous plug within the airway or by external compression due to fluid, tumor mass, exudate, or other matter in the area surrounding the airway.

■ OBSTRUCTIVE AIRWAY DISEASE

The term *obstructive airway disease* refers to a group of lung diseases that cause obstruction of the pulmonary airways. The airflow obstruction can be reversible as in bronchial asthma or irreversible as in chronic bronchitis and emphysema. The cardinal symptoms in both acute and chronic airflow obstruction are cough, wheeze, and dyspnea. The discussion in this section focuses on bronchial asthma, chronic bronchitis and emphysema, bronchiectasis, and cystic fibrosis.

Air moves through the upper airways (trachea and major bronchi) into the lower or pulmonary airways (bronchi and alveoli) that are located within the lung. It is in the pulmonary airways where the cartilaginous layer that provides support for the trachea and major bronchi gradually disappears and is replaced with crisscrossing strips of smooth muscle.

The contraction and relaxation of the smooth muscle layer, which is innervated by the autonomic nervous system, controls the resistance to airflow. Parasympathetic stimulation, via the vagus nerve, increases bronchial constriction and sympathetic stimulation, via beta$_2$-adrenergic receptors, bronchodilation. Normally, a slight vagal-mediated bronchoconstrictor tone predominates. When there is need for increased airflow, as during exercise, the bronchoconstrictor tone is inhibited and the bronchodilator effects of the sympathetic nervous system stimulated.

Bronchial smooth muscle also responds to inflammatory mediators, such as histamine, that act directly on smooth muscle to produce bronchial constriction and inflammation. Many of these inflammatory mediators are released from a special type of cell, called a *mast cell*, that is present in the airways. The binding of the IgE antibodies to specific receptors on mast cells prepares them for an allergic reaction when antigen appears.

BRONCHIAL ASTHMA

An estimated 10 million Americans suffer from bronchial asthma. In the general population, asthma prevalence rates have increased 29% between 1980 and 1987.[34] The disease affects people of all ages and is the most common cause of chronic illness in children under age 17. There has been a reported increase in deaths due to asthma.[35, 36, 37]

The Expert Panel of the National Heart, Lung, and Blood Institute's National Asthma Education Program has defined bronchial asthma as: "(1) airway obstruction that is reversible (but not completely so in some patients) either spontaneously or with treatment; (2) airway inflammation; and (3) increased airway responsiveness to a variety of stimuli."[34]

People with asthma typically react to low concentrations of agents that do not normally cause symptoms. An asthmatic attack can be triggered by a variety of stimuli. Based on their mechanism of response, these triggers can be divided into two types—bronchospastic or inflammatory.[38] *Bronchospastic triggers* depend on the existing level of airway responsiveness. They do not increase airway responsiveness, but produce symptoms in people who are already predisposed to bronchospasm. Bronchospastic triggers include cold air, exercise, emotional upset, and exposure to bronchial irritants such as cigarette smoke. This type of asthma has been referred as *intrinsic asthma*. *Inflammatory triggers* exert their effects through the inflammatory response. They not only cause inflammation, but they prime the sensitive airways so they are hyperresponsive to nonallergic stimuli. Asthma due to inflammatory triggers such as allergens has been referred to as *extrinsic asthma*. Many people with asthma respond to both types of triggers. The mechanisms whereby these two types of triggers produce an asthmatic attack can be further described as the early versus the late response.

The *early response* results in immediate bronchoconstriction on exposure to an inhaled antigen. Symptoms usually develop within 10 to 20 minutes, and spontaneous recovery occurs within 60 to 90 minutes.[38] The acute response is probably caused by the release of chemical mediators from IgE-coated mast cells. In the case of airborne antigens, the reaction occurs when antigen binds to sensitized mast cells on the mucosal surface of the airways. Although this type of response is caused by inflammatory mediators, it tends to cause bronchospasm but not inflammation of the airways. It can be completely inhibited or reversed by bronchodilators, such as β_2-adrenergic agonists, but not by the antiinflammatory actions of the corticosteroids. The early response is fairly uncommon in people with severe asthma, probably because it is blocked by the regular use of bronchodilator drugs.

In contrast to the early response, the *late response* usually develops 3 to 5 hours after exposure to an asthmatic trigger.[34] The late response involves inflammation as well as increased airway responsiveness that serves to prolong the attack and cause a vicious cycle of exacerbations. It often, but not always, follows an early response. Typically, the response reaches a maximum within a few hours and may last for days or even weeks. An initial trigger in the late response causes the release of inflammatory mediators from mast cells, macrophages, and epithelial cells. These substances induce the migration and activation of other inflammatory cells (basophils, eosinophils, and neutrophils), which then produce epithelial injury and edema, changes in mucociliary function and reduced clearance of respiratory tract secretions, and increased airway responsiveness. In addition, there is often a heightened responsiveness to cholinergic mediators suggesting changes in parasympathetic control of airway function.[34]

CAUSES OF ASTHMA

A number of factors contribute to an asthmatic attack including allergens, respiratory tract infections, hyperventilation, cold air, exercise, drugs and chemicals, emotional upsets, and airborne pollutants.

Inhalation of allergens is a common cause of asthma. Generally, this form of asthma has its onset in childhood or adolescence and is seen in people with a family history of atopic allergy (see Chapter 14). People with allergic asthma often have other allergies, such as hay fever, hives, and eczema. Attacks are related to exposure to specific allergens. Skin tests for the offending allergens are usually positive.

Respiratory tract infections, especially those caused by viruses, may produce their effects by causing epithelial damage and stimulating the production of IgE antibodies directed toward the viral antigens. In addition to precipitating an asthmatic attack, viral respiratory infections increase airway responsiveness to other asthma triggers that may persist for weeks beyond the original infection.

Exercise-induced asthma occurs in 70% to 80% of people with bronchial asthma.[39] The cause of exercise-induced asthma is unclear. It has been suggested that during exercise, bronchospasm is due to increased airway cooling caused by an increased minute ventilation or, alternatively, by water loss from the airway mucosa.[39, 40] The response is commonly exaggerated when the person exercises in a cold environment; wearing a mask over the nose and mouth often minimizes the attack or prevents it. It appears that the proper selection of a mask could be important for people subject to exercise-induced asthma, because it has been shown that increasing the humidity of the inhaled air is more important than simply heating the air.[41] A proper warm-up period is also important.

Inhaled irritants include tobacco smoke and strong odors. These irritants are thought to induce bronchospasm by way of irritant receptors and a vagal reflex. Passive parenteral smoking has been reported to increase asthma severity in children.[42] High doses of irritant gases such as sulfur dioxide, nitrogen dioxide, and ozone may induce inflammatory exacerbations of airway responsiveness (*e.g.*, smog-related asthma). Occupational asthma is stimulated by fumes and gases (*e.g.*, epoxy resins, plastics, toluene), organic and chemical dusts (wood, cotton, platinum), and other chemicals (formaldehyde) that are present in the workplace.

Emotional factors exert bronchospasm by way of vagal pathways. They can act as a bronchospastic trigger, or they can serve to increase airway responsiveness to other triggers by way of noninflammatory mechanisms.

Several types of drugs and chemicals stimulate asthma. There is a small group of asthmatics in whom aspirin sensitivity is associated with severe asthmatic attacks, presence of nasal polyps, and recurrent episodes of rhinitis. In addition, the yellow food dye tartrazine, aspirin, and other NSAIDs, such as aminopyrine, phenylbutazone, ibuprofen, and indomethacin, may provoke attacks. A recent addition to the list of chemicals that can provoke an asthmatic attack are the sulfites used in food processing and as an additive to beer, wine, and fresh vegetables.

MANIFESTATIONS

People with asthma exhibit a wide range of signs and symptoms, from episodic wheezing and feelings of chest tightness to an acute immobilizing attack. The attacks differ from person to person, and between attacks many people are symptom-free. Attacks may occur spontaneously or in response to various triggers, respiratory infections, emotional stress, or weather changes. Asthma is often worse at night. Nocturnal asthma attacks usually occur at about 4 AM, due to the occurrence of late responses to allergens inhaled during the evening and because of circadian variations in bronchial reactivity.[32]

During an asthmatic attack, the airways narrow because of bronchospasm, edema of the bronchial mucosa, and mucus plugging. Expiration becomes prolonged due to progressive airway obstruction. The amount of air that can be forcibly expired in 1 second ($FEV_{1.0}$) and the peak expiratory flow rate (PEFR) are decreased. A fall in the $FEV_{1.0}$ or PEFR to levels below 25% of the predicted value during an acute asthmatic attack is suggestive of respiratory failure. Air also becomes trapped behind the occluded and narrowed airways, causing hyperinflation of the lungs. The functional residual capacity increases and both inspiratory reserve capacity and forced vital capacity (FVC) diminish so that the person breathes close to his or her total lung capacity (see Chapter 26). As a result, more energy is needed

to overcome the tension already present in the lungs and the accessory muscles (the sternocleidomastoid muscles) are used to maintain gas exchange. This causes dyspnea and fatigue. Because air is trapped in the alveoli and inspiration is occurring at higher residual lung volumes, the cough becomes less effective. As the condition progresses, the effectiveness of alveolar ventilation declines and mismatching of ventilation and perfusion causes hypoxemia and hypercapnia. Pulmonary vascular resistance may increase as a result of the hypoxemia and hyperinflation, causing pulmonary hypertension and increasing the work demands of the right heart.

The physical signs vary with the severity of the attack. A mild attack may produce a slight increase in respiratory rate, with prolonged expiration and mild wheezing. A cough may accompany the wheezing. More severe attacks are associated with use of the accessory muscles, distant breath sounds, and loud wheezing. As the condition progresses, fatigue develops, the skin becomes moist, and anxiety and apprehension are obvious. Dyspnea may be severe, and often the person is able to speak only one or two words before taking a breath. At the point where airflow is markedly decreased, breath sounds become inaudible with diminished wheezing and the cough becomes ineffective despite being repetitive and hacking. This point often marks the onset of respiratory failure.

Also, with increased air-trapping, a greater negative intrapleural pressure is needed to inflate the lungs. This negative pressure, which is transmitted to the heart and blood vessels, causes the systolic blood pressure to fall during inspiration, a condition called *pulsus paradoxus*. It can be detected using a blood pressure cuff (see Chapter 21). When pulsus paradoxus is present, it suggests that the $FEV_{1.0}$ is reduced to less than 50% of the predicated value.[34]

DIAGNOSIS

Diagnosis of asthma is based on a careful history, physical examination, and laboratory methods. Spirometry provides a means for measuring forced vital capacity (FVC), $FEV_{1.0}$, PEFR, tidal volume, expiratory reserve, and inspiratory capacity (see Chapter 26). The PEFR is the peak expiratory flow rate that can be generated during a forced expiratory maneuver. It is measured in liters per second. Small inexpensive portable meters that measure PEFR are available. These can be used in physicians' offices and in the home to provide frequent measures of flow rates. They provide objective measures that can be used as a guide for treatment. Day–night (circadian) variations in asthma and PEFR variability can be used to indicate the severity of bronchial hyperresponsiveness.

The level of airway responsiveness can be measured in the laboratory by inhalation challenge tests using metacholine (a cholingeric agonist) or histamine, or exposure to a nonpharmacologic agent such as cold air.

TREATMENT

The Expert Panel of the National Heart, Lung, and Blood Institute's National Asthma Education Program recommends two categories for treatment of asthma: nonpharmacologic and pharmacologic.[34]

The *nonpharmacologic methods* of treatment are aimed at prevention and appropriate early treatment of an asthmatic attack. They include education of the patient and family to avoid bronchial irritants and agents that are known to induce or trigger an attack. A careful history is often needed to identify all the contributory factors.

Relaxation techniques and controlled breathing help to allay the panic and anxiety that aggravate breathing difficulties. The hyperventilation that often accompanies anxiety and panic is known to act as an asthmatic trigger. In a child, measures to encourage independence as it relates to symptom control, along with those directed at helping to develop a positive self-concept, are essential.

When the offending agent cannot be avoided (*e.g.,* house dust), a program of desensitization may be undertaken. It involves the injection of selected antigens to stimulate the production of IgG antibodies that block the IgE response (see Chapter 14).

Pharmacologic treatment is used to prevent or treat reversible airway obstruction and airway hyperresponsiveness due to the inflammatory process. Medications include bronchodilators and antiinflammatory drugs. Some drugs have both bronchodilator and antiinflammatory actions.

Bronchodilators. Bronchodilators include β_2-adrenergic agonists, ipratropium, and theophylline. These drugs are most effective for treating asthmatic attacks that are caused by bronchiogenic triggers.

The *β-adrenergic agents* relax bronchial smooth muscle and relieve congestion of the bronchial mucosa. The selective β_2-adrenergic agonists (*e.g.,* albuterol, bitolterol, metaproterenol, terbutaline) are preferred over nonselective β-adrenergic agonists (*e.g.,* epinephrine and isoproterenol) that stimulate β_1 receptors in the heart as well as β_2 receptors in the lung. The β_2-agonists are usually administered by inhalation (metered-dose inhaler [MDI] or nebulizer) and are most effective in treating an isolated early response. Although they do not influence long-term airway responsiveness, they are often used to maintain bronchodilation in people with asthma due to a late response.

Ipratropium is an anticholinergic drug that blocks postganglionic efferent vagal pathways. It produces bronchodilation by direct action on the large airways and does not change the composition or viscosity of the bronchial mucus. The drug is administered by MDI.

Theophylline is a bronchodilator that acts by relaxing smooth muscle. It may also augment respiratory muscle activity, thus reducing muscle fatigue. Theophylline preparations can be administered by oral or intravenous route. Oral theophylline, until recently considered the cornerstone of treatment for asthma, is no longer used as frequently. Because drug metabolism and elimination vary widely among people, blood levels are used to determine the proper dosage.

Antiinflammatory Drugs. The antiinflammatory drugs include both steroidal and nonsteroidal agents. These drugs are often preferred in treating people with inflammatory-mediated asthma.

Cromolyn sodium is an NSAID used to prevent an asthmatic attack. The exact mechanism of action is not fully understood. It probably stabilizes mast cells, thereby preventing release of the inflammatory mediators that cause an asthmatic attack. Cromolyn is used prophylactically to prevent both early and late responses. It is of no benefit when taken during an attack. The drug comes in a powdered form and is administered by inhalation.

Corticosteroids are effective in inflammatory response associated with the late response. Inhaled corticosteroids (beclomethasone, triamcinolone, budesonide, and flunisolide), administered by MDI, are usually preferred because of minimal systemic absorption and degree of hypothalamic–pituitary–adrenal dysfunction. In severe cases, oral or parenterally administered corticosteroids may be necessary.

Aerosol Therapy. The MDI is usually the preferred method for delivery of sympathomimetic, anticholinergic, and corticosteroid drugs. Various extension devices (spacers) are available to facilitate use and enhance aerosol deposition in the lungs. This is difficult to achieve when the nebulizer is held at the level of the mouth. In this position, large droplets tend to be delivered to the oropharynx and throat, rather than moving down into the small airways. Optimal use of the extender requires one inhaler puff just after beginning a slow, deep breath from functional residual capacity, followed by holding the breath in inspiration for 10 seconds.

STATUS ASTHMATICUS AND FATAL ASTHMA

Status asthmaticus is severe, prolonged asthma that is refractory to conventional methods of therapy. The death rate from asthma in the United States during the years 1980 through 1987 has increased 31%, from 1.3 to 1.7 per 100,000. African-Americans have asthma-related mortality rates higher than those of whites, especially in young age groups.[36]

The majority of asthma deaths have occurred outside the hospital. People at highest risk are those with previous exacerbations resulting in respiratory failure, respiratory acidosis, and need for intubation. Although the cause of death during an acute asthmatic attack is largely unknown, both cardiac dysrhythmias and asphyxia due to severe airway obstruction have been implicated. β-agonist drugs and theophylline increase myocardial irritability. It has been suggested that an underestimation of the severity of the attack may be a contributing factor. Deterioration often occurs rapidly during an acute attack, and underestimation of its severity may lead to a life-threatening delay in seeking medical attention. Also, frequent and repetitive use of β-agonist inhalers far in excess of the recommended doses may temporarily blunt symptoms and mask the severity of the condition. Lack of access to medical care is another risk factor associated with asthma-related death. Either distance, as in rural areas, or lack of financial resources, as in the uninsured or underinsured, may limit access to emergency care.

BRONCHIAL ASTHMA IN CHILDREN

Asthma is a leading cause of chronic illness in children, responsible for a significant number of lost school days. It is the most frequent admitting diagnosis in children's hospitals. As many as 10% to 15% of boys and 7% to 10% of girls have asthma at some time in their childhood.[43] Asthma may have its onset at any age; 30% of children are symptomatic by 1 year of age; and 80% to 90% are symptomatic by 4 to 5 years of age. Data on inheritance of asthma are most consistent with polygenic or multifactorial determinants. A child with one affected parent has about a 25% risk of developing the disease, and this risk increases to 50% when both parents are affected.

As with adults, asthma in children is almost always associated with an IgE-related reaction.[44] It has been suggested that IgE directed against respiratory viruses may be important in the pathogenesis of wheezing illnesses in infants (bronchiolitis), which often precedes the onset of asthma. One of the suggested contributing factors to development of childhood asthma is exposure during early childhood to house-dust mite antigens.[45]

The signs and symptoms of asthma in children are fairly typical. Previously well infants and children develop what may seem to be a cold with rhinorrhea, rapidly followed by irritability, cough, tachypnea, and wheezing. The symptoms may progress rapidly and require a trip to the emergency room or hospitalization.[43]

As for adults, the Expert Panel of the National Heart, Lung, and Blood Institute's National Asthma Education Program has developed guidelines for management of asthma in children.[34] The committee suggests that children as young as 5 years of age can be taught to measure their PEFR and use an MDI. The medication of choice for mild and intermittent asthma in children is a β$_2$-agonist used as needed. In children over 5 years of age, the medication is usually administered by MDI. In children under 5 years of age, it is administered either orally or by nebulizer. For some children ages 3 to 5 years (and older children who have trouble with the MDI technique), a spacer device may eliminate the problem of synchronized activation and inhalation. These devices provide a holding chamber for the medication and allow the child to inhale when he or she is ready.[34] Therapy should be initiated when early symptoms occur or, if PEFR is monitored, when the PEFR declines more than 10% to 20%. For children under 5 years of age, symptoms of cough and dyspnea indicate need for treatment. Children with moderate asthma (those who have more than two acute attacks per week) should use a β$_2$-agonist two to four times daily as needed. To avoid β$_2$-agonist overuse, additional treatment with cromolyn sodium, or inhaled corticosteroids may be needed. The use of sustained-release theophylline is subject to debate. It is recommended that inhaled corticosteroids be added to the treatment protocol for children with chronic severe asthma (fluctuations in PEFR or FEV$_{1.0}$ between premedication and postmedication measures).

CHRONIC OBSTRUCTIVE PULMONARY DISEASE

The term *chronic obstructive pulmonary disease* (COPD) denotes a group of respiratory disorders characterized by chronic and recurrent obstruction of air flow in the pulmonary airways (*i.e.*, those within the lung). About 30 million Americans have some degree of airway obstruction and COPD. As a group, COPD and other allied conditions have become the fifth leading cause of death in the United States. The death rate is increasing, especially among older men.

There are multiple pathways to the final state of COPD, the most common being emphysema and chronic bronchitis. Other causes of COPD are cystic fibrosis and bronchiectasis. Because the final outcome in terms of disability is similar, the tendency is to lump all chronic, nonspecific, and progressive disease states of airflow obstruction under the heading of COPD.

The most common cause of COPD is smoking. Thus the disease is largely preventable. Unfortunately, clinical findings are almost absent during the early stages of COPD, and by the time symptoms appear the disease is usually far advanced. For smokers with early signs of airway disease, there is hope that early recognition, combined with appropriate treatment and smoking cessation, may prevent the usually relentless progression of the disease. Other risk factors for the development of COPD are exposure to inhaled toxins in the workplace and an inherited deficiency of α_1-antitrypsin.

PATHOGENESIS

The mechanisms involved in the pathogenesis of COPD are usually multiple and include (1) inflammation, edema, and fibrosis of the bronchial wall; (2) hypertrophy of the submucosal glands and hypersecretion of mucus; and (3) loss of elastic lung fibers and alveolar tissue.[46] Inflammation and excess mucus secretion obstruct airflow and cause mismatching of ventilation and perfusion. Loss of alveolar tissue decreases the surface area for gas exchange, and loss of elastic fibers impair expiratory flow rate and predispose to airway collapse. The recoil of the elastic fibers that were stretched during inspiration provide the pressure to move air out of the lung during expiration. Because the elastic fibers are attached to the airways, they also provide radial traction to hold the airways open during expiration. These three mechanisms are illustrated in Figure 27-4.

EMPHYSEMA

Emphysema, or type A COPD, is characterized by a loss of lung elasticity and abnormal, permanent enlargement of the air spaces distal to the terminal bronchioles with destruction of the alveolar walls and capillary beds without obvious fibrosis (Fig. 27-5).[47] Enlargement of the air spaces results in hyperinflation of the lungs and increased total lung capacity.

There are two commonly recognized types of emphysema—centrilobular and panlobular. The *centrilobular type* affects the bronchioles in the central part of respiratory lobule, with initial preservation of the alveolar ducts and sacs. It is the most common

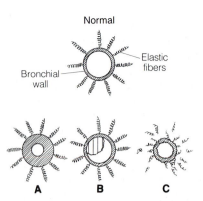

FIG. 27-4. Mechanisms of airflow obstruction in chronic obstructive lung disease. **(Top)** The normal bronchial airway with elastic fibers that provide traction and hold the airway open. **(Bottom)** Obstruction of the airway caused by (**A**) hypertrophy of the bronchial wall, (**B**) inflammation and hypersecretion of mucus, and (**C**) loss of elastic fibers that hold the airway open.

type of emphysema and is predominantly seen in male smokers. The *panlobular type* produces initial involvement of the peripheral alveoli and later extends to involve the more central bronchioles. It is the type of emphysema associated with an α_1-antitrypsin deficiency.

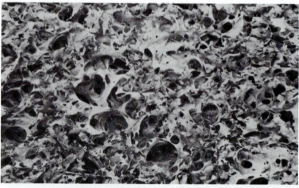

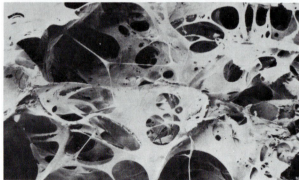

FIG. 27-5. Scanning electron micrographs of lung tissue. **(Top)** Normal tissue; **(bottom)** emphysematous tissue (both at same magnification). Note the enlargement of air spaces in the emphysematous lung. (Courtesy of Kenneth Siegesmund, PhD, Anatomy Department, The Medical College of Wisconsin, Milwaukee, WI)

Emphysema is thought to result from the breakdown of elastin and other alveolar wall components by enzymes, called *proteases*, that digest proteins. These proteases, particularly elastase, which is an enzyme that digests elastin, are released from polymorphonuclear leukocytes (neutrophils), alveolar macrophages, and other inflammatory cells. Normally, the lung is protected by an antiprotease enzyme called α_1-*antitrypsin*. With low levels of α_1-antitrypsin, the process of elastic tissue destruction goes unchecked. Normally, stimuli that increase the number of inflammatory cells in the lung or release of elastase also increase α_1-antitrypsin levels. One of the proposed mechanisms of emphysema development is an imbalance in protease/antiprotease activity (Fig. 27-6).[1]

Two of the recognized causes of emphysema are smoking and an inherited deficiency of α_1-antitrypsin. Smoking stimulates the recruitment of inflammatory cells to the alveoli, enhances the release of elastase from neutrophils, increases elastase activity in macrophages, and causes mast cell activation with release of mast cell elastases.[1]

An α_1-antitrypsin deficiency is inherited as an autosomal recessive disorder. Approximately 70% to 80% of people with a homozygous pattern of inheritance for α_1-antitrypsin deficiency (they inherit the recessive trait from both parents) have COPD.[48] However, the severity of the condition and age at onset may vary from person to person. There is evidence that cigarette smoking reduces body stores of α_1-antitrypsin over time and increases the number of macrophages in the alveolar walls. This influx of macrophages attracts increased numbers of neutrophils.[50] Therefore, smoking and repeated respiratory tract infections, which also decrease α_1-antitrypsin levels, contribute to the risk of emphysema in people with an α_1-antitrypsin deficiency. Laboratory

methods for measuring α_1-antitrypsin levels are available. Augmentation therapy is being studied as a means of preventing COPD in people with an α_1-antitrypsin deficiency.[49]

CHRONIC BRONCHITIS

In chronic bronchitis, or type B COPD, airway obstruction is caused by inflammation of both major and small airways. There is edema and hyperplasia of submucosal glands and excess mucus excretion into the bronchial tree.[47] A history of a chronic productive cough that has persisted for at least 3 months and for at least 2 consecutive years in the absence of other disease is necessary for diagnosis of chronic bronchitis. Typically, the cough has been present for many years, with a gradual increase in acute exacerbations that produce a frankly purulent sputum. Chronic bronchitis without airflow obstruction is often termed *simple bronchitis;* chronic bronchitis with airflow obstruction is termed *chronic obstructive bronchitis.* The outlook for people with simple bronchitis is good, compared with the premature morbidity and mortality associated with chronic obstructive bronchitis.

Chronic bronchitis is seen most commonly in middle-aged men and is associated with chronic irritation from smoking and recurrent infections. In the United States, smoking is the most important cause of chronic bronchitis. Viral and bacterial infections are common and are thought to be a result rather than a cause of the problem. Chronic asthmatic bronchitis is caused by increased bronchomotor tone and inflammatory triggers that cause bronchial asthma.

MANIFESTATIONS

The mnemonics "pink puffer" and "blue bloater" have been used to differentiate the clinical manifestations of emphysema and chronic obstructive bronchitis.[50] The important features of these two forms of COPD are described in Table 27-2. In actual practice the differentiation between the two types is not as vivid as presented here. Often people with COPD have both emphysema and chronic bronchitis.

A major difference between the pink puffers and the blue bloaters is the responsiveness to the hypoxic stimuli. With pulmonary emphysema, there is a proportionate loss of both ventilation and perfusion area in the lung. For whatever reason, these people are "pink puffers" or "fighters"—able to struggle and overventilate and thus maintain relatively normal blood gas levels until late in the disease. Chronic obstructive bronchitis is characterized by excessive bronchial secretions and airway obstruction that causes mismatching of ventilation and perfusion.

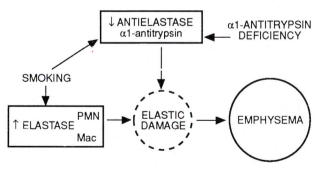

FIG. 27-6. Protease-antiprotease mechanisms of emphysema. Smoking inhibits antielastase and favors the recruitment of leukocytes and release of elastase. PMN = polymorphonuclear leukocyte; Mac = alveolar macrophage. (Cotran, R. S., Kumar, V., & Robbins, S. L. [1989]. *Robbins' pathologic basis of disease* (4th ed., p. 769). Philadelphia: W.B. Saunders)

TABLE 27-2. CHARACTERISTICS OF CHRONIC BRONCHITIS AND EMPHYSEMATOUS TYPES OF CHRONIC OBSTRUCTIVE LUNG DISEASE

CHARACTERISTIC	TYPE A PULMONARY EMPHYSEMA ("PINK PUFFERS")	TYPE B CHRONIC BRONCHITIS ("BLUE BLOATERS")
Smoking history	Usual	Usual
Age of onset	40 to 50 years of age	30 to 40 years of age; disability in middle age
Clinical features		
Barrel chest (hyperinflation of the lungs)	Often dramatic	May be present
Weight loss	May be severe in advanced disease	Infrequent
Shortness of breath	May be absent early in disease	Predominant early symptom, insidious in onset, exertional
Decreased breath sounds	Characteristic	Variable
Wheezing	Usually absent	Variable
Rhonchi	Usually absent or minimal	Often prominent
Sputum	May be absent or may develop late in the course	Frequent early manifestation, frequent infections, abundant purulent sputum
Cyanosis	Often absent, even late in the disease when there is low PO_2	Often dramatic
Blood gases	Relatively normal until late in the disease process	Hypercapnia may be present. Hypoxemia may be present
Cor pulmonale	Only in advanced cases	Frequent. Peripheral edema
Polycythemia	Only in advanced cases	Frequent
Prognosis	Slowly debilitating disease	Numerous life-threatening episodes due to acute exacerbations

People with chronic bronchitis do not compensate by increasing their ventilation; consequently, they develop hypoxemia, cyanosis, and eventually cor pulmonale with peripheral edema. These are the "blue bloaters" or "nonfighters."

People with emphysema have marked dyspnea and struggle to maintain normal blood gas levels with increased ventilatory effort, including prominent use of the accessory muscles. The work of breathing is greatly increased, and eating is often difficult. As a result, there is often considerable weight loss. An increase in the anterior-posterior dimensions of the chest due to hyperinflation of the lungs produces the so-called barrel chest that is typical of people with emphysema. Usually the seated position, which stabilizes chest structures and allows for maximum chest expansion, is preferred. Expiration is often accomplished through pursed lips. With loss of lung elasticity and hyperinflation of the lungs, the airways often collapse during expiration because the pressure in the surrounding lung tissues exceeds airway pressure. Pursed-lip breathing increases the resistance to outflow of air, producing a back pressure in the airways sufficient to prevent their collapse. Cough is not a prominent feature in emphysema.

Chronic obstructive bronchitis is characterized by shortness of breath with a progressive decrease in exercise tolerance. As the disease progresses, breathing becomes more labored, even at rest. The expiratory phase of respiration is prolonged, and expiratory rhonchi and rales can be heard on auscultation. Hypoxemia, hypercapnia, and cyanosis develop, reflecting an imbalance between ventilation and perfusion. Hypoxemia serves as stimulus for increased pulmonary vascular constriction and red blood cell production. As a result, people with chronic obstructive bronchitis also develop pulmonary hypertension, polycythemia, and right-sided heart failure with peripheral edema (cor pulmonale). In contrast to people with emphysema, those with chronic obstructive bronchitis do not increase their breathing effort to maintain blood gases. A common finding in chronic obstructive bronchitis is clubbing of the fingers, a condition in which the tips of the fingers become bulbous, resembling drumsticks.

Although emphysema and chronic bronchitis are diagnosed and treated as specific diseases, most people with COPD have features of both conditions. People with combined forms of COPD characteristically seek medical attention in the fifth or sixth decade of life complaining of cough, sputum production, and shortness of breath. Often the symptoms have been present to some extent for 10 years or more. The productive cough usually occurs in the morning. Dyspnea becomes more severe as the disease progresses. Frequent exacerbations of infection and respiratory insufficiency are common, with absence from work and eventual disability. The late stages of COPD are characterized by pulmonary hypertension, cor pulmonale, recurrent respiratory infections, and chronic respiratory failure. Death usually occurs during an exacerbation of illness associated with infection and respiratory failure.

DIAGNOSIS

The diagnosis of COPD is based on a careful history and physical examination, pulmonary function studies, chest x-rays, and laboratory tests.

Airway obstruction prolongs the expiratory phase of respiration and affords the potential for impaired gas exchange due to mismatching of ventilation and perfusion. The FVC is the amount of air that can be forcibly exhaled after maximal inspiration. In an adult with normal respiratory function, this should be achieved in 4 to 6 seconds. In chronic lung disease, the time required for FVC is increased and the $FEV_{1.0}$ and ratio of $FEV_{1.0}$ to FVC are decreased. In severe disease, the FVC is markedly reduced. Lung volume measurements reveal a marked increase in residual volume (RV) and an increase in total lung capacity (TLC) and elevation of the RV to TLC ratio. These and other measurements of expiratory flow are determined by spirometry and are used in the diagnosis of COPD (see Chapter 26).

TREATMENT

Maintaining or improving physical and psychosocial functioning is an essential part of the treatment plan for people with COPD. The treatment methods include discontinuance of cigarette smoking, education about the disease, measures to prevent and control environmental irritants and infection, maintenance of nutrition and fluid balance, use of bronchodilator drugs, and chest physiotherapy to mobilize secretions. Oxygen therapy is prescribed in selected people with significant hypoxemia. A long-term pulmonary rehabilitation program can significantly reduce episodes of hospitalization and add measurably to a person's ability to manage and cope with his or her impairment in a positive way. Breathing exercises and retraining focus on restoring the function of the diaphragm, reducing the work of breathing, and improving gas exchange. Physical conditioning, with a gradual increase in activity, improves exercise tolerance. Psychosocial rehabilitation must be individualized to meet the specific needs of people with COPD

and their families. These needs vary with age, occupation, financial resources, social and recreational interest, and interpersonal and family relationships. Work simplification strategies may be needed when impairment is severe.

Environmental Irritants and Infection. Avoidance of cigarette smoke and other environmental airway irritants is a must. Vocational counseling may be needed if there is occupational exposure. Monitoring of air pollution levels and adjusting activities accordingly aids in controlling shortness of breath. Wearing a cold weather mask often prevents dyspnea and bronchospasm due to cold air and wind exposure. Respiratory tract infections can prove fatal to people with severe COPD. A person with COPD should avoid exposure to others with known respiratory tract infections and should avoid attending large gatherings during periods of the year when influenza or respiratory tract infections are prevalent. Immunization for influenza and pneumococcal infections decreases the likelihood of their occurrence. People with COPD should be taught to monitor their sputum for signs of infection, so that treatment can be instituted at the earliest sign of infection.

Maintenance of Nutrition and Fluid Balance. Because people with COPD expend so much effort on breathing, many find it difficult to chew their food and manage the effort of a large meal. This situation, combined with impaired diaphragm descent, air-swallowing, and medications that cause anorexia and nausea, impairs nutrition and promotes weight loss. Small, frequent, nutritious, and easily swallowed feedings aid in maintaining good nutrition and preventing weight loss. Vitamin supplements may be called for. Water is the most readily available expectorant for liquefying secretions, so fluid intake should be encouraged, particularly in people who have thick, tenacious sputum. Fluid that is either too hot or too cold may aggravate breathing problems.

Pharmacologic Treatment. Bronchodilators, including adrenergic drugs, theophylline preparations, and anticholinergic drugs, are probably the most widely prescribed medications for use in treatment of COPD. Ipratropium produces bronchodilation by blocking parasympathetic cholinergic receptors that produce contraction of bronchial smooth muscle. In combination with other bronchodilators, the drug enhances and prolongs bronchodilation. β_2-specific agents have a more specific action than earlier adrenergic drugs and produce fewer cardiac effects. Theophylline preparations can be administered orally, rectally, or intravenously. As with bronchial asthma, maintenance therapy with oral theophylline drugs is controversial. When theophylline is prescribed, blood levels are used as a guide in arriving at an effective dose schedule.

Many adrenergic drugs are available in aerosol form for inhalation, and in this form they are particularly useful in controlling bronchospasm. Because they are convenient and effective, they can be abused by improper administration and overuse.

Although corticosteroid drugs are not routinely prescribed for long-term treatment of COPD, some people do require them. The corticosteroids are available for local use in aerosol form, minimizing the undesirable effects that often accompany systemic use.

Mobilization of Secretions. Postural drainage provides a means for removing excess secretions from the lungs. It is done by positioning the patient's body according to the distribution and configuration of the tracheobronchial tree so that gravity causes secretions to drain into the larger airways, from which they can be removed with relative ease. The effectiveness of postural drainage may be enhanced by percussion or vibration of the chest wall, done with vibrating or tapping motions of the hands or electronic vibrators or ultrasound generators. The reader is referred to other reference sources, some of which are listed at the end of this chapter, for a more complete description of these exercises and treatments.

Exercise and Breathing Retraining. Graded exercise programs help to prevent deterioration of physical condition and to improve the person's ability to carry out the activities of daily living. Most exercise programs use free or treadmill walking or stationary bicycling. The activities should be performed at least three to four times a week and should be limited by the person's dyspnea, not by a target heart rate. Pursed-lip breathing to prevent airway collapse, abdominal muscle assistance of expiration, and coordination of rib cage and abdominal compartment efforts improve ventilation, relieve fatigue of accessory muscles, and sometimes help prevent dyspnea.

Breathing exercises and retraining are designed to increase respiratory muscle strength and endurance, thereby improving exercise performance. In normal respiration, the diaphragm does 65% of the work of breathing, whereas the accessory muscles do about 35%.[51] In persons with COPD, the contribution of the diaphragm to the work of breathing is diminished because of loss of lung elasticity, with consequent air trapping, lung distention, and flattening of the diaphragm. Contracting this flattened diaphragm requires greater force generation. To compensate persons with COPD increasingly use their accessory muscles for breathing. This labored breathing pattern may progress to the point that the diaphragm contributes only about 30% to the effort of breathing, and the accessory muscles carry 70% of the load. Studies have shown that, although respiratory muscles may be weakened in COPD, it is possible to strengthen them through resistive loading inspiratory muscle training.[52, 53] Resistive loading is accomplished by having the person breathe through an inspiratory breathing device that increases the resistance to airflow during inspiration. Handheld devices that can be used at home are available for this purpose.

Oxygen Therapy. In advanced cases of COPD, the imbalance between ventilation and perfusion causes hypoxemia. Hypoxemia in which arterial Po_2 levels fall below 55 mmHg, causes polycythemia and reflex vasoconstriction of the pulmonary vessels, with resultant pulmonary hypertension and further impairment of gas exchange in the lung. Those affected are at risk for developing cor pulmonale.

In such severe cases, administration of continuous low-flow (1 to 2 L/min) oxygen to maintain Po_2 levels between 55 and 65 mmHg decreases dyspnea and pulmonary hypertension, and improves neuropsychological function and activity tolerance. Portable oxygen administration units, which allow for mobility and the performance of activities of daily living, are usually used. The Nocturnal Oxygen Therapy Trial Group study of people with advanced disease—particularly those with heart failure associated with COPD—performed at six centers in the United States and Canada has clearly shown that oxygen is more effective when given almost continuously than when it is given roughly 50% of the time.[54]

It has been found that people with COPD may have episodes of hypoxemia both at night and during daytime naps. These people do not, however, experience the daytime hypersomnolence and loud snoring that is usually associated with sleep apnea. The hypoxemia that occurs during sleep in people with COPD is usually associated with transient elevations of pulmonary artery pressure (pulmonary hypertension).[55, 56] These findings have been observed in persons with COPD before the chronic picture of cor pulmonale becomes evident. Sleep studies, in which arterial oxygen saturation is measured using an ear oximeter, may be done when nocturnal hypoxemia is suspected in a person with COPD. Although these people do not usually experience severe hypoxemia during waking hours and do not meet the criteria for continuous low-flow oxygen therapy, they may benefit from nocturnal oxygen therapy.[56]

Oxygen administration in people with severe

COPD must be undertaken with a certain amount of caution. The flow rate (in liters per minute) is usually titrated to provide an arterial P_{O_2} of 55 to 65 mmHg. Because the ventilatory drive associated with hypoxic stimulation of the peripheral chemoreceptors does not occur until the arterial P_{O_2} has been reduced to about 60 mmHg or less, increasing the arterial oxygen above that level tends to depress stimulation for ventilation and often leads to hypoventilation and carbon dioxide retention.

BRONCHIECTASIS

Bronchiectasis is an abnormal dilatation of the large bronchi associated with infection and destruction of the bronchial walls (Fig. 27-7). To be diagnosed as bronchiectasis the dilatation must be permanent, because reversible bronchial dilatation may accompany viral and bronchial pneumonias. There are a number of causes of bronchiectasis, including local airway obstruction due to conditions such as tumors and foreign bodies; congenital abnormalities associated with abnormal development of the bronchi; lung infection (tuberculosis, fungal infections, lung abscess); cystic fibrosis, in which airway obstruction is caused by impairment of normal mucociliary function; immunodeficiency states, which predispose to respiratory tract infections; and exposure to toxic gases, which cause airway obstruction. Two conditions, obstruction and infection, are present in all of these disorders, and both contribute to the development and progression of the disease. Bronchial obstruction causes atelectasis, which results in smooth muscle relaxation and dilatation of the walls of the airways that remain patent. Infection produces inflammation, impairs mucociliary function, and causes weakening and further dilatation of the walls of the bronchioles. Pooling of secretions produces a

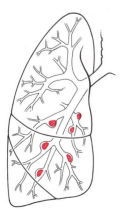

Bronchiectasis

FIG. 27-7. *Bronchiectasis showing abnormal dilations of the large bronchi that are filled with inflammatory exudate.*

vicious cycle of chronic inflammation and development of new infections. The disease is primarily a disease of children and young adults. Cystic fibrosis accounts for about half of all cases.[57]

Bronchiectasis is associated with an assortment of abnormalities that profoundly affect respiratory function, including atelectasis, obstruction of the smaller airways, and diffuse bronchitis. There is fever, recurrent bronchopulmonary infection, coughing, and production of copious amounts of foul-smelling, purulent sputum, and hemoptysis. Weight loss and anemia are common. The physiologic abnormalities that occur in bronchiectasis are similar to those seen in chronic bronchitis and emphysema. As in both of these conditions, chronic bronchial obstruction leads to marked dyspnea and cyanosis.

The basic therapy consists of early recognition and treatment of infection along with regular postural drainage and chest physical therapy. People with this disorder benefit from many of the rehabilitation and treatment measures used in the treatment of chronic bronchitis and emphysema.

CYSTIC FIBROSIS

Cystic fibrosis is an autosomal recessive exocrine gland disorder involving both the mucus-secreting and the eccrine sweat glands. Most of the clinical manifestations of the disease can be related to abnormal secretions that result in obstruction of organ passages such as the respiratory airways and pancreatic ducts. Because cystic fibrosis involves production of a thick tenacious mucus, it is sometimes referred to as *mucoviscidosis*. About 1 in 2500 whites are affected and about 1 in 25 are carriers. The gene is rare in African blacks and Asians. Homozygotes (people with two defective genes) have all, or substantially all, of the clinical symptoms of the disease, whereas heterozygotes are carriers of the disease but have no recognizable symptoms. The disease is the most common fatal hereditary disorder of whites in the United States and is the most common cause of chronic lung disease in children. About half of children with the disease live beyond age 20.

The cystic fibrosis gene was identified on the long arm of chromosome 7.[58, 59] In most cases of cystic fibrosis, the mutation consists of deletion of a single phenylalanine residue from the gene. The gene encodes the production of a single protein, the cystic fibrosis transmembrane conductance regulator (CFTR), which functions in chloride transport across membranes. In cystic fibrosis, chloride transport in airway epithelial cells is absent. Because of the defective chloride transport, there is a threefold increase in sodium reabsorption. Water moves out of the extracellular fluid with the sodium, causing the exocrine secretions to become exceedingly viscid.

Clinically, cystic fibrosis is manifested by a triad of chronic respiratory disease, pancreatic exocrine deficiency, and elevation of sodium chloride in the sweat.

Respiratory manifestations are due to an accumulation of viscid mucus in the bronchi, impaired mucociliary clearance, lung infections, bronchiectasis, and dilatation. Mucus plugs can result in the total obstruction of an airway, causing atelectasis.

Infection and ensuing inflammation are causes of lung destruction in cystic fibrosis. Both *Staphylococcus aureus* and *Pseudomonas* infections occur. With advanced disease, 80% of people harbor the *Pseudomonas* organism. New findings suggest that absence of the CFTR predisposes to *Pseudomonas* infections, and, once established, the *Pseudomonas* is not easily cleared from the lungs, producing a vicious cycle of chronic inflammation, tissue damage, and obstruction.

Abnormalities in pancreatic function are present in about 80% of affected children. The pancreatic insufficiency gives rise to malabsorption and steatorrhea. In the newborn, meconium ileus may cause intestinal obstruction.

DIAGNOSIS AND TREATMENT

Early diagnosis and treatment of cystic fibrosis are important in that they may delay the onset of chronic illness. The diagnosis is generally based on an abnormal pilocarpine iontophoresis sweat chloride test. The test is usually done on sweat obtained from a child's forearm or from an infant's thigh. A small electric current is used to carry the drug pilocarpine, which increases sweat production, into the skin. Sweat is collected using an absorbent paper or gauze sponge and then analyzed in the laboratory. The test is often inaccurate in newborns because the quantity of sweat produced is insufficient for testing. Newborns with cystic fibrosis can now be identified by determination of immunoreactive trypsin. The test can be done on blood spots collected for routine metabolic screening. It has been demonstrated that newborns with cystic fibrosis have elevated blood levels of immunoreactive trypsin, presumably due to secretory obstruction in the pancreas. Genetic testing methods to detect carriers of the cystic fibrosis gene have been developed. Unfortunately, current methods can only detect about 70% to 75% of carriers; hence, they are not recommended for general use.

The treatment of cystic fibrosis usually consists of replacement of pancreatic enzymes, physical measures to improve the clearance of tracheobronchial secretions (postural drainage and chest percussion),

and prompt treatment of respiratory tract infections. Progress of the disease is variable. Improved medical management has led to longer survival—to about age 20. Lung transplant is being used as a treatment for people with end-stage lung disease.

Treatment methods to manipulate the increased sodium reabsorption and decreased chloride secretion are being studied. Amiloride, a potassium-sparing diuretic that blocks sodium reabsorption, has been administered in aerosol form. In pilot studies that used the drug, there was a decrease in sputum viscosity and a slowing of the decline of pulmonary function. Agents (adenosine triphosphate and uridine triphosphate) that increase chloride secretion are also being studied.[60]

In summary, airway obstruction occurs in a number of reversible and chronic conditions. Bronchial asthma causes reversible bronchospasm, airway inflammation, and reversible airway responsiveness to a variety of stimuli. An asthmatic attack can be triggered by a variety of stimuli. Based on their mechanism of response, these triggers can be divided into two types—bronchospastic or inflammatory. *Bronchospastic triggers* depend on the existent level of airway responsiveness. There are two types of responses in people with asthma: the early response and late response. The early response results in immediate bronchoconstriction on exposure to an inhaled antigen and usually subsides within 90 minutes. The late response usually develops 3 to 5 hours after exposure to an asthmatic trigger; it involves inflammation as well as increased airway responsiveness that serves to prolong the attack and cause a vicious cycle of exacerbations.

COPD describes a group of conditions characterized by obstruction to airflow in the lungs. Among the conditions associated with COPD are emphysema, chronic bronchitis, and bronchiectasis. The condition is manifested by hyperinflation of the lungs, increased time required for the expiratory phase of respiration, and mismatching of ventilation and perfusion. As the condition advances, signs of respiratory distress and impaired gas exchange become evident, with development of hypercapnia and hypoxemia. Bronchiectasis is a form of COPD that is characterized by an abnormal dilatation of the large bronchi associated with infection and destruction of the bronchial walls. Cystic fibrosis is an autosomal recessive genetic disorder manifested by chronic lung disease, pancreatic exocrine deficiency, and elevation of sodium chloride in the sweat.

■ INTERSTITIAL LUNG DISEASES

The interstitial lung diseases are a diverse group of lung disorders that produce similar inflammatory and fibrotic changes in the interalveolar septum. They include sarcoidosis, the occupational lung diseases, and lung diseases caused by toxic drugs and radiation. In many cases no specific cause can be found.[61]

The interstitial lung diseases produce varying

TABLE 27-3. CAUSES AND EXAMPLES OF INTERSTITIAL LUNG DISEASES

CAUSES	EXAMPLES
Known	
Occupational and environmental inhalants	
Inorganic dusts	Silicosis
	Asbestosis
	Talcosis
	Coal miner's pneumoconiosis
	Berylliosis
Organic dusts	Farmer's lung (moldy hay)
	Pigeon breeder's lung (bird serum, excreta, and feathers)
	Air-conditioner lung (bacteria found in humidifiers and air conditioners)
	Bagassosis (contaminated sugarcane)
Gases, fumes, aerosols	Silo filler's lung (nitrogen dioxide, chlorine, ammonia, phosgene, sulfur dioxide)
Drugs	Cancer chemotherapeutic drugs (*e.g.,* bleomycin), nitrofurantoin
Radiation	External radiation, inhaled radioactive materials
Infections	Widespread tuberculosis
Poisons	Paraquat
Diseases of other organ systems	Chronic pulmonary edema
	Chronic uremia
Unknown	
	Sarcoidosis
	Idiopathic pulmonary fibrosis
	Connective tissue diseases, such as lupus erythematosus, scleroderma, and rheumatoid arthritis

degrees of inflammation, fibrosis, and disability. The disorders may be acute or insidious in onset; they may be rapidly progressive, slowly progressive, or static in their course. Because they result in a stiff and noncompliant lung, they are commonly classified as fibrotic or restrictive lung disorders. The most common of the interstitial lung diseases are those caused by exposure to occupational and environmental inhalants and sarcoidosis, the cause of which is unknown. Examples of interstitial lung diseases and their etiologies are listed in Table 27-3.

In contrast to the obstructive lung diseases, which primarily involve the airways of the lung, the interstitial lung disorders exert their effect on the collagen and elastic connective tissue found between the airways and the blood vessels of the lung. In addition, many of these diseases also involve the airways, arteries, and veins. In general, these lung diseases share a pattern of lung dysfunction that includes diminished lung volumes, reduced diffusing capacity of the lung, and varying degrees of hypoxemia.

Current theory suggests that most interstitial lung diseases, regardless of the cause, have a common pathogenesis. It is thought that these disorders are initiated by some type of injury to the alveolar epithelium, followed by an inflammatory process that involves the alveoli and interstitium of the lung.

An accumulation of inflammatory and immune cells causes continued damage of lung tissue and the replacement of normal, functioning lung tissue with fibrous scar tissue.

MANIFESTATIONS

Interstitial lung disease is characterized by an insidious onset of breathlessness that initially occurs during exercise and may progress to the point that the person is totally incapacitated. Typically, a person with a restrictive lung disease breathes with a pattern of rapid, shallow respirations. This tachypneic pattern of breathing, in which the respiratory rate is increased and the tidal volume is decreased, reduces the work of breathing. This is because it takes less work to move air through the airways at an increased rate than it does to stretch a stiff lung to accommodate a larger tidal volume. A nonproductive cough is also present in many people, particularly if there is continued exposure to the inhaled irritant. Clubbing of the fingers and toes may develop.

Lung volumes, including vital capacity and TLC, are reduced in interstitial lung disease. In contrast to COPD, in which expiratory flow rates are reduced, the $FEV_{1.0}$ is usually preserved, even though the ratio between the $FEV_{1.0}$ and the FVC may increase. Although resting arterial blood gases are usually normal early in the course of the disease, arterial oxygen levels may fall during exercise, and, in cases of advanced disease, hypoxemia is often present even at rest. In the late stages of the disease, hypercapnia and respiratory acidosis develop. The impaired diffusion of gases that occurs in people with interstitial lung disease is thought to be due primarily to an increase in physiologic dead space resulting from unventilated regions of the lung.

DIAGNOSIS AND TREATMENT

The diagnosis of interstitial lung disease requires a careful personal and family history, with particular emphasis on exposure to environmental, occupational, and other injurious agents. Chest x-rays may be used as an initial diagnostic method, and serial chest films are often used in following the progress of the disease. A biopsy specimen for histologic study and culture may be obtained by means of surgical incision or by bronchoscopy using a fiberoptic bronchoscope. In bronchoalveolar lavage, fluid is instilled into the alveoli through a bronchoscope and then removed by suction to obtain inflammatory and immune cells for laboratory study. Gallium lung scans are often used to detect and quantify the chronic alveolitis that occurs in interstitial lung disease. Gallium does not localize in normal lung tissue, but uptake of the radionuclide is increased in interstitial lung disease and other diffuse lung diseases.

The treatment goals for people with interstitial lung disease focus on identifying and removing the injurious agent, suppressing the inflammatory response, preventing progression of the disease, and providing supportive therapy for people with advanced disease. Generally, the treatment measures vary with the type of lung disease that is present. Corticosteroid drugs are frequently used to suppress the inflammatory response. Many of the supportive treatment measures used in the late stages of the disease, such as oxygen therapy and measures to prevent infection, are similar to those discussed for people with COPD.

OCCUPATIONAL LUNG DISEASES

The occupational lung diseases can be divided into two major groups: the pneumoconioses and the hypersensitivity diseases. The pneumoconioses are caused by the inhalation of inorganic dusts and particulate matter. The hypersensitivity diseases result from the inhalation of organic dusts and related occupational antigens. A third type of occupational lung disease, byssinosis, a disease that affects cotton workers, has characteristics of both the pneumoconioses and hypersensitivity lung disease.

Among the pneumoconioses are silicosis (found in hard-rock miners, foundry workers, sandblasters, pottery makers, and workers in the slate industry), coal miner's pneumoconiosis (coal miners), asbestosis (asbestos miners, manufacturers of asbestos products, and installers and removers of asbestos insulation), talcosis (talc miners or millers and infants and small children who accidentally inhale powder containing talc), and berylliosis (ore extraction workers and alloy production workers). The danger of exposure to asbestos dust is not confined to the workplace. The dust pervades the general environment because it was used in the construction of buildings and in other applications before its health hazards were realized. It has been mixed into paints and plaster, wrapped around water and heating pipes, used to insulate hair dryers, and woven into theater curtains, hot pads, and ironing-board covers.

Important etiologic determinants in the development of the pneumoconioses are (1) the size of the dust particle, its chemical nature, and its ability to incite lung destruction and (2) the concentration of dust and the length of exposure to it. The most dangerous particles are those in the range of 1 to 5 μm. These small particles are carried through the inspired air into the alveolar structures, whereas larger particles are trapped in the nose or mucous linings of the airways and removed by the mucociliary blanket. Exceptions are asbestos and talc particles, which range in size from 30 to 60 μm but find their way into the alveoli because of their density. All particles within the alveoli must be cleared by the lung macrophages. Macrophages are thought to transport engulfed particles from the small bronchioles and the alveoli, which have neither cilia nor mucus-secreting cells, to the mucociliary escalator or to the lymphatic channels for removal from the lung. This clearing function is hampered when the function of the macrophage is impaired by factors such as cigarette smoking, consumption of alcohol, and hypersensitivity reactions. This helps to explain the increased incidence of lung disease among smokers exposed to asbestos. In silicosis, the ingestion of silica particles leads to the destruction of the lung macrophages and the release of substances that produce fibrosis. Tuberculosis and other diseases caused by the mycobacteria are common in people with silicosis. Because the macrophages are responsible for protecting the lungs from tuberculosis, the destruction of macrophages accounts for the increased susceptibility of people with silicosis to tuberculosis.

With some dusts, the concentration of dust in the environment strongly influences the effect on the lung. For example, acute silicosis is seen only in people whose occupations entail intense exposure to silica dust over a short period. It is seen in sandblasters, who use a high-speed jet of sand to clean and polish bricks and the insides of corroded tanks, in tunnelers, and in rock drillers, particularly if they drill through sandstone. Acute silicosis is a rapidly progressive disease, usually leading to severe disability and death within 5 years of diagnosis. In contrast to acute silicosis, which is caused by exposure to extremely high concentrations of silica dust, the symptoms related to chronic low-level exposure to silica dust often do not begin to develop until after many years of exposure, and then the symptoms are often insidious in onset and slow to progress.

The hypersensitivity occupational lung disorders (hypersensitivity pneumonitis) are caused by intense and often prolonged exposure to inhaled organic dusts and related occupational antigens. Affected people have a heightened sensitivity to the antigen. Unlike bronchial asthma, this type of hypersensitivity reaction involves primarily the alveoli. These disorders cause progressive fibrotic lung disease, which can be prevented by the removal of the environmental agent. The most common forms of hypersensitivity pneumonitis are farmers' lung, which results from exposure to moldy hay; pigeon breeders' lung, provoked by exposure to the serum, excreta, or feathers of birds; bagassosis, from contaminated sugar cane; and humidifier or air-conditioner lung, caused by mold in the water reservoirs of these appliances.

SARCOIDOSIS

Sarcoidosis is a multisystem granulomatous disorder of unknown etiology characterized by exaggerated cellular immune response at the sites of involvement. The disease predominantly affects young adults, aged 20 to 40 years, although it may occur in older persons.[32, 61, 62] The annual incidence of sarcoidosis in the United States is about 22,500 cases; it is 10 to 20 times more common in African-Americans and is more prevalent in both African-Americans and whites living in the southeastern part of the country.

Sarcoidosis has variable manifestations and an unpredictable course of progression in which any organ system can be affected. The three systems that most commonly present symptoms are the lungs, the skin, and the eyes. More than 40% of people with sarcoidosis report nonspecific symptoms such as fever, sweating, anorexia, weight loss, fatigue, and myalgia. Although only about 60% of people with sarcoidosis have respiratory symptoms, almost all have abnormal chest x-rays. In about 25% of cases, the disease is first detected on a routine chest x-ray.

Overall, approximately 50% develop permanent pulmonary abnormalities and 5% to 15% have progressive pulmonary fibrosis.[62] Sarcoidosis is primarily an interstitial lung disease.

The diagnosis of sarcoidosis is usually made using the transbronchial lung biopsy, bronchial lavage, the Kveim-Siltzbach skin test, and serum angiotensin-converting enzyme (SACE) test. The Kveim-Siltzbach test is a skin test that uses antigen from human sarcoid tissue injected intradermally into the flexor surface of the forearm. The injection site is observed for the development of a nodule during the 6 weeks after injection of the antigen. If a nodule develops, it is examined through biopsy for sarcoid tissue. In active sarcoidosis, the SACE level is elevated. The SACE test is used to evaluate the progress of the disease and the effectiveness of treatment. When treatment is indicated, the corticosteroid drugs are used. These agents produce clearing of the chest x-ray and improve pulmonary function, but it is not known whether they affect the long-term outcome of the disease.

In summary, the interstitial lung diseases are characterized by fibrosis and decreased compliance of the lung. They include the occupational lung diseases, lung diseases caused by toxic drugs and radiation, and lung diseases of unknown etiology, such as sarcoidosis. These disorders are thought to result from an inflammatory process that begins in the alveoli and extends to involve the interstitial tissues of the lung. In contrast with COPDs, which affect the airways, interstitial lung diseases affect the supporting collagen and elastic tissues that lie between the airways and blood vessels. These lung diseases produce a decrease in lung volumes, a reduction in the diffusing capacity of the lung, and varying degrees of hypoxia. Because lung compliance is reduced, people with this form of lung disease have a rapid, shallow breathing pattern.

■ PULMONARY VASCULAR DISORDERS

As blood moves through the lung, blood oxygen levels are raised and carbon dioxide is removed. These processes depend on the matching of ventilation (gas exchange) and perfusion (blood flow). This section discusses two major problems of the pulmonary circulation, pulmonary embolism and pulmonary hypertension. Pulmonary edema, another major problem of the pulmonary circulation, is discussed in Chapter 24.

PULMONARY EMBOLISM

Pulmonary embolism develops when a bloodborne substance lodges in a branch of the pulmonary artery and obstructs the flow. The embolism may consist of a thrombus, air that has accidentally been injected during intravenous infusion, fat that has been mobilized from the bone marrow after a fracture or from a traumatized fat depot, or amniotic fluid that has entered the maternal circulation after rupture of the membranes at the time of delivery. This discussion is limited to the most common form of pulmonary embolism, thromboembolism.

In the United States, as many as 250,000 hospitalizations occur annually due to pulmonary emboli.[63] Mortality statistics range from 18% to 35% in undiagnosed and therefore untreated cases to as low as 8% to 10% in treated cases. Pulmonary embolism is uncommon before adulthood and increases in incidence with age, so that at age 80, about 70% of autopsied patients have emboli.[64]

Almost all pulmonary emboli are due to deep vein thrombosis. Therefore, people at risk for developing venous thrombosis are the same people who are at risk for developing thromboemboli. Among the physiologic factors that contribute to venous thrombosis are venous stasis, venous endothelial injury, and hypercoagulability states. Clinical risk factors include prolonged bedrest, trauma, surgery, childbirth, obesity, fractures of the hip and femur, advanced age, myocardial infarction and congestive heart failure, and spinal cord injury. People undergoing orthopedic surgery and gynecologic cancer surgery are at particular risk, as are bedridden patients in an intensive care unit.[65] An enlarged fibrillating right atrium often contains thrombosed blood. The presence of thrombosis in the deep veins of the legs or pelvis is often unsuspected until embolism occurs. Venous thrombosis is further discussed in Chapter 20.

The effects of emboli on the pulmonary circulation are related to mechanical obstruction of the pulmonary circulation and neurohumoral reflexes causing vasoconstriction. Obstruction of pulmonary blood flow causes reflex bronchoconstriction in the affected area of the lung, wasted ventilation and impaired gas exchange, and loss of alveolar surfactant. Pulmonary hypertension and right heart failure may develop when there is massive vasoconstriction due to a large embolus. Although small areas of infarction may occur, frank pulmonary infarction is uncommon.

MANIFESTATIONS

The manifestations of pulmonary embolism depend on the size and location of the obstruction. Chest pain, dyspnea, and increased respiratory rate are the most frequent signs and symptoms of pulmonary embolism. Pulmonary infarction often causes pleuritic pain that changes with respiration, being more severe on inspiration and less severe on expiration. Moderate hypoxemia without carbon dioxide retention occurs as a result of impaired gas exchange. Small emboli that become lodged in the peripheral branches of the pulmonary artery may exert little effect and go unrecognized. However, repeated small emboli gradually reduce pulmonary capillary bed, resulting in pulmonary hypertension. Moderate-sized emboli often present with breathlessness accompanied by pleuritic pain, apprehension, slight fever, and cough productive of blood-streaked sputum. Tachycardia is often present, and the breathing pattern is rapid and shallow. Massive emboli usually present with sudden collapse, crushing substernal chest pain, shock, and sometimes loss of consciousness. The pulse is rapid and weak, the blood pressure is low, the neck veins are distended, and the skin is cyanotic and diaphoretic. Massive pulmonary emboli are often fatal.

DIAGNOSIS AND TREATMENT

Diagnosis of pulmonary embolism is based on blood gases, lung scan (perfusion, ventilation, or both), chest x-ray films, electrocardiogram (ECG), and, in selected cases, angiography. The arterial oxygen tension (PO_2) is almost always decreased when emboli of significant size are present in the lung. This is because of the mismatching of ventilation and perfusion. The lung scan is a widely used diagnostic test. A perfusion lung scan uses radiolabeled albumin, which is injected intravenously and is distributed in proportion to blood flow in the pulmonary circulation. A scintillation (gamma) camera is used to scan the various lung segments for blood flow. A ventilation scan uses a radiolabeled gas (usually xenon-133).[66] The person inhales the gas by way of a mask and holds his or her breath (for as long as 20 seconds) while a scintillation (gamma) camera scans the lung and records the distribution of the radiolabeled gas. A ventilation scan may be done before a perfusion scan if there is concurrent lung disease. Use of both the ventilation and perfusion scans provides a means of evaluating ventilation–perfusion relationships in the lung. The laboratory studies and chest x-ray films are useful in ruling out other conditions that might give rise to similar symptoms. The ECG may show signs of right heart strain, because emboli can cause an increase in pulmonary vascular resistance. Angiography involves the passage of a venous catheter through the heart and into the pulmonary artery under fluoroscopy. An embolectomy is sometimes performed during this procedure.

The treatment goals for pulmonary emboli focus on (1) preventing deep vein thrombosis and the development of thromboemboli, (2) protecting the lungs from exposure to thromboemboli when they occur, and (3) in the case of large and life-threatening pulmonary emboli, sustaining life and restoring pulmonary blood flow.

Prevention focuses on (1) identification of people at risk, (2) avoidance of venous stasis and hypercoagulability states, and (3) early detection of venous thrombosis. Early detection of venous thrombosis can be accomplished through the use of compression ultrasonography, impedance plethysmography, and Doppler imaging.[65]

In patients at risk, graded-compression elastic stockings and intermittent pneumatic-compression (IPC) boots can be used to prevent venous stasis. Both of these devices are safe and practical ways to prevent venous thrombosis. IPC boots provide intermittent inflation of air-filled cuffs that prevent venous stasis. Some devices produce sequential gradient compression that moves blood upward in the leg (*e.g.*, pressure of 35, 30, and 20 mmHg in the ankle, calf, and thigh, respectively).[63]

Pharmacologic prophylaxis involves the use of anticoagulant drugs. Low-dose subcutaneous heparin may be administered to decrease the likelihood of deep vein thrombosis, thromboembolism, and fatal pulmonary embolism after major surgical procedures.[67] Warfarin, an oral anticoagulation drug, may be used for people with long-term risk of developing thromboemboli. Dextran is a glucose polymer that is given intravenously. It impairs platelet function by causing decreased platelet aggregability. Potential adverse effects include anaphylaxis, volume overload, and nephrotoxicity. It may be used in people who require pharmacologic prophylaxis but are unable to receive heparin prophylaxis because of bleeding or other adverse reactions.

There are two surgical procedures for protecting the lung from thromboemboli: venous ligation to prevent the embolus from traveling to the lung and vena caval plication. The plication, done with a suture or by insertion of a clip, filter, or sieve, permits blood to flow while trapping the embolus.

Restoration of blood flow in people with life-threatening pulmonary emboli can be accomplished through the surgical removal of the embolus or emboli. In the case of multiple pulmonary emboli, thrombolytic therapy using streptokinase, urokinase, or recombinant tissue plasminogen activator may be used. It is recommended that the thrombolytic therapy be administered through a peripheral vein rather than through a pulmonary artery because the latter approach is neither safer nor more effective.[65] Thrombolytic therapy is followed by administration of heparin and then warfarin.

PULMONARY HYPERTENSION

The term pulmonary hypertension describes the elevation of pressure in the pulmonary arterial system. The pulmonary circulation is a low-pressure system designed to accommodate varying amounts of blood delivered from the right heart and to facilitate gas exchange. The normal mean pulmonary artery pressure is about 15 mmHg (28 systolic/8 diastolic). Pulmonary artery hypertension can be caused by an elevation in left atrial pressure, by increased pulmonary blood flow, or by increased pulmonary vascular resistance. Although pulmonary hypertension can develop as a primary disorder, most cases develop secondary to some other condition.

In conditions such as mitral valve stenosis and left ventricular heart failure, the elevation in left atrial pressure is transmitted to the pulmonary circulation and results in a passive elevation of pulmonary arterial pressures. Continued increases in left atrial pressure can lead to medial hypertrophy and intimal thickening of the small pulmonary arteries, causing sustained hypertension.

Increased pulmonary blood flow results from increased flow through left-to-right shunts in congenital heart diseases such as atrial or ventricular septal defects and patent ductus arteriosus. If the high-flow state is allowed to continue, morphologic changes occur in the pulmonary vessels, leading to sustained pulmonary hypertension. The pulmonary vascular changes that occur with congenital heart disorders are discussed in Chapter 23.

Unlike the vessels in the systemic circulation, which generally dilate in response to hypoxemia and hypercapnia, the pulmonary vessels constrict. The stimulus for constriction seems to originate in the air spaces in the vicinity of the small branches of the pulmonary arteries. In situations in which certain regions of the lung are hypoventilated, the response is adaptive in that it diverts blood flow away from the poorly ventilated areas to more adequately ventilated portions of the lung. This effect, however, becomes less beneficial as more and more areas of the lung become poorly ventilated.

Pulmonary hypertension may develop at high altitudes in people with normal lungs. It is also a common problem in people with advanced chronic bronchitis and emphysema. In interstitial lung diseases, the fibrotic process may actually cause obliteration of pulmonary vessels, leading to pulmonary hypertension. People who experience marked hypoxemia during sleep (*i.e.*, those with sleep apnea) may experience marked elevations in pulmonary arterial pressure.

PRIMARY PULMONARY HYPERTENSION

Primary pulmonary hypertension is a rare, often lethal, form of pulmonary hypertension, the etiology of which is unknown. It is characterized by marked intimal fibrosis of the pulmonary arteries and arterioles. The disease can occur at any age, and familial occurrences have been reported. People with the disorder usually have a steadily progressive downhill course, with death occurring in 3 to 4 years. The recent use of the vasodilators hydralazine and diazoxide for the treatment of this form of pulmonary hypertension has met with some degree of success.

COR PULMONALE

The term *cor pulmonale* refers to heart failure resulting from primary lung disease and longstanding pulmonary hypertension. It involves hypertrophy and the eventual failure of the right ventricle. The manifestations of cor pulmonale include the signs and symptoms of the primary lung disease and the signs of right-sided heart failure. There is shortness of breath and a productive cough, which becomes worse during periods of heart failure. Failure of the right ventricle and elevation of intrathoracic pressure resulting from airway obstruction cause venous distention and peripheral edema. Plethora (redness) and cyanosis and warm, moist skin may be present because of the compensatory polycythemia and desaturation of arterial blood that accompany chronic lung disease. Drowsiness and altered consciousness may occur as the result of carbon dioxide retention. Management of cor pulmonale focuses on the treatment of both the lung disease and the heart failure. Low-flow oxygen therapy may be used to reduce the pulmonary hypertension and polycythemia associated with severe hypoxemia due to chronic lung disease.

In summary, pulmonary vascular disorders include pulmonary embolism and pulmonary hypertension. Pulmonary embolism develops when a bloodborne substance lodges in a branch of the pulmonary artery and obstructs blood flow. The embolus can consist of a thrombus, air, fat, or amniotic fluid. The most common form is a thromboemboli arising from the deep venous channels of the lower extremities. Pulmonary hypertension is the elevation of pulmonary arterial pressure. It can be caused by an elevated left atrial pressure, increased pulmonary blood flow, or increased pulmonary vascular resistance secondary to lung disease. The term *cor pulmonale* describes right heart failure caused by primary pulmonary disease and longstanding pulmonary hypertension.

■ CANCER OF THE LUNG

In the United States, lung cancer strikes an estimated 157,000 people every year, most commonly those between 50 and 75 years of age.[68] Lung cancer is the leading cause of cancer deaths among both men and women in the United States. The increases in lung cancer incidence and deaths over the past 50 years have coincided closely with the increase in cigarette smoking over the same span. It has been estimated that 85% of lung cancer cases are due to cigarette smoking. Many studies have shown that the risk of developing lung cancer increases with the number of cigarettes smoked and that the average male smoker is ten times more likely to develop lung cancer than the nonsmoker. Industrial hazards also contribute to the incidence of lung cancer. A commonly recognized hazard is exposure to asbestos, with the mean risk of lung cancer being significantly greater in asbestos workers than in the general population. Tobacco smoke contributes heavily to the development of lung cancer in people exposed to asbestos; the risk in this population group is estimated to be 55 times greater than that for nonsmokers.[69]

Because cancer of the lung is usually far advanced before it is discovered, the prognosis is generally poor. The overall 5-year survival rate is 13%, whereas it was 7% in 1963.[68]

Bronchogenic carcinoma is the cancer type seen in 90% to 95% of cases. These tumors can be further subdivided into non-small cell lung carcinoma (70% to 75%); small cell lung carcinoma (20% to 25%), and combined patterns (5% to 10%). Bronchiogenic carcinomas are aggressive, locally invasive, and widely metastatic tumors that arise from the epithelial lining of the major bronchi. All varieties of bronchiogenic carcinomas, especially small cell lung carcinoma, have the capacity to synthesize bioactive products and produce paraneoplastic syndromes. These tumors begin as small mucosal lesions that may follow one of several patterns of growth. They form intraluminal masses that invade the bronchial mucosa and infiltrate the peribronchial connective tissue or they may form large bulky masses that extend into the adjacent lung tissue. Some large tumors undergo central necrosis and develop local areas of hemorrhage and some invade the pleural cavity and chest wall, and spread to adjacent intrathoracic structures.[69]

There are three types of non-small cell lung carcinoma (NSLC): squamous cell carcinoma (25% to 30%), adenocarcinoma, including bronchioalveolar carcinoma (30% to 35%), and large cell carcinoma (10% to 15%).[69] Squamous cell carcinomas are more common in men than women; they tend to spread centrally into major bronchi and eventually spread to hilar nodes, but disseminate outside the thorax later than other types of NSLC. Adenocarcinomas are almost equally divided between men and women, and the association between cigarette smoking is weaker than for squamous cell carcinoma. They may occur as central lesions in the bronchi but are usually more peripherally located, many arising in relation to peripheral scars. Generally these tumors grow slowly and produce smaller masses than other types of NSLC. Bronchioalveolar carcinoma, a special category of adenocarcinoma, occurs as two variants: one that forms multifocal mucinous masses and a second that is evidenced by a single tumor that does not elaborate mucin. These tumors have a better prognosis than other bronchiogenic carcinomas; the multifocal variant has a 20% to 25% 5-year survival rate, and the localized single mass has a 50% to 70% 5-year survival rate. Large cell carcinomas constitute a group of neoplasms that are highly anaplastic and difficult to categorize as either squamous or adenocarcinoma. They have a poor prognosis because of their tendency to spread to distant sites early in their course. More than half have spread to the CNS at the time of diagnosis, and the 5-year survival rate is 2% to 3%.

The small cell lung carcinomas (SCLC) are rapidly growing tumors that tend to infiltrate widely, disseminate early in their course, and are rarely resectable by surgery. The 2-year survival rate is only 5% to 8%, although newer protocols have improved the outlook somewhat.[69] The SCLC is one form of cancer that has paraneoplastic properties (see Chapter 5). It has the ability to secrete a host of polypeptide hormones including adrenocorticotropic hormone (ACTH), antidiuretic hormone (ADH), parathormone-like hormone, and gastrin-releasing peptide.

MANIFESTATIONS

Cancer of the lung develops insidiously, often giving little or no warning of its presence. Because its symptoms are similar to those associated with smoking and chronic bronchitis, they are often disregarded.

The manifestations of lung cancer can be divided into four categories: (1) local respiratory disturbances, (2) the effects of local spread and metastasis, (3) nonspecific effects such as weight loss, and (4) the nonmetastatic endocrine, neurologic, and connective tissue disorders.

Lung cancers produce their local effects by irritation and obstruction of the airways and invasion of the mediastinum and pleural space. The earliest symptoms are chronic cough, shortness of breath, and wheezing due to airway irritation and obstruction. Hemoptysis (blood in the sputum) occurs when the lesion erodes blood vessels. Pain receptors in the chest are limited to the parietal pleura, mediastinum, larger blood vessels, and peribronchial afferent vagal fibers. Dull, intermittent, poorly localized retrosternal pain is common in tumors that involve the mediastinum. Pain becomes persistent, localized, and more severe when the disease invades the pleura.

Tumors that invade the mediastinum may cause hoarseness (because of the involvement of the recurrent laryngeal nerve) and difficulty in swallowing (due to compression of the esophagus). An uncommon complication called the *superior vena cava syndrome* can occur in some people with mediastinal involvement. Interruption of flow in this vessel usually results from compression by the tumor or involved lymph nodes. The disorder can interfere with venous drainage from the head, neck, and chest wall. The outcome is determined by the speed with which the disorder develops and the adequacy of the collateral circulation.

Tumors adjacent to the visceral pleura often insidiously produce pleural effusion. This effusion can compress the lung and cause atelectasis and dyspnea. It is less apt to cause fever, pleural friction rub, or pain than pleural effusion resulting from other causes.

Metastases already exist in 50% of patients presenting with evidence of lung cancer and develop eventually in the majority (90%) of patients. The most common sites of these metastases are the brain, bone, and liver.

Paraneoplastic disorders are those that are unrelated to metastasis. These include hypercalcemia (due to secretion of parathormone-like peptide), Cushing's syndrome (due to ACTH secretion), diabetes insipidus (due to inappropriate secretion of antidiuretic hormone), neuromuscular syndromes (myasthenic syndromes, peripheral neuropathy, and polymyositis), and hematologic disorders (migratory thrombophlebitis, nonbacterial endocarditis, and disseminated intravascular coagulation). Neurologic or muscular symptoms often develop 6 months to 4 years before the lung tumor is detected. One of the more common of these problems is weakness and wasting of the proximal muscles of the pelvic and shoulder girdles with decreased deep tendon reflexes, but without sensory changes. Hypercalcemia is seen most often in people with squamous cell carcinoma; hematologic syndromes in people with adenocarcinomas; and the remaining syndromes in people with small cell neoplasms.[69] Sometimes, manifestations of the paraneoplastic syndrome may precede the onset of other signs of lung cancer and may lead to discovery of an occult tumor.

DIAGNOSIS AND TREATMENT

The diagnosis of lung cancer is based on a careful history and physical examination and other tests such as chest radiography, bronchoscopy, cytologic studies (Papanicolaou's test) of the sputum or bronchial washings, percutaneous needle biopsy of lung tissue, and scalene lymph node biopsy. CT scans, magnetic resonance imaging (MRI), and ultrasound are used to locate lesions and evaluate the extent of the disease. The carcinoembryonic antigen (CEA) is produced by undifferentiated lung tumor cells; high CEA titers usually correlate with extensive disease. This test is often used to follow the progress of the disease and its response to treatment.

Like other types of cancer, lung cancers are classified according to cell type (squamous cell carcinoma, adenocarcinoma, small cell anaplastic carcinoma, and large cell carcinoma) and staged according to the TNM system (see Chapter 5). These classifications are used for treatment planning.

Treatment methods for lung cancer include surgery, radiotherapy, and chemotherapy.[68] These treatments may be used singly or in combination. Surgery is usually used for the removal of small localized tumors. It can involve a lobectomy, pneumonectomy, or segmental resection of the lung. Radiation can be used as a definitive or main treatment modality, as part of a combined treatment plan, or for palliation of symptoms. Because of the frequency of metastases, chemotherapy is often used in treating lung cancer. Combination chemotherapy, which uses a regimen of several drugs, is usually employed. Chemotherapy is the treatment of choice in SCLC. Recent advances in use of combination chemotherapy have improved the outlook for people with SCLC. National Cancer Institute studies report that 10% of people with limited stage disease and 5% of all people with SCLC treated with combination chemotherapy have survived 10 years or longer.[70]

In summary, cancer of the lung is a leading cause of death among men and women ages 50 to 75, and the death rate is increasing among women. In the United States, this increase in death rate has coincided with the increase in cigarette smoking. Industrial hazards, such as exposure to asbestos, increase the risk of developing lung cancer. Of all forms of lung cancer, bronchogenic carcinoma is the most common, accounting for 90% to 95% of cases. Because lung cancer develops insidiously, it is often far advanced before it is diagnosed, a fact that is used to explain the poor 5-year survival rate.

■ RESPIRATORY DISORDERS IN CHILDREN

Acute respiratory disease is the most common cause of illness in infancy and childhood, accounting for 50% of illness in children under 5 years of age and 30% of illness in children between 5 and 12 years of age.[71] The discussion in this chapter focuses on: (1) lung development with an emphasis on the developmental basis for lung disorders in children, (2) respiratory disorders in the neonate, and (3) respiratory infections in children. A discussion of bronchial asthma in children and cystic fibrosis is included in the section on obstructive lung disorders.

LUNG DEVELOPMENT

Although other body systems are physiologically ready for extrauterine life by as early as 25 weeks of gestation, the lungs require much longer. Immaturity of the respiratory system is a major cause of morbidity and mortality in infants born prematurely. Even at birth the lungs are not fully mature, and additional growth and maturation continue well into childhood.

Developmental Stages. Lung development may be divided into five stages: (1) embryonic period, (2) glandular period, (3) canicular period, (4) saccular period, and (5) alveolar period.[72,73,74,75] The development of the respiratory system begins with the *embryonic period* (weeks 4 to 6 of gestation), during which a rudimentary lung bud branches from the esophagus to begin formation of the airways and alveolar spaces (Fig. 27-8). The lung bud divides into two lung buds that grow laterally; the right bud giving rise to two secondary buds and the left bud to one secondary bud. Consequently, in the adult, there are three main (primary) bronchi and three lung lobes on the right and only two main bronchi and two lung lobes on the left. Each secondary lung bud subsequently undergoes continuous branching. The tertiary (segmental) bronchi (10 in the right lung and 8 or 9 in the left lung begin to form during the 7th week.

During the *glandular period* (weeks 5 to 16), the lungs resemble a gland; during this period the conducting airways are formed. At 17 weeks, all of the major elements of the lung have formed except the gas exchange structures. Respiration is not possible because the airways end in blind tubes. The *canicular period* (weeks 17 to 27) marks the formation of the primitive alveoli. During this period, the lumina of the bronchi and bronchioles become much larger and the lung tissue becomes more highly vascularized. By the 24th week, each bronchiole has given rise to two more respiratory bronchioles. Respiration is possible at this time because some primitive alveoli have developed at the ends of the bronchioles.[74] The *saccular period* (weeks 27 to 35) is devoted to the development of the terminal alveolar sacs, which facilitate gas exchange; during this period, the terminal sacs thin out and capillaries begin to bulge into the termi-

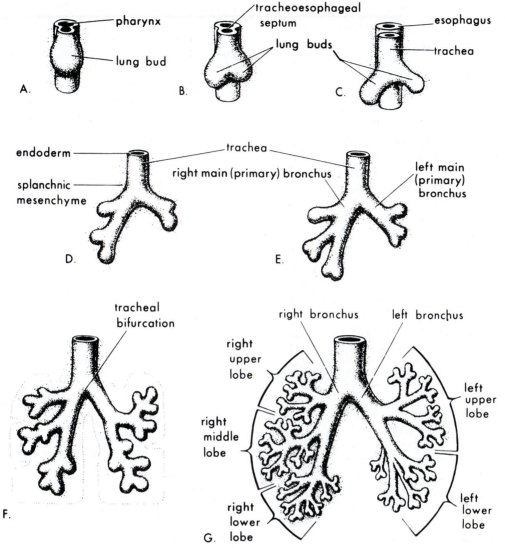

FIG. 27-8. Drawings of ventral views illustrating successive stages in the development of the bronchi and lungs: (**A–C**) 4 weeks, (**D, E**) 5 weeks, (**F**) 6 weeks, (**G**) 8 weeks. (Moore, K. [1993]. *The developing human* [5th ed.]. Philadelphia: W.B. Saunders)

nal sacs. These thin cells are known as *type I alveolar cells*. By the 25th to 28th week, sufficient terminal sacs are present to permit survival. Before this time, the premature lungs were incapable of adequate gas exchange. It is not so much the presence of the thin alveolar epithelium as it is adequate matching pulmonary vasculature that is critical to survival.[74] Type II alveolar cells begin to develop at about 24 weeks. These cells produce surfactant, a substance capable of lowering the surface tension of the air–alveoli interface (see Chapter 26). By the 25th to 28th week, the amount of surfactant that is available is sufficient to prevent alveolar collapse when breathing begins.

The *alveolar period* (late fetal to early childhood) marks the maturation and expansion of the alveoli. Starting as early as 30 weeks and nearly always by 36

weeks, the saccular structures become alveoli. Alveolation is characterized by thinning of the pulmonary interstitium and the appearance of a single capillary network, in which one capillary bulges into each terminal alveolar sac. By the late fetal period, the lungs are capable of respiration because the alveolar-capillary membrane is sufficiently thin to allow for gas exchange.

Although transformation of the lungs from glandlike structures to highly vascular alveolilike organs occurs during the late fetal period, mature alveoli do not form for some time after birth. The growth of the lung during infancy and early childhood involves an increase in the number rather than the size of the alveoli. Only one eighth to one sixth of the adult number of alveoli are present at birth. There is a relative slowing of alveolar growth during the first 3 months after birth; this is followed by a rapid increase in alveolar number during the first year of life, reaching approximately the adult number of 300 million alveoli by 5 to 6 years of age.

Lung Liquid. The fetal lung is a secretory organ, and fluids and electrolytes are secreted into the potential air spaces. This fluid appears to be important in stimulating alveolar development. For the fetus to complete the transition from intrauterine life to extrauterine life, this fluid must be cleared from the lung soon after birth. Presumably with the onset of labor, the secretion of fluid ceases; during the birth process, pressure on the thorax causes the fluid to be expelled from the mouth and nose. When the lungs expand after birth, the fluid moves into the tissues surrounding the alveoli and is then absorbed into the pulmonary capillaries or removed by the lymphatic system.

Fetal Breathing. It is established that fetal breathing movements occur in utero. These movements are irregular in rate and amplitude, ranging from 30 to 70 breaths per minute, and become more rapid as gestation advances. Because they are rapid and shallow, these movements do not result in movement of fluid either into or out of the fetal lung. These movements are thought to condition the respiratory muscles and stimulate lung development. The breathing movements in the fetus increase in response to hypercapnia (increased carbon dioxide levels) and decrease in response to hypoxia.

BREATHING IN THE INFANT AND SMALL CHILD

The major difference between respiration in the fetus and the neonate is that, in the fetus, there is complete separation between gas exchange and breathing movements. Both the gas supply and exchange are entirely dependent on maternal mechanisms controlling placental circulation. At birth, dependence on the placental circulation is terminated and the infant must integrate the two previously separate functions of gas exchange and respiratory movements. Within seconds of clamping the umbilical cord, the infant takes its first breath and rhythmic breathing begins and persists for life.

MECHANICS OF BREATHING

The diaphragm is the principal muscle of inspiration. When the chest wall is sufficiently stiff, as it is in the adult, contraction of the diaphragm increases chest volume in both longitudinal and transverse directions. Also in the adult, the ribs angle downward,

from front to back, so that contraction of the external intercostals elevate the rib cage. In contrast to the adult, the chest wall of the neonate is compliant; although this is advantageous during the birth process in that it allows for marked distortion to occur without damaging chest structures, it has implications for ventilation during the postnatal period. Not only is the infant's chest wall compliant, but the diaphragm inserts more horizontally, is flatter, and is less capable of moving downward to increase the volume of the chest cavity.[71] The external intercostals, rather than raising the rib cage, serve to stabilize the chest wall during inspiration.

A striking characteristic of neonatal breathing is the paradoxical inward movement of the upper chest during inspiration, especially during active sleep. This is because there is decreased activity of the intercostal muscles during active sleep, which allows the contracting diaphragm to pull the highly compliant chest wall inward. Under circumstances such as crying, the intercostal muscles of the neonate function together with the diaphragm.

Normally the infant's lungs are also compliant; this is advantageous to the infant with its compliant chest cage because it takes only small changes in inspiratory pressure to inflate a compliant lung. When respiratory disease develops, lung compliance is reduced and it takes more effort to inflate the lungs. The diaphragm must generate more negative pressure; as a result, the compliant chest wall structures are sucked inward. *Retractions* are abnormal inward movements of the chest wall during inspiration; they may occur intercostally (between the ribs), in the substernal or epigastric area, and the supraclavicular spaces. Because the chest wall of the infant is compliant, substernal retractions become more obvious with small changes in lung function. Increased retractions can indicate airway obstruction or atelectasis.

Also influencing the effectiveness of ventilation in the neonate is the intrinsic mechanical properties of the diaphragm. Although much uncertainty remains regarding the functioning of the respiratory muscles in the neonate, it seems that these muscles in the newborn, particularly in the preterm infant, are poorly adapted for high work loads. This is because they contain relatively few fatigue-resistant, slow-twitch, highly-oxidative fibers, have low glycogen and fat stores, and can easily become hypoxic.[75]

AIRWAY RESISTANCE

Normal lung inflation requires uninterrupted movement of air through the extrathoracic (nose, pharynx, larynx, and upper trachea) and intrathoracic (bronchi and bronchioles) airways. The neonate (0 to 4 weeks of age) breathes predominantly through the nose and does not adapt well to mouth breathing. Any obstruction of the nose or nasopharynx may increase upper airway resistance and increase the work of breathing.

The airways of the infant and small child are much smaller than those of the adult. Because the resistance to airflow is directly related to the fourth power of the radius (resistance = $1/\text{radius}^4$), relatively small amounts of mucus secretion, edema, or airway constriction can produce marked changes in airway resistance and airflow (Fig. 27-9). Nasal flaring is a method that infants use to take in more air. This method of breathing increases the size of the nares and decreases the resistance of the small airways.

Normally the extrathoracic airways in the infant narrow during inspiration and dilate during expiration, and the intrathoracic airways widen during inspiration and narrow during expiration.[76] This is because the pressure inside the extrathoracic airways reflects the intrapleural pressures of the thoracic cavity, whereas the pressure outside the intrathoracic airways is similar to atmospheric pressure or essentially zero; during inspiration, the pressure inside becomes more negative, causing the airways to narrow, and during expiration, it becomes more positive, causing them to widen. In contrast to the extrathoracic airways, the pressure outside the intrathoracic airways is equal to the intrapleural pressure; these airways widen during inspiration as the surrounding intrapleural pressure becomes more negative and pulls them open, and they narrow during expiration as the surrounding pressure becomes more positive.

LUNG VOLUMES AND GAS EXCHANGE

The functional residual capacity, air left in the lungs at the end of normal expiration, plays an important role in the gas exchange of the infant. In the infant, the functional residual capacity occurs at higher lung volumes than in the older child or adult.[77] This increased end-expiratory volume is caused by the more rapid respiratory rate and insufficient time available to the neonate for expiration. However, the increased residual volume is important to the neonate because it serves to hold the airways open throughout all phases of respiration; it favors the reabsorption of intrapulmonary fluids; and it maintains more uniform lung expansion and enhances gas exchange. During sleep, the tone of the upper airway muscles is reduced, so that the time spent in expiration is shorter and the intercostal activity that stabilizes the chest wall is less; this produces a lower end-expiratory volume and less optimal gas exchange.

CONTROL OF VENTILATION

The fetal oxygen (P_{O_2}) levels normally range from 25 to 30 mmHg, and carbon dioxide (P_{CO_2}) levels range from 45 to 50 mmHg, independent of any respiratory movements. Any decrease in oxygen levels induces quiet sleep in the fetus with subsequent cessation of breathing movements, both of which lead to a decrease in oxygen consumption. The switching from the placenta to the aerated lung immediately after

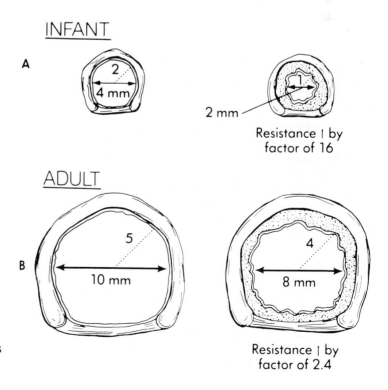

FIG. 27-9. The effect of edema on airway radius and airflow in the infant and adult.

birth causes an immediate increase in P_{O_2} to 50 mmHg; within a few hours it increases to 70 mmHg.[75] These levels, which greatly exceed fetal levels, cause the chemoreceptors (see Chapter 26) to become silent for several days. Although the infant's P_{O_2} may fluctuate during this critical time, the chemoreceptors do not respond appropriately. Within several days of birth, the chemoreceptors "reset" their P_{O_2} threshold; only then do the oxygen-sensitive chemoreceptors become the major controller of breathing.[74] However, the response seems to be biphasic with an initial hyperventilation, followed by a decreased respiratory rate and even apnea. Even in normal neonates, but particularly in preterm infants, breathing patterns and respiratory reflexes depend on the arousal state. Periodic breathing and apnea are characteristic of premature infants and reflect patterns of fetal breathing. The fact that they occur with sleep and disappear during wakefulness underscores the importance of arousal.

ALTERATIONS IN BREATHING

Most lung diseases in children produce decreased lung compliance and manifestations of restrictive lung disease, or they increase airway resistance.

Children with restrictive lung disease breathe at faster rates, and their respiratory excursions are shallow. Grunting is an audible noise emitted during expiration; it may be either intermittent or continuous. An expiratory grunt is common as the child tries to raise the functional residual capacity by closing the glottis at the end of expiration. It is a sign of labored breathing usually due to decreased lung compliance or lung volume; grunting may be a compensatory mechanism for lung dysfunction by increasing lung volume and improving arterial oxygenation.

The pressure needed to overcome airway resistance depends on the rate of airflow as it moves into and out of the lungs, the need being greatest during periods of high flow. Because airway resistance increases the work of breathing, children with obstructive disease take slower, deeper breaths. When the obstruction is extrathoracic, inspiration is more prolonged than expiration and an inspiratory stridor is commonly heard. When the obstruction is intrathoracic, expiration is prolonged and the child makes use of the accessory expiratory muscles.

When obstruction of the extrathoracic airways occurs, as in croup, the pressures distal (below) to the point of obstruction must become more negative to overcome the resistance; this causes collapse of the distal airways, and the increased turbulence of air moving through the obstructed airways produces an audible crowing sound called a *stridor*. With intra-thoracic airway obstruction as occurs with bronchiolitis and bronchial asthma, the intrapleural pressure becomes more positive during expiration due to air-trapping; this causes collapse of intrathoracic airways and produces an audible *wheezing* or whistling sound during expiration.

RESPIRATORY DISORDERS OF THE NEONATE

The neonatal period is one of transition from placental dependency to air breathing. This transition requires functioning of the surfactant system, the conditioning of the respiratory muscles, and establishment of parallel pulmonary and systemic circulations. Respiratory disorders develop in infants who are born prematurely or who have other problems that impair this transition. Among the respiratory disorders of the neonate are the respiratory distress syndrome, bronchopulmonary dysplasia, and persistent fetal circulation (delayed closure of the ductus arteriosus and foramen ovale).

RESPIRATORY DISTRESS SYNDROME

Respiratory distress syndrome (RDS), also known as hyaline membrane disease, is the one of most common causes of respiratory disease in premature infants. In these babies, pulmonary immaturity, together with surfactant deficiency, leads to alveolar collapse. The type II alveolar cells that produce surfactant do not begin to mature until about the 25th to 28th week of gestation, and, consequently, many premature babies are born with poorly functioning type II alveolar cells and have difficulty producing sufficient amounts of surfactant. Other perinatal conditions that predispose to RDS are asphyxia, maternal diabetes, and delivery by caesarean section (when performed before the 38th week of gestation). The incidence is higher in males than females. Surfactant synthesis is influenced by several hormones including insulin and cortisol. Insulin tends to inhibit surfactant production; this explains why infants of insulin-dependent diabetic mothers are at increased risk of developing RDS. A number of studies have shown that cortisol can accelerate maturation of type II cells and formation of surfactant.[78] The reason that premature babies born by caesarean section are presumably at greater risk of developing RDS is because they are not subjected to the stress of vaginal delivery thought to increase the babies' cortisol levels. These observations have led to administration of corticosteroid drugs before delivery in mothers with babies at high risk for developing RDS.

As discussed in Chapter 26, surfactant reduces the surface tension in the alveoli, thereby reducing the amount of pressure needed to inflate and hold the alveolus open. At birth, the first breath requires high inspiratory pressures to expand the lungs. With normal levels of surfactant, the lungs retain up to 40% of the residual volume after the first breath; and subsequent breaths require far lower inspiratory pressures.[1] With a surfactant deficiency, the lungs collapse between breaths so the infant must work as hard with each successive breath as with the first breath. The airless portions of the lungs becomes stiff and noncompliant. A hyaline membrane forms inside the alveoli as protein- and fibrin-rich fluids are pulled into the alveolar spaces. The fibrin-hyaline membrane constitutes a barrier to gas exchange, leading to hypoxemia and carbon dioxide retention. There is further impairment of surfactant production due to hypoxemia.

Infants with RDS present with multiple signs of respiratory distress, usually within the first 24 hours of birth. Central cyanosis is a prominent sign. Breathing becomes more difficult, and retractions occur as the infant's soft chest wall is pulled in as the diaphragm descends. Grunting sounds occur during expiration. As the tidal volume drops due to atelectasis, the respiration rate increases (usually to 60 to 120 breaths/min) in an effort to maintain normal minute ventilation. Fatigue may develop rapidly due to the increased work of breathing. The stiff lung of infants with RDS also increases resistance to blood flow in the pulmonary circulation. As a result, infants with RDS may develop a hemodynamically significant patent ductus arteriosus (see Chapter 23).

Infants with suspected RDS require continuous cardiorespiratory monitoring. Oxygen and carbon dioxide levels can be assessed through an arterial line (umbilical) or by way of transcutaneous oxygen sensor. Treatment includes administration of supplemental oxygen, continuous positive airway pressure (CPAP) by way of nasal prongs, and often mechanical ventilation. A neutral thermal environment and prevention of hypoglycemia are recommended. A number of surfactant preparations are available that have been effective in preventing or diminishing the severity of RDS.[79, 80]

BRONCHOPULMONARY DYSPLASIA

Bronchopulmonary dysplasia is a chronic pulmonary disease that develops in premature infants who were treated with mechanical ventilation mainly for RDS.[81] The disorder is thought to be a response of the premature lung to early injury. High inspired oxygen concentration and injury from positive pressure ventilation (barotrauma) have been implicated.

Infants with the disorder demonstrate reduced lung compliance, increased airway resistance, and severe expiratory flow limitation. There is mismatching of ventilation and perfusion with development of hypoxemia and hypercapnia. Pulmonary vascular resistance may be increased. The infant may develop pulmonary hypertension and cor pulmonale (right heart failure associated with lung disease).

The child may have tachycardia, dyspnea, chest retractions, barrel chest, and poor weight gain. Hypoxemia and compensated respiratory acidosis are present. Clubbing of the fingers is present in children with severe disease. Children with right heart failure develop tachycardia, tachypnea, hepatomegaly, and periorbital edema.

The treatment is mechanical ventilation and administration of adequate oxygenation. Weaning from ventilation is accomplished gradually, and some infants may require ventilation at home. Rapid lung growth occurs during the first year of life, and lung function usually improves. Adequate nutrition is essential for recovery of infants with bronchopulmonary dysplasia.

Most adolescents and young adults who had bronchopulmonary dysplasia during infancy have some degree of pulmonary dysfunction, consisting of airway obstruction, airway hyperreactivity, or hyperinflation.[82]

RESPIRATORY INFECTIONS IN CHILDREN

In children, respiratory tract infections are common; although they are troublesome, they are usually not serious. Frequent infections occur because the immune system of infants and small children has not been exposed to many common pathogens; consequently, they tend to develop infections with each new exposure. Although most such infections are not serious, the small size of an infant or child's airways tends to promote impaired airflow and obstruction. For example, an infection that causes only sore throat and hoarseness in an adult may result in serious airway obstruction in a small child.

UPPER AIRWAY INFECTIONS

Two serious upper respiratory tract infections are relatively common during early childhood—croup and epiglottitis. Croup is the more common one, and it is usually benign and self-limiting. Epiglottitis, on the other hand, is rapidly progressive and life-threatening. The characteristics of both infections are described in Table 27-4.

Obstruction of the upper airways secondary to infection tends to exert its greatest effect during the inspiratory phase of respiration. Movement of air

TABLE 27-4. CHARACTERISTICS OF EPIGLOTTITIS, CROUP, AND BRONCHIOLITIS IN SMALL CHILDREN

CHARACTERISTICS	EPIGLOTTITIS	CROUP	BRONCHIOLITIS
Common causative agent	*Hemophilus influenzae*, type B, bacterium	Parainfluenza virus	Respiratory syncytial virus
Most commonly affected age group	2–7 years (peak 3½ years)	3 months to 5 years	Less than 2 years (most severe in infants under 6 months)
Onset and preceding history	Sudden onset	Usually follows symptoms of a cold	Preceded by stuffy nose and other signs
Prominent features	Child appears very sick and toxic Sits with mouth open and chin thrust forward Low-pitch stridor, difficulty swallowing, fever, drooling, anxiety *Danger of airway obstruction and asphyxia*	Stridor and a wet, barking cough Usually occurs at night Relieved by exposure to cold or moist air	Breathlessness, rapid shallow breathing, wheezing, cough, and retractions of lower ribs and sternum during inspiration
Usual treatment	Hospitalization Intubation or tracheotomy Treatment with appropriate antibiotic	Mist tent or vaporizor Administration of oxygen	Supportive treatment, administration of oxygen and hydration

through an obstructed upper airway, particularly the vocal cords in the larynx, causes stridor. Impairment of the expiratory phase of respiration can also occur, causing wheezing. With mild to moderate obstruction, inspiratory stridor is more prominent than expiratory wheezing because the airways tend to dilate with expiration. When the swelling and obstruction become severe, the airways can no longer dilate during expiration and both stridor and wheezing occur.

Cartilaginous support of the trachea and the larynx is poorly developed in infants and small children. As a result, these structures are soft and tend to collapse when the airway is obstructed and the child cries, causing the inspiratory pressures to become more negative. When this happens, both the stridor and inspiratory effort are increased. The phenomenon of airway collapse in the small child is analogous to what happens when a thick beverage, such as a milkshake, is drunk through a soft paper straw. The straw collapses when the negative pressure produced by the sucking effort exceeds the flow of liquid through the straw.

Croup. Croup is a viral infection that affects the larynx, trachea, and bronchi. The parainfluenza viruses account for about 75% all cases; the remaining 25% of cases are caused by adenoviruses, respiratory syncytial virus, influenza A and B virus, and measles virus. Viral croup is generally seen in children aged 3 months to 5 years.[77] Because the subglottic area is normally the narrowest part of the respiratory tree in

this age group, the obstruction is usually greatest in this area.

Croup is characterized by inspiratory stridor, hoarseness, and a barking cough. The British use the term *croup* to describe the cry of the crow or raven, and this is undoubtedly how the term originated. One form of croup, spasmodic croup, characteristically occurs at night. The episode usually lasts several hours and may recur several nights in a row. Spasmodic croup tends to recur with subsequent respiratory infections.

Although the respiratory manifestations of croup often appear suddenly, they are usually preceded by upper respiratory infections that cause rhinorrhea (runny nose), coryza (common cold), hoarseness, and a low-grade fever. In most children, the manifestation of croup only advances to stridor and slight dyspnea, before they begin to recover. The symptoms usually subside when the child is exposed to moist air. For example, letting the bathroom shower run and then taking the child into the bathroom often brings prompt and dramatic relief of symptoms. A mist tent or vaporizer is used for more continuous treatment. Exposure to cold air also seems to relieve the airway spasm; often, the severe symptoms are relieved simply because the child is exposed to cold air on the way to the hospital emergency room.

However, airway obstruction may progress in some children. As obstruction increases, the stridor becomes continuous and is associated with nasal flaring with substernal and intercostal retractions. Agitation and crying aggravate the signs and symptoms, and the child prefers to sit up or be held upright. In the cyanotic, pale, or obstructed child, any manipulation of the pharynx, including use of tongue depressor can cause cardiorespiratory arrest and should only be done in a medical setting that has the facilities for emergency airway management.

Most children with spasmodic croup can be effectively managed at home. An environment of high cold humidity (mist tent or humidifier) serves to lessen irritation and prevent drying of secretions. The child should be disturbed as little as possible and carefully monitored for signs of respiratory distress. Other treatments may be required when a humidifier or mist tent is ineffective. One method is to administer a racemic mixture of epinephrine (L-epinephrine and D-epinephrine) by positive pressure breathing through a face mask. Establishment of an artificial airway may become necessary in severe airway obstruction. Viral and spasmodic croup do not respond to antibiotics; expectorants, bronchodilating agents, and antihistamines are not helpful.[76]

Epiglottitis. Acute epiglottitis is a dramatic, potentially fatal condition caused by *Hemophilus influenzae*, type B, bacterium. The condition usually occurs in children 2 to 7 years of age with a peak incidence at about 3 1/2 years.[76, 77] It is characterized by inflammatory edema of the supraglottic area, including the epiglottis and pharyngeal structures, that comes on suddenly, bringing danger of airway obstruction and asphyxia. Within a matter of hours, epiglottitis may progress to complete obstruction of the airway and death unless adequate treatment is instituted.

The child appears pale, toxic, and lethargic and assumes a distinctive position—sitting up with the mouth open and the chin thrust forward. Difficulty in swallowing, a muffled voice, drooling, fever, and extreme anxiety are present. Moderate-to-severe respiratory distress is evident. There are an inspiratory and sometimes expiratory stridor, flaring of the nares, and inspiratory retractions of the suprasternal notch, supraclavicular, and intercostal spaces. Usually no other family members are ill with acute respiratory disease.

The child with epiglottitis requires immediate hospitalization. Immediate establishment of an airway by either endotracheal tube or tracheotomy is usually needed. If epiglottitis is suspected, the child should never be forced to lie down because this causes the epiglottis to fall backward and may lead to complete airway obstruction. Examination of the throat with a tongue blade or other instrument may

cause cardiopulmonary arrest and should be done only by medical personnel experienced in intubation of small children. It is also unwise to attempt any procedure, such as drawing blood, that would heighten the child's anxiety because this, too, could precipitate airway spasm and cause death.

Recovery from epiglottitis is usually rapid and uneventful once an adequate airway has been established and appropriate antibiotic therapy has been initiated.

It should be pointed out that epiglottitis can occur in adults as well as children. At present, the incidence is small (an estimated 9.7 cases per million) but appears to be increasing. In adults, epiglottitis may present with acute respiratory compromise or as a milder form of disease. Although the causative agent or agents have not been identified, *Hemophilus influenzae* does not appear to be a primary causative agent in adults. Also, airway closure is less of a threat in adults; it does occur, however, and provision for emergency tracheotomy should be available.[83]

LOWER AIRWAY INFECTIONS

Lower airway infections produce air trapping with prolonged expiration. Wheezing results from bronchospasm, mucosal inflammation, and edema. The child presents with increased expiratory effort, increased respiratory rate, and wheezing. If the infection is severe, there are also marked intercostal retractions and signs of impending respiratory failure.

Bronchiolitis. Acute bronchiolitis is a viral infection of the lower airways, most commonly caused by the respiratory syncytial virus.[84] Other viruses, such as adenovirus, parainfluenza, and rhinovirus, have also been implicated as causative agents. The infection produces inflammatory obstruction of the small airways and necrosis of the cells lining the lower airways. It occurs during the first 2 years of life with a peak incidence at approximately 6 months of age.[76, 77] The source of infection is usually a family member with a minor respiratory illness. Older children and adults tolerate bronchiolar edema much better than infants and do not develop the clinical picture of bronchiolitis. Because the resistance to airflow in a tube is related to the fourth power of the radius, even minor swelling of bronchioles in an infant may produce profound changes in airflow.

Most affected infants who develop bronchiolitis have a history of a mild upper respiratory tract infection. These symptoms usually last several days and may be accompanied by fever and diminished appetite. There is then a gradual development of respiratory distress, characterized by a wheezy cough, dyspnea, and irritability. The infant is usually able to take in sufficient air but has trouble exhaling it. Air becomes trapped in the lung distal to the site of obstruction and interferes with gas exchange. Hypoxemia and, in severe cases, hypercapnia may develop. Airway obstruction may produce air trapping and hyperinflation of the lungs or collapse of the alveoli. Babies with acute bronchiolitis have a typical appearance, marked by breathlessness with rapid respirations, a distressing cough, and retractions of the lower ribs and sternum. Crying and feeding exaggerate these signs. Wheezing and rales may or may not be present depending on the degree of airway obstruction. In infants with severe airway obstruction, wheezing decreases as the airflow diminishes. Generally, the most critical phase of the disease is the first 24 to 72 hours. Cyanosis, pallor, listlessness, and sudden diminution or absence of breath sounds indicate impending respiratory failure. The characteristics of bronchiolitis are described in Table 27-4.

Infants with respiratory distress are usually hospitalized. Treatment is supportive and includes administration of humidified oxygen to relieve hypoxia. A position that facilitates respiratory movements (elevation of the head) and avoids airway compression is used. Handling is kept at a minimum to avoid tiring. Because the infection is viral, antibiotics are not effective and are given only for a secondary bacterial infection. Dehydration may occur as the result of increased insensible water losses because of the rapid respiratory rate and feeding difficulties, and measures to ensure adequate hydration are needed. Recovery begins after the first 48 to 72 hours and is usually rapid and complete.[14]

SIGNS OF IMPENDING RESPIRATORY FAILURE

Respiratory problems of infants and small children are often of sudden origin, and recovery is usually rapid and complete. However, children are at risk for development of airway obstruction and respiratory failure resulting from obstructive disorders or lung infection. The child with epiglottitis is at risk for development of airway obstruction; the child with bronchiolitis is at risk for development of respiratory failure resulting from impaired gas exchange. The signs and symptoms of impending respiratory failure are listed in Chart 27-1.

In summary, acute respiratory disease is the most common cause of illness in infancy and childhood, accounting for 50% of illness in children under 5 years of age and 30% of illness in children between 5 and 12 years of age. Although other body systems are physiologically ready for extrauterine life as early as 25 weeks of gestation, the lungs take longer.

CHART 27-1: SIGNS OF RESPIRATORY DISTRESS AND IMPENDING RESPIRATORY FAILURE IN THE INFANT AND SMALL CHILD

Severe increase in respiratory effort, including severe retractions or grunting, decreased chest movement
Cyanosis that is not relieved by administration of oxygen (40%)
Heart rate of 150 per minute or greater and increasing
Bradycardia
Very rapid breathing (rate 60 per minute in the newborn to 6 months or above 30 per minute in children 6 months to 2 years)
Very depressed breathing (rate 20 per minute or below)
Retractions of the supraclavicular area, sternum, epigastrium, and intercostal spaces
Extreme anxiety and agitation
Fatigue
Decreased level of consciousness

Immaturity of the respiratory system is a major cause of morbidity and mortality in premature infants.

Lung development may be divided into five stages: (1) embryonic period, (2) glandular period, (3) canicular period, (4) saccular period, and (5) alveolar period. The first three phases are devoted to development of the conducting airways, and the last two phases are devoted to development of the gas exchange portion of the lung. By the 25th to 28th week of gestation, sufficient terminal air sacs are present to permit survival. It is also during this period that type II alveolar cells that produce surfactant begin to function. Lung development is incomplete at birth; an infant is born with only one eighth to one sixth the adult number of alveoli. Alveoli continue to be formed during early childhood, reaching the adult number of 300 million alveoli by 5 to 6 years of age.

Children with restrictive lung disease breathe at faster rates, and their respiratory excursions are shallow. An expiratory grunt is common as the child tries to raise the functional residual capacity by closing the glottis at the end of expiration. Obstruction of the extrathoracic airways often produces turbulence of airflow and audible inspiratory crowing sound called a *stridor*, and obstruction of the intrathoracic airways produces an audible expiratory *wheezing* or whistling sound. Respiratory distress syndrome is the one of most common cause of respiratory disease in premature infants. In these babies, pulmonary immaturity, together with surfactant deficiency, leads to alveolar collapse. Bronchopulmonary dysplasia is a chronic pulmonary disease that develops in premature infants who were treated with mechanical ventilation.

Because of the smallness of the airway of infants and children, respiratory tract infections in these groups are often more serious. Infections that may cause only a sore throat and hoarseness in the adult may produce serious obstruction in the child. Among the respiratory tract infections that affect small children are croup, epiglottitis, and bronchiolitis. Epiglottitis is a life-threatening supraglottic infection carrying the danger of airway obstruction and asphyxia.

■ REFERENCES

1. Cotran, R.S., Kumar, V., Robbins, S.L. (1989). *Robbins' pathologic basis of disease* (4th ed., pp. 315, 375, 401, 524, 780–832). Philadelphia: W.B. Saunders.
2. Lowenstein, S.R., & Parrino, T.A. (1987). Management of the common cold. *Advances in Internal Medicine, 32,* 207.
3. Hendley, J.A., Gwaltney, J.M., Jr., & Jordon, W.S. (1969). Rhinovirus infections in an industrial population. IV. Infections within the families of employees during two fall peaks of respiratory illness. *American Journal of Epidemiology, 89,* 184.
4. Beem, M.O. (1969). Acute respiratory illness in nursery school children: A longitudinal study of occurrence of illness and respiratory viruses. *American Journal of Epidemiology, 90,* 30.
5. Hendley, J.O., Wenzel, R.P., & Gwaltney, J.M., Jr. (1973). Transmission of rhinovirus colds by self-inoculation. *New England Journal of Medicine, 288,* 1361.
6. Gwaltney, J.M., Jr., Moskalski, P.B., & Hendley, J.O. (1978). Hand-to-hand transmission of rhinovirus colds. *Annals of Internal Medicine, 88,* 464.
7. Cohen, S., Tyrerell, D.A.J., & Smith, A.P. (1991). Psychological stress and susceptibility to the common cold. *New England Journal of Medicine, 325,* 606–612.
8. Anderson, T.W., Reid, B.W., & Beaton, G.H. (1974). Vitamin C and the common cold: A double blind study. *Canadian Medical Association Journal, 107,* 503–508.
9. Miller, J.Z., Nance, W.E., Norton, J.A., et al. (1977). Therapeutic effect of vitamin C: A co-twin study. *Journal of the American Medical Association, 237,* 248–251.
10. Carr, B., Einstein, R., Lai, L.Y., Martin, N.G., & Starmer, G. A. (1981). Vitamin C and the common cold. *Medical Journal of Australia, 2,* 411–412.
11. Small, P.A., Jr. (1990). Influenza: Pathogenesis and host defense. *Hospital Practice, 25*(11A), 51–62.
12. Douglas, R.G. (1990). Prophylaxis and treatment of influenza. *New England Journal of Medicine, 322,* 443–450.
13. Prevention and control of influenza: Recommendations of the Immunization Practices Advisory Committee (ACIP). (1992). *Morbidity and Mortality Weekly Report, 40*(RR-6), 1–15.
14. Eickhoff, T.C. (1990). Current immunization practices in adults. *Hospital Practice,* (10A), 114–115.
15. Centers for Disease Control. (1991). Update on adult immunization. Recommendations of the Immunization Practices Advisory Committee (ACIP). *Morbidity and Mortality Weekly Report, 40*(RR-12), 42–44.
16. Andreoli, T.E., Carpenter, C.C.J., Plum, F., & Smith, L.H. (1986). *Cecil essentials of medicine* (pp. 164–165). Philadelphia: W.B. Saunders.
17. Murray, J.F., & Mills, J. (1990). Pulmonary infectious complications of human immunodeficiency virus infection. Part I. *American Review of Respiratory Disease, 141,* 1356–1372.
18. Henry, S.B., & Holzemr, W.L. (1992). Critical care management of the patient with HIV infection who has *Pneumocystis carinii. Heart & Lung, 21,* 243–249.
19. Hughes, W.T. (1990). The prevention of *P. carinii* pneumonia. *Hospital Practice, 25*(4A), 33–43.
20. Goldsmith, R. (1993). Infectious diseases: Protozoal. In S.A. Schroeder, L.M. Tierney, S.J. McPhee, et al. (Eds.). *Current diagnosis and treatment* (pp. 1133–1135). Norwalk, CT: Appleton & Lange.
21. Snider, D.E. (1991). Final 1990 tuberculosis cases and case rates. Atlanta Centers for Disease Control. *Morbidity and Mortality Weekly Report, 39*(10), 153–157.
22. Rieder, H.L., Gauthen, G.M., Kelly, G.D., et al. Tuberculosis in the United States. *Journal of the American Medical Association, 262,* 385–389.
23. Jereb, J.A., Kelly, G.D., Dooley, S.W., et al. (1991). Tuberculosis morbidity in the United States: Final data, 1990. *Morbidity and Mortality Weekly Report, 40* (No.SS-3), 24–26.
24. American Thoracic Society. (1990). Diagnostic standards and classification of tuberculosis. *American Review of Respiratory Disease, 142,* 725–735.
25. Bernardo, J. (1991). Tuberculosis: A disease of the 1990s. *Hospital Practice, 25*(10A), 195–222.
26. Centers for Disease Control. (1992). Management of people exposed to multidrug-resistant tuberculosis. *Morbidity and Mortality Weekly Report, 41*(RR-11), 61–71.
27. Davies, S.F., & Sarosi, G.A. (1983). Fungal infections of the lung. *Postgraduate Medicine, 73*(6), 242.
28. Hammarsten, J.E., & Hammarsten, J.F. (1990). Histoplasmosis: Recognition and treatment. *Hospital Practice, 25*(6A), 95–126.
29. Davis, S.F., & Sarosi, G.A. (1983). Fungal infections of the lung. *Postgraduate Medicine, 73*(6), 242.
30. Light, R.W. (1990). *Pleural diseases* (2nd ed.). Philadelphia: Lea & Febiger.
31. Sahn, S.A. (1981). Pleural manifestations of pulmonary disease. *Hospital Practice, 16*(3), 73–89.
32. Stauffer, J.L. (1993). Pulmonary diseases. In S.A. Schroeder, L.M. Tierney, S.J. McPhee, et al. (Eds.). *Current diagnosis and treatment* (pp. 189–201, 229–230, 232–238, 255–261). Norwalk, CT: Appleton & Lange.
33. Guenther, C.A., & Welch, M.H. (1982). *Pulmonary medicine* (2nd ed., pp. 524–526). Philadelphia: J.B. Lippincott.
34. National Heart, Lung and Blood Institute. (1991). National Asthma Education Program Expert Panel. Guidelines for diagnosis and management of asthma. *Pediatric Asthma Allergy and Immunology, 5*(2), 57–188.
35. Sly, R.M. (1984). Increases in deaths from asthma. *Annals of Allergy, 53,* 20–25.
36. Benatar, S.R. (1986). Fatal asthma. *New England Journal of Medicine, 314,* 423–428.
37. McFadden, E.R., Jr. (1991). Fatal and near-fatal asthma. *New England Journal of Medicine, 324,* 409–411.
38. Cockcroft, D.W. (1990). Airway hyperresponsiveness in asthma. *Hospital Practice, 25*(1A), 111–129.
39. Roberts, J.A. (1988). Exercise-induced asthma in athletes. *Sports Medicine, 6,* 193–195.
40. Haltom, J.R., & Strunk, R.C. (1986). Pathogenesis of exercise-induced asthma: Implications for treatment. *Annual Review of Medicine, 37,* 143–148.
41. McFadden, E.R., & Ingram, R.H., Jr. (1979). Exercise-induced asthma. *New England Journal of Medicine, 301,* 763–769.
42. Young, S., Le Souef, P.N., Geelhoed, G.C., et al. (1991). The influence of a family history of asthma and parental smoking on airway responsiveness in early infancy. *New England Journal of Medicine, 324,* 1168–1173.
43. Behrman, R.E. (1992). *Nelson textbook of pediatrics* (13th ed., pp. 587–596). Philadelphia: W.B. Saunders.
44. Larsen, G.L. (1992). Asthma in children. *New England Journal of Medicine, 326,* 1540–1545.
45. Sporik, R., Holgate, S.T., Platts-Mills, T.A.E., et al. (1990). Exposure to house dust mite antigen allergen (*Der p 1*) and the development of asthma in childhood. *New England Journal of Medicine, 323,* 502–507.

46. West, J.B. (1987). *Pulmonary pathophysiology: The essentials* (3rd ed., pp. 59–60, 125). Baltimore: Williams & Wilkins.

47. American Thoracic Society. (1987). Standards for the diagnosis and care of patients with chronic obstructive lung disease (COPD) and asthma. *American Review of Respiratory Disease, 136,* 225–228.

48. Kueppers, F., & Black, L.P. (1974). Alpha-antitrypsin and its deficiency. *American Review of Respiratory Disease, 110,* 176.

49. Crystal, R. (1991). α_1-Antitrypsin deficiency: Pathogenesis and treatment. *Hospital Practice, 26*(2A), 81–94.

50. Owens, G.R. (1992). Advances in the treatment of chronic obstructive pulmonary disease. *Hospital Formulary, 27,* 1012–1027.

51. Hodgkin, J.E., Balchum, O.J., Kass, I., et al. (1975). Chronic obstructive airway disease. *Journal of the American Medical Association, 232,* 1253–1260.

52. Kim, M.J. (1984). Respiratory muscle training: Implications for patient care. *Heart & Lung, 13,* 333–339.

53. Pardy, R.L., Rivington, R., Daspas, P.J., et al. (1981). Inspiratory muscle training compared with physiotherapy in patients with chronic airflow limitations. *American Review of Respiratory Disease, 123,* 421–425.

54. Nocturnal Oxygen Therapy Group Trial. (1980). Continuous or nocturnal oxygen therapy in hypoxemic chronic obstructive lung disease. *Annals of Internal Medicine, 93,* 391–398.

55. Tirlapur, D.T.M., & Mir, M.A. (1982). Nocturnal hypoxemia associated with electrocardiographic changes in patients with chronic obstructive airways disease. *New England Journal of Medicine, 306,* 125–130.

56. Fletcher, E.C., & Levin, D.C. (1984). Cardiopulmonary hemodynamics during sleep in subjects with chronic obstructive pulmonary disease. *Chest, 85,* 6–13.

57. Murray, J.F. (1991). New presentations of bronchiectasis. *Hospital Practice, 26*(3A), 55–74.

58. Collins, F.S., Riordran, J.R., & Lap-Chee, T. (1990). The cystic fibrosis gene: Isolation and significance. *Hospital Practice, 25*(10A), 47–57.

59. Davis, P.B. (1991). Cystic fibrosis from bench to bedside. *New England Journal of Medicine, 325,* 575–576.

60. Knowles, M.R., Church, N.L., Waltner, W.E., et al. (1990). A pilot study of aerosolized amiloride for the treatment of lung disease in cystic fibrosis. *New England Journal of Medicine, 322,* 1189–1194.

61. Crystal, R.G., Bitterman, P.B., Rennard, S.I., et al. (1984). Interstitial lung diseases of unknown cause. *New England Journal of Medicine, 310,* 154–166, 235–244.

62. Crystal, R.G. (1991). Sarcoidosis. In J.P. Wilson, E. Braunwald, & K.J. Isselbacher (Eds.). *Harrison's principles of internal medicine* (pp. 1463–1469). New York: McGraw-Hill.

63. Goldhaber, S.Z. (1991). Managing pulmonary embolism. *Hospital Practice, 26*(9A), 37–48.

64. Dalen, J.E., & Alpert, J.S. (1975). Natural history of pulmonary embolism. *Progress in Cardiovascular Diseases, 17,* 259.

65. Goldfaber, S.Z., & Morpurgo, M. (1992). Diagnosis, treatment and prevention of pulmonary embolism: Report of the WHO/International Society and Federation of Cardiology Task Force. *Journal of the American Medical Association, 268,* 1727–1733.

66. Stratton, M.B. (1990). Ventilation–perfusion scintigraphy in diagnosis of pulmonary thromboembolism. *AACN Focus on Critical Care, 17,* 287–293.

67. Collins, R., Scrimgeour, A., Yusuf, S., et al. (1988). Reduction in fatal pulmonary embolism and venous thrombosis by perioperative administration of subcutaneous heparin. *New England Journal of Medicine, 318,* 1162–1172.

68. Faber, L.P. (1991). Lung cancer. In A.I. Hollieb, D.J. Fink, & G.P. Murphy (Eds.). *Clinical oncology* (pp. 194–212). Atlanta: American Cancer Society.

69. Kumar, V., Cotran, R.S., & Robbins, S.L. (1992). *Basic pathology* (5th ed., pp. 428–332). Philadelphia: W.B. Saunders.

70. Lin, A.Y., & Ihde, D.C. (1992). Recent developments in the treatment of lung cancer. *Journal of the American Medical Association, 267,* 1661–1664.

71. Zander, J., & Hazinski, M.F. (1992). Pulmonary disorders. In M.F. Hazinski (Ed.). *Nursing care of the critically ill child* (2nd ed., pp. 395–407). Philadelphia: W.B. Saunders.

72. Hanson, T., & Corbet, A. (1991). Lung development and function. In H.W. Taeusch, R.A. Ballard, & M.E. Avery (Eds.). *Shaffer and Avery's diseases of the newborn* (6th ed., pp. 461–469). Philadelphia: W.B. Saunders.

73. Turner, B.S. (1990). Embryologic and physiologic basis for neonatal respiration. *AACN Clinical Issues in Critical Care Nursing, 1,* 389–398.

74. Moore, K. (1988). *The developing human* (4th ed., pp. 207–216). Philadelphia: W.B. Saunders.

75. Davis, G.M., & Bureau, M.A. (1987). Pulmonary and chest wall mechanics in the control of respiration in the newborn. *Clinics in Perinatology, 14,* 551–579.

76. Berhrman, R.E., Kliegman, R.M., Nelson, W.E., & Vaughan, V.C. (Eds.). (1992). *Nelson textbook of pediatrics* (13th ed., pp. 1049–1083). Philadelphia: W.B. Saunders.

77. Oski, F.A., DeAnglis, C.D., Feegor, R.D., et al. (1990). *Principles and practice of pediatrics* (pp. 330–335, 903–908, 1332–1334). Philadelphia: J.B. Lippincott.

78. Caminiti, S.P., & Young, S.L. (1991). The pulmonary surfactant system. *Hospital Practice, 26*(A), 87–100.

79. Merenstein, G.B. (Chairman). (1991). American Academy of Pediatrics: Committee on Fetus and Newborn: Surfactant replacement therapy for respiratory distress syndrome. *Pediatrics, 87,* 946–947.

80. Avery, M.E., & Merritt, T.A. (1991). Surfactant-replacement therapy. *New England Journal of Medicine, 324,* 910–911.

81. Monin, P. (1987). The management of bronchopulmonary dysplagia. *Clinics in Perinatology, 14,* 531–549.

82. Northwood, W.B., Moss, R.B., Carlisle, K.B., et al. (1990). Late pulmonary sequelae of bronchopulmonary dysplasia. *New England Journal of Medicine, 323,* 1793–1799.

83. Baker, A.S., & Eavey, R.D. (1986). Adult supraglottitis (epiglottitis). *New England Journal of Medicine, 314,* 1185.

84. Corey, M.A., & Clore, E.R. (1991). Management of the infant with respiratory syncytial virus. *Journal of Pediatric Nursing, 6,* 93–98.

■ BIBLIOGRAPHY

Ashcraft, C.K., & Steele, R.W. (1988). Epiglottitis: A pediatric emergency. *Journal of Respiratory Disease, 9,* 48.

Australian, R. (1986). Pneumococcal pneumonia: Diagnosis, epidemiologic, therapeutic, and prophylactic considerations. *Chest, 90,* 738.

Bass, J.B. (1989). The face of TB changes again. *Hospital Practice, 24*(4A), 81–100.

Bentley, D.W. (1988). Bacterial pneumonia in the elderly. *Hospital Practice, 23*(12A), 99–115.

Bjornsdottir, V.S., & Busse, W.W. (1992). Respiratory infections and asthma. *Medical Clinics of North America, 76,* 195–214.

Brouilletee, R.T., Weese-Mayer, D.E., & Hunt, C.E. (1990). Breathing control in infants and children. *Hospital Practice, 25*(8A), 82–103.

Cockcroft, D.W. (1990). Airway hyperresponsiveness in asthma. *Hospital Practice, 25*(1A), 111–129.

Corrigan, C.J., & Kay, A.B. (1991). The roles of inflammatory cells in the pathogenesis of asthma and chronic obstructive pulmonary disease. *American Review of Respiratory Disease, 143,* 1165–1168.

Finegold, S.M. (1991). Aspiration pneumonia. *Reviews of Infectious Diseases, 13*(Suppl 9), S737–742.

Goldhaber, S.Z. (1992). Recent advances in the diagnosis and lytic therapy for pulmonary embolism. *Chest, 101* (Suppl), 183S.

Hirsch, J. (Ed.). (1986). Venous thromboembolism: Prevention, diagnosis and treatment. *Chest, 89*(Suppl), 369 (entire issue).

Hughes, W. (1987). *Pneumocystis carinii* pneumonitis. *New England Journal of Medicine, 317,* 1021.

Insel, R.A., & Wasserman, S.I. (1990). Asthma: A disorder of adrenergic receptors. *FASEB Journal, 4,* 2732–2736.

Jones, D.B., & Deveau, D. (1991). Nasal prong CPAP: A proven method of reducing chronic lung disease. *Neonatal Network, 10*(4), 7–15.

Kendig, J.W., Notter, R.H., Cox, C., et al. (1991). A comparison of surfactant as immediate prophylaxis and as rescue therapy for newborns less than 30 weeks gestation. *New England Journal of Medicine, 324,* 865–871.

Lowenstein, S. R. (1987). Management of the common cold. *Advances in Internal Medicine 32,* 207.

Massaro, D. (1990). Regulation of alveolar formation. *Hospital Practice, 25*(9A), 81–88.

Matthay, R.A., Niederman, M.S., & Wiedeman, H.P. (1990). Cardiovascular-pulmonary interaction in chronic obstructive pulmonary disease with special reference to the pathogenesis and management of cor pulmonale. *Medical Clinics of North America, 74,* 571–578.

McFadden, E.R. (1987). Exercise and asthma. *New England Journal of Medicine, 317,* 502.

Moser, K.M. (1990). Venous thromboembolism. *American Review of Respiratory Disease, 141,* 235.

Nichols, D.G. (1991). Respiratory muscle performance in infants and children. *Journal of Pediatrics, 118,* 493–502.

O'Duffy, J.D. (1990). Screening for cystic fibrosis. *New England Journal of Medicine, 322,* 328–329.

Phelan, P.D. (1991). Hyperresponsiveness as a determinant of outcome in childhood asthma. *American Review of Respiratory Disease, 143,* 1463–1467.

Possmayer, F. (1991). The role of surfactant-associated proteins (editorial). *American Review of Respiratory Disease, 142,* 749–752.

Quinton, P.M. (1990). Cystic fibrosis: A disease of electrolyte transport. *FASEB Journal, 4,* 2709–2717.

Rochester, D.F. (1991). The diaphragm in COPD. *New England Journal of Medicine, 325,* 961–962.

Rubin, L.J. (1989). Approach to diagnosis and treatment of pulmonary hypertension. *Chest, 96,* 659.

Skoner, D., & Caliguiri, L. (1988). The wheezing infant. *Pediatric Clinics of North America, 35,* 101–129.

Thomas, P.D., & Hunninghake, G.W. (1987). Current concepts of the pathogenesis of sarcoidosis. *American Review of Respiratory Disease, 135,* 747.

Toogood, J.H. (1991). Inhaled steroids in chronic asthma. *Hospital Practice, 26*(4A), 1526.

Voelkel, N.F. (1986). Mechanisms of hypoxic pulmonary vasoconstriction: New perspectives. *Chest, 89,* 279.

Wilfert, C.M. (1990). Epidemiology of *Haemophilus influenza* type b infections. *Pediatrics* (Suppl), 631–634.

Wollschlager, C.M., & Khan, F. (1986). Secondary pulmonary hypertension. *Heart & Lung, 15,* 336.

Woolcock, A.J., Anderson, S.D., Peat, J.K., et al. (1991). Characteristics of bronchial hyperresponsiveness in chronic obstructive pulmonary disease and in asthma. *American Review of Respiratory Disease, 143,* 1438–1443.

ALTERATIONS IN VENTILATION, IMPAIRED GAS EXCHANGE, AND RESPIRATORY FAILURE

■ OBJECTIVES

After you have studied this chapter, you should be able to meet the following objectives:

■ Describe the type of periodic breathing known as *Cheyne-Stokes breathing*.

■ Define *dyspnea* and list three types of conditions in which dyspnea occurs.

■ Differentiate total and alveolar ventilation.

■ List at least three categories of drugs that can depress respiratory function.

■ Define *sleep apnea*.

■ Compare the respiratory activities in each of the four stages of sleep.

■ State the signs and symptoms of sleep apnea and differentiate between central and obstructive sleep apnea.

■ Describe methods that might be used in the diagnosis of sleep apnea.

■ Cite four general causes of hyperventilation syndrome.

■ State the signs and symptoms of hyperventilation syndrome.

■ Relate the alterations in arterial carbon dioxide levels to the production of altered body function in hyperventilation syndrome.

■ Describe the measures used in the treatment of hyperventilation syndrome.

■ Define the terms *hypoxia*, *hypoxemia*, and *hypercapnia*.

■ List the four types of hypoxia and cite causes of each.

■ Compare the manifestations of acute hypoxia and chronic hypoxia.

■ Explain why cyanosis may not be an accurate diagnostic criterion for hypoxemia.

■ State the four causes of hypercapnia.

■ Define the *respiratory quotient* and relate to the production of carbon dioxide with carbohydrate, fat, and protein metabolism.

■ State a general definition for *acute respiratory failure*.

■ Explain the pathology of respiratory failure by citing clinical examples.

■ Describe the pathologic lung changes that occur in adult respiratory distress syndrome (ARDS) and relate to the clinical manifestations of the disorder.

Carol Mattson Porth: PATHOPHYSIOLOGY: CONCEPTS OF
ALTERED HEALTH STATES, 4th ed. © 1994, 1990, 1986, 1982
J.B. Lippincott Company

The major function of the lungs is to oxygenate and remove carbon dioxide from the blood as a means of supporting the metabolic functions of body cells. Hypoventilation and respiratory failure result in hypoxia and hypercapnia, whereas hyperventilation causes hypocapnia. The content in this chapter has been organized into four sections: (1) alterations in breathing patterns, (2) alterations in control of ventilation, (3) impaired blood gases, and (4) acute respiratory failure.

■ ALTERATIONS IN BREATHING PATTERNS

The act of breathing normally is effortless and does not require conscious thought. In an adult, the normal rate of respiration is about 16 to 18 breaths per minute, with about one breath for every four heartbeats. The rate increases with exercise and other activities that raise the body's metabolism. In normal breathing, expiration is largely passive and accomplished within 4 to 6 seconds.

Respiratory movements are smooth, with equal expansion of both sides of the chest. In men, respiratory movements are primarily diaphragmatic, whereas in women, there is greater movement of the intercostal muscles. When breathing becomes labored, the accessory muscles of the neck come into play, and there may be flaring of the nostrils.

The suffix -pnea refers to breathing. *Tachypnea* is rapid breathing, and *hyperpnea* is an increase in both the rate and the depth of respiration. Hyperpnea is normal during exercise. *Bradypnea* is an abnormally slow respiratory rate. *Hyperventilation* is ventilation in excess of that needed for normal elimination of carbon dioxide. It is associated with decreased partial pressure of carbon dioxide (P_{CO_2}) in the arterial blood and respiratory alkalosis (see Chapter 29). Hypoventilation is ventilation that is inadequate for alveolocapillary exchange of carbon dioxide and oxygen. Hypoventilation causes an increase in P_{CO_2} and respiratory acidosis as well as a decrease in the partial pressure of oxygen (P_{O_2}) in the arterial blood.

Periodic breathing describes a breathing pattern in which there are episodes of apnea, or absence of breathing. *Cheyne-Stokes breathing* is a type of periodic breathing characterized by periods of slowly waxing and waning respirations separated by a period of apnea that lasts for up to 30 seconds. Cheyne-Stokes breathing is thought to be caused by impaired function of the central feedback mechanisms that buffer the respiratory center's response to carbon dioxide. For Cheyne-Stokes respirations to occur, the hyperpneic and apneic phases of the breathing pattern must be long enough for sufficient changes in the carbon dioxide content of the blood to occur. During the hyperpneic phase of Cheyne-Stokes breathing, carbon dioxide levels fall, leading to a decreased stimulus for ventilation and, finally, to apnea. The period of apnea in turn causes carbon dioxide to accumulate in the blood, and this leads to the hyperpneic phase of the respiratory pattern. Two types of disease conditions predispose to Cheyne-Stokes breathing. One is congestive heart failure, in which there is a great delay in moving blood with its altered carbon dioxide content from the lungs to the chemoreceptors in the brain that control ventilation. The other is impaired function of the brain centers that regulate the feedback mechanisms that control respiration. An area of the brain stem controls the feedback gain of the respiratory center in response to changes in the carbon dioxide level. Cheyne-Stokes respirations may be seen in people who have brain lesions that affect this area. They also occur in healthy people as an adaptive response to high altitudes, especially during sleep.

DYSPNEA

Dyspnea is a subjective sensation or a person's perception of difficulty in breathing that includes both the perception of labored breathing and the reaction to that sensation.[1] The terms *dyspnea, breathlessness,* and *shortness of breath* often are used interchangeably. Dyspnea is observed in at least three major cardiopulmonary disease states: (1) primary lung diseases such as pneumonia, asthma, and emphysema; (2) heart disease that is characterized by pulmonary congestion; and (3) neuromuscular disorders such as myasthenia gravis and muscular dystrophy that affect the respiratory muscles. Although dyspnea commonly is associated with respiratory disease, its presence does not necessarily imply pathology; dyspnea occurs during exercise, particularly in untrained people.

The cause of dyspnea is unknown. Four types of mechanisms have been proposed to explain the sensation: (1) stimulation of lung receptors; (2) increased sensitivity to changes in ventilation perceived through central nervous system mechanisms; (3) reduced ventilatory capacity or breathing reserve; and (4) stimulation of neural receptors in the muscle fibers of the intercostals and diaphragm and of receptors in the skeletal joints.[2] The first of the suggested mechanisms is stimulation of lung receptors. These receptors are stimulated by the contraction of bronchial smooth muscle, the stretch of the bronchial wall, pulmonary congestion, and conditions that decrease lung compliance. The second category of proposed mechanisms focuses on central nervous system (CNS) mechanisms that transmit information to the cortex regarding respiratory muscle weakness or a discrepancy between the increased effort of breathing and inadequate respiratory muscle contraction. The third type of mechanism focuses on a reduction in ventilatory capacity or breathing reserve. A reduction in breathing reserve (maximum voluntary ventilation not being used during a given activity) to less than 65% to 75% usually correlates well with dyspnea. The fourth possible mechanism is stimulation of muscle and joint receptors in the respiratory musculature because of a discrepancy in the tension generated by these muscles and the tidal volume that results. These receptors, once stimulated, transmit signals that bring about an awareness of the breathing discrepancy.

Like other subjective symptoms, such as fatigue and pain, dyspnea is difficult to quantify because it relies on a person's perception of the problem. The most common method for measuring dyspnea is a retrospective determination of the level of daily activity at which a person experiences dyspnea. A number of scales are available for this use. One of these uses four grades of dyspnea to evaluate disability (Table 28-1).[2] The visual analog scale is used to assess breathing difficulty that occurs with a given activity, such as walking a certain distance. It can also be used to assess dyspnea over time. The treatment of dyspnea depends on the cause. The techniques used clinically to reduce dyspnea include those used to reduce anxiety, breathing retraining, and energy conservation measures.

In summary, alterations in breathing patterns include tachypnea (rapid breathing), hyperpnea (increase in both the rate and the depth of respiration), bradypnea (abnormally slow respiratory rate), hyperventilation (respiration in excess of that needed to maintain a normal level of Pco_2), and hypoventilation (inadequate ventilation). Periodic breathing is manifested by periods of apnea. Dyspnea is a subjective sensation of difficulty in breathing.

■ ALTERATIONS IN CONTROL OF VENTILATION

The term ventilation refers to the movement of air into and out of the lungs. The lungs can be expanded by the upward and downward movement of the diaphragm or the elevation and depression of the ribs to increase or decrease the anterolateral diameter of the chest cavity. Alveolar ventilation represents the component of the total ventilation that reaches the perfused alveoli and is, therefore, effective in eliminating carbon dioxide. The amount or portion of expired ventilation that remains in the airways is wasted or dead-space ventilation (see Chapter 26).

The act of ventilation or breathing involves a smooth and regular sequence of inspiration and expiration at a rate and depth regulated to maintain the arterial Po_2 and Pco_2 at relatively constant levels. Unlike the action of the heart, which beats independently of the nervous system, the inflation and deflation of the lungs require continuous input from the nervous system (see Chapter 26). A number of differ-

TABLE 28-1. INSTRUMENT TO MEASURE DYSPNEA*

A. Degree of Shortness of Breath Graded From 0 to 3

Grade	Description
0	No unusual shortness of breath compared to other persons of same age, height, and sex
1	More shortness of breath than a person of same age when walking up hills or hurrying on level ground
2	Shortness of breath when walking on level ground
3	Shortness of breath at rest or while dressing

B. Visual Analog Scale

0 _____ 10

10 cm

No difficulty breathing   Unable to breathe

* For use in illness trajectory.
(Carrieri, V.K., Jansen-Bjerklie, S., & Jacobs, S. [1984]. The sensation of dyspnea: A review. *Heart and Lung, 13*(4), 441)

ent types of disorders may alter the effectiveness of ventilation. The ventilatory drive can be depressed by drugs, or ventilation can be impaired by disorders that affect the respiratory muscles. In sleep apnea, abnormalities in the coordination of ventilation occur during sleep; in hyperventilation syndrome, ventilation is in excess of that needed to maintain normal P_{CO_2} levels.

DRUG-INDUCED RESPIRATORY DEPRESSION

The function of the respiratory muscles can be impaired by drugs that depress the central nervous system and the respiratory center; by neuromuscular blocking drugs, such as *d*-tubocurarine and succinylcholine (used to effect muscle relaxation during surgery), that block the transmission of impulses at the level of the myoneural junction; or by drugs that act peripherally at a site beyond the myoneural junction, possibly by interfering with calcium release from the sarcoplasmic reticulum (Table 28-2).

Almost all the drugs known to cause depression

of the CNS have been associated with decreased alveolar ventilation. Overdoses of barbiturates, hypnotics, narcotics, and antidepressant drugs are common causes of admission to respiratory intensive care units. Airway obstruction caused by involvement of the muscles of the oropharynx and loss of the cough reflex precedes or accompanies loss of ventilatory drive and complicates the condition. Insertion of an endotracheal tube with mechanical ventilatory support may be needed when hypoventilation causes hypercapnia. Small doses of drugs that depress the respiratory center may further impair ventilation and lead to hypercapnia in people with preexisting respiratory disease. Therefore, these drugs should be used with great caution in people with chronic lung disease and respiratory muscle weakness.

WEAKNESS OF THE RESPIRATORY MUSCLES

Weakness of the respiratory muscles can result from conditions that interrupt innervation of the muscles (*e.g.*, spinal cord injury and poliomyelitis), affect the

TABLE 28-2. DRUGS WITH RESPIRATORY DEPRESSANT ACTIONS*

FUNCTIONAL DRUG GROUPS†	MECHANISMS OF ACTION
Anesthetic Agents	
General anesthesia	Depression of CNS function, including medullary respiratory center
Spinal anesthesia	Production of ascending muscle paralysis to level of respiratory muscles
Drugs Affecting Brain Stem Respiratory Mechanisms	
Opiates and narcotic analgesics	Depression of brain stem respiratory mechanisms, causing a decrease in ventilatory drive
Barbiturates and sedatives	
Tricyclic antidepressants	
Alcohol	
Drugs Affecting Myoneural Junction	
Muscle relaxants	Production of impulse blockade at level of myoneural junction in skeletal muscle, including respiratory muscles
Aminoglycoside antibiotics‡	
Polymyxin antibiotics‡	
Quinine‡	
Quinidine‡	
Drugs Affecting Muscle Contraction	
Dantrolene	Reduction of excitation–contraction coupling within skeletal muscle fiber, causing muscle weakness

* The respiratory effects of these drugs usually are dose dependent.
† This list of drugs is not inclusive.
‡ The respiratory effects of these drugs usually occur at toxic doses.

myoneural junction (*e.g.*, myasthenia gravis), or directly involve the muscles themselves (*e.g.*, muscular dystrophy). Disorders of the respiratory muscles are characterized by decreases in vital capacity and maximum voluntary ventilation, whereas measures of expiratory flow are well maintained. Many people with these disorders may be able to maintain adequate ventilation for brief periods, but sustaining normal minute ventilation (respiration rate × tidal volume) may impose an excessive load on the weakened and fatigued muscles, and hypoventilation may result. People with impaired respiratory muscle function show extreme sensitivity to respiratory depressant drugs.

SLEEP APNEA

Sleep apnea is the cessation of airflow through the nose and mouth for 10 seconds or longer. The diagnosis of sleep apnea depends on the occurrence of 30 or more apneic periods during 7 hours of sleep.[3] The apneic periods typically last for 15 to 120 seconds, and some people may have as many as 500 apneic periods per night.

SLEEP STAGES AND RESPIRATION

Sleep is not a constant, uniform state but rather a pattern of sequential stages with a periodicity of about 90 minutes. These stages are associated with electroencephalographic (EEG), behavioral, and physiologic changes that affect the control of breathing. Two sleep states have been defined: rapid-eye-movement (REM) sleep, also referred to as active sleep, and non-REM sleep, or quiet sleep.

Non-REM sleep is encountered when one first becomes drowsy; it has four stages reflecting an increasing depth of sleep. Stage 1 consists primarily of low-voltage, mixed-frequency EEG activity; it reflects the drowsy state. Stage 2 is a deeper sleep during which EEG activity is characterized by bursts of high-frequency (12 to 14 cycles per second) and high-amplitude waves called K complexes. Stages 1 and 2 of non-REM sleep are characterized by a pattern of breathing in which there is cyclic waning and waxing of tidal volume and respiratory rate, which may include brief periods (5 to 15 seconds) of apnea. Stages 3 and 4 are referred to as slow-wave sleep because the EEG is dominated by high-voltage, low-frequency (1 to 2 cycles per second) waves. This breathing pattern is called *periodic breathing*. Although the amount of periodic breathing that occurs during the first two stages of non-REM sleep differs among healthy people, it is more common in people over age 40.[4] Once sleep is stabilized during stages 3 and 4 of non-REM sleep, breathing becomes more regular. During slow-wave sleep, ventilation usually is 1 to 2 L/min less than during quiet wakefulness; the P_{CO_2} levels are 4 to 8 mmHg greater; the P_{O_2} levels are 3 to 10 mmHg less; and the *p*H is 0.03 to 0.05 units less.[4] Control of breathing during non-REM sleep is dominated by automatic (involuntary reflex) control mechanisms—responses to hypercapnia, hypoxia, and lung inflation are intact and critically important to maintaining ventilation.

REM sleep resembles wakefulness in many ways: the EEG displays unsynchronized, low-voltage, mixed-frequency waves, and there are frequent muscular and rapid eye movements. Autonomic nervous system activity changes during REM sleep: the heart rate and blood pressure may fluctuate rapidly and the cerebral blood flow and metabolic rate decrease. Respiration becomes irregular (but not periodic) and may include periods of apnea lasting as long as 15 to 20 seconds in healthy adults and 10 seconds in infants. Breathing during REM sleep has many of the features of the voluntary type of control that integrates breathing with voluntary acts such as talking, walking, and swallowing. Automatic control of breathing remains during REM sleep, but its influence is diminished.

In all stages of sleep, all skeletal muscles except the diaphragm undergo a decrease in tone.[5] This loss of muscle tone is most pronounced during REM sleep. In the awake state, intercostal muscle activity stiffens the rib cage. With the absence of this tone during sleep, the negative intrapleural pressure caused by contraction of the diaphragm can cause paradoxical motion of the rib cage (the rib cage moves inward during inspiration rather than outward) and a decrease in functional residual capacity. The loss of tone in the upper airways can cause airway obstruction. Negative airway pressure produced by the contraction of the diaphragm brings the vocal cords together, collapses the pharyngeal wall, and sucks the tongue back into the throat. Airway collapse is accentuated in people with conditions that cause narrowing of the upper airway or weakness of the throat muscles.

TYPES OF SLEEP APNEA

Sleep apnea can be classified into three types: obstructive, central, and mixed. Obstructive apnea is caused by the obstruction of the upper airway. With central apnea, the respiratory drive ceases and there is no movement of the rib cage or abdominal muscle. Mixed apnea constitutes a mixture of central and obstructive apnea. Because breathing seems to be controlled by different mechanisms during REM and non-REM sleep, different causes are associated with the different types of sleep apnea. Figure 28-1 shows

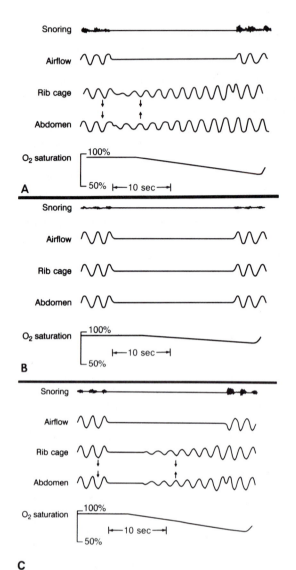

FIG. 28-1. Types of sleep apnea. (**A**) Obstructive apnea is characterized by loud intermittent snoring, complete cessation of airflow, paradoxic movement of the chest and abdomen, and moderate to severe oxygen desaturation. (**B**) In central apnea, snoring and simultaneous cessation of airflow and respiratory effort are absent. Only mild to moderate oxygen desaturation usually is present. (**C**) In mixed apnea, an initial central apnea is followed by an obstructive apnea that usually produces moderate to severe oxygen desaturation. (Burton, G. G., Hodgkin, J. E., & Ward, J. J. [Eds.]. [1991]. *Respiratory care: A guide to clinical practice* [3rd ed., p. 282]. Philadelphia: J.B. Lippincott.)

the variations in airflow and rib cage and abdominal movements in the three types of sleep apnea.

Obstructive Sleep Apnea. Obstructive sleep apnea typically is associated with obesity and disorders that compromise the patency of the airway. It is most common in middle-aged men. Although androgens are suspected of contributing to the disorder, their mechanism of action is unknown. The pick-

wickian syndrome, named after the fat boy in Charles Dickens' *The Posthumous Papers of the Pickwick Club*, published in 1837, is characterized by obesity, hypersomnolence, periodic breathing, hypoxemia, and right-sided heart failure. Alcohol and other drugs that depress the central nervous system seem to increase the severity of obstructive apneic episodes.

Obstructive sleep apnea is characterized by loud snoring interrupted by periods of silence. Abnormal gross motor movements during sleep are common. In many cases, the snoring precedes by many years the onset of other signs of sleep apnea. Many people complain of morning headache and nausea and persistent daytime sleepiness. Hypersomnolence can lead to occupational and driving accidents. Psychological problems associated with impotence, intellectual deterioration, and depression are also part of the symptom complex. The signs and symptoms of sleep apnea are summarized in Chart 28-1. In children, a decline in school performance may be the only indication of the problem.

In addition to the sleep disturbances, cardiovascular problems are associated with sleep apnea syndromes. A number of cardiac arrhythmias have been observed in people with sleep apnea. Frequent apneic periods may result in increased pulmonary and systemic blood pressures. More than two thirds of patients with sleep apnea in one study had daytime hypertension.[6] In severe cases, pulmonary hypertension, polycythemia, and cor pulmonale may develop.

Sleep apnea and sleep-related periodic leg movements appear to be more widespread among elderly people. One study reported a 24% prevalence of sleep apnea among subjects aged 60 to 95 years.[7] Sleep apnea usually is mild in elderly people, with few sleep-wake complaints and only small changes in heart rate (mean 10 beats or less) and oxygen desaturation (mean less than 5%). It is not known if this

CHART 28-1: SIGNS AND SYMPTOMS OF SLEEP APNEA

Noisy snoring
Insomnia
Abnormal movements during sleep
Morning headaches
Excessive daytime sleepiness
Intellectual and personality changes
Sexual impotence
Systemic hypertension
Pulmonary hypertension, cor pulmonale
Polycythemia

type of sleep apnea in elderly people contributes to conditions such as hypertension.

Central Sleep Apnea. Central sleep apnea is associated with disorders that affect the CNS and respiratory neurons, such as encephalitis, brain stem infarction, and bulbar poliomyelitis. With central sleep apnea, sleep is difficult to maintain and several awakenings occur during the night. There may be some daytime fatigue, depression, and impaired sexual functioning. In contrast to people with obstructive sleep apnea, people with central sleep apnea are of normal weight.

DIAGNOSIS AND TREATMENT

Sleep apnea usually is suspected from a history of snoring, disturbed sleep, and daytime sleepiness. A definitive diagnosis is accomplished with sleep studies done in a sleep laboratory using polysomnography.[8] This procedure consists of (1) EEG and electro-oculography to determine the sleep stages; (2) monitoring of the airflow; (3) electrocardiography (ECG) to detect arrhythmias; (4) impedance pneumography, intercostal electromyography, or esophageal manometry to monitor respiratory effort; and (5) ear oximetry or transcutaneous oxygen monitoring to detect changes in oxygen saturation. It is recommended that the evaluation of sleep apnea also include a multiple sleep latency test (MSLT). The MSLT determines the amount of daytime hypersomnolence that is present and rules out narcolepsy (a condition characterized by uncontrolled periods of daytime sleep).[8] The study is begun 1.5 to 2 hours after the person's usual nighttime sleep. Polysomnographic recordings are made during three to five naps spaced 2 hours apart during the day. Special attention is paid to how much time elapses from when the lights go out to the first evidence of sleep. This interval is termed sleep latency. The MSLT can be used along with nighttime polysomnography to monitor the response to therapy.

The treatment of sleep apnea is determined by the type of apnea that is present. Weight loss often is beneficial in people with obstructive apnea. In many instances, the disordered breathing events are confined to the supine sleeping position, so that training the person to sleep in the lateral position may help to alleviate the problem. The application of continuous positive airway pressure to the nasal airways at night has been reported to help in obstructive sleep apnea.[9] This method uses a soft, occlusive nasal mask held to the face by straps, an expiratory valve and tubing, and a blower system to generate positive pressure.[8] Protriptyline, a nonsedative tricyclic antidepressant that reduces REM sleep, has also been used suc-

cessfully to reduce apneic episodes in some people.[10] In cases of central sleep apnea, various medications have been used to increase the central respiratory drive, including theophylline, acetazolamide, clomipramine, and medroxyprogesterone. Several surgical procedures have been used to correct airway obstruction, including nasal septoplasty (repair of the nasal septum) and uvulopalatopharyngoplasty (excision of excess soft tissue on the palate, uvula, and posterior pharyngeal wall). Both of these procedures have met with limited success. Studies are now under way to determine which preoperative criteria will predict success.[8] Severe cases of sleep apnea may require a tracheostomy (surgical placement of a tube into the trachea for the purpose of maintaining an open airway). The tracheostomy tube remains stoppered during the day and is opened during the night.

HYPERVENTILATION SYNDROME

Hyperventilation syndrome involves overbreathing, reduction in P_{CO_2}, and respiratory alkalosis. In 1871, De Costa provided the first account of the syndrome in the medical literature when he reported on the cases of 300 Civil War soldiers affected with the disorder. The disorder subsequently has been labeled soldier's heart, irritable heart, De Costa's syndrome, and neurocirculatory asthenia. De Costa noted that the affected soldier ''got out of breath, could not keep up with his comrades, was annoyed with dizziness and palpitation, and with pain in the chest; his accouterments oppressed him, and all through this he appeared well and healthy.'' The nervous manifestations of the syndrome were ''headache, dizziness, and disturbed sleep.''[11] Removal from the stress of active duty along with enforced rest reduced the symptoms, but even with removal from active duty, the ''irritability of the heart remained.''[11]

CAUSES

The causes of hyperventilation syndrome have been categorized into four groups: organic, physiologic, emotional, and habitual (faulty breathing habits).[12] Organic causes include drug effects and central nervous system lesions, such as meningitis. Responses to high altitude, heat, and exercise constitute physiologic causes of hyperventilation. Emotional states that predispose to hyperventilation are hysteria, anxiety, depression, and anger. Faulty breathing habits such as rapid and shallow breathing are often linked to emotional states. Although stress may trigger the initial event, anxiety and fear over the symptoms may perpetuate the syndrome. Because the symptoms of hyperventilation syndrome commonly involve the heart and head, the person experiences intense anxiety, often accompanied by a fear of death or of losing control. The condition occurs in children as well as adults.[13]

MANIFESTATIONS

Hyperventilation syndrome commonly produces such symptoms as headache, dyspnea, numbness and tingling sensations, light-headedness, chest pain, palpitations, and, sometimes, syncope. Many people complain of dyspnea and of being unable to take a full deep breath. People with a full constellation of the syndrome breathe with rapid, shallow breaths marked by irregularity in the depth and rate of respiration. Sighing is common. Those who hyperventilate are primarily thoracic rather than abdominal breathers. They tend to use their upper chest wall intercostal muscles to breathe, which may cause dull aching soreness in the left precordial area, mimicking angina. It has been suggested that the alkalosis associated with hyperventilation syndrome can induce coronary artery spasm in people with Prinzmetal's angina[14, 15] and in some people with atherosclerotic coronary artery disease.[15, 16] It has also been observed that ST-wave changes can occur with hyperventilation.

Many people afflicted with hyperventilation syndrome do not have a continuously symptomatic state but rather recurrences of symptoms with or without recognizable provocative stresses. Others have a more chronic form of the disorder in which the respiratory center is reset to enable low levels of P_{CO_2} to persist despite a normal pH.[17] This may explain the chronicity of the disorder and the ease with which symptoms associated with hyperventilation can be provoked in people who are chronically hypocapnic. Sympathetic nervous system stimulation provokes a hyperventilatory response and may increase the occurrence of symptoms in people with chronic hyperventilation problems.

Panic disorder and hyperventilation syndrome have recently been observed to have similar manifestations. Hyperventilation has been demonstrated in people with panic episodes, and panic is a frequent manifestation of hyperventilation. It has been suggested that some people with either diagnosis have the same disorder and share a biologically and often genetically determined hypersensitivity of a central nervous system alarm system.[18]

DIAGNOSIS AND TREATMENT

A provocative test in which a person deliberately hyperventilates can be done to demonstrate occurrence of the symptoms.[12] Arterial blood gases may be obtained to study the pH and carbon dioxide levels. ECG monitoring is done during the test on people who have complained of chest pain, and caution should be used when performing the test on people with known or suspected coronary artery disease.

Treatment focuses on educating the person and his or her family about the disorder, relaxation therapy, and training to overcome faulty breathing patterns. Rebreathing into a paper bag can be used to control the symptoms. For many people, the realization that they can control their symptoms and nothing is seriously wrong reduces their anxiety and helps them to control the disorder. Adjunctive pharmacologic treatment may be useful in some cases. β-Adrenergic blocking agents lessen the peripheral symptoms of anxiety, such as palpitations and diaphoresis, and may lessen the respiratory stimulatory effect of the catecholamines released during periods of high anxiety.[19]

In summary, alterations in the control of ventilation include drug-induced disorders, respiratory muscle weakness, sleep apnea, and hyperventilation syndrome. Almost all the drugs known to cause depression of the respiratory system have been associated with impairment of ventilation. Drugs can act centrally to depress the respiratory center, or they may act peripherally at the level of the myoneural junction. Weakness of the respiratory muscles can result from conditions that denervate the muscles, affect the myoneural junction, or directly involve muscle tissue. Sleep apnea involves 30 or more apneic periods characterized by the cessation of airflow through the nose and mouth for 10 seconds or longer. It can result from disorders that compromise the patency of the airways during sleep (obstructive sleep apnea) or that affect the central nervous system. Hyperventilation syndrome consists of overbreathing, reduction in P_{CO_2}, and respiratory alkalosis. It can result from organic causes, such as drug effects and central nervous system lesions; physiologic changes caused by heat exposure and exercise; emotional states; or habit. It can cause headache, dyspnea, numbness and tingling sensations, light-headedness, palpitations, and, sometimes, syncope.

■ IMPAIRED GAS EXCHANGE

Impaired gas exchange is characterized by inadequate addition of oxygen to the blood and deficient removal of oxygen from the blood. It can result from environmental conditions, lung disease, neuromuscular problems that impair ventilation, or neural control of respiration. The term *hypoxia* refers to a reduction in oxygen supply to the tissues; *hypoxemia*, to a low level of oxygen in the blood; and *hypercapnia* (sometimes referred to as *hypercarbia*), to excess carbon dioxide in the blood. In this chapter, the term hypoxia is used to describe both the reduction in oxygen supply to the tissues and the low level of oxygen in the blood and the term hypercapnia is used to refer to excess carbon dioxide in the blood. Both hypoxia and hypercapnia may present as acute and chronic conditions, and hypoxia may exist without hypercapnia or the two conditions may coexist. Cyanosis reflects the presence of deoxygenated hemoglobin in the blood. Clubbing of the fingers may reflect the presence of chronic hypoxia.

HYPOXIA

The partial pressure of oxygen decreases as one ascends above sea level, and much of what is known about acute hypoxia has been learned from high-altitude and aviation studies. The partial pressure of oxygen, which constitutes 21% of the total gases in the air, falls from 159 mmHg at sea level (760 mmHg barometric pressure) to 110 mmHg at 10,000 ft to 73 mmHg at 20,000 ft.[20] Denver, Colorado, which has an altitude of 5250 ft, has partial pressure of oxygen of 121 mmHg. Water vapor and carbon dioxide are added to atmospheric air in the lungs; the partial pressure of oxygen is less since it makes up less of the total gases in the lung. As a result, alveolar oxygen pressure is less than that in the environment; it falls from about 104 mmHg at sea level to 67 mmHg at 10,000 ft to 40 mmHg at 20,000 ft. The ceiling for breathing air is about 23,000 ft; this can be doubled to about 47,000 ft when breathing pure oxygen. The use of pressurized cabins in aircraft allows for safe travel at high altitudes. In the clinical setting, acute hypoxia can occur at sea level in people with sudden blood loss,

carbon monoxide poisoning, acute circulatory disorders, respiratory disease, or other disorders that interfere with the exchange or transport of oxygen.

Hypoxia refers to a reduction in tissue oxygenation. It can result from an inadequate amount of oxygen in the air, disease of the respiratory system, alterations in circulatory function, anemia, or the inability of the cells to use oxygen. The causes of hypoxia can be divided into four categories: (1) hypoxemic hypoxia, in which the oxygen content of the blood is reduced; (2) stagnant, or ischemic, hypoxia, in which impaired blood oxygen interferes with transport; (3) anemic hypoxia, in which the ability to transport oxygen in the blood decreases; and (4) histotoxic hypoxia, in which the cells are unable to use oxygen (*e.g.*, cyanide poisoning). The categories, mechanisms of production, and causes of hypoxia are summarized in Table 28-3.

ACUTE AND CHRONIC HYPOXIA

Severe acute hypoxia causes cyanosis, cardiovascular signs such as tachycardia, and central nervous system signs such as mental clouding. The signs and symptoms of hypoxia usually are mild until the Po_2 falls below 60 mmHg and do not become severe until the Po_2 falls to 40 to 50 mmHg. One of the earliest signs of acute hypoxia is a chemoreceptor-mediated increase in ventilation. The chemoreceptors (see Chapter 26) are particularly sensitive to changes in Po_2 in the range of 60 to 30 mmHg. Important early

TABLE 28-3. TYPES, MECHANISMS OF PRODUCTION, AND CAUSES OF HYPOXIA

TYPE	MECHANISMS OF PRODUCTION	CAUSES
Hypoxemic hypoxia	Insufficient oxygen reaching the blood	Decreased oxygen in the atmosphere Pulmonary disease Airway obstruction Neuromuscular disease
Stagnant hypoxia	Failure to transport oxygen because of impaired blood flow	Heart failure Circulatory shock Local disruption of blood flow
Anemic hypoxia	Reduction in the oxygen-carrying capacity of the blood	Decrease in red blood cells Abnormal hemoglobin Carbon monoxide poisoning
Histotoxic hypoxia	Impaired utilization of oxygen by the cell	Cellular poisons such as cyanide Tissue edema Abnormal tissue needs

effects of acute hypoxia are decreases in judgment and motor proficiency. These manifestations become more acute with prolonged exposure to hypoxic conditions. For example, mental proficiency is decreased to one half of normal after 1 hour of sudden exposure to the barometric pressures at 15,000 ft and to one fifth after 18 hours.[20] Other signs and symptoms of acute hypoxia include dyspnea, fatigue, headache, nausea, vomiting, and decreased visual acuity. Cyanosis of the lips and nail beds usually is present in people with adequate hemoglobin levels. Cheyne-Stokes breathing and insomnia are common problems in unacclimated people during the first several days of exposure to high altitudes. Disorientation, hallucinations, seizures, and coma occur with extreme levels of hypoxia. It has been speculated that some of the symptoms associated with ascent to high altitudes, such as insomnia and Cheyne-Stokes breathing, are related to the decreased carbon dioxide levels that result from hyperventilation.

Chronic Hypoxia. Chronic hypoxia induces changes similar—albeit of a lesser degree—to those observed in acute hypoxia. Dyspnea, fatigue, and cyanosis are common problems associated with a long-term impairment in the oxygenation of tissues. In addition, there is evidence of adaptive mechanisms, such as pulmonary hypertension and polycythemia.

MANIFESTATIONS

In hypoxia, the blood oxygen level is insufficient to meet the oxidative requirements of body tissues. These tissues vary considerably in their vulnerability to hypoxia; those with the greatest need are the nervous system and heart. The signs and symptoms of hypoxia, which are listed in Chart 28-2, can be grouped into two categories: those resulting from impaired function of vital centers and those resulting from activation of compensatory mechanisms.

CHART 28-2: SIGNS AND SYMPTOMS OF HYPOXIA

Arterial PO$_2$ below 50 mmHg	Loss of judgment
Tachycardia	Euphoria
Mild increase in blood pressure	Unruly or combative behavior
Cool and moist skin	Sensory impairment
Confusion	Mental fatigue
Delirium	Drowsiness
Difficulty in problem solving	Stupor and coma (late)
	Hypotension (late)
	Bradycardia (late)

Acute hypoxia often produces central nervous system manifestations similar to those of acute alcohol intoxication. There may be personality changes, restlessness, agitated or combative behavior, muscle incoordination, euphoria, impaired judgment, delirium, and, eventually, coma. Tachycardia, cool skin (peripheral vasoconstriction), diaphoresis, and a mild increase in blood pressure result from the recruitment of sympathetic compensatory mechanisms. Although cyanosis may be evident, its presence cannot be relied on. When the hemoglobin concentration is normal, this means that the arterial saturation must be reduced to below 70% and the arterial PO$_2$ reduced to less than 35 mmHg before cyanosis develops; hence, it is a late sign of hypoxia. This is especially critical in people with anemia, since they may be severely hypoxic but lack the hemoglobin necessary for the development of cyanosis. Hypotension and bradycardia often are preterminal events in hypoxia, indicating the failure of compensatory mechanisms.

In conditions of chronic hypoxia, the manifestations may be insidious in onset and attributed to other causes, particularly in chronic lung disease. Decreased sensory function, such as impaired vision or fewer complaints of pain, may be an early sign of worsening hypoxia. This is probably because the involved sensory neurons have the same need for high levels of oxygen as do other parts of the nervous system.

The body adapts to hypoxia by increased ventilation, pulmonary vasoconstriction, and increased production of red blood cells. Hyperventilation results from the hypoxic stimulation of the chemoreceptors. The stimulus for the increased production of red blood cells results from the release of erythropoietin from the kidneys in response to hypoxia (see Chapter 18). Polycythemia increases the red blood cell concentration and the oxygen-carrying capacity of the blood. Pulmonary vasoconstriction occurs as a local response to alveolar hypoxia; it increases pulmonary arterial pressure and serves to improve the matching of ventilation and blood flow. Other adaptive mechanisms include a shift to the right in the oxygen dissociation curve as a means of increasing oxygen release to the tissues (see Chapter 26). An increase in oxidative enzymes in the cell serves as a means of increasing the efficiency of oxygen utilization.

Cyanosis. Cyanosis refers to the bluish discoloration of the skin and mucous membranes that results from an excessive concentration of reduced or deoxygenated hemoglobin in the small blood vessels. It usually is most marked in the lips, nail beds, ears, and cheeks. The degree of cyanosis is modified by the amount of cutaneous pigment, skin thickness, and the state of the cutaneous capillaries. Cyanosis is more difficult to distinguish in people with dark skin and in areas of the body where there is increased thickness of the skin. A concentration of about 5 g/dL of deoxygenated hemoglobin is required in the circulating blood for cyanosis. The absolute quantity of reduced hemoglobin, rather than the relative quantity, is important in producing cyanosis. Thus, people with anemia and low hemoglobin levels are less likely to exhibit cyanosis (because they have less hemoglobin to deoxygenate), even though they may be relatively hypoxic because of their decreased ability to transport oxygen, than people who have high hemoglobin concentrations. In fact, someone with a high hemoglobin level because of polycythemia may well be cyanotic without being hypoxic.

Cyanosis may be subdivided into two types: central and peripheral. In central cyanosis, there is an increased amount of deoxygenated hemoglobin or abnormal hemoglobin derivative in the arterial blood and the mucous membranes and skin are both affected. Abnormal hemoglobin derivatives include methemoglobin, in which the nitrite ion reacts with hemoglobin. Because methemoglobin has a low affinity for oxygen, large doses of nitrites can result in cyanosis and tissue hypoxia. Although nitrites are used in treating angina, the therapeutic dose is too small to cause cyanosis. Sodium nitrite is used as a curing agent for meat. In nursing infants, the intestinal flora is capable of converting significant amounts of inorganic nitrate (*e.g.*, from well water) into nitrite ion.[21]

Peripheral cyanosis is due to the slowing of blood flow to an area of the body with increased extraction of oxygen from the blood. It results from vasoconstriction and diminished peripheral blood flow, such as occurs with cold exposure, shock, congestive heart failure, and peripheral vascular disease. Acute arterial obstruction to an extremity, such as with an embolus or arterial spasm (Raynaud's phenomenon, discussed in Chapter 20), usually presents with pallor and coldness, although there may be cyanosis.

Clubbing of the Fingers. Clubbing of the fingers involves the bulbous enlargement of the distal segment of the digit because of an increase in soft tissue (Fig. 28-2). It may be hereditary or acquired. Acquired clubbing of the fingers is associated with various conditions that impair oxygen delivery, including cyanotic heart disease and chronic lung disease, as well as some gastrointestinal disorders, such as cirrhosis of the liver. Although the mechanisms of clubbing are unclear, it appears to occur secondary to the presence of a substance (presumably one that

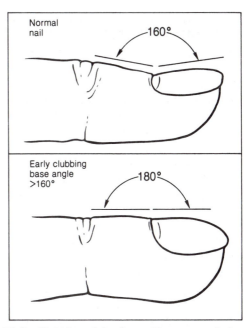

FIG. 28-2. Clubbing of the finger. There normally is an obtuse angle of about 160 degrees between the base of the nail and the adjacent dorsal surface of the finger; with clubbing, this angle exceeds 180 degrees.

circulates in the blood) that causes dilation of the vessels of the fingertips.

DIAGNOSIS AND TREATMENT

Diagnosis of hypoxia is based on clinical observation and diagnostic measures of oxygen levels. The analysis of arterial blood gases provides a direct measure of the oxygen content of blood and is a good indicator of the lungs' ability to oxygenate the blood. In the critical care unit, continuous mixed venous oxygen saturation (SVO_2) can be monitored using a special type of pulmonary artery catheter.[22] This method, which measures the mixed venous blood that is being returned to the lungs, reflects the utilization of oxygen by the peripheral tissues. Both arterial blood gases and SVO_2 are monitored in critically ill patients. Both measurements are invasive and require direct sampling of the patient's blood through either a peripheral arterial catheter (blood gases) or a pulmonary artery catheter (SVO_2). There are two noninvasive methods for oxygen assessment: the transcutaneous sensor method and the pulse oximeter.[23] Transcutaneous oxygen monitoring uses an oxygen electrode. The electrode and covering membrane allow oxygen to diffuse through the skin and be measured. The pulse oximeter uses light-emitting diodes and combines plethysmography (changes in light absorbance and vasodilatation) with spectrophotometry.[23] Spectrophotometry uses a red-wavelength light that passes through oxygenated hemoglobin and is absorbed by deoxygenated hemoglobin and an infrared-wavelength light that is absorbed by oxygenated hemoglobin and passes through deoxygenated hemoglobin. Sensors that can be placed on the ear, finger, toe, or forehead are now available. These methods, although not as accurate as the invasive methods, provide a means for monitoring oxygen levels and are useful indicators of respiratory and circulatory status.

The treatment of hypoxia focuses on correcting the problem causing impaired gas exchange and on oxygen administration. Oxygen may be delivered by nasal cannula or mask. It may also be administered directly into an endotracheal or tracheostomy tube. A high-flow administration system is one in which the flow rate and reserve capacity are sufficient to provide all the inspired air. A low-flow oxygen system delivers less than the total inspired air. The oxygen must be humidified as it is being administered. The flow rate (liters per minute) is based on the arterial P_{O_2}. The rate must be carefully monitored in people with chronic lung disease because marked increases in P_{O_2} (above 60 mmHg) are apt to depress the ventilatory drive. There is also the danger of oxygen toxicity with high concentrations of oxygen. Continuous breathing of oxygen at high concentrations can lead to diffuse parenchymal lung injury. People with healthy lungs begin to experience respiratory symptoms ranging from cough, sore throat, substernal distress, nasal congestion, and painful inspiration after breathing pure oxygen for 14 to 16 hours.[24]

HYPERCAPNIA

Hypercapnia refers to an increase in the carbon dioxide content of the blood. It is a well-recognized consequence of a number of diseases—not only those that involve the lungs but also those that involve the neuromuscular, chest wall, circulatory, and neural control components of the respiratory system.

MECHANISMS

The carbon dioxide level in the blood, or P_{CO_2}, is proportional to carbon dioxide production and inversely related to alveolar ventilation. In the clinical setting, four factors contribute to hypercapnia: (1) alterations in carbon dioxide production, (2) a disturbance in the gas exchange function of the lung, (3) abnormalities in the respiratory function of the chest wall and respiratory muscles, and (4) changes in the neural control of respiration.[25] The diffusing capacity of carbon dioxide is 20 times that of oxygen; therefore, hypercapnia is observed only in situations of hypoventilation sufficient to cause hypoxia.

Alterations in Carbon Dioxide Production. Changes in the metabolic rate resulting from an increase in activity level, fever, or disease can have profound effects on carbon dioxide production. For example, carbon dioxide production increases 13% for every 1° C increase in temperature above normal.[25] Alveolar ventilation usually rises proportionally with these changes, and hypercapnia occurs only when this increase is inappropriate.

Interest has recently been generated in the effect of carbohydrate metabolism on carbon dioxide production. The respiratory quotient (RQ), which is the ratio of carbon dioxide production to oxygen consumption (RQ = CO_2 production/O_2 consumption), varies with the type of food metabolized. A characteristic of carbohydrate metabolism is an RQ of 1.0, with equal carbon dioxide being produced and oxygen being consumed. Because fats contain less oxygen than carbohydrates, their oxidation produces less carbon dioxide (RQ = 0.7). The metabolism of pure proteins (RQ = 0.81) results in the production of more carbon dioxide than the metabolism of fat but less than the metabolism of carbohydrates. Thus, the type of food that is eaten or the types of nutrients that are delivered through enteral feedings (through a tube placed in the small intestine) or parenteral nutrition (through a venous catheter placed in the central vena cava) may impact on P_{CO_2} levels. Portable devices and metabolic carts that use indirect calorimetry to determine the RQ and energy requirements are available for use in the clinical setting.[26]

In people who receive a high glucose load in association with total parenteral nutrition, the RQ can rise to a level of 1 or more.[25] People with adequate respiratory function can increase their alveolar ventilation proportional to the increased P_{CO_2} production. On the other hand, hypercapnic respiratory failure can occur in people who cannot adequately increase their ventilation. It has been suggested that such people receive a larger proportion of nonprotein calories in the form of fat emulsions because these emulsions are associated with a lower rate of carbon dioxide production.[25]

Disturbances in the Gas Exchange Function of the Lungs. Lung disease contributes to the retention of carbon dioxide by reducing the effective alveolar ventilation, even when total ventilation is maintained. This is either because a region of lung is not perfused and, therefore, gas exchange cannot take place or because an area of the lung is not being ventilated. In people with chronic lung disease, ventilation–perfusion mismatch is an important contributing factor to hypercapnia. Maintaining a high ventilation rate effectively prevents hypercapnia but also increases the work of breathing.

Musculoskeletal Disorders. Respiratory muscle fatigue can contribute to carbon dioxide retention in people with various primary respiratory diseases as well as in those with neuromuscular disorders. In these people, respiratory muscle fatigue develops when energy requirements exceed the energy supply. A number of factors increase energy requirements or decrease the energy supply. The energy demands of the respiratory muscles are increased by high levels of ventilation or by factors that increase the work of breathing, such as high levels of airway resistance. On the other hand, the energy supply depends on blood flow and the oxygen content of the blood. Therefore, low cardiac output, anemia, and decreased oxygen saturation all contribute to a decreased energy supply and increase the likelihood of respiratory muscle fatigue.

With malnutrition, the energy stores of the muscles are diminished, and there may be structural changes in the muscle as well. Electrolyte imbalances, especially hypokalemia and hypophosphatemia, contribute to respiratory muscle weakness.[25]

Disorders of Neural Control of Respiration. The respiratory center, which activates the muscles of respiration, is a crucial determinant of ventilation and adequate elimination of carbon dioxide. It is composed of widely dispersed groups of neurons located in the medulla oblongata and pons (see Chap. 26). Carbon dioxide crosses the blood–brain barrier with ease. Carbon dioxide does not stimulate ventilation directly; instead, it does so by reacting with water to form carbonic acid; this in turn dissociates into hydrogen ions, which have a potent direct stimulatory effect. The excitation of the respiratory center by carbon dioxide is great during the first 1 to 2 days that blood levels are elevated but then gradually declines over the next 1 to 2 days, decreasing to about one fifth the initial effect.[20] Part of this decline results from renal compensatory mechanisms that readjust the hydrogen ion concentration by increasing blood bicarbonate levels. Thus, in people with respiratory problems that cause chronic hypoxia and hypercapnia, the peripheral chemoreceptors that monitor blood oxygen levels become the driving force for ventilation. Administration of high-flow oxygen to these people can abolish the input from these peripheral receptors, causing a decrease in alveolar ventilation and a further rise in PCO_2 levels.

MANIFESTATIONS

Hypercapnia affects the respiratory system as well as renal function, neural function, cardiovascular function, and acid–base balance (see Chap. 30). The body adapts to chronic increases in blood levels of carbon dioxide; hence, people with chronic hypercapnia may not develop symptoms until the PCO_2 is markedly elevated. Elevated levels of PCO_2 are characterized by respiratory acidosis, discussed in Chapter 30. The body adapts to increased PCO_2 levels by metabolic adjustments (renal bicarbonate retention). As long as the pH is in an acceptable range, the main complication is due to the associated hypoxia.

Carbon dioxide has a direct vasodilatory effect on many blood vessels and a sedative effect on the nervous system. When the cerebral vessels are dilated, headache develops. The conjunctiva are hyperemic and the skin flushed. Hypercapnia has nervous system effects similar to those of an anesthetic—hence the term *carbon dioxide narcosis*. There is progressive somnolence, disorientation, and, if the condition is untreated, coma. Mild to moderate increases in blood pressure are common. Air hunger and rapid breathing occur when alveolar PCO_2 levels rise to about 60 to 75 mmHg; as PCO_2 levels reach 80 to 100 mmHg, the person becomes lethargic and, sometimes, semicomatose. Anesthesia and death can result when PCO_2 levels reach 100 to 150 mmHg.[20] The signs and symptoms of hypercapnia are summarized in Chart 28-3.

DIAGNOSIS AND TREATMENT

Diagnosis of hypercapnia is based on blood gas measurements and end-tidal volume carbon dioxide tension (capnometry).

Therapy is directed at decreasing the work of breathing and improving the ventilation–perfusion balance. Intermittent rest therapy, such as nocturnal negative pressure ventilation, applied to hypercapnic patients with chronic obstructive disease or chest wall disease may be effective in increasing the strength and endurance of the respiratory muscle and improving the PCO_2. Respiratory muscle retrain-

---

CHART 28-3: SIGNS AND SYMPTOMS OF HYPERCAPNIA

Increased PCO_2
Headache
Conjunctival hyperemia
Flushed skin
Increased sedation
   Drowsiness
   Disorientation
   Coma
Tachycardia
Diaphoresis
Mild to moderate increase in blood pressure

ing aimed at improving the respiratory muscles, their endurance, or both has been used to improve exercise tolerance and diminish the likelihood of respiratory fatigue.

In summary, the lungs enable inhaled air to come in proximity to the blood flowing through the pulmonary capillaries, so that the exchange of gases between the internal environment of the body and the external environment can take place. Hypoxia refers to an acute or chronic reduction in tissue oxygenation. It can result from decreased oxygen content of the blood (hypoxemic hypoxia), impaired blood flow (stagnant hypoxia), reduced oxygen-carrying capacity of the blood (anemic hypoxia), or impaired cellular utilization of oxygen (histotoxic hypoxia). Hypoxia incites sympathetic nervous system responses such as tachycardia and produces symptoms that are similar to those of alcohol intoxication. Hypercapnia refers to an increase in carbon dioxide levels. In the clinical setting, four factors contribute to hypercapnia: (1) alterations in carbon dioxide production, (2) disturbance in the gas exchange function of the lungs, (3) abnormalities in respiratory function of the chest wall and respiratory muscles, and (4) changes in neural control of respiration. The manifestations of hypercapnia consist of those associated with the vasodilation of blood vessels, including those in the brain, and the depression of the central nervous system (carbon dioxide narcosis).

■ ACUTE RESPIRATORY FAILURE

Respiratory failure occurs when the lungs are unable to adequately oxygenate the blood or prevent undue retention of carbon dioxide even at rest. It can develop acutely in people whose lungs previously had been normal or may be superimposed on chronic disease of the lung or chest wall.

There is no absolute definition of the levels of arterial PO_2 and PCO_2 that indicate respiratory failure. As a general rule, *respiratory failure* refers to a PO_2 level of 50 mmHg or less, and a PCO_2 level greater than 50 mmHg. These values are not reliable when dealing with people who have chronic lung disease because many of these people are alert and functioning with blood gas levels outside this range. Table 28-4 compares the normal values for blood gases with those of respiratory failure.

CAUSES

Respiratory failure is not a specific disease. It is associated with a number of disorders in which the lungs fail to deliver sufficient oxygen to the arterial blood or to remove sufficient carbon dioxide. Three types of conditions contribute to the hypoxia in respiratory failure: hypoventilation, impaired diffusion across the alveolocapillary membrane, and mismatching of ventilation and perfusion. These conditions include impaired ventilation caused by upper airway obstruction, weakness or paralysis of the respiratory muscles, chest wall injury, and disease of the pulmonary airways and lungs. The causes of respiratory failure are summarized in Table 28-5; many are discussed in other parts of the text.

MANIFESTATIONS

Respiratory failure may be seen in previously healthy people as the result of acute disease or trauma involving the respiratory system, or it may develop in the course of a chronic respiratory disease. The presenting signs and symptoms are different in each of these situations. The common manifestations of respiratory failure are hypoxia and hypercapnia. Various types of respiratory failure are associated with different degrees of hypoxia and carbon dioxide retention. In respiratory disorders that impair diffusion across the alveolocapillary membrane, hypoxia becomes severe, whereas arterial PCO_2 decreases or remains normal because carbon dioxide is more soluble in the alveolocapillary membrane than oxygen. In conditions such as chronic obstructive pulmonary disease in which respiratory failure is superimposed on lung disease, severe mismatching of ventilation and perfusion often results in both hypoxia and hypercapnia.

TREATMENT

Treatment of respiratory failure is directed toward correcting the cause and relieving the hypoxia and hypercapnia; for this purpose, a number of treatment

TABLE 28-4. BLOOD GASES IN RESPIRATORY FAILURE COMPARED WITH NORMAL VALUES

ARTERIAL BLOOD GAS VALUE	NORMAL VALUE	RESPIRATORY FAILURE
PO_2	Above 80 mmHg	50 mmHg or less
PCO_2	35–45 mmHg	50 mmHg or above

TABLE 28-5. CAUSES OF RESPIRATORY FAILURE

CATEGORY OF IMPAIRMENT	EXAMPLES
Impaired Ventilation	
Upper airway obstruction	Laryngospasm
	Foreign-body aspiration
	Tumor of the upper airways
	Infection of the upper airways (*e.g.*, epiglottitis)
Weakness or paralysis of the respiratory muscles	Drug overdose
	Injury to the spinal cord
	Poliomyelitis
	Guillain-Barré syndrome
	Muscular dystrophy
	Disease of the brain stem
Chest wall injury	Rib fracture
	Burn eschar
Impaired Matching of Ventilation and Perfusion	
	Chronic obstructive lung disease
	Restrictive lung disease
	Severe pneumonia
	Atelectasis
Impaired Diffusion	
Pulmonary edema	Left heart failure
	Inhalation of toxic materials
Respiratory distress syndrome	Respiratory distress syndrome in the neonate
	Adult respiratory distress syndrome (shock lung)

modalities are available, including the establishment of an airway, use of bronchodilators, and antibiotics for respiratory infections. Controlled oxygen therapy and mechanical ventilation are used in treating blood gas abnormalities associated with respiratory failure.

MECHANICAL VENTILATION

When alveolar ventilation is inadequate to maintain Po_2 or Pco_2 levels because of either respiratory or neurologic failure, mechanical ventilation may be life-saving. There are two types of positive-pressure mechanical ventilators: pressure-controlled units and volume-controlled units. The pressure-controlled ventilator delivers a tidal volume determined by the airway pressure while the flow rate is being controlled. The volume-controlled ventilator delivers a preselected tidal volume while the pressure is monitored. The tidal volume and respiratory rate are adjusted to maintain ventilation at a given minute volume. A nasotracheal, orotracheal, or tracheotomy tube is inserted into the trachea to provide the patient with the airway needed for mechanical ventilation.

A third type of ventilator (iron lung, Cuirass, Poncho, and Body Wrap) uses negative pressure to expand the chest. These ventilators do not require an artificial airway. One of the disadvantages of negative-pressure ventilators is that the application of negative pressure to the abdominal cavity causes blood returning to the right atrium to pool in the large abdominal veins, causing a transient decrease in venous return and cardiac output.[27]

ADULT RESPIRATORY DISTRESS SYNDROME

Adult respiratory distress syndrome (ARDS), first described in 1967, is an extreme form of noncardiac pulmonary edema. It is the final common pathway through which many serious localized and systemic disorders produce diffuse lung injury. ARDS affects about 150,000 to 200,000 persons a year; at least 50% to 60% of these people die, despite the most sophisticated intensive medical care.

The exact cause of ARDS is unknown. It is

thought to result from injury to the microcirculation (small blood vessels and capillaries) of the lung. Numerous insults are associated with its development. The term *shock lung* (see Chapter 25) has been used to describe the respiratory distress syndrome associated with trauma and hypovolemic or septic shock. It may also result from aspiration of gastric contents, major trauma (with or without fat emboli), sepsis (secondary to pulmonary or nonpulmonary infections), acute pancreatitis, hematologic disorders, metabolic events, and reactions to drugs and toxins (Chart 28-4). It is not known whether ARDS results from several distinct pathogenic mechanisms that operate to cause a similar pattern of injury or whether a similar pattern of injury is triggered by different mechanisms. Many investigators believe that neutrophils play a central role in the pathogenesis of ARDS. Neutrophils can synthesize and release products that are capable of tissue injury, including proteolytic enzymes, toxic oxygen species (free radicals; see Chapter 2), and phospholipid products.[28]

Although a number of conditions may lead to ARDS, they all produce similar pathologic lung changes that include diffuse alveolocapillary injury with increased permeability and abnormal surfactant.[28, 29] The increased permeability of the alveolocapillary membrane permits fluid, protein, and blood cells to move out of the vascular compartment into the interstitium and alveoli of the lung. The resultant pulmonary edema leads to intrapulmonary shunting of blood and profound hypoxia. The mechanism of surfactant abnormality is less well known. It could be due either to inactivation of surfactant by the presence of plasma inhibitors or to injury to the surfactant-producing alveolar cells. The type II alveolar cells, which produce surfactant, have the capacity to transport sodium and thereby regulate the clearance of alveolar fluid. When the cells are injured, the clearance of fluid declines, with subsequent flooding of the alveolar space. As these changes take place, the lung stiffens and becomes more difficult to inflate and the work of breathing increases. Progression of the disease is characterized by formation of hyaline membranes and fibrotic thickening of the alveolar walls, compromising the diffusion of respiratory gases.

Clinically, the syndrome consists of progressive respiratory distress, an increase in respiratory rate, and signs of respiratory failure. Radiologic findings usually show extensive bilateral consolidation of the lung tissue. Severe hypoxia persists despite increased inspired oxygen levels.

The treatment goals in ARDS are to supply oxygen to vital organs and provide supportive care until the condition causing the pathologic process has

---

CHART 28-4: CONDITIONS IN WHICH ADULT RESPIRATORY DISTRESS SYNDROME CAN DEVELOP*

Aspiration

Gastric acid
Near-drowning

Reaction to Drugs and Toxins

Chlordiazepoxide
Heroin
Methadone
Propoxyphene
Chloroform
Colchicine
Barbiturates
Inhaled gases
  Ammonia
  Phosgene
  Ozone
  Oxygen (high concentrations)
  Smoke

Hematologic Disorders

Multiple blood transfusions
Disseminated intravascular clotting
Exposure to cardiopulmonary bypass

Infectious Causes

Bacterial pneumonia
Fungal and *Pneumocystis carinii* pneumonias
Gram-negative sepsis
Viral pneumonia

Immune Reactions

Anaphylactic shock
Allergic reactions to inhaled substances

Metabolic Disorders

Diabetic ketoacidosis
Uremia

Trauma

Burns
Fat embolus
Heat trauma
Chest trauma and lung injury
Shock

  * This list not intended to be inclusive.

---

been reversed and the lungs have had a chance to heal. Assisted ventilation using high concentrations of oxygen may be required to overcome the hypoxia. Positive end-expiratory pressure breathing, which increases the pressure in the airways during expiration, may be used to assist in reinflating the collapsed areas of the lung and to improve the matching of ventilation and perfusion. There has been recent interest in the use of nonsteroidal antiinflammatory agents (ibuprofen), surfactant replacement, antioxidant agents, and other blockers of potential mediators of injury. The use of corticosteroid therapy is controversial.

In summary, respiratory failure is a condition in which the lungs fail to adequately oxygenate the blood or to prevent undue retention of carbon dioxide. The causes of respiratory failure are many: it may arise acutely in people with previously healthy lungs, or it may be superimposed in chronic lung disease. Respiratory failure is defined as a Po_2 of 50 mmHg or less and a Pco_2 of 50 mmHg or more. ARDS is an extreme form of noncardiogenic pulmonary edema that results in respiratory failure. The condition can be caused by a number of serious localized and systemic disorders that damage the alveolocapillary membrane of the lung. It results in interstitial edema of lung tissue, an increase in surface tension caused by inactivation of surfactant, collapse of the alveolar structures, a stiff and noncompliant lung that is difficult to inflate, and impaired diffusion of the respiratory gases with severe hypoxia that is resistant to oxygen therapy.

■ REFERENCES

1. Howell, J.B.L. (Ed.). (1966). *Breathlessness*. Philadelphia: F.A. Davis.
2. Carrieri, V.K., & Jansen-Bjerklie, S. (1984). The sensation of dyspnea: A critical review. *Heart and Lung, 13,* 437.
3. Kales, A., Vela-Bueno, A., & Kales, J. (1987). Sleep disorders: Sleep apnea and narcolepsy. *Annals of Internal Medicine, 106,* 434.
4. Phillipson, E.A. (1979). Breathing disorders during sleep. *Basics of RD, 7*(3), 102.
5. Cherniack, N.A. (1981). Respiratory dysrhythmias during sleep. *New England Journal of Medicine, 305,* 325.
6. Guilleminault, C., Cummeninsky, J., & Dement, W.C. (1980). Sleep apnea: Recent advances. *Advances in Internal Medicine, 25,* 347.
7. Mosko, S.S., Dickel, M.J., Paul, T., et al. (1988). Sleep apnea and sleep-related periodic leg movements in community resident seniors. *Journal of the American Geriatrics Society, 36,* 502.
8. Kaplan, J. (1991). Diagnosis and therapy of sleep-disordered breathing. In G.G. Burton, J.E. Hodgkin, & J.J. Ward (Eds.). *Respiratory care: A guide to clinical practice* (3rd ed., pp. 279–287). Philadelphia: J.B. Lippincott.
9. Rapoport, D.M., Sorkin, B., Garay, S.M., et al. (1982). Reversal of the "Pickwickian syndrome" by long-term use of nocturnal nasal-airway pressure. *New England Journal of Medicine, 307,* 931.
10. Brownell, L.G., West, P., Sweatman, P., et al. (1982). Protriptyline in obstructive sleep apnea. *New England Journal of Medicine, 307,* 1038.
11. Kryger, M.H. (Ed.). (1981). *Pathophysiology of respiration* (p. 265). New York: John Wiley.
12. Magarian, G.J. (1982). Hyperventilation syndromes: Infrequently recognized common expression of anxiety and stress. *Medicine (Baltimore), 61,* 219.
13. Herman, S.P., Stickler, G.B., & Lucas, A.R. (1981). Hyperventilation syndromes in children and adolescents: Long-term follow-up. *Pediatrics, 67,* 183.
14. Mortenson, S.A., Vihelmson, R., & Sande, E. (1981). Prinzmetal's variant angina (PVA), circadian variation in response to hyperventilation. *Acta Medica Scandinavica, 644*(Suppl.), 38.
15. Yasue, H., Nagao, M., Omote, S., et al. (1978). Coronary artery spasm and Prinzmetal's variant form of angina induced by hyperventilation and tris-buffer infusion. *Circulation, 58,* 56.
16. Yasue, H., Omote, S., Takizawa, A., et al. (1981). Alkalosis-induced coronary vasoconstriction: Effects of calcium, diltiazem, nitroglycerin and propranolol. *American Heart Journal, 102,* 206.
17. Gennari, F.J., Goldstein, M.B., & Schwartz, W.B. (1972). The nature of renal adaptation to chronic hypocapnia. *Journal of Clinical Investigation, 51,* 1722.
18. Cowley, D.S., & Roy-Byrne, P.P. (1987). Hyperventilation and panic disorder. *American Journal of Medicine, 83,* 929.
19. Tavel, M.E. (1990). Hyperventilation syndrome: Hiding behind pseudonyms. *Chest, 97,* 1285–1288.
20. Guyton, A. (1991). *Textbook of medical physiology* (8th ed., pp. 444–453, 460, 464–467). Philadelphia: W.B. Saunders.
21. Katzung, B.G. (1989). *Basic and clinical pharmacology* (4th ed., p. 144). E. Norwalk, CT: Appleton Lange.
22. White, K.M., Winslow, E.H., Clark, A., et al. (1990). The physiologic basis for continuous mixed venous oxygen saturation. *Heart and Lung, 19*(5, part 2), 548–551.
23. Rueden, K.T. (1990). Noninvasive assessment of gas exchange in the critically ill patient. *AACN Clinical Issues in Critical Care Nursing, 1,* 239–247.
24. Brown, L.H. (1990). Pulmonary oxygen toxicity. *Focus on Critical Care, 17*(1), 68–75.
25. Weinberger, S.E., Schwartzstein, R.M., & Weiss, J.W. (1989). Hypercapnia. *New England Journal of Medicine, 321,* 1223–1230.
26. St. John, R.E., & Eisenberg, P. (1991). Nutrition and use of metabolic assessment in the ventilator-dependent patient. *AACN Clinical Issues in Critical Care Nursing, 2,* 453–462.
27. Vasbinder-Dillon, D. (1988). Understanding mechanical ventilation. *Critical Care Nurse, 8*(7), 42.
28. Beer, D.J. (1992). ARDS: Evolving concepts of a systemic disease. *Hospital Practice, 27,* 57–80.
29. Hudson, L.D. (1991). Adult respiratory distress syndrome. In G.G. Burton, J.E. Hodgkin, & J.J. Ward (Eds.), *Respiratory care: A guide to clinical practice* (3rd ed., pp. 857–873). Philadelphia: J.B. Lippincott.

■ BIBLIOGRAPHY

Ashworth, L.J. (1990). Pressure support ventilation. *Critical Care Nurse, 10,* 20–27.

Carpenter, K.D. (1991). Oxygen transport in the blood. *Critical Care Nurse, 11,* 20–33.

Cowley, D.S., & Roy-Byrne, P.P. (1987). Hyperventilation and panic disorder. *Medical Clinics of North America, 83,* 929.

Dettenmeirer, P.A., & Jackson, N.C. (1991). Chronic hypoventilation syndrome: Treatment with non-invasive mechanical ventilation. *ACCN Clinical Issues in Critical Care Nursing, 2,* 415–431.

Elliott, M.W., Adams, L., Cockcroft, A., et al. (1991). The language of breathlessness. *American Review of Respiratory Disease, 144,* 826–832.

Guilleminault, C., Quera-Salva, M.A., Nino-Murcia, G., et al. (1987). Central sleep apnea and partial obstruction of the upper airway. *Annals of Neurology, 21,* 465.

Harman, E., Wynne, J.W., Block, A.J., et al. Sleep-disordered breathing.

Hudgel, D.W. (1992). Mechanisms of obstructive sleep apnea. *Chest, 101,* 541–549.

Kelson, S.G. (1986). The effects of undernutrition on the respiratory muscles. *Clinics in Chest Medicine, 7,* 101.

Massaro, D. (1986). Oxygen: Toxicity and tolerance. *Hospital Practice, 21,* 95.

O'Donnel, D.E., & Webb, K.A. (1992). Breathlessness in patients with severe chronic airway limitation. *Chest, 102,* 824–831.

Reischman, R.R. (1988). Review of ventilation and perfusion physiology. *Critcial Care Nurse, 8,* 24–30.

Rochester, D.F. (1986). Malnutrition and the respiratory muscles. *Clinics in Chest Medicine, 7,* 91.

Schroeder, C.H. (1988). Pulse oximetry: A nursing care plan. *Critical Care Nurse, 8*(8), 50.

Vasbinder-Dillon, D. (1988). Understanding mechanical ventilators. *Critical Care Nurse, 8*(7), 42.

Wasserman, K., & Casaburi, R. (1988). Dyspnea: Physiological and pathophysiological mechanisms. *Annual Review of Medicine, 39,* 503.

ALTERATIONS IN FLUIDS AND ELECTROLYTES

CHAPTER 29

ALTERATIONS IN FLUIDS AND ELECTROLYTES

■ OBJECTIVES

After you have studied this chapter, you should be able to meet the following objectives:

■ Differentiate between the intracellular and extracellular compartments in terms of distribution of body fluids and electrolytes.

■ Define the term *electrolyte*.

■ Relate the concept of a concentration gradient to the processes of diffusion and osmosis.

■ List major sources of body water gain and loss.

■ State the function and stimuli of thirst.

■ Explain how ADH regulates the urine-concentrating ability of the kidneys.

■ Compare the pathology and manifestations of diabetes insipidus and the syndrome of inappropriate ADH.

■ Describe the causes of fluid volume deficit with reference to the skin, gastrointestinal tract, third spaces, and kidneys.

■ Describe the effects of fluid volume deficit on the skin, brain, and circulatory, nervous, urinary, and gastrointestinal systems.

■ Describe the effect of body water levels on the sodium concentration in the extracellular fluids.

■ Cite the causes of hyponatremia and hypernatremia in terms of altered intake, output, and regulation mechanisms.

■ Relate the functions of sodium to the clinical manifestations of hyponatremia and hypernatremia.

■ Explain the functions of potassium.

■ State the causes of hypokalemia and hyperkalemia in terms of altered intake, output, and intracellular versus extracellular distribution mechanisms.

■ Relate the functions of potassium to the clinical manifestations of hypokalemia and hyperkalemia.

■ Describe the function of vitamin D, parathyroid hormone, and calcitonin in terms of regulating serum calcium and phosphate levels.

■ Describe the causes of hypocalcemia in terms of altered gastrointestinal tract absorption, mobilization of bone stores, renal losses, and protein or citrate binding.

■ Relate the manifestations of hypophosphatemia and hyperphosphatemia to the functions of phosphate.

Carol Mattson Porth: PATHOPHYSIOLOGY: CONCEPTS OF
ALTERED HEALTH STATES, 4th ed. © 1994, 1990, 1986, 1982
J.B. Lippincott Company

■ List the major functions of magnesium.
■ Describe the role of the capillaries in regulating interstitial fluid volume.
■ Describe the factors that control fluid exchange at the capillary level and relate to the development of edema.

■ Describe the physiologic effects of edema.
■ Relate the principles of edema to the accumulation of fluids in serous cavities.

Body fluids contain water, electrolytes, proteins, and other substances. The precise regulation of these fluids within a narrow physiologic range is essential to life. The volume and composition of these fluids remain relatively constant in the presence of a wide range of changes in intake and output. Environmental stresses and disease conditions often increase losses, impair intake, and otherwise interfere with mechanisms that regulate body fluid volume, composition, and distribution. This chapter is divided into four sections: (1)physiology of body fluid composition and distribution, (2) alterations in fluid volume, (3) alterations in the electrolyte composition of body fluids, and (4) alterations in interstitial fluids and edema.

■ PHYSIOLOGY OF BODY FLUID COMPOSITION AND DISTRIBUTION

Body fluids are distributed between two body compartments: the intracellular compartment and the extracellular compartment. The *intracellular compartment* consists of the fluid contained within all the body's billions of cells (Fig. 29-1). The *extracellular compartment* contains all the fluid located outside the cells. Included in the extracellular compartment are interstitial fluids (fluids that surround the cells), intravascular fluids, cerebrospinal fluid, and fluid contained within the various body spaces, such as the pleural cavity and the joint spaces. Even the water contained in the anterior chamber of the eye is considered extracellular fluid.

The primary barrier to the movement of substances between the extracellular and intracellular compartments is at the level of the cell membrane. The ability to cross the cell membrane depends on the solubility of the substance in the cell membrane or its ability to pass through special openings in the cell membrane. Lipid-soluble substances such as gases (oxygen and carbon dioxide), which dissolve in the lipid matrix of the cell membrane, pass directly through the membrane using virtually the entire membrane surface. Other substances that are water-soluble rather than lipid-soluble, such as glucose and sodium chloride, must pass through special water-

filled channels in the membrane or be transported by special carrier systems. Movement through the membrane is determined by particle size, its electrochemical properties, and the osmotic forces that develop between the inside and the outside of the cell. Macromolecules such as proteins either cannot cross the membrane or do so slowly in comparison with small particles such as sodium and chloride. The size constraint is apparently related to the size and structure of the membrane channel. Some channels, such as the sodium channels, selectively permit the passage of certain electrolytes.

ELECTROCHEMICAL PROPERTIES

Body fluids contain both water and chemical compounds. In solution, these chemical compounds can either remain as an intact molecule or dissociate into smaller particles. Electrolytes are substances that dis-

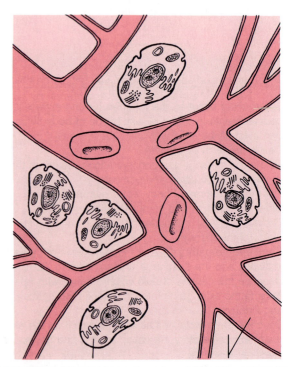

FIG. 29-1. Distribution of body water. The extracellular space includes the vascular compartment and the interstitial spaces.

sociate in solution to form *charged particles*, or *ions*. For example, a sodium chloride molecule dissociates to form a positively charged sodium (Na+) and a negatively charged chloride (Cl−) ion. Particles such as glucose and urea do not dissociate into ions and are called *nonelectrolytes*.

Positively charged ions are called *cations* because they are attracted to the cathode of a wet electric cell. Similarly, negatively charged ions are called *anions* because they are attracted to the anode. The ions found in body fluids carry either one charge (*a monovalent ion*) or two charges (*a divalent ion*). When cations and anions combine, they do so according to their ionic charge, not according to their atomic weight.

The distribution of electrolytes between the intracellular and extracellular compartments is influenced by their electrical charges. Ions with like charges repel, and ions with opposite charges attract. This repulsion or attraction can cause electrolytes to move from one body compartment to another. In other words, an excess of positively charged ions in a body compartment attracts negatively charged ions in an attempt to balance the electrical charge.

Electroneutrality requires that the total number of cations in the body equal the total number of anions. The unit that expresses the charge equivalency of a given weight of an electrolyte is a milliequivalent (mEq). Thus, 1 mEq of sodium has the same number of charges as 1 mEq of chloride, regardless of molecular weight (although sodium is positive and chloride is negative). The number of milliequivalents of an electrolyte in a liter of solution can be derived from the following formula:

$$mEq/L = \frac{mg/100 \text{ mL} \times 10 \times \text{valence}}{\text{atomic weight}}$$

The International System of Units expresses electrolytes as millimoles per liter (mmol/L).

$$mmol/L = \frac{mEq/L}{\text{valence}}$$

This means that 1 mEq equals 1 mmol of a monovalent electrolyte. Laboratory reports of serum electrolytes and electrolyte composition of intravenous solutions and other medications are expressed as either mEq/L or mmol/L. Some electrolytes, such as calcium, phosphate, and magnesium, are sometimes expressed in milligrams per deciliter (mg/dL).

DIFFUSION AND OSMOSIS

In a biologic system, the concentration of dissolved particles in a solution influences water movement and controls cell size. Diffusion is the movement of charged or uncharged particles along a concentration gradient. The behavior of sugar added to a container

of water is an example of diffusion. The concentration of sugar initially is greatest at the point where it comes in contact with the water. Moments later the sugar will have diffused, so that its concentration is equalized throughout the container. Many small molecules diffuse from one body compartment to another along a concentration gradient.

Most cell membranes are semipermeable. This means that they allow water and small uncharged particles to diffuse freely through their pores while partially or completely preventing the passage of charged ions and large molecules. In diffusing through a semipermeable membrane, water moves from the side with the lesser number of nondiffusible particles to the side that has the greater number (Fig. 29-2). The pressure caused by water movement is called the *osmotic pressure*.

The osmotic activity, or work potential, that the nondiffusible particles exert in drawing water from one side of the semipermeable membrane to the other is measured by a unit called an *osmole*. The osmole is the standard unit of osmotic pressure and is derived from the gram molecular weight (1 gram molecular weight of a nondiffusible and nonionizable substance is equal to 1 osmole). In the clinical setting, osmotic activity usually is expressed in milliosmoles (one thousandth of an osmole) per liter. Each nondiffusible particle, large or small, is equally effective in its ability to pull water through a semipermeable membrane. Thus, the osmotic activity of a solution is

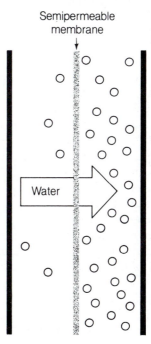

FIG. 29-2. Movement of water across a semipermeable membrane. Water movement is from the side that has the lesser number of nondiffusible particles to the side that has the greater number.

determined by the number, rather than the size, of the nondiffusible particles.

The osmotic activity of a solution may be expressed as either osmolarity or osmolality. Osmolarity refers to the osmolar concentration in 1 L of solution (mOsm/L), whereas osmolality refers to the osmoles dissolved in 1 kg of water (mOsm/kg H₂O). Although the terms *osmolarity* and *osmolality* often are used interchangeably, most clinical laboratories report osmotic activity as osmolality.

The predominant osmotically active particles within the cell are potassium and its attendant anions. In the extracellular fluid, sodium and its attendant anions account for 90% to 95% of the osmotic pressure. Blood urea nitrogen (BUN) and glucose account for less than 5% of the total osmotic pressure in the extracellular compartment. This can change, however, as when blood glucose levels are elevated in people with diabetes mellitus or when BUN levels rise in people with renal failure. Serum osmolality, which normally ranges between 275 and 295 mOsm/kg, can be calculated using the following formula (1 mOsm of glucose equals 180 mg/L; 1 mOsm of urea equals 28 mg/L):

$$\text{Osmolality (mOsm/kg)} = 2[\text{Na}^+ \text{ (mmol/L)}] + \frac{\text{Glucose (mg/dL)}}{18} + \frac{\text{BUN (mg/dL)}}{2.8}$$

The cell is enclosed in a flexible membrane; therefore, any change in its volume produces a change in cell size. The term *tonicity* refers to the tension or effect that the osmotic pressure of a solution exerts on cell size because of water movement across the cell membrane. By definition, a *hypertonic* solution is one that causes a cell to shrink or become *crenated* (Fig. 29-3). A *hypotonic* solution causes a cell to swell. An *isotonic* solution is one that does not cause a change in cell size.

The osmotic pressure in the extracellular and intracellular compartments usually is the same, except for momentary differences. This is because water moves freely across cell membranes in response to osmotic pressure changes. Body cells may shrink or swell, but the osmolality of the intracellular fluid remains the same as that of the extracellular fluid. When water is lost from the extracellular compartment, water diffuses out of the intracellular compartment into the extracellular compartment until an equilibrium is reached.

In summary, body fluids are distributed between the intracellular and extracellular compartments of the body. The extracellular fluid compartment contains intravascular fluid, interstitial fluid, and fluid contained in the extracellular spaces, such as the pleural cavity. Body fluids contain water, charged particles called *electrolytes*, and noncharged particles called *nonelectrolytes*. Electrolytes are measured in *milliequivalents*

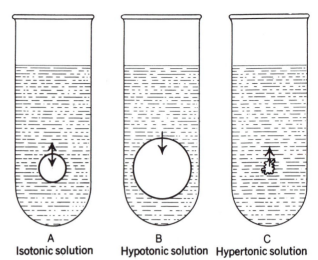

A — Isotonic solution B — Hypotonic solution C — Hypertonic solution

FIG. 29-3. Osmosis. (**A**) Red cells undergo no change in size in isotonic solutions. They increase in size in hypotonic solutions (**B**) and decrease in size in hypertonic solutions (**C**). (Chaffee, E. E., & Greisheimer, E. M. [1974]. *Basic physiology and anatomy* [3rd ed.]. Philadelphia: J.B. Lippincott.)

per liter or millimoles per liter, measurement units that express the charge equivalency of a given weight of an electrolyte. Diffusion is the movement of charged and noncharged particles along a concentration gradient. Both electrolytes and nonelectrolytes move between body compartments by diffusion. The movement of water across the semipermeable membranes of the body is controlled by the nondiffusible particles on either side of the membrane in a process called *osmosis*. Osmosis is regulated by the number, rather than the size, of the nondiffusible particles. The tension or effect that the osmotic pressure of a solution exerts on body cells is called tonicity. When cells are exposed to a hypotonic solution, they swell; when they are exposed to a hypertonic solution, they shrink.

■ ALTERATIONS IN FLUID VOLUME

Body water is distributed between the intracellular and extracellular compartments. The intracellular compartment contains about two thirds of the body's water and the extracellular compartment, about one third. In the adult, intracellular water constitutes about 45% of body weight and extracellular fluid, about 15% (Fig. 29-4). The distribution of body water is determined by the osmotic properties of body fluids and the concentration of electrolytes. Water provides about 90% to 93% of the volume in the extracellular fluid compartment.

The functions of water in the human body are many (Chart 29-1). Water adds to the structure of the body, acts as a transport vehicle, lubricates and cushions, acts to hydrolyze food in the digestive system, and is necessary for chemical reactions that occur within the cell.

Water gives the body its structure. One has only

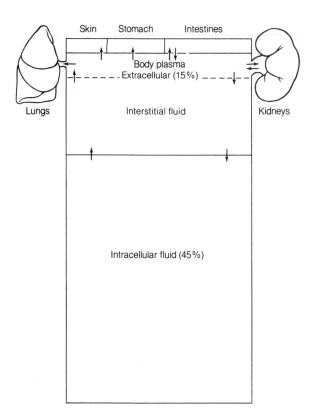

FIG. 29-4. Fluid compartments in the adult. Fluid in the intracellular compartment constitutes about 45% of body weight, whereas fluid in the extracellular compartment constitutes about 15% of body weight. Fluid from the extracellular compartment moves into the gastrointestinal tract, skin, lungs, and kidneys.

to compare the dry, wrinkled skin of an elderly person with the soft, smooth skin of a child to understand the extent to which water contributes to the body's overall form and appearance. Water adds a resiliency to the skin and underlying tissues that is referred to as *skin,* or *tissue, turgor.* Tissue turgor is assessed by pinching a fold of skin between the

---

CHART 29-1: FUNCTIONS OF WATER

Provides form for body structures
Acts as a transport vehicle for
   nutrients
   electrolytes
   blood gases
   metabolic wastes
   heat
   electric currents
Provides insulation
Aids in the hydrolysis of food
Acts as a medium and reactant for chemical reactions
Acts as a lubricant
Cushions and acts as a shock absorber

---

thumb and forefinger. The skin should immediately return to its normal configuration when the fingers are released. A loss of 3% to 5% of body water causes the resiliency of the skin to be lost, and the tissue remains raised for several seconds.

The transport of body nutrients, wastes, electrical impulses, and heat depends on fluid movement both in the interstitial spaces and in the vascular compartment. In relation to body temperature, water not only transports heat from the inner core of the body to the periphery where it can be released into the external environment but it also insulates the body against changes in the external temperature. Were it not for the insulation afforded the body by its water content, the body would be much like a rock, gaining heat during the day and losing it at night.

Water also lubricates and cushions. Synovial fluid lubricates the joints, and pericardial fluid prevents the heart from rubbing against the pericardial sac. The act of swallowing would be difficult, if not impossible, were it not for the lubricating properties of the mucus that lines the gastrointestinal tract. Cerebrospinal fluid cushions the brain. During pregnancy, amniotic fluid acts as a shock absorber and protects the delicate fetus.

Water hydrolyzes the food eaten, breaking it down into particles that can be digested and then absorbed across the gastrointestinal tract wall. In addition, many of the chemical reactions that occur within the body require water as a medium or reactant.

REQUIREMENTS

The body is largely water; therefore, body water usually is expressed as a percentage of body weight. Total body water varies with age, decreasing from infancy to old age. In a full-term infant, body water constitutes as much as 75% to 80% of body weight, whereas body water accounts for only 60% to 70% of body weight in an adult. A premature infant has even a greater amount of body water than a full-term infant; an elderly person has much less water in relation to body weight than a younger adult. Because fat essentially is water-free, obesity decreases the percentage of water that the body contains, sometimes reducing these levels to values as low as 45% of body weight.

Despite its greater body water content, an infant is more likely to develop fluid imbalances than is an adult. This is because an infant has both a higher metabolic rate and a larger surface area in relation to its body mass than an older child or an adult. Also, an infant has more difficulty concentrating its urine because its kidney structures are immature. This means that an infant has greater skin and urine losses and that more water is needed for metabolic processes. An infant, therefore, both ingests and excretes greater volumes of water in relation to its size than an adult. For example, an infant may exchange one half of its extracellular fluid volume in a single day, whereas an adult exchanges only about one sixth of this volume during the same period. By the 3rd year of life, the percentages and distribution of body water in a young child approach those of an adult.

Regardless of age, all healthy people require about 100 mL of water per 100 calories metabolized. This means that a person who expends 1800 calories for energy requires about 1800 mL of water for metabolic purposes. The metabolic rate increases with fever; it rises 12% for every 1°C (7% for every 1°F) increase in body temperature.

GAINS AND LOSSES

The main source of water gain is absorption from the gastrointestinal tract; the water gained in this manner includes that obtained from fluids, ingested foods, tube feedings, and parenterally administered fluids. Water is also derived from cellular oxidation of foodstuffs. The quantity gained in this manner varies from 150 to 250 mL, depending on the rate of metabolism.[1]

Water losses occur through the kidneys, skin, lungs, and gastrointestinal tract. Even when oral or parenteral intake has been withheld, the kidneys continue to produce urine as a means of ridding the body of metabolic wastes. The urine output that is required to eliminate these wastes is called the *obligatory urine output*. The obligatory urine loss is about 300 to 500 mL/day.

Water losses that occur from the skin and respiratory tract are termed *insensible water losses* because the person is not aware of them. Under normal conditions, water vapor lost from the skin and lungs approximates 500 mL/m^2 of surface area per day. Skin losses include the water that continually diffuses through the pores in the skin as well as the water lost in sweating. Respiratory losses consist of water vapor that is withdrawn from the mucous membranes to humidify the inspired air and then is lost to the environment during expiration. The frosty breath that one sees on a cold day is evidence of water losses that occur with respiration. Sources of water gain and loss are listed in Table 29-1.

REGULATION

Two physiologic mechanisms assist in regulating body water levels; one of these is thirst and the other is the kidneys' ability to concentrate urine. Thirst is

TABLE 29-1. SOURCES OF BODY WATER GAINS AND LOSSES IN THE ADULT

GAINS		LOSSES	
		Urine	1500 mL
Oral intake		Insensible losses	
As water	1000 mL	Lungs	300 mL
In food	1300 mL	Skin	500 mL
Water of oxidation	200 mL	Feces	200 mL
Total	2500 mL	Total	2500 mL

primarily a regulator of intake, and urine-concentrating mechanisms are regulators of output. Both mechanisms respond to changes in extracellular volume and osmolality.

THIRST

Thirst is the sensation associated with a craving to drink. It usually serves as the stimulus for drinking water or liquids that are high in water content.[2] The thirst center is located in the anterior hypothalamus (Fig. 29-5). Nerve cells called osmoreceptors, which are located in or near the thirst center, respond to changes in extracellular osmolality by either swelling or shrinking. Thirst occurs when an increase in extracellular osmolality causes these cells to shrink. Thirst normally develops when 0.5% of body water has been lost.

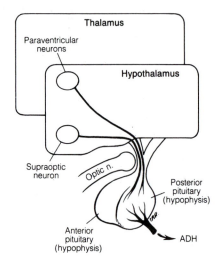

FIG. 29-5. Centers of the hypothalamus and pituitary gland, which are involved in water balance. Antidiuretic hormone (ADH) is synthesized by cells in the supraoptic and paraventricular nuclei of the hypothalamus; it travels along a neural pathway to the posterior pituitary where it is stored for future release. The thirst center also is located in the anterior hypothalamus.

There are two *main* stimuli for thirst: (1) cellular dehydration caused by an increase in extracellular osmolality and (2) a decrease in blood volume, which may or may not be associated with a decrease in serum osmolality. Thirst is one of the earliest symptoms of hemorrhage, often being present long before other signs of blood loss appear.

A third mechanism, the renin–angiotensin mechanism, contributes to nonosmotic thirst. The renin–angiotensin system is considered a backup system for thirst if other systems should fail. Because it is a backup system, it probably does not contribute to the regulation of normal thirst. Elevated levels of angiotensin II, however, may lead to thirst in some pathologic states, such as chronic renal failure and congestive heart failure, in which renin levels may be elevated. Thirst and elevated renin levels are also found in people with primary aldosteronism and in those with secondary hyperaldosteronism accompanying anorexia nervosa, hemorrhage, and sodium depletion.

Lastly, dryness of the mouth produces a sensation of thirst that is not necessarily associated with the body's state of hydration—for example, the thirst a lecturer experiences as the mouth dries out during speaking. Thirst sensation also occurs in those who breathe through their mouths, such as smokers and people with chronic respiratory disease or hyperventilation syndrome.

Liquids commonly are consumed with meals; more water is consumed when salty foods are ingested. As a result, thirst is basically an emergency response. It usually occurs only when the need for water has not been anticipated. Most people drink without being thirsty, and water is consumed before it is needed.

Polydipsia, or excessive thirst, is normal when it accompanies conditions of water deficit. Increased thirst and drinking behavior can be classified into three categories: (1) symptomatic thirst, (2) inappropriate or false thirst that occurs despite normal levels of body water and serum osmolality, and (3) compulsive water drinking. Symptomatic thirst develops when there is a loss of body water and resolves once the loss has been resolved. Among the most common causes of symptomatic thirst are diarrhea, vomiting, diabetes mellitus, and diabetes insipidus. Inappropriate or excessive thirst persists despite adequate hydration. It is a common complaint in people with renal failure and congestive heart failure. It is also a common complaint in people with dry mouth caused by decreased salivary function or treatment with pharmacologic agents that lead to decreased salivary flow. Compulsive water drinking, or psychogenic polydipsia, usually occurs in people with psychiatric disorders. People afflicted with this

disorder drink water in excess of what the kidneys can excrete. A 1977 news story related the fatal outcome of a 29-year-old woman with a diagnosis of chronic schizophrenia who was drinking 4 gal of water a day to "cleanse her body of cancer."[3] Compulsive water drinking can lead to water intoxication, a condition characterized by profound hyponatremia and hypo-osmolality of body fluids.

The thirst mechanism may also be impaired, resulting in inadequate water intake. There is evidence that thirst is decreased and water intake is reduced in elderly people, despite higher serum sodium and osmolality levels.[4, 5] Thirst and drinking are compounded in people who have had a stroke and may be further influenced by confusion and sensory disturbances.

RENAL CONCENTRATING MECHANISMS

The kidneys control the concentration of most of the constituents in body fluids, including water and electrolytes. Each kidney has about 1 million functional units called nephrons, each containing a glomerulus and tubule (see Chapter 31). Water and electrolytes are filtered from the blood in the glomeruli and then selectively reabsorbed in the tubules. The rate at which water and electrolytes can be removed from the body is determined by renal blood flow and the glomerular filtration rate. As the urine filtrate moves through the tubule, water and electrolytes that are needed for maintaining the volume and composition of body fluids are reabsorbed into the extracellular fluid and those that are not needed are excreted in the urine.

ANTIDIURETIC HORMONE

The reabsorption of water by the kidneys is regulated by the antidiuretic hormone (ADH), also known as *vasopressin*. ADH is synthesized by cells in the supraoptic and paraventricular nuclei of the hypothalamus (see Fig. 29-5). The hormone is transported along a neural pathway (the hypophysial tract) to the neurohypophysis (posterior pituitary) and then stored for future release. A rise in ADH levels produces an increase in water reabsorption from the distal tubules and collecting ducts of the kidneys. As with thirst, ADH levels are controlled by volume and osmolar changes in the extracellular fluids. Osmoreceptors in the hypothalamus sense changes in extracellular osmolality and stimulate the production and release of ADH. A small increase in serum osmolality of 1% to 2% is sufficient to cause ADH release. Likewise, stretch receptors in the great veins, atria, and carotid sinus area sense changes in blood volume or blood pressure, and input from these receptors aids in the regulation of ADH release.

A blood volume decrease of 10% to 15% produces a maximal increase in ADH levels, and blood pressure reductions of 5% to 10% are needed to increase ADH levels.[6] As with many other homeostatic mechanisms, acute conditions produce greater changes in ADH levels than do chronic conditions; long-term changes in blood volume or blood pressure may exist without affecting ADH levels.

Many stress situations increase the synthesis and release of ADH. Severe pain, nausea, trauma, surgery, certain anesthetic agents, and some analgesic drugs increase ADH levels. Nausea is the most potent stimulus of ADH secretion; it can increase ADH levels 10 to 1000 times those required for maximal diuresis.[6] The stimulus is mediated by way of the chemoreceptor trigger zone in the medulla, which then relays the impulse to the supraoptic and paraventricular nuclei in the hypothalamus. Afferent input from the gastrointestinal tract may be important in some circumstances. Among the drugs that affect ADH are nicotine, which stimulates its release, and alcohol, which inhibits it. Table 29-2 lists drugs that are known to affect ADH levels.

Two important conditions alter ADH levels: diabetes insipidus and inappropriate secretion of ADH. Because of their effects on water balance, both of these conditions are discussed in this chapter.

Diabetes Insipidus. Diabetes insipidus means "tasteless diabetes," as opposed to diabetes mellitus, or "sweet diabetes." A disorder of ADH availability or function, it is characterized by polyuria (excessive urination) and subsequent polydipsia triggered by plasma hyperosmolality.

There are two types of diabetes insipidus: (1) *central or neurogenic diabetes insipidus*, which occurs because of a defect in the synthesis or release of ADH, and (2) *nephrogenic diabetes insipidus*, which occurs because the kidneys do not respond to ADH. In neurogenic diabetes insipidus, loss of 75% of ADH-secretory neurons is necessary for clinically important polyuria.[7] Most people with neurogenic diabetes insipidus have an incomplete form of the disorder and retain some ability to concentrate their urine. Temporary diabetes insipidus can follow head injury or surgery near the hypophysial tract. Nephrogenic diabetes insipidus is characterized by impairment of urine-concentrating ability and free-water conservation. It may occur as an X-linked recessive trait or, more commonly, as a result of kidney disease, potassium depletion, or chronic hypercalcemia. Polyuria and polydipsia are frequent adverse effects of lithium therapy.

People with diabetes insipidus are unable to concentrate their urine during periods of water restriction; they excrete large volumes of urine, usually 3 to 20 L/day, depending on the degree of ADH deficiency or renal insensitivity to ADH. This large urine output is accompanied by excessive thirst; as long as the thirst mechanism is normal and fluid is readily available, there is little or no alteration in the fluid levels in people with diabetes insipidus. The danger arises when the condition develops in an unconscious person because an inadequate fluid intake rapidly leads to hypertonic dehydration and increased serum osmolality.

Diagnosis of diabetes insipidus is based on measurements of urine and serum osmolality. These tests may be used to evaluate the response to water deprivation, an infusion of a hypertonic saline solution, or pharmacologic preparations of ADH. People with nephrogenic diabetes insipidus do not respond to pharmacologic preparations of the hormone; this method is used to differentiate between the two forms of the disease. Diagnostic measures for diabetes insipidus include those that rule out psychogenic polydipsia as a reason for the excessive thirst and increased urine output. A recently developed radioimmunoassay for ADH can be used for this purpose. When central diabetes insipidus is suspected, diagnostic methods such as skull x-ray studies and computed tomographic (CT) scanning of the pituitary hypothalamic area are used to determine the cause of the disorder.

The management of central diabetes insipidus consists of treating any underlying disorder and supplying the body with pharmacologic preparations

TABLE 29-2. DRUGS THAT AFFECT ADH LEVELS

DRUGS THAT DECREASE ADH LEVELS/ACTION	DRUGS THAT INCREASE ADH LEVELS/ACTION
Demeclocycline	Acetaminophen
Ethanol	Analgesics (morphine and meperidine)
Glucocorticoids	Anesthetics (most)
Lithium carbonate	Antipsychotic tranquilizers
Morphine antagonists	Cancer drugs (vincristine and cyclophosphamide)
Norepinephrine	Carbamazepine
Phenytoin	Chlorpropamide
Reserpine, chlorpromazine	Clofibrate
	Isoproterenol
	Nicotine
	Phenobarbital
	Thiazide diuretics (chlorothiazide)
	Tricyclic antidepressants

that contain the missing hormone. These preparations must be administered parenterally or nasally; they are not given by mouth because they are destroyed in the gastrointestinal tract. The preferred drug for treating chronic diabetes insipidus is desmopressin acetate (DDAVP).[7] Desmopressin, which can be given by intranasal insufflation or spray, has a duration of action of 8 to 20 hours as a result of the removal of an amine group from the first amino acid of ADH. Many persons with incomplete neurogenic diabetes insipidus maintain near-normal water balance when permitted to ingest water in response to thirst. Sometimes other nonhormonal forms of therapy are used for cases in which ADH release is still present. The oral antidiabetic agent chlorpropamide may be used to stimulate ADH release in central diabetes insipidus. Other drugs that are used to treat this form of diabetes insipidus are carbamazepine and clofibrate. In nephrogenic diabetes insipidus, the thiazide diuretics are the specific form of therapy. These drugs probably act predominantly by causing an increase in sodium excretion by the kidneys, which lowers the glomerular filtration rate and increases reabsorption of fluid in the proximal tubule.

Syndrome of Inappropriate ADH. The syndrome of inappropriate ADH (SIADH) results from a failure of the negative feedback system that regulates the release and inhibition of ADH. When this syndrome is present, ADH secretion continues even when serum osmolality is decreased; this leads to marked retention of water in excess of sodium, causing dilutional hyponatremia. An increase in the glomerular filtration rate resulting from an increased plasma volume causes further increases in sodium loss. Urine osmolality is high and serum osmolality, low. Urine output decreases despite adequate or increased fluid intake, and the resultant water retention produces a rapid gain in body weight. Hematocrit and serum sodium and BUN levels are all decreased because of the expansion of the extracellular fluid volume.

SIADH can be caused by a number of conditions, including lung tumors, chest lesions, and central nervous system (CNS) disorders, and by various pharmacologic agents. The first report of SIADH was made in the late 1950s in association with lung cancer. Tumors, particularly bronchogenic carcinomas, are known to produce and release ADH independent of hypothalamic control mechanisms. Other intrathoracic conditions, such as advanced tuberculosis, severe pneumonia, and positive-pressure breathing, also cause SIADH. The suggested mechanism for SIADH in these cases is activation of intrathoracic baroreceptors that respond to marked changes in intrathoracic pressure. Disease and injury to the CNS can cause direct pressure on or direct involvement of the hypothalamic–posterior pituitary structures. Examples include brain tumors, hydrocephalus, head injury, meningitis, and encephalitis. Other stimuli, such as pain, stress, and temperature changes, are capable of stimulating ADH release through the limbic system. Drugs induce SIADH in different ways; some drugs are thought to increase hypothalamic production and release, whereas others are believed to act directly on the renal tubules to potentiate the action of ADH.

SIADH may occur as a transient condition, as in a stress situation, or as a chronic condition, resulting from such disorders as a lung tumor. The severity of symptoms usually is proportional to the extent of sodium depletion and water intoxication. Symptoms of mild SIADH (serum sodium levels around 130 mEq/L) include headache, anorexia, muscle cramps, general fatigue, and dulling of the sensorium. In severe SIADH (serum sodium levels below 126 mEq/L), neurologic symptoms of acute water intoxication begin to appear; they include nausea, vomiting, muscle twitching, seizures, and coma.

The treatment of SIADH depends on its severity. In mild cases, treatment consists of fluid restriction. If fluid restriction is not sufficient, diuretics such as mannitol and furosemide (Lasix) may be given to promote diuresis and free-water clearance. Lithium and the antibiotic demeclocycline inhibit the action of ADH on the renal collecting ducts and sometimes are used in treating the disorder. In cases of severe sodium depletion, a hypertonic (3% or 5%) sodium chloride solution may be administered intravenously.

FLUID VOLUME DEFICIT

The extracellular fluid compartment is the source of all body secretions, including sweat, urine, and gastrointestinal tract secretions. Fluid volume deficit occurs when the loss of body fluids exceeds fluid intake. Water moves rapidly between body compartments; because of this, an extracellular fluid volume deficit usually is accompanied by a deficit of intracellular fluids. Fluid deficit is a serious threat, especially in those with a limited ability to conserve water. Dehydration caused by diarrhea continues to be one of the leading causes of death among young children in some parts of the world.

CAUSES

There are two main causes of fluid volume deficit: inadequate intake and increased losses (Table 29-3).

Impaired Intake. Fluid intake may be reduced because of a lack of access to water, impaired thirst, unconsciousness, or neuromuscular problems that

TABLE 29-3. FLUID VOLUME DEFICIT

CAUSES	SIGNS AND SYMPTOMS
Inadequate Fluid Intake Unconsciousness or inability to express thirst Oral trauma or inability to swallow Impaired thirst mechanism Withholding of fluids for therapeutic reasons **Excessive Fluid Losses** Gastrointestinal losses Vomiting Diarrhea Gastrointestinal suction Fistula drainage Urine losses Diuretic therapy Osmotic diuresis (hyperglycemia) Adrenal insufficiency Salt-wasting renal disease Skin losses (salt and water) Fever Exposure to hot environment Burns and wounds that remove skin Third-space losses (sodium and water) Intestinal obstruction Edema Ascites Burns (first several days)	**Acute Weight Loss (% Body Weight)** Mild extracellular deficit: 2% loss Moderate extracellular deficit: 2%–5% loss Severe extracellular deficit: 6% or more loss **Thirst** Increased thirst **Decreased Urine Output** Increased urine osmolality Increased specific gravity **Increased Serum Osmolality** Increased hematocrit Increased BUN **Decreased Vascular Volume** Tachycardia Weak and thready pulse Postural hypotension Decreased vein filling and increased vein refill time Hypotension and shock **Decreased Extracellular Fluid Loss** Depressed fontanelle in an infant Sunken eyes and soft eyeballs **Intracellular Fluid Loss** Dry skin and mucous membranes Cracked and fissured tongue Decreased salivation and lacrimation Neuromuscular weakness Fatigue **Body Temperature** Increased body temperature

prevent water access or impair swallowing. Access to water commonly is taken for granted. For someone with impaired movement, however, water availability becomes a problem. With hypodipsia, or impaired thirst, the need for water intake does not activate the thirst stimulus. The inability to swallow impairs water intake.

Gastrointestinal Losses. In a single day, 8 to 10 L of extracellular fluid is secreted into the gastrointestinal tract; most of this fluid is reabsorbed as the bowel contents move toward the anus. Vomiting and diarrhea interrupt the reabsorption process and, in some situations, lead to increased secretion of fluid (in excess of 8 to 10 L) into the gastrointestinal tract. The presence of irritating or hypertonic contents increases the movement of fluid into the bowel, exaggerating fluid losses. In many forms of diarrhea, the rate of fluid secretion into the gastrointestinal tract is increased because of the osmotic or irritating effects of the causative agent. In Asiatic cholera, death can occur within a matter of hours as irritating substances formed by the cholera organism cause excessive amounts of fluid to be secreted into the bowel; these fluids are then lost as vomitus or diarrheal fluid.

Urine Losses. The kidneys regulate the volume and solute concentration of extracellular fluid—promoting diuresis in conditions of fluid excess and conserving water when extracellular fluid volume is decreased. Extracellular fluid deficit can result from osmotic diuresis or the injudicious use of diuretic therapy. In hyperglycemia, serum sodium is diluted as the osmotic effects of the elevated glucose level cause water to be pulled out of body cells. The presence of glucose in the urine filtrate prevents reabsorption of water by the renal tubules; this causes increased losses of both sodium and water. The degree of hyponatremia, or serum sodium decrease, resulting from hyperglycemia can be estimated by assuming a 1.6 mEq/L decrease in serum sodium for every 100 mg/mL rise in blood glucose above normal values.[8]

Skin Losses. The skin acts as an exchange surface for body heat and as a vapor barrier to prevent water from leaving the body. Body surface losses of sodium and water increase when there is excessive sweating or when large areas of the skin have been damaged. Hot weather and fever increase sweating. In hot weather, water losses through sweating may be increased by as much as 1.5 to 2.0 L/hr.[1] Both respiratory rate and sweating usually are increased as the body temperature rises. As much as 3 L of water may be lost in a single day as a result of fever. Burns are another cause of excess fluid loss. Evaporative losses range from 0.8 to 2.6 mL/kg for every percentage point of burn area. This loss can approach a level of 6 to 8 L/day.[9]

Third-Space Losses. Third-space losses refer to the sequestering of extracellular fluids in an area that is physiologically unavailable to the body—in the serous cavities, extracellular spaces in injured tissues, or lumen of the gut. For example, fluid deficits can develop in intestinal obstruction as water and electrolytes pool in the distended bowel. Third spacing results from increased capillary permeability; there is a concomitant movement of plasma proteins into the sequestered area. The osmotic gradient associated with the presence of these colloids causes additional water to move into the third-space area.

MANIFESTATIONS

The signs and symptoms of fluid volume deficit summarized in Table 29-3 are closely associated with the functions of water discussed earlier in the chapter. A discussion of the signs and symptoms associated with extracellular fluid deficit is complicated by the fact that fluid deficit may present as an isotonic depletion of fluid volume in which both water and sodium are lost or as a condition in which water losses exceed sodium loss. The signs and symptoms presented in this section apply in both circumstances.

Body Weight. An acute decrease in body weight is one of the best indicators of fluid loss. One liter of water weighs 1 kg (2.2 lb). A mild extracellular fluid deficit exists when weight loss equals 2% of body weight; in a person who weighs 68 kg (150 lb),

this percentage of weight loss equals 1.4 L of water. Severe fluid deficit exists when weight loss is in excess of 6% of body weight. To be accurate, weight must be measured at the same time each day with an equal amount of clothing being worn. Because extracellular fluid is trapped within the body in people with third-space losses, body weight may not decrease when extracellular fluid loss occurs for this reason.

Intake and Output. Intake and output measurements afford a second method for assessing fluid balance. Although these measurements provide insight into the causes of fluid imbalance, they often are inadequate in measuring actual losses and gains. This is because accurate measurements of intake and output often are difficult to obtain and insensible losses are difficult to estimate. Pflaum reported a mean error in intake and output calculations of 800 mL/day compared with daily weight measurements.[10]

Thirst is an early symptom of water deficit, occurring when water losses are equal to 0.5% of body water. Infants as well as people who are unconscious or cannot communicate are unable to express this need. Also, thirst is not always present in isotonic fluid deficit caused by sodium depletion.

Urine output usually decreases and urine osmolality and specific gravity increase during periods of water deficit. An exception to this rule occurs when the fluid deficit follows either an impairment in the kidneys' ability to concentrate urine or diuresis that occurs for other reasons. The ratio of urine osmolality to serum osmolality in a 24-hour urine sample normally exceeds 1:1 and after a period of overnight water deprivation should be greater than 3:1. A dehydrated patient (one who has a loss of water) may have a urine-serum ratio that approaches 4:1. In these patients, urine osmolality may exceed 1000 mOsm/kg H_2O. In people who have difficulty concentrating their urine—for example, those with diabetes insipidus or chronic renal failure—the urine-serum ratio often is less or equal to 1:1. Urine specific gravity compares the weight of urine with that of water, providing an index for solute concentration. A change in specific gravity of 1.010 to 1.020 (water is considered to be 1.000) is an increase of 400 mOsm/kg H_2O. In the sodium-depleted state, the kidneys usually try to conserve sodium; urine specific gravity is normal and urine sodium and chloride concentrations are low.

Serum Osmolality. The normal range for serum osmolality is 275 to 295 mOsm/kg. Because the serum in the extracellular compartment is roughly 90% to 93% water, the concentrations of blood cells and other solutes increase as extracellular water decreases. This is true of hematocrit and BUN levels. Serum sodium concentration also increases when fluid deficit is due primarily to a water loss.

Vascular Volume. Arterial and venous volumes decline during periods of fluid deficit. Both the pulse rate and the blood pressure change as the volume in the arterial system declines: the heart rate increases and the pulse becomes weak and thready. Postural hypotension is an early sign of fluid deficit, characterized by a blood pressure that is at least 10 mmHg lower when the patient is sitting or standing than when the patient is lying down. When volume depletion becomes severe, signs of shock and vascular collapse appear. On the venous side of the circulation, the veins become less prominent and venous refill time increases. A simple test to determine venous refill time consists of compressing the distal end of a vein on the dorsal aspect of the hand (when the hand is not in the dependent position). The vein is then emptied by "milking" the blood toward the heart. The vein should refill almost immediately when the occluding finger is removed. When venous volume is decreased, as occurs in fluid deficit, venous refill time increases.

The amount of fluid in all the body spaces decreases in fluid volume deficit. Although most body spaces are not visible, a decrease in cerebrospinal fluid in the infant causes depression of the anterior fontanelle. Likewise, the eyes assume a sunken appearance and feel softer than normal when the fluid content in the anterior chamber of the eye is decreased.

Cellular Dehydration. As fluid is lost from the extracellular compartment in excess of solute, the extracellular fluid becomes hypertonic in relation to the fluid in the intracellular compartment. When this happens, the water is pulled out of body cells. The skin and mucous membranes become dry, and there is a decrease in the activity of the cells in the salivary and lacrimal glands. The tongue becomes dry and fissured. Swallowing is difficult. A reliable method for testing for dryness of the mouth is to place your finger on the mucous membranes where the gums and the cheek meet. When a fluid deficit is present, your finger does not glide easily because of the dryness. This method works well in infants and in people who are unconscious.

One of the most serious aspects of a fluid deficit is the dehydration of brain and nerve cells. Generalized muscle weakness, muscle rigidity, and muscle tremors often occur in severe fluid deficit as water is removed from the cells in the nervous system. Delirium, hallucinations, and maniacal behavior may also develop when the fluid deficit is severe.

Body Temperature. Dehydration is known to produce a rise in body temperature. Part of this elevation in temperature probably results from a lack of available fluid for sweating. Loss of vascular volume impairs the transport of core body heat to the periphery for exchange with the external environment. It also appears that dehydration has a direct effect on the hypothalamus, because dehydration can cause fever even in a cold environment. Body temperature may reach 105°F when dehydration is severe.[11]

TREATMENT

The treatment of fluid deficit consists of replacement therapy, which includes replacing both the water and the electrolytes that have been lost. Replacement fluids can be given orally or intravenously. The oral route is preferable.

Oral glucose-electrolyte replacement solutions are available for the treatment of infants with diarrhea.[12, 13] Until recently, these solutions were prescribed either early in the diarrhea illness to prevent dehydration or as a first step in reestablishing oral intake after parenteral replacement therapy. These solutions are now being widely used as replacements for intravenous fluids in the treatment of dehydration caused by diarrhea in young children, especially in developing countries where the availability of intravenous fluids is limited and diarrhea is the leading cause of death. Although cola drinks commonly are recommended as folk remedies for dehydration caused by acute diarrhea, their electrolyte content often is inadequate for replacement purposes and their high sugar content may complicate the situation by inducing an osmotic diarrhea.[14] Intravenous replacement solutions continue to be the treatment of choice in severe fluid deficit.

FLUID VOLUME EXCESS

Fluid volume excess can result from retention of both sodium and water that produces an isotonic expansion of the extracellular fluid compartment or from water retention in excess of sodium (water intoxication). For purposes of clarification, an isotonic expansion of extracellular fluid volume is referred to here as *fluid volume excess* and water retention in excess of sodium, as *water volume excess*. Fluid volume excess involves an increase in both interstitial and vascular volumes. Water volume excess is accompanied by solute dilution and hypotonicity of the extracellular fluids.

CAUSES

An increase in body fluids usually results from decreased excretion, particularly if it is coupled with increased intake. With fluid volume excess, both sodium and water usually are retained. Among the causes of decreased sodium and water elimination are heart failure, cirrhosis of the liver, and decreased kidney function (Table 29-4). A condition called *circulatory overload* results from an increase in intravascular blood volume; it can occur during infusion of intravenous fluids or transfusion of blood if the amount or rate of administration is excessive. Elderly people and people with heart disease require careful observation because even small amounts of blood may overload the circulatory system. Although an increase in fluid volume typically accompanies disease, this is not always true. For example, a compensatory isotonic expansion of body fluids occurs during hot weather as a mechanism for increasing body heat loss. As discussed previously, water retention that occurs with SIADH can produce hyponatremia and a hypotonic expansion of body fluids.

MANIFESTATIONS

The manifestations of fluid or water excess depend on the effect of the excess fluid on serum osmolality. *Edema*, or excess fluid in the interstitial spaces, is characteristic of isotonic fluid excess. Just as weight loss is a good indicator of fluid volume deficit, so also is weight gain an indicator of fluid excess. In circumstances where the fluid excess accumulates gradually, edema fluid may mask weight loss that is due to actual loss of tissue mass; this often happens in debilitating disease conditions and in starvation. The edema associated with extracellular fluid excess may be generalized, or it may be confined to dependent areas of the body, such as the legs and feet. The eyelids often are puffy when the person awakens. When excess fluid accumulates in the lungs (*i.e.*, pulmonary edema), there is shortness of breath, complaints of difficult breathing, respiratory rales,

and a productive cough (see Chapter 24). An increase in vascular volume causes the pulse to have a full and bounding quality.

The manifestations of water volume excess are largely related to solute dilution, decreased serum osmolality, and cellular swelling. The signs and symptoms may be acute (severe water intoxication), or more insidious in onset and less severe. Severe water intoxication is manifested by headache, nausea, vomiting, abdominal cramps, weakness, and stupor. Seizures and coma may develop as a result of changes in the water content of brain cells. The manifestations of water volume excess are similar to those for hyponatremia summarized in Table 27-6.

TREATMENT

The treatment of fluid volume excess focuses on providing a more favorable balance between sodium and water intake and output. Diuretics commonly are used to increase sodium elimination. When there is need for intravenous fluid administration or transfusion of blood components, the procedure should be carefully monitored to prevent fluid overload.

The treatment of water excess depends on its cause and severity. Water restriction may be sufficient (see treatment for SIADH). Hypertonic saline solutions may be used to reduce cellular swelling in cases of severe water intoxication.

In summary, body water is distributed between the intracellular and extracellular fluid compartments. Body water levels are regulated by thirst (intake) and by renal mechanisms that control urine concentration (output). Renal mechanisms for concentrating urine are mediated by ADH. Diabetes insipidus is a condition of inadequate ADH levels (neurogenic diabetes insipidus) or inadequate renal responsiveness to the hormone (nephrogenic diabetes insipidus); SIADH is a condition of inappropriate secretion of the hormone. Fluid volume deficit is

TABLE 29-4. FLUID VOLUME EXCESS

CAUSES	SIGNS AND SYMPTOMS
Excessive Sodium and Water Intake	**Acute Weight Gain (% Body Weight) In Excess of 5%**
Excessive dietary intake	
Excessive ingestion of medications or home remedies containing sodium	**Increased Extracellular Fluid**
	Pitting edema of the extremities
Excessive administration of parenteral solutions containing sodium	Puffy eyelids
Inadequate Sodium and Water Losses	**Increased Vascular Volume**
Renal disease	Pulmonary edema
Increased corticosteroid levels	Shortness of breath
Aldosterone	Rales
Glucocorticoids	Dyspnea
Congestive heart failure	Cough
Cirrhosis of the liver	Full and bounding pulse
	Venous distention

characterized by a reduction in intracellular and extracellular fluids. It causes thirst, a decrease in vascular volume and circulatory function, decreased urine output and increased urine specific gravity, and signs related to loss of fluid from the cellular compartment. Fluid volume excess can exist as an isotonic expansion of body fluids or as a disproportionate increase in water volume. It is characterized by increases in both interstitial and intravascular fluids. Water volume excess (water intoxication), characterized by decreased serum osmolality and cellular swelling, occurs when water is retained in excess of sodium salts (as in SIADH).

■ ALTERATIONS IN THE ELECTROLYTE COMPOSITION OF BODY FLUIDS

Although water provides volume for the body fluids, the electrolytes contribute to the function of these fluids. Electrolytes serve many functions. They (1) assist in regulating fluid balance, (2) participate in acid–base regulation, (3) contribute to enzyme reactions, and (4) play an essential role in neuromuscular activity. This section focuses on the alterations in body function that are associated with disturbances in sodium, potassium, calcium, phosphate, and magnesium balance. Alterations in bicarbonate and chloride concentrations are discussed in Chapter 30.

There are marked differences in the composition of intracellular and extracellular electrolytes (Table 29-5). The reader will note that the sodium concentration is greatest in the extracellular compartment, whereas potassium is concentrated within the cells. Blood (serum) tests measure the concentration of electrolytes in the extracellular compartment rather than in the intracellular compartment. The suffix -emia refers to blood. Hyponatremia, for example, denotes a decreased sodium concentration in the blood. Although blood levels usually are representative of the total body levels of an electrolyte, this is not always the case, particularly with potassium, which

is about 28 times more concentrated inside the cell than outside.

ALTERATIONS IN SODIUM BALANCE

Sodium affects many body functions. Regulation of serum sodium is essential for maintaining (1) the osmolality of extracellular fluids, (2) normal neuromuscular function, (3) acid–base balance, and (4) numerous vital chemical reactions. As the major cation in the extracellular compartment, sodium and its attendant anions (chloride and bicarbonate) account for about 90% to 95% of the osmotic activity in the extracellular fluids. Sodium is a component of sodium bicarbonate and, as such, is important in regulating acid–base balance.

GAINS AND LOSSES

Sodium intake normally is derived from dietary sources. Body needs usually can be met by as little as 500 mg/day. In the United States, the average salt intake is about 6 to 15 g/day, or 12 to 30 times the daily requirement. Other sources of sodium are intravenous saline infusions and medications that contain sodium. An often-forgotten source of sodium is the sodium bicarbonate or other sodium-containing home remedies used to treat upset stomach or other ailments. Sodium ingestion in excess of what the kidneys can excrete is an unlikely occurrence in healthy people, probably because taste prohibits this from occurring and because of the kidneys' remarkable ability to regulate sodium. Sodium excess has occurred in patients receiving intravenous saline infusions and in those unable to monitor their oral intake.

The body loses sodium through the kidneys, skin, and gastrointestinal tract. Less that 10% of the

TABLE 29-5. CONCENTRATION OF EXTRACELLULAR ELECTROLYTES (ADULTS)*		
ELECTROLYTE	**EXTRACELLULAR CONCENTRATION**	
Sodium	135–148 mEq/L	135–148 mmol/L
Potassium	3.5–5.0 mEq/L	3.5–5.0 mmol/L
Chloride	98–106 mEq/L	98–106 mmol/L
Bicarbonate	24–31 mEq/L	24–31 mmol/L
Calcium	8.8–10.0 mg/dL	2.20–2.50 mmol/L
Phosphate/Phosphorus	2.7–4.5 mg/dL	0.87–1.45 mmol/L
Magnesium	1.7–2.7 mg/dL	0.70–1.11 mmol/L

* Values may vary among laboratories depending on the method of analysis used.

usual dietary sodium intake is lost by way of stools and sweat; the rest is excreted by the kidneys. The kidneys are extremely efficient in regulating sodium output, and when sodium intake is limited or conservation of sodium is needed, the kidneys are able to reabsorb almost all the sodium that has been filtered by the glomerulus. This results in an essentially sodium-free urine. Conversely, urinary losses of sodium increase as intake increases. For practical purposes, the 24-hour urinary excretion of sodium is assumed to be equal to sodium intake.

Alterations in kidney function can cause either an increase or a decrease in sodium losses. Sodium deficit with an accompanying loss of extracellular fluid occurs in salt-wasting kidney disease. On the other hand, many forms of kidney disease cause sodium retention. A decrease in renal blood flow causes increased sodium retention by means of the renin–angiotensin–aldosterone mechanism. For this reason, sodium retention is increased in nonrenal diseases that cause a decrease in renal blood flow. In congestive heart failure, renal blood flow is decreased because the heart does not pump properly.

Although skin losses of sodium usually are negligible, sweat losses can be extensive during exercise and periods of exposure to a hot environment. A person who sweats profusely can lose as much as 15 to 30 g of sodium per day; this amount decreases to as little as 3 to 5 g with acclimatization.[1] Loss of skin surface, such as occurs in extensive burns, also leads to excessive skin losses of sodium.

Sodium moves freely between the extracellular fluid and the contents of the gastrointestinal tract. In the upper part of the gastrointestinal tract, the concentration of sodium is similar to that of blood serum. Sodium is reabsorbed as the contents of the gut move through the lower part of the bowel, so that the concentration of sodium in the stool is only about 32 mEq/L. Sodium losses increase with vomiting, diarrhea, fistula drainage, and gastrointestinal suction. Irrigation of gastrointestinal tubes with distilled water removes sodium from the gastrointestinal tract, as do repeated tap water enemas.

REGULATION

The normal serum concentration of sodium ranges from 135 to 148 mEq/L (135 to 148 mmol/L). Serum sodium values reflect the concentration of sodium in the extracellular fluids, expressed as milliequivalents per liter, rather than an absolute amount. This means that dehydration causes the concentration of sodium to increase even though the total body sodium remains unchanged. Likewise, fluid excess causes sodium levels to decrease even though sodium has not been lost from the body.

Aldosterone Regulation. The reabsorption of sodium by the kidneys is largely regulated by aldosterone. Aldosterone is a mineralocorticoid hormone that is produced by the adrenal cortex. In the cortical collecting tubules of the kidneys, aldosterone promotes the reabsorption of sodium into the blood, and in exchange, potassium is secreted into the tubular fluid so that it can be eliminated in the urine. The aldosterone mechanism allows for fine tuning of serum sodium and potassium levels.

Three factors are known to stimulate the secretion of aldosterone: (1) a decrease in extracellular sodium levels, (2) an increase in extracellular potassium levels, and (3) angiotensin II. The second of these is important in regulating serum potassium levels. Angiotensin II levels are regulated by renal blood flow and the angiotensin-converting enzyme (see Chapter 21).

Although aldosterone increases sodium reabsorption by the kidneys and thereby contributes to what might be called short-term regulation of sodium balance, it is thought to play only a minor role in long-term regulation of sodium levels. This is because an increase in sodium reabsorption through the aldosterone mechanism ultimately leads to an increase in renal blood flow and glomerular filtration rate with a subsequent decrease in renin release.

In *Addison's disease* (see Chapter 45), a condition of chronic adrenocortical insufficiency, there is unregulated loss of sodium in the urine accompanied by increased potassium retention caused by impaired mineralocorticoid function.

The glucocorticoids are also synthesized in the adrenal cortex. *Cushing's syndrome* is a condition of glucocorticoid excess (see Chapter 45). Because cortisol, the most active of the glucocorticoids, has weak mineralocorticoid activity, Cushing's disease predisposes to increased sodium retention and increased potassium losses. The fact that cortisol increases salt and water retention also helps to explain why patients who are being treated with cortisol or related steroid drugs may develop edema and hypertension.

The pharmacologic inhibition of sodium reabsorption in the cortical collecting tubules can be achieved by blocking the actions of aldosterone (potassium-sparing diuretics, such as spironolactone, amiloride, and triamterene), by suppressing renin release (β-adrenergic blocking drugs), or by inhibiting the conversion of angiotensin I to angiotensin II (angiotensin-converting enzyme inhibitors).

HYPONATREMIA

Hyponatremia occurs when the sodium concentration in the blood falls below 135 mEq/L (135 mmol/L) and the serum osmolality is less than 280 mOsm/kg.[15]

Plasma sodium concentration represents the ratio of total body sodium to total body water. A reduction in this ratio might conceivably arise from (1) a decrease in total body sodium with a lesser decrease in body water or (2) normal body sodium with excess retention of body water.

Causes. Excessive sodium losses occur with excessive sweating, gastrointestinal losses, and diuresis. Iso-osmotic fluid loss, as in vomiting or diarrhea, cannot directly lower serum sodium concentration unless losses are replaced with ingested or administered water. Excessive sweating in hot weather, particularly during heavy exercise, leads to loss of sodium and water; hyponatremia develops when water rather than electrolyte-containing liquids is used to replace fluids lost in sweating. Repeated tap water enemas or frequent gastrointestinal irrigations with distilled water remove sodium chloride from the gastrointestinal tract. Salt depletion also occurs with adrenal insufficiency and with diuresis caused by vigorous use of diuretics (Table 29-6).

Hyperglycemia, too, depresses serum sodium concentration. Because sodium is largely an extracellular cation, it becomes diluted as water moves out of cells in response to the osmotic effects of the elevated blood glucose level. There is about a 1.6 mEq/L decrease in serum sodium for every 100 mg/dL rise in serum glucose above the normal level (100 mg/dL).[16] In this case, hyponatremia may occur despite serum hyperosmolality.

Another way that hyponatremia can arise is when there is ingestion or administration of more water than the kidneys can excrete. Homeostatic mechanisms make it almost impossible to produce an increase in body water when renal function is adequate and ADH and aldosterone levels are normal. Excess water can be retained, however, when water excretion is reduced because of abnormal kidney function or when ADH levels are elevated. Although uncommon, water excess can occur as the result of excessive water intake. As mentioned earlier, patients with psychogenic polydipsia drink water in excess of what the kidneys can excrete. Water intoxication in the psychiatric patient may be aggravated by treatment with antipsychotic drugs that increase ADH levels.

An artifactual hyponatremia caused by laboratory measurement methods can occur in hyperlipidemic and hyperproteinemic states. This is be-

TABLE 29-6. HYPONATREMIA

CAUSES	SIGNS AND SYMPTOMS
Excessive Sodium Losses	**Laboratory Values**
Sweating	Serum sodium below 135 mEq/L
Gastrointestinal losses	(135 mmol/L)
Diuresis	Decreased serum osmolality
Sodium Dilution	Dilution of other blood components,
Excess administration of sodium-free	including chloride, hematocrit, and
parenteral solutions	BUN
Psychogenic polydipsia	**Increased Water Content**
Ingestion of tap water during periods	**of Brain and Nerve Cells**
of sodium deficit	Headache
Repeated administration of tap water	Mental depression
enemas	Personality changes
Kidney disease that impairs water	Confusion
elimination	Apprehension and feeling of impend-
Increased ADH levels	ing doom
Trauma, stress, pain	Lethargy, weakness
SIADH	Stupor
Use of medications that increase	Coma
ADH	Seizures
Hypoglycemia	**Gastrointestinal Disturbances**
Hyperglycemia	Anorexia, nausea, vomiting
	Abdominal cramps
	Diarrhea
	Increased Intracellular Fluid
	Fingerprint edema

cause the modern autoanalyzer equipment used in most clinical laboratories includes the excess lipids or proteins in the water volume of the sample, causing an artifactual dilution of sodium.

Manifestations. In the absence of abnormal solute accumulation (*e.g.*, hyperglycemia), hyponatremia is associated with low serum osmolality. Water moves from the extracellular compartment into the cells. Urine osmolality is low in hyponatremia because of water intoxication, whereas urine osmolality is normal or elevated in chronic hyponatremia because of sodium loss.

Because of water movement, hyponatremia causes intracellular hypo-osmolality, which in turn is responsible for many of the *clinical* manifestations of the disorder.[17] Muscle cramps, weakness, and fatigue reflect the hypo-osmolality of skeletal muscle cells and are often early signs of hyponatremia. The signs and symptoms of hyponatremia depend on the rapidity of onset and the severity of the sodium dilution. If the condition develops slowly, signs and symptoms do not develop until serum sodium levels approach 125 mEq/L (125 mmol/L). The brain and nervous system are the most seriously affected by increases in intracellular water. Progressive neurologic symptoms occur once the serum sodium falls below this level. Symptoms include apathy, lethargy, and headache, which can progress to disorientation, confusion, and gross motor weakness. Seizures and coma occur when serum sodium levels reach extremely low levels (*e.g.*, less than 110 mEq/L). These severe changes, which are due to brain swelling, may be irreversible.

The effect of rapid changes in serum osmolality on the peripheral nervous system often is associated with muscle cramps and depression of deep tendon reflexes. These effects commonly are observed in the hyponatremia that occurs with heavy exercise during hot weather.

Fingerprint edema, a sign of intracellular water, may be present. This phenomenon is demonstrated by pressing the finger firmly over the bony surface of the sternum for 15 to 30 seconds.[18] On removal of the finger, a fingerprint that is similar to one that occurs when pressing on a piece of modeling clay is visible when excess intracellular water is present.

Treatment. The treatment of hyponatremia focuses on the underlying cause. When hyponatremia is due to water intoxication, simply limiting water intake or discontinuing medications that contribute to SIADH may be sufficient. The administration of saline solution either by mouth or intravenously may be needed when hyponatremia is due to sodium deficiency. Symptomatic hyponatremia (neurologic

manifestations) often is treated with hypertonic saline solution and furosemide, a diuretic that impairs the kidneys' ability to concentrate urine. This combination allows for rapid correction of serum sodium levels while ridding the body of excess water.

HYPERNATREMIA

Hypernatremia infers a serum sodium level above 148 mEq/L (148 mmol/L) and a serum osmolality greater than 295 mOsm/kg.[15] It represents an imbalance of total body sodium and water and can arise when there is (1) rapid hypertonic sodium ingestion with insufficient time or opportunity for water ingestion, (2) a defect in thirst or inability to drink water, or (3) water ingestion insufficient to keep pace with renal or extrarenal water losses (Table 29-7).

Causes. Serum sodium excess almost always follows a loss of body fluids that have a lower than normal concentration of sodium, so that water is lost in excess of sodium. This can result from excessive urinary losses as in diabetes insipidus, from increased losses from the respiratory tract during fever or strenuous exercise, from watery diarrhea, or when osmotically active tube feedings are given with inadequate amounts of water. Hypernatremia, with an accompanying water deficit, stimulates thirst and increases water intake. It is, therefore, more apt to occur in infants and in people who cannot express their thirst or obtain water to drink. The unconscious person is particularly at risk for developing hypernatremia.

The therapeutic administration of sodium-containing solutions may also cause hypernatremia. For example, the administration of sodium bicarbonate during cardiopulmonary resuscitation increases body sodium levels, since the sodium concentration of each 50-mL ampule of 7.5% sodium bicarbonate contains 892 mEq of sodium.[15] Hypertonic saline solution intended for intraamniotic instillation for therapeutic abortion may inadvertently be injected intravenously, causing hypernatremia. Rarely, there is rapid salt intake as in taking excess salt tablets or during near-drowning in salt water.

Manifestations. The clinical manifestations of hypernatremia are largely related to an increase in serum osmolality; this causes water to be pulled out of body cells. Urine output is decreased because of renal conserving mechanisms. Thirst is excessive. Body temperature frequently is elevated, and the skin becomes warm and flushed. The mucous membranes are dry and sticky, and the tongue is rough and dry. The subcutaneous tissues assume a firm, rubbery texture. The vascular volume decreases, the

TABLE 29-7. HYPERNATREMIA

CAUSES	SIGNS AND SYMPTOMS

Excessive Sodium Intake
    Rapid or excessive administration of
      parenteral sodium chloride or so-
      dium bicarbonate solutions
    Excessive oral intake
    Near-drowning in salt water
Decreased Extracellular Water
    Increased water losses
      Diuretic therapy
      Adrenocortical hormone excess
      Diabetes insipidus
      Tracheobronchitis
      Watery diarrhea
      Hypertonic tube feedings
    Decreased water intake
      Unconsciousness or inability to ex-
        press thirst
      Oral trauma or inability to swallow
      Impaired thirst mechanism
      Withholding of water for therapeutic
        reasons
	Laboratory Findings
	    Serum sodium above 148 mEq/L
	      (148 mmol/L)
	    Increased serum osmolality
	Thirst
	    Increased thirst
	Urine Output
	    Oliguria or anuria
	    High specific gravity
	Intracellular Dehydration
	    Skin and mucous membranes
	      Skin dry and flushed
	      Mucous membranes dry and sticky
	      Tongue rough and dry
	    Subcutaneous tissue
	      Firm and rubbery
	    Central nervous system
	      Agitation and restlessness
	      Decreased reflexes
	      Maniacal behavior
	      Seizures and coma
	    Increased body temperature
	Decreased vascular volume
	    Tachycardia
	    Decreased blood pressure
	    Weak and thready pulse

pulse rate becomes rapid, and the blood pressure drops. Most significantly, water is pulled out of the cells in the CNS; this causes decreased reflexes, agitation, headache, and restlessness. Coma and seizures may develop as hypernatremia progresses.

Because total body sodium content is the major determinant of extracellular fluid volume, it is important to determine if hypernatremia is accompanied by normal, decreased, or increased water volume. A dilute urine with an osmolality of less than 250 mOsm/kg is characteristic of diabetes insipidus.

Treatment. Treatment of hypernatremia focuses on the cause of the disorder. In situations of sodium excess, administration of water either orally or intravenously usually is sufficient.

Serum osmolality should be corrected slowly in cases of chronic hypernatremia. This is because brain cells synthesize amino acids and other osmotically active solutes that have been termed *idiogenic osmoles*.[15] These osmotically active solutes serve to produce a gradual increase in intracellular osmolality, allowing osmotic flow of water back into the cell and restoring cell volume. This response begins within

4 to 6 hours of increased serum osmolality and takes several days to become fully effective.[15] Thus, changes in brain water content are greatest during acute hypernatremia but only slightly reduced in chronic hypernatremia. If hypernatremia is corrected too rapidly, before the idiogenic osmoles have had a chance to dissipate, the plasma may become relatively hypotonic in relation to brain cell osmolality; water moves into the brain cells, causing cerebral edema and potentially severe neurologic impairment.

ALTERATIONS IN POTASSIUM BALANCE

Potassium is the second most abundant cation in body fluids. As the most abundant intracellular cation, potassium (1) contributes to maintenance of intracellular osmolality; (2) is necessary for neuromuscular control and the precise regulation of skeletal, cardiac, and smooth muscle activity; (3) influences acid–base balance; and (4) participates in many intracellular enzyme reactions. For example, potassium contributes to the intricate chemical reactions that transform carbohydrates into energy, change glucose into glycogen, and convert amino acids to proteins.

GAINS AND LOSSES

Potassium intake is derived from dietary sources. In healthy people, potassium balance usually can be maintained by a daily dietary intake of 50 to 100 mEq. Additional amounts of potassium are needed during periods of trauma and stress. The kidneys are the main source of potassium loss. Renal losses of potassium are influenced by the urine flow rate, serum sodium concentration, potassium intake, acid–base balance, and aldosterone levels. Potassium is filtered in the glomerulus, reabsorbed with sodium and water in the proximal tubule and with sodium and chloride in the descending limb of Henle, and secreted into the distal tubule and collecting duct for elimination in the urine. About 80% to 90% of potassium losses occur in the urine and the rest occur in the stool or sweat.

REGULATION

Potassium essentially is an intracellular cation; all but about 2% of body potassium is contained within body cells.[19] This means that serum levels of potassium, which normally range from 3.5 to 5.0 mEq/L (3.5 to 5.0 mmol/L), do not always accurately reflect intracellular levels. Serum levels of potassium are mainly regulated by renal mechanisms and redistribution between the intracellular and extracellular compartments. Insulin increases movement of potassium into body cells and plays a central role in maintaining normal extracellular-intracellular distribution of potassium. Although the serum insulin level does not rise unless serum potassium concentration increases by 1 mEq/L, it has been suggested that pancreatic insulin release and portal insulin levels increase in a feedback response to even small changes in serum potassium.[15]

When body cells are injured or when cellular activity becomes catabolic, potassium is released into the extracellular compartment and then lost in the urine. Subsequently, with chronic potassium deficiency, the kidneys' ability to conserve potassium improves and the urine loss is reduced to as little as 5 mEq/L (5 mmol/L). When this happens, serum levels of potassium are likely to remain within normal range even though total body potassium has decreased. Serum potassium levels fall when tissue breakdown ceases and cellular activity becomes anabolic, causing potassium to move back into the cellular compartment. This is because potassium is needed for glycogen storage and protein synthesis.

Magnesium deficiency causes intracellular potassium depletion, whether or not there is adequate potassium intake. This is discussed in the section on alterations in magnesium.

Aldosterone Regulation. Aldosterone plays an essential role in regulating the extracellular potassium concentration. Urinary losses of potassium increase under the influence of aldosterone, whereas sodium retention is increased. The feedback regulation of aldosterone levels, in turn, is strongly regulated by serum potassium levels; for example, an increase in potassium ion concentration of less than 1 mEq/L causes aldosterone levels to triple. Furthermore, this increased secretion continues for as long as the elevated potassium levels are present.

Potassium balance can be seriously affected by disorders of aldosterone secretion. *Primary aldosteronism* is caused by a tumor in the cells of the adrenal cortex (in the zona glomerulosa) that secrete aldosterone. Excess secretion of aldosterone by the tumor cells causes severe potassium losses and a decrease in serum potassium levels. Patients with this disorder may develop muscle paralysis as a result of the low serum levels of potassium. Adrenal insufficiency (Addison's disease) causes the opposite effect; people with this disorder have elevated serum potassium levels.

Potassium–Hydrogen Ion Exchange. The hydrogen ion concentration (pH) of the extracellular fluid contributes to compartmental shifts of potassium. In acidosis, the movement of hydrogen ions into body cells is used as a means of buffering pH changes in extracellular fluids. The serum potassium concentration rises 0.6 mEq/L for each 0.1 unit fall in serum pH. When a hydrogen ion moves into the cell, another positively charged ion (potassium) must move out into the extracellular fluid. This means that potassium moves out of the intracellular compartment in acidosis and into the intracellular compartment in alkalosis.

A potassium-hydrogen exchange also occurs in the distal tubules of the kidneys. When the extracellular concentration of potassium is high, tubular secretion of potassium into the urine is increased and hydrogen excretion is decreased, causing a decrease in serum pH (metabolic acidosis). Conversely, when extracellular concentrations of potassium are low, tubular secretion of potassium into the urine is decreased and hydrogen ion secretion is increased; this leads to metabolic alkalosis. Metabolic alkalosis exaggerates urine losses of potassium. This is because the excess negatively charged bicarbonate ions that are present in the urine must be accompanied by positively charged ions as they are eliminated. Some sodium ions are excreted with the bicarbonate, but some are reabsorbed in exchange for potassium ions, which are then lost in the urine.

HYPOKALEMIA

Hypokalemia refers to a decrease in serum potassium levels below 3.5 mEq/L (3.5 mmol/L). Because potassium moves freely between the intracellular and extracellular compartments, hypokalemia can occur as the result of a loss of total body potassium or because extracellular potassium has moved into the intracellular compartment. Intracellular and extracellular potassium concentrations usually decrease simultaneously.

Causes. The causes of potassium deficit can be grouped into three categories: (1) inadequate intake, (2) excessive losses, and (3) redistribution between the intracellular and extracellular fluid compartments (Table 29-8).

The kidneys are unable to conserve potassium during periods of acute potassium loss and continue to excrete it even in time of great need. This means that a potassium deficit can develop rather quickly if intake is inadequate. Intake frequently is impaired at the time potassium losses are increased—for example, after surgery or during prolonged diarrhea. Elderly people are particularly likely to develop a potassium deficit. This is because many have poor eating habits as a consequence of living alone; they may have limited income, which makes buying foods high in potassium difficult; they may have difficulty chewing many foods that have a high potassium content because of poorly fitting dentures; or they may have problems with swallowing. Furthermore, many

---

TABLE 29-8. HYPOKALEMIA

CAUSES	SIGNS AND SYMPTOMS

Inadequate Intake
Inability to eat
Diet deficient in potassium
Administration of potassium-free
  parenteral solutions
Excessive Gastrointestinal Losses
Vomiting
Diarrhea
Suction
Fistula drainage
Excessive Renal Losses
Diuretic phase of renal failure
Diuretic therapy (except aldosterone
  antagonists)
Increased mineralocorticoid levels
  Cushing's syndrome
  Primary aldosteronism
  Treatment with glucocorticoid
    hormones
Intracellular Shift
Treatment for diabetic acidosis
Alkalosis, either metabolic or
  respiratory
	Laboratory Values
	Serum potassium below 3.5 mEq/L
	  (3.5 mmol/L)
	Skeletal Muscle Manifestations
	Muscle tenderness, paresthesia, or
	  cramps
	Weakness
	Muscle flabbiness
	Paralysis
	Cardiovascular Manifestations
	Postural hypotension
	Increased sensitivity to digitalis
	Arrhythmias
	Gastrointestinal Manifestations
	Anorexia
	Vomiting
	Abdominal distention
	Paralytic ileus
	Respiratory Manifestations
	Shortness of breath
	Shallow breathing
	Urine Output
	Polyuria
	Low osmolality and specific gravity of
	  urine
	Nocturia
	Thirst
	Increased thirst
	Central Nervous System Function
	Confusion
	Depression
	Acid–Base Balance
	Metabolic alkalosis

medical problems in elderly people require treatment with drugs, such as diuretics, that increase potassium losses.

The kidneys are the main source of potassium loss. About 80% to 90% of potassium losses occur in the urine, with the remaining losses in the stool and sweat. The kidneys do not have the homeostatic mechanisms needed to conserve potassium during brief periods of insufficient intake. An adult on a potassium-free diet continues to lose about 5 to 15 mEq of potassium daily. After trauma and in stress situations, urinary losses of potassium are greatly increased, sometimes approaching levels of 150 to 200 mEq/d (150 to 200 mmol/L). Diuretic therapy (with the exception of potassium-sparing diuretics such as spironolactone) results in additional urinary losses of potassium. Some antibiotics, particularly amphotericin B and gentamicin, are impermeable anions that require the presence of positively charged cations for elimination in the urine; this causes potassium wasting.

Although potassium losses from the skin and the gastrointestinal tract usually are minimal, these losses can become excessive under certain conditions. For instance, burns increase surface losses of potassium, and sweat losses can become markedly increased in people who are acclimated to a hot climate. This is partly because increased secretion of aldosterone during heat acclimatization increases the loss of potassium in both urine and sweat.[1] Gastrointestinal losses can also become excessive; this occurs with vomiting and diarrhea and when gastrointestinal suction is being used. The potassium content of liquid stools, for example, is about 40 to 60 mEq/L (40 to 60 mmol/L).[19]

Because of the high ratio of intracellular to extracellular potassium, a redistribution of potassium from the extracellular to the intracellular compartment can produce a marked fall in serum levels. One cause of potassium redistribution is insulin. After insulin administration, there is increased movement of both glucose and potassium into cells. Potent β-adrenergic drugs such as epinephrine and albuterol have a similar effect on potassium distribution.

Manifestations. Potassium deficit causes altered renal function and produces changes in skeletal, cardiac, and smooth muscle function. Clinical signs seldom develop until the potassium level has fallen below 3.5 mEq/L (3.5 mmol/L). The signs and symptoms of potassium deficit typically are gradual in onset and for that reason go undetected for a long time.

Hypokalemia leads to impairment of the kidneys' ability to concentrate urine and to an increase in ammonia production. Urine output and serum osmolality are increased and urine specific gravity is decreased. There are complaints of polyuria, nocturia, and thirst. Increased ammonia production appears to be a compensatory mechanism that occurs in response to a decrease in intracellular pH resulting from a potassium-hydrogen exchange that occurs with hypokalemia. As the intracellular pH falls, renal synthesis of ammonia is increased. Because ammonia is obtained through the deamination of amino acids, nitrogen balance becomes negative and protein synthesis is impaired. For this reason, children who need proteins for growth and people who need amino acids for tissue repair are particularly vulnerable to prolonged periods of hypokalemia. Ammonia is eliminated through the liver. For patients with advanced liver disease, hypokalemia can lead to disturbing elevations in serum ammonia levels.

Hypokalemia causes numerous signs and symptoms associated with gastrointestinal function. These include anorexia, nausea, vomiting, abdominal distention, absence of bowel sounds, and paralytic ileus. When gastrointestinal symptoms occur gradually and are not severe, they often serve to impair potassium intake and exaggerate the condition.

At least three defects in skeletal muscle function occur with potassium deficiency: (1) alterations in the resting membrane potential (see Chapter 1), (2) alterations in glycogen synthesis and storage, and (3) impaired ability to increase blood flow during strenuous exercise.[20] With hypokalemia, there is hyperpolarization of neuromuscular tissue with decreased responsiveness to stimulation. Neuromuscular signs and symptoms appear when serum potassium levels fall to about 2.5 mEq/L (2.5 mmol/L).

Clinical manifestations include muscle weakness, fatigue, and cramps, particularly during exercise. Paralysis can occur with severe hypokalemia. Leg muscles, particularly the quadriceps, are most prominently affected. Some patients complain of muscle tenderness and paresthesias rather than weakness. In chronic potassium deficiency, actual muscle atrophy may occur and contribute to muscle weakness. In a rare condition called *hypokalemic familial periodic paralysis*, episodes of hypokalemia cause attacks of flaccid paralysis that last from 6 to 48 hours if untreated.[21] The paralysis may be precipitated by situations that cause severe hypokalemia by producing an intracellular shift in potassium, such as ingestion of a high-carbohydrate meal or administration of insulin, epinephrine, or glucocorticoid drugs. The paralysis often can be reversed by potassium replacement therapy.

Normal concentrations of intracellular potassium are necessary for glycogen synthesis in muscle cells. This means that potassium deficiency can interfere not only with the electrical activity of skeletal muscle but also with muscle metabolism, especially under exercise conditions that rely heavily on anaerobic pathways. The release of potassium from muscle is thought to contribute to the autoregulation of blood flow during exercise, and potassium deficiency can interfere with the release of potassium ions from exercising muscle. Thus, potassium deficiency can lead to impaired blood flow and consequent ischemic injury to muscle cells during intense physical exercise.[20]

Potassium deficiency also affects cardiovascular function. Postural hypotension is common. Serious cardiac arrhythmias can result from hypokalemia. Of particular importance is the fact that hypokalemia increases the risk of digitalis toxicity. The dangers associated with digitalis toxicity are compounded in patients who are receiving both digitalis and diuretics.

Treatment. When possible, hypokalemia caused by potassium deficit is treated by increasing the intake of foods high in potassium content—meats, dried fruits, fruit juices (particularly orange juice), and bananas. The reader is referred to a nutrition text for a description of foods high in potassium. Oral potassium supplements are prescribed for people whose intake of potassium is insufficient in relation to losses. This is particularly true of patients who are receiving diuretic therapy and those who are taking digitalis. Many of these supplements are caustic and bitter-tasting. Granules, liquids, and powders need to be adequately diluted before they are administered. A wax matrix, extended-release tablet form of the drug is available; it does not have a bitter taste and is less offensive to take.

Potassium is given intravenously when the oral route is not tolerated or when rapid replacement is needed. The rapid infusion of a concentrated potassium solution can cause death resulting from cardiac arrest. Health personnel who assume responsibility for administering intravenous solutions that contain potassium should be fully aware of all the precautions pertaining to their dilution and flow rate. Pharmacology texts, drug company package inserts, fluid and electrolyte texts, and pharmacists serve as useful resources for this information. Magnesium deficiency may impair potassium correction; in such cases, magnesium replacement is indicated.[22]

HYPERKALEMIA

Hyperkalemia refers to an increase in serum levels of potassium in excess of 5.0 mEq/L (5.0 mmol/L). It seldom occurs in healthy people because the body is extremely effective in preventing excess potassium accumulation in the extracellular fluid.

Causes. The major causes of potassium excess are (1) renal failure, (2) insufficient aldosterone activity, and (3) excess potassium gains caused by tissue trauma or administration of potassium (oral or intravenous) at a rate that exceeds the kidneys' ability to control serum potassium levels (Table 29-9). The most common cause of hyperkalemia is decreased renal function. Insufficient aldosterone activity can result from (1) depression of aldosterone release because of a decrease in renin or angiotensin II, (2) adrenal insufficiency (Addison's disease), or (3) impaired

TABLE 29-9. HYPERKALEMIA

CAUSES	SIGNS AND SYMPTOMS
Excessive Intake or Gain	**Laboratory Values**
Excessive oral intake	Serum potassium above 5.0 mEq/L
Excessive or rapid parenteral infusion	(5.0 mmol/L)
Tissue trauma, burns, and massive crushing injuries	**Neural and Skeletal Muscle Activity**
	Paresthesia
Inadequate Renal Losses	Weakness and dizziness
Renal failure	Muscle cramps
Adrenal insufficiency (Addison's disease)	**Gastrointestinal Manifestations**
Potassium-sparing diuretics	Nausea, diarrhea
	Intestinal colic and gastrointestinal distress
	Cardiac Electrophysiology
	Peaked T waves, depressed S-T segment
	Depressed P wave and widening of QRS segment
	Cardiac arrest

ability of the kidneys to respond to aldosterone. Potassium-sparing diuretics (*e.g.*, spironolactone, amiloride, and triamterene) can produce hyperkalemia by means of the latter mechanism.

It is difficult to increase potassium intake to the point of causing hyperkalemia when sufficient aldosterone is present and renal function is adequate. An exception to this rule is when potassium solutions are being infused intravenously. In some cases, severe and fatal incidents of hyperkalemia have resulted from the intravenous infusion of potassium. Intravenous solutions that contain potassium should never be started until urine output has been assessed and renal function has been deemed to be adequate. This is because the kidneys control potassium losses. The movement of potassium out of body cells into the extracellular fluids also can lead to elevated serum potassium levels. For example, burns and crushing injuries cause potassium to be liberated into the extracellular fluid. The same injuries often cause a decrease in renal function, which contributes to the development of hyperkalemia. Transient hyperkalemia may be induced during extreme exercise when muscle cells are permeable to potassium. In a rare autosomal dominant disorder called *hyperkalemic periodic paralysis*, hyperkalemia may cause transient periods of muscle weakness and paralysis after exercise, cold exposure, or other situations that cause potassium to move out of the cells. In contrast to hypokalemic periodic paralysis, the episodes are mild, with a duration of less than 2 hours.[21]

Manifestations. The signs and symptoms of potassium excess are closely related to the alterations in neuromuscular function that accompany potassium deficit. The rise in serum potassium depolarizes cells; although the mechanisms responsible for the altered neuromuscular function observed in hypokalemia and hyperkalemia are different, the end results are similar. The first symptom associated with hyperkalemia typically is paresthesia; this may appear when potassium levels reach 6 mEq/L (6 mmol/L). With serum levels less than 6 mEq/L, symptoms are minor or absent. The most serious effect of hyperkalemia is cardiac arrest. The electrocardiographic

changes that occur with alterations in serum potassium levels are described in Figure 29-6.

Treatment. The treatment of potassium excess focuses on (1) decreasing or curtailing intake, (2) increasing renal excretion, and (3) increasing cellular uptake. Decreased intake can be achieved by restricting dietary sources of potassium. The major ingredient in most salt substitutes is potassium chloride, and such substitutes should not be given to patients with renal problems. Increasing potassium output often is more difficult. Patients with renal failure may require hemodialysis or peritoneal dialysis to reduce serum potassium levels. Sodium polystyrene sulfonate (Kayexalate), a potassium-removing resin, may also be used to remove potassium ions from the colon. The sodium ions in the resin are exchanged for potassium ions and then the potassium-containing resin is eliminated in the stool.

Most emergency methods focus on measures that cause serum potassium to move into the cell. Sometimes the intravenous infusion of insulin and glucose is used for this purpose.

ALTERATIONS IN CALCIUM AND PHOSPHATE BALANCE

There is a close link between the regulation of the divalent calcium and phosphate ions in the body; a change in the concentration of one ion leads to a change in the concentration of the other. Therefore, calcium and phosphate are discussed together in this chapter.

Calcium and phosphate salts are deposited in the organic matrix of bone; bone essentially is 30% matrix and 70% salts. In the extracellular fluid, the concentrations of calcium and phosphate are reciprocally regulated; when calcium levels are high, phosphate levels are low and vice versa. Normal serum levels of calcium (8.8 to 10.0 mg/dL in adults and 9.2 to 11.0 mg/dL in children) and phosphate (2.7 to 4.5 mg/dL in adults and 4.5 to 5.5 mg/dL in children) are regulated so that their product (calcium × phosphate) is maintained at a value of about 35. Maintenance of this reciprocal relation is important in pre-

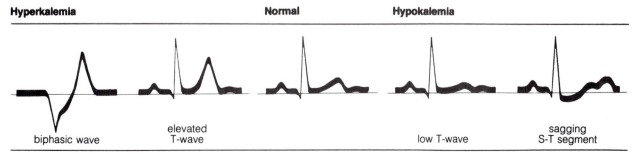

FIG. 29-6. Electrocardiographic changes with hyperkalemia and hypokalemia.

venting tissue precipitation. Precipitation of calcium and phosphate salts is also prevented by inhibitors that are present in most tissues.

GAINS AND LOSSES

Calcium and phosphate enter the body through the gastrointestinal tract and are stored in bone and excreted through the kidneys. The major sources of calcium are milk and milk products. Phosphate is derived from many sources, including milk and meats. Only about 30% to 50% of dietary calcium is absorbed into the body from the duodenum and upper jejunum; the remainder is eliminated in the stool. Phosphate, on the other hand, is absorbed exceedingly well.

The kidneys control calcium and phosphate losses. The two ions are filtered in the glomerulus and selectively reabsorbed in the renal tubules. Renal elimination of phosphate is regulated by an overflow mechanism in which the amount of phosphate lost in the urine is directly related to phosphate concentrations in the blood. When serum phosphate levels rise above a critical level, the rate of phosphate loss in the urine reflects the excess serum phosphate levels. Calcium excretion is reciprocally related to phosphate excretion. In renal failure, phosphate excretion is impaired, and as a result, serum calcium levels decline as serum phosphate levels rise.

REGULATION

Serum calcium and phosphate levels are regulated by vitamin D, parathyroid hormone, and calcitonin. The body contains a supply of exchangeable calcium that is in equilibrium with calcium in the extracellular fluids. Most of this exchangeable calcium is found in bone. This exchangeable pool serves as a storage site for calcium. The movement of calcium between the extracellular fluids and the exchangeable pool is rapid, usually occurring within minutes to 1 hour. The phosphate ion is freely absorbed from the intestine, and changing the serum phosphate levels to as high as three to four times the normal value does not seem to have an immediate effect on body function. Bone metabolism and the actions of vitamin D, parathyroid hormone, and calcitonin are discussed in Chapter 57.

EXTRACELLULAR CALCIUM LEVELS

Calcium can be found in several forms in the body. About 99% of body calcium is found in bone, where it provides the strength and stability for the collagen and ground substance that form the structural matrix of the skeletal system. The remaining 1% is located in the tissues and extracellular fluids. The calcium salts in bone serve as a reservoir of tissue and serum calcium.

Extracellular calcium exists in three forms. About 40% of serum calcium is bound to plasma proteins and cannot diffuse or pass through the capillary wall to leave the vascular compartment. About 10% of serum calcium is complexed with substances such as citrate, phosphate, and sulfate. This form is not ionized. The remaining 50% of serum calcium is ionized. This form of calcium, which can leave the vascular compartment and participate in cellular functions, is the physiologically active form.

Most of the nondiffusible calcium is bound to albumin; only about 10% to 15% of the protein-bound fraction is associated with globulin. Thus, total serum calcium changes with alterations in serum albumin. As a rule, the total serum calcium level is decreased 0.75 to 1.0 mg/dL for every 1 g/dL decrease from normal in the serum albumin level and by 0.16 mg/dL for each 0.10 unit rise in pH.[15] Hypocalcemia associated with decreased serum albumin levels results in a decrease in protein-bound, rather than ionized, calcium and usually is asymptomatic. A change in pH shifts the balance of ionized calcium to bound and complexed calcium. An alkaline pH increases binding of calcium to protein, lowering the ionized calcium while the total serum calcium remains unchanged. Hyperventilation causing respiratory alkalosis can produce an effective hypocalcemia with tetany by increasing the protein binding of calcium without altering the total calcium concentrations.[23]

Ionized calcium serves a number of functions; it (1) participates in many enzyme reactions; (2) exerts an important effect on cell membrane potentials and permeability; (3) is necessary for contraction in skeletal, cardiac, and smooth muscle; (4) controls the synaptic release of acetylcholine; (5) influences cardiac contractility and automaticity by way of slow calcium channels; and (6) is essential for blood clotting. The use of calcium-channel blocking drugs in circulatory disorders demonstrates the importance of the calcium ion in the normal function of the heart and blood vessels. Calcium is required for all but the first two steps of the intrinsic pathway for blood coagulation. Because of its ability to bind calcium, citrate often is used to prevent clotting in blood that is to be used for transfusions.

HYPOCALCEMIA

Hypocalcemia represents a serum calcium level of less than 8.5 mg/dL.[15] The biologically active component of the serum calcium is the free or ionized calcium.

Thus the onset and severity of hypocalcemia may be influenced by factors that change the fraction of calcium that is complexed or protein-bound.

Causes. The causes of hypocalcemia, or a deficit in ionized calcium, are (1) impaired ability to mobilize calcium from bone stores, (2) abnormal binding of calcium so that greater proportions of calcium are in the un-ionized form, (3) abnormal losses of calcium from the kidneys, and (4) decreased absorption of calcium from the intestine (Table 29-10).

The ability to mobilize calcium from bone stores is impaired in hypoparathyroidism. A parathyroid hormone (PTH) deficiency occurs with primary hypoparathyroidism; it can occur secondary to neck surgery, particularly if the surgery involves removal of a parathyroid adenoma, thyroidectomy, and bilateral neck resection for cancer. PTH deficiency may result from parathyroid gland suppression (after parathyroid surgery) or from interference with the blood supply. Hypocalcemia may occur immediately or from 1 to 2 days after surgery and usually is transient.

The electrolyte or ionized form of calcium is decreased as serum calcium binds to plasma proteins or complexes with other substances. For example, serum pH affects the ionization of calcium; ionization is decreased in alkalosis. Free fatty acids (FFA) increase binding of calcium to albumin.[24] Elevations in FFA sufficient to alter calcium binding may occur during stressful situations that cause elevations of epinephrine, glucagon, growth hormone, and adrenocorticotropic hormone. Heparin, β-adrenergic drugs (epinephrine, isoproterenol, and norepinephrine), and alcohol can also produce elevations in FFA sufficient to increase calcium binding. As mentioned previously, citrate complexes with calcium and often is used as an anticoagulant for blood transfusions. Theoretically, excess citrate in donor blood could combine with the calcium in a recipient's blood, causing hypocalcemia and tetany. This normally does not occur because the liver removes the citrate within a matter of minutes. Therefore, when blood transfusions are administered at a slow rate (less than 1 L/hr in the adult), there is little danger of hypocalcemia caused by citrate binding.[1] Hypocalcemia is a common finding in acute pancreatitis. It is not known whether the calcium is precipitated in the pancreas as a result of fat necrosis or sequestered elsewhere.

There is an inverse relation between calcium and phosphate excretion by the kidneys. Phosphate is retained in renal failure, causing serum calcium levels to decrease and PTH levels to rise. Hypocalcemia and hyperphosphatemia occur when the glomerular filtration rate falls below 25 to 30 mL/min, the normal being 100 to 120 mL/min.

Intestinal absorption of calcium decreases with a deficiency of vitamin D. Vitamin D deficiency stemming from low intake is seldom seen today because many foods are fortified with vitamin D. Vitamin D

TABLE 29-10. HYPOCALCEMIA	
CAUSES	**SIGNS AND SYMPTOMS**
Impaired Ability to Mobilize Calcium from Bone Hypoparathyroidism **Abnormal Calcium Binding** Decreased serum albumin Increased pH Increased free fatty acids Rapid transfusion of citrated blood Acute pancreatitis **Abnormal Losses** Renal failure **Decreased Absorption from the Intestine** Vitamin D deficiency or inactivity	**Laboratory Values** Serum calcium below 8.5 mg/dL **Increased Nerve Excitability** Paresthesia, especially numbness or tingling Skeletal muscle cramps Abdominal spasms and cramps Hyperactive reflexes Carpopedal spasm Tetany Laryngeal spasm Positive Chvostek's test Positive Trousseau's test **Cardiovascular Manifestations** Hypotension Cardiac insufficiency Failure to respond to drugs that act by means of calcium-mediated mechanisms

deficiency is more apt to occur in malabsorption states, such as biliary obstruction, pancreatic insufficiency, and celiac disease, in which the ability to absorb fat and fat-soluble vitamins is impaired. Vitamin D (inactivated form) is stored in the liver. In subsequent steps the liver and the kidneys convert inactive vitamin D to the activated form (1,25-dihydroxycholecalciferol). Vitamin D remains in the body only a short time once it has been activated. This means that patients with renal failure will have problems with the absorption of calcium because of impaired activation of vitamin D. Fortunately, the activated form of the hormone (calcitriol) has been synthesized and is now available for use in the treatment of calcium deficit in persons with renal failure.

Manifestations. The manifestations of acute hypocalcemia relate to increased neural excitability and cardiovascular effects. Ionized calcium stabilizes neuromuscular excitability. In severe hypocalcemia, increased neuromuscular excitability can cause tetany, laryngeal spasm, seizures, and death. Both Chvostek's and Trousseau's signs are used in checking for an increase in neuromuscular excitability and tetany. Chvostek's sign is elicited by tapping the face just below the temple at the point where the facial nerve emerges. Tapping the face over the facial nerve causes spasm of the lip, nose, or face when the test is positive. An inflated blood pressure cuff is used to test for Trousseau's sign. The cuff is inflated to a point where it temporarily occludes the circulation of the hand, usually for 1 to 5 minutes. Contraction of the fingers and hands (carpopedal spasm) indicates the presence of tetany. Cardiovascular effects of acute hypocalcemia include hypotension, cardiac insufficiency, cardiac dysrhythmias, and failure to respond to drugs such as digitalis, norepinephrine, and dopamine that act through calcium-mediated mechanisms.

Treatment. The treatment of calcium deficit is directed toward increasing the intake or absorption from the intestine. One glass of milk contains about 300 mg of calcium. An intravenous infusion containing calcium (calcium gluconate, calcium gluceptate, calcium chloride) is used when tetany or acute symptoms are present or anticipated because of a decrease in serum calcium. The active form of vitamin D is administered when the liver or kidney mechanisms needed for hormone activation are impaired.

HYPERCALCEMIA

Hypercalcemia represents a total serum calcium greater than 10.5 mg/dL. Falsely elevated levels of calcium can result from prolonged drawing of blood with an excessively tight tourniquet. Increased plasma proteins (*e.g.*, hyperalbuminemia and hyperglobulinemia) may elevate the total serum calcium but not affect the ionized calcium concentration.

Causes. A serum calcium excess (hypercalcemia) results when calcium influx into the circulation overwhelms the calcium regulatory hormones (PTH and vitamin D) or the ability of the kidney to excrete the excess calcium ions (Table 29-11). The most common causes of hypercalcemia are increased bone resorption (or destruction) due to neoplasms, hyperparathyroidism, and prolonged immobility. A number of malignant tumors, including carcinoma of the lungs, have been associated with hypercalcemia. Some tumors actually destroy the bone, whereas others produce an osteoclast-activating factor, and some are sites of ectopic PTH production. Hyperparathyroidism may be mild or severe. It is more common in postmenopausal women because estrogen increases the effect of PTH on bone. Lithium is associated with increased levels of PTH.

Intestinal absorption of calcium increases with excessive doses of vitamin D. The liver can store vitamin D, and it is reported that 1000 times the normal quantities can be ingested with only a threefold increase in serum levels of the active hormone.[1] Granulomatous conditions such as sarcoidosis, tuberculosis, silicosis, and histoplasmosis produce an increase in vitamin D. In such conditions, vitamin D is produced by the monocytes that compose the granuloma. Another cause of excessive calcium absorption is the milk–alkali syndrome. The condition is thought to be caused by mild hypercalcemia that leads to increased sodium excretion and decreased extracellular fluid volume, followed by bicarbonate retention (alkalosis) and a resultant increase in renal calcium retention. The syndrome is due to excessive ingestion of calcium (often in the form of milk) and absorbable antacids. Discontinuance of the antacid repairs the alkalosis and calcium retention.

Thiazide diuretics can produce an increase in total serum calcium of 0.5 to 1.0 mg/dL in otherwise healthy people.[23] This reflects the indirect effects of hemoconcentration and the direct effects of bone resorption. In most people, calcium levels return to normal after several weeks of therapy. Thiazide diuretics may cause hypercalcemia in patients with underlying bone disorders and increased bone resorption.

Manifestations. The signs and symptoms associated with calcium excess originate from three sources: (1) a decrease in neuromuscular activity, (2) resorption of calcium from bone, and (3) exposure of the kidneys to high concentrations of calcium.

TABLE 29-11. HYPERCALCEMIA

CAUSES	SIGNS AND SYMPTOMS

Excessive Gains
  Increased intestinal absorption
    Excessive vitamin D
    Excessive calcium in diet
    Milk–alkali syndrome
Increased Bone Resorption
  Immobility
  Increased levels of parathyroid hormone
  Malignant neoplasms
  Thiazide diuretics
	Laboratory Values
	  Serum calcium above 10.5 mg/dL
	Altered Neural and Muscular Activity
	  Muscle weakness and atrophy
	  Ataxia, loss of muscle tone
	  Lethargy
	  Stupor and coma
	  Personality or behavioral changes
	Associated with Increased Bone Resorption
	  Deep bone pain
	  Pathologic fractures
	Renal Manifestations
	  Signs of renal insufficiency (acute reversible)
	  Polyuria
	  Flank pain
	  Signs of kidney stones
	  Increased losses of sodium and potassium
	Cardiovascular Manifestations
	  Hypertension
	  Shortening of the QT interval, AV block on electrocardiogram
	Gastrointestinal Manifestations
	  Anorexia
	  Nausea
	  Vomiting
	  Constipation

Neural excitability is decreased in hypercalcemia. There may be a dulling of consciousness, stupor, weakness, and muscle flaccidity. Acute psychoses are common when calcium levels rise above 16 mg/dL. The heart responds to elevated levels of calcium with increased contractility and ventricular arrhythmias. Digitalis causes these responses to be accentuated. High calcium concentrations in the urine impair the ability of the kidneys to concentrate urine by interfering with the action of ADH. This causes salt and water diuresis and an increased sensation of thirst. Hypercalciuria also predisposes to the development of renal calculi.

Hypercalcemic crisis describes an acute increase in serum calcium. Malignant disease and hyperparathyroidism are major causes of hypercalcemic crisis. In hypercalcemic crisis, polyuria, excessive thirst, volume depletion, fever, altered levels of consciousness, azotemia (nitrogenous wastes in the blood), and a disturbed mental state accompany other signs of calcium excess. Symptomatic hypercalcemia is associated with a high mortality rate; death often is due to cardiac arrest.

Treatment. The treatment of calcium excess usually is directed toward correcting or controlling the condition that is causing the disorder. The excretion of sodium is accompanied by calcium excretion. Diuretics and sodium chloride can be administered in emergency treatment of hypercalcemia. Corticosteroids and plicamycin (Mithramycin) are used to treat hypercalcemia associated with cancer. Diphosphonates, which are bone crystal formation inhibitors, are being investigated as a treatment method.[25]

EXTRACELLULAR PHOSPHATE LEVELS

Phosphate is an integral part of all body tissues. About 85% of phosphorus is located in bone; the remainder is predominantly (14%) in body cells. Only about 10% is in the extracellular fluid. In the adult, the normal serum phosphate level ranges from 2.7 to 4.5 mg/dL. These values are slightly higher in children (4.5 to 5.5 mg/dL).

Phosphorous is the fourth most abundant element in the body after carbon, nitrogen, and calcium. Total body phosphorous in a 70-kg man is about 700 g. About 90% of intracellular phosphorous is in the organic rather than the inorganic form. The phosphate-containing organic form includes the nucleic acids, adenosine triphosphate (ATP), phosphoproteins, and membrane proteins. Cell injury or atrophy leads to a loss of cell components that contain organic phosphate; regeneration of these cellular components results in withdrawal of inorganic phosphate from the extracellular compartment.

The functions of phosphate can be grouped into four categories: (1) it plays a major role in bone formation; (2) it is essential to certain metabolic processes, including the formation of ATP and the enzymes needed for metabolism of glucose, fat, and protein; (3) it is a necessary component of several vital parts of the cell, being incorporated into the nucleic acids and the cell membrane; and (4) it serves as an acid–base buffer in the extracellular fluid and in the renal excretion of hydrogen ions. Delivery of oxygen by the red blood cell depends on organic phosphates in ATP and 2,3-diphosphoglycerate (2,3-DPG). Phosphate is also needed for normal function of other blood cells, including the white cells and platelets.

HYPOPHOSPHATEMIA

Hypophosphatemia is commonly defined by a serum phosphorus level of less than 2.7 mg/dL.

The most common causes of hypophosphatemia are (1) depletion of phosphorus due to insufficient intestinal absorption, (2) a redistribution between the intracellular and extracellular compartments, and (3) increased renal losses (Table 29-12). Antacids that contain aluminum hydroxide, aluminum carbonate, and calcium carbonate bind with phosphate, causing increased phosphate losses in the stool. Sometimes aluminum hydroxide is used therapeutically to decrease phosphate levels in chronic renal failure. Alcoholism is recognized as a cause of hypophosphatemia. The mechanisms underlying hypophosphatemia in the person addicted to alcohol are not clearly understood; they may be related to malnutrition or to hypomagnesemia. Hypophosphatemia can occur during prolonged courses of in-

TABLE 29-12. HYPOPHOSPHATEMIA

CAUSES	SIGNS AND SYMPTOMS
Decreased Intestinal Absorption	**Laboratory Values**
Antacids (aluminum and calcium)	Serum levels below 2.7 mg/dL in adults
Severe diarrhea	and 4.5 mg/dL in children
Lack of vitamin D	**Neural Manifestations**
Increased Renal Excretion	Intention tremor
Alkalosis	Ataxia
Hyperparathyroidism	Paresthesia
Diabetic ketoacidosis	Hyporeflexia
Renal tubular defects	Confusion
Malnutrition and Intracellular Shift	Stupor
Alcoholism	Coma
Total parenteral nutrition	Seizures
Recovery from malnutrition	**Musculoskeletal Manifestations**
Administration of insulin and recovery	Muscle weakness
from diabetic ketoacidosis	Joint stiffness
	Bone pain
	Osteomalacia
	Gastrointestinal Manifestations
	Anorexia
	Dysphagia
	Hematologic Disorders
	Hemolytic anemia
	Platelet dysfunction with bleeding disorders
	Impaired function of white blood cells

travenous therapy or nutritional repletion.[26] Like potassium, only a small amount of total body phosphorus is in the extracellular compartment; hence, even a small redistribution between the extracellular and intracellular compartments can cause hypophosphatemia without a change in total body phosphorus. Malnutrition and diabetic ketoacidosis increase phosphate excretion and phosphate loss from the body. Refeeding of malnourished patients increases the incorporation of phosphate into nucleic acids and phosphorylated compounds in the cell. The same thing happens when diabetic ketoacidosis is reversed with insulin therapy. The intracellular shift of phosphate causes the serum phosphate levels to drop. PTH decreases serum phosphate levels through a different mechanism: it increases the renal excretion of phosphate. Alkalosis has an indirect effect on serum phosphate levels. The increase in pH causes increased binding of calcium, which in turn leads to a decrease in ionized calcium and an increase in the release of PTH, causing phosphate excretion.

Manifestations. Hypophosphatemia causes signs and symptoms related to altered neural function, disturbed musculoskeletal function, and hematologic disorders. Neural manifestations include intentional tremors, paresthesia, hyporeflexia, stupor, coma, and seizures (see Table 29-12). Anorexia and dysphagia can occur. There may be muscle weakness, joint stiffness, bone pain, and osteomalacia. Red cell metabolism is impaired in phosphate deficiency; the cells become rigid and have increased hemolysis and diminished ATP and 2,3-DPG levels. Chemotaxis and phagocytosis by white blood cells are impaired. Platelet function is also disturbed. Respiratory insufficiency resulting from impaired function of the respiratory muscles can develop in severe hypophosphatemia.[27]

Treatment. The treatment of hypophosphatemia includes replacement therapy. This may be accomplished with dietary sources high in phosphate (one glassful of milk contains about 250 mg of phosphate) or with oral or intravenous replacement solutions. Phosphate supplements usually are contraindicated in hypercalcemia and renal failure. Treatment with phosphate supplements can lead to disseminated calcification.

HYPERPHOSPHATEMIA

Hyperphosphatemia represents a serum phosphorus concentration in excess of 4.5 mg/dL.

In contrast to hypophosphatemia, hyperphosphatemia results from (1) failure of the kidneys to excrete excess phosphate, (2) rapid redistribution of intracellular phosphate to the extracellular compartment, and (3) excessive intake of phosphate. The most common cause of hyperphosphatemia is impaired renal function. It is a common electrolyte disorder in patients with end-stage renal disease. PTH deficiency decreases renal losses of phosphate. Intracellular release of phosphate can result from conditions such as tissue injury, heatstroke, potassium deficiency, and seizures. Chemotherapy can raise serum phosphate levels because of the rapid destruction of tumor cells. The administration of excess phosphate-containing antacids, laxatives, or enemas can be another cause of hyperphosphatemia, especially when there is a decrease in vascular volume and a reduced glomerular filtration rate. Phosphate-containing laxatives and enemas predispose to hypovolemia and a decreased glomerular filtration rate by inducing diarrhea, thereby increasing the risk of hypophosphatemia. Hyperphosphatemia has been reported in children after the use of a single sodium phosphate–biphosphate enema.[28]

Hyperphosphatemia is associated with a decrease in serum calcium; thus, many of the signs and symptoms of a phosphate excess may be related to a calcium deficit (see Table 29-10).

The treatment of hyperphosphatemia is directed at the cause of the disorder. Dietary restriction of foods that are high in phosphate may be used. Calcium-, magnesium-, and aluminum-based phosphate binders are useful in chronic hyperphosphatemia. Magnesium-based phosphate binders must be used cautiously in patients with renal failure because of the danger of hypermagnesemia.

ALTERATIONS IN MAGNESIUM

Magnesium is the second most abundant intracellular cation. Of the total, 50% is stored in bone, 49% is contained in the body cells, and the remaining 1% is dispersed in the extracellular fluids. The normal serum concentration of magnesium is 1.7 to 2.7 mg/dL.

Only recently has the importance of magnesium to the overall function of the body been recognized. Magnesium acts as a cofactor in many enzyme reactions. It is essential in all enzyme systems known to be catalyzed by ATP, so that profound disruption of cell function occurs in magnesium-deficient tissues. Magnesium is necessary for protein and DNA synthesis, DNA and RNA transcription, and translation of RNA. Maintenance of normal intracellular levels of potassium depends on magnesium: magnesium deficiency causes intracellular potassium depletion. Magnesium can bind to calcium receptors; it has been suggested that alterations in magnesium levels may exert their effects through calcium-mediated mechanisms. Magnesium may bind competitively to calcium binding sites, producing the appropriate response; it may compete with calcium for a binding site but not exert an effect; or it may alter the distribution of calcium by interfering with its movement across the cell membrane.[29]

REGULATION

The average American consumes about 180 to 300 mg of magnesium daily. All green vegetables contain abundant amounts of magnesium. Although some controversy exists, it is generally agreed that the minimum daily requirement for magnesium in the adult is about 3.6 mg/kg.[18]

Magnesium is absorbed from the intestine and excreted by the kidneys. Intestinal absorption is not closely regulated, and about 25% to 65% of dietary magnesium is absorbed. Calcium and magnesium compete for reabsorption in both the intestines and the renal tubules; factors that increase calcium absorption cause a decrease in magnesium absorption. PTH is thought to enhance renal reabsorption of magnesium, although this action often is outweighed by the effects of hypercalcemia, which act to inhibit reabsorption.

HYPOMAGNESEMIA

Hypomagnesemia represents a serum magnesium concentration of less than 1.7 mg/dL. Hypomagnesemia can be expected in 6.9% to 11% of hospitalized patients in whom serum electrolyte determinations are routinely performed,[30] and 38% to 42% of patients with hypokalemia have concurrent hypomagnesemia.[31, 32]

Magnesium deficiency usually results from impaired absorption in the intestine or from increased urinary losses. Although the kidneys are able to defend against hypermagnesemia, they are less able to conserve magnesium and prevent hypomagnesemia. Urine losses of magnesium are increased with diuresis, and diuretics are the most common cause of increased renal losses (Table 29-13).

Another common cause of magnesium deficiency is chronic alcoholism.[23] Many factors contribute to hypomagnesemia in alcoholism, including low intake and gastrointestinal losses from diarrhea. The effects of hypomagnesemia are exaggerated by other electrolyte disorders, such as hypokalemia, hypocalcemia, and metabolic acidosis, often seen in chronic alcoholism.

Magnesium levels are also decreased in conditions that cause malabsorption, in malnutrition, and in patients receiving total parenteral nutrition in which the magnesium content is inadequate. Prolonged diarrhea or laxative abuse may also lead to severe magnesium deficiency. Excessive calcium intake impairs magnesium absorption by competing for the same transport site. Magnesium losses are increased in diabetic ketoacidosis, diuretic therapy, hyperparathyroidism, and hyperaldosteronism.

Magnesium deficit is characterized by personality change; neuromuscular irritability; tremors; athetoid or choreiform movements; positive Babinski's, Chvostek's, or Trousseau's signs; tachycardia; hypertension; and ventricular dysrhythmias. The loss of potassium from cardiac and skeletal muscle

---

TABLE 29-13. HYPOMAGNESEMIA

CAUSES	SIGNS AND SYMPTOMS
Impaired Intake or Absorption	**Laboratory Findings**
Alcoholism	Serum magnesium less than 1.7 mg/dL
Malabsorption	**Neuromuscular Hyperirritability**
Small bowel bypass surgery	Personality change
Malnutrition or starvation	Athetoid or choreiform movements
Parenteral hyperalimentation of inadequate magnesium	Positive Babinski's sign
High dietary intake of calcium without concomitant increase in magnesium	Nystagmus
	Tetany
	Positive Chvostek's or Trousseau's sign
Increased Losses	**Cardiovascular Manifestations**
Diabetic ketoacidosis	Tachycardia
Diuretic therapy	Hypertension
Hyperparathyroidism	Ventricular arrhythmias
Hyperaldosteronism	
Magnesium-wasting renal disease	

fibers is accelerated. Hypokalemia has long been associated with diuretic therapy and digitalis toxicity. More recently, magnesium deficiency has been implicated in aggravating potassium deficiency and interfering with potassium repletion. Electrocardiographic changes are associated with both hypomagnesemia and hypokalemia.

HYPERMAGNESEMIA

Magnesium excess (serum concentration in excess of 2.7 mg/dL) is rare. When it does occur, it usually is related to renal insufficiency or the injudicious use of magnesium sulfate as a laxative. Magnesium sulfate is also used to treat toxemia of pregnancy and premature labor; in these cases, careful monitoring for signs of hypermagnesemia is essential.

The signs and symptoms occur only when serum magnesium levels exceed 4.9 mg/dL (2 mmol/L).[26] Hypermagnesemia causes sedation of the nervous system with hyporeflexia, muscle weakness, confusion, and respiratory paralysis. Blood pressure is decreased, and the electrocardiogram shows an increase in the PR interval, a broadening of the QRS complex, and elevation of the T wave. Hypotension and cardiac dysrhythmias can occur with moderate hypermagnesemia (<10 mg/dL) and confusion and coma with several hypermagnesemia (>10 mg/dL). Very severe hypermagnesemia (>15 mg/dL) may cause cardiac arrest.[15] The treatment of hypermagnesemia includes cessation of magnesium administration. Calcium is a direct antagonist of magnesium, and intravenous administration of calcium may be used. Peritoneal dialysis or hemodialysis may be required.

In summary, electrolytes serve many functions. They (1) assist in regulating body water balance, (2) participate in acid–base balance, (3) contribute to enzyme reactions, and (4) play an essential role in neuromuscular activity. Serum levels of an electrolyte represent its concentration (milliequivalents per liter) in the extracellular compartment.

Sodium is the major cation in the extracellular fluid. Serum sodium levels are strongly affected by extracellular water levels: sodium concentration is increased in water deficit and decreased in water excess. Normal levels of sodium are essential to maintaining the osmolality of the extracellular fluids; many of the manifestations of altered sodium balance are caused by swelling (hyponatremia) or shrinking (hypernatremia) of body cells, including those of the CNS. Sodium also contributes to neuromuscular excitability, acid–base balance, and numerous chemical reactions that occur in the body.

Potassium is the major intracellular cation. It contributes to the maintenance of intracellular osmolality, is necessary for normal neuromuscular function, and influences acid–base balance. Because potassium is poorly conserved by the body, adequate daily intake is needed. Most of the body's potassium loss occurs through the kidneys; hence, potassium imbalances can occur rapidly in diuresis (hypokalemia) or renal failure (hyperkalemia). Alterations in potassium balance affect skeletal, cardiac, and smooth muscle function.

There is a close link between the regulation of calcium and the regulation of phosphate in the body (*e.g.*, an elevation of serum phosphate produces a decrease in serum calcium). Of the three forms of extracellular calcium (protein-bound, citrate-bound, and ionized), only the ionized form can cross the cell membrane and contribute to cellular function. Ionized calcium has a number of functions: it contributes to neuromuscular function, plays a vital role in the blood clotting process, and participates in a number of enzyme reactions. Alterations in ionized calcium levels produce neural effects: neural excitability is increased in hypocalcemia and decreased in hypercalcemia. Phosphate is largely an intracellular anion. It is incorporated into the nucleic acids and ATP. A phosphate deficit causes signs and symptoms of altered neural function, disturbed musculoskeletal function, and hematologic disorders. Phosphate excess occurs with renal failure and PTH deficit; it is associated with decreased serum calcium levels. Magnesium is the second most abundant intracellular cation. It acts as a cofactor in many enzyme reactions and affects neuromuscular function in the same manner as the calcium ion.

■ ALTERATIONS IN INTERSTITIAL FLUIDS AND EDEMA

About 25% of the total body water is contained in the interstitial, or tissue, spaces. This water acts as a transport vehicle for gases, nutrients, wastes, and other materials that move between the vascular compartment and body cells. Interstitial fluid also provides a reservoir from which vascular volume can be maintained during periods of hemorrhage or loss of vascular volume. A tissue gel, or sponge-like material composed of large quantities of mucopolysaccharides, fills the tissue spaces and aids in the even distribution of interstitial fluid. The decrease in tissue gel that occurs with age is thought to account in part for the wrinkles that accompany aging.

REGULATION OF INTERSTITIAL FLUID VOLUME

The interchange of cellular and vascular fluid occurs at the capillary level, with fluid leaving the capillary bed, traversing the interstitial spaces, and entering the cell and vice versa. Capillary pressure pushes fluid out of the capillary and into the interstitial spaces, and the plasma colloidal osmotic pressure pulls fluid back into the capillaries from the tissue spaces. Normally a small amount of fluid that moves into the tissues is not pulled back into the capillaries. This fluid is returned to the circulation via the lymphatic system. The movement of fluid between the capillary bed and the interstitial spaces is continuous. A state of equilibrium exists as long as equal amounts of fluid enter and leave the interstitial spaces.

Fluid leaving the capillary =
fluid reentering the capillary + lymphatic flow

Capillaries are microscopic vessels one layer thick that connect the arterioles of the arterial system with the venules of the venous system (Fig. 29-7). Small cuffs of smooth muscle, the precapillary sphincters, are positioned at the arterial end of the capillary. The smooth muscle tone of the arterioles, venules, and precapillary sphincters serves to control blood flow through the capillary bed.

Two types of mechanisms control the exchange of fluid through the capillary membrane—the outward forces that cause fluid to leave the capillary and enter the interstitial spaces and the inward forces that pull fluid back into the capillary from the interstitial spaces. The major outward force is the capillary filtration pressure that pushes fluid out of the capillary. There is also evidence of a negative interstitial fluid pressure that contributes to the outward movement of fluid into the tissue spaces. Also, when osmotically active particles are present in the interstitial spaces, they pull fluid out of the capillary and into the tissue spaces. The inward movement of fluid is controlled largely by the plasma colloidal osmotic pressure. The plasma colloidal osmotic pressure causes about nine-tenths of the fluid that has been filtered out of capillaries to be reabsorbed. The other one-tenth flows into the lymphatic channel.

CAPILLARY FILTRATION PRESSURE

Capillary filtration pressure is the force that pushes water through the capillary pores into the interstitial spaces. It reflects the arterial pressure, the venous pressure, and the hydrostatic effects of gravity (Fig. 29-8).

The arterial pressure decreases as blood moves away from the heart. Nevertheless, the pressure at the arterial end of the capillary normally is higher than the pressure at its venous end. This pressure difference, or gradient, contributes to the exchange of fluid at the capillary level. Venous pressure can also be transmitted back to the capillary because there are no sphincters at this end of the capillary. This means that an increase in venous pressure, such as that which occurs with heart failure, eventually leads to an increase in intracapillary pressure. Capillary pressure also reflects changes in capillary volume. Capillary volume is controlled by the precapillary flow (the tone of the precapillary sphincters and the arterioles that supply the capillary) and the postcapillary (venule and small vein) resistances. Constriction of the arterioles and precapillary sphincters leads to a decrease in capillary pressure, whereas an increase in resistance to venous outflow leads to an increase in pressure.

The pressure caused by gravity is called *hydrostatic pressure*. In a person who is standing, the weight of the blood in the vascular column causes an increase of 1 mmHg in pressure for every 13.6 mm of distance below the level of the heart. Dependent upon height,

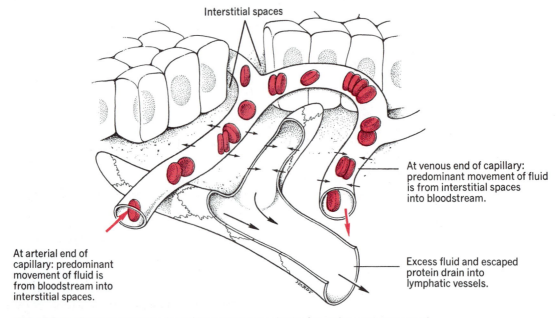

Interstitial spaces

At venous end of capillary: predominant movement of fluid is from interstitial spaces into bloodstream.

At arterial end of capillary: predominant movement of fluid is from bloodstream into interstitial spaces.

Excess fluid and escaped protein drain into lymphatic vessels.

FIG. 29-7. Exchanges through capillary membranes in the formation and removal of interstitial fluid. (Chaffee, E. E., and Lytle, I. M. [1980]. *Basic physiology and anatomy* [4th ed.]. Philadelphia: J.B. Lippincott.)

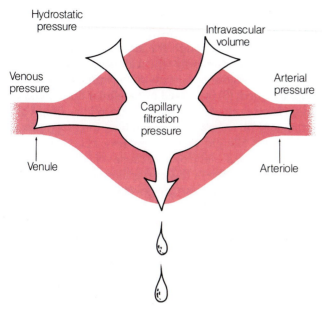

FIG. 29-8. Forces that influence capillary filtration pressure.

this means that the hydrostatic pressure in the veins of a tall standing adult can reach a level of 90 mmHg. Gravity has no effect on blood pressure in a person in the recumbent position because the blood vessels are then at the level of the heart. The terms *capillary pressure* and *hydrostatic pressure* often are used interchangeably; this is because of the passive nature of pressure in the capillary bed. In this chapter, for purposes of discussion, hydrostatic pressure is considered the result of gravity and is presented separately from other factors that affect capillary pressure.

COLLOIDAL OSMOTIC PRESSURE

A colloid solution is one in which there are evenly dispersed particles, much as cream particles become dispersed when milk is homogenized. The term *colloidal osmotic pressure* is used to distinguish the osmotic effects of the particles in a colloidal solution from those of the dissolved crystalloids such as sodium. The plasma proteins are large molecules that disperse in the blood and occasionally escape into the tissue spaces. Because the capillary membrane is almost impermeable to the plasma proteins, these particles exert a force that draws fluid into the capillary and offsets the pushing force of the capillary filtration pressure. The plasma contains a mixture of plasma proteins, including albumin, the globulins, and fibrinogen. Albumin, which is the smallest and most abundant of the plasma proteins, accounts for about 70% of the total osmotic pressure. The reader is reminded that it is the number and not the size of the particles in solution that controls the osmotic pres-

sure. One gram of albumin (molecular weight 69,000) contains almost six times as many molecules as 1 g of fibrinogen (molecular weight 400,000). Because of its smaller size and larger quantity, albumin (normal value of about 4.5 g/dL) has a much greater influence on the plasma colloidal osmotic pressure than the other plasma proteins (globulins, 2.5 g/dL and fibrinogen, 0.3 g/dL).

LYMPH FLOW

Slightly more fluid leaves the capillary than can be reabsorbed at the venous end. This excess fluid is returned to the circulation by way of the lymph channels; almost all body tissues have lymph channels. Also, white blood cells, plasma proteins, and other large molecules enter the interstitial spaces; these cells and molecules, which are too large to reenter the capillary, rely on the loosely structured wall of the lymphatic vessels for return to the vascular compartment. If allowed to accumulate, these osmotically active particles would hold fluid in the tissue spaces.

The structure of the lymph capillary is unique in that the junctions between the endothelial cells of the vessels are loosely connected to form valves and are attached by anchoring filaments to the surrounding tissue (Fig. 29-9). These valves allow fluid to enter the lymph channel. The anchoring filaments serve to pull the valves open when tissue fluid increases. Once the fluid has entered the lymph channel it cannot leave because the valve prevents backward flow. Contraction of smooth muscles in the lymph channels (lymph pump) causes the lymph fluid to empty into the veins in the chest. Compression of tissues and muscle movements contribute to the movement of fluid in the lymph channels.

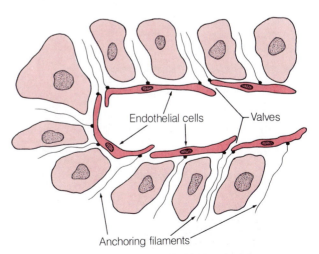

FIG. 29-9. Special structure of the lymphatic capillaries that permits passage of substances of high molecular weight back into the circulation. (Guyton, A. C. [1981]. *Textbook of medical physiology* [6th ed.]. Philadelphia: W.B. Saunders.)

EDEMA

Edema refers to excess interstitial fluid in the tissues. Edema is not a disease but rather the manifestation of altered physiologic function.

CAUSES

The alterations in physiologic function that lead to edema are (1) increases in capillary filtration pressure, (2) decreases in capillary colloidal osmotic pressure, (3) increases in capillary permeability, and (4) obstruction to lymph flow. Edema can occur in healthy as well as sick people—for example, the swelling of the hands and feet that occurs during hot weather. The causes of edema are summarized in Chart 29-2.

Increased Capillary Pressure. Edema develops when an increase in capillary pressure causes excess movement of fluid from the capillary bed into the

---

CHART 29-2: CAUSES OF EDEMA

Increased Capillary Pressure

Arteriolar dilatation
   Allergic responses (hives and angioneurotic edema)
   Inflammation
Venous obstruction
   Hepatic obstruction
   Heart failure
   Thrombophlebitis
Increased vascular volume
   Heart failure
   Increased levels of adrenocortical hormones
   Premenstrual sodium retention
   Pregnancy
   Environmental heat stress
Effects of gravity
   Prolonged standing

Decreased Colloidal Osmotic Pressure

Decreased production of plasma proteins
   Liver disease
   Starvation or severe protein deficiency
Increased loss of plasma proteins
   Protein-losing kidney diseases
   Extensive burns

Increased Capillary Permeability

Inflammation
Immune responses
Neoplastic disease
Tissue injury and burns

Obstruction of Lymphatic Flow

Infection or disease of the lymphatic structures
Surgical removal of lymph nodes

---

interstitial spaces. Among the factors that cause an increase in capillary pressures are (1) decreased resistance to flow through the arterioles and capillary sphincters that supply the capillary bed; (2) increased resistance to outflow at the venous end of the capillary bed; (3) increased extracellular fluid volume associated with an increase in intracellular fluid volume; and (4) increased gravitational forces. In hives and other allergic or inflammatory conditions, localized edema develops because of a histamine-induced dilatation of the precapillary sphincters and arterioles that supply the swollen area. Impaired venous outflow from the capillary causes a retrograde increase in capillary pressure. Thrombophlebitis, or the presence of venous blood clots, leads to edema of the affected part. In right-sided heart failure, blood dams up throughout the entire systemic venous system, causing organ congestion and edema of the dependent extremities. Increased reabsorption of sodium and water by the kidneys leads to an increase in extracellular volume with an increase in capillary pressure and subsequent movement of fluid into the tissue spaces. In hot weather, the superficial blood vessels dilate and sodium and water retention increases, which causes swelling of the hands and feet. Because of the effects of gravity, edema resulting from increased capillary pressure commonly causes fluid to accumulate in the dependent parts of the body, a condition referred to as *dependent edema*. For example, edema of the ankles and feet becomes more pronounced during prolonged periods of standing, due to the forces of gravity.

Decreased Colloidal Osmotic Pressure. The plasma proteins exert the osmotic force that is needed to move fluid back into the capillary from the tissue spaces. Edema develops when plasma protein levels become inadequate because of abnormal losses or inadequate production. Because the plasma proteins are equally distributed throughout the circulatory system, a decrease in plasma colloidal osmotic pressure causes generalized edema that affects both dependent and nondependent parts of the body. The glomerulus of the kidney nephron is a network of capillaries. In certain conditions, these capillaries become permeable to the plasma proteins. When this happens, large amounts of plasma proteins are filtered out of the blood and then lost in the urine. Generalized edema is common in persons with protein-losing kidney disease. An excess loss of plasma proteins also occurs when large areas of skin are injured or destroyed. Edema is a common problem during the early stages of a burn, resulting from both capillary injury and loss of plasma proteins.

Plasma proteins are synthesized from amino acids. In starvation and malnutrition, edema develops because of a lack of amino acids for use in plasma protein production. In starvation, edema may mask the loss of tissue mass. Finally, because plasma proteins are synthesized in the liver, severe liver dysfunction causes decreased plasma protein synthesis with the development of edema and ascites. Liver disease also contributes to edema formation by causing obstruction to venous flow through the portal circulation and through impaired metabolism of hormones, such as aldosterone, which increase sodium retention.

It is possible to measure the colloidal osmotic pressure of the plasma (25.4 mmHg is normal).[33] Infusion of albumin can be used to raise colloidal osmotic pressure as a means of restoring intravascular volume or reversing interstitial fluid losses.

Increased Capillary Permeability. When the capillary pores become enlarged or the integrity of the capillary wall is destroyed, capillary permeability is increased. Burn injury, mechanical distention, inflammation, and immune responses increase capillary permeability. Once an increase in capillary permeability has been established, plasma proteins and other osmotically active particles leak into the interstitial spaces and perpetuate the accumulation of tissue fluid.

Obstruction of Lymphatic Flow. The osmotically active plasma proteins and other large particles rely on the lymphatics for movement back into the circulatory system from the interstitial spaces. When lymph flow is obstructed, lymphedema occurs. Malignant involvement of lymph structures and removal of lymph nodes at the time of cancer surgery are common causes of lymphedema. Another cause of lymphedema is infection. Elephantiasis (filariasis) is a tropical infection in which nematodes of the superfamily Filarioidea invade the lymph nodes, causing massive swelling of a body part. This infection has been reported to cause a single leg to swell to such proportions that it weighs almost as much as the rest of the body.

MANIFESTATIONS

The effects of edema are determined largely by its location. Edema of the brain, larynx, or lungs is an acute, life-threatening condition. On the other hand, swelling of the ankles and feet often is insidious in onset and may or may not be associated with disease. Edema may interfere with movement, limiting motion or making opening of the eyes difficult. Edema can also be disfiguring. In terms of psychologic effects and self-concept, edema often causes a distortion of body features, creating problems in obtaining proper-fitting clothing and shoes.

At the tissue level, edema increases the distance for diffusion of oxygen, nutrients, and wastes. Edematous tissues usually are more susceptible to injury and to development of ischemic tissue damage, including pressure sores. The skin of a severely swollen finger can act as a tourniquet, shutting off the blood flow to the finger.

In chronic edema, the intercellular fibers in the tissue spaces become stretched out like an old balloon so that less filtration pressure is needed to push fluids into the interstitial spaces. The stretching of the tissue spaces makes correction or permanent reversal of edema difficult.

Pitting edema occurs when the accumulation of interstitial fluid exceeds the absorptive capacity of the tissue gel. In this form of edema, the tissue water is mobile and can be translocated with pressure exerted by a finger. To test for pitting edema, the observer applies firm finger pressure to the edematous areas. If an indentation remains after the finger has been removed, pitting edema is present.

Nonpitting edema usually reflects a condition in which serum proteins have accumulated in the tissue spaces and coagulated. The area often is firm and discolored. Brawny edema is a type of nonpitting edema in which the skin thickens and hardens. Nonpitting edema most frequently is seen after local infection or trauma.

ASSESSMENT AND TREATMENT

Methods for assessing edema include visual inspection, using finger pressure to determine the degree of pitting that is present. Pitting edema is evaluated on a scale of +1 to +4. Daily weight is also a useful index of interstitial fluid gain. A third assessment measure involves measuring the circumference of an extremity (or the abdomen).

Treatment of edema usually is directed toward (1) maintaining life when the swelling involves vital structures, (2) correcting or controlling the cause, and (3) preventing tissue injury. Diuretic therapy commonly is used to treat edema. The reader is again reminded that edema is not always associated with disease and that normal compensatory increases in tissue fluid may respond to such simple measures as elevating the feet.

Elastic support stockings and sleeves increase tissue pressure and resistance of the capillary walls to outward movement of fluid, and thus decrease the movement of fluid from the capillary into the tissue spaces. These support devices typically are prescribed in conditions such as lymphatic or venous obstruction and are most efficient if applied before the tissue spaces have filled with fluid—in the morning, for example, before the effects of gravity have caused fluid to move into the ankles.

ACCUMULATION OF FLUID IN THE SEROUS CAVITIES

The serous cavities are potential spaces located in strategic body areas where there is continual movement of body structures—the joints, the pericardial sac, and the pleural cavity. The exchange of extracellular fluid between the capillaries, the interstitial spaces, and the potential space of the serous cavity resembles capillary exchange elsewhere in the body. The potential spaces are closely linked with lymphatic drainage systems. The milking action of the moving structures continually forces fluid and plasma proteins back into the circulation, keeping these cavities empty. Any obstruction to lymph flow causes fluid accumulation in the serous cavities.

The prefix *hydro-* may be used to indicate the presence of excessive fluid, as in *hydrothorax*, which means excessive fluid in the pleural cavity. Or the term *effusion* may be used, as in *pleural effusion*, referring to an accumulation of fluid in the pleural cavity.

The fluid accumulated in a serous cavity may be either serous or exudative. A common cause of fluid accumulation in serous cavities is infection. In infection, white blood cells and cellular debris collect and obstruct lymph flow, causing osmotically active proteins to accumulate. A second cause of fluid accumulation is a malignant tumor; malignant tumors may invade the lymph channels that drain the serous cavity, and thus contribute to fluid accumulation.

Ascites is an accumulation of fluid in the peritoneal cavity. Because of its proximity to the portal circulation, the peritoneal cavity is more susceptible to excess fluid accumulation than are other body cavities. This is because anytime pressure in the liver sinusoids increases significantly, serum exudes through the capillaries on the surface of the liver and passes into the peritoneal cavity. Congestive heart failure, cirrhosis, and carcinoma of the liver are examples of conditions that obstruct hepatic blood flow and cause fluid to move into the peritoneal cavity. Because the portal vein receives blood from the peritoneal surface, portal hypertension creates an increase in the filtration pressure of the capillaries that line the peritoneal cavity.

Excess fluid may be aspirated or removed from a serous cavity. The term *paracentesis* refers to puncture of a cavity for removal of fluid. A needle or similar instrument is inserted into the cavity and the fluid is withdrawn. Analysis of the fluid for the presence of infectious organisms and malignant cells aids in the diagnosis of the disease responsible for the fluid accumulation.

In summary, exchange of fluids between the vascular compartment and the interstitial spaces occurs at the capillary level. The capillary filtration pressure pushes fluids out of the capillaries, and the colloidal osmotic pressure exerted by the plasma proteins pulls fluids back into the capillaries. Albumin, which is the smallest and most abundant of the plasma proteins, provides the major osmotic force for return of fluid to the vascular compartment. Slightly more fluid leaves the capillary bed than can be reabsorbed. This excess fluid is returned to the circulation by way of the lymphatic channels.

Edema occurs in healthy as well as sick people. The physiologic mechanisms that predispose to edema formation are (1) increased capillary pressure, (2) decreased capillary colloidal osmotic pressure, (3) increased capillary permeability, and (4) obstruction of lymphatic flow. The effect that edema exerts on body function is determined by its location; cerebral edema can be a life-threatening situation, whereas swollen feet can be a normal discomfort that accompanies hot weather.

■ REFERENCES

1. Guyton, A. (1991). *Textbook of medical physiology* (8th ed., pp. 274-285, 398, 801). Philadelphia: W.B. Saunders.
2. Porth, C.J.M., & Erickson, M. (1992). Physiology of thirst and drinking: Implications for nursing practice. *Heart and Lung, 21,* 273-284.
3. Lawrence, S. (1977). Woman's death by water intoxication ruled suicide. *Clinical Psychiatric News, 5,* 3.
4. Miller, P.D., Krebs, R.A., Neal, B.J., et al. (1983). Hypodipsia in geriatric patients. *American Journal of Medicine, 73,* 354-356.
5. Phillips, P.A., Rolls, B.J., Ledingham, J.G.G., et al. (1984). Reduced thirst after water deprivation in healthy men. *New England Journal of Medicine, 73,* 753-759.
6. Robertson, G.L. (1983). Thirst and vasopressin function in normal and disordered states of water balance. *Journal of Laboratory and Clinical Medicine, 101*(3), 351.
7. Blevins, L.S., & Wand, G.S. (1992). Diabetes insipidus. *Critical Care Medicine, 20,* 69-79.
8. Narins, R.G., Jones, E.R., & Stom, M.C. (1982). Diagnostic strategies in disorders of fluid, electrolyte, and acid–base disorders. *American Journal of Medicine, 72,* 496.
9. Pruit, B.A. (1979). Other complications of burn injury. In C.P. Artz, et al. (Eds.). *Burns* (p. 518). Philadelphia: W.B. Saunders.
10. Pflaum, S.S. (1979). Investigation of intake-output as a means of assessing body fluid balance. *Heart and Lung, 8,* 498.
11. Goldberger, E. (1980). *A primer on water, electrolytes, and acid–base syndromes* (6th ed., p. 34). Philadelphia: Lea & Febiger.
12. Snyder, J.D. (1982). From Pedialyte to Popsicles: A look at oral rehydration therapy in the United States. *American Journal of Clinical Nutrition, 35,* 157.
13. Casteel, H.B., & Fiedorek, S.C. (1990). Oral rehydration therapy. *Pediatric Clinics of North America, 37,* 295–311.

14. Weisman, Z. (1986). Cola drinks and rehydration in acute diarrhea (letter). *New England Journal of Medicine, 315,* 768.
15. Cogan, M.G. (1991). *Fluid and electrolytes* (pp. 100–111, 112–123, 129, 242, 251). E. Norwalk, CT: Appleton & Lange.
16. Katz, M.A. (1975). Hyperglycemic-induced hypernatremia—calculations of expected serum sodium depression. *New England Journal of Medicine, 293,* 843.
17. Oh, M.S., & Carroll, H.J. (1992). Disorders of sodium metabolism: Hypernatremia and hyponatremia. *Critical Care Medicine, 20,* 94–103.
18. Methaney, N.M. (1987). *Fluid and electrolyte balance: Nursing considerations* (pp. 54, 90–101). Philadelphia: J.B. Lippincott.
19. Knockel, J.F. (1987). Etiology and management of potassium deficiency. *Hospital Practice, 22*(1), 153.
20. Knockel, J.P. (1982). Neuromuscular manifestations of electrolyte disorders. *American Journal of Medicine, 72,* 521.
21. Rose, B.D. (1989). *Clinical physiology of acid–base and electrolyte disorders* (3rd ed., pp. 119–120, 764). New York: McGraw-Hill.
22. Whang, G., Whang, G.G., & Ryan, M.P. (1992). Refractory potassium repletion: A consequence of magnesium deficiency. *Archives of Internal Medicine, 152,* 40.
23. Agus, L.S., Wasserstein, A., & Goldfarb, S. (1982). Disorders of calcium and magnesium homeostasis. *American Journal of Medicine, 72,* 473.
24. Zaloga, G.P., & Chennow, B. (1986). Hypocalcemia in critical illness. *Journal of the American Medical Association, 256,* 1924.
25. Harinck, H., Plantingh, A.S.T., Elte, J.W., et al. (1987). Role of bone and kidney in tumor-induced hypercalcemia and its treatment with bisphosphate and sodium chloride. *American Journal of Medicine, 82*(6), 1133.
26. Knockel, J.P. (1985). The clinical status of hypophosphatemia. *New England Journal of Medicine, 313,* 447.
27. Aubier, M., Murciano, D., Lecocquic, Y., et al. (1985). Effect of hypophosphatemia on diaphragmatic contractility in patients with acute respiratory failure. *New England Journal of Medicine, 313,* 420.
28. Davis, R.F., Eichner, J., Archie, W., et al. (1977). Hypocalcemia, hyperphosphatemia and dehydration following a single hypertonic phosphate enema. *Journal of Pediatrics, 90,* 484.
29. Levine, B.S., & Coburn, J.W. (1984). Magnesium, the mimic/agonist of calcium. *New England Journal of Medicine, 310,* 1253.
30. Whang, R. (1987). Magnesium deficiency: Pathogenesis, prevalence, and clinical complications. *American Journal of Medicine, 82*(Suppl. 3A), 24.
31. Whang, R., Oei, T.O., Aikawa, J., et al. (1984). Predictors of clinical hypomagnesemia—hypokalemia, hypophosphatemia, hyponatremia, hypocalcemia. *Archives of Internal Medicine, 144,* 1794.
32. Boyd, J.C., Bruns, D.E., & Wills, M.R. (1983). Frequency of hypomagnesemia in hypokalemic states. *Clinical Chemistry, 29,* 178.
33. Morisette, M.P. (1977). Colloid osmotic pressure: Its measurement and clinical value. *Canadian Medical Association Journal, 116,* 897.

▪ BIBLIOGRAPHY

Arief, A.I. (1987). Hyponatremia associated with permanent brain damage. *Advances in Internal Medicine, 32,* 325.

Arieff, A.I. (1988). Osmotic failure: Physiology and strategies for treatment. *Hospital Practice, 23*(6), 173.

Berry, P.L., & Belsa, C.W. (1990). Hyponatremia. *Pediatric Clinics of North America, 37,* 351–363.

Bilezikian, J.P. (1992). Management of acute hypercalcemia. *New England Journal of Medicine, 326,* 1196–1203.

Brem, A.S. (1990). Disorders of potassium homeostasis. *Pediatric Clinics of North America, 37,* 419–427.

Cannon-Babb, M.L., & Schwartz, A.B. (1986). Drug-induced hyperkalemia. *Hospital Practice, 21*(9), 99.

Casteel, H.B., & Fiedorek, S.C. (1990). Oral rehydration therapy. *Pediatric Clinics of North America, 37,* 295–311.

Clive, D.M., & Stoff, J.S. (1988). Hyperkalemia: The potential for harm. *Journal of Intensive Care Medicine, 3*(1), 1.

Cronin, R.E. (1987). Psychogenic polydipsia with hyponatremia: Report of eleven cases. *American Journal of Kidney Diseases, 9,* 410.

Friday, B.A., & Reinhart, R.A. (1991). Magnesium metabolism: A case report and literature review. *Critical Care Nurse, 11,* 62–71.

Gumz, J.G. (1987). Clinical significance of magnesium: A review. *Drug Intelligence and Clinical Pharmacy, 21,* 240.

Khilnani, P. (1992). Electrolyte abnormalities in critically ill children. *Critical Care Medicine, 20,* 241–250.

Kobrin, S.M., & Goldfarb, S. (1990). Magnesium deficiency. *Seminars in Nephrology, 10,* 525–535.

Kuhn, M.M. (1991). Colloids vs crystalloids. *Critical Care Nurse, 11,* 37–51.

Levine, M.M., & Kleeman, C.R. (1987). Hypercalcemia: Pathophysiology and treatment. Hospital Practice, 22(7), 93.

Lynch, R.E. (1990). Ionized calcium: Pediatric perspective. *Pediatric Clinics of North America, 37,* 373–389.

Robertson, G.L., & Harris, A. (1989). Clinical use of vasopressin analogs. *Hospital Practice, 24*(10A), 114–139.

Schrier, R.W., & Briner, V.A. (1990). The differential diagnosis of hypernatremia. *Hospital Practice, 25* (9A), 29–37.

Solomon, L.R., & Lye, M. (1990). Hypernatremia in the elderly patient. *Gerontology, 36,* 171–179.

Stein, J.H. (1988). Hypokalemia: Common and uncommon causes. *Hospital Practice, 23*(3), 55.

Williams, M.E., & Rosa, R.M. (1988). Hyperkalemia: Disorders of internal and external potassium balance. *Journal of Intensive Care Medicine, 3*(1), 52.

Workman, M.L. (1992). Magnesium and phosphorous: The neglected electrolytes. *Clinical Issues in Critical Care Nursing, 3,* 653–663.

Zaloga, G.P. (1992). Hypercalcemia in critically ill patients. *Critical Care Medicine, 20,* 62.

CHAPTER 30

ALTERATIONS IN ACID–BASE BALANCE

■ OBJECTIVES

After you have studied this chapter, you should be able to meet the following objectives:

- Define _acid_ and _base_.
- Cite the source of the body's volatile and metabolic acids.
- Describe the three forms of carbon dioxide transport and their contribution to acid–base balance.
- Compare the role of the kidneys and respiratory system in regulation of acid–base balance.
- Use the Henderson-Hasselbalch equation to calculate _p_H.
- Describe the blood buffer systems.
- Describe the renal phosphate buffer system and the ammonia buffer system.
- Compare corrective and compensatory mechanisms for regulating body _p_H.
- Explain how potassium ions and hydrogen ions interact in _p_H regulation.

- Define _metabolic acidosis_, _metabolic alkalosis_, _respiratory acidosis_, and _respiratory alkalosis_.
- List the common causes of metabolic acidosis, metabolic alkalosis, respiratory acidosis, and respiratory alkalosis.
- Compare the neurologic manifestations of acidosis and alkalosis.
- Explain the use of the plasma anion gap in differentiating types of metabolic acidosis.
- Describe a clinical situation involving an acid–base disorder in which both primary and compensatory mechanisms might be active.
- Contrast and compare the clinical manifestations of acidosis and alkalosis.

Carol Mattson Porth: PATHOPHYSIOLOGY: CONCEPTS OF
ALTERED HEALTH STATES, 4th ed. © 1994, 1990, 1986, 1982
J.B. Lippincott Company

Normal body function depends on acid–base balance being regulated within a narrow physiologic range. The metabolic activities that take place in the body require the precise regulation of pH so that membrane excitability, enzyme systems, and chemical reactions can function in an optimal way. Many conditions, pathologic or otherwise, can alter body pH. This chapter has been organized into two sections: (1) mechanisms of acid–base balance and (2) alterations in acid–base balance.

■ MECHANISMS OF ACID–BASE BALANCE

An *acid* is a molecule that can contribute a hydrogen ion (H^+), and a *base* is a molecule that can accept or remove a H^+ ion. The concentration of H^+ in body fluid is low compared with other ions. For example, sodium (Na^+) is present at a concentration approximately 1 million times that of H^+. Because of the low H^+ concentration in body fluids, it is commonly expressed as the pH. Specifically, the pH represents the negative logarithm (p) of the H^+ concentration in equivalents per liter (pH of 7.0 implies a hydrogen concentration of 10^{-7} equivalents per liter). The pH of extracellular body fluids is normally maintained within the narrow range of 7.35 to 7.45.

The degree to which an acid dissociates and acts as a hydrogen donor determines whether it is a strong or weak acid. The same is true of a base and its ability to dissociate and accept a hydrogen ion. Most of the body's acids and bases are weak; the most important of these are carbonic acid (derived from carbon dioxide), which is a weak acid, and bicarbonate, which is a weak base.

METABOLIC ACID AND BICARBONATE PRODUCTION

Hydrogen and bicarbonate are by-products of metabolic processes. These metabolic processes are unique in that they result in the production of both *volatile* and *nonvolatile* acids. By far the largest source of metabolic acids is the oxidation of glucose and other carbohydrates that yield the carbon dioxide and the volatile acid, carbonic acid, which is eliminated through the lungs. The oxidation of other fuels such as proteins and fats produce nonvolatile acids. The kidneys must excrete these nonvolatile acids.

CARBON DIOXIDE AND BICARBONATE PRODUCTION

Body metabolism results in the production of about 15,000 mmol of carbon dioxide (CO_2) each day.[1] The carbon dioxide in the blood is transported in three

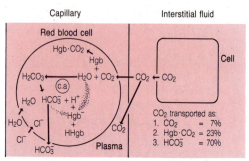

FIG. 30-1. Mechanisms of carbon dioxide transport. (After Guyton, A. C. [1986]. *Textbook of medical physiology* (7th ed.). Philadelphia: W.B. Saunders)

forms: (1) attached to hemoglobin, (2) as dissolved carbon dioxide, and (3) as bicarbonate (Fig. 30-1). Collectively, dissolved carbon dioxide and HCO_3^- constitute about 77% of the carbon dioxide that is transported in the extracellular fluid; the remaining CO_2 travels attached to hemoglobin. Although CO_2 is not an acid, a small percentage of it combines with water in the bloodstream resulting in the formation of carbonic acid (H_2CO_3):

$$CO_2 + H_2O \rightleftharpoons H_2CO_3 \rightleftharpoons H^+ + HCO_3^-$$

The reaction between CO_2 and water is catalyzed by an enzyme called *carbonic anhydrase*, which is present in large quantities in red blood cells, renal tubular cells, and other tissues in the body. The rate of the reaction between carbon dioxide and water is increased about 5000 times by the presence of carbonic anhydrase. Were it not for this enzyme, the reaction would occur too slowly to be of any significance.

The dissolved CO_2 content of the blood, which is the source of H_2CO_2, can be calculated using the partial pressure of CO_2 (PCO_2) and its solubility coefficient. Under normal physiologic conditions, the solubility coefficient for CO_2 is 0.03. This means that the dissolved CO_2 in venous blood, which normally has a PCO_2 of about 45 mmHg, will be 1.35 mEq/L or 1.35 mmol/L (45 × 0.03 = 1.35). The dissolved CO_2 and H_2CO_2 in a solution are in a reversible equilibrium state, with the amount of carbonic acid being proportional to the amount of dissolved CO_2. Because it is almost impossible to measure undissociated H_2CO_2, estimates of dissolved CO_2 using PCO_2 measurements are commonly substituted for H_2CO_2 when calculating pH.

NONVOLATILE ACID PRODUCTION

The catabolism of proteins yields two strong inorganic acids–sulfuric acid and phosphoric acid. Incomplete oxidation of glucose results in the formation of lactic acid and oxidation of fats in ketoacids. In all, the average diet yields about 50 to 100 mmol of nonvolatile acids each day.

The production of these nonvolatile acids is off-set by the production of bicarbonate through the metabolism of certain amino acids such as aspartate and glutamate, as well as the metabolism of certain organic anions (*e.g.*, citrate). Acid production exceeds bicarbonate production, with the net effect being the addition of approximately 1 mmol/kg body weight of nonvolatile acid to the body each day. These acids do not circulate throughout the body but are immediately buffered forming the sodium salt of the acid (*e.g.*, $H_2SO_4 + 2\,NaHCO_3 \rightleftharpoons 2\,NaSO_4 + 2\,CO_2 + 2\,H_2O$). In this situation, bicarbonate is removed from the extracellular fluid, and two sodium salts of the strong anion are added to the extracellular fluid. The kidney must excrete the sodium salts and replenish the bicarbonate.

CALCULATION OF *P*H

The *p*H of the extracellular fluid is determined by the ratio of bicarbonate to carbonic acid and the degree to which carbonic acid dissociates to form a hydrogen ion and a bicarbonate ion. The dissociation constant (*K*) is used to describe the degree to which an acid or base dissociates. The symbol *p*K refers to the negative logarithm of the dissociation constant. The use of a negative logarithm for the dissociation constant allows *p*H to be expressed as a positive value. At normal body temperature, the *p*K for the bicarbonate buffer system is 6.1.

The serum *p*H can be calculated using an equation called the *Henderson-Hasselbalch equation*. This equation uses the logarithms of the dissociation constant and ratio of bicarbonate to dissolved CO_2 to calculate *p*H. In its simplest form, this equation states that

$$pH = pK + \log \frac{HCO_3^-}{CO_2}$$

Importantly, it is the ratio rather than the absolute values for bicarbonate and dissolved CO_2 (carbonic acid) that determines *p*H. Let us consider two examples to emphasize this point. The first situation uses normal serum values, and the second uses increased concentrations of both bicarbonate and dissolved CO_2.

Situation 1

$$pH\ 7.4 = 6.1 + \log \frac{27\ \text{mEq/L}\ HCO_3^-}{1.35\ \text{mEq/L}\ CO_2}$$

$$\text{ratio}\ 27:1.35 = 20:1$$

Situation 2

$$pH\ 7.4 = 6.1 + \log \frac{48\ \text{mEq/L}\ HCO_3^-}{2.40\ \text{mEq/L}\ CO_2}$$

$$\text{ratio}\ 48:2.4 = 20:1$$

These examples demonstrate that *p*H remains relatively stable over a wide range of changes in bicarbonate and dissolved CO_2 concentrations as long as the two concentrations approach a ratio value of 20 to 1. Plasma *p*H decreases when the ratio is less than 20 to 1 (*e.g.*, the log of 10 is 1; when the ratio of bicarbonate to dissolved CO_2 is equal to 10, the *p*H of the blood will be 7.1), and it increases when the ratio is greater than 20 to 1.

REGULATION OF *P*H

The *p*H of body fluids is regulated by (1) intracellular and extracellular buffering systems that prevent large moment-to-moment changes in the extracellular *p*H, (2) respiratory mechanisms that eliminate carbon dioxide, and (3) renal mechanisms that conserve bicarbonate and eliminate hydrogen ions. The *p*H is further influenced by the electrolyte composition of the intracellular and extracellular compartments.

ACID–BASE BUFFER SYSTEMS

The moment-by-moment regulation of *p*H depends on buffer systems. These buffer systems are immediately available to combine with excess acids or alkalis and thus prevent large changes in *p*H from occurring while respiratory and renal mechanisms are being recruited.

A buffer system consists of a weak acid and the alkali salt of that acid, or a weak base and its acid salt. In the process of preventing large changes in *p*H, the system trades a strong acid for a weak acid or a strong base for a weak base. Three major buffer systems protect the *p*H of body fluids: (1) the bicarbonate buffer system, (2) the phosphate buffer system, and (3) protein buffers.

The *bicarbonate buffer system* uses carbonic acid as its weak acid and bicarbonate as its weak base. It substitutes the weak carbonic acid for a strong acid such as hydrochloric acid ($HCl + NaHCO_3 \rightleftharpoons H_2CO_3 + NaCl$) or the weak bicarbonate base for a strong base such as sodium hydroxide ($NaOH + H_2CO_3 \rightleftharpoons NaHCO_3 + H_2O$).

The *phosphate buffer system* consists of two elements, $H_2PO_4^-$ and HPO_4^{--}. When a strong acid such as hydrochloric acid is added to a mixture of these two phosphates, a weak acid is formed and the *p*H changes only slightly ($HCl + Na_2HPO_4 \rightleftharpoons NaH_2PO_4 + NaCl$). Likewise, if a strong base such as sodium hydroxide is added to the solution, a weak base is formed ($NaOH + NaH_2PO_4 \rightleftharpoons Na_2HPO_4 + H_2O$). Because phosphate is eliminated in the urine, this system is particularly important in buffering fluids in the kidney tubules.

Proteins are composed of amino acids, some of which have free acidic radicals that can dissociate into a base plus H^+. The protein buffers are largely located within cells. Both hydrogen and CO_2 can diffuse across cell membranes for buffering by intracellular proteins. The protein buffer system is particularly plentiful and hence it is an important and powerful system.

RESPIRATORY CONTROL MECHANISMS

The respiratory system provides for the elimination of CO_2 into the air and plays a major role in acid–base regulation. Carbon dioxide crosses the blood–brain barrier with ease and, in the process, reacts with water to form carbonic acid, which dissociates into hydrogen and bicarbonate ions; it is the hydrogen ions that stimulate the respiratory center. Thus, increased levels of CO_2 in the blood induce an almost immediate increase in ventilation, causing an increase in the amount of CO_2 exhaled and a rapid correction in CO_2 level.

RENAL CONTROL MECHANISMS

The kidneys regulate acid–base balance by excreting either an acidic or an alkaline urine. Excreting an acidic urine reduces the amount of acid in the extracellular fluid, whereas excreting an alkaline urine removes base from the extracellular fluid. The renal mechanisms for regulating acid–base balance cannot adjust the *p*H within minutes, as respiratory mechanisms can, but they keep on functioning for days until the *p*H has returned to normal or near-normal range.

Hydrogen Ion Elimination and Bicarbonate Conservation. The kidneys contribute to acid–base balance by regulating hydrogen ion secretion so bicarbonate levels remain within the appropriate limits. They do this by eliminating metabolic acids and reabsorbing bicarbonate ions. Bicarbonate reabsorption can be regarded as a recycling process in which the filtered bicarbonate is reabsorbed and returned to the blood. The process of bicarbonate reabsorption begins when CO_2 moves into a tubular cell and combines with water, in a carbonic anhydrase-mediated reaction, to form a bicarbonate ion and hydrogen ion (Fig. 30-2). The hydrogen ion is secreted into the tubular fluid, and a sodium ion is then reabsorbed in a coupled transport process. The reabsorbed sodium ion and the newly generated bicarbonate ion move from the tubular cell into the extracellular fluid. In the tubular fluid, the

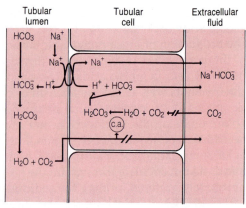

FIG. 30-2. Hydrogen ion (H^+) secretion and bicarbonate ion (HCO_3^-) retrieval in a renal tubular cell. Carbon dioxide (CO_2) diffuses into the tubular cell from the blood or urine filtrate where it combines with water in a carbonic anhydrase... catalyzed reaction that yields carbonic acid (H_2CO_3). The H_2CO_3 dissociates to form H^+ and HCO_3^-. The H^+ is secreted into the tubular fluid in exchange for Na^+. The Na^+ and HCO_3^- enter the extracellular fluid.

secreted hydrogen ion combines with a filtered bicarbonate ion to yield CO_2 and water. The water is eliminated in the urine, and the CO_2 diffuses into the tubular cell and combines with water to form another bicarbonate and hydrogen ion.

Normally, only a few of the hydrogen ions remain in the tubular fluid as it moves from the proximal to the distal and collecting tubules to become urine. This is because the secretion of hydrogen ions into the tubular fluid is usually roughly equivalent to the number of bicarbonate ions that are filtered in the glomerulus. When excess CO_2 is present, as occurs during respiratory acidosis, hydrogen ion secretion exceeds bicarbonate ion filtration and the urine becomes acidic. On the other hand, filtration of bicarbonate in excess of hydrogen ion secretion results in production of an alkaline urine.

Tubular Buffering Systems. The *p*H of the urine can range from 4.5 to 8.0. An extremely acidic urine would be damaging to structures in the urinary tract; this limits the number of unbuffered hydrogen ions that can be excreted by the kidneys. When the number of free hydrogen ions secreted into the renal tubules threatens to cause the *p*H of the urine to become too acidic, the hydrogen ions must be carried in some other form. This is accomplished by the hydrogen ions first combining with intratubular buffers and then being excreted in the urine. There are two important intratubular buffers: (1) the phosphate buffer and (2) the ammonia buffer.

The phosphate buffer uses monohydrogen phosphate (HPO_4^{--}) and dihydrogen phosphate ($H_2PO_4^-$) that are present in the urine. The combination of H^+ with HPO_4^{--} to form $H_2PO_4^-$ allows the kidneys to increase their excretion of hydrogen ions (Fig. 30-3). Because they are poorly absorbed, the phosphates become more concentrated as they move through the tubules. Importantly, this system works best when the renal tubular fluid contains a high concentration of hydrogen ions.

Another but more important, complex buffer system is the ammonia buffer system. Renal tubular cells are able to use amino acids to synthesize ammonia (NH_3) and secrete it into the tubular fluid; hydrogen ions then combine with the NH_3 to form an ammonium ion (NH_4^+). The NH_4^+ ions combine with chloride (Cl^-) ions, which are present in the tubular fluid and are excreted in the urine as ammonium chloride (NH_4Cl; Fig. 30-4). Most of the negative ions in the tubular fluid are chloride ions; only a few hydrogen ions could be transported in direct combination with chloride, because hydrochloric acid would rapidly cause the pH of the urine to fall below the critical value of 4.5, below which hydrogen ion secretion ceases. The ammonia buffer system allows for elimination of both chloride and hydrogen ions without effecting a change in urine pH. The ammonia buffer system requires large amounts of an enzyme that deaminates the amino acids that are used in ammonia synthesis; therefore, it takes 2 or 3 days for the tubular cells to increase enzyme synthesis and for this buffer system to become efficient.

ION EXCHANGE MECHANISMS AND THEIR EFFECT ON PH

Because of their electrolyte properties, the positively charged hydrogen ion and the negatively charged bicarbonate ion can be exchanged for other similarly charged ions, thereby affecting acid–base balance.

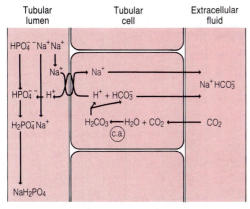

FIG. 30-3. The renal phosphate buffer system. The monohydrogen phosphate ion (HPO_4^{--}) enters the renal tubular fluid in the glomerulus. A H^+ combines with the HPO_4^{--} to form $H_2PO_4^-$ and is then excreted into the urine in combination with Na^+. The HCO_3^- moves into the extracellular fluid along with the Na^+ that was exchanged during secretion of the H^+.

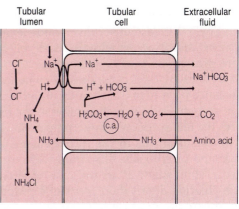

FIG. 30-4. The ammonia buffer system in a renal tubular cell. The tubular cell synthesizes ammonia (NH_3) from amino acids. The NH_3 is secreted into the tubular fluid, where it combines with a H^+ to form an ammonium ion (NH_4^+). The ammonium ion combines with chloride for excretion in the urine. The HCO_3^- moves into the extracellular fluid along with the NA^+ that was exchanged during secretion of the H^+.

Potassium–Hydrogen Exchange. The potassium ion interacts in important ways with the hydrogen ion. Both ions are positively charged, and both ions move freely between the intracellular and extracellular compartments; when excess hydrogen ions are present in the extracellular fluid, they move into the intracellular compartment for buffering. When this happens, another cation—in this case potassium—must leave the cell and move into the extracellular fluid. When extracellular potassium levels fall, potassium moves out of the cell and is replaced by hydrogen ions.

The reciprocity between hydrogen and potassium ion exchange extends to the kidneys. When plasma potassium levels decrease, fewer potassium ions are available for secretion in the urine by the renal tubular cells and, consequently, hydrogen ion secretion is increased. As hydrogen ion secretion continues, metabolic alkalosis develops. An elevation in plasma potassium has the opposite effect. Likewise, acidosis (elevated hydrogen ion concentration) causes a decrease in potassium secretion, and alkalosis causes an increase in potassium secretion.

Chloride–Bicarbonate Exchange. One of the mechanisms that the kidneys use in regulating the pH of the extracellular fluids is to conserve or eliminate bicarbonate ions; in the process, it is often necessary to shuffle anions. Chloride is the most abundant anion in the extracellular fluid and can substitute for bicarbonate when an anion shift is needed. As an example, serum bicarbonate levels normally increase as hydrochloric acid is secreted into the stomach after a heavy meal, causing what is termed the *postprandial alkaline tide*. Later, as the chloride is reabsorbed in the small intestine, the pH returns to normal. *Hypo-*

chloremic alkalosis refers to an increase in *p*H that is induced by a decrease in serum chloride levels. *Hyperchloremic acidosis* occurs when excess levels of chloride are present.

Body sodium levels can indirectly influence acid–base balance by way of the chloride–bicarbonate exchange system. Sodium reabsorption in the kidneys requires the reabsorption of an accompanying anion. The two major anions in the extracellular fluid are chloride and bicarbonate. If sodium reabsorption is markedly stimulated, as in the case of prolonged sodium chloride deprivation or volume contraction, an accompanying increase in bicarbonate reabsorption can result in alkalosis.

LABORATORY TESTS

The terms *acidemia* and *alkalemia* refer only to the *p*H of the blood as measured by a *p*H meter or electrode and give little information about the cause of the acid–base disorder. It was pointed out earlier that *p*H can be relatively normal within a wide range of dissolved CO_2 and base bicarbonate levels. Laboratory tests that are used in assessing acid–base balance include carbon dioxide and bicarbonate levels, base excess or deficit, and the anion gap.

Carbon Dioxide and Bicarbonate Levels. The dissolved CO_2 levels can be determined from blood gas measurements using the P_{CO_2} and the solubility coefficient for CO_2 (normal arterial P_{CO_2} is 38 to 42 mmHg). A measure of the total CO_2 content of blood, including that contained in bicarbonate, can be obtained by adding a strong acid to a plasma sample and measuring the amount of CO_2 generated.

More than 70% of the CO_2 in the blood is in the form of bicarbonate. The serum bicarbonate concentration can be determined from the total CO_2 content of the blood. The normal range of values for venous bicarbonate is 24 mEq/L to 33 mEq/L (24 mmol/L to 33 mmol/L).

Base Excess or Deficit. Base excess or deficit measures the level of all the buffer systems of the blood—hemoglobin, protein, phosphate, and bicarbonate. The base excess or deficit describes the amount of a fixed acid or base that must be added to a blood sample to achieve a *p*H of 7.4 (normal ±3.0 mEq/L).[1] For practical purposes, base excess/deficit is a measurement of bicarbonate excess or deficit. A base excess indicates metabolic alkalosis, and a base deficit indicates metabolic acidosis.

Anion Gap. The anion gap describes the difference between the plasma concentration of the major measured cation (sodium) and the sum of the mea-sured anions (Cl^- and HCO_3^-). This difference represents the concentration of unmeasured anions, such as phosphates, sulfates, organic acids, and proteins, that is present (Fig. 30-5). Normally, the anion gap ranges between 8 and 12 mEq/L (a value of 16 mEq is normal if both sodium and potassium concentrations are used in the calculation). The anion gap is increased in conditions such as lactic acidosis and ketoacidosis that result from elevated levels of metabolic acids. A low anion gap is found in conditions that produce a fall in unmeasured anions (primarily albumin) or rise in unmeasured cations. The latter can occur in hyperkalemia, hypercalcemia, hypermagnesemia, lithium intoxication, or multiple myeloma (see Chapter 16) in which a cationic IgG paraprotein is produced.

The anion gap of urine can also be measured. It uses values for the measurable cations (Na^+ and K^+) and measurable anion (Cl^-) to provide an estimate of ammonium (NH_4^+) excretion. Because ammonium is a cation, the value of the anion gap becomes more negative as the ammonium level increases. In normal people secreting 20 to 40 mmol of ammonium/L, the urine anion gap is close to zero. In metabolic acidosis, amount of unmeasurable NH_4^+ should increase if renal excretion of H^+ is intact; as a result, the urine anion gap should become more negative.

In summary, normal body function depends on the precise regulation of acid–base balance. The *p*H of the extracellular fluid is normally maintained within the narrow physiologic range of 7.35 to 7.45. Metabolic processes produce both volatile and nonvolatile metabolic acids that must be buffered and eliminated from the body. The volatile acid, H_2CO_3, is in equilibrium with dissolved CO_2, which is eliminated from the lungs. The nonvolatile metabolic acids, most of which are excreted by

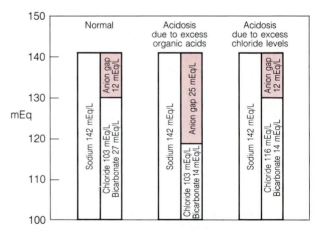

FIG. 30-5. The anion gap in acidosis due to excess metabolic acids and excess serum chloride levels. Unmeasured anions such as phosphates, sulfates, and organic acids increase the anion gap because they replace bicarbonate (this assumes there is no change in sodium content).

the kidneys, are derived mainly from protein and fat metabolism. It is the ratio of the bicarbonate ion concentration to dissolved CO_2 (carbonic acid concentration) that determines body pH. When this ratio is 20:1, the pH is 7.4. The ability of the body to maintain pH within the normal physiologic range depends on respiratory and renal mechanisms as well as blood buffer systems; the most important of these is the bicarbonate buffer system. Potassium and hydrogen ions are interchangeable cations; excess potassium can affect acid–base balance, and alterations in acid–base balance can affect potassium levels. Likewise, the bicarbonate and chloride anions can produce changes in acid–base balance as they are interchanged.

CHART 30-1: PRIMARY DEFECTS IN ACID-BASE BALANCE	
$\downarrow HCO_3^-$	Metabolic acidosis represents a decrease in bicarbonate (HCO_3^- deficit)
$\uparrow H_2CO_3$	Respiratory acidosis represents an increase in carbonic acid (H_2CO_3 excess)
$\uparrow HCO_3^-$	Metabolic alkalosis represents an increase in bicarbonate (HCO_3^- excess)
$\downarrow H_2CO_3$	Respiratory alkalosis represents a decrease in carbonic acid (H_2CO_3 deficit)

■ ALTERATIONS IN ACID–BASE BALANCE

The terms *acidosis* and *alkalosis* describe the clinical conditions that arise as a result of changes in dissolved CO_2 and bicarbonate concentration. An *alkali* represents a combination of one or more alkali metals such as sodium or potassium with a highly basic ion such as a hydroxyl ion (OH^-). Sodium bicarbonate is the main alkali in the extracellular fluid. Although the definitions differ somewhat, the terms *alkali* and *base* are often used interchangeably. Hence the term *alkalosis* has come to mean the opposite of acidosis.

Metabolic Versus Respiratory Acid–Base Disorders. Metabolic acid–base disorders are those in which the primary disturbance is in the concentration of bicarbonate. Because the bicarbonate occurs in the numerator of the Henderson-Hasselbalch equation, increased bicarbonate levels produce an increase in pH and metabolic alkalosis and decreased bicarbonate levels produce a decrease in pH and metabolic acidosis (Chart 30-1). Respiratory acid–base disorders are those that arise primarily from changes in the concentration of carbon dioxide; because carbon dioxide appears in the denominator of the Henderson-Hasselbalch equation, an increase in carbon dioxide concentration causes a decrease in pH and respiratory acidosis, and a decrease in carbon dioxide concentration causes an increase in pH and respiratory alkalosis. Because compensatory measures can minimize or prevent a change in hydrogen ion concentration, the terms *acidemia* and *alkalemia* may be used to indicate those situations in which in which plasma pH is measured.

Primary Versus Compensatory Mechanisms. Acidosis and alkalosis typically involve both a *primary* or initiating event and a *compensatory* state that results from homeostatic mechanisms that attempt to correct or prevent large changes in pH. For example, a person may have a primary metabolic acidosis as a result of overproduction of ketoacids and a compen-

satory respiratory alkalosis because of a compensatory increase in ventilation. Compensatory mechanisms adjust the pH toward a more normal level without actually correcting the underlying cause of the disorder. The respiratory mechanisms, which compensate by either increasing or decreasing ventilation, are rapid but seldom able to return the pH to normal. This is because, as the pH returns toward normal, the respiratory stimulus is lost. The kidneys compensate by conserving bicarbonate and secreting hydrogen ions. It normally takes longer to recruit renal compensatory mechanisms than it does to recruit respiratory compensatory mechanisms. Renal mechanisms are more efficient, however, because they continue to operate until the pH has returned to normal or a near-normal value.

Compensatory mechanisms provide a means to control pH in situations where correction is impossible or cannot be immediately achieved. Often, compensatory mechanisms are interim measures that permit survival while the body attempts to correct the primary disorder. It is important to recognize that compensation requires the use of mechanisms that are different from those that caused the primary disorder. In other words, the lungs cannot compensate for respiratory acidosis that is caused by lung disease, nor can the kidneys compensate for metabolic acidosis that occurs because of renal failure. The body can, however, use renal mechanisms to compensate for respiratory-induced changes in pH, and it can use respiratory mechanisms to compensate for metabolically induced changes in acid–base balance.

Compensatory mechanisms often become more effective with time; thus, there are differences between the level of pH change that occurs with acute and chronic acid–base disorders. Fig. 30-6 is a pH–bicarbonate diagram that can be used to determine the acute or chronic nature of an acid–base disorder and the compensation that has occurred. From the diagram, it can be seen that a given increase in PCO_2 is associated with a lesser fall in pH in chronic compensated respiratory acidosis than in acute uncompensated respiratory acidosis.

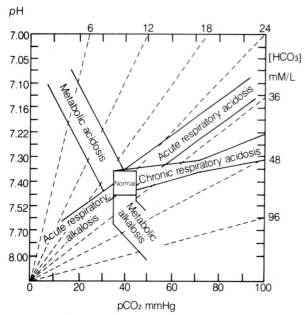

FIG. 30-6. Acute and chronic acid–base disorders as determined by Pco₂, bicarbonate, and pH values. (Adapted from Masoro, E. J., & Siegel, P. D. [1977]. *Acid–base regulation: Its physiology, pathophysiology and interpretation of blood gas analysis.* Philadelphia: W.B. Saunders)

Manifestations of Acid–Base Disorders. Most of the manifestations of acid–base disorders fall into three categories: (1) those associated with the primary disorder that caused the *p*H disturbance, (2) those related to the altered *p*H, and (3) those that occur because of the body's attempt to compensate for the altered *p*H.

Many of the alterations in body function associated with acid–base disturbances are related to the *p*H change and its effect on membrane potentials of nerve cell membranes and those of other excitable tissue. The hydrogen ion tends to stabilize membranes of excitable tissues, rendering them less excitable. When the *p*H falls below 7.0, for example, the nervous system becomes depressed to the extent that confusion and coma develop. Alterations in *p*H also affect calcium ionization and thus affect neural excitability, which also contributes to the neurologic manifestations that occur with acid–base disorders (see Chapter 29).

METABOLIC ACIDOSIS

Metabolic acidosis refers to a primary deficit in base bicarbonate. It can be caused by one of three mechanisms: (1) increased production of nonvolatile acids, (2) decreased acid secretion by the kidney, or (3) excessive loss of bicarbonate[2] (Table 30-1).

INCREASED METABOLIC ACID GAIN

Metabolic acids increase when there is: (1) accumulation of lactic acid, (2) overproduction of ketoacids, (3) drug and chemical anion ingestion, or (4) inability of the kidneys to excrete metabolic acids or conserve bicarbonate. The presence of excess metabolic acids leads to a replacement of sodium bicarbonate by the sodium salt of the offending acid (*e.g.*, sodium lactate); this produces an increase in the anion gap.

Lactic Acidosis. Acute acidosis is one of the most common types of metabolic acidosis. Metabolic production and consumption of lactate are normally balanced. Under normal conditions, the liver and kidney consume lactate produced by tissues such as red blood cells, intestine, and skeletal muscle. However, if oxygen delivery is inadequate, any tissue can produce lactate. Most cases of lactic acidosis are due to poor tissue perfusion as in shock or cardiac arrest. These conditions not only increase lactic acid production, but, more importantly, hepatic metabolism and clearance of lactic acid are also reduced due to poor liver perfusion. Mortality is high with lactic acidosis due to shock and tissue hypoxia. During vigorous exercise or grand mal seizures (convulsions), local disproportion between oxygen supply and demand in contracting muscles may lead to transient lactic acidosis.

Lactic acidosis is also associated with disorders in which tissue hypoxia does not appear to be present. It has been reported in people with leukemia, lymphomas, and other cancers; with poorly controlled diabetes mellitus; and with severe liver failure. Mechanisms causing lactic acidosis in these conditions are poorly understood. Some conditions such as neoplasms may produce local increases in tissue metabolism and lactate production, others may impair blood flow, and still others may interfere with lactate metabolism. Ethanol produces a slight elevation in lactic acid, but clinically significant lactic acidosis does not occur in alcohol intoxication unless other problems such as liver failure are present. Lactic acidosis may also complicate the severe acidosis that occurs in salicylate poisoning.

Ketoacidosis. Ketoacids are produced in the liver from fatty acids; they are the source of fuel for many body tissues, and it is only when production exceeds utilization that acidosis develops. An overproduction of ketoacids occurs when carbohydrate stores are inadequate or when the body cannot use available carbohydrates as a fuel. Under these conditions, fatty acids are converted to ketones by the liver. When the ketone production by the liver exceeds the body tissue utilization, ketoacidosis develops.

TABLE 30-1. METABOLIC ACIDOSIS	
CAUSES	**MANIFESTATIONS**

Excess Metabolic Acids (Increased Anion Gap)
    Excessive production of metabolic acids
        Lactic acidosis
        Diabetic ketoacidosis
        Fasting and starvation
        Alcoholic ketoacidosis
        Poisoning (salicylate, methanol, ethylene glycol)
    Decreased loss of metabolic acids
        Kidney failure or dysfunction
Excessive Bicarbonate Loss (Normal Anion Gap)
    Loss of intestinal secretions
        Diarrhea
        Intestinal suction
        Intestinal or biliary fistula
    Increased renal losses
        Renal tubular acidosis
        Treatment with carbonic anhydrase inhibitors
        Hyoaldosteronism
Increased Chloride Levels (Normal Anion Gap)
    Abnormal chloride reabsorption by the kidney
    Sodium chloride infusions
    Treatment with ammonium chloride
    Parenteral hyperalimentation
	Blood pH, HCO_3^-, Pco_2
	    pH ↓
	    HCO_3^- ↓ (primary)
	    Pco_2 ↓ (compensation)
	Altered Gastrointestinal Function
	    Anorexia
	    Nausea and Vomiting
	    Abdominal pain
	Depression Neural Function
	    Weakness
	    Lethargy
	    General malaise
	    Confusion
	    Stupor
	    Coma
	    Depression of vital functions
	Cardiovascular Manifestations
	    Cardiac dysrhythmias
	    Heart unresponsive to catecholamines
	    Decreased cardiac output
	Skin
	    Warm and flushed
	Signs of Compensation
	    Kussmaul's breathing
	    Acid urine
	    Increased ammonia in urine

The most common cause of ketoacidosis is uncontrolled diabetes mellitus, in which an insulin deficiency leads to the release of fatty acids from adipose cells with subsequent production of excess ketoacids (see Chapter 46). During periods of fasting or food deprivation, the lack of carbohydrates produces a self-limited state of ketoacidosis. This is because the fall in blood sugar that accompanies fasting promotes the release of insulin, which, in turn, acts to suppress the release of fatty acids from fat cells. A ketogenic diet is one that is low in carbohydrate and favors ketoacid production. Over the years, various ketogenic diets have been used for weight reduction; part of the success of these diets derives from symptoms such as anorexia that occur with metabolic acidosis.

Ketones are formed during the oxidation of alcohol, a process that occurs in the liver. A condition called *alcoholic ketoacidosis* can develop in people who engage in excess alcohol consumption. It usually follows prolonged alcohol ingestion, particularly if accompanied by decreased food intake and vomiting.[3, 4]

The ketoacids responsible for alcoholic ketoacidosis are, in part, formed as a result of alcohol metabolism. Failure to eat and extracellular fluid volume depletion caused by vomiting, decreased fluid intake, and the inhibition of antidiuretic hormone by alcohol (see Chapter 29) often contribute to alcoholic ketoacidosis. Ketone formation may be further enhanced by the hypoglycemia that results from alcohol induced inhibition of glucose synthesis (gluconeogenesis) by the liver and impaired ketone elimination by the kidneys due to dehydration. Numerous other factors, such as elevations in cortisol, growth hormone, glucagon, and catecholamines, mediate free fatty acid release and thereby contribute to the development of alcoholic ketoacidosis.

Drug or Chemical Anion Ingestion. Several drugs or chemicals can produce metabolic acidosis. These include methanol, ethylene glycol, and salicylates (when ingested as an overdose). Methanol (wood alcohol) is a component of shellac, varnish, deicing solutions, sterno, and other commercial products. It is metabolized to formic acid.[1] Early complaints include weakness, nausea, headache, and decreased vision, which can progress to blindness, coma, and death. Ethylene glycol is a component of antifreeze and solvents that is metabolized to a number of toxic metabolites including glycolic acid and oxalic acid.[1] Both methanol and ethylene glycol are metabolized by way of the enzyme alcohol dehydrogenase into toxic metabolites. This is the same enzyme that is used in the metabolism of ethanol. Because the enzyme has more than a 10 times greater affinity for ethanol, intravenous or oral ethanol is used as an antidote for methanol and ethylene glycol poisoning.[1]

Salicylate overdose produces serious toxic effects, including death. A fatal overdose can occur with as little as 10 to 30 g in adults and 3 g in children.[1] The diagnosis can only be made with certainty by measurement of serum salicylate concentration.

Aspirin (acetylsalicylic acid) is converted to salicylic acid in the body. Increasing doses of aspirin cause a progressively greater risk of toxicity because of the saturation of protective mechanisms. At therapeutic levels, much of salicylate is protein bound so that it remains in the vascular compartment; the drug is partially changed in the liver to salicyluric acid, which is both less toxic and more rapidly excreted by the kidney than salicylate. With salicylate toxicity, these mechanisms become saturated and renal elimination is decreased and more salicylate is able to reach the tissues.

A variety of acid–base disturbances can occur with salicylate toxicity. The salicylates cross the blood–brain barrier and directly stimulate the respiratory center, causing hyperventilation and respiratory alkalosis. The kidneys compensate by excreting increased amounts of bicarbonate, potassium, and sodium. This contributes to the development of metabolic acidosis. Salicylates also interfere with carbohydrate metabolism, which results in increased production of metabolic acids.

One of the treatments for salicylate toxicity is alkalinization of the plasma. Salicylic acid, which is a weak acid, exists in equilibrium with the alkaline salicylate anion. It is the salicylic acid that is toxic because of its ability to cross cell membranes and enter brain cells. The salicylate anion crosses membranes poorly and is less toxic. With alkalinization of the extracellular fluids, the ratio of salicylic acid to salicylate is greatly reduced. This allows cellular salicylic acid to move out of cells into the extracellular fluid along a concentration gradient. The renal elimination of salicylates follows a similar pattern when the urine is alkalinized. Hemodialysis (use of the artificial kidney) may be used to increase the removal of salicylates from the body when salicylate toxicity is life-threatening.

Decreased Renal Function. Renal disease is the most common cause of chronic metabolic acidosis. The *kidneys* conserve bicarbonate and secrete hydrogen ions into the urine for elimination from the body. In renal failure there is loss of both glomerular and tubular function with retention of nitrogenous wastes and metabolic acids. In a condition called *renal tubular acidosis*, there is normal glomerular function, but the tubular secretion of hydrogen ions or reabsorption of bicarbonate is abnormal. Renal tubular acidosis is discussed in Chapter 32.

INCREASED BICARBONATE LOSSES

Increased bicarbonate losses occur with loss of bicarbonate-rich body fluids or when there is an excess of chloride ions.

Intestinal secretions have a high bicarbonate concentration. Consequently, excessive losses of bicarbonate occur with severe diarrhea; small bowel, pancreatic, or biliary fistula drainage; iliostomy drainage; and intestinal suction. In diarrhea of microbial origin, bicarbonate is secreted into the bowel to neutralize the metabolic acids produced by the microorganisms causing the diarrhea. Creation of an ileal bladder, which is done for conditions such as neurogenic bladder and in surgical removal of the bladder due to cancer, involves the implantation of the ureters into a short loop of ileum. With this procedure, contact time between the urine and intestine is normally too short for significant anion exchange.[1]

Hyperchloremic acidosis occurs when there is a increase in extracellular chloride concentration; because both chloride and bicarbonate are anions, bicarbonate ion concentration decreases when there is an increase in chloride ions. Hyperchloremic acidosis can occur as the result of abnormal absorption of chloride by the kidneys or as a result of treatment with chloride-containing medications (sodium chloride, amino acid–chloride hyperalimentation solutions, and ammonium chloride). Ammonium chloride is broken down into an ammonium (NH_4^+) and a chloride ion. The ammonium ion is converted to urea in the liver, leaving the chloride ion free to react with hydrogen to form hydrochloric acid. The administration of intravenous sodium chloride or parenteral hyperalimentation solutions that contain an amino acid–chloride combination can cause acidosis in a similar manner.

With hyperchloremic acidosis, the anion gap is within the normal range; however, the chloride levels are increased and bicarbonate levels are decreased.

MANIFESTATIONS

Metabolic acidosis is characterized by an increase in extracellular H^+ ion concentration and a decrease in bicarbonate levels: the pH falls below 7.35 and the serum bicarbonate decreases to less than 24 mEq/L. Extracellular bicarbonate is reduced by reaction with hydrogen ions or by loss of bicarbonate in urine or stool. Hydrogen ions move into the cell for buffering, replacing potassium that moves out of the cell, tending to elevate plasma levels of potassium.

The anion gap is often useful in determining the cause of the metabolic acidosis (Chart 30-2). It is increased in situations where acidosis is due to increased production of nonvolatile acids, but remains within normal limits when it is caused by an increase in chloride levels (hyperchloremic acidosis).

The manifestations of metabolic acidosis fall into three categories: (1) signs and symptoms of the disorder causing the acidosis, (2) alterations in function resulting from the decreased pH, and (3) changes in body function related to recruitment of compensatory mechanisms. The signs and symptoms of metabolic acidosis usually begin to appear when the plasma bicarbonate concentration falls to 20 mEq/L or less.

CHART 30-2: THE ANION GAP IN DIFFERENTIAL DIAGNOSIS OF METABOLIC ACIDOSIS

Decreased Anion Gap (<8 mEq/L)

Hypoalbuminemia (decrease in unmeasured anions)
Multiple myeloma (increase in unmeasured cationic IgG paraproteins)
Increased unmeasured cations (hyperkalemia, hypercalcemia, hypermagnesemia, lithium intoxication)

Increased Anion Gap (>12 mEq/L)

Presence of unmeasured metabolic anion
    Diabetic ketoacidosis
Alcoholic ketoacidosis
    Lactic acidosis
    Starvation
    Renal insufficiency
Presence of drug or chemical anion
    Salicylate poisoning
    Methanol poisoning
    Ethylene glycol poisoning

Normal Anion Gap (8–12 mEq/L)

Loss of bicarbonate
    Diarrhea
    Pancreatic fluid loss
    Ileostomy (unadapted)
Chloride retention
    Renal tubular acidosis
    Ileal loop bladder
    Parenteral nutrition (arginine and lysine)

Metabolic acidosis is seldom a primary disorder. Rather, it usually develops during the course of another disease. Hence, the manifestations of metabolic acidosis are frequently superimposed on the symptoms of the contributing health problem. With diabetic ketoacidosis, which is a common cause of metabolic acidosis, there is an increase in blood and urine glucose and a characteristic smell of ketones to the breath. In metabolic acidosis that accompanies renal failure, blood urea nitrogen levels are elevated and tests of renal function yield abnormal results.

Changes in pH have a direct effect on body function that can produce signs and symptoms that are common to all types of metabolic acidosis, regardless of cause. A person with metabolic acidosis often complains of weakness, fatigue, general malaise, and a dull headache. There may also be anorexia, nausea, vomiting, and abdominal pain. As mentioned earlier, the anorexia associated with mild metabolic acidosis may be viewed as an advantage to someone on a weight loss ketogenic diet. On the other hand, the gastrointestinal symptoms may be misleading in a person with undiagnosed diabetes mellitus. In this case, the person may be thought to have gastrointestinal flu or other abdominal pathology, such as appendicitis.

Neural activity becomes depressed as body pH declines. The hydrogen ion crosses the blood–brain barrier with ease; as acidosis progresses, the level of consciousness declines and stupor and coma develop. The skin is often warm and flushed because skin vessels become less responsive to the vasoconstrictor input from the sympathetic nervous system. Tissue turgor is impaired and the skin is dry when fluid deficit accompanies acidosis. When the pH falls to 7.0, cardiac dysrhythmias, including fatal ventricular dysrhythmias, can develop and the heart becomes unresponsive to the catecholamines (norepinephrine and epinephrine). At this point, both heart rate and cardiac output decrease. A decrease in ventricular function may be particularly important in perpetuating of shock-induced lactic acidosis, and partial correction of the acidemia may be necessary before tissue perfusion can be restored.[1]

Metabolic acidosis is also accompanied by signs and symptoms related to the recruitment of compensatory mechanisms. In situations of acute metabolic acidosis, the respiratory system compensates for a decrease in pH by increasing ventilation in order to reduce Pco_2; this is accomplished through deep and rapid respirations. In diabetic ketoacidosis, this breathing pattern is referred to as *Kussmaul's breathing*. For descriptive purposes, it can be said that Kussmaul's breathing resembles the hyperpnea of exercise—the person breathes as though he or she had been running. There may be complaints of difficult breathing or dyspnea with exertion; with severe acidosis, dyspnea may be present even at rest. Respiratory compensation for acute acidosis tends to be somewhat greater than for chronic metabolic alkalosis.

When kidney function is normal, net acid excretion increases promptly in response to acidosis and the urine becomes more acid. Net acid excretion may increase 5 to 10 times above normal. Most of the initial acid secretion is accomplished through use of the phosphate buffer system. Over several days, ammonia production by the kidney increases and becomes the most important mechanism for excreting excess H^+ ions.

Chronic acidemia, as in renal failure, can lead to a variety of skeletal problems that are probably due in part to release of calcium and phosphate during bone buffering of excess hydrogen ions. Of particular importance is impaired growth in children. In infants and children, acidemia may be associated with a variety of nonspecific symptoms such as anorexia, weight loss, muscle weakness, and listlessness.[1] Muscle weakness and listlessness may result from alterations in muscle metabolism.

TREATMENT

The treatment of metabolic acidosis focuses on correcting the condition that caused the disorder and restoring the fluids and electrolytes that have been lost from the body. The treatment of diabetic ketoacidosis is discussed in Chapter 46.

The use of supplemental sodium bicarbonate may be indicated in the treatment of some forms of normal anion gap acidosis. However, its use in treatment of increased anion gap types of metabolic acidosis is controversial, particularly in lactic acidosis. In most people with cardiac arrest, shock or sepsis, impaired oxygen delivery is the primary cause of lactic acidosis. In these situations, the administration of large amounts of sodium bicarbonate does not improve oxygen delivery and may produce hypernatremia, hyperosmolality, and decreased oxygen release by hemoglobin due to a shift in the oxygen dissociation curve.[5]

METABOLIC ALKALOSIS

Metabolic alkalosis refers to a primary increase in serum base bicarbonate. Metabolic alkalosis occurs in conditions that produce: (1) a loss of hydrogen ions, (2) increased retention of bicarbonate by the kidneys, or (3) contraction of the extracellular fluid compartment (Table 30-2). Metabolic alkalosis can also be produced by ingestion or administration of excess bicarbonate or other alkali (carbonate, citrate, acetate).

LOSS OF HYDROGEN IONS

Vomiting, removal of gastric secretion through use of nasogastric suction, and low potassium levels due to diuretic therapy are the most common causes of metabolic alkalosis in hospitalized patients.[3] Gastric secretions contain high concentrations of hy-

---

TABLE 30-2. METABOLIC ALKALOSIS

CAUSES	MANIFESTATIONS
Increased Loss Hydrogen Ions	**Blood pH, HCO_3^-, and Pco_2**
Vomiting	pH ↑
Gastric suction	HCO_3^- ↑ (primary)
Bulimia	Pco_2 ↑ (compensation)
Potassium deficit	**Increased Neural Excitability**
Diuretic therapy	(develops late because HCO_3 crosses
Hyperaldosteronism	blood–brain barrier slowly)
Increased Retention Bicarbonate	Confusion
Loss of chloride with bicarbonate retention	Hyperactive reflexes
	Muscle hypertonicity
Bicarbonate ingestion or administration	Tetany
Milk-alkali syndrome	Convulsions
Volume Contraction	**Signs of Compensation**
Loss body fluids	Decreased rate and depth respirations
Diuretic therapy	Increased urine pH

drochloric acid and lesser concentrations of potassium chloride. Under normal conditions, each mEq of H^+ that is secreted into the stomach generates 1 mEq of serum HCO_3.[6] Normally the increase in serum bicarbonate is only transient since the entry of acid into the duodenum stimulates an equal amount of pancreatic bicarbonate secretion. Vomiting and gastric suction remove both hydrogen and chloride ions, thereby disrupting balance between acid secretion and bicarbonate generation. Bulimia, or self-induced vomiting, is often associated with metabolic alkalosis.[5] Metabolic alkalosis is also associated with low potassium levels, such as that caused by certain diuretics (*e.g.*, thiazides and furosemide) and excessive adrenocorticosteroid hormones (as in hyperaldosteronism or Cushing's syndrome). In situations of low potassium levels, renal excretion of H^+ ions is increased as the kidneys focus on conserving potassium. The hormone aldosterone increases sodium reabsorption and increases potassium loss (see Chapter 29). Thus, primary hyperaldosteronism can promote H^+ secretion and development of metabolic alkalosis.

INCREASED BICARBONATE RETENTION

Most of the body's serum bicarbonate is obtained either from CO_2 that is produced during metabolic processes or from recycling of bicarbonate by the kidneys. Usually bicarbonate production and renal reabsorption are balanced in a manner that prevents alkalosis from occurring. It is only when new bicarbonate is added to the body or excessive amounts of bicarbonate are retained that metabolic alkalosis develops. Excessive alkali ingestion, as in use of bicarbonate-containing antacids (*e.g.*, Alka-Seltzer), or sodium bicarbonate administration during cardiopulmonary resuscitation can cause metabolic alkalosis.

Hydrogen and chloride losses are associated with increased bicarbonate retention by the kidneys. Chloride is the major anion in the extracellular fluid, and, when it is lost from the body, bicarbonate is conserved as a replacement anion.

Renal H^+ secretion and HCO_3 reabsorption are increased by hypercalcemia. A condition called the *milk alkali syndrome* may develop in people who consume excessive amounts of milk along with alkaline antacids.

Chronic respiratory acidosis produces a compensatory loss of hydrogen and chloride ions in the urine along with bicarbonate retention. When respiratory acidosis is corrected abruptly as with mechanical ventilation, metabolic alkalosis may develop due to a rapid drop in P_{CO_2}, whereas plasma HCO_3 remains elevated.

VOLUME CONTRACTION

Sudden decreases in extracellular fluid volume, known as *volume contraction*, produce a decrease in glomerular filtration rate and a resultant increase in renal reabsorption of sodium and bicarbonate. In vomiting or gastric suction, the loss of hydrochloric acid initiates metabolic alkalosis, but volume contraction from loss of chloride sustains the alkalosis. Volume contraction can also occur in the course of diuretic therapy. Diuretics that block chloride reabsorption in the kidney (*e.g.*, chlorothiazide and furosemide) produce a bicarbonate retention through both volume contraction and loss of the chloride ion.

MANIFESTATIONS

In metabolic alkalosis, blood pH is above 7.45, plasma bicarbonate is above 29 mEq/L (29 mmol/L), and base excess is above +3.0 mEq/L (3 mmol/L).

People with metabolic alkalosis are often asymptomatic or have signs related to volume depletion or hypokalemia. The neurologic signs (hyperexcitability) occur less frequently with metabolic alkalosis than with other acid–base disorders. This is because the bicarbonate ion crosses the blood–brain barrier more slowly than hydrogen or CO_2; therefore, it produces a lesser change in cerebral spinal fluid pH. When neurologic manifestations do occur, as in acute and severe metabolic alkalosis, they include mental confusion, hyperactive reflexes, tetany, and carpopedal spasm. Metabolic alkalosis also leads to a compensatory hypoventilation with development of varying degrees of hypoxemia and respiratory acidosis. Significant morbidity occurs with severe metabolic alkalosis (pH above 7.55), including respiratory failure, dysrhythmias, seizures, and coma.[3]

TREATMENT

The treatment of metabolic alkalosis is usually directed toward correcting the cause of the condition. A chloride deficit requires correction. Potassium chloride is usually the treatment of choice for metabolic alkalosis when there is an accompanying potassium deficit. When potassium chloride is used as a therapy, the chloride anion replaces the bicarbonate anion, and the administration of potassium not only allows for correction of the potassium deficit but also allows the kidneys to conserve hydrogen ions while eliminating the potassium ions. Fluid replacement with normal saline or one half normal saline is often used in the treatment of people with volume contraction alkalosis.

RESPIRATORY ACIDOSIS

Respiratory acidosis refers to a primary increase in carbon dioxide. Respiratory acidosis occurs in conditions that decrease ventilation and cause an accumulation of dissolved CO_2 (Table 30-3). It can occur as an acute or chronic disorder. Because renal compensatory mechanisms take time to exert their effects, blood pH can drop sharply in people with acute respiratory acidosis.

Acute respiratory acidosis can be caused by impaired function of the respiratory center in the medulla (as in narcotic overdose), chest injury, weakness of the respiratory muscles, or airway obstruction. Acute respiratory acidosis can also result from breathing air with a high CO_2 content. Almost all people with acute respiratory acidosis will be hypoxemic if they are breathing room air. In many cases, signs of hypoxemia develop before those of respiratory acidosis. This is because CO_2 diffuses across the alveolar capillary membrane 20 times more rapidly than oxygen. In many lung disorders, there are some areas of the lung that have more severely compromised gas-exchange function than others. In these circumstances, either the respiratory acidosis or hypoxemia stimulates ventilation so that elimination of CO_2 from the relatively normal areas of the lung is increased, whereas oxygen uptake from the same area is limited by a hemoglobin saturation that approaches 100%.

Chronic respiratory acidosis is a relatively common disturbance in people with chronic obstructive lung disease (see Chapter 27). In these people, the persistent elevation of PCO_2 stimulates renal H^+ ion secretion and HCO_3 reabsorption. The effectiveness of these compensatory mechanisms can often return the pH to near-normal values as long as oxygen levels are maintained within a range that does not unduly stimulate or suppress respirations.

An acute episode of respiratory acidosis can develop in people with chronic lung disease who have chronically elevated PCO_2 levels. This is sometimes called *CO_2 narcosis*. In these people, the medullary respiratory center has become adapted to the elevated levels of CO_2 and no longer responds to increases in PCO_2. Instead, the oxygen content of their blood becomes the major stimulus for respiration. If oxygen is administered at a flow rate that is sufficient to suppress this stimulus, the rate and depth of respiration decrease and the CO_2 content of the blood increases.

TABLE 30-3. RESPIRATORY ACIDOSIS

CAUSES	MANIFESTATIONS
Impaired Ventilation	**Blood pH, PCO_2, HCO_3^-**
Depression of the central nervous system	pH ↓
Drug overdose	PCO_2 ↑ (primary)
Head injury	HCO_3^- ↑ (compensatory)
Diseases of the airways or lungs	**Cerebral Vasodilatation and**
Bronchial asthma	**Depression Neural Function**
Emphysema	Headache
Chronic bronchitis	Weakness
Respiratory distress in the newborn	Behavioral changes
Pneumonia	Confusion and disorientation
Pulmonary edema	Depression
Disorders of Chest Wall and	Paranoia
Respiratory Muscles	Hallucinations
Paralysis of respiratory muscles	Tremors
Chest injuries	Paralysis
Kyphoscoliosis	Stupor and coma
Extreme obesity	**Skin**
Treatment with curare-type drugs	Warm and flushed
Upper airways obstruction	**Signs of Compensation**
Aspiration of foreign body	Acid urine
Obstructive sleep apnea	
Increased CO_2 Inhalation	
Breathing air with high CO_2 CONTENT	

MANIFESTATIONS

In respiratory acidosis, blood pH is below 7.35 and arterial P_{CO_2} is above 50 mmHg. Acute respiratory failure is associated with severe acidosis and only a small change in serum bicarbonate. Within a day, renal compensatory mechanisms become effective in generating more HCO_3; at this point, bicarbonate levels rise. In chronic respiratory acidosis, there is a compensatory increase in bicarbonate levels.

The signs and symptoms of respiratory acidosis depend on the rapidity of onset and on whether the condition is acute or chronic. Because respiratory acidosis is often accompanied by hypoxemia, the manifestations of respiratory acidosis are often inter-mixed with those of oxygen deficit. Carbon dioxide readily crosses the blood–brain barrier, exerting its effects by changing the pH of brain fluids. It produces an increase in cerebral blood flow. If the condition is severe and prolonged, it can cause an increase in cerebral spinal fluid pressure and papilledema. Head-ache, blurred vision, irritability, muscle twitching, and psychological disturbances can occur with acute respiratory acidosis. Impairment of consciousness, ranging from lethargy to coma, develops as the P_{CO_2} rises. Paralysis of extremities may occur, and there may be respiratory depression. Less severe forms of acidosis are often accompanied by warm and flushed skin, weakness, and tachycardia.

TREATMENT

The treatment of acute and chronic respiratory acidosis is directed toward improving ventilation. In severe cases, mechanical ventilation may be neces-sary. The treatment of respiratory acidosis due to respiratory failure is discussed in Chapter 28.

RESPIRATORY ALKALOSIS

Respiratory alkalosis represents a decrease in dis-solved CO_2 or a carbonic acid deficit. Respiratory alka-losis is caused by conditions that cause hyperventila-tion or respiratory rate in excess of that needed to maintain normal P_{CO_2} levels (Table 30-4).

One of the most common causes of respiratory alkalosis is the hyperventilation syndrome, which is characterized by recurring episodes of overbreathing (see Chapter 28). Other causes of hyperventilation are fever, oxygen deficiency, early salicylate toxicity, and encephalitis. Hypoxemia exerts its effect through the peripheral chemoreceptors. Salicylate toxicity and encephalitis produce hyperventilation by di-rectly stimulating the medullary respiratory center. Hyperventilation can also occur during anesthesia or with use of mechanical ventilatory devices.

MANIFESTATIONS

In respiratory alkalosis, the pH is above 7.45, arterial P_{CO_2} is below 35 mmHg, and serum bicarbonate levels are below 24 mEq/L (24 mmol/L). Because res-piratory alkalosis can occur suddenly, bicarbonate acute level may not change before respiratory correc-tion has been accomplished. The increase in pH is less in chronic compensated respiratory alkalosis and the fall in bicarbonate is greater.

The signs and symptoms of respiratory alkalosis are associated with hyperexcitability of the nervous

TABLE 30-4. RESPIRATORY ALKALOSIS	
CAUSES	**MANIFESTATIONS**
Excessive Ventilation	**Blood pH, P_{CO_2}, and HCO_3^-**
Anxiety and psychogenic	pH ↑
hyperventilation	P_{CO_2} ↓ (primary)
Reflex stimulation of ventilation due to	HCO_3^- ↓ (compensation)
hypoxia	**Cerebral Vasoconstriction and**
Lung disease that reflexly stimulates	**Increased Neural Excitability**
ventilation	Numbness and tingling of fingers and
Local lung lesions	toes
Stimulation respiratory center	Dizziness, panic, and lightheadedness
Elevated blood ammonia	Tetany
Salicylate toxicity	Positive Chvostek's and Trousseau's
Encephalitis	signs
Fever	Convulsions
Mechanical ventilation	**Cardiovascular Manifestations**
	Cardiac dysrhythmias

system and a decrease in cerebral blood flow. There is often a feeling of lightheadedness, dizziness, tingling, and numbness of the fingers and toes. There may also be sweating, palpitations, panic, air hunger, and dyspnea. Chvostek's and Trousseau's signs may be positive, and tetany and convulsions may occur. Because CO_2 provides the stimulus for short-term regulation of respiration, short periods of apnea may occur in people with acute episodes of hyperventilation.

TREATMENT

The treatment of respiratory alkalosis focuses on measures to increase the P_{CO_2}. Attention is directed toward correcting the disorder that caused the over-breathing. Rebreathing of small amounts of expired air (breathing into a paper bag) may prove useful in restoring P_{CO_2} levels in people with anxiety-produced respiratory alkalosis.

In summary, acidosis describes a decrease in *pH*, and alkalosis describes an increase in *pH*. Acid–base disorders may be caused by alterations in the body's volatile acids (respiratory acidosis or respiratory alkalosis) or nonvolatile acids (metabolic acidosis or metabolic alkalosis). Metabolic acidosis is defined as a decrease in bicarbonate, and metabolic alkalosis is defined as an increase in bicarbonate. Metabolic acidosis is caused by either an excessive production and accumulation of metabolic acids or an excessive loss of bicarbonate. Metabolic alkalosis is caused by an increase in bicarbonate or a decrease in hydrogen ion or chloride ion levels. Respiratory acidosis reflects an increase in CO_2 levels and is caused by conditions that produce hypoventilation. Respiratory alkalosis is caused by conditions that cause hyperventilation and a reduction in CO_2 levels. The signs and symptoms of acidosis and alkalosis reflect (1) alterations in body function associated with the disorder causing the acid–base disturbance, (2) the effect of the *pH* change on body function, and (3) the body's attempt to correct and maintain the *pH* within a normal physiologic range. In general, neuromuscular excitability is decreased in acidosis and increased in alkalosis.

■ REFERENCES

1. Rose, B.D. (1989). *Clinical physiology of acid–base and electrolyte disorders* (3rd ed., pp. 485, 520–527, 540, 557). New York: McGraw-Hill.
2. Levinsky, N.G. (1991). Acidosis and alkalosis. In J.D. Wilson, E. Braunwald, & K.J. Isselbacher (Eds.). *Harrison's principles of internal medicine* (12th ed., pp. 289–295). Philadelphia: W.B. Saunders.
3. Duffens, K., & Marx, J.A. (1987). Alcoholic ketoacidosis— A review. *Journal of Emergency Medicine, 5,* 399.
4. Williams, H.E. (1984). Alcoholic hypoglycemia and ketoacidosis. *Medical Clinics of North America, 68,* 33.
5. Arieff, A.I. (1991). Indications for use of bicarbonate in patients with metabolic acidosis. *British Journal of Anaesthesiology, 65,* 165–177.
6. Galla, J.H., & Luke, R.G. (1987). Pathophysiology of metabolic alkalosis. *Hospital Practice, 22*(10), 123.
7. Mennen, M. (1988). Severe metabolic alkalosis in the emergency department. *Annals of Emergency Medicine, 17,* 354.

■ BIBLIOGRAPHY

Atkinson, D.E., & Bourke, E. (1987). Metabolic aspects of regulation of systemic *pH. American Journal of Physiology, 252,* F947.

Brewer, E.D. (1990). Disorders of acid–base balance. *Pediatric Clinics of North America, 37,* 429–447.

Duffens, K., & Marx, J.A. (1987). Alcoholic ketoacidosis. *Journal of Emergency Medicine, 5,* 399.

Haber, R.J. (1991). A practical approach to acid–base disorders. *Western Journal of Medicine, 155,* 146–151.

Hamm, L.L., & Simon, E.E. (1987). Roles and mechanisms of urinary buffer excretion. *American Journal of Physiology, 253,* F595–605.

Jenkins, J.K., Best, T.R., & Nicks, S.A. (1987). Milk-alkali syndrome with a serum calcium level of 22 mg/dl and J waves on the ECG. *Southern Medical Journal, 80,* 1444.

Koch, S.M., & Taylor, R.W. (1992). Chloride ion in intensive care medicine. *Critical Care Medicine, 20,* 227–240.

Lorenz, A. (1989). Lactic acidosis: A nursing challenge. *Critical Care Nursing, 9*(4):64–73.

Mizock, B.A., & Falk, J.L. (1992). Lactic acidosis in critical illness. *Critical Care Medicine, 20,* 80–93.

Oster, J.R. (1987). The binge-purge syndrome: A common albeit unappreciated cause of acid–base and fluid-electrolyte disturbances. *Southern Medical Journal, 80,* 58.

Perez, G.O., Oster, J.R., & Rogers, A. (1987). Acid–base disturbances in gastrointestinal disease. *Digestive Disease and Science, 32,* 1033–1043.

Salem, M.M., & Mujais, S.K. (1992). Gaps in the anion gap. *Archives of Internal Medicine, 152,* 1625–1629.

CHAPTER 31

CONTROL OF RENAL FUNCTION

■ OBJECTIVES

After you have studied this chapter, you should be able to meet the following objectives:

■ Describe the anatomy of a normal kidney.

■ Describe the structure and function of the glomerular capillary membrane, including the endothelial layer, basement membrane, and epithelial layer.

■ List the parts of the tubule.

■ Differentiate between glomerular filtration, tubular reabsorption, and tubular secretion.

■ Describe the determinants of blood flow in the kidneys.

■ Define renal clearance.

■ Explain how the kidneys produce a concentrated urine.

■ Describe the role of aldosterone in regulating sodium and potassium.

■ Explain the endocrine functions of the kidneys.

■ Describe the characteristics of normal urine.

■ Explain the significance of casts in the urine.

■ Explain the value of urine specific gravity in evaluating renal function.

■ Explain the concept of the glomerular filtration rate.

■ Explain the value of serum creatinine levels in evaluating renal function.

■ State the relation between urine pH and drug elimination.

■ Describe the methods used in cystoscopic examination of the urinary tract, ultrasound studies of the urinary tract, computed tomographic scans, magnetic resonance imaging studies, excretory urography, and renal angiography.

It is no exaggeration to say that the composition of the blood is determined not so much by what the mouth takes in as by what the kidneys keep.[1]

The kidneys are remarkable organs. Each is smaller than a person's fist, yet in a single day they process about 1700 L of blood and combine its waste products into about 1.5 L of urine. As part of their function, the kidneys filter physiologically essential substances, such as sodium and potassium ions, from the blood and selectively reabsorb those substances that are needed to maintain the normal composition of internal body fluids. Substances that are not needed for this purpose pass into the urine. In regulating the volume and composition of body fluids, the kidneys perform both excretory and endocrine functions. The renin–angiotensin mechanism participates in the regulation of blood pressure and the maintenance of circulating blood volume, and erythropoietin stimulates red blood cell production. The discussion in this chapter focuses on the structure and function of the kidneys, tests of renal function, and the action of diuretics.

■ KIDNEY STRUCTURE AND FUNCTION

The kidneys are paired, bean-shaped organs that lie outside the peritoneal cavity in the back of the upper abdomen, one on each side of the vertebral column at the level of the 12th thoracic to 3rd lumbar vertebrae (Fig. 31-1). The right kidney normally is situated lower than the left, presumably because of the position of the liver. In the adult, each kidney measures about 10 to 12 cm in length, 5 to 6 cm in width, and 2.5 cm in depth and weighs about 113 to 170 g. Only the lower edge of the right kidney usually is palpable on abdominal examination. Alterations in kidney size and shape frequently are associated with disease states.

The medial border of the kidneys is indented by a deep fissure called the *hilus*. It is here that blood vessels and nerves enter and leave the kidneys. The ureters, which connect the kidneys with the bladder, also enter the kidneys at the hilus.

The kidneys are multilobular structures. Each is composed of up to 18 lobes. On longitudinal section, a kidney can be divided into an outer cortex and an inner medulla (Fig. 31-2). The cortex, which is reddish brown, contains the glomeruli and convoluted tubules of the nephron and blood vessels. The medulla consists of light-colored, cone-shaped masses—the renal pyramids—which are divided by the columns of the cortex (columns of Bertin) that extend into the medulla. Each pyramid, topped by a region of cortex, forms a lobe of the kidney. The apices of the pyramids form the papillae (8 to 18 per

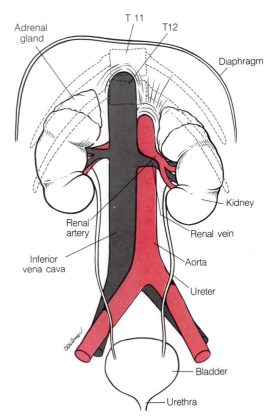

FIG. 31-1. Kidneys, ureters, and bladder.

kidney, corresponding to the number of lobes), which are perforated by the openings of the collecting ducts. The renal pelvis is a wide, funnel-shaped structure at the upper end of the ureter. It is made up of the calyces or cup-like structures that drain the upper and lower halves of the kidney.

Each kidney is ensheathed in a fibrous external capsule and surrounded by a mass of fatty connective tissue, especially at its ends and borders. The adipose tissue protects the kidney from mechanical blows and assists, together with the attached blood vessels and fascia, in holding the kidney in place. Although the kidneys are relatively well protected, they may be bruised by blows to the loin or by compression between the lower ribs and the ilium. Because the kidneys are outside the peritoneal cavity, injury and rupture do not produce the same threat of peritoneal involvement as does the rupture of organs such as the liver or spleen.

Each kidney is composed of more than 1 million tiny, closely packed functional units called *nephrons*. Each nephron consists of a vascular component (a glomerulus) and a tubular component (Fig. 31-3). The nephron is supplied by two capillary systems, the glomerulus and the peritubular capillary network. The glomerulus is a unique high-pressure filtration system located between two arterioles—the afferent and the efferent arterioles—which can selec-

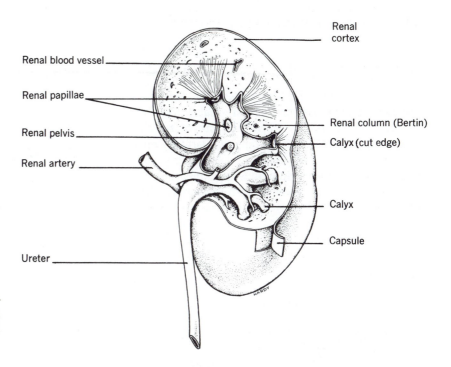

FIG. 31-2. Internal structure of the kidney. (Chaffee, E. E., & Lytle, I. M. [1980]. *Basic physiology and anatomy* [4th ed.]. Philadelphia: J.B. Lippincott)

Renal cortex
Renal blood vessel
Renal papillae
Renal pelvis
Renal artery
Renal column (Bertin)
Calyx (cut edge)
Calyx
Capsule
Ureter

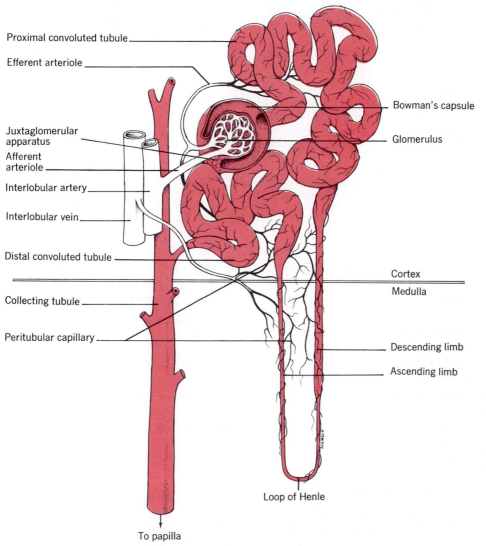

Proximal convoluted tubule
Efferent arteriole
Juxtaglomerular apparatus
Afferent arteriole
Interlobular artery
Interlobular vein
Distal convoluted tubule
Collecting tubule
Peritubular capillary
Bowman's capsule
Glomerulus
Cortex
Medulla
Descending limb
Ascending limb
Loop of Henle
To papilla

FIG. 31-3. Nephron, showing the glomerular and tubular structures along with the blood supply. (Chaffee, E. E., & Greisheimer, E. M. [1974]. *Basic physiology and anatomy* [3rd ed.]. Philadelphia: J.B. Lippincott)

tively dilate or constrict to regulate the glomerular capillary pressure.

The peritubular capillary network is a low-pressure reabsorptive system that originates from the efferent arteriole. These capillaries are distributed around all portions of the tubules, an arrangement that permits rapid movement of solutes and water between the tubular lumen and the capillaries. The peritubular capillaries rejoin to form the venous channels by which blood ultimately leaves the kidneys.

GLOMERULAR STRUCTURE AND FUNCTION

The glomerulus consists of a network of capillaries encased in a thin-walled sac, *Bowman's capsule*. Fluid and particles from the blood are filtered through the membrane of the glomerulus into Bowman's capsule, which extends to form the tubules of the nephron. The mass of capillaries and its surrounding epithelial capsule are collectively referred to as the *renal corpuscle* (Fig. 31-4A).

The glomerular capillary membrane is composed of three layers: (1) the capillary endothelial layer, (2) the basement membrane, and (3) the single-celled capsular epithelial layer (Fig. 31-4B). The endothelial layer lines the glomerulus and interfaces with blood as it moves through the capillary. This layer contains many small perforations, called *fenestrations*. The basement membrane consists of a homogeneous acellular meshwork of collagen fibers, glycoproteins, and mucopolysaccharides (Fig. 31-4C). The epithelial layer that covers the glomerulus is continuous with the epithelium that lines Bowman's capsule. The epithelial layer that covers the glomerulus is called the *visceral epithelium* to differentiate it from the *parietal layer* that lines Bowman's capsule. The visceral epithelial cells have unusual octopus-like structures that possess a large number of extensions, or foot processes (podocytes), which are embedded in the basement membrane (Fig. 31-5). These foot processes form slit pores through which the glomerular filtrate passes.

Because both the endothelial and the epithelial layers of the glomerular capillary have porous structures, the basement membrane determines the permeability of the glomerular capillary membrane. The spaces between the fibers that make up the basement membrane represent the pores of a filter and determine the size-dependent permeability barrier of the glomerulus. The size of the pores in the basement membrane normally prevents red blood cells and plasma proteins from passing through the glomerular membrane into the urine filtrate. There is evidence that the epithelium plays a major role in forming the basement membrane components, and it is

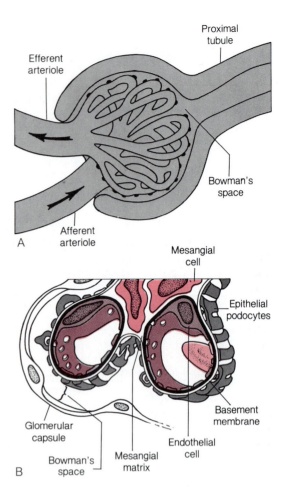

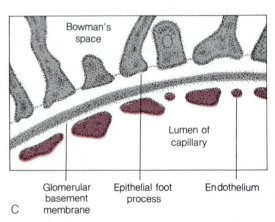

FIG. 31-4. Renal corpuscle. (**A**) Structures of the glomerulus. (**B**) Position of the mesangial cells in relation to the capillary loops and Bowman's capsule. (**C**) Cross section of the glomerular membrane showing the position of the endothelium, basement membrane, and epithelial foot processes.

probable that the epithelial cells are active in forming new basement membrane material throughout life. Because material is being added to the exterior of the basement membrane, it seems reasonable to assume that equal amounts are being removed from the inner surface to keep it from becoming unduly thick.[2] Al-

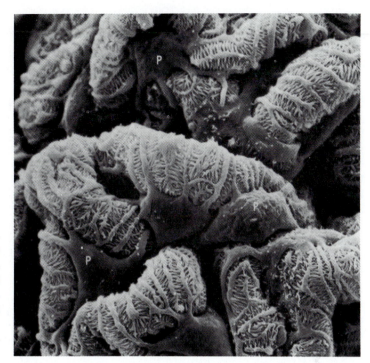

FIG. 31-5. Scanning electron micrograph of a glomerulus from the kidney of a normal rat. The visceral epithelial cells, or podocytes (*P*), extend multiple processes outward from the main cell body to wrap around individual capillary loops. Immediately adjacent pedicels, or foot processes, arise from different podocytes (magnification × 4800). (Brenner, B. M., & Rector, F. C. [1981]. *The kidney.* Philadelphia: W.B. Saunders. Reprinted by permission)

terations in the structure and composition of the glomerular basement membrane are responsible for the leakage of proteins and blood cells that occurs with many forms of glomerular disease.

Another important component of the glomerulus is the mesangium. In some areas, the capillary endothelium and the basement membrane do not completely surround each capillary. Mesangial cells, which lie between the capillary tufts, provide support for the glomerulus in these areas (see Fig. 31-4B). They produce an intercellular substance similar to that of the basement membrane. This substance covers the endothelial cells where they are not covered by epithelially derived basement membrane. The mesangial cells possess (or can develop) phagocytic properties and remove macromolecular materials that enter the intercapillary spaces. Mesangial cells also exhibit contractile properties in response to neurohumoral substances and are thought to contribute to the regulation of blood flow through the glomerulus. In normal glomeruli, the mesangial area is narrow and contains only a small number of cells. Mesangial hyperplasia and increased mesangial matrix occur in a number of glomerular diseases.

TUBULAR STRUCTURE AND FUNCTION

Although the plasma is filtered in the glomerulus, it is the tubular structures that transform the filtered fluid into urine. The nephron tubule is divided into four segments: (1) a highly coiled segment called the *proximal convoluted tubule*, which originates in Bowman's capsule; (2) a thin, looped structure called the *loop of Henle;* (3) a distal coiled portion called the *distal convoluted tubule;* and (4) the final segment called the *collecting tubule*, which joins with several tubules to collect the urine filtrate. The filtrate passes through each of these segments before reaching the pelvis of the kidney.

Nephrons can be roughly grouped into two categories. About 85% of the nephrons originate in the superficial part of the cortex and are called *cortical nephrons*. They have short, thick loops of Henle that penetrate only a short distance into the medulla. The remaining 15% are called *juxtamedullary nephrons*. They originate deeper in the cortex and have longer and thinner loops of Henle that penetrate the entire length of the medulla. The juxtamedullary nephrons are largely concerned with urine concentration.

Throughout its course, the tubule is composed of a single layer of epithelial cells resting on a basement membrane. The structure of the epithelial cells varies with tubular function. The cells of the proximal tubule have a fine villous structure that increases the surface area for reabsorption; they are also rich in mitochondria, which support active transport processes. The epithelial layer of the thin segment of the loop of Henle has few mitochondria, indicating minimal metabolic activity and active reabsorptive function.

About 65% of all reabsorptive and secretory processes that occur in the tubular system take place in the proximal tubule.[3] There is almost complete reabsorption of nutritionally important substances, such as glucose, amino acids, and vitamins; electrolytes, such as sodium, potassium, chloride, and bicarbonate, are 65% to 80% reabsorbed in this tubular segment. As solutes are transported out of the tubular cells, their concentration within the lumen decreases and their concentration outside the tubule increases, providing a concentration gradient for the osmotic reabsorption of water. The proximal tubule is highly permeable to water, and the osmotic movement of water occurs so rapidly that the concentration difference of solutes on either side of the membrane seldom is more than a few milliosmoles.

The *thin segment* of the loop of Henle is important in maintaining the concentrating capabilities of the nephron. As its name implies, the epithelial cells of this tubular segment are very thin, which contributes to their permeability characteristics. The descending limb is highly permeable to water and moderately permeable to urea, sodium, and other ions. The ascending limb, in contrast to the descending limb, is only slightly permeable to urea and water but is capable of active sodium transport. As explained later, these differences in permeability and sodium transport are responsible for the production of a countercurrent mechanism that concentrates solutes in the interstitial fluids that surround the collecting ducts, a condition necessary for the antidiuretic hormone (ADH)–mediated reabsorption of water.

The *thick segment* of the loop of Henle begins in the ascending limb of the loop where the epithelial cells become thickened. This segment extends all the way back to the glomerulus from which the tubule originated and then passes between the afferent and efferent arteriole, forming the *juxtaglomerular complex* (Fig. 31-6). Because of its location, the juxtaglomerular complex is thought to play an essential feedback role in linking the functioning of the afferent and efferent arterioles to the composition of the distal tubular fluid. This hypothesis is supported by the presence in the distal tubule of macula densa cells that appear to secrete substances toward the arterioles. In addition, juxtaglomerular cells in the afferent and efferent arterioles contain granules of inactive renin, suggesting that the composition of the distal tubular fluid contributes to the control of sodium and water reabsorption through the renin–angiotensin–aldosterone mechanism (discussed later in this chapter and in Chapter 21).

The distal tubule begins at the juxtaglomerular complex, continuing from the thick segment of the ascending loop of Henle. The distal tubule is divided into two segments: the *diluting segment* and the *late distal tubule*. The diluting segment includes the entire thick portion of the loop of Henle and about half the convoluted portion of the distal tubule. The cells of

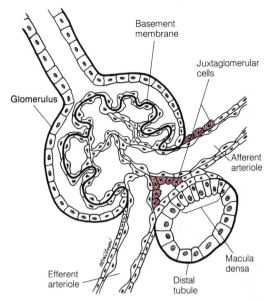

FIG. 31-6. Juxtaglomerular apparatus showing the close contact of the distal tubule with the afferent arteriole and the macula densa and the juxtaglomerular cells.

the thick segment are specifically adapted to reabsorb chloride from the tubular lumen into the extracellular fluid for return to the bloodstream. The reabsorption of the negative chloride ions creates an electrical gradient, which results in the passive reabsorption of sodium. Certain diuretic drugs act by inhibiting this transport system. The diluting segment is almost entirely impermeable to water and urea. Consequently, the outward transport of sodium and chloride dilutes the tubular fluid, a condition that is necessary for production of a dilute urine. The later distal tubule is adapted for the active transport of sodium and other positive ions. It is here and in the collecting tubule that potassium ions are secreted into the tubular fluid and aldosterone exerts its effects on sodium and potassium reabsorption.

Like the distal tubule, the collecting duct is divided into two segments: the *cortical collecting tubule* and the *inner medullary collecting duct*. The cortical segment begins in the renal cortex at the termination of the convoluted distal tubule. It fuses with cortical tubules from several other nephrons before it turns down from the cortex toward the renal papillae. As the cortical collecting duct passes through the medullary portion of the kidneys, it becomes the inner medullary collecting duct. The epithelium of the collecting duct is well designed to resist extreme changes in the osmotic or pH characteristics of tubular fluid, and it is here that the urine becomes highly concentrated, highly diluted, highly alkaline, or highly acidic. The permeability of the epithelium to water in both portions of the collecting duct is determined mainly by the concentration of ADH. When large quantities of the hormone are present, the tubular epithelium becomes very permeable to water, and most of the water in the tubular fluid is reabsorbed from the tubule and returned to the blood. Little water is reabsorbed in the absence of the hormone. Alterations in body fluids caused by disorders of ADH levels are discussed in Chapter 29.

URINE FORMATION

Urine formation begins with the filtration of essentially protein-free plasma through the glomerular capillaries into Bowman's capsule. The movement of fluid through the glomerular capillaries is determined by the same factors (capillary pressure and colloidal osmotic pressure) that affect fluid movement through other capillaries in the body (see Chapter 29). About 125 mL of fluid is filtered each minute. This is called the *glomerular filtration rate (GFR)*. This rate can vary from a few milliliters per minute to as high as 200 mL/minute.

The location of the glomerulus, between two arterioles, allows for the maintenance of a high-pressure filtration system. The capillary filtration pressure (about 60 mmHg) in the glomerulus is about two to three times higher than that of other capillary beds in the body. The filtration pressure and the GFR are regulated by the constriction and relaxation of the afferent and efferent arterioles. Constriction of the efferent arteriole increases resistance to outflow from the glomeruli and increases the glomerular pressure and the GFR. On the other hand, constriction of the afferent arteriole causes a reduction in the renal blood flow, glomerular filtration pressure, and GFR. Both the afferent and the efferent arteriole are innervated by the sympathetic nervous system. During periods of strong sympathetic stimulation, such as occurs during shock, renal blood flow and the glomerular filtration pressure can be temporarily decreased to as little as 10% to 30% and urine output can fall to almost zero.[3]

From Bowman's capsule, the glomerular filtrate moves into the tubular segments of the nephron. In its movement through the lumen of the tubular segments, the glomerular filtrate is changed considerably by the transtubular transport of water and solutes. Tubular transport can result in *secretion* of substances into the tubular fluid from the blood or in *reabsorption* of substances from the tubular fluid into the blood (Fig. 31-7). The basic mechanisms of transport across the tubular epithelial cell membrane are similar to those of cell membranes in the body and include both passive and active transport. Water and urea are passively absorbed along concentration gradients. Sodium, potassium, chloride, calcium, phos-

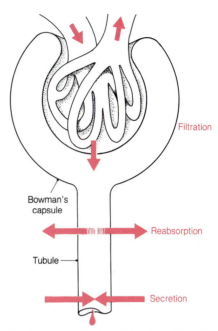

FIG. 31-7. Mechanisms of urine formation. The plasma is filtered in the glomerulus, and urine is formed as substances are reabsorbed or secreted into the filtrate.

phate, and urate ions as well as glucose molecules and amino acids are actively transported across the tubular membrane. Some substances, such as hydrogen, potassium, and urate ions, are actively secreted into the tubular fluids. Under normal conditions, only about 1 mL of the 125 mL of glomerular filtrate that is formed each minute is excreted in the urine. The other 124 mL is reabsorbed in the tubules. This means that the average output of urine is about 60 mL/hour.

GLOMERULAR FILTRATION AND TUBULAR REABSORPTION BALANCE

One of the most remarkable features of the kidneys is their feedback regulation between glomerular filtration and the rate of tubular reabsorption. Although the mechanism is unclear, there is a feedback mechanism that produces a decrease in the GFR when tubular reabsorption is reduced. Likewise, a reduction in tubular reabsorption occurs when the GFR falls. This feedback mechanism ensures a constant proportionality between filtration and reabsorption.

RENAL CLEARANCE

Renal clearance is the volume of plasma that is completely cleared each minute of any substance that finds its way into the urine. It is determined by the ability of the substance to be filtered in the glomeruli and the capacity of the renal tubules to reabsorb or secrete the substance. Every substance has its own clearance rate, the units of which are always in volume of plasma per unit time. It can be determined by measuring the amount of a substance that is excreted in the urine (urine concentration × urine flow rate in milliliters per minute) and dividing by its plasma concentration. Inulin, a large polysaccharide, is freely filtered in the glomeruli and neither reabsorbed nor secreted by the tubular cells. After intravenous injection, the amount that appears in the urine is equal to the amount that is filtered in the glomeruli (*e.g.*, the clearance rate is equal to the GFR). Because of these properties, inulin can be used as a laboratory measure of the GFR. Some substances, such as urea, are freely filtered in the glomeruli, but the volume that is cleared from the plasma is less than the GFR, indicating that at least some of the substance is being reabsorbed. At normal plasma levels, glucose has a clearance of 0 because it is reabsorbed in the tubules, so that none appears in the urine.

RENAL THRESHOLD (TRANSPORT MAXIMUM)

Many substances, such as glucose, are freely filtered in the glomerulus and reabsorbed by special energy-dependent tubular transport systems. The maximum amount of substances that these transport systems can reabsorb, called the *transport maximum*, usually is sufficient for all the filtered substance to be reabsorbed and none to appear in the urine. The point at which the substance appears in the urine is also called the *renal threshold*. Under some circumstances, the amount of substance filtered in the glomerulus exceeds the transport maximum for the substance. For example, when the blood glucose level is elevated in uncontrolled diabetes mellitus, the amount that is filtered in the glomerulus often exceeds the transport maximum (about 320 mg/minute) for glucose, and glucose spills into the urine.

CONTROL OF URINE CONCENTRATION

The kidneys can produce either a concentrated or a dilute urine, depending on the composition and volume of the extracellular fluids. The concentration or dilution of the urine occurs in the collecting tubules and depends on (1) the increased solute concentration in the medullary area surrounding the collecting ducts and (2) the selective permeability of the collecting tubules, which is controlled by ADH.

In about one fifth of the nephrons (juxtamedullary nephrons), the loops of Henle and special peri-

tubular capillaries called the *vasa recta* descend into the renal medulla. Here a countercurrent mechanism controls water and solute flow. As a result, water is kept out of the peritubular area and sodium and urea are retained. A consequence of these processes is that a high concentration of the osmotically active particles collect in the interstitium of this portion of the kidney (Fig. 31-8). It is here, where the kidney interstitium surrounds the collecting tubules, that the presence of these osmotically active particles facilitates the ADH-mediated reabsorption of water.

During periods of dehydration, the kidneys play a major role in maintaining water balance. Osmoreceptors in the hypothalamus sense the increase in osmolality of extracellular fluids and stimulate the release of ADH (see Chapter 29). The collecting tubules, under the influence of ADH, become permeable to water. Once the permeability of the collecting tubules has been established, water moves out of the tubular lumen and into the interstitium of the medullary area, where it enters the peritubular capillaries for return to the vascular system. This serves to maintain extracellular volume by returning water to the vascular compartment and leads to the production of a concentrated urine by removing water from the tubular filtrate. In the absence of ADH, the renal

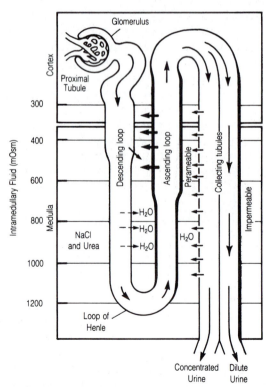

FIG. 31-8. Countercurrent mechanism for concentrating urine. Antidiuretic hormone controls the permeability of the collecting tubule. The urine is concentrated when ADH levels are increased and dilute when ADH is decreased.

tubules remain impermeable to water, and a dilute urine is formed.

SODIUM AND POTASSIUM ELIMINATION

The excretion of sodium by the kidneys is highly variable. The sodium in the blood is freely filtered, so that its concentration in the glomerular filtrate approximates that of plasma; it is then actively transported back into the plasma as fluid moves through the tubules. It is important that the tubular reabsorption varies with the GFR. For example, when additional sodium filtration occurs because of an increase in the GFR, reabsorption must increase to maintain serum sodium levels. About 65% of sodium reabsorption takes place in the proximal tubule, 27% in the loop of Henle, and 8% in the distal tubule.

Sodium reabsorption in the distal tubule is highly variable and depends on the presence of aldosterone, a hormone secreted by the adrenal gland. In the presence of aldosterone, almost all the sodium from the distal tubular fluid is reabsorbed, and the urine essentially becomes sodium-free. In the absence of aldosterone, virtually no sodium is reabsorbed from the distal tubule. The remarkable ability of the distal tubular cells to alter sodium reabsorption in relation to changes in aldosterone allows the kidneys to excrete urine with sodium levels that range from a few tenths of a gram to 40 grams.

Like sodium, potassium is freely filtered in the glomerulus; but unlike sodium, potassium is both reabsorbed from and secreted into the tubular fluid. The secretion of potassium into the tubular fluid occurs in the distal tubule and, like that of sodium, is regulated by aldosterone. Only about 70 mEq of potassium is delivered to the distal tubule each day, yet the average person consumes this much and more potassium in the diet. Excess potassium that is not filtered in the glomerulus and delivered to the distal tubule must, therefore, be secreted (transported from the blood) into the tubular fluid for elimination from the body. In the absence of aldosterone (as in Addison's disease; see Chapter 29), potassium secretion becomes minimal. In these circumstances, potassium reabsorption exceeds secretion and blood levels of potassium increase.

REGULATION OF *p*H

The kidneys regulate body *p*H by conserving base bicarbonate or eliminating hydrogen ions. Neither the blood buffer systems nor the respiratory control mechanisms for carbon dioxide elimination can eliminate hydrogen ions (H^+) from the body. This is accomplished by the kidneys. The average North American diet results in the liberation of 40 to 80 mmol of hydrogen ions each day. Virtually all the hydrogen ions excreted in the urine are secreted into the tubular fluid by means of tubular secretory mechanisms. The lowest tubular fluid *p*H that can be achieved is 4.4.[4] The ability of the kidneys to excrete hydrogen ions depends on buffers in the urine that combine with the hydrogen ion. The three major urine buffers are bicarbonate (HCO_3^-), phosphate (HPO_4^{--}), and ammonia (NH_3). Bicarbonate, which is present in the urine filtrate, combines with hydrogen ions that have been secreted into the tubular fluid; this results in the formation of carbon dioxide and water. The carbon dioxide is then absorbed into the tubular cells and bicarbonate is regenerated. The phosphate ion is a metabolic end product that is filtered into the tubular fluid; it combines with a secreted hydrogen ion and is not reabsorbed. Ammonia is synthesized in tubular cells by deamination of the amino acid glutamine; it diffuses into the tubular fluid and combines with the hydrogen ion. An important aspect of this buffer system is that the deamination process increases whenever the body's hydrogen ion concentration remains elevated for 1 to 2 days. These mechanisms for *p*H regulation are described more fully in Chapter 30.

*p*H-DEPENDENT ELIMINATION OF ORGANIC IONS

The proximal tubule actively secretes large amounts of different organic anions. Both foreign anions (*e.g.*, drugs such as salicylates and penicillin) and endogenously produced anions (*e.g.*, bile acids and uric acid) are actively secreted into the tubular fluid. Most of the anions that are secreted use the same transport system, allowing the kidneys to rid the body of many different drugs and environmental agents. Because the same transport system is shared by different anions, there is competition for transport such that elevated levels of one substance tends to inhibit the secretion of other anions. The proximal tubules also possess an active transport system for organic cations that is analogous to that for organic ions.

URIC ACID ELIMINATION

Uric acid is a product of purine metabolism (see Chapter 58). Excessively high blood levels (hyperuricemia) can cause gout, and excessive levels in the urine can cause kidney stones. Uric acid is freely filtered in the glomerulus and is both reabsorbed and secreted into the proximal tubules. Uric acid is one of the anions that uses the previously described anion transport system in the proximal tubule. Tubular reabsorption normally exceeds secretion, so that the net effect is removal of uric acid from the filtrate. Although the rate of reabsorption exceeds secretion, the secretory process is homeostatically controlled to maintain a constant plasma level. Many people with elevated uric acid levels secrete less uric acid than do people with normal uric acid levels.

Uric acid uses the same transport systems as other anions, such as aspirin, sulfinpyrazone, and probenecid. Small doses of aspirin compete with uric acid for secretion into the tubular fluid and reduce uric acid secretion, whereas large doses compete with uric acid for reabsorption and increase uric acid excretion in the urine. Because of its effect on uric acid secretion, aspirin is not recommended for treatment of gouty arthritis. Thiazide and loop diuretics (furosemide and ethacrynic acid) can also cause hyperuricemia (and gouty arthritis), presumably through a decrease in extracellular fluid volume and enhanced uric acid reabsorption.

UREA ELIMINATION

Urea is an end product of protein metabolism. The normal adult produces 25 to 30 g/day; the quantity rises when a high-protein diet is consumed, when there is excessive tissue breakdown, or in the presence of gastrointestinal bleeding. In the presence of gastrointestinal bleeding, the blood proteins are broken down to form ammonia in the intestine; the ammonia is then absorbed into the portal circulation and converted to urea by the liver before being released into the bloodstream. The kidneys, in their role as regulators of blood urea nitrogen (BUN) levels, filter urea in the glomeruli and then reabsorb it in the tubules. This allows for maintenance of a normal BUN, which is in the range of 8 to 25 mg/dL (2.9 to 8.9 mmol/L). During periods of dehydration, the blood volume and GFR drop and BUN levels increase. The renal tubules are permeable to urea, which means that the longer the tubular fluid remains in the kidneys, the greater the reabsorption of urea into the blood. Hence, only small amounts of urea are reabsorbed into the blood when the GFR is high, whereas relatively large amounts of urea are returned to the blood when the GFR is reduced.

DRUG ELIMINATION

Many drugs are eliminated in the urine. These drugs are selectively filtered in the glomerulus and reabsorbed or secreted into the tubular fluid. Most drugs are either weak acids or weak bases and are present in the renal tubular fluid partly as a water-soluble ion or partly as an undissociated lipid-soluble acid or base.[5] Because the renal tubular cells behave like a lipid

layer, the undissociated lipid-soluble form of the drug diffuses back into the blood more rapidly that the ionized form. The ratio of ionized to un-ionized drug depends on the pH of the urine. For example, aspirin is mainly ionized in alkaline urine and in this form is rapidly excreted in the urine, whereas it is largely un-ionized in acid urine and much of the drug is reabsorbed rather than excreted.

Alkaline or acid diuresis may be used to increase elimination of drugs in the urine, particularly in situations of drug overdose. Alkaline diuresis enhances the elimination of phenobarbital and salicylates, including aspirin. Acid diuresis enhances the elimination of amphetamines, cocaine, quinidine, quinine, and the sympathomimetic drugs. Because urine pH changes the amount of drug that is eliminated in the urine, pH should be measured in urine specimens used for drug testing.

RENAL BLOOD FLOW

Each kidney is supplied by a renal artery that arises on either side of the aorta. On entering the kidney, the renal artery divides into the segmental and then the lobar arteries that supply the upper, middle, and lower parts of the kidney. The lobar arteries further subdivide to form the interlobular arteries at the level of the cortical medullary junction (Fig. 31-9). These arteries arch across the pyramids to form the arcuate arteries, which give rise to the intralobular arteries. The afferent arterioles that supply the glomeruli arise from the intralobular arteries.

In the adult, the kidneys are perfused with about 1300 mL of blood per minute, or 20% to 25% of the cardiac output. This large blood flow is needed not

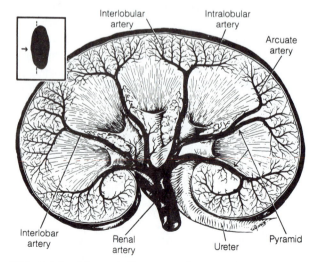

FIG. 31-9. Schematic illustration of the arterial supply of the kidney, simplified for clarity. (Ham, A. W., & Cormack, D. H. [1987]. *Histology* [9th ed., p. 583]. Philadelphia: J.B. Lippincott)

for renal metabolism, but to ensure sufficient glomerular filtration for the removal of waste products from the blood. Blood flow to the kidneys remains relatively constant within a mean arterial blood pressure range of 80 to 180 mmHg.

The renal blood flow is controlled by a number of neural and humoral influences. As previously described, input from the sympathetic nervous system can drastically decrease renal blood flow by increasing the resistance of the afferent and efferent arterioles. The constancy of flow is further maintained by a process called autoregulation (discussed in Chapter 19). For autoregulation to occur, the resistance to flow through the kidneys must be varied in direct proportion to the arterial pressure. The exact mechanisms responsible for the intrarenal regulation of blood flow are still unclear. One of the proposed mechanisms is that of direct stimulation of arteriolar smooth muscle that causes the blood vessels to relax when there is an increase in blood pressure and constrict when there is a decrease in pressure. Renal blood flow may also be regulated by prostaglandins, which enhance renal blood flow. Prostaglandin release by the kidneys is stimulated by angiotensin II, and renin release is inhibited by prostaglandins. Thus, it has been proposed that prostaglandins may protect the kidneys against the vasoconstricting effects of angiotensin II.[6]

Although nearly all the blood flow to the kidneys passes through the cortex, less than 10% is directed to the medulla and only about 1% goes to the papillae. Under conditions of decreased renal blood flow or increased sympathetic nervous system stimulation, blood flow is redistributed away from the cortex toward the medulla. This redistribution of blood flow decreases glomerular filtration while maintaining the urine concentrating ability of the kidneys, a factor that is important during conditions such as shock.

ENDOCRINE FUNCTION

In addition to their function in regulating body fluids and electrolytes, the kidneys function as an endocrine organ in that they produce chemical mediators that travel through the blood to distant sites where they exert their actions. The kidneys participate in control of blood pressure by way of the renin–angiotensin mechanism, in calcium metabolism by activating vitamin D, and in regulating red blood cell production through the synthesis of erythropoietin.

RENIN–ANGIOTENSIN MECHANISM

The renin–angiotensin–aldosterone mechanism plays an important part in both short- and long-term regulation of blood pressure (see Chapter 21).

Renin is synthesized and stored in the juxtaglomerular cells of the kidney (see Fig. 31-6). This enzyme is thought to be released in response to a decrease in renal blood flow or a change in the composition of the distal tubular fluid or as the result of sympathetic nervous system stimulation. Renin itself has no direct effect on blood pressure. Rather, it acts enzymatically to convert a circulating plasma protein called *angiotensinogen* to angiotensin I. Angiotensin I, which has few vasoconstrictor properties, leaves the kidneys and enters and the circulation; as it is circulated through the lungs, *angiotensin-converting enzyme* catalzyes the conversion of angiotensin I to angiotensin II. Angiotensin II is a potent vasoconstrictor and it acts directly on the kidneys to decrease salt and water excretion. Both of these mechanisms have a relatively short period of action. Angiotensin II also stimulates aldosterone secretion by the adrenal gland. Aldosterone acts on the distal tubule to increase sodium reabsorption and exerts a more long-term effect on the maintenance of blood pressure.

ERYTHROPOIETIN

Eighty to 95% of erythropoietin is formed in the kidneys. It regulates red blood cell production and is released in response to hypoxia. It is believed that the kidneys respond to hypoxia by producing erythropoietin. This hormone acts on the bone marrow to stimulate production and release of red blood cells (see Chapter 18). As a result, many people with chronic hypoxia have increased red blood cell levels (polycythemia). This occurs in conditions such as congestive heart failure and chronic lung disease.

VITAMIN D

Vitamin D increases calcium absorption from the gastrointestinal tract and helps to regulate calcium deposition in bone. It exists in several forms: natural vitamin D (cholecalciferol), which results from ultraviolet irradiation of the skin, and synthetic vitamin D (ergocalciferol), which is derived from irradiation of ergosterol. The active form of vitamin D is 1,25-dihydroxycholecalciferol; both cholecalciferol and ergocalciferol must undergo chemical transformation to become active: first to 25-hydroxycholecalciferol in the liver and then to 1,25-dihydroxycholecalciferol in the kidneys.

In summary, the kidneys perform both excretory and endocrine functions. In the process of excreting wastes, the kidneys filter the blood and then selectively reabsorb those materials that are needed to maintain a stable internal environment. The kidneys (1) rid the body of metabolic wastes, (2) regulate fluid volume, (3) regulate the composition of electrolytes, (4) assist in maintaining acid–base balance, (5) aid in regulation of blood pressure through the renin–angiotensin–aldosterone mechanism and control of extracellular fluid volume, (6) regulate red blood cell production through erythropoietin, and (7) aid in calcium metabolism by activating vitamin D.

■ TESTS OF RENAL FUNCTION

The function of the kidneys is to filter the blood, selectively reabsorb those substances that are needed to maintain the constancy of body fluid, and excrete metabolic wastes. Therefore, the composition of urine and blood provides valuable information about the adequacy of renal function. Radiologic tests, endoscopy, and renal biopsy afford a means of viewing the gross and microscopic structures of the kidneys and urinary system.

URINALYSIS

Urine is a clear, amber-colored fluid that is about 95% water and 5% dissolved solids. The kidneys normally produce about 1.5 L of urine a day. Normal urine contains metabolic wastes and few, if any, plasma proteins, blood cells, or glucose molecules. Urine tests can be performed on a single urine specimen or on a 24-hour urine specimen. First-voided morning specimens are useful for qualitative protein and specific gravity testing. A freshly voided specimen is most reliable. Urine specimens that have been left standing may contain lysed red blood cells, disintegrating casts, and rapidly multiplying bacteria. Table 31-1 describes urinalysis values for normal urine.

Casts are molds of the distal nephron lumen. A gel-like substance called Tamm-Horsfall mucoprotein, which is formed in the tubular epithelium, is the major protein constituent of urinary casts. Casts composed of this gel but devoid of cells are called hyaline casts. These casts develop when the protein

concentration of the urine is high (as in nephrotic syndrome), urine osmolality is high, and urine pH is low. The inclusion of granules or cells in the matrix of the protein gel leads to the formation of various other types of casts.

The specific gravity (or osmolality) of urine varies with its concentration of solutes. Urine specific gravity provides a valuable index of the hydration status and functional ability of the kidneys. Although there are more sophisticated methods for measuring specific gravity, it can be easily measured using an inexpensive piece of equipment called a urinometer. Healthy kidneys can produce a concentrated urine with a specific gravity of 1.030 to 1.040. During periods of marked hydration, the specific gravity can approach 1.000. With diminished renal function, there is a loss of renal concentrating ability, and the urine specific gravity may fall to levels of 1.006 to 1.010 (usual range is 1.015 to 1.025 with normal fluid intake). These low levels are particularly significant if they occur during periods that follow a decrease in water intake (e.g., during the first urine specimen on arising in the morning).

BLOOD TESTS

Blood tests can provide valuable information about the kidneys' ability to remove metabolic wastes from the blood and to maintain normal electrolyte and pH composition of the blood. Normal blood values are listed in Table 31-2. Serum levels of potassium, phosphate, BUN, and creatinine increase in renal failure. Serum pH, calcium, and bicarbonate levels decrease in renal failure. The effect of renal failure on the concentration of serum electrolytes and metabolic end products is discussed in Chapter 33.

Blood Urea Nitrogen. Urea is formed in the liver as a by-product of protein metabolism and elimi-

---

TABLE 31-1. NORMAL VALUES FOR ROUTINE URINALYSIS

GENERAL CHARACTERISTICS AND MEASUREMENTS	CHEMICAL DETERMINATIONS	MICROSCOPIC EXAMINATION OF SEDIMENT
Color: yellow-amber—indicates a high specific gravity and small output of urine	Glucose: negative	Casts negative: occasional hyaline casts
Turbidity: clear to slightly hazy	Ketones: negative	Red blood cells negative or rare
Specific gravity: 1.010–1.025 with a normal fluid intake	Blood: negative	Crystals negative
pH: 4.6–4.8—average person has a pH of about 6 (acid)	Protein: negative	White blood cells: negative or rare
	Bilirubin: negative	Epithelial cells: few
	Urobilinogen: 0.1–1	
	Nitrate for bacteria: negative	
	Leukocyte esterase: negative	

(Fishbach, F. [1992]. *A manual of laboratory diagnostic tests* [p. 148]. Philadelphia: J.B. Lippincott)

TABLE 31-2. NORMAL BLOOD CHEMISTRY LEVELS

SUBSTANCE	NORMAL VALUE
BUN	8.0–25.0 mg/dL (2.9–8.9 mmol/L)
Creatinine	0.7–1.5 mg/dL (60–130 μmol/L)
Sodium	137–147 mEq/L (137–147 mmol/L)
Chloride	100–106 mEq/L (100–106 mmol/L)
Potassium	3.5–5 mEq/L (3.5–5 mmol/L)
Carbon dioxide (CO_2 content)	24–29 mEq/L (24–29 mmol/L)
Calcium	8.5–10.3 mg/dL (2.1–2.6 mmol/L)
Phosphate	3–4.5 mg/dL (1–1.5 mmol/L)
Uric acid	2.6–7.2 mg/dL (0.154–0.42 mmol/L)
pH	7.35–7.45

nated entirely by the kidneys. BUN is, therefore, related to the GFR but, unlike creatinine, is also influenced by protein intake, gastrointestinal bleeding, and hydration status. Both increased protein intake and gastrointestinal bleeding increase urea by way of protein metabolism. In gastrointestinal bleeding, the blood is broken down by the intestinal flora and the nitrogenous waste is absorbed into the portal vein and transported to the liver where it is converted to urea. During dehydration, elevated BUN levels result from increased concentration. About two thirds of renal function must be lost before a significant rise in the BUN level occurs.[6] Therefore, BUN is less specific for renal insufficiency than creatinine. The BUN-creatinine ratio, however, may provide useful diagnostic information. The ratio normally is about 10:1. Ratios greater than 15:1 represent prerenal conditions such as in congestive heart failure and upper gastrointestinal tract bleeding that produce an increase in BUN but not creatinine. A ratio of less than 10:1 occurs in people with liver disease and in those who receive a low-protein diet or chronic dialysis, since BUN is more readily dialyzable than creatinine.

GLOMERULAR FILTRATION RATE

The GFR provides a gauge of renal function. It can be measured clinically by collecting timed samples of blood and urine. Creatinine, a product of creatine metabolism by the muscle, is filtered by the kidneys but not reabsorbed in the renal tubule. Therefore, creatinine values in the blood and urine can be used to measure GFR. The clearance rate for creatinine is the amount that is completely cleared by the kidneys in 1 minute. The formula is expressed as

$$C = UV/P$$

where C = clearance rate (mL/minute), U = urine concentration (mg/dL), V = urine volume excreted (mL/minute or 24 hour), and P = plasma concentration (mg/dL).

Normal creatinine clearance is 115 to 125 mL/minute. This value is corrected for body surface area, which reflects the muscle mass where creatinine metabolism takes place. The test may be done on a 24-hour basis, with blood being drawn at the time the urine collection is completed. In another method, two 1-hour urine specimens are collected and a blood sample is drawn in between.

Serum Creatinine. Serum creatinine levels reflect the glomerular filtration rate. They are easily obtained and relatively inexpensive; therefore, they are often used as a screening measure of renal function. *Creatinine* is a product of *creatine* metabolism in muscles; therefore, its formation and release are relatively constant and proportional to the amount of muscle mass present. Because creatinine is filtered in the glomeruli but not secreted into the tubules from the blood or reabsored from the tubules into the blood, its blood values depend closely on the GFR. The normal creatinine value is about 0.7 mg/dL of blood for a woman with a small frame, about 1.0 mg/dL of blood for a normal adult man, and about 1.5 mg/dL of blood (60 to 130 mmol/L) for a muscular man. There is an age-related decline in creatinine clearance in many elderly people because both muscle mass and the GFR decline with age (see Chapter 33).

A normal serum creatinine level usually is indicative of normal renal function. In addition to its use in calculating the GFR, the serum creatinine level is used in estimating the functional capacity of the kidneys (Fig. 31-10). If the value doubles, the GFR—and renal function—probably has fallen to half its normal state. A rise in the serum creatinine level to three times its normal value suggests that there is a 75%

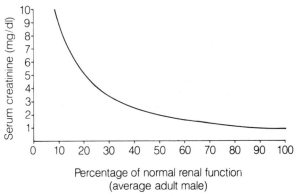

FIG. 31-10. Relation between percentage of renal function and serum creatinine levels. (From data in Mitch, W. E., & Walser, M. [1976]. A simple method of estimating progression of chronic renal failure. *Lancet, 2,* 1326)

loss of renal function, and with creatinine values of 10 mg/dL or more, it can be assumed that about 90% of renal function has been lost.

CYSTOSCOPY

Cystoscopy provides a means for direct visualization of the urethra, bladder, and ureteral orifices. It relies on the use of a cystoscope, an instrument with a lighted lens. The cystoscope is inserted through the urethra into the bladder. Biopsy specimens, lesions, small stones, and foreign bodies can be removed from the bladder. Urethroscopy may be used to remove stones from the ureter and aid in the treatment of ureteral disorders such as ureteral strictures.

ULTRASONOGRAPHY

Ultrasound studies use the reflection of ultrasonic (high-frequency) waves to visualize the deep structures of the body. The procedure is painless and noninvasive and requires no patient preparation. Ultrasonography is used to visualize the structures of the kidneys and has proved useful in the diagnosis of many urinary tract disorders, including congenital anomalies, renal abscesses, hydronephrosis, and kidney stones. It can differentiate between a renal cyst and a renal tumor. The use of ultrasonography also enables accurate placement of needles for renal biopsy and catheters for percutaneous nephrostomy.

RADIOLOGIC AND OTHER IMAGING STUDIES

Radiologic studies include a simple flat plate (x-ray) of the kidneys, ureters, and bladder that can be used to determine the size, shape, and position of the kidneys and to note any radiopaque stones that may be in the kidney pelvis or ureters. In excretory urography, or intravenous pyelography, a radiopaque dye is injected into a peripheral vein; the dye is then filtered by the glomerulus and excreted into the urine, and x-ray films are taken as it moves through the kidneys and ureters. Urography is used to detect space-occupying lesions of the kidneys, pyelonephritis, hydronephrosis, vesicoureteral reflux, and kidney stones. Some people are allergic to the dye used for urography and may develop an anaphylactic reaction after its administration. Therefore, every person undergoing urography studies should be questioned about previous reactions to the dye or to similar dyes. If the test is considered essential in such people, premedication with antihistamines and corticosteroids may be used. The dye also reduces renal blood flow; acute renal failure can occur, particularly in people with vascular disease or preexisting renal insufficiency.

Other diagnostic tests include computed tomographic (CT) scans, magnetic resonance imaging (MRI), radionuclide imaging, and renal angiography. CT scans may be used to outline the kidneys and detect renal masses and tumors. *MRI* is becoming readily available. It is used in imaging the kidneys, retroperitoneum, and urinary bladder and is particularly useful in evaluating vascular abnormalities in and around the kidneys. *Radionuclide imaging* involves the injection of a radioactive material that subsequently is detected externally by a scintillation camera, which detects the radioactive emissions. Radionuclide imaging is used to evaluate renal function and structures as well as the ureters and bladder. It is particularly useful in evaluating the function of kidney transplants. *Renal angiography* provides x-ray pictures of the blood vessels that supply the kidneys. It involves the injection of a radiopaque dye directly into the renal artery. A catheter usually is introduced through the femoral artery and advanced under fluoroscopic view into the abdominal aorta; the catheter tip is then maneuvered into the renal artery and the dye is injected. This test is used in evaluating people suspected of having renal artery stenosis, abnormalities of renal blood vessels, or vascular damage to the renal arteries after trauma.

In summary, urinalysis and blood tests that measure levels of by-products of metabolism and electrolytes provide information about renal function. Cystoscopic examinations can be used for direct visualization of the urethra, bladder, and ureters. Ultrasonography can be used to determine kidney size, and renal radionuclide imaging can be used to evaluate the kidney structures. Radiologic methods such as excretory urography provide a means by which kidney structures such as the renal calyces, pelvis, ureters, and bladder can be outlined.

■ ACTION OF DIURETICS

In some disease states, it is desirable to increase urine output through the use of diuretics. Diuresis is the rapid passage of urine through the kidneys. Water reabsorption in the kidneys is largely passive and depends on sodium reabsorption. Therefore, most diuretics exert their action by interfering with sodium reabsorption. Only those substances that have a direct impact on the kidneys are regarded as diuretics. For example, digitalis preparations increase urine output in people with heart failure by increasing cardiac output, renal blood flow, and the GFR but are not diuretics. Because of diuretics' mechanism of action, it is logical to include a discussion of them in this chapter. There are four types of diuretics: (1) osmotic, (2) inhibitors of urine acidification, (3) inhibitors of sodium transport, and (4) aldosterone antagonists.

OSMOTIC DIURETICS

Osmotic diuretics, such as mannitol, are filtered in the glomerulus but not reabsorbed in the tubules. Because these substances are not reabsorbed, they serve to increase the osmolality of the tubular filtrate and cause a decrease in water reabsorption. The osmotic diuretics maintain a high urine volume after a hemolytic reaction or the ingestion of toxic substances, such as salicylates or barbiturates, which are excreted in the urine. These diuretics have a dehydrating effect on body tissues and may be useful in reducing intracranial or intraocular pressure. In diabetes mellitus, the renal tubular cells cannot reabsorb all the glucose that is filtered in the glomerulus, and the excess glucose acts as an osmotic diuretic.

INHIBITORS OF URINE ACIDIFICATION

Acetazolamide (Diamox), a carbonic anhydrase inhibitor, impairs the reaction that converts carbon dioxide and water to bicarbonate and hydrogen ions. Bicarbonate is poorly absorbed in the renal tubules; rather, it combines with hydrogen that is secreted into the tubule to form carbon dioxide and water. The carbon dioxide is then reabsorbed into the tubular cells, where it combines with water in a carbonic anhydrase–catalyzed reaction to form bicarbonate and hydrogen ions. When hydrogen ion secretion is blocked by the action of acetazolamide, both the bicarbonate ion and the sodium ion that accompany it are lost in the urine. The loss of bicarbonate results in a mild systemic acidosis. As this occurs, the kidneys resume the secretion of hydrogen ions, overcoming the effect of the carbonic anhydrase inhibition. Therefore, the action of acetazolamide is of short duration. This drug has been largely replaced by more effective diuretics, such as the thiazides. Acetazolamide also decreases the formation of aqueous humor and cerebrospinal fluid and continues to be used for that purpose.

INHIBITORS OF SODIUM TRANSPORT

Sodium reabsorption occurs in the proximal tubule, the thick ascending loop of Henle, and the distal tubule where aldosterone regulates sodium and potassium exchange. Diuretics that alter sodium transport can act at any of these levels.

Thiazide diuretics (*e.g.*, chlorothiazide [Diuri],

chlorthalidone [Hygroton], and hydrochlorothiazide [HydroDIURIL]) exert their action by preventing the reabsorption of chloride in the section of the tubule that is located between the thick ascending loop of Henle and the distal tubule. A decrease in sodium reabsorption follows the blocking of chloride reabsorption. The thiazides produce increased losses of potassium in the urine, uric acid retention, and some impairment in glucose tolerance. They are given orally and are suitable for long-term therapy.

Furosemide (Lasix), *ethacrynic acid* (Edecrin), and *bumetanide* (Bumex) are called *loop diuretics* because they exert their major effect on sodium chloride reabsorption that occurs in the thick ascending loop of Henle. About three fourths of the sodium that remains after passage through the proximal tubule is absorbed in the ascending loop of Henle. This means that diuretics that act at these sites can cause potent diuresis. Impairment of sodium reabsorption in the loop of Henle causes a decrease in the osmolarity of the interstitial fluid surrounding the collecting ducts and further impedes the kidneys' ability to concentrate urine. The loop diuretics cause potassium loss, increase uric acid retention, and impair glucose tolerance. These drugs also can cause hypovolemia. Ethacrynic acid is associated with eighth cranial nerve damage and deafness. Because of its ability to produce arteriolar vasodilatation and diuresis when given intravenously, furosemide often is administered in emergency treatment of pulmonary edema.

POTASSIUM-SPARING DIURETICS

The potassium-sparing diuretics increase the loss of sodium in the urine while enhancing potassium retention. There are two types of potassium-sparing diuretics: (1) those that act as direct aldosterone antagonists and (2) those that act independent of aldosterone. The first type (*e.g.*, spironolactone) act as competitive antagonists to aldosterone, thus increasing the loss of sodium in the urine while enhancing potassium retention. The second type (*e.g.*, triamterene, amiloride) act by interfering with the transport of sodium in the collecting tubule; they increase sodium excretion and decrease potassium excretion, particularly when potassium losses are high because of administration of another diuretic or an excess of aldosterone. These diuretics are used during states of mineralocorticoid excess and because of their effects on potassium excretion. Combination products that combine thiazide and potassium-sparing diuretics (hydrochlorothiazide/triamterene [Dyazide], hydrochlorothiazide/amiloride [Moduretic], hydrochlorothiazide/spironolactone [Aldactazide]) are available. Because of their mechanism of action, these diuretics may cause severe hyperkalemia. Spironolactone in particular has the potential for causing hyperkalemia.

In summary, diuretics are drugs that increase urine output. With the exception of osmotic diuretics, they exert their action by altering sodium transport. Osmotic diuretics are filtered in the glomerulus and reabsorbed in the tubules. They act by increasing the osmolarity of tubular fluid. Inhibitors of urine acidification, such as acetazolamide, prevent bicarbonate reabsorption and the accompanying sodium reabsorption. Loop diuretics block sodium reabsorption in the thick ascending loop of Henle and thiazide diuretics in the section of the tubule between the thick ascending loop of Henle and the distal tubule. The potassium-sparing diuretics decrease sodium reabsorption while causing potassium retention.

■ **REFERENCES**

1. Smith, H. (1953). *From fish to philosopher* (p. 4). Boston: Little, Brown.
2. Cormack, D.H. (1987). *Ham's histology* (9th ed., pp. 575–576). Philadelphia: J.B. Lippincott.
3. Guyton, A. (1991). *Textbook of medical physiology* (8th ed., pp. 343–356, 400). Philadelphia: W.B. Saunders.
4. Johnson, L.R. (1992). *Essentials of medical physiology* (pp. 342–356). New York: Raven Press.
5. Reidenberg, M.M. (1985). Kidney function and drug action. *New England Journal of Medicine, 313,* 816–817.
6. Vander, A.J. (1991). *Renal physiology* (4th ed.). New York: McGraw-Hill.

CHAPTER 32

ALTERATIONS IN RENAL FUNCTION

■ OBJECTIVES

After you have studied this chapter, you should be able to meet the following objectives:

■ Cite the effect of urinary obstruction in the fetus.

■ Describe the effects of urinary tract obstruction on renal structure and function.

■ Cite three theories that are used to explain the formation of kidney stones.

■ Explain the mechanisms of pain and infection that occur with kidney stones.

■ State the difference between the methods of ureterorenoscopy, percutaneous nephrostomy, and extracorporeal lithotripsy for removal of kidney stones.

■ Cite the organisms most responsible for urinary tract infections.

■ List three physiologic mechanisms that protect against urinary tract infections.

■ Describe factors that predispose to urinary tract infections in children, sexually active women, pregnant women, and older adults.

■ State common signs and symptoms of urinary tract infections in different age groups, including infants, toddlers, adolescents, adults, and older adults.

■ Describe measures used to reduce urinary tract infections caused by urinary catheters.

■ Use the terms *proliferation, sclerosis, membranous, diffuse, focal, segmental*, and *mesangial* to explain changes in glomerular structure that occur with glomerulonephritis.

■ Relate the proteinuria, hematuria, pyuria, oliguria, edema, hypertension, and azotemia that occur with glomerulonephritis to changes in glomerular structure.

■ Differentiate between the signs and symptoms that occur with the nephrotic syndrome, nephritic syndromes, rapidly progressive glomerulonephritis, and chronic glomerulonephritis in terms of clinical manifestations and prognosis.

■ Describe the genetic basis for renal cystic disease and the pathology of the disorder to the production of signs and symptoms.

■ Explain the fluid and electrolyte disorders that occur in renal tubular acidosis.

■ Explain the vulnerability of the kidneys to injury caused by drugs and toxins.

■ List the major manifestations of renal cancer.

More than 20 million North Americans suffer from diseases of the kidneys and urinary tract; about 80,000 die each year because of these diseases. Kidney and urinary tract diseases are a major cause of work loss among men and women: about 10% of America's outpatient visits result from such problems.[1] The number of people with chronic and disabling kidney disease has increased, in part because recent advances in dialysis and kidney transplantation methods are now keeping people alive who formerly would have died.

The kidneys are subject to many of the same types of disorders that affect other body structures, including developmental defects, infections, altered immune responses, and neoplasms. The kidneys filter blood from all parts of the body, and although many forms of kidney disease originate in the kidneys, referred to as primary kidney disorders, others develop secondary to disorders such as diabetes mellitus and systemic lupus erythematosus. The discussion in this chapter focuses on congenital disorders of the kidneys, obstructive disorders, urinary tract infections (UTIs), disorders of glomerular function, tubulointerstitial disorders, and neoplasms of the kidneys. Acute and chronic renal failure are discussed in Chapter 33, and the effects of other disease conditions, such as hypertension, shock, and diabetes mellitus, are discussed in other sections of the book.

■ CONGENITAL DISORDERS OF THE KIDNEYS

About 10% of people are born with potentially significant malformations of the urinary system. Congenital defects of the kidneys can take several forms. They can present as a decrease in the amount of kidney tissue (agenesis or hypoplasia) or as alterations in the form and position of the kidneys (kidney displacement or horseshoe kidney). Developmental anomalies of the fetal urinary tract are among the most commonly recognized congenital anomalies. The incidence of lethal anomalies is between 0.3 and 0.7 per 1000 births.[2]

AGENESIS AND HYPOPLASIA

The kidneys begin to develop early in the 5th week of gestation and start to function about 3 weeks later. Formation of urine is thought to begin in the 9th to 12th week of gestation; by the 32nd week, the fetal production of urine reaches about 28 mL/hour.[3] Urine is the main constituent of amniotic fluid. The relative amount of amniotic fluid can provide information about the status of fetal renal function.

The term *agenesis* refers to the absence of an organ because of failure to develop. *Dysgenesis* is the failure to develop normally. Unilateral agenesis of the kidneys is relatively common, and many people with this defect are unaware of its presence as long as the single kidney functions normally. Dysgenesis or agenesis of both kidneys is relatively rare; when either does occur, it often is accompanied by pulmonary hypoplasia. These defects are incompatible with life, and infants that have them are stillborn or die shortly after birth of either pulmonary or renal complications. In renal *hypoplasia*, the kidneys do not develop to normal size. Like agenesis, hypoplasia more commonly affects only one kidney. When both kidneys are affected, there is progressive development of renal failure. In pregnancies that involve babies with nonfunctional kidneys or outflow obstruction of the kidneys, the amount of amniotic fluid is small—a condition called *oligohydramnios*. The cause of fetal death in these babies is thought to be cord compression caused by the oligohydramnios.[2]

Recent animal experiments have shown that ureteral or bladder outlet obstruction causes renal dysgenesis or agenesis and pulmonary hypoplasia. Obstructions in fetal urinary outflow can now be diagnosed with ultrasound imaging. In the normal fetus, the kidneys can be visualized as early as 12 weeks. The sensitivity with which fetal obstructive uropathy can be diagnosed is low before 20 weeks and high between 35 and 40 weeks. In utero surgery has been done to relieve outflow obstructions with the hope of preventing pulmonary hypoplasia and renal dysgenesis. The procedure is experimental, and its success rate is still being determined.[4]

ALTERATIONS IN KIDNEY POSITION AND FORM

The developmental process can result in kidneys that lie outside their normal position, usually just above the pelvic brim or within the pelvis. Because of the abnormal position, kinking of the ureters and obstruction of urine flow may occur.

One of the most common alterations in kidney form is horseshoe kidney. This abnormality occurs in about 1 out of every 500 to 1000 persons.[5] In this disorder, the upper or lower poles of the two kidneys are fused, producing a horseshoe-shaped structure that is continuous along the midline of the body anterior to the great vessels. Most horseshoe kidneys are fused at the lower pole. The condition does not cause problems unless there is an associated defect in the renal pelvis or other urinary structures that favors obstruction of urine flow.

In summary, about 10% of infants are born with potentially significant malformations of the urinary system. These abnormalities can range from bilateral renal agenesis, which is incompatible with life, to hypogenesis of one kidney, which usually causes no problems unless the function of the single kidney is impaired. The developmental process can result in kidneys that lie outside their normal position. Because of the abnormal position, kinking of the ureters and obstruction of urine flow can occur.

■ OBSTRUCTIVE DISORDERS

Urinary obstruction can occur in people of any age and can involve any level of the urinary tract from the urethra to the renal pelvis. The conditions that cause urinary tract obstruction include developmental defects, calculi (stones), normal pregnancy, benign prostatic hyperplasia, scar tissue resulting from infection and inflammation, tumors, and neurologic disorders such as spinal cord injury and diabetic neuropathy (Fig. 32-1). The causes of urinary tract obstructions are summarized in Table 32-1.

MECHANISMS OF RENAL DAMAGE

The destructive effects of urinary obstruction on kidney structures are determined by the degree of obstruction (partial versus complete, unilateral versus bilateral) and the duration of obstruction. The two

TABLE 32-1. CAUSES OF URINARY TRACT OBSTRUCTION	
LEVEL OF OBSTRUCTION	**CAUSE**
Renal pelvis	Renal calculi
	Papillary necrosis
Ureter	Renal calculi
	Pregnancy
	Tumors that compress the ureter
	Ureteral stricture
	Congenital disorders of the ureterovesical junction and ureteropelvic junction strictures
Bladder and urethra	Bladder cancer
	Neurogenic bladder
	Bladder stones
	Prostatic hyperplasia or cancer
	Urethral strictures
	Congenital urethral defects

most damaging effects of urinary obstruction are (1) stasis of urine, which predisposes to infection and stone formation, and (2) development of a back pressure, which interferes with blood flow and destroys renal tissue.

A common complication of urinary tract obstruction is infection. Stagnation of urine predisposes to infection, which may spread throughout the urinary tract. When present, urinary calculi serve as foreign bodies and contribute to the infection. Once established, the infection is difficult to treat. It often is caused by urea-splitting organisms (*e.g.*, *Proteus*, staphylococci) that increase ammonia production and cause the urine to become alkaline. Calcium salts precipitate more readily in stagnant alkaline urine; thus, urinary tract obstructions also predispose to stone formation.

In situations of marked or complete obstruction, a back pressure develops because of a combination of continued glomerular filtration and impedance to urinary flow. Prolonged or severe partial obstruction causes irreversible kidney damage. Depending on the degree of obstruction, pressure builds up beginning at the site of obstruction and moving backward from the renal pelvis and calices. The severest effects typically occur at the level of the papillae because these structures are subjected to the greatest pressure. Damage to the nephrons and other functional components of the kidneys are due to compression atrophy from increased intrapelvic pressure and ischemic atrophy from disturbances in blood flow. Experimental studies have shown recovery of renal

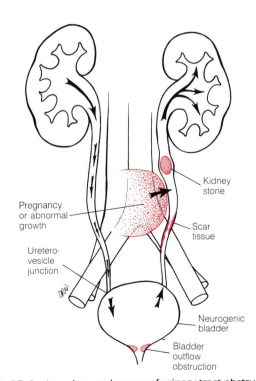

Pregnancy or abnormal growth

Uretero-vesicle junction

Kidney stone

Scar tissue

Neurogenic bladder

Bladder outflow obstruction

FIG. 32-1. Locations and causes of urinary tract obstruction.

function after release of complete obstruction of up to 4 weeks' duration.[6] Irreversible damage can, however, begin as early as 7 days.[6]

Hypertension is an occasional complication of urinary tract obstruction. It is more common in cases of unilateral obstruction in which renin secretion is enhanced, probably secondary to impaired renal blood flow. In these circumstances, removal of the obstruction often leads to a reduction in blood pressure. When hypertension accompanies bilateral obstruction, renin levels usually are normal and the elevated blood pressure probably is volume-related. The relief of bilateral obstruction leads to loss of volume and a fall in blood pressure.[7] In some cases, relieving the obstruction does not correct the hypertension.

Dilatation of the ureters and renal pelvis occurs with prolonged urinary tract obstruction. When the obstruction is in the distal ureter, the increased pressure dilates the proximal ureter, a condition called *hydroureter* (Fig. 32-2). Hydroureter is also a complication of bladder outflow obstruction owing to prostatic hyperplasia (see Chapter 36). With increasing

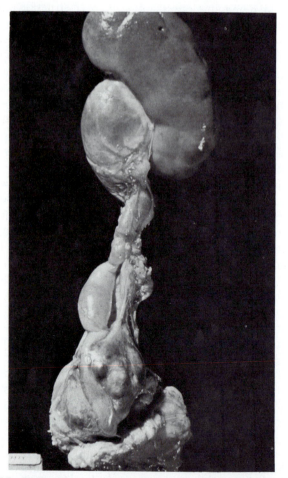

FIG. 32-2. Hydroureter caused by ureteral obstruction in a woman with cancer of the uterus.

pressure, the ureteral wall becomes severely stretched and loses its ability to undergo peristaltic contractions. In extreme cases, the ureter may become so dilated that it resembles a loop of bowel. *Hydronephrosis* refers to urine-filled dilatation of the renal pelvis and calices. The degree of hydronephrosis depends on the duration, degree, and site of obstruction. Bilateral hydronephrosis occurs only when the obstruction is below the level of the ureters. If the obstruction occurs at the level of the ureters or above, hydronephrosis is unilateral. Only in unilateral hydronephrosis are the advanced stages of hydronephrotic atrophy seen. The kidney eventually is destroyed and appears as a thin-walled shell that is filled with fluid.

MANIFESTATIONS

The manifestations of urinary obstruction depend on the site of obstruction, the cause, and the rapidity with which the condition developed. Most commonly there is pain, signs and symptoms of urinary tract infection, and manifestations of renal dysfunction, such as impaired ability to concentrate urine. Changes in urine output may be misleading, since output may be normal or even high in partial obstruction.

Pain, which often is the factor that causes a person to seek medical attention, is the result of distention of the bladder, collecting system, or renal capsule. Its severity is most closely related to the rate rather than the degree of distention.[7]

Pain most often occurs with acute obstruction, in which the distention of urinary structures is rapid. This is in contrast to chronic obstruction, in which distention is gradual and may not cause pain. Instead, gradual obstruction may produce only vague abdominal or back discomfort. When pain occurs, it is related to the site of obstruction. Obstruction of the renal pelvis or upper ureter causes pain and tenderness over the flank area. With lower levels of obstruction, the pain may radiate to the testes in the male or the labia in the female. With partial obstruction, particularly of the ureteropelvic junction, pain may occur during periods of high fluid intake, when a high rate of urine flow causes an acute hydronephrosis. Because of its visceral innervation, ureteral obstruction may produce reflex impairment of gastrointestinal tract peristalsis and motility with abdominal distention and, in severe cases, paralytic ileus.

DIAGNOSIS AND TREATMENT

Early diagnosis of urinary tract obstruction is important because the condition usually is treatable and a delay in therapy may result in permanent damage to the kidneys. Diagnostic methods vary with the symptoms. For example, a distended bladder suggests prostatic hyperplasia in the male. Radiologic methods commonly are used. The opaque kidney stones often are visible on x-ray films. Excretory urography, computed tomography (CT), and renal scanning using a radiopharmaceutical agent such as gallium may be used. Ultrasonography has proved to be the single most useful noninvasive diagnostic modality for urinary obstruction. Other diagnostic methods, such as urinalysis, are used to determine the extent of renal involvement and the presence of infection.

Treatment of urinary obstruction depends on the cause. Urinary stone removal may be necessary or surgical treatment of structural defects indicated.

RENAL CALCULI

The most common cause of urinary tract obstruction is urinary calculi. The term *nephrolithiasis* refers to kidney stones. Although stones can form in any part of the urinary tract, most develop in the kidneys. About 1 million North Americans are hospitalized each year with kidney stones, and an equal number are treated for stones without hospitalization.

Kidney stones are crystalline structures made up of materials that the kidneys normally excrete in the urine. They require a nidus, or nucleus, to form and a urinary environment that supports continued precipitation of stone components to grow. It is thought that the urine normally contains substances that inhibit precipitation of stone components. Three major theories are used to explain stone formation: the saturation theory, the inhibitor deficiency theory, and the matrix theory.[8] One or more of these theories may apply to stone formation in the same person. The saturation theory states that the risk of stone formation is increased when the urine is supersaturated with stone components (calcium salts, uric acid, magnesium ammonium phosphate, or cystine). The inhibitor theory suggests that people who have a deficiency of endogenous compounds that inhibit stone formation in their urine are at increased risk for stone formation. One such compound has recently been identified and termed *nephrocalcin*.[9] The matrix theory proposes that organic materials, such as mucopolysaccharides derived from the epithelial cells that line the tubules, act as a nidus for stone formation. This theory is based on the observation that organic matrix materials can be found in all layers of kidney stones. It is not known whether the matrix material contributes to the initiation of stone formation or the material is merely entrapped as the stone forms.

TYPES OF STONES

There are four basic types of kidney stones: calcium stones (oxalate or phosphate), magnesium ammonium phosphate stones, uric acid stones, and cystine stones. The causes and treatment measures for each of these types of renal stones are described in Table 32-2.

Most kidney stones (80% to 90%) are calcium stones—calcium oxalate, calcium phosphate, or a combination of the two materials. Calcium stones usually are associated with increased concentrations of calcium in the blood and urine. Excessive bone resorption caused by immobility, bone disease, hyperparathyroidism, and renal tubular acidosis are all contributing conditions. High oxalate concentrations in the blood and urine predispose to formation of oxalate stones.

Magnesium ammonium phosphate stones, also called *struvite stones*, form only in alkaline urine and in the presence of bacteria that possess an enzyme called urease, which splits the urea the kidneys secrete in large amounts to ammonia and carbon dioxide. The ammonia that is formed takes up a hydrogen ion to become an ammonium ion, increasing the *pH* of the urine so it becomes more alkaline. Phosphate levels are increased in alkaline urine, and because magnesium is always present, struvite stones form. These stones enlarge as the bacterial count grows and can increase in size until they fill an entire renal pelvis. Because of their shape, they are called *staghorn stones*. Staghorn stones are almost always associated with urinary tract infections and a persistently alkaline urine.

Uric acid stones develop in the presence of gout and high concentrations of uric acid in the urine. Unlike radiopaque calcium stones, uric acid stones are not visible on x-ray films. Hyperuricosuria may also contribute to calcium stone formation by acting as a nucleus for calcium oxalate stone formation. Cystine stones are rare. They are seen in cystinuria, which results from a genetic defect in renal transport of cystine.

MANIFESTATIONS

Renal colic is the term used to describe the colicky pain that accompanies urinary obstruction caused by kidney stones. The symptoms of renal colic are caused by stones 1 to 5 mm in diameter that can move into the ureter and obstruct flow. Classic ureteral colic is manifested by acute, intermittent, and excruciating pain in the flank and upper outer quadrant of the abdomen on the affected side. The pain may radiate to the lower abdominal quadrant, bladder area, perineum, or scrotum in the male. The skin may be cool

TABLE 32-2. COMPOSITION, CONTRIBUTING FACTORS, AND TREATMENT OF KIDNEY STONES

TYPE OF STONE	CONTRIBUTING FACTORS	TREATMENT
Calcium (oxalate and phosphate)	Hypercalcemia and hypercalciuria Immobilization Hyperparathyroidism Vitamin D intoxication Diffuse bone disease Milk-alkali syndrome Renal tubular acidosis	Treatment of underlying conditions Thiazide diuretics Increased fluid intake
	Hyperoxaluria Intestinal bypass surgery	Dietary restriction of foods high in oxalate
Magnesium ammonium phosphate (struvite)	Urea-splitting urinary tract infections	Treatment of urinary tract infection Acidification of the urine Increased fluid intake
Uric acid (urate)	Formed in acid urine with pH of about 5.5 Gout High-purine diet	Increased fluid intake Allopurinol for hyperuricuria Alkalinization of urine
Cystine	Cystinuria (inherited disorder of amino acid metabolism)	Increased fluid intake Alkalinization of urine

and clammy, and nausea and vomiting often are present.

DIAGNOSIS AND TREATMENT

Patients with kidney stones often present with acute renal colic, and the diagnosis is based on symptomatology and diagnostic tests, which include urinalysis, abdominal radiology, and excretory urography. Urinalysis provides information related to hematuria, infection, the presence of stone-forming crystals, and urine pH. At least 90% of stones are radiopaque and are readily visible on a plain film of the abdomen. Excretory urography uses a contrast medium that is filtered in the glomeruli to visualize the collecting system and the ureters of the kidneys. Retrograde urography, ultrasonography, CT scanning, and magnetic resonance imaging may also be used.

Treatment of acute renal colic usually is supportive. Pain relief may be needed during acute phases of obstruction, and antibiotic therapy may be necessary to treat urinary infections. Most stones that are less than 5 mm in diameter pass spontaneously. All urine should be strained during an attack in the hope of retrieving the stone for chemical analysis and determination of type. This information, along with a careful history and laboratory tests, affords the basis for long-term preventive measures.

A major goal of treatment in people who have passed kidney stones or have had them removed is to prevent their recurrence. Prevention requires investigation into the cause of stone formation using urine tests, blood chemistries, and stone analysis. Underlying disease conditions, such as hyperparathyroidism, are treated. Adequate fluid intake reduces the saturation of stone-forming crystals and needs to be encouraged. Depending on the type of stone that is formed, dietary changes or medications or both may be used to alter the concentration of stone-forming elements in the urine. For example, people who form calcium oxalate stones may need to decrease their intake of foods that are high in oxalate (*e.g.*, spinach, Swiss chard, cocoa, chocolate, pecans, and peanuts). Thiazide diuretics lower urinary calcium excretion by increasing the fractional absorption of calcium and reducing intestinal calcium absorption.[9] Measures to change the pH of the urine can also influence kidney stone formation. In people who lose the ability to lower the pH of or acidify their urine, there is an increase in the divalent and trivalent forms of urine phosphate that combines with calcium to form calcium phosphate stones. The formation of uric acid stones, on the other hand, is increased in acid urine;

stone formation can be reduced by raising the *p*H of urine to 6.0 to 6.5 with potassium alkali salts. Table 32-2 summarizes measures for preventing the recurrence of different types of kidney stones.

In some cases, stone removal may be necessary. Several methods are available for removing kidney stones: ureteroscopic removal, percutaneous removal, and extracorporeal lithotripsy. All these procedures eliminate the need for an open surgical procedure, which is another form of treatment. Struvite stones cannot be passed and require removal; extracorporeal lithotripsy and percutaneous removal can be used to reduce the damage incurred by these stones.

Ureteroscopic removal involves the passage of an instrument through the urethra into the bladder and then into the ureter. The development of high-quality optics has improved both the ease with which this procedure is performed and its outcome. The procedure, which is performed under fluoroscopic guidance, involves the use of various instruments for dilating the ureter and for grasping and removing the stone. Preprocedure radiologic studies using a contrast medium (excretory urography) are done to determine the position of the stone and direct the placement of the ureteroscope.[9]

Percutaneous nephrostomy involves the insertion through the flank of a small-gauge needle into the collecting system of the kidney; the needle tract is then dilated and an instrument called a *nephroscope* is inserted into the renal pelvis.[9] The procedure is performed under fluoroscopic guidance. Preprocedure radiologic and ultrasound examinations of the kidney and ureter are used in determining the placement of the nephroscope. Stones up to 1 cm can be removed through this method. Larger stones must be broken up with an electrohydraulic or ultrasonic lithotriptor (stone-breaker).

A nonsurgical treatment called *extracorporeal shock wave lithotripsy*, introduced in Germany in 1980, received U.S. Food and Drug Administration approval in 1984 for treatment of stones primarily in the renal calix and pelvis and the upper third of the ureter.[10] The procedure uses acoustic shock waves to fragment calculi into sand-like particles that are passed in the urine over the next few days. Because of the large amount of stone particles that are generated during the procedure, a ureteral catheter may be inserted to ensure adequate urine drainage. The catheter may be left in place for several weeks, depending on the stone burden and likelihood of ureteral obstruction.

In summary, obstruction of urine flow can occur at any level of the urinary tract. Among the causes of urinary tract obstruction are developmental defects, normal pregnancy, infection and inflammation, kidney stones, neurologic defects, and prostatic hypertrophy. Obstructive disorders produce

stasis of urine, thereby increasing the risk of infection and calculi formation, and result in back pressure that is damaging to kidney structures. There are four types of kidney stones: calcium (oxalate and phosphate) stones, which are associated with increased serum calcium levels; magnesium ammonium phosphate (struvite) stones, which are associated with UTIs; uric acid stones, which are related to elevated uric acid levels; and cystine stones, which are seen in cystinuria.

■ URINARY TRACT INFECTIONS

Urinary tract infections (UTIs) are the second most common type of bacterial infections seen by the physician (respiratory tract infections are first). The term *urinary tract infection* can refer to several distinct entities, including asymptomatic bacteriuria, symptomatic UTIs, lower UTIs such as cystitis, and upper UTIs such as pyelonephritis. Because of their ability to cause renal damage, upper UTIs are considered more serious than lower UTIs.

UTIs affect people of all ages. In infants, they occur more often in boys than in girls. After the first year of life, however, UTIs are more frequent in females because of the short urethra and because the vaginal vestibule can be easily contaminated with fecal flora. About 20% of all adult women develop at least one UTI during their lifetime. In men, the length of the urethra and the antibacterial properties of the prostatic fluid provide some protection from ascending UTIs until about age 50. After this age, prostatic hypertrophy becomes more common, and with it may come obstruction and UTI.

There are two routes by which bacteria can enter the kidneys: through the bloodstream and as an ascending infection from the lower urinary tract. Most infections are of the ascending type. Although the distal portion of the urethra often contains pathogens, the urine formed in the kidneys and found in the bladder normally is sterile or free of bacteria. This is because of the washout phenomenon, in which urine from the bladder normally washes bacteria out of the urethra. When a UTI occurs, the bacteria that have colonized the urethra, vagina, or perineal area often are responsible. *Escherichia coli* is by far the most common urinary pathogen. Other common pathogens include *Proteus, Klebsiella, Enterobacter,* and *Serratia* species.[11]

HOST–AGENT INTERACTIONS

Because certain people seem to be predisposed to developing UTIs, considerable interest has been focused on studies that relate host–agent interactions and identify factors that increase the risk of UTI. Studies have shown an increased risk of UTI in people with urinary obstruction and reflux, in pregnant and nonpregnant women, and in elderly people.[12] Furthermore, some conditions, including diabetes mellitus, pregnancy, immunosuppression, and upper urinary tract obstruction, are associated with serious morbidity from UTIs. Instrumentation and urinary catheterization are the most common predisposing factors in nosocomial UTIs.[13]

Host Defenses. In the development of a UTI, host defenses are matched against the virulence of the pathogen. The host defenses of the bladder have several components, including the washout phenomenon (in which bacteria are removed from the bladder and urethra during voiding), the protective mucin layer that lines the bladder and protects against bacterial invasion, and local immune responses. In the ureters, peristaltic movements facilitate the movement of urine from the renal pelvis through the ureters and into the bladder. Immune mechanisms, particularly secretory IgA immunoglobulins, are considered to provide an important antibacterial defense. Phagocytic blood cells further assist in the removal of bacteria from the urinary tract.

There has been a growing appreciation of the protective function of the bladder's mucin layer. It is thought that the epithelial cells that line the bladder synthesize protective substances that subsequently become incorporated into the mucin layer that adheres to the bladder wall. One theory proposes that the mucin layer acts by binding water, which then constitutes a protective barrier between the bacteria and the epithelium. Elderly and postmenopausal women produce less mucin than younger women, suggesting that estrogen may play a role in its secretion.

Pathogen Virulence. Investigations are focusing on the adherence properties of the bacteria that infect the urinary tract. These bacteria have fine protein filaments that help them adhere to receptors on the lining of urinary tract structures. These filaments are called *fimbriae* or *pili*. Among the factors that contribute to bacterial virulence, the type of fimbriae that the bacteria possess may be the most important. Bacteria with certain types of fimbriae are associated primarily with cystitis, and those with other types are associated with a high incidence of pyelonephritis. The bacteria associated with pyelonephritis are thought to have fimbriae that bind to carbohydrates that are specific to the surfaces of epithelial cells in this part of the urinary tract.

Obstruction and Reflux. Obstruction and reflux are important contributing factors in the development of UTIs. Any microorganisms that enter the bladder normally are washed out during voiding. When outflow is obstructed, urine remains in the bladder and acts as a medium for microbial growth;

the microorganisms in the contaminated urine can then ascend along the ureters to infect the kidneys. The presence of residual urine correlates directly with bacteriuria and with its recurrence after treatment.[14] Another aspect of bladder outflow obstruction and bladder distention is increased intravesicular pressure, which compresses blood vessels in the bladder wall, leading to a decrease in the mucosal defenses of the bladder.

In UTIs associated with stasis of urine flow, the obstruction may be either anatomic or functional. Anatomic obstructions include urinary tract stones, prostatic hyperplasia in elderly men, pregnancy, and obstructions of the posterior urethral valve, ureteropelvic junction, or ureterovesical junction. The latter types of obstruction have been reported in 3% to 21% of children who present with UTIs.[15] Functional obstructions include neurogenic bladder, infrequent voiding, detrusor (bladder) muscle instability, and constipation.

Reflux occurs when urine from the urethra moves into the bladder (urethrovesical reflux) or from the bladder into the ureters (vesicoureteral reflux). In women, a urethrovesical reflux can occur during activities such as coughing or squatting, in which an increase in intraabdominal pressure causes the urine to be squeezed into the urethra and then to flow back into the bladder as the pressure decreases. This can also happen when the act of voiding is abruptly interrupted. Because the urethral orifice frequently is contaminated with bacteria, the reflux mechanism may cause bacteria to be drawn back into the bladder.

A second type of reflux mechanism can occur at the level of the bladder and ureter. This reflux mechanism is called the *vesicoureteral reflux*. Peristaltic movements propel urine from the kidneys to the bladder. In vesicoureteral reflux, urine is propelled from the bladder through the ureters into the kidneys. It most commonly is seen in children with UTIs and is believed to result from congenital defects in length, diameter, muscle structure, or innervation of the submucosal segment of the ureter. It is also seen in adults with obstruction to bladder outflow.

URINARY TRACT INFECTIONS IN WOMEN

In women, the urethra is short and in proximity to the vagina and rectum, offering little protection against entry of microorganisms into the bladder. There is a peak incidence of these infections in the 15- to 24-year-old age group, suggesting that hormonal and anatomic changes associated with puberty as well as sexual activity contribute to UTIs.

The role of sexual activity in the development of urethritis and cystitis is controversial. The well-documented "honeymoon cystitis" suggests that sexual activity may contribute to such infections in susceptible women. The anterior urethra usually is colonized with bacteria; urethral massage or sexual intercourse can force these bacteria back into the bladder. A nonpharmacologic approach to the treatment of frequent UTIs associated with sexual intercourse is to increase fluid intake before intercourse and to void soon after intercourse. This procedure uses the washout phenomena to remove bacteria from the bladder.

UTIs are more common during pregnancy. This is particularly true of those women who have bacteriuria during their initial prenatal visit. Normal changes in the functioning of the urinary tract that occur during pregnancy predispose to UTIs. These changes involve the collecting system of the kidneys and include dilatation of the renal calices, pelves, and ureters that begins during the first trimester and becomes most pronounced during the third trimester. This dilatation of the upper urinary system is accompanied by a reduction in the peristaltic activity of the ureters that is thought to result from the muscle-relaxing effects of progesterone-like hormones and the mechanical obstruction from the enlarging uterus. In addition to the changes in the kidneys and ureters, the bladder becomes displaced from its pelvic position to a more abdominal position, producing further alterations in ureteral position.[16]

The complications of UTI during pregnancy include acute pyelonephritis, persistent bacteriuria, chronic pyelonephritis, toxemia of pregnancy, and premature delivery. Evidence suggests that few women become bacteriuric during pregnancy. Rather, it would appear that symptomatic UTIs during pregnancy reflect preexisting asymptomatic bacteriuria; that changes that occur during pregnancy simply permit the prior urinary colonization to lead to symptomatic infection and invasion of the kidneys.[17] About 20% to 40% of women with bacteriuria detected early in pregnancy and not treated will develop symptomatic UTIs later in pregnancy.[17] Because bacteriuria may occur as an asymptomatic condition in pregnant women, it is recommended that women be screened for bacteriuria during their first prenatal visit. Women with bacteriuria should be followed closely, and infections should be properly treated to prevent complications.

URINARY TRACT INFECTIONS IN CHILDREN

UTIs occur in as many as 5% of female and 1% to 2% of male children.[18] As many as 80% of children with uncomplicated UTI have recurrences. Children who are at increased risk for bacteriuria or symptomatic UTIs are premature babies discharged from neonatal intensive care units; children with systemic or immunologic disease or urinary tract abnormalities

such as neurogenic bladder or vesicoureteral reflux; those with a family history of UTI or anomalies with reflux; and girls younger than age 5 with a history of UTI.[18]

Many neonates with UTI have bacteremia and may show signs and symptoms of septicemia, including fever, hypothermia, apneic spells, poor skin perfusion, abdominal distention, diarrhea, vomiting, lethargy, and irritability. Older infants may present with feeding problems, failure to thrive, diarrhea, vomiting, fever, and foul-smelling urine. Many toddlers present with abdominal pain, vomiting, diarrhea, abnormal voiding patterns, foul-smelling urine, fever, and poor growth. In older children with lower UTI, the classic features of UTI (enuresis, frequency, dysuria, and suprapubic discomfort) are more common. Fever, chills, nausea, vomiting, and flank pain occur in children with upper UTI.

Diagnosis is based on a careful history of the symptomatology and voiding patterns; physical examination to determine fever, hypertension, abdominal or suprapubic tenderness, and other manifestations of UTI; and urinalysis to determine bacteriuria, pyuria, proteinuria, and hematuria. A positive urine culture that is obtained correctly is essential for the diagnosis. Additional diagnostic methods may be needed to determine the cause of the disorder. The presence of urinary symptoms in the absence of bacteriuria suggests vaginitis, urethritis, sexual molestation, the use of irritating bubble baths, pinworms, or viral cystitis. In adolescent girls, a history of dysuria and vaginal discharge makes vaginitis or vulvitis a consideration.

The approach to treatment is based on the clinical severity of the infection, the site of infection (lower versus upper urinary tract), the risk of sepsis, and the presence of structural abnormalities. The immediate treatment of infants and young children is essential. Most infants with symptomatic UTI and children with clinical evidence of acute upper UTIs require hospitalization and intravenous antibiotic therapy. Most children with uncomplicated UTIs are treated with antibiotics for 7 to 10 days.

Although most children respond to treatment, severe infection can result in renal scarring, hypertension, and compromised renal function. Children with reflux have a much higher incidence of pyelonephritis and renal scarring than those without reflux.[18]

URINARY TRACT INFECTIONS IN ELDERLY PEOPLE

UTIs are relatively common in elderly people. It has been reported that 20% of elderly women and 10% of elderly men living at home have bacteriuria. These numbers increase to about 25% of women and 20% of men living in nursing homes or extended-care facilities.[19] The vast majority of these infections follow invasion of the urinary tract by the ascending route. Several factors predispose elderly people to UTIs: (1) immobility resulting in poor bladder emptying, (2) bladder outflow obstruction caused by prostatic hyperplasia or kidney stones, (3) bladder ischemia caused by urine retention, (4) senile vaginitis, (5) constipation, and (6) diminished bactericidal activity of urine and prostatic secretions.[20] Added to these risks are other health problems that necessitate instrumentation of the urinary tract. UTIs have been shown to develop in 1% of ambulatory patients after a single catheterization and within 3 to 4 days in essentially all patients with indwelling catheters.[19]

Furthermore, elderly people may not present with the usual symptoms of UTI. Even when symptoms of lower UTIs are present, they may be difficult to interpret because uninfected elderly people commonly experience urgency, frequency, and incontinence. Typical signs and symptoms of upper UTIs (*e.g.*, pyelonephritis) include fever, chills, flank pain, and tenderness, but these features may be altered or absent in elderly people.[19] Sometimes no symptoms occur until the infection is far advanced.

LOWER URINARY TRACT INFECTIONS

Lower UTIs include the presence of bacteria in the urine, cystitis, and catheter-induced infections. Pyelonephritis and upper UTI are discussed with tubulointerstitial disorders.

CYSTITIS

An acute episode of cystitis or bladder infection is characterized by frequency of urination (sometimes as often as every 20 minutes), lower abdominal discomfort, and burning and pain on urination (dysuria). There also may be systemic signs of infection, with fever and generalized malaise. If there are no complications, the symptoms disappear within 48 hours. This type of cystitis is mainly a disorder of young women. The symptoms of cystitis may also represent urethritis or vaginitis attributable to *Trichomonas*, bacterial vaginosis, chlamydial infection, or gonorrhea.

CATHETER-INDUCED INFECTIONS

Urinary catheters are tubes made of latex or plastic. They are inserted through the urethra into the bladder for the purpose of draining urine. They are a source of urethral irritation and provide a means for entry of microorganisms into the urinary tract. Indwelling catheters are used in about 10% of patients admitted to general hospitals.[21] A closed drainage system (closed to air and other sources of contamination) and careful attention to perineal hygiene (cleansing of the area around the urethral meatus) help to prevent infections in people who require an indwelling catheter. Careful hand washing and early detection and treatment of UTIs are also essential. When an indwelling catheter is used, the risk of infection is increased with the use of broad-spectrum antibiotics and catheter irrigations; in fact, hospital patients themselves are cited as the most common reservoir of infection.

DIAGNOSIS AND TREATMENT

Early diagnosis and treatment of UTI are essential for preventing permanent kidney damage. Screening of high-risk groups and attention to care of patients with indwelling catheters are important measures. Pregnant women and people with diabetes or renal problems who are at risk for developing UTIs usually can be managed in the physician's office.

The diagnosis of UTI usually is based on symptoms and on examination of the urine for the presence of microorganisms. Bacteriuria, or the presence of bacteria in the urine, often is used in diagnosing UTIs. The source of bacteria in the urine can be contamination of the urine specimen, simple colonization of the urinary tract, or bacterial invasion of urinary structures. Colonization usually is defined as the multiplication of microorganisms in or on a host without apparent evidence of invasiveness or tissue injury. A commonly accepted criterion for diagnosis of a UTI is the presence of more than 100,000 (10^5) organisms per milliliter of urine. The accuracy of the diagnosis is strengthened if such numbers are found in two consecutive urine specimens and if the bacteria are of a single type. Contaminated urine specimens commonly contain several types of microorganisms.

Care is needed in collecting urine specimens representative of bladder urine. Specimens that are kept for longer than 1 hour must be refrigerated to prevent the contaminating organisms from multiplying. Catheterized urine specimens, once common, have largely been replaced with clean voided specimens. To obtain a clean voided specimen, the area around the urethra is carefully cleansed and a midstream specimen is obtained by having the person void directly into a sterile container. This method usually is adequate and eliminates the risk of introducing microorganisms into the bladder during insertion of a catheter. In infants and sometimes in other age groups, suprapubic aspiration may be done to obtain a sample of bladder urine.

In addition to the bacterial count, the urine leukocyte count is used; the presence of pyuria (more than 10 leukocytes per microliter of uncentrifuged urine) indicates host injury as opposed to asymptomatic bacterial colonization. When necessary, x-ray films, ultrasound, and CT and renal scans are used to identify contributing factors, such as obstruction.

Immunofluorescence studies may be done to determine whether the infection involves the upper urinary tract. These tests are expensive and usually are not done routinely. Detailed identification and antibiotic sensitivity tests often are done in cases of chronic infection. The treatment of UTI is based on the type of infection that is present (lower or upper UTI) and the presence of contributing host–agent factors.

Antibiotics typically are used to treat acute infection. The forcing of fluids may relieve signs and symptoms and is used as an adjunct to antibiotic treatment.

Most lower UTIs are treated successfully with antimicrobial therapy and increased fluid intake. Acute cystitis usually is treated with a 3-day course of trimethoprim with sulfamethoxazole or ampicillin. With pyelonephritis, there is risk of permanent kidney damage, so these infections are treated more aggressively. Treatment with an appropriate antimicrobial agent usually is continued for 10 to 14 days. Hospitalization may be recommended during the early stages of infection until a response to treatment is observed.

Chronic infection is more difficult to treat. Because it often is associated with obstructive uropathy or reflux flow of urine, diagnostic tests usually are performed to detect such abnormalities. When possible, the condition causing the reflux flow or obstruction is corrected. Most people with recurrent UTIs are treated with antibiotics for 10 to 14 days in doses sufficient to maintain high urine levels and investigated for obstruction or other causes of infection. Men in particular should be investigated for obstructive disorders or a prostatic focus of infection.

In summary, UTI is the second most common type of bacterial infection seen by the practicing physician. Infections can range from simple bacteriuria to severe kidney infections that cause irreversible kidney damage. Most UTIs ascend from the urethra and bladder. A number of factors interact in determining the predisposition to development of UTIs, including urinary tract obstruction, urine stasis and reflux, pregnancy-induced changes in urinary tract function, age-related changes in the urinary tract, changes in the protective mechanisms of the bladder and ureters, impaired immune function, and virulence of the pathogen. Urinary tract catheters and urinary instrumentation contribute to the incidence of UTIs. Early diag-

nosis and treatment of UTI are essential to preventing permanent kidney damage.

■ DISORDERS OF GLOMERULAR FUNCTION

The glomeruli are tufts of capillaries that lie between the afferent and efferent arterioles. The capillaries of the glomeruli are arranged in lobules and supported by a stalk consisting of mesangial cells and a basement membrane–like extracellular matrix (Fig. 32-3). The glomerular membrane is composed of three layers: an endothelial layer lining the capillary, a basement membrane, and a layer of epithelial cells forming the outer surface of the capillary and also lining Bowman's capsule. The epithelial cells are attached to the basement membrane by discrete cytoplasmic extensions, the foot processes (podocytes).

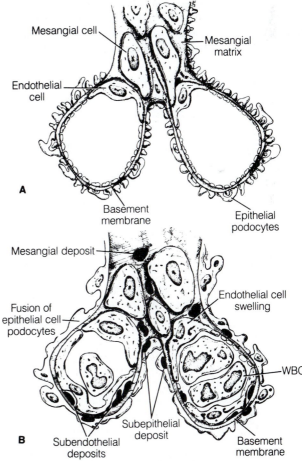

FIG. 32-3. Schematic representation of glomerulus. (**A**) Normal; (**B**) localization of immune deposits (mesangial, subendothelial, subepithelial) and changes in glomerular architecture associated with injury. (Whitley, K., Keane, W. F., & Vernier, R. L. [1984]. Acute glomerulonephritis: A clinical overview. *Medical Clinics of North America, 68*(2), 263)

Within the glomeruli, blood is filtered and the urine filtrate formed. The capillary membrane is selectively permeable: it allows water, electrolytes, and dissolved particles, such as glucose and amino acids, to leave the capillary and enter Bowman's space and prevents larger particles, such as plasma proteins and blood cells, from leaving the blood.

Glomerulonephritis, an inflammatory process that involves glomerular structures, is the leading cause of chronic renal failure in the United States, accounting for one half of people who need dialysis. The disorder causes 12,000 deaths a year and is responsible for $20 million in work loss.[1] There are many causes of glomerular disease. The disease may occur as a primary condition in which the glomerular pathology is the only disease present, or it may occur as a secondary condition in which the glomerular pathology occurs secondary to another disease, such as vasculitis or systemic lupus erythematosus. An understanding of the various forms of glomerular pathology has emerged only recently. Much of this understanding can be attributed to advances in immunobiology and electron microscopy, development of animal models, and increased use of renal biopsy during the early stages of glomerular disease.

Although little is known about the causative agents or triggering events that produce glomerular disease, it is clear that most cases of primary glomerular disease and many cases of secondary disease have an immune origin.[22, 23] Two types of immune mechanisms have been implicated from research studies: (1) injury resulting from deposition of soluble circulating antigen–antibody complexes in the glomeruli and (2) injury resulting from antibodies reacting with insoluble fixed glomerular antigens. With circulating immune complexes, the kidneys are the "innocent bystanders" because the antigen is not of glomerular origin and the kidneys do not initiate the event.[7] The antigen of the immune complexes may be of endogenous origin, such as DNA in systemic lupus erythematosus, or it may be of exogenous origin, such as streptococcal membrane antigens in poststreptococcal glomerulonephritis. The antigen frequently is unknown. Whatever the inciting antigen, the antigen–antibody complex is formed in the circulation and becomes trapped in the glomerular membrane as blood is being filtered. The antigen–antibody complexes probably produce injury through complement-mediated mechanisms such as cell lysis or chemotaxis, which draws leukocytes to the area.[23] Once deposited, the immune complexes eventually are degraded by infiltrating monocytes and phagocytic mesangial cells. If the inciting antigen is short-lived, as in poststreptococcal glomerulonephritis, the inflammatory changes cause an acute response and then subside. If the antigen is continu-

ously being produced, repeated inflammatory reactions may occur, leading to chronic glomerulonephritis.

The fixed antigens that cause glomerular disease may have their origin in the glomerulus or may be planted there from another source. The best-known model is the so-called antiglomerular membrane antibodies implicated in Goodpasture's syndrome. With this type of injury, antibodies are directed against glomerular basement membrane antigens. Damage to the glomeruli probably is complement- and leukocyte-mediated, although other mechanisms may be involved. Activation of complement initiates the generation of chemotactic agents and the recruitment of neutrophils. The neutrophils release proteases that cause breakdown of the glomerular basement membrane and release of free radicals that cause cell damage. Injury may also occur without complement involvement. In these cases, other factors, such as platelet interactions, arachidonic acid metabolites, and free radicals, have been suggested as injurious agents. There is also evidence that intraglomerular hemodynamic changes, such as increased intracapillary pressures or filtration rates, may contribute to glomerular injury and the progression of glomerulonephritis.

The cellular changes that occur with glomerular disease include proliferative, sclerotic, and membranous changes. The term *proliferative* refers to an increase in the cellular components of the glomerulus, regardless of origin; *sclerotic*, to an increase in the noncellular components of the glomerulus (primarily collagen); and *membranous*, to an increase in the thickness of the glomerular capillary wall, often caused by immune complex deposition. Glomerular changes can be *diffuse*, involving all glomeruli and all parts of the glomeruli; *focal*, where only some glomeruli are affected and others are essentially normal; *segmental*, involving only a certain segment of each glomeruli; or *mesangial*, affecting only the mesangial cell.[7] Figure 32-3 shows changes associated with glomerular disease.

Diseases of the glomeruli disrupt glomerular filtration and alter the capillary membrane so that it becomes permeable to plasma proteins and blood cells. Increased glomerular capillary permeability leads to proteinuria, hematuria, pyuria, oliguria, edema, hypertension, and azotemia (increased levels of nitrogenous wastes in the blood). In many cases, early glomerular disease is asymptomatic, and the condition often is discovered incidentally through abnormal findings on urinalysis (primarily proteinuria, azotemia) or elevated blood pressure.

Proteinuria, predominantly albuminuria, provides the most important evidence of glomerular injury. With progression from mild to severe glomerular injury, progressively increased amounts of larger plasma proteins, such as gamma globulins, are found in the urine. Hematuria can result from bleeding anywhere in the urinary tract. With glomerular disease, hematuria develops because of active inflammatory disease and damage to the capillary membrane. The hematuria may be minimal and detected only on microscopic examination, or it may be sufficient to discolor the urine. The red blood cells are either entrapped in casts or degraded by tubular enzymes so that the urine is smoke- or cola-colored. Red blood cells in the urine sediment are pathognomonic of glomerular inflammation (glomerulonephritis). The passage of polymorphonuclear leukocytes through the glomerular membrane causes pyuria.

Oliguria, edema, hypertension, and azotemia commonly accompany glomerular injury. Oliguria occurs when glomerular injury is severe enough to produce a marked decrease in glomerular filtration. The edema of glomerular disease has two causes: loss of albumin in the urine and dilution of albumin caused by retention of sodium and water. The effect is to lower plasma colloidal osmotic pressure, causing edema (see Chapter 29). The hypertension is due to the increase in vascular volume caused by sodium and water retention and, possibly, to increased synthesis of vasoconstrictor substances by the kidneys. Azotemia results from both a reduction in the filtration of urea and other nitrogenous wastes in the glomeruli and an increase in tubular reabsorption of these substances because of renal hypoperfusion.

Glomerular pathologies have been grouped into two categories: (1) nephrotic syndrome, which affects the integrity of the glomerular capillary membrane, and (2) nephritic syndrome, which evokes an inflammatory response within the glomeruli.

NEPHROTIC SYNDROME

Nephrotic syndrome is not a specific glomerular disease but a constellation of clinical findings that result from increased glomerular permeability to protein. It is characterized by massive proteinuria (a daily loss of 3.5 g or more) and lipiduria (free fat, oval bodies, fatty casts). There is an associated hypoalbuminemia (less than 3 g/dL), generalized edema, and hyperlipidemia (cholesterol >300 mg/dL).

The generalized edema, which usually is the first manifestation and can be so severe as to be incapacitating, results from the decrease in colloidal osmotic pressure that accompanies the loss of plasma proteins. Other factors, such as increased sodium and water retention, may also play a role in edema formation. The hyperlipidemia is characterized by

elevated levels of both triglycerides and cholesterol. It is believed that hyperlipidemia results when a compensatory increase in albumin synthesis by the liver serves as a stimulus for increased synthesis of low-density lipoproteins. Because of the elevated levels of low-density lipoproteins, people with nephrotic syndrome are at increased risk of developing atherosclerosis. The loss of immunoglobulins in the urine is believed to increase susceptibility to infection, especially those caused by staphylococci and pneumococci. Another problem that arises in people with nephrosis is thrombosis (arterial and venous), presumably from an imbalance in coagulation factors that accompanies loss of plasma proteins in the urine. In general, low-molecular-weight plasma proteins, such as factors IX, X, XI, and XII as well as prothrombin, plasminogen, antiplasmin, antithrombin III, and α-antitrypsin, are lost in the urine. In contrast, those of high molecular weight (factors V, VII, and VIII and von Willebrand's factor) remain in the circulation.[24] It is thought that an imbalance between procoagulation and anticoagulation factors may be responsible for the high incidence of thrombosis.

Nephrosis can occur as a primary disorder or secondary to glomerular changes caused by systemic diseases such as diabetes mellitus and systemic lupus erythematosus. The relative frequency of these causes varies with age. In children under age 15, nephrotic syndrome is almost always caused by primary glomerular disease, whereas in adults, it often occurs as a secondary disorder.

Among the primary glomerular lesions leading to nephrotic syndrome are (1) minimal change disease, characterized by diffuse loss (fusion) of foot processes from the epithelial layer of the glomerular membrane; (2) focal sclerosis, in which there is sclerosis (increased collagen deposition) of some of the tufts within a glomerulus; (3) membranous glomerulopathy, in which there is diffuse thickening of the glomerular basement membrane because of deposition of immune complexes; and (4) membranoproliferative glomerulonephritis, in which there is both basement membrane thickening and cellular proliferation.

NEPHRITIC SYNDROME

Nephritic syndrome is a clinical complex characterized by hematuria with red cell casts in the urine, a diminished glomerular filtration rate (GFR), azotemia, oliguria, and hypertension. Although there may also be proteinuria and edema, these are not sufficient to cause nephrotic syndrome.

Nephritic syndrome is caused by diseases that provoke a proliferative inflammatory response of the endothelial, mesangial, or epithelial cells of the glomeruli. The inflammatory process damages the capillary wall, permitting red blood cells to escape into the urine (hematuria) and producing hemodynamic changes that cause a decrease in the GFR. The disorder may result from primary disease of the glomerulus or as a secondary effect of another disease condition, such as vasculitis or systemic lupus erythematosus. It can be initiated by immune complexes, antiglomerular basement antibodies, cellular mechanisms alone, or blood-borne leukocytes (neutrophils, monocytes, and lymphocytes). One of the most common primary nephritic disorders is acute proliferative glomerulonephritis, especially poststreptococcal glomerulonephritis.

ACUTE PROLIFERATIVE GLOMERULONEPHRITIS

The most commonly recognized form of acute nephritic syndrome is diffuse proliferative glomerulonephritis, which follows infections caused by strains of group A β-hemolytic streptococci. Diffuse proliferative glomerulonephritis may also occur after infections by other organisms, including staphylococci and a number of viral agents, such as those responsible for mumps, measles, and chickenpox. With this type of nephritis, the inflammatory response is caused by an immune reaction that occurs when circulating immune complexes become entrapped in the glomerular membrane. Proliferation of the endothelial cells lining the glomerular capillary (endocapillary form of the disease) and the mesangial cells lying between the endothelium and the epithelium follows (see Fig. 32-3). The capillary membrane swells and becomes permeable to plasma proteins and blood cells. Although the disease is seen primarily in children, adults of any age can also be affected.

The classic case of poststreptococcal glomerulonephritis follows a streptococcal infection by about 10 days to 2 weeks—the time needed for the development of antibodies. Oliguria, which develops as the GFR decreases, is one of the first symptoms. Proteinuria and hematuria follow because of increased glomerular capillary wall permeability. The blood is degraded by materials in the urine, and a cola-colored urine may be the first sign of the disorder. Sodium and water retention give rise to edema (particularly of the face and hands) and hypertension. Important laboratory findings include an elevated streptococcal exoenzyme (antistreptolysin-O) titer, a decline in C3 complement (see Chapter 13), and the presence of cryoglobulins (large immune complexes) in the serum.

Treatment for acute poststreptococcal glomerulonephritis is largely symptomatic. The acute symptoms usually begin to subside in about 10 days to 2 weeks, although in some children, the proteinuria may persist for several months. The immediate prognosis is favorable, and about 95% of children recover spontaneously. The outlook for adults is less favorable; about 60% recover completely. In the remainder of cases, the lesions eventually resolve, but there may be permanent kidney damage.

RAPIDLY PROGRESSIVE GLOMERULONEPHRITIS

Like nephrotic syndrome and nephritic disorders, rapidly progressive glomerulonephritis does not have a single, specific cause. As its name implies, this type of glomerulonephritis is rapidly progressive: it involves a 50% decrease in the GFR within 3 months. About 90% of those affected develop renal failure and require dialysis or transplantation.[7] The disorder is characterized by focal and segmental proliferation of glomerular cells as well as activation and recruitment of monocytes (macrophages) with formation of crescent-shaped structures that obliterate the Bowman's space. Most people with this disorder have evidence of antibodies directed against the basement membrane. Among the systemic diseases associated with this form of glomerulonephritis are vasculitis, systemic lupus erythematosus, acute poststreptococcal glomerulonephritis (usually in adults), and primary glomerular diseases, such as Goodpasture's syndrome.

CHRONIC GLOMERULONEPHRITIS

Chronic glomerulonephritis represents the end stage of the many types of glomerulonephritis. Histologically, it is characterized by small kidneys with sclerosed glomeruli. It seldom develops in children with acute poststreptococcal glomerulonephritis and frequently is seen in people who survive the acute phase of rapidly progressive glomerulonephritis. In about one fourth of the people who present with chronic glomerulonephritis, there is no history of glomerular disease.[4] In most cases, chronic glomerulonephritis develops insidiously and is characterized by signs and symptoms of chronic renal failure (see Chapter 33). The disease is progressive but at widely varying rates.

DIABETIC GLOMERULOSCLEROSIS

Diabetic nephropathy, or kidney disease, is a major complication of diabetes mellitus. About 55% of people with type I insulin-dependent diabetes and 30% of people with type II non–insulin-dependent diabetes develop end-stage kidney disease.[7] The glomerulus is the most commonly affected structure in diabetic nephropathy, thickening of the glomerular basement membrane and development of diffuse or nodular glomerulosclerosis being the most prominent types of pathology. Widespread thickening of the glomerular capillary basement membrane occurs in almost all people with diabetes and can occur without evidence of proteinuria.[5] Diffuse glomerulosclerosis involves an increase in mesangial matrix and a thickening of the glomerular basement membrane. In nodular glomerulosclerosis, also known as *Kimmelstiel-Wilson syndrome*, there is nodular deposition of hyaline in the mesangial portion of the glomerulus. As the sclerotic process progresses in both the diffuse and the nodular form of glomerulosclerosis, there is complete obliteration of the glomerulus with impairment of renal function. Although the mechanisms of glomerular changes in diabetes are uncertain, they are thought to represent enhanced or defective synthesis of the basement membrane and mesangial matrix with an inappropriate incorporation of glucose into the noncellular components of these glomerular structures.

The manifestations of diabetic glomerulosclerosis include recurrent proteinuria with slow but steady progression to renal failure. The condition occurs more frequently in people with poorly controlled diabetes, which emphasizes the need for adherence to treatment methods that improve metabolic control.

HYPERTENSIVE GLOMERULAR DISEASE

Renal failure and azotemia occur in 1% to 5% of people with long-standing hypertension.[4] Hypertension is associated with a number of changes in glomerular structures, including sclerotic changes. As the glomerular vascular structures thicken and perfusion diminishes, the blood supply to the nephron decreases, causing the kidneys to lose some of their ability to concentrate the urine. This may be evidenced by nocturia. Blood urea nitrogen levels may also become elevated, particularly during periods of water deprivation. Proteinuria may occur as a result of changes in glomerular structure.

In summary, diseases of the glomerulus disrupt glomerular filtration and alter the permeability of glomerular capillary membrane to plasma proteins and blood cells. Glomerulonephritis is a term used to describe a group of diseases that cause inflammation and injury of the glomerulus. These diseases disrupt the capillary membrane and cause proteinuria, hematuria, pyuria, oliguria, edema, hypertension, and azote-

mia. Almost all types of glomerulonephritis are due to immune mechanisms.

Glomerular pathologies have been grouped into four categories: (1) nephrotic syndrome, which affects the integrity of the glomerular capillary membrane and is characterized by massive proteinuria, hypoalbuminemia, generalized edema, lipiduria, and hyperlipidemia; (2) nephritic syndrome, which evokes an inflammatory response within the glomeruli and is characterized by hematuria with red cell casts in the urine, a diminished GFR, azotemia, oliguria, and hypertension; (3) rapidly progressive glomerulonephritis, characterized by rapid and progressive loss of renal function; and (4) chronic glomerulonephritis, in which there is an insidious onset of uremia or renal failure. Glomerulosclerosis is a major complication of diabetes mellitus and hypertension.

■ TUBULOINTERSTITIAL DISORDERS

A number of disorders affect renal tubular structures, including the proximal and distal tubules. Most also affect the interstitial tissue that surrounds the tubules; thus, the disorders often are called *tubulointerstitial diseases*. These disorders include acute tubular necrosis (see Chapter 33), renal tubular acidosis, pyelonephritis, renal cystic disease, and the effects of drugs and toxins.

Tubulointerstitial renal diseases may be divided into acute and chronic disorders. The acute disorders are characterized by their sudden onset and by signs and symptoms of interstitial edema; they include acute pyelonephritis and acute hypersensitivity reaction to drugs. The chronic disorders produce interstitial fibrosis, atrophy, and mononuclear infiltrates; most people are asymptomatic until late in the course of the disease. In the early stages, tubulointerstitial diseases commonly are manifested by fluid and electrolyte imbalances that reflect subtle changes in tubular function. These manifestations can include inability to concentrate urine, as evidenced by polyuria and nocturia; interference with acidification of urine, resulting in metabolic acidosis; and diminished tubular reabsorption of sodium and other substances.[25]

RENAL TUBULAR ACIDOSIS

Renal tubular acidosis refers to a group of tubular disorders that result in acidosis and its subsequent complications, including metabolic bone disease, kidney stones, and growth failure in children. There are two main types of renal tubular acidosis: proximal tubular disorders that affect bicarbonate reabsorption and distal tubular defects that affect the secretion of fixed metabolic acids.[26, 27]

The proximal tubule is the site where 90% to 95%

of the filtered bicarbonate is reabsorbed. With the onset of impaired tubular bicarbonate absorption, there is a loss of bicarbonate in the urine that reduces plasma bicarbonate levels. There is a concomitant loss of sodium in the urine that accompanies the bicarbonate loss; this leads to contraction of the extracellular fluid volume with increased aldosterone secretion and a resultant decrease in serum potassium levels (see Chapter 29). With proximal tubular defects in acid–base regulation, the distal tubular sites for secretion of the fixed acids into the urine continue to function, and the reabsorption of bicarbonate by the proximal cells eventually resumes, albeit at a lower level of serum bicarbonate. Whenever serum levels rise above this decreased level, bicarbonate is lost in the urine. The proximal tubular defect in bicarbonate reabsorption can extend to other substances, such as glucose, amino acids, and phosphate. Defects in calcium and phosphate reabsorption may accentuate bicarbonate losses.

Distal tubular acidosis involves a defect in the secretion of fixed acids that leads to failure to acidify the urine. The secretion of hydrogen ions in the distal tubules is linked to sodium reabsorption; failure to secrete hydrogen ions results in a loss of sodium bicarbonate in the urine. The extracellular fluid volume compartment contracts, aldosterone production increases, and hypokalemia develops. The persistent acidosis causes calcium to be released from bone. Increased losses of calcium in the urine lead to increased levels of parathyroid hormone, resorption of bone, bone pain, and development of kidney stones.

The treatment of renal tubular acidosis depends on the defect and may require administration of bicarbonate and potassium. The selective use of diuretics may also be indicated.

RENAL CYSTIC DISEASE

A renal cyst is a fluid-filled sac or segment of a dilated nephron. Renal cystic disease may be inherited or acquired. The cysts may be single or multiple and can vary in size from microscopic to several centimeters in diameter. Renal cystic disease is thought to result from tubular obstructions that increase intratubular pressure or from changes in the basement membrane of the renal tubules that predispose to cystic dilatation. Once the cyst begins to form, continued fluid accumulation contributes to its persistent growth. Renal cystic diseases probably exert their effects by compressing renal blood vessels, producing degeneration of functional renal tissue and obstructing tubular flow.

There are essentially four types of renal cystic disease: polycystic kidney disease, medullary sponge kidney, acquired cystic disease, and single or multiple kidney cysts.[28] Polycystic disease develops as an inherited trait. Medullary sponge kidney is a congenital lesion that affects the distal and collecting ducts. Medullary sponge kidney does not cause progressive renal failure; it does, however, produce urinary stasis and predisposes to kidney infections and kidney stones. Acquired renal cystic disease occurs in people with advanced renal failure and is caused by degenerative changes in the kidney. Simple cysts are the most common cystic disease of the kidney. These can be single or multiple, unilateral or bilateral, and usually are less than 1 cm in diameter, although they may grow larger. Most simple cysts do not produce signs or symptoms or compromise renal function. When they are symptomatic, they may cause flank pain, hematuria, UTI, and hypertension related to ischemia-produced stimulation of the renin–angiotensin system. They are most common in older people.

Polycystic Kidney Disease. The most common form of renal cystic disease is polycystic kidney disease that develops as a hereditary trait. It is one of the most common hereditary diseases in the United States, affecting more than 500,000 Americans.[29] There are two types of inherited polycystic disease: autosomal recessive and autosomal dominant. Autosomal recessive polycystic disease is relatively rare. Because the condition often is present at birth, it formerly was called infantile polycystic disease. Significant renal dysfunction usually is present, accompanied by variable degrees of liver fibrosis and portal hypertension. The disorder can be diagnosed by ultrasonography. There is no known treatment for the disease, and death usually occurs in infancy. Some children may present with less severe kidney problems and more severe liver disease. The disorder is transmitted as a recessive trait, meaning that there is a one-in-four chance of the parents having another child with the disorder.

Autosomal dominant polycystic kidney disease affects children and adults in the prime of life and accounts for 10% of people who require treatment for end-stage renal disease. The disorder is transmitted as a dominant trait, which means that there is a 50% chance of children of an affected parent developing the disorder. The mutant gene responsible for the defect is located on the short arm of chromosome 16. There is a high degree of penetrance for the defect; people who inherit the gene are likely to develop the disorder. There is considerable variability in gene expression, however, so that many affected people do not develop clinical symptoms, or if they do, the symptoms occur late in life.

The kidneys of people with polycystic disease eventually become enlarged because of the presence of multiple cysts. Cysts may also be found in the liver and, less commonly, the pancreas and spleen. Additionally, there may be a weakness in the walls of the cerebral arteries that could lead to aneurysm formation. Subarachnoid hemorrhage occurs in about 10% to 15% of people with polycystic kidney disease.

The manifestations of polycystic kidney disease include pain from the enlarging cysts that may reach debilitating levels, episodes of gross hematuria from bleeding into a cyst, infected cysts from ascending UTI, and hypertension resulting from compression of intrarenal blood vessels with activation of the renin–angiotensin mechanism. People with polycystic kidney disease are also at risk for development of renal cell carcinoma. The progress of the disease is slow, and end-stage renal failure is uncommon before age 40.

The diagnosis of autosomal polycystic kidney disease can be made by radiologic studies, such as excretory urography, and ultrasonography or CT scans. Ultrasonography and CT scans have largely replaced excretory urography because they are better able to detect small cysts. Ultrasonography is particularly useful as a screening test for the disease. It is recommended that first-degree relatives of affected people be screened for polycystic disease if they are at least age 20. The sensitivity of ultrasonography in this age group is about 95%; before that age, false negatives may occur because the cysts are too small to detect.[30]

The treatment of polycystic kidney disease is largely supportive. Control of hypertension and prevention of ascending UTI are important. The cysts may be surgically removed if refractory pain is present.[28] Dialysis and kidney transplantation are reserved for those people who progress to end-stage renal disease.

PYELONEPHRITIS

Pyelonephritis refers to an infection of the kidneys and renal pelvis. In its earliest stages, it is characterized by inflammatory foci that are interspersed throughout the renal interstitium. Small abscesses may form on the surface of the kidneys. In time, the lesions are replaced by scar tissue. There are two forms of pyelonephritis: acute and chronic. Because pyelonephritis affects the tubules and interstitium of the kidneys, it is classified as a tubulointerstitial kidney disease.

Acute pyelonephritis represents an acute suppurative inflammation of renal tubulointerstitial tissues caused by bacterial infection. Infection may occur through the bloodstream or ascend from the bladder. Factors that contribute to the development of acute pyelonephritis are catheterization and urinary tract instrumentation, vesicoureteral reflux, preg-

nancy, increased susceptibility to infection, and neurogenic bladder.

The onset of acute pyelonephritis typically is abrupt, with chills, fever, headache, back pain, tenderness over the costovertebral angle, and general malaise. It usually is accompanied by symptoms of bladder irritation, such as dysuria, frequency, and urgency. Pyuria occurs but is not diagnostic because it also occurs in lower UTIs. It is now possible to determine whether an infection involves the upper or lower urinary tract through detection of the antibody coating on the bacteria. Antibody coating is an immune response that occurs in the kidneys during upper UTIs and is easily detected by the immunofluorescence test. Also, the finding of leukocyte casts in the urine indicates that the infection is in the kidneys rather than the lower urinary tract.

Acute pyelonephritis is treated with appropriate antimicrobial drugs. Unless obstruction or other complications are present, the symptoms usually disappear within several days. Hospitalization during initial treatment may be necessary. Depending on the cause, recurrent infections are possible.

Chronic pyelonephritis is both chronic and progressive. There is scarring and deformation of the renal calices and pelvis. The disorder appears to involve a bacterial infection superimposed on obstructive abnormalities or the vesicoureteral reflux. Although the mechanisms by which the urinary obstruction interacts to produce kidney damage in chronic pyelonephritis are unknown, observations suggest that some component of the urine may serve as an antigenic determinant to induce an immune response. One of the suspected urine components is the Tamm-Horsfall proteins, which are synthesized in the tubular epithelial cells of the thick ascending loop of Henle and the distal convoluted tubules.[31]

Chronic pyelonephritis may cause many of the same symptoms as acute pyelonephritis, or its onset may be insidious. Loss of tubular function and of the ability to concentrate urine give rise to polyuria and nocturia, and mild proteinuria is common. Severe hypertension often is a contributing factor in the progress of the disease. Chronic pyelonephritis is a significant cause of renal failure. It is thought to be responsible for 25% of all cases of renal insufficiency and end-stage renal disease.

DRUG-RELATED NEPHROPATHIES

Drug-related nephropathies involve functional or structural changes in the kidneys that occur after exposure to a drug. The kidneys are exposed to a high rate of delivery of any substance in the blood because of their large blood flow and high filtration pressure. The kidneys are also active in the metabolic transformation of drugs and are, therefore, exposed to a number of toxic metabolites. Some drugs and toxic substances damage the kidneys by causing a decrease in blood flow; others directly damage tubulo-interstitial structures; and still others cause damage by producing hypersensitivity reactions. The tolerance to drugs varies with age and depends on renal function, state of hydration, blood pressure, and the *p*H of the urine. Because of a decrease in physiologic function, elderly people are particularly susceptible to kidney damage caused by drugs and toxins. The dangers of nephrotoxicity are increased when two or more drugs capable of producing kidney damage are given at the same time.

Acute drug-related hypersensitivity reactions produce tubulointerstitial nephritis, with damage to the tubules and interstitium. It was initially observed in people who were sensitive to the sulfonamide drugs; currently, it more often results from the use of methicillin and other synthetic antibiotics as well as furosemide and the thiazide diuretics by people who are sensitive to these drugs. The condition begins about 15 days after exposure to the drug (the period may vary from 2 to 40 days).[7] At the onset, there is fever, eosinophilia, hematuria, mild proteinuria, and, in about one fourth of cases, a rash. In about 50% of cases, signs and symptoms of acute renal failure develop. Withdrawal of the drug commonly is followed by complete recovery, but there may be permanent damage in some cases, usually in older people. Drug nephritis may not be recognized in its early stage because it is uncommon.

Chronic analgesic nephritis, seen in association with analgesic abuse, causes interstitial nephritis with renal papillary necrosis.[7] When first observed, it was attributed to phenacetin, a then-common ingredient of over-the-counter medications containing aspirin, phenacetin, and caffeine. Although phenacetin is no longer contained in these preparations, it has been suggested that other ingredients, such as aspirin and acetaminophen, may also contribute to the disorder. How much analgesic it takes to produce papillary necrosis is not known; ingestion of 2 to 30 kg of these analgesic compounds over a period of years has been known to result in papillary necrosis.[7] Headache, anemia, gastrointestinal tract symptoms, and hypertension are associated with the condition.

In summary, tubulointerstitial diseases affect both the tubules and the surrounding interstitium of the kidneys. These disorders include renal tubular acidosis, chronic pyelonephritis, renal cystic disease, and the effects of drugs and toxins. Renal tubular acidosis describes a form of systemic acidosis that results from tubular defects in bicarbonate reabsorption or hydrogen ion secretion. Renal cystic disease is a condition in which there is dilatation of tubular structures to form a cyst. Cysts may be single or multiple. Polycystic kidney disease is an inherited form of renal cystic disease; it can be inherited as an autosomal recessive or an autosomal dominant trait. Autosomal recessive polycystic kidney disease is rare and usually presents as severe renal dysfunction during infancy. Autosomal dominant polycystic disease usually does not become symptomatic until later in life, often after age 40. Pyelonephritis can occur as an acute or a chronic condition. Acute pyelonephritis typically is caused by ascending bladder infections or infections that come from the bloodstream; it usually is successfully treated with appropriate antimicrobial drugs. Chronic pyelonephritis is a progressive disease that produces scarring and deformation of the renal calices and pelvis. Drug-induced impairment of tubulointerstitial structure and function usually is the result of hypersensitivity reactions.

■ NEOPLASMS

There are two major groups of renal neoplasms: embryonic kidney tumors (Wilms' tumor) that occur during childhood and adult kidney cancers.

WILMS' TUMOR

Wilms' tumor (nephroblastoma) is one of the most common malignant tumors in children (see Chapter 5); 75% of cases occur in children under age 5.[32] Epithelial, muscle, and bone tissue are components of the tumor. The common presenting signs are a large abdominal mass and hypertension. Treatment involves surgery, chemotherapy, and radiotherapy (the tumor is radiosensitive). Two-year survival rates for children under age 2 have increased to about 73% with this aggressive plan of treatment. The survival rate for older children is lower.[32]

ADULT KIDNEY CANCERS

Adult kidney cancer accounts for 2% of all cancers. Each year an estimated 24,000 new cases of kidney cancer are diagnosed and about 10,300 persons die of this type of cancer.[32] The availability of CT scanning has contributed significantly to earlier diagnosis and more accurate staging of kidney cancers.

Renal cell carcinoma (hypernephroma) accounts for about 80% of kidney tumors, with transitional or squamous cell cancers of the renal pelvis accounting for most of the remaining cancers. The cause of renal cell carcinoma remains unclear. It occurs most often in older people in the 6th to 7th decade. Men are affected twice as frequently as women. Some of these tumors may occur as a result of chronic irritation associated with kidney stones. Epidemiologic evidence suggests a correlation between smoking and kidney cancer.[32]

Kidney cancer is largely a silent disorder during its early stages, and symptoms usually denote advanced disease. Presenting features include hematuria, costovertebral pain, presence of a palpable mass, polycythemia, and fever. Hematuria, which occurs in 70% to 90% of cases, is the most reliable sign. It is, however, intermittent and may be microscopic; as a result, the tumor may reach considerable size before it is detected. In about one third of cases, metastases are present at the time of diagnosis.

Kidney cancer is suspected when there are findings of hematuria and a renal mass. Ultrasonography, CT scanning, excretory urography, and renal angiography are used to confirm the diagnosis. Surgery (radical nephrectomy with lymph node dissection) is the treatment of choice for all resectable tumors. Single-agent and combination chemotherapy have been used with limited success. The 5-year survival rate for early-stage disease ranges from 30% to 50% and is less favorable for more advanced stages.

In summary, there are two major groups of renal neoplasms: embryonic kidney tumors (Wilms' tumor) that occur during childhood and adult kidney cancers. Wilms' tumor is the most common malignant tumor of children. The most common presenting signs are a large abdominal mass and hypertension. The 2-year survival rate for children with Wilms' tumor is about 90% with an aggressive plan of treatment.

Adult kidney cancers account for 2% of all cancers. The most common manifestation of kidney cancer is hematuria. Ultrasonography has contributed significantly to earlier diagnosis and more accurate staging of kidney cancers.

■ REFERENCES

1. National Kidney Foundation. (1988). Facts about transplantation and kidney and urologic diseases. In *KF News*. New York: National Kidney Foundation.
2. Manning, F.A. (1987). Fetal surgery for obstructive uropathy: Rationale considerations. *American Journal of Kidney Diseases, 10*, 259–267.
3. Stewart, C.L., & Jose, P.A. (1991). Transitional nephrology. *Urologic Clinics of North America, 18*, 143–149.
5. Glassberg, K.I. (1988). Summary of the annual meeting of the section of pediatric urology. *Pediatrics, 81*, 588.
5. Cotran, R.S., Kumar, V., & Robbins, S.L. (1989). *Pathologic basis of disease* (4th ed., pp. 1011–1081). Philadelphia: W.B. Saunders.
6. Tanagho, E.A. (1992). Urinary obstruction and stasis. In E.A. Tanagho & J.W. McAninch (Eds.). *Smith's general urology* (13th ed., pp. 165–194). E. Norwalk, CT: Appleton & Lange.
7. Rose, B.D. (1987). *Pathophysiology of renal disease* (2nd ed., pp. 387–437, 447–467). New York: McGraw-Hill.
8. Abraham, P.A., & Smith, C.L. (1984). Medical evaluation and management of calcium nephrolithiasis. *Medical Clinics of North America, 68*, 281.
9. Coe, F.L., Parks, J.H., & Asplin, J.R. (1992). The pathogenesis and treatment of kidney stones. *New England Journal of Medicine, 327*, 1141–1152.
10. Rotolo, J.E., O'Brien, W.M., & Pahira, J.J. (1988). Urinary tract calculi: Three new procedures to replace open surgery. *Consultant, 28*(3), 110.
11. Ludy, J.P. (1982). Urologic sepsis. *Urologic Clinics of North America, 9*, 259.
12. Andriole, V.T. (1987). Urinary tract infections: Recent developments. *Journal of Infectious Diseases, 156*, 865.
13. Kunin, C.M. (1984). Genitourinary infections in the patient at risk: Extrinsic risk factors. *American Journal of Medicine, 76*, 141.
14. Lindberg, U., Bjure, J., Haugstvedt, S., et al. (1975). Asymptomatic bacteriuria in schoolgirls: III. Relation between residual urine volume and recurrence. *Acta Paediatrica Scandinavica, 64*, 437.
15. Spencer, J.R., & Schaeffer, A.J. (1986). Pediatric urinary tract infections. *Urologic Clinics of North America, 13*, 661–672.
16. Krieger, J.N. (1986). Complications and treatment of urinary tract infections during pregnancy. *Urologic Clinics of North America, 13*, 685–693.
17. Andriole, V.T., & Patterson, T.F. (1991). Epidemiology, natural history, and management of urinary tract infections during pregnancy. *Medical Clinics of North America, 75*, 359–373.
18. Zelikovic, I., Adelman, R.D., & Nancarrow, R.A. (1992). Urinary tract infections in children—an update. *Western Journal of Medicine, 157*, 554–556.
19. Baldassare, J.S., & Kaye, D. (1991). Special problems of urinary tract infection in the elderly. *Medical Clinics of North America, 75*, 375–390.
20. Zweig, S. (1987). Urinary tract infections in the elderly. *American Family Practice, 35*(5), 123–130.
21. Glassock, R.J. (1988). Pathology of acute glomerulonephritis. *Hospital Practice, 23*(2A), 163–178.
22. Wilson, C.B., & Dixon, F.J. (1986). The renal response to immunologic injury. In B.M. Brenner & F.C. Rector, Jr. (Eds.). *The kidney* (3rd ed., pp. 800–805). Philadelphia: W.B. Saunders.
23. Micheal, A.F. (1985). Immunologic mechanisms in immune complex disease. *Kidney International, 28*, 569.
24. Cameron, J.S. (1987). The nephrotic syndrome and its complications. *American Journal of Kidney Diseases, 10*, 163–171.
25. Cotran, R. (1982). Tubulointerstitial nephropathies. *Hospital Practice, 1*, 79–96.
26. Davidman, M., & Schmitz, P. (1988). Renal tubular acidosis: A pathophysiologic approach. *Hospital Practice, 23*(1), 77–96.
27. Kurtzman, N.A. (1987). Renal tubular acidosis: A constellation of syndromes. *Hospital Practice, 22*(11), 173.
28. Bennett, W.M., Elzinga, L.W., & Barry, J.M. (1992). Polycystic kidney disease: II. Diagnosis and management. *Hospital Practice, 27*(4A), 61–72.
29. Grantham, J.J. (1992). Polycystic kidney disease: I. Etiology and pathogenesis. *Hospital Practice, 27*(3A), 51–59.
30. Thompson, C. (1988). The spectrum of renal cystic diseases. *Hospital Practice, 23*(4), 165.
31. Andriole, V.T. (1985). The role of Tamm-Horsfall protein in the pathogenesis of reflux nephropathy and chronic pyelonephritis. *Yale Journal of Biology and Medicine, 58*, 91.
32. Frank, I., Graham, S.D., & Nabors, W.L. (1991). Urological and male genital cancers. In A.I. Hollieb, D.J. Fink, & G.P. Murphy (Eds.). *Clinical oncology* (pp. 270–272). Atlanta: American Cancer Society.

■ BIBLIOGRAPHY

Allen, T.D. (1992). Commentary: Voiding dysfunction and reflux. *Journal of Urology, 148,* 1706–1707.

Bernard, D.B. (1990). Nephrotic syndrome. *Hospital Practice, 25*(9A), 114–129.

Burgener, S. (1987). Justification of closed intermittent urinary catheter irrigation/instillation: A review of current research and practice. *Journal of Advanced Nursing, 12,* 229.

Coe, F.L. (Chairperson). (1988). Consensus Conference: Prevention and treatment of kidney stones. *Journal of the American Medical Association, 260,* 977–981.

Couser, W.G. (1988). Rapidly progressive glomerulonephritis: Classification, pathogenesis, mechanisms, and therapy. *American Journal of Kidney Diseases, 11,* 449–464.

Davison, J.M. (1987). Overview: Kidney function in pregnant women. *American Journal of Kidney Diseases, 14,* 248–252.

Exelby, P.R. (1991). Wilms' tumor 1991. *Urologic Clinics of North America, 15,* 539–597.

Gardner, K.D. (1988). Pathogenesis of human cystic renal disease. *Annual Review of Medicine, 39,* 185.

Hooten, T.M., & Stamm, W.E. (1991). Management of uncomplicated urinary tract infections in adults. *Medical Clinics of North America, 75,* 339–357.

Koff, A. (1992). Relationship between dysfunctional voiding and reflux. *Journal of Urology 148,* 1703–1705.

Remis, R.S., Gurwith, M.J., Gurwith, D., et al. (1987). Risk factors for urinary tract infections. *American Journal of Epidemiology, 126,* 685–694.

Richardson, K., & Gennon, C. (1991). Renal function in the preterm neonate: An overview. *Neonatal Network, 10* (4), 17–23.

Robillar, J.E., Nakamura, K.T., & Jose, P.A. (1988). Renal hemodynamics and functional adjustments to postnatal life. *Seminars in Perinatology, 12,* 143–150.

See, W., & Williams, R.D. (1992). Tumors of the kidney, ureter, and bladder. *Western Journal of Medicine, 156,* 523–534.

Sherbotie, J.R., & Cornfield, D. (1991). Management of urinary tract infections in children. *Medical Clinics of North America, 75,* 327–337.

Sobel, J.D., & Reinhart, H. (1991). Antibacterial host factors in the urinary tract. *Advances in Internal Medicine,* 131–151.

Stamm, W.E., Johnson, J.R., Johnson, C., et al. (1988). Urinary tract infections: From pathogenesis to treatment. *Journal of Infectious Diseases, 159,* 400–406.

Stull, T., & LiPuma, J.J. (1991). Epidemiology and natural history of urinary tract infections in children. *Medical Clinics of North America, 75,* 287–297.

Warren, J.W. (1991). The catheter and urinary tract infections. *Medical Clinics of North America, 75,* 481–493.

CHAPTER 33

RENAL FAILURE

SUSAN GALLAGHER-LEPAK

Acute Renal Failure
Prerenal Conditions
Postrenal Conditions
Intrarenal Conditions
Treatment

Chronic Renal Failure
Clinical Manifestations
Effect of Renal Failure
   on Elimination of Drugs
Treatment

Renal Failure in Children
and Elderly People
Chronic Renal Failure in Children
Chronic Renal Failure
   in Elderly People

■ OBJECTIVES

After you have studied this chapter, you should be able to meet the following objectives:

■ Differentiate between acute and chronic renal failure in terms of onset, cause, and outcome.

■ Classify the following conditions as prerenal, intrarenal, or postrenal: acute glomerulonephritis, prostatic hypertrophy, hemorrhage, septicemia, hemolytic reaction.

■ Describe the clinical manifestations of the oliguric and diuretic phases of acute tubular necrosis.

■ Compare the renal dysfunction that occurs with renal impairment, renal insufficiency, and end-stage renal disease.

■ Compare the clinical manifestations of azotemia and uremia.

■ List the manifestations of end-stage renal disease and state their physiologic significance.

■ State the possible rationale for neurologic manifestations that occur in end-stage renal disease.

■ Define the term *osteodystrophy* and relate it to the altered calcium and phosphate balance that occurs in end-stage renal disease.

■ List the skin disorders that develop in people with end-stage renal disease.

■ State the possible alterations in sexual function that occur in end-stage renal disease.

■ State the basis for adverse drug reactions in people with end-stage renal disease.

■ Describe the scientific principles underlying dialysis treatment.

■ Compare hemodialysis with peritoneal dialysis.

■ Cite the complications of kidney transplantation.

■ State the goals for dietary management of people with end-stage renal disease as they relate to protein restrictions; carbohydrate, fat, and caloric needs; and potassium, sodium, and fluid intake.

■ Describe the special needs of children and elderly people as they relate to chronic renal failure.

Carol Mattson Porth: PATHOPHYSIOLOGY: CONCEPTS OF
ALTERED HEALTH STATES, 4th ed. © 1994, 1990, 1986, 1982
J.B. Lippincott Company

Renal failure is a condition in which the kidneys fail to remove metabolic end products from the blood and to regulate the fluid, electrolyte, and pH balance of the extracellular fluids. The underlying cause may be renal pathology, systemic disease, or urologic defects of nonrenal origin. Renal failure can occur as an acute or a chronic disorder. Acute renal failure is abrupt in onset and often is reversible if recognized early and treated appropriately. By contrast, chronic renal failure is the end result of irreparable damage to the kidneys. It develops slowly, usually over the course of a number of years.

Azotemia refers to an abnormally high level of nitrogenous wastes (urea nitrogen, uric acid, and creatinine) in the blood largely related to a decrease in the glomerular filtration rate (GFR). Its presence results from the inability of the kidneys to filter these waste products from the blood. Azotemia is present in both acute and chronic renal failure. *Uremia* is a clinical syndrome that comprises the signs and symptoms associated with end-stage renal disease.

■ ACUTE RENAL FAILURE

A clinical syndrome of diverse causes, acute renal failure is characterized by an acute reduction of renal function. About 5% of all hospitalized patients develop acute renal failure; in some settings, such as intensive care units, it occurs in up to 20% of patients.[1] The manifestations of acute renal failure frequently are superimposed on the signs and symptoms of the condition that caused the renal failure—heart failure, shock, prostatic hyperplasia, and others. Because acute renal failure is potentially reversible, it is important that early signs be recognized so that appropriate treatment measures can be instituted promptly.

The causes of acute renal failure can be categorized as prerenal, postrenal, and intrarenal (Chart 33-1). This classification aids in identifying and treating the disorder.

PRERENAL FAILURE

Prerenal failure results from impaired renal blood flow. Causes of prerenal failure include severe hemorrhage, profound volume depletion, cardiogenic shock, increased vascular capacity caused by anaphylaxis or sepsis, and operative procedures associated with interrupted renal blood flow. The most common form of acute renal failure, it is considered reversible if the cause of renal hypofunction can be identified and corrected within 24 hours.

As a rule, the blood supply to a normal kidney can be interrupted for about 30 minutes without

---

CHART 33-1: CAUSES OF ACUTE RENAL FAILURE

Prerenal

Hypovolemia
  Dehydration
  Loss of gastrointestinal tract fluid
  Hemorrhage
  Fluid sequestration (*e.g.*, burns)
Septicemia
  Septic shock
Heart failure
Interruption of renal blood flow caused by surgery and other causes

Intrarenal

Acute tubular necrosis
  Prolonged renal ischemia
  Exposure to nephrotoxic agents
    Aminoglycosides (*e.g.*, gentamicin, kanamycin, colistin)
    Heavy metals (*e.g.*, lead, mercury)
    Organic solvents (*e.g.*, carbon tetrachloride, ethylene glycol)
    Radiopaque contrast media
Intratubular obstruction
  Uric acid crystals
  Hemolytic reactions (*e.g.*, blood transfusion reactions)
  Precipitated proteins resulting from multiple myelomas
  Rhabdomyolysis
  Acute glomerulonephritis

Postrenal

Ureteral obstruction (*e.g.*, calculi, tumors)
Bladder outlet obstruction (*e.g.*, prostatic hyperplasia, urethral strictures)

---

damaging the kidney,[2] but in conditions such as acute trauma, sepsis, and heart failure, the interruption in blood flow often is more severe and lasts longer. Improperly treated, prolonged renal hypoperfusion can lead to ischemic tubular necrosis with significant morbidity and mortality.

The kidneys normally filter about 20% to 25% of the cardiac output. With a loss of blood volume or impaired cardiac function, the percentage of cardiac output that flows through the kidneys is reduced. When the pressure in the afferent arterioles in the kidneys falls much below 60 to 70 mmHg, glomerular filtration ceases and little or no urine is formed. Thus, one of the early manifestations of prerenal failure is a sharp decrease in urine output. The ratio of blood urea nitrogen (BUN) to serum creatinine normally is about 10:1, but in acute prerenal failure, there is a disproportionate elevation in the BUN level compared with that of serum creatinine. This is because the low GFR allows more time for smaller particles, such as urea, to be reabsorbed back into the blood. Creatinine, being larger and nondiffusible, remains in the tubular fluid, and the total amount of creatinine that is filtered, although small, is excreted in the urine.

POSTRENAL FAILURE

Postrenal failure results from obstruction of urine outflow from the kidneys. The obstruction can occur in the ureter (calculi and strictures), bladder (tumors or neurogenic bladder), or urethra (prostatic hypertrophy). Prostatic hyperplasia is the most common underlying problem. Obstructive uropathy is responsible for about 10% of cases of acute renal failure.[1] The treatment of acute postrenal failure consists of treating the underlying cause of obstruction so that urine flow can be reestablished before permanent nephron damage occurs.

INTRARENAL FAILURE

Acute intrarenal failure is caused by primary damage to the nephrons. The major cause of intrarenal failure is a condition called *acute tubular necrosis*, which results from an ischemic or toxic insult to the nephron. Intratubular obstruction and specific diseases such as acute glomerulonephritis and acute pyelonephritis are also intrarenal causes of acute renal failure.

ACUTE TUBULAR NECROSIS

Acute tubular necrosis is characterized by destructive changes in the tubular epithelium owing to ischemia or exposure to nephrotoxic agents. The most common cause of acute tubular necrosis is prolonged acute prerenal failure, whereas the most common causes of toxic acute tubular necrosis are nephrotoxic drugs and toxic products of microorganisms responsible for septicemia.[3] Several drugs and other chemicals, including organic solvents and heavy metals such as lead and mercury, can injure the renal tubular structures. The aminoglycosides, a group of antibiotics of which gentamicin, kanamycin, and colistin are examples, are all capable of impairing renal function. Several factors contribute to aminoglycoside toxicity, including a decrease in the GFR, which commonly occurs in elderly people, preexisting renal disease, hypovolemia, and concurrent administration of other drugs that have a nephrotoxic effect.[1] Contrast media used during cardiac catheterization and intravenous cholangiography, for example, may also be nephrotoxic. The risk of renal damage caused by radiopaque contrast media is greatest in elderly people, in people with diabetes mellitus, and in people

who, for one reason or another, are susceptible to kidney disease.

Acute tubular necrosis usually follows four successive phases: (1) onset or initiating phase, (2) oliguric or anuric phase, (3) diuretic phase, and (4) recovery or convalescent phase.[3] The onset or initiating phase is the time from the onset of the precipitating event (*e.g.*, ischemic phase of prerenal failure) until tubular injury occurs. The oliguric phase is represented by a decrease in urine output. Oliguria (urine output less than 400 mL/day) is more common in postischemic forms of acute tubular necrosis, and nonoliguria (urine output greater than 400 mL/day) is more common in toxic tubular necrosis. When oliguria occurs, it starts shortly after the initiating event and lasts an average of 10 to 14 days.

Formerly, most patients with acute tubular necrosis were oliguric. During the past two decades, however, a nonoliguric form of renal failure has become increasingly prevalent.[4] This is probably the result of new approaches to the treatment of poor cardiac performance and circulatory failure that focus on vigorous plasma volume expansion, vasodilator therapy, and the use of dopamine for treatment of hypotensive patients. Dopamine has renal vasodilator properties and inhibits sodium reabsorption in the proximal tubule, thereby increasing urinary excretion of solute. Early reports suggest that people with nonoliguric acute renal failure have a better prognosis than those with the oliguric (classic) form.[4]

The oliguric phase of acute tubular necrosis is characterized by a marked decrease in GFR, causing sudden retention of endogenous metabolites, urea, potassium, sulfate, and creatinine that normally are cleared by the kidneys. Fluid retention gives rise to edema, water intoxication, and pulmonary congestion. If the period of oliguria is prolonged, hypertension frequently develops and with it signs of uremia. When untreated, uremia's neurologic manifestations progress from neuromuscular irritability to seizures, somnolence, and, finally, coma and death. Hyperkalemia usually is asymptomatic until serum levels of potassium rise above 6.0 to 6.5 mEq/L, at which point characteristic electrocardiographic changes and symptoms of muscle weakness are seen. People with nonoliguric failure have higher levels of glomerular filtration and excrete more nitrogenous waste, water, and electrolytes in their urine. Hence, abnormalities in blood chemistry levels usually are milder and cause fewer complications.

The diuretic phase of acute renal failure typically begins within a few days to 6 weeks after oliguria, indicating that the nephrons have recovered to the point where urine excretion is possible. Diuresis usually occurs before renal function has returned to normal. Consequently, BUN and serum creatinine, potassium, and phosphate levels may remain elevated or continue to rise even though urine output is increased. In some cases, the diuresis may be due to impaired nephron function and may cause excessive loss of water and electrolytes.

During the convalescent phase, renal function recovers slowly. The GFR returns to 70% to 80% of normal within 1 to 2 years. In some cases, mild to moderate kidney damage persists.

INTRATUBULAR OBSTRUCTIONS

Intratubular obstructions are caused by the accumulation of casts and cellular debris that accompanies severe hemolytic reactions or myoglobinuria. Skeletal and cardiac muscles contain myoglobin, which accounts for their rubiginous color. Myoglobin corresponds to hemoglobin in function, serving as an oxygen reservoir within the muscle fibers. Myoglobin normally is not found in the serum or urine. It has a low molecular weight of 17,000; if it escapes into the circulation, it is rapidly filtered in the glomerulus. Myoglobinuria most commonly is due to muscle trauma but may result from extreme exertion, hyperthermia, sepsis, prolonged seizures, potassium or phosphate depletion, and alcoholism or drug abuse. Hemoglobin may also escape into the glomerular filtrate when serum levels are markedly increased as a result of a severe hemolytic reaction. Both myoglobin and hemoglobin discolor the urine, ranging from the color of tea to red, brown, or black.

TREATMENT

A major concern in the treatment of acute renal failure is identifying and correcting the cause (*e.g.*, by improving renal perfusion or discontinuing nephrotoxic drugs). Fluids are carefully regulated in an effort to maintain normal fluid volume and electrolyte concentrations. Adequate caloric intake is needed to prevent the breakdown of body proteins, which increases nitrogenous wastes. Parenteral hyperalimentation may be used for this purpose. Because secondary infections are a major cause of death in people with acute renal failure, constant vigilance is needed to detect and prevent such infection. Dialysis or continuous renal replacement therapy (CRRT) may be indicated when nitrogenous wastes and the water and electrolyte balance cannot be kept under control by other means. CRRT, which is used to treat acute renal failure in patients too hemodynamically unstable to tolerate hemodialysis, provides slow, continuous (8 to 24 hours) ultrafiltration and clearance of uremic wastes.[5]

In summary, acute renal failure is an acute reversible suppression of kidney function. It is classified as prerenal, intrarenal, or postrenal in origin. It typically progresses through an oliguric phase during which urine output is markedly diminished and fluid as well as metabolic end products accumulate. During the second phase, that of diuresis, urine output increases as renal function begins to return. Correction of azotemia usually follows diuresis.

■ CHRONIC RENAL FAILURE

Unlike acute renal failure, chronic renal failure represents progressive and irreversible destruction of kidney structures. As recently as 20 years ago, many people with chronic renal failure progressed to the final stages of the disease and then died. The high mortality rate was associated not only with the limitations in the treatment of renal disease but also with the tremendous cost of ongoing treatment. In 1972, federal support for dialysis and transplantation through a Medicare entitlement program began. Technologic advances in dialysis therapy and transplantation have improved the outcomes for people with renal disease.

Chronic renal failure can result from a number of conditions that cause permanent loss of nephrons, including uncontrolled hypertension, urinary tract obstruction and infection, hereditary defects of the kidneys, disorders of the glomeruli, and systemic diseases such as diabetes mellitus and systemic lupus erythematosus. Regardless of the cause, chronic renal failure results in progressive deterioration of glomerular filtration, tubular reabsorption, and endocrine functions of the kidneys. All forms of renal failure are characterized by a reduction in the GFR, reflecting a corresponding reduction in functional nephrons.

The signs and symptoms of renal failure typically occur gradually and do not become evident until the disease is far advanced. This is because of the amazing compensatory ability of the kidneys. As kidney structures are destroyed, the remaining nephrons undergo structural and functional hypertrophy, each increasing its function as a means of compensating for those that have been lost (Fig. 33-1). It is only when the few remaining nephrons are destroyed that the manifestations of renal failure become evident.

The rate of nephron destruction differs from case to case, ranging from several months to many years. The progression of chronic renal failure usually occurs in four stages: (1) diminished renal reserve, (2) renal insufficiency, (3) renal failure, and (4) end-stage renal disease.[6]

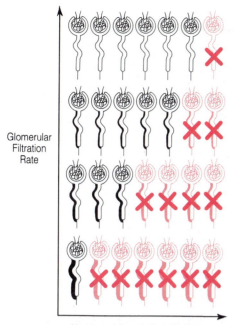

Glomerular
Filtration
Rate

Number of Functioning Nephrons

FIG. 33-1. Relation of renal function and nephron mass. Each kidney contains 1 million tiny nephrons. A proportional relation exists between the number of nephrons affected by disease and the resulting glomerular filtration rate.

Diminished renal reserve occurs when the GFR is about 50% of normal. Serum BUN and creatinine levels are normal, and no symptoms of impaired renal function are evident. Because of the diminished reserve, the risk of developing azotemia increases with an additional renal insult.

Renal insufficiency represents a reduction in the GFR of about 20% to 35% of normal. During this stage, azotemia, anemia, and hypertension appear. Signs and symptoms of renal insufficiency do not begin to appear until more than half the function in both kidneys is lost. This is supported by the fact that many people survive an entire lifetime with only one kidney. The kidneys initially have tremendous adaptive capabilities. As nephrons are destroyed, the remaining nephrons undergo changes to compensate for those that are lost. In the process, each of the remaining nephrons must filter more solute particles from the blood. Because the solute particles are osmotically active, they cause additional water to be lost in the urine. One of the earliest symptoms of renal failure is *isosthenuria*—polyuria that is almost isotonic with plasma. Nocturia occurs for the same reasons.

Conservative treatment during this stage includes measures to retard deterioration of renal function and assist the body in managing the effects of impaired function. Because the kidneys have diffi-culty eliminating the waste products of protein metabolism, a restricted-protein diet usually produces fewer uremic symptoms and slows progression of renal failure. The few remaining nephrons that constitute the functional reserve of the kidneys can be easily disrupted; at that point, renal failure progresses rapidly.

Renal failure develops when the GFR is less than 20% to 25% of normal. The kidneys cannot regulate volume and solute composition; edema, metabolic acidosis, and hypercalcemia develop. Overt uremia may ensue with neurologic, gastrointestinal, and cardiovascular complications.

End-stage renal disease occurs when the GFR is less than 5% of normal. Histologic findings of an end-stage kidney include a reduction in renal capillaries and scarring in the glomeruli. Atrophy and fibrosis are evident in the tubules. The mass of the kidneys usually is reduced. At this final phase of renal failure, treatment with either dialysis or transplantation is necessary for survival.

CLINICAL MANIFESTATIONS

Azotemia is an early sign of renal failure, usually occurring before other symptoms become evident. Urea is one of the first nitrogenous wastes to accumulate in the blood. The BUN level becomes increasingly elevated as renal failure progresses. The normal concentration of urea in the plasma is about 26 mg/dL. In renal failure, this level may rise to as high as 800 mg/dL. Creatinine, a by-product of muscle metabolism, is freely filtered in the glomerulus and is not reabsorbed in the renal tubules. Because creatinine is produced at a relatively constant rate, and because any creatinine that is filtered in the glomerulus is lost in the urine rather than being reabsorbed into the blood, serum creatinine can be used as an indirect method for assessing the GFR and the extent of renal damage that has occurred in renal failure (see Chapter 31).

Uremia, which literally means "urine in the blood," is the term used to describe the clinical manifestations of end-stage renal disease. Few symptoms of uremia appear until at least two thirds of the nephrons have been destroyed. Uremia differs from azotemia, which merely indicates the accumulation of nitrogenous wastes in the blood and can occur without symptoms. The uremic condition includes signs and symptoms of altered fluid, electrolyte, and acid–base balance; alterations in regulatory functions (*e.g.*, hypertension, anemia, osteodystrophy); and accumulation of waste products (*e.g.*, uremic encephalopathy, neuropathy, pruritus). At this stage, virtually every organ and structure in the body is affected. The symptoms at the onset of uremia (*e.g.*, weakness, fatigue, nausea, and apathy) often are subtle. More severe symptoms include extreme weakness, frequent vomiting, lethargy, and confusion. Without treatment, coma and death follow. These changes are summarized in Table 33-1.

FLUID, ELECTROLYTE, AND ACID–BASE BALANCE

Either dehydration or fluid overload can be seen in chronic renal failure, depending on the pathology of the renal disease. In addition to these defects in volume regulation, the kidneys do not correctly filter the

TABLE 33-1. ALTERATIONS IN BODY FUNCTION THAT OCCUR WITH CHRONIC RENAL FAILURE

BODY SYSTEM	CHANGE IN FUNCTION	MANIFESTATION
Body fluids	Compensatory changes in tubular functions	Fixed specific gravity of urine; polyuria and nocturia
	Decreased ability to synthesize ammonia and conserve bicarbonate	Metabolic acidosis
	Inability to excrete potassium	Hyperkalemia
	Inability to regulate sodium excretion	Salt wasting or sodium retention
	Impaired ability to excrete phosphate	Hyperphosphatemia
	Hyperphosphatemia and inability to activate vitamin D	Hypocalcemia and increased levels of parathyroid hormone
Hematologic	Impaired synthesis of erythropoietin and effects of uremia	Anemia
	Impaired platelet function	Bleeding tendencies
Cardiovascular	Activation of renin–angiotensin mechanism, increased vascular volume, and failure to produce vasopressor substances	Hypertension
	Fluid retention and hypoalbuminemia	Edema
	Excess extracellular fluid volume, anemia	Congestive heart failure; pulmonary edema
	Elevated BUN	Uremic pericarditis
Gastrointestinal	Increased metabolic wastes	Anorexia, nausea, vomiting
	Decreased platelet function and increased gastric acid secretion due to hyperparathyroidism	Gastrointestinal bleeding
Neurologic	Fluid and electrolyte imbalance	Headache
	Increase in metabolic acids and other small, diffusible particles, such as urea	Signs of uremic encephalopathy: lethargy, decreased alertness, loss of recent memory, delirium, coma, seizures, asterixis, muscle twitching, and tremulousness
		Signs of neuropathy: restless leg syndrome, paresthesias, muscle weakness, and paralysis
Osteodystrophy	Hyperphosphatemia	Osteomalacia
	Hypocalcemia	Osteoporosis
	Hyperparathyroidism	Bone pain and tenderness
		Spontaneous fractures
	Calcium × phosphate product greater than 60	Metastatic calcifications
Skin	Salt wasting	Dry skin and mucous membranes
	Anemia	Pale, sallow complexion
	Hyperparathyroidism	Pruritus
	Decreased platelet function and bleeding tendencies	Ecchymosis and subcutaneous bruises
	High concentration of metabolic end products in body fluids	Uremic frost and odor of urine on skin and breath
Genitourinary	Impaired general health	
	Decreased testosterone	Impotence and loss of libido
	Decreased estrogen	Amenorrhea and loss of libido

blood, reabsorb necessary electrolytes, or concentrate urine. When the glomerular capillary membrane is damaged, larger particles, such as plasma proteins and blood cells, enter the renal tubules and are excreted into the urine.

An early sign of impaired renal function is the inability of the kidneys to regulate the concentration of urine. In renal failure, the specific gravity of the urine becomes fixed (1.008 to 1.012) and varies little from voiding to voiding. Polyuria and nocturia are common.

As renal function declines, the ability to regulate sodium excretion is reduced. The kidneys normally tolerate large variations in sodium intake (from 1 to 900 mEq) while maintaining normal serum sodium levels. In chronic renal failure, they lose the ability to regulate sodium excretion. There is impaired ability to adjust to a sudden reduction in sodium intake and poor tolerance of an acute sodium overload. Volume depletion with an accompanying decrease in the GFR can occur with a restricted sodium intake or excess sodium loss caused by diarrhea or vomiting. Salt wasting is a common problem in advanced renal failure because of impaired tubular reabsorption of sodium. Increasing sodium intake in people with chronic renal failure often improves the GFR and whatever renal function remains. In people with associated hypertension, the possibility of increasing blood pressure or producing congestive heart failure often rules out supplemental sodium intake.

About 90% of potassium excretion is through the kidneys. In renal failure, potassium excretion by each nephron increases as the kidneys adapt to a decrease in the GFR. As a result, hyperkalemia usually does not develop until renal function is severely compromised. Because of this adaptive mechanism, it usually is not necessary to restrict potassium intake in chronic renal failure until the GFR has dropped below 5 mL/minute.[7] In people with chronic renal failure, hyperkalemia often results from failure to follow dietary potassium restrictions and ingestion of medications that contain potassium or from endogenous release of potassium, as in trauma or infection.

The kidneys are largely responsible for maintaining body *p*H by eliminating hydrogen ions produced in metabolic processes. This is achieved through hydrogen ion secretion, sodium and bicarbonate reabsorption, and the production of ammonia, which acts as a buffer for titratable acids. With a decline in renal function, these mechanisms become impaired and metabolic acidosis results. In chronic renal failure, acidosis seems to stabilize as the disease progresses, probably as a result of the tremendous buffering capacity of bone. This buffering action is thought to increase bone resorption and contribute to skeletal defects present in chronic renal failure.

CALCIUM, PHOSPHATE, AND BONE METABOLISM

Abnormalities of calcium, phosphorus, and vitamin D metabolism occur early in the course of chronic renal failure. The regulation of serum phosphate levels requires a daily urinary excretion of an amount equal to that ingested in the diet. With deteriorating renal function, phosphate excretion is impaired and, as a result, serum phosphorus levels rise; conversely, serum calcium levels, which are inversely regulated in relation to serum phosphorus levels, fall (discussed in Chapter 29). The drop in serum calcium, caused by hyperphosphatemia, stimulates parathyroid hormone release with a resultant increase in calcium resorption from bone. Although serum calcium levels are maintained through increased parathyroid function, this adjustment is accomplished at the expense of the skeletal system and other body organs. Most people with chronic renal failure develop secondary hyperparathyroidism, the result of chronic stimulation of the parathyroid glands.

The hypocalcemia of chronic renal failure is aggravated by impaired vitamin D function. The kidneys control vitamin D activity by converting the inactive form of vitamin D (25-hydroxycholecalciferol) to its active form (1,25-dihydroxycholecalciferol). Chronic renal failure impairs the ability to convert vitamin D to its active form. With reduced levels of activated vitamin D, calcium absorption from the small intestine is decreased, causing further stimulation of parathyroid function and demineralization of bone.

Renal osteodystrophy occurs in chronic renal failure because of abnormalities of the calcium and phosphorus balance. Sometimes the condition is called *renal rickets* because its manifestations in children resemble those of a vitamin D deficiency. The primary changes in renal osteodystrophy are osteomalacia and osteoporosis, in which the calcium and phosphate contents of the bone decrease and loss of the supporting structural matrix occurs. Increased parathyroid function causes excessive reabsorption of calcium from long bones, distal ends of the clavicle, and smaller bones, which can be seen on x-ray films. In advanced osteodystrophy, cysts may develop in the bone, a condition called *osteitis fibrosa cystica*. The symptoms of renal osteodystrophy include tenderness, pain, and, sometimes, spontaneous fractures.

Soft tissue calcification, or *metastatic calcification* of the cornea, arteries, subcutaneous tissues, and muscle, can occur when the phosphate times calcium product rises higher than 60. This is seen after dialysis has been instituted and usually is associated with a rapid rise in the calcium level, which precedes a fall in the phosphate level. Calcium deposits in the eyes cause conjunctivitis and often are evidenced by "band" keratopathy. Calcium deposits in the skin cause intense itching.

HEMATOLOGIC AND IMMUNE FUNCTION

Chronic anemia is the most profound hematologic alteration that accompanies renal failure. People with renal failure experience a gradual reduction in hematocrit as renal function deteriorates. An untreated hematocrit for a person on hemodialysis may stabilize at about 20%.[8] The kidneys are the primary site for the production of the hormone erythropoietin, which controls red blood cell production. In renal failure, erythropoietin production usually is insufficient to stimulate adequate red blood cell production by the bone marrow. The accumulation of uremic toxins further suppresses red cell production in the bone marrow, and the cells that are produced have a shortened life span. Both of these factors contribute to anemia in chronic renal failure.

An estimated 17% to 20% of people with chronic renal failure have a bleeding tendency.[3] Although platelet production is normal in number, platelet function is impaired, causing bleeding problems. Epistaxis, gastrointestinal bleeding, and bruising of the skin and subcutaneous tissues are seen.

Immunologic abnormalities accompany chronic renal disease, decreasing the efficiency of the immune response to infection. All leukocyte cell types may be affected adversely by the high levels of urea and metabolic wastes in people with renal failure.[7] This includes decreases in lymphocyte function, cell-mediated immunity, and granulocyte count. There is impairment of the acute inflammatory response and decreased delayed hypersensitivity. In people with uremia, less fever occurs in response to infection and infections are more difficult to recognize. Mucosal barriers to infection may also be defective, and in people who are maintained on dialysis, vascular access devices are common portals of entry for pathogens. Thus, infection is a common complication and cause of hospitalization and death in chronic renal failure.

CARDIOVASCULAR FUNCTION

Cardiovascular disorders, including hypertension, congestive heart failure, and pericarditis, are common among people with chronic renal failure. Hyperkalemia, which often accompanies renal failure, can contribute to cardiovascular problems.

Hypertension frequently is an early manifestation of renal failure. It is caused in part by increased renin production (renin–angiotensin mechanism) by the kidneys coupled with excess extracellular fluid volume.[7] Even in advanced renal failure, enough functioning renal tissue is present to produce renin in quantities sufficient to raise blood pressure. Most people with renal insufficiency need to take several antihypertensive medications to control blood pressure. A diuretic and a β-adrenergic blocking drug, such as propranolol, are prescribed. In the later stage of renal failure, dialysis is needed to maintain the extracellular fluid volume.

Increased extracellular fluid volume resulting from sodium and water retention, proteinuria, and hypoalbuminemia is clinically identified by the presence of edema. This condition can lead to congestive heart failure and pulmonary edema, especially in the later stages of renal failure.

Pericarditis, which results from metabolic toxins, was once a common complication of chronic renal failure. It is now seen infrequently because of the early initiation of dialysis.[7] When it does occur, it usually is related to a viral infection or systemic disease.

GASTROINTESTINAL FUNCTION

Anorexia, nausea, and vomiting are common in uremia, along with a metallic taste in the mouth that further depresses the appetite. Early-morning nausea commonly occurs. Ulceration and bleeding of the gastrointestinal mucosa may develop, and hiccoughs are common. A possible cause of nausea and vomiting is the decomposition of urea by intestinal flora, resulting in a high concentration of ammonia. Parathyroid hormone increases gastric acid secretion and, thus, contributes to gastrointestinal problems. Nausea and vomiting often improve with restriction of dietary protein and after initiation of dialysis and usually disappear with transplantation.

NEUROLOGIC FUNCTION

Neurologic disorders, common in uremia, can be categorized as peripheral neuropathies and uremic encephalopathy.

Neuropathy, or involvement of the peripheral nerves, affects the lower limbs more frequently than the upper limbs. It is symmetric and affects both sensory and motor function. Neuropathy is caused by atrophy and demyelination of nerve fibers, possibly caused by uremic toxins.[9] Restless legs syndrome is a manifestation of peripheral nerve involvement and can be seen in up to two thirds of people who are on dialysis.[9] This syndrome is characterized by creeping, prickling, and itching sensations that typically are more intense at rest. Temporary relief is obtained by moving the legs. A burning sensation of the feet, which may be followed by muscle weakness and atrophy, is a manifestation of uremia.

Uremic encephalopathy is poorly understood and may result, at least in part, from an excess of toxic organic acids that alter normal mechanisms, preventing their crossing of the blood–brain barrier and entering neural tissue. Electrolyte abnormalities, such as sodium shifts, may also contribute.

The central nervous system disturbances in uremia are similar to those caused by other metabolic and toxic disorders, such as portal-systemic encephalopathy, hypoxia, and water intoxication. The manifestations are more closely related to the progress of the uremic disorder than to the level of the metabolic end products.[10] Profound encephalopathy is common in acute renal failure and less common in chronic renal failure, despite the marked blood chemistry abnormalities seen in the latter. Reductions in alertness and awareness are the earliest and most significant indications of uremic encephalopathy. This often is followed by an inability to fix attention, loss of recent memory, and perceptual errors in identifying people and objects. Delirium and coma occur late in the course; seizures are the preterminal event.

Disorders of motor function commonly accompany the neurologic manifestations of uremic encephalopathy. During the early stages, there often is difficulty in performing fine movements of the extremities; the gait becomes unsteady and clumsy with *tremulousness* of movement. *Asterixis*, dorsiflexion movements of the hands and feet, typically occurs as the disease progresses. It can be elicited by having the person hyperextend his or her arms at the elbow and wrist with the fingers spread apart. If asterixis is present, this position causes side-to-side flapping movements of the fingers.

SKIN INTEGRITY

The skin is pale in renal failure because of anemia and may have a sallow, yellow-brown hue. The skin and mucous membranes are dry, and subcutaneous bruising is common. Skin dryness is caused by a reduction in perspiration owing to the decreased size of sweat glands and the diminished activity of oil glands. Pruritus is common; it is secondary to the high serum phosphate levels and the development of phosphate crystals, which occurs with hyperparathyroidism. Severe scratching or repeated needlesticks, especially with hemodialysis, break the skin integrity and increase the risk for infection. In the advanced stages of untreated renal failure, urea crystals may precipitate on the skin—the result of high urea concentration present in body fluids. The fingernails may become thin and brittle with a dark

band just behind the leading edge of the nail, followed by a white band. This appearance is known as *Terry's nails*.

SEXUAL FUNCTIONING

The cause of sexual dysfunction in both men and women with chronic renal failure is unclear. The cause probably is multifactorial and may result from high levels of uremic toxins, neuropathy, altered endocrine function, psychological factors, and medications (*e.g.*, antihypertensive drugs). Alterations in physiologic sexual responses, reproductive ability, and libido are common.

Impotence occurs in as many as 56% of male dialysis patients.[11] Derangements of the pituitary and gonadal hormones, such as decreases in testosterone levels and increases in prolactin and luteinizing hormone levels, are common and cause erectile difficulties and decreased spermatocyte counts. Loss of libido may result from chronic anemia as well as decreased testosterone levels. Several drugs, such as exogenous testosterone and bromocriptine, have been used in an attempt to return hormone levels to normal.

Impaired sexual function in women is manifested by abnormal levels of progesterone, luteinizing hormone, and prolactin. Hypofertility, menstrual abnormalities, decreased vaginal lubrication, and various orgasmic problems have been described.[12] Amenorrhea is common among women who are on dialysis therapy.

EFFECT OF RENAL FAILURE ON ELIMINATION OF DRUGS

The incidence of adverse drug reactions increases in people with renal failure. In considering the effect of various drugs and medications on people with renal disease, several factors about the drugs need to be taken into account: their absorption, distribution, metabolism, and excretion. The administration of large quantities of phosphate-binding antacids to control hyperphosphatemia and hypocalcemia in people with advanced renal failure interferes with the absorption of some drugs. Many drugs are bound to plasma proteins, such as albumin, for transport in the body; the unbound portion of the drug is available to act at the various receptor sites and is free to be metabolized. In many people, there is a decrease in the level of plasma proteins, which are used for the binding and transport of drugs.

In the process of metabolism, some drugs form intermediate metabolites that are toxic if not eliminated. This is true of meperidine (Demerol); it is metabolized to the toxic intermediate normeperidine, which causes excessive sedation, nausea, and vomiting. Some pathways of drug metabolism, such as hydrolysis, are slowed with uremia. This results in decreased insulin requirements for diabetics as renal function deteriorates.[13]

Decreased elimination by the kidneys allows drugs or their metabolites to accumulate in the body and requires that drug dosages be adjusted accordingly. Some drugs contain unwanted nitrogen, sodium, potassium, and magnesium and must be avoided in people with renal failure. Penicillin, for example, contains potassium. Nitrofurantoin and ammonium chloride add to the body's nitrogen pool. Many antacids contain magnesium. Patients with renal failure should be cautioned against the use of over-the-counter remedies.

TREATMENT

A notable trend over the past several decades has been an increasing number of people who require renal replacement therapy with dialysis or transplantation. The growing volume is largely attributable to the improvement in treatment as well as more liberal policies regarding who is treated. About 30,000 Americans begin dialysis therapy each year, compared with 18,000 new patients during 1980.[14] Each year, a total of 85,000 persons are maintained by dialysis therapy in the United States. The average cost of maintenance hemodialysis is about $30,000 per year. In comparison, about 9900 kidney transplantation operations were performed in 1991, and more than 20,000 patients remained on the waiting list for such operations. The cost of transplantation is $35,000 to $40,000, with a cost of $4,000 to $10,000 during subsequent years.[14]

MEDICAL MANAGEMENT

The treatment of chronic renal failure can be divided into two types: conservative management of renal insufficiency and renal replacement therapy with dialysis or transplantation. Conservative treatment consists of measures to prevent or retard deterioration in remaining renal function and to assist the body in compensating for the existing impairment. Interventions that have been shown to significantly retard the progression of chronic renal insufficiency include dietary protein restriction and blood pressure normalization.[15] Various interventions are used to compensate for reduced renal function and to correct the resulting anemia, hypocalcemia, and acidosis. These interventions often are used in conjunction with dialysis therapy for patients with renal insufficiency.

The most remarkable advance in medical management over the past decade has been the development of recombinant human erythropoietin (r-HuEPO) to treat profound anemia in patients with renal disease. Erythropoietin, which is primarily produced by the kidneys, acts on the bone marrow by stimulating erythroblast maturation to maintain the hematocrit level. Since its approval by the Food and Drug Administration in June 1989, r-HuEPO therapy has been used to maintain hematocrit levels in the range of 28% to 33%.[16] Secondary benefits of the therapy, previously attributed to uremia, include improvement in appetite, energy level, sexual function, skin color, and hair and nail growth as well as reduced cold intolerance.[16] The regular use of this medication has reduced the need among dialysis patients for regular blood transfusions to treat anemia.

Early treatment of hypocalcemia and hyperphosphatemia is important to prevent or slow long-term bone complications, such as osteodystrophy. Phosphate-binding antacids frequently are prescribed that act by increasing fecal losses of phosphate, thereby reducing its absorption from the gastrointestinal tract. Magnesium-containing antacids (*e.g.*, Maalox, Mylanta) are contraindicated because the kidneys regulate the excretion of this mineral. Additionally, milk products and other foods high in phosphorus content are restricted in the diet. Calcitriol (1,25-dihydroxycholecalciferol) and calcium supplements often are used to facilitate intestinal absorption of calcium and increase serum calcium levels. Metabolic acidosis, which occurs as a result of the kidneys' inability to appropriately regulate body *p*H, is treated with sodium bicarbonate.

DIALYSIS AND TRANSPLANTATION

Dialysis or renal replacement therapy is indicated when advanced uremia or serious electrolyte imbalances are present. The choice between dialysis and transplantation is dictated by age, related health problems, donor availability, and personal preference. Although transplantation often is the treatment preference, dialysis plays a critical role as a treatment method for end-stage renal disease. It is life-sustaining for people who are either not candidates for transplantation or awaiting transplantation and as a backup treatment if transplantation is unsuccessful.

Hemodialysis. The basic principles of hemodialysis have remained unchanged over the years. New technology has improved both the efficiency and the speed of dialysis. A hemodialysis system, or artificial kidney, consists of three parts: a blood compartment, a dialysis fluid compartment, and a cellophane mem-

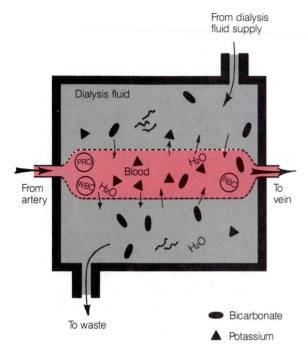

FIG. 33-2. Schematic diagram of a hemodialysis system. The blood compartment and dialysis solution compartment are separated by a cellophane membrane. This membrane is porous enough to allow all the constituents, except the plasma proteins and blood cells, to diffuse between the two compartments.

From dialysis fluid supply

Dialysis fluid

PRO

Blood H_2O

WBC H_2O

RBC

From artery

To vein

H_2O

H_2O

To waste

● Bicarbonate

▲ Potassium

brane that separates the two compartments. There are several types of dialyzers; all incorporate these parts and all function in a similar manner. The cellophane membrane is semipermeable, permitting all molecules except blood cells and plasma proteins to move freely in both directions—from the blood into the dialyzing solution and from the dialyzing solution into the blood. The direction of flow is determined by the concentration of the substances contained in the two solutions. The waste products and excess electrolytes in the blood normally diffuse into the dialyzing solution. If there is a need to replace or add substances, such as bicarbonate, to the blood, these can be added to the dialyzing solution (Fig. 33-2).

During dialysis, blood moves from an artery through the tubing and blood chamber in the dialysis machine and then back into the body through a vein. Access to the vascular system is through an external arteriovenous (AV) shunt (tubing implanted into an artery and a vein) or, more commonly, through an internal AV fistula (anastomosis of a vein to an artery, usually in the forearm). Heparin is used to prevent clotting during the dialysis treatment; it can be administered continuously or intermittently. Problems that may occur during dialysis, depending on the blood flow rate and rate of solute removal, include

hypotension, nausea, vomiting, muscle cramps, headache, chest pain, and disequilibrium syndrome. Most people are dialyzed three times a week for 3 to 4 hours. Many dialysis centers provide the option for people to learn how to perform hemodialysis at home.

Peritoneal Dialysis. The same principles of diffusion, osmosis, and ultrafiltration that apply to hemodialysis also apply to peritoneal dialysis. The thin serous membrane of the peritoneal cavity serves as the dialyzing membrane. A Silastic catheter is surgically implanted in the peritoneal cavity below the umbilicus to provide access. The catheter is tunneled through subcutaneous tissue and exits on the side of the abdomen (Fig. 33-3). The dialysis process involves instilling a sterile dialyzing solution (usually 2 L) through the catheter over 10 minutes. The solution is then allowed to remain, or dwell, in the peritoneal cavity for a prescribed amount of time, during which the metabolic end products and extracellular fluid diffuse into the dialysis solution. Commercial dialysis solution is available in 1.5%, 2.5%, and 4.25% dextrose concentrations. Solutions with higher dextrose levels increase osmosis, causing more fluid to be removed. At the end of the dwell time, the dialysis fluid is drained out of the peritoneal cavity by gravity into a sterile bag.

Peritoneal dialysis can be performed in a number of ways—at home versus in a center, automated versus manual system, intermittent versus continuous—all with variations in the number of exchanges

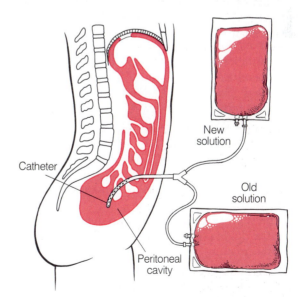

Catheter

New solution

Old solution

Peritoneal cavity

FIG. 33-3. Peritoneal dialysis. A semipermeable membrane, richly supplied with small blood vessels, lines the peritoneal cavity. With dialysate dwelling in the peritoneal cavity, waste products diffuse from the network of blood cells into the dialysate.

and in dwell time. Individual preference, manual ability, life-style, knowledge of the procedure, and physiologic response to treatment influence the dialysis schedule.

The most common method is continuous ambulatory peritoneal dialysis (CAPD). It is a self-care procedure in which the person manages the dialysis procedure and the type of solution (dextrose concentration) used at home. CAPD involves instilling dialysate into the peritoneal cavity and rolling up the bag and tubing and securing them under clothing during the dwell. After the dwell time is completed (4 to 6 hours during the day), the bag is unrolled and lowered, allowing the waste-containing dialysis solution to drain from the peritoneal cavity into the bag. Each exchange, which involves draining the solution and infusing a new solution, requires about 30 to 45 minutes. Four exchanges usually are performed each day. The continuous rather than intermittent nature of CAPD ensures that the rapid fluctuations in extracellular fluid volume associated with hemodialysis are avoided, and dietary restrictions can be liberalized somewhat.

Potential problems with peritoneal dialysis include infection, catheter malfunction, dehydration caused by excessive fluid removal, hyperglycemia, and hernia. The most serious complication is infection, which can occur at the catheter exit site, in the subcutaneous tunnel, or in the peritoneal cavity (peritonitis).

Transplantation. Greatly improved success rates have made kidney transplantation the treatment of choice for many people with chronic renal failure. Graft rates at 1 year are about 80% after cadaver transplantation and 90% after living-related transplantation.[17] At 5 years after cadaver transplantation, results show that about 60% have functional transplants. Living-related donors account for about 30% of all transplants in the United States; the remainder are cadaver transplants. Donor (cadaver) availability continues to limit the number of transplantations performed each year. Transplants from living nonrelated donors (*e.g.*, spouse) have been used in cases where suitable ABO and tissue compatibility were present.

The success of transplantation depends primarily on the degree of histocompatibility, adequate organ preservation, and immunologic management. Maintenance immunosuppression therapy typically consists of prednisone, azathioprine (Imuran), and cyclosporine (Sandimmune). Because of the increased number of effective immunosuppressants that have become available over the past decade, lower prednisone doses are used, resulting in reduced cushingoid effects after transplantation.

Among children in particular, alternate-day prednisone therapy often is used.[18] Rejection, which is categorized as acute and chronic, can occur at any time. Acute rejection most commonly occurs during the first several months post transplantation and involves a cellular response with the proliferation of T lymphocytes. Chronic rejection can occur later, months to years after transplantation. Because chronic rejection is caused by both cellular and humoral immunity, it does not respond to increased immunosuppressant therapy.

Maintenance immunosuppression and increased use of immunosuppression to treat rejection predispose the person to a spectrum of infectious complications. Prophylactic antibiotics are prescribed to decrease the incidence of common infections, such as candidiasis, herpes, and *Pneumocystis carinii* pneumonia. Other infections, such as cytomegalovirus and aspergillosis, are seen with chronic immunosuppression.

DIETARY MANAGEMENT

A major component in the treatment of chronic renal failure is dietary management. The goal of dietary treatment is to provide optimum nutrition while maintaining tolerable levels of metabolic wastes. The specific diet prescription depends on the type and severity of renal disease and the dialysis modality. Because of the severe restrictions placed on food and fluid intake, these diets may be complicated and unappetizing. After kidney transplantation, a less restrictive diet may be necessary, even when renal function is normal, to control the adverse effects from immunosuppressive medication. Common diet prescriptions are shown in Table 33-2.

Protein. Dietary restriction of protein is necessary with renal insufficiency and dialysis because proteins are broken down to form nitrogenous wastes. Considerable controversy exists over the degree of restriction needed. A protein restriction with 70% or more of high biologic value (containing more essential amino acids) is used with renal insufficiency. Proteins with a high biologic value are believed to promote the reuse of endogenous nitrogen, decreasing the amount of nitrogenous wastes that are produced and, thus, ameliorating the symptoms of uremia. In reusing nitrogen, the proteins ingested in the diet are broken down into their constituent amino acids to be used in the synthesis of protein required by the body. A 70-kg man synthesizes at least 150 g of protein daily while ingesting only 60 g.[19] For this to be accomplished, amino acids must be recycled; the ingestion of proteins that have a high

TABLE 33-2. COMMON DAILY DIET RECOMMENDATIONS FOR ADULTS

NUTRIENT	RENAL INSUFFICIENCY	MAINTENANCE HEMODIALYSIS	MAINTENANCE CAPD	INITIAL POSTTRANSPLANTATION
Protein	0.6–0.8 g/kg	0.8–1.0 g/kg	1.2–1.5 g/kg	1.3–2.0 g/kg
Carbohydrate	Unrestricted	Unrestricted	Unrestricted	1.0–1.5 g/kg
Fat	Unrestricted	Unrestricted	Unrestricted	<35% of calories
Calories	40–50 kcal/kg	40–50 kcal/kg	Restricted by dialysate	30–35 kcal/kg or to maintain ideal body weight
Potassium	40–70 mEq	40–70 mEq	Unrestricted	Unrestricted
Sodium	Variable	750–1500 mg	750–1500 mg	2000 mg
Phosporus	800–1200 mg	600–1200 mg	600–1200 mg	Unrestricted

CAPD, continuous ambulatory peritoneal dialysis.
(Data from Foulks, C.J. [1988]. Nutritional evaluation of patients on maintenance dialysis therapy. *American Nephrology Nurses' Journal, 15*, 13; Gammarino, M. [1987]. Renal transplant diet: Recommendations for the acute phase. *Dialysis and Transplantation, 16*, 497; Harum, P. [1984]. Renal nutrition for the renal nurse. *American Nephrology Nurses' Journal, 8*, 38; and Lancaster, L.E. [1982]. Renal failure: Pathophysiology, assessment, and intervention. *Critical Care Nursing, 1*, 50)

biologic value makes it possible. Almost all the amino acids in a whole egg are used in the synthesis of essential body proteins; hence, eggs are said to have a high biologic value. In contrast, fewer than half the amino acids in cereal proteins are reused. Amino acids that are not reused to build body proteins are broken down and form the end product of protein metabolism, such as urea.

People who are on peritoneal dialysis require a greater protein intake because of significant protein losses, ranging from 4 to 13 g/day, through dialysis.[20] Even higher protein losses can occur with peritonitis. With kidney transplantation, high doses of prednisone, especially during the immediate postoperative period or during acute rejection episodes, accelerate protein catabolism.[21] Diets that are high in protein content can reverse steroid-induced negative nitrogen balance.[22]

Carbohydrates, Fat, and Calories. With renal failure, adequate calories in the form of carbohydrates and fat are required to meet energy needs. This is particularly important when the protein content of the diet is severely restricted. If sufficient calories are not available, either the limited protein in the diet goes into energy production or body tissue itself is used for energy purposes.

Caloric intake for people on CAPD includes food intake as well as calories absorbed from the dialysis solution. A 2-L bag of 1.5% dialysate solution equals 105 calories, and a 4.25% solution delivers 289 calories.[23] Therefore, a 70-kg man on CAPD with an ideal caloric intake of 40 kcal/kg, or 2800 calories, who uses two bags of 1.5% solution and two bags of 4.25% solution per day only needs to ingest about 2000 calories (788 calories from dialysate).

Calories often need to be limited with kidney transplantation, since weight gain is common. Lowering the carbohydrate intake reduces the cushingoid effects caused by the corticosteroid drugs used to prevent transplant rejection. Reducing the intake of dietary fats and increasing the percentage of polyunsaturated fats can reduce hyperlipidemia after transplantation.[24]

Potassium. When the GFR falls to extremely low levels and when undergoing hemodialysis therapy, dietary restriction of potassium becomes mandatory. Using salt substitutes that contain potassium or ingesting fruits, fruit juice, chocolate, potatoes, or other high-potassium foods can cause hyperkalemia. Most people on continuous peritoneal dialysis do not need to limit potassium intake and often may need to increase intake.

Sodium and Fluid Intake. The sodium and fluid restrictions depend on the kidneys' ability to excrete sodium and water and must be individually determined. Renal disease of glomerular origin is more likely to contribute to sodium retention, whereas tubular dysfunction causes salt wasting.

Fluid intake in excess of what the kidneys can excrete causes circulatory overload, edema, and water intoxication. Thirst is a common problem among hemodialysis patients, often resulting in large weight gains between treatments. Increased thirst appears to be related to elevated renin levels and the production of angiotensin II.[25] Inadequate intake, on the other hand, causes volume depletion and hypotension and can cause further decreases in the already compromised GFR. It is common practice to allow a daily fluid intake of 500 to 800 mL, which is equal to insensible water loss, plus a quantity equal to the 24-hour urine output.

EXERCISE

The many medical problems that result from renal failure lead to reductions in physical functioning, energy level, and exercise capacity. Variables that strongly affect rehabilitation include age, diabetic status, and treatment mode. With the initiation of dialysis, younger adults usually have higher activity levels than older adults.[26] The physical activity level is much lower among people with diabetes who are on dialysis than among people the same age who do not have diabetes and are on dialysis.[27]

The exercise capacity, as measured by maximal oxygen consumption, for people treated with hemodialysis or peritoneal dialysis is below that of sedentary healthy people and people who have had successful kidney transplantations.[28] Factors that have been suggested as causes of reduced exercise capacity are anemia, altered peripheral metabolism of lactate, cardiac changes caused by uremia, and general physical deconditioning. Because of this, some dialysis centers have exercise training programs (*e.g.*, cycling) during hemodialysis treatments.

RENAL FAILURE IN CHILDREN AND ELDERLY PEOPLE

Although the spectrum of renal disease among children and elderly people is similar to that of adults, several unique issues that warrant further discussion are present among these groups.

CHRONIC RENAL FAILURE IN CHILDREN

Chronic renal failure in children, estimated at a 2% incidence per year, most frequently results from glomerulonephritis and congenital malformation (*i.e.*, renal dysgenesis).[29] Features of renal disease that are marked during childhood include growth impairment, delay in sexual maturation, and more extensive bone abnormalities. Critical growth periods occur during the first 2 years of life and during adolescence. Growth retardation as well as development at a slower rate are consequences of renal disease, especially among children with congenital renal disease. Factors related to impaired growth include deficient nutrition, anemia, renal osteodystrophy, chronic acidosis, and cases of nephrotic syndrome that require high-dose glucocorticoid therapy.[30] Puberty usually occurs at a later age in children with renal failure partly because of endocrine abnormalities. Renal osteodystrophy is more common and extensive in children than in adults because of the presence of open epiphyses.[30] As a result, metaphyseal fractures, bone pain, impaired bone growth and short stature, and osteitis fibrosa cystica occur with greater frequency. In addition, some hereditary renal diseases, such as medullary cystic disease, have skeletal involvement that further complicates the problems of renal osteodystrophy.

All forms of renal replacement therapy can be safely and reliably used for children. In fact, hemodialysis of a premature infant as small as 1500 g has been reported with only modest difficulties.[31] Children typically are treated with CAPD or transplantation to optimize growth and development. Early transplantation in young children is regarded as the best way to promote age-appropriate development.

CHRONIC RENAL FAILURE IN ELDERLY PEOPLE

Older adults (age 65 and over) account for about 42% of new patients each year with end-stage renal disease. In particular, the over-74 age group has shown a four-fold increase in incidence over the past decade.[23] Among elderly people, the presentation and course of renal failure may be altered because of the presence of age-related changes in the kidneys as well as concurrent medical conditions.

Normal aging is associated with a decline in the GFR and, subsequently, reduced homeostatic regulation under stressful conditions. This reduction in GFR makes elderly people more susceptible to the detrimental effects of nephrotoxic drugs, such as x-ray contrast compounds. The reduction in GFR related to aging is not accompanied by a parallel rise in the serum creatinine level. This occurs because the serum creatinine level, which results from muscle metabolism, is significantly reduced in elderly people because of diminished muscle mass and other age-related changes. For this reason, evaluation of renal function in elderly people should include a measurement of creatinine clearance along with the serum creatinine level. The Cockcoft and Gault equation is gaining popularity as an estimate of renal function with allowance for age.[32] Using the equation, an indirect estimate of creatinine clearance in mL/minute is:

$$\frac{(140 - age) \times (body\ weight\ in\ kg)}{72 \times serum\ creatinine\ in\ mg/dL}$$

(The equation should be multiplied by .085 for women.) The prevalence of chronic disease that affects the cerebrovascular, cardiovascular, and skeletal systems is higher in this age group.

Because of the presence of concurrent disease, the presenting symptoms of renal disease in elderly people may be less typical that those observed in younger adults. For example, congestive heart failure and hypertension may be more prevailing clinical features with the onset of acute glomerulonephritis, whereas oliguria and cola-colored urine are more often the first signs in younger adults.[33] Additionally, the course of renal failure may be more complicated in people with numerous chronic diseases.

Treatment options for chronic renal failure in elderly patients include hemodialysis, peritoneal dialysis, transplantation, and acceptance of death from uremia. The general reduction in T-cell function with age has been suggested as a beneficial effect that increases transplant graft survival.

In summary, chronic renal failure results from the destructive effects of many forms of renal disease. Regardless of the cause, the consequences of nephron destruction present in end-stage renal disease are alterations in the filtration, reabsorption, and endocrine functions of the kidneys. In the advanced stages, renal failure affects almost every body system. It causes azotemia as well as alterations in sodium and water excretion and body levels of potassium, phosphate, calcium, and magnesium. It also causes anemia, alterations in cardiovascular function, neurologic disturbances, gastrointestinal dysfunction, and discomforting skin changes. Within the past 20 years, dialysis and transplantation have allowed people with what was once a fatal disease to survive and lead relatively normal and productive lives.

■ REFERENCES

1. Anderson, R.J., & Schrier, R.W. (1991). Acute renal failure. In J.D. Wilson, E. Braunwald, K.J. Isselbacher, et al. (Eds.). *Harrison's principles of internal medicine* (12th ed., pp. 1144–1150). New York: McGraw-Hill.
2. Leaf, A., & Cotran, R. (1985). *Renal pathophysiology* (2nd ed., pp. 174–211). New York: Oxford University Press.
3. Lancaster, L. (1990). Renal response to shock. *Critical Care Clinics of North America, 2*(2), 221–233.
4. Myers, B.D., & Moran, S.M. (1986). Hemodynamically mediated acute renal failure. *New England Journal of Medicine, 314,* 97–105.
5. Price, C.A. (1991). Continuous renal replacement therapy: The treatment of choice for acute renal failure. *American Nephrology Nurses' Association Journal, 18*(3), 239.
6. Cotran, R.S., Kumar, V., & Robbins, S.L. (1989). *Robbins' pathologic basis of disease* (4th ed., pp. 1016–1017). Philadelphia: W.B. Saunders.
7. Brenner, B.M., & Lazarus, J.M. (1991). Chronic renal failure. In J.D. Wilson, E. Braunwald, K.J. Isselbacher, et al. (Eds.). *Harrison's principles of internal medicine* (12th ed., pp. 1150–1156). New York: McGraw-Hill.
8. Lancaster, L.E. (1982). Renal failure: Pathophysiology, assessment, and intervention. *Critical Care Nurse, 1,* 47, 45.
9. Van Stone, J.C. (1983). *Dialysis and the treatment of renal insufficiency* (pp. 1–31). New York: Grune & Stratton.
10. Raskin, N.H., & Fisherman, R.A. (1976). Neurological disorders in renal failure. *New England Journal of Medicine, 294,* 143, 147.
11. Foulks, C.J., & Cushner, H.M. (1986). Sexual dysfunction in the male dialysis patient: Pathogenesis, evaluation, and therapy. *American Journal of Kidney Diseases, 8,* 211, 212.
12. Rickus, M.A. (19870. Sexual dysfunction in the female ESRD patient. *American Nephrology Nurses' Association Journal, 14*(3), 185, 186.
13. Rennett, W.M., & McCarron, D.A. (1987). *Pharmacotherapy of renal disease and hypertension* (p. 5). New York: Churchill Livingston.
14. Health Care Financing Administration. (1987). *U.S. transplant statistics.* Washington, D.C.: U.S. Department of Health and Human Services.
15. Zeller, K.R. (1991). Low-protein diets in renal disease. *Diabetes Care, 14*(9), 859, 861.
16. Lundin, A.P. (1991). Recombinant erythropoietin and chronic renal failure. *Hospital Practice, 26*(4A), 62.
17. Morris, P.J. (1991). Kidney transplantation, 1960–1990. *Advances in Nephrology 20,* 14.
18. McEnery, P.T., Stablein, D.M., Arbus, G., & Tejani, A. (1992). Renal transplantation in children. *New England Journal of Medicine, 326*(26), 1730.
19. Giordano, C. (1977). The role of diet in renal disease. *Hospital Practice, 12*(11), 115–119.
20. Blumenkrantz, M.J., Gahl, G.M., Kopple, J.D., Kamdar, A.V., Jones, M.R., Kessel, M., & Coburn, J.W. (1981). Protein loss during peritoneal dialysis. *Kidney International, 19,* 593.
21. Hoy, W.E., Sargent, J.A., Hall, D., McKenna, B.A., Pabico, R.C., Freeman, R.B., Yarger, J.M., & Byer, B.M. (1985). Protein catabolism during the postoperative course after renal transplantation. *American Journal of Kidney Diseases, 5,* 187.
22. Cogan, M.G., Sargent, J.A., Yarbrough, S.G., Vincenti, F., & Amend, W.J. (1981). Prevention of prednisone-induced negative nitrogen balance. *Annals of Internal Medicine, 95,* 160.
23. Harum, P. (1984). Renal nutrition for the renal nurse. *American Nephrology Nurses' Association Journal 8,* 39.
24. Disler, P.B., Goldberg, R.B., Kuhn, L., Meyers, A.M., Joffe, B.I., & Seftel, H.C. (1981). The role of diet in the pathogenesis and control of hyperlipidemia after renal transplantation. *Clinical Nephrology, 16,* 31.
25. Porth, C.M., & Erickson, M. (1992). Physiology of thirst and drinking: Implication for nursing practice. *Heart & Lung, 21*(3), 275.
26. Carlson, D.M., Johnson, W.J., & Kjellstrand, C.M. (1987). Functional status of patients with end-stage renal disease. *Mayo Clinic Proceedings, 62,* 340.
27. Gutman, R.A., Stead, W.W., & Robinson, R.R. (1981). Physical activity and employment status of patients on maintenance dialysis. *New England Journal of Medicine, 304,* 310.
28. Painter, P., Messer-Rehak, D., Hanson, P., Zimmerman, S.W., & Glass, N.R. (1986). Exercise capacity in hemodialysis, CAPD, and renal transplant patients. *Nephron, 42,* 48.
29. U.S. Renal Data System. (1991). ESRD in children. *American Journal of Kidney Diseases, 18*(5), 83.
30. Chesney, R.W., & Friedman, A.L. (1984). The medical management of chronic renal failure. In B.M. Tune & S.A. Mendoza (Eds.). *Pediatric nephrology* (p. 322). New York: Churchill Livingstone.
31. Nevins, T.E., & Mauer, S.M. (1984). Infant hemodialysis. In R.N. Fine & A.B. Gruskin (Eds.). *End stage renal disease in children* (p. 39). Philadelphia: W.B. Saunders.
32. Levin, M.L. (1989). The elderly patient with advanced renal failure. *Hospital Practice, 24*(3A), 35–44.
33. Burkart, J.M., & Beck, L.H. (1990). Renal diseases in

the elderly. In W.R. Hazzard, R. Andres, E.L. Bierman, & J.P. Blass (Eds.). *Principles of geriatric medicine and gerontology* (2nd ed., p. 565). New York: McGraw-Hill.

■ BIBLIOGRAPHY

Badr, K., & Ichikawa, I. (1988). Prerenal failure: A deleterious shift from renal compensation to decompensation. *New England Journal of Medicine, 319*, 623.

Coburn, J.W., & Salusky, I.B. (1990). Control of serum phosphorus in uremia. *New England Journal of Medicine, 320*, 1140–1142.

Eckhardt, K., & Kurtz, A. (1992). The biological role, site, and regulation of erythropoietin production. *Advances in Nephrology from the Necker Hospital, 21*, 203–233.

Epstein, F.H., & Brown, R.S. (1988). Acute renal failure: A collection of paradoxes. *Hospital Practice, 23*(1), 171.

Feldman, H.I. (1991). Protein restriction in chronic renal failure. *Hospital Practice, 26*(6), 220–225.

Fine, L.G. (1991). How much kidney tissue is enough. *New England Journal of Medicine, 325*, 1097–1099.

Fraser, C.L., & Arieff, A.I. (1988). Nervous system complications of uremia. *Annals of Internal Medicine, 109*, 143.

Hatch, F.E. (1990). Reversing the anemia of renal failure. *Hospital Practice, 25*(2A), 25–34.

Ihle, B.U., Becker, J.A., Whitworth, R.A., et al. (1989). The effect of protein restriction on progression of renal insufficiency. *New England Journal of Medicine, 321*, 1773–1777.

Klahr, S., Schreiner, G., & Ichikawa, I. (1988). The progression of renal failure. *New England Journal of Medicine, 318*, 1663, 1657.

Lee, D.B., Goodman, W.G., & Coburn, J.W. (1988). Renal osteodystrophy: Some questions on an old disorder. *American Journal of Kidney Diseases, 11*, 365.

Levey, A.S., Perrone, R.D., & Madias, N.E. (1988). Serum creatinine and renal function. *Annual Review of Medicine, 39*, 465.

Malluche, H.H., & Faugere, M.C. (1989). Renal osteodystrophy. *New England Journal of Medicine, 321*, 317–319.

Nolph, K.D., Lindblad, A.S., & Novak, J.W. (1988). Continuous ambulatory peritoneal dialysis. *New England Journal of Medicine, 318*, 1595.

Price, C.A. (1989). Continuous arteriovenous ultrafiltration: A monitoring guide for nurses. *Critical Care Nurse 9*(1), 12–19.

Sherwood, L.M. (1987). Vitamin D, parathyroid hormone, and renal disease. *New England Journal of Medicine, 316*, 1601.

Stapleton, S., & Wright, J. (1992). Continuous arteriovenous hemofiltration: An alternative dialysis therapy in infants. *Neonatal Network 11*(4), 17–25.

Tolkiff-Rubin, N.E., & Rubin, R.H. (1990). Uremia and host defenses. *New England Journal of Medicine, 322*, 770–772.

ALTERATIONS IN GENITOURINARY FUNCTION

CHAPTER 34

ALTERATIONS IN URINE ELIMINATION

■ OBJECTIVES

After you have studied this chapter, you should be able to meet the following objectives:

■ Trace the innervation of the bladder from the afferent stretch receptors to reflex control of detrusor muscle contraction and voluntary control of the external sphincter.

■ Explain the mechanism of low-pressure urine storage in the bladder.

■ List at least three classes of autonomic drugs and explain their potential effect on bladder function.

■ Describe at least three urodynamic studies that can be used to assess bladder function.

■ State the signs of urine retention.

■ Explain the common cause, symptoms, and dangers of autonomic hyperreflexia in a patient with spinal cord injuries.

■ Differentiate between lesions that produce spastic bladder dysfunction and those that produce flaccid bladder dysfunction in terms of the level of the lesions and their effects on bladder function.

■ Cite the pathology and causes of nonrelaxing external sphincter.

■ Describe the symptoms of diabetic bladder neuropathy.

■ State the rationale for the use of clean self-catheterization in terms of preventing bladder infections.

■ Describe the difference between bladder training methods used for a neurogenic bladder caused by a lesion of the spinal cord micturition reflex center and one caused by a lesion above the level of the reflex center.

■ Define *incontinence* and list the categories of this condition.

■ Describe Kegel's exercises and explain their use in the control of stress incontinence.

■ List at least four special problems of elderly people that contribute to the development of incontinence.

■ Discuss the difference between superficial and invasive bladder cancer in terms of bladder involvement, extension of the disease, and prognosis.

■ State the most common sign of bladder cancer.

Carol Mattson Porth: PATHOPHYSIOLOGY: CONCEPTS OF
ALTERED HEALTH STATES, 4th ed. © 1994, 1990, 1986, 1982
J.B. Lippincott Company

Although the kidneys control the formation of urine and regulate the composition of body fluids, it is the bladder that stores urine and controls its elimination from the body.[1] Alterations in the storage and expulsion functions of the bladder can result in incontinence, with its accompanying social and hygienic problems, or obstruction of urinary flow, which has deleterious effects on ureteral and, ultimately, renal function. The discussion in this chapter focuses on normal control of urine elimination, urine retention, neurogenic bladder, incontinence, and bladder cancer. Urinary tract infections are discussed in Chapter 32.

■ CONTROL OF URINE ELIMINATION

The bladder (also known as the urinary vesicle) is a freely movable organ located behind the pelvic bone in the male and in front of the vagina in the female. It consists of two parts: the fundus, or body, and the neck, or posterior urethra. In the male, the urethra continues anteriorly through the penis. Urine passes from the kidneys to the bladder through the ureters, which are 4 to 5 mm in diameter and about 30 cm in length. The ureters enter the bladder bilaterally at a location toward its base and close to the urethra (Fig. 34-1). The triangular area that is bounded by the ureters and the urethra is called the *trigone*. There are no valves at the ureteral openings, but as the pressure of the urine within the bladder rises, the ends of the ureters are compressed against the bladder wall to prevent the backflow of urine.

BLADDER STRUCTURE

The bladder is composed of four layers: (1) an outer serosal layer, which covers the upper surface and is continuous with the peritoneum; (2) a network of smooth muscle fibers called the detrusor muscle; (3) a

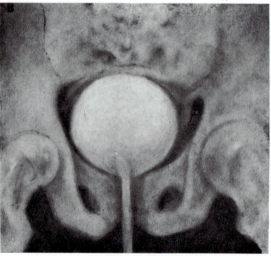
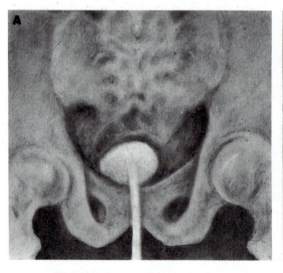
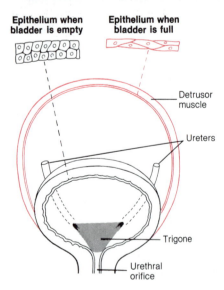

FIG. 34-1. (**Top**) Cystogram of male bladder, showing position and filling. (**Bottom**) Diagram of the bladder, showing the detrusor muscle, ureters, trigone area, and urethral orifice. Note the flattening of epithelial cells when the bladder is full and the wall is stretched. (Chaffee, E. E., & Lytle, I. M. [1980]. *Basic physiology and anatomy* [4th ed.]. Philadelphia: J.B. Lippincott)

submucosal layer of loose connective tissue; and (4) an inner mucosal lining of transitional epithelium.

The tonicity of the urine often is quite different from that of the blood, and the transitional epithelial lining of the bladder acts as an effective barrier to prevent the passage of water between the blood and the bladder contents. The inner elements of the bladder form smooth folds, or rugae. As the bladder expands during filling, these rugae spread out to form a single layer without disrupting the integrity of the epithelial lining.

The detrusor muscle is the muscle of micturition. When it contracts, urine is expelled from the bladder. The abdominal muscles play a secondary role in micturition. Their contraction increases intraabdominal pressure, which further increases intravesicular pressure.

Muscles in the bladder neck, sometimes referred to as the internal sphincter, are a continuation of the detrusor muscle. They run down obliquely behind the proximal urethra, forming the posterior urethra in males and the entire urethra in females. When the bladder is relaxed, these circular muscle fibers are closed and act as a sphincter. When the detrusor muscle contracts, the sphincter is pulled open simply by the changes that occur in bladder shape. In the female, the urethra (2.5 to 3.5 cm) is shorter than in the male (16.5 to 18.5 cm) and usually affords less resistance to urine outflow.

Another muscle important to bladder function is the external sphincter, a circular muscle composed of striated muscle fibers that surrounds the urethra distal to the base of the bladder. The external sphincter operates as a reserve mechanism to stop micturition when it is occurring and to maintain continence in the face of unusually high bladder pressure. The skeletal muscle of the pelvic floor also contributes to the support of the bladder and the maintenance of continence.

NEURAL CONTROL OF BLADDER FUNCTION

The innervation of the bladder consists of a peripheral autonomic nervous system reflex that is subject to facilitation or inhibition by higher neurologic centers. There are three main levels of neurologic control for bladder function: (1) the spinal cord reflex centers, (2) the micturition center in the brain stem, and (3) the cortical and subcortical centers.

Spinal Cord Centers. The centers for reflex control of micturition (passage of urine) are located in the sacral (S2 through S4) and thoracolumbar (T11 through L1) segments of the spinal cord (Fig. 34-2).

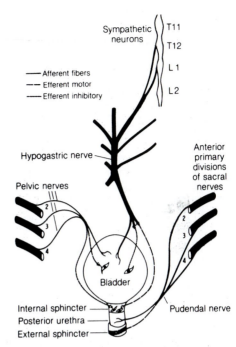

FIG. 34-2. Nerve supply to the bladder and the urethra. (Chaffee, E. E., & Lytle, I. M. [1980]. *Basic physiology and anatomy* [4th ed.]. Philadelphia: J.B. Lippincott)

Motor neurons for the detrusor muscle are located in the sacral cord; their axons travel to the bladder through the pelvic nerve. Lower motor neurons for the external sphincter are also located in the sacral segments of the spinal cord. These motor neurons communicate with the cerebral cortex by way of the pyramidal tracts and send impulses to the external sphincter by way of the pudendal nerve. The trigonal area of the bladder (because of its different embryology) receives its innervation from sympathetic outflow from the thoracolumbar (T11–L2) segments of the spinal cord. The bladder neck, along with the seminal vesicles, ampula of the vas, and vas deferens, also receives sympathetic innervation from the thoracolumbar segments of the cord.

The afferent input from the bladder and urethra is carried to the central nervous system by means of fibers that travel with the parasympathetic (pelvic), somatic (pudendal), and sympathetic (hypogastric) nerves. The pelvic nerve carries sensory fibers from the stretch receptors in the bladder wall; the pudendal nerve carries sensory fibers from the external sphincter and pelvic muscles; and the hypogastric nerve carries sensory fibers from the trigone area.

Brain Stem Micturition Center. The immediate coordination of the normal micturition reflex occurs in the micturition center of the brain stem, facilitated by ascending and descending pathways from the reflex centers in the spinal cord (Fig. 34-3). This center is thought to coordinate the activity of the detrusor

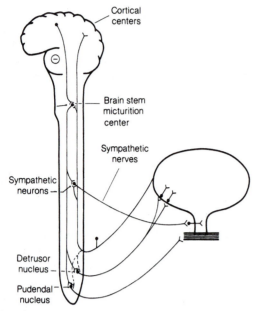

FIG. 34-3. Neuronal interactions between lower urinary tract and nervous system. Before micturition, the bladder afferents ascend to the micturition center, which normally is inhibited by higher centers. Efferents from the micturition center descend to the thoracolumbar sympathetic center and the detrusor and pudendal nuclei to coordinate vesical contraction with relaxation of the smooth muscle and striated muscle sphincters. (Krane, R. J., & Sirosky, M. B. [Eds.] [1979]. *Clinical neuro-urology* [p. 145]. Boston: Little, Brown. Used with permission)

muscle and the external sphincter. The detrusor motor neurons of the sacral cord do not respond directly to afferent information generated by bladder filling. Instead, bladder emptying occurs only after afferent generation of a brain stem–integrated micturition response.

Cortical and Subcortical Centers. Cortical brain centers allow for inhibition of the micturition center in the brain stem and conscious control of urination. Neural influences from the subcortical centers in the basal ganglia, which are conveyed by extrapyramidal pathways, modulate the contractile response. They modify and delay the detrusor contractile response during filling and then modulate the expulsive activity of the bladder to facilitate complete emptying.[2]

MICTURITION

When the bladder is distended to 150 to 300 mL, the sensation of fullness is transmitted to the spinal cord and then to the cerebral cortex, allowing for conscious inhibition of the micturition reflex. During the act of micturition, the detrusor muscle of the bladder fundus and bladder neck contract down on the urine

in the fundus; the ureteral orifices are forced shut; the bladder neck is widened and shortened as it is pulled up by the globular muscles in the bladder fundus; and the resistance of the internal sphincter in the bladder neck is decreased as urine moves out of the bladder.

In infants and young children, micturition is an involuntary act that is triggered by a spinal cord reflex; when the bladder fills to a given capacity, the detrusor muscle contracts and the external sphincter relaxes. As the bladder grows and increases in capacity, the tonicity of the external sphincter increases. At ages 2 to 3, the child becomes conscious of the need to urinate and can learn to briefly contract the pelvic muscles to inhibit contraction of the detrusor muscle and, thus, delay urination. As the central nervous system continues to mature, inhibition of involuntary detrusor muscle activity takes place. Once the child achieves continence, micturition becomes voluntary.

To maintain continence, or retention of urine, the bladder must function as a low-pressure storage system; that is, the pressure within the bladder must remain lower than urethral pressure. To ensure that this condition is met, the increase in intravesicular pressure that accompanies bladder filling is almost imperceptible. An increase in bladder volume from 10 to 400 mL may be accompanied by only a 5- to 10-cm H_2O increase in pressure.[3] Sustained elevations in intravesicular pressures (greater than 40 to 50 cm H_2O) often are associated with vesicoureteral reflux (a backward movement of urine from the bladder into the ureter) and the development of ureteral dilatation. Although the pressure within the bladder is maintained at low levels, sphincter pressure remains high (45 to 65 cm H_2O) as a means of preventing loss of urine as the bladder fills.

PHARMACOLOGY OF MICTURITION

The autonomic nervous system plays a central role in micturition. Both sympathetic and parasympathetic neurotransmitters contribute to the micturition reflex. Parasympathetic innervation of the bladder is mediated by the neurotransmitter acetylcholine. Two types of acetylcholine receptors affect various aspects of micturition: nicotinic and muscarinic. Nicotinic receptors are found in the synapses between the preganglionic and postganglionic neurons of both the sympathetic and the parasympathetic system as well as in the neuromuscular end plates of the striated muscle fibers of the external sphincter and pelvic muscles. Muscarinic receptors are found in the postganglionic parasympathetic endings of the detrusor muscle.

Although sympathetic innervation is not essential to the act of micturition, it allows the bladder to store a large volume without the involuntary escape of urine—a mechanism that is consistent with the fight-or-flight function subserved by the sympathetic nervous system. The bladder is supplied with both α- and β (β$_2$)-adrenergic receptors. The β-receptors are found in the detrusor muscle; they produce relaxation of the detrusor muscle, increasing the bladder volume at which the micturition reflex is triggered.[4] α-Receptors are found in the trigone area, including the intramural ureteral musculature, bladder neck, and internal sphincter. The activation of α-receptors produces contraction of these muscles. Sympathetic activity ceases when the micturition reflex is activated. During ejaculation, which is mediated by the sympathetic nervous system, the musculature of the trigone area as well as that of the bladder neck and prostatic urethra contracts and prevents the backflow of seminal fluid into the bladder.

Because of their effect on bladder function, drugs that selectively activate or block autonomic nervous system outflow or receptor activity can alter urine elimination. Table 34-1 describes the action of drugs that can impair bladder function or be used in the treatment of micturition disorders. Many of the nonprescription cold preparations contain α-adrenergic agonists and antihistamine agents that have anticholinergic properties. These drugs can cause urinary retention. Many of the antidepressant and antipsychotic drugs have anticholinergic actions that influence urination.

DIAGNOSTIC METHODS OF EVALUATING BLADDER FUNCTION

Bladder structure and function can be assessed by a number of methods. Reports or observations of frequency, hesitancy, straining to void, and a weak or interrupted stream are suggestive of outflow obstruction. Palpation and percussion provide information about bladder distention.

Post-voided residual urine volume (PVR) provides information about bladder emptying. It can be estimated by abdominal palpation and percussion. Catheterization and ultrasonography can be used to obtain specific measurements of PVR. A PVR of less

TABLE 34-1. BLADDER FUNCTION AND DRUG ACTIONS

FUNCTION	DRUG GROUPS	EXAMPLES
Detrusor Muscle		
Increased tone and contraction	Cholinergic drugs (stimulate parasympathetic receptors that cause detrusor muscle contraction)	Bethanechol (Urecholine)
	Anticholinesterase drugs (inhibit acetylcholine destruction)	Neostigmine (Prostigmin)
Inhibition of detrusor muscle relaxation during filling	β-Adrenergic blocking drugs (block β-receptors that cause detrusor muscle relaxation)	Propranolol (Inderal)
Decreased tone	Anticholinergic drugs (block parasympathetic receptors that cause detrusor muscle contraction)	Atropine Methantheline (Banthine) Propantheline (Pro-Banthine) Oxybutynin (Ditropan)
	Adrenergic agonists (activate β-sympathetic receptors that cause detrusor muscle relaxation)	Isoproterenol (Isuprel) Nifedipine (Adalat, Procardia)
	Calcium-channel blocking drugs (may interfere with influx of calcium to support detrusor muscle tone)	Virapamil (Calan, Isoptin) Diltiazem (Cardizem)
Internal Sphincter		
Increased tone	α-Adrenergic agonists (activate α-receptors that cause contraction of muscles of the internal sphincter)	Phenylephrine (generic) Ephedrine (generic) Phenylpropanolamine (generic) Phenoxybenzamine (Dibenzyline) Prazosin (Minipress)
Decreased tone	α-Adrenergic blocking drugs	
External Sphincter		
Decreased tone	Skeletal muscle relaxants	Baclofen (Lioresal) Dantrolene (Dantrium) Diazepam (Valium)

than 50 mL is considered adequate bladder emptying and more than 200 mL, inadequate bladder emptying.[5]

Urine tests provide information about kidney function and urinary tract infections. The presence of bacteriuria or pyuria suggests urinary tract infection and the possibility of urinary tract obstruction. Blood tests (blood urea nitrogen and creatinine) provide information about renal function.

Pelvic examination is used in women to assess perineal skin condition, perivaginal muscle tone, genital atrophy, pelvic prolapse (cystocele, rectocele, uterine prolapse), pelvic mass, or other conditions that might impair bladder function. Bimanual examination (pelvic and abdominal palpation) can be used to assess PVR. Rectal examination is used to test for perineal sensation, sphincter tone, fecal impaction, and rectal mass. It is used to assess the contour of the prostate in men.

Bladder structures can be visualized indirectly by taking x-ray films of the abdomen and by using excretory urography (which involves the use of a radiopaque dye [see Fig. 34-1]), computed tomographic (CT) scanning, magnetic resonance imaging (MRI), or ultrasonography. Cystoscopy enables direct visualization of the urethra, bladder, and ureteral orifices.

URODYNAMIC STUDIES

Urodynamic studies are used to study bladder function and voiding problems. Three aspects of bladder function can be assessed by urodynamic studies: (1) bladder, urethral, and intraabdominal pressure changes; (2) characteristics of urine flow; and (3) the activity of the striated muscles of the external sphincter and pelvic floor. Specific urodynamic tests include uroflometry, cystometrography, urethral pressure profile, sphincter electromyography, and uroflow studies.

Uroflometry. Uroflometry measures the flow rate (milliliters per minute) during urination. It commonly is done using a weight-recording device located at the bottom of a commode receptacle unit. As the person being tested voids, the weight of the commode receptacle unit increases. This weight change is electronically recorded and then analyzed using both weight (converted to milliliters) and time.

Cystometrography. Cystometrography (CMG) is used to measure bladder pressure during both filling and voiding. It provides valuable information about total bladder capacity, intravesicular pressures during bladder filling, the ability to perceive bladder fullness and the desire to urinate, the ability of the bladder to contract and sustain a contraction, unin-

hibited bladder contractions, and the ability to inhibit urination. The test uses either a gas (carbon dioxide) or sterile water (instilled through an indwelling catheter) to fill the bladder and some means for continuous recording of pressure during bladder filling and voiding. Gas cystometers originally became popular because they were simpler and faster to use, but they have proved less reliable and less informative than water cystometers.[6]

In a normally functioning bladder, the pressure remains constant at 8 to 15 cm H_2O until 350 to 450 mL of fluid has been instilled in the bladder. At this point, a definite sensation of fullness occurs, the pressure rises sharply to 40 to 100 cm H_2O, and voiding around the catheter occurs. Urinary continence requires that urethral pressure exceed bladder pressure. Bladder pressure usually rises 30 to 40 cm H_2O during voiding. If the urethral resistance is high because of obstruction, greater pressures is required, a condition that can be detected by the CMG.

Urethral Pressure Profile. The urethral pressure profile (UPP) is used to evaluate the intraluminal pressure changes along the length of the urethra with the bladder at rest. It provides information about smooth muscle activity along the length of the urethra. This test can be done using the infusion method (the most commonly used), the membrane catheter method, or the microtip transducer. The infusion method involves inserting a small double-lumen urethral catheter, infusing fluid or carbon dioxide into the bladder, and measuring the changes in urethral pressure as the catheter is slowly withdrawn.

Sphincter Electromyography. Sphincter electromyography (EMG) allows the activity of the striated (voluntary) muscles of the perineal area to be studied. Activity is recorded using anal (catheter or plug), urethral (catheter), or perineal (cup or paste) electrodes. Electrode placement is based on the muscle groups that need to be tested. The test usually is done along with urodynamic tests such as the CMG and uroflow studies.

It often is advantageous to evaluate several components of bladder function simultaneously. The most common combinations of studies are CMG, urethral sphincter EMG, and abdominal pressure; UPP and urethral sphincter EMG; and uroflometry, urethral sphincter EMG, and abdominal and bladder pressure (often referred to as a micturition study).[7] Rectal pressure commonly is used as a measure of abdominal pressure.

In summary, although the kidneys function in the formation of urine and the regulation of body fluids, it is the bladder that stores and controls the elimination of urine. Micturition basically is a function of the peripheral autonomic nervous system, subject to facilitation or inhibition from higher neurologic centers. The parasympathetic nervous system controls the motor function of the bladder detrusor muscle and the tone of the internal sphincter; its cell bodies are located in the sacral spinal cord and communicate with the bladder through the pelvic nerve. Efferent sympathetic control originates at the level of segments T11 through L1 of the spinal cord and produces relaxation of the detrusor muscle and contraction of the internal sphincter. Skeletal muscle found in the external sphincter and the pelvic muscles that support the bladder are supplied by the pudendal nerve, which exits the spinal cord at the level of segments S2 through S4. The micturition center in the brain stem coordinates the action of the detrusor muscle and the external sphincter, whereas cortical centers permit conscious control of micturition. Bladder function can be evaluated using urodynamic studies that measure bladder, urethral, and abdominal pressures; urine flow characteristics; and skeletal muscle activity of the external sphincter.

■ ALTERATIONS IN BLADDER FUNCTION

Alterations in bladder function include both urinary obstruction with retention of urine and urinary incontinence with involuntary loss of urine. Although the two conditions have almost opposite effects on urination, they can have similar causes. Both can result either from structural changes in the bladder, urethra, or surrounding organs or from impairment of neurologic control of bladder function.

URINE RETENTION

In urine retention, urine is produced normally by the kidneys but is retained in the bladder. The condition has a number of causes, including urethral obstruction, impaired innervation of the bladder (neurogenic bladder), and the effects of drug actions on the control of bladder function. Because it has the potential to produce vesicoureteral reflux and cause kidney damage, urine retention is a serious disorder.

URETHRAL OBSTRUCTION

Major structural urinary obstruction most often is due to processes that cause intrinsic narrowing or external compression of the urinary meatus or bladder outlet structures. In males, the most important cause of urinary obstruction is external compression of the urethra caused by enlargement of the prostate gland (see Chapter 36). External obstructive processes are less common in females. When they do occur, they typically are caused by a cystocele of the bladder (see Chapter 38). Bladder tumors and secondary invasion of the bladder by tumors arising in structures that surround the bladder and urethra can compress the bladder neck or urethra and cause obstruction. Narrowing of the urethra owing to congenital deformities or scar tissue from injury or infection can also obstruct urine flow. Congenital narrowing of the urinary meatus (meatal stenosis) is more common in boys, and obstructive disorders of the posterior urethra are more common in girls. Gonorrhea and other sexually transmitted diseases contribute to the incidence of infection-produced urethral strictures.

Constipation and fecal impaction can compress the urethra and produce urethral obstruction. This is a particular problem in elderly people.

Compensatory Changes. The body compensates for the obstruction of urine outflow with mechanisms designed to prevent urine retention. These mechanisms can be divided into three stages: an irritability stage, a compensatory stage, and a decompensatory stage. The degree to which these changes occur and their effect on bladder structure and urinary function depend on the extent of the obstruction, the rapidity with which it occurs, and the presence of other contributing factors, such as neurologic impairment and infection.

During the early stage of obstruction, the bladder begins to hypertrophy and becomes hypersensitive to afferent stimuli arising from bladder filling. The ability to suppress urination is diminished, and bladder contraction can become so strong that it virtually produces bladder spasm. There is urgency, sometimes to the point of incontinence, and frequency both during the day and at night.

With continuation and progression of the obstruction, compensatory changes begin to occur. There is further hypertrophy of the bladder muscle, the thickness of the bladder wall may double, and the pressure generated by detrusor contraction can increase from a normal 20 to 40 cm H_2O to 50 to 100 cm H_2O to overcome the resistance from the obstruction. As the force needed to expel urine from the bladder increases, compensatory mechanisms may become ineffective, causing muscle fatigue before complete emptying can be accomplished. After a few minutes, voiding can again be initiated and completed, accounting for the frequency of urination.

The inner bladder surface forms smooth folds. With continued outflow obstruction, this smooth surface is replaced with coarsely woven structures (hypertrophied smooth muscle fibers) called trabeculae. Small pockets of mucosal tissue, called cellules, commonly develop between the trabecular ridges. These pockets form diverticula when they extend between the actual fibers of the bladder muscle (Fig. 34-4). Because the diverticula have no muscle, they are unable to contract and expel their urine into the

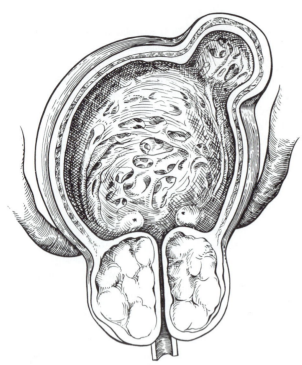

FIG. 34-4. Destructive changes of the bladder wall with development of diverticula caused by benign prostatic hypertrophy.

bladder, and secondary infections caused by stasis are common.

Along with hypertrophy of the bladder wall, there is hypertrophy of the trigone area and the interureteric ridge, which is located between the two ureters. This causes back pressure on the ureters, the development of hydroureters (dilated, urine-filled ureters), and, eventually, kidney damage. In addition, stasis of urine predisposes to urinary tract infections.

When compensatory mechanisms are no longer effective, signs of decompensation begin to occur. The period of detrusor muscle contraction becomes too short to completely expel the urine, and residual urine remains in the bladder. At this point, the symptoms of obstruction—frequency of urination, hesitancy, a need to strain to initiate urination, a weak and small stream, and termination of the stream before the bladder is completely emptied—become pronounced. The amount of residual urine may increase up to 1000 to 3000 mL, and overflow incontinence occurs. There may also be acute or sudden complete retention of urine. The signs of urine retention are summarized in Chart 34-1.

Treatment. The immediate treatment of outflow obstruction is directed toward relief of bladder distention. This usually is accomplished through uri-

nary catheterization (discussed later in this chapter). If constipation or fecal impaction is present, this should be corrected. Long-term treatment is directed toward correcting the problem causing the obstruction.

NEUROGENIC BLADDER DISORDERS

The innervation of the bladder can be interrupted at any level and can selectively involve either sensory or motor innervation or both. Neurogenic disorders of the bladder commonly are manifested in one of two ways: by spastic bladder dysfunction or by flaccid bladder dysfunction. Spastic bladder dysfunction usually results from neurologic lesions that are above the level of the sacral micturition reflex center, whereas flaccid bladder dysfunction results from lesions at the level of sacral micturition reflexes or peripheral innervation of the bladder. In addition to detrusor muscle dysfunction, disruption of micturition occurs when the neurologic control of external sphincter function is impaired. Some disorders, such as Parkinson's disease, cause mixed spastic and semiflaccid bladder dysfunction. Table 34-2 describes the characteristics of neurogenic bladder according to the level of the lesion.

SPASTIC BLADDER DYSFUNCTION

The terms *reflex neurogenic bladder*, *spastic neurogenic bladder*, *cord bladder*, and *uninhibited bladder* have been variously used to describe a neurogenic disorder that causes spastic bladder dysfunction. This condition can be caused by any neurologic condition above the level of the voiding reflex arc. The degree of spasticity and dysfunction depends on the level and extent of neurologic dysfunction. Common lesions above the level of the brain stem micturition center that affect voiding are cerebrovascular accident (stroke), dementia, multiple sclerosis, and brain tumors. Spinal cord lesions are the single most important causes of

CHART 34-1: SIGNS OF URETHRAL OBSTRUCTION AND URINE RETENTION

Bladder distention
Hesitancy
Straining with initiating urination
Small and weak stream
Frequency
Feeling of incomplete bladder emptying
Overflow incontinence

TABLE 34-2. CHARACTERISTICS AND TYPES OF NEUROGENIC BLADDER

LEVEL OF LESION	CHANGE IN BLADDER FUNCTION	COMMON CAUSES
Cortex or pyramidal tract	Loss of cortical ability to perceive bladder filling results in low volume; physiologically normal micturition occurs suddenly and is difficult to inhibit	Stroke and advanced age
Basal ganglia or extra-pyramidal tract	Detrusor contractions are elicited suddenly without warning and are difficult to control; bladder contraction is shorter than normal and does not produce full bladder emptying	Parkinson's disease
Brain stem micturition center or communicating tracts in the spinal cord	Storage reflexes are provoked during filling, and external sphincter responses are heightened; uninhibited bladder contractions occur at a lower volume than normal and do not continue until the bladder is emptied; antagonistic activity occurs between the detrusor muscle and the external sphincter	Spinal cord injury
Sacral cord or nerve roots	Areflexic bladder fills but does not contract; loss of external sphincter tone occurs when the lesion affects the α-adrengic motor neurons or pudendal nerve	Injury to sacral cord or spinal roots
Pelvic nerve	Increased filling and impaired sphincter control cause increased intravesicular pressure	Radical pelvic surgery
Autonomic peripheral sensory pathways	Bladder overfilling occurs with lack of appreciation of bladder events	Diabetic neuropathies, multiple sclerosis

spastic bladder dysfunction caused by lesions below the level of the micturition center. Spinal cord lesions include trauma (spinal cord injury), herniated intervertebral disk, vascular lesions, multiple sclerosis, tumors, and myelitis.

Uninhibited Neurogenic Bladder. A mild form of reflex neurogenic bladder, sometimes called uninhibited bladder, can develop after a stroke, during the early stages of multiple sclerosis, or as a result of lesions located in the inhibitory centers of the cortex or the pyramidal tract. With this type of disorder, the sacral reflex arc and sensation are retained, the urine stream is normal, and there is no residual urine. Bladder capacity is diminished, however, because of increased detrusor muscle tone and spasticity.

Detrusor–Sphincter Dyssynergy. Depending on the level of the lesion, the coordinated activity of the detrusor muscle and the external sphincter may be affected. Lesions that affect the micturition center in the brain stem or impair communication between this center and spinal cord centers interrupt the coordinated activity of the detrusor muscle and the external sphincter. This is called detrusor–sphincter dyssynergy. Instead of relaxing during micturition, the external sphincter becomes more constricted. This condition can lead to elevated intravesicular pressures and vesicoureteral reflux.

Bladder Dysfunction Caused by Spinal Cord Injury. One of the most common types of spinal cord lesions is spinal cord injury (see Chapter 50).

The immediate and early effects of spinal cord injury on bladder function are quite different from those that follow recovery from the impact of the initial injury. During the period immediately after spinal cord injury, a state of spinal shock develops during which all the reflexes, including the micturition reflex, are depressed. During this stage, the bladder becomes atonic and cannot contract. Catheterization is necessary to prevent injury to urinary structures associated with overdistention of the bladder. Aseptic intermittent catheterization is the preferred method of catheterization. Depression of reflexes lasts for about 1 to 2 months, after which time the spinal reflexes return and become hyperactive.

After the acute stage of spinal cord injury, the micturition response changes from a long-tract reflex to a segmental reflex. Because the sacral reflex arc remains intact, stimuli generated by bladder stretch receptors during filling produce frequent spontaneous contractions of the detrusor muscle. This creates a small, hyperactive bladder subject to high-pressure and short-duration uninhibited bladder contractions. Voiding is interrupted, involuntary, or incomplete. Hypertrophy of the trigone develops, often leading to vesicoureteral reflux and renal damage. Dilation of the internal sphincter and spasticity of the perineal muscles innervated by upper motor neurons occur, producing resistance to bladder emptying.

FLACCID BLADDER DYSFUNCTION

Detrusor muscle areflexia, or flaccid neurogenic bladder, occurs when there is injury to the micturition center of the sacral cord, the cauda equina, or the sacral roots that supply the bladder. Atony of the detrusor muscle and loss of the perception of bladder fullness permit the overstretching of the detrusor muscle that contributes to weak and ineffective bladder contractions. External sphincter tone and perineal muscle tone are diminished. Voluntary urination does not occur, but fairly efficient emptying can be achieved by increased intraabdominal pressure or manual suprapubic pressure. Among the causes of flaccid neurogenic bladder are meningomyelocele and spina bifida.

BLADDER DYSFUNCTION CAUSED BY PERIPHERAL NEUROPATHIES

In addition to central nervous system lesions and conditions that disrupt bladder function, disorders of the peripheral (pelvic, pudendal, and hypogastric) neurons that supply the bladder can occur. These neuropathies can selectively interrupt sensory or motor pathways for the bladder or involve both pathways. One of the most common causes of bladder neuropathies is diabetes mellitus.

Epidemiologic studies indicate that diabetic bladder neuropathy occurs in 43% to 87% of people with insulin-dependent diabetes, with no age or sex difference.[9] The disorder initially affects the sensory axons of the urinary bladder without involvement of the pudendal nerve. There is an insidious onset of bladder dysfunction during which time voidings gradually decrease until urine is passed only once or twice a day.[10] There frequently is need for straining, accompanied by hesitation, weakness of the stream, dribbling, and a sensation of incomplete bladder emptying. The chief complications are vesicoureteral reflux and ascending urinary tract infection. Because people with diabetes are already at risk for developing glomerular disease (see Chapter 32), reflux can have serious effects on kidney function. Treatment consists of surgical creation of a temporary urinary diversion, bladder training, and pharmacologic manipulation of bladder function with parasympathetic drugs.[11] To compensate for the decreased contractile properties of the detrusor muscle, the bladder neck may be resected to decrease the resistance to outflow of urine from the bladder. Because the innervation of the external sphincter is not disturbed, continence is maintained.

NONRELAXING EXTERNAL SPHINCTER

Another condition that affects the peripheral innervation of micturition is *nonrelaxing external sphincter*.[12] This condition usually is related to a delay in maturation, developmental regression, psychomotor disorders, or locally irritative lesions. Inadequate relaxation of the external sphincter can be the result of anxiety or depression. Any local irritation can produce spasms of the sphincter by means of afferent sensory input from the pudendal nerve; included are vaginitis, perineal inflammation, and inflammation or irritation of the urethra. In men, chronic prostatitis contributes to the impaired relaxation of the external sphincter.

TREATMENT

The goals of treatment for neurogenic bladder disorders center on preventing bladder overdistention, urinary tract infections, and renal damage that can be life-threatening and on reducing the undesirable social and psychological effects of the disorder. Treatment is based on the type of neurologic lesion that is involved; information obtained through the health history, including fluid intake; report or observation of voiding patterns; presence of other health problems; urodynamic studies when indicated; and the ability of the person to participate in the treatment. Treatment methods include catheterization, bladder training, pharmacologic manipulation of bladder function, and surgery.

Catheterization. Catheterization involves the insertion of a small-diameter latex or silicon tube into the bladder through the urethra. The catheter may be inserted on a one-time basis to relieve temporary bladder distention, left indwelling (retention catheter), or inserted intermittently. With acute overdistention of the bladder, no more than 1000 mL of urine is removed from the bladder at one time. The theory behind this limitation is that removing more than this amount at one time releases pressure on the pelvic blood vessels and predisposes to shock. Sometimes permanent indwelling catheters are used when there is urine retention or incontinence in people who are ill or debilitated or when conservative or surgical methods for the correction of incontinence are not feasible. The use of permanent indwelling bladder catheters in patients with spinal cord injury has been shown to produce a number of complications, including urinary tract infections, urethral irritation and injury, epididymoorchitis, pyelonephritis, and kidney stones.[13]

Intermittent catheterization is used to treat urine

retention or incomplete emptying secondary to various neurologic or obstructive disorders. Properly used, it prevents bladder overdistention and urethral irritation, allows for more freedom of activity, and provides for periodic distention of the bladder to prevent muscle atony. It often is used with pharmacologic manipulation to achieve continence; when possible, it is learned and managed as a self-care procedure (intermittent self-catheterization). It may be carried out as either an aseptic (sterile) or a clean procedure. Aseptic intermittent catheterization is used in people with spinal shock and in those who need short-term catheterization. The clean procedure usually is followed for self-catheterization. It is performed at 3- to 4-hour intervals to prevent overdistention of the bladder. The best results are obtained if only 300 to 400 mL is allowed to collect in the bladder between catheterizations. The use of the clean as opposed to the sterile procedure has been defended on the basis that most urinary tract infections are due to some underlying abnormality of the urinary tract that leads to impaired tissue resistance to bacterial infection, the most common cause of which is decreased blood flow because of overdistention.[14] Overdistention has also been shown to decrease the mucin layer that protects the mucosal surface of the bladder.[15] Studies have shown up to a 48% decrease in bacteriuria after the institution of intermittent self-catheterization.[14] This treatment has proved particularly effective in children with meningomyelocele.

Bladder Training. Bladder training differs with the type of disorder that is present. Training includes the use of body positions that facilitate micturition and the monitoring of fluid intake to prevent urinary tract infections and control urine volume and osmolality.

Among the considerations when monitoring fluid intake is the need to ensure adequate fluid intake to prevent unduly concentrated urine that may serve to stimulate afferent neurons of the micturition reflex. In hyperreflexive bladder or detrusor–sphincter dyssynergy, the stimulation of afferent nerve endings by irritating constituents of the urine results in increased vesicular pressures, vesicoureteral reflux, and overflow incontinence. On the other hand, fluid intake must be balanced to prevent bladder overdistention from occurring during the night. Adequate fluid intake is also needed to prevent urinary tract infections, the irritating effects of which increase bladder irritability and the risk of urinary incontinence and renal damage.

The methods used for bladder retraining depend on the type of lesion that is present. In spastic neurogenic bladder, methods designed to trigger the sacral micturition reflex are used; in flaccid neuro-genic bladder, manual methods that increase intravesicular pressure are used. *Trigger voiding methods* include manual stimulation of the afferent loop of the micturition reflex through such maneuvers as tapping the suprapubic area, pulling on the pubic hairs, stroking the glans penis, or rubbing the thighs. *Credé's method*, which is done with the person in a sitting position, consists of applying pressure (with four fingers of one hand or both hands) to the suprapubic area as a means of increasing intravesicular pressure. The use of Valsalva's maneuver (bearing down by exhaling against a closed glottis) increases intraabdominal pressure and aids in bladder emptying. This maneuver is repeated until the bladder is empty. For the best results, the patient must cooperate fully with the procedures or, if possible, learn to perform them independently.

Biofeedback methods have been useful for teaching some aspects of bladder control. They involve the use of EMG or cystometry as a feedback signal for training a person to control the function of the external sphincter or raise intravesicular pressure enough to overcome outflow resistance.

Pharmacologic Manipulation. Pharmacologic manipulation includes the use of drugs to alter the contractile properties of the bladder, decrease the outflow resistance of the internal sphincter, and relax the external sphincter. The usefulness of drug therapy often is evaluated during cystometric studies. Anticholinergic drugs, such as propantheline (Pro-Banthine), decrease detrusor muscle tone and increase bladder capacity in people with spastic bladder dysfunction. Parasympathomimetic drugs, such as bethanechol chloride (Urecholine), provide increased bladder tonus and may prove helpful in the symptomatic treatment of milder forms of flaccid neurogenic bladder. Muscle relaxants, such as diazepam (Valium) and baclofen (Lioresal), may be used to decrease the tone of the external sphincter. Table 34-1 describes the drugs that affect bladder function.

Surgical Procedures. Among the surgical procedures used in the management of neurogenic bladder are sphincterectomy or transurethral resection of the bladder neck in men with prostatic hypertrophy, reconstruction of the sphincter, nerve resection (the sacral reflex nerves that cause spasticity or the pudendal nerve that controls the external sphincter), and urinary diversion. Urinary diversion can be done by creating an ileal or a colon loop into which the ureters are anastomosed; the distal end of the loop is brought out and attached to the abdominal wall. Other procedures include the attachment of the ureters to the skin of the abdominal wall or the attachment of the ureters to the sigmoid colon with the rectum serving as a receptacle for the urine.

Extensive research is being conducted on methods of restoring voluntary control of the storage and evacuation functions of the bladder through the use of implanted electrodes. Single and multiple electrodes can be placed on selected nerves and then coupled to a subcutaneous receiver.[6]

URINARY INCONTINENCE

The Urinary Incontinence Guideline Panel defines urinary incontinence as an involuntary loss of urine that is sufficient to be a problem.[5] This panel was convened by the Agency for Health Care Policy and Research for the purpose of developing specific guidelines to improve the care of people with urinary incontinence.

Urinary incontinence affects about 10 million Americans. Many body functions decline with age, and incontinence, although not a normal accompaniment of the aging process, is seen with increased frequency in elderly people. Ten percent of men and 17% of women over age 65 have problems with incontinence. The increase in health problems often seen in elderly people probably contributes to the greater frequency of incontinence. Despite the prevalence of incontinence, most affected people do not seek help for it primarily because of embarrassment or because they are not aware that help is available.

Incontinence can be caused by a number of conditions. It can occur without the person's knowledge, and at other times, the person may be aware of the condition but be unable to prevent it. The Urinary Incontinence Guideline Panel has identified three main types of incontinence: stress, urge, and overflow.[5] Table 34-3 summarizes the characteristics of each of these types of incontinence. The condition may occur as a transient and correctable phenome-

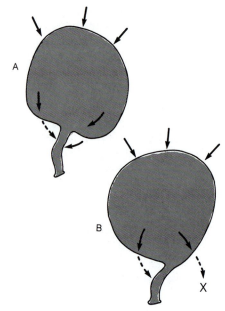

FIG. 34-5. Importance of the posterior urethrovesical (PU-V) angle to the continence mechanism. (**A**) In the presence of the normal PU-V angle, sudden changes in intraabdominal pressure are transmitted optimally (indicated by the *arrows* with dotted lines) to all sides of the proximal urethra. In this way, intraurethral pressure is maintained higher than the simultaneously elevated intravesicular pressure. This prevents loss of urine with sudden stress. (**B**) Loss of the PU-V angle results in displacement of the vesicle neck to the most dependent portion of the bladder, preventing the equal transmission of sudden increases in intraabdominal pressure to the lumen of the proximal urethra. Thus, the pressure in the region of the vesical neck rises considerably more than the intraurethral pressure just beyond it, and stress incontinence occurs. (Green, J. T., Jr. [1968]. *Obstetrical and Gynecological Survey, 23,* 603. Reprinted with permission)

non, or it may not be totally correctable and occur with varying degrees of frequency. Among the transient causes of urinary incontinence are confusional states; medications that alter bladder function or perception of bladder filling and the need to urinate; diuretics and conditions that increase bladder filling; restricted mobility; and stool impaction.

STRESS INCONTINENCE

Stress incontinence is the involuntary loss of urine during coughing, laughing, sneezing, or lifting that increases intraabdominal pressure. The most common cause is hypermobility and significant displacement of the urethra during exertion. In women, the angle between the bladder and the posterior proximal urethra (urethrovesical junction) is important to continence. This angle normally is 90 to 100 degrees, with at least one third of the bladder base contributing to the angle when not voiding (Fig. 34-5).[16] Dur-

TABLE 34-3. TYPES AND CHARACTERISTICS OF URINARY INCONTINENCE

TYPE	CHARACTERISTICS
Stress	Involuntary loss of urine associated with activities, such as coughing, that increase intraabdominal pressure
Urge	Involuntary loss of urine associated with strong desire to void
Overflow	Involuntary loss of urine when intravesicular pressure exceeds maximal urethral pressure in the absence of detrusor activity

ing the first stage of voiding, this angle is lost as the bladder descends. In women, diminution of muscle tone associated with normal aging, childbirth, or surgical procedures can cause weakness of the pelvic floor muscles and result in stress incontinence by obliterating the critical posterior urethrovesical angle. In these women, loss of the posterior urethrovesical angle, descent and funneling of the bladder neck, and backward and downward rotation of the bladder occur, so that the bladder and urethra are already in an anatomic position for the first stage of voiding. Therefore, any activity that causes downward pressure on the bladder is sufficient to allow the urine to escape involuntarily.

Another cause of stress incontinence is intrinsic urethral deficiency, which may be due to congenital sphincter weakness, such as occurs with myelomeningocele. It may also be acquired as a result of prostatectomy, trauma, radiation, or sacral cord lesion.

URGE INCONTINENCE

Urge, or urgency, incontinence is the involuntary loss of urine associated with a strong desire to void. It often is associated with involuntary and hyperreflexive detrusor contractions. Although hyperreflexive detrusor contractions occur in people with neurogenic bladder dysfunction (*e.g.*, spastic bladder dysfunction), they can also occur in people who have no evidence of neurologic dysfunction.

Among the causes of urge incontinence are those conditions in which a partial upper motor neuron lesion makes movement difficult, so that the interval between knowing the bladder needs to be emptied and being able to stop it from emptying may be less than the time needed to reach the lavatory. Multiple sclerosis is a common cause of this type of incontinence. Musculoskeletal disorders, such as arthritis and joint instability, may also prevent an otherwise continent person from reaching the toilet in time.

Drugs such as hypnotics, tranquilizers, and sedatives can interfere with the conscious inhibition of voiding, leading to urge incontinence. Diuretics, particularly in elderly people, increase the flow of urine and may contribute to incontinence, particularly in people with diminished bladder capacity and in those who have difficulty reaching the toilet. Urinary infections, increased bladder irritability, urgency, and frequency occur in people of all ages. In elderly people, these conditions often precipitate incontinence.

OVERFLOW INCONTINENCE

Overflow incontinence is an involuntary loss of urine that occurs when intravesicular pressure exceeds the maximal urethral pressure because of bladder disten-

tion in the absence of detrusor activity. It can occur with retention of urine owing to nervous system lesions or obstruction of the bladder neck. With this type of incontinence, the bladder is distended and small amounts of urine are passed, particularly at night. In males, one of the most common causes of obstructive incontinence is enlargement of the prostate gland. Another cause that commonly is overlooked is fecal impaction (the presence of dry, hard feces in the rectum). When a large amount (bolus) of stool forms in the rectum, it can push against the urethra and block the flow of urine.

OTHER CAUSES OF INCONTINENCE

Another cause of incontinence is decreased bladder compliance. This abnormal bladder condition may result from radiation therapy, radical pelvic surgery, or interstitial cystitis. Many people with this disorder have severe urgency related to bladder hypersensitivity that results in loss of bladder elasticity such that any small increase in bladder volume or detrusor function causes a sharp rise in bladder pressure and severe urgency.

Incontinence may also be caused by factors outside the lower urinary tract, such as the inability to locate, reach, or receive assistance in reaching an appropriate place to void.[17] This may be a particular problem in elderly people, who may have problems with mobility and manual dexterity or find themselves in unfamiliar surroundings. It occurs when a person cannot find or reach the bathroom or manipulate clothing quickly enough. Failing vision may contribute to the problem. Embarrassment in front of other people at having to use the bathroom, particularly if the timing seems inappropriate, may cause a person to delay emptying the bladder and may lead to incontinence. Treatment with drugs such as diuretics may cause the bladder to fill more rapidly than usual, making it difficult to reach the bathroom in time if there are problems with mobility or if a bathroom is not readily available. Night sedation may cause a person to sleep through the signal that normally would waken a person so he or she could get up and empty the bladder and avoid wetting the bed.

DIAGNOSIS AND TREATMENT

Urinary incontinence is a frequent and major health problem. It increases social isolation, frequently leads to institutionalization in elderly people, and predisposes to infections and skin breakdown.

Urinary incontinence is not a single disease but a symptom with many possible causes. As a symptom, it requires full investigation to establish its cause. This usually is accomplished through a careful history, physical examination, blood tests, and urinalysis. A voiding record (diary) may be used to determine the frequency, timing, amount of voiding, and other factors associated with the incontinence.[5] Because many drugs affect bladder function, a full drug history is essential. Estimation of PVR volume is recommended for all people with incontinence. Provocative stress testing is done when stress incontinence is suspected. This test is done by having the person relax and then cough vigorously while the examiner observes for urine loss. The test usually is done in the lithotomy position; if no leakage is observed, it is repeated in the standing position.[5] Urodynamic studies may be needed to provide information about urinary pressures and urine flow rates.

Treatment or management depends on the type of incontinence that is present, accompanying health problems, and the person's age. Exercises to strengthen the pelvic muscles and surgical correction of pelvic relaxation disorders often are used in women with stress incontinence. Noncatheter devices to obstruct urine flow or collect urine as it is passed may be used when urine flow cannot be controlled. Urinary incontinence is a major problem in elderly people, who have special treatment needs. Indwelling catheters (discussed earlier in the chapter), although a solution to the problem of urinary incontinence, usually are considered only after all other treatment methods have failed. In some types of incontinence, such as that associated with spinal cord injury or meningomyelocele, self-catheterization provides the means for controlling urine elimination.

Treatment of Stress Incontinence. Stress incontinence can be treated by physiotherapeutic measures, surgery, or a combination of the two. Surgical correction of cystocele and pelvic relaxation disorders in the female may be needed.

Active muscle-tensing exercises of the pelvic muscles may prove effective. These exercises were first advocated by Kegel; hence, they commonly are called *Kegel's exercises.*[18] Two groups of muscles are strengthened: (1) those of the back part of the pelvic floor (these are the muscles used to contract the anus and control the passing of stool) and (2) the front muscles of the pelvic floor (these are the muscles used to stop the flow of urine during voiding). In learning the exercises, a woman concentrates on identifying the muscle groups and learning how to control contraction. Once this has been accomplished, she can start an exercise program that consists of slowly contracting the muscles, beginning at the front and working to the back while counting to four and then releasing. The exercises can be done while sitting or standing and should be performed in repetitions of 10, three times a day.

α-Adrenergic agonist drugs, such as phenylpropanolamine, increase sympathetic relaxation of the detrusor muscle as well as internal sphincter tone and may be used in treating stress incontinence.[5]

Noncatheter Devices. Two types of noncatheter devices commonly are used in the management of urinary incontinence: one obstructs flow and the other collects urine as it is passed. Obstruction of urine flow is achieved by compressing the urethra or stimulating the contraction of the pelvic floor muscles. Penile clamps are available that occlude the urethra without obstructing blood circulation to the penis. Clamps must be removed at 3-hour intervals to empty the bladder. Complications such as penile and urethral erosion can occur if clamps are used incorrectly. In females, compression of the urethra usually is accomplished by intravaginal devices. Surgically implanted artificial sphincters are available for use in both males and females.[19] These devices consist of an inflatable cuff that surrounds the proximal urethra. The cuff is connected by tubing to an implanted fluid reservoir and an inflation bulb. Pressing the bulb, which is placed in the scrotum in males, inflates the cuff. It is emptied in a similar manner. Another method of occluding the bladder outlet in both males and females is the use of battery-operated electrodes that cause contraction of the pelvic floor muscles. This treatment is most effective in women with stress incontinence caused by weakness of the pelvic floor muscles. Implantable electrodes have largely been replaced by those that can be worn in the vagina or in the anus.

When urinary incontinence cannot be prevented, various types of urine collection devices or protective pads are used. Men can be fitted with collection devices (condom or sheath urinals) that are worn over the penis and attached to a container at the bedside or fastened to the body. There are no effective external collection devices for women. Pants and pads usually are used. Dribbling bags (males) and pads (females) in which the urine changes to a nonpourable gel are available for occasional dribbling but are unsuitable for considerable wetting.

SPECIAL NEEDS OF ELDERLY PEOPLE

Urinary incontinence is a common problem in elderly people. The incidence is reported to vary from 11% to 42%, depending on whether the survey is taken in the community or in the hospital.[20] Many factors contribute to incontinence in elderly people, a number of which can be altered. Pelvic relaxation disorders are more frequent in older than in younger females, and prostatic hypertrophy is more common in older than in younger males. Many elderly people have difficulty getting to the toilet in time. This can be caused by arthritis that makes walking or removing clothing difficult or by failing vision that makes trips to the bathroom precarious, especially in new and unfamiliar surroundings. Medication prescribed for other health problems may prevent a healthy bladder from functioning normally. Potent, fast-acting diuretics are known for their ability to cause urge incontinence. Psychoactive drugs, such as tranquilizers and sedatives, may diminish normal attention to bladder clues. Impaired thirst or limited access to fluids predisposes to constipation with urethral obstruction and overflow incontinence and to concentrated and infected urine, which increases bladder excitability.

According to Stanton, "there are two guiding principles in management of incontinence in the elderly. First, growing old does not imply becoming incontinent and, second, incontinence should not be left untreated just because the patient is old."[21] Treatment may involve changes in the physical environment so that the older person can reach the bathroom more easily or remove clothing more quickly. Habit training with regularly scheduled toileting—usually every 2 to 4 hours—often is effective. Many elderly people who void on a regular schedule can gradually increase the interval between toileting while improving their ability to suppress bladder instability.[22] The treatment plan may require dietary changes to prevent constipation or a plan to promote adequate fluid intake to ensure adequate bladder filling and prevent urinary stasis and symptomatic urinary tract infections.

In summary, alterations in bladder function include both urinary obstruction with retention of urine and urinary incontinence with involuntary loss of urine. Urine retention occurs when the outflow of urine from the bladder is obstructed because of either urethral obstruction or impaired bladder innervation. Urethral obstruction causes bladder irritability, detrusor muscle hypertrophy, trabeculation and the formation of diverticula, development of hydroureters, and, eventually, renal failure.

Neurogenic bladder is caused by interruption in the innervation of the bladder. It can cause spastic bladder dysfunction or flaccid bladder dysfunction, depending on the level of the lesion. Spastic bladder dysfunction usually results from neurologic lesions that are above the level of the sacral micturition reflex center; flaccid bladder dysfunction results from lesions at the level of sacral micturition reflexes or peripheral innervation of the bladder.

Urinary incontinence is the involuntary loss of urine that is sufficient to be a problem. It may present as stress incontinence, in which the loss of urine occurs as a result of coughing, sneezing, laughing, or lifting; urge incontinence, characterized by a strong desire to void that often is associated with strong hyperreflexive bladder contraction; or overflow, or reflex, incontinence, which results when intravesicular pressure exceeds the maximal urethral pressure because of bladder distention. Other causes of incontinence include a small, contracted bladder or external environmental conditions that make it difficult to access proper toileting facilities.

The treatment of urinary obstruction, neurogenic bladder, and incontinence requires careful diagnosis to determine the cause and contributing factors. Treatment methods include correction of the underlying cause, such as obstruction due to prostatic hyperplasia; behavior methods that focus on bladder and habit training; exercises to improve pelvic floor function; pharmacologic methods; and the use of catheters and urine collection devices.

■ CANCER OF THE BLADDER

Bladder cancer is the most frequent form of urinary tract cancer in the United States, accounting for about 51,600 new cases and 9,500 deaths each year.[23] It most commonly occurs in the 50-to-70-year age group and is twice as frequent in men as in women.[24]

Bladder cancers fall into two major groups: superficial and invasive, according to their natural history.[25] About 80% of superficial bladder cancers remain confined to the mucosa and submucosa throughout their natural history, whereas most invasive bladder cancers have penetrated the deep bladder layers at the time of presentation and are associated with metastasis and a worse prognosis. About 70% to 75% of bladder cancers present as superficial noninvasive tumors. With traditional methods of therapy (*e.g.*, transurethral resection, electrocautery removal, and cystectomy), the long-term survival of people with this type of bladder cancer is more than 80%. These tumors frequently recur, however, and the apparent rate of cure is less than 50%.[25] The remaining 25% to 30% of bladder cancers are highly invasive. These tumors may present as in situ lesions that progress rapidly to invasive lesions or as advanced invasive disease. The most common sites of metastasis are the pelvic lymph nodes, lungs, bones, and liver.

Although the cause of bladder cancer is unknown, evidence suggests that its origin is related to local influences, such as carcinogens that are excreted in the urine and stored in the bladder. This includes the breakdown products of aniline dyes used in the rubber and cable industries. Smoking also deserves attention: it may be responsible for as many as 50% of cases of cancer in men and 33% in women. About 3 mg of 2-naphthylamine, one of the first bladder carcinogens to be identified, is absorbed from the smoke of 20 unfiltered cigarettes.[26] Chronic bladder infections and bladder stones also increase the risk of bladder cancer. Although earlier studies have suggested an association between bladder cancer and artificial sweeteners such as saccharin and cyclamates, this association has not been proved. Bladder cancer occurs among people harboring the parasite *Schistosoma haematobium* in their bladders. In Egypt, where the infection is common, bladder tumors represent 10% to 40% of all cancers.[27] It is not known whether the parasite excretes a carcinogen or produces its effects through irritation of the bladder.

DIAGNOSIS AND TREATMENT

The most common sign of bladder cancer is hematuria. Gross hematuria is a presenting sign in 75% of people with the disease, and microscopic hematuria is present in most others.[23–25] Frequency, urgency, and dysuria occasionally accompany the hematuria. Because hematuria often is intermittent, the diagnosis may be delayed. Periodic urine cytology is recommended for all people who are at high risk for the development of bladder cancer because of exposure to urinary tract carcinogens. Ureteral invasion leading to bacterial and obstructive renal disease and dissemination of the cancer are potential complications and ultimate causes of death. The prognosis depends on the histologic grade of the cancer and the stage of the disease at the time of diagnosis.

Diagnostic methods include cytologic studies, excretory urography, cystoscopy, and biopsy. Ultrasonography and CT scans are used as an aid for staging the tumor. Other imaging techniques, such as MRI, are being evaluated.

Cytologic studies performed on biopsy tissues or cells obtained from bladder washings may be used to detect the presence of malignant cells. A technique called *flow cytometry* is helpful in screening people at high risk for the disease and for follow-up of therapy. In flow cytometry, the interaction between fluorochromes or dyes with DNA causes the emission of high-intensity light similar to that produced by a laser.[25] Flow cytometry can be carried out on biopsy specimens, bladder washings, or cytologic preparations. There appears to be a correlation between the DNA content (ploidy) and the level of differentiation (the grade), depth of invasion (the stage), and response to treatment. The expression of blood group antigens on the surface of bladder cancer cells has proved to be a useful prognostic determinant. Tumors that express the A, B, or H antigens have a better prognosis than tumors that do not express these antigens.[25]

The treatment of bladder cancer depends on the extent of the lesion and the health of the patient. Endoscopic resection usually is done for diagnostic purposes and may be used as a treatment for superficial lesions. Diathermy (electrocautery) may be used to remove the tumors. Segmental surgical resection may be used for removing a large single lesion. When the tumor is invasive, cystectomy with resection of the pelvic lymph nodes frequently is the treatment of choice. In males, the prostate and seminal vesicles often are removed as well. Until the 1980s, nearly all men who underwent radical cystectomy became impotent.[25] Newer surgical approaches designed to preserve erectile function are now being used. Cystectomy requires urinary diversion, an alternative reservoir, usually created from the ileum (*e.g.*, an ileal loop, discussed earlier), that is designed to collect the urine. Traditionally, the ileostomy reservoir drains urine continuously into an external collecting device. Methods of urinary diversion that provide continence and eliminate the need to wear an external collection bag are being explored.[25]

Although a number of chemotherapeutic drugs have been used in the treatment of bladder cancer, no chemotherapeutic regimens for the disease have been established. Perhaps of more importance is the increasing use of intravesicular chemotherapy, in which the cytotoxic drug is instilled directly into the bladder. These drugs can be instilled prophylactically (after surgical resection of all demonstrable tumor) or therapeutically in the presence of residual disease. Among the chemotherapeutic drugs that have been used for this purpose are thiotepa, mitomycin C, and doxorubicin (Adriamycin). The intervesicular administration of *bacillus Calmette-Guérin* (BCG), a vaccine made from *Mycobacterium bovis* that formerly was used to protect against tuberculosis, causes a significant reduction in the rate of relapse and prolongs relapse-free interval in people with cancer in situ. The vaccine is thought to act as an nonspecific stimulator of cell-mediated immunity. It is not known whether the effects of BCG are immunologic or include a component of direct toxicity. Several strains of this agent exist, and it is not known which is the most active and least toxic.[25]

In summary, cancer of the bladder is the most common cause of urinary tract cancer in the United States, accounting for about 51,600 new cases and 9,500 deaths each year. It most frequently occurs in the 50- to 70-year age group and is twice as common in men as in women. Bladder cancers fall into two major groups: superficial tumors that remain confined to the mucosa and submucosa and invasive cancers that have penetrated the deep bladder layers at the time of presentation and are associated with metastasis and a worse prognosis. Even the superficial tumors tend to recur after removal, and the apparent rate of cure in less than 50%. Although the cause of cancer of the bladder is unknown, evidence suggests that carcinogens excreted in the urine may play a role. Gross hematuria is the most common sign of bladder cancer, occurring in 75% of people with the disease. Treatment of bladder cancer depends on the cytologic grade of the tumor and the extent of the invasiveness of the lesion.

■ REFERENCES

1. McGuire, E.J. (1983). Physiology of the lower urinary tract. *American Journal of Kidney Diseases, 2,* 402.
2. McGuire, E.J. (1980). Urinary dysfunction in the aged: Neurological considerations. *Bulletin of the New York Academy of Medicine, 56,* 275.
3. Berne, R.M., & Levy, M.N. (1988). *Physiology* (2nd ed., p. 814). St. Louis: C.V. Mosby.
4. Mahoney, D.T., Laferte, R.L., & Blias, D.J. (1977). Integral storage function and voiding reflexes. *Urology, 9,* 95.
5. Urinary Incontinence Guideline Panel. (1992). *Urinary incontinence in adults: Clinical practice guidelines.* APCPR Pub. No 92-0038. Rockville, MD: Agency for Health Care Policy and Research, Public Health Service, U.S. Department of Health and Human Services.
6. McConnell, E.A., & Zimmerman, M.F. (1983). *Care of patients with urologic problems* (p. 32). Philadelphia: J.B. Lippincott.
7. Tanagho, E.A., & Schmidt, R.A. (1992). Neuropathic bladder disorders. In E.A. Tanagho & J.W. McAninch (Eds.). *Smith's general urology* (13th ed., pp. 454–472). Los Altos, CA: Lange Medical Publishers.
8. Trop, C.S., & Bennett, C.J. (1991). Autonomic dysreflexia and its urological implications. *Journal of Urology, 146,* 1461.
9. Frimodt-Miller, C. (1980). Diabetic cystopathy: Epidemiology and related disorders. *Annals of Internal Medicine, 92,*(2), 318.
10. Ellenberg, M. (1980). Development of urinary bladder dysfunction in diabetes mellitus. *Annals of Internal Medicine, 92*(2), 321.
11. Frimodt-Miller, C., & Mortenson, S. (1980). Treatment of diabetic cystopathy. *Annals of Internal Medicine, 92,*(2), 327.
12. Thon, W., & Altwein, J.E. (1984). Voiding dysfunction. *Urology, 23,* 323.
13. Jacobs, S.C., & Kaufman, J.M. (1978). Complications of permanent bladder catheter drainage in spinal cord injury patients. *Journal of Urology, 119,* 740.
14. Lapides, J., Diokno, A.C., & Silber, S.J. (1971). Clean, intermittent self-catheterization in treatment of urinary tract disease. *Transactions of the American Association of Genitourinary Surgeons, 63,* 92.
15. Perlow, D.L., Gikas, P.W., & Horwitz, E.M. (1981). Effects of vesicle overdistention on bladder mucin. *Urology, 18,* 380.
16. Green, T.H. (1975). Urinary stress incontinence: Differential diagnosis, pathophysiology, and management. *American Journal of Obstetrics and Gynecology, 122,* 368.
17. Robison, J. (1982). Incontinence is not a disease. *Community Care, 399,* 20.
18. Kegel, A.H. (1948). Progressive resistance exercises in the functional restoration of the perineal muscles. *American Journal of Obstetrics and Gynecology, 56,* 238.
19. Brocklehurst, J.C. (1982). Noncatheter devices for urinary incontinence in the elderly. *Medical Instrumentation, 16,* 167.
20. Palmer, M.H. (1988). Incontinence: The magnitude of the problem. *Nursing Clinics of North America, 23,* 139.
21. Stanton, S.L. (1984). Surgical management of female incontinence. In J.C. Brocklehurst (Ed.). *Urology in the elderly* (p. 93). New York: Churchill Livingstone.
22. Rousseau, P., & Fuentevilla-Clifton, A. (1992). Urinary incontinence in the aged. Pt 2: Management strategies. *Geriatrics, 47*(6), 37.
23. American Cancer Society. (1992). *Cancer facts and figures—1992.* Atlanta: American Cancer Society.
24. Frank, I.N., Graham, S.D., & Nabors, W.L. (1991). Urologic and male genital cancers. In A.I. Hollieb, D.J. Fink, & G.P. Murphy (Eds.). *Clinical oncology* (pp. 276–280). Atlanta: American Cancer Society.
25. Raghavan, D., Shipley, W.U., Garnick, M.B., et al. (1990). Biology and management of bladder cancer. *New England Journal of Medicine, 322,* 1129.
26. Murphy, W.M. (1983). Current topics in the pathology of bladder cancer. *Pathology Annual, 18*(Pt1), 1.
27. Cotran, R.S., Kumar, V., & Robbins, S.L. (1989). *Pathologic basis of disease* (4th ed., pp. 1090–1094). Philadelphia: W.B. Saunders.

■ BIBLIOGRAPHY

Burgener, S. (1987). Justification of closed intermittent urinary catheter irrigation/instillation: A review of current research and practice. *Journal of Advanced Nursing, 12,* 229.

Burgio, K.L., Robinson, C., & Engel, B.T. (1986). The role of biofeedback in Kegel exercise training for stress urinary incontinence. *American Journal of Obstetrics and Gynecology, 154,* 58.

Burns, P.A., Pranikoff, K., Nochajski, T., et al. (1990). Treatment of stress incontinence with pelvic floor exercise and biofeedback. *Journal of the American Geriatric Society, 38,* 314.

deGroat, W.C., & Booth, A.M. (1980). Physiology of the urinary bladder and urethra. *Annals of Internal Medicine, 92,* 312.

Fantl, J.A., Hurt, W.G., Bump, R.C., et al. (1986). Urethral axis and sphincteric function. *American Journal of Obstetrics and Gynecology, 155,* 554.

Fantl, J.A., Wyman, J.F., Harkins, S.W., et al. (1990). Bladder training in the management of lower urinary tract dysfunction in women. *Journal of the American Geriatric Society, 38,* 329.

Hadley, E.C. (1986). Bladder training and related therapies for urinary incontinence in older people. *Journal of the American Medical Association, 256,* 372.

Kunin, C.M. (1988). Can we build a better urinary catheter? *New England Journal of Medicine, 319,* 365.

National Institutes of Health Consensus Development Conference. (1990). Urinary incontinence in adults. *Journal of the American Medical Association, 38,* 265.

Ouslander, J.G. (1989). Disorders of micturition in the aging patient. *Advances in Internal Medicine, 34,* 165.

Ouslander, J.G., & Sier, H.C. (1986). Drug therapy for geriatric urinary incontinence. *Geriatric Clinical Medicine, 2,* 789.

Resnick, N.M., & Yalla, S.V. (1985). Management of urinary incontinence in the elderly. *New England Journal of Medicine, 313,* 800.

Resnick, N.M., Yalla, S.V., & Laurino, E. (1989). The pathophysiology of urinary incontinence among institutionalized elderly persons. *New England Journal of Medicine, 320,* 1.

Rousseau, P., & Fuentevilla-Clifton, A. (1992). Urinary incontinence in the aged. Pt 1: Patient evaluation. *Geriatrics, 47*(6), 22.

Sier, H., Ouslander, J., & Orzeck, S. (1986). Urinary incontinence among geriatric patients in an acute-care hospital. *Journal of the American Medical Association, 257,* 1767.

Webb, R.J., Lawson, A.L., & Neal, D.E. (1990). Clean intermittent self-catheterization in 172 adults. *British Journal of Urology, 65,* 20.

Wyman, J.F. (1988). Nursing assessment of the incontinent geriatric outpatient. *Nursing Clinics of North America, 23*(1), 169.

STRUCTURE AND FUNCTION OF THE MALE GENITOURINARY SYSTEM

STEPHANIE M. STEWART

Genitourinary Structures
 Embryonic Development
 Testes and Scrotum
 Penis

Reproductive Function
 Spermatogenesis
 Hormonal Control of Male
 Reproductive Function

Neural Control of Sexual Function
 Aging Changes

■ OBJECTIVES

After you have studied this chapter, you should be able to meet the following objectives:

■ Describe the anatomy of the testes and scrotum.
■ Describe the process of spermatogenesis.
■ State the name of the testicular cells that produce testosterone.
■ State the functions of testosterone.
■ Draw a diagram illustrating the secretion, site of action, and feedback control of GnRH, LH, and FSH.

■ Describe the function of FSH in terms of spermatogenesis.
■ Describe the autonomic nervous system control of erection and ejaculation.
■ Describe changes in the male reproductive system that occur with aging.

The male genitourinary system consists of a pair of gonads, the testes, a system of excretory ducts, and the accessory organs. The accessory organs include the penis, the bulbourethral glands, the prostate gland, and the seminal vesicles. The system has two basic functions—urine elimination and reproduction. This chapter focuses on the embryonic development of the male reproductive structures, the structure of the male genitourinary system, spermatogenesis, sexual performance, hormonal regulation of reproductive function in the male, and changes in genitourinary function that occur at puberty and as a result of the aging process.

■ GENITOURINARY STRUCTURES

EMBRYONIC DEVELOPMENT

The sex of a person is determined at the time of fertilization by the sex chromosomes. In the early stages of embryonic development, the tissues from which the male and female reproductive organs develop are undifferentiated. Until approximately the seventh week of gestation, it is impossible to determine whether the embryo is male or female unless the chromosomes are studied. Until this time, the genital tracts of both the male and the female consist

Carol Mattson Porth: PATHOPHYSIOLOGY: CONCEPTS OF
ALTERED HEALTH STATES, 4th ed. © 1994, 1990, 1986, 1982
J.B. Lippincott Company

of two wolffian ducts, from which the male genitalia develop, and two müllerian ducts, from which the female genital structures develop. During this period of gestation, the gonads (ovaries and testes) are also undifferentiated.

In the seventh week of embryonic life, the gonadal ridge of an embryo with XY chromosomes differentiates to form testes and that of an embryo with XX chromosomes differentiates to form into ovaries. The fetal testes produce two hormones: one stimulates development of the wolffian ducts into structures that form seminal vesicles, vas deferens, and epididymis; the other suppresses the development of female genital structures from the müllerian ducts. Development of the external male genital structures begins during the twelfth week of embryonic life. The presence or absence of the androgen testosterone determines whether an embryo develops male or female genital structures. In the absence of tes-

tosterone, a male embryo with an XY chromosomal pattern develops female genitalia. It has been hypothesized that the Y chromosome contains a gene that codes for a substance called the H-Y antigen. In the presence of the H-Y antigen, the embryonic gonads develop into testes and in its absence the gonads develop into ovaries.[7]

TESTES AND SCROTUM

The testes, or male gonads, are two egg-shaped structures located outside the abdominal cavity in the scrotum, where they are suspended by the spermatic cord (Fig. 35-1). The spermatic cord is composed of the arteries, veins, lymphatics, and excretory ducts that supply the testes. The cremaster muscle that suspends the testes and forms the muscle of the scrotum is also contained in the spermatic cord.

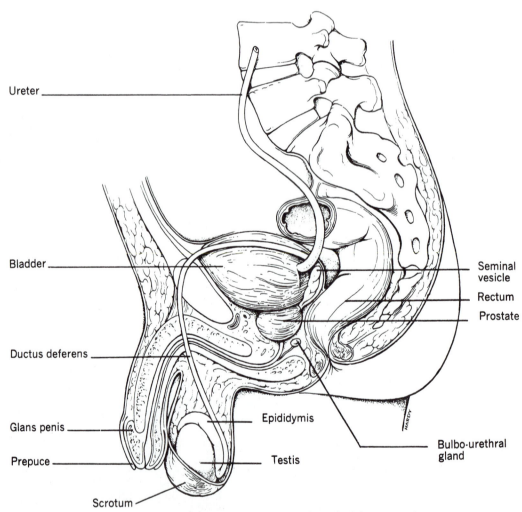

FIG. 35-1. The structures of the male reproductive system, including the testes, the scrotum, and the excretory ducts. (Chaffee, E. E., & Greisheimer, E. M. [1974]. *Basic physiology and anatomy* [3rd ed.]. Philadelphia: J.B. Lippincott)

The testes are responsible for both testosterone and sperm production.

The scrotum, which houses the testes, is made up of an outer skin layer, which forms rugae or folds and is continuous with the perineum and outer skin layer, which is continuous with that of the thighs. Under the outer skin lies a thin layer of muscle and fascia, the *tunica dartos*. This layer contains a septum that separates the two testes.

A function of the scrotum is to regulate the temperature of the testes. The optimal temperature for sperm production is about 2°F to 3°F below body temperature. If the testicular temperature is too low, the muscles within the scrotum contract, causing the testes to be brought up tight against the body. On the other hand, when the testicular temperature rises, the muscles relax, which allows the scrotal sac to fall away from the body. Some tight-fitting undergarments hold the testes against the body and are thought to contribute to infertility by interfering with the thermoregulatory function of the scrotum. Cryptorchidism, the failure of the testes to descend into the scrotum, also exposes the testes to the higher temperature of the body.

The testes and epididymis are enclosed in a double-layered membrane, the *tunica vaginalis*, which is derived embryologically from the abdominal peritoneum. An outer covering, the *tunica albuginea*, is a tough white fibrous sheath that resembles the sclera of the eye. The tunica albuginea protects the testes and gives them their ovoid shape.

Embryologically, the testes do not develop within the scrotal sac; they develop in the abdominal cavity and descend through the inguinal canal into a long pouch of peritoneum (which becomes the tunica vaginalis) in the scrotum during the seventh to the ninth month of fetal life. The descent of the testes is thought to be caused by the male hormone, testosterone, which is active during this stage of development. Just before birth, the inguinal canal closes almost completely. Failure of this canal to close predisposes to the development of an inguinal hernia later in life.

Duct System. Internally, the testes are composed of several hundred compartments or lobules (Fig. 35-2). Each lobule contains one or more coiled *seminiferous* tubules. These tubules are the site of sperm production. As the tubules lead into the *efferent ducts*, the seminiferous tubules become the *rete testis*. From the rete testis, 10,000 to 20,000 efferent ducts emerge to join the epididymis, which is the final site for sperm maturation. Interspersed in the connective tissue that fills the spaces between the seminiferous tubules are the epithelial cells—*Leydig's cells*—which produce *testosterone*.

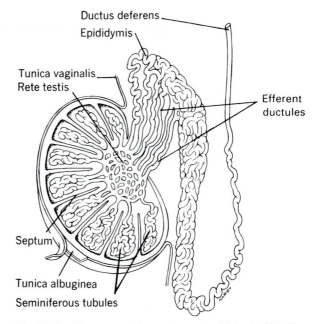

FIG. 35-2. The parts of the testes and epididymis. (Chaffee, E. E., & Lytle, I. M. [1980]. *Basic physiology and anatomy* [4th ed.]. Philadelphia: J.B. Lippincott)

Accessory Organs. Sperm are transported through the reproductive structures by movement of the seminal fluid, which is combined with secretions from the accessory sex glands, epididymis, seminal vesicles, prostate, and Cowper's glands. When sperm is combined with the seminal plasma, it is called *semen*.

The sperm enters the epididymis from the efferent ductules in the testes. Because the sperm are not motile at this stage of development, peristaltic movements of the ductal walls of the epididymis aid in sperm movement. The sperm continue their migration through the *ductus deferens*, or vas deferens, and enter the *ampulla*, where they are stored until they are released through ejaculation (Fig. 35-3). Sperm can be stored in the genital ducts for as long as 42 days and still maintain their fertility.

From the ampulla, the sperm moves to the seminal vesicles, which secrete a fluid containing fructose and other substances required to nourish the sperm. The seminal vesicles are primarily secretory organs. Each of the paired seminal vesicles is lined with secretory epithelium containing an abundance of fructose, prostaglandins, and fibrinogens. The fructose provides nutrients for the ejaculated sperm. The prostaglandins are thought to assist in fertilization by making the cervical mucus more receptive to sperm and by causing reverse peristaltic contractions in the uterus and fallopian tubes to move the sperm toward the ovaries.[2]

Each seminal vesicle joins its corresponding vas deferens to form the ejaculatory duct, which enters

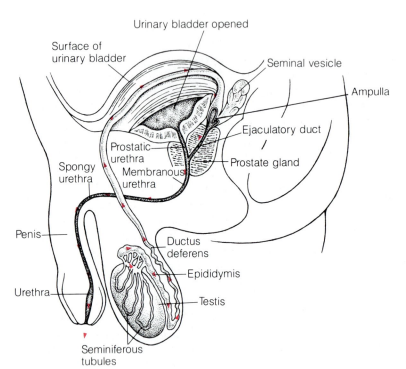

FIG. 35-3. The excretory ducts of the male reproductive system and the path that sperm follows as it leaves the testis and travels to the urethra. (Chaffee, E. E., & Greisheimer, E. M. [1974]. *Basic physiology and anatomy* [3rd ed.]. Philadelphia: J.B. Lippincott)

the posterior part of the prostate and continues through until it ends in the prostatic portion of the urethra. During emission, each vesicle empties fluid into the ejaculatory duct, which adds bulk to the semen. The prostate gland, in turn, secretes a thin milky alkaline fluid containing citric acid, calcium, acid phosphate, a clotting enzyme, and a pro-fibrinolysin. During emission, the capsule of the prostate contracts, and the added fluid increases the bulk of the semen. The alkaline nature of these secretions is essential for successful fertilization of the ovum, because sperm mobilization occurs at a *p*H of 6.0 to 6.5. Both vaginal secretions and the fluid from the vas deferens are strongly acidic. The bulbo-urethral or Cowper's glands lie on either side of the membranous urethra and secrete an alkaline mucus, which probably aids in neutralizing acids from the urine that remain in the urethra.

A man usually ejaculates about 2 mL to 5 mL of semen. The ejaculate may vary with frequency of intercourse. It is less with frequent ejaculation and may increase two to four times its normal amount during periods of abstinence. The semen that is ejaculated is largely fluid—98% fluid and about 2% sperm.

PENIS

The penis is the external genital organ through which the urethra passes. Anatomically, the external penis consists of a shaft that ends in a tip called the *glans*

(Fig. 35-4). The loose skin of the penis shaft folds to cover the glans, forming the *prepuce*, or *foreskin*. It is this cuff of skin that is removed during circumcision. There has been mounting opposition to the once routine practice of neonatal circumcision from the medical community and the public alike, based on the argument that the small risks of death and mutilation do not justify circumcision. The American College of Obstetrics and Gynecologists and the American Academy of Pediatrics have concluded that there is no absolute medical indication for routine circumcision. Those supporting the practice contend, on the other hand, that the higher rates of infection and penile problems among uncircumcised boys after infancy indicate continued use of the procedure. It is argued that uncircumcised male children have more balanitis and irritation after infancy.[3, 4]

The glans of the penis contains many sensory nerves, making this the most sensitive portion of the penile shaft. The cylindrical body or shaft of the penis is composed of three masses of erectile tissue held together by fibrous strands and covered with skin. The two lateral masses of tissue are called the *corpora cavernosa*. The third ventral mass is called the *corpus spongiosum*. The cavernous masses are composed of erectile tissue that distends with blood during penile erection.

In summary, the male genitourinary system functions in both urine elimination and reproduction. The reproductive system consists of a pair of gonads (the testes), a system of

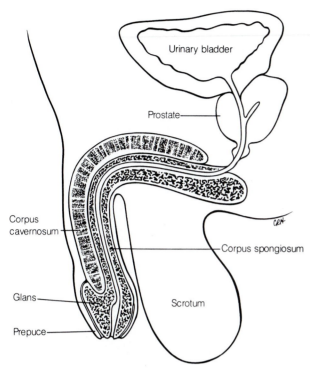

FIG. 35-4. *Sagittal section of the penis, showing the prepuce, glans, corpus cavernosum, and corpus spongiosum.*

excretory ducts (seminiferous tubules and efferent ducts), the accessory organs (epididymis, seminal vesicles, prostate, and Cowper's glands), and the penis. The sex of a person is determined by the sex chromosomes at the time of fertilization. During the seventh week of gestation, the XY chromosome pattern in the male is responsible for the development of the testes with the subsequent production of testosterone and testosterone-stimulated development of the internal and external male genital structures. Before this period of embryonic development, the tissues from which the reproductive structures of the male and female develop are undifferentiated. In the absence of testosterone production, the male embryo with an XY chromosomal pattern develops female genitalia.

■ REPRODUCTIVE FUNCTION

At puberty, the male gonads and testes begin to mature and to carry out spermatogenesis and hormone production. Sometime around the age of 10 or 11, the adenohypophysis, or anterior pituitary, begins to secrete the gonadotropins that stimulate testicular function and cause the interstitial cells to begin producing testosterone. About the same time, hormonal stimulation induces mitotic activity of the germ cells that develop in sperm. Once cell maturation has begun, the testes begin to enlarge rapidly as the individual tubules grow. Full maturity and spermatogenesis are usually attained by age 15 or 16.

SPERMATOGENESIS

Spermatogenesis refers to the generation of sperm. It begins at an average age of 13 and continues throughout the reproductive years of a man's life. Spermatogenesis occurs in the seminiferous tubules of the testes. These tubules, if placed end to end, would measure about 750 feet. The outer layer of the seminiferous tubules are made up of connective tissue and smooth muscle; the inner lining is composed of Sertoli's cells, within which are embedded the spermatogonia and sperm in various stages of development. Sertoli's cells secrete a special fluid that contains nutrients to bathe and nourish the immature germ cells; they provide digestive enzymes that play a role in spermiation (converting the spermatocytes to sperm); and they are thought to play a role in shaping the head and tail of the sperm. In addition, Sertoli's cells secrete several hormones, including müllerian inhibitory factor (MIF), which is secreted by the testes during fetal life to inhibit development of fallopian tubes; estradiol, the principal feminizing sex hormone, which seems to be required in the male for spermatogenesis; and inhibin, which serves to control the function of Sertoli's cells through feedback inhibition of follicle-stimulating hormone (FSH) from the anterior pituitary gland.[5]

In the first stage of spermatogenesis, small unspecialized germinal cells located immediately adjacent to the tubular wall, called the *spermatogonia*, undergo rapid mitotic division and provide a continuous source of new germinal cells. As these cells multiply, the more mature spermatogonia divide into two daughter cells, which grow in size and become the *primary spermatocytes*—the precursors of sperm. Over a period of several weeks, large primary spermatocytes divide by meiosis to form two smaller secondary spermatocytes. Each of the secondary spermatocytes, in turn, divide to form two *spermatids*, or infant sperm.

The spermatid elongates into a *spermatozoon*, or mature sperm cell, with a head and tail (Fig. 35-5). The outside of the anterior two thirds of the head, called the *acrosome*, contains enzymes necessary for penetration and fertilization of the ovum. To-and-fro (flagellar) motion of the tail provides movement for the sperm. The energy for this process is supplied by the mitochondria in the tail. Normal sperm move in a straight line at a velocity of 1 mm to 4 mm per minute. This allows them to move through the female genital tract.

When the sperm grow to full size, they move to the epididymis to further mature and gain mobility. A small quantity of sperm can be stored in the epididymis but most are stored in the vas deferens or the ampulla of the vas deferens. With excessive sexual

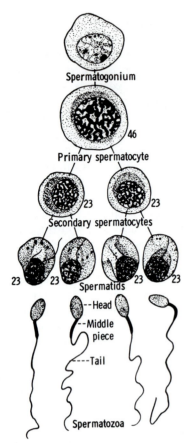

FIG. 35-5. The various stages of spermatogenesis. (Chaffee, E. E., & Lytle, I. M. [1980]. *Basic physiology and anatomy* [4th ed.]. Philadelphia: J.B. Lippincott)

activity, storage may be no longer than a few days. The sperm can live for many weeks in the male genital tract; however, in the female genital tract, their life expectancy is 1 or 2 days. Frozen sperm have been preserved for years.

The entire process of spermatogenesis takes about 60 to 70 days. The sperm count in a normal ejaculate is about 100 million to 400 million. Infertility may occur when insufficient numbers of motile, healthy sperm are present.

HORMONAL CONTROL OF MALE REPRODUCTIVE FUNCTION

The male sex hormones are called androgens. Testosterone is the main androgen produced in the testes. The adrenal cortex also produces androgens, but in much smaller quantities than the testes. Over 95% of the testosterone is secreted by the testes; the remainder is secreted by the adrenals.

Testosterone is secreted by the interstitial Leydig's cells in the testes. It is metabolized in the liver and excreted by the kidneys. In the bloodstream, testosterone exists in a free or a bound form.

The bound form is attached to plasma proteins, including albumin and the sex-hormone binding protein produced by the liver. About 2% is not bound and is able to enter the cell and exert its metabolic effects. Testosterone exerts a variety of biologic effects in the male (Chart 35-1). In the male embryo, testosterone is essential for the appropriate differentiation of the internal and external genitalia. Testosterone is essential to the development of primary and secondary male sex characteristics during puberty and for the maintenance of these characteristics during adult life. In addition, androgens function as anabolic agents in both males and females to promote metabolism and musculoskeletal growth.

The hypothalamus and the anterior pituitary gland play an essential role in promoting spermatogenic activity in the testes and maintaining endocrine function of the testes by means of the gonadotropic hormones. The release of gonadotropic hormones from the pituitary gland is regulated by the gonadotropin-releasing factor (GnRH), which is synthesized by the hypothalamus and secreted into the hypothalamohypophyseal portal blood (Fig. 35-6). Two gonadotropic hormones are secreted by the pituitary gland: follicle-stimulating hormone (FSH) and luteinizing hormone (LH). In the male, LH is also called interstitial cell-stimulating hormone (ICSH).

The production of testosterone by the interstitial Leydig's cells is regulated by LH (see Fig. 35-6). FSH binds selectively to Sertoli's cells, where it functions in the initiation of spermatogenesis. Although FSH is necessary for the initiation of spermatogenesis, full maturation of the spermatozoa requires testosterone. Sertoli's cells produce an androgen-binding protein that binds testosterone; one of the major actions

---

CHART 35-1: MAIN ACTIONS OF TESTOSTERONE

Induces differentiation of the male genital tract during fetal development
Induces development of primary and secondary sex characteristics:
  Gonadal function
  External genitalia and accessory organs
  Male voice timbre
  Male skin characteristics
  Male hair distribution
Anabolic effects
  Promotes protein metabolism
  Promotes musculoskeletal growth
  Influences subcutaneous fat distribution
Promotes spermatogenesis (in FSH-primed tubules) and maturation of sperm

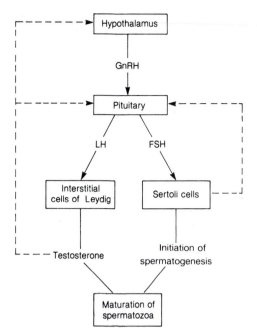

FIG. 35-6. Hypothalamic-pituitary feedback control of spermatogenesis and testosterone levels in the male.

of FSH may be the regulation of androgen-binding protein production by Sertoli's cells as a means of maintaining high intratubular concentrations of testosterone.

Circulating levels of the gonadotropic hormones are regulated in a negative feedback manner by testosterone. High levels of testosterone produce a negative feedback suppression of LH secretion through a direct action on the pituitary and an inhibitory effect on the hypothalamus. FSH is thought to be inhibited by a substance called *inhibin*, which is produced by Sertoli's cells. Inhibin appears to act mainly at the level of the pituitary gland.[1] Unlike the cyclic hormonal pattern in the female, in the male FSH, LH, and testosterone secretion and spermatogenesis occur at relatively unchanging rates during adulthood.

▪ NEURAL CONTROL OF SEXUAL FUNCTION

In the male, sexual function requires both erection and ejaculation. The physiology of penile erection involves a complex interaction between three systems of the body: the vascular system, the nervous system, and the endocrine system. Although much research has been done on erectile function and dysfunction, many aspects of function remain unclear.

The most important source of impulse stimulation for initiating the male sexual act is the glans penis, which contains a highly organized sensory system. Afferent impulses from sensory receptors in the glans penis pass through the pudendal nerve to ascending fibers in the spinal cord by way of the sacral plexus. Stimulation of other perineal areas, such as the anal epithelium, the scrotum, and the testes, can transmit signals to the cord, adding to sexual satisfaction. Ascending fibers from the spinal pathways communicate with undefined areas of the cerebrum. There is a psychic element to sexual stimulation, because thinking sexual thoughts can cause erection and ejaculation. Although psychic involvement and higher-center functions contribute to the sex act, they are not necessary for sexual performance. Genital stimulation can produce erection and ejaculation in men with complete transection of the spinal cord (this is discussed in Chapter 50).

Erection results from dilation of the arteries in the penis and an increase in intracavernous pressure to levels above the systolic blood pressure. This causes arterial blood under high pressure to build up in erectile tissue of the penis. This erectile tissue consists of large cavernous venous sinusoids, which normally are relatively empty but which fill up rapidly when blood flows into them under high pressure. Various neurotransmitters that control erection are being studied. Several have been identified in penile tissue, including vasoactive intestinal polypeptide (VIP), acetylcholine, and norepinephrine. Erection most likely involves several neurotransmitters. One possibility is that VIP and acetylcholine act synergistically to relax arteriolar and trabecular smooth muscle. Detumescence, or loss of erection, is probably due to the recovery of vascular smooth muscle tone and reactivation of norepinephrine release, which causes contraction of the trabecular muscles and penile arterioles and thereby decreases vascular inflow and increases outflow.[6]

Emission and ejaculation constitute the culmination of the male sexual act. With increasing intensity of the sexual stimulus, the reflex centers of the spinal cord begin to emit sympathetic impulses that leave the cord at the L1 and L2 level and pass through the hypogastric plexus to the genital organs to initiate emission, which is the forerunner of ejaculation. Fluid from the vas deferens, the ampulla, the prostate, and the seminal vesicles is mixed with secretions from the bulbourethral glands and propelled into the internal urethra by contractions of the ischiocavernous and bulbocavernous muscles. The filling of the internal urethra elicits signals that are transmitted through the pudendal nerves from the spinal cord. Increases in pressure in the urethra cause the semen to be propelled to the exterior, resulting in ejaculation. The period of emission and ejaculation is termed *male orgasm*. After ejaculation, erection ceases within 1 to 2 minutes.[7]

The role of circulating androgens in regard to

sexual function remains unclear. It is apparent that sexual desire and performance depend on some threshold level of testosterone; however, this level varies from man to man. Studies of hypogonadal and castrated males show a variety of sexual behavior ranging from complete loss of libido to normal sexual activity. It may be that the role of testosterone in male sexuality is in the area of sexual interest motivation, with individual intrapsychic factors playing a significant role.[8]

AGING CHANGES

Like other body systems, the male reproductive system undergoes degenerative changes as a result of the aging process; it becomes less efficient with age. The declining physiologic efficiency of male reproductive function occurs gradually and involves the endocrine, circulatory, and neuromuscular systems. Compared with the marked physiologic change in aging females, the changes in the aging male are more gradual and less drastic. Gonadal and reproductive failure are not generally related directly to age, because a male remains fertile into advanced age. Eighty- and 90-year-olds have been known to father children.

Contrary to popular belief, many investigators consider that there is no physiologic basis for what has been termed the male climacteric. Instead, they attribute its symptomatology to psychological mechanisms. An aging man may experience midlife crisis with concomitant psychosomatic manifestations that mimic the symptomatology of menopause. Most experts agree that decline in male sexual desire parallels decline in physical vigor and represents the aging of all the body tissues and neural structures.

As the male ages, his reproductive system differs measurably in both structure and function from that of the younger male. Male sex hormone levels, particularly of testosterone, decrease with age, the decline starting later, on the average, than in women. The sex hormones play a part in the structure and function of the reproductive system and other body systems from conception to old age; they affect protein synthesis, salt and water balance, bone growth, and cardiovascular function. Decreasing levels of testosterone affect sexual energy, muscle strength, and the genital tissues. The testes become smaller and lose their firmness. The seminiferous tubules, which produce spermatozoa, thicken and begin a degenerative process that finally inhibits sperm production, resulting in a decrease of viable spermatozoa.[9] The prostate gland enlarges, and its contractions become weaker. The force of ejaculation decreases because of a reduction in the volume and viscosity of the semi-

nal fluid. The seminal vesicle changes little from childhood to puberty. The pubertal increases in the fluid capacity of the gland remain throughout adulthood and decline after age 60. After age 60, the walls of the seminal vesicles thin, the epithelium decreases in height, and the muscle layer is replaced by connective tissue. Age-related changes in the penis consist of fibrotic changes in the trabeculae in the corpus spongiosum, with progressive sclerotic changes in both arteries and veins. Sclerotic changes also follow in the corpora cavernosa, the condition becoming generalized in the 55- to 60-year-old age group.[10]

As a sexual partner, the aging male exhibits some differences in responsiveness and activity from his younger counterpart. Masters and Johnson studied the significant aging changes in the physiology of the sex act.[11] They noted that frequency of intercourse, intensity of sensation, speed of attaining erection, and force of ejaculation are all reduced.

Many social and cultural practices do not support or encourage sexual activity in the elderly. Research, however, indicates that not only does sexual thought and feeling continue into old age but sexual activity also continues for most healthy older people. Most gerontologists agree that continued sexual interest and activity can be therapeutic for the elderly.

Sexual dysfunction in the elderly male is often directly related to the general physical condition of the person. Diseases that accompany aging can have direct bearing on male reproductive organs. Various cardiovascular, respiratory, hormonal, neurologic, and hematologic disorders can be responsible for secondary impotence. For example, vascular disease affects male potency because it may impair blood flow to the pudendal arteries or their tributaries, resulting in loss of blood volume with subsequent poor distention of the vascular spaces of erectile tissue. Other diseases affecting potency include hypertension, diabetes, cardiac disease, and malignancies of the reproductive organs.[12–14]

One of the greatest inhibitors of sexual functioning in older males is loss of self-esteem and development of a negative self-image. The emphasis on youth pervades much of our society both in terms of physical attractiveness and sexuality. The image of success for a man often involves qualities of masculinity and sexual attractiveness. When queried about success, men often mentioned such things as work, managing money well, participating in sports or other activities, discussing politics or world events, advising younger people, and being attractive to women. When a man feels good about himself and expresses self-confidence, sexual attractiveness is communicated regardless of age. Many older men live in environments that are not sensitive to the importance of helping them maintain a positive self-image. Premature cessation of the aforementioned esteem-building activities can contribute to loss of libido and zest for life in the elderly male.[3]

In summary, the function of the male reproductive system is under the negative feedback control of the hypothalamus and the anterior pituitary gonadotropic hormones FSH and LH. Spermatogenesis is initiated by FSH, and the production of testosterone is regulated by LH. Testosterone, the major sex hormone in the male, is produced by the interstitial Leydig's cells in the testes. In addition to the differentiation of the internal and external genitalia in the male embryo, testosterone is essential for the development of secondary male characteristics during puberty, the maintenance of these characteristics during adult life, and spermatozoa maturation.

Like other body systems, the male reproductive system undergoes changes as a result of the aging process. The changes occur gradually and involve parallel changes in endocrine, circulatory, and neuromuscular function. Testosterone levels decrease, the size and firmness of the testes decrease, sperm production declines, and the prostate gland enlarges. There is usually a decrease in frequency of intercourse, intensity of sensation, speed of attaining erection, and force of ejaculation. However, sexual thought, interest, and activity usually continue into old age.

■   REFERENCES

1. Greenspan, F.S., & Forshan, P.H. (1991). *Basic and clinical endocrinology* (pp. 411–413). Norwalk, CT: Appleton-Lange.

2. Guyton, A.C. (1991). *Textbook of medical physiology* (8th ed., pp. 885–893). Philadelphia: W.B. Saunders.

3. Fergusson, D.M., Lawton, J.M., & Shannon, J.T. (1988). Neonatal circumcision and penile problems: An 8-year longitudinal study. *Pediatrics, 81,* 537.

4. Herzog, L.W., & Álvarez, S.R. (1986). The frequency of foreskin problems in uncircumcised children. *American Journal of Diseases of Children, 140,* 254.

5. West, J.B. (1985). *Best and Taylor's physiologic basis of medical practice* (11th ed., pp. 907–920). Baltimore: Williams & Wilkins.

6. Lue, T.F. (1992). Male sexual dysfunction. In D.R. Smith (Ed.). *General urology* (13th ed., pp. 696–711). Norwalk, CT: Appleton and Lange.

7. Aboseif, S.R. (1988). Hemodynamics of penile erection. *Urologic Clinics of North America, 15,* 1.

8. Blackmore, C. (1988). The impact of orchiectomy upon the sexuality of the man with testicular cancer. *Cancer Nursing, 11,* 33.

9. Weg, R.B. (1981). Normal aging changes in the reproductive system. In I.M. Burnside (Ed.). *Nursing and the aged* (pp. 362–374). New York: McGraw-Hill.

10. Croft, L.H. (1982). *Physiology of aging* (pp. 47–65). Boston: John Wright.

11. Masters, W.H., & Johnson, V. (1970). *Human sexual inadequacy* (pp. 337–338). Boston: Little, Brown.

12. Steinke, E.E., & Bergen, M.B. (1986). Sexuality and aging: A review of the literature from a nursing perspective. *Journal of Gerontological Nursing, 12,* 6.

13. Carnevali, D.L., & Patrick, M. (1986). *Nursing management of the elderly* (pp. 60–61). Philadelphia: J.B. Lippincott.

14. Breitiung, J.C. (1987). *Caring for the older adult* (pp. 100–111). Philadelphia: W.B. Saunders.

C H A P T E R   3 6

ALTERATIONS IN STRUCTURE AND FUNCTION OF THE MALE GENITOURINARY SYSTEM

STEPHANIE M. STEWART

Disorders of the Penis
  Hypospadias and Epispadias
  Phimosis and Paraphimosis
  Priapism
  Peyronie's Disease
  Balanitis/Balanoposthitis
  Cancer of the Penis

Disorders of the Scrotum and Testes
  Cryptorchidism
  Hydrocele
  Hematocele
  Spermatocele
  Varicocele

Testicular Torsion
Epididymitis
Orchitis
Neoplasms
Disorders of the Prostate
  Prostatitis
  Benign Prostatic Hyperplasia
  Prostatic Cancer

■ OBJECTIVES

After you have studied this chapter, you should be able to meet the following objectives:

■ State the difference between hypospadias and epispadias.

■ Cite the significance of phimosis.

■ Describe the pathology of priapism.

■ Describe the anatomic changes that occur with Peyronie's disease.

■ Describe the appearance of balanitis xerotica obliterans.

■ List the signs of penile cancer.

■ State the physical manifestations of cryptorchidism.

■ Describe the potential risks associated with cryptorchidism.

■ Compare the etiology, appearance, and significance of hydrocele, hematocele, spermatocele, and varicocele.

■ State the difference between extravaginal and intravaginal testicular torsion.

■ Describe the symptoms of epididymitis.

■ State the manifestations and possible complications of mumps orchitis.

■ Relate environmental factors to development of scrotal cancer.

■ State the cell types involved in seminoma, embryonal carcinoma, teratoma, and choriocarcinoma tumors of the testes.

■ Compare the pathology and symptoms of acute bacterial prostatitis, chronic bacterial prostatitis, nonbacterial prostatitis, and prostatodynia.

■ Describe the urologic manifestations of benign prostatic hyperplasia.

■ List the methods used in the diagnosis and treatment of prostatic cancer.

Carol Mattson Porth: PATHOPHYSIOLOGY: CONCEPTS OF ALTERED HEALTH STATES, 4th ed. © 1994, 1990, 1986, 1982 J.B. Lippincott Company

The male genitourinary system is subject to structural defects, inflammation, and neoplasms, all of which can affect urine elimination, sexual function, and fertility. This chapter discusses disorders of the penis, the scrotum and testes, and the prostate.

■ DISORDERS OF THE PENIS

The penis is the external male genitalia through which the urethra passes to the exterior of the body. It is involved in both urinary and sexual function. Disorders of the penis include congenital and acquired defects, inflammatory conditions, and neoplasms.

HYPOSPADIAS AND EPISPADIAS

Both hypospadias and epispadias are congenital disorders of the penis resulting from embryologic defects in development of the urethral groove and penile urethra (Fig. 36-1). In hypospadias, which is present in about 1 out of every 400 to 500 male infants, the termination of the urethra is on the ventral surface of the penis. Epispadias, in which the opening of the urethra is on the dorsal surface of the penis, is a less common defect. Both of these abnormalities are often accompanied by other congenital urogenital defects. Testes are undescended in 10% of boys born with hypospadias, and the incidence of chordee

(ventral bowing of the penis) and inguinal hernia is also common. In the newborn with severe hypospadias and undescended testes, the differential diagnosis should include consideration of ambiguous genitalia and masculinization that is seen in females with congenital adrenal hyperplasia. Because many chromosomal aberrations result in ambiguity of the external genitalia, chromosomal studies are often recommended for male infants with hypospadias and cryptorchidism.[1]

Surgery is the treatment of choice for hypospadias and epispadias. Circumcision is avoided because the foreskin is used for surgical repair. In mild cases, the surgery is done for cosmetic reasons only. In more severe cases, however, repair becomes essential for normal sexual functioning and the psychological sequelae of having malformed genitalia. The ideal age for repair is controversial, but most surgeries are performed before 18 months of age. Even with associated chordee, these anomalies can be repaired in a single operation, often with return home on the day of surgery.[2]

PHIMOSIS AND PARAPHIMOSIS

Phimosis refers to a tightening of the penile foreskin that prevents its retraction over the glans. Embryologically the foreskin begins to develop during the eighth week of gestation, as a fold of skin at the distal edge of the penis that eventually grows forward over the base of the glans. By the 16th week of gestation, the prepuce and the glans are adherent. Only a small percentage of newborns have a fully retractable foreskin. With growth, a space develops between the glans and foreskin, and, by 3 years of age, about 90% of male children have a retractable foreskin.

Because the foreskin of many males cannot be fully retracted in early childhood, it is important that the area be cleansed thoroughly. There is no need to retract the foreskin forcibly, because this could lead to infection, scarring, or paraphimosis. As the child grows, the foreskin becomes retractable, and the glans and foreskin should be cleansed routinely. If symptomatic phimosis occurs after childhood, it can cause difficulty with voiding or sexual activity. Circumcision is then the treatment of choice.[3]

In a related condition called *paraphimosis*, the foreskin is so tight and constricted that it cannot cover the glans. A tight foreskin can constrict the blood supply to the glans and lead to ischemia and necrosis. Many cases of paraphimosis occur secondary to the foreskin being retracted for an extended period, as in the case of uncircumcised catheterized males.

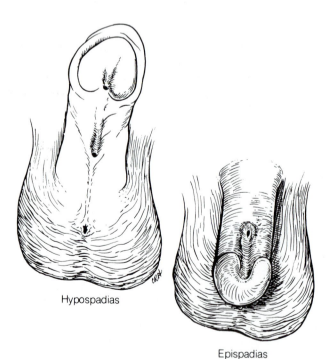

Hypospadias

Epispadias

FIG. 36-1. Hypospadias and epispadias.

PRIAPISM

Priapism is an involuntary prolonged and painful erection that can persist for hours or days and is not associated with sexual excitement. Priapism is a true urologic emergency with significant risk of subsequent impotence.

The condition is caused by impaired blood flow in the corpora cavernosa of the penis. Two mechanisms for priapism have been proposed: (1) low-flow (ischemic) priapism in which there is stasis of blood flow in the corpora cavernosa with a resultant failure of detumescence and (2) high-flow (nonischemic) priapism, which involves persistent arterial flow into the corpora cavernosa. In high-flow priapism, there is no hypoxia of local tissue, the penis is less rigid, and the pain is less than in stasis priapism.

Priapism can occur at any age. It is classified as primary (idiopathic) or secondary to a disease or drug effect. Primary priapism is the result of conditions such as trauma, infection, and neoplasms. Secondary causes include hematologic conditions such as leukemia, sickle cell disease, and thrombocytopenia; neurologic conditions such as stroke, spinal cord injury, and other central nervous system (CNS) lesions; and renal failure. Various medications, such as antihypertensive drugs, anticoagulant drugs, antidepressant drugs, alcohol, and marijuana, can also contribute to the development of priapism.

The diagnosis of priapism is usually based on clinical findings. Blood gas studies using intracaveranal aspirate may be helpful in distinguishing ischemic low-flow priapism from nonischemic high-flow priapism. Doppler studies of penile blood flow, penile ultrasound, and computed tomography (CT) scans may be used to determine intrapelvic pathology.

Initial treatment measures include analgesics, sedation, and hydration. Urinary retention may necessitate catheterization. Local measures include ice packs and cold saline enemas, aspiration and irrigation of the corpus cavernosum with plain or heparinized saline, or instillation of α-adrenergic drugs. If less aggressive treatment does not produce detumescence, a temporary surgical shunt may be established between the corpus cavernosum and the corpus spongiosum.

The prognosis of whether fibrosis or erectile failure will occur is determined by the severity and duration of blood stasis. In high-flow priapism, the damaging effects of decreased oxygen tension and intracavernal blood pressure are less pronounced than in stasis priapism. Normal erectile potency can be restored even after a long duration of high-flow priapism. Persistent stasis priapism, in contrast, is known to result in impaired erectile function and tissue fibrosis unless resolved within 24 hours of onset.[4]

PEYRONIE'S DISEASE

Peyronie's disease involves a localized and progressive fibrosis of unknown etiology that affects the tunica albuginea (tough whitish layer of tissue) at the top of the penile shaft (Fig. 36-2). It is characterized initially by an inflammatory process that results in dense fibrous plaque formation. This plaque may become calcified and bony. The fibrous tissue prevents lengthening of the involved area during erection, making intercourse difficult and painful. There is no pain when the penis is in the nonerect state. The disease usually occurs in middle-aged or elderly men. Although the cause of the disorder is unknown, the dense microscopic plaques are consistent with findings of severe vasculitis.[5]

The erectile dysfunction associated with Peyronie's disease may be due to the disease or impaired erection. It is often difficult to determine whether it is

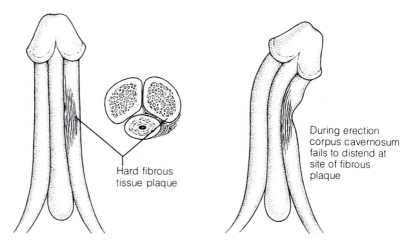

FIG. 36-2. A hard, fibrous plaque occurs with Peyronie's disease. (Adapted from Blandy, J. [1977]. *Lecture notes on urology* [2nd ed.]. Oxford: Blackwell Scientific Publications)

Hard fibrous tissue plaque

During erection corpus cavernosum fails to distend at site of fibrous plaque of arterial, venous, or functional origin. Doppler ultrasound may be used to assess causation of the disorder. Although surgical interventions can be used to correct the disorder, it is often delayed because in many cases the disorder is self-limiting.[6] Less invasive treatments include injecting hydrocortisone into the fibrous area, administering vitamin E, using ultrasound wave therapy, or administering fibrolytic agents such as potassium para-aminobenzoate.

BALANITIS/BALANOPOSTHITIS

Balanitis is an acute or chronic inflammation of the glans penis. Balanoposthitis refers to inflammation of the glans and prepuce. It is usually encountered in males with phimosis or a large redundant prepuce that interferes with cleanliness and predisposes to bacterial growth within the accumulated secretions and smegma (debris from the desquamated epithelia). If left untreated, the condition may cause ulcerations of the mucosal surface of the glans; these ulcerations may lead to inflammatory scarring of the phimosis and further aggravate the condition.

Acute superficial balanoposthitis is characterized by erythema of the glans and prepuce. An exudate in the form of malodorous discharge may be present. Extension of the erythema and edema may result in phimosis. The condition may originate due to infection, trauma, or irritation. Infective balanoposthitis may be caused by a wide variety of organisms. *Chlamydia* and *Mycoplasma* are being identified as causative organisms in this disease. The inflammatory reaction is nonspecific, and correct identification of the specific agent requires bacterial smears and cultures.

Balanitis xerotica obliterans is a chronic sclerosing, atrophic process of the glans penis that occurs in uncircumcised males. It is clinically and histologically similar to lichen sclerosus that is seen in females. Typically, the lesions consist of whitish plaques on the surface of the glans penis and the prepuce. The foreskin is thickened and fibrous and is not retractable. Treatment measures include circumcision and topical or intralesional injections of corticosteroids.[7]

CANCER OF THE PENIS

Squamous cell cancer of the penis is most common in men between 45 and 60 years of age. In the United States, it accounts for less than 1% of male genital tumors; however, in other countries of the world, it accounts for 10% to 20% of male cancers.[8] The cause of penile cancer is unknown. There is an association between penile cancer and poor genital hygiene and phimosis. This type of cancer is rare in Jewish and Muslim men who are circumcised routinely. Phimosis is found in about 75% of the males with squamous cell carcinoma of the penis and is the most common abnormality associated with the tumor.[9] Although studies have yielded conflicting results, it has been hypothesized that smegma may serve as a carcinogenic agent. However, there is increasing evidence of a viral role in the development of cancer of the penis; studies have shown that certain types of papillomavirus may be implicated. Ultraviolet radiation may also have a carcinogenic effect on the penis. Males who were treated for psoriasis with ultraviolet A or B (PUVAA, PUVAB) therapies have had a reported increased incidence of genital squamous cell carcinomas. Because of this observation, it is suggested that men should shield their genital area when using tanning salons.[9]

The tumor begins as a small lump or ulcer on the penis. If phimosis is present, there may be painful swelling, purulent drainage, or difficulty in urinating. Palpable lymph nodes may be present in the inguinal region. Cavernsonagraphy, CT scans, and magnetic resonance imaging (MRI) may be used in the diagnostic work-up.

Penile cancer tends to be slow growing. When it is diagnosed early, it is highly curable. The greatest hindrance to early diagnosis is delay in seeking medical attention. Treatment options vary according to stage, size, location, and invasiveness of the tumor. Surgery remains the mainstay of treatment. Superficial primary lesions that are freely movable, do not invade the corpora, and show no evidence of metastatic disease can be treated with sleeve resection. Partial or total penectomy is indicated for invasive lesions. About 65% of invasive penile cancer are stage III, with lymph node involvement. For these men, bilateral lymph node dissection is indicated.

Cumulative data reveal that males with penile cancer have an overall 5-year survival rate that ranges from 65% to 90%. The most important prognostic indicator is the lymph node status. For men with positive lymph nodes, the 5-year survival rate ranges from 3% to 50%.[10]

In summary, disorders of the penis can be either congenital or acquired. Hypospadias and epispadias are congenital defects in which there is a malposition of the urethral opening: it is located on the ventral surface in hypospadias and on the dorsal surface in epispadias. Phimosis is the condition in which the opening of the foreskin is too tight to permit retraction over the glans. Prolonged, painful, and nonsexual erection that can lead to thrombosis with ischemia and necrosis is called priapism. Peyronie's disease is characterized by the growth of a band of fibrous tissue on top of the penile shaft. Balanitis is an acute or chronic inflammation of the glans penis and balanoposthitis is an inflammation of the glans and prepuce. Cancer of the penis accounts for less than 1% of male genital cancers. Although the tumor is slow growing and highly curable when diagnosed early, the greatest hindrance to successful treatment is delay in seeking medical attention.

■ DISORDERS OF THE SCROTUM AND TESTES

The scrotum is a skin-covered pouch that contains the testes and their accessory organs. Defects of the scrotum and testes include cryptorchidism, disorders of the scrotal sac, vascular disorders, inflammation of the scrotum and testes, and neoplasms.

CRYPTORCHIDISM

The testes develop intraabdominally in the fetus and usually descend into the scrotum through the inguinal canal during the eighth or ninth month of gestation. Cryptorchidism, or undescended testes, occurs when one or both of the testicles fail to move down into the scrotal sac. The undescended testes may remain within the lower abdomen or at a point of descent within the inguinal canal (Fig. 36-3). The cause of cryptorchidism is poorly understood. It may be due to anatomic factors, such as a short spermatic cord or a narrow inguinal ring; or genetic or hormonal factors.[11] The incidence of cryptorchidism is directly related to birth weight and gestational age; infants

who are born prematurely or are small for gestational age have the highest incidence of the disorder. In 75% of full-term infants and 95% of premature infants born with cryptorchidism, spontaneous testicular descent occurs within the first year of life. Spontaneous descent rarely occurs before the age of 1 year.

In children with cryptorchidism, histologic abnormalities of the testes occur secondarily to intrinsic defects in the testicle or to adverse effects of the extrascrotal environment. Temperatures in the inguinal canal are 1°C to 2°C higher than in the scrotum. This increased temperature may damage the undescended testicle. It may also produce morphologic changes in the contralateral testis, possibly reflecting autosensitization through the production of antibodies against spermatozoa, germinal epithelium, or Sertoli's cells. These testicular changes may cause infertility and increase the risk of testicular cancer in later life.

Males with unilateral or bilateral cryptorchidism usually have decreased sperm counts in both the undescended testis and the contralateral testis. Spermatogonia counts in males with cryptorchidism never reach the normal counts that are found in males whose testes have descended in the usual manner. Studies have shown abnormalities in the sperm density and hormonal levels of men who underwent orchiopexy (surgical fixation of the testes in the scrotum) between the ages of 4 and 12 years. The increased risk of testicular cancer is not significantly affected by orchiopexy, hormonal therapy, or late spontaneous descent after the age of 2 years.[12]

The major manifestation of cryptorchidism is the absence of one or more of the testes from the scrotum. The testis either is not palpable (lying within or proximal to the inguinal ring) or can be felt external to the inguinal ring. The testes are not palpable in 15% to 20% of males with cryptorchidism. Improved techniques for testicular localization include ultrasonography (visualization of the testes by recording the pulses of ultrasonic waves directed into the tissues), gonadal venography and arteriography (x-ray of the veins and arteries of the testes after the injection of a contrast medium), and laparoscopy (examination of the interior of the abdomen using a visualization instrument).

The treatment goals for the male with cryptorchidism include measures to (1) enhance fertility, (2) place the gonad in a favorable place for cancer detection, and (3) improve cosmetic appearance. Regardless of the type of treatment that is employed, it should be carried out before the child reaches 2 years of age.[1] Treatment modalities for children with unilateral or bilateral cryptorchidism include initial hormone therapy with human chorionic gonadotropin (HCG). The gonadotropin-releasing hormone (Gn-

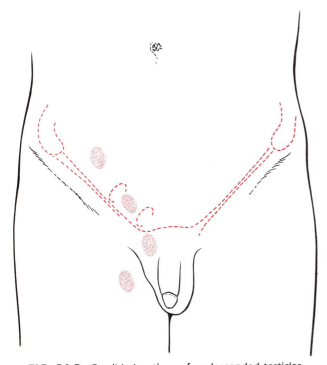

FIG. 36-3. Possible locations of undescended testicles.

RH), a hypothalamic hormone that stimulates production of the gonadotropic hormones by the anterior pituitary gland, has been used with considerable success in Europe and has recently been introduced in the United States.[13] For children who do not respond to hormonal treatment, surgical placement and fixation of the testes in the scrotum have proved effective.

HYDROCELE

The testes and epididymis are completely surrounded by the tunica vaginalis, a serous pouch derived from the peritoneum during the fetal descent of the testes from the abdomen into the scrotum. The tunica vaginalis has an outer parietal layer as well as a deeper visceral layer that adheres to the dense fibrous covering of the testes, the tunica albuginea. A space exists between these two layers that typically contains a few milliliters of clear fluid.

A hydrocele forms when excess fluid collects within the layers of the tunica vaginalis (Fig. 36-4). It may be bilateral or unilateral and can develop as a primary congenital defect or as a secondary condition. Acute hydrocele may develop secondary to local injury, epididymitis or orchitis, gonorrhea, lymph obstruction, germ cell testicular tumor, or as a side effect of radiation therapy. Chronic hydrocele is more common. Fluid collects about the testis, and the mass grows gradually. Its cause is unknown, and it usually develops in men past 40 years.

Most cases of hydrocele in male infants and children are caused by a patent processus vaginalis, which is continuous with the peritoneal cavity. It is also a form of indirect inguinal hernia. Most hydroceles of infancy close spontaneously; therefore, they are not repaired before age one. If the hydrocele

persists beyond 18 months of age, surgical treatment is usually indicated.

Hydroceles are palpated as cystic masses that may attain massive proportions. If there is enough fluid, the mass may be mistaken for a solid tumor. Transillumination (shining a light through the scrotum for the purposes of visualizing its internal structures) or ultrasonography can help to determine whether the mass is solid or cystic and whether the testicle is normal.

A tense hydrocele that does not illuminate should be differentiated from a testicular tumor. If a hydrocele develops in a young man without apparent cause, careful evaluation is needed to rule out cancer or infection.

In an adult male, a hydrocele is a relatively benign condition. The condition is often asymptomatic, and no treatment is necessary. When symptoms do occur, the feeling may be that of heaviness in the scrotum or pain in the lower back. In cases of secondary hydrocele, the primary condition is treated. If the hydrocele is painful or cosmetically undesirable, surgical correction is indicated. Surgical repair may be done either inguinally or transcrotally.[14]

HEMATOCELE

A hematocele is an accumulation of blood in the tunica vaginalis, which, in turn, causes the scrotal skin to become dark red or purple. It may develop as a result of an abdominal surgical procedure, scrotal trauma, bleeding disorder, or testicular tumor.

SPERMATOCELE

A spermatocele is a painless, sperm-containing cyst that forms at the end of the epididymis. It is located above and posterior to the testis, is attached to the epididymis, and is separate from the testes. Spermatoceles may be solitary or occur in groups and are usually less than 1 cm in size. They are freely movable and should transilluminate. Spermatoceles rarely cause problems; however, a large one may become painful and require excision.

VARICOCELE

Varicocele is characterized by varicosities of the pampiniform plexus, a network of veins supplying the testes, with the left side being more commonly affected. This is because the left internal spermatic vein inserts into the left renal vein at a right angle, whereas the right spermatic vein usually enters the inferior vena cava. Incompetent valves are more com-

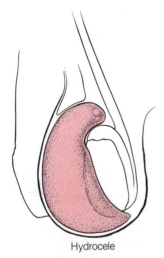

Hydrocele

FIG. 36-4. Hydrocele.

mon in the left internal spermatic veins, causing a reflux of blood back into the veins of the pampiniform plexus. The force of gravity resulting from the upright position also contributes to venous dilatation. If the condition persists, there is damage to the elastic fibers and hypertrophy of the vein walls the same as occurs in formation of varicose veins in the leg.

The presence of a varicocele may be associated with male infertility. Although the exact mechanism whereby varicocele produces infertility is not fully understood, several theories of pathogenesis exist. One theory suggests that because a varicocele may be caused by a retrograde flow of blood down the internal spermatic vein, metabolites may be refluxed down the vein, producing adverse effects on sperm production. A second theoretical mechanism involves the effect of heat on the testes. This theory proposes that a varicocele can cause an increase in scrotal temperature, a factor that is thought to impair spermatogenesis. A third theory links epididymal conditions within the epididymis with infertility. Several factors in the epididymis determine motility and maturation of the spermatozoa, including blood supply, tissue androgens, and electrolyte composition. The retrograde flow of blood in the pampiniform plexus could adversely affect environmental conditions in the epididymis and thereby impair the maturation of the spermatozoa leading to disturbances in motility. There is also the possibility that occult epididymal obstruction accounts for impaired spermatogenesis and infertility. It is possible that several of these factors may interact and impair fertility in the presence of varicocele.

Varicoceles are rarely found before puberty, and the incidence is highest in men between 15 and 35 years of age. Symptoms of varicocele include an abnormal feeling of heaviness in the left scrotum, although many varicoceles are asymptomatic. Usually the presence of varicocele is readily diagnosed on physical examination in both the standing and recumbent positions. Classically, the varicocele disappears in the lying position due to venous decompression into the renal vein. Scrotal palpation of a varicocele has been compared to feeling a "bag of worms." Small varicoceles are sometimes difficult to identify. Valsalva's maneuver (forced expiration against a closed glottis) may be used to accentuate small varicosities. A hand-held Doppler stethoscope is used while the patient performs Valsalva's maneuver. If the varicocele is present, a distinct venous rush is heard because of the sudden retrograde blood flow. Other diagnostic aids include realtime ultrasound, radioisotope scanning, spermatic venography,[15] and scrotopenogram.[16]

Treatment options include surgical ligation or embolization or sclerosing by way of a percutaneous

transvenous catheter under fluoroscopic guidance. Both can be performed as outpatient procedures. The benefits of the percutaneous technique include a slightly lower recurrence rate and more rapid return to full physical activity.[15] It has been shown that 40% of men with abnormalities in their semen and a varicocele show some degree of improvement in fertility after obliteration of the dilated veins. Aside from improving fertility, other reasons for surgery include the relief of the sensation of "heaviness" and cosmetic improvement.

TESTICULAR TORSION

Testicular torsion is a twisting of the spermatic cord, which suspends the testis (Fig. 36-5). It is the most common acute scrotal disorder in the pediatric and young-adult population. Testicular torsion can be divided into two distinct clinical entities depending on the level of spermatic cord involvement: extravaginal and intravaginal torsion.

In extravaginal torsion, the less common form of testicular torsion, the testicle and the fascial tunicae that surround it rotate around the spermatic cord at a level well above the tunica vaginalis. Extravaginal torsion occurs almost exclusively in neonates. The torsion probably occurs during fetal or neonatal descent of the testes before the tunica adheres to the scrotal wall. At birth or shortly thereafter, a firm, smooth, painless scrotal mass is identified. The scrotal skin appears red, and some edema is present. Differential diagnosis is relatively easy because testicular tumors, epididymitis, and orchitis are exceedingly rare in neonates; hydrocele is softer and can be transilluminated, and physical examination excludes the presence of hernia. Treatment includes elective unilateral surgical exploration and orchiectomy (removal of the testis).[17]

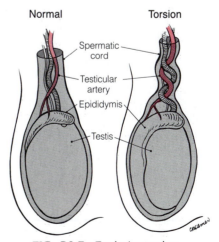

FIG. 36-5. Testicular torsion.

Intravaginal torsion is considerably more common than extravaginal torsion. It occurs when the testis rotates on the long axis within the tunica vaginalis. In most cases, congenital abnormalities of the tunica vaginalis or spermatic cord exist. The tunica vaginalis normally surrounds the testes and epididymis, allowing the testicle to rotate freely within the tunica. Although anomalies of suspension vary, the epididymal attachment may be loose enough to permit torsion between the testis and the epididymis. More commonly, however, the testis rotates about the distal spermatic cord. Because this abnormality is developmental, bilateral anomalies are common.

Intravaginal torsion occurs most frequently in males aged 8 to 18 years and is rarely seen after age 30. Males usually present in severe distress within hours of onset. Often nausea, vomiting, and tachycardia are present. The affected testis is large and tender with pain radiating to the inguinal area. Extensive cremaster muscle contraction causes a thickening of the spermatic cord.

Testicular torsion must be differentiated from epididymitis orchitis and trauma to the testis. On physical examination, the testicle is often high in the scrotum and in an abnormal orientation. These changes are caused by the twisting and shortening of the spermatic cord. Depending on the duration of symptoms, there will be a variable amount of scrotal swelling and redness. The testis will be firm and tender. The cremasteric reflex, normally elicited by stroking the medial aspect of the thigh and observing testicular retraction, is frequently absent. Urinalysis should be performed because pyuria indicates an infectious process rather than torsion. A Doppler ultrasound and testicular radionuclide scanning aid in diagnosis.[18]

Testicular torsion is a true surgical emergency, and early recognition and treatment are necessary if the testicle is to be saved. Treatment includes surgical detorsion and orchiectomy. Orchiectomy is carried out when the testis is deemed nonviable after surgical detorsion.

Testicular salvage rates are directly related to the duration of torsion. Studies have shown a more than 80% testicular salvage rate if detorsion is performed in less than 3 hours, but only a 20% testicular salvage rate if more than 12 hours have elapsed before detorsioning. Because the opposite testicle usually is affected by the same abnormal attachments, prophylactic fixation of that testis should be performed.

EPIDIDYMITIS

Epididymitis is an inflammation of the epididymis, the elongated cordlike structure that lies along the posterior border of the testis, whose function is the storage, transport, and maturation of spermatozoa. There are two major types of epididymitis: (1) sexually transmitted infections associated with urethritis and (2) primary nonsexually transmitted infections associated with urinary tract infections and prostatitis. Most cases of epididymitis are caused by bacterial pathogens.

In primary nonsexual infections, the pressure associated with voiding or physical strain may force urine containing pathogens from the urethra or prostate up the ejaculatory duct and through the vas deferens and into the epididymis. Infections may also reach the epididymis through the lymphatics of the spermatic cord. In rare cases, organisms from other foci of infection reach the epididymis through the bloodstream. In children, the disorder is usually associated with congenital urinary tract abnormalities and infection with gram-negative rods.

Sexually transmitted acute epididymitis occurs mainly in young men without underlying genitourinary disease and is most commonly caused by *Chlamydia trachomatis* and *Neisseria gonorrhoeae* (singly or in combination). In men over 35 years of age, epididymitis is often associated with pathogens such as *E. coli*, *Pseudomonas*, and gram-positive cocci.

Epididymitis is characterized by unilateral pain and swelling, accompanied by erythema and edema of the overlying scrotal skin that develops over a period of 24 to 48 hours. Initially the swelling and induration are limited to the epididymis. However, the distinction between the testis and epididymis becomes less evident as the inflammation progresses, and the testis and epididymis become one mass. There may be tenderness over the groin (spermatic cord) or in the lower abdomen. Fever and complaint of dysuria occur in about half of the cases. Whether urethral discharge is present or not depends on the organism causing the infection; it usually accompanies gonorrheal infections, is common in chlamydial infections, and is less common in infections due to gram-negative organisms.

Laboratory findings usually reveal an elevated white blood cell count. Urinalysis and urine culture are important in the diagnosis of epididymitis with bacteriuria and pyuria suggestive of the disorder. The cause of epididymitis can be differentiated by Gram's stain examination or culture of a midstream urine specimen or a urethral specimen.

Treatment during the acute phase (which usually lasts for 3 to 4 days) includes bedrest, scrotal elevation and support, and antibiotics. Bedrest with scrotal support improves lymphatic drainage. The choice of antibiotics is determined by age, physical findings, urinalysis, Gram's stain, cultures, and sexual history. Oral analgesics and antipyretics are usually indicated. Sexual activity or physical strain may exacerbate the infection and worsen the symptoms and should be avoided.

ORCHITIS

Orchitis, an infection of the testes, can be precipitated by a primary infection in the genitourinary tract, such as urethritis, cystitis, or seminal vesiculitis. Many infections from other parts of the body spread to the testes through the bloodstream or the lymphatics. Orchitis can develop as a complication of a systemic infection, such as parotitis (mumps), scarlet fever, or pneumonia. Probably the best known of these complications is orchitis caused by the mumps virus. Interestingly, mumps orchitis does not occur in prepubertal males. However, about 25% to 33% of males 10 years of age or older with mumps develop this form of orchitis.[12]

The onset of mumps orchitis is sudden; it usually occurs about 3 to 4 days after the onset of the parotitis and is characterized by fever, painful enlargement of the testes, and small hemorrhages into the tunica albuginea. Unlike epididymitis, the urinary symptoms are absent. The symptoms usually run their course in 7 to 10 days. Microscopically, an acute inflammatory response is seen in the seminiferous tubules with proliferation of neutrophils, lymphocytes, and histiocytes, causing distention of the tubules. The residual effects that are seen after the acute phase include hyalinization of the seminiferous tubules and atrophy of the testes. Spermatogenesis is irreversibly damaged in about 30% of testes damaged by mumps orchitis. If both testes are involved, permanent sterility results, but androgenic hormone function is usually maintained.[19]

NEOPLASMS

Tumors can develop in either the scrotum or the testes. Benign scrotal tumors are common and often do not require treatment. Carcinoma of the scrotum is rare and is usually associated with exposure to carcinogenic agents. On the other hand, almost all solid tumors of the testes are malignant.

CANCER OF THE SCROTUM

Cancer of the scrotum was the first cancer directly linked to a specific occupation when in the 1800s it was associated with chimney sweeps.[20] Studies have linked this cancer to exposure to tar, soot, and oils. Today, most squamous cell cancers of the scrotum are due to poor hygiene and chronic inflammation. Exposure to ultraviolet A radiation (PUVA) or human papillomavirus has also been associated with the disease.

Malignant tumors of the scrotum are rare in the United States but are 20 times more common in the United Kingdom. The mean age of presentation with the disease is 60 years; often preceded by 20 to 30 years of chronic irritation.

In the early stages, it may appear as a small tumor or wartlike growth that eventually ulcerates. The thin scrotal wall lacks the tissue reactivity needed to block the malignant process; over half of the cases seen involve metastasis to the lymph nodes. Because this tumor does not respond well to chemotherapy or radiation, the treatment includes wide local excision of the tumor with inguinal and femoral node dissection.[21] The prognosis correlates with the presence or absence of lymph node involvement.

TESTICULAR CANCER

Approximately 5000 men are diagnosed with testicular cancer each year. This accounts for 1% of all male cancers and 3% of male urogenital cancers. Although relatively rare, it is the most common cause of cancer in the 15- to 35-year-old age group. In the past, testicular cancer has been a leading cause of death among males entering their most productive years. However, over the past 20 years, advances in therapy have transformed an almost invariably fatal disease into one that is highly curable. With the exception of men with advanced metastatic disease at the time of presentation or those who relapse after primary chemotherapy, the vast majority of men with these tumors are cured with available therapy.

Although the etiology of testicular cancer is unknown, both congenital and acquired factors have been implicated as contributing factors. The strongest association has been with cryptoid testis. The incidence of testicular cancer is 35 times higher in males with cryptoid testis.[22] Administration of exogenous estrogen to the mother during pregnancy has been associated with an increased relative risk of testicular tumors ranging from 2.8% to 5.3% over the expected incidence.[10] Other acquired factors such as trauma and infection have also been implicated, although a causal relationship has not been established.

Often the first sign of testicular cancer is a slight enlargement of the testicle that may be accompanied by some degree of discomfort. This may be an ache in the abdomen or groin or a sensation of dragging or heaviness in the scrotum. Frank pain may be experienced in the later stages when the tumor is growing rapidly and hemorrhaging occurs. Testicular cancer can spread when the tumor may be barely palpable.

The prognosis and extent of treatment required for testicular cancer are related to the stage of the disease at the time of presentation. A delay in seeking medical attention is related to increased stage of the disease and decreased treatment effectiveness. Recognition of the importance of prompt diagnosis and treatment has resulted in development of a procedure for testicular self-examination and an emphasis on public education programs about this type of cancer. The American Cancer Society strongly advocates that every young adult male examines his testes at least once a month as a means of early detection of testicular cancer. The examination should be done after a warm bath or shower when the scrotal skin is relaxed. To do this self-examination, each testicle is examined with the fingers of both hands by rolling the testicle between the thumb and fingers to check for the presence of any lumps. If any lump, nodule, or enlargement is noted, it should be brought immediately to the attention of a physician.

The diagnosis of testicular cancer requires a thorough urologic history and physical examination. A painless testicular mass is highly suspicious of cancer. Conditions that produce an intrascrotal mass similar to testicular cancer include epididymitis, orchitis, hydrocele, or hematocele. The examination for masses should include palpation of the testes and surrounding structures, transillumination of the scrotum, and abdominal palpation. Testicular ultrasound can be used to differentiate testicular masses. The intravenous pyelogram (IVP) may be used to evaluate kidney structure. CT scans and MRI are used in assessing metastatic spread.

There are several systems for classification of testicular cancer. The Armed Forces Institute of Pathology (AFIP) classification system divides testicular cancer into germinal (germ cell) tumors arising from the spermatozoa and their derivatives and nongerminal cell tumors arising from other cellular components of the testes.

Germ cell tumors, which constitute about 95% of all testicular tumors, can be divided into two groups: seminomas and nonseminomas. The peak incidence of seminoma occurs in men between 30 and 40 years of age and nonseminoma in men between ages 20 and 30 years.

Seminomas are thought to arise from the seminiferous epithelium of the testes. They are the most common type of testicular cancer, accounting for approximately 40% of all germ cell tumors. Nonseminoma germ cell tumors are classified into three histologic types: (1) embryonal carcinoma, (2) teratoma, and (3) choriocarcinoma. Embryonal carcinomas represent about 10% to 20% of all germ cell tumors. They are less differentiated and more aggressive than seminomas. Teratomas are derived from totipotential germ cells that have the capacity to differentiate into tissues representing any of the three germ layers of the embryo—ectoderm, mesoderm, or endoderm. They constitute less than 10% of germ cell tumors and can occur at any age from infancy to old age. They usually behave as benign tumors in children; in adults, they often contain minute foci of cancer cells. Choriocarcinoma, a highly malignant form of cancer that is identical to tumors that arise in the placental tissue, accounts for 1% of testicular cancers. Each of these basic histologic types can occur as a pure form or as a combination of cell types. Forty percent of testicular cancers are of mixed tissue types.[10] The most common mixture is teratocarcinoma, which contains both embryonal carcinoma and teratoma elements. The peak incidence of nonseminoma occurs between 20 and 30 years of age.

The clinical staging (TNM classification) for testicular cancer is as follows: stage I, tumor confined to testes; stage II, tumor spread to retroperitoneal lymph nodes; stage III, distant metastases (see Chapter 5). Staging procedures include CT scans of the chest, abdomen, and pelvis; ultrasonography for detection of bulky inferior nodal metastases; venacavography; and lymphangiography. Radiographic methods are used to detect metastatic spread. Tumor markers, radioimmunoassay studies that measure protein antigens produced by malignant cells, provide information about both the existence of a tumor and the type of tumor present and may detect tumors that are too small to be detected on physical examination or x-ray.

Three tumor markers are useful in evaluating the tumor response: α-*fetoprotein* (AFP), a glycoprotein that is normally present in fetal serum in large amounts; *HCG*, a hormone that is normally produced by the placenta in pregnant women; and *lactic acid dehydrogenase* (LDH), a cellular enzyme normally found in muscle, liver, kidney, and brain.[10] During embryonic development, the totipotential germ cells of the testes travel down normal differentiation pathways and produce different protein products. The reappearance of these protein markers in the adult suggests activity of the undifferentiated cells in a testicular germ cell tumor.

The basic treatment of all testicular cancers includes orchiectomy, which is done at the time of diagnostic exploration. The widely used surgical procedure is the unilateral radical orchiectomy by way of an inguinal incision. Surgical therapy is advantageous because it enables precise staging of the disease. Recommendations for further therapy (retroperitoneal dissection, chemotherapy, radiation therapy) are based on the pathologic findings from the surgical procedure.

Seminomas are radiosensitive; the treatment of stage I or II seminoma is irradiation of the retroperitoneal and homolateral lymph nodes to the level of the diaphragm. Patients with bulky retroperitoneal or distant metastases are often treated with multiagent chemotherapy. Seminoma is probably the most curable of all solid tumors. Retroperitoneal lymph node dissection is widely used after orchiectomy to treat stage II and nonseminomatous germ cell tumors. Patient who have extensive retroperitoneal or chest metastasis are best treated with multiagent chemotherapy after orchiectomy.

With appropriate treatment, the prognosis of men with testicular cancer is excellent. The 5-year survival rate for patients with stage I and II disease exceeds 90%. Patients with stage III tumors have an overall survival rate of approximately 70%, with prognosis related to the amount of distant metastases present. Even patients with mild or moderate lung metastases have excellent chances for long-term survival.

Therapy for testicular cancer can have potentially adverse effects on sexual functioning. It has been reported that up to 50% of men who had been treated for testicular cancer had some type of sexual dysfunction. Men who have retroperitoneal lymph node dissection may experience retrograde ejaculation or failure to ejaculate because of severing of the sympathetic plexus. A nerve-sparing technique can be used in cases without extensive disease and can preserve seminal emission and fertility in 90% of these men.

In summary, disorders of the scrotum and testes include cryptorchidism (undescended testicles), hydrocele, hematocele, spermatocele, varicocele, and testicular torsion. Inflammatory conditions can involve the scrotal sac, epididymis, or testes. Tumors can arise in either the scrotum or the testes. Scrotal cancers are usually associated with exposure to petroleum products such as tar, pitch, and soot. Testicular cancer accounts for 3% of cancers of the male genitourinary system. With present treatment methods, a large percentage of men with these tumors can be cured. Testicular self-examination is recommended as a means of early detection of this form of cancer.

■ DISORDERS OF THE PROSTATE

The prostate is a firm glandular structure that surrounds the urethra. It produces a thin, milky alkaline secretion that aids sperm motility by helping to maintain an optimum pH. The contraction of the smooth muscle in the gland promotes semen expulsion during ejaculation.

PROSTATITIS

Prostatitis refers to a variety of inflammatory disorders of the prostate gland, some bacterial in nature and some not. It may occur spontaneously, as a result of catheterization or instrumentation, or secondary to other diseases of the male genitourinary system. There are four types of prostatitis: (1) acute bacterial, (2) chronic bacterial, (3) nonbacterial, and (4) prostatodynia.

ACUTE BACTERIAL PROSTATITIS

Acute bacterial prostatitis is relatively rare but dramatic in its presentation. Symptoms include high fever, chills, malaise, myalgia, and arthralgia. Further symptoms include frequent and urgent urination, dysuria, and urethral discharge. Dull aching pain is present in the perineum, rectum, or sacrococcygeal region. Rectal examination reveals a swollen, tender, warm prostate with soft scattered areas. Prostatic massage produces a thick discharge with white blood cells that grow large numbers of pathogens on culture. These pathogens often include gram-negative enteric bacteria such as *Pseudomonas*, as well as gram-positive staphylococci and streptococci.

Treatment of acute bacterial prostatitis depends on the severity of symptoms. It usually includes bedrest, adequate hydration, antipyretics, analgesics (often narcotics) or spasmolytic drugs to alleviate pain, and stool softeners. Hospitalization may be necessary. A suprapubic catheter may be indicated if voiding is difficult or painful.

Usually acute prostatitis responds to appropriate antimicrobial therapy chosen in accordance with the sensitivity of the causative agents in the urethral discharge. Depending on the urine culture, antibiotic therapy is usually continued for at least 4 weeks. Because acute prostatitis is often associated with anatomic abnormalities, a thorough urologic examination is usually performed after treatment is completed.

A persistent fever indicates the need for further investigation for an additional site of infection or development of a prostatic abscess. CT scans and transrectal ultrasound of the prostate are useful in the diagnosis of prostatic abscesses. Prostatic abscesses, which are relatively uncommon since the advent of effective antibiotic therapy, are found more commonly in males with diabetes mellitus. Prostatic abscesses are usually associated with bacteremia; prompt drainage by transperitoneal or transurethral incision followed by appropriate antimicrobial therapy is usually indicated.[19]

CHRONIC BACTERIAL PROSTATITIS

In contrast to acute bacterial prostatitis, chronic bacterial prostatitis is a subtle disorder that is difficult to treat. The symptoms of chronic prostatitis are variable and include frequent and urgent urination, dysuria, perineal discomfort, and low-back pain. Occasionally myalgia and arthralgia accompany the other symptoms. Secondary epididymitis is sometimes associated with the disorder. Many men suffer relapsing lower or upper urinary tract infections because of recurrent invasion of the bladder by the prostatic bacteria. Bacteria may continue to be present in the prostate gland even when the prostatic fluid is sterile. Organisms responsible for chronic bacterial prostatitis are usually the gram-negative enterobacteria (*Escherichia coli, Proteus mirabilis,* or *Klebsiella pneumoniae*) or *Pseudomonas aeruginosa.* Occasionally, a gram-positive organism such as *Streptococcus faecalis* is the causative organism. Infected prostatic calculi may develop and contribute to the chronic infection.

The most accurate method of establishing a diagnosis is by localizing cultures. It is based on sequential collections of the initially voided urine (urethral specimen), midstream specimen (bladder specimen), the expressed prostatic secretion (obtained by prostatic massage), and the urine voided after prostatic massage. The last two specimens are considered prostatic urine. A positive expressed prostatic specimen establishes the diagnosis of bacterial prostatitis, ruling out nonbacterial prostatitis and prostatodynia.

Even after an accurate diagnosis has been established, treatment for chronic prostatitis is often difficult and frustrating. Unlike their action in the acutely inflamed prostate, antibacterial drugs penetrate poorly into the chronically inflamed prostate. Long-term therapy (4 to 6 months) with an appropriate low-dose oral antimicrobial agent such as trimethoprim-sulfamethoxazole, carbenicillin indanyl sodium, minocycline, or erythromycin is often used to treat the infection. Transurethral prostatectomy may be indicated when the infection is not cured or adequately controlled by medical therapy, particularly when prostate stones are present.

NONBACTERIAL PROSTATITIS

A large group of men with prostatitis suffer from pains along the penis, testicles, and scrotum; painful ejaculation, low-back pain; rectal pain along the inner thighs; urinary symptoms; decreased libido, and impotence but have no bacteria present in the urinary system. Men with nonbacterial prostatitis often have inflammation of the prostate with an elevated white blood cell count and abnormal inflammatory cells in their prostatic secretions. The cause of the disorder is unknown, and efforts to prove the presence of unusual pathogens (*e.g.,* mycoplasmas, chlamydiae, trichomonads, and viruses) have been largely unsuccessful. Some researchers believe nonbacterial prostatitis is an autoimmune disorder. Those affected may be treated with tetracycline, with erythromycin, or, if mycosis is present, with an antifungal treatment. Because nonbacterial prostatitis does not usually respond to antibiotic therapy, treatment is often

directed toward symptom control. Antiinflammatory agents such as ibuprofen may be used to provide symptom relief.

PROSTATODYNIA

Men with prostatodynia have symptoms resembling those of nonbacterial prostatitis but have negative urine cultures and no evidence of prostatic inflammation (negative leukocyte counts). The cause of prostatodynia is unknown, but, because of the absence of inflammation, the search for the cause of symptoms associated with prostatodynia has been directed toward extraprostatic sources. In some cases, there is an apparent functional obstruction of the bladder neck and near the external urethral sphincter during voiding this results in higher than normal pressures within the prostatic urethra that cause intraprostatic urine reflux and chemical irritation of the prostate by urine. In other cases, there is an apparent myalgia (muscle pain) associated with prolonged tension of the pelvic floor muscles. Emotional stress has been implicated in still other cases.

BENIGN PROSTATIC HYPERPLASIA

Benign prostatic hyperplasia is an age-related nonmalignant enlargement of the prostate gland. It is one of the most common diseases of aging men. In one study of men 50 years of age and older, 75% had some symptoms of prostate enlargement, 50% were symptomatic to a moderate or large degree, and 25% had symptoms severe enough to require surgery.[23]

Benign prostatic hyperplasia is characterized by the formation of large discrete lesions in the periurethral region of the prostate. Although the condition has traditionally been referred to as benign prostatic hypertrophy (BPH), the basic process is one of hyperplasia rather than hypertrophy. The exact cause of benign prostatic hyperplasia is unknown. The fact that the condition occurs largely in older men suggests a relationship to changes in hormone balance associated with aging. Both androgens (testosterone) and estrogens appear to contribute to the process. Dihydrotestosterone, believed to be the biologically active metabolite of testosterone, is thought to be the ultimate mediator of hyperplasia, with estrogen serving to sensitize the prostatic tissue to the growth-producing effects of dihydrotestosterone. Although the exact source is uncertain, small amounts of estrogen are produced in the male. It has been postulated that the increase in levels of estrogen that occurs with aging may facilitate the action of androgens within the prostate despite a decline in testicular output of testosterone.[12]

The symptoms of benign prostatic hyperplasia are related to the compression of the urethra with accompanying bladder distention and hypertrophy, urinary tract infection, and renal disease. The typical picture includes outflow obstruction with a decreased caliber and force of the urinary stream. As the obstruction increases, acute retention with overdistention of the bladder may occur. The presence of residual urine in the bladder causes frequency of urination and a constant desire to empty the bladder, which becomes worse at night. With marked bladder distention, overflow incontinence may occur with the slightest increase in intraabdominal pressure.

The clinical significance of benign prostatic hyperplasia resides in its tendency to compress the urethra and cause partial or complete obstruction of urinary outflow. The resulting obstruction to urinary flow can give rise to urinary tract infection, destructive changes of the bladder wall, hydroureter, and hydronephrosis. Hypertrophy and changes in bladder-wall structure develop in stages. At first, the exaggerated criss-cross fibers form trabeculations and then herniations, or sacculations; finally, diverticula develop as the herniations extend through the bladder wall (see Chapter 34, Fig. 34-3). Because urine is seldom completely emptied from them, these diverticula are readily infected. Back pressure on the ureters and collecting system of kidneys promotes hydroureter, hydronephrosis, and danger of eventual renal failure.

The diagnosis of benign prostatic hyperplasia is based on a history and observation of urinary retention. The bladder may be seen and palpated as retention of urine increases. On digital rectal examination, a smooth rubbery enlargement of the prostate is usually detected. Hardened areas of the prostate gland suggest cancer and should be biopsied. An enlarged prostate found during a rectal examination does not always correlate with the degree of urinary obstruction. Some males can have greatly enlarged prostate glands with no urinary obstruction, whereas others may have severe symptoms without a palpable enlargement of the prostate. The reason for this occurrence is that symptoms are produced by compression of the urethra. A man may have an enlarged gland that protrudes into the soft surrounding tissue without compressing the urethra, thus no symptoms are produced.

Among the objective signs of benign prostatic hyperplasia are a large residual volume and reduced urine flow rate. A postvoiding catheterization for residual urine volume is often useful in determining the extent of urinary obstruction. Residual urines greater than 100 mL are considered high. Uroflowmetry provides an objective measure of urine flow rate. The patient is asked to void with a relatively full bladder (at least 150 mL) into a device that electronically measures the force of the stream and urine flow rate. A urinary flow rate of greater than 14 mL per second is considered "normal," and less than 10 mL per second is indicative of obstruction.

In the past, intravenous urography (IVU) was used extensively for visualization of the urinary tract; however, with new imaging techniques, routine urography should no longer be considered necessary. Diagnostic ultrasound, either transabdominal or transrectal, offers the ability to evaluate the kidneys, ureters, and bladder.[24] Abdominal x-rays may be used to reveal the size of the gland. Cystourethroscopy gives the length and diameter of the urethra, the size and configuration of the prostate, and the bladder capacity. It also detects the presence of trabeculations, bladder stones, and small bladder cancers. CT scans, MRI studies, and radionuclide scanning are not used routinely and are reserved for rare instances of tumor detection or staging.[24] Blood and urine analyses are used as adjuncts to determine benign prostatic hyperplasia complications. Urinalysis is done to detect bacteria, white blood cells, or microscopic hematuria in the presence of infection and inflammation. Elevations in serum creatinine and blood urea nitrogen (BUN) suggest renal damage.

When a man develops mild symptoms related to BPH, a "watch and wait" stance is often taken by the physician. The condition does not always run a predictable course. It may remain stable or even improve. However, when more severe signs of obstruction develop, treatment is indicated to provide comfort and to avoid serious renal damage.[25]

Until the 1980s, surgery was the only method of treatment to alleviate the obstruction. Transurethral resection of the prostate (TURP) or an open approach (suprapubic, retropubic, or perineal prostatectomy) is also done in the case of urethral stricture, bladder diverticuli, or bladder calculi that necessitate removal.[26] After a TURP, one of the major complaints of men is impairment of sexual function. About a 10% chance for impotence exists because of neurologic damage. Retrograde ejaculation is another problem that may occur because of resection of bladder neck tissue. Incontinence rarely occurs except for a transient urge incontinence immediately after surgery.[27]

Several alternative procedures for treatment of benign prostatic hyperplasia have been developed. A new surgical approach is the transurethral incision of the prostate (TUIP). This procedure involves making one or two incisions in the bundle of smooth muscle where the prostate gland is attached to the bladder. The gland is split to reduce pressure on the urethra. This procedure is helpful for smaller prostate glands that cause obstruction.[28]

A balloon dilation approach for removing the obstruction is another new technique. This procedure may be performed on an outpatient basis with recovery in 2 to 10 days versus 6 to 12 weeks after surgical procedures. The procedure is not done if the postvoiding residual urine exceeds 500 mL, if prostate cancer is suspected, if the prostatic urethra is longer than 8 cm, or if the prostate is larger than 40 g.[26] Transrectal ultrasound is used to monitor balloon dilation of the prostate. Because this procedure is still relatively new, studies are needed to evaluate long-term results.

Laser treatment can also be used to eliminate prostate tissue. This procedure is called a transurethral ultrasound-guided laser-induced prostatectomy (TULIP). An instrument with an inflatable beam is inserted into the urethra. The beam destroys the prostate gland while sparing the surrounding tissue. Laser surgery involves a one-night hospital stay and a less traumatic recovery with fewer side effects than traditional surgery.[28]

For men who have heart or lung disease or a condition that precludes major surgery, a stent may be used to widen and keep open the urethra. A stent is a device made up of tubular mesh. The insertion of a stent is done under local or regional anesthesia. Afterward, the lining of the urethra grows into the tube, allowing free passage of urine.[28]

Pharmacologic methods may also be used as a therapeutic option to relieve urinary obstruction. The presence of α-adrenergic receptors in prostatic smooth muscle has stimulated the use of α-adrenergic blocking drugs to relieve prostatic obstruction and increase urine flow. Three selective α-blockers have been used for this purpose: prozosin, doxazosin, and terazosin. Orthostatic hypotension can be a side effect of the α-adrenergic blocking drugs. Doxazosin and terazosin are thought to cause less orthostatic hypotension and can be given in a single daily dose. Also under investigation are drugs that block the action of androgen stimulation of the prostate gland. Of the commercially available drugs, two offer hope of success with minimal side effects. Flutamide, which is an antiandrogen, blocks androgens at the prostate cellular level. Finasteride exerts its effect by blocking the conversion of testosterone to dihydrotestosterone.

PROSTATIC CANCER

Prostatic cancer is the most common male cancer in the United States and is second to lung cancer as a cause of cancer-related deaths in men. It has been estimated that 1 out of every 11 men will develop prostate cancer at some point in his lifetime.[29] The incidence increases with age; over 80% of all prostate cancers are diagnosed in men over the age of 65. The 5-year survival rate for all stages of prostatic cancer combined have steadily improved, increasing from 50% to 74% over the past 30 years.

The incidence of prostate cancer varies markedly from country to country and varies among races in the same country. African-American males have the highest reported incidence and mortality rates, being 50% higher than white males.[30] Japanese-American men have the lowest. It has been noted that immigrants to the United States from low-risk countries such as Japan have incidence figures that are somewhere between that of their original country and that of the United States, suggesting that environmental factors may play a role in the disease.

The precise etiology of prostatic cancer is unknown, although there appears to be some hormonal relationship. Genetic and environmental factors may also be involved. In terms of hormonal influence, higher serum levels of testosterone have been proposed as a major risk determinant of prostatic cancer. Evidence favoring a hormonal influence include the presence of steroid receptors in the prostate, the requirement of sex hormones for normal growth and development of the prostate, and the fact that prostate cancer almost never develops in men who have been castrated. The response of prostatic cancer to estrogen administration or androgen deprivation further supports a relationship between the disease and testosterone levels. There is evidence that genetic factors are also important in the etiology of the disease. Familial clustering of the disease has been observed, but no genetic markers have been described. It has been estimated that men who have both an affected first-degree relative (father, brother) and an affected second-degree relative (grandfather, uncle) have an eightfold increase in risk.[31] Furthermore, the mortality of prostate cancer has been reported to be up to three times greater in relatives of men with prostate cancer as compared with men without a family history of the disease. Certain industries have an excess mortality due to prostatic cancer, suggesting an environmental influence. A higher incidence of prostate cancer has been observed among men who have had prolonged occupational exposure to cadmium through welding, alkaline battery production, or electroplating. Other work-related exposures include farmers, typesetters, shipfitters, and those involved in horticulture.

The majority of prostate cancers are asymptomatic and are incidentally discovered on rectal examination. The American Cancer Society recommends that every man 40 years of age and older should have a rectal examination as part of his annual physical examination.[29] It has been suggested that 12,000 prostatic cancers are detected at a curable stage every year by this method.[32] A new approach, transrectal ultrasonography, may detect cancers that are too small to be detected by physical examination. This method may be of benefit to men who are at high risk.[29]

Depending on the size and location of prostatic cancer at the time of diagnosis, there may be changes associated with the voiding pattern similar to those found in benign prostatic hyperplasia. These include urgency, frequency, nocturia, hesitancy, dysuria, hematuria, or blood in the ejaculate.[31] On physical examination, the prostate is nodular and fixed. Bone metastasis, when present, is often characterized by low-back pain. Pathologic fractures can occur at the site of metastasis. In addition, men with metastatic disease may have experienced weight loss, anemia, or shortness of breath.

Diagnosis of prostate cancer is confirmed through biopsy methods. Two new biopsy techniques, fine needle aspiration and automated core biopsy, are available for this purpose. Both of these methods can be done without anesthesia, cause little discomfort, and can be done on an outpatient basis. The fine needle aspiration technique is done either transrectally or transperitoneally and uses a flexible aspiration needle guide, and aspiration syringe. The aspirated material is placed on slides, dried, and stained for microscopic study. The automated core biopsy method is done transrectally; it uses a spring-powered device that on activation allows an inner trocar needle to cut through the tissue in a fraction of a second. This method has the advantage of obtaining tissue samples for histologic examination.

Transrectal ultrasonography, a continuously improving method of imaging, has become a proven method for detecting prostatic cancers as small as 5 mm in diameter. It is credited with detecting lesions that are out of the range of the examining finger in digital examinations. It is also used to guide a biopsy needle and document the exact location of the biopsied tissue. Newly developed small probes for transrectal MRI have been shown to be sensitive indicators of the presence of cancer within the prostate. This method may prevent unnecessary biopsies and can be expected to be used increasingly in the early diagnosis of prostatic cancer. Radiologic examination of the bones of the skull, ribs, spine, and pelvis can be used to reveal metastases, although radionuclide bone scans are more sensitive. Excretory urograms are used to delineate changes due to urinary tract obstruction and renal involvement. Lymphangiography is often done to determine pelvic node metastases.

Cancer of the prostate, like other forms of cancer, is both graded and staged (see Chapter 5). Well-differentiated tumors are assigned a grade of 1, and poorly differentiated tumors are assigned a grade of 5. Stage A cancers are asymptomatic and discovered on histologic examination of prostatectomy specimens.[34] The incidence of stage A tumors increases with age and approaches 60% in men over age 80. Stage B cancers are palpable on digital examination but are confined to the prostate gland. Stage C tumors have extended beyond the prostate but have not produced clinically evident metastases. Stage D cancers are those with distant metastasis.

Two tumor markers, prostate-specific antigen (PSA) and serum prostatic acid phosphatase, are important in the staging and management of prostatic cancer. Both markers are produced in normal prostatic tissue as well as malignant prostatic tissue. PSA is a glycoprotein secreted into the cytoplasm of both benign and malignant prostatic cells and is found in no other normal tissues or tumors. Gram for gram, the average prostatic cancer produces about 10 times the amount of PSA produced by normal prostatic tissue.[33] Detectable levels of PSA after prostatectomy suggest persistent local or metastatic disease. Because PSA is also elevated in benign prostatic hyperplasia and is often elevated after prostate manipulations, it is usually considered suitable for pretreatment screening. Elevated levels of serum prostatic acid phosphatase are associated with poor prognosis in both local and disseminated disease.

Cancer of the prostate is treated by surgery, radiotherapy, and hormonal manipulations. Men with stage A_1 are usually treated with watchful waiting unless they are relatively young. Radical prostatectomy and radiation therapy are used as curative methods of treatment in early disease that is limited to the prostate (stages A_2 and B). The use of nerve-sparing methods of radical prostatectomy has improved the outcomes of surgical intervention. Radiation therapy is being used increasingly in the treatment of stage C disease. Systemic chemotherapy has not proven beneficial in this disease.

Metastatic disease (stage D) is usually treated with antiandrogen therapy. Orchiectomy or estrogen therapy is often effective in reducing symptoms and extending survival. Blocking testosterone production with leutinizing hormone-releasing hormone (LH-RH) analogue (leuprolide) that inhibits LH release from the pituitary has proved effective and avoids the side effects of estrogen therapy, including gynecomastia, voice changes, cardiovascular complications, and nausea and vomiting. However, they are expensive and are often associated with a flare phenomenon characterized by an increase in bone pain and outlet obstruction.[35] Flutamide is a nonsteroidal antiandrogen approved in the United States for use with a LH-RH analogue; it blocks the uptake and actions binding of androgens in the target tissues. Combined use of an LH-RH analogue and flutamide has provided better results, particularly in men with minimal disease.[35]

In summary, the prostate is a firm glandular structure that surrounds the urethra. Inflammation of the prostate occurs as either an acute or a chronic process. Chronic prostatitis is probably the most common cause of relapsing urinary tract infections in the male. Benign prostatic hyperplasia is a common disorder in men over 50 years of age. Because the prostate encircles the urethra, benign prostatic hyperplasia exerts its effect through obstruction of urinary outflow from the bladder. Advances in the treatment of benign prostatic hyperplasia include laser surgery, balloon dilation, prostatic stents, and pharmacologic treatment using α-adrenergic receptor blockers and agents that block the effects of androgens on the prostate. Prostatic cancer is one of the most common cancers in men; it is second to lung cancer as a cause of cancer-related deaths in men. The incidence increases with age; over 80% of all prostate cancers are diagnosed in men over the age of 65. The majority of prostate cancers are asymptomatic and are incidentally discovered on rectal examination. The American Cancer Society suggests that every man 40 years of age and older should have a rectal examination as part of his annual physical examination. Transrectal ultrasonography and prostate specific antigen (PSA) have become recognized methods in the diagnosis, staging, and management of prostatic cancer. The treatment of prostatic cancer includes surgery, radiotherapy, and hormonal manipulation. With diagnosis and treatment, there is a 74% combined 5-year survival rate for all stages of prostatic cancer.

■ REFERENCES

1. Behrman, R., Kleigman, R.M., & Nelson, W. (1992). *Nelson's textbook of pediatrics* (14th ed., p. 1377). Philadelphia: W.B. Saunders.
2. Spiro, S.A., & Seitzinger, J.W. (1992). Hypospadias with dorsal chordee. *Urology, 39*(4), 389–392.
3. Duckett, J.W., & Snow, B.W. (1986). Disorders of the urethra and penis. In P.C. Walsh, R.F. Gittes, & A.D. Permutter (Eds.). *Campbell's urology* (5th ed., pp. 200–239). Philadelphia: W.B. Saunders.
4. Bakht, F.R. (1989). Genitourinary emergencies in the male patient. *Primary Care, 16*(4), 905–923.
5. McAninch, J.W. (1992). Disorders of the penis and male urethra. In E.A. Tanagho & J.W. McAninch (Eds.). *Smith's general urology* (13th ed., pp. 594–607). Norwalk, CT: Appleton & Lange.
6. Ralph, D.J., Hughes, T., Lees, W.R., et al. (1992). Preoperative assessment of Peyronie's disease using colour Doppler sonography. *British Journal of Urology, 69*, 629–631.
7. Vohra, S., & Badlani, G. (1992). Balanitis and balanoposthitis. *Urological Clinics of North America, 19*, 143–147.
8. Burgers, J.K., Badalament, R.A., & Drago, J.R. (1992). Penile cancer, clinical presentation, diagnosis and staging. *Urologic Clinics of North America, 79*(2), 247–255.
9. Grossman, H.B. (1992). Premalignant and early carcinomas of the penis and scrotum. *Urologic Clinics of North America, 19*(2), 221–225.
10. Presti, J.C., & Herr, H.W. (1992). Genital tumors. In E.A. Tanagho & J.W. McAninch (Eds.), *Smith's general urology* (13th ed., pp. 413–425). Norwalk, CT: Appleton & Lange.
11. Kumar, V., Cotran, R.S., & Robbins, S.L. (1992). *Basic pathology* (5th ed., p. 591). Philadelphia: W.B. Saunders.
12. Gillenwater, J.Y., Grayhoch, J.T., Howards, S.S., et al. (1991). *Adult and pediatric urology* (2nd ed.). St. Louis: C.V. Mosby.
13. Raufer, J., Handelsman, D.J., & Swerdloff, R.S., et al. (1986). Hormonal therapy of cryptorchidism. *New England Journal of Medicine, 314*, 466–470.
14. Derkson, D.J., & Smith, A.Y. (1989). Genitourinary problems in the male patient. *Primary Care, 16*(4), 981–995.
15. Thomas, A.J., & Geisinger, M.A. (1990). Current management of varicoceles. *Urologic Clinics of North America, 17*(4), 893–895.
16. Kim, Y.C., & Choi, H.K. (1992). Clinical value of scrotopenogram for evaluating varicocele and erectile dysfunction. *Urology, 29*(2), 150–156.
17. Fontanarosa, P.M., & Hellman, M.G. (1991). The acute scrotum. *Topics in Emergency Medicine, 3*(1), 84–92.
18. Tonetti, J.A., & Tonetti, F.W. (1990). Testicular torsion or acute epididymitis: Diagnosis and treatment. *Journal of Emergency Nursing, 16*(2), 96–98.
19. Meares, E.M. (1992). Nonspecific infections of the genitourinary tract. In E.A. Tanagho & J.W. McAninch (Eds.), *Smith's general urology* (13th ed., pp. 231–232). Norwalk, CT: Appleton & Lange.
20. Mebcow, M.M. (1975). Percivall Pott (1713–1788): 200th anniversary of first report of occupation-induced cancer of the scrotum in chimney sweepers (1745). *Urology, 6*, 745.
21. Lowe, F.C. (1992). Squamous cell carcinoma of the scrotum. *Urologic Clinics of North America, 19*(2), 297–405.
22. Lasater, S.J. (1990). Testicular cancer: A perioperative challenge. *AORN Journal, 51*(2), 513–523.
23. Smith, R.H., Wake, R., & Soloway, M.S. (1988). Benign prostatic hyperplasia: A universal problem among aging men. *Postgraduate Medicine, 83*(6), 79.
24. Narayan, P. (1992). Neoplasms of the prostate gland. In E.A. Tanagho & J.W. McAninch (Eds.). *Smith's general urology* (13th ed., pp. 378–412). Norwalk, CT: Appleton & Lange.
25. Christensen, M.M., & Bruskewitz, R.C. (1990). Clinical manifestations of benign prostatic hyperplasia and indications for therapeutic interventions. *Urologic Clinics of North America, 17*, 509–515.
26. Willis, D. (1992). Taming the overgrown prostate. *American Journal of Nursing, 92*(2), 35–39.
27. Tafelski, T.J., & Navarre, R. (1989). Benign diseases of the prostate. *Primary Care, 16*(4), 997–1011.
28. Tafelski, T.J., & Navarre, R. (1992). Prostate gland enlargement. *Mayo Clinic Health Letter, 10*(7), 4–5.
29. American Cancer Society. (1992). *Cancer Facts and Figures—1992.* Atlanta: American Cancer Society.
30. Wilson, P. (1991). Testicular, prostate and penile cancers in primary care settings: The importance of early detection. *The Nurse Practitioner, 16*(11), 18–27.
31. Steinber, G.D., Carter, B.S., Beaty, T.L., et al. (1990). The familial aggregation of prostate cancer: A case control study [abstract]. *Journal of Urology, 143*, 131A.
32. Chodek, G.W., Keller, P., & Schoenberg, H.W. (1989). Assessment screening for prostate cancer using digital examination. *Journal of Urology, 141*, 1136–1137.
33. Gittes, R.F. (1991). Carcinoma of the prostate. *New England Journal of Medicine, 324*, 236–245.

34. Catalona, W.J. (1987). Diagnosis, staging, and surgical treatment of prostatic cancer. *Archives of Internal Medicine, 147,* 361.
35. Frank, I.N., Graham, S.D., & Nabors, W.L. (1991). Urologic and male genital cancers. In A.I. Hollieb, D.J. Fink, G.P. Murphy (Eds.). *Clinical oncology* (pp. 280–283). Atlanta: American Cancer Society.

■ BIBLIOGRAPHY

Barry, M.J. (1990). Epidemiology and natural history of benign prostatic hyperplasia. *Urologic Clinics of North America, 17*(3): 495–505.

Bostwick, D.G. (1989). The pathology of early prostate cancer. *CA: A Cancer Journal for Clinicians, 39*(6): 376–392.

Boyer, M.Y., & Raghoven, D. (1992). Toxicity of treatment of germ cell tumors. *Seminars in Oncology, 19*(2), 128–142.

Brower, M.K., & Lange, P.H. (1989). Prostate-specific antigen and premalignant change: Implications for early detection. *CA: A Cancer Journal for Clinicians, 39*(6): 361–375.

Catalona, W.J., Smith, D.S., Ratliff, T.L., et al. (1991). Measurement of prostatic specific antigen in serum as a screening test for prostate cancer. *New England Journal of Medicine, 324,* 1156–1161.

Collens, P.M. (1990). Tumor markers and screening tools in cancer detection. *Nursing Clinics of North America, 25,* 283–289.

Drago, J.R. (1989). The role of new modalities in the early detection and diagnosis of prostate cancer. *CA: A Cancer Journal for Clinicians, 39*(6), 326–334.

Droz, J-P., Kramer, A., & Rey, A. (1992). Prognostic factors in metastatic disease. *Seminars in Oncology, 19*(2), 181–187.

Foster, R.S., & Donahue, J.P. (1992). Surgical treatment of clinical stage A nonseminomatous testis cancer. *Seminars in Oncology, 19*(2), 166–170.

Garrow, G.C., & Johnson, D.H. (1992). Treatment of "good risk" metastatic testicular cancer. *Seminars in Oncology, 19*(2), 159–165.

Higgs, D. (1990). The patient with testicular cancer: Nursing management of chemotherapy. *Oncology Nursing Forum, 17*(2), 243–249.

Horwich, A., & Dearnaley, D.P. (1992). Treatment of seminoma. *Seminars in Oncology, 19*(2), 171–179.

Kabalin, J.N. (1992). Prostate specific antigen: Clinical use in the diagnosis and management of prostatic cancer. *Geriatrics, 47*(9), 26–32.

Lee, F., Torp-Pederson, S.T., & Siders, D.B. (1989). The role of transurethral ultrasound in the early detection of prostate cancer. *CA: A Cancer Journal for Clinicians, 39*(6), 337–358.

Martin, J.P. (1990). Male cancer awareness: Impact of an employee education program. *Oncology Nursing Forum, 17*(1), 59–64.

Meares, E.M. (1991). Prostatitis. *Medical Clinics of North America, 75,* 405–424.

Mizrahi, S., & Shtamler, B. (1992). Surgical approach and outcome in torsion of testes. *Urology, 39*(1), 52–54.

Paola, A.S., & Khan, S.A. (1989). Clinical evaluation of scrotal masses: An overview. *Hospital Practice, 24*(3A), 255–264.

Reid, D.L., & Goldman, G.E. (1991). Genitourinary infections. *Topics in Emergency Medicine, 13*(1), 55–65.

Rotolo, J.E., & Lynch, J.H. (1991). Penile cancer: Curable with early detection. *Hospital Practice, 26*(6A), 131–138.

Stone, N.N. (1992). Treatment options in benign prostatic hypertrophy. *Hospital Practice, 27*(10A), 85–92.

Vogelzang, N.J., & Kennealy, G.T. (1992). Recent development in endocrine treatment of prostate cancer. *Cancer, 70,* 966–976.

Walther, T.R., & Weigard, J.V. (1991). The acute scrotum. *Topics in Emergency Medicine, 13*(1), 15–24.

Wein, A.J. (1990). Evaluation of treatment response to drugs in benign prostatic hyperplasia. *Urologic Clinics of North America, 17,* 631–640.

STRUCTURE AND FUNCTION OF THE FEMALE REPRODUCTIVE SYSTEM

PATRICIA McCOWEN MEHRING

Reproductive Structures
External Genitalia
Internal Genitalia
Menstrual Cycle
Hormonal Control

Ovarian Follicle Development
  and Ovulation
Endometrial Changes
Cervical Mucus
Menopause

Breasts
Structure
Pregnancy
Lactation
Changes with Menopause

■ OBJECTIVES

After you have studied this chapter, you should be able to meet the following objectives:

■ Describe the anatomic relation of the structures of the external genitalia.

■ Cite the location of the ovaries in relation to the uterus, fallopian tubes, broad ligaments, and ovarian ligaments.

■ Explain the function of the fallopian tubes.

■ State the function of endocervical secretions.

■ Describe the feedback control of estrogen and progesterone levels by means of gonadotropin-releasing hormone, luteinizing hormone (LH), follicle-stimulating hormone (FSH), and ovarian follicle function.

■ List the actions of estrogen and progesterone.

■ Describe the four functional compartments of the ovary.

■ Relate FSH and LH levels to the stages of follicle development and to estrogen and progesterone production.

■ Describe the endometrial changes that occur during the menstrual cycle.

■ Describe the composition of normal cervical mucus and the changes that occur during the menstrual cycle.

■ Describe the physiology of normal menopause.

■ Describe the anatomy of the female breast.

■ Describe the influence of hormones on breast development.

The female genitourinary system consists of internal paired ovaries, uterine tubes, uterus, vagina, external mons pubis, labia majora, labia minora, clitoris, urethra, and perineal body. Although the female urinary structures are anatomically separate from the genital structures, their anatomic proximity provides a means for cross-contamination and shared symptomatology between the two systems (Fig. 37-1). This chapter focuses on the internal and external genitalia. It includes a discussion of hormonal and physical changes that occur throughout the life cycle in response to the gonadotropic hor-

Carol Mattson Porth: PATHOPHYSIOLOGY: CONCEPTS OF ALTERED HEALTH STATES, 4th ed. © 1994, 1990, 1986, 1982 J.B. Lippincott Company

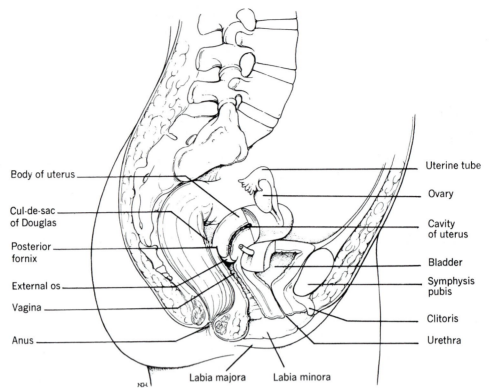

FIG. 37-1. Female reproductive system as seen in sagittal section. (Chaffee, E. E., & Greisheimer, E. M. [1974]. *Basic physiology and anatomy* [3rd ed.]. Philadelphia: J.B. Lippincott)

mones. The reader is referred to a specialty text for a discussion of pregnancy.

■ REPRODUCTIVE STRUCTURES

EXTERNAL GENITALIA

The external genitalia are located at the base of the pelvis in the perineal area and include the mons pubis, labia majora, labia minora, clitoris, and perineal body. The urethra and anus, although not genital structures, usually are considered in a discussion of the external genitalia. The external genitalia, also known collectively as the vulva, are diagrammed in Figure 37-2.

The *mons pubis* is a rounded, skin-covered fat pad located anterior to the symphysis pubis. Puberty stimulates an increase in the amount of fat and the development of darker and coarser hair over the mons. Normal pubic hair distribution in the female follows an inverted triangle with the base centered over the mons. Hair color and texture varies from person to person and among racial groups. There is an abundance of sebaceous glands in the skin that can become infected owing to normal variations in glandular secretions or poor hygiene. The mons

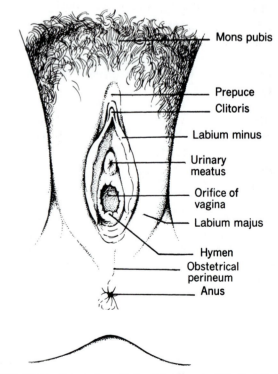

FIG. 37-2. External genitalia of the female. (Chaffee, E. E., & Lytle, I. M. [1980]. *Basic physiology and anatomy* [4th ed.]. Philadelphia: J.B. Lippincott)

pubis is the most common site of pubic lice infestation in the female.

The *labia majora* (singular, labium majus) are analogous to the male scrotum. These structures are the outermost lips of the vulva, beginning anteriorly at the base of the mons pubis and ending posteriorly at the anus. The labia majora are composed of folds of skin and fat and become covered with hair at the onset of puberty. Before puberty, the labia majora have a skin covering similar to that covering the abdomen. With sufficient hormonal stimulation, the labia of a mature woman close over the urethral and vaginal openings; this can change after childbirth or surgery.

The *labia minora* (singular, labium minus) are located between the labia majora. These delicate cutaneous structures are smaller than the labia majora and are made up of skin, fat, and some erectile tissue. Unlike the skin of the labia majora, that of the labia minora is hairless and usually light pink. The labia minora begin anteriorly at the hood of the clitoris and end posteriorly at the base of the vagina. The area between them is called the vestibule. Within the vestibule are located the urethral and vaginal openings as well as the *Bartholin's lubricating glands.* During sexual arousal, the labia minora become distended with blood; with resolution, the labia throb and then return to normal size. The sebaceous glands secrete odoriferous fluid in both the presence and the absence of sexual arousal.

The *clitoris* is located below the clitoral hood, or prepuce, which is formed by the joining of the two labia minora. The female clitoris is an erectile organ, rich in blood and nerve supply. Analogous to the male penis, it is a highly sensitive organ that becomes distended during sexual stimulation.

The *urethra*, or urinary meatus, is the external opening of the internal urinary bladder. The urethra is posterior to the clitoris and usually is closer to the vaginal opening than to the clitoris. The urethra, vaginal opening, and Bartholin's glands lie within the vestibule. The urethral opening is the site of the Skene's glands, which have a lubricating function.

The vaginal orifice, commonly known as the *introitus*, is the opening between the external and internal genitalia. The size and shape of the opening are determined by a connective tissue membrane called the hymen that surrounds the introitus. The opening may be oval, circular, or sieve-like and may be partially or completely occluded. Occlusion may occur because of the presence of an intact or partially intact hymen. Contrary to popular notion, an intact hymen does not indicate virginity because this tissue can be stretched without tearing. At puberty, an intact hymen may require surgical intervention to permit discharge of menstrual fluids.

The *perineal body* is that tissue located posterior to the vaginal opening and anterior to the anus. It is composed of fibrous connective tissue and is the site of insertion of several perineal muscles.

INTERNAL GENITALIA

VAGINA

Connecting the internal and external genitalia is a fibromuscular tube called the *vagina*. The vagina, which is essentially free of nerve-sensation fibers, is located behind the urinary bladder and urethra and anterior to the rectum. The uterine cervix projects into the vagina at its upper end, forming recesses called *fornices*. The vagina functions as a route for discharge of menses and other secretions. It also serves as an organ of sexual fulfillment and reproduction.

The membranous vaginal wall forms two longitudinal folds and several transverse folds, or rugae. The vagina is lined with mucus-secreting stratified squamous epithelial cells. Vaginal tissue usually is moist, with a *p*H maintained within the bacteriostatic range of 3.8 to 4.2. The epithelial cells of the vagina, like other tissues of the reproductive system, respond to changing levels of the ovarian sex hormones. Estrogen stimulates the proliferation and maturation of the vaginal mucosa; this results in a thickening of the vaginal mucosa and an increased glycogen content of the epithelial cells. The glycogen is fermented to lactic acid by the lactobacilli (Döderlein's bacilli) that are part of the normal vaginal flora, accounting for the mildly acid *p*H of vaginal fluid. The vaginal ecology can be disrupted at many levels, rendering it susceptible to infection. Pregnancy and the use of oral contraceptive agents increase the amount of estrogen within the system. Diabetes or a prediabetic state may increase the glycogen content of the cells. The use of systemic antibiotics may decrease the number of lactobacilli within the vagina. Decreased estrogen stimulation after menopause causes the vaginal mucosa to become thin and dry, often resulting in dyspareunia (painful intercourse), atrophic vaginitis, and, occasionally, vaginal bleeding. During a routine pelvic examination, the estrogen level can be estimated by examining the cellular structure and configuration of the vaginal epithelial cells. This test is known as the *maturation index.*

UTERUS AND CERVIX

The uterus is a thick-walled muscular organ. This pear-shaped hollow structure is located between the bladder and the rectum. The uterus can be divided into three parts: the portion above the insertion of the fallopian tubes, called the *fundus*; the lower constricted part, called the *cervix;* and the portion between the fundus and the cervix, called the *body* of the uterus (Fig. 37-3). The uterus is supported on both sides by four sets of ligaments: the broad ligaments, which run laterally from the body of the uterus to the pelvic side walls; the round ligaments, which run from the fundus laterally into each labium majus; the uterosacral ligaments, which run from the uterocervical junction to the sacrum; and the cardinal or transverse cervical ligaments.

The wall of the uterus is composed of three layers: the perimetrium, the myometrium, and the endometrium. The *perimetrium* is the outer serous covering that is derived from the abdominal peritoneum. This outer layer merges with the peritoneum that covers the broad ligaments. Anteriorly, the perimetrium is reflected over the bladder wall, forming the vesicouterine pouch; posteriorly, it extends to form the *cul-de-sac,* or *pouch of Douglas.* Because of the proximity of the perimetrium to the urinary bladder, infection of this organ often causes uterine symptoms, particularly during pregnancy.

The middle muscle layer, the *myometrium,* forms the major portion of the uterine wall. It is continuous with the myometrium of the fallopian tubes and the vagina and extends into all the supporting ligaments with the exception of the broad ligaments. The inner fibers of the myometrium run in various directions, giving it an interwoven appearance. Contractions of these muscle fibers help to expel menstrual flow and the products of conception during miscarriage or childbirth. When pain accompanies the contractions associated with menses, it is called *dysmenorrhea.* The myometrium has an amazing ability to change length during pregnancy and labor, increasing the uterine capacity more than 4000 times.[1]

The *endometrium,* the inner layer of the uterus, is continuous with the lining of the fallopian tubes and vagina. The endometrium is made up of a basal and a superficial layer. The superficial layer is shed during menstruation and regenerated by cells of the basal layer. Ciliated cells promote the movement of tubal–uterine secretions out of the uterine cavity into the vagina.

The round cervix is the neck of the uterus that projects into the vagina. The cervix is a firm structure, composed of a connective tissue matrix of glands and muscular tissue elements, that becomes soft and pliable under the influence of hormones produced during pregnancy. Glandular tissue provides a rich supply of protective mucus that changes in character and quantity during the menstrual cycle as well as during pregnancy. The cervix is richly supplied with blood from the uterine artery and can be a site of significant blood loss during delivery.

The opening of the cervix, the *os,* forms a pathway between the uterus and the vagina. The vaginal opening is called the external os and the uterine opening, the internal os. The space between these two openings is the endocervical canal. Secretions from the columnar epithelium of the endocervix protect the uterus from infection, alter receptivity to

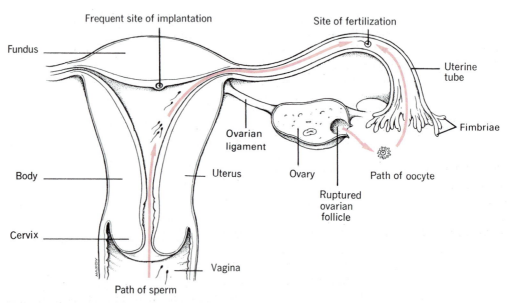

FIG. 37-3. Schematic drawing of female reproductive organs, showing the path of the oocyte as it moves from the ovary into the fallopian (uterine) tube; the path of sperm is also shown, as is the usual site of fertilization. (Chaffee, E. E., & Lytle, I. M. [1980]. *Basic physiology and anatomy* [4th ed.]. Philadelphia: J.B. Lippincott)

sperm, and form a mucoid "plug" during pregnancy. The endocervical canal provides a route for menstrual discharge and sperm entrance.

FALLOPIAN TUBES

The fallopian, or uterine, tubes are slender, cylindrical structures attached bilaterally to the uterus and supported by the upper folds of the broad ligament. The end of the fallopian tube nearest the ovary forms a funnel-like opening with fringed finger-like projections, called *fimbriae*, that pick up the ovum after its release into the peritoneal cavity after ovulation (see Fig. 37-3). The fallopian tubes are formed of smooth muscle and lined with a ciliated, mucus-producing epithelial layer. The beating of the cilia, along with contractile movements of the smooth muscle, propels the nonmobile ova toward the uterus. If coitus has been recent, fertilization normally occurs in the middle to outer portion of the fallopian tube. Besides providing a passageway for ova and sperm, the fallopian tubes provide for drainage of tubal secretions into the uterus.

OVARIES

By the 3rd month of fetal life, the ovaries of the female have fully developed and descended to their permanent pelvic position. Remnants of the primitive genital system provide lateral supporting attachments to the uterus; in the mature female, these supporting structures evolve into the round and suspensory ligaments. Remnants that do not evolve may also form cysts, which may become symptomatic later in life.

Oogenesis is the process of generation of ova by mitotic division that begins at the 6th week of fetal life. These primitive germ cells ultimately provide the 1 to 2 million or so oocytes that are present in the ovaries at birth. At puberty, this number is reduced through cell death to about 300,000.[2]

The neonate's ovaries are smooth, pale, and elongated. They become shorter, thicker, and heavier before the onset of menarche, which is initiated by pituitary influence. The initial hormonal stimulus for this development is believed to come from ovarian rather than systemic estrogen.

In the adult, the ovaries are flat, almond-shaped structures that measure 3 to 5 cm in length and weigh 2 to 3 g. They are located on either side of the uterus below the fimbriated ends of the two oviducts, or fallopian tubes. The ovaries are attached to the posterior surface of the broad ligament and to the uterus by the ovarian ligament. They are covered with a thin layer of surface epithelium that is continuous with

the lining of the peritoneum. The integrity of this covering is periodically broken at the time of ovulation.

The ovaries, like the male testes, have a dual function: they store the female germ cells, or ova, and produce the female sex hormones estrogen and progesterone. Unlike the male gonads, which produce sperm throughout a man's reproductive life, the female gonads contain a fixed number of ova at birth that diminishes throughout a woman's life.

Structurally, the mature ovary is divided into a highly vascular inner medulla, which contains supporting connective tissue, and an outer cortex of stroma and epithelial follicles (vesicles), which contain the primary oocytes, or germ cells. After puberty, the pituitary gonadotropic hormones—follicle stimulating hormone (FSH) and luteinizing hormone (LH)—stimulate primordial follicles to develop into mature graafian follicles. The graafian follicle produces estrogen, which begins to stimulate the development of the endometrium in the uterus. Although several follicles begin to develop during each ovulatory cycle, only one or two complete the entire developmental process and rupture to release a mature ovum. After ovulation, the follicle becomes luteinized; as the corpus luteum, it produces both estrogen and progesterone to support the endometrium until conception occurs or the cycle begins again.

In summary, the female genitourinary system consists of the external and internal genitalia. The genitourinary system as a whole serves both sexual and reproductive functions throughout the life cycle. The gonads, or ovaries, which are internal in the female (unlike the testes in the male) have the dual function of storing the female germ cells, or ova, and producing the female sex hormones. Through the regulation and release of sex hormones, the ovaries influence the development of secondary sexual characteristics, regulation of menstrual cycles, maintenance of pregnancy, and advent of menopause.

▪ MENSTRUAL CYCLE

Between menarche (first menstrual bleeding) and menopause (last menstrual bleeding), the female reproductive system undergoes cyclic changes termed the menstrual cycle. This includes the maturation and release of oocytes from the ovary during ovulation and periodic vaginal bleeding resulting from the shedding of the endometrial lining. It is not necessary for a woman to ovulate in order to menstruate; anovulatory cycles do occur. The menstrual cycle produces changes in the breasts, uterus, skin, ovaries, and perhaps other, unidentified tissues. The maintenance of the cycle affects biologic and social aspects of a woman's life, including fertility, reproduction, sexuality, and femaleness.

HORMONAL CONTROL

Normal menstrual function results from interactions among the central nervous system, hypothalamus, anterior pituitary, ovaries, and associated target tissues. Although each part of the system is essential to normal function, the ovaries are primarily responsible for controlling the cyclic changes and the length of the menstrual cycle. In most women in the middle reproductive years, menstrual bleeding occurs every 25 to 35 days, with a median length of 28 days.[3]

The hormonal control of the menstrual cycle is complex. For example, the biosynthesis of estrogens that occurs in adipose tissue may be a significant source of the hormone. There is evidence that a certain minimum body weight (48 kg) and fat content (17%) are necessary for menarche to occur and for the menstrual cycle to be maintained.[2] Although menarche is variable, this is supported by the observation of amenorrhea in women with anorexia nervosa, chronic disease, and malnutrition and in those who are long-distance runners. In women with anorexia nervosa, gonadotropin and estriol secretion, including LH release and responsiveness to gonadotropin-releasing hormone (GnRH), can revert to prepubertal levels.[4] With resumption of weight gain and attainment of sufficient body mass, the normal hormonal pattern usually is reinstated. Obesity or significant weight gain is also associated with oligomenorrhea or amenorrhea and infertility, although the mechanism is not well understood.

HYPOTHALAMIC AND PITUITARY HORMONES

Growth, prepubertal maturation, reproductive cycle, and sex hormone secretion in both males and females are regulated by FSH and LH from the anterior pituitary gland (Fig. 37-4). Because these hormones promote the growth of cells in the ovaries and testes as a means of stimulating the production of sex hormones, they are called the gonadotropic hormones. The secretion of both LH and FSH is stimulated by GnRH from the hypothalamus.

In addition to LH and FSH, the anterior pituitary secretes a third hormone—prolactin. Its primary function is the stimulation of lactation in the postpartum period. During pregnancy, prolactin, along with other hormones (estrogen, progesterone, insulin, and cortisol), contributes to breast development in preparation for lactation. Although prolactin does not appear to play a physiologic role in ovarian function, hyperprolactinemia leads to hypogonadism. This may include an initial shortening of the luteal phase with subsequent anovulation, oligomenorrhea or amenorrhea, and infertility. Prolactin production

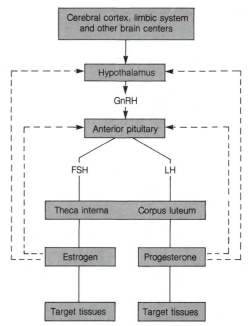

FIG. 37-4. Hypothalamic-pituitary feedback control of estrogen and progesterone levels in the female.

by the pituitary normally is inhibited by a hypothalamic inhibiting factor. Hyperprolactinemia may occur as an adverse effect of drug treatment using phenothiazine derivatives (antipsychotic drugs). These drugs are thought to act at the level of the hypothalamus to increase prolactin release by the pituitary.

OVARIAN HORMONES

The ovaries produce estrogens, progesterone, and androgens. Ovarian hormones are secreted in a cyclic pattern as a result of the interaction between the hypothalamic-releasing factors and the pituitary gonadotropic hormones.

The steroid sex hormones enter cells by passive diffusion, bind to specific receptor proteins in the cytoplasm, and then move to the nucleus where they bind to specific sites on the chromosomes. These hormones exert their effects through gene–hormone interactions, which stimulate the synthesis of specific messenger ribonucleic acid (see Chapter 3). The number of hormonal receptor sites on a cell is not fixed; evidence suggests that they are constantly being removed and replaced. An increase or a decrease in the number of receptors can serve as a mechanism for regulating hormonal activity. For example, estrogen may induce the development of an increased number of estrogen receptors in some tissues and may also stimulate the synthesis of progesterone receptors. In contrast, progesterone may cause a reduction in the number of estrogen and progesterone receptors.

Estrogens. Estrogens are a family of structurally related female sex hormones synthesized and secreted by cells in the ovaries and, in small amounts, by cells in the adrenal cortex. In addition, androgens can be converted to estrogens peripherally, especially in fat tissue. Three estrogens occur naturally in humans: estrone (E_1), estradiol (E_2), and estriol (E_3). Of these, estradiol is the most biologically potent and the most abundantly secreted product of the ovary. Estrogens are secreted throughout the menstrual cycle. Two peaks occur: one before ovulation and one in the middle of the luteal phase. Estrogens are transported in the blood bound to specific plasma globulins (which can also bind testosterone), inactivated and conjugated in the liver, and then excreted in the bile.

Estrogens are necessary for the normal physical maturation of the female. In concert with other hormones, estrogens provide for the reproductive processes of ovulation, implantation, pregnancy, parturition, and lactation by stimulating the development and maintaining the growth of the accessory organs. In the absence of androgens, estrogens stimulate the intrauterine development of the vagina, uterus, and uterine tubes from the embryonic müllerian system. They also stimulate the stromal development and ductal growth of the breasts at puberty; are responsible for the accelerated pubertal skeletal growth phase and for closure of the epiphyses of the long bones; contribute to the growth of axillary and pubic hair; and alter the distribution of body fat to produce the typical female body contours, including the accumulation of body fat around the hips and breasts. Larger quantities stimulate pigmentation of the skin in the nipple, areolar, and genital regions.

In addition to their effects on the growth of uterine muscle, estrogens play an important role in the development of the endometrial lining. During anovulatory cycles, continued exposure to estrogens for prolonged periods leads to abnormal hyperplasia of the endometrium and abnormal bleeding patterns. When estrogen production is poorly coordinated during the normal menstrual period, inappropriate bleeding and shedding of the endometrium can also occur.

Estrogens have a number of important extragenital metabolic effects. They are responsible for maintaining the normal structure of skin and blood vessels in women. Estrogens decrease the rate of bone resorption by antagonizing the effects of parathyroid hormone on bone; for this reason, osteoporosis is a common problem in estrogen-deficient postmenopausal women. In the liver, estrogens increase the synthesis of transport proteins for thyrox-ine, estrogen, testosterone, and other hormones. Estrogens affect the composition of the plasma lipoproteins; they produce an increase in high-density lipoproteins, a slight reduction in low-density lipoproteins, and a reduction in cholesterol levels. Plasma triglyceride levels are increased. Estrogens enhance the coagulability of blood by effecting increased circulating levels of plasminogen and factors II, VII, IX, and X.

The estrogens cause moderate retention of sodium and water. Most women retain sodium and water and gain weight just before menstruation. This occurs because the estrogens facilitate the loss of intravascular fluids into the extracellular spaces, producing edema and increased sodium and water retention by the kidneys because of the decreased plasma volume. The actions of estrogens are summarized in Table 37-1.

Progesterone. Although the word *progesterone* refers to a substance that maintains pregnancy, progesterone is secreted as part of the normal menstrual cycle. The corpus luteum of the ovary secretes large amounts of progesterone after ovulation, and the adrenal cortex secretes small amounts. The hormone circulates in the blood attached to a specific plasma protein. It is metabolized in the liver and conjugated for excretion in the bile.

The local effects of progesterone on reproductive organs include the glandular development of the lobular and alveolar tissue of the breasts and the cyclic glandular development of the endometrium. Progesterone can also compete with aldosterone at the level of the renal tubule, causing a decrease in sodium reabsorption with a resultant increase in secretion of aldosterone by the adrenal cortex (such as occurs in pregnancy).[3] Although the mechanism is uncertain, progesterone increases basal body temperature and is, therefore, responsible for the increase in body temperature that occurs with ovulation.

Smooth muscle relaxation under the influence of progesterone plays an important role in maintaining pregnancy by decreasing uterine contractions and is responsible for many of the common discomforts of pregnancy, such as edema, nausea, constipation, flatulence, and headaches. The increased progesterone present during pregnancy and the luteal phase of the menstrual cycle enhances the ventilatory response to carbon dioxide, leading to a measurable change in arterial and alveolar P_{CO_2}.

Androgens. The normal female produces androgens as well as estrogens and progesterone. About 25% of these androgens are secreted from the ovaries, 25% from the adrenal cortex, and 50% from either ovarian or adrenal precursors. In the female,

TABLE 37-1. ACTIONS OF ESTROGENS

GENERAL FUNCTION	SPECIFIC ACTIONS
Growth and Development	
Reproductive organs	Stimulate development of vagina, uterus, and fallopian tubes *in utero* and of secondary sex characteristics during puberty
Skeleton	Accelerate growth of long bones and closure of epiphyses at puberty
Reproductive Processes	
Ovulation	Promote growth of ovarian follicles
Fertilization	Alter the cervical secretions to favor survival and transport of sperm
	Promote motility of sperm within the fallopian tubes by decreasing mucus viscosity
Implantation	Promote development of endometrial lining in the event of pregnancy
Vagina	Proliferate and cornify vaginal mucosa
Cervix	Increase mucus consistency
Breasts	Stimulate stromal development and ductal growth
General Metabolic Effects	
Bone resorption	Decrease rate of bone resorption
Plasma proteins	Increase production of thyroid and other binding globulins
Lipoproteins	Increase high-density lipoproteins

androgens contribute to normal hair growth at puberty and may have other important metabolic effects.

OVARIAN FOLLICLE DEVELOPMENT AND OVULATION

The tissues of the adult ovary can be conveniently divided into four compartments, or units: (1) the stroma, or supporting tissue; (2) the interstitial cells; (3) the follicles; and (4) the corpus luteum. The stroma is the connective tissue substance of the ovary in which the follicles are distributed. The interstitial cells are estrogen-secreting cells that resemble the Leydig's cells, or interstitial cells, of the testes.

Beginning at puberty, a cyclic rise in the anterior pituitary gonadotropic hormones FSH and LH stimulate the development of several graafian, or mature, follicles. Follicles at all stages of development can be found in both ovaries, except in menopausal women (Fig. 37-5).

The vast majority of follicles exist as primary follicles, each of which consists of a round oocyte surrounded by a single layer of flattened epithelial-derived granulosa cells and a basement membrane. The primary follicles constitute an inactive pool of follicles from which all the ovulating follicles develop. Under the influence of endocrine stimulation, 6 to 12 primary follicles develop into secondary follicles once every ovulatory cycle. During the development of the secondary follicle, the primary oocyte increases in size and the granulosa cells proliferate to form a multilayered wall around it. During this time, a membrane called the zona pellucida develops and surrounds the oocyte and small pockets of fluid begin to appear between the granulosa cells. Blood vessels, however, do not penetrate the basement membrane; the granulosa cell layer remains avascular until after ovulation has occurred.[3]

As the follicles mature, FSH stimulates the development of the cell layers. Cells from the surround-

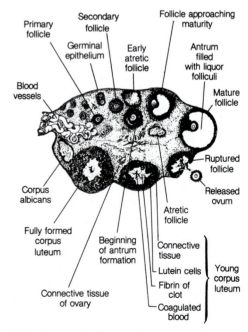

FIG. 37-5. Schematic diagram of an ovary, showing the sequence of events in the origin, growth, and rupture of an ovarian follicle and the formation and retrogression of a corpus luteum. The atretic follicles are those that show signs of degeneration and death. (Patten, B.M. *Human embryology.* New York: Blakiston)

ing stromal tissue align themselves to form a cellular wall called the theca. The cells of the theca become differentiated into two layers: an inner theca interna, which lies adjacent to the follicular cells, and an outer theca externa. As the follicle enlarges, a single large cavity, or antrum, is formed and a portion of the granulosa cells and the oocytes are displaced to one side of the follicle by the fluid that accumulates. The secondary oocyte remains surrounded by a crown of granulosa cells, the corona radiata. As the follicle ripens, ovarian estrogen is produced by the granulosa cells. Selection of a dominant follicle occurs with the conversion to an estrogen microenvironment; the lesser follicles, although continuing to produce some estrogen, atrophy or become atretic. The dominant follicle accumulates a greater mass of granulosa cells and the theca becomes richly vascular, giving the follicle a hyperemic appearance.[2] High levels of estrogen exert a negative feedback on FSH, inhibiting multiple follicular development and causing an increase in LH levels. This represents the follicular stage of the menstrual cycle. As estrogen suppresses FSH, the actions of LH predominate and the mature follicle (measuring about 20 mm) bursts; the oocyte, along with the corona radiata, is ejected from the follicle.[5] The ovum normally is then picked up and transported through the fallopian tube toward the uterus.

After ovulation, the follicle collapses and the luteal stage of the menstrual cycle begins. The granulosa cells are invaded by blood vessels and yellow lipochrome-bearing cells from the theca layer. A rapid accumulation of blood and fluid forms a mass called the *corpus luteum*. Leakage of this blood onto the peritoneal surface that surrounds the ovary is thought to contribute to the *mittelschmerz* (middle, or intermenstrual, pain) of ovulation. During the luteal stage, progesterone is secreted from the corpus luteum. If fertilization does not take place, the corpus luteum atrophies and is replaced by white scar tissue (corpus albicans); the hormonal support of the endometrium is withdrawn and menstruation occurs. In the event of fertilization, human chorionic gonadotropin is produced by the trophoblastic cells within the blastocyst and prevents luteal regression. The corpus luteum remains functional for 3 months and provides hormonal support for pregnancy until the placenta is fully functional. Figure 37-6 shows the hormonal changes that occur during the development of the ovarian follicle and ovulation.

ENDOMETRIAL CHANGES

The endometrium consists of two distinct layers, or zones, that are responsive to hormonal stimulation: a basal layer and a functional layer. The basal layer lies

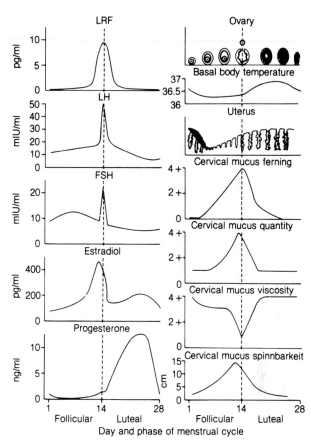

FIG. 37-6. Hormonal and morphologic changes during the normal menstrual cycle. (Hershman, J. M. [1982]. *Endocrine pathophysiology* [2nd ed.]. Philadelphia: Lea & Febiger)

adjacent to the myometrium and is not sloughed during menstruation. The functional layer arises from the basal layer and undergoes proliferative changes and menstrual sloughing. It can be subdivided into two components: a thin, superficial, compact layer and a deeper spongiosa layer that makes up most of the secretory and fully developed endometrium. The endometrial cycle can be divided into three phases: (1) the proliferative, or preovulatory, phase, during which the glands and stroma of the superficial layer grow rapidly under the influence of estrogen; (2) the secretory, or postovulatory, phase, during which progesterone produces glandular dilation and active mucus secretion and the endometrium becomes highly vascular and edematous; and (3) the menstrual phase, during which the superficial layer degenerates and sloughs off.

CERVICAL MUCUS

Cervical mucus is a complex heterogeneous secretion produced by the glands of the endocervix. It is composed of 92% to 98% water and 1% inorganic salts, mainly sodium chloride. The mucus also contains simple sugars, polysaccharides, proteins, and glycoproteins. Its *p*H usually is alkaline, ranging from 6.5 to 9.0.[3] Its characteristics are strongly influenced by serum levels of estrogen and progesterone. Estrogen stimulates the production of large amounts of clear, watery mucus through which sperm can penetrate most easily. Progesterone, even in the presence of estrogen, reduces the secretion of mucus. During the luteal phase of the menstrual cycle, mucus is scant, viscous, and cellular (see Fig. 37-6).

Two methods are used to examine the properties of cervical mucus and correlate them with hormonal activity. *Spinnbarkeit* is the property that allows cervical mucus to be stretched or drawn into a thread. Spinnbarkeit can be estimated by stretching a sample of cervical mucus between two glass slides and measuring the maximum length of the thread before it breaks. At midcycle, spinnbarkeit usually exceeds 10 cm.[3] A second method of estimating hormonal levels is ferning, or arborization. *Ferning* refers to the characteristic microscopic pattern that results from the crystallization of the inorganic salts in the cervical mucus when it is dried. As the estrogen levels increase, the composition of the cervical mucus changes, so that dried mucus begins to demonstrate ferning in the latter part of the follicular phase. The absence of ferning can indicate inadequate estrogen stimulation of the endocervical glands or inhibition of the endocervical glands by increased secretion of progesterone. Persistent ferning throughout the menstrual cycle suggests anovulatory cycles or insufficient progesterone secretion.

MENOPAUSE

Menopause is the cessation of menstrual cycles. It is as much a process as menstruation—not an event. The process at first takes the form of less frequent and lighter menses, culminating in cessation of menses. Also known as the climacteric, menopause may go on for 1 to several years. The usual age at menopause is 45 to 50 years. With improved nutrition, menopause may occur later in life, so that a woman may have a longer reproductive period. A woman who has not menstruated for a full year is said to have completed menopause.

Menopause is due to the gradual cessation of ovarian function and the resultant diminished levels of estrogen. Although estrogens derived from the adrenal cortex continue to circulate in a woman's body, they are insufficient to maintain the secondary sexual characteristics in the same manner as ovarian estrogens. As a result, breast tissue, body hair, skin elasticity, and subcutaneous fat decrease; the ovaries and uterus diminish in size; and the cervix and vagina become pale and friable. The woman may find

intercourse painful and traumatic, although some type of vaginal lubrication may be helpful.

Systemically, a woman may experience significant vasomotor instability secondary to the decrease in estrogens and the relative increase in pituitary FSH. This instability may give rise to "hot flashes," palpitations, dizziness, and headaches as the blood vessels dilate. A woman may feel anxious or depressed about these uncontrollable and unpredictable events.

Societal mores influence behaviors. A society that emphasizes youthfulness, fitness, and vigor does not look on aging as a positive process, and menopause is regarded as a hallmark of advancing age. A woman who focuses her energy on beauty and youth may feel frustrated or depressed by the natural aging process. On the other hand, a woman who values her other, nonphysical attributes may welcome advancing age as a time when she may more fully develop as a person.

In summary, between the menarche and menopause, the female reproductive system undergoes cyclic changes termed the menstrual cycle. Normal menstrual function results from complex interactions among the hypothalamus, anterior pituitary gland, ovaries, and associated target tissues, such as the endometrium and the vaginal mucosa. Although each component of the system is essential for normal function, the ovaries are largely responsible for controlling the cyclic changes and length of the menstrual cycle.

■ BREASTS

Although anatomically separate, the breasts are functionally related to the female genitourinary system, in that they respond to the cyclic changes in sex hormones and produce milk for infant nourishment. The breasts are also important for their sexual function and for cosmetic appearance. Breast cancer represents one fifth of all female cancers. The high rate of breast cancer has drawn even greater attention to the importance of the breasts throughout the life span.

STRUCTURE

The breasts, or mammary tissues, are located between the third and seventh ribs of the anterior chest wall, supported by the pectoral muscles and superficial fascia. They are specialized glandular structures that have an abundant shared nerve, vascular, and lymphatic supply (Fig. 37-7). What we commonly call breasts are actually two parts of a single anatomic breast. This contiguous nature of breast tissue is important in both health and illness. Men and women

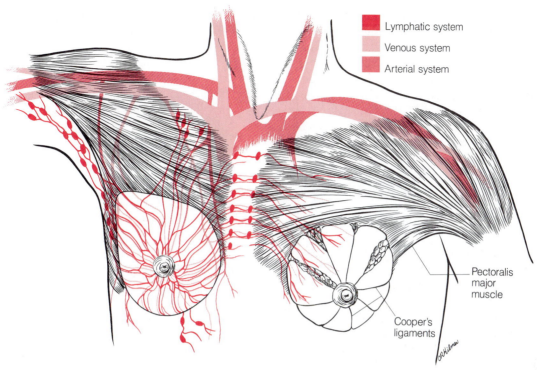

Lymphatic system
Venous system
Arterial system

Pectoralis
major
muscle

Cooper's
ligaments

FIG. 37-7. The breasts, showing the shared vascular and lymphatic supply as well as the pectoral muscles.

alike are born with rudimentary breast tissue, the ducts lined with epithelium. In women, the pituitary release of FSH, LH, and prolactin at puberty stimulates the ovary to produce and release estrogen. This estrogen stimulates the growth and proliferation of the ductile system. With the onset of ovulatory cycles, progesterone release stimulates the growth and development of ductile and alveolar secretory epithelium. By adolescence, the breasts have developed characteristic fat deposition patterns and contours.

Structurally, the breast consists of fat, fibrous connective tissue, and glandular tissue. The superficial fibrous connective tissue is attached to the skin, a fact that is important in the visual observation of skin movement over the breast during breast self-examination. The breast mass is supported by the fascia of the pectoralis major and minor muscles and by the fibrous connective tissue of the breast. Fibrous tissue ligaments, called *Cooper's ligaments*, extend from the outer boundaries of the breast to the nipple area in a radial manner, like the spokes on a wheel (see Fig. 37-7). These ligaments further support the breast and form septa that divide the breast into 15 to 25 lobes. Each lobe consists of grapelike clusters, alveoli or glands, which are interconnected by ducts. The alveoli are lined with secretory cells capable of producing milk or fluid under the proper hormonal conditions (Fig. 37-8). The route of descent of milk and other breast secretions is from alveoli to duct, to

intralobar duct, to lactiferous duct and reservoir, to nipple. Breast milk is produced secondary to complex hormonal changes associated with pregnancy. Fluid is produced and reabsorbed during the menstrual cycle. The breasts respond to the cyclic changes in the menstrual cycle with fullness and discomfort.

The nipple is made up of epithelial, glandular, erectile, and nervous tissue. Areolar tissue surrounds the nipple and is recognized as the darker smooth skin between the nipple and the breast. The small bumps or projections on the areolar surface are Montgomery's tubercles, sebaceous glands that keep the nipple area soft and elastic. At puberty and during pregnancy, increased levels of estrogen and progesterone cause the areola and nipple to become darker and more prominent and Montgomery's glands to become more active. The erectile tissue of the nipple is responsive to psychological and tactile stimuli, which contributes to the sexual function of the breasts.

There are many individual variations in breast size and shape. The shape and texture vary with hormonal, genetic, nutritional, and endocrine factors as well as with muscle tone, age, and pregnancy. A well-developed set of pectoralis muscles will support the breast mass higher on the chest wall. Poor posture, significant weight loss, and lack of support may cause the breasts to droop.

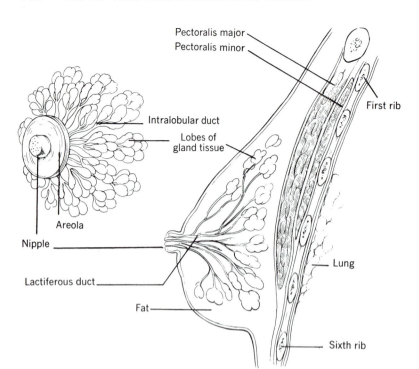

FIG. 37-8. The breast, showing the glandular tissue and ducts of the mammary glands. (Chaffee, E. E., & Lytle, I. M. [1980]. *Basic physiology and anatomy* [4th ed.]. Philadelphia: J.B. Lippincott)

PREGNANCY

During pregnancy, the breasts are significantly altered by increased levels of estrogen and progesterone. Estrogen stimulates increased vascularity of the breasts as well as growth and extension of the ductile structures, causing "heaviness" of the breasts. Progesterone causes marked budding and growth of the alveolar structures. The alveolar epithelium assumes a secretory state in preparation for lactation. The progesterone-induced changes that occur during pregnancy may confer some protection against cancer. Cellular changes that occur within the alveolar lining are thought to change the susceptibility of these cells to estrogen-mediated changes later in life.

LACTATION

During lactation, milk is secreted by alveolar cells, which are under the influence of the anterior pituitary hormone prolactin. Milk ejection from the ductile system occurs in response to the release of oxytocin from the posterior pituitary. The suckling of the infant provides the stimulus for milk ejection. Suckling produces feedback to the hypothalamus, stimulating the release of oxytocin from the posterior pituitary. Oxytocin in turn causes contraction of the myoepithelial cells lining the alveoli and ejection of milk into the ductal system. A woman may have breast leakage for 3 months to 1 year after the termination of breastfeeding as breast tissue and hormones regress to the nonlactating state. Overzealous

breast stimulation with or without pregnancy can likewise cause breast leakage.

CHANGES WITH MENOPAUSE

At the onset of menopause, the levels of estrogen and progesterone are gradually reduced and the breasts regress secondary to the loss of glandular tissue. The lobular–alveolar structures atrophy, leaving fat, connective tissue, and ducts. The breasts become pendulous with the decrease in tissue mass.

In summary, the breast is a complex structure of variable size, consistency, and composition. Although anatomically distinct, the breasts are functionally related to the female genitourinary system, in that they respond to cyclic changes in sex hormones and produce milk for infant nourishment. Breast tissue is not static but changes throughout the life cycle.

■ REFERENCES

1. Benson, R.C. (1983). *Handbook of obstetrics and gynecology* (8th ed., p. 20). Los Altos, CA: Lange Medical Publications.
2. Speroff, L., Glass, R.H., & Kase, N.G. (1989). *Clinical gynecologic endocrinology and infertility* (4th ed., pp. 83, 98, 124). Baltimore: Williams & Wilkins.
3. Greenspan, F.S., & Forsham, P.H. (1991). *Basic and clinical endocrinology* (pp. 449–460). Norwalk, CT: Appleton & Lange.
4. Hershman, J.M. (1982). *Endocrine pathophysiology* (2nd ed., p. 146). Philadelphia: Lea & Febiger.
5. Austin, C.R., & Short, R.V. (1984). *Hormonal control of reproduction* (2nd ed., p. 107). New York: Cambridge Press.

C H A P T E R 3 8

ALTERATIONS IN STRUCTURE AND FUNCTION OF THE FEMALE REPRODUCTIVE SYSTEM

PATRICIA McCOWEN MEHRING

■ OBJECTIVES

After you have studied this chapter, you should be able to meet the following objectives:

■ Compare the extragenital pathologies associated with vulvitis, Bartholin's cyst, epidermal cysts, nevi, vulvar dystrophy, and cancer of the vulva.

■ Describe the conditions that predispose to vaginal infections and methods used to prevent and treat these infections.

■ Define the terms *dysplasia* and *metaplasia*.

■ Describe the importance of the cervical transformation zone in the development of cervical cancer.

■ Compare the lesions associated with nabothian cysts and cervical polyps.

■ Relate the importance of Papanicolaou's test in early detection and decreased incidence of deaths from cervical cancer.

■ Define the terms *conization, biopsy, local cautery, cryosurgery*, and *laser therapy* as they relate to the diagnosis and treatment of cervical cancer.

■ List the complications of untreated cervicitis.

■ Compare the early signs and symptoms of cancer of the vulva, vagina, cervix, endometrium, fallopian tubes, and ovaries.

■ Describe the pathology associated with endometriosis.

■ Compare the age distribution for cervical and endometrial cancer.

■ Compare the risk factors for development of cervical and endometrial cancer.

■ Compare the intramural and subserosal leiomyomas.

Carol Mattson Porth: PATHOPHYSIOLOGY: CONCEPTS OF
ALTERED HEALTH STATES, 4th ed. © 1994, 1990, 1986, 1982
J.B. Lippincott Company

■ List the common causes of pelvic inflammatory disease (PID).

■ List the common symptoms of PID.

■ State the causative factors associated with tubal pregnancy.

■ Describe the symptoms of a tubal pregnancy.

■ State the underlying cause of ovarian cyst.

■ Differentiate benign ovarian cyst from the Stein-Leventhal syndrome.

■ List the hormones produced by the three types of functioning ovarian tumors.

■ State the one reason that ovarian cancer may be difficult to detect in an early stage.

■ Describe the three types of dysfunction that can result from disorders of pelvic support.

■ Explain how uterine anteflexion, retroflexion, and retroversion differ from normal uterine position.

■ Define the terms *amenorrhea, hypomenorrhea, oligomenorrhea, menorrhagia, metrorrhagia,* and *menometrorrhagia.*

■ State the general cause of most dysfunctional menstrual cycles.

■ Compare the symptoms of primary dysmenorrhea with those of secondary dysmenorrhea.

■ Define the condition known as *premenstrual syndrome (PMS).*

■ List at least 10 possible symptoms of PMS.

■ Describe the purpose of treatment methods for PMS.

■ Name and describe four or more benign disorders of the female breast.

Disorders of the female genitourinary system have widespread effects on both physical and psychological function, affecting both sexuality and reproductive function. The reproductive structures are located close to other pelvic structures, particularly those of the urinary system. Therefore, disorders of the reproductive system may also affect urinary function. This chapter focuses on infection and inflammation, benign conditions, and neoplasms of the female reproductive structures; disorders of pelvic support and uterine position; and alterations in menstruation. An overview of infertility is also included.

■ DISORDERS OF THE EXTERNAL GENITALIA

VULVITIS AND FOLLICULITIS

Vulvitis is characterized by inflammation and pruritus (itching) of the vulva. It is not considered a specific disease but typically develops subsequent to other local and systemic disorders. The cause often is an irritating vaginal discharge. *Candida albicans* (yeast) is the most common cause of chronic vulvar pruritus, particularly in women with diabetes mellitus. Vulvitis may also be a component of sexually transmitted diseases such as herpes genitalis and human papilloma virus (HPV) infection (condyloma). Local dermatologic reactions to chemical irritants, such as laundry products, perfumed soaps or sprays, and spermicides, or to allergens, such as poison ivy, can also cause inflammation. Finally, vulvar itching may be due to atrophy that is part of the normal aging process. The management of vulvitis focuses on appropriate treatment of underlying causes and comfort measures to relieve the irritation. These include keeping the area clean and dry; using warm sitz baths with baking soda, wet dressings, or Burow's solution soaks (a mild astringent); or applying a mild hydrocortisone cream for the immediate relief of symptoms.

Folliculitis is an infection that involves the hair follicles of the mons or labia majora. The infection, characterized by small red papules or pustules surrounding the hair shaft, is relatively common because of the density of bacteria in this area as well as the occlusive nature of clothing covering the genitalia. Treatment includes thorough cleansing of the area with germicidal soap followed by the application of a mild bacterial ointment, such as Neosporin or Polysporin.

BARTHOLIN'S CYST AND BARTHOLIN ABSCESS

A cyst is a fluid-filled sac. Bartholin's cyst results from the occlusion of the duct system within Bartholin's gland. When the cyst becomes infected, the contents become purulent; if the infection goes untreated, a bartholinian abscess can result. The obstruction that causes cyst and abscess formation most commonly follows a bacterial, chlamydial, or gonococcal infection. Cysts can attain the size of an orange and frequently recur (Fig. 38-1). Abscesses can be extremely tender and painful. Asymptomatic cysts require no treatment. The treatment of symptomatic cysts consists of the administration of appropriate antibiotics, local application of moist heat, and incision and drainage. Cysts that frequently are abscessed or are large enough to cause blockage of the

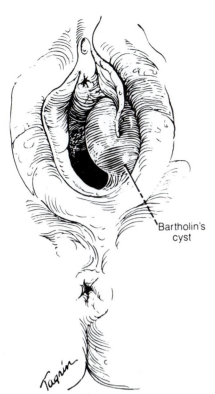

FIG. 38-1. Bartholin's cyst. (Green, T. H., Jr. [1977]. *Gynecology: Essentials of clinical practice* [3rd ed.]. Boston: Little, Brown)

introitus may require surgical intervention (marsupialization).

EPIDERMAL CYSTS

Epidermal cysts (sebaceous or inclusion cysts) are common semisolid tumors of the vulva. These small nodules are lined with keratinizing squamous epithelium and contain cellular debris with a sebaceous appearance and odor. Epidermal cysts may be solitary or multiple and have a yellow appearance when stretched or compressed. They usually resolve spontaneously, and treatment is unnecessary unless they become infected or significantly enlarged.[1]

NEVI

Nevi (moles) occur on the vulva as elsewhere on the body. They can be singular or multiple, flat or raised, and may vary in degree of pigmentation from flesh-colored to dark brown or black. Nevi are asymptomatic but should be observed for changes that could indicate cancer. Nevi may resemble melanomas or basal cell carcinomas, and excisional biopsy is recommended when doubt exists.

VULVAR DYSTROPHY

Vulvar dystrophy, characterized by white lesions of the vulva, is a common condition once considered to be precancerous. The lesions may be categorized as lichen sclerosus, hyperplastic dystrophy, or a mixed classification, depending on clinical and histologic characteristics. Clinically, lichen sclerosus patches are thin, parchment-like, and "atrophic," whereas hyperplastic areas are thick, gray-white plaques. Both can be pruritic. Vulvar biopsy is needed for accurate diagnosis. Lichen sclerosus responds best to topical application of testosterone propionate in petroleum jelly; hyperplastic dystrophy, to a combination steroid (betamethasone valerate) and antipruritic (crotamiton [Eurax]) cream. Lichen sclerosus frequently recurs, and lifetime maintenance therapy is suggested. Hyperplastic dystrophy is less common. Mixed dystrophy requires combination therapy over a longer period.[1]

CANCER OF THE VULVA

Carcinoma of the vulva accounts for about 5% of all cancers of the female genitourinary system. Invasive carcinoma most frequently is seen in women who are age 60 or older; almost one half are over age 70. The mean age for carcinoma in situ is 10 years younger than for invasive carcinoma.[2] Certain sexually transmitted diseases, such as condyloma accuminatum, predispose to vulvar cancer, which may account for the recent rise in incidence of vulvar intraepithelial neoplasia among women in their 20s and 30s.

About 85% to 90% of invasive cancers of the vulva are epidermoid carcinomas. The initial lesion may appear as an inconspicuous thickening of the skin, a small raised area or lump, or an ulceration that fails to heal. These lesions often resemble eczema or dermatitis and may produce few symptoms, other than pruritus, local discomfort, and exudation. A recurrent, persistent, pruritic vulvitis may be the only complaint. Therefore, the symptoms frequently are treated with various home remedies before medical treatment is sought. The lesion often becomes secondarily infected, and this causes pain and discomfort. The malignant lesion gradually spreads superficially or as a deep furrow involving all of one labial side. Because there are many lymph channels around the vulva, the cancer metastasizes freely to the regional lymph nodes. The most common extension is to the superficial inguinal, deep femoral, and external iliac lymph nodes.

Other types of cancer found on the vulva include intraepithelial cancer (Bowen's disease, erythroplasia of Queyrat, and carcinoma in situ simplex), extramammary Paget's disease (intraepithelial or invasive), carcinoma of Bartholin's gland (5% of vulvar cancer), basal cell carcinoma (2% to 3% of vulvar cancer), and malignant melanoma (8% to 11% of vulvar cancer).[2]

Early diagnosis is important in the treatment of vulvar carcinoma. Because malignant lesions can vary in appearance and commonly are mistaken for other conditions, biopsy and treatment often are delayed. Treatment is primarily wide surgical excision of the lesion for noninvasive cancer and vulvectomy with node resection for invasive cancer. Local chemotherapeutic agents (fluorouracil [5-FU]) and colposcopically guided laser therapy are used to treat focal areas of cancer in cases where surgery is contraindicated. The 5-year survival rate for women with lesions less than 3 cm in diameter and minimal node involvement is about 65% after surgical treatment. Follow-up visits every 3 months for the first 2 years after surgery and then every 6 months thereafter are important to detect recurrent disease or a second primary cancer. The 5-year survival rate for patients who have larger lesions in conjunction with three or more positive nodes is less than 15% after surgical treatment.[2] Once pelvic lymphadenopathy is established, the prognosis is poor.

In summary, the surface of the vulva is affected by disorders that affect skin on other parts of the body. These disorders include inflammation (vulvitis and folliculitis), epidermal cysts, and nevi. Although these disorders are not serious, they can be distressing, in that they produce severe discomfort and itching. Bartholin's cysts are the result of occluded ducts within the Bartholin's glands. They often are painful and can become infected. Vulvar dystrophies are characterized by thinning and hyperplastic thickening of vulvar tissues. Cancer of the vulva, which accounts for 3% to 5% of all female genitourinary cancers, is associated with genital herpes infections and HPV.

■ DISORDERS OF THE VAGINA

The normal vaginal ecology depends on the delicate balance of hormones and bacterial flora. Normal estrogen levels maintain a thick protective squamous epithelium that contains glycogen. *Döderlein's bacilli*, part of the normal vaginal flora, metabolize glycogen and, in the process, produce the lactic acid that normally maintains the vaginal *p*H below 4.5. Disruptions in these normal environmental conditions predispose to infection.

VAGINITIS

Vaginitis is an inflammation of the vagina; it is characterized by vaginal discharge and burning, itching, redness, and swelling of vaginal tissues. Pain often occurs with urination and with sexual intercourse. Vaginitis may be caused by chemical irritants, foreign bodies, and infectious agents. The causes of vaginitis differ in various age groups. In premenarchal girls, most vaginal infections are due to nonspecific causes, such as poor hygiene, intestinal parasites, or the presence of foreign bodies. *C. albicans, Trichomonas vaginalis*, and bacterial vaginosis are the most common causes of vaginal discharge in the childbearing years and can be transmitted sexually (see Chapter 39). In postmenopausal women, atrophic vaginitis is the most common form.

Atrophic vaginitis is an inflammation of the vagina that occurs after menopause or removal of the ovaries and their estrogen supply. Estrogen deficiency results in a lack of regenerative growth of the vaginal epithelium, rendering these tissues more susceptible to infection and irritation. Furthermore, Döderlein's bacilli disappear, so that the vaginal secretions become less acidic. The symptoms of atrophic vaginitis include itching, burning, and painful intercourse. These symptoms usually can be reversed by local application of estrogen creams or by vaginal suppositories.

Every woman has a normal vaginal discharge during the menstrual cycle, but it should not cause burning or itching or have an unpleasant odor. These symptoms are suggestive of inflammation or infection. Because these symptoms are common to the different types of vaginitis, precise identification of the organism is essential for proper treatment. A careful history should include information about systemic disease conditions, the use of drugs—such as antibiotics—that foster the growth of yeast, dietary habits, stress, and other factors that alter the resistance of vaginal tissue to infections. A physical examination usually is done to evaluate the nature of the discharge and its effects on the genital structures. Microscopic examination of a saline wet-mount smear (prepared by dipping a cotton-tipped applicator into a test tube of saline solution and transferring a small amount to a slide) is the primary means of identifying the organism responsible for the infection. A small amount of potassium hydroxide (KOH) is added to the solution on the slide to aid in the identification of *C. albicans*. Culture methods may be needed when the organism is not apparent on the wet-mount preparation.

The prevention and treatment of vaginal infections depend on proper health habits and accurate diagnosis and treatment of ongoing infections. Measures to prevent infection include development of daily hygiene habits that keep the genital area clean and dry, maintenance of normal vaginal flora and healthy vaginal mucosa, and avoidance of contact with organisms known to cause vaginal infections. Perfumed products, such as feminine deodorant sprays, douches, bath powders, soaps, and even toilet paper, can be irritating and may alter the normal vaginal flora. Tight clothing prevents the dissipation of body heat and evaporation of skin moisture and, thus, promotes favorable conditions for the growth of pathogens as well as irritation. Nylon and other synthetic undergarments, pantyhose, and swimsuits hold body moisture next to the skin and harbor infectious organisms, even after they have been washed. Cotton undergarments that withstand hot water and bleach (a fungicide) may be preferable for women to prevent such infections. Swimsuits and other garments that cannot withstand hot water or bleaching should be hung in the sunlight to dry. Women should be taught to wipe the perineal area from front to back to avoid bringing rectal contamination into the vagina. Avoiding sexual contact whenever an infection is known to exist or suspected should limit that route of transmission.

CANCER OF THE VAGINA

Primary cancers of the vagina are extremely rare. They account for about 1% to 2% of all cancers of the female reproductive system. Like vulvar carcinoma, carcinoma of the vagina is largely a disease of older women, with a peak incidence between ages 50 and 70. The exception to that is clear cell adenocarcinoma associated with diethylstilbestrol (DES) exposure in utero, which has an age range of 7 to 29 years.[3] Vaginal cancers may result from local extension of cervical cancer, from local irritation such as occurs with prolonged use of a pessary, or from exposure to sexually transmitted herpes virus or papillomaviruses.

About 85% of vaginal cancers are epidermoid carcinomas, with other common types being adenocarcinomas, sarcomas, and melanomas.[2] Maternal ingestion of DES in early pregnancy has clearly been associated with the development of clear cell adenocarcinoma in female offspring who were exposed in utero. Between 1940 and 1975, DES, a nonsteroidal synthetic estrogen, commonly was prescribed to prevent miscarriage. Its association with adenocarcinoma of the vagina was not discovered until the late 1960s. A tumor registry of clear cell adenocarcinoma of the genital tract in young women was established in 1971, and more than 500 cases have now been reported. The incidence of clear cell adenocarcinoma of the vagina is quite low, about 0.1% in young women who were exposed in utero to synthetic estrogen. This is fortunate, since at the time of the banning of DES, an estimated 4 million American women had taken the drug. Although only a small percentage of girls exposed to estrogen actually develop clear cell adenocarcinoma, 75% to 90% of them do develop benign adenosis (ectopic extension of cervical columnar epithelium into the vagina, which normally is

stratified squamous epithelium), which may predispose to cancer. Any girl exposed to DES should be encouraged to have semiannual gynecologic examinations beginning at age 14 or menarche with an initial examination that includes careful colposcopic inspection of the cervix and vagina.

The most common symptom of vaginal carcinoma is abnormal bleeding. Twenty percent of women are asymptomatic, with the cancer being discovered during a routine pelvic examination. The anatomic proximity of the vagina to other pelvic structures (urethra, bladder, and rectum) permits early spread to these areas. Pelvic pain, dysuria, constipation, and vaginal discharge can be associated symptoms. Vaginal epidermoid carcinoma most often is detected in the upper anterior one third of the vagina, with adenocarcinoma more often found on the lower anterior and lateral vaginal vault.[4] Cancer can develop anywhere within the vagina, however, and visualization during physical examination should always cover the entire vault. Women should continue to have vaginal cytology studies (Papanicolaou's test [Pap smear]) at least every 2 years after hysterectomy to rule out development of vaginal cancer. Diagnosis requires a biopsy of suspicious lesions or areas.

Treatment of vaginal cancer must take into consideration the size, location, and spread of the lesion as well as the woman's age. Radical surgery and radiation therapy are both curative. When there is upper vaginal involvement, radical surgery includes a total hysterectomy, pelvic lymph node dissection, and placement of a graft from the buttock to the area from which the vagina was excised. The ovaries usually are preserved unless they are diseased. Extensive lesions and those located in the middle or lower vaginal area usually are treated by radiation therapy. Newer therapies for isolated lesions include vaporization with the carbon dioxide laser or intravaginal application of a cream incorporating 5-FU (Efudex).[2,5] The prognosis depends on the stage of the disease, the involvement of lymph nodes, and the degree of mitotic activity of the tumor. With appropriate treatment and follow-up, the 5-year survival rate for stage I or II disease is 70% to 75%. This drops to 20% to 30% for stage III disease. Few survive stage IV disease.[2] For DES-related cancers, the survival rate is about 80%.[6]

■ DISORDERS OF THE CERVIX

The cervix is composed of two distinct types of tissue. The exocervix, or visible portion, is covered with stratified squamous epithelium, which also lines the vagina. The endocervical canal is lined with columnar epithelium. The junction of these two tissue types (the squamocolumnar junction) appears at various locations on the cervix at different points in a woman's life (Fig. 38-2). During periods of high estrogen production, particularly fetal existence, menarche, and the first pregnancy, the cervix everts or turns outward, exposing the columnar epithelium to the vaginal environment. The combination of estrogen and low vaginal *pH* leads to a gradual transformation from columnar to squamous epithelium—a process called *metaplasia*. The dynamic area of change where metaplasia takes place is called the *transformation zone*.[7]

The transformation zone is a critical area for the development of cervical cancer. During metaplasia, the newly developed squamous epithelial cells are vulnerable to genetic change if exposed to carcinogenic agents (cancer-producing substances). *Dysplasia* literally means disordered growth or development. Although initially a reversible cell change, untreated dysplasia can develop into carcinoma.

Metaplasia can result in retention cysts, called *nabothian cysts*, that develop when mucus becomes trapped within the deeper clefts of the columnar epithelial cells. These are benign cysts that require no treatment unless they become so numerous that they cause cervical enlargement. The nabothian cyst farthest away from the external cervical os indicates the outer aspect of the transformation zone. The transformation zone is the area of the cervix that must be sampled to have an adequate Pap smear and the area most carefully examined during colposcopy.

CERVICITIS AND CERVICAL POLYPS

Cervicitis is an acute or chronic inflammation of the cervix. Acute cervicitis may result from the direct infection of the cervix or may be secondary to a vaginal or uterine infection. It may be caused by a variety of infective agents, including *C. albicans, T. vaginalis, Neisseria gonorrhoeae, Gardnerella vaginalis, Chlamydia trachomatis, Ureaplasma urealyticum*, and herpes simplex virus. *Chlamydia* is the organism most commonly associated with mucopurulent cervicitis.[8] Chronic cervicitis represents a low-grade inflammatory process. It is common in parous women and may be a sequela to minute lacerations that occur during childbirth, instrumentation, or other trauma. The organisms usually are of a nonspecific type, often staphylococcus, streptococcus, or coliform bacteria.

With acute cervicitis, the cervix becomes reddened and edematous. Irritation from the infection results in copious mucopurulent drainage and leukorrhea. The symptoms of chronic cervicitis are less well defined: the cervix may be ulcerated or normal in appearance; it may contain nabothian cysts; the cervical os may be distorted by old lacerations or everted to expose areas of columnar epithelium; and a mucopurulent drainage may be present.

Untreated cervicitis may extend to include the development of pelvic cellulitis, low back pain, painful intercourse, cervical stenosis, dysmenorrhea, and further infection of the uterus or fallopian tubes. Depending on the causative agent, acute cervicitis is treated with appropriate antibiotic therapy. Diagnosis of chronic cervicitis is based on vaginal examination, colposcopy, cytologic smears, and, occasionally, biopsy to rule out malignant changes. The treatment usually involves cryosurgery or cauterization, which causes the tissues to slough and, thus, leads to eradication of the infection. Colposcopically guided laser vaporization of abnormal epithelium is the newest but most expensive treatment for cervicitis.

Polyps are the most common lesions of the cervix. They can be found in women of all ages, but their incidence is higher during the reproductive years. The polyps are soft, velvety-red lesions; they usually are pedunculated and often are found protruding through the cervical os. They usually develop as a result of inflammatory hyperplasia of the endocervical mucosa. Polyps typically are asymptomatic but may have associated postcoital bleeding. Most are benign, but they should be removed and examined by a pathologist to rule out malignant change.

CANCER OF THE CERVIX

Cervical cancer is the most readily detected and, if detected early, the most easily cured of all the cancers of the female reproductive system. The incidence of invasive cervical cancer has steadily decreased over the years, whereas that of cancer in situ has risen. About 13,500 cases of cancer of the cervix were diagnosed in 1992; there were about 4400 deaths from

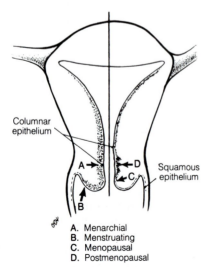

Columnar epithelium

Squamous epithelium

A. Menarchial
B. Menstruating
C. Menopausal
D. Postmenopausal

FIG. 38-2. Location of squamocolumnar junction in menarchial, menstruating, menopausal, and postmenopausal women.

cervical cancer during the same period. The death rate has steadily declined over the past 40 years with the introduction of more sensitive and readily available screening methods (Pap smear, colposcopy, cervicography), consistent use of a standardized grading system that guides treatment, and more effective treatment methods. The 5-year survival rate for all cervical cancer patients is 66%. With early diagnosis, the rate is 80% to 90%, and for cancer in situ, the rate approaches 100%.[9]

Carcinoma of the cervix is considered a sexually transmitted disease. It is rare among celibate women. Risk factors include early age at first intercourse, multiple sexual partners, a promiscuous male partner, smoking, and a history of sexually transmitted diseases.[10] An uncircumcised male partner, multiple pregnancies, and the use of oral contraceptives— once considered predisposing factors—have all been eliminated from the list of factors that place women at risk for cervical cancer. A relation between herpes simplex virus 2 (HSV-2) and HPV with cancer of the cervix has been demonstrated. An HSV antigen (AG) has been identified in 90% of cervical carcinoma biopsy samples, and HSV DNA sequences have been identified within the DNA molecule of malignant cells. Certain strains of HPV have been identified in invasive carcinoma of the cervix, whereas others are more often associated with dysplasia or cancer in situ.[11, 12] Because these viruses are spread by sexual contact, their association with cervical cancer provides a tempting hypothesis to explain the relation between sexual practices and cervical cancer.

One of the most important advances in the early diagnosis and treatment of cancer of the cervix was made possible by the observation that this cancer arises from precursor lesions, which begin with the development of atypical cervical cells. These gradually progress to cancer in situ and, finally, to invasive cancer of the cervix. Atypical cells differ from normal cervical squamous epithelium. There are changes in the nuclear and cytoplasmic parts of the cell and more variation in cell size and shape (dysplasia). Cancer in situ is localized to the epithelial layer, whereas invasive cancer of the cervix spreads. A system of grading devised to describe the dysplastic changes of cancer precursors involves the use of the term *cervical intraepithelial neoplasia (CIN)*. The CIN system grades according to extent of involvement of the epithelial thickness of the cervix: CIN grade I (mild dysplasia) involves the initial one third of the epithelial layer and the lesion is well differentiated; CIN grade II (moderate dysplasia) involves one third to two thirds of the epithelial layer and is less well differentiated; and CIN grade III is an undifferentiated intraepithelial lesion with two thirds (severe dysplasia) to full-thickness (carcinoma in situ) involvement. Once cancer has been diagnosed, the

general preference is to use the International Federation of Gynecology and Obstetrics (FIGO) classification system to describe the histologic and clinical extent of the disease (staging). The development of an internationally accepted grading system has significantly increased the data base for cervical cancer and the consistency of that data base.

The atypical cellular changes that precede frank neoplastic changes consistent with cancer of the cervix can be recognized by a number of direct and microscopic techniques, including the Pap smear, colposcopy, and cervicography. The precursor lesions can exist in a reversible form, which may regress spontaneously or may progress and undergo malignant change. Cancers of the cervix have a long latent period; untreated dysplasia gradually progresses to carcinoma in situ, which may remain static for 7 to 10 years before it becomes invasive.[2] After the preinvasive period, growth is rapid, and if the cancer is untreated, death follows within 2 to 5 years of the onset of symptoms.

The purpose of the Pap smear (also discussed in Chapter 5) is to detect the presence of abnormal cells on the surface of the cervix or within the endocervix. This test detects both precancerous and cancerous lesions. Although the American Cancer Society has suggested that the Pap smear need not be done annually if there have been three normal tests in succession, most clinicians maintain that performing an annual test is the safest course to follow. If the woman has risk factors, such as previous herpes or HPV infection, DES exposure in utero, or a strong family history of cervical cancer, more frequent Pap smears may be recommended. There are several methods for classifying the Pap smear. The older method divides the results into the following five classes:

> Class I: Normal, or no abnormal cells
> Class II: Atypical cells below the level of neoplasia (benign atypia, or inflammatory)
> Class III: Abnormal cells typical of dysplasia (mild or moderate; CIN 1 or CIN 2)
> Class IV: Cells consistent with cancer in situ (severe dysplasia; CIN 3)
> Class V: Abnormal cells consistent with invasive squamous cell carcinoma

Sometimes these classifications were thought to be ambiguous and resulted in confusion about the clinical implications of the report. A new system for reporting cervical and vaginal cytologic diagnoses, the *Bethesda System*, was developed during a National Cancer Institute Workshop in 1989. The Bethesda System includes a statement of specimen adequacy, general categorization (within normal limits or other), and a descriptive diagnosis of findings, including infection, reactive and reparative changes, hormonal evaluation, and epithelial cell abnormalities, using the terms low-grade and high-grade squamous intra-epithelial lesion (SIL). These two terms encompass the spectrum of terms previously used to delineate squamous cell precursors to invasive carcinoma. Low-grade SIL includes cellular changes associated with HPV and mild dysplasia (CIN 1). High-grade SIL includes moderate and severe dysplasia (CIN 2 and 3) and carcinoma in situ.[12]

Pap smears are only about 80% to 90% accurate in diagnosing CIN even under optimal circumstances. Care must be taken to obtain an adequate smear from the transformation zone that includes endocervical cells and to ensure that the cytologic examination is done by a competent laboratory. The presence of normal endometrial cells in a cervical cytologic sample during the luteal phase of the menstrual cycle or in the postmenopausal period has been associated with endometrial disease and warrants further evaluation.[13] This demonstrates that even shedding of normal cells at an inappropriate time may indicate disease.

Diagnosis of cancer requires pathologic confirmation. If a Pap smear shows atypical cells, a colposcopic study usually is done. This is a vaginal examination that is done using a colposcope, an instrument that affords a well-lighted and magnified stereoscopic view of the cervix. During colposcopy, the cervical tissue may be stained with an iodine solution (Schiller's test) or acetic acid solution to accentuate topographic or vascular changes that can differentiate normal from abnormal tissue. A biopsy sample may be obtained from suspicious areas and examined microscopically. With the availability of colposcopy, many women with abnormal Pap smears have been able to avoid surgical cone biopsy. Cone biopsy involves the removal of a cone-shaped wedge of cervix including the entire transformation zone and at least 50% of the endocervical canal. Postoperative hemorrhage, infection, cervical stenosis, infertility, and incompetent cervix are possible sequelae that warrant avoidance of this procedure unless it is truly necessary. Diagnostic conization is indicated when a lesion is partly or completely beyond colposcopic view or colposcopically directed biopsy fails to explain the cytology.

The *loop electrode excision procedure (LEEP)*, a refinement of loop diathermy techniques dating back to the 1940s, is quickly becoming the first-line management for SIL. This outpatient procedure allows for the simultaneous diagnosis and treatment of dysplastic lesions found on colposcopy. It uses a thin, rigid, wire loop electrode attached to a generator that blends high-frequency, low-voltage current for cutting and a modulated higher voltage for coagulation.

In skilled hands, this wire can remove the entire transformation zone, thus providing adequate treatment for the lesion while providing a specimen for further histologic evaluation. The width and depth of the tissue excised are controlled by the size and shape of the loop as well as the speed and pressure that is applied during the procedure. To avoid the problems that can occur after surgical cone biopsy (*e.g.*, stenosis and incompetent cervix), it is imperative that the depth of the excision does not exceed the regenerative capacity of the cervix.[14] Bleeding can be minimized by fulguration of the base with electrocoagulation or by applying a thin layer of Monsel's gel (chemical cautery). Although long-term results are not available, this procedure, which requires only local anesthesia, appears to provide a lower-cost, office-based alternative to cone biopsy.

A final diagnostic tool in areas where colposcopy is not readily available is cervicography, a noninvasive photographic technique that provides permanent objective documentation of normal and abnormal cervical patterns. Acetic acid (5%) is applied to the cervix, a cervicography camera is used to take photos, and the projected cervicogram (slide after film developing) can be sent for expert evaluation. In a recent study, the cervicogram was found to give a greater yield of CIN than Pap smear alone.[15]

Early treatment of cervical cancer involves removal of the lesion by one of various techniques. Biopsy or local cautery may be therapeutic in and of itself. Electrocautery, cryosurgery, or carbon dioxide laser therapy may be used to treat moderate to severe dysplasia that is limited to the exocervix (squamocolumnar junction clearly visible). Therapeutic conization becomes necessary if the lesion extends into the endocervical canal and can be done surgically or with LEEP in the physician's office. Depending on the stage of involvement of the cervix, invasive cancer is treated with radiation therapy, surgery, or both. Both external beam irradiation and intracavitary cesium irradiation (insertion of a closed metal cylinder containing cesium) can be used in the treatment of cervical cancer. Intracavitary radiation is most effective when the tumor is small. The larger the tumor, the greater the reliance on external beam radiation to shrink the tumor to a size at which it can be effectively irradiated by intracavitary irradiation. Surgery can include (1) extended hysterectomy (removal of the uterus, fallopian tubes, ovaries, and upper portion of the vagina) without pelvic lymph node dissection, (2) radical hysterectomy with pelvic lymph node dissection, or (3) pelvic exenteration (removal of all pelvic organs, including the bladder, rectum, vulva, and vagina). The choice of treatment usually is influenced by the patient's age and health.

■ DISORDERS OF THE UTERUS

ENDOMETRITIS

Inflammation or infection of the endometrium is an ill-defined entity that produces variable symptoms. The presence of plasma cells is required for diagnosis. Endometritis can occur as a postpartum or postabortal infection, with gonococcal or chlamydial salpingitis, after instrumentation or surgery or secondary to the presence of an intrauterine device or tuberculosis.[16] Causative organisms, in addition to *N. gonorrhoeae, Chlamydia,* and *Mycobacterium tuberculosis,* include *Escherichia coli, Proteus, Pseudomonas, Klebsiella, Bacteroides,* and *Mycoplasma* species. Abnormal vaginal bleeding, mild to severe uterine tenderness, fever, malaise, and foul-smelling discharge have been associated with endometritis, but the clinical picture is variable. Treatment involves either oral or intravenous antibiotic therapy, depending on the severity of the condition.

ENDOMETRIOSIS

Endometriosis is the condition in which functional endometrial tissue is found in ectopic sites outside the uterus. The site may be the ovaries, broad ligaments, pouch of Douglas (cul-de-sac), pelvis, vagina, vulva, perineum, or intestines. Rarely, endometrial implants have been found in the nostrils, umbilicus, lungs, and limbs.

The cause of endometriosis is not known. There appears to have been an increase in its incidence in the developing Western countries during the past four to five decades. About 10% to 15% of premenopausal women have some degree of endometriosis. It can be found in up to 50% of women undergoing diagnostic laparoscopy for infertility.[17] It is more common in women who have postponed childbearing. Risk factors for endometriosis may include early menarche, regular periods with shorter cycle interval (27 days or less), longer duration (greater than 7 days), heavier flow, and increased menstrual pain.[18] There are several theories that attempt to account for endometriosis. One theory suggests that menstrual blood containing fragments of endometrium is forced upward through the fallopian tubes into the peritoneal cavity. Retrograde menstruation is not an uncommon phenomenon, however, and it is unknown why endometrial cells implant and grow in some women but not in others. Another proposal is that dormant, immature cellular elements spread over a wide area during embryonic development persist into adult life and that the ensuing metaplasia accounts for the development of ectopic endometrial

tissue. Yet another theory suggests that the endometrial tissue may metastasize through the lymphatics or vascular system.

The gross pathologic changes that occur in endometriosis differ with location and duration. In the ovary, the endometrial tissue may form cysts (endometriomas filled with old blood that resembles chocolate syrup [*chocolate cysts*]). Rupture of these cysts can cause peritonitis and adhesions. Elsewhere in the pelvis, the tissue may take the form of small hemorrhagic lesions called *mulberry spots* or *powder burn spots,* which are surrounded by scar tissue. These ectopic implants respond to hormonal stimulation in the same way normal endometrium does, becoming proliferative, then secretory, and finally undergoing menstrual breakdown. Bleeding into the surrounding structures can cause pain and the development of significant pelvic adhesions. Extensive fibrotic tissue occasionally may mimic carcinoma and cause bowel obstruction.

Endometriosis may be difficult to diagnose because its symptoms mimic those of other pelvic disorders. Furthermore, the severity of the symptoms does not always reflect the extent of the disease. The classic triad of dysmenorrhea, dyspareunia, and infertility strongly suggests endometriosis. Accurate diagnosis can be accomplished only through laparoscopy.

The treatment modalities for endometriosis fall into three categories: (1) pain relief, (2) endometrial suppression, and (3) surgery. In young, unmarried women, simple observation and antiprostaglandin analgesics may be sufficient treatment. The use of hormones to induce physiologic amenorrhea is based on the observation that pregnancy affords temporary relief by inducing atrophy of the endometrial tissue. This can be accomplished through administration of estrogen or progesterone alone, combined oral contraceptive pills, danazol (a testosterone derivative), or long-acting gonadotropin-releasing hormone (GnRH) analogues that inhibit the pituitary gonadotropins and suppress ovulation.[19]

Surgery is the most definitive therapy for many women with endometriosis. In the past, laparoscopic use of cautery was limited to mild endometriosis without extensive adhesions. With the advent of carbon dioxide or potassium-titanyl-phosphate (KTP) lasers, in-depth treatment of endometriosis or pelvic adhesions can be accomplished by means of laparoscopy. Advantages of laser surgery include better hemostasis, more precision in vaporizing lesions with less damage to surrounding tissue, and better access to areas that are not well visualized or would be difficult to reach with cautery. The KTP laser is particularly useful for endometriosis because of its flexible fiberoptic delivery system, which allows tissue incision and vaporization in addition to photocoagulation, and its green beam, which makes visualization and fine focusing easier.[20] Radical treatment involves total hysterectomy and bilateral salpingo-oophorectomy (removal of the fallopian tubes and ovaries) when the symptoms are unbearable or the woman's childbearing is completed. Treatment offers relief but not cure. Recurrence of endometriosis is not uncommon, regardless of the treatment (except for radical surgery). According to one source, recurrence rates confirmed by surgery were 10% after 3 years and 35% after 5 years.[2] Pregnancy may delay but does not preclude recurrence.

ADENOMYOSIS

Adenomyosis is the condition in which endometrial glands and stroma are found within the myometrium interspersed between the smooth muscle fibers. In contrast to endometriosis, which usually is a problem of young, infertile women, adenomyosis typically is found in multiparous women in their late 30s or 40s. It is thought that events associated with repeated pregnancies, deliveries, and uterine involution may cause the endometrium to be displaced throughout the myometrium. Adenomyosis frequently coexists with uterine myomas or endometrial hyperplasia. The diagnosis of adenomyosis often occurs as an incidental finding in a uterus removed for symptoms suggestive of myoma or hyperplasia.[16] Adenomyosis resolves with menopause. Hysterectomy (with preservation of the ovaries in premenopausal women) is the treatment of choice. Efforts to control this condition with pelvic irradiation or medication to suppress ovarian stimulation have been largely unsuccessful.[2]

ENDOMETRIAL CANCER

Endometrial cancer is the most common cancer found within the female pelvis—occurring more than twice as often as cervical cancer. In 1988, the American Cancer Society estimated that there were 32,000 cases diagnosed and 5600 deaths from endometrial cancer.[9] Endometrial cancer is primarily a disease of older women (peak ages 55 to 65), suggesting that the high frequency of occurrence may reflect a demographic shift—that is, an increase in the elderly population. Estrogen stimulation has been suggested as a causative factor. A sharp rise in endometrial cancer was noted in the 1970s among middle-aged women who had received estrogen therapy for menopausal symptoms. In fact, most women who develop endometrial cancer have a history consistent with exposure to abnormal hormone levels. Many of these women are obese, have diabetes or other evidence of endocrine disturbances, are hypertensive,

have Stein-Leventhal syndrome, or have a history of previous use of sequential birth control pills (estrogen for 15 to 16 days followed by 6 to 7 days of combined estrogen and progesterone). Sequential birth control pills were withdrawn in the early 1970s when the association between the use of unopposed estrogen and endometrial cancer was observed. Some of the women took DES during pregnancy; others took estrogen for menopausal symptoms; many are nulliparous or infertile, have had menstrual irregularities and ovulation failure, have had breast cancer, or have been treated with hormone therapy. Numerous case control studies have demonstrated a 2- to 10-fold increase in the incidence of endometrial cancer in women who have received exogenous estrogen. This risk appears to be neutralized with the addition of cyclic progestin each month; in fact, the use of combined oral contraceptives appears to decrease the risk of developing endometrial cancer by about half.[21]

As with cervical cancer, it is believed that precancerous abnormalities of the endometrium precede endometrial cancer. These precancerous changes include endometrial hyperplasia or an abnormal pattern of growth in the cells that line the uterus. These cellular changes may be spontaneous, or they may develop secondary to exposure to unopposed exogenous estrogens. Hyperplasia often causes abnormal bleeding and spotting and can be diagnosed with an endometrial biopsy (tissue sample obtained in an office procedure) or by dilatation and curettage (D&C), which consists of dilating the cervix and scraping the uterine cavity.

The major symptom of endometrial cancer is abnormal, painless bleeding. Any postmenopausal bleeding is abnormal and warrants investigation to rule out endometrial cancer or its precursor stages. Because bleeding is such an early warning sign of the disease and because endometrial cancer tends to be rather slow-growing, particularly in its early stages, the chances of cure are good if prompt medical attention is sought. Later signs of uterine cancer may include cramping, pelvic discomfort, postcoital bleeding, lower abdominal pressure, and enlarged lymph nodes. As a screening test, the Pap smear may not be effective in detecting endometrial cancer: it is falsely negative in about 40% to 50% of cases. Endometrial sampling obtained by direct aspiration of the endometrial cavity is far more accurate: 80% to 90% of endometrial cancers are identified if adequate tissue is obtained. D&C is the definitive procedure for diagnosis because it provides a more thorough evaluation.

Surgery and radiation therapy are the most successful methods of treatment for endometrial cancer. Combination therapy often is recommended if metastases are present. Controversy exists over which is the most appropriate form of irradiation therapy. Treatment may involve a short course of external beam or internal irradiation followed by total abdominal hysterectomy and bilateral salpingo-oophorectomy. A 4-to-6-week rest period after irradiation therapy may precede surgical treatment. In cases of advanced disease, surgery may be followed by external beam irradiation or application of radium to the vaginal vault. With early diagnosis and treatment, the 5-year survival rate ranges from 83% to almost 100%. Once the cancer has metastasized to the para-aortic and abdominal lymph nodes, the survival rate decreases to less than 5%.

LEIOMYOMAS

Leiomyomas are benign neoplasms of smooth muscle origin. They are also known as *myomas* or, colloquially, *fibroids*. These are the most common form of pelvic tumor and are believed to occur in one out of every four or five women over age 35. They are seen more often and their rate of growth is more rapid in black women than in white women. Leiomyomas usually develop in the corpus of the uterus; they may be submucosal, subserosal, or intramural (Fig. 38-3). Intramural fibroids are embedded within the myometrium. They are the most common type of fibroids, taking the form of a symmetric enlargement of the nonpregnant uterus. *Subserosal* tumors are located beneath the perimetrium of the uterus. These tumors

are recognized as irregular projections on the uterine surface; they may become pedunculated, displacing or impinging on other genitourinary structures and causing hydroureter or bladder problems. *Submucosal* fibroids displace endometrial tissue and are more likely to cause bleeding, necrosis, and infection than either of the other types.

Leiomyomas may be manifested as follows: they may be asymptomatic and be discovered during a routine pelvic examination, or they may cause bleeding, particularly at the time of the menstrual period. Their rate of growth is variable, but they may increase in size during pregnancy or with exogenous estrogen stimulation (oral contraceptives or menopausal estrogen replacement therapy). Interference with pregnancy is rare unless the tumor is submucosal and interferes with implantation or obstructs the cervical outlet. These tumors may outgrow their blood supply, become infarcted, and undergo degenerative changes. Most leiomyomas regress with menopause, but if bleeding, pressure on the bladder, pain, or other problems persist, hysterectomy may be required. Myomectomy (removal of just the tumors) can be done to preserve the uterus for future childbearing. Cesarean section may be recommended if the uterine cavity is entered during myomectomy. If the woman is not a good surgical risk, danazol (Danocrine) or GnRH antagonists (leuprolide [Lupron]) may be used to suppress leiomyoma growth.

■ DISORDERS OF THE FALLOPIAN TUBES AND OVARIES

PELVIC INFLAMMATORY DISEASE

Pelvic inflammatory disease (PID) is an inflammation of the upper reproductive tract that involves the uterus (endometritis), fallopian tubes (salpingitis), or ovaries (oophoritis). About 80% of women with acute salpingitis have either *N. gonorrhoeae* or *C. trachomatis* identified within the reproductive tract.[22] At one time, the gonococcus was thought to be the only organism responsible for nonpuerperal PID. The etiology appears to be changing, however, and *Chlamydia* as well as other opportunistic bacteria in the *Bacteroides* and *Peptostreptococcus* groups are now involved. The organisms ascend through the endocervical canal to the endometrial cavity and then to the tubes and ovaries. The endocervical canal is slightly dilated during menstruation; thus, bacteria can gain entrance to the uterus and other pelvic structures. Once inside the upper reproductive tract, the organisms multiply rapidly in the favorable environment of the sloughing endometrium and ascend to the fallopian tube. Factors that predispose women to the de-

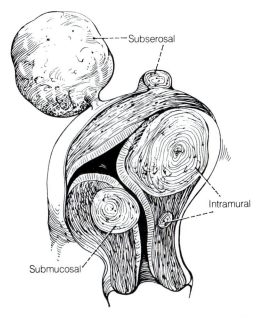

FIG. 38-3. Submucosal, intramural, and subserosal leiomyomas. (Green, T H., Jr. [1977]. *Gynecology: Essentials of clinical practice* [3rd ed.]. Boston: Little, Brown)

velopment of PID include ages 16 to 24, unmarried status, nulliparity, history of multiple sexual partners, and previous history of PID. The use of an intrauterine contraceptive device (IUD) increases the risk of developing PID three- to five-fold. A recent study, however, indicates that women with only one sexual partner who are at low risk of acquiring sexually transmitted diseases have no significant risk of developing PID from using an IUD.[23]

The symptoms of PID include lower abdominal pain, which may start just after a menstrual period; purulent cervical discharge; adnexal tenderness; and an exquisitely painful cervix. Fever (greater than 100.4°F [41°C]), increased erythrocyte sedimentation rate, and an elevated white blood cell count (greater than 10,000) commonly are seen, even though the woman may not appear acutely ill. A newer test involves measurement of C reactive protein (CRP) in the blood. Elevated CRP levels equate with inflammation.

Treatment may involve hospitalization with intravenous administration of antibiotics. Bed rest in the Fowler's position (head and knees elevated) facilitates pelvic drainage. If the condition is diagnosed early, outpatient antibiotic therapy may be sufficient. The Centers for Disease Control recommend doxycycline plus cefoxitan intravenously for at least 4 days followed by oral doxycycline for 10 to 14 days. Ambulatory treatment involves an initial dose of cefoxitan, amoxicillin, ampicillin, or aqueous procaine penicillin followed by 10 to 14 days of oral doxycycline.[24] Treatment is aimed at preventing complications, which can include pelvic adhesions, infertility, ectopic pregnancy, chronic abdominal pain, and tubo-ovarian abscesses. Accurate diagnosis and appropriate antibiotic therapy may decrease the severity and frequency of PID sequelae.

ECTOPIC PREGNANCY

Although pregnancy is not discussed in detail in this text, it is reasonable to mention ectopic pregnancy because it represents a true gynecologic emergency and should be considered when a woman of reproductive age presents with the complaint of pelvic pain. Ectopic pregnancy occurs when a fertilized ovum implants outside the uterine cavity. The most common site for ectopic pregnancy is the fallopian tube. According to the Centers for Disease Control, between 1970 and 1987, the number of ectopic pregnancies increased from 17,800 to 88,000; the rate of occurrence among females aged 15 to 44 rose from 4.5 per 1000 to 14.3 per 1000 reported pregnancies (live births, abortions, and ectopics). Although complications from ectopic pregnancy are one of two leading causes of maternal death in the United States, the death rate has steadily declined to its current rate of 3.4 per 10,000 ectopic pregnancies.[25]

The cause of ectopic pregnancy is delayed ovum transport, which may, in turn, be caused by decreased tubal motility or distorted tubal anatomy (narrowed lumen, convolutions, or diverticuli). Factors that may predispose to the development of an ectopic pregnancy include PID, therapeutic abortion, tubal ligation or tubal reversal, previous ectopic pregnancy, infertility, and the use of clomiphene citrate to induce ovulation.[26] Contraceptive failure with progestin-only birth control pills or the "morning-after pill" has also been associated with ectopic pregnancy.

The site of implantation within the tube (*e.g.*, isthmus, ampulla) may determine the onset of symptoms and the timing of diagnosis. As the tubal pregnancy progresses, the surrounding tissue is stretched. The pregnancy eventually outgrows its blood supply, at which point the pregnancy either terminates or the tube itself ruptures because it can no longer contain the growing pregnancy. Symptoms can include lower abdominal discomfort—diffuse or localized to one side—which progresses to severe pain caused by rupture, spotting, syncope, referred shoulder pain from bleeding into the abdominal cavity, and amenorrhea. Physical examination usually reveals adnexal tenderness; an adnexal mass is found in only 50% of cases. Culdocentesis (needle aspiration from the cul-de-sac) may reveal blood if rupture has occurred. Quantitative β-human chorionic gonadotropin (hCG) pregnancy tests may detect lower than normal hCG production. Pelvic ultrasound studies after 5 weeks' gestation may demonstrate an empty uterine cavity or presence of the gestational sac outside the uterus. Definitive diagnosis requires laparoscopy. Differential diagnosis for this type of pelvic pain includes ruptured ovarian cyst, threatened or incomplete abortion, PID, acute appendicitis, and degenerating fibroid.

Treatment is surgical, usually a laparoscopic salpingostomy to remove the ectopic pregnancy if the fallopian tube has not ruptured or salpingectomy if it has. Salpingostomy preserves fertility but requires careful surgical technique to minimize the risk of recurrent ectopic pregnancies. Laparoscopic treatment of ectopic pregnancy is well tolerated and more cost-effective than laparotomy because of shorter convalescence and the reduced need for postoperative analgesia. When possible, it is the preferred method of treatment. Laparotomy becomes necessary when there is internal bleeding, when the ectopic site cannot be visualized through the laparoscope, or when performance of a salpingectomy becomes necessary.[26] Methotrexate, a chemotherapeutic agent, has been successfully used to eliminate residual ectopic pregnancy tissue after laparoscopy or in cases where the pregnancy is unruptured and surgery is contraindicated. The drug is given for 1 to 8 days and is better tolerated when given orally. Adverse effects can include oral lesions, transient elevation of liver enzyme levels, and anemia.

CANCER OF THE FALLOPIAN TUBE

Cancer of the fallopian tube is rare, accounting for less than 1% of all female genital tract cancers. Fewer than 3000 cases have been reported. Diagnosis of this cancer is extremely difficult, and the disease may be well advanced when found. Most primary tubal cancers are papillary adenocarcinomas, and these tumors develop bilaterally in 40% to 50% of cases.[2]

Symptoms are uncommon, but intermittent serosanguineous vaginal discharge, abnormal vaginal bleeding, and colicky low abdominal pain have been reported. An adnexal mass may be present; however, preoperative diagnosis in most cases is leiomyoma or ovarian tumor.

Treatment is total hysterectomy, bilateral salpingo-oophorectomy, and pelvic lymph node dissection. More extensive procedures may be warranted, depending on the stage of the disease. The 5-year survival rates vary from 0% to 44%; if metastasis has occurred, the prognosis is poor.

BENIGN OVARIAN CYSTS AND TUMORS

The ovaries have a dual function: they produce germ cells, or ova, and they synthesize the female sex hormones. Therefore, disorders of the ovaries frequently cause menstrual and fertility problems. Benign conditions of the ovaries can present as primary lesions of the ovarian structures or as secondary disorders related to hypothalamic, pituitary, or adrenal dysfunction.

OVARIAN CYSTS

Cysts are the most common form of ovarian tumor. Many are benign. A follicular cyst is one that results from occlusion of the duct of the follicle. Each month several follicles begin to develop and are blighted at various stages of development. These follicles form cavities that fill with fluid, producing a cyst. The dominant follicle normally ruptures to release the egg (ovulation) but occasionally persists and continues growing. Likewise, a luteal cyst is a persistent cystic enlargement of the corpus luteum that is formed after ovulation and does not regress in the absence of pregnancy. Functional cysts are asymptomatic unless there is substantial enlargement or bleeding into the

cyst. This can cause considerable discomfort or a dull, aching sensation on the affected side. The cyst may become twisted or may rupture into the intraabdominal cavity. These cysts usually regress spontaneously.

POLYCYSTIC OVARIAN (STEIN-LEVENTHAL) SYNDROME

Ovarian dysfunction associated with infrequent or absent menses in obese infertile women was first reported in the 1930s by Stein and Leventhal, for whom the syndrome was originally named. Once thought to be relatively rare, it now appears that this clinical entity is one of the most common endocrinologic disorders among women in the reproductive years. The syndrome characterized by hirsutism, obesity, and infertility is just one manifestation of this condition. Anovulation, causing amenorrhea or irregular menses, commonly accompanies the finding of bilaterally enlarged polycystic ovaries. Whether this condition is a primary ovarian defect or a result of hypothalamic-pituitary dysfunction is still being debated. Most women with polycystic ovarian disease have elevated luteinizing hormone (LH) levels with normal estrogen and follicle-stimulating hormone (FSH) production. Elevated levels of testosterone, dehydroepiandrosterone sulfate (DHAS), or androstenedione are not uncommon, and hyperprolactinemia or hypothyroidism occasionally is present. The diagnosis can be suspected from the clinical picture and confirmed with ultrasound or laparoscopic visualization of the ovaries. The condition usually is treated by the administration of the hypothalamic-pituitary–stimulating drug clomiphene citrate (Clomid) to induce ovulation. This drug is used carefully because it can induce extreme enlargement of the ovaries. If fertility is not desired, oral contraceptives can induce regular menses and prevent the development of endometrial hyperplasia caused by unopposed estrogen. When medication is ineffective, laser surgery to puncture the multiple follicles can be helpful. Bilateral wedge resection seldom is performed today.

BENIGN OVARIAN TUMORS

Serous cystadenoma and mucinous cystadenoma are the most common benign ovarian neoplasms. Some of these adenomas, however, are considered to have low malignant potential. They are asymptomatic unless the size is sufficient to cause abdominal enlargement. Treatment is surgical oophorectomy.

Endometriomas are the chocolate cysts that develop secondary to ovarian endometriosis (see the section on endometriosis earlier in this chapter). *Ovar-*

ian fibromas are connective tissue tumors composed of fibrocytes and collagen. They range in size from 6 to 20 cm and are treated by surgical excision. *Cystic teratomas*, or *dermoid cysts*, are derived from primordial germ cells and are composed of varying combinations of well-differentiated ectodermal, mesodermal, and endodermal elements. Not uncommonly, they contain sebaceous material, hair, or teeth. Treatment is surgical excision.

FUNCTIONING OVARIAN TUMORS

Functioning ovarian tumors are of three types: estrogen-secreting, androgen-secreting, and mixed estrogen-androgen–secreting. These tumors may be either benign or cancerous. One such tumor, the granulosa cell tumor, is associated with excess estrogen production. When it develops during the reproductive period, the persistent and uncontrolled production of estrogen interferes with the normal menstrual cycle, causing irregular and excessive bleeding, endometrial hyperplasia, or amenorrhea and fertility problems. When it develops after menopause, it causes postmenopausal bleeding, stimulation of the glandular tissues of the breast, and other signs of renewed estrogen production. Androgen-secreting tumors (Sertoli-Leydig cell tumor or androblastoma) inhibit ovulation and estrogen production. They tend to cause hirsutism and development of masculine characteristics, such as baldness, acne, oily skin, breast atrophy, and deepening of the voice. The treatment is surgical removal of the tumor.

OVARIAN CANCER

Ovarian cancer is the second most common female genitourinary cancer and the most lethal. In 1992, 21,000 new cases of ovarian cancer were reported in the United States, two thirds of which were in advanced stages of the disease. Most of these women die of the disease (13,000 women in 1992).[9] The incidence of ovarian cancer increases with age, being greatest between ages 65 and 84. Ovarian cancer is difficult to diagnose, and 60% to 70% of women have metastatic disease before the time of discovery. The most significant risk factor for ovarian cancer appears to be ovulatory age—the length of time during a woman's life when her ovarian cycle is not suppressed by pregnancy, lactation, or oral contraceptive use. The incidence of ovarian cancer is much lower in countries where women bear numerous children than in the United States.

Cancer of the ovary is complex because of the diversity of tissue types that originate in the ovary. As a result of this diversity, there are a number of different types of ovarian cancers. Malignant neo-plasms of the ovary can be divided into three categories: epithelial tumors, germ cell tumors, and gonadal stromal tumors. Epithelial tumors account for about 90% of cases.[16] These different cancers display various degrees of virulence, depending on the type of tumor and degree of differentiation involved. A well-differentiated cancer of the ovary may have produced symptoms for many months and still be found operable at the time of surgery. On the other hand, a poorly differentiated tumor may have been clinically evident for only a few days but found to be widespread and inoperable. Often no correlation exists between the duration of symptoms and the extent of the disease.

No good screening tests or other early methods of detection exist for ovarian cancer. Ovarian tumor antigen (CA-125) is an antigenic determinant expressed by more than 80% of nonmucinous ovarian epithelial cancers.[27] Although not tumor-specific for ovarian cancer (levels also are elevated in the presence of endometriosis), it has been suggested as a possible screening test for ovarian cancer. In a postmenopausal woman with a pelvic mass, an elevated CA-125 has a positive predictive value greater than 70% for cancer. It can also be used in monitoring therapy and recurrences when preoperative levels have been elevated. Although CA-125 clearly has a role in the management of ovarian cancer, its value as a cost-effective screening test has yet to be established. Transvaginal ultrasonography has also been shown to be useful in evaluating ovarian masses for malignant potential. However, the cost of universal screening for ovarian cancer using this technology has been estimated at $1 million to save one woman. The combined use of sonography and CA-125 to screen all women over age 45 would cost about $14 billion annually.[28] Further evaluation of both tests for use as screening techniques is ongoing.

Most cancers of the ovary are asymptomatic, or the symptoms are so vague that the woman seldom seeks medical care until the disease is far advanced. These vague discomforts include abdominal distress, flatulence, and bloating (especially after ingesting food). These gastrointestinal manifestations may precede other symptoms by months. Many women take antacids or bicarbonate of soda for a time before consulting a physician. The physician may also dismiss the woman's complaints as being caused by other conditions, causing a further delay in diagnosis and treatment. It is not fully understood why the initial symptoms of ovarian cancer are manifested as gastrointestinal disturbances. It is thought that biochemical changes in the peritoneal fluids may irritate the bowel or that pain originating in the ovary may be referred to the abdomen and be interpreted as a gastrointestinal disturbance. Clinically evident ascites (fluid in the peritoneal cavity) is seen in about one fourth of women with malignant ovarian tumors and is associated with worsened prognosis.

Early methods of ovarian cancer treatment consisted of homogeneous surgery, assessment of response, and subsequent chemotherapy. Current treatment methods include cytoreductive and de-bulking surgery to reduce the size of the tumor followed by immediate irradiation or chemotherapy. Chemotherapy may be given before surgery. At the time of surgery, the uterus, fallopian tubes, ovaries, and omentum are removed; the liver, diaphragm, retroperitoneal and aortic lymph nodes, and peritoneal surface should be examined. Cytologic washings commonly are done to test for cancerous cells in the peritoneal fluid. The type and sequence of treatment depend on the stage of the disease. Women with limited disease (stage Ia) do not require adjuvant treatment; women with intermediate disease (stage Ib, II) can be cured by radiotherapy after surgery; and women with advanced disease (stage III, IV) may require extensive chemotherapy.

The lack of accurate diagnostic tools and previously inconsistent staging techniques have contributed to incomplete knowledge and treatment of the disease. In addition, the resistant nature of ovarian cancers significantly affects the success of treatment and, thus, survival. Five-year survival is 85% in women whose ovarian cancer is detected and treated early; however, only 23% of all cases are detected at the localized stage. Overall, the 5-year survival rate is 39%.[9]

■ DISORDERS OF PELVIC SUPPORT AND UTERINE POSITION

The uterus and the pelvic structures are maintained in proper position by the uterosacral ligaments, round ligaments, broad ligament, and cardinal ligaments. The two cardinal ligaments maintain the cervix in its normal position. The uterosacral ligaments normally hold the uterus in a forward position (Fig. 38-4). The broad ligament suspends the uterus, fallopian tubes, and ovaries within the pelvis. The vagina is encased in the semirigid structure of the strong investing fascia. The muscular floor of the pelvis is a strong slinglike structure that supports the uterus, vagina, urinary bladder, and rectum (Fig. 38-5).

In the female anatomy, nature is faced with the problems of supporting the pelvic viscera against the force of gravity and increases in intraabdominal pressure associated with coughing, sneezing, defecation, laughing, and so on, while at the same time allowing for urination, defecation, and normal reproductive tract function (in particular, the delivery of a baby).

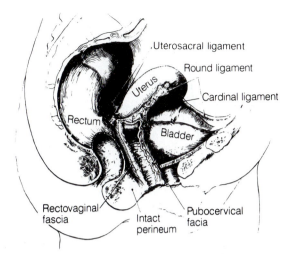

FIG. 38-4. Normal support of the uterus and vagina. (Mattingly, R. F. [1985]. *TeLinde's operative gynecology* [6th ed., p. 39]. Philadelphia: J.B. Lippincott)

Three supporting structures are provided for the abdominal pelvic diaphragm. The bony pelvis provides support and protection for parts of the digestive tract and genitourinary structures, and the peritoneum holds the pelvic viscera in place. The main support for the viscera, however, is the pelvic diaphragm, made up of muscles and connective tissue that stretch across the bones of the pelvic outlet. The openings that must exist for the urethra, rectum, and vagina cause an inherent weakness in the pelvic diaphragm. Congenital or acquired weakness of the pelvic diaphragm results in widening of these openings, particularly the vagina, with the possible herniation of pelvic viscera through the pelvic floor (prolapse).

Relaxation of the pelvic outlet usually comes about because of overstretching of the perineal supporting tissues during pregnancy and childbirth. Although the tissues are stretched only during these times, there may be no difficulty until later in life, such as the fifth or sixth decade, when further loss of elasticity and muscle tone occurs. Even in a woman who has not borne children, the combination of aging and postmenopausal changes may give rise to problems related to relaxation of the pelvic support structures. The three most common conditions associated with this relaxation are cystocele, rectocele, and uterine prolapse. These may occur separately or in association with one another.

CYSTOCELE

Cystocele is a herniation of the bladder into the vagina. It occurs when the normal muscle support for the bladder is weakened, so that the bladder sags below the uterus. The vaginal wall stretches and

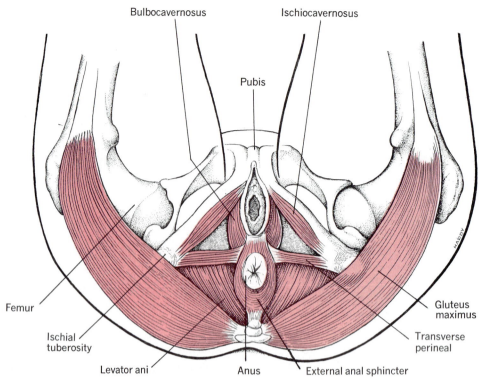

FIG. 38-5. Muscles of the pelvic floor (female perineum). (Chaffee, E. E., & Lytle, I. M. [1980]. *Basic physiology and anatomy* [4th ed.]. Philadelphia: J.B. Lippincott)

bulges downward because of the force of gravity and the pressure from coughing, lifting, straining at stool, and so on. Finally, the bladder herniates through the anterior vaginal wall, and a cystocele forms (Fig. 38-6). The symptoms include an annoying bearing-down sensation, difficulty in emptying the bladder, frequency and urgency of urination, and cystitis. Stress incontinence may occur at times of increased abdominal pressure, such as during squatting, straining, coughing, sneezing, laughing, or lifting.

RECTOCELE AND ENTEROCELE

Rectocele is the herniation of the rectum into the vagina. It occurs when the posterior vaginal wall and underlying rectum bulge forward, ultimately protruding through the introitus as the pelvic floor and perineal muscles are weakened. The symptoms include discomfort because of the protrusion of the rectum and difficulty in defecation (see Fig. 38-6). Digital pressure (splinting) on the bulging posterior wall of the vagina may become necessary for defecation.

The area between the uterosacral ligaments just posterior to the cervix may weaken and form a hernial sac into which the small bowel protrudes when the woman is standing. This defect, called an *enterocele*, may extend into the rectovaginal septum. It may

be congenital or acquired through birth trauma. Enterocele can be asymptomatic or cause a dull, dragging sensation and, occasionally, low backache.

UTERINE PROLAPSE

Uterine prolapse is the bulging of the uterus into the vagina that occurs when the primary supportive ligaments (cardinal ligaments) are stretched. Prolapse is ranked as first, second, or third degree, depending on how far the uterus protrudes through the introitus. First-degree prolapse shows some descent, but the cervix has not reached the introitus. In second-degree prolapse, the cervix or part of the uterus has passed through the introitus. The entire uterus protrudes through the vaginal opening in third-degree prolapse (procidentia).

The symptoms associated with uterine prolapse are due to irritation of the exposed mucous membranes of the cervix and vagina and the discomfort of the protruding mass. Prolapse often is accompanied by perineal relaxation, cystocele, or rectocele. Like cystocele, rectocele, and enterocele, it most commonly occurs in multiparous women, since childbearing is accompanied by injuries to pelvic structures and uterine ligaments. It may also result from pelvic tumors and neurologic conditions, such as spina bifida and diabetic neuropathy, that interrupt

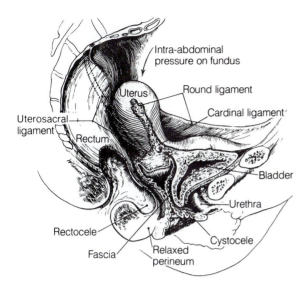

FIG. 38-6. Relaxation of pelvic support structures with descent of the uterus as well as formation of cystocele and rectocele. (Mattingly, R. F. [1985]. *TeLinde's operative gynecology* [6th ed., p. 43]. Philadelphia: J.B. Lippincott)

the innervation of pelvic muscles. A pessary may be inserted to hold the uterus in place and may stave off surgical intervention in women who want to have children or in older women for whom the surgery might pose a significant health risk.

TREATMENT OF PELVIC SUPPORT DISORDERS

Most of the disorders of pelvic relaxation require surgical correction. These are elective surgeries and usually are deferred until after the childbearing years. The symptoms associated with the disorders often are not severe enough to warrant surgical correction. In other cases, the stress of surgery is contraindicated because of other physical disorders; this is particularly true of older women, in whom many of these disorders occur.

There are a number of surgical procedures for the conditions that result from relaxation of pelvic support structures. Removal of the uterus through the vagina (vaginal hysterectomy) with appropriate repair of the vaginal wall (colporrhaphy) often is done when uterine prolapse is accompanied by cystocele or rectocele. A vesicourethral suspension may be done to alleviate the symptoms of stress incontinence. Finally, repair may involve abdominal hysterectomy along with anterior-posterior repair. Kegel exercises, which strengthen the pubococcygeus muscle, may be helpful in cases of mild cystocele or rectocele or after surgical repair to help maintain the improved function.

VARIATIONS IN UTERINE POSITION

Variations in the position of the uterus are common. Some variations are innocuous; others, which may be the result of weakness and relaxation of the perineum, give rise to various problems that compromise the structural integrity of the pelvic floor, particularly after childbirth.

The uterus usually is flexed about 45 degrees anteriorly with the cervix positioned posteriorly and downward in the anteverted position. When the female is standing, the angle of the uterus is such that it lies practically horizontal, resting lightly on the bladder. Asymptomatic normal variations in the axis of the uterus in relation to the cervix (flexion) and physiologic displacements that arise after pregnancy or with cul-de-sac pathology include anteflexion, retroflexion, and retroversion (Fig. 38-7). An anteflexed uterus is flexed forward on itself. Retroflexion is flexion backward at the isthmus. Retroversion describes the condition in which the uterus inclines posteriorly while the cervix remains tilted forward. Simple retroversion of the uterus is the most common displacement, being found in 30% of normal women. It usually is a congenital condition caused by a short anterior vaginal wall and relaxed uterosacral ligaments; together these force the uterus to fall back into the cul-de-sac of Douglas. Retroversion can also follow certain diseases, such as endometriosis and PID, which produce fibrous tissue adherence with retraction of the fundus posteriorly. Large leiomyomas may also cause the uterus to move into a posterior position. Dyspareunia with deep penetration or low back pain with menses can be associated with retro-

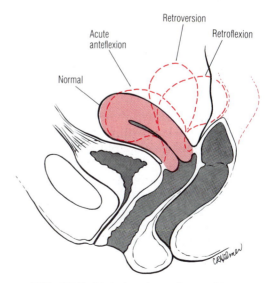

FIG. 38-7. Variations in uterine position.

version. Most symptoms in these women are due to the associated condition (*e.g.*, adhesions, fibroids) rather than to congenital retroversion.

In summary, alterations in pelvic support frequently occur because of weaknesses and relaxation of the pelvic floor and perineum. Cystocele and rectocele involve herniation of the bladder or rectum into the vagina. Uterine prolapse occurs when the uterus bulges into the vagina. Pelvic relaxation disorders typically result from overstretching of the perineal supporting muscles during pregnancy and childbirth. The loss of elasticity in these structures that is a normal accompaniment of aging contributes to these problems. Variations in uterine position are common; they include anteflexion, retroflexion, and retroversion. These disorders, which often are innocuous, can be the result of a congenital shortness of the vaginal wall, development of fibrous adhesions secondary to endometriosis or PID, or displacement caused by large uterine leiomyomas.

■ MENSTRUAL DISORDERS

DYSFUNCTIONAL MENSTRUAL CYCLES

Although unexplained uterine bleeding can occur for many reasons, such as pregnancy, abortion, blood dyscrasias, and neoplasms, the most frequent cause in the nonpregnant female is what are commonly called dysfunctional menstrual cycles or bleeding. Dysfunctional cycles may take the form of *amenorrhea* (absence of menstruation), *hypomenorrhea* (scanty menstruation), *oligomenorrhea* (infrequent menstruation, periods more than 35 days apart), *menorrhagia* (excessive menstruation), or *metrorrhagia* (bleeding between periods). *Menometrorrhagia* is heavy bleeding both during and between menstrual periods.

Dysfunctional menstrual cycles are related to alterations in the hormones that support normal cyclic endometrial changes. Estrogen deprivation causes retrogression of a previously built-up endometrium and bleeding. Such bleeding often is irregular in amount and duration, the flow varying with the time and degree of estrogen stimulation as well as the degree of estrogen withdrawal. A lack of progesterone can cause abnormal menstrual bleeding; in its absence, estrogen induces development of a much thicker endometrial layer with a richer blood supply. The absence of progesterone results from the failure of any of the developing ovarian follicles to mature to the point of ovulation with the subsequent formation of the corpus luteum and production and secretion of progesterone. Periodic bleeding episodes alternating with amenorrhea are caused by variations in the number of functioning ovarian follicles present. If a number are present and active, and if new follicles assume functional capacity, high levels of estrogen will develop, causing the endometrium to proliferate

for weeks or even months. In time, estrogen withdrawal and bleeding will develop. This can occur for two reasons: (1) an absolute estrogen deficiency may develop when several follicles simultaneously degenerate or (2) a relative deficiency may develop as the needs of the enlarged endometrial tissue mass exceed the capabilities of the existing follicles, even though estrogen levels remain constant. Both estrogen and progesterone deficiency are associated with the absence of ovulation, hence the term *anovulatory bleeding*. Because the vasoconstriction and myometrial contractions that normally accompany menstruation are caused by progesterone, anovulatory bleeding seldom is accompanied by cramps, and the flow frequently is heavy.

Anovulatory cycles are common among adolescents during the first several years after menarche, when ovarian function is becoming established, and among perimenopausal women, whose ovarian function is beginning to decline.

Dysfunctional menstrual cycles can originate as a primary disorder of the ovaries or as a secondary defect in ovarian function related to hypothalamic-pituitary stimulation. The latter can be initiated by emotional stress, marked variation in weight (sudden gain or loss), or nonspecific endocrine or metabolic disturbances. Organic causes of irregular menstrual bleeding include endometrial polyps, submucous myoma (fibroid), blood dyscrasia, infection, endometrial cancer, polycystic ovarian disease, and pregnancy.

The treatment of dysfunctional bleeding depends on what is identified as the probable cause. A detailed history with emphasis on bleeding pattern and a physical examination should be the minimum evaluation that is done. Endocrine studies (FSH-LH ratio, prolactin, testosterone, DHAS), β-hCG pregnancy test, endometrial biopsy, D&C with or without hysteroscopy, and progesterone withdrawal tests may be needed for diagnosis. If organic problems are ruled out and alterations in hormone levels are the primary cause, treatment may include the use of oral contraceptives, cyclic progesterone therapy, or long-acting progesterone injections.[29]

AMENORRHEA

There are two types of amenorrhea: primary and secondary. Primary amenorrhea is the failure to menstruate by age 16, or by age 14 if failure to menstruate is accompanied by absence of secondary sex characteristics. Secondary amenorrhea is the cessation of menses for at least 6 months in a woman who has established normal menstrual cycles. Primary amenorrhea usually is due to gonadal dysgenesis, congenital müllerian agenesis, testicular feminization, or a hypothalamic-pituitary-ovarian axis disorder. Causes of secondary amenorrhea include ovarian, pituitary, or hypothalamic dysfunction; intrauterine adhesions (Asherman's syndrome); infections (tuberculosis, schistosomiasis); pituitary tumor; anorexia nervosa; or strenuous physical exercise, which can alter the critical body fat–muscle ratio needed for menses to occur.[29] Diagnostic evaluation resembles that for dysfunctional uterine bleeding, with the possible addition of a computed tomographic (CT) scan to rule out a pituitary tumor. Treatment is based on correcting the underlying cause and inducing menstruation with cyclic progesterone or combined estrogen-progesterone regimens.

DYSMENORRHEA

Dysmenorrhea is pain or discomfort with menstruation. Although not usually a serious medical problem, it causes some degree of monthly disability for a significant number of women. There are two forms of dysmenorrhea: primary and secondary.

Primary dysmenorrhea is menstrual pain that is not associated with a physical abnormality or pathology. It usually occurs with ovulatory menstruation beginning 6 months to 2 years after menarche. Symptoms may begin 1 to 2 days before menses, peak on the first day of flow, and subside within several hours to several days. Severe dysmenorrhea may be associated with systemic symptoms such as headache, nausea, vomiting, diarrhea, fatigue, irritability, dizziness, and syncope. The pain typically is described as dull, lower abdominal aching or cramping, spasmodic or colicky in nature, often radiating to the lower back, labia majora, or upper thighs.

Secondary dysmenorrhea is menstrual pain caused by specific organic conditions, such as endometriosis, uterine fibroids, adenomyosis, pelvic adhesions, IUDs, or PID. Laparoscopy often is required for diagnosis of secondary dysmenorrhea if medication for primary dysmenorrhea is ineffective.

Treatment for primary dysmenorrhea is directed at symptom control. Although analgesic agents such as aspirin and acetaminophen may relieve minor uterine cramping or low back pain, prostaglandin synthetase inhibitors, such as ibuprofen, naproxen, mefanamic acid, and indomethacin, are more specific for dysmenorrhea and the treatment of choice if contraception is not a concern. Ovulation suppression and symptomatic relief of dysmenorrhea can be instituted simultaneously with the use of oral contraceptives. Relief of secondary dysmenorrhea depends on identifying the cause of the problem. Medical or surgical intervention may be needed to eliminate the problem.

PREMENSTRUAL SYNDROME

The premenstrual syndrome (PMS) is a distinct clinical entity characterized by a cluster of physical and psychological symptoms limited to 3 to 14 days preceding menstruation that are relieved by onset of the menses. According to recent surveys, 30% to 40% of the adult female population in the United States experience some monthly symptoms that they attribute to PMS.[30] How many of these women have symptoms that are severe enough to warrant treatment is unknown. The incidence of PMS seems to increase with age. It is less common in women in their teens and 20s, with the highest number of women seeking help for the problem being in their mid-30s. There is some dispute about whether PMS occurs more frequently in women who have not had children or in those who have had children. The disorder is not culturally distinct; it affects non-Westerners as well as Westerners.

The physical symptoms of PMS include painful and swollen breasts, bloating, abdominal pain, headache, and backache. Psychologically, there may be depression, anxiety, irritability, and behavioral changes. In some cases, there are puzzling alterations in motor function, such as clumsiness and altered handwriting. Women with PMS may report one or several symptoms, with symptoms varying from woman to woman and from month to month in the same patient. Signs and symptoms associated with this disorder are summarized in Table 38-1.

PMS can significantly affect a woman's ability to perform at normal levels. She may lose time from or function ineffectively at work. Family responsibilities and relationships may suffer. Students have been known to have lower grades during the premenstrual period. More crimes are committed by females during the premenstrual phase of the cycle, and more lives are lost to suicide during this period.

Although the causes of PMS are poorly documented, they are probably multifactorial. Like dysmenorrhea, only recently has PMS become recognized as a bona fide disorder rather than merely a psychosomatic illness.

There has been a tendency to link the disorder with endocrine imbalances such as hyperprolactinemia, estrogen excess, and alteration in estrogen-progesterone ratio. Prolactin concentration affects sodium and water retention, is higher in the luteal phase than in the follicular phase, and can be increased by estrogens, stress, and hypoglycemia as well as by pregnancy and oral contraceptives.[30] Estrogens stimulate anxiety and nervous tension, while increased progesterone levels may produce depression. The role of hormonal factors in the etiology of PMS is supported by two well-established phenom-

TABLE 38-1. SYMPTOMS OF PREMENSTRUAL SYNDROME (PMS) BY SYSTEM

BODY SYSTEM	SYMPTOMS
Cerebral	Irritability, anxiety, nervousness, fatigue, and exhaustion; increased physical and mental activity; lability; crying spells; depressions; inability to concentrate
Gastrointestinal	Craving for sweets or salts, lower abdominal pain, bloating, nausea, vomiting, diarrhea, constipation
Vascular	Headache, edema, weakness, or fainting
Reproductive	Swelling and tenderness of the breasts, pelvic congestion, ovarian pain, altered libido
Neuromuscular	Trembling of the extremities, changes in coordination, clumsiness, backache, leg aches
General	Weight gain, insomnia, dizziness, acne

ena: first, women who have undergone a hysterectomy but not an oophorectomy may have cyclic symptoms that resemble PMS; second, PMS symptoms are rare in postmenopausal women. Research has failed to confirm these theories. Other hypotheses suggest that increased aldosterone may contribute to symptoms associated with fluid retention (headache, bloating, breast tenderness, and weight gain); that pyridoxine (vitamin B_6) deficiency may lead to estrogen excess or decrease production of the neurotransmitters dopamine and serotonin, which in turn may contribute to PMS symptoms; or that decreased prostaglandin E_1 (PGE_1) concentrations can lead to abnormal sensitivity to prolactin, with associated fluid retention, irritability, and depression. In addition, increased appetite, binge eating, fatigue, and depression have been associated with altered endorphin activity and subclinical hypoglycemia.[30–32] There is also evidence that learned beliefs about menstruation can contribute to the production of PMS or at least affect the woman's response to the symptoms.

Diagnosis centers on identification of the symptom clusters by means of prospective charting for at least 3 months. A complete history and physical examination are necessary to rule out other physical causes of the symptoms. Depending on the symptom pattern, blood studies, including thyroid hormones, glucose, and prolactin assays, may be done. Psychosocial evaluation is helpful to rule out emotional illness that is merely exacerbated premenstrually.

In the past, the treatment of PMS has been largely symptomatic. Attempts have been made to effect weight loss and reduce fluid retention through the use of diuretics. Tranquilizer drugs were used to treat mood changes, and pain was treated with mild analgesics. The current treatment is still, to some extent, directed toward somatic complaints. Relief of somatic pain does not, however, totally resolve PMS suffering. The latest approach is to recommend an integrated program of personal assessment by diary, regular exercise, avoidance of caffeine, and a diet low in simple sugars and high in lean proteins. Additional therapeutic regimens include vitamin or mineral supplements (particularly pyridoxine, vitamin E, and magnesium), natural progesterone supplements, low-dose monophasic oral contraceptives, GnRH agonists, bromocriptine for prolactin suppression, danazol (a synthetic androgen), spironolactone (an aldosterone antagonist and steroidogenesis inhibitor), evening primrose oil (contains linoleic acid, a precursor of prostaglandin PGE_1), and lithium for marked functional impairment from affective symptoms.[31] The daily use of prescribed relaxation techniques during the premenstrual period have been shown to improve both physical and emotional symptoms.[32] Management includes education and support directed toward life-style changes. Drug therapy should be used cautiously until well-controlled studies establish criteria for use and effective treatment results. Placebo effect may account for symptom relief in a significant number of women. It is unlikely that a single cause or treatment for PMS will ever be found. Evaluation and management should focus on identifying and controlling the individual symptom clusters when possible.

In summary, menstrual disorders include dysfunctional menstrual cycles, dysmenorrhea, and premenstrual syndrome. Dysfunctional menstrual cycles occur when the hormonal support of the endometrium is altered. These cycles produce amenorrhea, oligomenorrhea, metrorrhagia, or menorrhagia. Dysmenorrhea is characterized by pain or discomfort during menses. It can occur as a primary or secondary disorder. Primary dysmenorrhea is not associated with other disorders and begins soon after menarche. Secondary dysmenorrhea is caused by a specific organic condition, such as endometriosis or pelvic adhesions. It occurs in women with previously painless menses. PMS represents a cluster of physical and psychological symptoms that precede menstruation by 1 to 2 weeks. The true incidence and nature of PMS has only recently been recognized, and its cause and methods for treatment are still under study.

■ DISORDERS OF THE BREAST

Most breast disease may be described as either benign or cancerous. Breast tissue is never static; the breast is constantly responding to changes in hormonal, nutritional, psychological, and environmental stimuli that cause continual cellular changes. Benign breast conditions are nonprogressive; some forms of benign disease, however, increase the risk of malignant disease. In light of this, strict adherence to a dichotomy of benign versus malignant disease may not always be appropriate. This dichotomy is, however, useful for the sake of simplicity and clarity.

GALACTORRHEA

Galactorrhea is the secretion of breast milk in a nonlactating breast. Galactorrhea may result from vigorous nipple stimulation during lovemaking, exogenous hormones, internal hormonal imbalance, or local chest infection or trauma. A pituitary tumor may produce large amounts of prolactin and cause galactorrhea. Galactorrhea occurs in both men and women and usually is benign. Observation may be continued for several months before diagnostic hormonal screening.

MASTITIS

Mastitis is an inflammation of the breast. It most frequently occurs during lactation but may also result from other conditions.

In the lactating woman, inflammation results from an ascending infection that travels from the nipple to the ductile structures. The offending organisms originate from either the suckling infant's nasopharynx or the mother's hands. During the early weeks of nursing, the breast is particularly vulnerable to bacterial invasion because of minor cracks and fissures that occur with vigorous suckling. Infection and inflammation cause obstruction of the ductile system; the breast area becomes hard, inflamed, and tender if not treated early. Without treatment, the area becomes walled off and may abscess, requiring incision and drainage. It is advisable for the mother to continue breastfeeding during antibiotic therapy to prevent this. Mastitis is not confined to the postpartum period; it can occur as a result of hormonal fluctuations, tumors, trauma, or skin infection. Cyclic inflammation of the breast occurs most frequently in adolescents, who commonly have a fluctuating hormone level. Tumors may cause mastitis secondary to skin involvement or lymphatic obstruction. Local trauma or infection may develop into mastitis because of ductal blockage of trapped blood, cellular debris, or the extension of superficial inflammation.

The treatment for mastitis symptoms may include application of heat or cold, excision, aspiration, mild analgesics, antibiotics, and a supportive brassiere or breast binder.

DUCTAL DISORDERS

Ductal ectasia presents in older women as a spontaneous, intermittent, usually unilateral, grayish green nipple discharge. Palpation of the breast increases the discharge. Ectasia occurs during or after menopause and is symptomatically associated with burning, itching, pain, and a pulling sensation of the nipple and areola. The disease results in inflammation of the ducts with subsequent thickening. The treatment requires removal of the involved ductal mass.

Intraductal papillomas are benign epithelial tissue tumors that range in size from 2 mm to 5 cm. Papillomas usually present with a bloody nipple discharge. The tumor may be palpated in the areolar area. The papilloma is probed through the nipple, and the involved duct is thus removed.

FIBROADENOMA AND FIBROCYSTIC DISEASE

Fibroadenoma is seen in premenopausal women (most commonly in the third and fourth decade). The clinical findings include a firm, rubbery, sharply defined round mass. On palpation, the mass "slides" between the fingers and is easily movable. These masses usually are singular; only 15% are multiple or bilateral. Fibroadenoma is asymptomatic and usually found by accident. It is not believed to be precancerous. The treatment involves simple excision.

Fibrocystic breast disease (mammary dysplasia) is a condition typified by the development of fibrosis and cystic tissue formation. It is the single most common disorder of the breast and accounts for 50% to 75% of the surgical procedures on the female breast. The term *fibrocystic disease* has become a catchall for breast irregularities that occur bilaterally, change cyclically, and, in younger women, are accompanied by dull, aching pain and heaviness. Some clinicians believe that the term is overused and that the breast changes associated with this process are a result of hormonally modulated proliferative activity with incomplete resolution. This incomplete resolution may be a result of excess hormonal stimulation or hypersensitive breast epithelium.[33] On the other hand, some clinicians believe that fibrocystic disease is part of a continuum of breast pathology related to cancer. This is particularly true when the fibrocystic disease includes epithelial hyperplasia or demonstrable calcifications.

Fibrocystic disease usually presents as nodular ("shotty"), granular breast masses that are more prominent and painful during the luteal or progesterone-dominant portion of the menstrual cycle. Discomfort ranges from heaviness to exquisite tenderness, depending on the degree of vascular engorgement and cystic distention. Diagnosis is made by physical examination, biopsy (either aspiration or tissue sample), and mammography. The use of mammography for diagnosis in high-risk groups under age 35 on a routine basis is still controversial. Mammography may be helpful in establishing the diagnosis, but increased breast tissue density in women with fibrocystic disease may make an abnormal or cancerous mass difficult to discern among the other structures. Hand-held sonography (ultrasound) can be useful in clarifying inconclusive mammographic densities.

The treatment for fibrocystic breast disease usually is symptomatic. Aspirin, mild analgesics, and local heat or cold may be recommended. Some physicians attempt to aspirate prominent or persistent cysts and send any fluid obtained to the laboratory for cytologic analysis. Women are advised to avoid foods that contain the xanthines (coffee, cola, chocolate, and tea) in their daily diets, particularly premenstrually. Vitamin E may be helpful in reducing mastalgia (breast pain), and women should be encouraged to wear a good supporting brassiere. Danazol can be used for women with severe pain, although the potential for adverse effects warrants trying other methods first.

There is controversy regarding the relation between fibrocystic disease and cancer of the breast. It appears that the catchall term "fibrocystic disease" encompasses several disorders, some of which may undergo malignant changes. Nonproliferative lesions (70%) do not demonstrate added risk for cancer; proliferative lesions without atypia (26%) may have a slightly increased risk for cancer. The remaining 4% of women with "fibrocystic" disease per biopsy show proliferative lesions with atypia and have a four times increased risk of cancer.[33] Suffice it to say that any discrete mass or lump on the breast should be viewed as possible carcinoma, and cancer should be ruled out before the conservative measures used to treat fibrocystic disease are used.

BREAST CANCER

Cancer of the breast is second only to lung cancer as a cause of cancer-related death in women. One in nine women in the United States will have breast cancer in her lifetime. In 1992, breast cancer affected 180,000 American women and killed almost 46,000 women. An additional 300 deaths occurred from breast cancer in males. Risk factors for breast cancer include being female, being over age 50, having a personal or family history of breast cancer, and having had no full-term pregnancies or a first child after age 30.[9]

Almost all breast cancers (90%) are found by women themselves, often through breast self-examination (BSE). Cancer may present clinically as a mass, a puckering, nipple retraction, or an unusual discharge. Some women identify cancer when only a thickening or subtle change in breast contour is noted. The variety of symptoms and the high self-discovery rate underscore the need for regular, systematic self-examination.

BSE should be done routinely by women over age 20. Premenopausal women should conduct the examination right after the cessation of menses. This time is most appropriate in relation to the cyclic breast changes that occur in response to changes in hormone levels. Postmenopausal women and women who have had a hysterectomy should perform the examination on about the same day of every month. A woman can choose a day relative to her past menstrual history. Examination may conveniently be done in the shower or bath or at bedtime. The most important thing is to devise a regular, systematic, convenient, and consistent method of examination.

X-ray mammography is the only effective screening technique for the early detection of clinically inapparent lesions. A generally slow-growing form of cancer, breast cancer may have been present for 2 to 9 years before it reaches 1 cm, the smallest size mass normally detected by palpation. Mammography can disclose lesions as small as 1 mm as well as clustering of calcifications that may warrant biopsy to exclude cancer. The American Cancer Society recommends a baseline mammogram between ages 35 and 40, studies every 1 to 2 years between 40 and 49 years, and annual evaluation for women over age 50.

Procedures used in the diagnosis of breast cancer include physical examination, mammography, thermography, ultrasonography, percutaneous needle aspiration, and excisional biopsy. Breast cancer often presents as a solitary, painless, firm, fixed lesion with poorly defined borders. It can be found anywhere in the breast but is most common in the upper outer quadrant. Because of the variability in presentation, any suspicious change in breast tissue warrants further investigation. The diagnostic use of mammography enables additional definition of the clinically suspicious area (*e.g.*, appearance, character, calcification). Placement of a wire marker under radiographic guidance can ensure accurate surgical biopsy of nonpalpable suspicious areas. Ultrasonography is useful as a diagnostic adjunct to differentiate cystic from tumor tissue in women with nonspecific thickening. Fine-needle aspiration is a simple in-office procedure that can be performed repeatedly in multiple sites and with minimal discomfort. When performed in conjunction with hand-held sonography, it can be useful in defining cystic masses or fibrocystic changes and in providing cytologic evaluation.[34] Excisional biopsy provides the only definitive diagnosis of breast cancer. Thermography (temperature detection), CT mammography, and diaphanography (transillumination) are still considered experimental, since their diagnostic capabilities for breast cancer detection remain unproven. Tumors are classified histologically according to tissue characteristics and staged clinically according to tumor size, nodal involvement, and presence of metastasis. It is recommended that estrogen and progesterone receptor analysis be performed on surgical specimens. Information about the presence or absence of estrogen and progesterone receptors can be used in predicting tumor responsiveness to hormonal manipulation. High levels of both receptors improve the prognosis and increase the likelihood of remission.

The treatment methods for breast cancer are controversial. They may include surgery, chemotherapy, radiation therapy, and hormonal manipulation. Radical mastectomy (removal of the entire breast, underlying muscles, and all axillary nodes) has fallen into disfavor as a primary surgical therapy for breast cancer. Modified surgical techniques (mastectomy plus axillary dissection or lumpectomy) accompanied by chemotherapy or radiation therapy have achieved outcomes comparable to radical surgical methods. The prognosis is related more to the extent of nodal involvement than to the extent of breast involvement. Greater nodal involvement requires more aggressive postsurgical treatment; therefore, many cancer specialists believe that a diagnosis of breast cancer is not complete until dissection and testing of the axillary lymph nodes has been accomplished. The 5-year survival rate for localized cancer is 92%; with nodal involvement, it is about 71%. Reconstructive breast surgery, done simultaneously with mastectomy or as a delayed procedure, offers improved quality of life. Early detection, however, is still the best bargain.

PAGET'S DISEASE

Paget's disease accounts for 2% to 3% of all breast cancers. The disease presents as an eczemoid lesion localized to the nipple and areola. Paget's disease is treated locally but may indicate systemic disease. Complete examination is, therefore, recommended

in cases of Paget's disease, including a mammogram and, usually, biopsy.

In summary, the breasts are subject to both benign and malignant disease. Mastitis is inflammation of the breast, occurring most frequently during lactation. Galactorrhea is an abnormal secretion of milk that may occur as a symptom of increased prolactin secretion. Both ductal ectasia and intraductal papilloma cause abnormal drainage from the nipple. Fibroadenoma and fibrocystic disease are characterized by abnormal masses in the breast that are benign. By far the most important disease of the breast is breast cancer, which is a significant cause of death in women. BSE affords a woman the best protection against breast cancer. It provides the means for early detection of breast cancer and, in many cases, allows for early treatment and cure.

■ INFERTILITY

Infertility—the inability to conceive a child after 1 year of unprotected intercourse—affects about 15% of couples in the United States. *Primary infertility* refers to situations in which there has been no prior conception. *Secondary infertility* is infertility that occurs after one or more previous pregnancies. *Sterility* is the inability to father a child or, for a woman, to become pregnant because of congenital anomalies, disease, or surgical intervention. About 1% to 2% of U.S. couples are affected by sterility.

The complexity of the process that must occur to achieve a pregnancy is taken for granted by most couples. For some couples, pregnancy occurs far too easily, whereas for others, no amount of money, hard work, love, patience, or medical resources seems to be able to bring about this amazing, desired event. Although a full discussion of the diagnosis and treatment of infertility is beyond the scope of this book, an overview of the areas in which problems can occur is presented. The causes of infertility are almost equally divided between male factors (30% to 40%), female factors (30% to 40%), and combined factors (30% to 40%). In about 10% to 15% of infertile couples, the cause remains unknown even after a full work-up.

MALE FACTORS

For pregnancy to occur, the male must be able to provide sperm in sufficient quantity, delivered to the upper end of the vagina, with adequate motility to traverse the female reproductive tract. The male contribution to this process is assessed by means of a semen analysis, which evaluates volume of semen (normally 2 to 5 mL), sperm density (greater than 20 million/mL), motility (greater than 50% good progressive), viability (greater than 50%), morphology (greater than 60% normal), and viscosity (full liquefaction within 20 minutes). The specimen is best collected by masturbation into a sterile container after 3 days of abstinence. Because of variability in specimens, abnormal results should lead to a repeat test before the need for treatment is presumed. *Azoospermia* is the absence of sperm; *oligospermia* refers to decreased numbers of sperm; and *asthenospermia* refers to poor motility of sperm. Tests of sperm function include a cervical mucus penetration test (postcoital test, Penetrak), sperm penetration assay (Hamster Zona Free Ovum test), and sperm antibody testing.

The causes of male infertility include varicocele, ejaculatory dysfunction, hyperprolactinemia, hypogonadotropic hypogonadism, infection, immunologic problems (sperm antibodies), obstruction, and congenital anomalies. Risk factors for sperm problems include history of mumps orchitis, cryptorchidism (undescended testes), testicular torsion, hypospadias, previous urologic surgery, infection, and exposure to known gonadotoxins.[35] Treatment depends on the cause and may include surgery, medication, or the use of artificial insemination to deliver a more concentrated specimen directly to the cervical canal or uterine fundus. Artificial insemination with donor sperm can be offered if the male is sterile and this is an acceptable alternative to both husband and wife.

FEMALE FACTORS

The female contribution to pregnancy is more complex, requiring production and release of a mature ovum capable of being fertilized; production of cervical mucus that assists in sperm transport and maintains sperm viability within the female reproductive tract; patent fallopian tubes with the motility potential to pick up and transfer the ovum to the uterine cavity; development of an endometrium that is suitable for the implantation and nourishment of a fertilized ovum; and a uterine cavity that allows for growth and development of a fetus. Each of these factors is discussed briefly, along with an overview of diagnostic tests and treatment.

OVULATORY DYSFUNCTION

In a normally menstruating female, ovulatory cycles begin several months to a year after menarche. Release of FSH from the pituitary causes the development of several primordial follicles within the ovary. At some point, a dominant follicle is selected and the remaining follicles undergo atresia. When the dominant follicle has become large enough to contain a mature ovum (16 to 20 mm in diameter) and is producing sufficient estradiol to ensure adequate prolif-

eration of the endometrium, production of LH increases—the LH surge—and the increased LH level induces release of the ovum from within the follicle (ovulation). After ovulation, under the influence of LH, the former follicle luteinizes and begins producing progesterone in addition to estradiol. The progesterone stimulates the development of secretory endometrium, which has the capability to nourish a fertilized ovum if one should implant. The presence of progesterone after ovulation causes a rise in the woman's basal body temperature (BBT). This thermogenic property of progesterone provides the basis for the simplest, most inexpensive beginning test of ovulatory function—the measurement of BBT. Women should be able to detect at least a 0.4°F rise in their BBT (at rest) after ovulation that should be maintained throughout the luteal phase. This biphasic temperature pattern not only demonstrates that ovulation has taken place but also where in the cycle it occurred and the length of the luteal phase. BBT can be influenced by many other factors, including restless sleep, alcohol intake, drug use, fever due to illness, and change in usual rising time. However, as an initial step in the infertility investigation, it can provide useful information to direct other forms of testing.

Endometrial biopsy (removal of a sample of the endometrium during an office procedure) provides histologic evidence of secretory endometrium and the level of maturation of the lining. The luteal phase should be consistently 14 days in length because without pregnancy and the subsequent secretion of hCG, the corpus luteum begins to degenerate. LH is produced by the pituitary only for 7 to 10 days after the initial surge. The luteal phase of the cycle, therefore, is so consistent that a pathologist can tell by evaluating a section of endometrium that it is representative of a particular day of the luteal phase. The pathologist's assessment of maturation is compared with the arrival of the next menses. If a discrepancy of more than 2 days exists, the woman is said to have a luteal phase defect (LPD). This diagnosis indicates that although ovulation is occurring, endometrial development is insufficient and implantation may not be possible. Pregnancy requires both fertilization and implantation. LPD can also be suggested by an abnormal serum progesterone level 7 days after ovulation. It can be treated directly with supplemental progesterone after ovulation or with the use of clomiphene citrate to stimulate increased pituitary production of FSH and LH.

Anovulation (no ovulation) and oligo-ovulation (irregular ovulation) are other forms of ovulatory dysfunction. These problems can be identified by the tests for LPD previously described. Ovulatory problems can be primary problems of the ovary or secondary problems related to endocrine dysfunction. Therefore, when disturbances in ovulation are confirmed, it is reasonable to evaluate other endocrine function before initiating treatment. If pituitary hormone (FSH, LH, prolactin) tests, thyroid studies, and tests of adrenal function (DHAS, androstanedione) are normal, then ovulatory dysfunction is primary and should respond to treatment. Abnormalities in any of the other endocrine areas should be further evaluated as needed and treated appropriately. Hyperprolactinemia responds well to bromocriptine, but pituitary microadenoma may need to be ruled out first; hypothyroidism requires thyroid replacement; hyperthyroidism requires suppressive therapy and, sometimes, surgical intervention with thyroid replacement later; adrenal suppression can be instituted with dexamethasone, a glucocorticoid analogue. Normal ovulatory function may resume without further intervention; if not, treatment can be concurrent with management of other endocrine problems.

CERVICAL MUCUS PROBLEMS

High preovulatory levels of estradiol stimulate the production of large amounts of clear, stretchy cervical mucus that aids the transport of sperm into the uterine cavity and helps to maintain an environment that keeps the sperm viable for up to 72 hours. Insufficient estrogen production (inherent or secondary to treatment with clomiphene citrate, an antiestrogen), cervical abnormalities from disease or invasive procedures (DES exposure, stenosis, conization), and cervical infection (chlamydial or mycoplasmal infection, gonorrhea) can adversely affect the production of healthy cervical mucus. A postcoital test (Sims-Huhner) involves evaluation of the cervical mucus 1 to 8 hours after intercourse within the 48 hours before ovulation. A sample of cervical mucus is obtained using a special syringe and evaluated grossly for amount, clarity, and stretch (spinnbarkeit) and microscopically for cellularity, for number and quality of motile sperm, and for the presence of ferning after the sample has air-dried on the slide. To obtain good-quality mucus, it is essential to obtain the sample within the 48 hours before ovulation. Tests may have to be repeated within the same cycle or in subsequent cycles to ensure appropriate timing. If inadequate estrogen effect is seen (poor-quality mucus), supplemental oral estrogen can be given in the first 9 days of the next cycle and the test can be repeated. Administration of mucolytic expectorants (1 tsp four times daily starting day 10 until ovulation is confirmed) may also improve the quality of the mucus. If mucus is good but sperm are inadequate in number or motility, further evaluation of the male may be needed. Both the male and the female should be tested for sperm antibodies when repeated postcoital tests reveal that the sperm are all dead or agglutinated. Artificial insemination with the husband's sperm may be helpful to bypass the cervical mucus. Cervical cultures for gonorrhea and chlamydial and mycoplasmal infection should be obtained with the postcoital test if they have not already been acquired. If the cultures give positive results, treatment should be instituted as needed.

UTERINE CAVITY ABNORMALITIES

Alterations within the uterine cavity can occur secondary to DES exposure, submucous fibroids, cervical polyps, synechiae or bands of scar tissue, or congenital anomalies (e.g., bicornuate septum, single horn). These defects may be suspected from history or pelvic examination but require hysterosalpingography (an x-ray study in which dye is placed through the cervix to outline the uterine cavity and demonstrate tubal patency) or hysteroscopy (a study in which a lighted fiberoptic scope placed through the cervix under general anesthesia allows direct visualization of the uterine cavity) for confirmation. Treatment is surgical when possible.

TUBAL FACTORS

Tubal patency is required for fertilization and can be disrupted secondary to PID, ectopic pregnancy (salpingectomy or salpingostomy), large myomas, endometriosis, pelvic adhesions, and previous tubal ligation. Hysterosalpingography can reveal the location and type of any blockage present (fimbrial, cornual, hydrosalpinx). Sometimes microsurgical repair is possible.

Even when tubal patency is demonstrated, it is possible for tubal disease to make ovum pick up impossible. Contrary to popular belief, the ovum is not extruded directly into the fallopian tube. Rather, the tube must be free to move to engulf the ovum after release. Pelvic adhesions from previous infection, surgery, or endometriosis can interfere with the tube's mobility. Laparoscopic evaluation of the pelvis is needed for diagnosis. Laser surgery or cautery can be used for the lysis of adhesions and removal of endometriosis either through the laparoscope or, if severe, with laparotomy.

NEW TECHNOLOGIES

In vitro fertilization (IVF) was developed in 1978 for women with significantly damaged or absent tubes to provide them an opportunity for pregnancy where none normally exists. The ovaries are superstimulated to produce multiple follicles using clomiphene citrate, human menopausal menotropins (Pergonal), pure FSH (Metrodin), or a combination of these drugs. Follicular maturation is monitored by means of ultrasonography and assay of serum estradiol levels. When preovulatory criteria are met, an injection of hCG is given to simulate an LH surge; 34 hours later, the follicles are aspirated either laparoscopically or by the newer ultrasound-guided transvaginal route. The follicular fluid is evaluated microscopically for the presence of ova, which, when found, are removed and placed into culture media in an incubator. The eggs are inseminated with semen from the husband that has been prepared by a washing technique that removes the semen, begins the capacitation process, and allows the strongest sperm to be used for fertilization. Then, 12 to 24 hours after insemination, the ova are evaluated for signs of fertilization. If signs are present, the ova are returned to the incubator. Finally, 48 to 72 hours after egg retrieval, the fertilized eggs are placed back into the woman's uterus by means of a transcervical catheter. Hormonal supplementation of the luteal phase often is used to increase the possibility of implantation. The overall live delivery rate for 1990, as reported by the National IVF-ET registry, was 14% per egg retrieval.[36] By mid-1992, more than 30,000 babies had been born worldwide using IVF technology, and future research will no doubt be focused on understanding and improving the implantation process. Indications for IVF have been expanded to include male factors (severe oligospermia or asthenospermia), immunologic infertility, severe endometriosis, and idiopathic or unknown infertility. The substantial risk of multiple births with IVF procedures has been reduced with the availability of cryopreservation, which allows freezing of excess embryos and limits the number of fresh embryos transferred.

An outgrowth of IVF technology is gamete intrafallopian transfer (GIFT), which uses similar ovarian stimulation protocols and laparoscopic egg retrieval and involves placing ovum and sperm directly into the fallopian tube during the same laparoscopy procedure. This procedure requires at least one patent fallopian tube and was developed primarily to try to increase the pregnancy rate in women with idiopathic infertility. The basic premises are that if a transportation problem is interfering with ovum pick up, GIFT would solve that problem, and that implantation might result more often if fertilization occurs within the body. The live delivery rate for 1990 was 22%.[35] The multiple birth rate with GIFT is similar to that with IVF.

Newer advanced reproductive technologies include zygote intrafallopian transfer (ZIFT) and tubal embryo transplant (TET). With ZIFT, the zygote is placed laparosopically into the fallopian tube after the traditional IVF procedure. With TET, the embryos are transferred into the fallopian tubes transcervically using ultrasound guidance or by means of hysteroscopy. The theoretical advantages of these procedures involve tubal factors that may facilitate implantation. Live delivery rate for ZIFT-related procedures in 1990 was 16%.[35]

In summary, infertility affects about 15% of couples in the United States and often is a multifactorial problem. The evaluation can be lengthy and highly stressful for the couple. Options for therapy continue to expand, but newer treatment modalities, such as IVF and GIFT, are expensive, and financial resources can be strained while couples seek their sometimes elusive dream of having a child.

■ REFERENCES

1. Friedrich, E.G. (1983). *Vulvar disease* (2nd ed., pp. 130–140, 200). Philadelphia: W.B. Saunders.
2. Pernoll, M.L., & Benson, R.C. (1991). *Current obstetric and gynecologic diagnosis and treatment* (pp. 740, 922, 926, 931, 932, 934, 943, 952, 991). E. Norwalk, CT: Appleton & Lange.
3. Van Nagell, J.R., Powell, D.F., & Gay, E.C. (1983). Cancer of the vagina–Part 1. *Female Patient, 8*(5), 15.
4. Manetta, A., Pinto, J.L., Larson, J.E., et al. (1988). Primary invasive carcinoma of the vagina. *Obstetrics and Gynecology, 72*(1), 77.
5. Van Nagell, J.R., Powell, D.F., & Gay, E.C. (1983). Cancer of the vagina—Part 2. *Female Patient, 8*(6), 24.
6. Robbins, S.L., Cotran, R.S., & Kumar, V. (1984). *Pathologic basis of disease* (2nd ed., p. 1121). Philadelphia: W.B. Saunders.
7. Nichols, D.H., & Evrard, J.R. (1985). *Ambulatory gynecology* (pp. 319–322). Philadelphia: Harper & Row.
8. Paavonen, J., Critchlow, C.W., DeRouen, T., et al. (1986). Etiology of cervical inflammation. *American Journal of Obstetrics and Gynecology, 154*, 556.
9. American Cancer Society. (1992). *Cancer facts and figures 1992* (pp. 11, 13). New York: American Cancer Society.
10. Schaffer, S.D., & Philput, C.B. (1990). Predictors of abnormal cervical cytology: Statistical analysis of HPV and cofactors. *Nurse Practitioner, 17*(3), 21.
11. Rubin, M.M., & Lauver, D. (1990). Assessment and management of cervical intraepithelial neoplasia. *Nurse Practitioner, 15*(9), 23.
12. Fullerton, J.T., & Barger, M.K. (1989). Papanicolaou smear—an update on classification and management. *Journal of the American Academy of Nurse Practitioners, 1*(3), 84.
13. Cherkis, R.C., Patten, S.F., Andrews, T.J., et al. (1988). Significance of normal endometrial cells detected by cervical cytology. *Obstetrics and Gynecology, 71*, 242.
14. Baggish, M.S., Campion, M.J., & Ferenczy, A.S. (1992). Exploring excision technique with LEEP. *Contemporary OB-GYN, Special issue—Technology*, 81.
15. Tawa, K., Forsythe, A., et al. (1988). A comparison of Papanicolaou smear and the cervigram: Sensitivity, specificity, and cost analysis. *Obstetrics and Gynecology, 71*, 242.

16. Danforth, D.N., & Scott, J.R. (1986). *Obstetrics and gynecology* (5th ed., pp. 918, 1080). Philadelphia: J.B. Lippincott.
17. Malinak, L.R., & Wheeler, J.M. (1985). A practical approach to endometriosis—Part 1: Diagnosis. *Female Patient, 10*(5), 39.
18. Cramer, D.W., Wilson, E., et al. (1986). The relationship of endometriosis to menstrual characteristics, smoking and exercise. *Journal of the American Medical Association, 255*, 1904.
19. Steingold, K.A., Cedars, M., Lu, J.K., et al. (1987). Treatment of endometriosis with a long-acting gonadotropin-releasing hormone agonist. *Obstetrics and Gynecology, 69*, 403.
20. Daniell, J.F., Miller, W., & Tosh, R. (1986). Initial evaluation of the use of potassium-titanyl-phosphate (KTP/532) laser in gynecologic laparoscopy. *Fertility and Sterility, 46*(3), 373.
21. Centers for Disease Control Cancer and Steroid Hormone Study. (1983). Oral contraceptive use and risk of endometrial cancer. *Journal of the American Medical Association, 249*, 1600.
22. Centers for Disease Control. (1991). Pelvic inflammatory disease—guidelines for prevention and management. *Morbidity and Mortality Weekly Report, 40*, RR-5.
23. Lee, N.C., Rubin, G.l., & Borucki, R. (1988). The intrauterine device and PID revisited: New results from the Women's Health Study. *Obstetrics and Gynecology, 72*, 1.
24. Centers for Disease Control. (1989). STD treatment guidelines 1989. *Morbidity and Mortality Weekly Report, 38*, S-8.
25. Centers for Disease Control. (1990). Ectopic pregnancy mortality 1970–1987. *Morbidity and Mortality Weekly Report, 39*(24).
26. Catlin, A.J., & Wetzel, W.S. (1991). Ectopic pregnancy—clinical evaluation, diagnostic measures and prevention. *Nurse Practitioner, 16*(1), 38, 43.
27. Potsner, B. (1991). How serum Ca-125 serves as tumor marker. *Contemporary OB-GYN, 3*, 37.
28. Pierce, C. (1992). MDs pressured to provide ovarian cancer screening. *OB-GYN News, 27*(8), 1.
29. Murata, J.M. (1991). Abnormal genital bleeding and secondary amenorrhea. *Journal of Obstetric, Gynecologic, and Neonatal Nursing, 19*(1), 31, 33.
30. Severino, S.K., Anderson, M., Hurt, S.W., et al. (1987). Premenstrual syndrome: An update. *Female Patient, 12*(1), 69.
31. Magos, A. (1990). Advances in the treatment of the premenstrual syndrome. *British Journal of Obstetrics and Gynaecology, 97*(1), 7–10.
32. Goodale, I.L., Domar, A.D., & Benson, H. (1990). Alleviation of premenstrual syndrome symptoms with relaxation response. *Obstetrics and Gynecology, 75*(4), 649–655.
33. Norwood, S.L. (1990). Fibrocystic breast disease—an update and review. *Journal of Obstetric, Gynecologic, and Neonatal Nursing, 19*(2), 116.
34. Nyirjesy, I., & Billingsley, F. (1992). Management of breast problems in gynecologic office practice using sonography and fine needle aspiration. *Obstetrics and Gynecology, 79*(5), 699.
35. Jarow, J.P., & Lipschultz, L.I. (1987 September). Urologic evaluation of male infertility. *Contemporary OB-GYN, Special Issue*, 85.
36. Medical Research International Society for Assisted Reproductive Technology. (1992). In vitro fertilization/embryo transfer in the United States: 1990 results from the National IVF/ET Registry. *Fertility and Sterility, 57*(1), 15.

■ BIBLIOGRAPHY

Boyd, M.E. (1985). Endometriosis. *Canadian Journal of Surgery, 28*, 471.

Bullen, B.A., Skrinar, G.S., Butins, I.Z., et al. (1985). Induction of menstrual disorders by strenuous exercise in untrained women. *New England Journal of Medicine, 312*, 1349.

Bullough, B., Hindi-Alexander, M., & Fetouh, A. (1990). Methylxanthines and fibrocystic breast disease—a study of correlations. *Nurse Practitioner, 15*(3), 135.

Cowan, B.D., & Morrison, J.C. (1991). Management of genital bleeding in girls and women. *New England Journal of Medicine, 324*, 1710–1714.

Fayez, J.A., & Taylor, R.B. (1984). Endometriosis: Staging and management. *Hospital Physician, 11*, 26.

Fehrer, T.L. (1985). Chronic pain—Part 1: Primary dysmenorrhea and cryptic pelvic pain. *Female Patient, 10*(6), 44.

Hamwi, D.A. (1990). Screening mammography—increasing the effort toward breast cancer detection. *Nurse Practitioner, 15*(12), 21.

Hansen, A.M., Immordino, K.F., & Farber, M. (1984). The diagnostic evaluation and therapy of secondary amenorrhea. *Journal of Obstetric, Gynecologic, and Neonatal Nursing, 3*, 180.

Harris, J.R., Lipman, M.E., Veronesi, U., et al. (1992). Medical progress: Breast cancer. Parts I, II, III. *New England Journal of Medicine, 327*, 319–328, 390–398, 473–480.

Hewitt, J., Plisse, M., & Paniel, B.J. (1991). *Diseases of the vulva*. New York: McGraw-Hill.

Kossoff, M.M. (1992). Clinical role of breast ultrasonography. *Female Patient, 17*(4), 130.

Laube, D.W. (1986). Premenstrual syndrome. *Female Patient, 11*(1), 107.

McKenna, T.J. (1988). Pathogenesis and treatment of polycystic ovary syndrome. *New England Journal of Medicine, 318*, 558–562.

Mirecki, D.M., & Jordan, V.C. (1985). Steroid hormone receptors and human breast cancer. *Laboratory Medicine, 16*, 287.

Molgaard, C.A., Golbeck, A.L., & Gresham, L. (1985). Current concepts in endometriosis. *Western Journal of Medicine, 145*(7), 42.

Nettles-Carlson, B. (1989). Early detection of breast cancer. *Journal of Obstetric, Gynecologic, and Neonatal Nursing, 9*, 373.

(1992). Panel recommendations on silicone gel-filled breast implants follow moratorium. *FDA Medical Bulletin, 22*(1), 3.

Pinsonneault, O., & Goldstein, D.P. (1986). Gynecologic disorders in adolescents—Part 1: Pain syndromes. *Female Patient, 11*(4), 26.

Pinsonneault, O., & Goldstein, D.P. (1986). Gynecologic disorders in adolescents—Part 2: Dysfunctional uterine bleeding and breast masses. *Female Patient, 11*(5), 30.

Reid, R. (1991). Premenstrual syndrome. *New England Journal of Medicine, 324,* 208–210.

Seltzer, V. (1985). Pitfalls of Pap smear and colposcopy. *Medical Digest, 2,* 1.

Vaitukaitis, J.L. (1983). Polycystic ovary syndrome—what is it? *New England Journal of Medicine, 309,* 1245.

Weiss, R.M. (1992). Treatment options of abnormal uterine bleeding. *Hospital Practice, 27*(10A), 55–78.

CHAPTER 39

SEXUALLY TRANSMITTED DISEASES

PATRICIA McCOWEN MEHRING

■ OBJECTIVES

After you have studied this chapter, you should be able to meet the following objectives:

■ Define what is meant by a *sexually transmitted disease (STD)*.

■ Give a reason why the reported incidences of STDs may not accurately reflect the true incidence.

■ List common portals of entry for STDs.

■ Name the organisms responsible for condyloma acuminata, genital herpes, molluscum contagiosum, chancroid, granuloma inguinale, lymphogranuloma venereum, candidiasis vaginal infections, trichomonal vaginal infections, bacterial vaginosis (nonspecific vaginitis), chlamydial urogenital infections, gonorrhea, nonspecific urogenital infection, and syphilis.

■ List the STDs that pose a threat to the unborn child either in utero or during childbirth.

■ State the significance of condyloma acuminata.

■ Explain the recurrent infections in genital herpes.

■ State the difference between wet-mount slide and culture methods of diagnosis of STDs.

■ Compare the signs and symptoms of infections caused by *Chlamydia trachomatis, Candida albicans, Trichomonas vaginalis*, and bacterial vaginosis.

■ Compare the signs and symptoms of gonorrhea in the male and female.

■ Describe the three stages of syphilis.

■ State the genital and nongenital complications that can occur with chlamydial infections, gonorrhea, nonspecific urogenital infection, and syphilis.

■ Compare the treatments for condyloma acuminata, genital herpes, molluscum contagiosum, chancroid, granuloma inguinale, lymphogranuloma venereum, vaginal candidiasis, trichomonal vaginal infections, bacterial vaginosis, chlamydial urogenital infections, gonorrhea, nonspecific urogenital infections, and syphilis.

Carol Mattson Porth: PATHOPHYSIOLOGY: CONCEPTS OF
ALTERED HEALTH STATES, 4th ed. © 1994, 1990, 1986, 1982
J.B. Lippincott Company

The incidence and types of sexually transmitted diseases (STDs), as reported in the professional literature and public health statistics, are increasing. It must be recognized, however, that the incidence of disease is based on clinical reports, and many STDs are either not reportable or not reported. The agents of transmission include bacteria, chlamydiae, viruses, fungi, protozoa, parasites, and unidentified microorganisms (see Chapter 12). Portals of entry include the mouth, genitalia, urinary meatus, rectum, and skin. All STDs are more common in people who have more than one sexual partner, and it is not uncommon for a person to be concurrently infected with more than one type of STD. This chapter discusses the manifestations of STDs in both men and women and has been divided into three sections: infections of the external genitalia, vaginal infections, and infections that have systemic effects as well as genitourinary manifestations. Human immunodeficiency virus (HIV) infection is presented in Chapter 15.

▪ INFECTIONS OF THE EXTERNAL GENITALIA

Some STDs primarily affect the mucocutaneous tissues of the external genitalia. These include human papillomavirus infection, genital herpes, molluscum contagiosum, chancroid, granuloma inguinale, and lymphogranuloma venereum.

HUMAN PAPILLOMAVIRUS (CONDYLOMATA ACUMINATA)

Condylomata acuminata, or genital warts, are the most common manifestation of the human papillomavirus (HPV). Although recognized for centuries, HPV-induced genital warts have become one of the fastest rising STDs of the past decade. The Centers for Disease Control (CDC) estimate that the number of visits to private physicians for genital warts increased from 169,000 in 1966 to 1 million in 1981 and to 2 million in 1983.[1,2] The current prevalence of HPV is difficult to determine because it is not a reportable disease and estimates are based only on visible HPV lesions.[3]

The incubation period for HPV ranges from 6 weeks to 8 months. Although HPV infections often are asymptomatic, they can be detected by the presence of characteristic warty lesions. Structurally, there are four types of condylomas or warts: (1) papillous, (2) flat, (3) spiked, and (4) exophytic.[4] Papillous condylomas are soft, pink, fleshy growths of external genitalia. They often are difficult to distinguish from normal genital tissue and may require biopsy for definitive diagnosis. Until recently, papillous condylomas were the only type of condyloma recognized. The flat condyloma, discovered in 1977, is the most virulent type. The flat condyloma, which is a macular, flat, granular lesion, typically is found on the cervix or introitus in women and on the frenulum or upper shaft of the penis in men. The lesions, which frequently are invisible to the naked eye, become readily apparent when the affected area is soaked with a 5% acetic acid solution. Biopsy may be required to differentiate these lesions from other hyperkeratotic or precancerous lesions. Spiked condylomas, which are less common, are small, pointed projections found primarily in the vagina. Exophytic or inverted condylomas grow only within the glands of the cervix and can mimic carcinoma in situ.

A relation between HPV and genital neoplasms has become increasingly apparent over the past 10 years.[3,5,6] Sixty types of HPV have been identified.[5] Several of these have been associated with genital neoplasms. Types 16 and 18 are present in more than 80% of invasive squamous cell carcinomas of the cervix, vulva, and penis and in higher grades of intraepithelial neoplasms of the cervix and vulva.[3] Types 31 and 33 have been detected, to a lesser degree, in cervical dysplasias and neoplasms.[5] In contrast, types 6 and 11 more often are associated with benign warts and mild forms of dysplasia. Numerous studies have demonstrated that HPV infection is common—affecting about 50% of the normal adult population and 40% of children—and that its presence alone is not sufficient to induce neoplasia. Cofactors that increase the risk for cancer include smoking, immunosuppression, other STDs—particularly herpes—and exposure to exogenous hormones (oral contraceptives).[3,5] This association with premalignant and malignant changes has increased the concern for diagnosis and treatment of this virus.

Genital condylomas should be considered in any woman who presents with the primary complaint of vulvar pruritus or who has had an abnormal Papanicolaou test (Pap smear). Microscopic examination of a wet-mount slide preparation and cultures are used to rule out associated vaginitis. Acetic acid soaks are used before inspecting the vulva under magnification, and specimens for biopsy are taken from questionable areas. Colposcopic examination of the cervix and vagina is advised as a follow-up measure when there is an abnormal Pap smear or when HPV lesions are identified on the vulva. The presence of koilocytes (hollow cells) on the Pap smear or pathology report is diagnostic of HPV. Because the male sexual partner may be the primary reservoir for this virus, examination of the penis using acetic acid soaks is recommended.

In the past, the primary treatment for condyloma acuminata was podophyllin 25% in tincture of benzoin. With multiple applications, this cytotoxic agent produced resolution of the lesions. This treatment was contraindicated in pregnancy because the medication could be absorbed systemically. Currently, the first line of treatment for vulvar, vaginal, or penile condylomas is the topical application of a 50% to 80% solution of trichloroacetic acid. This weak destructive agent produces an initial burning in the affected area followed in several days by a sloughing of the superficial tissue. Several applications 1 to 2 weeks apart may be necessary to eradicate the virus. Vulvar, vaginal, and penile condylomas may also be treated with electrocautery. Topical 5-fluorouracil (5-FU, Efudex) and laser therapy have been used successfully in the treatment of vaginal condylomas.[7] Because it can penetrate deeper than other forms of therapy, cryotherapy (freezing therapy) is the treatment of choice for cervical HPV lesions. Laser surgery can be used to remove large or widespread lesions of the cervix or lesions of the cervix that have failed to respond to other first-line methods of treatment. The results of laser treatment have been excellent, but the equipment is expensive and the method requires extensive training for safe and effective use. Interferon, either in the form of a topical application or as an intralesional injection, is under investigation as a possible form of treatment but has not shown any advantage over other available forms of treatment. Sexual abstinence is necessary during any type of treatment.

Recurrence of HPV is high, sometimes occurring as early as 3 to 6 weeks after treatment. Originally, it was assumed that reinfection from sexual partners was the primary cause. It is now believed that the recurrences are due to a persistent HPV infection existing in a latent state in the apparently normal tissue near the treated lesions.[2] Stress and trauma appear to be two possible factors in the reactivation of the latent virus. Extending the area of treatment 5 mm beyond the lesion border is recommended as a method for preventing recurrences. Research eventually may lead to the prevention or eradication of this form of what appears to be a sexually transmitted precursor to neoplasia.

GENITAL HERPES

Genital herpes is caused by the herpes simplex virus (HSV). Because herpesvirus infection is not reportable in all states, reliable data on its true incidence and prevalence are lacking. Estimates indicate that 500,000 to 1 million new cases occur each year. A study evaluating the prevalence of genital herpes in private physician practices determined that the number of physician's office visits for herpes increased 15-fold between 1966 and 1984.[8]

There are five types of herpesviruses that cause infections in humans: two types of HSV—HSV-I, which causes cold sores, and HSV-II, which causes genital herpes; varicella-zoster virus, which causes chickenpox and shingles; Epstein-Barr virus, which causes infectious mononucleosis and Burkitt's lymphoma; and the cytomegalovirus, which causes cytomegalic inclusion disease. The herpesviruses are neurotropic: that is, they grow within neurons and share the biologic property of latency. *Latency* refers to the ability to maintain disease potential in the absence of clinical signs and symptoms. In genital herpes, the virus ascends through the peripheral nerves to the sacral dorsal root ganglia (Fig. 39-1). The virus can remain dormant in the dorsal root ganglia, or it can reactivate, in which case the viral particles are transported back down the nerve root to the skin, where they multiply and cause a lesion to develop. During the dormant or latent period, the virus replicates in a different manner so that the immune system or available treatments have no effect on it. It is not known what reactivates the virus. It may be that the body's defense mechanisms are altered. Numerous studies have shown that host responses to infection influence initial development of the disease, severity of infection, development and maintenance of latency, and frequency of HSV recurrences.[9]

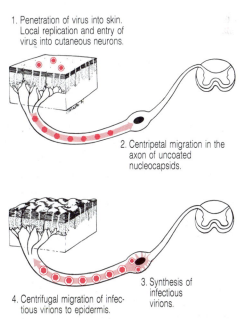

1. Penetration of virus into skin. Local replication and entry of virus into cutaneous neurons.

2. Centripetal migration in the axon of uncoated nucleocapsids.

3. Synthesis of infectious virions.

4. Centrifugal migration of infectious virions to epidermis.

FIG. 39-1. Pathogenesis of primary mucocutaneous herpes simplex virus infection. (Corey, L., & Spear, P. G. [1986]. Infections with herpes simplex viruses. Pt. 1. *New England Journal of Medicine, 314*, 686)

Both HSV-I and HSV-II can cause genital lesions. HSV is shed from active lesions and usually is transmitted by contact with infectious lesions or genital secretions. HSV-I often is transmitted by kissing. When one has a cold sore on the mouth, HSV-I may be spread to the genital area by autoinoculation secondary to poor hand-washing or through oral intercourse. HSV-II usually is transmitted by sexual contact but can be passed to an infant during childbirth if the virus is actively being shed from the genital tract.

The incubation period for HSV is 2 to 10 days. Genital HSV may present as either a primary or a nonprimary form of infection. Primary infections are infections that occur in a person who is seronegative for antibody to HSV-I or HSV-II. Nonprimary infections refer to the clinical appearance of genital herpes in a person who is seropositive for antibodies to HSV-I or HSV-II, implying a previous asymptomatic exposure.

The initial symptoms of primary genital herpes infections include tingling, itching, and pain in the genital area followed by eruption of small pustules and vesicles. These lesions rupture on about the 5th day to form wet ulcers that are excruciatingly painful to touch and can be associated with dysuria, dyspareunia, and urine retention. Involvement of the cervix and urethra is seen in more than 80% of women with primary infections.[10] In men, the infection can cause urethritis as well as lesions of the penis and scrotum. Rectal and perianal infections are possible with anal intercourse. Systemic symptoms associated with primary infections include fever, headache, malaise, muscle ache, and lymphadenopathy. Primary infections may be debilitating enough to require hospitalization, particularly in women. Untreated primary infections typically are self-limiting and last for about 2 to 4 weeks. The symptoms usually worsen for the first 10 to 12 days. This period is followed by a 10- to 12-day interval during which the lesions crust over and gradually heal. Nonprimary episodes of genital herpes present with similar symptoms—albeit less severe—that usually are of shorter duration and have fewer systemic manifestations. Except for the greater tendency of HSV-II to recur, the clinical manifestations of HSV-II and genital HSV-I are similar. Genital HSV-II infections are twice as likely to be reactivated and recur 8 to 12 times more often than genital HSV-I.[10]

Recurrent HSV infections result from reactivation of the virus stored in the dorsal root ganglia of the infected dermatomes. Actual outbreaks may be preceded by a prodrome of itching, burning, or tingling at the site of future lesions. Because patients have already developed immune lymphocytes from the primary infection, recurrent episodes have fewer lesions, fewer systemic symptoms, less pain, and a shorter duration (7 to 10 days). Frequency and severity of recurrences vary from person to person. Numerous factors, including emotional stress, lack of sleep, overexertion, other infections, vigorous or prolonged coitus, and premenstrual or menstrual distress, have been identified as triggering mechanisms.

Asymptomatic disease is possible. Some people possess antibodies to HSV-I or HSV-II without any history of clinical disease. Asymptomatic shedding of the virus can occur from these people as well as from those whose recurrences result in viral excretion into saliva or cervical secretions without development of overt lesions. Little is known about the frequency or quantity of asymptomatic shedding, but it appears that transmission of the disease is more likely during symptomatic periods of viral excretion.[9]

Diagnosis of genital herpes is based on the symptoms, appearance of the lesions, and identification of the virus from a Tzanck smear or cultures taken from the lesions. Depending on the laboratory, a preliminary report on cultures takes from 2 to 5 days, and a final negative report takes from 10 to 12 days. The stability of the virus in transport media is good for 48 to 72 hours, making mail transport possible. The likelihood of obtaining a positive culture decreases with each day that has elapsed after a lesion develops. The chance of obtaining a positive culture from a crusted lesion is slight, and patients suspected of having genital herpes should be instructed to have a culture within 24 hours of developing new lesions. A Tzanck smear is done by scraping a debrided lesion with a cytology spatula and smearing the exudate on a slide, allowing the slide to dry, and sending it to a laboratory for microscopic identification of multinucleated giant cells. About 50% of Tzanck smear results are falsely negative. They are, however, available in 24 to 48 hours, as opposed to the 2 to 5 days required for culture tests. Newer tests for HSV-I and HSV-II include immunofluorescence assays that use monoclonal antibodies, DNA-hybridization procedures, and combined tissue culture and immunologic detection (modified viral culture). These methods provide faster, cheaper diagnosis but require special equipment and training to perform and are less specific than viral culture techniques. These types of testing are continually being improved and should be in wider use in the near future.

There is no known cure for genital herpes, and the methods of treatment are largely symptomatic. The antiviral drug acyclovir has become a significant component of the management of genital herpes. By interfering with viral DNA replication, acyclovir decreases the frequency of recurrences, shortens the duration of active lesions, reduces the number of new lesions formed, and decreases viral shedding with primary infections. The drug is most useful in people with depressed immune function and in those experiencing an initial outbreak. Originally available only for topical application or intravenous administration, oral acyclovir is now the more common treatment form. Oral acyclovir reduces the duration of viral shedding and the healing time for recurrent lesions but is not needed unless the recurrences are severe. Although acyclovir is well tolerated with few adverse effects, its use beyond 12 months is not recommended until further studies of its long-term effects have been completed. Long-term suppressive therapy does not limit latency, and reactivation of the disease occurs after the drug is discontinued. Topical treatment with antibacterial soaps, lotions, dyes, ultrasonography, and ultraviolet light has been tried with little success. Sometimes symptomatic relief can be obtained with cool compresses (Burow's soaks), sitz baths, topical anesthetic agents, and oral analgesic drugs.

Good hygiene is essential to prevent secondary infection with HSV infections. Fastidious handwashing is recommended to avoid hand-to-eye spread of the infection. HSV infection of the eye is the most frequent cause of corneal blindness in the United States.[10] To prevent spread of the disease, intimate contact should be avoided until lesions are completely healed. Because up to 65% of infected neonates die if they contract herpes infections during vaginal delivery, active infection during labor may necessitate cesarean delivery. Recommendations from the American College of Obstetrics and Gynecologists direct care providers to obtain cultures when a pregnant woman has active lesions, but vaginal delivery is acceptable if visable lesions are not present at the onset of labor. Weekly surveillance cultures from women with a history of human immunodeficiency virus are no longer suggested.[8] Finally, because women with HSV-II appear to be at increased risk for developing cervical cancer, it is recommended that they obtain annual Pap smears and be alert to the development of suspicious vulvar lesions that might warrant biopsy.

MOLLUSCUM CONTAGIOSUM

Molluscum contagiosum is a common viral disease of the skin that gives rise to multiple umbilicated papules. The disease is mildly contagious; it is transmitted by skin-to-skin contact, fomites, and autoinoculation. Lesions are domelike and have a dimpled appearance. A curdlike material can be expressed from the center of the lesion. Necrosis and secondary infection are possible. Diagnosis is based on the appearance of the lesion and microscopic identification of intracytoplasmic molluscum bodies. Molluscum is a benign and self-limiting disease. The goal of treatment is to prevent its spread for cosmetic reasons.[11]

When indicated, treatment consists of unroofing the papule with a sterile needle or scalpel, expressing the contents of each lesion, and applying alcohol or silver nitrate to the base. Electrodesiccation, cryosurgery (freezing), and surgical biopsy are alternative treatments but seldom are needed unless lesions are large.[11]

CHANCROID

Chancroid (soft chancre) is a disease of the external genitalia and lymph nodes. The causative organism is the gram-negative bacterium *Haemophilus ducreyi*, which causes acute ulcerative lesions with profuse discharge. This disease is somewhat uncommon in the United States.[11] It is more prevalent in Southeast Asia, the West Indies, and North Africa. A highly infectious disease, chancroid usually is transmitted by sexual intercourse or through skin and mucous membrane abrasions. Autoinoculation may lead to multiple chancres.

Lesions begin as macules, progress to pustules, and then rupture. This painful ulcer has a necrotic base and jagged edges. In contrast, the syphilitic chancre is nontender and indurated. Subsequent discharge can lead to further infection of self or others. On physical examination, lesions and regional lymphadenopathy may be found. Secondary infection may cause significant tissue destruction. Diagnosis is confirmed through the use of Gram stain and culture. The organism has shown resistance to treatment with sulfamethoxazole alone and to tetracycline. The CDC recommend treatment with erythromycin, ceftriaxone, or an alternative regimen of sulfamethoxazole and trimethoprim.[12]

GRANULOMA INGUINALE

Granuloma inguinale (granuloma venereum) is caused by a gram-negative bacillus, *Calymmatobacterium donovani*, which is a tiny, encapsulated, intracellular parasite. This disease is almost nonexistent in the United States. It most frequently is found in India, Brazil, the West Indies, and parts of China, Australia, and Africa. Granuloma inguinale causes ulceration of the genitalia, beginning with an innocuous papule. The papule progresses through nodular or vesicular stages until it begins to break down as pink granulomatous tissue. At this final stage, the tissue becomes thin and friable and bleeds easily. There are complaints of swelling, pain, and itching. Extensive inflammatory scarring may cause late sequelae, such as lymphatic obstruction with the development of enlarged and elephantoid external genitalia. The liver, bladder, bone, joint, lung, and bowel tissue may become involved. Genital complications include tubo-ovarian abscess, fistula, vaginal stenosis, and occlusion of vaginal or anal orifices. Lesions may become neoplastic. Diagnosis is made through the identification of Donovan bodies (large mononuclear cells filled with intracytoplasmic gram-negative rods) in tissue smears, biopsy samples, or culture. A 2- to 3-week period of treatment with tetracycline, erythromycin, or gentamicin is used in treating the disorder.

LYMPHOGRANULOMA VENEREUM

Lymphogranuloma venereum is an acute and chronic venereal disease caused by *Chlamydia trachomatis* (types L1, L2, P3). The disease, although found worldwide, has a low incidence outside the tropics. Most cases reported in the United States are in men.

The lesions of lymphogranuloma can incubate for a few days to several weeks and thereafter cause small painless papules or vesicles that may go undetected. An important characteristic of the disease is the early (1 to 4 weeks later) development of large, tender, and sometimes fluctuant inguinal lymph nodes called buboes. There may be flulike symptoms with joint pain, rash, weight loss, pneumonitis, tachycardia, splenomegaly, and proctitis. In later stages of the disease, a small percentage of people develop elephantiasis of the external genitalia; this is due to lymphatic obstruction or fibrous strictures of the rectum or urethra caused by the inflammation and scarring. Urethral involvement may cause pyuria and dysuria. Anorectal structures may be compromised to the point of incontinence. Complications of lymphogranuloma infection may be minor or extensive, involving compromise of whole systems or progression to a cancerous state. Diagnosis usually is by means of a complement fixation test for *Chlamydia* group antibody. High titers for this antibody differentiate this group from other chlamydial subgroups. Treatment involves 2 weeks of tetracycline or erythromycin. Surgery may be required to correct sequelae such as strictures or fistulas.

In summary, STDs that primarily affect the external genitalia include HPV (condyloma acuminata), genital herpes (HVS-II), molluscum contagiosum, chancroid, granuloma inguinale, and lymphogranuloma venereum. The lesions of these infections occur on the external genitalia of both male and female sexual partners. Of current concern is the relation between HPV and genital neoplasms. Genital herpes is caused by a neurotropic virus (HVS-II) that ascends through the peripheral nerves to reside in the sacral dorsal root ganglia. The herpes virus can be reactivated and produce recurrent lesions in genital structures that are supplied by the peripheral nerves of the affected ganglia. There is no permanent cure for herpes infections. Molluscum contagiosum is a benign and self-limiting infection that is only mildly contagious. Chancroid, granuloma inguinale, and lymphogranuloma venereum produce external genital lesions with varying degrees of inguinal lymph node involvement. These diseases are uncommon in the United States.

■ VAGINAL INFECTIONS

Candidiasis, trichomoniasis, and bacterial vaginosis are vaginal infections that can be sexually transmitted. Although these infections can be transmitted sexually, the male partner usually is asymptomatic.

CANDIDIASIS

Also called yeast infection, thrush, and moniliasis, candidiasis is the leading cause of vulvovaginitis in the United States.[13] The causative organism is *Candida*, a genus of yeastlike fungi. The species most commonly identified is *Candida albicans* (Fig. 39-2), but other candidal species, such as *C. glabrata* and *C. tropicalis*, have also been shown to cause clinical symptomatology. Additionally, 18 separate strains of *C. albicans* with varying levels of virulence have been identified.[14] These organisms often are present in healthy people without causing symptoms, and the decision of the CDC to classify candidiasis as an STD is controversial. The possibility of sexual transmission has been recognized for many years; however,

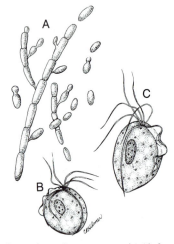

FIG. 39-2. Organisms that cause vaginal infections. (**A**) *Candida albicans* (blastospores and pseudohyphae). (**B, C**) *Trichomonas vaginalis*.

candidiasis requires a favorable environment for its growth. The gastrointestinal tract also serves as a reservoir for this organism, and candidiasis can develop through autoinoculation in women who are not sexually active. Although studies have documented the presence of *Candida* on the penis of male partners of women with vulvovaginal candidiasis, few men develop balanoposthitis that requires treatment.[15]

Causes for the overgrowth of *C. albicans* include (1) antibiotic therapy, which suppresses the normal protective bacterial flora; (2) high hormone levels owing to pregnancy or the use of oral contraceptives, which cause an increase in vaginal glycogen stores; and (3) diabetes mellitus, which may increase the sugar levels in the vaginal mucosa but more likely causes candidiasis because it compromises the immune system of the host.[15] Food allergies, hypothyroidism, endocrine disorders, and altered immune status have also been suggested as possible contributors to the development of vulvovaginal candidiasis.

In obese people, *Candida* may grow in skin folds underneath the breast tissue, the abdominal flap, and the inguinal folds. Vulvar pruritus accompanied by irritation, dysuria, dyspareunia, erythema, and an odorless, thick, cheesy vaginal discharge are the predominant symptoms of the infection. Accurate diagnosis is made by identification of budding yeast filaments (hyphae) or spores on a wet-mount slide using 20% potassium hydroxide (see Fig. 39-2). The *p*H of the discharge (checked with litmus paper) typically is less than 4.5. When the wet-mount technique is negative but the clinical manifestations are suggestive of candidiasis, a culture may be necessary.

Antifungals such as clotrimazole, miconazole, butaconazole, and terconazole, in various forms, are effective in treating candidiasis. Oral fluconazole has been shown to be as safe and effective as the standard intravaginal regimens.[16] Gentian violet solution (1%) applied to the vagina by swabs or tampon, potassium sorbate douches, or boric acid soaks to the vulva are treatment adjuncts. Tepid sodium bicarbonate baths, clothing that allows adequate ventilation, and the application of corn starch to dry the area may increase comfort during treatment. Chronic vulvovaginal candidiasis represents a challenge to researchers to find a means of eradicating this nonserious but aggravating affliction.

Candidiasis can be confused with Döderlein cytolysis—an excess of lactobacilli—which can present with a similar clinical picture. In the case of Döderlein cytolysis, both wet-mount and culture techniques show only excessive lactobacilli—no yeast. Treatment for Döderlein cytolysis involves use of a sodium bicarbonate douche two to three times a week to raise the vaginal *p*H and decrease the symptoms.[13]

TRICHOMONIASIS

An anaerobic protozoan that can be transmitted sexually, *Trichomonas vaginalis* is shaped like a turnip and has three or four anterior flagellae (see Fig. 39-2). Trichomonads can reside in the paraurethral glands of both sexes. Males harbor the organism in the urethra and prostate and are asymptomatic. Although 10% to 25% of women are asymptomatic, trichomoniasis is a common cause of vaginitis when some imbalance allows the protozoan to proliferate. This extracellular parasite feeds on the vaginal mucosa and ingests bacteria and leukocytes. The infection causes a copious, frothy, malodorous green or yellow discharge. There commonly is erythema and edema of the affected mucosa with occasional itching and irritation. Sometimes small hemorrhagic areas, called strawberry spots, appear on the cervix.

Diagnosis is made microscopically by identification of the protozoan on a wet-mount slide preparation. The *p*H of the discharge usually is greater than 6.0. Special culture media are available for diagnosis but are costly and not needed for diagnosis.

Because the organism resides in other urogenital structures besides the vagina, systemic treatment is recommended. The treatment of choice is oral metronidazole (Flagyl), a medication that is effective against anaerobic protozoans. Metronidazole is chemically similar to disulfiram (Antabuse), a drug used in the treatment of alcohol addiction that causes nausea, vomiting, flushing of the skin, headache, palpitations, and lowering of the blood pressure when alcohol is ingested. Therefore, alcohol should be avoided during and for 24 to 48 hours after treatment. Gastrointestinal disturbances and a metallic taste in the mouth are potential adverse effects of the drug. Metronidazole has not been proved safe for use during pregnancy and is used only after the first trimester for fear of potential teratogenic effects. Trichomoniasis may be alternatively treated with acidification of the environment with Aci-jel therapeutic jelly, povidone-iodine vaginal gel or douche, or clotrimazole vaginal suppositories. If the female is in a monogamous relationship, both sexual partners are treated simultaneously to decrease the incidence of reinfection. If the woman has more than one sexual partner, abstinence during therapy and for 1 week after completing therapy or the use of condoms is recommended.

BACTERIAL VAGINOSIS (NONSPECIFIC VAGINITIS)

Considerable controversy exists regarding the organisms responsible for a vaginal infection that produces a characteristic fishy or ammonia-smelling discharge yet fails to produce an inflammatory response that is characteristic of most infections. A number of terms have been used to describe the nonspecific vaginitis that cannot be attributed to one of the accepted pathogenic organisms, such as *T. vaginalis* or C. *albicans*. In 1955, Gardner and Dukes isolated an organism from women with this vaginitis and proposed the name *Haemophilus vaginalis*, apparently because the organism was gram-negative and required blood for growth.[17] In 1963 gram-positive isolates were found, and the organism was renamed *Corynebacterium vaginale*. Because the organism did not meet all the criteria of corynebacteria, it was renamed *Gardnerella vaginalis* in 1980, after its original discoverer, and admitted to a taxonomic genus of its own.[18] The development of a special agar on which *G. vaginalis* could be cultured led to the discovery that 40% to 70% of women harbor this organism as part of their normal vaginal flora. Further study revealed that abnormal discharge frequently contained highly motile, crescent-shaped rods called mobiluncus and many more anaerobic than aerobic bacteria.[19] It has been suggested that the presence of anaerobes, which produce ammonia or amines from amino acids, favors the growth of *G. vaginalis* by raising vaginal pH. Because of the presence of anaerobic bacteria and the lack of an inflammatory response, a new term, *bacterial vaginosis*, was proposed.[20]

Bacterial vaginosis is thought to be sexually transmissible and may be carried asymptomatically by both the male and the female. Reinfection is common and greatly affected by vaginal pH in women. The predominant symptom of bacterial vaginosis is a thin, grayish white discharge that has a foul, fishy odor. Burning, itching, and erythema usually are absent because the bacteria has only minimal inflammatory potential.

The diagnosis is made when at least three of the following characteristics are present: (1) homogeneous discharge, (2) production of a fishy amine odor when a 10% potassium hydroxide solution is dropped onto the secretions, (3) vaginal pH above 4.5 (usually 5.0 to 6.0), and (4) appearance of characteristic "clue cells" on wet-mount microscopic studies. Clue cells are squamous epithelial cells covered with masses of coccobacilli, often with large clumps of organisms floating free from the cell. Because *G. vaginalis* can be a normal vaginal flora, cultures should not be done routinely. They are of limited clinical value, since it is believed that the condition is caused by a combination of *G. vaginalis* and anaerobic bacteria.

The mere presence of *G. vaginalis* in an asymptomatic woman is not an indication for treatment. When indicated, treatment is aimed at eradicating the anaerobic component of bacterial vaginosis. The CDC recommends metronidazole, although failure rates may range from 30% to 70%. Alternative therapies include clindamycin, ampicillin or amoxicillin, vaginal sulfonamides, and povidone preparations.

In summary, candidiasis, trichomoniasis, and bacterial vaginosis are vaginal infections that can be spread through sexual contact. Although these infections are sexually transmitted, the male partner usually is asymptomatic. Candidiasis, also called a yeast infection, is the leading cause of vulvovaginitis in the United States. *Candida* can be present without producing symptoms; usually some host factor, such as altered immune status or increased sugar levels in the vaginal mucosa caused by diabetes mellitus, contributes to the development of vulvovaginitis. Trichomoniasis is caused by an anaerobic protozoan. The infection incites the production of a copious, frothy, yellow or green, malodorous discharge. Bacterial vaginosis is a nonspecific type of infection that produces a characteristic fishy-smelling discharge. The infection is thought to be caused by the combined presence of *G. vaginalis* and anaerobic bacteria. The anaerobe raises the vaginal pH, thereby favoring the growth of *G. vaginalis*.

■ VAGINAL–UROGENITAL–SYSTEMIC INFECTIONS

Some STDs infect both genital and extragenital structures. Among the infections of this type are chlamydial infections, gonorrhea, nonspecific urogenital infection, and syphilis. Many of these infections also pose a risk to babies born to infected mothers. Some infections, such as syphilis, may be spread to the infant while in utero; others, such as chlamydial and gonorrheal infections, can be spread to the infant during the birth process.

CHLAMYDIAL INFECTIONS

C. trachomatis is an obligate intracellular bacterial pathogen that is closely related to gram-negative bacteria. It resembles a virus in that it requires tissue culture for isolation, but like a bacteria it has both RNA and DNA and is susceptible to some antibiotics. *C. trachomatis* can be serologically subdivided into types A, B, and C, which are associated with trachoma; types L1, L2, and L3, which are associated with lymphogranuloma venereum; and types D through K, which are associated with genital infections and their complications. The organism causes a wide variety of genitourinary infections, including nongonococcal urethritis in men and pelvic inflammatory disease in women. *Chlamydia* can cause significant ocular disease in neonates; it is a leading cause of blindness in underdeveloped countries. In these countries, the organism is spread primarily by flies, fomites, and nonsexual personal contact. In industrial countries, the organism is spread almost exclusively by sexual contact and, therefore, affects primarily the genitourinary structures. Although chlamydial infections are not reportable in all states, their incidence is estimated to be more than twice that of gonorrhea. The most prevalent STD in the United States, chlamydial infections occur at an annual rate of 3 to 10 million, according to CDC estimates.[21]

The chlamydial organism exists in two forms: (1) the elementary body, which is the infectious particle capable of entering uninfected cells, and (2) the initiator or reticulate body, which multiplies by binary fission to produce the inclusions identified in stained cells. The 48-hour growth cycle starts with attachment of the elementary body to the susceptible host cell, following which it is ingested by a process that resembles phagocytosis (Fig. 39-3). Once within the cell, the elementary body is organized into the reticulate body, the metabolically active form of the organism, which is capable of reproduction. The reticulate body is not infectious and cannot survive outside the body. The reticulate bodies divide within the cell for up to 36 hours and then condense to form new elementary bodies, which are released when the infected cell bursts.

The signs and symptoms of chlamydial infections resemble those produced by gonorrhea. In women, chlamydial infections may cause urinary frequency, dysuria, and vaginal discharge. The most common symptom is a mucopurulent cervical discharge. The cervix itself frequently hypertrophies and becomes erythematous, edematous, and extremely friable. The organism may cause pelvic in-flammatory disease, which in turn can result in infertility (11,000 women per year) or ectopic pregnancy (3,600 women per year).[21] The most significant difference between chlamydial and gonococcal salpingitis is that chlamydial infections may be asymptomatic or subclinically nonspecific. This can lead to greater fallopian tube damage as well as increase the reservoir for further chlamydial infections. Between 25% and 50% of infants born to mothers with cervical chlamydial infections develop ocular disease (inclusion conjunctivitis), and 10% to 20% develop chlamydial pneumonitis.

In men, chlamydial infections cause urethritis, including meatal erythema and tenderness, urethral discharge, dysuria, and urethral itching. Prostatitis and epididymitis with subsequent infertility may develop. The most serious complication that can develop with nongonococcal urethritis is Reiter's disease (see Chapter 58). In one study, two thirds of men with untreated acute Reiter's disease were found to have a chlamydial infection of the urethra.[11]

Diagnosis of chlamydial infections takes several forms. The identification of polymorphonuclear leukocytes on Gram stain of male discharge or cervical discharge is presumptive evidence. The two available serologic tests can be misleading. Complement fixation tests are the most useful in diagnosing lymphogranuloma venereum. The microimmunofluorescent test is more sensitive for *C. trachomatis* types D through K but does not distinguish among acute, chronic, or carrier states. The high rates of antichlamydial antibodies in sexually active populations renders serodiagnosis inconclusive.[11] Tissue cultures

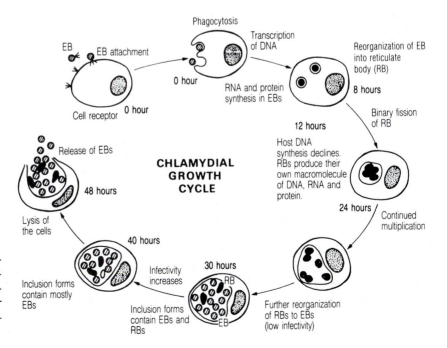

FIG. 39-3. Chlamydial growth cycle. EB, elementary body; RB, reticulate body. (Thompson, S. E., & Washington, A. E. [1983]. Epidemiology of sexually transmitted *Chlamydia trachomatis* infections. *Epidemiologic Reviews, 5,* 96–123)

are definitive but slow (requiring at least 3 days), costly, and not always available. Newer nonculture methods, such as direct fluorescent antibody test (DFA; Microtrak) and an enzyme-linked immunosorbent assay (ELISA; Chlamydiazyme), which uses antibodies against an antigen present in the *Chlamydia* cell wall, have been developed. These are less expensive, rapid tests that require less sophisticated laboratory techniques but have a lower sensitivity than culture (DFA, 90% sensitivity and 96% specificity; ELISA, 67% to 90% sensitivity and 92% to 98% specificity).[22] The positive predictive value of these tests is excellent among high-risk groups, but false-positive results occur more often in populations with lower risks. The DFA test appears to be the most effective screening test available but may require follow-up with culture if the validity of the positive result is questioned.[23]

The CDC recommends the use of tetracycline or doxycycline in the treatment of chlamydial infection; penicillin is ineffective. Antibiotic treatment of both sexual partners simultaneously is recommended. Abstinence from sexual activity is encouraged to facilitate cure.

GONORRHEA

Gonorrhea is a reportable disease caused by the bacterium *Neisseria gonorrhoeae*. In 1990, there were 600,169 reported cases of gonorrhea in the United States.[21] Of these reported cases, 90% involved the 15-to-39 age group, with the heaviest concentration among young adults (ages 20 to 24). Although the incidence of gonorrhea has continued to decline since its peak in 1975, there has been an increase in infections caused by antibiotic-resistant strains, which in 1990 reached almost 9% of all cases reported.[21]

The gonococcus is a pyogenic (pus-forming), gram-negative diplococcus that evokes inflammatory reactions characterized by purulent exudates. Humans are the only natural host for *N. gonorrhoeae*. The organism grows best in warm, mucus-secreting epithelia. The portal of entry can be the genitourinary tract, eyes, oropharynx, anorectum, or skin. Transmission usually is by sexual intercourse, either heterosexual or homosexual. Autoinoculation of the organism to the conjunctiva is possible. Neonates born to infected mothers can acquire the infection during passage through the birth canal and are in danger of developing gonorrheal conjunctivitis, with resultant blindness, unless treated promptly. An amniotic infection syndrome characterized by premature rupture of the membranes, premature delivery, and increased risk of infant morbidity and mortality has been identified as an additional complication of

gonococcal infections in pregnancy.[11] Genital gonorrhea in young children should raise the possibility of sexual abuse.

The infection commonly becomes manifest 2 to 7 days after exposure. It typically begins in the anterior urethra, accessory urethral glands, Bartholin's or Skene's glands, and the cervix. If untreated, gonorrhea spreads from its initial sites upward into the genital tract. In males, it spreads to the prostate and epididymis; in females, it commonly moves to the fallopian tubes. Pharyngitis may follow oral–genital contact.

The organism can also invade the bloodstream (disseminated gonococcal infection), causing serious sequelae such as bacteremic involvement of joint spaces, heart valves, meninges, and other body organs and tissues.[11]

People with gonorrhea may be asymptomatic and, thus, may unwittingly spread the disease to their sexual partners. Men are more likely to be symptomatic than women. In men, the initial symptoms include urethral pain and a creamy, yellow, sometimes bloody discharge. The disorder may become chronic and affect the prostate, epididymis, and periurethral glands. Rectal infections are common in homosexual men. In women, recognizable symptoms include unusual genital or urinary discharge, dysuria, dyspareunia, pelvic pain or tenderness, unusual vaginal bleeding (including bleeding after intercourse), fever, and proctitis. Symptoms may occur or increase during or immediately after menses, since the bacterium is an intracellular diplococcus that thrives in menstrual blood but cannot survive long outside the human body. There may be infections of the uterus and development of acute or chronic infection of the fallopian tubes (salpingitis) with ultimate scarring and sterility.

Diagnosis is based on the history of sexual exposure and symptoms. It is confirmed by identification of the organism on Gram stain or culture. A Gram stain usually is an effective means of diagnosis in symptomatic males (*i.e.*, those with discharge). In women and asymptomatic men, a culture usually is preferred since the Gram stains often are unreliable. A specimen should be collected from the appropriate site (endocervix, urethra, anal canal, or oropharynx), plated onto selective Thayer-Martin media, and placed in a carbon dioxide environment. *N. gonorrhoeae* is a fastidious organism with specific nutrient and environmental needs. Optimal growth requires a *p*H of 7.4, temperature of 35.5° C, and an atmosphere that contains 2% to 10% carbon dioxide.[11] The accuracy of culture results is affected if transport is delayed or growth requirements are not available. The search for methods to provide rapid and accurate diagnosis of *N. gonorrhoeae* continues. An enzyme immunoassay for detecting gonococcal antigens (Gonozyme) is available but has several requirements that limit its usefulness. Testing for other STDs, particularly syphilis and chlamydial infections, is suggested at the time of examination. Pregnant women are routinely screened at the time of their first prenatal visit; high-risk populations should have repeat cultures during the third trimester. Neonates are routinely treated with various antibacterial agents applied to the conjunctiva within 1 hour of birth to protect against undiagnosed gonorrhea as well as other diseases.

The standard treatment of gonorrhea has been with the use of injectable penicillin and oral probenecid, a drug that delays the renal excretion of penicillin. Patients who were allergic to penicillin were treated with oral tetracycline for 7 days instead. The current treatment recommendation to combat tetracycline- and penicillin-resistant strains of *N. gonorrhea* is ceftriaxone in a single injection. In the presence of symptoms, particularly in the male partner, it is common practice to treat both partners before culture results are available because of potential loss of reproductive capacity. People with the disease, particularly pregnant women, should be followed with repeat cultures to determine the effectiveness of treatment. Patients are instructed to refrain from intercourse or to use condoms until cultures show negative results. Because of the high rate of concomitant chlamydial infections (30% to 50%) in women with gonococcal pelvic inflammatory disease, the CDC now recommends a treatment regimen for gonorrhea that treats both infections. The combination regimen supplements the single-dose ceftriaxone treatment with a 7-day treatment of oral doxycycline. Another alternative is a single injection of spectinomycin and 7-day treatment with doxycycline. In pregnant women, erythromycin can be substituted for tetracycline.[12]

NONSPECIFIC UROGENITAL INFECTION

Nonspecific urogenital infection is chiefly a disease of the male urethra but may involve the cervix, urethra, Bartholin's glands, vagina, and fallopian tubes in the female. In about 50% of cases, the disease is secondary to chlamydial infection. As discussed earlier, *Chlamydia* is a formidable pathogen because of its long-term effects and ability to affect the neonate. This disease entity, like nonspecific vaginitis, will probably be named more specifically as the causative agents are identified. Diagnosis is made through the use of cultures. The treatment is by various antibiotic regimens and dictated by the organism and antibiotic sensitivity.

SYPHILIS

Syphilis is a reportable disease caused by a spirochete, *Treponema pallidum*. During 1990, 50,223 new cases of primary and secondary syphilis were reported in the United States. This demonstrates a steady rise since 1985 and is the highest rate of occurrence (140 per 100,000) since 1948. The populations that are experiencing the largest rise in incidence of syphilis are blacks and Hispanics in urban areas and women of all racial and ethnic backgrounds. The reasons for the reversal in the trend of decreasing incidence that characterized the years prior to 1985 are unknown. Budget reductions in syphilis control programs, the practice of trading sex with multiple partners for illegal drugs, and the increased use of cocaine among women of childbearing age may be contributing factors.[24]

T. pallidum is spread by direct contact with an infectious moist lesion, usually through sexual intercourse. Bacteria-laden secretions may transfer the organism during kissing or intimate contact. Skin abrasions provide another possible portal of entry. There is rapid transplacental transmission of the organism from the mother to the fetus after 16 weeks' gestation, so that active disease in the mother during pregnancy can produce congenital syphilis in the fetus. Untreated syphilis can cause prematurity, stillbirth, and congenital defects as well as active infection in the infant. Once treated for syphilis, a pregnant woman usually is followed throughout pregnancy by repeat testing of serum titers.

The clinical disease is divided into three stages: primary, secondary, and tertiary. Primary syphilis is characterized by the appearance of a chancre at the site of exposure. Chancres typically appear within 3 weeks of exposure but may incubate for 1 week to 3 months. The primary chancre begins as a single, indurated, button-like papule up to several centimeters in diameter that erodes to create a clean-based ulcerated lesion on an elevated base. These lesions usually are painless and located at the site of sexual contact.

Primary syphilis is readily apparent in the male, where the lesion is on the penis or scrotum. Although chancres can develop on the external genitalia in females, they are more common on the vagina or cervix, and primary syphilis may, therefore, go untreated. There usually is an accompanying regional lymphadenopathy. The disease is highly contagious at this stage, but because the symptoms are mild, it frequently goes unnoticed. The chancre usually heals within 3 to 12 weeks, with or without treatment.

The timing of the second stage of syphilis varies even more than that of the first, ranging in duration from 1 week to 6 months. The symptoms of a rash (especially on the palms and soles), fever, sore throat, stomatitis, nausea, loss of appetite, and inflamed eyes may come and go for a year but usually last for 3 to 6 months. Secondary manifestations may include alopecia and genital condylomata lata. Condylomata lata are elevated red-brown lesions that may ulcerate and produce a foul discharge. They range from 2 to 3 cm in diameter, contain many spirochetes, and are highly contagious. After the second stage, syphilis frequently enters a latent phase that may last the lifetime of the person or progress to tertiary syphilis at some point. People can be infective during the first 1 to 2 years of latency.

Tertiary syphilis is a delayed response of the untreated disease. It can occur as long as 20 years after the initial infection. Only about one third of those with untreated syphilis progress to the tertiary stage of the disease, and about one half of these develop symptoms. About one third undergo spontaneous cure, and the remaining one third continue to have positive serologic tests but do not develop structural lesions.[11] When syphilis does progress to the symptomatic tertiary stage, it commonly takes one of three forms: (1) development of localized destructive lesions called gummas, (2) development of cardiovascular lesions, or (3) development of central nervous system lesions. The syphilitic gumma is a peculiar rubbery, necrotic lesion that is caused by noninflammatory tissue necrosis. Gummas can occur singly or multiply and vary in size from microscopic lesions to large, tumorous masses. They most commonly are found in the liver, testes, and bone. Central nervous system lesions can produce dementia, blindness, or injury to the spinal cord with ataxia and sensory loss (tabes dorsalis). Cardiovascular manifestations usually result from scarring of the medial layer of the thoracic aorta with aneurysm formation (see Chapter 20). These aneurysms produce enlargement of the aortic valve ring with aortic valve insufficiency.

T. pallidum does not produce either endotoxins or exotoxins but evokes a humoral immune response that provides the basis for serologic tests. Two types of antibodies—nonspecific and specific—are produced. The nonspecific antibodies can be detected by flocculation (Venereal Disease Research Laboratory [VDRL]) tests and complement fixation (Wasserman and Kahn) tests. Because these tests are nonspecific, positive results can also occur with diseases other than syphilis. The VDRL test is easy to perform, rapid, and inexpensive and frequently is used as a screening test for syphilis. The results become positive 4 to 6 weeks after infection or 1 to 3 weeks after the appearance of the primary lesion. The VDRL titer usually is high during the secondary stage of the

disease and becomes less so during the tertiary stage. A falling titer during treatment suggests a favorable response. The fluorescent treponemal antibody absorption (FTA-ABS) test is used to detect specific antibodies to *T. pallidum*. The FTA-ABS test is used to determine whether a positive result on a nonspecific test such as the VDRL is due to syphilis.

T. pallidum cannot be cultured. Therefore, diagnosis of syphilis is based on serologic tests or darkfield microscopic examination with identification of the spirochete in specimens collected from lesions. Because the disease's incubation period may delay test sensitivity, serologic tests usually are repeated after 6 weeks when the initial test results are negative.

The treatment of choice for syphilis is penicillin. Because of the spirochetes' long generation time, effective tissue levels of penicillin must be maintained for several weeks. For this reason, long-acting injectable forms of penicillin are used. Tetracycline or erythromycin is used for treatment in people who are sensitive to penicillin. Sexual partners should be evaluated and treated prophylactically even though they may show no sign of infection.

In summary, the vaginal–urogenital–systemic STDs—chlamydial infections, gonorrhea, nonspecific urogenital infection, and syphilis—can severely involve the genital structures and also manifest as systemic infection. Both gonorrheal and chlamydial infections can cause a wide variety of genitourinary complications in men and women, and both can cause ocular disease and blindness in neonates born to infected mothers. Nonspecific urogenital infection is primarily a disease of the male urethra but may involve the cervix, urethra, Bartholin's glands, vagina, and fallopian tubes in the female. Syphilis is caused by a spirocete, *T. pallidum*. It can produce widespread systemic effects and is transferred to the fetus of infected mothers by way of the placenta.

■ REFERENCES

1. Centers for Disease Control. (1983). Condyloma acuminatum—United States 1966–1981. *Morbidity and Mortality Weekly Report*, 32(23), 306.
2. Ferenczy, A., Silverstein, S., & Crum, P.C. (1987). Importance of latency in HPV infections. *Contemporary OB Gyn*, 11, 71.
3. Tinkle, M.B. (1990). Genital human papillomavirus infection—a growing risk. *Journal of Obstetric, Gynecologic, and Neonatal Nursing*, 19(6), 501.
4. Story, B. (1987). Condylomata acuminata—an epidemic with malignant potential. *Physicians Assistant*, 12, 13.
5. Koss, L. G. (1992). Human papillomaviruses and genital cancer. *Female Patient*, 17(2), 25.
6. Schneider, A., Sawada, E., Gissman, L., et al. (1987). Human papillomaviruses in women with a history of abnormal Papanicolaou smears and in their male partners. *Obstetrics and Gynecology*, 169, 555.

7. Ferenczy, A. (1984). Comparison of 5-FU and CO$_2$ laser for treatment of vaginal condylomas. *Obstetrics and Gynecology, 64,* 773.
8. Davies, K. (1990). Genital herpes—an overview. *Neonatal Nursing, 19*(5), 401.
9. Corey, L., & Spear, P.G. (1986). Infections with herpes simplex viruses—Part 1. *New England Journal of Medicine, 314,* 686.
10. Corey, L., & Spear, P.G. (1986). Infections with herpes simplex viruses—Part 2. *New England Journal of Medicine, 314,* 749.
11. Sweet, R.L., & Gibbs, R.S. (1985). *Infectious diseases of the female genital tract* (pp. 17–26, 27–29, 35, 39–40, 103–122). Baltimore: Williams & Wilkins.
12. Centers for Disease Control. (1989). STD treatment guidelines 1989. *Morbidity and Mortality Weekly Report, 38*(S-8), 4, 22–28.
13. Cibley, L.J., & Cibley, L.J. (1986). Vulvovaginitis: Current approach to diagnosis and treatment. *Female Patient, 11*(2), 41.
14. Robertson, W.H. (1988). Mycology of vulvovaginitis. *American Journal of Obstetrics and Gynecology, 158,* 989.
15. Sobel, J.B. (1992). Pathogenesis and treatment of recurrent vulvovaginal candidiasis. *Clinics in Infectious Diseases, 14*(suppl 1), S148.
16. Patel, H.S., Peters, M.D., & Smith, C.L. (1992). Is there a role for fluconazole in the treatment of vulvovaginal candidiasis. *Annals of Pharmacotherapy, 26*(3), 350.
17. Gardner, H.L., & Dukes, C.D. (1955). *Haemophilus vaginalis* vaginitis. *American Journal of Obstetrics and Gynecology, 69,* 962.
18. Jones, B.M. (1983). *Gardnerella* vaginitis. *Medical Laboratory Sciences, 40,* 53.
19. Thomason, J.L., Schreckenberger, P.C., Spellacy, W.N., et al. (1984). Clinical and microbiological characterization of patients with nonspecific vaginosis associated with motile, curved anaerobic rods. *Journal of Infectious Diseases, 149,* 814.
20. Eschenback, D.A. (1984). Diagnosis of bacterial vaginosis (nonspecific vaginitis): Role of the laboratory. *Clinical Microbiology Newsletter, 6,* 18.
21. Centers for Disease Control. (1991). Summary of notifiable diseases—United States 1990 (formerly entitled Annual Summary). *Morbidity and Mortality Weekly Report, 39*(53), 5, 8, 22–24.
22. Addiss, D.G., Davis, J.P., & Katcher, M.L. (1987). Testing for *Chlamydia trachomatis*: Objective criteria for recommendations for screening using nonculture techniques. *Wisconsin Medical Journal, 86*(9), 25.
23. Nettleman, M.D., & Jones, R.B. (1988). Cost effectiveness of screening women at moderate risk for genital infections caused by *Chlamydial trachomatis*. *Journal of the American Medical Association, 260,* 207.
24. Buckley, H.B. (1992). Syphilis—a review and update of the "new" infection of the 90s. *Nurse Practitioner, 17*(8), 25.

■ BIBLIOGRAPHY

Breslin, E. (1988). Genital herpes simplex. *Nursing Clinics of North America, 23,* 907.

Fogel, C.I. (1988). Gonorrhea: Not a new problem but a serious one. *Nursing Clinics of North America 23,* 885.

Freund, K. (1992). Chlamydial disease in women. *Hospital Practice, 27*(2), 175–186.

Holmesk, K., March, P., Sparling, P.F., et al. (1990). *Sexually transmitted diseases.* New York: McGraw-Hill.

Lucas, V.A. (1988). Human papillomavirus infection: A potentially carcinogenic sexually transmitted disease (condylomata acuminata, genital warts). *Nursing Clinics of North America, 23,* 917.

Maccato, M., Estrada, R., Hammill, H., et al. (1992). Prevalence of active *Chlamydia trachomatis* infection at the time of exploratory laparotomy for ectopic pregnancy. *Obstetrics and Gynecology, 79*(2), 211–213.

Nettina, S.L., & Kauffman, R.H. (1990). Diagnosis and management of sexually transmitted genital lesions. *Nurse Practitioner, 15*(1), 20.

Roddy, R.E. (1988). Genital herpes. *Physician Assistant, 7,* 21.

Schiffman, M.H. (1992). Recent progress in defining the epidemiology of human papillomavirus infections and cervical neoplasia. *Journal of the National Cancer Institute, 84*(6), 394.

Secor, M.C. (1988). Bacterial vaginosis. *Nursing Clinics of North America, 23,* 865.

Smith, L.S., & Lauver, D. (1986). Assessment and management of vaginitis and cervicitis. *Nurse Practitioner, 6,* 34.

Tillman, J. (1992). Syphilis—an old disease, a contemporary perinatal problem. *Journal of Obstetric, Gynecologic, and Neonatal Nursing, 21*(3), 209.

Whalen, M. (1988). Nursing management of the patient with *Chlamydia trachomatis* infection. *Nursing Clinics of North America, 23*(4), 877.

ALTERATIONS IN METABOLISM, ENDOCRINE FUNCTION, AND NUTRITION

CHAPTER 40

CONTROL OF GASTROINTESTINAL FUNCTION

■ OBJECTIVES

After you have studied this chapter, you should be able to meet the following objectives:

■ Describe the physiologic function of the four parts of the digestive system.

■ Describe the function of the intramural neural plexuses in control of gastrointestinal function.

■ Compare the effect of parasympathetic and sympathetic activity on the motility and secretory function of the gastrointestinal tract.

■ Describe the physiology of peristalsis.

■ Trace a bolus of food through the stages of swallowing.

■ Describe the action of the internal and external sphincters in control of defecation.

■ State the source of water and electrolytes in digestive secretions.

■ Explain the protective function of saliva.

■ Describe the function of the gastric secretions in the process of digestion.

■ List three major gastrointestinal hormones and cite their function.

■ Describe the site of gastric acid and pepsin production and secretion in the stomach.

■ Describe the function of the gastric mucosal barrier.

■ Name the secretions of the small and the large intestine.

■ Relate the characteristics of the small intestine to its absorptive function.

■ Explain the function of intestinal brush border enzymes.

■ Compare the absorption of carbohydrates, fats, and proteins.

Carol Mattson Porth: PATHOPHYSIOLOGY: CONCEPTS OF
ALTERED HEALTH STATES, 4th ed. © 1994, 1990, 1986, 1982
J.B. Lippincott Company

The process of digestion and absorption of nutrients requires an intact and healthy gastrointestinal tract epithelial lining that can resist the effects of its own digestive secretions. The process involves the movement of materials through the gastrointestinal tract at a rate that facilitates absorption, and it requires the presence of enzymes for the digestion and absorption of nutrients. Structurally, the gastrointestinal tract is a long, hollow tube with its lumen inside the body and its wall acting as an interface between the internal and external environments. The wall does not normally allow harmful agents to enter the body, nor does it permit body fluids and other materials to escape.

The digestive system is truly an amazing structure. In this system, enzymes and hormones are produced, vitamins are synthesized and stored, and food is dismantled and then reassembled. Finally, wastes are collected and eliminated efficiently. Although this chapter cannot cover gastrointestinal function in its entirety, it is designed to provide the reader with an overview that is deemed essential to an understanding of subsequent chapters.

Nutrients, vitamins, minerals, electrolytes, and water enter the body through the gastrointestinal tract. As a matter of semantics, it should be pointed out that the gastrointestinal tract is also referred to as the digestive tract, the alimentary canal, and, at times, the gut. The intestinal portion may also be called the bowel. For our purposes, the salivary glands, the liver, and the pancreas, which produce secretions that aid in digestion, are considered accessory structures.

STRUCTURE AND ORGANIZATION OF THE GASTROINTESTINAL TRACT

In the digestive tract, food and other materials move slowly along its length as they are systematically broken down into ions and molecules that can be absorbed into the body itself. In the large intestine unabsorbed nutrients and wastes are collected for later elimination. What is important for the reader to recognize is that although the gastrointestinal tract is located within the body, it is really a long, hollow tube, the lumen (hollow center) of which is an extension of the external environment. Thus, nutrients do not become part of the internal environment until they have passed through the intestinal wall and have entered the blood or lymph channels.

For simplicity and understanding, the digestive system can be divided into four parts (Fig. 40-1). The *upper part*—the mouth, esophagus, and stomach—acts as an intake source and receptacle through which food passes and in which initial digestive processes take place. The *middle portion* consists of the small intestine—the duodenum, jejunum, and ileum. Most digestive and absorptive processes occur in the small intestine. The *lower segment*—the cecum, colon, and rectum—serves as a storage channel for the efficient elimination of waste. The *fourth part* consists of the accessory structures—the salivary glands, liver, and pancreas. These structures produce digestive secretions that help dismantle foods and regulate the use and storage of nutrients. The discussion in this chapter focuses on the first three parts of the gastrointestinal tract. The liver and pancreas are discussed in Chapter 42.

UPPER GASTROINTESTINAL TRACT

The mouth forms the entryway into the gastrointestinal tract for food; it contains the teeth, used in the mastication of food, and the tongue and other structures needed to direct food toward the pharyngeal structures and the esophagus.

The esophagus begins at the lower end of the pharynx. It receives food from the pharynx, and in the process of swallowing a series of peristaltic contractions moves the food into the stomach. The esophagus is a muscular, collapsible tube, about 25 cm (10 in) long, that lies behind the trachea. The muscular walls of the upper third of the esophagus are striated muscle; these muscle fibers are gradually replaced by smooth muscle fibers until at the lower third of the esophagus the muscle layer is entirely smooth muscle. The striated muscle of the upper esophagus is supplied by autonomic nervous system fibers that travel in the glossopharyngeal and vagus nerves and supply the smooth muscle. The upper and lower ends of the esophagus act as sphincters. The upper sphincter is formed by a thickening of the striated muscle; it prevents air from entering the esophagus during respiration. The lower sphincter, which is not identifiable anatomically, occurs at a point 1 cm to 2 cm from where the esophagus joins the stomach. The lower sphincter prevents gastric reflux into the esophagus.

The stomach is a pouchlike structure that lies in the upper part of the abdomen and serves as a food storage reservoir during the early stages of digestion. Although the luminal volume of the stomach is only about 50 mL, it can increase its volume to almost 1000 mL before intraluminal pressure begins to rise. The esophagus opens into the stomach through an opening called the cardiac orifice, so named because of its proximity to the heart. The part of the stomach that lies above and to the left of the cardiac orifice is called the fundus, the central portion is called the body, the

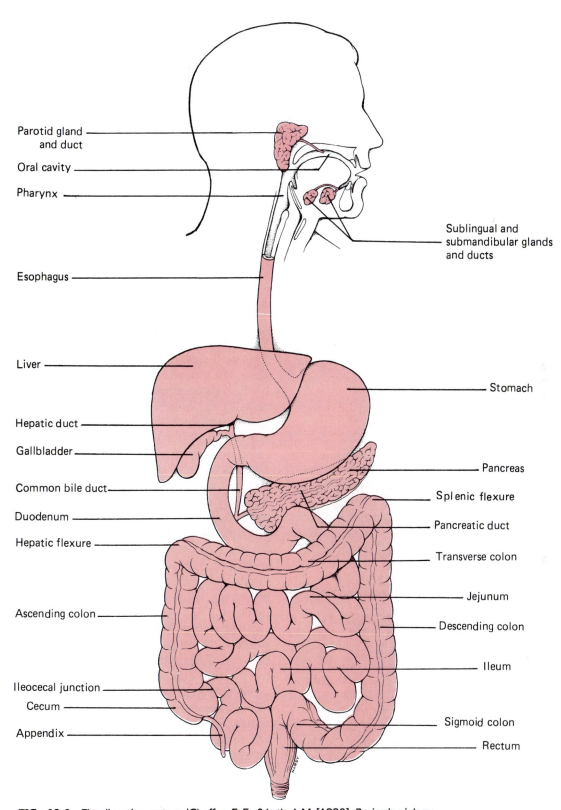

FIG. 40-1. The digestive system. (Chaffee, E. E., & Lytle, I. M. [1980]. *Basic physiology and anatomy* [4th ed.]. Philadelphia: J.B. Lippincott)

orifice encircled by a ringlike muscle that opens into the small intestine is called the pylorus, and the portion between the body and pylorus called the antrum (Fig. 40-2). The presence of a true pyloric sphincter is controversial. Whether or not an actual sphincter is present, contractions of the smooth muscle in the pyloric area control gastric emptying.

MIDDLE GASTROINTESTINAL TRACT

The small intestine, which forms the middle portion of the digestive tract, consists of three subdivisions: the duodenum, the jejunum, and the ileum. The duodenum, which is about 22 cm (10 in) in length, connects the stomach to the jejunum and contains the opening for the common bile duct and the main pancreatic duct. Bile and pancreatic juices enter the intestine through these ducts. It is in the jejunum and ileum, which are about 7 m (23 ft) in length and must be folded on themselves, that food is digested and absorbed.

LOWER GASTROINTESTINAL TRACT

The large intestine is about 1.5 m (4.5–5 ft) in length and 6 cm to 7 cm (2.5 in) in diameter. It is divided into the cecum, colon, rectum, and anal canal. The cecum is a blind pouch that hangs down at the junction of the ileum and the colon. The ileocecal valve lies at the upper border of the cecum and prevents the return of feces from the cecum into the small intestine. The

appendix arises from the cecum about 2.5 cm (1 in) from the ileocecal valve. The colon is further divided into ascending, transverse, descending, and sigmoid portions. The ascending colon extends from the cecum to the undersurface of the liver, where it turns abruptly to form the right colic (hepatic) flexure. The transverse colon crosses the upper half of the abdominal cavity from right to left and then curves sharply downward beneath the lower end of the spleen, forming the left colic (splenic) flexure. The descending colon extends the colic flexure to the rectum. The rectum extends from the sigmoid colon to the anus. The anal canal passes between the two medial borders of the levator ani muscles. Powerful sphincter muscles guard against fecal incontinence.

GASTROINTESTINAL WALL STRUCTURE

The digestive tract, once it leaves the upper third of the esophagus, is essentially a five-layered tube (Fig. 40-3). The inner luminal layer, or *mucosa*, is so named because its cells produce mucus that lubricates and protects the inner surface of the alimentary canal. The epithelial cells in this layer have a rapid turnover rate, being replaced every 4 to 5 days. Approximately 250 g of these cells are shed each day in the stool. Because of the regenerative capabilities of the mucosal layer, injury to this layer of tissue heals rapidly without leaving scar tissue. The *submucosal layer* is made up of connective tissue. This layer contains blood vessels, nerves, and structures responsible for secreting digestive enzymes. Movement in the gastrointestinal tract is facilitated by the *circular* and *longitudinal* smooth muscle layers. The fifth layer, the *peritoneum*, is loosely attached to the outer wall of the intestine.

The *peritoneum* is the largest serous membrane in the body, having a surface area about equal to that of the skin. The peritoneal membrane is composed of two layers, a thin layer of squamous cells resting on a layer of connective tissue. If the squamous layer is injured because of surgery or inflammation, there is danger that adhesions (fibrous scar-tissue bands) will form, causing sections of the viscera to heal together. Unfortunately, adhesions may alter the position and movement of the abdominal viscera.

The *peritoneal cavity* is a potential space formed between what is called the *parietal peritoneum* and the *visceral peritoneum*. The parietal peritoneum comes in contact with and is loosely attached to the abdominal wall, whereas the abdominal organs are in contact with the visceral peritoneum. The two layers of the peritoneum can be compared to a deflated balloon.[1] If

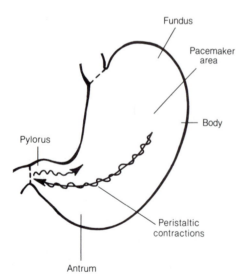

FIG. 40-2. Structures of the stomach, showing the pacemaker area and the direction of chyme movement resulting from peristaltic contractions.

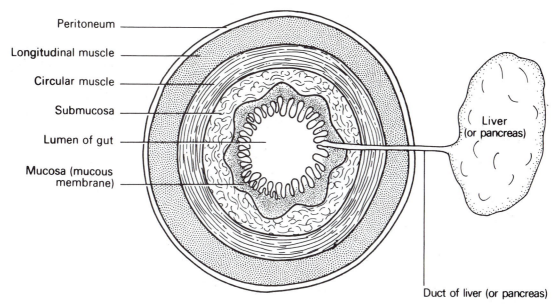

FIG. 40-3. Transverse section of the digestive system. (Thompson, J. S. [1977]. *Core textbook of anatomy*. Philadelphia: J.B. Lippincott)

one makes a fist into the balloon, the outer surface can be equated with the parietal peritoneum and the fist interfaces with the visceral peritoneum (Fig. 40-4). In this case, the area within the balloon represents the peritoneal cavity. The connective tissue layer of the peritoneum forms both the parietal and the visceral peritoneum, whereas the smooth, squamous-cell layer of the membrane lines the cavity. The adjacent membrane layers within the peritoneal cavity are separated by a thin layer of serous fluid. This fluid prevents friction between continuously moving abdominal structures. In certain pathologic states the amount of fluid in the potential space of the peritoneal cavity is increased, causing a condition called *ascites*. The *mesentery* is a double fold of peritoneum that encloses and supports the abdominal organs

(Fig. 40-5). The mesentery is no more than 20 cm to 25 cm deep, about 15 cm long in the small intestine and 7 cm long in the large intestine.

In summary, the gastrointestinal tract is a long, hollow tube, the lumen of which is an extension of the external environment. The digestive tract can be divided into four parts: an upper part consisting of the mouth, esophagus, and stomach; a middle part consisting of the small intestine; a lower part consisting of the cecum, colon, and rectum; and the accessory organs consisting of the salivary glands, the liver, and the pancreas. Throughout its length, except for the mouth, throat, and upper esophagus, the gastrointestinal tract is composed of five layers: an inner mucosal layer, a submucosal layer, a layer of circular smooth muscle fibers, a layer of longitudinal smooth muscle fibers, and an outer serosal layer that forms the peritoneum and is continuous with the mesentery.

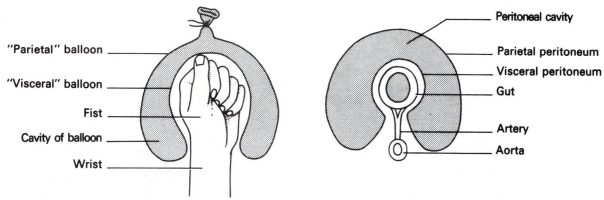

FIG. 40-4. Comparison of the peritoneal cavity with a balloon. (Thompson, J. S. [1977]. *Core textbook of anatomy*. Philadelphia: J.B. Lippincott)

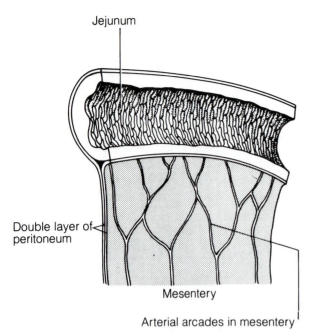

Jejunum

Double layer of peritoneum

Mesentery

Arterial arcades in mesentery

FIG. 40-5. The attachment of the mesentery to the small bowel. (Thompson, J. S. [1977]. *Core textbook of anatomy.* Philadelphia: J.B. Lippincott)

■ MOTILITY

The motility of the gastrointestinal tract propels food products and fluids along its length, from mouth to anus, in a manner that facilitates digestion and absorption. Except in the pharynx and upper third of the esophagus, smooth muscle provides the contractile force for gastrointestinal motility. The rhythmic movements of the digestive tract are self-perpetuating, much like the activity of the heart, and are influenced by local, humoral (blood-borne), and neural influences. The ability to initiate impulses is a property of the smooth muscle itself. Contractions occur in sheets or tubes of completely denervated muscle. Impulses are conducted from one muscle fiber to another.

The movements of the gastrointestinal tract are both tonic and rhythmic. The *tonic movements* are continuous movements that last for long periods of time—minutes or even hours. Tonic contractions occur at *sphincters.* The rhythmic movements consist of intermittent contractions that are responsible for mixing and moving food along the digestive tract. *Peristaltic movements* are rhythmic propulsive movements that occur when the smooth muscle layer constricts, forming a contractile band that forces the intraluminal contents forward. During peristalsis the segment that lies distal to, or ahead of, the contracted portion relaxes, so that the contents move forward with ease. Normal peristalsis always moves in the direction from the mouth toward the anus.

NEURAL CONTROL MECHANISMS

Gastrointestinal motility is controlled by neurons contained within the wall of the gastointestinal tract and by the parasympathetic and sympathetic divisions of the autonomic nervous system (ANS). The intramural neurons (those contained within the gastrointestinal tract) consist of two networks, the myenteric and submucosal plexuses. These intramural plexuses extend along the length of the gastrointestinal wall. The myenteric (Auerbach's) plexus is located between the outer muscle layers, and the submucosal (Meissner's) plexus is located between the circular muscle and the submucosal layers (Fig. 40-6). The activity of the neurons in the myenteric and submucosal plexuses is regulated both by local influences and by input from the ANS. Both plexuses are aggregates of ganglionic cells, most of which receive synaptic input from the vagus nerve. The sympathetic postganglionic fibers synapse directly with the muscle fibers. The myenteric plexus primarily influences motility, whereas the submucosal plexus affects both motility and secretion. Nerve impulses initiated in one ganglionic cell spread through multiple intramural pathways, mainly in a longitudinal direction.

Nerves of the digestive tract contain many visceral afferent fibers, which can be divided into two classes: (1) those whose cell bodies are located in the nervous system and (2) those whose cell bodies are within the intramural plexuses. The first group has receptors in the mucosal epithelium and in the muscle layers; their fibers pass centrally in vagal and sympathetic fibers. The second group exerts local control over motility by means of activity in the intramural plexus.

Efferent parasympathetic innervation to the stomach, small intestine, cecum, ascending colon, and transverse colon is by way of the vagus nerve (Fig. 40-7). The rest of the colon is innervated by parasympathetic fibers in the pelvic nerve that exits from the sacral segments of the spinal cord. Preganglionic parasympathetic fibers can synapse with intramural plexus neurons, or they can act directly on intestinal smooth muscle. Most parasympathetic fibers are excitatory. Numerous vagovagal reflexes, whose afferent and efferent fibers are both vagal nerves, influence motility as well as secretions of the digestive tract.

Efferent sympathetic innervation of the gastrointestinal tract is through the thoracic chain of sympathetic ganglia and the celiac, superior mesenteric, and inferior mesenteric ganglia. The sympathetic nervous system exerts several effects on gastrointestinal function. It controls the extent of mucus secretion by the mucosal glands, reduces motility by

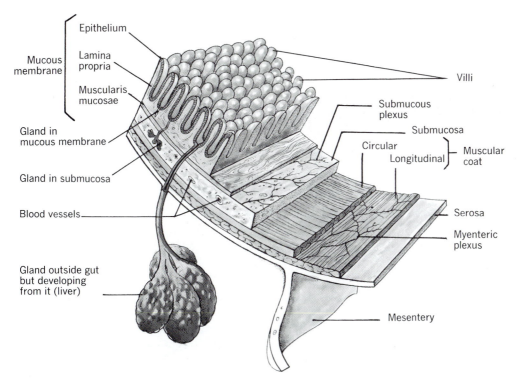

FIG. 40-6. Diagram of the four main layers of the wall of the digestive tube: mucosa, submucosa, muscular, and serosa (below the diaphragm). (Chaffee, E. E., & Lytle, I. M. [1980]. *Basic physiology and anatomy* [4th ed., p. 433]. Philadelphia: J.B. Lippincott)

inhibiting the activity of intramural plexus neurons, enhances sphincter function, and increases the vascular smooth muscle tone of the blood vessels that supply the gastrointestinal tract. The effect of the sympathetic stimulation is to block the release of the excitatory neuromediators in the intramural plexuses, inhibiting gastrointestinal motility. Sympathetic control of gastrointestinal function is largely mediated by activity within the intramural plexuses. For example, when gastric motility is enhanced because of increased vagal activity, stimulation of sympathetic centers in the hypothalamus promptly and often completely inhibits motility. The sympathetic fibers that supply the lower esophageal, pyloric, and internal and external anal sphincters are largely excitatory, but their role in controlling these sphincters is poorly understood.[2]

Intramural plexus neurons also communicate with receptors in the mucosal and muscle layers. Mechanoreceptors monitor the stretch and distention of the gastrointestinal tract wall, and chemoreceptors monitor the chemical composition (osmolality, *p*H, and digestive products of protein and fat metabolism) of its contents. These receptors can communicate directly with ganglionic cells in the intramural plexuses or with afferent fibers of the sympathetic or parasympathetic nervous system.

CHEWING AND SWALLOWING

Chewing begins the digestive process; it breaks the food into particles of a size that can be swallowed, lubricates it by mixing it with saliva, and mixes starch-containing food with salivary amylase. Although chewing is usually considered a voluntary act, it can be carried out involuntarily by a person who has lost the function of the cerebral cortex.

The swallowing reflex is a rigidly ordered sequence of events that results in the propulsion of food from the mouth to the stomach through the esophagus. Although swallowing is initiated as a voluntary activity, it becomes involuntary. Sensory impulses for the reflex begin at tactile receptors in the pharynx and esophagus and are integrated with the motor components of the response in an area of the reticular formation of the medulla and lower pons called the swallowing center. Diseases that disrupt these brain centers disrupt the coordination of swallowing and predispose an individual to food and fluid lodging in the trachea and bronchi, leading to risk of asphyxiation or aspiration pneumonia.

Swallowing consists of three phases: an oral, or voluntary phase; a pharyngeal phase; and an esophageal phase. During the oral, or voluntary, phase the bolus is collected at the back of the mouth so that the

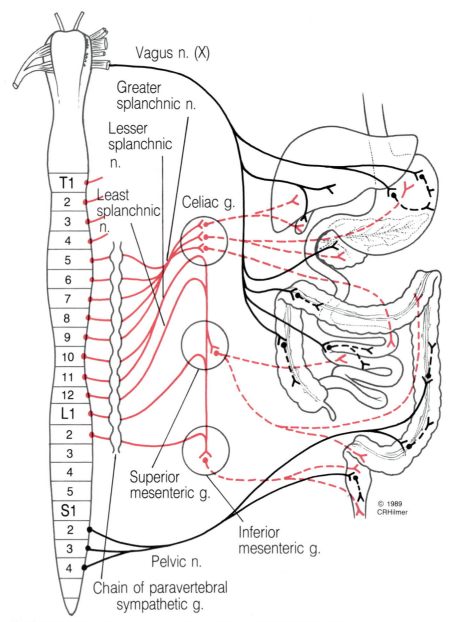

FIG. 40-7. The autonomic innervation of the gastrointestinal tract.

tongue can lift the food upward until it touches the posterior wall of the pharynx. At this point, the second stage of swallowing is initiated: the soft palate is pulled upward, the palatopharyngeal folds are pulled together so that food does not enter the nasopharynx; the vocal cords are pulled together, and the epiglottis is moved so that it covers the larynx; respiration is inhibited; and the bolus is moved backward into the esophagus by constrictive movements of the pharynx. Although the striated muscles of the pharynx are involved in the second stage of swallowing, it is an involuntary stage.

The third stage of swallowing is the esophageal stage. As food enters the esophagus and stretches its walls, both local and central nervous system reflexes that initiate peristalsis are triggered. There are two types of peristalsis—primary and secondary. Primary peristalsis is controlled by the swallowing center in the brain stem and begins when food enters the esophagus. Secondary peristalsis is partially mediated by smooth muscle fibers in the esophagus and occurs when primary peristalsis is inadequate to move food through the esophagus.[3] Peristalsis begins at the site of distention and moves downward. Before the peristaltic wave reaches the stomach, the lower esophageal sphincter relaxes to allow the bolus of food to enter the stomach. The pressure in the lower esophageal sphincter normally is greater than that in the stomach, an important factor in preventing the reflux of gastric contents. The opening of the lower esophageal sphincter is mediated vagally. Increased levels of the parasympathetic neuromediator acetylcholine increase the constriction of the sphincter. The hormone gastrin also increases constriction of the sphincter. Gastrin provides the major stimulus for stomach acid production, and its action on the lower esophageal sphincter serves to protect the esophageal mucosa when gastric acid levels are elevated.

GASTRIC MOTILITY

The stomach serves as a reservoir for ingested solids and liquids. Motility of the stomach results in the churning and grinding of solid foods and regulates the emptying of the gastric contents, or chyme, into the duodenum. Peristaltic mixing and churning contractions begin in a pacemaker area in the middle of the stomach and move toward the antrum (see Fig. 40-2). They occur at a frequency of 3 to 5 contractions per minute, with a duration of 2 seconds to 20 seconds. As the peristaltic wave approaches the antrum it speeds up, and the entire terminal 5 cm to 10 cm of the antrum contracts, occluding the pyloric opening. Contraction of the antrum reverses the movement of the chyme, returning the larger particles to the body of the stomach for further churning and kneading. Because the pylorus is contracted during antral contraction, the gastric contents are emptied into the duodenum between contractions.

Although the pylorus does not contain a true anatomic sphincter, it does function as a physiologic sphincter to prevent the backflow of gastric contents and allow them to flow into the duodenum at a rate commensurate with the ability of the duodenum to accept them. This is important because the regurgitation of bile salts and duodenal contents can damage the antrum and lead to gastric ulcers. Likewise, the duodenum can be damaged by the rapid influx of highly acid gastric contents.

Like other parts of the gastrointestinal tract, the stomach is richly innervated by both intrinsic and extrinsic nerves. Axons from the intramural plexuses innervate the smooth muscles and glands of the stomach. Extrinsic parasympathetic innervation is provided by the vagus, and sympathetic innervation by the celiac ganglia. The emptying of the stomach is regulated by both hormonal and neural mechanisms. The hormones cholecystokinin and gastric inhibitory peptide, which are thought to control gastric emptying, are released in response to pH and the osmolar and fatty acid composition of the chyme. Both local and central circuitry are involved in the neural control of gastric emptying. Afferent receptor fibers either synapse with the neurons in the intramural plexus or trigger intrinsic reflexes by means of vagal or sympathetic pathways that participate in extrinsic reflexes.[3]

Disorders of gastric motility can occur when the rate is too slow or too fast (see Chapter 41). A rate that is too slow causes gastric retention. It can be caused by either obstruction or gastric atony. Obstruction can result from the formation of scar tissue following a peptic ulcer. Another example of obstruction is hypertrophic pyloric stenosis, which can occur in infants with an abnormally thick muscularis layer in the terminal pylorus. Myotomy, or surgical incision of the muscular ring, is usually done to relieve the obstruction. Gastric atony can occur as a complication of visceral neuropathies in diabetes mellitus. Surgical procedures that disrupt vagal activity can also result in gastric atony. Abnormally fast emptying occurs in the dumping syndrome, which is a consequence of certain types of gastric surgeries. This condition is characterized by the rapid dumping of highly acidic and hyperosmotic gastric secretions into the duodenum and jejunum.

SMALL INTESTINE MOTILITY

The small intestine is the major site for the digestion and absorption of food; its movements are both mixing and propulsive. Regular peristaltic movements begin in the duodenum near the entry sites of the common duct and the main hepatic duct. A series of local pacemakers function to maintain the frequency of intestinal contraction. The peristaltic movements (about 12 per minute in the jejunum) become less frequent as they move further from the pylorus, becoming about 9 per minute in the ileum. The contractions produce both segmentation waves and propulsive movements through the muscles of the small intestine. With segmentation waves, slow contractions of circular muscle occlude the lumen and drive the contents forward and backward. Most of the contractions that produce segmentation waves are local events involving only 1 cm to 4 cm at a time. They function mainly to mix the chyme with the digestive enzymes from the pancreas and to ensure adequate exposure of all parts of the chyme to the mucosal surface of the intestine, where absorption takes place. The frequency of segmenting activity increases after a meal. Presumably it is stimulated by receptors in the stomach and intestine, because the activity does not occur following denervation of the intestine. Propulsive movements occur with synchronized activity in a section 10 cm to 20 cm in length. They are accomplished by contraction of the proximal, or orad, portion of the intestine with the sequential relaxation of its distal, or anal, portion.

Once material has been propelled to the ileocecal junction by peristaltic movement, stretching of the distal ileum produces a local reflex that relaxes the sphincter and allows fluid to squirt into the cecum.

Motility disturbances of the small bowel are common, and auscultation of the abdomen can be used to assess bowel activity. Inflammatory changes increase motility. In many instances it is not certain whether changes in motility occur because of inflammation or secondary to toxins or secreted and unabsorbed materials. Delayed passage of materials in the small intestine can also be a problem. Transient interruption of intestinal motility often occurs following gastrointestinal surgery. Intubation with suction is required to remove the accumulating intestinal contents and gases until activity is resumed.

COLONIC MOTILITY

As might be expected, the storage function of the *colon* dictates that movements within this section of the gut be different from those in the small intestine. Basically, movements in the colon are of two types. First are the segmental mixing movements, called *haustrations*, so named because they occur within sacculations called *haustra*. These movements produce a local digging-type action, which ensures that all portions of the fecal mass are exposed to the intestinal surface. Second are the *propulsive mass movements*, in which a large segment of the colon (20 cm or more) contracts as a unit, moving the fecal contents forward as a unit. Mass movements last about 30 seconds, followed by a 2- to 3-minute period of relaxation, after which another contraction occurs. A series of mass movements lasts for only 10 to 30 minutes and may only occur several times a day. Defecation is normally initiated by the mass movements.

DEFECATION

Defecation is controlled by the action of two sphincters, the *internal* and *external anal sphincters*. The internal sphincter is controlled by the autonomic nervous system, and the external sphincter is under the conscious control of the cerebral cortex.

The defecation reflex is integrated in the sacral segment of the spinal cord. In this reflex arc, afferent fibers from the rectum communicate with nerves in the sacral cord and with parasympathetic efferent fibers that move back to the bowel (see Fig. 40-7). The efferent signals from this reflex produce increased activity along the entire length of the large bowel. Other actions associated with defecation, such as abdominal pushing movements, are simultaneously integrated in the spinal cord. To prevent involuntary

defecation from occurring, the external anal sphincter is under the conscious control of the cortex. Thus, as afferent impulses arrive at the sacral cord, signaling the presence of a distended rectum, messages are transmitted to the cortex. If defecation is inappropriate, the cortex initiates impulses that constrict the external sphincter and inhibit efferent parasympathetic activity. Normally, the afferent impulses in this reflex loop fatigue easily and the urge to defecate soon dies out. At a more convenient time, contraction of the abdominal muscles compresses the contents in the large bowel, reinitiating afferent impulses to the cord.

In summary, motility of the gastrointestinal tract propels food products and fluids along its length from mouth to anus. Although the activity of gastrointestinal smooth muscle is self-propagating and can continue without input from the nervous system, its rate and strength of contractions are regulated by a network of intramural neurons that receive input from the autonomic nervous system and local receptors that monitor wall stretch and the chemical composition of its luminal contents. Parasympathetic innervation occurs by means of the vagus nerve and nerve fibers from sacral segments of the spinal cord; it serves to increase gastrointestinal motility. Sympathetic activity occurs by way of thoracolumbar output from the spinal cord, its paravertebral ganglia, and celiac, superior mesenteric, and inferior mesenteric ganglia. Sympathetic stimulation enhances sphincter function and reduces motility by inhibiting the activity of intramural plexus neurons.

■ SECRETORY FUNCTION

Each day about 7000 mL of fluid is secreted into the gastrointestinal tract (Table 40-1). Only about 50 mL to 200 mL of this fluid leaves the body in the stool; the remainder is reabsorbed in the small and large intestines. These secretions are mainly water and have a sodium and potassium concentration similar to that of extracellular fluid. Because water and electrolytes for digestive tract secretions are derived from the extracellular fluid compartment, excessive secretion

TABLE 40-1. SECRETIONS OF THE GASTROINTESTINAL TRACT	
SECRETIONS	**AMOUNT DAILY (mL)**
Salivary	1200
Gastric	2000
Pancreatic	1200
Biliary	700
Intestinal	2000
Total	7100

TABLE 40-2. MAJOR GASTROINTESTINAL HORMONES AND THEIR ACTIONS

HORMONE	SITE OF SECRETION	STIMULUS FOR SECRETION	ACTION
Cholecystokinin	Duodenum, jejunum	Amino acids	Stimulates contraction of gall-bladder; stimulates secretion of pancreatic enzymes; slows gastric emptying
Gastrin	Antrum of the stomach, duodenum	Vagal stimulation; epinephrine; neutral amino acids; solutions of calcium salts, including milk; and alcohol. Secretion inhibited by acid contents in the antrum of the stomach (below pH 2.5)	Stimulates secretion of gastric acid and pepsinogen; increases gastric blood flow; stimulates gastric smooth muscle contraction; stimulates growth of gastric mucosa, small intestine mucosa, and exocrine pancreas
Secretin	Duodenum	Acid pH or chyme entering duodenum (below pH 3.0)	Stimulates secretion of bicarbonate-containing solution by pancreas and liver

or impaired absorption can lead to extracellular fluid deficit.

CONTROL OF SECRETORY FUNCTION

The secretory activity of the gut is influenced by local, humoral, and neural influences. Neural control of gastrointestinal secretory activity is mediated through the autonomic nervous system. Secretory activity, like motility, is increased with parasympathetic stimulation and inhibited with sympathetic activity. Many of the local influences, including pH, osmolality, and chyme, consistently act as stimuli for neural and humoral mechanisms.

GASTROINTESTINAL HORMONES

The gastrointestinal tract is the largest endocrine organ in the body. It produces hormones that pass from the portal circulation into the general circulation and then back to the digestive tract, where they exert their action. Among the hormones produced by the gastrointestinal tract are *gastrin*, *secretin*, and *cholecystokinin*. These hormones influence motility and the secretion of electrolytes, enzymes, and other hormones. It has been observed that gastrin also influences the growth of the exocrine pancreas and the mucosa of the stomach and small intestine. It is reported that removal of the tissue that produces gastrin results in atrophy of these structures. This atrophy can be reversed by the administration of exogenous gastrin. The gastrointestinal tract hormones and their functions are summarized in Table 40-2.

SALIVARY SECRETIONS

Saliva is secreted in the mouth. The salivary glands consist of the parotid, submaxillary, sublingual, and buccal glands. Saliva has three functions. The first of these is protection and lubrication. Saliva is rich in mucus, which serves to protect the oral mucosa and to coat the food as it passes through the mouth, pharynx, and esophagus. The sublingual and buccal glands produce only mucous-type secretions. The second function of saliva is its protective antimicrobial action. The saliva not only cleanses the mouth but contains the enzyme lysozyme, which has an antibacterial action. Third, saliva contains ptyalin and amylase, which initiate the digestion of dietary starches. Secretions from the salivary glands are primarily regulated by the autonomic nervous system. Parasympathetic stimulation increases flow and sympathetic stimulation decreases flow. The dry mouth that accompanies anxiety attests to the effects of sympathetic activity on salivary secretions.

Mumps, or *parotitis*, is an infection of the parotid glands. Although most of us associate mumps with the contagious viral form of the disease, inflammation of the parotid glands can occur in the seriously ill person who does not receive adequate oral hygiene and who is unable to take fluids orally. Potassium iodide increases the secretory activity of the salivary glands, including the parotid glands. In a small percentage of persons, parotid swelling may occur in the course of treatment with this drug.

GASTRIC SECRETIONS

Three types of gastric glands in the stomach produce secretions: the cardiac, gastric, and pyloric glands. These glands are closely packed and oriented perpendicular to the mucosa, with one end opening into the surface epithelium. Both the cardiac glands (located in the vicinity of the esophageal orifice) and the pyloric glands (located in the distal 4 cm to 5 cm of the antrum) produce a protective mucus. The gastric glands, which are located in the fundic area of the stomach, contain chief cells, parietal cells, mucus-producing cells, and argentaffin cells. The parietal cells produce hydrochloric acid. There are about a billion parietal cells in the stomach; together they produce and secrete about 20 mEq of hydrochloric acid in several hundred milliliters of gastric juice each hour. The chief cells secrete pepsinogen, which is rapidly converted to pepsin when exposed to the low pH of the gastric juices. Some of the argentaffin cells produce serotonin (5-hydroxytryptamine). Similar cells, located in the antrum, produce gastrin. Gastric intrinsic factor, which is produced by the parietal cells, is necessary for the absorption of vitamin B_{12}.

One of the important characteristics of the gastric mucosa is its resistance to the highly acid secretions that it produces, a property derived from the mucosa's impermeability to hydrogen ions. When the gastric mucosa is damaged by aspirin, indomethacin, ethyl alcohol, or bile salts, this impermeability is disrupted and the hydrogen ions move into the tissue. This is called breaking the mucosal barrier, and substances that alter the permeability are called barrier breakers. As the hydrogen ions accumulate in the mucosal cells, intracellular pH decreases, enzymatic reactions become impaired, and cellular structures are disrupted. The result is local ischemia, vascular stasis, hypoxia, and tissue necrosis. The mucosal surface is further protected by prostaglandins. Aspirin and indomethacin inhibit prostaglandin synthesis, which also impairs the integrity of the mucosal surface.

Both parasympathetic stimulation (via the vagus nerve) and gastrin increase gastric secretions. It has long been known that histamine increases gastric-acid secretions. Recent research and clinical use of the histamine$_2$-receptor antagonists suggest that histamine may be the final common pathway for gastric-acid production. Gastric-acid secretion and its relationship to peptic ulcer are discussed in Chapter 41.

INTESTINAL SECRETIONS

The *small intestine* both secretes digestive juices and receives secretions from the liver and pancreas (see Chapter 42). Mucus-producing glands are concentrated in the duodenum at the site where the contents from the stomach and secretions from the liver and pancreas enter. These glands, called *Brunner's glands*, serve to protect the duodenum from the acid content in the gastric chyme and from the action of the digestive enzymes. The activity of Brunner's glands is strongly influenced by autonomic factors. For example, sympathetic stimulation causes a marked decrease in mucus production, leaving this area more susceptible to irritation. Interestingly, 75% to 80% of peptic ulcers occur at this site.

In addition to mucus, the intestinal mucosa produces two other types of secretions. The first is a serous fluid (pH 6.5–7.5) secreted by specialized cells (crypts of Lieberkühn) in the intestinal mucosal layer. This fluid, which is produced at the rate of 2000 mL/day, acts as a diluent for absorption. The second type consists of surface enzymes that aid absorption. These enzymes are the peptidases—enzymes that separate amino acids—and the disaccharidases—enzymes that split sugars.

The *large intestine* usually secretes only mucus. Autonomic nervous system activity strongly influences mucus production in the bowel, as in other parts of the digestive tract. During intense parasympathetic stimulation, mucus secretion may increase to the point where the stool contains large amounts of obvious mucus. Although the bowel normally does not secrete water or electrolytes, these substances are lost in large quantities when the bowel becomes irritated or inflamed.

In summary, the secretions of the gastrointestinal tract include saliva, gastric juices, bile, and pancreatic and intestinal secretions. Each day more than 7000 mL of fluid is secreted into the digestive tract; all but 50 mL to 200 mL of this fluid is reabsorbed. Water, derived from the extracellular fluid compartment, is the major component of gastrointestinal tract secretions. Neural, humoral, and local mechanisms contribute to the control of these secretions. The parasympathetic nervous system increases secretion, whereas sympathetic activity exerts an inhibitory effect. In addition to secreting fluids containing digestive enzymes, the gastrointestinal tract produces and secretes hormones, such as gastrin, secretin, and cholecystokinin, that contribute to the control of gastrointestinal function.

■ DIGESTION AND ABSORPTION

Digestion and absorption occur mainly in the small intestine. *Digestion* is the process of dismantling foods into their constituent parts. Digestion requires hydrolysis, enzyme cleavage, and fat emulsification. Hydrolysis is breakdown of a compound that involves a chemical reaction with water. The importance of hydrolysis to digestion is evidenced by the amount of water (7–8 liters) that is secreted into the gastrointestinal tract daily. *Absorption* is the process of moving nutrients and other materials from the external environment of the gastrointestinal tract into the internal environment. The intestinal mucosa is impermeable to most large molecules. Therefore, most proteins, fats, and carbohydrates must be broken down into smaller particles before they can be absorbed. Although some digestion of carbohydrates and proteins begins in the stomach, digestion takes place mainly in the small intestine. The hydrolysis of fats to free fatty acids and monoglycerides takes place entirely in the small intestine. The liver, with its production of bile, and the pancreas, which supplies a number of digestive enzymes, also play important roles in digestion.

Absorption is accomplished by active transport and diffusion. The stomach is a poor absoptive structure, and only a few lipid-soluble substances, including alcohol, are absorbed from the stomach. The absoptive function of the large intestine focuses mainly on water reabsorption. A number of substances require a specific transport carrier or system. For example, vitamin B_{12} is not absorbed in the absence of intrinsic factor. Transport of amino acid and glucose occurs mainly in the presence of sodium. Water is absorbed passively, obeying the usual laws of osmosis.

The distinguishing characteristic of the small intestine is its large surface area, which in the adult is estimated to be about 250 m^2. Anatomic features that contribute to this enlarged surface area are the circular folds that extend into the lumen of the intestine and the villi, which are finger-like projections of mucous membrane numbering as many as 25,000, that line the entire small intestine (Fig. 40-8). Each villus

is equipped with an artery, vein, and lymph vessel (lacteal), which bring blood to the surface of the intestine and transport the nutrients and other materials that have passed into the blood from the lumen of the intestine (Fig. 40-9). Fats rely largely on the lymphatics for absorption.

Each villus is covered with cells called *enterocytes* that contribute to the absorptive and digestive functions of the small bowel and goblet cells that provide mucus. The crypts of Lieberkühn are glandular structures that open into the spaces between the villi. The enterocytes have a life span of about 4 to 5 days, and it is believed that replacement cells differentiate from cells located in the area of the crypts. The maturing enterocytes migrate up the villus and are eventually extruded from the tip.

The enterocytes secrete a number of enzymes that aid in the digestion of carbohydrates and proteins. These enzymes are called *brush border enzymes* because they adhere to the border of the villus structures. In this way they have access to the carbohydrates and protein molecules as they come in contact with the absorptive surface of the intestine. This mechanism of secretion places the enzymes where they are needed and eliminates the need to produce enough enzymes to mix with the entire contents that fill the lumen of the small bowel. The digested molecules either diffuse through the membrane or are actively transported across the mucosal surface to enter the blood or, in the case of fatty acids, the lacteal. These molecules are then transported through the portal vein or lymphatics into the systemic circulation.

CARBOHYDRATE ABSORPTION

Carbohydrates must be broken down into monosaccharides, or single sugars, before they can be absorbed from the small intestine. The average daily

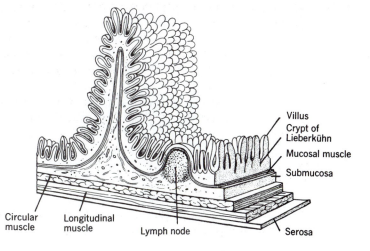

FIG. 40-8. The mucous membrane of the small intestine. Note the numerous villi on a circular fold. (Chaffee, E. E., & Lytle, I. M. [1980]. *Basic physiology and anatomy* [4th ed.]. Philadelphia: J.B. Lippincott)

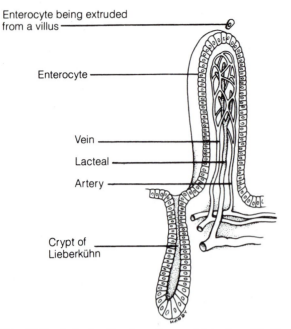

FIG. 40-9. A single villus from the small intestine. (Chaffee, E. E., & Lytle, I. M. [1980]. *Basic physiology and anatomy* [4th ed.]. Philadelphia: J.B. Lippincott)

intake of carbohydrate in the American diet is about 350 g to 400 g. Starch makes up about 50% of this total, sucrose (table sugar) about 30%, lactose (milk sugar) about 6%, and maltose about 1.5%. Digestion of starch begins in the mouth with the action of amylase. Pancreatic secretions also contain an amylase. As a result of the action of amylase, starch is broken down into several disaccharides, including maltose, isomaltose, and α-dextrins. It is the brush border enzymes that convert the disaccharides into monosaccharides that can be absorbed (Table 40-3). Sucrose yields glucose and fructose, lactose is converted to glucose and galactose, and maltose is changed to glucose. When the disaccharides are not broken down to monosaccharides, they cannot be absorbed but remain as osmotically active particles in the contents of the digestive system, causing diarrhea.

Fructose is transported across the intestinal mucosa by facilitated diffusion, which does not require energy expenditure. In this case, fructose moves along a concentration gradient. Glucose and galactose, on the other hand, are transported by way of a sodium-dependent carrier system that uses adenosine triphosphate (ATP) as an energy source (Fig. 40-10). Water absorption from the intestine is linked to absorption of osmotically active particles, such as glucose and sodium. It follows that an important consideration in facilitating the transport of water across the intestine (and decreasing diarrhea) following temporary disruption in bowel function is to include both sodium and glucose in the fluids that are taken. A number of carbonated soft drinks can be used for this purpose.

FAT ABSORPTION

The average adult eats about 60 g to 100 g of fat daily, principally as triglycerides containing long-chain fatty acids. These triglycerides are broken down by pancreatic lipase. Bile salts act as a carrier system for the fatty acids and fat-soluble vitamins A, D, E, and K by forming micelles, which transport these substances to the surface of intestinal villi where they are absorbed. The major site of fat absorption is the upper jejunum. Medium-chain triglycerides, with 6 to 10 carbon atoms, are absorbed better than longer chains of fatty acids because they are more completely hydrolyzed by pancreatic lipase and they form micelles more easily. Because they are easily absorbed, medium-chain triglycerides are often used in the treatment of persons with malabsorption syndrome. The absorption of vitamins A, D, E, and K, which are fat-soluble vitamins, requires bile salts.

TABLE 40-3. ENZYMES USED IN DIGESTION OF CARBOHYDRATES

DIETARY CARBOHYDRATES	ENZYME	MONOSACCHARIDES PRODUCED
Lactose	Lactase	Glucose and galactose
Sucrose	Sucrase	Fructose and glucose
Starch	Amylase	Maltose, maltotriase, and α-dextrins
Maltose and maltotriose	Maltase	Glucose and glucose
α-Dextrins	Isomaltase	Glucose and glucose

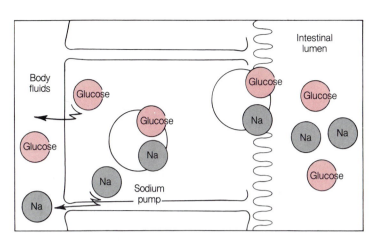

FIG. 40-10. The hypothetical sodium-dependent transport system for glucose. Both sodium and glucose must attach to the transport carrier before either can be transported into the cell. The concentration of glucose builds up within the intestinal cell until a diffusion gradient develops, causing glucose to move into the body fluids. Sodium is transported out of the cell by the energy-dependent (ATP) sodium pump. This creates the gradient needed to operate the transport system.

Fat that is not absorbed in the intestine is excreted in the stool. *Steatorrhea* is the term used to describe fatty stools. It usually indicates that there are 20 g or more of fat in a 24-hour stool sample.[2] Normally, a chemical test is done on a 72-hour stool collection, during which time the diet is restricted to 80 g to 100 g of fat per day.

PROTEIN ABSORPTION

Proteins are broken down by pancreatic enzymes, such as trypsin, chymotrypsin, carboxypeptidase, and elastase. The amino acids are liberated either intramurally or on the surface of the villi by brush border enzymes that degrade proteins into one-, two-, and three-amino-acid peptides. These amino acids are transported across the mucosal membrane in a sodium-linked process that uses ATP as an energy source.

In summary, the digestion and absorption of foodstuffs take place in the small intestine. Proteins, fats, carbohydrates, and other components of the diet are broken down into molecules that can be transported from the intestinal lumen into the body fluids.

■ REFERENCES

1. Thompson, J.S. (1990). *Core textbook of anatomy* (2nd ed., p. 111). Philadelphia: J.B. Lippincott.
2. Davenport, H.W. (1982). *Physiology of the digestive tract* (5th ed., pp. 4, 229). Chicago: Year Book Medical Publishers.
3. Berne, R.M., & Levy, M.N. (1988). *Physiology* (pp. 662, 671). St. Louis: C.V. Mosby.
4. Kosek, M.S. (1984). Medical genetics. In Krupp, M.A., & Chatton, M.J. (Eds.). *Medical diagnosis and treatment* (p. 1045). Los Altos, CA: Lange Medical Publications.
5. Kolars, J.C., Levitt, M.D., Motafa, A., et al. (1984). Yogurt—an autodigesting source of lactose. *New England Journal of Medicine, 310*, 1.

C H A P T E R   4 1

ALTERATIONS IN GASTROINTESTINAL FUNCTION

◼ OBJECTIVES

After you have studied this chapter, you should be able to meet the following objectives:

◼ Describe the physiologic mechanisms involved in anorexia, nausea, and vomiting.

◼ Define *dysphagia, odynophagia*, and *achalasia*.

◼ Relate the causes of gastroesophageal reflux to measures used in treatment of the condition.

◼ State the reason for poor prognosis in esophageal cancer.

◼ Cite the proposed role of the *Helicobacter pylori* in the development of chronic gastritis and peptic ulcer.

◼ Describe the factors that contribute to the gastric mucosal barrier.

◼ Differentiate between the causes and manifestations of acute and chronic gastritis.

◼ Describe the predisposing factors in development of peptic ulcer and cite the three complications of peptic ulcer.

◼ Compare the pharmacologic actions of antacids, histamine$_2$-receptor antagonists, and mucosal protective agents as they relate to the treatment of peptic ulcer.

◼ State the diagnostic criteria for irritable bowel syndrome.

◼ Compare the characteristics of Crohn's disease and ulcerative colitis.

◼ List at least four systemic manifestations of inflammatory bowel disease.

◼ Relate the use of a high-fiber diet in the treatment of diverticular disease to the etiologic factors involved in the development of the condition.

◼ Describe the rationale for the symptoms associated with appendicitis.

◼ List the risk factors associated with colorectal cancer.

◼ State the American Cancer Society screening methods for colorectal cancer.

◼ Compare the causes and manifestations of small-volume diarrhea and large-volume diarrhea.

◼ Explain why a failure to respond to the defecation urge may result in constipation.

◼ List five causes of fecal impaction.

Carol Mattson Porth: PATHOPHYSIOLOGY: CONCEPTS OF ALTERED HEALTH STATES, 4th ed. © 1994, 1990, 1986, 1982 J.B. Lippincott Company

■ Differentiate between mechanical and paralytic intestinal obstruction in terms of cause and manifestations.
■ List conditions that cause malabsorption by impaired intraluminal malabsorption, mucosal malabsorption, and lymphatic obstruction.

■ Describe the characteristics of the peritoneum that increase its vulnerability and protect it against the effects of peritonitis.

Gastrointestinal (GI) disorders are not cited as the leading cause of death in the United States, nor do they receive the same publicity as heart disease and cancer. Yet, according to government reports, digestive diseases rank third in the total economic burden of illness, causing considerable human suffering, personal expenditures for treatment, lost working hours, and a drain on the nation's economy. It has been estimated that 20 million Americans, one out of every nine people in the United States, have digestive disease. Even more important is the fact that proper nutrition or a change in health practices could prevent or minimize many of these disorders. The content of this chapter has been organized into five sections: (1) manifestations of GI disorders: (2) disorders of the esophagus, (3) disorders of the stomach, (4) disorders of the small and large intestine, and (5) disorders of the peritoneum.

■ MANIFESTATIONS OF GASTROINTESTINAL DISORDERS

Several signs and symptoms are common to many types of GI disorders. These include anorexia, nausea, vomiting, and GI bleeding. Because they occur with so many of the disorders, they are discussed separately as an introduction to the content that follows.

ANOREXIA, NAUSEA, AND VOMITING

Anorexia, nausea, and vomiting are physiologic responses that are common to many GI disorders. These responses are protective to the extent that they signal the presence of disease and, in the case of vomiting, remove noxious agents from the GI tract. They can also contribute to impaired intake or loss of fluids and nutrients.

Anorexia. Anorexia is loss of appetite. A number of factors influence appetite. One of these factors is hunger, which is stimulated by contractions of the empty stomach. Appetite or the desire for food intake is also regulated by the hypothalamus and other associated centers in the brain. Smell plays an important role, as evidenced by the fact that appetite can be stimulated or suppressed by the smell of food. Loss of appetite is associated with emotional situations, such as fear, depression, frustration, and anxiety. Many drugs and disease states cause anorexia. In uremia, for example, the accumulation of nitrogenous wastes in the blood contributes to the development of anorexia. Anorexia is often a forerunner of nausea, and most conditions that cause nausea and vomiting also produce anorexia.

Nausea. Nausea is an ill-defined and unpleasant subjective sensation. It is basically a conscious recognition of stimulation of the medullary vomiting center. Nausea is usually preceded by anorexia, and stimuli such as foods and drugs that cause anorexia in small doses will usually produce nausea when given in larger doses. A common cause of nausea is distention of the duodenum, or upper small intestinal tract. Nausea is frequently accompanied by autonomic responses such as watery salivation and vasoconstriction with pallor, sweating, and tachycardia. Nausea may function as an early warning signal of pathology.

Vomiting. Vomiting or emesis is the sudden and forceful oral expulsion of the contents of the stomach. It is usually, but not always, preceded by nausea. The contents that are vomited are called *vomitus*. Vomiting appears to involve two functionally distinct medullary centers: the vomiting center and the chemoreceptor trigger zone. The act of vomiting is integrated by the vomiting center, which is located in the dorsal portion of the reticular formation of the medulla near the sensory nuclei of the vagus. The act of vomiting consists of taking a deep breath, closing the airways, and producing a strong, forceful contraction of the diaphragm and abdominal muscles along with relaxation of the gastroesophageal sphincter. Respiration ceases during the act of vomiting. Vomiting may be accompanied by dizziness, lightheadedness, decrease in blood pressure, and bradycardia.

The vomiting center may receive stimuli from

the GI tract and other organs, from the cerebral cortex, from the vestibular apparatus responsible for motion sickness, and from the chemoreceptor trigger zone activated by many drugs and endogenous and exogenous toxins. The phenothiazine derivatives, such as chlorpromazine (Thorazine) and prochlorperazine (Compazine), depress vomiting caused by stimulation of the chemoreceptor trigger zone. Hypoxia exerts a direct effect on the vomiting center, producing nausea and vomiting. This direct effect probably accounts for the vomiting that occurs during periods of decreased cardiac output, shock, environmental hypoxia, and brain ischemia caused by increased intracranial pressure. Inflammation of any of the intraabdominal organs, including the liver, gallbladder, or urinary tract, can cause vomiting because of stimulation of the visceral afferent pathways that communicate with the vomiting center. Distention or irritation of the GI tract also causes vomiting through stimulation of visceral afferent neurons.

Vomiting, as a basic physiologic protective mechanism, limits the possibility of damage from ingested noxious agents by emptying the contents of the stomach and portions of the small intestine. Nausea and vomiting may represent a total-body response to drug therapy, including overdosage, cumulative effects, toxicity, and side effects.

GASTROINTESTINAL TRACT BLEEDING

Bleeding from the GI tract can be evidenced by blood that appears in either the vomitus or the feces. It can result from disease or trauma to the GI structures, as a result of primary diseases of the blood vessels (*i.e.*, esophageal varices or hemorrhoids), or because of disorders in blood clotting.

Hematemesis. The presence of blood in the stomach is usually irritating and causes vomiting. Hematemesis refers to blood in the vomitus. It may be bright red or have a "coffee-ground" appearance because of the action of the digestive enzymes.

Melena. Blood that appears in the stool may range in color from bright red to tarry black. Bright red blood usually indicates that the bleeding is from the lower bowel. When it coats the stool, it is often the result of bleeding hemorrhoids. The word *melena* means black and refers to the passage of black and tarry stools. These stools have a characteristic odor that is not easily forgotten. The presence of tarry stools usually indicates that the source of bleeding is above the level of the ileocecal valve, although this is not always the case. Approximately 60 mL of blood

are required to produce a single tarry stool; acute blood loss may produce melena for up to 3 days.[1] With hypermotility of the GI tract, bright red blood may be present in the stools even though the bleeding is from the upper GI tract. *Occult* (hidden) blood is blood that can only be detected by chemical means. It can be caused by gastritis, peptic ulcer, or lesions of the intestine. Occult bleeding can be detected by the use of a simple card test for hemoglobin peroxidase. A positive test can be due to upper or lower GI bleeding, dietary peroxidases, or vitamin C.

Blood urea nitrogen (BUN) is frequently elevated after hematemesis or melena. This results from breakdown of the blood by the digestive enzymes and the absorption of the nitrogenous end-products into the blood. The BUN usually reaches a peak within 24 hours after the GI hemorrhage. It does not appear when the bleeding is in the colon, because digestion does not take place at this level of the digestive system. An elevation in body temperature may also follow GI hemorrhage. It usually occurs within 24 hours and may last for a few days to a few weeks.

In summary, the signs and symptoms of many GI tract disorders are manifested by anorexia, nausea, and vomiting. Anorexia, or loss of appetite, may occur alone or may accompany nausea and vomiting. Nausea, which is an ill-defined, unpleasant sensation, signals the stimulation of the medullary vomiting center. It often precedes vomiting and is frequently accompanied by autonomic responses such as salivation and vasoconstriction with pallor, sweating, and tachycardia. The act of vomiting, which is integrated by the vomiting center, involves the forceful oral expulsion of the gastric contents. It is a basic physiologic mechanism that rids the GI tract of noxious agents. Disorders that disrupt the integrity of the GI tract often cause bleeding, which can be manifested as blood in the vomitus (hematemesis) or as blood in the stool (melena).

■ DISORDERS OF THE ESOPHAGUS

The esophagus is a tube that connects the oropharynx with the stomach. It lies posterior to the trachea and larynx and extends through the mediastinum, intersecting the diaphragm at the level of the 11th thoracic vertebra. The esophagus functions primarily as a conduit for passage of food from the pharynx to the stomach, and the structures of its walls are designed for this purpose: the smooth muscle layers provide the peristaltic movements needed to move food along its length, whereas the epithelial layer secretes mucus, which protects its surface and aids in lubricating food. There are sphincters at either end of the esophagus: an upper esophageal sphincter and a lower esophageal sphincter. The upper esophageal (or pharyngoesophageal) sphincter consists of a circular layer of striated muscle, the cricopharyngeal muscle. The lower esophageal (or gastroesophageal) sphincter is a 1- to 2-cm zone of increased pressure that is maintained at a level greater than that of the stomach. The anatomic structure of the lower esophageal sphincter is no different from the rest of the esophagus; however, physiologically, it remains tonically constricted, in contrast to the middle and upper portions of the esophagus.[2]

DYSPHAGIA

The act of swallowing depends on the coordinated action of the tongue and pharynx. These structures are innervated by the 5th, 9th, 10th, and 12th cranial nerves. *Dysphagia* refers to difficulty in swallowing. If swallowing is painful, it is referred to as *odynophagia*. Dysphagia can result from altered nerve function or from disorders that produce narrowing of the esophagus. Lesions of the central nervous system, such as a stroke, often involve the cranial nerves that control swallowing. Strictures and cancer of the esophagus and strictures resulting from scarring reduce the size of the esophageal lumen and make swallowing difficult.

In a condition called *achalasia*, the lower esophageal sphincter fails to relax; food that has been swallowed has difficulty passing into the stomach, and the esophagus above the sphincter becomes enlarged. One or several meals may lodge in the esophagus and pass slowly into the stomach over a period of time. There is danger of aspiration of esophageal contents into the lungs when the person lies down. Treatment is mechanical dilatation or surgical procedures to weaken the sphincter.

ESOPHAGEAL DIVERTICULUM

A diverticulum of the esophagus is an outpouching of the esophageal wall caused by a weakness of the muscularis layer. An esophageal diverticulum tends to retain food. Complaints that the food stops before it reaches the stomach are common, as are reports of gurgling, belching, coughing, and foul-smelling breath. Additionally, the trapped food may cause esophagitis and ulceration. Because the condition is usually progressive, correction of the defect requires surgical intervention.

GASTROESOPHAGEAL REFLUX

The term *reflux* refers to backward or return movement. In terms of gastroesophageal reflux, it refers to backward movement of gastric contents into the esophagus, a condition that causes heartburn. It is probably the most common disorder originating in

the GI tract. Most people experience heartburn occasionally as a result of reflux. Such symptoms usually occur soon after eating, are short-lived, and seldom cause more serious problems. However, for some people, persistent heartburn can represent reflux disease with esophagitis.

Reflux esophagitis involves mucosal injury to the esophagus, hyperemia, and inflammation. A hiatal hernia may or may not be present. Although once thought to be the primary cause of gastroesophageal reflux, hiatal hernia is no longer considered to play a major role in the pathology of the disorder.[3] Instead, it is currently thought that the condition results from a weak or incompetent lower esophageal sphincter that allows reflux to occur and factors such as decreased esophageal peristalsis and salivary function that impair clearance of the refluxed acid from the esophagus once it has occurred. Findings indicate that swallowed saliva contributes to acid neutralization and its clearance from the esophagus after reflux.[4] Thus, esophageal acid clearance may be delayed by impaired peristalsis, an abnormality in swallowed saliva, or both.

The most frequent symptom of gastroesophageal reflux is heartburn. It is frequently severe occurring 30 to 60 minutes after eating and is often made worse by bending at the waist and recumbency and is usually relieved by sitting upright. The severity of heartburn is not indicative of the extent of mucosal injury; only 30% to 40% of people who complain of heartburn have mucosal injury.[5] Often the heartburn occurs during the night. Antacids give prompt, although transient relief. Drinking of water or other liquids may afford relief, probably because they wash the gastric contents back into the stomach. Other symptoms include belching and sometimes chest pain. The pain is usually located in the epigastric or retrosternal area and often radiates to the throat, shoulder, or back. Because of its location, the pain may be confused with angina. The reflux of gastric contents may also produce respiratory symptoms such as wheezing, chronic cough, and hoarseness.

Complications can result from persistent reflux, producing a cycle of mucosal damage that causes hyperemia, edema, and erosion of the luminal surface. These complications include strictures and a condition called *Barrett's esophagus*. Strictures are caused by a combination of scar tissue, spasm, and edema. They produce narrowing of the esophagus and cause dysphagia when the lumen becomes sufficiently constricted. Barrett's esophagus is characterized by a reparative process in which the squamous mucosa of the esophagus is gradually replaced by columnar epithelium resembling that in the stomach or intestines. It is associated with increased risk of developing esophageal cancer.

DIAGNOSIS AND TREATMENT

Diagnosis of gastroesophageal reflux depends on history and selective use of diagnostic methods including radiographic studies using a contrast medium such as barium, esophagoscopy, and 24-hour pH monitoring. Esophagoscopy involves the passage of a flexible fiberoptic endoscope into the esophagus for the purpose of visualizing the lumen of the upper GI tract. It also permits performance of a biopsy, should that be indicated. For the 24-hour pH monitoring, a small tube with a pH electrode is passed through the nose and down into the esophagus. Data from the electrode are recorded in a small lightweight box worn on a belt around the waist and later are analyzed by computer. The box has a button that the person can press to indicate episodes of heartburn or pain; these can be correlated with episodes of acid reflux.

The treatment of gastroesophageal reflux generally focuses on conservative measures. These measures include avoidance of positions and conditions that increase gastric reflux. Frequent, small feedings are preferred to large meals because they prevent gastric distention. It is recommended that meals be eaten sitting up and that the recumbent position be avoided for several hours after a meal. Bending for long periods should be avoided, because it tends to increase intraabdominal pressure and cause gastric reflux. Sleeping with head elevated helps to prevent reflux during the night. This is best accomplished by placing blocks under the head of the bed or by using a wedge-shaped bolster to elevate the head and shoulders by at least 6 inches. Antacids or a combination of antacids and alginic acid is also recommended for mild disease. Alginic acid produces a foam when it comes in contact with gastric acid; if reflux occurs, the foam rather than acid rises into the esophagus. For some people, drinking of water dilutes the gastric acid and washes it back into the stomach. Histamine$_2$ blocking drugs, which inhibit gastric acid production, are often recommended when additional treatment is needed. A newer drug, omeprazole, acts by inhibiting the gastric proton pump, which regulates the final pathway for acid secretion. This drug may be used for people who continue to have daytime symptoms, recurrent strictures, or large esophageal ulcerations. The safety of long-term use of the drug has not been established; the drug can only be given for 3 months at a time.[4]

CANCER OF THE ESOPHAGUS

Carcinoma of the esophagus accounts for 1% to 2% of all cancer deaths. This disease is more common in men over the age of 50 with the male-to-female ratio being approximately 3:1.[6] It is reported that environmental factors contribute to the development of esophageal cancers. These environmental factors include conditions that cause food or drink to remain in the esophagus for prolonged periods of time and continued exposure to irritants such as alcohol and tobacco. Certain precancerous conditions such as achalasia and history of caustic injury to the esophagus increase the risk of esophageal cancer, as does Barrett's esophagus.

Dysphagia is by far the most frequent complaint of people with esophageal cancer. It is apparent first with ingestion of bulky food, later with soft food, and finally with liquids. Unfortunately, it is a late manifestation of the disease. Weight loss, anorexia, fatigue, and pain on swallowing may also be present.

Treatment includes surgical resection, which provides a means of cure when done in early disease and palliation when done in late disease. Radiation is used as a palliative treatment. Chemotherapy is sometimes used preoperatively to decrease the size of the tumor, and it may used along with radiation and surgery in an effort to increase survival.[7]

The prognosis for people with cancer of the esophagus, although poor, has improved.[7] Even with modern forms of therapy, however, the long-term survival is limited because, in many cases, the disease has already metastasized by the time the diagnosis is made. This indicates that better methods of early diagnosis are needed.

In summary, the esophagus is a tube that connects the oropharynx with the stomach; it functions primarily as a conduit for passage of food from the pharynx to the stomach. Dysphagia refers to difficulty in swallowing; it can result from altered nerve function or from disorders that produce narrowing of the esophagus. A diverticulum of the esophagus is an outpouching of the esophageal wall caused by a weakness of the muscularis layer. Gastrointestinal reflux refers to backward movement of gastric contents into the esophagus, a condition that causes heartburn. Although most people experience occasional esophageal reflux and heartburn, persistent reflux can cause esophagitis. Carcinoma of the esophagus, which accounts for 1% to 2% of all cancer deaths, is more common in men over the age of 50 with the male-to-female ratio being approximately 3:1. It is commonly linked to environmental factors including conditions that cause food or drink to remain in the esophagus for prolonged periods of time and continued exposure to irritants such as alcohol and tobacco.

■ DISORDERS OF THE STOMACH

The stomach is a reservoir for contents entering the digestive tract; it lies in the upper abdomen, anterior to the pancreas, splenic vessels, and left kidney. Anteriorly, the stomach is bounded by the anterior abdominal wall and the left inferior lobe of the liver. While in the stomach, food is churned and mixed with hydrochloric acid and pepsin before being released into the small intestine. Normally, the mucosal surface of the stomach provides a barrier that protects it from the hydrochloric acid and pepsin contained in gastric secretions. Disorders of the stomach include gastritis, peptic ulcer, and gastric carcinoma.

GASTRIC MUCOSAL BARRIER

Normally, the stomach lining is impermeable to the acid it secretes, a property that allows the stomach to contain acid and pepsin without having its wall digested. Several factors contribute to the protection of the gastric mucosa including: (1) an impermeable epithelial cell surface covering, (2) mechanisms for the selective transport of hydrogen and bicarbonate ions, and (3) the characteristics of gastric mucus.[8] These mechanisms are collectively referred to as the *gastric mucosal barrier.*

The gastric epithelial cells are connected by tight junctions that prevent acid penetration, and they are covered with an impermeable hydrophobic lipid layer that prevents diffusion of ionized water-soluble molecules. Aspirin, which is nonionized and lipid-soluble in acid solutions, rapidly diffuses across this lipid layer increasing mucosal permeability and damaging epithelial cells. Occult bleeding due to gastric irritation occurs in a significant number of people who take aspirin on a regular basis (*e.g.,* as a treatment for arthritis). Aspirin becomes ionized in neutral or basic solutions; therefore, buffered aspirin is less likely to penetrate the cell surface covering and cause gastric irritation. Alcohol, which is also lipid-soluble, is known to disrupt the mucosal barrier; when aspirin and alcohol are taken in combination, as they often are, there is increased risk of gastric irritation. Bile acids also attack the lipid components of the mucosal barrier and afford the potential for gastric irritation when there is reflux of duodenal contents into the stomach.

Normally, the secretion of hydrochloric acid secretion by the parietal cells of the stomach is accompanied by secretion of bicarbonate ions. For every hydrogen ion that is secreted, a bicarbonate ion is produced and diffuses out of the cell. The bicarbonate ion serves to buffer the hydrogen ions, and, as long as bicarbonate ion production is equal to hydrogen ion secretion, mucosal injury does not occur. Changes in gastric blood flow, as in shock, tend to decrease bicarbonate production. This is particularly true in situations in which decreased blood flow is accompanied by acidosis. Aspirin and the nonsteroi-

dal antiinflammatory drugs (NSAIDs) such as indomethacin and ibuprofen also impair bicarbonate secretion.

The mucus that protects the gastric mucosa is of two types: water-insoluble and water-soluble.[8] Water-insoluble mucus forms a thin stable gel that adheres to the gastric mucosal surface and provides protection from the proteolytic (protein-digesting) actions of pepsin. It also forms an unstirred layer that traps bicarbonate, forming an alkaline interface between the luminal contents of the stomach and its mucosal surface. The water-insoluble mucus is washed from the mucosal surface and mixes with the luminal contents; its viscid nature makes it a lubricant that prevents mechanical damage to the mucosal surface. In addition to their effects on mucosal permeability and bicarbonate production, damaging agents such as aspirin and the NSAIDs inhibit and modify the characteristics of gastric mucus.

It is becoming increasingly evident that the prostaglandins play an important role in protecting the GI mucosa from injury. The prostaglandins (chemical messengers derived from cell membrane lipids) probably exert their effect through improved blood flow, increased bicarbonate ion secretion, and improved mucus production and characteristics. The fact that drugs such as aspirin and the NSAIDs inhibit prostaglandin synthesis may contribute to their ability to produce gastric irritation. Smoking and older age have been associated with reduced gastric and duodenal prostaglandin concentrations; these observations may explain the predisposition to ulcer disease in smokers and older people.[9]

The S-shaped bacterium called *Helicobacter pylori* (formerly *Campylobacter pylori*) can colonize the mucus-secreting epithelial cells of the stomach and disrupt the barrier.[10] The *H. pylori* have multiple flagella, which allow them to move through the mucous layer of the stomach, and they secrete urease, which enables them to produce sufficient ammonia to buffer the acidity of their immediate environment. These properties help to explain why the organism is able to survive in the acidic environment of the stomach. Because the organism will only adhere to the mucus-secreting cells of the stomach, it does not usually colonize other parts of the GI tract. The exceptions are areas such as Barrett's esophagus and a duodenal ulcer site in which the normal epithelial layer has been replaced with gastric mucosa. The organism produces an enzyme that degrades mucin and has the capacity to interfere with the local protection of the gastric mucosa against acid. It may also produce toxins that directly damage the mucosa and produce ulceration in other ways. There is increasing evidence that the organism contributes to the development of both chronic gastritis (type B) and peptic ulcer. Ingestion of *H. pylori* has been shown to cause gastritis; eradication of the organism by means of antimicrobial agents resolves the disorder.[10]

GASTRITIS

Gastritis refers to inflammation of the gastric mucosa. There are many causes of gastritis, most of which can be grouped under the headings of acute or chronic gastritis.

ACUTE GASTRITIS

Acute gastritis refers to a transient inflammation of the gastric mucosa. It is most commonly associated with local irritants such as bacterial endotoxins, caffeine, alcohol, and aspirin. Depending on the severity of the disorder, the mucosal response may vary from moderate edema and hyperemia to hemorrhagic erosion of the gastric mucosa.

The complaints of people with acute gastritis vary. Often, people with aspirin-related gastritis are totally unaware of the condition or may complain only of heartburn or sour stomach. Gastritis associated with excessive alcohol consumption is a different situation: it often causes transient gastric distress, which may lead to vomiting and, in more severe situations, to bleeding and hematemesis. Gastritis caused by infectious organisms, such as the staphylococcal endotoxins, usually has an abrupt and violent onset, with gastric distress and vomiting about 5 hours after the ingestion of a contaminated food source. Acute gastritis is usually a self-limiting disorder; complete regeneration and healing usually occur within several days.

CHRONIC GASTRITIS

Chronic gastritis is a separate entity from that of acute gastritis. It is characterized by the absence of grossly visible erosions and the presence of chronic inflammatory changes leading eventually to atrophy of the glandular epithelium of the stomach. The changes may become dysplastic and possibly be transformed into carcinoma. There are two major forms of chronic gastritis, type A and type B, based on their distribution and their pathogenesis.

Type A gastritis is the least common form of chronic gastritis. It typically involves the fundus and the body of the stomach and is associated with pernicious anemia. This form of chronic gastritis is considered to be of autoimmune origin, and most people with the disorder have circulating antibodies to parietal cells and intrinsic factor. Autoimmune destruction of the parietal cells leads to hypo- or achlorhydria, a high intragastric *p*H, and hypergastrinemia. Because of decreased secretion of intrinsic factor, some people go on to develop pernicious anemia (see Chapter 18). This type of chronic gastritis is frequently associated with other autoimmune disorders such as Hashimoto's thyroiditis and Addison's disease.

Type B gastritis is the more common form of chronic gastritis and is of nonimmune origin. The incidence of chronic gastritis increases with age. Many people with peptic ulcer have an associated chronic gastritis. This form of gastritis can be further subdivided into hypersecretory antral gastritis and environmental gastritis.[11] People with hypersecretory gastritis generally secrete excess acid, have a lower intragastric *p*H, and frequently have an associated duodenal ulcer. Environmental gastritis has a worldwide distribution and in any country is the most common form of gastritis in all age groups, particularly in the elderly. Therefore, it is believed to be related to environmental factors that have not been clearly defined. *H. pylori* has been implicated as a major causative agent. Colonization with *H. pylori* is common in the general population, and its increasing prevalence with age could explain the increased prevalence of chronic gastritis in the elderly. Other factors such as chronic alcohol abuse, cigarette smoking, and chronic use of NSAIDs may contribute to development of the disease.

Chronic gastritis causes few symptoms related directly to gastric changes. People with type A chronic gastritis may develop pernicious anemia. More important is the development of peptic ulcer and increased risk of gastric carcinoma. Approximately 2% to 4% of people with atrophic gastritis eventually develop gastric carcinoma.[6]

PEPTIC ULCER DISEASE

Peptic ulcer is a term used to describe a group of ulcerative disorders that occur in areas of the upper GI tract that are exposed to acid–pepsin secretions. The most common forms of peptic ulcer are duodenal and gastric ulcers.

Peptic ulcer disease, with its remissions and exacerbations, represent a chronic health problem. At present, 10% of the population has or will develop a peptic ulcer. In terms of location, duodenal ulcers are two to three times more common than gastric ulcers. Ulcers in the duodenum occur at any age and are frequently seen in early adulthood. Gastric ulcers, on the other hand, tend to affect the older age group with peak incidence in the sixth and seventh decades. Both types of ulcers affect men three to four times as frequently as they do women.

PREDISPOSING FACTORS

A peptic ulcer represents a break in the continuity of the mucosal layer. Although knowledge is incomplete, it is generally assumed that peptic ulcer formation reflects an imbalance between (1) acid and pepsin production and (2) the ability of the affected gastric mucosal barrier to resist the destructive action of these digestive agents. Seldom can ulcer development be traced to a single cause. It is more likely that both factors contribute to the development of a peptic ulcer. Nevertheless, it seems helpful, in terms of understanding ulcer development, to view these differences in causation in terms of the function that the mucosal surface affords the stomach and the duodenum.

Increased Acid–Pepsin Production. Hydrochloric acid production is influenced by several factors, including neural and hormonal stimulation. The hormone gastrin, which is produced in the antrum of the stomach, is a potent stimulus for hydrochloric acid secretion. Increased levels of gastric acid have also been attributed to (1) increased numbers of acid–pepsin producing cells in the stomach, (2) increased sensitivity of the parietal cells to food and other stimuli (*e.g.*, both alcohol and caffeine are potent stimulators of hydrochloric acid secretion), (3) excessive vagal stimulation, and (4) impaired inhibition of gastric secretions as food moves into the intestine.

The intractable peptic ulcers observed in a condition called the *Zollinger-Ellison syndrome* are caused by a gastrin-secreting tumor of the pancreas. Normally, gastrin secretion is inhibited as food moves into the intestine. It has been postulated that this reflex inhibition of gastrin may be impaired in certain types of ulcers. For example, *Cushing's ulcer* is a special type of stress ulcer that occurs in association with severe brain injury or neurosurgery. It results from increased central stimulation of the vagus nerve and is unresponsive to reflex mechanisms that normally control gastric secretions.

Resistance of the Mucosal Surface. The defenses of the mucosal surface depend on an adequate blood flow and an intact mucosal barrier. It can be assumed that any disruption in the mucosal barrier reduces these defenses and renders the mucosal surface more susceptible to the destructive effects of the hydrogen ion.

It has been suggested that a basic abnormality in people with gastric peptic ulcers is an increased permeability of the epithelial lining of the stomach to hydrogen ions, which causes injury to the mucosal surface and reduces its resistance to further injury. It

also is possible that a chronically diseased mucosal membrane is unable to secrete sufficient mucus to form an effective barrier. Reflux of bile from the intestine into the stomach has been implicated in peptic ulcer. In addition to bile, a number of drugs are recognized as "barrier breakers." Both aspirin and alcohol are known to damage this barrier.

The duodenum, which acts as a passageway for digestive enzymes and acid-laden chyme, is a common site of peptic ulcers. Brunner's glands, located between the pylorus and the site where bile and pancreatic enzymes enter the duodenum, produce a large amount of viscid mucus, which serves to protect this area. The activity of these glands is inhibited by sympathetic stimulation; this may help to explain why anxiety and stress contribute to duodenal ulcer development.

In addition to the erosiveness of acid and pepsin, *H. pylori* is strongly suspected of playing a role in the development of peptic ulcer. Since its identification in 1982, the organism has generated worldwide interest. It has been reported that up to 90% of people with duodenal ulcer and 70% of people with gastric ulcer have *H. pylori* infection and active chronic gastritis. Eradication of the organism can result in resolution of gastritis, with subsequent ulcer healing. Furthermore, treatment trials have shown that eradication of *H. pylori* with bismuth preparations, antibiotics, or both leads to marked reduction in the recurrence rate of peptic ulcer when compared with standard acid-suppression methods. It is not known if *H. pylori* infection can cause peptic ulcer. Some people may have a bout of acute gastritis, but their immune system is able to eradicate the organism; others may be left with permanently damaged gastric mucosa that is susceptible to erosion and ulcer. The role that *H. pylori* plays in the development of gastritis and peptic ulcer is expected to become clearer as more definitive information becomes available.

MANIFESTATIONS AND COMPLICATIONS

The clinical manifestations of uncomplicated peptic ulcer focus on discomfort and pain. The pain, which is described as burning, gnawing, or cramplike, is usually rhythmic and frequently occurs when the stomach is empty—between meals and at 1 o'clock or 2 o'clock in the morning. The pain is usually located over a small area near the midline in the epigastrium near the xiphoid and may radiate below the costal margins, into the back, or rarely, to the right shoulder. Characteristically, the pain is relieved by food or antacids. Superficial and deep epigastric tenderness and voluntary muscle guarding may occur with more extensive lesions.

A peptic ulcer can affect one or all layers of the stomach or duodenum. The ulcer may penetrate only the mucosal surface, or it may extend into the smooth muscle layers. Occasionally, an ulcer will penetrate the outer wall of the stomach or duodenum. Spontaneous remissions and exacerbations are common. Healing of the muscularis layer involves replacement with scar tissue; although the mucosal layers that cover the scarred muscle layer regenerate, the regeneration is often less than perfect, which contributes to repeated episodes of ulceration. Precipitating factors include local injury, infections, and physical or emotional stress.

The complications of peptic ulcer include hemorrhage, obstruction, and perforation. Hemorrhage is caused by bleeding from granulation tissue or from erosion of an ulcer into an artery or vein. It occurs in 10% to 15% of people with peptic ulcer. Evidence of bleeding may consist of hematemesis or melena. Bleeding may be sudden, severe, and without warning, or it may be insidious, producing only occult (hidden) blood in the stool. Acute hemorrhage is evidenced by the sudden onset of weakness, dizziness, thirst, cold moist skin, the desire to defecate, and the passage of loose tarry or even red stools, and coffee-ground emesis. Signs of circulatory shock develop depending on the amount of blood that is lost.

Obstruction is caused by edema, spasm, or contraction of scar tissue and interference with the free passage of gastric contents through the pylorus or adjacent areas. There is a feeling of epigastric fullness and heaviness after meals; with severe obstruction, there is vomiting of undigested food.

Perforation occurs when an ulcer erodes through all the layers of the stomach or duodenum wall. With perforation, GI contents enter the peritoneum and cause peritonitis, or penetrate adjacent structures such as the pancreas. Radiation of the pain into the back, severe night distress, inadequate pain relief from eating foods or taking antacids in people with a long history of peptic ulcer may signify perforation. Peritonitis is discussed as a separate topic at the end of this chapter.

DIAGNOSIS AND TREATMENT

Diagnostic procedures for peptic ulcer include history, laboratory findings, radiologic imaging, and endoscopic examination. Laboratory findings of hypochromic anemia and occult blood in the stools indicate bleeding. Radiographic (x-ray) studies using a contrast media such as barium are used to detect the presence of an ulcer crater and to rule out gastric carcinoma. Endoscopy (gastroscopy and duodenoscopy) can be used to visualize the ulcer area.

Treatment of peptic ulcer focuses on measures to (1) decrease or neutralize the hydrochloric acid, (2) increase the resistance of the mucosal layer, and (3) promote healing.

Conservative treatment measures include (1) efforts to relieve stress and anxiety, (2) dietary management, and (3) medications that act to buffer or reduce gastric-acid secretion. Smoking has been shown to decrease the rate of ulcer healing and should be discouraged.

Although in the past the conservative treatment of peptic ulcers has usually included use of a bland diet, at present there is considerable controversy over its value. Most physicians would agree that coffee and alcoholic beverages should be avoided. Most physicians would agree, too, that the use of food as an antacid should also be avoided, because such feedings are generally accompanied by a rebound increase in gastric acid secretion.

Medications used in the treatment of peptic ulcers include antacids, mucosal protective agents, anticholinergic drugs, histamine₂ (H₂)-receptor antagonists, proton-pump inhibitors, and sedatives or tranquilizers. Anticholinergic drugs are less effective inhibitors of gastric acid secretions than antacids and H₂-receptor antagonists, and, therefore, they are usually used in combination with other methods of treatment. Sedatives and tranquilizers are individualized forms of treatment used for people in whom stress is a large contributing factor.

Antacids. Antacids, either self-prescribed or physician-prescribed, represent a large business in the United States, with millions of dollars spent each year for these medications. Essentially three types of antacids are used to relieve gastric acidity: calcium carbonate, aluminum hydroxide, and magnesium hydroxide. Many antacids contain a combination of ingredients, such as magnesium aluminum hydroxide. *Calcium preparations* are constipating and may cause hypercalcemia and the milk-alkali syndrome (see Chapter 30). There is also evidence that oral calcium preparations increase gastric-acid secretion after their buffering effect has been utilized. *Magnesium hydroxide* is a potent antacid that also has laxative effects. Approximately 5% to 10% of the magnesium in this preparation is absorbed from the intestine; because magnesium is excreted through the kidneys, it should not be used in people with renal failure. *Aluminum hydroxide* reacts with hydrochloric acid to form aluminum chloride. It combines with phosphate in the intestine, and prolonged use may lead to phosphate depletion and osteoporosis. Sodium bicarbonate, sometimes used as a home remedy, is not recommended as an antacid. Because of its water-solubility, it leaves the stomach rapidly and produces a transient effect, and it tends to cause metabolic alkalosis. It also contains large amounts of sodium. Antacids can alter the absorption, bio-availability, and renal elimination of a number of drugs; this should be considered when antacids are administered with other medications.

Mucosal Protective Agents. The drug sucralfate (Carafate), or aluminum sucrose sulfate, selectively binds to necrotic ulcer tissue and serves as a barrier to acid, pepsin, and bile. In addition, sucralfate may directly absorb bile salts. It is not absorbed systemically. The drug requires an acid pH for activation and should not be administered with antacids or a histamine$_2$ antagonist.

H$_2$-Receptor Antagonists. Histamine is the major physiologic mediator for hydrochloric acid secretion. The H$_2$-receptor antagonists, cimetidine (Tagamet), ranitidine (Zantac), famotidine (Pepcid), and nizatidine (Axid), block gastric acid secretion stimulated by histamine, gastrin, and acetylcholine. The volume of both gastric secretion and concentration of pepsin is also reduced. These drugs are relatively well-tolerated. Cimetidine can reduce liver blood flow and interfere with the oxidative metabolism of drugs such as the warfarin-type anticoagulants, phenytoin, propranolol, chlordiazepoxide, diazepam, and theophylline. Cimetidine also binds to androgen receptors and can cause gynecomastia in men and galactorrhea in women.

Proton Pump Inhibitors. Omeprazole inhibits the final stage of hydrogen ion secretion by blocking the action of the gastric parietal cell proton pump (H$^+$-, K$^+$-ATPase).

Surgical Treatment. When the conservative management of peptic ulcer is ineffective, surgical intervention may be indicated. Four types of surgical procedures are done: (1) subtotal gastrectomy, in which 75% to 80% of the stomach is removed and the remaining portion is attached to the jejunum; (2) parietal cell vagotomy; (3) truncal vagotomy and drainage, in which the vagus nerve trunks are cut and the outlet of the stomach is enlarged; and (4) truncal vagotomy and antrectomy, in which the vagus nerve trunks are cut and the distal 50% of the stomach is removed.

One of the complications after surgery for peptic ulcers is the *dumping syndrome*. It occurs to some extent in about 20% of people who have this type of operation. It is believed to be caused by the rapid entry of hyperosmolar liquids into the intestine and is characterized by symptoms such as nausea, vomiting, diarrhea, diaphoresis, palpitations, tachycardia, lightheadedness, and flushing that occur either while eating or shortly after. It is often followed (in about 2 hours) by an episode of hypoglycemia, resulting from the rapid absorption of glucose, which acts as a stimulus for insulin release by the beta cells of the pancreas. Treatment consists of limiting the diet to small, frequent feedings, which are taken without liquids and which are low in simple sugars (these are the most osmotically active parts of the diet). Symptoms usually diminish with time.

ZOLLINGER-ELLISON SYNDROME

The Zollinger-Ellison syndrome is a rare condition caused by a gastrin-secreting tumor. In people with this disorder, gastric acid secretion reaches such levels that ulceration becomes inevitable. The tumors may be single or multiple; although most tumors are located in the pancreas, a few develop in the submucosa of the stomach or duodenum. About two thirds of these tumors are malignant.[12] The increased gastric secretions cause symptoms related to peptic ulcer. Diarrhea may occur secondary to hypersecretion or as a result of inactivation of intestinal lipase and impaired fat digestion that occurs with a decrease in intestinal pH. The diagnosis of the Zollinger-Ellison syndrome is based on elevated serum gastrin levels and elevated basal gastric acid levels. H$_2$-receptor blocking drugs are used to control gastric acid secretion. Computed tomography (CT) scan, abdominal ultrasonography, and selective angiography are used to localize the tumor. Surgical removal is indicated in situations in which the tumor is malignant and has not undergone metastasis. Gastrectomy surgery and vagotomy may be done in selected cases.

STRESS ULCERS

A stress ulcer, sometimes called a *Curling's ulcer*, refers to GI ulcerations that develop in relation to major physiologic stress. These lesions occur most often in the gastric fundus and are thought to result from ischemia, tissue acidosis, and bile salts entering the stomach in critically ill people with decreased GI tract motility.[13, 14] They are usually manifested by painless upper GI tract bleeding. People at high risk for developing stress ulcers include those with large surface area burns, trauma, sepsis, acute respiratory distress syndrome, severe liver failure, and major surgical procedures. Monitoring and maintaining gastric pH >3.5 helps to prevent the development of stress ulcers. Antacids, H$_2$-receptor antagonists, and sucralfate are used in both prevention and treatment of stress ulcers. Prostaglandins have been used experimentally to promote ulcer healing.

CANCER OF THE STOMACH

Cancer of the stomach strikes approximately 23,000 people each year and accounts for 14,000 cancer deaths.[15] It is found more commonly in people between 50 and 70 years of age. Although its incidence has decreased over the past 50 years, it remains the seventh leading cause of death in the United States.

Among the factors that increase the risk of gastric cancer are a genetic predisposition, carcinogenic factors in the diet (*e.g.*, nitrates, smoked foods), atrophic gastritis, and gastric polyps. Fifty percent of gastric cancers occur in the pyloric region or adjacent to the antrum. Compared with a benign ulcer, which has smooth margins and is concentrically shaped, gastric cancers tend to be larger, are irregularly shaped, have irregular margins, and are usually located in the greater curvature of the stomach.

Unfortunately, stomach cancers are often asymptomatic until late in their course. Symptoms, when they do occur, are usually vague and include indigestion, anorexia, weight loss, vague epigastric pain, vomiting, and an abdominal mass. Diagnosis of gastric cancer is accomplished by means of a variety of techniques, including barium x-ray studies, gastroscopy studies with biopsy, and cytologic studies (Pap smear) of gastric secretions. Cytologic studies can prove particularly useful as a routine screening test in people with atrophic gastritis or gastric polyps.

Surgery in the form of radical subtotal gastrectomy is usually the treatment of choice.[15] Radiation and chemotherapy have not proved particularly useful as primary treatment modalities in stomach cancer. When these methods are used, it is usually for palliative purposes or to control metastatic spread of the disease.

In summary, disorders of the stomach include gastritis, peptic ulcer, and cancer of the stomach. Gastritis refers to inflammation of the gastric mucosa. Acute gastritis refers to a transient inflammation of the gastric mucosa; it is most commonly associated with local irritants such as bacterial endotoxins, caffeine, alcohol, and aspirin. Chronic gastritis is characterized by the absence of grossly visible erosions and the presence of chronic inflammatory changes leading eventually to atrophy of the glandular epithelium of the stomach. Type A chronic gastritis is the least common form of chronic gastritis; it involves the fundus and the body of the stomach and is associated with pernicious anemia. Type B gastritis is the more common form of chronic gastritis, it is of nonimmune origin, and its incidence increases with age. Peptic ulcer is a term used to describe a group of ulcerative disorders that occur in areas of the upper GI tract that are exposed to acid–pepsin secretions, most commonly the duodenum and stomach. Peptic ulcers are thought to result from an imbalance between (1) acid and pepsin production and (2) the ability of the affected gastric

mucosal barrier to resist the destructive action of these digestive agents. Of recent interest is the identification of a S-shaped bacterium, called *H. pylori* which colonizes the mucus-secreting epithelial cells of the stomach. This organism has been associated with both chronic (type B) gastritis and peptic ulcer. Cancer of the stomach is often asymptomatic until late in its course; although its incidence has decreased over the past 50 years, it remains the seventh leading cause of death in the United States.

■ DISORDERS OF THE SMALL AND LARGE INTESTINES

There are many similarities in conditions that disrupt the integrity of the small and large intestines. The wall of both the small and large intestines consists of five layers (see Chapter 40, Fig. 40-2): an outer serosal layer; a muscularis layer, which is divided into a layer of circular and a layer of longitudinal muscle fibers; a submucosal layer; and an inner mucosal layer, which lines the lumen of the intestine. Among the conditions that cause altered intestinal function are irritable bowel disease, inflammatory bowel disease, diverticulitis, appendicitis, alterations in bowel motility (diarrhea, constipation, and bowel obstruction), cancer of the colon and rectum, and malabsorption syndrome.

IRRITABLE BOWEL SYNDROME

The term *irritable bowel syndrome* is used to describe a functional GI disorder characterized by a variable combination of chronic and recurrent intestinal symptoms not explained by structural or biochemical abnormalities. There is evidence to suggest that 15% to 20% of people in Western countries suffer from the disorder, although most do not seek medical attention.[16]

The condition is characterized by abdominal pain, altered bowel function, and varying complaints of flatulence, bloatedness, nausea and anorexia, and anxiety or depression. Various stimuli including stress alter colonic and small intestine motor activity; it is presumed that the pain symptoms of people with irritable bowel syndrome are produced by the motor hyperreactivity. Although changes in intestinal activity are normal responses to stress, these responses are exaggerated in people with irritable bowel syndrome. Diagnosis of irritable bowel syndrome is based on continuous or recurrent symptoms for at least 3 months of abdominal pain or discomfort relieved by defecation, or associated with a change in the frequency or consistency of stool and the presence of three or more varying patterns of altered defecation that are present at least 25% of the time.

These patterns of defecation include: (1) altered stool frequency, (2) altered stool form (hard or loose, watery stool), (3) altered stool passage (straining, urgency, or feeling of incomplete evacuation), (4) passage of mucus, and (5) bloating or feeling of abdominal discomfort.[17] A history of lactose intolerance should be considered, because intolerance to lactose and other sugars may be a precipitating factor in some people. The role psychological factors play in the etiology of the disease is uncertain.

The treatment of irritable bowel syndrome focuses on methods of stress management, particularly those related to symptom production. Reassurance is important. Usually no special diet is indicated, although adequate fiber intake is usually recommended. Avoidance of GI stimulants such as caffeine-containing beverages may be beneficial.

INFLAMMATORY BOWEL DISEASE

The term *inflammatory bowel disease* is used to designate two inflammatory conditions: Crohn's disease and ulcerative colitis. Although the peak occurrence for both diseases is between ages 15 and 35, they occur in all age groups. Ulcerative colitis and Crohn's disease are prominent causes of chronic illness among children and adolescents. There is evidence to suggest that the incidence of ulcerative colitis, which is an inflammatory disorder of the rectum and colon, has reached a plateau, whereas that of Crohn's disease, which can affect either the large or small bowel, has increased steadily over the past 20 years.

The causes of both Crohn's disease and ulcerative colitis are largely unknown. The diseases appear to have a familial occurrence, which suggests a hereditary predisposition. There is increased preva-lence of the disease among first-degree relatives as well as increased incidence among certain population, most notably the Ashkenazi Jews.[18] One of the common beliefs is that genetic factors predispose to some form of autoimmune reaction, possibly triggered by some relatively innocuous environmental agent such as a dietary antigen or microbial agent. Although psychogenic factors may contribute to the severity and onset of both conditions, it seems unlikely that they are the primary cause.

Both Crohn's disease and ulcerative colitis are characterized by remissions and exacerbations of diarrhea, fecal urgency, and weight loss. Acute complications such as intestinal obstruction may develop during periods of fulminant disease. Both diseases may be accompanied by extraintestinal manifestations such as arthritis. Although the two diseases share many common features, they can be distinguished based on clinical, radiologic, endoscopic, and histologic features. The distinguishing characteristics of Crohn's disease and ulcerative colitis are summarized in Table 41-1.

CROHN'S DISEASE

Crohn's disease is a recurrent granulomatous type of inflammatory response that can affect any area of the GI tract from the mouth to the anus. It is a slowly progressive, relentless, and often disabling disease. The disease usually strikes in early adulthood and affects both men and women equally. In spite of the substantial increase in the prevalence of Crohn's disease in the early 1980s, the distribution of affected sites has not changed substantially. In nearly 40% of people with disease, the lesions are restricted to the small intestine; in 30% only the large bowel is affected, and in the additional 30% both the large and small bowel are affected.[18]

TABLE 41-1. DIFFERENTIATING CHARACTERISTICS OF CROHN'S DISEASE AND ULCERATIVE COLITIS

CHARACTERISTIC	CROHN'S DISEASE	ULCERATIVE COLITIS
Types of inflammation	Granulomatous	Ulcerative and exudative
Level of involvement	Primarily submucosal	Primarily mucosal
Extent of involvement	Skip lesions	Continuous
Areas of involvement	Primarily ileum Secondarily colon	Primarily rectum and left colon
Diarrhea	Common	Common
Rectal bleeding	Rare	Common
Fistulas	Common	Rare
Strictures	Common	Rare
Perianal abscesses	Common	Rare
Development of cancer	Rare	Relatively common

A characteristic feature of Crohn's disease is the sharply demarcated granulomatous lesions that occur and that are surrounded by normal-appearing mucosal tissue. When the lesions are multiple, they are often referred to as skip lesions because they are interspersed between what appear to be normal segments of the bowel. All the layers of the bowel are involved, the submucosal layer being affected to the greatest extent. The surface of the inflamed bowel usually has a characteristic "cobblestone" appearance resulting from the fissures and crevices that develop and surround areas of submucosal edema. There is usually a relative sparing of the smooth muscle layers of the bowel with marked inflammatory and fibrotic changes of the submucosal layer. The bowel wall, after a time, often becomes thickened and inflexible; its appearance has been likened to a lead pipe or rubber hose. The adjacent mesentery may become inflamed, and the regional lymph nodes and channels may become enlarged. In addition, Crohn's disease is often accompanied by the formation of fistulas, or tubelike passages that form pathologic connections between different sites in the GI tract. They may develop between the bowel and other sites, including the bladder, vagina, urethra, and skin. Perineal fistulas that originate in the ileum are relatively common.[19] Fistulas in the GI tract may lead to malabsorption, syndromes of bacterial overgrowth, and diarrhea. They can also become infected and cause abscess formation.

The clinical course of Crohn's disease is variable; often there are periods of exacerbations and remissions, with symptoms being related to the location of the lesions. The principal symptoms include intermittent diarrhea, colicky pain (usually in the lower right quadrant), weight loss, fluid and electrolyte disorders, malaise, and low-grade fever. Because Crohn's disease affects the submucosal layer to a greater extent than the mucosal layer, there is less bloody diarrhea than with ulcerative colitis. Ulceration of the perianal skin is common, largely due to the severity of the diarrhea. The absorptive surface of the intestine may be disrupted; nutritional deficiencies may occur, related to the specific segment of the intestine that is involved. Complications include intestinal obstruction, abdominal abscess formation, and fistula formation.

ULCERATIVE COLITIS

Ulcerative colitis is a nonspecific inflammatory condition of the colon. The disease begins most often in the second and third decade of life, has no predominant sex difference, and affects whites more often than nonwhites. Unlike Crohn's disease, which can affect various sites in the GI tract, ulcerative colitis is confined to the rectum and colon. The disease usually begins in the rectum and spreads proximally, affecting primarily the mucosal layer, although it can extend into the submucosal layer. The length of proximal extension varies. It may involve the entire colon. The inflammatory process tends to be confluent and continuous instead of skipping areas, as it does in Crohn's disease.

Characteristic of the disease are the lesions that form in the crypts of Lieberkühn in the base of the mucosal layer (see Figure 40-10). The inflammatory process causes pinpoint mucosal hemorrhages to occur, which, in time, suppurate and develop into *crypt abscesses*. These inflammatory lesions may become necrotic and ulcerate. Although the ulcerations are usually superficial, they often extend, causing large, denuded areas. As a result of the inflammatory process, the mucosal layer often develops tonguelike projections that resemble polyps and are therefore called *pseudopolyps*. With repeated episodes of colitis, there is thickening of the bowel wall.

Ulcerative colitis usually follows a course of remissions and exacerbations. The severity of the disease varies from mild to fulminating. Accordingly, the disease has been divided into three types depending on its severity: mild chronic, chronic intermittent, and acute fulminating. The most common form is the mild chronic form of the disease, in which bleeding and diarrhea are mild and systemic signs are minimal or absent. This form of the disease can usually be managed by conservative means. The chronic intermittent form continues after the initial attack. Compared with the milder form, usually more of the colon surface is involved with the chronic intermittent form and the presence of systemic signs and complications is greater. In about 15% of people, the disease assumes a more fulminant course, involves the entire colon, and presents with severe bloody diarrhea, fever, and acute abdominal pain. These people are at risk to develop toxic megacolon and perforation.

Diarrhea, which is the characteristic manifestation of ulcerative colitis, will vary according to the severity of the disease. There may be up to 30 to 40 bowel movements a day. Because ulcerative colitis affects the mucosal layer of the bowel, the stools typically contain both blood and mucus. Nocturnal diarrhea is usually present when daytime symptoms are severe. There may be mild abdominal cramping and incontinence of stools. Anorexia, weakness, and fatigability are common.

COMPLICATIONS

Both Crohn's disease and ulcerative colitis are associated with a wide variety of complications encompassing the secondary effects of the inflammatory process of the GI tract and associated extraintestinal manifestations.

Fistulas can develop between the bowel and other sites, including the bladder, vagina, and skin, in Crohn's disease. One potentially dangerous life-threatening complication of both Crohn's disease and ulcerative colitis is *toxic megacolon*. It is characterized by dilatation of the colon and signs of systemic toxicity. It results from extension of the inflammatory response, with involvement of neural and vascular components of the bowel. Contributing factors include use of laxatives, narcotics, and anticholinergic drugs and the presence of hypokalemia.

A number of extraintestinal manifestations have been identified in people with Crohn's disease and ulcerative colitis. These include axial arthritis affecting the spine and sacroiliac joints, as well as oligoarticular arthritis affecting the large joints of the arms and legs; inflammatory conditions of the eye, usually uveitis; skin lesions, especially erythema nodosum; stomatitis; autoimmune anemia, hypercoagulability of blood, and sclerosing cholangitis. Occasionally, these systemic manifestations may herald the recurrence of intestinal disease. In children, growth retardation may occur, particularly if the symptoms are prolonged and nutrient intake has been poor.

Cancer of the colon is one of the feared complications of ulcerative colitis. The risk of developing cancer among people who have had the disease for 20 years is about 2% for left-sided disease and 10% for total colon involvement; after 30 years, the risk becomes 3% to 4% and 15% to 25%, respectively.[6]

DIAGNOSIS AND TREATMENT

The diagnosis of inflammatory bowel disease requires a thorough history and physical examination. Sigmoidoscopy is used for direct visualization of the affected areas and to obtain biopsies. Measures are taken to rule out infectious agents as the cause of the disorder. This is usually accomplished by the use of stool cultures and examination of fresh stool specimens for ova and parasites. In people suspected of having Crohn's disease, radiologic contrast studies provide a means for determining the extent of involvement of the small bowel and establishing the presence and nature of fistulas. CT scans may be used to determine whether an inflammatory mass or abscess is present.

Treatment methods focus on terminating the inflammatory response and promoting healing, maintaining adequate nutrition, and preventing and treating complications.

Sulfasalazine (Azulfidine), a poorly absorbed drug with antiinflammatory action, and the corticosteroid drugs are frequently prescribed to treat the acute disease. Sulfasalazine reduces both the frequency and severity of recurrent ulcerative colitis. In contrast, no beneficial effect has been demonstrated after acute disease activity has been controlled in Crohn's disease.[20] Unfortunately, hypersensitivity reactions prevent its use in many people. The beneficial effects of the sulfasalazine are attributable to one component of the drug (5-aminosalicylic acid); efforts are being made to develop orally active forms of this component. Topical 5-aminosalicylic acid, given as an enema, is available in the United States. The corticosteroids are used selectively to lessen the acute inflammatory response. These drugs can be given by enema or in the form of a suppository. Immunosuppressive drugs such as azathioprine, and its active derivative, mercaptopurine, may be used to treat people with refractory Crohn's disease.

Surgical treatment (removal of the rectum and entire colon) with the creation of an ileostomy or ilioanal anastomosis may be required for those people with ulcerative colitis who do not respond to conservative methods of treatment.

Nutritional deficiencies are common in Crohn's disease because of diarrhea, steatorrhea, and other malabsorption problems. A nutritious diet that is high in calories, vitamins, and proteins is recommended. Fats often aggravate the diarrhea, and it is generally recommended that they be avoided. Elemental diets, which are nutritionally balanced yet are residue free and bulk free, may be given during the acute phase of the illness. These diets are largely absorbed in the jejunum and allow the inflamed bowel to rest. Total parenteral nutrition (parenteral hyperalimentation) consists of intravenous administration of hypertonic glucose solutions to which amino acids and fats may be added. This form of nutritional therapy may be needed when food cannot be absorbed from the intestine. Because of the hypertonicity of these solutions, they must be administered through a large-diameter central vein.

DIVERTICULAR DISEASE

Diverticular disease is a condition in which the mucosal layer of the colon herniates through the muscularis layer. Often there are multiple diverticuli, and most occur in the sigmoid colon (Fig. 41-1). Diverticular disease is common in the United States. It is one of the most common disorders of aging, affecting 50% of the population by age 90.[20] Although the disorder is prevalent in the developed countries of the world, it is almost nonexistent in many of the African nations and other underdeveloped countries. This suggests that dietary factors (lack of fiber content), a decrease in physical activity, and poor bowel habits

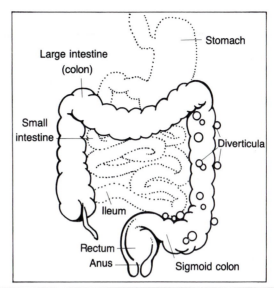

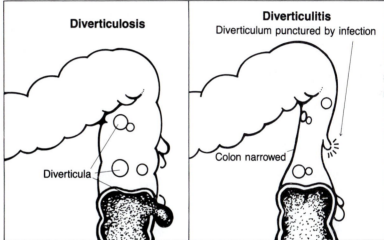

FIG. 41-1. (**Top**) Location of diverticula in the sigmoid colon. (**Bottom left**) Diverticulosis. (**Bottom right**) Diverticulitis. (National Digestive Diseases Information Clearinghouse. [1989]. Clearinghouse fact sheet: Diverticulosis and diverticulitis. NIH publication 90-1163. Washington, DC: US Department of Health and Human Services)

(in which the urge to defecate is neglected), along with the effects of aging, contribute to the development of the disease.

In the colon, the longitudinal muscle does not form a continuous layer, as it does in the small bowel. Instead there are three separate longitudinal bands of muscle called the teniae coli. In a manner similar to the small intestine, bands of circular muscle cause constriction in the large intestine. At each of these constrictive points (about every 2.5 cm), the circular muscle contracts, sometimes constricting the lumen of the bowel so that it is almost occluded. The combined contraction of the circular muscle and lack of a continuous longitudinal muscle layer causes the unstimulated intestine to bulge outward into pouches called *haustra* (Fig. 41-2). Diverticula develop between the longitudinal muscle band of the haustra, in the area where the blood vessels pierce the circular muscle layer to bring blood to the mucosal layer. An increase in intraluminal pressure within the haustra provides the force for creating these herniations. The

increase in pressure is thought to be related to the volume of the colonic contents. The more scanty the contents, the more vigorous the contractions and the greater the pressure within the haustra.

The vast majority of people with diverticular disease remain asymptomatic. The disease is often found when x-ray studies are done for other purposes. When symptoms do occur, they are often attributed to irritable bowel syndrome or other causes. Ill-defined lower abdominal discomfort, a change in bowel habits such as diarrhea and constipation, bloating, and flatulence are often present.

Diverticulitis is a complication of diverticular disease in which there is inflammation and gross or microscopic perforation of the diverticulum. One of the most common complaints of diverticulitis is pain in the lower left quadrant, accompanied by nausea and vomiting, tenderness in the lower left quadrant, a slight fever, and elevation in white blood cell count. These symptoms usually last for several days, unless complications occur, and are usually caused by

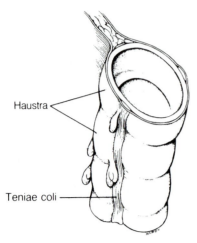

FIG. 41-2. A portion of the sigmoid colon, showing the haustra and teniae coli.

localized inflammation of the diverticulitis with perforation and development of a small localized abscess. Complications include perforation with peritonitis, hemorrhage, and bowel obstruction. Fistula formation can occur; it usually involves the bladder (vesicosigmoid fistula) but can also be to skin, perianal area, or small bowel. Pneumaturia (air in the urine) is a sign of vesicosigmoid fistula.

DIAGNOSIS AND TREATMENT

The diagnosis of diverticular disease is based on history and presenting clinical manifestations. The disease may be confirmed by barium enema x-ray studies or colonoscopy. Because of the risk of peritonitis, barium enema studies should be avoided in people who are suspected of having acute diverticulitis. Flat abdominal x-rays may be used to detect complications associated with acute diverticulitis.

The usual treatment for diverticular disease is to prevent symptoms and complications. This includes increasing the bulk in the diet and bowel retraining so that the person has at least one bowel movement a day. The increased bulk not only promotes regular defecation but it also increases colonic contents and colon diameter, thereby decreasing intraluminal pressure. Acute diverticulitis is treated by withholding solid food and use of a broad-spectrum antibiotic. Surgical treatment is reserved for complications.

APPENDICITIS

Acute appendicitis is extremely common. It is seen most frequently in the 5- to 30-year age group, but it can occur at any age. The appendix becomes inflamed, swollen, and gangrenous, and it eventually perforates if not treated. Although the cause of appendicitis is not known, it is thought to be related to intraluminal obstruction due to a fecalith (hard piece of stool) or twisting.

Appendicitis usually has an abrupt onset, with pain referred to the epigastric or periumbilical area. This pain is due to stretching of the appendix during the early inflammatory process. At about the same time that the pain appears, there are one or two episodes of nausea. Initially the pain is vague, but over a period of 2 to 12 hours it gradually increases and may become colicky in nature. When the inflammatory process has extended to involve the serosal layer of the appendix and the peritoneum, the pain becomes localized to the lower right quadrant. There is usually an elevation in temperature and a white blood cell count of over 10,000 per mm^3 with 75% or more polymorphonuclear cells. Palpation of the abdomen usually reveals a deep tenderness in the lower right quadrant, which is confined to a small area about the size of the fingertip. It is usually located at about the site of the inflamed appendix. Many times, the person with appendicitis will be able to place his or her finger directly over the tender area. Rebound tenderness, pain that occurs when pressure is applied to the area and then released, and spasm of the overlying abdominal muscles are common. Treatment consists of surgical removal of the appendix. Complications include peritonitis, localized periappendiceal abscess formation, and septicemia.

COLORECTAL CANCER

More than 61,000 people in the United States die each year of colorectal cancer.[21] It is the second most common site of fatal cancer. The main drawback to successful treatment is the fact that most lesions do not produce symptoms until late in the course of the disease.

Almost all cancers of the colon and rectum are carcinomas. There has been a shift in location of colorectal cancers to the right colon; 25% occur in the cecum and ascending colon, 25% in the descending and proximal sigmoid colon, 25% in the rectum and distal sigmoid colon, and the remainder are scattered elsewhere.[6] The cause of cancer of the colon and rectum is largely unknown. Its incidence increases with age, as evidenced by the fact that about 80% of people who develop this form of cancer are over age 50. Its incidence is increased in people with a family history of cancer, in people with ulcerative colitis, and in those with familial multiple polyposis of the colon. Genetic as well as environmental factors are thought to be involved. Attention has focused on (1) dietary fat intake, (2) refined sugar intake, (3) fiber intake, and (4) the adequacy of such protective micronutrients as vitamins A, C, and E in the diet.[6] It has been hypothesized that high fat in the diet increases the synthesis of bile acids in liver, which may be converted to potential carcinogens by the bacterial flora in the colon. Bacteroid organisms in particular are suspected of converting bile acids to carcinogens; their proliferation is enhanced by a high dietary level of refined sugars. Dietary fiber is thought to increase stool bulk and thereby dilute and remove potential carcinogens.

Most, if not all, colorectal carcinomas arise in preexisting adenomatous polyps. The frequency of polyps increases with age, and presence of adenomatous polyps is about 20% to 30% before age 40, rising to 40% to 50% after age 60.[6] Both males and females are equally affected. Importantly, the peak incidence of adenomatous polyps precedes by some years the peak for colorectal cancer. Programs that provide careful follow-up for people with adenomatous polyps and remove all that are suspicious have substantially reduced the incidence of colorectal cancer.[6]

Usually, cancer of the colon and rectum is present for a long time before it produces symptoms. Bleeding is a highly significant early symptom, and it is usually the one that causes people to seek medical care. Other symptoms include a change in bowel habits, either diarrhea or constipation, and sometimes a sense of urgency or incomplete emptying of the bowel. Pain is usually a late symptom.

The prognosis for people with colorectal cancer depends largely on the extent of bowel involvement and on the presence of metastasis at the time of diagnosis. This form of cancer can be divided into four categories according to the classification system by Duke. A stage A tumor is limited to invasion of the mucosal and submucosal layers of the colon and has a 5-year survival rate of almost 100%. A stage B tumor involves the entire wall of the colon but without lymph node involvement and has a 5-year survival rate of about 43% to 65%. With a stage C tumor, there is invasion of the serosal layer, with involvement of the regional lymph nodes. The 5-year survival rate is approximately 15%. Stage D colorectal cancer involves far-advanced metastasis.[6]

DIAGNOSIS AND TREATMENT

Among the methods used in the diagnosis of colorectal cancers are stool occult blood tests and digital rectal examination, usually done during routine physical examinations; x-ray studies using barium (barium enema); and proctosigmoidoscopy and colonoscopy. Digital rectal examinations are most helpful in detecting neoplasms of the rectum. Rectal examination should be considered a routine part of a good physical examination. The American Cancer Society recommends that all asymptomatic men and women over age 40 should have a digital rectal examination performed annually as a part of their physical examination and that those over age 50 should have an annual stool test for occult blood and a proctosigmoidoscopy examination done every 3 to 5 years as recommended by their physician.[22]

Almost all cancers of the colon and rectum bleed intermittently even though the amount of blood is small and usually not apparent in the stools. It is therefore feasible to screen for colorectal cancers using commercially prepared tests for occult blood in the stool that are available. This method uses a guaiac-impregnated filter paper. The technique involves preparing two slides per day from different portions of the same stool for 3 to 4 days while the patient follows a high-fiber diet that is free of meat and ascorbic acid. Although the diet is not particularly appealing, this stool test has been shown to be a relatively reliable and inexpensive method of screening for colorectal cancer. People with a positive stool occult blood test should be referred to their physicians for further study. Usually a physical examination, rectal examination, barium enema, and proctosigmoidoscopy or colonoscopy are done.

Proctosigmoidoscopy involves examination of the rectum and sigmoid colon with a hollow, lighted tube that is inserted through the rectum. Polyps can be removed or tissue can be obtained for biopsy during the procedure.

Colonoscopy provides a means for direct visualization of the rectum and colon. The colonoscope consists of a flexible 4-cm glass bundle that has some 250,000 glass fibers with a lens at either end to focus and magnify the image. Light from an external source is transmitted by the fiberoptic viewing bundle. Instruments are available that afford direct examination of the sigmoid colon or the entire colon. This method is used for screening people at high risk for developing cancer of the colon (*e.g.*, those with ulcerative colitis) and for those with symptoms. Colonoscopy is also useful for obtaining a biopsy and for removing polyps. Although this method is one of the most accurate for detecting early colorectal cancers, it is not suitable for mass screening because it is expensive and time-consuming and must be done by a person who is highly trained in the use of the instrument.

The carcinoembryonic antigen (CEA) can be used as marker for colorectal cancer. However, blood levels are of little screening or diagnostic value because they become elevated only after the tumor has reached considerable size. Moreover, CEA is produced by other types of cancers as well as noncancerous conditions such as alcoholic cirrhosis, pancreatitis, and ulcerative colitis. This marker is of greatest value for monitoring tumor recurrence in people after resection of the primary tumor.[6]

The only recognized *treatment* for cancer of the colon and rectum is surgical removal.[22] Preoperative radiation may be used and has in some cases demonstrated increased 5-year survival rates. Postoperative adjuvant therapy with 5-fluorouracil (5-FU) has had some success. Radiation and chemotherapy are palliative treatment methods.

ALTERATIONS IN INTESTINAL MOTILITY

The movement of contents through the GI tract is controlled by neurons located in the submucosal and myenteric plexus of the gut (see Chapter 40). The axons from the cell bodies in the myenteric plexus innervate both the circular and longitudinal smooth muscle layers of the gut. These neurons receive impulses from local receptors located in the mucosal and muscle layers of the gut and extrinsic input from the parasympathetic and sympathetic nervous systems. As a general rule, the parasympathetic nervous system tends to increase the motility of the bowel, whereas sympathetic stimulation tends to slow its activity.

The colon, which has sphincters at both ends—the ileocecal sphincter, which separates it from the small intestine, and the anal sphincter, which prevents the movement of feces to the outside of the body—acts as a reservoir for fecal material. Normally, about 400 mL of water, 55 mEq of sodium, 30 mEq of chloride, and 15 mEq of bicarbonate are absorbed each day in the colon. At the same time, about 5 mEq of potassium is secreted into the lumen of the colon. The amount of water and electrolytes that remains in the stool reflects the absorption or secretion that occurs in the colon. The average adult ingesting a "typical" American diet evacuates about 200 to 300 g of stool each day.

DIARRHEA

The usual definition of *diarrhea* is excessively frequent passage of stools. Diarrhea can be acute or chronic. Diarrhea is considered to be chronic when the symptoms persist for 3 weeks in children or adults and 4 weeks in infants. Acute diarrhea affects 500 million children throughout the world and is the leading cause of death in children under 4 years of age.[23]

The complaint of diarrhea is a general one and can be related to a number of factors pathologic or otherwise. Diarrhea is usually divided into two types: large-volume and small-volume. Large-volume diarrhea results from an increase in the water content of the stool, and small-volume diarrhea re-

sults from an increase in the propulsive activity of the bowel. Some of the common causes of small- and large-volume diarrhea are summarized in Chart 41-1. Often diarrhea is a combination of these two types.

Large-Volume Diarrhea. Large-volume diarrhea can be classified as secretory or osmotic, according to the cause of the increased water content in the feces. Water is either pulled into the colon along an osmotic gradient (osmotic diarrhea) or is secreted into the bowel by the mucosal cells (secretory diarrhea). The large-volume form of diarrhea is usually a painless, watery type without blood or pus in the stools.

In osmotic diarrhea, water is pulled into the bowel by the hyperosmotic nature of its contents. It occurs when osmotically active particles are not absorbed. In lactase deficiency, the lactose present in milk cannot be broken down and absorbed. Magnesium salts, which are contained in milk of magnesia and many antacids, are poorly absorbed and cause diarrhea when taken in sufficient quantities. Another cause of osmotic diarrhea is decreased transit time, which interferes with absorption. This happens in the dumping syndrome, which was discussed earlier in relation to the surgical treatment of peptic ulcer. Osmotic diarrhea usually disappears with fasting.

Secretory diarrhea occurs when the secretory processes of the bowel are increased. Most acute infectious diarrheas are of this type. Enteric organ-

---

CHART 41-1: CAUSES OF LARGE- AND SMALL-VOLUME DIARRHEA

Large-Volume Diarrhea

Osmotic diarrhea
   Saline cathartics
   Dumping syndrome
   Lactase deficiency
Secretory diarrhea
   Failure to absorb bile salts
   Fat malabsorption
   Chronic laxative abuse
   Carcinoid syndrome
   Zollinger-Ellison syndrome
   Fecal impaction
   Acute infectious diarrhea

Small-Volume Diarrhea

Inflammatory bowel disease
   Crohn's disease
   Ulcerative colitis
Infectious disease
   Shigellosis
   Salmonellosis
Irritable colon

isms cause diarrhea by several ways. Some are noninvasive but secrete toxins that stimulate fluid secretion (*e.g.*, pathogenic *Escherichia coli* or *Vibrio cholerae*). Others invade and destroy intestinal epithelial cells, thereby altering fluid transport so secretory activity continues while absorption activity is halted.[24] Secretory diarrhea also occurs when excess bile acids are present in the gut contents as they enter the colon. This often happens with disease processes of the ileum, because bile salts are absorbed here. It may also occur when bacterial overgrowth occurs in the small bowel, which also interferes with bile absorption. Some tumors, such as Zollinger-Ellison syndrome and carcinoid syndrome, produce hormones that cause increased secretory activity of the bowel.

Small-Volume Diarrhea. Small-volume diarrhea is commonly associated with acute or chronic inflammation or intrinsic disease of the colon, such as ulcerative colitis or Crohn's disease. Diarrhea with vomiting and fever suggests food poisoning, often due to staphylococcal enteroxin. Small-volume diarrhea is usually evidenced by frequency and urgency and colicky abdominal pain. It is commonly accompanied by tenesmus (painful straining at stool), fecal soiling of clothing, and awakening during the night with the urge to defecate.

Diagnosis and Treatment. The diagnosis of diarrhea is based on complaints of frequent stools and a history of accompanying factors such as concurrent illnesses, medication use, and exposure to potential intestinal pathogens. Disorders such as inflammatory bowel disease need to be considered. If the onset of diarrhea is related to travel outside the United States, the possibility of travelers' diarrhea needs to be considered.

Although most acute forms of diarrhea are self-limited and require no treatment, diarrhea can be particularly serious in infants and small children, people with other illnesses, the elderly, and even previously healthy people if it continues for any length of time. Fluid and electrolyte corrections are therefore considered to be a primary therapeutic goal in the treatment of diarrhea. Oral electrolyte replacement solutions can be given in situations of uncomplicated diarrhea that can be treated at home. Complete oral rehydration solutions contain carbohydrate, sodium, potassium, chloride, and base to replace that lost in the diarrheal stool. The effectiveness of oral rehydration therapy is based on the coupled transport of sodium and glucose or other actively transported small organic molecules (see Chapter 40).

Oral rehydration therapy can be particularly effective in treating dehydration associated with diar-

rheal disease in infants and small children. However, the cost may be a factor. The oral rehydration products for infants and children that are available in the United States range in price from $2.50 to $4.00 per liter.[25] In severe cases of diarrhea, a child may require several liters per day. Thus, the cost can be a sizable burden on socioeconomically disadvantaged families, which are the same families that are at greatest risk for a poor outcome from diarrhea. Also, the use of oral rehydration therapy is labor intensive, requiring frequent feeding, sometimes using a spoon.[26] More importantly, the diarrhea does not promptly cease once oral rehydration has been instituted; this can be discouraging for parents and caregivers who desire early results from their efforts. When oral rehydration is not feasible or adequate, intravenous fluid replacement may be needed.

Restricting oral foods may be helpful in acute diarrhea, because this decreases peristalsis. When intake is resumed after diarrhea, the diet should consist of bland foods that will not stimulate GI motility. Cold liquids that move rapidly from the stomach to the small intestine and stimulate peristalsis should be avoided.

Drugs used in the treatment of diarrhea include camphorated tincture of opium (paregoric), diphenoxylate (Lomotil), and loperamide (Imodium), which are opiumlike drugs. These drugs decrease GI motility and stimulate water and electrolyte absorption. Adsorbents, such as kaolin and pectin, adsorb irritants and toxins from the bowel. These ingredients are included in many over-the-counter antidiarrheal preparations because they adsorb toxins responsible for certain types of diarrhea. Antibiotics are reserved for people with identified enteric pathogens.

CONSTIPATION

Constipation can be defined as the infrequent passage of stools. The difficulty with this definition arises from the many individual variations of a function that are normal. In other words, what might be considered normal for one person (two or three bowel movements per week) might well be considered evidence of constipation by another.

Some common causes of constipation are failure to respond to the urge to defecate, inadequate fiber in the diet, inadequate fluid intake, weakness of the abdominal muscles, inactivity and bedrest, pregnancy, hemorrhoids, and GI disease. Drugs such as narcotics, belladonna derivatives, diuretics, calcium, iron and aluminum hydroxide, and phosphate gels tend to cause constipation. The sudden onset of constipation may indicate serious disease (*e.g.*, one sign of cancer of the colon and rectum is a change in bowel habits).

Treatment. The treatment of constipation is usually directed toward relieving the cause. A conscious effort should be made to respond to the defecation urge. A time should be set aside after a meal, when mass movements in the colon are most apt to occur, for a bowel movement. Adequate fluid intake and bulk in the diet should be encouraged. Moderate exercise is essential, and people on bedrest benefit from passive and active exercises. Laxatives and enemas should be used judiciously. They should not be used on a regular basis to treat simple constipation because they interfere with the defecation reflex and may actually damage the rectal mucosa.

FECAL IMPACTION

Fecal impaction is the retention of hardened or puttylike stool in the rectum and colon, which interferes with normal passage of feces. If not removed, it can cause partial or complete bowel obstruction. It may occur in any age group, but is more common in incapacitated elderly people. Fecal impaction may be due to painful anorectal disease, tumors, or neurogenic disease, use of constipating antacids, bulk laxatives, low-residue diet, drug-induced colonic stasis, or prolonged bedrest and debility. In children, a habitual neglect of the urge to defecate because it interferes with play may promote impaction.[27] The manifestations may be those of severe constipation, but frequently there is a history of watery diarrhea and fecal incontinence. This is caused by increased secretory activity of the bowel, representing the body's attempt to break up the mass so that it can be evacuated. The abdomen may be distended, and there may be blood and mucus in the stool. The fecal mass may compress the urethra, giving rise to urinary incontinence. Fecal impaction should be considered in an elderly or immobilized person who develops watery stools with fecal or urinary incontinence.

Digital examination of the rectum is done to assess for the presence of a fecal mass. The mass may need to be broken up and dislodged manually or with the use of a sigmoidoscope. Oil enemas are often used to soften the mass before removal. The best treatment is prevention.

INTESTINAL OBSTRUCTION

Intestinal obstruction designates an impairment of movement of intestinal contents in a cephalocaudal direction. The causes of intestinal obstruction can be categorized under two headings: mechanical and paralytic obstruction. Strangulation with necrosis of the bowel may occur and lead to perforation, peritonitis, and sepsis. It is a serious complication and may increase the mortality rate of intestinal obstruction to about 25%.[28]

Mechanical obstruction can result from a number of conditions, either intrinsic or extrinsic, which encroach on the patency of the bowel lumen. Major inciting causes include external hernia (inguinal, femoral, or umbilical) and postoperative adhesions. Less common causes are strictures, tumor, foreign bodies, intussusception, and volvulus. Intussusception involves the telescoping of bowel into the adjacent segment (Fig. 41-3). It is the most common cause of intestinal obstruction in children under 2 years of age.[29] The most common form is the intussusception of the terminal ileum into the right colon, but other areas of the bowel may be involved. In most cases, the cause of the disorder is unknown. The condition can also occur in adults, when an intraluminal mass or tumor acts as traction force and pulls the segment along as it telescopes into the distal segment. Volvulus refers to a complete twisting of the bowel on an axis formed by its mesentery (Fig. 41-4). Volvulus of the colon accounts for 5% to 10% of large bowel obstruction.[29] Mechanical bowel obstructions may present as a simple obstruction in which there is no alteration in blood flow or as a strangulated obstruction in which there is impairment of blood flow and necrosis of bowel tissue.

Paralysis (adynamic) obstruction results from neurogenic or muscular impairment of peristalsis. *Paralytic ileus* is seen most commonly after abdominal surgery. It is also accompanies inflammatory conditions of the abdomen, intestinal ischemia, pelvic frac-

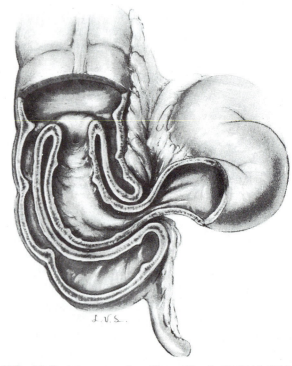

FIG. 41-3. Intussusception. (From Way, L. W. [Ed.]. [1991]. *Current surgical diagnosis & treatment* [p. 1192]. Norwalk, CT: Appleton Lange.)

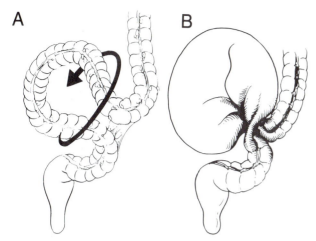

FIG. 41-4. Volvulus of the sigmoid colon. (From Way, L. W. [Ed.]. [1991]. *Current surgical diagnosis & treatment* [p. 664]. Norwalk, CT: Appleton Lange.)

tures, and back injuries. It occurs early in the course of peritonitis and can result from chemical irritation caused by bile, bacterial toxins, electrolyte imbalances as in hypokalemia, and vascular insufficiency.

The major effects of both types of intestinal obstruction are abdominal distention and loss of fluids and electrolytes. Gases and fluids accumulate within the area. If untreated, the distention resulting from bowel obstruction tends to perpetuate itself by causing atony of the bowel and further distention. Distention is further aggravated by the accumulation of gases. About 70% of these gases are estimated to be due to swallowed air. As the process continues, the distention moves proximally (toward the mouth), involving additional segments of bowel.

Either form of obstruction may eventually lead to strangulation (interruption of blood flow), gangrenous changes, and ultimately perforation of the bowel. The increased pressure within the intestine tends to compromise mucosal blood flow, leading to necrosis and movement of blood into the luminal fluids. This promotes rapid growth of bacteria within the obstructed bowel. Anaerobes grow rapidly in this favorable environment and produce a lethal endotoxin.

The manifestations of intestinal obstruction depend on the degree of obstruction and its duration. With acute obstruction, the onset is usually sudden and dramatic. With chronic conditions, the onset is often more gradual. The cardinal symptoms of intestinal obstruction are pain, absolute constipation, abdominal distention, and vomiting. With mechanical obstruction, the pain is severe and colicky, in contrast with the continuous pain and silent abdomen seen with paralytic ileus. There is also borborygmus (rumbling sounds made by propulsion of gas in the intestine), audible high-pitched peristalsis, and peristaltic rushes. Visible peristalsis may appear along the course of the distended intestine. Extreme restlessness and conscious awareness of intestinal movements are present along with weakness, perspiration, and anxiety. Should strangulation occur, the symptoms change. The character of the pain shifts from the intermittent colicky pain caused by the hyperperistaltic movements of the intestine to a severe and steady type of pain. Vomiting and fluid and electrolyte disorders occur with both types of obstruction.

Diagnosis of intestinal obstruction is usually based on history and physical findings. Abdominal x-ray studies will reveal a gas-filled bowel.

Treatment depends on the cause and type of obstruction. Most cases of adynamic obstruction respond to decompression of the bowel through nasogastric suction and correction of fluid and electrolyte imbalances. Strangulation and complete bowel obstruction require surgical intervention.

ALTERATIONS IN INTESTINAL ABSORPTION

Malabsorption is the failure to transport dietary constituents, such as fats, carbohydrates, proteins, vitamins, and minerals, from the lumen of the intestine to the extracellular fluid compartment for transport to the various parts of the body. It can selectively affect a single component, such as vitamin B_{12} or lactose, or its effects can extend to all the substances absorbed in a specific segment of the intestine. When one segment of the intestine is affected, another may compensate. For example, the ileum may compensate for malabsorption in the proximal small intestine by absorbing substantial amounts of fats, carbohydrates, and amino acids. Similarly, the colon, which normally absorbs water, sodium, chloride, and bicarbonate, can compensate for small intestine malabsorption by absorbing 50% or more of some of the end-products of bacterial carbohydrate metabolism.[30]

The conditions that impair one or more steps involved in digestion and absorption of nutrients can be divided into three broad categories: (1) intraluminal maldigestion, (2) mucosal malabsorption, and (3) lymphatic obstruction. Intraluminal maldigestion involves a defect in processing of nutrients within the intestinal lumen. The most common causes are pancreatic insufficiency, hepatobiliary disease, and intraluminal bacterial growth. Mucosal malabsorption is caused by mucosal lesions that impair uptake and transport of available intraluminal nutrients across the mucosal surface of the intestine. They include disorders such as celiac disease, tropical sprue, and Crohn's disease. Lymphatic obstruction interferes with the transport of the products of fat digestion to the systemic circulation once they have been absorbed by the intestinal mucosa. The process can be interrupted by congenital defects, neoplasms, trauma, and selected infectious diseases.

MALABSORPTION SYNDROME

The term *syndrome* implies a common constellation of symptoms arising from multiple causes. People with conditions that diffusely affect the small intestine and reduce its absorptive functions share certain common features referred to as malabsorption syndrome. Among the causes of malabsorption syndrome are sprue, Crohn's disease, and resection of large segments of the small bowel.

Sprue syndromes are diseases of disturbed small intestine function characterized by impaired absorption. Celiac sprue is an intolerance to dietary gluten found in wheat, barley, and rye. There is convincing evidence that the disorder is caused by an immunologic response to the gliadin fraction of gluten. The condition results in loss of absorptive villi from the small intestine. When the resulting lesions are extensive, they may impair absorption of virtually all nutrients. In about one third of cases, symptoms begin in childhood. The effects of celiac sprue are usually reversed after removal of all wheat, rye, barley, and oat gluten from the diet. Corn and rice products are not toxic and can be used as a substitute. In a condition called *tropical sprue*, the changes that occur in the villi resemble those seen in celiac sprue. The cause of this disorder is unclear, although administration of folic acid is known to be helpful in treatment.

People with intestinal malabsorption usually have symptoms directly referable to the GI tract that include diarrhea, steatorrhea, flatulence, bloating, abdominal pain, and cramps. Weakness, muscle wasting, weight loss, and abdominal distention are often present. Weight loss often occurs despite normal or excessive caloric intake. Steatorrhea stools contain excess fat. The fat content causes bulky, yellow-gray malodorous stools that float in the toilet and are difficult to dispose of by flushing. In a person consuming a diet containing 80 to 100 g of fat a day, excretion of 7 to 9 g of fat indicates steatorrhea.

Along with loss of fat in the stools, there is failure to absorb the fat-soluble vitamins. This can lead to easy bruising and bleeding (vitamin K deficiency), bone pain, predisposition to develop fractures and tetany (vitamin D and calcium deficiency), macrocytic anemia, and glossitis (folic acid deficiency). Neuropathy, atrophy of the skin, and peripheral edema may be present. Table 41-2 describes the signs and symptoms of impaired absorption of dietary constituents.

In summary, disorders of the small and large intestines include irritable bowel syndrome, inflammatory bowel disease, *diverticular disease, colorectal cancer, disorders of motility (diarrhea, constipation, fecal impaction, and intestinal obstruction), and alterations in intestinal absorption.*

Irritable bowel disease is a functional disorder characterized by a variable combination of chronic and recurrent intestinal symptoms not explained by structural or biochemical abnormalities. The term inflammatory bowel disease is used to designate two inflammatory conditions: Crohn's disease, which affects both the small and large bowel, and ulcerative colitis, which affects the colon and rectum. Both are chronic diseases characterized by remissions and exacerbations of diarrhea, weight loss, fluid and electrolyte disorders, and systemic signs of inflammation. Diverticular disease includes diverticulosis, which is a condition in which the mucosal layer of the colon herniates through the muscularis layer, and diverticulitis in which there is inflammation and gross or microscopic perforation of the diverticulum. Colorectal cancer, the second most common fatal cancer, is seen most commonly in people over age 50. Most, if not all, cancers of the colon and rectum arise in preexisting adenomatous polyps.

Diarrhea and constipation represent disorders of intestinal motility. Diarrhea, characterized by excessively frequent passage of stools, can be divided into large-volume diarrhea (characterized by the increased water content in the feces) and small-volume diarrhea (associated with intrinsic bowel disease and frequent passage of small stools). Constipation can be defined as the infrequent passage of stools; it is commonly caused by failure to respond to the urge to defecate, inadequate fiber or fluid intake, weakness of the abdominal muscles, inactivity and bedrest, pregnancy, hemorrhoids, and GI disease. Fecal impaction is the retention of hardened or puttylike stool in the rectum and colon, which interferes with normal passage of feces. Intestinal obstruction designates an impairment of movement of intestinal contents in a cephalocaudal direction as the result of either mechanical or paralytic mechanisms.

Malabsorption results from the impaired absorption of nutrients and other dietary constituents from the intestine. It can involve a single dietary constituent such as vitamin B_{12} or extend to involve all of the substances absorbed in a particular part of the small intestine. Malabsorption can result from disease of the small bowel and disorders that impair digestion and can (in some cases) obstruct the lymph flow by which fats are transported to the general circulation.

■ PERITONITIS

Peritonitis is an inflammatory response of the serous membrane that lines the abdominal cavity and covers the visceral organs. It can be caused by either bacterial invasion or chemical irritation. Most commonly, enteric bacteria enter the peritoneum because of a defect in the wall of one of the abdominal organs. The most common causes of peritonitis are perforated peptic ulcer, ruptured appendix, perforated diverticulum, gangrenous bowel, pelvic inflammatory disease, and gangrenous gallbladder. Other causes are abdominal trauma and wounds. Generalized peritonitis, although no longer the overwhelming problem

TABLE 41-2. SITES OF AND REQUIREMENTS FOR ABSORPTION OF DIETARY CONSTITUENTS AND MANIFESTATIONS OF MALABSORPTION

DIETARY CONSTITUENT	SITE OF ABSORPTION	REQUIREMENTS	MANIFESTATIONS
Water and electrolytes	Mainly small bowel	Osmotic gradient	Diarrhea Dehydration Cramps
Fat	Upper jejunum	Pancreatic lipase Bile salts Functioning lymphatic channels	Weight loss Steatorrhea Fat-soluble vitamin deficiency
Carbohydrates			
Starch	Small intestine	Amylase Maltase Isomaltase α-dextrins	Diarrhea Flatulence Abdominal discomfort
Sucrose	Small intestine	Sucrase	
Lactose	Small intestine	Lactase	
Maltose	Small intestine	Maltase	
Fructose	Small intestine		
Protein	Small intestine	Pancreatic enzymes (trypsin, chymotrypsin, elastin, and so forth)	Loss in muscle mass Weakness Edema
Vitamins			
A	Upper jejunum	Bile salts	Night blindness Dry eyes Corneal irritation
Folic acid	Duodenum and jejunum	Absorptive; may be impaired by some drugs (*i.e.,* anticonvulsants)	Cheilosis Glossitis Megaloblastic anemia
B_{12}	Ileum	Intrinsic factor	Glossitis Neuropathy Megaloblastic anemia
D	Upper jejunum	Bile salts	Bone pain Fractures Tetany
E	Upper jejunum	Bile salts	Uncertain
K	Upper jejunum	Bile salts	Easy bruising and bleeding
Calcium	Duodenum	Vitamin D and parathyroid hormone	Bone pain Fractures Tetany
Iron	Duodenum and jejunum	Normal *p*H (hydrochloric acid secretion)	Iron-deficiency anemia Glossitis

it once was, is still a leading cause of death after abdominal surgery.

The peritoneum has several characteristics that either increase its vulnerability to or protect it against the effects of peritonitis. One weakness of the peritoneal cavity is that it is a large, unbroken space that favors the dissemination of contaminants. For the same reason, it has a large surface that permits rapid absorption of bacterial toxins into the blood. On the other hand, the peritoneum is particularly well adapted for producing an inflammatory response as a means of controlling infection. It tends, for example, to exude a thick, sticky, and fibrinous substance that adheres to other structures, such as the mesen-

tery and omentum, and that serves to seal off the perforated viscus and aid in localizing the process. Localization is enhanced by sympathetic stimulation that limits intestinal motility. Although the diminished or absent peristalsis that occurs tends to give rise to associated problems, it does inhibit the movement of contaminants throughout the peritoneal cavity.

One of the most important manifestations of peritonitis is the translocation of extracellular fluid into the peritoneal cavity (through weeping or serous fluid from the inflamed peritoneum) and into the bowel as a result of bowel obstruction. Nausea and vomiting cause further losses of fluid. The fluid loss may encourage development of hypovolemia and shock.

The onset of peritonitis may be acute, as in a ruptured appendix, or it may have a more gradual onset such as occurs in progressive inflammatory disease. Pain and tenderness are common symptoms. The pain is usually more intense over the inflamed area. The person with peritonitis usually lies still because any movement aggravates the pain. Breathing is often shallow to prevent movement of the abdominal muscles. The abdomen is usually rigid and sometimes described as boardlike, because of reflex muscle guarding. Vomiting is common. Fever, elevation in white blood cell count, tachycardia, and frequently hypotension are present. Hiccups may develop because of irritation of the phrenic nerve. Paralytic ileus occurs shortly after the onset of widespread peritonitis and is accompanied by abdominal distention. Peritonitis that progresses and is untreated leads to toxemia and shock.

TREATMENT

Treatment measures for peritonitis are directed toward (1) preventing the extension of the inflammatory response, (2) correcting the fluid and electrolyte imbalances that develop, and (3) minimizing the effects of paralytic ileus and abdominal distention. Surgical intervention may be needed to remove an acutely inflamed appendix or to close the opening in a perforated peptic ulcer. Oral fluids are forbidden. Nasogastric suction, which entails the insertion of a tube (placed through the nose) into the stomach or intestine, is employed to decompress the bowel and relieve the abdominal distention. Fluid and electrolyte replacement is essential. These fluids are prescribed on the basis of frequent blood chemistry determinations. Antibiotics are given to combat infection. Narcotics are often needed for pain relief.

> In summary, peritonitis is an inflammatory response of the serous membrane that lines the abdominal cavity and covers the visceral organs. It can be caused by either bacterial invasion or chemical irritation caused by perforation of the viscera or abdominal organs. It is characterized by severe pain, fluid and electrolyte disorders, paralytic intestinal obstruction, and sepsis. The treatment of peritonitis focuses on preventing the extension of the inflammatory response, correcting the fluid and electrolyte imbalances that develop, and minimizing the effects of bowel obstruction.

■ REFERENCES

1. Richter, J.M., & Isselbacher, K.J. (1991). Gastrointestinal bleeding. In J. Wilson, E. Braunwald, K.J. Isselbacher (Eds.). *Harrison's principles of internal medicine* (12th ed., p. 261). New York: McGraw-Hill.

2. Guyton, A. (1991). *Textbook of medical physiology* (8th ed., p. 700). Philadelphia: W.B. Saunders.

3. Gelfand, G. (1991). Gastroesophageal reflux disease. *Medical Clinics of North America, 75,* 923–941.

4. Helm, J.F., Dodds, N.J., Pile, L.R., et al. (1984). Effect of esophageal emptying and saliva on clearance of acid from the esophagus. *New England Journal of Medicine, 310,* 284–288.

5. Richter, J.E. (1992). Gastroesophageal reflux: Diagnosis and management. *Hospital Practice, 27,* (1A), 59–66.

6. Kumar, V.S., Cotran, R.S., & Robbins, S.L. (1992). *Basic pathology* (5th ed., pp. 284–290, 482–483, 510–517). Philadelphia: W.B. Saunders.

7. Ellis, F.H., Levitan, N., & Lo, T.C.M. (1991). Cancer of the esophagus. In A.I. Hollieb, D.J. Fink, & G.P. Murphy (Eds.). *Clinical oncology* (pp. 254–262). Atlanta: American Cancer Society.

8. Fromm, D. (1987). Mechanisms involved in gastric mucosal resistance to injury. *Annual Review of Medicine, 38,* 119.

9. Cryer, B., Lee, E., & Feldman, M. (1992). Factors influencing mucosal prostaglandin concentrations: Role of smoking and aging. *Annals of Internal Medicine, 116,* 636–640.

10. Lind, C.D., & Blaser, M.J. (1991). *Helicobacter pylori* and duodenal ulcers. *Hospital Practice, 26*(2), 45–63.

11. Cotran, S., Kumar, V., & Robbins, S.L. (1989). *Pathologic basis of disease* (4th ed., pp. 844). Philadelphia: W.B. Saunders.

12. Wolfe, M.M., & Jensen, R.T. (1987). Zollinger-Ellison syndrome. *New England Journal of Medicine, 317,* 1200.

13. Zuckerman, G.R., Cort, D., & Schuman, R.B. (1988). Stress ulcer syndrome. *Journal of Intensive Care Medicine, 3,* 21.

14. Konopad, E., & Noseworthy, T. (1988). Stress ulceration: A serious complication in critically ill patients. *Heart & Lung, 17,* 339.

15. Lawrence, W. (1991). Gastric neoplasms. In A.I. Hollieb, D.J. Fink, & G.P. Murphy (Eds.). *Clinical oncology* (pp. 245–253). Atlanta: American Cancer Society.

16. Drossman, D.A., Funch-Jensen, P., Janssens, J., et al. (1990). Identification of subgroups of functional bowel disorders. *Gastroenterol Int, 3,* 159–172.

17. Drossman, D.A., & Thompson, W.G. (1992). The irritable bowel syndrome: Review and graduated multicomponent treatment approach. *Annals of Internal Medicine, 116,* 1009–1016.

18. Podolsky, D.K. (1991). Inflammatory bowel disease (first of two parts). *New England Journal of Medicine, 325,* 1008–1016.

19. Podolsky, D.K. (1991). Inflammatory bowel disease (second of two parts). *New England Journal of Medicine, 325,* 1008–1016.

20. Van Ness, M., & Peller, C. (1991). Acute diverticular disease: Diagnosis and management. *Hospital Practice, 26*(3A), 83–91.

21. Beart, R.W., Jr. (1991). Colorectal cancer. In A.I. Hollieb, D.J. Fink, & G.P. Murphy (Eds.). *Clinical oncology* (pp. 213–218). Atlanta: American Cancer Society.

22. American Cancer Society. (1992). *Cancer facts and figures* (p. 8). Atlanta: American Cancer Society.

23. Bruckstein, A.H. (1988, October). Acute diarrhea. *American Family Practice, 20,* 217.

24. Field, M., Rao, M.C., & Chang, E.B. (1989). Intestinal electrolyte transport and diarrheal disease (part 2). *New England Journal of Medicine, 321,* 879–883.

25. Oral therapy for diarrhea. (1991). *Hospital Practice, 26*(5), 86–88.
26. Avery, M.E., & Snyder, J.D. (1990). Oral therapy for acute diarrhea. *New England Journal of Medicine, 323,* 891–894.
27. Knauer, C.M. (1993). Alimentary tract. In L.M. Tierney, S.J. McPhee, M.A. Papadakis, et al. (Eds.). *Current medical diagnosis and treatment* (pp. 483–484). Norwalk, CT: Appleton Lange.
28. Schrock, T.R. (1991). Large intestine. In L.W. Way (Ed.). *Current surgical diagnosis and treatment* (9th ed., pp. 664, 1192). Norwalk, CT: Appleton Lange.
29. Wren, K. (1989). Fecal impaction. *New England Journal of Medicine, 321,* 658–662.
30. Trier, J.S. (1988). Intestinal malabsorption: Differentiation of cause. *Hospital Practice, 23* (May 13), 195.

■ **BIBLIOGRAPHY**

Bayless, T.M. (1990). Inflammatory bowel disease and irritable bowel disease. *Medical Clinics of North America, 74,* 21–28.

Bayless, T.M. (1989). Chronic diarrhea: Newly appreciated syndromes. *Hospital Practice, 24*(1A), 117–135.

Camilleri, M., & Prather, C.M. (1992). The irritable bowel syndrome: Mechanisms and a practical approach to management. *Annals of Internal Medicine, 116,* 1001–1008.

Geier, D.L., & Miner, P.B. (1992). New therapeutic agents in treatment of inflammatory bowel disease. *American Journal of Medicine, 93,* 199–208.

Gelfand, M.D. (1990). Gastroesophageal reflux disease. *Medical Clinics of North America, 75,* 923–941.

Gryboski, J.D. (1990). Peptic ulcer disease in children. *Medical Clinics of North America, 75,* 889–903.

Levinson, M.J. (1989). Gastric stress ulcers. *Hospital Practice, 24*(3), 59–63.

Littman, A. (1987). Lactose deficiency. *Hospital Practice, 22*(1), 111.

Makhlouf, G.M. (1990). Neural and hormonal regulation of function in the gut. *Hospital Practice, 25*(2A), 79–98.

Peterson, W.L. (1991). *Helicobacter pylori* and peptic ulcer disease. *New England Journal of Medicine, 324,* 104348.

Ransohoff, D.F., & Lang, C.A. (1991). Screening for colorectal cancer. *New England Journal of Medicine, 325,* 37–41.

Rudderman, W.B. (1990). Newer pharmacologic agents for the therapy of inflammatory bowel disease. *Medical Clinics of North America, 75,* 133–153.

Shamburek, R.D., & Farrar, J.T. (1990). Disorders of the digestive system in the elderly. *New England Journal of Medicine, 322,* 438–442.

Snyder, J.D. (1991). Oral therapy for diarrhea. *Hospital Practice, 26*(5), 86–89.

Soll, A.H. (Moderator UCLA Conference). (1991). Nonsteroidal anti-inflammatory drugs and peptic ulcer disease. *Annals of Internal Medicine, 114,* 307–319.

Soll, A.H. (1990). Pathogenesis of peptic ulcer and implications for therapy. *New England Journal of Medicine, 322,* 90916.

Spechler, S.J., & Goval, R.K. (1986). Barrett's esophagus. *New England Journal of Medicine, 315,* 362–371.

Tremaine, W.J. (1990). Chronic constipation: Causes and management. *Hospital Practice, 25*(4), 89–100.

Trier, J.S. (1991). Celiac sprue. *New England Journal of Medicine, 325,* 170919.

Vargas, J. (1988, February 15). Sorting out the causes of vomiting and diarrhea. *Emergency Medicine, 20,* 139.

Wolfe, M.M., & Soll, A.H. (1988). The physiology of gastric acid secretion. *New England Journal of Medicine, 319,* 1707–1715.

ALTERATIONS IN FUNCTION OF THE HEPATOBILIARY SYSTEM AND EXOCRINE PANCREAS

■ ## OBJECTIVES

After you have studied this chapter, you should be able to meet the following objectives:

■ List the functions of the liver and the signs of disruption of these functions.

■ State the two ways by which drugs and other substances are metabolized or inactivated in the liver.

■ Diagram the mechanism of bilirubin formation, transport, and elimination.

■ Compare hemolytic jaundice and obstructive jaundice with reference to their clinical manifestations.

■ State the origin of ammonia and describe the function of the liver in terms of its detoxification.

■ Explain the rationale for the use of laboratory measures of serum aminotransferase activity in diagnosis and management of persons with liver disease.

■ Compare hepatitis A, B, C, D, and E in terms of source of infection, incubation period, development of chronic disease, and the carrier state.

■ Characterize postnecrotic cirrhosis and biliary cirrhosis.

■ Summarize the three stages of alcoholic cirrhosis.

■ Describe the physiologic basis for portal hypertension and relate to the development of ascites, esophageal varices, and spenogmegaly.

■ Characterize hepatic-systemic encephalopathy.

■ State the reason for the poor prognosis in persons with hepatocellular cancer.

■ Explain the function of the gall bladder in regulating the flow of bile into the duodenum.

■ Describe the formation of gallstones.

■ Describe the clinical manifestations of acute pancreatitis.

■ Compare chronic calcifying pancreatitis and chronic obstructive pancreatitis.

■ State the reason for the poor prognosis in pancreatic cancer.

Carol Mattson Porth: PATHOPHYSIOLOGY: CONCEPTS OF
ALTERED HEALTH STATES, 4th ed. © 1994, 1990, 1986, 1982
J.B. Lippincott Company

The liver, the gallbladder, and the exocrine pancreas are classified as accessory organs of the gastrointestinal tract. In addition to producing digestive secretions, both the liver and the pancreas have other important functions. The endocrine pancreas, for example, supplies the insulin and glucagon needed in cell metabolism, whereas the liver synthesizes glucose, plasma proteins, and blood clotting factors and is responsible for the degradation and elimination of drugs and hormones, among other functions. The content of this chapter focuses on functions and disorders of the liver, the biliary tract and gallbladder, and the exocrine pancreas.

■ THE LIVER AND BILIARY SYSTEM

The liver is the largest internal organ in the body, weighing about 1.3 kg, or 3 lb, in the adult. It is located below the diaphragm and occupies much of the right hypochondrium. The falciform ligament, which extends from the peritoneal surface of the anterior abdominal wall between the umbilicus and diaphragm, divides the liver into two lobes, a large right lobe and a small left lobe (Fig. 42-1). There are two additional lobes on the visceral surface of the liver, the caudate and quadrate lobes. Except for that portion that is in the epigastric area, the liver is contained within the rib cage and in healthy persons cannot normally be palpated. The liver is surrounded by a tough fibroelastic capsule called *Glisson's capsule*.

The liver is unique among the abdominal organs in having a dual blood supply—the hepatic artery and the portal vein. About 400 mL per minute of blood enters the liver through the hepatic artery; another 1000 mL per minute enters by way of the valveless portal vein, which carries blood from the stomach, the small and the large intestines, the pancreas, and the spleen (Fig. 42-2). Although the blood from the portal vein is incompletely saturated with oxygen, it supplies about 60% to 70% of the oxygen needs of the liver. The venous outflow from the liver is carried by the valveless hepatic veins, which empty into the inferior vena cava just below the level of the diaphragm. The pressure difference between the hepatic vein and the portal vein is normally such that the liver stores about 200 mL to 400 mL of blood. This blood can be shifted back into the general circulation during periods of hypovolemia and shock. In congestive heart failure, in which the pressure within the vena cava increases, blood backs up and accumulates in the liver.

The lobules are the functional units of the liver. Each lobule is a cylindrical structure that measures about 0.8 mm to 2 mm in diameter and is several millimeters in length. There are about 50,000 to 100,000 lobules in the liver. Each lobule is organized around a central vein that empties into the hepatic veins and from there into the vena cava. The terminal bile ducts and small branches of the portal vein and hepatic artery are located at the periphery of the lobule. Plates of hepatic cells radiate centrifugally from the central vein like spokes on a wheel (Fig. 42-3). These hepatic plates are separated by wide thin-walled channels, called *sinusoids*, that extend from the periphery of the lobule to its central vein. There are also small tubular channels, called *bile canaliculi*, that lie between the cell membranes of adjacent hepatocytes. The sinusoids are supplied by blood from both the portal vein and hepatic artery. The plates of hepatic cells are no more than two layers thick so that every cell is exposed to the blood that travels through the sinusoids. The hepatic cells remove substances from the blood and excrete them into the canaliculi. The hepatic cells can also release substances into the blood.

The venous sinusoids are lined with two types of cells: the typical endothelial cells and the Kupffer's cells. The Kupffer's cells are reticuloendothelial cells that are capable of removing and phagocytizing old and defective blood cells, bacteria, and other foreign material from the portal blood as it flows through the sinusoid. This phagocytic action removes the colon bacilli and other harmful substances that filter into the blood from the intestine.

The bile produced by the hepatocytes flows into the canaliculi, and then to the periphery of the lobules, which drain into larger ducts, until it reaches the right and left hepatic ducts. The intrahepatic and extrahepatic bile ducts are often collectively referred to as the *hepatobiliary tree*. These ducts unite to form the common duct (Fig. 42-4). The common duct, which is about 10 cm to 15 cm in length, descends and passes behind the pancreas and enters the descending duodenum. The pancreatic duct joins the common duct in the ampulla of Vater, which empties into the duodenum through the duodenal papilla. Muscle tissue at the junction of the papilla, called the *sphincter of Oddi*, regulates the flow of bile into the duodenum. A second sphincter (sphincter of Boyden), which is just above the point where the pancreatic duct fuses with the common duct, controls the flow of bile into this area of the common duct. When this sphincter is closed, bile moves back into the gallbladder.

FUNCTIONS OF THE LIVER

The liver is one of the most versatile and active organs in the body. It produces bile; metabolizes hormones and drugs; synthesizes proteins, glucose, and clot-

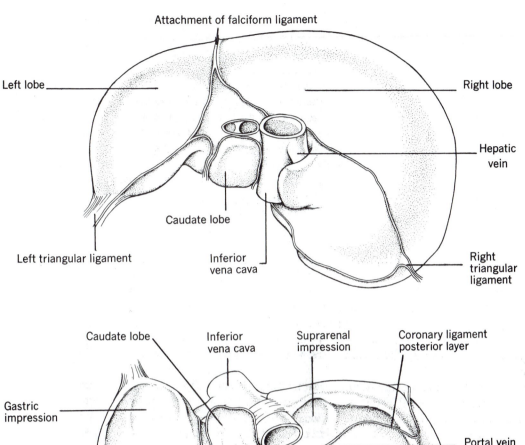

FIG. 42-1. Superior posterior view (**top**) and inferior view (**bottom**) of the liver. (Chaffee, E. E., & Lytle, I. M. [1980]. *Basic physiology and anatomy* [4th ed.]. Philadelphia: J.B. Lippincott)

ting factors; stores vitamins and minerals; changes ammonia produced by deamination of amino acids to urea; converts fatty acids to ketones; and has other functions as well. In this process, the liver degrades excess nutrients and converts them into substances essential to the body. It builds carbohydrates from proteins, converts sugars to fats that can be stored, and interchanges protein molecules so that they can be used for a number of purposes. In its capacity for metabolizing drugs and hormones, the liver serves as an excretory organ. In this respect, the bile, which carries the end-products of substances metabolized by the liver, is much like the urine, which carries the body wastes filtered by the kidneys. The functions of the liver are summarized in Table 42-1.

DRUG AND HORMONE METABOLISM

By virtue of its many enzyme systems that are involved in biochemical transformations and modifications, the liver has an important role in the metabolism of many drugs, hormones, and endogenous

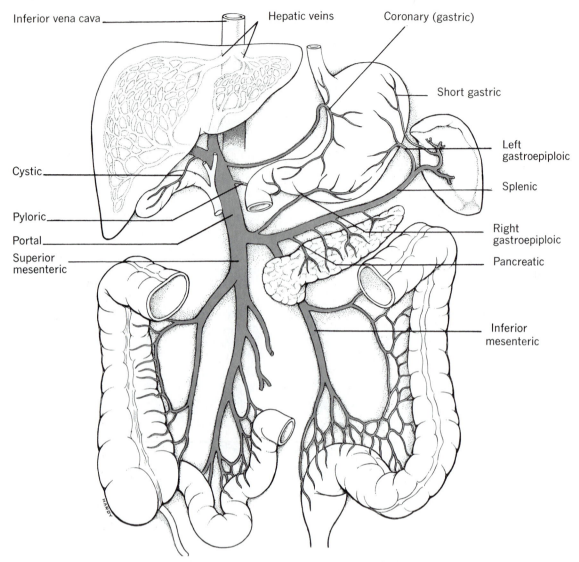

FIG. 42-2. The portal circulation. Blood from the gastrointestinal tract, spleen, and pancreas travels to the liver by way of the portal vein before moving into the vena cava for return to the heart. (Chaffee, E. E., & Lytle, I. M. [1980]. *Basic physiology and anatomy* [4th ed.]. Philadelphia: J.B. Lippincott)

substances such as bilirubin. The liver is particularly important in terms of metabolizing lipid soluble substances that cannot be directly excreted by the kidneys. There are two major types of reactions involved in the detoxification and metabolism of drugs and other chemicals: (1) phase I, reactions which involve chemical modification or inactivation of a substance, and (2) phase II, reactions which involve conversion of lipid-soluble substances to water-soluble derivatives.[1] Often the two types of reactions are linked. Many phase I reactants are not soluble and must therefore undergo a subsequent phase II reaction to be eliminated. These reactions, which are called *biotransformations*, are important considerations in drug therapy.

Phase I reactions result in chemical modification of reactive drug groups by oxidation, reduction, hydroxylation, or other chemical reactions. Most drug-metabolizing enzymes are located in the lipophilic membranes of the smooth endoplasmic reticulum of liver cells (see Chapter 1). When these membranes are broken down and separated in the laboratory, they reform into vesicles called *microsomes*. Hence, the enzymes that are present in these membranes are often referred as microsomal enzymes. Most oxidative reactions are carried out by a large family of microsomal isoenzymes called cytochromes *P-450*.[2] An increase in microsomal enzyme levels can be induced by drugs such as alcohol and barbiturates. Such induction usually results in acceleration of drug

Cross section of liver lobule

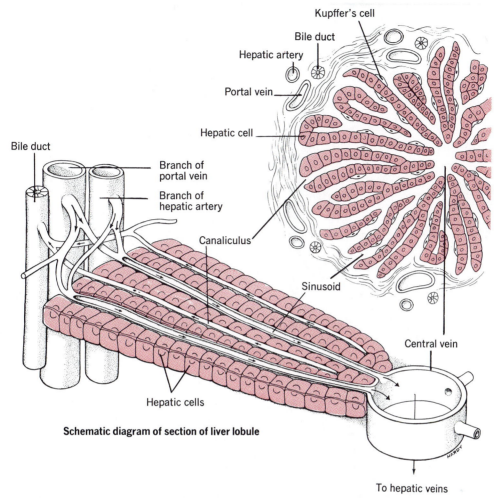

FIG. 42-3. A section of liver lobule showing the location of the hepatic veins, hepatic cells, liver sinusoids, and branches of the portal vein and hepatic artery. (Chaffee, E E., & Lytle, I. M. [1980]. *Basic physiology and anatomy* [4th ed.]. Philadelphia: J.B. Lippincott)

metabolism and a decrease in pharmacologic action of the drug and also of coadministered drugs that are metabolized by the same enzyme system. In the case of drugs metabolically transformed to reactive intermediates, enzyme induction may exacerbate drug-mediated tissue toxicity. Environmental pollutants are also capable of inducing cytochromes P-450. For example, exposure to benzo(a)pyrene, present in tobacco smoke, charcoal-broiled meat, and other organic pyrolysis products, is known to induce cytochromes P-450 and alter the rates of metabolism of some drugs. Enzymes in the cytochrome system can also be inhibited by drugs. For example, imidazole-containing drugs such as cimetidine and ketoconazole effectively inhibit the metabolism of testosterone.[1]

Phase II reactions, which involve the conversion of water- soluble derivatives to lipid-soluble sub-

stances, may follow phase I reactions or proceed independently. Conjugation, catalyzed by endoplasmic reticulum enzymes that couple the drug with another chemical compound to render it water soluble, is one of the most common phase II reactions. Although many water-soluble drugs and endogenous substances are excreted unchanged in the urine or bile, lipid-soluble substances tend to accumulate in the body unless they are converted to less active compounds or water-soluble metabolites. In general, the conjugates are more soluble than the parent compound and are pharmacologically inactive.

In addition to its role in metabolism of drugs and chemicals, the liver is also responsible for hormone inactivation or modification. Insulin and glucagon are inactivated by proteolysis or deamination. Thyroxine and triiodothyronine are metabolized by reac-

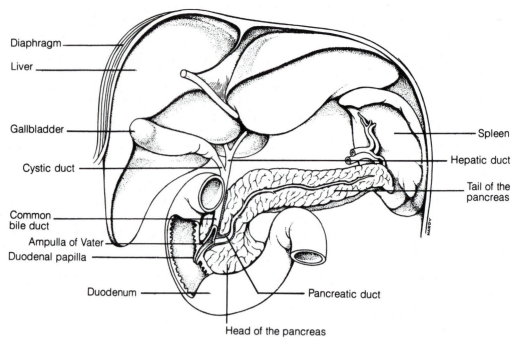

FIG. 42-4. The liver and biliary system, including the gallbladder and bile ducts. (Chaffee, E. E., & Lytle, I. M. [1980]. *Basic physiology and anatomy* [4th ed.]. Philadelphia: J.B. Lippincott)

tions involving deiodination. Steroid hormones such as the glucocorticoids are first inactivated by a phase I reaction and then conjugated by a phase II reaction.

Alcohol Metabolism. Alcohol is absorbed readily from the gastrointestinal tract, being one of the few substances that can be absorbed from the stomach. As a substance, alcohol fits somewhere between a food and a drug. It supplies calories but cannot be broken down or stored as protein, fat, or carbohydrate. As a food, alcohol yields 7.0 kcal/g compared with the 4.0 kcal/g produced by metabolism of an equal amount of carbohydrate. Between 80 to 90 percent of the alcohol a person drinks is metabolized by the liver. The rest is excreted through the lungs, kidneys, and skin. The average person can metabolize about 18 g of alcohol per hour (it takes about 2 hours to metabolize one mixed drink).

Alcohol metabolism proceeds simultaneously by two pathways, one involving alcohol dehydrogenase and the other the microsomal ethanol-oxidizing system (MEOS).[3–5] The alcohol dehydrogenase pathway, which takes place in the cytoplasm, produces acetaldehyde and hydrogen ions. The acetaldehyde is subsequently converted to acetate by acetaldehyde dehydrogenase, a reaction that occurs primarily in the mitochondria.

The MEOS pathway, which occurs in the smooth endoplasmic reticulum, produces acetaldehyde and free radicals. Prolonged and excessive alcohol inges-

tion results in enzyme induction and increased activity of the MEOS. One of the most important enzymes of the MEOS, a cytochrome P-450, also oxidizes a number of other compounds including various drugs (acetaminophen, isoniazid, and many others), toxins (carbon tetrachloride, halothane), vitamins A and D, and carcinogenic agents (aflatoxin, nitrosamines). Thus, increased activity of this system enhances the susceptibility of persons with heavy alcohol consumption to the hepatotoxic effects of industrial toxins, anesthetic agents, chemical carcinogens, vitamins, and over-the-counter analgesics such as acetaminophen. For example, acetaminophen is generally safe when taken in recommended doses. However, a small fraction is metabolized by the microsomal system to an active product that is highly toxic to the liver; this fraction increases with chronic alcohol use.[3]

The metabolic end-products of alcohol metabolism (*e.g.*, acetaldehyde and free radicals) are responsible for a variety of metabolic alterations that play a major role in the development of liver injury. Acetaldehyde, for example, has multiple toxic effects on liver cells and liver function.

Alcohol metabolism requires a cofactor, nicotinamide adenine dinucleotide (NAD), that is required for many other metabolic processes, including the metabolism of pyruvates, urates, and fatty acids. Because alcohol competes for utilization of intracellular cofactors normally needed for other metabolic

TABLE 42-1. FUNCTIONS OF THE LIVER AND MANIFESTATIONS OF ALTERED FUNCTION

FUNCTION	MANIFESTATIONS OF ALTERED FUNCTION
Production of bile salts	Malabsorption of fat and fat-soluble vitamins
Elimination of bilirubin	Failure to eliminate bilirubin causes elevation in serum bilirubin and jaundice
Metabolism of steroid hormones	
Estrogens and progesterone	Disturbances in gonadal function, including gynecomastia in
Testosterone	the male
Glucocorticoids	Signs of Cushing's syndrome
Aldosterone	Sodium retention and edema; hypokalemia
Metabolism of drugs	Decreased plasma binding of drugs owing to a decrease in albumin production
	Decreased removal of drugs that are metabolized by the liver
Carbohydrate metabolism	Hypoglycemia may develop when glycogenolysis and gluconeogenesis are impaired
Stores glycogen	
Synthesizes glucose from	Abnormal glucose tolerance curve may occur because of impaired uptake and release of glucose by the liver
Amino acids	
Lactic acid	
Glycerol	
Fat metabolism	
Formation of lipoproteins	Impaired synthesis of lipoproteins
Conversion of carbohydrates and proteins to fat	
Synthesis of cholesterol	
Formation of ketones from fatty acid	
Protein metabolism	
Deamination of proteins	
Formation of urea from ammonia	Elevated blood ammonia levels
Synthesis of plasma proteins	Decreased levels of plasma proteins, particularly albumin, which contributes to edema formation
Synthesis of clotting factors	Bleeding tendency
Fibrinogen	
Prothrombin	
Factors V, VII, IX, X	
Storage of mineral and vitamins	Signs of deficiency of fat-soluble and other vitamins that are stored in the liver
Filtration of blood and removal of bacteria and particulate matter by Kupffer cells	Increased exposure of the body to colon bacilli and other foreign matter

processes, it tends to disrupt other metabolic functions of the liver. The preferential utilization of NAD for alcohol metabolism can result in increased production and accumulation of lactic acid in the blood. The increased lactate levels tend to impair uric acid excretion by the kidney, which probably explains why excessive alcohol consumption may aggravate or precipitate gout. Alcohol also appears to stimulate production of uric acid. By reducing the availability of the cofactor NAD, alcohol also impairs the liver's ability to form glucose from amino acids and other glucose precursors. Thus, alcohol-induced hypoglycemia can develop when excessive alcohol ingestion occurs during periods of depleted liver glycogen stores. This may become a particular problem for the alcoholic who has been vomiting and has not eaten for several days. The combination of excess alcohol

consumption and starvation can also result in metabolic acidosis from accumulation of lactate and keto-acids. The situation begins with starvation, which causes mobilization of free fatty acids from fat stores. Because of the scarcity of glucose, insulin levels fall and levels of glucagon, cortisol, and growth hormone rise to promote gluconeogenesis and ketogenesis.

BILE PRODUCTION

The secretion of bile is essential for digestion of dietary fats and absorption of fats and fat-soluble vitamins from the intestine. The liver produces about 600 mL to 800 mL of yellow-green bile daily. Bile contains water, bile salts, bilirubin, cholesterol, and certain products of organic metabolism. Of these, only bile salts, which are formed from cholesterol, are important in digestion. The other components of bile depends on the secretion of sodium, chloride, bicarbonate, and potassium by the bile ducts.

Bile Salts. The liver forms about 0.5 g of bile salts daily. Bile salts serve an important function in digestion: they aid in emulsifying dietary fats, and they are necessary for the formation of the micelles that transport fatty acids and fat-soluble vitamins to the surface of the intestinal mucosa for absorption. About 94% of bile salts that enter the intestine are reabsorbed into the portal circulation by an active transport process that takes place in the distal ileum. From the portal circulation, the bile salts pass into the liver where they are recycled. Normally, bile salts travel this entire circuit about 18 times before being expelled in the feces.[6] This system for recirculation of bile is called the *enterohepatic circulation*.

BILIRUBIN ELIMINATION

Bilirubin is the substance that gives bile its color. It is formed from senescent red blood cells. In the process of degradation, the hemoglobin from the red blood cell is broken down to form biliverdin, which is rapidly converted to free bilirubin (Fig. 42-5). Free bilirubin, which is insoluble in plasma, is transported in the blood attached to plasma albumin. Even when it is bound to albumin, this bilirubin is still called *free bilirubin*. As it passes through the liver, free bilirubin is released from the albumin-carrier molecule and absorbed by the hepatocytes. Once inside the hepatocyte, free bilirubin is converted to *conjugated bilirubin*, making it soluble in bile. Conjugated bilirubin is secreted as a constituent of bile, and in this form it

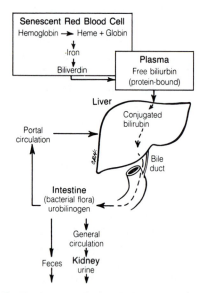

FIG. 42-5. The process of bilirubin formation, circulation, and elimination.

passes through the bile ducts into the small intestine. Once in the intestine, about half of the bilirubin is converted into a highly soluble substance called *urobilinogen* by the intestinal flora. Urobilinogen is either reabsorbed into the portal circulation or excreted in the feces. Most of the urobilinogen that is reabsorbed is returned to the liver to be re-excreted into the bile. A small amount of urobilinogen, about 5%, is reabsorbed into the general circulation and is then excreted by the kidneys.

Usually, only a small amount of bilirubin is found in the blood, the normal level of total serum bilirubin being 0.1 to 1.2 mg/dL. Laboratory measurements of bilirubin usually measure both free and conjugated bilirubin as well as the total bilirubin. These are reported as the *direct* or conjugated bilirubin and the *indirect* or free bilirubin.

MANIFESTATIONS OF DYSFUNCTION

JAUNDICE

Jaundice (icterus) is due to an abnormally high accumulation of bilirubin in the blood, as a result of which there is a yellowish discoloration to the skin and deep tissues. Jaundice develops when the plasma contains about twice the normal amount of bilirubin. Normal skin has a yellow cast, and therefore early signs of jaundice are often difficult to detect. This is especially true in persons with dark skin. Because bilirubin has a special affinity for elastic tissue, the sclera of the eye, which contains considerable elastic fibers, is usually one of the first structures in which jaundice can be detected. The four chief causes of jaundice are (1) excessive destruction of red blood cells, (2) impaired uptake of bilirubin by the liver cells, (3) decreased conjugation of bilirubin, and (4) obstruction of bile flow, either in the canaliculi of the liver or in the intra- or extrahepatic bile ducts. From an anatomic standpoint, jaundice can be categorized as prehepatic, hepatic, and posthepatic.[7] Chart 42-1 lists the common causes of prehepatic, hepatic, and posthepatic jaundice.

The major cause of *prehepatic jaundice* is excessive hemolysis of red blood cells. Hemolytic jaundice occurs when red blood cells are destroyed at a rate in excess of the liver's ability to remove the bilirubin from the blood. It may follow a hemolytic blood transfusion reaction or may occur in diseases such as hereditary spherocytosis, in which the red cell membranes are defective, or in hemolytic disease of the newborn (see Chapter 18). There is normal stool and urine color, mild jaundice, and indirect hyperbilirubinemia, with no bilirubin in the urine.

Intrahepatic or hepatocellular jaundice is caused by

CHART 42-1. CAUSES OF JAUNDICE

Prehepatic (Excessive Red Blood Cell Destruction)

Hemolytic blood transfusion reaction
Hereditary disorders of the red blood cell
    Sickle cell anemia
    Thalassemia
    Spherocytosis
Acquired hemolytic disorders
Hemolytic disease of the newborn
Autoimmune hemolytic anemias

Intrahepatic

Decreased bilirubin uptake by the liver
Gilbert's disease
Decreased conjugation of bilirubin
Hepatocellular liver damage
    Hepatitis
    Cirrhosis
    Cancer of the liver
Drug-induced cholestasis

Posthepatic (Obstruction of Bile Flow)

Structural disorders of the bile duct
Cholelithiasis
Congenital atresia of the extrahepatic bile ducts
Bile duct obstruction caused by tumors

disorders that directly affect the ability of the liver to remove bilirubin from the blood and/or conjugate it so it can be eliminated in the bile. *Gilbert's disease* is inherited as a dominant trait and results in a reduced uptake of bilirubin; the disorder is benign and fairly common. Affected persons have no symptoms other than a slightly elevated unconjugated bilirubin and mild jaundice. Conjugation of bilirubin is impaired whenever liver cells are damaged, when transport of bilirubin into liver cells becomes deficient, or when the enzymes needed to conjugate the bile are lacking. Liver disease, drugs—especially the anesthetic halothane—oral contraceptives, estrogen, anabolic steroids, isoniazid, and chlorpromazine are all possible causative factors. Hepatitis and cirrhosis are the most common causes of this form of jaundice. Hepatocellular jaundice usually interferes with all phases of bilirubin metabolism—uptake, conjugation, and excretion. It is associated with dark urine and elevated alkaline phosphate. Alkaline phosphatase is produced by the liver and excreted with the bile; thus when bile flow is obstructed, the blood alkaline phosphatase becomes elevated.

Posthepatic or obstructive jaundice (also called cholestatic jaundice) is seen when there is obstruction to bile flow between the liver and the intestine, with the obstruction located at any point between the junction of the right or left hepatic duct and the point where the bile duct opens into the intestine. Among the causes are strictures of the bile duct, gallstones, and tumors of the bile duct or the pancreas. Both conjugated and unconjugated bilirubin levels are usually elevated; the stools are clay colored because of the lack of bilirubin in the bile; the urine is dark because of the increased elimination of bilirubin in the urine; and serum levels of alkaline phosphatase are elevated and aspartate aminotransferase slightly increased. Blood levels of bilirubin are often elevated in obstructive jaundice. As the bile acids accumulate in the blood, pruritus (itching) develops. A history of pruritus preceding jaundice is common in obstructive jaundice.

ALTERED PROTEIN SYNTHESIS AND CONVERSION OF AMMONIA TO UREA

The most important functions of the liver in terms of protein metabolism are (1) protein synthesis, (2) interconversion of amino acids, and (3) conversion of ammonia to urea.

Protein Metabolism and Conversion of Ammonia to Urea. The liver is an important site for protein synthesis and degradation. Amino acids utilized for protein synthesis are derived from dietary proteins, metabolic turnover of endogenous proteins (mainly muscle), and direct hepatic synthesis.

Athough the body muscle produces the greatest amount of protein, the liver has the greatest rate of protein synthesis per gram of tissue. It produces not only the proteins for its own cellular needs but also secretory proteins that are released into the circulation. The most important of these secretory proteins is albumin. The liver produces about 12 grams of albumin per day, representing 25 percent of its total protein synthesis.[8] Albumin contributes significantly to the plasma colloidal osmotic pressure (see Chapter 29) and to the binding and transport of numerous substances including some hormones, fatty acids, bilirubin, and other anions. The liver also produces other important secretory proteins, such as fibrinogen and most of the blood clotting factors.

Interconversion of Amino Acid and Ammonia Metabolism. Through a variety of anabolic and catabolic processes, the liver is the major site of amino acid interconversion. Hepatic catabolism and degradation involves two major reactions: transamination and deamination. In transamination an amino group of an amino acid is transferred to an acceptor substance. As a result of transamination, amino acids can participate in the intermediary metabolism of carbohydrates and lipids. During periods of fasting

$$2NH_3 + CO_2 \rightarrow H_2N - \underset{\underset{O}{\|}}{C} - NH_2 + H_2O$$

Ammonia   Carbon dioxide   Urea   Water

FIG. 42-6. Formation of urea from ammonia.

or starvation, amino acids are used for producing glucose (gluconeogensis). Most of the nonessential amino acids are synthesized in the liver by transamination. The process of transamination is catalyzed by aminotransferases, enzymes that are found in high amounts in the liver. Oxidative deamination results in conversion of amino acids to keto acids and ammonia. Ammonia is very toxic to body tissues, particularly neurons. The ammonia that is released during deamination is removed from the blood almost immediately and converted to urea, a process in which two amino groups combine with carbon dioxide to form urea (Fig. 42-6). Essentially all urea formed in the body is synthesized in the liver and is then excreted by the kidneys. The average excretion of urea changes with the amount of protein in the diet but averages about 13 g/day.

Although urea is mostly excreted by the kidneys, some diffuses into the intestine where it is converted to ammonia by enteric bacteria. The intestinal production of ammonia also results from bacterial deammination of unabsorbed amino acids and protein derived from the diet, exfoliated cells, or blood in the gastrointestinal tract. This ammonia is absorbed into the portal circulation and transported to the liver where it is converted to urea before being released into the blood. Intestinal production of ammonia is increased following ingestion of high-protein foods and gastrointestinal bleeding.

In advanced liver disease urea synthesis is often depressed, leading to an accumulation of ammonia and subsequent reduction in blood urea nitrogen (BUN).

TESTS OF HEPATOBILIARY FUNCTION

The history and physical examination will, in most instances, provide clues about liver function. Diagnostic tests help to assess liver function and the extent of liver disease.

Laboratory tests commonly used to confirm the diagnosis of liver disease include measurements of serum bilirubin levels and of liver enzyme (aminotransferase and alkaline phosphatase) activity, along with determinations of prothrombin time and albumin levels. Aminotransferase activities are highly sensitive to hepatocellular (liver cell) damage. Alanine aminotransferase (ALT or SGPT) is liver specific, whereas aspartate aminotransferase (AST or SGOT) is derived from organs other than the liver. In

most cases of liver damage, there are parallel rises in both ALT and AST. The most dramatic rise is seen in cases of acute hepatocellular injury such as occurs with viral hepatitis, hypoxic or ischemic injury, acute toxic injury, or Reye's syndrome. Gamma-glutamyl-transpepsidase (GGT) is thought to function in the transport of amino acids and peptides into cells; it is a sensitive indicator of hepatobiliary disease. Hepatic synthetic activities are reflected in measures of serum protein levels and prothrombin time (synthesis of coagulation factors). Hypoalbuminemia due to depressed synthesis may complicate severe liver disease. Deficiencies of coagulation factor V and vitamin K–dependent factors (II, VII, IX, and X) may occur. Serum levels of bile acids are sensitive indicators of hepatobiliary function.

Ultrasound provides information about the size, composition, and blood flow of the liver. It has largely replaced cholangiography in detecting stones in the gallbladder or biliary tree. Computed tomography (CT) scanning provides information similar to that obtained by ultrasound. Magnetic resonance imaging (MRI) has proved to be useful in some disorders. Selective angiography of the celiac, superior mesenteric, or hepatic artery may be used to visualize the hepatic or portal circulation. A liver biopsy affords a means of examining liver tissue without necessitating surgery.

In summary, the hepatobiliary system consists of the liver, gallbladder, and bile ducts. The liver is the largest and, in function, one of the most versatile organs in the body. It is located between the gastrointestinal tract and the systemic circulation; venous blood from the intestine flows through the liver before it is returned to the heart. In this way, nutrients can be removed for processing and storage, and bacteria and other foreign matter can be removed by the Kupffer's cells before the blood is returned to the systemic circulation. The liver synthesizes bile salts, fats, glucose, and plasma proteins. It metabolizes drugs and alcohol and removes, conjugates, and secretes bilirubin into the bile. Because alcohol competes for utilization of intracellular cofactors normally needed by the liver for other metabolic processes, it tends to disrupt the metabolic functions of the liver. Jaundice occurs when bilirubin accumulates in the blood. It can occur because of excessive red blood cell destruction, failure of the liver to remove and conjugate the bilirubin, or obstructed biliary flow. Other important functions of the liver include deamination of amino acids, conversion of ammonia to urea, and the interconversion of amino acids and other compounds that are important to the metabolic processes of the body.

■ ALTERATIONS IN HEPATIC AND BILIARY FUNCTION

The structures of the hepatobiliary system are subject to many of the same pathologic conditions that affect other body systems: inflammation and immune responses, metabolic disorders, toxic injury, and neoplasms. This section focuses on alterations in liver function due to hepatitis, cirrhosis, portal hypertension and liver failure, cancer of the liver, and gallbladder disease.

HEPATITIS

Hepatitis refers to inflammation of the liver. It can be caused by reactions to drugs and toxins; by infectious disorders such as malaria, infectious mononucleosis, salmonellosis, and amebiasis that cause primary infections of extrahepatic tissues and secondary hepatitis; and by hepatotropic viruses that primarily affect liver cells or hepatocytes.

VIRAL HEPATITIS

The known hepatotropic viruses include hepatitis A virus, hepatitis B virus, the hepatitis B–associated delta virus, hepatitis C virus, and hepatitis E virus. Although all of these viruses cause acute hepatitis, they differ in mode of transmission and incubation period; mechanism, degree, and chronicity of liver damage; and ability to evolve to a carrier state. The presence of viral antigens and antigen antibodies can be determined through laboratory tests.

Hepatitis A. *Hepatitis A*, formerly called *infectious hepatitis*, is caused by the small, unenveloped, RNA-containing hepatitis A virus (HAV). Antibodies to HAV (anti-HAV) appear early in the disease and tend to persist in the serum (Fig. 42-7). The IgM antibodies (see Chapter 13) usually appear during the first week of symptomatic disease and begin to decline in a few months. Their presence coincides with a decline in fecal shedding of the virus. Peak levels of IgG antibodies occur after 1 month of illness and may persist for years; they provide long-term protective immunity against reinfection. The presence of IgM anti-HAV is indicative of acute hepatitis A, whereas IgG anti-HAV merely documents past exposure.

Hepatitis A has a brief incubation period (15 to 45 days) and is usually transmitted by the fecal–oral route. It is usually a benign, self-limiting disease, although it can cause acute fulminant hepatitis and death due to liver failure in very rare cases. It does not cause chronic hepatitis or the carrier state. The fecal shedding of HAV occurs up to 2 weeks before the development of symptoms and ends as the IgM levels rise.[7] The disease often occurs sporadically or in epidemics. Drinking contaminated milk or water and eating shellfish from infected waters are fairly common routes of transmission. At special risk are persons traveling abroad who have not previously been exposed to the virus. Institutions housing large numbers of people (usually children) are sometimes stricken with an epidemic of hepatitis A. Oral behavior and lack of toilet training promote viral infection among children attending preschool day-care centers, who then carry the virus home to older siblings and parents. Sexual transmission of HAV is common among homosexual men, especially those having oral–anal contact.[9] Hepatitis A is not usually transmitted by transfusion of blood or plasma derivatives, presumably because its short period of viremia usually coincides with clinical illness, so that the disease is apparent and blood donations are not accepted.

Gamma globulin is usually administered to close personal contacts of persons with hepatitis A. It may be advisable for persons traveling to countries where hepatitis A is endemic to receive a protective dose of gamma globulin within 2 weeks of arrival in that country and to receive booster doses if their stay is an extended one. An inactivated purified hepatitis A vaccine has been developed and is being tested.[10]

Hepatitis B. *Hepatitis B*, formerly referred to as *serum hepatitis*, has a longer incubation period and represents a more serious health problem than hepatitis A. Hepatitis B can produce acute hepatitis, chronic hepatitis, progression of chronic hepatitis to cirrhosis, fulminant hepatitis with massive necrosis, and the carrier state.[7] It also contributes to the development of hepatitis D (delta hepatitis). The Centers for Disease Control (CDC) estimate that there are 200,000 to 300,000 new cases of hepatitis B each year and 1 to 1.25 million chronic carriers in the United States.[11] At particular risk of becoming carriers are infants born to hepatitis B–infected mothers. The

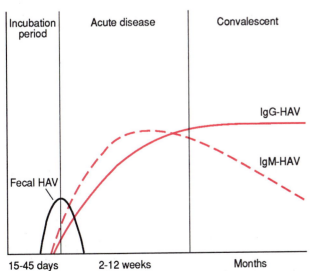

FIG. 42-7. The sequence of serologic changes in acute hepatitis A. (Redrawn from Kumar, V., Cotran, R. S., & Robbins, S. L. [1993]. *Basic pathology* [5th ed., p. 532]. Philadelphia: W.B. Saunders)

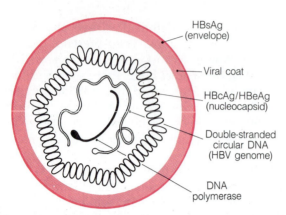

FIG. 42-8. The hepatitis B virus. The HBsAg is found in the viral envelope and the HBcAg and HBeAg in the nucleocapsid. The HBV-DNA and DNA polymerase are contained within the core of the virus.

CDC also estimates that each year in the United States there are 4000 to 5000 deaths due to hepatitis B–related cirrhosis and hepatocellular carcinoma. These figures are dwarfed by a much higher frequency of hepatitis B on a global scale. For example, the infection is endemic in regions of Africa and Southeast Asia.

The hepatitis B virus (HBV) is a double-stranded DNA virus. The complete viron, also called a *Dane particle*, consists of an outer envelope and an inner nucleocapsid that contains HBV-DNA and DNA polymerase (Fig. 42-8). Three well-defined antigens are associated with the virus: two core antigens, *HBcAg* and *HBeAg*, which are contained in the nucleocapsid, and a third surface antigen, *HBsAg*, which is found in the outer envelope of the virus. The HBV antigens evoke specific antibodies: anti-HBs, anti-HBc, and anti-HBe. These antigens and their antibodies serve as serologic markers to follow the course of the disease (Fig. 42-9).

The presence of *HBV-DNA* in the serum is the most certain indicator of hepatitis B infection. It is transiently present during the presymptomatic period and for a brief time during the acute illness. *DNA polymerase* activity usually is transient but may persist for years in persons who are chronic carriers and is an indication of continued infectivity.

HBsAg is the antigen most routinely measured in blood. It is produced in abundance by infected liver cells and released into the serum. In the past HBsAg was called the *Australian antigen* because it was first identified in an Australian aborigine. HBsAg is the earliest serologic marker to appear; it appears before the onset of symptoms and is an indicator of active infection, either acute or chronic. The HBsAg level begins to decline after the onset of the illness and is usually undetectable in 3 to 6 months. Persistence beyond 6 months indicates continued viral replication, infectivity, and risk of chronic hepatitis. *Anti-HBs*, a specific antibody to HBsAg, occurs in most individuals after clearance of HBsAg and after successful immunization for hepatitis B. There is usu-

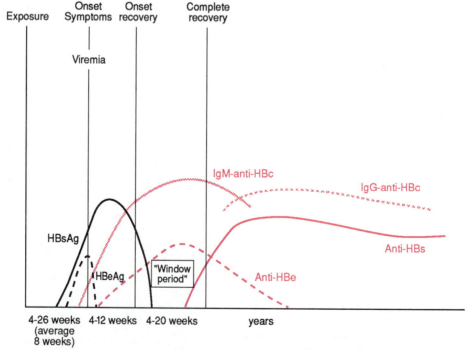

FIG. 42-9. The sequence of serologic changes in acute resolving hepatitis B. (Redrawn from Kumar, V., Cotran, R. S., & Robbins, S. L. [1993]. *Basic pathology* [5th ed., p. 533]. Philadelphia: W.B. Saunders)

ally a delay in appearance of anti-HBs following clearance of HBsAg. During this period of serologic gap, called the *window period*, infectivity has been demonstrated. Development of anti-HBs signals recovery from HBV, noninfectivity, and protection from HBV infection.

HbeAg is thought to be a cleavage product of the viral core antigen; it may be found in the serum as a soluble protein and is an active marker for the disease and shedding of complete virons into the blood stream. It appears during the incubation period, shortly after the appearance of HBsAg, and is found only in the presence of HBsAg. HBeAg usually disappears before HBsAg. *Anti-HBe* begins to appear in the serum at about the time that HBeAg disappears; its appearance signals the onset of resolution of the acute illness. The clinical usefulness of the antigen and its antibody lies in its predictive value for infectivity.

HbcAg does not circulate in the blood; therefore, it is not a useful marker for the disease. Although the antigen is not found in the blood, its antibodies (*Anti-HBc*) are the first to be detected. They appear toward the end of the incubation period and persist during the acute illness and for several months to years after that. The initial HBcAg antibody is IgM; it serves a marker for recent infection and is followed in 6 to 18 months by IgG antibodies. These antibodies are not protective and are detectable in the presence of chronic disease.

Hepatitis B has a long incubation period ranging from 4 to 26 weeks (average, 1.5 to 2 months).[7] This is followed by the acute disease, lasting weeks to months. For persons who recover from the acute infection there is a definable pattern of disappearance of antigen and appearance of antibodies. HBeAg and HBV-DNA and DNA polymerase disappear first, usually at the time of peak illness or early convalescence, and antibody to HBeAg (anti-HBe) can be detected. As convalescence continues, HBsAg disappears and anti-HBs can be detected. Anti-HBe persists for several years and anti-HBs for life. Persistence of HBsAg and failure to develop anti-HBs, along with the presence of anti-HBe, suggests development of chronic hepatitis.

The HBV virus is usually transmitted through inoculation with infected blood or serum. However, the viral antigen can be found in most body secretions and can be spread by oral or sexual contact. In the United States most persons with hepatitis B acquire the infection as adults or adolescents. The disease is highly prevalent among homosexuals and intravenous drug abusers. Health care workers are at risk owing to blood exposure and accidental needle injuries. Although the virus can be spread through transfusion or administration of blood products, routine screening methods have appreciably reduced transmission through this route.

The risk of hepatitis B infection among infants born to HBV- infected mothers ranges from 10% to 85%, depending on the mother's HBeAg status. Infants who become infected have a 90% risk of becoming chronic carriers, and up to 25% will die of chronic liver disease as adults.[11] Also, there is a high risk of horizontal spread of HBV from mother to child during the first 5 years of life.

Two types of products are available for prophylaxis against hepatitis B: hepatitis B immune globulin and hepatitis B vaccine. Hepatitis B immune globulin (HBIG) is prepared from plasma known to contain a high titer of antibody against HBsAG (Anti-HBs). It provides temporary (*i.e.*, 3 to 6 months) protection against HBV. Hepatitis B vaccine provides long-term protection against HBV infection and is recommended for both pre- and postexposure prophylaxis. The currently available hepatitis B vaccine is produced by recombinant DNA technology. Hepatitis B vaccine is highly recommended for all persons who are at high risk for exposure to the virus, including persons with occupational risk (health care workers and public safety workers), clients and staff of institutions for the developmentally disabled, hemodialysis patients, recipients of certain blood products, household contacts and sexual partners of HBV carriers, adoptees from countries where HBV is endemic, international travelers, injecting drug users, sexually active homosexual and bisexual men, sexually active heterosexual men and women, and inmates of long-term correctional agencies. It is recommended that persons with end-stage renal disease be vaccinated before they require hemodialysis and that universal hepatitis B vaccination of teenagers be implemented in communities where injecting drug use, pregnancy among teenagers, and sexually transmitted diseases are common.[11]

The CDC also recommends that all pregnant women be routinely tested for HBsAG during an early prenatal visit and that infants born to HBsAG mothers receive appropriate doses of both HBIG and hepatitis B vaccine.[11] Women admitted for delivery who have not been tested should have blood drawn for testing, and their infants should receive hepatitis B vaccine while test results are pending. If the mother is found to be HBsAG positive, the infant should receive HBIG as soon as possible and within 7 days. If the mother is found to be HBsAG negative, the infant should continue to receive hepatitis B vaccine as part of his or her vaccination schedule. The CDC further recommends that all infants be vaccinated, regardless of the HBsAg status of the mother; special efforts should be made to ensure that high levels of hepatitis vaccination are achieved in populations in which

HBV infection occurs at high rates among children (Alaskan natives, Pacific Islanders, and infants of immigrants from countries where HBV is endemic).[11]

Hepatitis C. The development of markers for HAV and HBV infections led to the awareness that about 90% of transfusion-related hepatitis was not caused by either of these viruses. The term *non-A, non-B hepatitis* was initially used to designate such cases. In 1989, the hepatitis C virus (HCV) was characterized, and it was subsequently discovered that this virus was responsible for the vast majority of cases of non-A, non-B post-transfusion hepatitis. The HCV virus is a single-stranded RNA virus that is distantly related to the viruses that cause yellow fever and dengue fever. Like HBV, HCV causes acute and chronic hepatitis and chronic carrier states and is also linked as a cause of hepatocellular cancer.[12] Exposure to blood products is the most common mode of transmission. Although body secretions may transmit the virus, this form of transmission is less of a risk than with HBV. Thus, the high-risk groups are persons who receive blood transfusions, intravenous drug abusers, and medical personnel exposed to blood products. With current methods of testing, HCV antibodies cannot be detected for several months after an acute infection. Although blood banks routinely screen for HCV, the delayed development of detectable antibodies has not completely eliminated the risk of post-transfusion hepatitis.[13] Investigation continues regarding development of tests for HCV.

Hepatitis D. Hepatitis D virus (HDV), or the delta hepatitis agent, is a defective RNA virus. It can cause either acute or chronic hepatitis. Infection is dependent upon concomitant infection with hepatitis B, specifically the presence of HBsAg. Acute hepatitis D occurs in two forms: coinfection that occurs simultaneously with acute hepatitis B and as a superinfection in which hepatitis B is imposed on chronic hepatitis B or hepatitis B carrier state.[14] The delta agent often increases the severity of HBV. It may convert mild HBV into severe fulminating hepatitis, cause acute hepatitis in asymptomatic carriers, or increase the tendency to chronic progressive hepatitis and cirrhosis.

The routes of transmission of hepatitis D are similar to those for hepatitis B. In the United States, infection is largely restricted to persons at high risk for HBV infection, particularly injecting drug users and persons receiving clotting factor concentrates. The greatest risk is in HBsAG carriers; these persons should be informed about the dangers of HDV superinfection. Laboratory methods are available to detect delta infection. Currently there is no treatment for hepatitis D. Because the infection is linked to hepatitis B, prevention of hepatitis D should begin with prevention of hepatitis B through vaccination.

Hepatitis E. The hepatitis E virus (HBE) is an unenveloped, single-stranded RNA virus. It is transmitted by the fecal–oral route and causes manifestations of acute hepatitis that are similar to hepatitis A. It does not cause chronic hepatitis or the carrier state. Its distinguishing feature is the high mortality rate (about 20%) among pregnant women, owing to the development of fulminant hepatitis. The infection occurs primarily in developing countries such as India, other Southeast Asian countries, parts of Africa, and Mexico. At present, the only reported cases in the United States have been in persons who have recently been in an endemic area.

Pathogenesis. The cellular changes that occur with hepatitis A, B, C, and D are those involving varying degrees of liver cell injury and necrosis. There are two mechanisms of liver cell injury in viral hepatitis: (1) direct cellular injury and (2) the induction of immune responses against the viral antigens. There is evidence that HDV and HCV are directly cytotoxic, whereas HBV and possibly HAV are immune mediated.[7]

The mechanisms of injury have been most closely studied in HBV. It is thought that the extent of inflammation and necrosis depends on the individual immune response. Accordingly, a prompt immune response during the acute phase of the infection would be expected to cause cell injury but at the same time eliminate the virus. Fulminant hepatitis would be explained in terms of an accelerated immune response with severe liver necrosis. This has been supported by the observation that persons who survive massive liver damage caused by fulminant hepatitis seldom become carriers. In contrast, persons who respond with a marginal immune response would fail to eliminate the virus and hepatocytes expressing viral antigens would persist, leading to low-level continued destruction expressed as chronic hepatitis. Finally, the carrier state would be expressed as failure of the immune response.

Clinical Manifestations. The clinical manifestations of viral hepatitis are extremely variable, ranging from asymptomatic infection without jaundice to fulminating disease (less than 1% to 3%) and death in a few days.

The *incubation period* for viral hepatitis ranges from weeks to months, depending on the virus that is involved. The manifestations of acute hepatitis have been divided into three phases: (1) the preicterus or prodromal period, (2) the icterus period, and (3) the convalescent period. Serologic tests are available with which to establish a diagnosis of hepatitis A, B, C, or D.

The *preicterus* or *prodromal* phase varies from abrupt to insidious with general malaise, myalgia, arthralgia, easy fatigability, upper respiratory symptoms (nasal discharge and pharyngitis), and severe anorexia out of proportion to the degree of illness. Gastrointestinal symptoms such as nausea, vomiting, and diarrhea or constipation may occur. Abdominal pain is usually mild and in the upper right quadrant. Chills and fever may mark an abrupt onset. Upper abdominal pain may occur. In persons who smoke, there may be a distaste for smoking that parallels that of anorexia. The serum transaminases aspartate aminotransferase (AST) and alanine aminotransferase (ALT) show variable increases during the preicterus phase of acute viral hepatitis and precede a rise in bilirubin.

The *icteric phase* is characterized by the development of jaundice (although some persons do not develop jaundice). It may follow the prodromal manifestations by 5 to 10 days or occur at the same time. The prodromal symptoms may become worse with the onset of jaundice, followed by progressive clinical improvement. Severe pruritis is common during the icteric phase. The serum bilirubin level typically rises when jaundice appears. Liver tenderness is common. Liver enlargement (hepatomegaly) and spleen enlargement (splenomegaly) may occur.

The *convalescent phase* is characterized by a gradual increase in sense of well-being, return of appetite, and disappearance of jaundice. The acute illness usually subsides rapidly over a 2- to 3-week period, with complete clinical recovery by 9 weeks for hepatitis A and by 16 weeks for hepatitis B and C.

Diagnosis and Treatment. Diagnosis is based on signs and symptoms. An elevation in serum bilirubin often precedes the appearance of jaundice, and enzyme tests that reflect hepatocellular damage such as the serum ALT and AST are elevated. Differentiation among the various viruses responsible for hepatitis requires the use of serologic markers.

The treatment of hepatitis is largely symptomatic. Bedrest, which at one time was a mainstay in treatment, has now largely been replaced by a more liberal program that permits patients to pace their own activity. Most patients will elect to limit activity because of fatigue. Dietary restrictions are usually minimal. If oral intake becomes inadequate, glucose solutions may be administered intravenously. Patients are instructed to avoid strenuous exercise, alcohol, and other hepatotoxic agents.

Carrier State. Hepatitis B and C can also produce a carrier state in which the person does not have symptoms but harbors the virus and can therefore transmit the disease. Evidence also indicates a carrier state for HDV. There is no carrier state for HAV. There are two types of carriers: healthy carriers who have few if any ill effects, and those with chronic disease who may or may not have symptoms. Factors that increase the risk of becoming a carrier are age at time of infection and immune status. Infections early in life, as in infants of HBV-infected mothers, may be as high as 90% to 95% as compared with 1% to 10% of adults who become carriers.[7] This is more common in African and Asian countries in which the carrier rates are 5% and 15%, respectively. Other persons at high risk for becoming carriers are those with impaired immunity, those who have received multiple transfusions or blood products, those who are on hemodialysis, and drug addicts.

CHRONIC HEPATITIS

Chronic hepatitis is defined as the continuation of hepatitis inflammation and necrosis for longer than 6 months. The causes of chronic hepatitis are diverse and include alcoholic hepatitis, drug-induced hepatitis, hepatitis due to metabolic disorders, and autoimmune hepatitis. Most cases of chronic hepatitis are caused by HBV and HCV. Chronic HBV develops in about 90% of acutely infected infants but in only about 5% to 10% of acutely infected adults.[15] There are two forms of chronic viral hepatitis: chronic persistent hepatitis and chronic active hepatitis.

Chronic persistent hepatitis is evidenced by minimal necrosis and a relatively benign course. It is characterized by elevated levels of aminotransferase enzymes (AST and ALT) and alkaline phosphatase. Usually there are no symptoms, but some persons may experience episodes of malaise, loss of appetite, nausea, and mild jaundice. Although usually benign, it is now thought that chronic persistent hepatitis may progress to chronic active hepatitis.

In contrast to chronic persistent hepatitis, chronic active hepatitis is characterized by progressive liver destruction, often leading to cirrhosis, chronic liver failure, and eventual death. It is associated with highly variable clinical features. About 30% of persons who develop chronic active hepatitis have a history of acute hepatitis. In these persons, the signs and symptoms of acute liver disease persist. The progress of the disease varies. Some persons progress to cirrhosis in a few years, and there is evidence to suggest that some may revert to chronic persistent hepatitis. Corticosteroid drugs may be used in the treatment of HCV but, because of the risk of increased viral replication, are not usually used in the treatment of HBV. Immunosuppressant drugs may also be used. Recombinant alpha-interferon has been shown to produce remission in some cases of chronic HBV and HBC. The agent has been shown to produce improvement in about 35% to 50% of persons with chronic HCV.[12] However, experience with the agent is still limited, treatment is costly, and side effects are common.

Autoimmune chronic hepatitis is mainly a disease of young women, although it can occur at any age and in either males or females. The absence of HBV and HCV suggests a diagnosis of autoimmune hepatitis. A biopsy is used to confirm the diagnosis. Corticosteroid drugs and immunosuppressant drugs are the treatment of choice for this type of hepatitis.

CIRRHOSIS

Cirrhosis is characterized by diffuse fibrosis and conversion of normal liver architecture into structurally abnormal nodules. Although cirrhosis is usually associated with alcoholism, it can develop in the course of other disorders, including viral hepatitis, toxic reactions to drugs and chemicals, biliary obstruction, and cardiac disease. Cirrhosis also accompanies metabolic disorders that cause the deposition of minerals in the liver; two of these disorders are hemochromatosis (iron deposition) and Wilson's disease (copper deposition).

At present the classification of cirrhosis is controversial. Some authorities use a morphologic system, classifying the disease as either micronodular or macronodular based on the size of the nodules. Other authorities use the cause of the disorder as a means of classification. This discussion focuses on three of the most common types of cirrhosis: postnecrotic cirrhosis, biliary cirrhosis, and cirrhosis caused by alcohol abuse. Although each of these types has a different etiology, the clinical findings, including portal vein hypertension and eventual liver failure, are much the same.

POSTNECROTIC CIRRHOSIS

Postnecrotic cirrhosis is characterized by the replacement of liver tissue with small to large nodules of fibrous tissue, with a resultant markedly deformed and nodular liver. Postnecrotic cirrhosis accounts for 10% to 30% of cases of cirrhosis. It may follow viral hepatitis (type B or type C) or an autoimmune disease, or it may be a toxic response to drugs and other chemicals. It is a predisposing factor in hepatic cancer when it is caused by hepatitis type B.

BILIARY CIRRHOSIS

Biliary cirrhosis develops as a primary or secondary disorder that starts in the bile ducts with obstruction of bile flow (cholestasis). There is initial localized injury to biliary structures with gradual scarring and formation of bands of fibrous tissue that extend to adjacent lobular structures. Primary biliary cirrhosis accounts for 5% to 10% of cases of cirrhosis.[7]

Primary biliary cirrhosis involves inflammation and scarring of the septal and interlobular bile ducts. The disease is seen most commonly in women 30 to 55 years of age. Abnormalities of both cell-mediated and humoral immunity suggest an autoimmune causation. There is an association between biliary cirrhosis and other autoimmune diseases such as scleroderma, Hashimoto's thyroiditis, and Sjögren's syndrome. The disorder is characterized by an insidious onset and progressive scarring and destruction of liver tissue. The liver becomes enlarged and takes on a green hue due to the accumulated bile. The earliest symptoms are pruritus, followed by dark urine and pale stools. Once symptoms become clinically evident, life expectancy is about 5 years. Treatment is largely symptomatic. Some success has been reported with liver transplantation (discussed later).

Secondary biliary cirrhosis develops as the result of prolonged obstruction to bile flow. It is most commonly due to gallstones, stricture of the bile duct, or neoplasms that obstruct bile flow. Complete obstruction to outflow produces back-pressure throughout the biliary system, and the interlobular bile ducts are damaged as the bile becomes thick and impacted. Subtotal obstruction often leads to cholangitis and ascending infection of the biliary system. Treatment methods focus on correcting the cause of the obstruction.

ALCOHOLIC LIVER DISEASE AND CIRRHOSIS

The spectrum of alcoholic liver disease includes fatty liver disease, alcoholic hepatitis, and cirrhosis. Alcoholic cirrhosis is the eighth leading cause of death among adult Americans and the third leading cause among men 29 to 59 years of age. It is estimated that there are 10 million alcoholics in the United States. Interestingly, not all alcoholics develop cirrhosis, suggesting that other conditions such as genetic and environmental factors contribute to its occurrence. The prevalence of cirrhosis is only about 15% among heavy consumers of alcohol and known alcoholics. The lifetime incidence of cirrhosis approaches only 50% among persons who have consumed excess alcohol for over 20 years.[16] Most deaths from alcoholic cirrhosis are attributable to liver failure, bleeding esophageal varices, or kidney failure.

The metabolism of alcohol leads to chemical attack on certain membranes of the liver, but whether the damage is done by the first metabolite of alcohol oxidation, acetaldehyde, or other metabolites is unknown. Acetaldehyde impedes the mitochondrial electron transport system, which is responsible for oxidative metabolism and generation of ATP; as a result, the hydrogen ions that are generated in the mitochondria are shunted into lipid synthesis and ketogenesis. Abnormal accumulations of these substances are notable in hepatocytes (fatty liver) and blood. Binding of acetaldehyde to other molecules impairs the detoxification of free radicals and synthesis of proteins. Acetaldehyde also promotes collagen synthesis and fibrogenesis. The lesions of hepatocellular injury tend to be most prevalent in the centrilobular area, the part immediately surrounding the central vein.[3] This is the part of the lobule that has the lowest oxygen tension; it is thought that the lack of oxygen in this area of the liver may contribute to the damage. Also, the activity of the pathways for alcohol metabolism is greatest in this area.

Even after alcohol intake has stopped and all alcohol has been metabolized, processes that damage liver cells continue for many weeks and months.[16] In fact, clinical and chemical effects often become worse before the disease resolves. Usually, the accumulation of fat disappears within a few weeks, and cholestasis and inflammation also subside. However, fibrosis and scarring remain. The liver lobules become distorted as new liver cells regenerate and form nodules. With repeated bouts of drinking and hepatitis, liver injury may progress to cirrhosis. The gross appearance of the early cirrhotic liver is one of fine, uniform nodules on its surface. The condition has traditionally been called *micronodular* or *Laennec* cirrhosis. With more advanced cirrhosis, regenerative processes cause the nodules to become larger and more irregular in size and shape. As this happens, the nodules cause the liver to become relobulized through the formation of new portal tracts and venous outflow channels. The nodules may compress the hepatic veins, curtailing blood flow out of the liver and producing portal hypertension, extrahepatic portosystemic shunts, and cholestasis.

Stages of Development. Although the mechanism by which alcohol exerts its toxic effects on liver structures is somewhat unclear, the changes that develop can be divided into three stages: (1) fatty changes, (2) alcoholic hepatitis, and (3) cirrhosis. Because these three patterns of hepatocellular injury may occur independently of one another and occur in other types of end-stage liver disease, they are discussed separately.

Fatty Liver. One of the main effects of alcohol is the accumulation of fat within the liver, causing liver enlargement. When alcohol is present, it becomes the preferred fuel for the liver, displacing substrates such as fatty acids and impairing mitochondrial oxi-

dization of fats. Triglycerides accumulate in the liver, probably as a result of increased production and because of increased trapping of fatty acids within the liver cells.

During the fatty changes stage, the liver enlarges because of excessive accumulation of fat within the liver cells. There is evidence that high ingestion of alcohol can cause fatty liver changes even in the presence of an adequate diet. For example, young nonalcoholic volunteers had fatty liver changes after 2 days of consuming 18 oz to 24 oz of alcohol, even though adequate carbohydrates, fats, and proteins were included in the diet. The fatty changes that occur with ingestion of alcohol do not usually produce symptoms and are reversible once the alcohol intake has been discontinued.

Alcoholic Hepatitis. Alcoholic hepatitis is the intermediate stage between fatty changes and cirrhosis. It is characterized by inflammation and necrosis of liver cells and thus is always serious and sometimes fatal. The necrotic lesions are generally patchy but may involve an entire lobe. Although reversible, it is the most common cause of cirrhosis. It is often seen after an abrupt increase in alcohol intake and is common in "spree" drinkers. "Ballooning" of hepatocytes and the toxic effects of the intermediates of alcohol metabolism, such as acetaldehyde, are believed to be contributory factors. This stage is usually characterized by hepatic tenderness, pain, anorexia, nausea, fever, jaundice, ascites, and liver failure, but some patients may be asymptomatic.

The long-term prognosis depends on whether alcohol consumption ceases. Acute alcoholic hepatitis superimposed on cirrhosis is dangerous, accounting for much of the mortality.[16]

Cirrhosis. Cirrhosis designates the onset of end-stage alcoholic liver disease. The liver becomes yellow-orange, fatty, and diffusely scarred. Its normal structure is distorted by bands of fibrous tissue, which separate areas of regenerated cells. As the disease progresses, the liver shrinks. As normal tissue is replaced by scar tissue, blood flow through the liver is obstructed and extrahepatic shunts form, which serve as alternative routes for the return of portal blood to the heart.

The most common signs and symptoms of cirrhosis are weight loss (sometimes masked by ascites), weakness, and anorexia. Hepatomegaly and jaundice are also common signs of cirrhosis. Splenomegaly, ascites, and portosystemic shunts (esophageal varices, anorectal varices, and caput medusae) occur secondary to portal hypertension. Other complications include bleeding (due to abnormal clotting factors and thrombocytopenia due to splenomegaly), gynecomastia and feminizing pattern of pubic hair distribution in males due to testicular atrophy, spider angiomas, palmar erythema, and encephalopathy (with asterixis and neurologic signs).

CLINICAL MANIFESTATIONS

The manifestations of cirrhosis are variable, ranging from asymptomatic hepatomegaly to hepatic failure. Often there are no symptoms until the disease is far advanced; when symptoms do appear, they are vague at first, with complaints of fatigability and weight loss. At this point, the liver is often palpable and hard. Diarrhea is frequently present, although some persons may complain of constipation. There may be abdominal pain because of liver enlargement or stretching of Glisson's capsule. This pain is located in the epigastric area or in the upper right quadrant and is described as dull, aching, and causing a sensation of fullness. The late manifestations of cirrhosis are related to portal hypertension and liver cell failure. Portal hypertension causes complications such as esophageal varices and ascites; in hepatocellular

failure, there is decreased production of bile, plasma proteins, and blood-clotting factors and interference with removal of bilirubin, ammonia, and other substances. The manifestations of cirrhosis are discussed in the section that follows and are summarized in Table 42-2.

PORTAL HYPERTENSION

Venous blood, returning to the heart from the abdominal organs, collects in the portal vein and travels through the liver before entering the vena cava. Portal hypertension is characterized by increased resistance to flow and increased pressure in the portal venous system. It can be caused by a variety of conditions that affect hepatic blood flow, including (1) prehepatic conditions such as portal vein thrombosis or external compression due to cancers or enlarged lymph nodes that cause obstruction the portal vein before it enters the liver; (2) intrahepatic conditions that obstruct the flow of blood within the liver; and (3) posthepatic conditions such as severe right-sided

TABLE 42-2. MANIFESTATIONS OF PORTAL CIRRHOSIS

PRIMARY ALTERATION IN FUNCTION	MANIFESTATION
Portal Hypertension	
Development of collateral vessels	Esophageal varices
	Hemorrhoids
	Caput medusae (dilated cutaneous veins around the umbilicus)
Portal vein obstruction and decreased levels of serum albumin	Ascites
	Peripheral edema
Splenomegaly	Anemia
	Leukopenia
	Thrombocytopenia
Hepatorenal syndrome	Elevated serum creatinine
	Azotemia
	Oliguria
Portal–systemic shunting of blood	Hepatic–systemic encephalopathy
Hepatocellular Dysfunction	
Impaired metabolism of sex hormones	Female: menstrual disorders
	Male: testicular atrophy, gynecomastia, decrease in secondary sex characteristics
	Skin disorders: vascular spiders and palmar erythema
Impaired synthesis of plasma proteins	Decreased levels of serum albumin with development of edema and ascites
	Decreased synthesis of carrier proteins for hormones and drugs
Decreased synthesis of blood-clotting factors	Bleeding tendencies
Failure to remove and conjugate bilirubin from the blood	Jaundice
Impaired bile synthesis	Malabsorption of fats and fat-soluble vitamins
Impaired metabolism of drugs cleared by the liver	Risk of drug reactions and toxicities
Impaired gluconeogenesis	Abnormal glucose tolerance
Decreased ability to convert ammonia to urea	Elevated blood ammonia levels, encephalopathy

heart failure that obstruct the outflow of venous blood from the liver. The dominant intrahepatic causes of portal hypertension are the various types of cirrhosis; they account for 90% of cases of portal hypertension. The normal liver offers little resistance to portal venous flow. In cirrhosis, bands of fibrous tissue and fibrous nodules distort the architecture of the liver and increase the resistance to portal blood flow, which leads to portal hypertension. The pathologic consequences of portal hypertension include (1) ascites, (2) the formation of bypass channels from the portal to systemic circulations, and (3) splenomegaly.

ASCITES

Ascites is an accumulation of fluid within the peritoneal cavity. This fluid is a transudate of plasma, constantly being exchanged with fluid from the vascular compartment, and composed of electrolytes and albumin similar in composition to plasma. In cirrhosis, the two major factors contributing to ascites are (1) impaired synthesis of albumin by the liver, so that the plasma colloidal osmotic pressure falls, and (2) obstruction of venous flow through the liver. This obstruction causes increased accumulation of lymph, with oozing of serous fluid from the liver surface. The decreased colloidal osmotic pressure causes fluid to leak out of the capillaries in the splanchnic (visceral) circulation. Additionally, there is a rise in aldosterone, which augments retention of sodium and water by the kidneys. Among the causes postulated to be responsible for the increased aldosterone levels are impairment of aldosterone inactivation by the liver and production by the liver of a humoral substance that stimulates aldosterone secretion. The increased aldosterone levels also result in increased elimination of potassium by the kidneys and decreased serum potassium levels. Because of the fall in serum albumin and the retention of sodium and water, peripheral edema develops, particularly in the dependent parts of the body such as the feet.

Treatment of ascites usually focuses on dietary restriction of sodium and administration of diuretics. Water intake may also need to be restricted. To counteract the rise in aldosterone, an aldosterone-blocking diuretic, along with another diuretic such as furosamide, is administered. Oral potassium supplements are often given to prevent hypokalemia. Paracentesis may be done for diagnostic purposes but is seldom done to treat the ascites, because its effects are only temporary and it may cause a shift in fluid from the vascular compartment to the peritoneal cavity, along with complications such as infection and hemorrhage.

A surgical procedure called a peritoneovenous shunt may be used for severe cases. In this procedure the peritoneal fluid is shunted from the abdominal cavity through a one-way pressure-sensitive valve into a silicone tube that is inserted into the superior jugular vein and advanced so that the fluid empties into the superior vena cava. Although effective, these shunts carry a considerable complication risk from conditions such as disseminated intravascular coagulation, bacterial infections, and congestive heart failure.

PORTOSYSTEMIC SHUNTS

With the gradual obstruction of venous blood flow in the liver, the pressure in the portal vein increases and large collateral channels develop between the portal and systemic veins that supply the lower rectum and esophagus and in the umbilical veins of the falciform ligament that attaches to the anterior wall of the abdomen. The presence of collaterals between the inferior and internal iliac veins may give rise to hemorrhoids. In some persons, the fetal umbilical vein is not totally obliterated; it forms a channel on the anterior abdominal wall (Fig. 42-10). Dilated veins around the umbilicus are called *caput medusae*. Portopulmonary shunts may also develop, causing blood to bypass the pulmonary capillaries, thereby interfering with blood oxygenation and producing cyanosis.

Clinically, the most important collateral channels are those connecting the portal and coronary veins that lead to reversal of flow and formation of thin-walled varicosities in the submucosa of the gastric fundus and esophagus (Fig. 42-11). Being thin-walled, these varicosities are subject to rupture, with massive and sometimes fatal hemorrhage. Impaired hepatic synthesis of coagulation factors and decreased platelets (thrombocytopenia) due to splenomegaly may further complicate the control of esophageal bleeding.

Several methods are used in the control of variceal bleeding including administration of vasopressin, balloon tamponade, percutaneous transhepatic obliteration, endoscopic injection sclerotherapy, and portosystemic shunt surgery. *Vasopressin*, a hormone from the posterior pituitary, produces constriction of the splanchnic arterioles and a reduction in blood flow and pressure when given intravenously. Vasopressin can also cause coronary vasoconstriction; therefore, nitroglycerin may be given along with vasopressin. *Balloon tamponade* provides compression of the varices and is accomplished through the insertion of a tube with inflatable gastric and esophageal balloons. Once the tube has been inserted, the balloons are inflated (the esophageal balloon compresses the bleeding esophageal veins, and the gastric balloon helps to maintain the position of the tube). *Percutaneous transhepatic obliteration* entails the passage of a

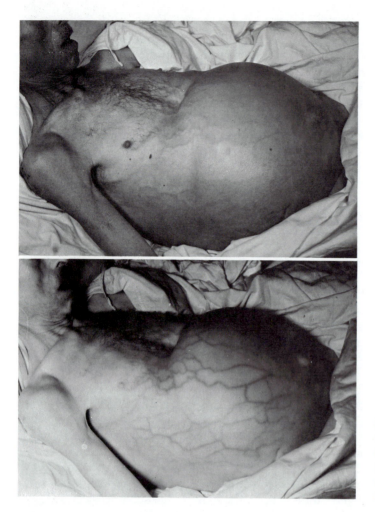

FIG. 42-10. Collateral abdominal veins on the anterior abdominal wall in a patient with alcoholic liver disease as recorded by black and white photography (**top**) and infrared photography (**bottom**). (Schiff, L. [1982]. *Diseases of the liver* [5th ed., p. 408]. Philadelphia: J.B. Lippincott)

catheter into the portal vein under fluoroscopic visualization. The catheter is threaded into the main portal vein and then selectively advanced into the individual collaterals supplying the varices, and a sclerosing solution is injected to obliterate the vessel. The procedure is repeated until all visible collaterals have been obliterated. During *endoscopic sclerotherapy*, the varices are injected with a sclerosing solution that causes obliteration of the vessel lumen.

Surgical treatment of portal hypertension consists of creating a portal–systemic shunt (an opening between the portal and a systemic vein). Although this procedure does not improve liver function, it does reduce the pressure within the esophageal veins and thus prevents esophageal hemorrhage. The two procedures that are done most frequently are portacaval shunt and splenorenal shunt. In a *portacaval* shunt, an opening is created between the portal vein and the vena cava. A *splenorenal* shunt involves removal of the spleen and anastomosis of the splenic vein to the left renal vein. It is often done when the spleen is enlarged, and it prevents further thrombocytopenia and leukopenia. One untoward sequela that develops in about 10% of persons with a

portal–systemic shunt is hepatic–systemic encephalopathy. As will be discussed, the neurologic manifestations of this disorder are believed to result from absorption of ammonia and other neurotoxic substances from the gut directly into the systemic circulation without going through the liver.

SPLENOMEGALY

The splenomegaly observed in portal hypertension results from the shunting of blood into the splenic vein, which gives rise to such hematologic disorders as anemia, thrombocytopenia, and leukopenia.

LIVER FAILURE

Although the liver is among the organs most frequently damaged, only about 10% of hepatic tissue is required for the liver to remain functional. The manifestations of liver failure reflect the various functions of the liver, including hematologic disorders, endocrine disorders, skin disorders, hepatorenal syndrome, and hepatic–systemic encephalopathy. *Fetor*

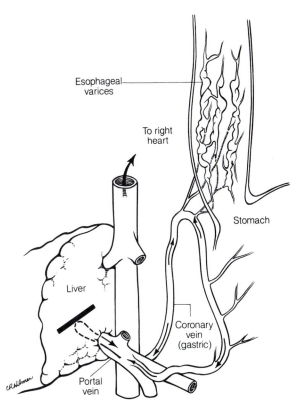

Esophageal
varices

To right
heart

Stomach

Liver

Coronary
vein
(gastric)

Portal
vein

FIG. 42-11. *Obstruction of blood flow in the portal circulation, with portal hypertension and diversion of blood flow to other venous channels, including the gastric and esophageal veins.*

hepaticus refers to a characteristic musty, sweetish odor of the breath in the patient in advanced liver failure, resulting from the products of metabolism of the intestinal bacteria.

HEMATOLOGIC DISORDERS

Anemia, thrombocytopenia, coagulation defects, and leukopenia may arise in the presence of cirrhosis. Anemia may be due to blood loss, excessive red blood cell destruction, and impaired formation of red blood cells. A folic acid deficiency may lead to severe megaloblastic anemia. Changes in the lipid composition of the red cell membrane increase hemolysis. Because factors V, VII, IX, X, prothrombin, and fibrinogen are synthesized by the liver, their decline in liver disease contributes to bleeding disorders. Malabsorption of the fat-soluble vitamin K contributes further to the impaired synthesis of these clotting factors. Often a thrombocytopenia occurs as the result of splenomegaly. Thus, the person with liver failure is subject to purpura, easy bruising, hematuria, and abnormal menstrual bleeding (women) and is vulnerable to bleeding from the esophagus and other segments of the gastrointestinal tract.

ENDOCRINE DISORDERS

The liver metabolizes the sex hormones. Endocrine disorders, particularly disturbances in gonadal function, are common accompaniments of cirrhosis and liver failure. In women there may be menstrual irregularities (usually amenorrhea), loss of libido, and sterility. In men the testosterone level usually falls, the testes atrophy, and loss of libido, impotence, and gynecomastia occur.

SKIN DISORDERS

Liver failure brings on numerous skin disorders. These lesions, called variously *vascular spiders, telangiectasia, spider angiomas,* and *spider nevi,* most often are seen in the upper half of the body. They consist of a central pulsating arteriole from which smaller vessels radiate. (It should be kept in mind that spider angiomas may be seen in pregnancy even when liver function is normal.) *Palmar erythema* is redness of the palms, probably because of an increased blood flow resulting from higher cardiac output. Clubbing of the fingers may be seen in persons with cirrhosis. Jaundice is usually a late manifestation of liver failure.

HEPATORENAL SYNDROME

The hepatorenal syndrome refers to a functional state of renal failure sometimes seen during the terminal stages of liver failure and ascites. It is characterized by progressive azotemia, increased serum creatinine levels, and oliguria. Although the basic cause is not known, a decrease in renal blood flow is believed to play a part. Ultimately, when renal failure is superimposed on liver failure, azotemia and elevated levels of blood ammonia occur; this is thought to contribute to hepatic encephalopathy and coma.

HEPATIC–SYSTEMIC ENCEPHALOPATHY

Hepatic–systemic encephalopathy refers to the totality of central nervous system manifestations of liver failure. It is characterized by neural disturbances ranging from a lack of mental alertness to confusion, coma, and convulsions. A very early sign of hepatic encephalopathy is a flapping tremor called *asterixis*. Loss of memory of varying degrees may occur, coupled with personality changes such as euphoria, irritability, anxiety, and lack of concern about personal appearance and self. There may also be impairment of speech and inability to perform certain purposeful movements. The encephalopathy may progress to decerebrate rigidity and, finally, to a terminal deep coma.

The cause of hepatic encephalopathy is not yet known. The presence of neurotoxins, which appear in the blood because the liver has lost its detoxifying capacity, is believed to be a related factor. As has been stated, hepatic encephalopathy develops in about 10% of persons having a portal–systemic shunt.

One of the suspected neurotoxins is ammonia. One function of the liver is to convert ammonia, a by-product of protein metabolism, to urea. Also, bacterial flora in the intestine convert proteins to ammonia. The ammonia diffuses back into the portal blood and is transported to the liver, where it is converted to urea before entering the general circulation. In situations in which the blood from the intestine bypasses the liver or in which the liver is unable to convert ammonia to urea, ammonia moves directly into the general circulation and from there to the cerebral circulation. Hence, hepatic encephalopathy may become worse following a large protein meal or gastrointestinal tract bleeding. When hypokalemic alkalosis is present, it causes increased renal production of ammonia. Narcotics and tranquilizers are poorly metabolized by the liver, and administration of these drugs may cause central nervous system depression and precipitate hepatic encephalopathy.

A nonabsorbable antibiotic, such as neomycin, may be given to eradicate bacteria from the bowel and thus prevent this cause of ammonia production. Another drug that may be given is lactulose. It is not absorbed from the small intestine but moves directly to the large intestine, where it is catabolized by colonic bacteria to small organic acids that cause production of large, loose stools with a low *p*H. The low *p*H favors the conversion of ammonia to ammonium ions, which are not absorbed by the blood. The acid *p*H also inhibits the degradation of amino acids, proteins, and blood.

TREATMENT

The treatment of liver failure is directed toward elimination of alcohol intake (when due to alcoholic cirrhosis); providing sufficient carbohydrate and calories to prevent protein breakdown; correcting fluid and electrolyte imbalances, particularly hypokalemia; and decreasing ammonia production in the gastrointestinal tract by limiting protein intake.

Liver Transplantation. Liver transplantation is rapidly becoming a realistic form of treatment for persons with end-stage liver disease.[17] The introduction of cyclosporine in 1980 has markedly improved the survival rate of persons with liver transplants. Careful selection of potential recipients and improved preoperative management have further contributed to the improved transplant results. In 1983,

the National Institutes of Health consensus conference concluded that liver transplantation had become a therapeutic modality, prompting many states and private insurance companies to pay for the procedure. The liver can be transplanted as an extra (auxiliary) organ at an ectopic site or in the orthoptic location after removal of the host liver.

Criteria for liver transplantation include the presence of a chronic liver disease for which all forms of therapy have failed. Conditions for which liver transplantation has been done are metabolic diseases of the liver such as Wilson's disease, primary biliary cirrhosis, chronic active hepatitis, sclerosing cholangitis, and biliary atresia in children. The use of liver transplantation for persons with alcoholic liver disease remains controversial, largely because of the scarcity of donor organs.[18, 19] The agents used to prevent liver transplant rejection—cyclosporine, corticosteroid drugs, and azathioprine—are the same ones used to maintain other whole-organ grafts such as heart and kidney transplants.

CANCER OF THE LIVER

Cancers of the liver include both metastatic and primary neoplasms. Metastatic implants from primary cancers arising in areas drained by the portal vein are the most common form of neoplastic involvement of the liver. Although the metastatic lesions may produce gross distortion of liver structure, functional insufficiency is rare because sufficient intervening tissue is spared.

Primary liver tumors are relatively rare in the United States, accounting for about 2% of all cancers. The average age of onset is 60 to 70 years. There are three primary types of liver cancer: (1) hepatocellular carcinoma, which arises from the liver cells; (2) cholangiocarcinoma, which is a primary cancer of bile duct cells; and (3) a mixed hepatocholangiocarcinoma.[7] Cirrhosis of the liver is present in 60% to 80% of persons with hepatocellular carcinoma. By contrast, cholangiocarcinoma has no association with cirrhosis. Three factors are thought to contribute to hepatocellular carcinoma: (1) chronic hepatitis B virus infection, (2) cirrhosis of the liver, and (3) possible hepatocarcinogens in food. Aflatoxin from moldy peanuts has been implicated.

The initial symptoms are weakness, anorexia, weight loss, fatigue, bloating, a sensation of abdominal fullness, and a dull, aching abdominal pain. Ascites, which often obscures weight loss, is common. Jaundice, if it is present, is usually mild. There may be a rapid increase in liver size and worsening of ascites in persons with preexisting cirrhosis. Usually, the liver is enlarged at the time these symptoms appear, and there is a low fever without apparent cause. Serum alpha-fetoprotein, a serum protein present in fetal life, normally is barely detectable in the serum after the age of 2 years, but it is present in some 50% to 90% of cases of hepatocarcinoma.[7]

Primary cancers of the liver are usually far advanced at the time of diagnosis; the 5-year survival rate is about 1%, and most patients die within 6 months. The treatment of choice is subtotal hepatectomy, if conditions permit.

GALLBLADDER DISEASE

The gallbladder is a distensible, pear-shaped, muscular sac located on the ventral surface of the liver. It has a smooth muscle wall and is lined with a thin layer of absorptive cells. The cystic duct joins the gallbladder to the common duct. The function of the gallbladder is to store and concentrate bile. When full, it can hold 20 mL to 50 mL of bile.

Entrance of food into the intestine causes contraction of the gallbladder and relaxation of the sphincter of Oddi. The stimulus for gallbladder contraction is primarily hormonal. Products of food digestion, particularly lipids, stimulate cholecystokinin release from the mucosa of the duodenum. Cholecystokinin, a gastrointestinal hormone, provides a strong stimulus for gallbladder contraction. The role of other gastrointestinal hormones in bile release is less clearly understood. Passage of bile into the intestine is regulated largely by the pressure within the common duct. Normally, the gallbladder serves to regulate this pressure: it collects and stores bile as it relaxes and the pressure in the common bile duct decreases, and it empties bile into the intestine as it contracts and causes an increase in common duct pressure. Following gallbladder surgery, the pressure in the common duct changes, causing the common duct to dilate. The flow of bile is then regulated by the sphincters in the common duct.

Two very common disorders of the biliary system are *cholelithiasis* (gallstones) and *cholecystitis* (inflammation of the gallbladder). At least 10% of adults have gallstones. About twice as many women as men have gallstones, and there is increased prevalence with age—after age 60, 10% to 15% in men and 20% to 40% in women.[20]

COMPOSITION OF BILE AND FORMATION OF GALLSTONES

Gallstones are due to the precipitation of substances contained in bile, mainly cholesterol and bilirubin. Bile contains bile salts, cholesterol, bilirubin, lecithin, fatty acids, and water as well as electrolytes normally found in the plasma. The cholesterol found in bile has no known function; it is assumed to be a by-product of bile salt formation, and its presence is linked to the excretory function of bile. Normally insoluble in water, cholesterol is rendered soluble by the action of bile salts, which combine with it to form micelles. In the gallbladder, water and electrolytes are absorbed from the liver bile, causing the bile to become more concentrated. Because neither lecithin nor bile salts are absorbed in the gallbladder, their concentration increases along with that of cholesterol; in this way the solubility of cholesterol is maintained.

The bile of which gallstones are formed is usually supersaturated with either cholesterol or bilirubinate. The majority of gallstones, about 75%, are composed primarily of cholesterol; the other 25% are pigment or calcium bilirubinate stones. Many stones have a mixed composition. Three factors contribute to the formation of gallstones: (1) abnormalities in the composition of bile, (2) stasis of bile, and (3) inflammation of the gallbladder. The formation of cholesterol stones is associated with obesity and is seen more frequently in women, especially women who have had multiple pregnancies or who are taking oral contraceptives. All of these factors cause the liver to excrete more cholesterol into the bile. Estrogen treatment also reduces the synthesis of bile acid in women. Drugs that lower serum cholesterol levels, such as clofibrate, also cause increased cholesterol excretion into the bile. Malabsorption disorders stemming from ileal disease or intestinal bypass surgery, for example, tend to interfere with the absorption of bile salts, which is needed to maintain the solubility of cholesterol. Inflammation of the gallbladder alters the absorptive characteristics of the mucosal layer, allowing for excessive absorption of water and bile salts. Cholesterol gallstones are extremely common among Native Americans, which suggests that a genetic component may have a role in gallstone formation. Pigment stones containing bilirubin are seen in persons with hemolytic disease (*e.g.*, sickle cell disease) and hepatic cirrhosis.

Many persons with gallstones have no symptoms. Gallstones cause symptoms when they obstruct bile flow. Small stones not more than 8 mm in diameter pass into the common duct, producing symptoms of indigestion and biliary colic. Larger stones are more likely to obstruct flow and cause jaundice. The pain of biliary colic is generally abrupt in onset, increasing steadily in intensity until it reaches a climax in 30 to 60 minutes. The upper right quadrant, or epigastric area, is the usual location of the pain, often with referred pain to the back, above the waist, the right shoulder, and the right scapula or the midscapular region. A few persons will experience pain on the left side. The pain usually persists for 2 to 8 hours and is followed by soreness in the upper right quadrant.

CHOLECYSTITIS AND CHOLELITHIASIS

The term cholecystitis refers to inflammation of the gallbladder. It may be either acute or chronic; both types are associated with cholelithiasis. Acute cholecystitis may be superimposed on chronic cholecystitis.

Acute cholecystitis is almost always associated with complete or partial obstruction of bile flow. It is believed that the inflammation is caused by chemical irritation from the concentrated bile, along with mucosal swelling and ischemia resulting from venous congestion and lymphatic stasis. The gallbladder is usually markedly distended. Bacterial infections may arise secondary to the ischemia and chemical irritation. The bacteria reach the injured gallbladder through the blood, lymphatics, or bile ducts or from adjacent organs. Among the common pathogens are staphylococci and enterococci. The wall of the gallbladder is most vulnerable to the effects of ischemia, as a result of which mucosal necrosis and sloughing occur. The process may lead to gangrenous changes and perforation of the gallbladder.

Manifestations. The signs and symptoms of acute cholecystitis vary with the severity of obstruction and inflammation. Pain, initially similar to that of biliary colic, is characteristic of acute cholecystitis. It is often precipitated by a fatty meal and may initiate with complaints of indigestion. It does not, however, subside spontaneously and responds poorly or only temporarily to potent analgesics. When the inflammation progresses to involve the peritoneum, the pain becomes more pronounced in the right upper quadrant. The right subcostal region is tender, and there is spasm of the muscles that surround the area. Vomiting occurs in about 75% of patients and jaundice in some 25%. Fever and an abnormally high white blood cell count attest to the presence of inflammation. Total serum bilirubin, serum transaminase, and alkaline phosphatase levels usually are elevated.

The manifestations of chronic cholecystitis are more vague than those of acute cholecystitis. There may be intolerance to fatty foods, belching, and other indications of discomfort. Often there are episodes of colicky pain with obstruction of biliary flow caused by gallstones. The gallbladder, which in chronic cholecystitis usually contains stones, may be enlarged, shrunken, or of normal size. The passage of a stone into the common duct causes obstruction of bile flow and may contribute to carcinoma of the gallbladder.

Diagnosis and Treatment. The current methods used in diagnosis of gallbladder disease include oral cholecystography, ultrasonography, and cholescintigraphy.[21, 22] Oral cholecystography is a radiologic technique that uses oral tablets containing a radiopaque contrast medium, which is absorbed from the gut, excreted in the bile, and becomes concentrated in the gallbladder. The patient must follow a fat-free diet for 1 to 2 days before the test. The dye must be taken 10 to 14 hours before the examination; it may produce nausea and vomiting in 5% to 10% of persons and diarrhea in up to 25%. Ultrasound is a widely used diagnostic method in gallbladder disease and has largely replaced the oral cholecystogram in many medical centers. Its overall accuracy in detecting gallbladder disease is high. In addition to stones, ultrasound can detect other findings such as wall thickening, which indicates inflammation. Cholescintigraphy, also called a *gallbladder scan*, relies on the ability of the liver to extract a rapidly injected radionuclide, technetium-99m bound to one of several iminodiacetic acids, that is excreted into the bile ducts. Serial scanning images are obtained within several minutes of the injection of the tracer and every 10 to 15 minutes during the next hour. The gallbladder scan is highly accurate in detecting acute cholecystitis. Other methods, such as computed tomographic scanning and magnetic resonance imaging, are being evaluated for their possible roles in diagnosing gallbladder disease.

Gallbladder disease is usually treated by removing the gallbladder or by dissolving or fragmenting the stones. The usual treatment of choice for symptomatic cholelithiasis and cholecystitis is surgical removal of the gallbladder (cholecystectomy). Unless complications demand immediate action, surgery is delayed if the inflammation is acute. This allows time for the inflammatory process to subside. The gallbladder serves to store and concentrate bile; as discussed earlier, its removal does not usually interfere with digestion.

Laparoscopic cholecystectomy is rapidly replacing open surgical procedures in which the gallbladder is removed through an open incision in the upper abdomen. The procedure involves insertion of a lapraoscope through a small incision near the umbilicus, and surgical instruments are inserted through several stab wounds in the upper abdomen. Although the procedure requires more time than the open procedure, it usually requires only one night in the hospital. A major advantage of the procedure is that patients can return to work in 1 to 2 weeks as compared with 4 to 6 weeks after open cholecystectomy.[20]

The bile acids—chenodeoxycholic acid and ursodeoxycholic acid—have proved capable of dissolving gallstones and may be used to treat asymptomatic cholelithiasis.[23] They act by desaturating cholesterol in solution in the bile. For the treatment to be effective, the stones must be predominantly cholesterol and not calcified. The treatment dissolves most stones within 1 or 2 years. Chenodeoxycholic acid is associated with elevation of low-density lipoproteins (LDL) and dose-related diarrhea and elevated liver enzymes (SGOT and SGPT). The drug is not recommended for women of childbearing years since they may adversely affect the fetal liver. Ursodeoxycholic acid appears to have less effect on liver enzymes and produces less diarrhea.

Extracorporeal shock wave lithotripsy uses sound waves to pulverize gallstones so that they can be passed through the bile duct.[24] The procedure is only suitable for radiolucent stones because the shock waves must be focused on each stone. Although not a common complication, stone fragments can become trapped in the bile duct. Adjunctive bile-acid therapy is often used to speed dissolution of stone fragments.[24]

CANCER OF THE GALLBLADDER

Cancer of the gallbladder occurs in approximately 2% of persons operated on for biliary tract disease. The onset of symptoms is usually insidious and resembles cholecystitis; the diagnosis is often made unexpectedly at the time of gallbladder surgery. Because of their ability to produce chronic irritation of the gallbladder mucosa, it is believed that gallstones play a role in the development of gallbladder cancer. The 5-year survival rate is low—only about 3%.

In summary, the liver is subject to most of the disease processes that affect other body structures, such as vascular disorders, inflammation, metabolic diseases, toxic injury, and neoplasms. Two of the most common liver diseases are hepatitis and cirrhosis. Hepatitis is characterized by inflammation of the liver. Acute viral hepatitis is caused by hepatitis viruses A, B, C, D, and E. Hepatitis can present as acute or fulminant. Hepatitis B, C, and D may progress to chronic hepatitis or a carrier state. Cirrhosis is the third leading cause of death in the United States. It is characterized by fibrosis and conversion of the normal hepatic architecture into structurally abnormal nodules. There are three types of cirrhosis—postnecrotic, biliary, and alcoholic—of which the most common is alcoholic cirrhosis. Regardless of cause, the manifestations of end-stage cirrhosis are similar and result from portal hypertension and liver failure. Portal hypertension is characterized by increased resistance to flow and increased pressure in the portal venous system; the pathologic consequences of the disorder include: (1) ascites, (2) the formation of bypass channels (*e.g.*, esophageal varices) from the portal–systemic circulations, and (3) splenomegaly. The manifestations of liver failure reflect the various functions of the liver, including hematologic disorders, endocrine disorders, skin disorders, hepatorenal syndrome, and hepatic–systemic encephalopathy. Cancers of the liver include both metastatic and primary neoplasms. Metastatic neoplasms are the most common form of liver cancer. Primary liver neoplasms are rare, accounting for only 2% of cancers, and those involving the hepatocytes or liver cells are commonly associated with cirrhosis of the liver. With the introduction of the immunosuppressant agent cyclosporine, liver transplantation is becoming a more realistic form of treatment for end-stage liver disease.

The biliary tract serves as a passageway for the delivery of bile from the liver to the intestine. This tract consists of the bile ducts and gallbladder. The most common causes of biliary tract disease are cholelithiasis and cholecystitis. Three factors contribute to the development of cholelithiasis: (1) abnormalities in the composition of bile, (2) stasis of bile, and (3) inflammation of the gallbladder. Cholelithiasis predisposes to obstruction of bile flow, causing biliary colic and acute or chronic cholecystitis. Cancer of the gallbladder, which has a poor 5-year survival rate, occurs in 2% of persons with biliary tract disease.

■ DISORDERS OF THE EXOCRINE PANCREAS

The pancreas lies transversely in the posterior part of the upper abdomen. The head of the pancreas is at the right of the abdomen; it rests against the curve of the duodenum in the area of the ampulla of Vater and its entrance into the duodenum. The body of the pancreas lies beneath the stomach. The tail touches the spleen. The pancreas is virtually hidden because of its posterior position; unlike many other organs, it cannot be palpated. Because of the position of the pancreas and its large functional reserve, symptoms of disease do not usually appear until the disorder is far advanced. This is particularly true of cancer of the pancreas.

The pancreas is both an endocrine and an exocrine organ. Its function as an endocrine organ is discussed in Chapter 46. The exocrine pancreas is made up of lobules that consist of acinar cells, which secrete digestive enzymes into a system of microscopic ducts. These ducts are terminal branches of larger ducts that drain into the main pancreatic duct, which extends from left to right through the substance of the pancreas (see Fig. 42-4). In most persons, the main pancreatic duct empties into the ampulla of Vater, although in some it empties directly into the duodenum. The pancreatic ducts are lined with epithelial cells that secrete water and bicarbonate and thereby modify the fluid and electrolyte composition of the pancreatic secretions. The pancreatic secretions contain proteolytic enzymes that break down dietary proteins, including trypsin, chymotrypsin, carboxypolypeptidase, ribonuclease, and deoxyribonuclease. The pancreas also secretes pancreatic amylase, which breaks down starch, and lipase, which hydrolyzes neutral fats into glycerol and fatty acids. The pancreatic enzymes are secreted in the inactive form and become activated once in the intestine. This is important because the enzymes would digest the tissue of the pancreas itself if they were secreted in the active form. The acinar cells secrete a trypsin inhibitor, which prevents trypsin activation. Because trypsin activates other proteolytic enzymes, the trypsin inhibitor prevents subsequent activation of those other enzymes. Two types of pancreatic disease are discussed here: acute and chronic pancreatitis and cancer of the pancreas.

ACUTE HEMORRHAGIC PANCREATITIS

Acute pancreatitis is a severe, life-threatening disorder associated with the escape of activated pancreatic enzymes into the pancreas and surrounding tissues. These enzymes cause fat necrosis, or autodigestion, of the pancreas and produce fatty deposits in the abdominal cavity with hemorrhage from the necrotic vessels. Although a number of factors are associated with the development of acute pancreatitis, the two most important are biliary tract disease with reflux of bile into the pancreas and alcoholism.[25] Biliary reflux is believed to activate the pancreatic enzymes within the ductile system of the pancreas. The precise mechanisms whereby alcohol exerts its action are largely unknown. Alcohol is known to be a potent stimulator of pancreatic secretions; at the same time, it often causes partial obstruction of the sphincter of Oddi. Acute pancreatitis is also associated with hyperlipidemia, hyperparathyroidism, infections (particularly viral), abdominal and surgical trauma, and drugs such as steroids and thiazide diuretics.

The onset of acute pancreatitis is usually abrupt and dramatic, and it may follow a heavy meal or an alcoholic binge. The most common initial symptom is severe epigastric and abdominal pain that radiates to the back. The pain is aggravated when the person is lying supine; it is less severe when the person is sitting and leaning forward. Abdominal distention accompanied by hypoactive bowel sounds is common. An important disturbance related to acute pancreatitis is the loss of a large volume of fluid into the retroperitoneal and peripancreatic spaces and the abdominal cavity. Tachycardia, hypotension, cool, clammy skin, and fever are often evident. Signs of hypocalcemia may develop, probably as a result of the precipitation of serum calcium in the areas of fat necrosis. Mild jaundice may appear after the first 24 hours because of biliary obstruction.

The serum amylase level becomes elevated within the first 24 hours and remains elevated for 48 to 72 hours. Serum lipase also becomes elevated during the first 24 to 48 hours but remains elevated for 5 to 14 days. Urinary clearance of amylase is increased. Because the serum amylase may be elevated as a result of the presence of other serious illnesses, the urinary amylase may be measured. The white blood cell count may be increased, and hyperglycemia and an elevated serum bilirubin level may be present. About 5% of persons with acute pancreatitis die of the acute effects of peripheral vascular collapse. Serious complications include acute respiratory distress syndrome and acute tubular necrosis. Hypocalcemia occurs in about 25% of patients. Age greater than 55 years and the presence of an elevated white blood cell count (above 16,000/uL), blood glucose (above 200 mg/dL), serum lactate dehydrogenase (above 350 IU/L), and aspartate aminotransferase (above 250 IU/L) at the time of diagnosis are associated with a poorer prognosis, as are a fall in hematocrit and serum calcium, increased fluid sequestration (greater than 6 L), an arterial oxygen tension less than 60 mmHg, and base deficit greater than 4 mEq/L that develop within the first 48 hours.[25]

The treatment consists of measures directed at pain relief, "putting the pancreas to rest," and restoration of lost plasma volume.[25] Meperidine (Demerol) rather than morphine is usually given for pain relief because it causes fewer spasms of the sphincter of Oddi. Papaverine, nitroglycerin, barbiturates, or anticholinergic drugs may be given as supplements to provide smooth muscle relaxation. Oral foods and fluids are withheld, and gastric suction is instituted to treat distention of the bowel and prevent further stimulation of the secretion of pancreatic enzymes. Intravenous fluids and electrolytes are administered to replace those lost from the circulation and to combat hypotension and shock. Intravenous colloid solutions are given to replace the fluid that has become sequestered in the abdomen and retroperitoneal space. Percutaneous peritoneal lavage has been tried as an early treatment of acute pancreatitis with encouraging results. Should a pancreatic abscess develop, it must be drained, usually through the flank.

A *pseudocyst* is a collection of pancreatic fluid in the peritoneal cavity, enclosed in a layer of inflammatory tissue. Autodigestion or liquefaction of pancreatic tissue may be the cause. The pseudocyst is most often connected to a pancreatic duct, so that it continues to increase in mass. The symptoms depend on its location; for example, jaundice may occur when a cyst develops near the head of the pancreas close to the common duct. Pseudocysts may resolve or, if they persist, may require surgical intervention.

CHRONIC PANCREATITIS

Chronic pancreatitis is characterized by progressive destruction of the pancreas. It can be divided into two types: *chronic calcifying pancreatitis* and *chronic obstructive pancreatitis*.[7] In chronic calcifying pancreatitis, calcified protein plugs (calculi) form in the pancreatic ducts. This form is seen most often in alcoholics. Chronic obstructive pancreatitis is associated with stenosis of the sphincter of Oddi. The lesions are prominent in the head of the pancreas. It is usually due to cholelithiasis and is sometimes relieved by removal of the sphincter of Oddi.

Chronic pancreatitis is manifested in episodes that are similar, albeit of lesser severity, to those of acute pancreatitis. There are persistent, recurring episodes of epigastric and upper left quadrant pain; the attacks are often precipitated by alcohol abuse or overeating. Anorexia, nausea, vomiting, constipation, and flatulence are common. Eventually the disease progresses to the extent that both endocrine and exocrine pancreatic functions become deficient. At this point, signs of diabetes mellitus and the malabsorption syndrome (*e.g.*, weight loss and fatty stools [steatorrhea]) become apparent.

Treatment consists of measures to treat coexisting biliary tract disease. A low-fat diet is usually prescribed. The signs of malabsorption may be treated with pancreatic enzymes. When diabetes is present, it is treated with insulin. Alcohol is forbidden because it frequently precipitates attacks. Because of the frequent pain episodes, narcotic addiction is a potential problem in persons with chronic pancreatitis. Surgical intervention is sometimes needed to relieve the pain and usually focuses on relieving any obstruction that may be present. In advanced cases, a subtotal or total pancreatectomy may be necessary.[26]

CANCER OF THE PANCREAS

The incidence of pancreatic cancer has remained fairly stable over the past 25 years. At present it is the fifth leading cause of cancer death in the United States. The risk of pancreatic cancer increases after the age of 50 years, with most cases occurring between ages 65 and 79. Cancer of the pancreas is usually far advanced when diagnosed, and the 5-year survival rate is less than 3%.[27]

The cause of pancreatic cancer is unknown. Smoking appears to be a major risk factor.[28] The incidence of pancreatic cancer is twice as high in smokers than in nonsmokers. The second most important factor appears to be diet. A high intake of fat, meat, or both is linked with the disease. A protective effect has been ascribed to a diet containing fresh fruits and vegetables. Diabetes and chronic pancreatitis also are associated with pancreatic cancer, although neither the nature nor the sequence of the possible cause–effect relation has been established.[28]

Cancer of the pancreas usually has an insidious onset. Pain, jaundice, or both are present in over 90% of patients and, along with weight loss, constitutes the classic presentation of the disease.

Because of the proximity of the pancreas to the common duct and the ampulla of Vater, cancer of the head of the pancreas tends to obstruct bile flow; this causes distention of the gallbladder and jaundice. Jaundice is frequently the presenting symptom in cancer of the head of the pancreas, and it is usually accompanied by complaints of pain and pruritus. Cancer of the body of the pancreas generally impinges on the celiac ganglion, causing pain. The pain usually worsens with ingestion of food or with assumption of the supine position. Cancer of the tail of the pancreas has usually metastasized before symptoms appear.

Ultransonography and computed tomography (CT) scans are the most frequently used diagnostic methods to confirm the disease. A wide variety of tumor markers have been proposed for use in the diagnosis and follow-up of persons with pancreatic cancer. The most extensively studied as been CA 19-9, which is currently available and used in many centers. However, levels are usually normal at the early stages of pancreatic cancer; hence, it cannot be used as a screening method. Also, CA 19-9 is elevated in other types of gastrointestinal cancers, such as those of the bile duct and colon; thus, it is not specific for pancreatic cancer. Carcinoembryonic antigen is also widely used as a marker, but it has low sensitivity and is elevated in many other malignant and benign conditions (see Chapter 5 for a discussion of cancer markers). Percutaneous fine-needle aspiration cytology of the pancreas has been one of the major advances in diagnosis of pancreatic cancer. Unfortunately, the smaller and more curable tumors are most likely missed by this procedure.

Most cancers of the pancreas have metastasized by the time of diagnosis. Surgical resection of the tumor is done when the tumor is localized or as a palliative measure. Radiation therapy may be useful in treatment when the disease is not resectable but still appears to be localized. The use of chemotherapy for pancreatic cancer continues to be investigated.

In summary, the pancreas is both an endocrine and an exocrine organ. Diabetes mellitus is the most common disorder of the endocrine pancreas, and it occurs independently of disease of the exocrine pancreas. The exocrine pancreas produces digestive enzymes that are secreted in an inactive form and transported to the small intestine through the main pancreatic duct, which usually empties into the ampulla of Vater and then into the duodenum through the sphincter of Oddi. The most common diseases of the exocrine pancreas are acute and chronic pancreatitis and cancer. Both acute and chronic pancreatitis are associated with biliary reflux and chronic alcoholism. Acute pancreatitis is a dramatic and life-threatening disorder in which there is autodigestion of pancreatic tissue. Chronic pancreatitis causes progressive destruction of both the endocrine and the exocrine pancreas. It is characterized by episodes of pain and epigastric distress that are similar to but less severe than that which occurs with acute pancreatitis. Cancer of the pancreas has remained relatively stable over the past 25 years. It is usually far advanced at the time of diagnosis, and as a result the 5-year survival rate is less than 3%.

■ REFERENCES

1. Katzung, B.G. (1989). *Basic and clinical pharmacology* (4th ed., pp. 42–46). Norwalk, CT: Appleton Lange.
2. Gilman, A.G., Rall, T.W., Nies, A.S., et al. (1990). *Goodman and Gilman's pharmacological basis of therapeutics* (8th ed., p. 16). New York: Pergamon Press, 1990.
3. Lieber, C.S. (1988). Biochemical and molecular basis of alcohol-induced injury to liver and other tissues. *New England Journal of Medicine, 319,* 1639.
4. Johnston, D.E., & Kaplan, M.M. (1989). Alcholic liver disease. In S. Chopra, & R.J. May (Eds.). *Pathophysiology of gastrointestinal disease* (pp. 360–368). Boston: Little Brown, 1989.
5. Lieber, C.S., & Guadagnini, K.S. (1990). The spectrum of alcoholic liver disease. *Hospital Practice, 25*(2), 51–69.
6. Guyton, A. (1991). *Textbook of medical physiology* (8th ed., p. 722). Philadelphia: W.B. Saunders.
7. Kumar, V., Cotran, R.S., & Robbins, S.L. (1993). *Basic pathology* (5th ed., pp. 530–541). Philadelphia: W.B. Saunders.
8. Podolsky, D.K., & Isselbacher, K.J. (1991). Derangements of hepatic metabolism. In J.D. Wilson, E. Braunwald, & K.J. Isselbacher (Eds.). *Harrison's principles of internal medicine* (12th ed., pp. 1311—1315). Philadelphia: W.B. Saunders.
9. Lemon, S.M. (1985). Type A hepatitis. *New England Journal of Medicine, 313,* 1059.
10. Werzberger, A., Mensch, B., Kuter, B., et al. (1992). A controlled trial of formalin-inactivated hepatitis A vaccine in healthy children. *New England Journal of Medicine, 327,* 453–457.
11. Hepatitis B virus: A comprehensive strategy for eliminating transmission in the United States through universal childhood vaccination. *Morbidity and Mortality Weekly Reports, 40* (RR-13), 1–25.
12. Tang, E. (1991). Hepatitis C: A review. *Western Journal of Medicine, 155,* 164-168.
13. Knauer, M. (1993). Liver, biliary tract, and pancreas. In L.M. Tierney Jr., S.J. McPhee, M.A. Papadakis, et al. (Eds.). *Current medical diagnosis and treatment* (p. 506). Norwalk, CT: Appleton Lange.
14. Hoffnagle, J.H. (1989). Type D (delta) hepatitis. *Journal of the American Medical Association, 261,* 1321–1325.
15. Kaplan, M.M. (1989). Chronic liver diseases: Current therapeutic options. *Hospital Practice, 24*(3A), 111–130.
16. U.S. Department of Health and Human Services. (1988). *Alcoholic hepatitis: A practical guide for physicians and other health care workers.* Washington, DC: DHHS Publication No. (ADM) 88-1547.
17. Starzl, T.E., Demetris, A.J., & Van Thiel, D. (1989). Liver transplantation (Part 1). *New England Journal of Medicine, 321,* 1014–1020.
18. Moss, A.H., & Siegler, M. (1991). Should alcoholics compete equally for liver transplantation? *Journal of the American Medical Association, 265,* 1295–1298.
19. Knechtle, S.J., Flemming, M.F., Barry, K.L., et al. (1992). Liver transplantation in alcholic liver disease. *Surgery, 112,* 694–701.
20. Johnston, D.E., & Kaplan, M.M. (1993). Pathogenesis and treatment of gallstones. *New England Journal of Medicine, 328,* 412–421.
21. Marton, K.I. (1988). How to image the gallbladder in suspected cholecystitis. *Annals of Internal Medicine, 109,* 722.
22. Health and Policy Committee, American College of Physicians. (1988). How to study the gallbladder. *Annals of Internal Medicine, 109,* 752.
23. Schuman, B.M. (1988). New weapons in the war against gallstones. *Emergency Medicine, 20,* 81.
24. Mulley, A.G. (1986). Shock-wave lithotripsy. *New England Journal of Medicine, 314,* 845.
25. Frey, C.F., Gerzof, S.G., & Vennes, J.A. (1992). Progress in acute pancreatitis. *Patient Care, June 15,* 258–290.
26. Knauer, C.M. (1993). Liver, biliary tract, and pancreas. In L.M. Tierney, S.J. McPhee, M.A. Papaakis, et al. (Eds.). *Current medical diagnosis and treatment* (pp. 535–536). Norwalk, CT: Appleton Lange.
27. American Cancer Society. (1992). *Cancer facts.* Atlanta: American Cancer Society.
28. Warshaw, A.I., & Castillo, C.F. (1992). Pancreatic carcinoma. *New England Journal of Medicine, 326,* 455–465.

■ BIBLIOGRAPHY

Aach, R.D. (1992). The emerging clinical significance of hepatitis C. *Hospital Practice, 26*(5), 19-22.

Bancroft, W.H. (1992). Hepatitis A vaccine. *New England Journal of Medicine, 327,* 488–490.

Bisceglie, A.M., Rustgi, V.K., Hoofnagle, J.H., et al. (Moderators) (1988). NIH Conference. Hepatocellular carcinoma. *Annals of Internal Medicine, 108,* 390–401.

Burns, S.M., & Martin, M.J. (1989). VP/NTG therapy in the patient with variceal bleeding. *Critical Care Nurse, 10*(9), 42-49.

Dewar, T.N. (1990). Non-A, non-B hepatitis. *Western Journal of Medicine, 153,* 173–179.

Dimangno, E.P., Rich, T.A., & Steele, G.D. (1992). Pancreatic cancer: What you need to know. *Patient Care, March 30,* 151-70.

Duane, W.C. (1990). Pathogenesis of gallstones: Implications for management. *Hospital Practice, 25*(3A), 65–80.

Epstein, M. (1992). The hepatorenal syndrome—newer perspectives. *New England Journal of Medicine, 327,* 1810–1811.

Fain, J.A., & Amato-Vealey, E. (1988). Acute pancreatitis: A gastrointestinal emergency. *Critical Care Nurse, 8*(5), 47.

Gocke, D.J. (1986). Hepatitis A revisited. *Annals of Internal Medicine, 105*, 960.

Hoofnagle, J.H. (1990). Chronic hepatitis B. *New England Journal of Medicine, 323*, 337–39.

Hsia, P.C., & Seeff, L.B. (1991). Non-A, non-B hepatitis: Impact on the emergence of the hepatitis C virus. *Advances in Internal Medicine, 37*, 197–221.

Pierce, J.D., Wilkerson, E., & Griffiths, S.A. (1989). Acute esophageal bleeding and endoscopic injection sclerotherapy. *Critical Care Nurse, 10*(9), 67–72.

Poovorawan, Y., Sanpavat, S., & Pongpynglert, W. (1992). Long term efficacy of hepatitis B vaccine in infants born to hepatitis B antigen–positive mothers. *Pediatric Infectious Disease Journal, 11*, 816–821.

Regan, L. (1989). Screening for hepatocellular carcinoma in high-risk individuals: A clinical review. *Archives of Internal Medicine, 149*, 1741–1744.

Sampliner, R.E. (1989). The recognition of early liver disease. *Hospital Practice, 24*(3), 53–56.

Sherman, K.E. (1991). Alanine aminotransferase in clinical practice: A review. *Archives of Internal Medicine, 151*, 260–265.

Steinberg, W.M. (1992). Acute pancreatitis. *New England Journal of Medicine, 326*, 635–637.

Terblanche, J., Burroughs, A.K., & Hobbs, K.E.F. (1989). Controversies in the management of esophageal varices (Parts 1 and 2). *New England Journal of Medicine, 320*, 1393–1398, 1469–1474.

Vierling, J.M., & Howell, C.D. (1990). Disappearing bile ducts: Immunologic mechanisms. *Hospital Practice, 25*(7A), 141–150.

Wilson, F.A. (1990). Modern approaches to bile transport proteins. *Hospital Practice, 25*(4A), 95–110.

Zimmiak, P. (1990). The pathogenesis of cholestasis. *Hospital Practice, 25*(8A), 107–125.

ALTERATIONS IN NUTRITIONAL STATUS

JOAN PLEUSS

◼ OBJECTIVES

After you have studied this chapter, you should be able to meet the following objectives:

◼ Define *nutritional status*.
◼ Define *calorie* and state the number of calories derived from the oxidation of 1 g of protein, fat, and carbohydrate.
◼ Describe the location and function of adipocytes in the body.
◼ Explain the difference between anabolism and catabolism.
◼ Relate the processes of glycogenolysis and gluconeogenesis to the regulation of blood glucose by the liver.
◼ Discuss the use of amino acids from body proteins as an energy source.
◼ Cite the effect of age on metabolic rate.
◼ State the purpose of the recommended daily allowance (RDA) of calories, proteins, fats, carbohydrates, vitamins, and minerals.
◼ State information for nutritional assessment that can be obtained from diet history, health assessment, body weight, skinfold and body circumference measurements, densiometry, bioelectrical impedance, computed tomographic scans, and laboratory studies.

◼ Compare relative body weight, the Metropolitan Life Insurance Table, and body mass index as methods for evaluating body weight in terms of undernutrition and overnutrition.
◼ Define and discuss the causes of obesity and health risks associated with obesity.
◼ Differentiate upper and lower body obesity and their implications in terms of health risk.
◼ Discuss the treatment of obesity as it relates to diet, behavior modification, exercise, social support, and surgical methods.
◼ List the major causes of malnutrition and starvation.
◼ State the difference between protein-calorie starvation (marasmus) and protein malnutrition (kwashiorkor).
◼ Explain the effect of malnutrition on muscle mass, respiratory function, acid–base balance, wound healing and immune function, bone mineralization, and the menstrual cycle in the female or testicular function in the male.

Carol Mattson Porth: PATHOPHYSIOLOGY: CONCEPTS OF
ALTERED HEALTH STATES, 4th ed. © 1994, 1990, 1986, 1982
J.B. Lippincott Company

■ State the causes of malnutrition in the hospitalized patient.

■ Compare the eating disorders and complications associated with anorexia nervosa and the binge–purge syndrome.

"You are what you eat" is often said. To a great extent, nutrition determines how a person looks, feels, and acts. The need for adequate nutrition begins at the time of conception and continues throughout life. Nutrition provided by food or supplements in the proper proportions enables the body to maintain life, to grow both physically and intellectually, to heal and repair tissue, and, in general, to maintain the stamina necessary for well-being. The content presented in this chapter has been divided into three parts: nutritional status, overnutrition and obesity, and undernutrition.

■ NUTRITIONAL STATUS

Nutritional status describes the condition of the body as it relates to the availability and use of nutrients. Nutrients provide the energy and materials necessary for performing the activities of daily living; for maintaining healthy skin, muscles, and other body tissues; for replacing and healing tissues; and for the effective functioning of all body systems including the immune and respiratory systems. Not only can poor nutritional status cause illness, but it can also make it impossible for the person to recuperate from illness.

Nutrients are derived from the digestive tract through the ingestion of foods or, in some cases, through liquid feedings that are delivered directly into the gastrointestinal tract by a synthetic tube (tube feedings). The exception occurs in people with certain illnesses in which the digestive tract is bypassed and the nutrients are infused directly into the circulatory system. Once inside the body, nutrients are used for energy or as the building blocks for tissue growth and repair. When excess nutrients are available, they frequently are stored for future use. If the required nutrients are unavailable, the body adapts by conserving and using its nutrient stores.

ENERGY METABOLISM

Energy is measured in heat units called *calories*. A calorie, spelled with a small *c* and also called a *gram calorie*, is the amount of heat or energy required to raise the temperature of 1 g of water 1°C. A *kilocalorie* (kcal), or *large calorie*, is the amount of energy needed to raise the temperature of 1 kg of water 1°C. Because a calorie is so small, kilocalories are often used in nutritional and physiologic studies. The oxidation of proteins provides 4 kcal/g; fats, 9 kcal/g; carbohydrates, 4 kcal/g, and alcohol, 7 kcal/g.

All body activities require energy whether they involve an individual cell, a single organ, or the entire body. Metabolism is the organized process through which nutrients such as carbohydrates, fats, and proteins are broken down, transformed, or otherwise converted into cellular energy. The process of metabolism is unique in that it not only allows for the continual release of energy, but it couples this energy release with physiologic functioning. For example, the energy used for muscle contraction is derived largely from energy sources that are stored in muscle cells. This energy is released as the muscle contracts. Because most of our energy sources come from the nutrients in the food that is eaten, the ability to store energy and control its release is important.

ADIPOSE (FAT) TISSUE

More than 90% of body energy is stored in the adipose tissues of the body.[1] Adipocytes, or fat cells, occur either singly or in small groups in loose connective tissue. In many parts of the body, they cushion body organs such as the kidneys. In addition to isolated groups of fat cells, entire regions of fat tissue are committed to fat storage. Collectively, fat cells constitute a large body organ that is metabolically active in the uptake, synthesis, storage, and mobilization of lipids, which are the main source of fuel storage for the body. Some tissues, such as liver cells, are able to store small amounts of lipids, but when these lipids accumulate, they begin to interfere with cell function. Adipose tissue not only serves as a storage for body fuels, but it provides insulation for the body, fills body crevices, and protects body organs.

Studies of adipocytes in the laboratory have shown that fully differentiated cells do not divide. However, such cells have a long life span, and anyone born with large numbers of adipocytes runs the risk of becoming obese. Some immature adipocytes capable of division are present in postnatal life; these cells respond to estrogen stimulation and are the potential source of additional fat cells during postnatal life.[2] Fat deposition results from a proliferation of these existing immature adipocytes and can occur as a consequence of excessive caloric intake when a woman is breast-feeding or during estrogen stimulation around the time of puberty. An increase in fat cells may also occur during late adolescence and in middle-aged people who are already fat.[2]

There are two types of adipose tissue: white fat and brown fat. White fat, which, despite its name, is cream colored or yellow, is the prevalent form of adipose tissue in postnatal life. It constitutes 10% to 20% of body weight in adult males and 15% to 25% in adult females.[2] At body temperature, the lipid content of fat cells is present as oil. It consists of triglycerides—three molecules of fatty acids esterified to a glycerol molecule. Triglycerides, which contain no water, have the highest caloric content of all nutrients and are an efficient form of energy storage. Fat cells synthesize triglycerides, the major fat storage form, from dietary fats and carbohydrates. Insulin is required for transport of glucose into fat cells. When calorie intake is restricted for any reason, fat cell triglycerides are broken down and the resultant fatty acids and glycerol are released as energy sources.

Brown fat, as the name implies, is brown in color. It differs from white fat in terms of its thermogenic capacity or ability to produce heat. Brown fat, the site of both diet-induced thermogenesis and nonshivering thermogenesis, is found primarily in early neonatal life in humans and in animals that hibernate. It has been suggested that the presence of brown fat allows animals to eat large quantities of poor-quality diets to obtain essential nutrients while avoiding weight gain. The presence and role of brown fat in older children and adults are controversial at present. It has been suggested that brown fat may have a thermogenic role in humans and that the sympathetic nervous system may play a role in its activation.[3]

ANABOLISM AND CATABOLISM

There are two phases of metabolism—anabolism and catabolism. *Anabolism* is the phase of metabolic storage and synthesis of cell constituents. Anabolism does not provide energy for the body; rather, it requires energy. *Catabolism*, on the other hand, involves the breakdown of complex molecules into substances that can be used in the production of energy. The chemical intermediates for anabolism and catabolism are called *metabolites* (*e.g.*, lactic acid is one of the metabolites formed when glucose is broken down in the absence of oxygen).

Both anabolism and catabolism are catalyzed by *enzyme systems* located within body cells. A *substrate* is a substance on which an enzyme acts. Enzyme systems selectively transform fuel substrates into cellular energy and facilitate the use of energy in the process of assembling molecules to form energy substrates and storage forms of energy.

Because body energy cannot be stored as heat, the cellular oxidative processes that release energy are flameless and have low temperature reactions. Instead of releasing only heat—as occurs when the same fuel is burned in the environment—the free energy released from the oxidation of foods is converted to chemical energy that can be stored. The body transforms carbohydrates, fats, and proteins into the intermediary compound, adenosine triphosphate (ATP). Adenosine triphosphate is often called the energy currency of the cell because almost all body cells use ATP as their energy source (see Chapter 1). The metabolic events involved in ATP formation allow cellular energy to be stored, used, and replenished.

GLUCOSE METABOLISM

Glucose is a six-carbon molecule; it is an efficient fuel that, when metabolized in the presence of oxygen, breaks down to form carbon dioxide and water (Fig. 43-1). Although many tissues and organ systems are able to use other forms of fuel, such as fatty acids and ketones, the brain and nervous system rely almost exclusively on glucose as a fuel source. The nervous system can neither store nor synthesize glucose; rather, it relies on the minute-by-minute extraction of glucose from the blood to meet its energy needs. In the fed and early fasting state, the nervous system requires about 100 to 115 g of glucose per day to meet its metabolic needs.[4, 5]

The liver regulates the entry of glucose into the blood. Glucose ingested in the diet is transported from the gastrointestinal tract, through the portal vein, to the liver before it gains access to the circulatory system (Fig. 43-2). The liver both stores and synthesizes glucose. When blood sugar is increased, the liver removes glucose from the blood and stores it for future use. Conversely, the liver releases its glucose stores when blood sugar drops. In this way, the liver acts as a buffer system to regulate blood sugar levels. Generally speaking, blood sugar levels reflect the difference between the amount of glucose released into the circulation by the liver and the amount of glucose removed from the blood by body cells.

Excess glucose is stored in two forms: (1) it can be converted to fatty acids and stored in fat cells as triglycerides, or (2) it can be stored in the liver and skeletal muscle as glycogen. Small amounts of gly-

H
|
H — C — OH
|
H — C — OH
|
H — C — OH
|
HO — C — H
|
H — C — OH
|
H — C
‖
O

Glucose
(Straight Chain)

$$
\begin{array}{c}
O \\
\| \\
CH - O - C - R_1 \\
O \qquad | \\
\| \qquad | \qquad O \\
R_2 - C - O - C \qquad \| \\
| \qquad CH_2 - O - C - R_3
\end{array}
$$

Triglyceride

H
|
R — C — COOH
|
NH₂

Amino Acid

FIG. 43-1. Glucose, triglyceride, and amino acid structure.

cogen are also stored in the skin and in some of the glandular tissues.

Glycogenolysis. Glycogenolysis, or the breakdown of glycogen, is controlled by the action of two hormones: glucagon and epinephrine. Epinephrine is more effective in stimulating glycogen breakdown in muscle. The liver, on the other hand, is more responsive to glucagon. The synthesis and degradation of glycogen are important because they help maintain blood sugar levels during periods of fasting and strenuous exercise. Only the liver, in contrast with other tissues that store glycogen, is able to release its glucose stores into the blood for use by other tissues, such as the brain and nervous system. This is because glycogen breaks down to form a phosphorylated glucose molecule. Glucose is too large, in its phosphorylated form, to pass through the cell membrane. The liver, but not skeletal muscle, has the enzyme glucose-6-phosphatase, which is needed to

remove the phosphate group and to allow the glucose molecule to enter the bloodstream.

Although they are rare, a number of genetic disorders exist in which glycogen breakdown is impaired. All of these disorders result in excessive accumulation of glycogen. *Von Gierke's disease* involves a genetic deficiency of glucose-6-phosphatase. Children with this disease have stunted growth, liver enlargement, hypoglycemia, and hylipidemia resulting from mobilization of fatty acids. McArdle's disease is characterized by a deficiency in the enzyme muscle phosphorylase. The disorder, which is limited to skeletal muscle, causes muscle cramps during strenuous exercise.

Gluconeogenesis. The synthesis of glucose is referred to as *gluconeogenesis*, or the building of glucose from new sources. The process of gluconeogenesis converts amino acids, lactate, and glycerol into glucose. Most of the gluconeogenesis occurs in the liver. Although fatty acids can be used as fuel by many body cells, they cannot be converted to glucose.

Glucose produced through the process of gluconeogenesis is either stored in the liver as glycogen or released into the general circulation. During periods of food deprivation or when the diet is low in

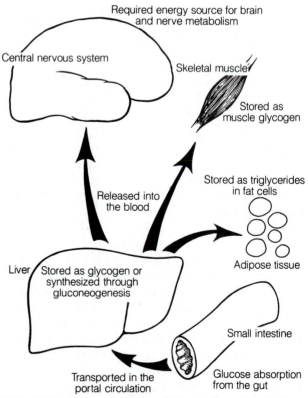

FIG. 43-2. Figure regulation of blood glucose by the liver.

carbohydrates, gluconeogenesis provides the glucose that is needed to meet the metabolic needs of the brain and other glucose-dependent tissues.

Several hormones stimulate gluconeogenesis, including glucagon, glucocorticoid hormones from the adrenal cortex, and thyroid hormone.

FAT METABOLISM

The average American diet provides 37% to 40% of calories in the form of fats. In contrast to glucose, which yields only 4 kcal/g, each gram of fat yields 9 kcal. Additionally, another 30% to 50% of the carbohydrates consumed in the diet are converted to triglycerides for storage.

A triglyceride contains three fatty acids linked by a glycerol molecule (see Fig. 43-1). Fatty acids and triglycerides can be derived from dietary sources, they can be synthesized in the body, or they can be mobilized from fat depots. Excess carbohydrate is converted to triglyceride and is transported by lipoproteins in the blood to adipose cells for storage. One gram of anhydrous (water-free) fat stores more than six times as much energy as one hydrated gram of glycogen. One reason weight loss is greatest at the beginning of a fast or weight-loss program is that this is when the body uses its glycogen stores. Later, when the body begins to use energy stored as triglycerides, water losses are decreased and weight loss tends to plateau.

The mobilization of fat for use in energy production is facilitated by the action of enzymes, or lipases, that break the triglycerides into three fatty acids and a glycerol molecule. After triglyceride breakdown, both the fatty acids and the glycerol molecule leave the fat cell and enter the circulation. Once in the circulation, many of the fatty acids are transported to the liver, where they are removed from the blood and are either used by liver cells as a source of energy or converted to ketones.

The efficient burning of fatty acids requires a balance between carbohydrate and fat metabolism. The ratio of fatty acid and carbohydrate utilization is altered in situations that favor fat breakdown, such as diabetes mellitus and fasting. In these situations, the liver produces more ketones than it can use; this excess is released into the bloodstream. Ketones can be an important source of energy, because even the brain adapts to the use of ketones during prolonged periods of starvation. A problem arises, however, when fat breakdown is accelerated and the production of ketones exceeds tissue use. Because ketone bodies are organic acids, they cause *ketoacidosis* when they are present in excessive amounts. The activation of lipases and the subsequent mobilization of fatty acids are stimulated by epinephrine, glucocorticoid hormones, growth hormones, and glucagon.

PROTEIN METABOLISM

About three fourths of body solids are proteins. Proteins are essential for the formation of all body structures, including genes, enzymes, contractile proteins in muscle, matrix of bone, and hemoglobin of red blood cells.

Amino acids are the building blocks of proteins. Twenty amino acids are present in body proteins in significant quantities. Each amino acid has an acidic group (COOH) and an amino group (NH_2; see Fig. 43-1). Unlike glucose and fatty acids, there is only a limited facility for the storage of excess amino acids in the body. Most of the stored amino acids are contained in body proteins. Amino acids in excess of those needed for protein synthesis are converted to fatty acids, ketone bodies, or glucose and are stored or used as metabolic fuel. Each gram of protein yields 4 kcal. Because fatty acids cannot be converted to glucose, the body must break down proteins and use the amino acids as a major source of substrate for gluconeogenesis during periods when metabolic needs exceed food intake. The liver has the enzymes and transfer mechanisms needed to deaminate and to convert the amino groups (NH_2) from the amino acid to urea. Thus, the breakdown or degradation of proteins and amino acids occurs primarily in the liver, which is also the site of gluconeogenesis.

ENERGY EXPENDITURE

The expenditure of body energy results from four mechanisms of heat production (thermogenesis): (1) basal metabolic rate (BMR) or basal energy equivalent (BEE), (2) diet-induced thermogenesis, (3) exercise-induced thermogenesis, and (4) thermogenesis in response to changes in environmental conditions. The amount of energy used varies with age, body size, rate of growth, and state of health.

METABOLIC RATE

The basal, or resting metabolism, refers to the chemical reactions occurring when the body is at rest. These reactions are necessary to provide energy for maintenance of normal body temperature, cardiovascular and respiratory function, muscle tone, and other essential activities of tissues and cells in the resting body. The resting metabolic rate constitutes 65% to 70% of body energy needs. The BMR can be determined by placing a person in a special chamber

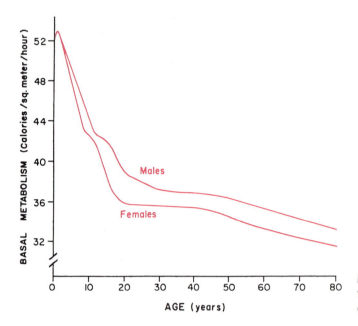

FIG. 43-3. Normal basal metabolic rates at different ages for each sex. (Guyton, A. [1986]. *Medical physiology* [7th ed.]. Philadelphia: W.B. Saunders)

and measuring the total quantity of heat liberated from the body in a given period of time. Because most of the energy expended by the body is derived from oxidative reactions involving dietary nutrients, the BEE measurement can be determined indirectly by measuring oxygen use. The BMR and BEE are measured after 12 hours of fasting while the person is awake and at rest in a warm room. Several factors that affect BMR are age, sex, physical state, and pregnancy. A progressive decline in the normal BMR occurs with aging. Women generally have a 5% to 10% lower BMR than men because of their higher percentage of adipose tissue. The BMR decreases by 2% each new decade of life after growth has ceased (Fig. 43-3).

The BEE can be estimated using the Harris-Benedict equation (Table 43-1). The Harris-Benedict equation correctly predicts the BEE for 90% of healthy adults.[6] Multiplying the BEE by a factor of 1.2 usually adequately predicts the calorie needs for maintenance of nutrition during health. A factor of 1.5 usually provides the needed nutrients during repletion and during illnesses such as pneumonia, long-bone fractures, cancer, peritonitis, and recovery from most types of major surgery.

DIET-INDUCED THERMOGENESIS

The diet-induced thermogenesis, or specific dynamic action of food, describes the energy used by the body for the digestion, absorption, and assimilation of food after its ingestion. It is energy expended over and above the caloric value of the food. It varies from 10% to 35% depending on the type and quantity of food consumed and accounts for 6% to 10% of the total calories expended.[6] When food is eaten, the metabolic rate rises and then returns to normal within a few hours. One explanation for the thermogenic response to a meal is that it results from enhanced activity of the sympathetic nervous system and its effect on brown adipose tissue. If this is true, decreased sympathetic activity in obese people could account for an enhanced metabolic efficiency that allows calories to be stored rather than expended.[1]

TABLE 43-1. EQUATION FOR CALCULATING BASAL ENERGY EXPENDITURE (BEE)

Men
  BEE = 66 + (13.7 × weight (kg)) + (5 × height (cm)) − (6.8 × age (yr))
Women
  BEE = 655 + (9.5 × weight (kg)) + (1.7 × height (cm)) − (4.7 × age (yr))

(Krause, M.V., & Mahan, L.K. [1984]. *Food, nutrition and diet therapy*. Philadelphia: W.B. Saunders)

EXERCISE-INDUCED THERMOGENESIS

The amount of energy expended for physical activity is determined by the type of activity performed, the length of participation, and the person's weight. Table 43-2 gives the energy expenditure for various activities.

NUTRITIONAL NEEDS AND RECOMMENDED DAILY ALLOWANCES

Nutritional status reflects the continued daily intake of nutrients over time and the deposition and use of these nutrients within the body. The body requires over 40 nutrients on a daily basis. Several of these have had a recommended daily allowance (RDA) established. The RDA is the level of intake of essential nutrients considered to be adequate to meet the known nutrient needs of practically all healthy people. The RDA is not the minimum requirement; it is usually two to six times the minimum daily requirement. Most people could have 80% of the RDA in their diet and still be well nourished.

The RDA amounts are set by determining the entire range of needs, selecting the numbers at the high end, and adding a safety factor without risking toxicity. Experts from universities and government comprise the Food and Nutrition Board of the National Research Council under the National Academy of Sciences. They continuously evaluate the current research and periodically determine and revise the RDA.[7] The latest RDA was published in 1989 (Table 43-3).

There are 17 age and sex classifications in the RDA. It is to be used as a standard for feeding programs, school lunch programs, penal institutions, hospital and health-care facilities, and computer software used to analyze diets and recipes. The RDA is intended to be met by a variety of foods versus supplements or extensive fortification.

The United States RDA (USRDA) was established for the purpose of labeling foods. It takes the highest value of each nutrient for people 4 years of age to adult (excluding pregnancy and lactation); therefore, the USRDA sometimes provides a margin of nutritional safety higher than the RDA.

Proteins, fats, carbohydrates, vitamins, and minerals each have their own function in providing the body with what it needs to maintain life and health. Recommended allowances have not been established for every nutrient; some are given as a safe and adequate intake, whereas others, such as carbohydrates and fats, are expressed as a percentage of the calorie intake. The function of each of these nutrients is presented, along with the suggested daily consumption of each.

TABLE 43-2. ENERGY EXPENDITURE PER HOUR DURING DIFFERENT TYPES OF ACTIVITY FOR A 70-KG MAN

FORM OF ACTIVITY	CALORIES PER HOUR
Sleeping	65
Awake lying still	77
Sitting at rest	100
Standing relaxed	105
Dressing and undressing	118
Tailoring	135
Typewriting rapidly	140
"Light" exercise	170
Walking slowly (2.6 mph)	200
Carpentry, metal working, industrial painting	240
"Active" exercise	290
"Severe" exercise	450
Sawing wood	480
Swimming	500
Running (5.3 mph)	570
"Very severe" exercise	600
Walking very fast (5.3 mph)	650
Walking up stairs	1100

(Extracted from data compiled by Professor M.S. Rose. Guyton, A. [1986]. *Medical physiology* [7th ed.]. Philadelphia: W.B. Saunders)

CALORIES

Energy requirements are greater during growth periods. Infants require approximately 115 kcal/kg at birth, 105 kcal/kg at 1 year, and 80 kcal/kg body weight from ages 1 to 10 years. During adolescence, boys require 45 kcal/kg body weight and girls require 38 kcal/kg body weight. During pregnancy, a woman needs an extra 300 kcal per day above her usual requirement, and, during the first 3 months of breast-feeding, she requires an additional 500 kcal.[7] Table 43-4 gives a simple formula for determining caloric intake in healthy adults.

PROTEINS

Proteins are required for growth and maintenance of body tissues, enzymes and antibody formation, fluid and electrolyte balance, and nutrient transport. Proteins are composed of amino acids, nine of which are essential to the body. These are leucine, isoleucine, methionine, phenylalanine, threonine, tryptophan, valine, lysine, and histidine. The foods that provide

TABLE 43-3. FOOD AND NUTRITION BOARD, NATIONAL ACADEMY OF SCIENCES—NATIONAL RESEARCH COUNCIL RECOMMENDED DIETARY ALLOWANCES,* REVISED 1989 DESIGNED FOR THE MAINTENANCE OF GOOD NUTRITION OF PRACTICALLY ALL HEALTHY PEOPLE IN THE UNITED STATES

CATEGORY	AGE (YEARS) OR CONDITION	WEIGHT† (kg)	WEIGHT† (lb)	HEIGHT† (cm)	HEIGHT† (in)	PROTEIN (G)	FAT-SOLUBLE VITAMINS Vitamin A (µg RE)‡	Vitamin D (µg)§	Vitamin E (mg α-TE)‖	Vitamin K (µg)
Infants	0.0–0.5	6	13	60	24	13	375	7.5	3	5
	0.5–1.0	9	20	71	28	14	375	10	4	10
Children	1–3	13	29	90	35	16	400	10	6	15
	4–6	20	44	112	44	24	500	10	7	20
	7–10	28	62	132	52	28	700	10	7	30
Males	11–14	45	99	157	62	45	1000	10	10	45
	15–18	66	145	176	69	59	1000	10	10	65
	19–24	72	160	177	70	58	1000	10	10	70
	25–50	79	174	176	70	63	1000	5	10	80
	51 +	77	170	173	68	63	1000	5	10	80
Females	11–14	46	101	157	62	46	800	10	8	45
	15–18	55	120	163	64	44	800	10	8	55
	19–24	58	128	164	65	46	800	10	8	60
	25–50	63	138	163	64	50	800	5	8	65
	51 +	65	143	160	63	50	800	5	8	65
Pregnant						60	800	10	10	65
Lactating	1st 6 months					65				
	2nd 6 months					62	1200	10	11	65

* The allowances, expressed as average daily intakes over time, are intended to provide for individual variations among most normal persons as they live in the United States under usual environmental stresses. Diets should be based on a variety of common foods to provide other nutrients for which human requirements have been less well defined. See text for detailed discussion of allowances and of nutrients not tabulated.

† Weights and heights of Reference Adults are actual medians for the U.S. population of the designated age, as reported by NHANES II. The median weights and heights of those under 19 years of age were taken from Hamill et al. (1979) (see pages 16–17). The use of these figures does not imply that the height-to-weight ratios are ideal.

these essential amino acids are milk, eggs, meat, fish, and poultry. These foods are referred to as complete proteins. The incomplete proteins are those that do not provide all nine essential amino acids. These include dried peas and beans, nuts, seeds, and grains. These need to be combined with each other or with complete proteins to meet the amino acid requirements. Diets that are inadequate in protein can result in kwashiorkor. If both calories and protein are inadequate, protein-calorie malnutrition occurs.

Unlike carbohydrates and fats, which are composed of hydrogen, carbon, and oxygen, proteins contain 16% nitrogen; therefore, nitrogen excretion is an indicator of protein intake. If the amount of nitrogen taken in by way of protein is equivalent to the nitrogen excreted, the person is said to be in *nitrogen balance*. A person is in positive nitrogen balance when the nitrogen consumed by way of protein is greater than the amount excreted. This occurs during growth, pregnancy, or healing after surgery or injury. A negative nitrogen balance often occurs during fever, illness, infection, trauma, or burns when more nitrogen is excreted than is consumed. Tissue wasting ensues.

FATS

Dietary fats are composed primarily of triglycerides (a mixture of fatty acids and glycerol). The fatty acids are either saturated (no double bonds), monounsaturated (one double bond), or polyunsaturated (two or more double bonds). The saturated fatty acids elevate blood cholesterol, whereas the monounsaturated and polyunsaturated fats lower blood cholesterol. Research indicates that dietary fat should be divided equally between the three types of fatty acids.[8] Saturated fats are generally from animal sources and remain solid at room temperature. With the exception

WATER-SOLUBLE VITAMINS							MINERALS						
Vitamin C (mg)	Thiamin (mg)	Riboflavin (mg)	Niacin (mg NE)	Vitamin B₆ (mg)	Folate (µg)	Vitamin B₁₂ (µg)	Calcium (mg)	Phosphorus (mg)	Magnesium (mg)	Iron (mg)	Zinc (mg)	Iodine (µg)	Selenium (µg)
30	0.3	0.4	5	0.3	25	0.3	400	300	40	6	5	40	10
35	0.4	0.5	6	0.8	35	0.5	600	500	60	10	5	50	15
40	0.7	0.8	9	1.0	50	0.7	800	800	80	10	10	70	20
45	0.9	1.1	12	1.1	75	1.0	800	800	120	10	10	90	20
45	1.0	1.2	13	1.4	100	1.4	800	800	170	10	10	120	30
50	1.3	1.5	17	1.7	150	2.0	1200	1200	270	12	15	150	40
60	1.5	1.8	20	2.0	200	2.0	1200	1200	400	12	15	150	50
60	1.5	1.7	19	2.0	200	2.0	1200	1200	350	10	15	150	70
60	1.5	1.7	19	2.0	200	2.0	800	800	350	10	15	150	70
60	1.2	1.4	15	2.0	200	2.0	800	800	350	10	15	150	70
50	1.1	1.3	15	1.4	150	2.0	1200	1200	280	15	12	150	45
60	1.1	1.3	15	1.5	180	2.0	1200	1200	300	15	12	150	50
60	1.1	1.3	15	1.6	180	2.0	1200	1200	280	15	12	150	55
60	1.1	1.3	15	1.6	180	2.0	800	800	280	15	12	150	55
60	1.0	1.2	13	1.6	180	2.0	800	800	280	10	12	150	55
70	1.5	1.6	17	2.2	400	2.2	1200	1200	320	30	15	175	65
95	1.6	1.8	20	2.1	280	2.6	1200	1200	355	15	19	200	75
90	1.6	1.7	20	2.1	260	2.6	1200	1200	340	15	16	200	75

‡ Retinol equivalents. 1 retinol equivalent = 1 µg retinol or 6 µg β-carotene. See text for calculation of vitamin A activity of diets as retinol equivalents.

§ As cholecalciferol. 10 µg cholecalciferol = 400 IU of vitamin D.

‖ α-Tocopherol equivalents. 1 mg d-α tocopherol = 1 α-TE. See text for variation in allowances and calculation of vitamin E activity of the diet as α-tocopherol equivalents.

¶ 1 NE (niacin equivalent) is equal to 1 mg of niacin or 60 mg of dietary tryptophan.

of coconut and palm oils (which are saturated), unsaturated fats are found in plant oils and are usually liquid at room temperature.

Dietary fats provide energy, serve as carriers for the fat-soluble vitamins, are precursors of prostaglandins, and are a source of fatty acids. The polyunsaturated fatty acid linoleic acid is the only fatty acid that is required. A deficiency of linoleic acid results in dermatitis. The daily requirement is 5 g or 1% to 2% of the total daily calories. Because vegetable oils are rich sources of linoleic acid, this level can be met by including one tablespoon of oil.

Other than the requirement for linoleic acid, there is no specific requirement for dietary fat, provided there is adequate nutrition available for energy. Fat is the most concentrated source of energy. It is recommended that only 30% of the calories in the diet should come from fats.[8]

Cholesterol is the major constituent of cell membranes and is synthesized by the body. Cholesterol metabolism and transport are discussed in Chapter 18. The daily dietary recommendation for cholesterol is 300 mg; however, many Americans have diets that contain about 600 mg.[9]

CARBOHYDRATES

Dietary carbohydrates are composed of simple sugars, complex carbohydrates, and undigested carbohydrates (fiber). Because of their vitamin, mineral, and fiber content, it is recommended that the bulk of the carbohydrate content in the diet be in the complex form rather than as simple sugars that contain few nutrients. Sucrose (table sugar) is implicated in the development of dental caries.

There is no specific dietary requirement for carbohydrates. All of the energy requirements can be met by dietary fats and proteins. Although some

TABLE 43-4. CALORIC REQUIREMENTS BASED ON BODY WEIGHT AND ACTIVITY LEVEL

	SEDENTARY	MODERATE	ACTIVE
Overweight	20–25 kcal/kg	30 kcal/kg	35 kcal/kg
Normal	30 kcal/kg	35 kcal/kg	40 kcal/kg
Underweight	30 kcal/kg	40 kcal/kg	45–50 kcal/kg

(Adapted from Goodhart, R.S., & Shils, M.E. [1980]. *Modern nutrition in health and disease* [6th ed.]. Philadelphia: Lea and Febiger.)

tissues, such as the nervous system, require glucose as an energy source, this need can be met through the conversion of amino acids and the glycerol part of the triglyceride molecule to glucose. The fatty acids from triglycerides are converted to ketones and used for energy by other body tissues. Thus, a carbohydrate-deficient diet usually results in the loss of tissue proteins and the development of ketosis. Because protein and fat metabolism increases the production of osmotically active metabolic wastes that must be eliminated through the kidneys, there is danger of dehydration and electrolyte imbalances. The amount of carbohydrate needed to prevent tissue wasting and ketosis is 50 to 100 g/day. In practice, the majority of the daily energy requirement should be from carbohydrate because protein is an expensive source of calories and because it is recommended that only 30% of the calories in the diet be derived from fat. The current recommendation is that the diet should provide 50% to 60% of the calories as carbohydrates.[8] The actual intake for most Americans is closer to 45%; hence, the average American diet is too low in carbohydrates and too high in fats and proteins.

VITAMINS

Vitamins are a group of organic compounds that act as catalysts in various chemical reactions. A compound cannot be classified as a vitamin unless it is shown that a deficiency of it causes disease. Contrary to popular belief, vitamins do not provide energy directly. As catalysts they are part of the enzyme systems required for the release of energy from protein, fat, and carbohydrates. Vitamins are also necessary for the formation of red blood cells, hormones, genetic materials, and the nervous system. They are essential for normal growth and development.

There are two types of vitamins: fat-soluble and water-soluble. The four fat-soluble vitamins are vitamins A, D, E, and K. The nine required water-soluble vitamins are thiamine, riboflavin, niacin, pyridoxine, pantothenic acid, B_{12}, folic acid, biotin, and vitamin C. Because the water-soluble vitamins are excreted in the urine, it is less likely that they will become toxic to

the body; but the fat-soluble vitamins are stored in the body, and they may reach toxic levels. See Table 43-5 for sources and functions of vitamins.

MINERALS

Minerals serve many functions. They are involved in acid–base balance and in the maintenance of osmotic pressure within body compartments. Minerals are components of vitamins, hormones, and enzymes. They maintain normal hemoglobin levels, have functions within the nervous system, and are involved in muscle contraction and skeletal development and maintenance. Minerals that are present in relatively large amounts in the body are called *macrominerals*. These include calcium, phosphorus, sodium, chloride, potassium, magnesium, and sulfur. The remainder are classified as *trace minerals*; they include iron, manganese, copper, iodine, zinc, cobalt, fluorine, and selenium. Table 43-6 lists mineral sources and functions.

FIBER

Fiber, the portion of food that cannot be digested by the human intestinal tract, increases stool bulk and facilitates bowel movements. Several studies have indicated that fiber decreases the incidence of digestive diseases and some cancers and lowers blood sugar and cholesterol.[10, 11]

NUTRITIONAL ASSESSMENT

The nutritional status of a person can be assessed by evaluation of the person's dietary intake, anthropometric measurements, physical examination, and laboratory tests. The nutritional assessment can provide information regarding the adequacy of the diet, the person's body size compared to normal ranges, and the possibility of overnutrition or undernutrition.

Nutritional assessment remains more of an art than a science. A global assessment obtains information about many facets of nutrition including current

TABLE 43-5. SOURCES AND FUNCTIONS OF VITAMINS

VITAMIN	MAJOR FOOD SOURCES	FUNCTIONS
Fat-Soluble Vitamins		
Vitamin A (retinol, provitamin, carotenoids)	Retinol: liver, butter, whole milk, cheese, egg yolks; Pro-vitamin A: carrots, leafy green vegetables, sweet potatoes, pumpkin, winter squash, apricots, cantaloupe, fortified margarine	Essential for normal retinal function; plays an essential role in cell growth and differentiation, particularly epithelial cells. Epidemiologic evidence suggests a role in preventing certain cancers
Vitamin D (calciferol)	Vitamin D–fortified dairy products, fortified margarine, fish oils, egg yolk	Increases intestinal absorption of calcium and promotes ossification of bones and teeth
Vitamin E (tocopherol)	Vegetable oil, margarine, shortening, green and leafy vegetables, wheat germ, whole grain products, egg yolk, butter, liver	Functions as an antioxidant protecting vitamins A and C and fatty acids; prevents cell membrane injury
Water-Soluble Vitamins		
Vitamin C (ascorbic acid)	Broccoli, sweet and hot peppers, collards, brussel sprouts, kale, potato, spinach, tomatoes, citrus fruits, strawberries	Potent antioxidant involved in many oxidation-reduction reactions; required for synthesis of collagen; increases absorption of nonheme iron; is involved in wound healing and drug metabolism
Thiamin (vitamin B_1)	Pork, liver, meat, whole grains, fortified grain products, legumes, nuts	Coenzyme required for several important biochemical reactions in carbohydrate metabolism. Thought to have an independent role in nerve conduction
Riboflavin (vitamin B_2)	Liver, milk, yogurt, cottage cheese, meat, fortified grain products	Coenzyme that participates in a variety of important oxidation-reduction reactions and important component of a number of enzymes
Niacin (nicotinamide, nicotinic acid)	Liver, meat, poultry, fish, peanuts, fortified grain products	Essential component of the coenzymes nicotinamide adenine dinucleotide (NAD) and nicotineamide dinucleotide diphosphate (NADP), which are involved in many oxidative reduction reactions
Folacin (Folic acid)	Liver, legumes, green leafy vegetables	Coenzyme in amino acid and nucleoprotein metabolism; promotes red cell formation
Vitamin B_6 (pyridoxine)	Meat, poultry, fish, shellfish, green and leafy vegetables, whole grain products, legumes	A major coenzyme involved in the metabolism of amino acids. Required for synthesis of heme
Vitamin B_{12}	Meat, poultry, fish, shellfish, eggs, diary products	Coenzyme involved in nucleic acid synthesis; assists in development of red cells and maintenance of nerve function
Biotin	Kidney, liver, milk, egg yolks, most fresh vegetables	Coenzyme in fat synthesis, amino acid metabolism, and glycogen formation
Pantothenic acid	Liver, kidney, meats, milk, egg yolk, whole grain products, legumes	Coenzyme involved in energy metabolism

(Data from *Vitamin facts*, National Dairy Council and other sources.)

physical symptoms, history of acute and chronic illnesses, and a detailed physical examination. Global assessment is probably one of the most valid methods of making a nutritional diagnosis and planning nutritional care.[12, 13]

DIET HISTORY

A nutritional assessment begins with evaluation of the person's diet. This can be accomplished by recording the food consumed by actual observation or

TABLE 43-6. SOURCES AND FUNCTIONS OF MINERALS

MINERAL	MAJOR SOURCES	FUNCTIONS
Calcium	Milk and milk products, fish with bones, greens	Bone formation and maintenance; tooth formation, vitamin B absorption, blood clotting, nerve and muscle function
Chloride	Table salt, meats, milk, eggs	Regulates pH of stomach, acid–base balance, osmotic pressure of extracellular fluids
Cobalt	Organ meats, meats	Aids in maturation of red blood cells (as part of B_{12} molecule)
Copper	Cereals, nuts, legumes, liver, shellfish, grapes, meats	Catalyst for hemoglobin formation, formation of elastin and collagen, energy release (cytochrome oxidase and catalase), formation of melanin, formation of phospholipids for myelin sheath of nerves
Fluoride	Fluorinated water	Strengthens bones and teeth
Iodine	Iodized salt, fish (saltwater and anadromous)	Thyroid hormone synthesis and its function in maintenance of metabolic rate
Iron	Meats, heart, liver, clams, oysters, lima beans, spinach, dates, dried nuts, enriched and whole-grain cereals	Hemoglobin synthesis, cellular energy release (cytochrome pathway), killing bacteria (myeloperoxidase)
Magnesium	Milk, green vegetables, nuts, bread, and cereals	Catalyst of many intracellular nerve impulses, retention of reactions, particularly those related to intracellular enzyme reactions; low magnesium levels produce an increase in irritability of the nervous system, vasodilatation, and cardiac dysrhythmias
Phosphorus	Meats, poultry, fish, milk and cheese, cereals, legumes, nuts	Bone formation and maintenance; essential component of nucleic acids and energy exchange forms such as adenosine triphosphate (ATP)
Potassium	Oranges, dried fruits, bananas, meats, potatoes, peanut butter, coffee	Maintenance of intracellular osmolality, acid–base balance, transmission of nerve impulses, catalyst in energy metabolism, formation of proteins, formation of glycogen
Sodium	Table salt, cured meats, meats, milk, olives	Maintenance of osmotic pressure of extracellular fluids, acid–base balance, neuromuscular function; absorption of glucose
Zinc	Whole-wheat cereals, eggs, legumes	Integral part of many enzymes including carbonic anhydrase, which facilitates combination of carbon dioxide with water in red blood cells; component of lactic dehydrogenase, important in cellular metabolism; component of many peptidases; important in digestion of proteins in gastrointestinal tract

by personal recall and through the administration of a questionnaire such as a diet history. Each technique has its own shortcomings, such as the tendency to alter behavior when it is known that the behavior is being observed or reported.

HEALTH ASSESSMENT

Health assessment, including a health history and physical examination, reveals weight changes, muscle wasting, fat stores, functional status, and nutritional status. Comparison of the person's current weight to previous weights identifies whether the person's weight is stable, changed drastically, or tends to fluctuate. For example, recent rapid weight loss can be a sign of cancer, a malfunctioning thyroid gland, or self-imposed starvation. A history of fluctuating weight could be associated with bulimia. Degradation of muscle, or muscle wasting, is a serious sign of malnutrition. A decrease in ability to initiate or complete activities of daily living could result from a decrease in energy caused by a poor diet, a neurologic malfunction such as multiple sclerosis, or a result of symptoms related to chronic obstructive pulmonary disease. Quality of the hair, absence of body hair, condition of gums, and skin lesions could signal poor nutritional status.

ANTHROPOMETRIC MEASUREMENTS

Anthropometric measurements provide a means for assessing body composition, particularly fat stores and skeletal muscle; it is done by measuring height, weight, circumferences and thickness of various skinfolds. These measurements are used to determine growth patterns in children and appropriateness of current weight in adults. Body weight is the most frequently used method of assessing nutritional status; it is usually used in combination with measurements of body height to establish whether a person is underweight or overweight.

Relative weight is the actual weight divided by the desirable weight multiplied by 100. A relative weight greater than 120% is indicative of obesity. Recent changes in weight are probably a better indication of undernutrition than a low relative weight. A loss of 10% of body weight or more within a 1- to 2-month period is usually considered predictive of a poor clinical outcome in many disease states.[14]

The Metropolitan Life Insurance Table is the most widely used standard for defining levels of underweight and overweight (Table 43-7). This table, which is based on life insurance statistics relating height and weight to the likelihood of survival, provides an index of desirable weight. The upper and lower frame sizes appear to be based on the upper and lower quartiles of the population, with the medium frame representing the two middle quartiles. Using this table, obesity is defined as the condition in which body weight is greater than 30% of the weight for the specific height and frame.[14] There are some problems with the insurance table: weight ranges define lowest mortality and not necessarily ideal body weight; it is based on an ill-defined concept of frame size; it may not be representative of the U.S.

population due to possible sampling biases; and it does not differentiate between weight gain due to increased muscle mass and weight gain due to increased fat content.

The body mass index (BMI) uses both height and weight to determine obesity. It is calculated by dividing the weight in kilograms by the height in meters squared (BMI = weight (kg)/height (m²)). The normal BMI is 19 to 27. People with a BMI greater than 30 are considered obese, and those with a BMI that exceeds 40 are classified as morbidly obese.[15] The National Institute of Health (NIH) Consensus Conference on the Health Implications of Obesity has recommended the use of height and weight measurements, together with the BMI and calculations of relative weight, in defining obesity.[16]

Body weight reflects both lean body mass and adipose tissue and cannot be used as a method for describing body composition or the percentage of fat tissue present. The proper body–fat ratio is age specific. For young adults under age 30, the recommended range for males is 12% to 15% and for females, 19% to 23%. The upper limit for a 50-year-old male is 19% and, for a female, about 27%.[1] During physical training, body fat usually decreases and lean body mass increases.

Several types of anthropometric measurements can be used to estimate body fat. Skinfold measurement, although difficult to perform and subject to

TABLE 43-7. 1983 METROPOLITAN HEIGHT AND WEIGHT TABLES*

MEN						WOMEN				
Height		Small Frame	Medium Frame	Large Frame		Height		Small Frame	Medium Frame	Large Frame
Feet	Inches					Feet	Inches			
5	2	128–134	131–141	138–150		4	10	102–111	109–121	118–131
5	3	130–136	133–143	140–153		4	11	103–113	111–123	120–134
5	4	132–138	135–145	142–156		5	0	104–115	113–126	122–137
5	5	134–140	137–148	144–160		5	1	106–118	115–129	125–140
5	6	136–142	139–151	146–164		5	2	108–121	118–132	128–143
5	7	138–145	142–154	149–168		5	3	111–124	121–135	131–147
5	8	140–148	145–157	152–172		5	4	114–127	124–138	134–151
5	9	142–151	148–160	155–176		5	5	117–130	127–141	137–155
5	10	144–154	151–163	158–180		5	6	120–133	130–144	140–159
5	11	146–157	154–166	161–184		5	7	123–136	133–147	143–163
6	0	149–160	157–170	164–188		5	8	126–139	136–150	146–167
6	1	152–164	160–174	168–192		5	9	129–142	139–153	149–170
6	2	155–168	164–178	172–197		5	10	132–145	142–156	152–173
6	3	158–172	167–182	176–202		5	11	135–148	145–159	155–176
6	4	162–176	171–187	181–207		6	0	138–151	148–162	158–179

*Weights at ages 25–59 based on lowest mortality. Weight in pounds according to frame (in indoor clothing weighing 5 lb for men and 3 lb for women; shoes with 1-in heels).

(Data from *1979 build study. Society of Actuaries and Association of Life Insurance Medical Directors of America.* [1983]. Metropolitan Life Insurance Company Health and Safety Education Division.)

error when used on obese people, can be used together with equations and tables to estimate the percentage of lean body mass and fat tissue.[17-21] Body circumferences are usually a more objective measurement and provide the information needed to calculate waist and hip ratio.[21, 22]

Densitometry by underwater weighing is more accurate than either skinfold thickness or body circumference measurements in determining the percentage of body fat; however, there are limitations. It requires access to special equipment; assumes a constant density of lean body mass, which is subject to error; and necessitates an estimation of residual gas volumes in the lungs, which is often difficult.

Another method of estimating body fat is bioelectrical impedance. This method is performed by attaching electrodes at the wrist and ankle that send a harmless current through the body. The flow of the current is affected by the amount of water within the body. Because fat-free tissue contains virtually all the water and the conducting electrolytes, measurements of the resistance (impedance) to current flow can be used to estimate the percentage of body fat present. Bioelectrical impedance may become one of the most widely available techniques for assessing body fat once its accuracy has been established.[22-24] The method is relatively inexpensive, easy to use, and portable.

Computed tomographic (CT) scans and magnetic resonance imaging (MRI) can be used to provide quantitative pictures from which the thickness of fat can be determined. A CT scan can be used to provide quantitative estimates of regional fat and give a ratio of intraabdominal to extraabdominal fat.[1]

LABORATORY STUDIES

Various laboratory tests on blood can aid in evaluating nutritional status. Some of the most commonly performed tests are serum albumin to assess the protein status, total lymphocyte count and delayed hypersensitivity reaction to assess cellular immunity, and creatinine–height index to assess skeletal protein. Vitamin and mineral deficiencies can be determined by measurements of their levels in blood, saliva, and other body tissues or by measuring nutrient-specific chemical reactions. All of these tests are limited by confounding factors and, therefore, need to be evaluated along with other clinical data.

In summary, nutritional status describes the condition of the body as it relates to the availability and use of nutrients. Nutrients provide the energy and materials necessary for performing the activities of daily living and for the growth and repair of body tissues. Metabolism is the organized process whereby nutrients such as carbohydrates, fats, and proteins are broken down, transformed, or otherwise converted to cellular energy. *Glucose, fats, and amino acids from proteins serve as fuel sources for cellular metabolism. These fuel sources are ingested during meals and stored for future use. Glucose is either stored as glycogen or converted to triglycerides in fat cells for storage. Fats are stored in adipose tissue as triglycerides. Amino acids are the building blocks of proteins, and most of the stored amino acids are contained in body proteins and as fuel sources for cellular metabolism. Energy is measured in heat units called kilocalories.*

The expenditure of body energy and need for metabolism are largely determined by heat production (thermogenesis) associated with: (1) the basal metabolic rate or basal energy equivalent, (2) diet-induced thermogenesis, (3) exercise-induced thermogenesis, and (4) thermogenesis in response to changes in environmental conditions.

The body requires over 40 nutrients on a daily basis. Nutritional status reflects the continued daily intake of nutrients over time and the deposition and use of these nutrients within the body. The RDA is the recommended daily intake of essential nutrients considered to be adequate to meet the known nutritional needs of healthy people. The RDA has 17 age and sex classifications and includes recommendations for calories, protein, fat, carbohydrates, vitamins, and minerals. The nutritional status of a person can be assessed by evaluation of dietary intake, anthropometric measurements, health assessment, and laboratory tests. Health assessment includes a health history and physical examination to determine weight changes, muscle wasting, fat stores, functional status, and nutritional status. Anthropometric measurements are used for assessing body composition; they include height and weight measurements and measurements (e.g., skinfold thickness, body circumferences, densitometry, bioelectrical impedance, and CT scans) to determine the composition of the body in relation to lean body mass and fat tissue.

■ OVERNUTRITION AND OBESITY

"Nicotine in the lungs is invisible, alcoholism may be hidden, but the results of addiction to food . . . cannot be concealed. Fat on the hips is irrevocably public."[25] Obesity is a major health problem in affluent countries. Estimates of its prevalence range from 10% to 50% of the adult population.[26] These differing estimates reflect the definitions and standards used to identify the population at risk.[1] The massively obese are easy to recognize and represent only a small segment of the population—5.8% of men and 8.3% of women in the United States using the 95th percentile for the BMI.[26] Because body weight measures muscle mass as well as body fat, overweight does not necessarily indicate obesity. To be obese, a person must have an abnormally high proportion of body fat.

CAUSES OF OBESITY

Obesity has been defined as an excess of body fat frequently resulting in a significant impairment of health.[9] This excess body fat is generated when the calories consumed exceed those expended through exercise and activity. Factors contributing to this imbalance are numerous and probably exist in differing combinations among obese people. Heredity, socioeconomic, culture, environmental factors, psychological influences, and activity levels have all been implicated as causative or contributing factors in the development of obesity. Contrary to popular belief, endocrine disorders are rarely a cause of obesity.

Epidemiologic surveys indicate that the prevalence of overweight is related to social and economic conditions. The second (1976 through 1980) National Health and Nutrition Examination Survey has shown that if American women were divided into two groups according to economic status, the prevalence of obesity is much higher among those in the poverty level.[27] In contrast, men above the poverty level had a higher prevalence of overweight than men below the poverty level.

Obesity is known to run in families, suggesting a hereditary component. The question that surrounds this observation is whether the disorder arises because of genetic endowment or environmental influences. Studies of twin and adopted children have provided evidence that heredity contributes to the disorder.[28] In a large study of 3580 male and female adoptees and their biologic and adoptive parents, a strong relationship was found between the BMI of the adoptees and those of their biologic parents and a lack of correlation between the BMI of the adoptees and those of their adoptive parents.[29] The amount of internal fat is influenced by heredity more than the amount of subcutaneous fat.[28]

Although genetic factors may explain much of the individual variations in terms of excess weight, environmental influences also must be taken into account. These influences include family dietary patterns, decreased level of activity due to labor-saving devices, reliance on the automobile for transportation, and easy access to food. The obese may be greatly influenced by the availability of food, its flavor, time of day, and other cues. The composition of the diet may also be a causal factor, and the percent-

age of dietary fat independent of total calorie intake may play a part in the development of obesity.[30] Psychological factors include using food as a reward, comfort, or means of getting attention. Two thirds of obese people, in one study, reported that they ate to cope with tension, anxiety, and mental fatigue.[31] Some people may overeat and use obesity as a means of avoiding threatening situations.

It is still uncertain whether obese people are less active or use calories more efficiently than lean people. It has been suggested that the increased prevalence of obesity in the United States has resulted from increased caloric intake together with a sedentary lifestyle and energy-saving conveniences. For example, the extension telephone can save 70 miles of walking each year—the equivalent of 2 to 3 lb of fat gain.[32] A review of the literature reveals that the obese are consistently more sedentary when compared with their normal-weight counterparts. They float more when swimming, play less tennis, and walk less per day. Even when a reasonable number of calories are consumed, fewer are expended because of inactivity.[33] A low rate of energy expenditure may contribute to the prevalence of obesity in some families.[33, 34] A recent study has shown that infants who become overweight by 3 months of age have a lower energy expenditure than normal-weight infants.[35]

TYPES OF OBESITY

Two types of obesity based on distribution of fat have been described: upper body obesity and lower body obesity. Upper body obesity is also referred to as *abdominal, android,* or *male obesity*. Lower body obesity is also known as *gluteal-femoral, gynoid, or female obesity*.[36] The obesity type is determined by dividing the waist by the hip circumference. A waist–hip ratio greater than 0.95 in men and 0.8 in women indicates upper body obesity (Fig. 43-4). Research suggests that fat distribution may be a more important factor for morbidity and mortality than overweight or obesity.[1]

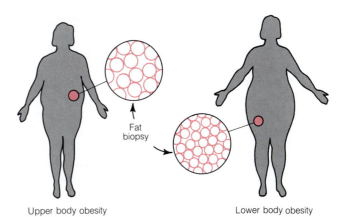

FIG. 43-4. Distribution of body fat and size of fat cells in persons with upper and lower body obesity. (Courtesy of Ahmed Kissebah, M.D., Ph.D., Medical College of Wisconsin, Milwaukee)

Fat biopsy

Upper body obesity

Lower body obesity

Upper body obesity is characterized by larger fat cells and is typically more predominant in men than women.[37] CT scans have shown that these people have a greater ratio of intraabdominal or visceral fat to subcutaneous fat.[38] Women are more likely to have abdominal obesity because of increased number of fat cells in this region. Triglycerides accumulate more readily in the gluteal-femoral adipocytes than in the abdominal fat cells. However, the abdominal cells are more lipolytically active. This places people with upper body obesity at greater risk for ischemic heart disease, stroke, and death independent of total body fat. They also tend to exhibit hypertension, elevated levels of triglycerides and decreased levels of high-density lipoproteins, hyperinsulinemia and diabetes mellitus, gallbladder disease, menstrual irregularities, and infertility.[38-43] Visceral fat is also associated with abnormalities of metabolic and sex hormone levels.[44-48] Weight loss causes a loss of visceral fat and has resulted in improvements in metabolic and hormonal abnormalities.[49, 52]

In terms of weight reduction, some studies have shown that people with upper body obesity are easier to treat than those with lower body obesity. Other studies have shown no difference in terms of success with weight-reduction programs between the two types of obesity.[53-58]

HEALTH RISKS ASSOCIATED WITH OBESITY

Social ostracism and isolation are not the only complications of obesity. Obese people are more likely to develop high blood pressure, hyperlipidemia, cardiovascular disease, glucose intolerance, insulin resistance, diabetes, infertility, and cancer of the endometrium, breast, prostate, and colon.[59] Obese women between 20 and 30 years of age have a sixfold increase in the risk of gallbladder disease; by age 60 years, nearly one third of obese women can expect to develop gallbladder disease.[59] In massively obese men, there may be a decrease in free testosterone.[60] Obese women often show less regularity in menstrual cycles, greater frequency of menstrual abnormalities, and infertility problems.[61]

The increased weight associated with obesity stresses the bones and joints, increasing the likelihood of arthritis. Because some drugs are lipophilic and exhibit increased distribution in fat tissue, the administration of these drugs, including some anesthetic agents, can be more dangerous in obese people.[62] If surgery is required, the obese person heals slower than the same age nonobese person.

It is only with morbid obesity that respiratory function is usually impaired. Sleep apnea and respiratory impairment are prevalent in the morbidly obese population (see Chapter 28). Other respiratory derangements include increased oxygen need to supply the increased body mass, increased respiratory rate to compensate for the resistance offered by chest and body fat, and decreased ventilation to the lower lungs.[63]

TREATMENT OF OBESITY

Studies have shown that weight reduction in obese people is beneficial to health. Data from the Framingham study showed a 10% reduction in weight for men was associated with a fall in serum glucose of 2.5 mg/dL, a fall in serum cholesterol of 11.3 mg/dL, a fall in systolic blood pressure of 6.6 mmHg, and a fall in uric acid of 0.33 mg/dL.[64] For each 10% reduction in body weight in men, these data predict an anticipated 20% decrease in coronary heart disease. Two factors that determine the need for treatment to produce weight loss are the health risk associated with total body fatness and the distribution of body fat. People with a BMI of 25 to 30 kg/m^2 have a low risk of health problems, those with a BMI of 30 to 35 kg/m^2 have a moderate risk, and those with a BMI above 40 kg/m^2 have a high risk.[65] The higher the proportion of upper body fat, the greater the risk of health problems. The risk of obesity is increased in people who are less than 40 years of age, who are of the male sex, or who have associated health problems such as diabetes mellitus, hypertension, or hyperlipidemia.

Treatment should be actively pursued in men with upper body obesity, even if no complications are present.[66] However, obese women who are at low risk do not require such pursuit. Most health benefits are achieved with a modest weight loss; achievement of ideal body weight as a goal is not necessary.[66]

There is no single effective treatment for obesity. Treatment methods should include nutritionally adequate weight-loss diets, behavior modification, exercise, social support,[67, 68] and, in situations of morbid obesity, surgical methods. Appetite suppressant medications are being investigated.[66]

With conventional techniques, 20% of participants lose 20 lb (9.1 kg) and maintain that loss over 2 years, whereas only 5% lose 40 lb (18.2 kg).[69] As a result, the success rate is discouraging. Some factors have been shown to be predictors of better outcomes. Close caregiver–client contact and length of that contact appear to be more important than the specific features of the weight-loss program. Careful client selection is necessary to include only those people who are sufficiently motivated.[70] Treatment matching is also possible if the clients are screened for health risk, motivation, previous attempts at weight loss, and eating disorders.[71] Because 25% to 50% of people who seek treatment for obesity are binge eaters, it is imperative that they receive treatment designed to help them with this problem.[66] This decreases frustration for the caregiver and the client and increases the likelihood of success. In addition, people who have better self-concepts, exercise more, and have greater social support are usually more successful in losing weight.

Weight-loss diets should have a reduced fat content and contain more complex carbohydrates with an emphasis on a wide variety of unprocessed foods.[9] Increasing the fiber content of the diet decreases caloric density, allowing a larger volume of food. Empty calories, such as fat, sucrose, and alcohol, should be limited. Diets that advocate large amounts of protein or fat or eating one food at a time provide no advantage and may even be harmful. A decrease of 500 to 1000 cal from maintenance usually produces a 1- to 2-lb (0.5- to 0.9-kg) weight loss per week.

Behavior modification focuses on new behaviors. These are achieved through record keeping, stimulus control, cognitive restructuring, and use of support systems. It has proven successful for achieving and maintaining weight loss and has also reported the lowest attrition rates. However, the average loss of any behavioral program reported in the literature is 1 lb per week, with 16 lb being the average total achieved.

Because many people need to lose a great deal more than 16 lb, newer forms of treatment have evolved. Very low-calorie diets are often used for severely obese people in conjunction with behavior modification techniques. The very low-calorie diets usually contain 400 to 800 cal of a liquid protein fortified with electrolytes and vitamins.[72, 73] Weight loss averages 2 to 4 lb (0.9 to 1.8 kg) per week. Because of the severe calorie restriction, these diets require medical supervision and frequent laboratory testing. Side effects include fatigue, orthostatic hypotension, and fluid and electrolyte disorders. Because severe calorie restriction is undesirable for pregnant and lactating women, these diets are contraindicated for that group, as well as for children, who still require protein for growth.

Exercise is an important part of a weight-loss program. It increases energy expenditure and helps preserve lean body tissue during weight loss. Continued exercise after weight loss predicts a greater chance of long-term success.[31] Exercise may also help to prevent the compensatory decrease in metabolic rate occurring with a reduction in calories that often makes weight loss difficult.[74] However, there is a high dropout rate from exercise programs. Many overweight people feel self-conscious, and some types of activities may prove to be uncomfortable or painful. For this reason, many weight-loss programs encourage walking for 10 to 15 minutes three to four times a week. The effect of this simple prescription may have long-lasting effects and may encourage other forms of exercise. Recommendations such as using the stairs versus the elevator and walking instead of using the car for short distances are encouraged. More strenuous types of exercise may require cardiovascular screening for establishing risk and developing an individualized exercise program.

The surgical treatment for obesity is usually reserved for people who meet the criteria for being extremely overweight (more than 100 lb or 45 kg).[75] Gastric surgeries intended to limit food intake but maintain normal digestion and absorption have proven to be relatively safe and effective.[58] Two types of gastric surgeries, gastric bypass and gastroplasty, are used for treating obesity.[65] Gastric bypass procedures establish a direct connection between the stomach and the small intestine. In one procedure, the stomach immediately adjacent to the esophagus is connected by way of a loop of intestine to the jejunum closing the larger portion of the stomach so that the stomach contents bypass part of the upper intestine. The smaller upper portion of the stomach is designed to hold 50 to 60 mL of food, causing a feeling of fullness with a small amount of food. Gastroplasty procedures are designed to reduce the size of the stomach and consist of banding or wrapping procedures. Complications of gastric surgeries can include anemia due to iron and vitamin B_{12} deficiency, as well as thiamine deficiency and its associated neuropathy. The use of intestinal bypass surgeries has largely been abandoned because of the high incidence of serious complications such as wound infections, pulmonary emboli, serious fluid and electrolyte disorders, liver disease, severe diarrhea, and malnutrition.[74]

CHILDHOOD OBESITY

Obesity is the most prevalent nutritional disorder affecting the pediatric population in the United States.[76] This is of concern because it is increasing rapidly, is accompanied by substantial morbidity, and there are few clinics equipped to treat it. A diagnosis of obesity is made when the triceps skinfold is greater than 85% or the weight for height is greater than 120% of ideal when controlled for age and sex.[77] In the United States, 25% and 30% of 6- to 12-year-old boys and girls, respectively, and 18% and 25% of 12- to 17-year-old boys and girls, respectively, are obese.[78] This is an increase of 54% in the 6- to 11-year-old age group and a 39% increase in the 12- to 17-year-old age group over a 15-year period.[76]

Childhood obesity is determined by a combination of hereditary and environmental factors. Children with one or two overweight parents are at highest risk; those with two overweight parents have a 70% risk of becoming obese. Television viewing is associated with consumption of calorie-dense snacks and decreased physical activity; time spent watching television has been directly related to obesity. Obese children appear to have a deficit in recognizing hunger sensations, stemming perhaps from parents who use food as gratification. These children may also have been exposed to an overprotected and perhaps rigid environment.[79]

Because adolescent obesity is predictive of adult obesity, treatment of childhood obesity is desirable.[80] Each child should be assessed and treated individually. Group treatment should only be used for those with less serious problems. The focus, however, should be on normalizing food intake, particularly fat intake, and increasing physical activity.[81] If weight gain can be slowed or maintained during growth, lean body mass increases and some of the abnormal metabolic effects of obesity may be reversed.[81] Family members need to be involved so they can learn to provide appropriate support and assist the child in taking responsibility for his or her own actions.

In summary, obesity is defined as excess body fat resulting from consumption of calories in excess of those expended for exercise and activities. Heredity, socioeconomic, culture, environmental factors, psychological influences, and activity levels have been implicated as causative factors in the development of obesity. The health risks associated with obesity include hyperlipidemia and cardiovascular disease including hypertension; insulin resistance, glucose intolerance, and diabetes mellitus; menstrual irregularities and infertility; cancer of the endometrium, breast, prostate, and colon; and gallbladder disease. There are two types of obesity—upper body and lower body obesity. Upper body obesity is associated with a higher incidence of complications. The treatment of obesity focuses on adequate weight-loss diets; behavior modification; exercise; social support; and, in situations of marked obesity, surgical methods. Obesity is the most prevalent nutritional disorder affecting the pediatric population in the United States.

■ UNDERNUTRITION

Undernutrition ranges from the selective deficiency of a single nutrient to starvation in which there is deprivation of all ingested nutrients. Undernutrition can result from willful eating behaviors as in anorexia nervosa and the binge–purge syndrome, lack of food availability, or health problems that impair food intake and decrease its absorption and use. There is general agreement that malnutrition is the most widespread cause of morbidity and mortality throughout the world. In the United States, poverty, homelessness, and hunger promote malnutrition among all age groups. Weight loss and malnutrition are common during illness, recovery from trauma, and hospitalization.

MALNUTRITION AND STARVATION

Malnutrition and starvation are conditions in which a person does not receive or is unable to use an adequate amount of calories and nutrients for body function. There is a wide range of causes of starvation. Some causes are willful (*e.g.*, the person with anorexia nervosa who does not consume enough food to maintain weight and health). People who are unable to absorb their food, such as those with Crohn's disease, are also at risk. Most cases of food deprivation result in semistarvation. Malnutrition can occur in people with chronic obstructive lung disease when their air hunger interferes with their ability to eat; eventually, the resultant malnutrition further complicates their respiratory status and food consumption. Studies indicate that 30% to 40% of people with chronic lung disease are significantly undernourished as determined by body weight and anthropometric estimates of body fat and muscle mass.[82, 83]

In malnutrition and starvation, the amount of food consumed and absorbed is drastically reduced. Most of the literature on malnutrition and starvation has dealt with infants and children of underdeveloped countries. The classic approach to the study of this population commonly divides cases into marasmus and kwashiorkor, with intermediate cases of marasmic kwashiorkor combining certain features of each condition. Marasmus is characterized by progressive wasting due to inadequate food intake that is equally deficient in calories and protein. The child with marasmus has a wasted appearance with stunted growth and loss of subcutaneous fat, but with relatively normal skin, hair, liver function, and affect. Kwashiorkor results from a protein deficiency. The term *kwashiorkor* comes from the African word meaning *the disease suffered by the displaced child*, because the condition develops soon after a child is displaced from the breast and placed on a starchy gruel feeding after the arrival of a new baby.[84] The child with kwashiorkor is characterized by edema, desquamating skin, discolored hair, hepatic enlargement, anorexia, and extreme apathy.

Depending on the prestarvation state, the metabolic events of starvation permit life to continue for months without caloric intake. In healthy, normally fed people, there is fuel enough to last for more than

80 days, assuming previous use of 2000 kcal/day; about 85% of these calories are stored in fat tissue, 14% in body proteins, and 1% in stored carbohydrate sources.[4] Despite the limited carbohydrate stores, which are depleted within 12 to 24 hours without food, a continuing supply of glucose is essential for survival. The central nervous system uses about 115 g of glucose a day, and red blood cells, bone marrow, kidneys, and peripheral nervous system use another 36 g of glucose.[4] One of the critical adaptive mechanisms in starvation is the production of new glucose (gluconeogenesis). The liver uses glycerol, lactate, and amino acids in the synthesis of glucose. The glycerol skeleton, obtained from triglycerides released from fat cells, plays a significant role in glucose synthesis. The predominant fuel for other tissues is fatty acids and ketones. For this reason, a state of ketosis is common during starvation.

Proteins have vital enzymatic and structural functions, and the body avoids using them as a fuel source until the late stages of starvation. Eventually, protein wasting ensues, with substantial weight loss, the most well-known and easily recognized sign of starvation. This weight loss is caused by loss of lean body tissue and fat along with diuresis. The importance of protein conservation to survival has been demonstrated in animal studies, in which a premorbid increase in nitrogen excretion due to protein use heralded the final stages of starvation.[4] Death from starvation rather than from hypoglycemia occurs when one third to one half of the body's protein is lost.[4]

Daily weight loss can range from 1 lb to several pounds depending on the stage of starvation.[4] Wound healing is poor, and the body is unable to fight off infection because of multiple immunologic malfunctions throughout the body.[5] The muscles used for breathing become weakened, and respiratory function becomes compromised as muscle proteins are used as a fuel source. A reduction in respiratory function has many implications, especially for people with burns, trauma, infection, chronic respiratory disease, or people who are being mechanically ventilated because of respiratory failure.[85, 86]

Although intellectual functioning remains intact despite the ketosis that occurs during starvation, depression and emotional lability are common. There is a diminished appetite and decreased desire for fluids due to altered hypothalamic function that occurs with ketosis. A marked decrease in libido is observed with starvation. The female experiences anovulation and amenorrhea, whereas the male experiences decreased testicular function.[5] The kidney does not go untouched by starvation. Calcium and phosphate are excreted as bone is dissolved, and uric acid is retained, which can cause gout.[4]

MALNUTRITION IN HOSPITALIZED PATIENTS

Malnutrition is much more prevalent in hospitalized patients than previously estimated. It has been estimated to occur in 30% to 50% of hospitalized people, despite socioeconomic status or illness experienced.[87] This malnutrition increases morbidity, mortality, incidence of complications, and length of hospital stay.

People may enter the hospital in a malnourished state. This malnutrition may be caused by poverty, inadequate food storage and preparation facilities, addiction to drugs or alcohol, adherence to fad diets, or even poorly fitting dentures. Furthermore, the hospitalized patient often finds eating a healthful diet difficult; they often have restrictions on food and water intake in preparation for tests and surgery. Pain, medications, special diets, and stress can decrease appetite. Even when the patient is well enough to eat, eating alone in a room where unpleasant treatments may be given is not conducive to eating.

Although hospitalized patients may appear to need fewer calories because they are on bedrest, their actual need for caloric intake may be higher because of other energy expenditures. For example, more calories are expended during fever when the metabolic rate is increased. There may also be an increased need for protein to support tissue repair after trauma or surgery.

Two types of malnutrition occur in the hospitalized patient: protein-calorie malnutrition and protein malnutrition.[88] Protein-calorie malnutrition is indicated when there is an unplanned weight loss of 10% in less than 2 weeks. It is characterized by loss of fat stores and muscle atrophy. Appetite is diminished, and diarrhea is a common complaint. There is little or no edema with protein-calorie malnutrition. Protein malnutrition is characterized by depressed visceral and endogenous protein synthesis. Plasma protein levels, particularly albumin, are decreased; this results in a decreased plasma colloidal pressure and development of edema (see Chapter 29). A hallmark of protein malnutrition is general apathy.[88] There may be an expression of appetite, yet often the foods that are eaten are high in carbohydrate and low in protein.

Cachexia is a state in which a person who is malnourished has marked wasting of body mass. The malnutrition that frequently accompanies heart failure is known as cardiac cachexia.[89] It is thought that this cachexia is caused by a decrease in the quality and quantity of food ingested, abnormal metabolism, and loss of nutrients by way of stool and urine. Decreased food intake could easily be influenced by the difficulty experienced in breathing, which is much more pronounced during eating. In addition, vascular congestion could influence stomach emptying and intestinal motility, causing abdominal distress. Medications used to manage congestive heart failure can also cause a decreased appetite (anorexia) or actually deplete the body of needed minerals. The fact that the person with heart disease seems to lose weight quicker than a person experiencing starvation suggests that more than just a decrease in the quality and quantity of food is taking place. A hypermetabolic state seems to be in process. More energy is expended to accomplish the respiratory work needed for survival.[88]

EATING DISORDERS

An eating disorder is a gross disturbance in eating behavior that jeopardizes a person's physical and psychological health. Eating disorders develop despite a normally functioning gastrointestinal tract and appetite. Anorexia nervosa and the binge–purge syndrome are chronic problems in which there is a preoccupation with food, eating, and weight loss.

ANOREXIA NERVOSA

Anorexia nervosa was first described in the scientific literature over a hundred years ago by Sir William Gull.[90] Anorexia nervosa is a self-starvation syndrome in which a person willingly loses an excessive amount of weight (20% or more of original body weight), exhibits muscle wasting, suffers from disturbances in body image, and experiences unreasonable fears about becoming obese. In actuality, the term *anorexia*, meaning loss of appetite, is a misnomer because hunger is actually felt; but, in this case, it is denied.

Anorexia nervosa is more prevalent in young women than men. The disorder typically begins in teenage women who are either obese or perceive themselves as being obese. An interest in weight reduction becomes an obsession with severely restricted caloric intake and, frequently, excessive physical exercise.

Many organ systems are affected by the malnutrition that occurs in people with anorexia nervosa. The severity of the abnormalities tends to be related to the degree of malnutrition and reversed with refeeding. The most frequent complication of anorexia is amenorrhea and loss of secondary sex characteristics with decreased levels of estrogen, which can eventually lead to osteoporosis. Constipation, cold intolerance and failure to shiver in the cold, bradycardia, hypotension, decreased heart size, electrocardiographic changes, blood abnormalities, and dry skin with lanugo (increased amounts of fine hair) are

common. Unexpected sudden deaths have been reported; the risk appears to increase as weight drops to less than 35% to 40% of ideal weight. It is believed that these deaths are due to myocardial degeneration and heart failure rather than heart dysrhythmias.[91]

The most exasperating aspect of the treatment of anorexia is the inability of the anorexic to recognize that there is a problem. Because anorexia is a form of starvation, it can lead to death if left untreated. Research suggests that anorexics can achieve a weight gain by way of treatment, although they may not reach ideal weight.[91] Frequently their abnormal eating pattern of avoiding high-calorie foods continues. There is no preferred single form of treatment. Psychological interventions are often helpful.

BINGE–PURGE SYNDROME

The binge–purge syndrome is an eating disorder that encompasses an array of distinctive behaviors, feelings, and thoughts. *Bulimia*, a term that literally means ox hunger, is characterized by secretive episodes or binges of eating large quantities of easily consumed high-calorie foods, such as doughnuts or ice cream. There are also periods of severe food restriction by way of dieting or fasting and purging to prevent weight gain. The purging behaviors that accompany binge eating distinguish bulimarexia from bulimia. Purging behaviors include self-induced vomiting, diuretic-induced diuresis, and laxative-induced diarrhea. Vomiting can be induced through the use of ipecac or self-stimulation of the gag reflex. Diuretics are used to reduce weight by increasing urinary excretion. An excessive intake of sorbitol-containing foods or abuse of laxatives causes weight loss through diarrhea.

People who experience the binge–purge syndrome are usually women in their late teens through the mid-thirties. Their weights may fluctuate but not to the dangerously low levels seen in people with anorexia nervosa. The thoughts and feelings of people with bulimia or bulimarexia range from fear of not being able to stop eating to a concern about gaining too much weight. They also experience feelings of sadness, anger, guilt, shame, and low self-esteem.

The complications of the binge–purge syndrome include those resulting from overeating, self-induced vomiting, and cathartic and diuretic abuse.[92] Among the complications of self-induced vomiting are dental disorders, fluid and electrolyte disorders, and parotitis. Dental abnormalities, such as sensitive teeth, increased dental caries, and periodontal disease, occur with frequent self-induced vomiting. This is because the frequent presence of vomitus with its high-acid content causes tooth enamel to dissolve. Esophagitis, dysphagia, and esophageal strictures are also common. With frequent vomiting, there is often reflux of gastric contents into the lower esophagus due to relaxation of the lower esophageal sphincter. Vomiting may lead to aspiration pneumonia, especially in intoxicated or debilitated people. Potassium, chloride, and hydrogen are lost in the vomitus, and frequent vomiting also predisposes to metabolic alkalosis with hypokalemia (see Chapters 29 and 30). An unexplained physical response to bulimarexia is the development of benign, painless parotid gland enlargement.

Use of emetic drugs and cathartics is associated with problems of drug overdose and abuse. Excessive doses of syrup of ipecac, which is sometimes used to induce vomiting, can produce serious cardiac disorders including conduction defects, dysrhythmias, and myocarditis. Chronic laxative use disrupts intestinal motility and normal bowel habits and causes higher stool electrolyte concentrations—the most frequent complication of potassium deficiency.

The primary goal of therapy for the binge–purge syndrome is to establish a regular healthful eating pattern. Unlike those who suffer from anorexia nervosa, the person with bulimia or bulimarexia is upset by the behaviors practiced and the thoughts and feelings experienced and is more willing to accept help. People with bulimia or bulimarexia who have been successfully treated for their eating disorder have reported that making meal plans, eating a balanced diet of three regular meals a day, avoiding high sugar foods and other binge foods, recording food intake, recording binge/vomit episodes, exercising regularly, finding alternative activities, and avoiding alcohol and drugs are helpful in maintaining their more healthful eating behaviors after treatment.[93]

In summary, undernutrition can range from a selective deficiency of a single nutrient to starvation in which there is a deprivation of all ingested nutrients. Malnutrition and starvation are among the most widespread causes of morbidity and mortality in the world. The body adapts to starvation through the use of fat stores and glucose synthesis to supply the energy needs of the central nervous system. Malnutrition is common during illness, recovery from trauma, and hospitalization. The effects of malnutrition and starvation on body function are widespread. They include loss of muscle mass, impaired wound healing, impaired immunologic function, decreased appetite, loss of calcium and phosphate from bone, anovulation and amenorrhea in women, and decreased testicular function in men. A reduction in respiratory muscle function that occurs with starvation has many implications for people with lung disease, infection, and trauma. Anorexia nervosa and the binge–purge syndrome are eating disorders that result in malnutrition. In anorexia nervosa, distorted attitudes about eating lead to serious weight loss and malnutrition. Bulimia is characterized by binge eating; bulimarexia is characterized by binge eating and purging with self-induced vomiting and use of laxatives or diuretics.

■ REFERENCES

1. Bray, G.A., & Gray, D.S. (1988). Obesity. Part 1—Pathogenesis. *Western Journal of Medicine, 149,* 429.
2. Cormack, D.H. (1987). *Ham's histology* (9th ed., pp. 181, 183). Philadelphia: J.B. Lippincott.
3. Timms-Hagen, J. (1984). Thermogenesis in brown adipose tissue as an energy buffer. *New England Journal of Medicine, 311,* 1549.
4. Sauded, K., & Felig, P. (1976). The metabolic events of starvation. *American Journal of Medicine, 60,* 117.
5. Cahill, C.F., Jr. (1976). Starvation in man. *Clin Endocrinol Metab, 5*(2), 405.
6. Krause, M.W., & Mahan, L.K. (1984). *Food, nutrition and diet therapy.* Philadelphia: WB Saunders.
7. Committee on Dietary Allowances, Food Nutrition Board (1980). *Recommended dietary allowances* (9th ed.). National Academy of Sciences—National Research Council. Washington, DC: National Academy Press.
8. Report of the National Cholesterol Education Program Expert Panel on Detection, Evaluation, and Treatment of High Blood Cholesterol in Adults. (1988). *Archives of Internal Medicine, 148,* 36.
9. U.S. Department of Agriculture, U.S. Department of Health and Human Services. (1985, August). *Nutrition and your health: Dietary guidelines for Americans* (2nd ed.). Home and Garden Bulletin No, 232, Washington DC: USDA/USDHHS.
10. Schneeman, B.O. (1987). Dietary fiber: Comments on interpreting recent research. *Journal of the American Dietetic Association, 87,* 1163.
11. Trowell, H. (1986). Physiologic role of dietary fiber: A ten year review. *Contemporary Nutrition, 11*(7), 1.
12. Grant, J.P. (1986). Nutritional assessment in clinical practice. *Nutr Clin Prac, 1,* 3.
13. Baker, J.P., Detsky, A.S., Wesson, D.E., et al. (1982). Nutritional assessment: A comparison of clinical judgement and objective measures. *New England Journal of Medicine, 306,* 969.
14. Blackburn, G.L. (1987). Guest editorial. *Topics in Clinical Nutrition, 2,* 1.
15. Blackburn, G.L. (1987). Obesity and weight loss. *Topics in Clinical Nutrition, 2,* viii.
16. Burton, B.T., Foster, W.R., Hirsh, J., et al. (1985). Health implications of obesity. An NIH Consensus Development Conference. *International Journal of Obesity, 9,* 155.
17. Johnson, F.E. (1982). Relationship between body composition and anthropometry. *Human Biology, 54,* 221.
18. Lohman, T.G. (1987). Skinfolds and body density and their relationship to body fatness: A review. *American Journal of Clinical Nutrition, 46,* 537.
19. Womersley, J., & Durnin, J.V.G.A. (1977). A comparison of skinfold method with extent of "overweight" and various weight–height relationships in the assessment of obesity. *British Journal of Nutrition, 38,* 271.
20. Mueller, W.H., Wear, M.L., Hanis, C.L., et al. (1986). Body circumferences as alternatives to skinfold measurements of body fat distribution in Mexican-Americans. *International Journal of Obesity, 11,* 309.
21. Fanelli, M.T., Kuzmarski, R.J., & Hirsch, M. (1988). Estimation of body fat from ultrasound measurements of subcutaneous fat and circumferences in obese women. *International Journal of Obesity, 12,* 125.
22. Lukaski, H.C., Bolonchuk, W.W., & Hall, C.B. (1986). Validation of tetrapolar bioelectrical impedance method to assess body composition. *Journal of Applied Physiology, 60,* 1327.

23. Segal, K.R., VanLoan, M., & Fitzgerrald, P.I. (1988). Lean body mass estimation by bioelectrical impedance analysis: A four-site cross-validation study. *American Journal of Clinical Nutrition, 47*, 7.

24. Coh, S.H. (1985). How valid are bioelectrical impedance measurements of body composition studies? *American Journal of Clinical Nutrition, 42*, 889.

25. Epstein, L.H., Wing, R.R., & Voloski, A. (1985). Childhood obesity. *Pediatric Clinics of North America, 32*(April), 2.

26. Bray, G.A. (1987). Overweight is risking fate. *Annals of the New York Academy of Sciences, 499*, 14.

27. *Plan and operation of the National Health and Nutrition Examination Survey, 1976–1980.* (1981). DDHS Publication (PHS) 81–1317, Vital and Health Statistics, Series 1, No. 15. Hyattsville, MD: National Center for Health Statistics.

28. Bouchard, C., Perusse, L., LeBlanc, C., et al. (1988). Inheritance and the amount and distribution of body fat. *International Journal of Obesity, 12*, 205.

29. Stunkard, A.J., Throkild, I.A., Sorenson, T., et al. (1986). An adoption study of human obesity. *New England Journal of Medicine, 314*, 193.

30. Romieu, I., Willett, W.C., Stamfler, M.J., et al. (1988). Energy intake and other determinants of human body fat. *American Journal of Nutrition, 47*, 406.

31. Foreyt, J.P., & Goodrich, G.K. (1991). Factors common to successful therapy for the obese patient. *Medicine and Science in Sports and Exercise, 23*, 292.

32. Ruvissin, E., Lillioja, A., Knowler, W.C., et al. (1988). Reduced rate of energy expenditure for body-weight gain. *New England Journal of Medicine, 318*, 467.

33. Stern, J.S. (1984). Is obesity a disease of inactivity? In A.J. Stunkard & E. Stellar (Eds.). *Eating and its disorders.* New York: Raven Press.

34. Bogardus, C., Lillioja, S., & Ravussin, E., et al. (1987). Familial dependence of the resting metabolic rate. *New England Journal of Medicine, 315*, 96.

35. Roberts, S.B., Savage, J., Coward, W., et al. (1988). Energy expenditure and intake in infants born to lean and overweight mothers. *New England Journal of Medicine, 318*, 461.

36. Bistrian, B.R. (1981). The medical treatment of obesity. *Archives of Internal Medicine, 141*, 429.

37. Krotkiewski, M., Bjorntorp, P., & Sjostrom, P. (1983). Impact of obesity on metabolism in men and women. *Journal of Clinical Investigation, 72*, 1150.

38. Ashwell, M., Cole, T.J., & Dixon, A.K. (1985). Obesity: New insight into the anthropometric classification of fat distribution shown by computed tomography. *British Journal of Medicine, 290*, 1692.

39. Bjorntorp, P. (1985). Adipose tissue in obesity. In J. Hirsch & T.B. Van Itallie (Eds.). *Recent advances in obesity research* (4th ed., p. 163). London: John Libby.

40. Kissebah, A.H., Vydelingum, N., Murray, R., et al. (1982). Relationship of body fat distribution to metabolic consequences of obesity. *Journal of Clinical Endocrinology and Metabolism, 54*, 254.

41. Kalkhoff, R.K., Hartz, A.H., Rupley, D., et al. (1983). Relationship of body fat distribution to blood pressure, carbohydrate tolerance, and plasma lipids in healthy obese women. *Journal of Laboratory and Clinical Medicine, 102*, 621.

42. Ohlson, L.O., Larsson, B., & Svardsudd, K. (1985). The influence of body fat distribution on the incidence of diabetes mellitus. *Diabetes, 34*, 1055.

43. Kissebah, A.H., Freedman, D.S., & Peiris, A.N. (1989). Health risks of obesity. *Medical Clinics of North America, 73*(1), 111.

44. Fujoka, S., Matsuzawa, Y., Tokunga, K., et al. (1987). Contribution of intra-abdominal fat accumulation to the impairment of glucose and lipid metabolism in human obesity. *Metabolism, 36*, 54.

45. Despres, J.P., Nadeau, A., Tremblay, A., et al. (1989). Role of deep abdominal fat in the association between regional adipose tissue distribution and glucose tolerance in obese women. *Diabetes, 38*, 304.

46. Peiris, A.N., Sothmann, M.S., Hennes, M.I., et al. (1989). Relative contribution of obesity and body fat distribution to alterations in glucose and insulin homeostasis: Predictive values of selected indices in premenopausal women. *American Journal of Clinical Nutrition, 49*, 758.

47. Gillum, R.F. (1987). The association of body-fat distribution with hypertension, hypertensive heart disease, cardiovascular heart disease, diabetes, and cardiovascular risk factors in men and women ages 18 to 79 years. *Journal of Chronic Diseases, 40*, 421.

48. Seidell, J.C., Bjornstrop, P., Sjostrom, L., et al. (1989). Regional distribution of muscle and fat mass in men—new insight into the risk of abdominal obesity using computed tomography. *International Journal of Obesity, 13*, 289.

49. Fujoka, S., Matsuzawa, Y., Tounaja, K., et al. (1991). Improvement of glucose and lipid metabolism associated with selective reduction of intra-abdominal fat in premenstrual women with visceral fat obesity. *International Journal of Obesity, 15*, 853.

50. Stallone, D.D., Stunkard, A.J., Wadden, T.A., et al. (1991). Weight loss and body fat distribution: A feasibility study using computerized tomography. *International Journal of Obesity, 15*, 775.

51. Pleuss, J.A., Goldstein, M.D., Hoffman, R.G., et al. (1991). Factors differentially affecting regional fat loss with diet. *International Journal of Obesity, 15*(Suppl 3), 37.

52. Pleuss, J.A., Hoffman, R.G., Sonnenberg, C.E., et al. (1993). Effects of abdominal fat loss on insulin and androgen levels. *Obesity Research, 1*(Suppl. 1), 25F.

53. Wadden, T.A., Stunkard, A.J., Johnston, F.E., et al. (1988). Body fat distribution in adult obese women. II. Changes in fat distribution accompanying weight reduction. *American Journal of Clinical Nutrition, 47*, 229.

54. den Besten, C., Vansant, G., Westrate, J.A., et al. (1988). Resting metabolic rate and diet-induced thermogenesis in abdominal and gluteal-femoral women before and after weight reduction. *American Journal of Clinical Nutrition, 47*, 840.

55. Krotkiewski, M., Sjostrom, L., Bjorntorp, P., et al. (1975). Adipose tissue cellularity in relation to prognosis for weight reduction. *International Journal of Obesity, 1*, 395.

56. Vansant, G., den Besten, C., Westrate, J., et al. (1988). Body fat distribution and the prognosis for weight reduction: Preliminary observations. *International Journal of Obesity, 12*, 133.

57. Brownell, K.D. (1984). The psychology and physiology of obesity: Implications for screening and treatment. *Journal of the American Dietetic Association, 84*, 406.

58. Kissebah, A.K., Freedman, D.S., & Peiris, A.N. (1989). Health risks of obesity. *Medical Clinics of North America, 73*(1), 111.

59. Hartz, A.J., Rupley, D.C., & Rimm, A.A. (1984). The association of girth measurements with disease in

32,856 women. *American Journal of Epidemiology, 119,* 71.

60. Kley, H.K., Solbach, H.G., McKinnan, J.C., et al. (1979). Testosterone decrease and estrogen increase in male patients with obesity. *Acta Endocrinologica, 91,* 553.

61. Hartz, A.J., Barboriak, P.N., Wong, A., et al. (1979). The association of obesity with infertility and associated menstrual abnormalities in women. *International Journal of Obesity, 3,* 57.

62. Abernethy, D.R., & Greenblatt, D.J. (1986). Drug disposition in humans: An update. *Clinical Pharmacokinetics, 11,* 199.

63. Wittels, E.H. (1985). Obesity and hormonal factors in sleep and sleep apnea. *Medical Clinics of North America, 69,* 6.

64. Ashley, F.W., Jr., & Kannel, W.B. (1974). Relation of weight change to changes in atherosclerotic traits: The Framingham Study. *Journal of Chronic Diseases, 27,* 103.

65. Bray, G.A., & Gray, D.S. (1988). Obesity. Part 2—Treatment. *Western Journal of Medicine, 149,* 555.

66. Stunkard, A.J. (1992). Changes in the indications for the treatment of obesity. *International Journal of Obesity, 16*(Suppl 1), vii.

67. Council on Scientific Affairs. (1988). Treatment of obesity in adults. *Journal of the American Medical Society, 260*(17), 2547.

68. Position of the American Dietetic Association: Optimal weight as a healthy promotion strategy. (1989). *Journal of the American Dietetic Association, 89,* 1814.

69. Leiter, L.A. (1986). Obesity: Overview of pathogenesis and treatment. *Canadian Journal of Physiology and Pharmacology, 64,* 824.

70. Brownell, K. (1982). Obesity: Understanding and treating a serious, prevalent, and refractory disorder. *Journal of Consulting and Clinical Psychology, 50,* 820.

71. Brownell, K.D., & Kramer, F.M. (1989). Behavioral management of obesity. *Medical Clinics of North America, 73*(1), 185.

72. Wadden, T.A., Van Itallie, T.B., & Blackburn, G.L. (1990). Responsible and irresponsible use of very low-calorie diets in the multidisciplinary treatment of obesity. *Journal of the American Medical Society, 263,* 83.

73. *The Medical Letter on Drugs and Therapeutics, 31*(787), 22, 1989.

74. Ackerman, S. (1983). The management of obesity. *Hospital Practice, 18,* 117.

75. Gastrointestinal surgery for severe obesity. (1992). National Institutes of Health Consensus Development Conference Statement. *American Journal of Clinical Nutrition, 55,* 6155.

76. Gormaker, S.L., Dietz, W.H., Sobol, et al. (1987). Increasing pediatric obesity in the United States. *American Journal of Diseases of Children, 141,* 535.

77. Dietz, W.H. (1983). Childhood obesity: Susceptibility, cause, and management. *Journal of Pediatrics, 103,* 676.

78. Dietz, W.H. (1986). Prevention of childhood obesity. *Pediatric Clinics of North America, 33,* 823.

79. Brone, R.J., & Fisher, C.B. (1988). Determinants of adolescent obesity: A comparison with anorexia nervosa. *Adolescence, 23,* 155.

80. Eck, L.H., Klesges, R.C., Hanson, C.L., et al. (1992). Children at familial risk for obesity: An examination of dietary intake, physical activity and weight status. *International Journal of Obesity, 16,* 71.

81. Rees, J.M. (1990). Managment of obesity in adolescence. *Medical Clinics of North America, 74,* 1275.

82. Braun, S.R., Keim, N.L., Dixon, R.M., et al. (1984). The prevalence and determinants of nutritional changes in chronic obstructive lung disease. *Chest, 86,* 559.

83. Hunter, A.M.B., Carey, M.A., & Larsh, H.W. (1981). The nutritional status of patients with chronic obstructive lung disease. *American Review of Respiratory Disease, 124,* 376.

84. Kinney, J.M., & Weisman, C. (1986). Forms of malnutrition in stressed and unstressed patients. *Clinics in Chest Medicine, 7,* 19.

85. Dudely, D.F. (1986). Malnutrition and respiratory muscles. *Clinics in Chest Medicine, 7,* 91.

86. Openbrier, D.R., & Covey, M. (1987). Ineffective breathing pattern related to malnutrition. *Nursing Clinics of North America, 22,* 225.

87. Mullen, J.L. (1981). Consequences of malnutrition in the surgical patient. *Surgical Clinics of North America, 61*(June), 3.

88. Dougherty, S. (1988). The malnourished respiratory patient. *Critical Care Nurse, 8,* 13.

89. Pittman, J.G., & Cohen, P. (1964). The pathogenesis of cardiac cachexia. *New England Journal of Medicine, 271,* 403.

90. Gull, W.W. (1974). Anorexia nervosa. *Trans Clin Soc London, 7,* 22.

91. Drossman, D.A. (1983). Anorexia nervosa: A comprehensive approach. *Advances in Internal Medicine, 28,* 339.

92. Halmi, K.A., Falk, J.R., & Schwartz, E. (1981). Binge-eating and vomiting: A survey of a college population. *Psychological Medicine, 11,* 695.

93. Gannon, M.A., & Mitchell, J.E. (1986). Subjective evaluation of treatment by patients treated for bulimia. *Journal of the American Dietetic Association, 86,* 4.

MECHANISMS OF ENDOCRINE CONTROL

■ OBJECTIVES

After you have studied this chapter, you should be able to meet the following objectives:

■ Characterize a hormone.
■ State a difference between the synthesis of protein hormones and that of steroid hormones.
■ Describe four mechanisms of hormone delivery to target cells.
■ State three ways in which hormones are inactivated or metabolized.
■ State the function of a hormone receptor.
■ Describe two alterations in hormone receptors that could be used to explain changes in hormone action.

■ State the difference between fixed hormone receptor interactions and mobile hormone receptor interactions.
■ Describe the role of the hypothalamus in regulating pituitary control of endocrine function.
■ State the major difference between positive and negative feedback control mechanisms.
■ Compare endocrine hypofunction and endocrine hyperfunction.
■ Describe the radioimmunoassay method of measuring hormone levels.

The endocrine system is involved in all of the integrative aspects of life, including growth, sex differentiation, metabolism, and adaptation to an ever-changing environment. This chapter focuses on general aspects of endocrine function, organization of the endocrine system, hormone receptors and hormone actions, and regulation of hormone levels.

■ THE ENDOCRINE SYSTEM

The endocrine system uses hormones as a means of integrating body functions. Although the endocrine system was once thought to consist solely of discrete *endocrine glands* and their hormones, termed the *classic endocrine system*, it is now known that a number of

Carol Mattson Porth: PATHOPHYSIOLOGY: CONCEPTS OF ALTERED HEALTH STATES, 4th ed. © 1994, 1990, 1986, 1982 J.B. Lippincott Company

other chemical messengers modulate the body processes. Hormones of the classic endocrine system are synthesized by endocrine glands, secreted into the bloodstream, and then transported to distant sites, or target cells, where they exert their action.

In addition to the hormones of the classic endocrine system, a number of hormonal peptides have now been identified; these peptides are produced by what is sometimes referred to as the *diffuse endocrine system*. Unlike the well-defined glands of the classic endocrine system, the diffuse endocrine system is dispersed throughout various organs and cells and is intermingled with nonendocrine cells. A great deal of mystery still surrounds these hormonal peptides. A number of them have been found in both brain and peripheral tissues, and their wide range of actions suggests that they act locally in a number of ways, depending on the tissues that they serve. Perhaps the most interesting of these peptides are the endorphins and enkephalins (see Chapter 48). The neurotransmitters (neurohormones), such as the catecholamines (epinephrine, norepinephrine, and dopamine), are also chemical mediators that are synthesized by nerve cells and released from nerve endings.

HORMONES

Hormones are generally thought of as *chemical messengers* that are transported in body fluids. Hormones do not initiate reactions; rather, they are modulators of body and cellular responses. Most hormones are present in the blood at all times, but in greater or lesser amounts depending on the needs of the body. Hormones can produce either a generalized or a localized effect.

A characteristic of hormones is that a single hormone can exert its various effects in different tissues, or, conversely, a single function can be regulated by several hormones. For example, estradiol, which is produced by the ovary, can act on the ovarian follicles to promote their maturation, on the uterus to stimulate its growth and maintain the cyclic changes in the uterine mucosa, on the mammary gland to stimulate ductal growth, on the hypothalamic-pituitary system to regulate the secretion of gonadotrophins and prolactin, and on general metabolic processes to affect adipose tissue distribution. Lipolysis—the release of free fatty acids from adipose tissue—is an example of a single function that is regulated by several hormones, including the catecholamines, glucagon, secretin, and prolactin. Table 44-1 lists the major functions and sources of body hormones.

STRUCTURAL CLASSIFICATION

Hormones have diverse structures ranging from single amino acid to complex proteins and lipids. Hormones are generally divided in three categories according to their structure: (1) amines and amino acids, (2) peptides and polypeptides, and (3) steroids. The first category, the amines, includes norepinephrine, epi-

TABLE 44-1. CLASSES OF HORMONES BASED ON STRUCTURE

| Amines and Amino Acids | PEPTIDES AND PROTEINS | |
	Peptides, Polypeptides, and Protein	STEROIDS
Epinephrine	Adrenocorticotropic hormone (ACTH)	Aldosterone
Norepinephrine	Angiotensin	Glucocorticoids
Dopamine	Calcitonin	Estrogens
Thyroid hormones	Cholecystokinin	Progesterone
	Erythropoietin	Testosterone
	Follicle-stimulating hormone (FSH)	
	Gastrin	
	Glucagon	
	Growth hormone	
	Insulin	
	Luteinizing hormone (LH)	
	Oxytocin	
	Parathyroid hormone	
	Prolactin	
	Secretin	
	Thyroid-stimulating hormone (TSH)	
	Antidiuretic hormone (ADH)	

nephrine, and dopamine, which are derived from a single amino acid (tyrosine), and the thyroid hormones, which derive from two iodinated tyrosine amino acid residues. The second category, the peptides and polypeptides, can be as small as a thyroid-releasing hormone, which contains three amino acids, and as large and complex as growth hormone and follicle-stimulating hormone, which have about 200 amino acids. The third category comprises the steroid hormones, which are derivatives of cholesterol. Table 44-2 presents a listing of hormones according to structure.

SYNTHESIS

The mechanisms for hormone synthesis vary with hormone structure. Protein and peptide hormones are synthesized and stored in granules or vesicles within the cytoplasm of the cell until secretion is required. The lipid-soluble steroid hormones are released as they are synthesized.

Protein and peptide hormones are synthesized in the rough endoplasmic reticulum in a manner similar to the synthesis of other proteins (see Chapter 1). The appropriate amino acid sequence is dictated by messenger RNAs from the nucleus. Usually synthesis involves the production of a precursor hormone, which is modified by the addition of peptides or sugar units. These precursor hormones often contain extra peptide units that ensure proper folding of the molecule and insertion of essential linkages. If extra amino acids are present, as in insulin, the precursor hormone is called a *prohormone*. Following synthesis and sequestration in the endoplasmic reticulum, the protein and peptide hormones move into the Golgi complex where they are packaged in granules or vesicles. It is in the Golgi complex that prohormones are converted into hormones.

TABLE 44-2. FUNCTIONAL CLASSIFICATION OF HORMONES

FUNCTION	HORMONE	MAJOR SOURCE
Control of water and electrolyte metabolism	Aldosterone	Adrenal cortex
	Antidiuretic hormone (ADH)	Posterior pituitary
	Calcitonin	C cells, thyroid
	Parathyroid hormone	Parathyroid
	Angiotensin	Kidney
Control of gastrointestinal function	Cholecystokinin	Gastrointestinal tract
	Gastrin	Gastrointestinal tract
	Secretin	Gastrointestinal tract
Regulation of energy, metabolism, and growth	Glucagon	α cells, pancreatic islets
	Insulin	β cells, pancreatic islets
	Growth hormone	Anterior pituitary
	Thyroid hormones	Thyroid gland
Neurotransmitters	Dopamine	CNS
	Epinephrine	Adrenal medulla
	Norepinephrine	Adrenal medulla and nervous system
Reproductive function	Chorionic gonadotropins	Placenta
	Estrogens	Ovary
	Oxytocin	Posterior pituitary
	Progesterone	Ovary
	Prolactin	Anterior pituitary
	Testosterone	Testes
Stress and control of inflammation	Glucocorticoids	Adrenal cortex
Tropic hormones (regulation of other hormone levels)	Adrenocorticotropic hormone (ACTH)	Anterior pituitary
	Follicle-stimulating hormone (FSH)	Anterior pituitary
	Luteinizing hormone (LH)	Anterior pituitary
	Thyroid-stimulating hormone (TSH)	Anterior pituitary

Steroid hormones are synthesized within the smooth endoplasmic reticulum, and steroid-secreting cells can be identified by their large amounts of smooth endoplasmic reticulum. Certain steroids serve as precursors for the production of other hormones. In the adrenal cortex, for example, progesterone and other steroid intermediates are enzymatically converted into either aldosterone, cortisol, or androgens (see Chapter 45).

Hormones that are released into the bloodstream circulate either as free molecules or as hormones attached to transport carriers. Peptide hormones and protein hormones generally circulate unbound in the blood. Steroid hormones and thyroid hormone are carried by specific proteins synthesized in the liver. The extent of carrier binding influences the rate at which hormones leave the blood and enter the cells. The half-life of a hormone—the time it takes for the body to reduce the concentration of the hormone by one-half—is positively correlated with its percentage of protein binding. Thyroxine, which is more than 99% protein bound, has a half-life of 6 days. Aldosterone, which is only 15% bound, has a half-life of only 25 minutes. Drugs that compete with a hormone for binding with the transport carrier molecules increase hormone action by increasing the availability of the active unbound hormone. For example, aspirin competes with thyroid hormone for binding to transport proteins; when the drug is administered to persons with excessive levels of circulating thyroid hormone (*i.e.*, thyroid crisis), serious effects occur.

METABOLISM AND RATE OF REACTION

Hormones secreted by endocrine cells must be continuously inactivated to prevent their accumulation. Both intracellular and extracellular mechanisms participate in the termination of hormone function. Some hormones are enzymatically inactivated at receptor sites where they exert their action. Peptide hormones have a short life span and are inactivated by enzymes that split peptide bonds. They are inactivated mainly in the liver and kidneys. As was previously mentioned, steroid hormones are bound to protein carriers for transport and are inactive in the bound state. Their activity depends on the availability of transport hormones. Unbound adrenal and gonadal steroid hormones are conjugated in the liver, which renders them inactive, and then excreted in the bile or urine. Thyroid hormones are also transported by carrier molecules. The free hormone is rendered inactive by the removal of amino acids (deamination) in the tissues and is also conjugated in the liver and eliminated in the bile.

Hormones react at different rates. The neurotransmitters, such as epinephrine, have a reaction time of milliseconds. Thyroid hormone, on the other hand, requires days for its effect to occur. Hormones are continually being metabolized or inactivated and removed from the body.

MECHANISMS OF ACTION

Hormones exert their action by binding to specific receptor sites located on the surfaces of the target cells. The function of these receptors is to recognize a specific hormone and translate the hormonal signal into a cellular response. The structure of these receptors varies in a manner that allows target cells to respond to one hormone and not to others. For example, receptors in the thyroid are specific for the thyroid-stimulating hormone, whereas receptors on the gonads respond to the gonadotropic hormones.

The response of a target cell to the action of a hormone will vary with the *number* of receptors present and with the *affinity* of these receptors for hormone binding. A variety of factors influence the number of receptors that are present on target cells and their affinity for hormone binding (Fig. 44-1).

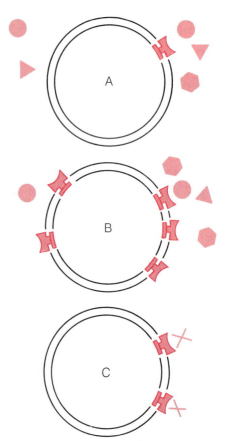

FIG. 44-1. (**A**) The role of cell-surface receptors in mediating the action of hormones. Hormone action is affected by (**B**) the number of receptors that are present and by (**C**) the affinity of these receptors for hormone binding.

There are generally 2,000 to 10,000 hormone receptor molecules per cell. The number of hormone receptors on a cell may be altered for any of several reasons. Antibodies may destroy the receptor proteins. Sustained levels of excess hormone may decrease the number of receptors per cell in a process called *down regulation*. This acts to modify the effect of chronic exposure to a given hormone. In some instances, the reverse effect occurs, and an increase in hormone levels appears to recruit its own receptors (*up regulation*), increasing the sensitivity of the cell to the hormone. Obesity has been shown to cause a decrease in the number of insulin receptors that are present on fat cells, and it is speculated that this may influence impaired glucose tolerance in the obese noninsulin-dependent diabetic. On the other hand, it has been shown that the oral hypoglycemic drugs, the sulfonylureas, cause an increase in the number of insulin receptors on body cells.

The affinity of receptors for binding hormones is also affected by a number of conditions. For example, the *pH* of the body fluids plays an important role in the affinity of insulin receptors. In ketoacidosis, the lowering of the *pH* reduces insulin binding.

Hormone–receptor interactions go about the process of modulating cell activity in one of two ways. One type of response occurs with the peptide hormones, which circulate in the blood in their free state. These hormones interact with fixed membrane receptors in a manner that incites the release of a *second messenger* (primarily cyclic AMP), which in turn activates a series of enzyme reactions that serve to alter cell function (Fig. 44-2). Glucagon, for example, incites glycogen breakdown by way of the second messenger system.

A second type of receptor mechanism is involved in mediating the action of hormones, such as the steroid and the thyroid hormones, which are transported in body fluids attached to carrier proteins (see Fig. 44-2). These hormones, being lipid-soluble, pass freely through the cell membrane and then attach to intracellular messengers that alter processes within the cell. For many hormones this second messenger is unknown. This hormone–messenger complex causes activation or repression of intracellular mechanisms such as gene activity with subsequent production of messenger RNA and protein synthesis. Chart 44-1 lists hormones that act by the two types of receptors.

CONTROL OF HORMONE LEVELS

Hormone secretion varies widely over a 24-hour period. Some hormones, such as growth hormone and adrenocorticotropic hormone (ACTH), have diurnal fluctuations that vary with the sleep–awakening cy-

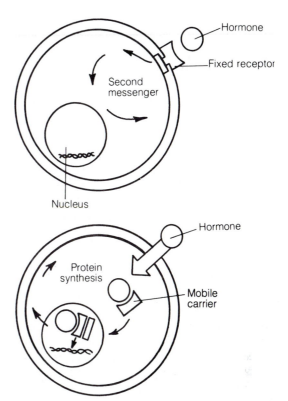

FIG. 44-2. The two types of hormone–receptor interactions: the fixed membrane receptor (**top**) and the intracellular mobile receptor (**bottom**).

cle. Others, such as the female sex hormones, are secreted in a complicated cyclic manner. The levels of hormones like insulin and antidiuretic hormone (ADH) are regulated by feedback mechanisms that monitor the amount of organic and inorganic substances present in the body. The levels of many of the

---

CHART 44-1: HORMONE–RECEPTOR INTERACTIONS

Fixed Messenger Interactions

Glucagon
Insulin
Epinephrine
Parathyroid hormone
Thyroid-stimulating hormone (TSH)
Adrenocorticotropic hormone (ACTH)
Follicle-stimulating hormone (FSH)
Luteinizing hormone (LH)
Antidiuretic hormone (ADH)
Secretin

Mobile Hormone–Carrier–Nuclear Interactions

Estrogens
Testosterone
Progesterone
Adrenal cortical hormones
Thyroid hormones

hormones are regulated by feedback mechanisms that involve the hypothalamic–pituitary–target cell system.

HYPOTHALAMIC–PITUITARY REGULATION

Because the integration of body function relies on input from both the nervous system and the endocrine system, it seems logical that input from the nervous system would participate in the regulation of hormone levels. In this respect, the hypothalamus and the pituitary (hypophysis) act as an integrative link between the central nervous system and the many endocrine-mediated functions of the body. These two structures are connected by blood flow in the hypophyseal portal system, which begins in the hypothalamus and drains into the anterior pituitary gland, and by the nerve axons that connect the supraoptic and paraventricular nuclei of the hypothalamus with the posterior pituitary gland (Fig. 44-3). Embryologically, the anterior pituitary gland developed from glandular tissue and the posterior pituitary developed from neural tissue.

The Endocrine Hypothalamus. The synthesis and release of anterior pituitary hormones are largely regulated by the action of releasing or inhibiting hormones from the hypothalamus, which is the coordinating center of the brain for endocrine, behavioral, and autonomic nervous system function. It is at the level of the hypothalamus that emotion, pain, body temperature, and other neural input are communicated to the endocrine system. The posterior pituitary hormones, ADH and oxytocin, are synthesized in the cell bodies of neurons in the hypothalamus with axons that travel to the posterior pituitary. The release and function of ADH are discussed in Chapter 29.

Anterior Pituitary Gland. The pituitary gland has been called the "master gland" because its hormones control the function of a number of target glands or cells. Hormones produced by the anterior pituitary control body growth and metabolism (growth hormone), function of the thyroid gland (thyroid-stimulating hormone), glucocorticoid hormone levels (adrenocorticotropic hormone), function of the gonads (follicle-stimulating and luteinizing

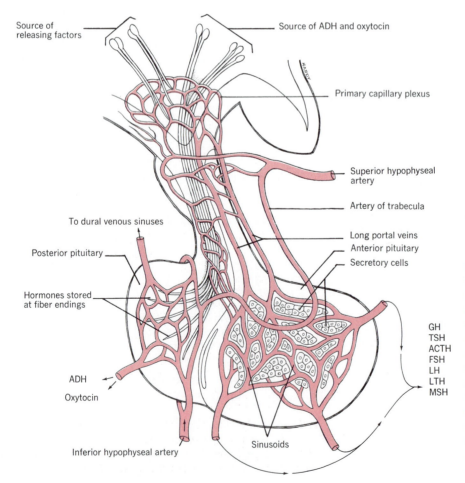

FIG. 44-3. The hypothalamus and the anterior and posterior pituitary. Hypothalamus releasing or inhibiting hormones are transported to the anterior pituitary by way of the portal vessels. ADH and oxytocin are produced by nerve cells in the supraoptic and paraventricular nuclei of the hypothalamus and then transported through the nerve axon to the posterior pituitary, where they are released into the circulation. (Chaffee, E. E., & Greisheimer, E. M. [1974]. *Basic physiology and anatomy* [3rd ed.]. Philadelphia: J.B. Lippincott)

hormones), and breast growth and milk production (prolactin). Melanocyte-stimulating hormone, which controls pigmentation of the skin, is produced by the pars intermedia of the pituitary gland.

FEEDBACK REGULATION

The level of many of the hormones in the body is regulated by negative feedback mechanisms. The function of this type of system is similar to that of the thermostat in a heating system. In the endocrine system, sensors detect a change in the hormone level and adjust hormone secretion so that body levels are maintained within an appropriate range. When the sensors detect a decrease in hormone levels, they initiate changes that cause an increase in hormone production; when hormone levels rise above the set point of the system, the sensors cause hormone production and release to decrease. For example, an increase in thyroid hormone is detected by sensors in the hypothalamus or anterior pituitary gland, and this causes a reduction in the secretion of thyroid-stimulating hormone with a subsequent decrease in the output of thyroid hormone from the thyroid gland. The feedback loops for the hypothalamic–pituitary feedback mechanisms are illustrated in Figure 44-4. Exogenous forms of hormones (given as drug preparations) can influence the normal feedback control of hormone production and release. One of the most common examples of this influence occurs with the administration of the adrenal cortical hormones, which causes suppression of the hypothalamic–pituitary–target cell system that regulates the production of these hormones.

Although the levels of most hormones are regulated by negative feedback mechanisms, a small number are under positive feedback control in which rising levels of a hormone cause another gland to release a hormone that is stimulating to the first. There must, however, be a mechanism for shutting off the release of the first hormone, or its production would continue unabated. An example of such a system is that of the female ovarian hormone estradiol. Increased estradiol production during the follicular stage of the menstrual cycle produces increased gonadotropin (FSH) production by the anterior pituitary gland. This stimulates further increases in estradiol levels until the demise of the follicle, which is the source of estradiol, results in a fall in gonadotropin levels.

In summary, the endocrine system acts as a communications system that uses chemical messengers, or hormones, for the transmission of information from cell to cell and from organ to organ. Hormones act at the level of the cell membrane, which has surface receptors that are specific for the different types of hormones. Many of the endocrine glands are under the regula-

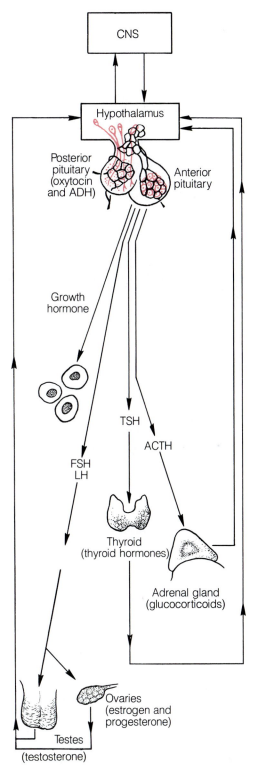

FIG. 44-4. Control of hormone production by hypothalamic–pituitary–target cell feedback mechanism. Hormone levels from the target glands regulate the release of hormones from the anterior pituitary by means of a negative feedback system.

tory control of other parts of the endocrine system. The hypothalamus and the pituitary gland form a complex integrative network that joins the nervous system and the endocrine system; this central network controls the output from many of the other glands in the body.

■ GENERAL ASPECTS OF ALTERED ENDOCRINE FUNCTION

HYPOFUNCTION AND HYPERFUNCTION

Disturbances of endocrine function can usually be divided into two categories: hypofunction and hyperfunction.

Hypofunction of an endocrine gland can occur for a variety of reasons. Congenital defects can result in the absence or impaired development of the gland or the absence of an enzyme needed for hormone synthesis. Destruction of the gland may occur because of disruption in blood flow, infection or inflammation, autoimmune responses, or neoplastic growth. There may be a decline in function with aging, or the gland may atrophy as the result of drug therapy or for unknown reasons. Some endocrine-deficient states are associated with receptor defects: hormone receptors may be absent, the receptor binding of hormones may be defective, or the cellular responsiveness to the hormone may be impaired. It is suspected that in some cases a gland may produce a biologically inactive hormone, or an active hormone may be destroyed by circulating antibodies before it can exert its action.

Hyperfunction is generally associated with excessive hormone production. This can result from excessive stimulation and hyperplasia of the endocrine gland or from a hormone-producing tumor of the gland. Sometimes an ectopic tumor will produce hormones; for example, certain bronchogenic tumors produce hormones such as antidiuretic hormone (ADH) and adrenocorticotropic hormone (ACTH).

PRIMARY AND SECONDARY DISORDERS

Endocrine disorders can generally be divided into two groups: primary and secondary. *Primary defects* in endocrine function originate within the target gland responsible for producing the hormone. In *secondary disorders* of endocrine function, the target gland is essentially normal, but its function is altered by defective levels of stimulating hormones or releasing factors from the hypothalamic–pituitary system. For example, adrenalectomy produces a primary deficiency of adrenal corticosteroid hormones. Removal or destruction of the pituitary gland, on the other hand, eliminates ACTH stimulation of the adrenal cortex and brings about a secondary deficiency.

DIAGNOSTIC METHODS

There are a number of techniques for assessing endocrine function and hormone levels. One technique measures the effect of a hormone on body function. Measurement of blood glucose, for example, reflects insulin levels and is an indirect method of assessing insulin availability. Another method is to measure hormone levels.

Hormones circulating in the plasma were first detected by bioassays using the intact animal or a portion of tissue from the animal. At one time, female rats or male frogs were used to test women's urine for the presence of human chorionic gonadotropin, which is produced by the placenta during pregnancy. Unfortunately, most bioassays lack the precision, sensitivity, and specificity to measure low concentrations in plasma and are inconvenient to perform.

Real progress in measuring plasma hormone levels came over 30 years ago with the use of competitive binding and the development of radioimmunoassay methods. This method uses a radiolabeled form of the hormone and a hormone antibody that has been prepared by injecting an appropriate animal with a purified form of the hormone. The unlabeled hormone in the sample being tested competes with the radiolabeled hormone for attachment to the binding sites of the antibody. Measurement of the radiolabeled hormone–antibody complex then provides a means of arriving at a measure of hormone level in the sample. Because hormone binding is competitive, the amount of radiolabeled hormone–antibody complex that is formed will decrease as the amount of unlabeled hormone in the sample is increased. Radioimmunoassay methods can be used to measure blood hormone levels or urinary hormone excretion or to perform dyanmic tests of endocrine function (stimulation and suppression tests).

Blood hormone levels provide information about hormone blood levels at a specific time. For example, blood insulin levels can be measured along with blood glucose following administration of a challenge dose of glucose to measure the time-course of change in blood insulin levels.

Measurements of urinary hormone or hormone metabolite excretion are often done on a 24-hour urine sample and provide a better measure of hormone levels during that period of time than hormones measured in an isolated blood sample. The use of urine samples has both advantages and disadvantages.

The advantages include the fact that urine samples are relatively easy to obtain and do not require blood sampling. The disadvantages are that reliable timed urine collections are often difficult to obtain. For example, a person may be unable to urinate at specific timed intervals, and urine samples may be accidentally discarded or inaccurately preserved. Also, since many urine tests involve the measure of a hormone metabolite rather than the hormone itself, drugs or disease states that alter hormone metabolism may interfere with the test. In addition, some urinary hormone metabolite measurements include hormones from more than one source and thus are of little value in measuring hormone secretion from a specific source. For example, urinary 17-ketosteroids are a measure of both adrenal and gonadal androgens.

Stimulation tests are usually used when hypofunction of an endocrine organ is suspected. A trophic hormone can be administered to test the capacity of an endocrine organ to increase hormone product. The capacity of the target gland to respond is measured by an increase in the appropriate hormone. For example, the function of the hypothalamic–pituitary–thyroid system could be evaluated through stimulation tests using thyrotropin-releasing factor (TRF) and thyroid-stimulating hormone (TSH). The failure to effect an increase in thyroid hormone after a stimulation using TRF would suggest inadequate production of TSH, and a failure to effect an increase in thyroid hormone following stimulation with TSH

would suggest, a defect in production of thyroid hormone by the thyroid gland.

Suppression tests are used when hyperfunction is suspected. They are used to determine if negative feedback control mechanisms are intact. For example, a glucocorticoid hormone can be administered to persons suspected of having hypercortisonism to assess the capacity to inhibit adrenal corticotrophin-releasing hormone (ACTH).

In summary, endocrine disorders are the result of hypo- or hyperfunction of an endocrine gland. They can occur as a primary defect in hormone production by a target gland or as a secondary disorder resulting from a defect in the hypothalamic–pituitary system that controls a target gland's function. Laboratory tests that measure hormone levels or assess the effect of a hormone on body function (*e.g.*, assessment of insulin function through blood sugar levels) are used in the diagnosis of endocrine disorders.

■ **BIBLIOGRAPHY**

Berne, R.M., & Levy, M.N. (1988). *Physiology* (2nd ed., pp. 832–837). St. Louis: C.V. Mosby.

Giffin, J.E., & Sergio, R.O. (Eds.). (1992). *Textbook of endocrine physiology* (2nd ed.). New York: Oxford University Press,

Greenspan, F.S. (1991). *Basic and clinical endocrinology* (3rd ed.). Norwalk, CT: Appleton-Lange.

Hanley, R.M., & Steiner, A.L. (1989). The second-messenger system for peptide proteins. *Hospital Practice*, 24(8A), 59–70.

CHAPTER 45

ALTERATIONS IN ENDOCRINE CONTROL OF GROWTH AND METABOLISM

CAROL MATTSON PORTH
LINDA S. HURWITZ

■ OBJECTIVES

After you have studied this chapter, you should be able to meet the following objectives:

■ State the effects of a deficiency in growth hormone.

■ Differentiate between genetic short stature and constitutional short stature.

■ State the mechanisms of short stature in hypothyroidism, poorly controlled diabetes mellitus, treatment with adrenal glucocorticosteroid hormones, malnutrition, and psychosocial dwarfism.

■ List three causes of tall stature.

■ Explain why children with isosexual precocious puberty are tall-statured as children but short-statured as adults.

■ Relate the functions of growth hormone to the manifestations of acromegaly.

■ Relate the functions of thyroid hormone to hypothyroidism and hyperthyroidism.

■ Diagram the hypothalamic–pituitary–thyroid feedback system.

■ Describe the effects of congenital hypothyroidism.

■ State the underlying cause of the adrenogenital syndrome.

■ Describe the function of the adrenal cortical hormones and their feedback regulation.

■ Relate the functions of the adrenal cortical hormones to Addison's disease (adrenal insufficiency) and Cushing's syndrome (cortisol excess).

Carol Mattson Porth: PATHOPHYSIOLOGY: CONCEPTS OF
ALTERED HEALTH STATES, 4th ed. © 1994, 1990, 1986, 1982
J.B. Lippincott Company

■ GROWTH DISORDERS

A number of hormones are essential for normal body growth and maturation including pituitary growth hormone, insulin, thyroid hormone, and androgens. In addition to its actions on carbohydrate and fat metabolism, insulin plays an essential role in growth processes. Children with diabetes, particularly those with poor control, often fail to grow normally even though GH levels are normal. When levels of thyroid hormone are lower than normal, bone growth and epiphyseal closure are delayed. Androgens such as testosterone and dihydrotestosterone exert anabolic growth effects through their actions on protein synthesis. Glucocorticoids, at excessive levels, are inhibitory to growth, apparently because of their antagonistic effect on GH secretion.

GROWTH HORMONE

Growth hormone, also called *somatotropin*, is a 191-amino-acid polypeptide hormone synthesized and secreted by special cells in the anterior pituitary called somatotropes. For many years it was thought that GH was produced primarily during periods of growth. However, this has proved to be incorrect because the rate of GH production in adults is almost as great as in children. It is now known that GH is not only necessary for growth but also contributes to the regulation of metabolic functions.[1,2] All aspects of cartilage growth are stimulated by GH; one of the most striking effects of GH is on linear bone growth resulting from its action on the epiphyseal cartilage plates of long bones. The width of bone increases because of enhanced periosteal growth; visceral and endocrine organs, skeletal and cardiac muscle, skin, and connective tissue all undergo increased growth in response to GH. In many instances, the increased growth of visceral and endocrine organs is accompanied by enhanced functional capacity. For example, increased growth of cardiac muscle is accompanied by an increase in cardiac output.

Aside from its effects on growth, GH facilitates the rate of protein synthesis by all of the cells of the body; it enhances fatty acid mobilization and increases the utilization of fatty acids for fuel; and it maintains or increases blood glucose levels by decreasing the utilization of glucose for fuel. Growth hormone has an initial effect of increasing insulin levels. However, the predominant effect of prolonged GH excess is to increase glucose levels despite an insulin increase. This occurs because GH induces a resistance to insulin in the peripheral tissues, thereby inhibiting the uptake of glucose by muscle and adipose tissues.

Many of the effects of GH depend on a family of peptides called *insulin-like growth factors* (IGF; also called somatomedins), which are produced mainly by the liver. Growth hormone cannot directly produce bone growth; instead it acts indirectly by causing the liver to produce the IGF. These peptides, in turn, act on cartilage and bone to promote their growth. Two human IGF, IGF-I and IGF-II, have been sequenced, and both have structures that are similar to proinsulin.[3] This undoubtedly explains the insulinlike activity of the IGF as well as the weak action of insulin on growth. Of the two IGF, IGF-I appears to be the more important in terms of growth and it is the one that is usually measured in laboratory tests.

Growth hormone is carried unbound in the plasma and has a half-life of about 20 to 50 minutes. The secretion of GH is regulated by two hypothalamic hormones: growth hormone releasing hormone (GH-RH) and somatostatin, which inhibits GH release. Somatostatin is also produced by delta cells in the islets of Langerhans in the pancreas where it influences glucagon and insulin release. These hypothalamic influences (GH-RH and somatostatin) are tightly regulated by neural, metabolic, and hormonal factors. The secretion of GH fluctuates over a 24-hour period with peak levels occurring 1 to 4 hours after onset of sleep (during sleep stages 3 and 4). The nocturnal sleep bursts, which account for 70% of daily GH secretion, are greater in children than adults.[3]

Growth hormone secretion is stimulated by hypoglycemia, fasting, starvation, increased blood levels of amino acids (particularly arginine), and stress conditions such as trauma, excitement and emotional stress, and heavy exercise. Growth hormone is inhibited by increased glucose levels, free fatty acid release, cortisol, and obesity. Impairment of secretion, leading to growth retardation, is not uncommon in children with severe emotional deprivation.

SHORT STATURE

Short stature is a condition in which the attained height is well below the fifth percentile or linear growth is below normal for age and sex. Short stature, or growth retardation, has a variety of causes, including chromosomal abnormalities such as Turner's syndrome (see Chapter 4), GH deficiency, hypothyroidism, and panhypopituitarism. Other conditions known to cause short stature include protein-calorie malnutrition, chronic diseases such as renal failure and poorly controlled diabetes mellitus, malabsorption syndromes, and certain therapies such as corticosteroid administration. Emotional disturbances can lead to functional endocrine disorders causing psychosocial dwarfism. The causes of short stature are summarized in Chart 45-1.

Two forms of short stature, genetic short stature and constitutional short stature, are not disease states but variations from population norms. Genetically short children tend to be well proportioned and to have a height close to the mean height of their parents. *Constitutional short stature* is a term used to describe children (particularly boys) who have moderately short stature, thin build, delayed skeletal and sexual maturation, and absence of other causes of decreased growth.

Catch-up growth is a term used to describe an abnormally high growth rate that occurs as a child approaches normal height for age. It occurs after the initiation of therapy for GH deficiency and hypothyroidism and the correction of chronic diseases.

Psychosocial dwarfism involves a functional hypopituitarism and is seen in some emotionally deprived children. These children usually present with poor growth, potbelly, and poor eating and drinking habits. Typically, there is a history of disturbed family relationships in which the child has been severely neglected or disciplined. Often the neglect is confined to one child in the family. Growth hormone function usually returns to normal after the child is removed from the home. The diagnosis depends on improvement in behavior and catch-up growth. Family therapy is usually indicated, and foster care may be necessary.

Accurate measurement of height is an extremely important part of the physical examination of children. Completion of the developmental history and growth charts is essential. Growth curves and growth velocity studies are also needed. Diagnosis of short stature is not made on a single measurement but is based on actual height as well as velocity of growth and parental height.

The diagnostic procedures for short stature include tests to rule out nonendocrine causes. If the cause is hormonal, extensive hormonal testing procedures are initiated. Usually both GH and IGF levels are determined. Tests can be performed using insulin (to induce hypoglycemia), levodopa, and arginine, all of which stimulate and evaluate GH reserve. Because administration of such agents can result in false-negative responses, two or more tests are usually performed. If a prompt rise in GH is realized, the child is considered normal. Levels of IGF usually reflect those of GH and may be used to indicate GH deficiency. Radiologic films are used to assess bone age, which is most often delayed. The size and shape of the sella turcica (depression in the sphenoid bone that contains the pituitary gland) are studied to determine if a pituitary tumor exists. Once the cause of short stature has been determined, treatment can be initiated.

CHART 45-1: CAUSES OF SHORT STATURE

Variants of Normal

Genetic short stature
Constitutional short stature

Endocrine Disorders

Growth hormone deficiency
  Primary growth hormone deficiency
    Idiopathic growth hormone deficiency
    Pituitary agenesis
  Secondary growth hormone deficiency
    Hypothalamic–pituitary tumors
    Postcranial radiation
    Head injuries
    Brain infections
    Hydrocephalus
  Biologically inactive growth hormone production
Hypothyroidism
Diabetes mellitus in poor control
Glucocorticoid excess
  Endogenous (Cushing's disease)
  Exogenous glucocorticoid drug treatment

Chronic Illness Malnutrition

Nutritional deprivation
Malabsorption syndrome

Functional Endocrine Disorders

Psychosocial dwarfism

Chromosomal Disorders

Turner's syndrome

GROWTH HORMONE DEFICIENCY

There are several forms of GH deficiency. Children with idiopathic GH deficiency lack GH-RH but have adequate somatotropes, whereas children with pituitary tumors or agenesis of the pituitary lack somatotropes. The term *panhypopituitarism* refers to conditions that cause a deficiency of all of the anterior pituitary hormones. In a rare condition called Laron type dwarfism, GH levels are normal or elevated but there is a hereditary defect in IGF receptors.

Congenital GH deficiency is associated with normal birth length, followed by a decrease in growth rate that can be identified by careful measurement during the first year and becomes obvious by 1 to 2 years of age. People with classic GH deficiency have normal intelligence, short stature, obesity with immature facial features, and some delay in skeletal maturation. Puberty is often delayed, and males with the disorder have microphallus, especially if the condition is accompanied by gonadotropin-releasing hormone (Gn-RH) deficiency. In the neonate, GH deficiency can lead to hypoglycemia and seizures; if adrenocorticotropic hormone (ACTH) deficiency is also present, the hypoglycemia is often more severe. Acquired GH deficiency develops in later childhood; it may be due to a hypothalamic–pituitary tumor, particularly if it is accompanied by other pituitary deficiencies. Cranial irradiation of the hypothalamic–pituitary region for brain tumors or acute lymphoblastic leukemia may result in GH deficiency 6 to 24 months later.[3]

When short stature is caused by a GH deficiency, GH replacement therapy is the treatment of choice. GH is species specific, and only human GH is effective in humans. GH was previously obtained from human cadaver pituitaries but now is produced by recombinant DNA (rDNA) technology and is available in adequate supply. In 1985, the National Hormone and Pituitary Program halted the distribution of human GH derived from cadaver pituitaries in the United States after receiving reports that three people died of Creutzfeldt-Jakob disease. The disease, which is caused by a neurotropic virus, was thought to be transmitted by cadaver GH preparations. GH is administered subcutaneously in multiple weekly doses during the period of active growth. Children with constitutional short stature and Turner's syndrome are also being treated with GH in clinical studies. It is still too early to predict the outcome of treatment for these children. There are concerns over misuse of the drug to produce additional growth in children with normal GH function who are of near-normal height. Guidelines for use of the hormone continue to be established.

TALL STATURE

Just as there are children who are short for their age and sex, there are also children who are tall for their age and sex. Normal variants of tall stature include genetic tall stature and constitutional tall stature. As with short stature, children with exceptionally tall parents tend to be taller than children with short parents. The term *constitutional tall stature* is used to describe a child who is taller than his or her peers and is growing at a velocity that is within the normal range for bone age. Other causes of tall stature are genetic or chromosomal disorders such as Marfan's syndrome or XYY syndrome (see Chapter 4). Endocrine causes of tall stature include sexual precocity because of early onset of estrogen and androgen secretion and excessive GH.

Exceptionally tall children (genetic tall stature and constitutional tall stature) can be treated with sex hormones (estrogens in girls and testosterone in boys) to effect early epiphyseal closure. Such treatment is undertaken only after full consideration of the risks involved. To be effective, such treatment must be instituted 3 to 4 years before expected epiphyseal fusion.

GIGANTISM

GH excess occurring before puberty and before the fusion of the epiphyses of the long bones results in gigantism. Excessive secretion of GH by somatotrope adenomas causes gigantism in the prepubertal child. It occurs when the epiphyses are not fused and high levels of IGF stimulate excessive skeletal growth. Fortunately, the condition is rare because of early recognition and treatment of the adenoma.

ISOSEXUAL PRECOCIOUS PUBERTY

Precocious sexual development may be idiopathic or may be caused by gonadal, adrenal, or hypothalamic tumors. Isosexual precocious puberty is defined as early activation of the hypothalamic–pituitary–gonadal axis, resulting in the development of appropriate sexual characteristics and fertility. Sexual development is considered precocious and warrants investigation when it occurs before 8 years of age for girls and before 9 years of age for boys. Tumors of the central nervous system (CNS), both benign and malignant, can cause precocious puberty. These tumors are thought to remove the inhibitory influences normally exerted on the hypothalamus during childhood.[4] CNS tumors are found more often in boys with precocious puberty than in girls. In girls, most cases are idiopathic.

Diagnosis of precocious puberty is based on physical findings of early thelarche (beginning of breast development), adrenarche (beginning of augmented adrenal androgen production), and menarche (beginning of menstrual function) in girls. The most common sign in boys is early genital enlargement. Radiologic findings may indicate advanced bone age. People with precocious puberty are usually tall for their age as children but are short as adults because of the early closure of the epiphyses. Computed tomography (CT) scans or magnetic resonance imaging (MRI) may be used to rule out intracranial lesions.

Depending on the cause of precocious puberty, the treatment may involve surgery, medication, or no treatment. The treatment of choice is administration of a long-acting Gn-RH agonist.[4] Constant levels of the hormone cause a decrease in pituitary responsiveness to Gn-RH, leading to decreased secretion of gonadotropic hormones and sex steroids. Parents often need education, support, and anticipatory guidance in dealing with their feelings and the child's physical needs and in relating to a child who appears older than his or her years.

ACROMEGALY

When GH excess occurs in adulthood or after the epiphyses of the long bones have fused, a condition known as acromegaly develops. Acromegaly is a chronic and debilitating disorder of body growth and metabolic derangements in the adult caused by excess levels of GH. The mean age at the time of diagnosis is about 40 in men and 45 in women.[5] Most cases of acromegaly are caused by pituitary adenoma. The disorder usually has an insidious onset, and symptoms are often present for a considerable period of time before a diagnosis is made.

When the production of excessive GH occurs after the epiphyses of the long bones have closed, as in the adult, the person cannot grow taller, but the soft tissues continue to grow. Enlargement of the small bones of the hands and feet and in the membranous bones of the face and skull results in a pronounced enlargement of the hands and feet, a broad and bulbous nose, a protruding lower jaw, and a slanting forehead (Fig. 45-1). The teeth become splayed, causing a disturbed bite and difficulty in chewing. The cartilaginous structures in the larynx and respiratory tract also become enlarged, resulting

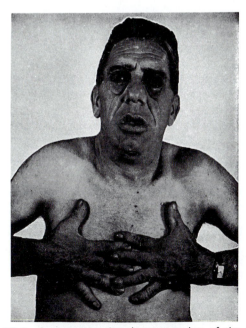

FIG. 45-1. Acromegaly, showing protrusion of the lower jaw, heavy lips, and "spade" hands. (Chaffee, E. E., & Lytle, I. M. [1980]. *Basic physiology and anatomy* [4th ed., p. 527]. Philadelphia: J.B. Lippincott)

in a deepening of the voice and tendency to develop bronchitis. Vertebral changes often lead to kyphosis, or hunchback. Bone overgrowth often leads to arthralgias and degenerative arthritis of the spine, hips, and knees. Virtually every organ of the body is increased in size. Enlargement of the heart and accelerated atherosclerosis may lead to an early death.

The metabolic effects of excess levels of GH include alterations in fat and carbohydrate metabolism. Increased levels of GH have a diabetogenic effect. GH acts as an insulin antagonist; in excess, it decreases carbohydrate utilization and it impairs glucose uptake into cells. This leads to glucose intolerance, which, in turn, stimulates the beta cells of the pancreas to produce additional insulin. In addition, GH also increases the ability of the beta cells to respond to insulinogenic stimuli. Long-term elevation of GH results in overstimulation of the beta cells, literally causing them to "burn out," predisposing to the development of diabetes mellitus. Impaired glucose tolerance is present in up to 50% to 70% of people with acromegaly; overt diabetes mellitus develops in a small number of these.[3]

The pituitary gland is located in the pituitary fossa of the sphenoid bone (sella turcica), which lies directly below the optic nerve. Almost all people with acromegaly have a recognizable adenohypophyseal tumor. Enlargement of the pituitary gland eventually causes erosion of the surrounding bone, and, because of its location, this can lead to headaches, visual field defects resulting from compression of the optic nerve, and cranial nerve palsies (III, IV, VI). Compression of other pituitary structures can cause secondary hypothyroidism, hypogonadism, and adrenal insufficiency. Other manifestations include excessive sweating with an unpleasant odor, oily skin, heat intolerance, moderate weight gain, muscle weakness and fatigue, menstrual irregularities, and decreased libido. Hypertension is relatively common. Paresthesias may develop because of nerve entrapment and compression caused by excess soft tissue and accumulation of subcutaneous fluid.

The disease often develops insidiously, and only a small number of people (about 13%) seek medical care because of change in appearance.[5] The diagnosis of acromegaly is facilitated by the typical features of the disorder (enlargement of the hands and feet and coarsening of facial features). Laboratory tests to detect elevated levels of GH not suppressed by a glucose load are used to confirm the diagnosis. CT scans and nuclear MRI may be done to detect and localize the pituitary lesions. Because most of the effects of GH are mediated by the IGF-I, IGF-I levels may provide information related to disease activity.

The goals of treatment in acromegaly are the rapid normalization of GH to prevent or reverse progression of the disorder; prevention or reversal of the pressure effects of the tumor on structures surrounding the sella turcica; and preservation or restoration of normal pituitary function. Pituitary tumors can be removed surgically using the transsphenoidal approach, or their size can be reduced with irradiation. Bromocriptine, a long-acting dopamine antagonist, reduces GH levels and has been used with some success in the medical management of acromegaly. However, high doses are often required, and side effects may be troublesome. A long-acting analogue of somatostatin, octreotide, can be used to suppress GH production and provides clinical improvement in acromegaly.[5]

In summary, a number of hormones are essential for normal body growth and maturation, including GH, insulin, thyroid hormone, and androgens. GH exerts its growth effects through a group of IGF. GH also exerts an effect on metabolism and is excreted in the adult as well as in the child. Its metabolic effects include a decrease in peripheral utilization of carbohydrates and an increased mobilization and utilization of fatty acids. In children, alterations in growth include short stature, isosexual precocious puberty, and tall stature. Short stature is a condition in which the attained height is well below the fifth percentile or the linear growth velocity is below normal for a child's age or sex. Short stature can occur as a variant of normal growth (genetic short stature or constitutional short stature) or as the result of endocrine disorders, chronic illness, malnutrition, emotional disturbances, or chromosomal disorders. Short stature resulting from GH deficiency can be treated with human GH preparations. Isosexual precocious puberty defines a condition of early activation of hypothalamic–pituitary–gonadal axis (before 8 years of age in girls and 10 years of age in boys) resulting in the development of appropriate sexual characteristics and fertility. It causes tall stature during childhood but results in short stature in adulthood because of the early closure of the epiphyses. Tall stature describes the condition in which children are tall for their age and sex. It can occur as a variant of normal growth (genetic tall stature or constitutional tall stature) or as the result of a chromosomal abnormality or GH excess. GH excess in adults results in acromegaly, which involves proliferation of bone, cartilage, and soft tissue along with the metabolic effects of excessive hormone levels.

■ THYROID DISORDERS

CONTROL OF THYROID FUNCTION

The thyroid gland is a shield-shaped structure located immediately below the larynx in the anterior middle portion of the neck. The thyroid gland is composed of a large number of tiny saclike structures called follicles (Fig. 45-2). These are the functional cells of the thyroid. Each follicle is formed by a single layer of epithelial (follicular) cells and is filled with a secretory substance called *colloid*, which consists largely of a glycoprotein–iodine complex, thyroglobulin.

The thyroglobulin that fills the thyroid follicles is a large glycoprotein molecule that contains 140 tyrosine amino acids. In the process of thyroid synthesis, iodine is attached to these tyrosine amino

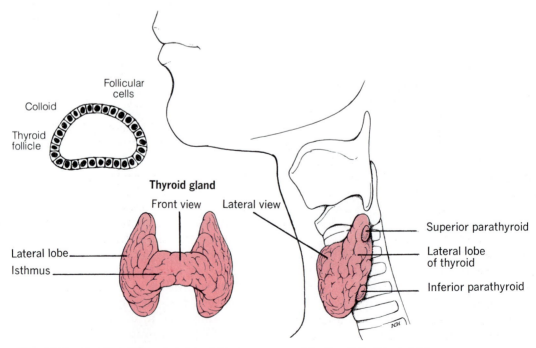

FIG. 45-2. The thyroid gland and the follicular structure. (Chaffee, E. E., & Lytle I. M. [1980]. *Basic physiology and anatomy* [4th ed., p. 434]. Philadelphia: J.B. Lippincott)

HO⟨○⟩ CH2 CH COOH
         |
         NH2

Tyrosine

HO⟨○⟩ CH2 CH COOH
  I |
         NH2

Monoiodotyrosine

HO⟨○⟩—O—⟨○⟩ CH2 CH COOH
  I   I |
           I   NH2

Triiodothyronine (T3)

HO⟨○⟩ CH2 CH COOH
  I |
  I   NH2

Diiodotyrosine

HO⟨○⟩—O—⟨○⟩ CH2 CH COOH
  I   I   I |
                    NH2

Thyroxine (T4).

FIG. 45-3. Chemistry of thyroid hormone production.

acids. Both thyroglobulin and iodide (I^-) are secreted into the colloid of the follicle by the follicular cells.

The thyroid is remarkably efficient in its utilization of iodide. A daily absorption of 100 to 200 μg of dietary iodide is sufficient to form normal quantities of thyroid hormone. In the process of removing iodide from the blood and storing it for future use, iodide is pumped into the follicular cells against a concentration gradient. As a result, the concentration of iodide within the normal thyroid gland is about 40 times that in the blood. Once inside the follicle, most of the iodide is oxidized by the enzyme peroxidase in a reaction that facilitates combination with a tyrosine molecule to form *monoiodotyrosine* and then *diiodotyrosine* (Fig. 45-3). In time, two diiodotyrosine residues become coupled to form *thyroxine* (T_4), or a monoiodotyrosine and a diiodotyrosine become coupled to form *triiodothyronine* (T_3). Only T_4 (90%) and T_3 (10%) are secreted into the circulation.

There is evidence that T_3 is the active form of the hormone and that T_4 is converted to T_3 before it can act physiologically. Thyroid hormones are bound to thyroid-binding globulin and other plasma proteins for transport in the blood. Only the free hormone enters cells and regulates the pituitary feedback mechanism. Thus protein-bound thyroid hormone forms a large storage reservoir pool that is slowly drawn on as free thyroid hormone is needed. There are three major thyroid-binding proteins: thyroid hormone binding globulin, thyroxine-binding prealbumin, and albumin. About 70% of T_4 is carried bound to thyroid-binding globulin; thyroxine-binding prealbumin binds essentially no T_3 and carries about 20% of T_4; albumin, which has the lowest affinity for T_4, carries about 10% of T_4 and 30% of T_3.[3] A number of disease conditions and pharmacologic agents can either decrease the amount of binding protein present in the plasma or influence the binding of hormone.

The secretion of thyroid hormone is regulated by the hypothalamic–pituitary–thyroid feedback system (Fig. 45-4). In this system, thyrotropin-releasing hormone (TRH), which is produced by the hypothalamus, controls the release of thyroid-stimulating hormone (TSH) from the anterior pituitary gland. TSH increases the overall activity of the thyroid gland by (1) increasing the thyroglobulin breakdown and release of thyroid hormone from follicles into the bloodstream, (2) activating the iodide pump, (3) increasing the oxidation of iodide and coupling of iodide to tyrosine, and (4) increasing the number of follicle cells and the size of the follicles. The effect of TSH on the release of thyroid hormones occurs within about 30 minutes, whereas the other effects require days or weeks. Increased levels of thyroid hormone act in the feedback mechanism by inhib-

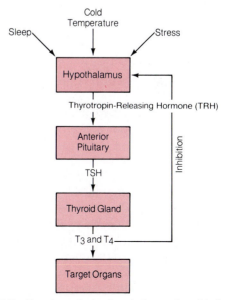

FIG. 45-4. The hypothalamic–pituitary–thyroid feedback system, which regulates the body levels of thyroid hormone.

iting TRH or TSH. High levels of iodide cause a temporary decrease in thyroid activity that lasts for several weeks, probably through a direct inhibition of TSH on the thyroid. Lugol's solution, which is an iodide preparation, is sometimes given to hyperthyroid patients in preparation for surgery as a means of decreasing thyroid function. Cold exposure is one of the strongest stimuli for increased thyroid hormone production and is probably mediated through TRH from the hypothalamus.

ACTIONS OF THYROID HORMONE

All the major organs in the body are affected by altered levels of thyroid hormone. Thyroid hormone has two major effects: (1) it increases metabolism and protein synthesis and (2) it is necessary for growth and development in children, including mental development and attainment of sexual maturity.

Metabolic Rate. Thyroid hormone increases the metabolism of all body tissues except the retina, spleen, testes, and lungs. The basal metabolic rate (BMR) can increase by 60% to 100% above normal when large amounts of thyroxine are secreted.[1] As a result of this higher metabolism, the rate of glucose, fat, and protein utilization increases. Lipids are mobilized from adipose tissue, and the catabolism of cholesterol by the liver is increased. As a result, blood levels of cholesterol are decreased in hyperthyroidism and increased in hypothyroidism. Muscle proteins are broken down and used as fuel, probably accounting for some of the muscle fatigue that occurs with hyperthyroidism. The absorption of glucose from the gastrointestinal tract is increased. Because vitamins are essential parts of metabolic enzymes and coenzymes, an increase in metabolic rate "speeds up the use" of vitamins and tends to cause vitamin deficiency.

Cardiovascular Function. Cardiovascular and respiratory functions are strongly affected by thyroid function. With an increase in metabolism, there is a rise in oxygen consumption and production of metabolic end-products with an accompanying increase in vasodilatation. Blood flow to the skin, in particular, is augmented as a means of dissipating the body heat that results from the higher metabolism. Blood volume, cardiac output, and ventilation are all increased as a means of maintaining blood flow and oxygen delivery to body tissues. Heart rate and cardiac contractility are enhanced as a means of maintaining the needed cardiac output. Blood pressure, on the other hand, is apt to change little, because the increase in vasodilatation tends to offset the increase in cardiac output.

Gastrointestinal Tract Function. Thyroid hormone enhances gastrointestinal function with an increase in both motility and production of gastrointestinal secretions often resulting in diarrhea. An increase in appetite and food intake accompanies the higher metabolic rate. At the same time, weight loss occurs because of the increased utilization of calories.

Neuromuscular Effects. Thyroid hormone produces marked effects on muscle function and tone. Slight elevations in hormone levels cause skeletal muscles to react more vigorously, and a drop in hormone levels causes muscles to react more sluggishly. In the hyperthyroid state, a fine muscle tremor is present. The cause of this tremor is unknown, but it may represent an increased sensitivity of the neural synapses in the spinal cord that control muscle tone.

In the infant, thyroid hormone is necessary for normal brain development. The hormone enhances cerebration; in the hyperstate, it causes extreme nervousness, anxiety, and difficulty in sleeping.

Evidence suggests a strong interaction between thyroid hormone and the sympathetic nervous system. As is discussed later, many of the signs and symptoms of hyperthyroidism suggest overactivity of the sympathetic division of the autonomic nervous system, for example, tachycardia, palpitations, and sweating. In addition, tremor, restlessness, anxiety, and diarrhea may reflect autonomic nervous system imbalances. Drugs that block sympathetic activity have proved to be valuable adjuncts in the treatment of hyperthyroidism because of their ability to relieve some of these undesirable symptoms.

TESTS OF THYROID FUNCTION

Various tests aid in diagnosing thyroid disorders. Direct measures of T_3, T_4, TSH, and thyroid-binding globulin have been made available through radioimmunoassay methods. The resin uptake test for T_3 measures the unsaturated binding sites of the thyroid hormones. Measurement of either T_3 or T_4 by radioimmunoassay plus T_3 resin uptake can be used to provide an estimate of free T_3 or T_4. Abnormalities of thyroid-binding globulin (TBG) can be detected through direct measurement of TBG. The *TSH test* differentiates primary and secondary thyroid disorders. The *radioactive iodide uptake test* measures the ability of the thyroid gland to remove and concentrate iodide from the blood. The *TRH stimulation test* is used to differentiate between hypothalamic and pituitary causes of secondary hypothyroidism. A test dose of TRH is given, and serum levels of TSH are measured. The thyroid scan detects thyroid nodules and active thyroid tissue. Ultrasonography can be used to differentiate between cystic and solid thyroid lesions, and CT scans and MRI are used to demonstrate tracheal compression or impingement on other neighboring structures.

ALTERATIONS IN THYROID FUNCTION

An alteration in thyroid function can represent either a hypofunctional or a hyperfunctional state. The manifestations of these two altered states are summarized in Table 45-1. Disorders of the thyroid may represent a congenital defect in thyroid development or they may develop later in life, with a gradual or a sudden onset.

Goiter is an increase in the size of the thyroid gland. It can occur in hypothyroid, euthyroid, and hyperthyroid states. Goiters may be diffuse, involving the entire gland without evidence of nodularity, or they may contain nodules. Diffuse goiters usually become nodular. Goiters may be toxic, producing signs of extreme hyperthyroidism, or *thyrotoxicosis*, or they may be nontoxic. Diffuse nontoxic and multinodular goiters are the result of compensatory hy-

pertrophy and hyperplasia of follicular epithelium secondary to some derangement that impairs thyroid hormone output. The degree of thyroid enlargement is usually proportional to the extent and duration of thyroid deficiency. Multinodular goiters produce the largest thyroid enlargements and are often associated with thyrotoxicosis. When sufficiently enlarged, they may compress the esophagus and trachea, causing difficulty in swallowing, a choking sensation, and inspiratory stridor. Such lesions may also compress the superior vena cava, producing distention of the veins of the neck and upper extremities, edema of the eyelids and conjunctiva, and syncope with coughing.

HYPOTHYROIDISM

Hypothyroidism can occur as a congenital or an acquired defect. The absence of thyroid function at birth is called *cretinism*. When the condition occurs later in life it is called *myxedema*. The term *cretin* hardly seems appropriate for describing the normally developing infant in whom replacement thyroid hormone therapy was instituted shortly after birth.

TABLE 45-1. MANIFESTATIONS OF HYPOTHYROID AND HYPERTHYROID STATES

LEVEL OF ORGANIZATION	HYPOTHYROIDISM	HYPERTHYROIDISM
Basal metabolic rate	Decreased	Increased
Sensitivity to catecholamines	Decreased	Increased
General features	Myxedematous features	Exophthalmos
	Deep voice	Lid lag
	Impaired growth (child)	Decreased blinking
Blood cholesterol levels	Increased	Decreased
General behavior	Mental retardation (infant)	Restlessness, irritability, anxiety
		Hyperkinesis
	Mental and physical sluggishness	Wakefulness
	Somnolence	
Cardiovascular function	Decreased cardiac output	Increased cardiac output
	Bradycardia	Tachycardia and palpitations
Gastrointestinal function	Constipation	Diarrhea
	Decreased appetite	Increased appetite
Respiratory function	Hypoventilation	Dyspnea
Muscle tone and reflexes	Decreased	Increased, with tremor and fibrillatory twitching
Temperature tolerance	Cold intolerance	Heat intolerance
Skin and hair	Decreased sweating	Increased sweating
	Coarse and dry skin and hair	Thin and silky skin and hair
Weight	Gain	Loss

CONGENITAL HYPOTHYROIDISM

Congenital hypothyroidism is perhaps one of the most common causes of preventable mental retardation. It affects about 1 out of 4000 infants. Hypothyroidism in the infant may result from a congenital lack of the thyroid gland or from abnormal biosynthesis of thyroid hormone or deficient TSH secretion. With congenital lack of the thyroid gland, the infant usually appears normal and functions normally at birth because hormones have been supplied *in utero* by the mother.

Thyroid hormone is essential for normal brain development and growth, almost half of which occurs during the first 6 months of life. If untreated, congenital hypothyroidism causes mental retardation and impairment of growth. Long-term studies show that closely monitored thyroxine supplementation begun in the first 6 weeks of life results in normal intelligence.[6,7] However, if treatment is delayed to between 3 and 7 months, 85% of these infants will have definite retardation.[8] Fortunately, neonatal screening tests have been instituted to detect congenital hypothyroidism during early infancy. Screening is usually done in the hospital nursery between the first and fifth days of life. In this test, a drop of blood is taken from the infant's heel and analyzed for T_4 and TSH.

Transient congenital hypothyroidism has become more frequently recognized since the introduction of neonatal screening.[9] It is characterized by high TSH levels and low thyroid hormone levels. The fetal and infant thyroids are sensitive to iodine excess. Iodine crosses the placenta and mammary glands and is readily absorbed by infant skin. Transient hypothyroidism may be caused by maternal ingestion of substances such as potassium iodide (for asthma), use of povidone-iodine as a disinfectant (as a vaginal douche or skin disinfectant), or povidone-iodine may be used as a skin disinfectant in the nursery. The use of iodine-containing radiographic contrast media may be another cause of excess iodine exposure. Also, antithyroid drugs such as propylthiouracil, methimazole, and carbimazole can easily cross the placenta and block fetal thyroid function.

Congenital hypothyroidism is treated by hormone replacement. Evidence indicates that it is important to normalize T_4 levels as rapidly as possible because a delay is accompanied by poorer psychomotor and mental development. Dosage levels are adjusted as the child grows.[9] Infants with transient hypothyroidism can usually have the replacement therapy withdrawn at 6 to 12 months. When early and adequate treatment regimens are followed, the risk of mental retardation in infants detected by screening programs is essentially nonexistent.[9]

MYXEDEMA (ACQUIRED HYPOTHYROIDISM)

When hypothyroidism occurs in older children or adults it is called myxedema. The term *myxedema* implies the presence of a nonpitting mucous type of edema caused by an accumulation of a hydrophilic mucopolysaccharide substance in the connective tissues throughout the body. The hypothyroid state may be mild, with only a few signs and symptoms, or it may progress to a life-threatening condition called *myxedematous coma*. It can result from destruction or dysfunction of the thyroid gland (primary hypothyroidism) or as a secondary disorder caused by impaired hypothalamic or pituitary function.

Primary hypothyroidism is much more common than secondary hypothyroidism. It may result from thyroidectomy (surgical removal) or ablation of the gland with radiation. Certain goitrogenic agents, such as lithium carbonate (used in the treatment of manic-depressive states) and the antithyroid drugs propylthiouracil and methimazole in continuous dosage, can block hormone synthesis and produce hypothyroidism with goiter. Large amounts of iodine (ingestion of kelp tablets or iodide-containing cough syrups or administration of iodide-containing radiographic contrast media) can also block thyroid hormone production and cause goiter, particularly in people with autoimmune thyroid disease. Iodine deficiency, which can cause goiter and hypothyroidism, is rare in the United States because of the widespread use of iodized salt and other iodide sources.

The most common cause of hypothyroidism is *Hashimoto's thyroiditis*, an autoimmune disorder in which the thyroid gland may be totally destroyed by an immunologic process. It is the major cause of goiter and hypothyroidism in children. Hashimoto's thyroiditis is predominantly a disease of women, with a female-to-male ratio of 10:1.[10] The course of the disease varies. At the onset, only a goiter may be present. In time, hypothyroidism usually becomes evident. Although the disorder generally causes hypothyroidism, a hyperthyroid state may develop midcourse in the disease. The transient hyperthyroid state is due to leakage of preformed thyroid hormone from damaged cells of the gland.

Myxedema affects almost all of the organ systems in the body. The manifestations of the disorder are largely related to two factors: (1) the hypometabolic state resulting from thyroid hormone deficiency and (2) myxedematous involvement of body tissues. Although the myxedema is most obvious in the face and other superficial parts, it also affects many of the body organs and is responsible for many of the manifestations of the hypothyroid state (Fig. 45-5).

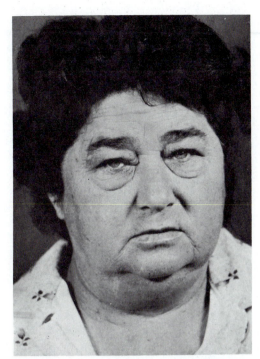

FIG. 45-5. Patient with myxedema. (Courtesy of Dr. Herbert Langford. From Guyton, A. [1981]. *Medical physiology* [6th ed., p. 941]. Philadelphia: W.B. Saunders. Reprinted by permission)

The hypometabolic state associated with myxedema is characterized by a gradual onset of weakness and fatigue, a tendency to gain weight despite a loss in appetite, and cold intolerance. As the condition progresses, the skin becomes dry and rough and acquires a pale yellowish cast, which is due primarily to carotene deposition, and the hair becomes coarse and brittle. There is loss of the lateral one third of the eyebrows. Gastrointestinal motility is decreased, giving rise to constipation, flatulence, and abdominal distention. Nervous system involvement is manifested in mental dullness, lethargy, and impaired memory.

As a result of fluid accumulation, the face takes on a characteristic puffy look, especially around the eyes. The tongue is enlarged, and the voice is hoarse and husky. Myxedematous fluid can collect in the interstitial spaces of almost any organ system. Pericardial or pleural effusion may develop. Mucopolysaccharide deposits in the heart cause generalized cardiac dilatation, bradycardia, and other signs of altered cardiac function. The signs and symptoms of hypothyroidism are summarized in Table 45-1.

Diagnosis of hypothyroidism is based on history, physical examination, and laboratory tests. A low serum T_4, low resin T_3, and elevated TSH are characteristic of primary hypothyroidism. The tests for antithyroid antibodies may be done when Hashimoto's thyroiditis is suspected. In secondary hypo-

thyroidism, a TRH stimulation test is helpful in differentiating between pituitary and hypothalamic disease. Hypothyroidism is treated by replacement therapy with synthetic preparations of T_3, T_4, or a mixture of T_3 and T_4. Thyroid hormones obtained from domestic animals are also available.

MYXEDEMATOUS COMA

Myxedematous coma is a life-threatening end-stage expression of hypothyroidism. It is characterized by coma, hypothermia, cardiovascular collapse, hypoventilation, and severe metabolic disorders that include hyponatremia, hypoglycemia, and lactic acidosis. It occurs most often in the elderly women who have chronic hypothyroidism from a spectrum of causes.[11] The fact that it occurs more frequently in winter months suggests that cold exposure may be a precipitating factor. The severely hypothyroid person is unable to metabolize sedatives, analgesics, and anesthetic drugs, and these agents may precipitate coma.

Treatment includes aggressive management of precipitating factors; supportive therapy such as management of cardiorespiratory status, hyponatremia and hypoglycemia; and thyroid replacement therapy. Prevention is preferable to treatment and entails special attention to high-risk populations such as women with a history of Hashimoto's thyroiditis. Such people should to be informed about the signs and symptoms of severe hypothyroidism and the need for early medical treatment.

HYPERTHYROIDISM

Hyperthyroidism, or *thyrotoxicosis*, results from excessive delivery of thyroid hormone to the peripheral tissue. The most common cause of hyperthyroidism is Graves' disease, which is accompanied by exophthalmos (bulging of the eyeballs) and goiter. Other causes of hyperthyroidism are multinodular goiter, adenoma of the thyroid, and occasionally the ingestion of an overdose of thyroid hormone. Thyroid crisis, or storm, is an acutely exaggerated manifestation of the hyperthyroid state.

Many of the manifestations of hyperthyroidism are related to the increase in oxygen consumption and increased utilization of metabolic fuels associated with the hypermetabolic state as well as the increase in sympathetic nervous system activity that occurs. The fact that many of the signs and symptoms of hyperthyroidism resemble those of excessive sympathetic activity suggests that the thyroid hormone may heighten the sensitivity of the body to the catecholamines or that thyroid hormone may act as a pseudocatecholamine. With the hypermetabolic state, there are frequent complaints of nervousness, irritability, and fatigability. Weight loss is common despite a large appetite. Other manifestations include tachycardia, palpitations, shortness of breath, excessive sweating, muscle cramps, and heat intolerance. The person appears restless and has a fine muscle tremor. Even in people without exophthalmos there is an abnormal retraction of the eyelids and infrequent blinking so that they appear to be staring. The hair and skin are usually thin and have a silky appearance. The signs and symptoms of hyperthyroidism are summarized in Table 45-1.

The treatment of hyperthyroidism is directed toward reducing the level of thyroid hormone. This can be accomplished through surgical removal of part or all of the thyroid gland, eradication of the gland with radioactive iodine, or the use of drugs that decrease thyroid function and thereby the effect of the thyroid hormone on the peripheral tissues. The β-adrenergic blocking drug propranolol is often administered to block the effects of the hyperthyroid state on sympathetic nervous system function. It is given in conjunction with other antithyroid drugs such as propylthiouracil and methimazole. These drugs prevent the thyroid gland from converting iodine to its organic (hormonal) form in the thyroid and block the conversion of T_4 to T_3 in the tissues. *Lugol's solution* (iodide) may be given to depress the thyroid gland in preparation for surgery. Unfortunately, this action is short-lived, and, in a few weeks, the symptoms reappear and may be intensified.

GRAVES' DISEASE

Graves' disease is a state of hyperthyroidism, goiter, and exophthalmos. The onset is usually between ages 20 and 40, and women are five times more likely to develop the disease than men. Grave's disease is an autoimmune disorder characterized by abnormal stimulation of the thyroid gland by thyroid-stimulating antibodies that act through the normal TSH receptors. It may be associated with other autoimmune disorders such as myasthenia gravis and pernicious anemia. The disease is associated with HLA-DR3 and HLA-B8, and a familial tendency is evident. The exophthalmos is thought to result from a separate antibody called *exophthalmos-producing factor* resulting in lymphocytic infiltration of the extraocular muscles. The ophthalmopathy of Graves' disease can cause severe eye problems, including paralysis of the extraocular muscles, involvement of the optic nerve with some visual loss, and corneal ulceration because the lids do not close over the protruding eyeball. The exophthalmos usually tends to stabilize after treatment of the hyperthyroidism. Unfortunately, not all

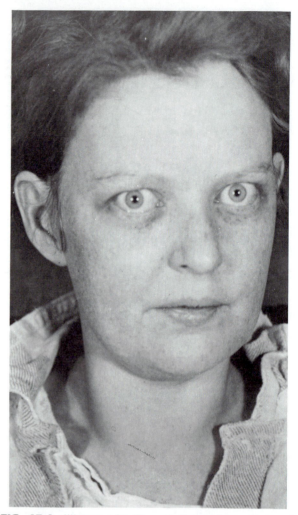

FIG. 45-6. Woman with Graves' disease. Note the exophthalmos and enlarged thyroid gland. (Chaffee, E. E., & Lytle, I. M. [1980]. *Basic physiology and anatomy* [4th ed.]. Philadelphia: J.B. Lippincott)

of the ocular changes are reversible. Figure 45-6 depicts a woman with Graves' disease.

THYROID STORM

Thyroid storm (crisis) is an extreme and life-threatening form of thyrotoxicosis, rarely seen today because of improved diagnosis and treatment methods. When it does occur, it is seen most often in undiagnosed cases or in people with hyperthyroidism who have not been adequately treated. It is often precipitated by stress, such as an infection (usually respiratory), by diabetic ketoacidosis, by physical or emotional trauma, or by manipulation of a hyperactive thyroid gland during thyroidectomy. Thyroid storm is manifested by a very high fever, extreme cardiovascular effects (tachycardia, congestive failure, and angina), and severe CNS effects (agitation, restlessness, and delirium). The mortality rate is high.

Thyroid storm requires rapid diagnosis and implementation of treatment. Peripheral cooling is initiated with cold packs and a cooling mattress. For cooling to be effective, the shivering response must be prevented. General supportive measures to replace fluids, glucose, and electrolytes are essential during the hypermetabolic state. A β-adrenergic blocking drug, such as propranolol, is given to block the undesirable effects of thyroxine on cardiovascular function. Glucocorticoids are used to correct the relative adrenal insufficiency resulting from the stress imposed by the hyperthyroid state and to inhibit the peripheral conversion of T_4 to T_3. Propylthiouracil or methimazole may be given to block thyroid synthesis. A saturated solution of potassium iodide is used to inhibit thyroid hormone release. Lithium also inhibits thyroid hormone release and is used for people who are iodine-sensitive. Aspirin increases the levels of free thyroid by displacing the hormones from their protein carriers and should not be used to reduce fever during thyroid storm.

In summary, thyroid hormones play a role in the metabolic process of almost all body cells and are necessary for normal physical and mental growth in the infant and small child. Alterations in thyroid function can present as either a hypostate or a hyperstate. Hypothyroidism can occur as either a congenital or an acquired defect. When it is present at birth, it is called cretinism; when it occurs later in life, it is termed myxedema. Congenital hypothyroidism leads to mental retardation and impaired physical growth unless treatment is initiated during the first months of life. Hypothyroidism leads to a decrease in metabolic rate and an accumulation of a mucopolysaccharide substance within the intercellular spaces; this substance attracts water and causes a mucous type of edema called myxedema. Hyperthyroidism causes an increase in metabolic rate and alterations in body function similar to those produced by enhanced sympathetic nervous system activity. Graves' disease is characterized by the triad of hyperthyroidism, goiter, and exophthalmos.

■ DISORDERS OF ADRENAL CORTICAL FUNCTION

CONTROL OF ADRENAL CORTICAL FUNCTION

The adrenal glands are small, bilateral structures that weigh about 5 g each and lie retroperitoneally at the apex of each kidney (Fig. 45-7). The medulla, or inner, portion of the gland secretes epinephrine and norepinephrine and is part of the sympathetic nervous system. The cortex forms the bulk of the adrenal gland and is responsible for secreting three types of hormones: the glucocorticoids, the mineralocorticoids, and the adrenal sex hormones. Because the sympathetic nervous system also secretes epinephrine and norepinephrine, adrenal medullary function is

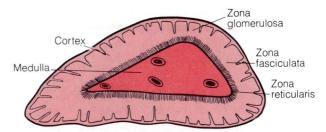

FIG. 45-7. The adrenal gland, showing the medulla and the three layers of the cortex. The zona glomerulosa is the outer layer of the cortex and is primarily responsible for mineralocorticoid production. The middle layer, the zona fasciculata, and the inner layer, the zona reticularis, produce the glucocorticoids and the adrenal sex hormones.

not essential for life, but adrenal cortical function is. The total loss of adrenal cortical function is fatal in 3 to 10 days if untreated.[1] This section of the chapter describes the synthesis and function of the adrenal cortical hormones and the effects of adrenal cortical insufficiency and excess.

BIOSYNTHESIS OF ADRENAL CORTICAL HORMONES

More than 30 hormones are produced by the adrenal gland. Of these hormones, aldosterone is the principal mineralocorticoid, cortisol (hydrocortisone) is the major glucocorticoid, and androgens are the chief sex hormones. All of the adrenal cortical hormones have a similar structure in that all are steroids and are synthesized from acetate and cholesterol; thus, the glucocorticoid drugs are often called steroids. Each of the steps involved in the synthesis of the various hormones requires a specific enzyme (Fig. 45-8). The secretion of both the glucocorticoids and the adrenal androgens are controlled by ACTH secreted by the anterior pituitary gland.

ADRENAL SEX HORMONES

The adrenal sex hormones are synthesized primarily by the zona reticularis and the zona fasciculata of the cortex (see Fig. 45-8). These sex hormones probably exert little effect on normal sexual function. There is evidence, however, that the adrenal sex hormones contribute to the pubertal growth of body hair, particularly pubic and axillary hair in women. They may also play a role in the steroid hormone economy of the pregnant woman and the fetal-placental unit.

MINERALOCORTICOIDS

The mineralocorticoids play an essential role in regulating potassium and sodium levels and water balance. They are produced in the zona glomerulosa,

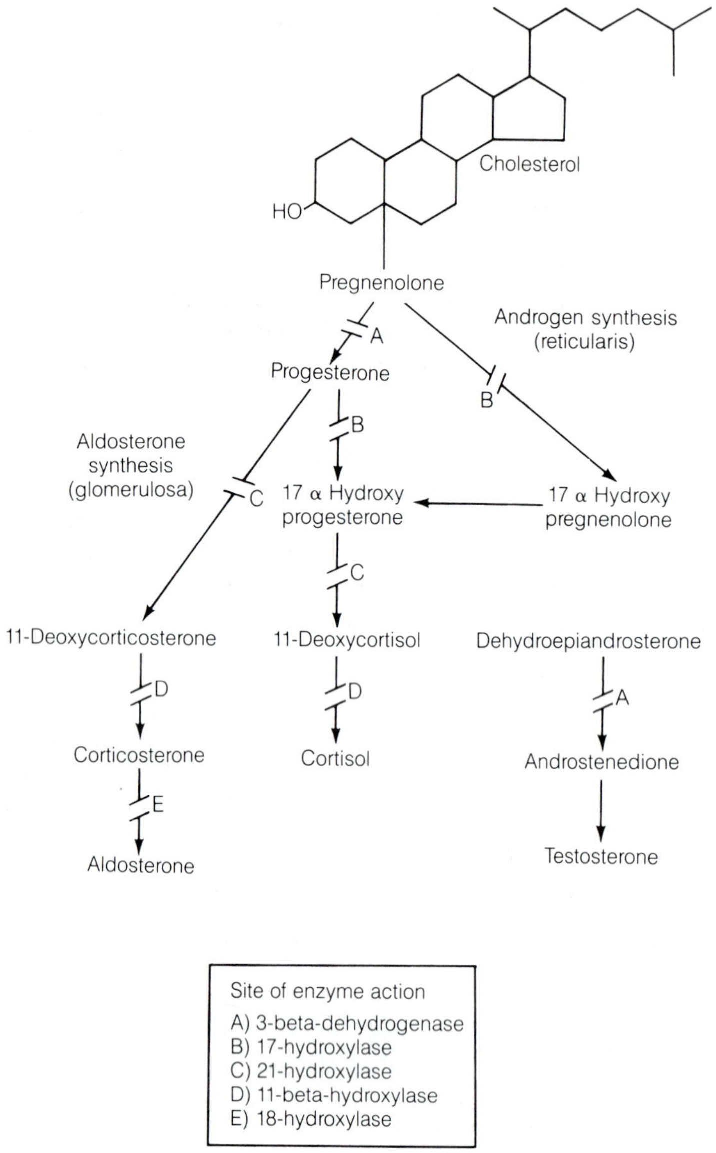

Site of enzyme action

A) 3-beta-dehydrogenase
B) 17-hydroxylase
C) 21-hydroxylase
D) 11-beta-hydroxylase
E) 18-hydroxylase

FIG. 45-8. Predominant biosynthetic pathways of the adrenal cortex. Critical enzymes in the biosynthetic process include 11-beta-hydroxylase and 21-hydroxylase. A deficiency in one of these enzymes blocks the synthesis of these hormones dependent on that enzyme and routes the precursors into alternative pathways.

the outer layer of cells of the adrenal cortex. Aldosterone secretion is regulated by the renin–angiotensin mechanism and by blood levels of potassium. Increased levels of aldosterone promote sodium retention by the distal tubules of the kidney while increasing urinary losses of potassium. The influence of aldosterone on fluid and electrolyte balance is discussed in Chapter 29.

GLUCOCORTICOIDS

The glucocorticoid hormones are synthesized in the zona fasciculata and the zona reticularis. The blood levels of these hormones are regulated by negative feedback mechanisms of the hypothalamic–pituitary–adrenal (HPA) system (Fig. 45-9). In the same manner that other pituitary hormones are controlled by releasing factors from the hypothalamus, the cortico-

tropin-releasing factor (CRF) is important in controlling the release of ACTH. Cortisol levels, in turn, increase as ACTH levels rise. There is considerable diurnal variation in ACTH levels, which reach their peak in the early morning (around 6 A.M. to 8 A.M.) and decline as the day progresses. As is discussed later, one of the earliest signs of Cushing's syndrome is loss of this diurnal variation. Increased plasma cortisol levels act in a negative feedback manner on receptors in the hypothalamus to decrease CRF and on the anterior pituitary to decrease ACTH. The stimulation of hypothalamic receptors and the release of CRF serve to integrate neural influences with the function of the adrenal cortex.

The glucocorticoids perform a necessary function in response to stress and are essential for survival. When produced as part of the stress response, these hormones aid in regulating the metabolic func-

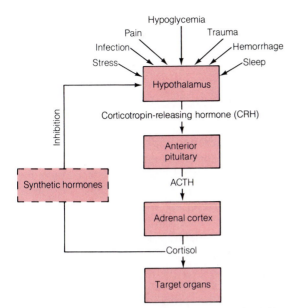

FIG. 45-9. The hypothalamic–pituitary–adrenal (HPA) feedback system that regulates glucocorticoid (cortisol) levels. Cortisol release is regulated by ACTH. Stress exerts its effects on cortisol release through the HPA system and the corticotropin-releasing factor (CRF), which controls the release of ACTH from the anterior pituitary gland. Increased cortisol levels incite a negative feedback inhibition of ACTH release. Pharmacologic doses of synthetic steroids inhibit ACTH release by way of the hypothalamic CRF.

tions of the body and in controlling the inflammatory response. The actions of cortisol are summarized in Table 45-2. Many of the antiinflammatory actions attributed to cortisol result from the administration of pharmacologic levels of the hormone.

Metabolic Effects. Cortisol stimulates glucose production by the liver, promotes protein breakdown, and causes mobilization of fatty acids. As body proteins are broken down, amino acids are mobilized and transported to the liver, where they are used in the production of glucose (gluconeogenesis). The mobilization of fatty acids serves to convert cell metabolism from the utilization of glucose for energy to the utilization of fatty acids instead.

As glucose production by the liver rises and peripheral glucose utilization falls, there is moderate insulin resistance. In persons with diabetes and those who are diabetes-prone, this has the effect of raising the blood sugar.

Psychic Effects. The glucocorticoid hormones appear to be involved either directly or indirectly in emotional behavior. Receptors for these hormones have been identified in brain tissue, which suggests that they play a role in the regulation of behavior.[12] It has been noted that people treated with adrenal cor-

TABLE 45-2. ACTIONS OF CORTISOL	
MAJOR INFLUENCE	**EFFECT ON BODY**
Glucose metabolism	Stimulates gluconeogenesis
	Decreases glucose utilization by the tissues
Protein metabolism	Increases breakdown of proteins
	Increases plasma protein levels
Fat metabolism	Increases mobilization of fatty acids
	Increases utilization of fatty acids
Antiinflammatory action (pharmacologic levels)	Stabilizes lysosomal membranes of the inflammatory cells, preventing the release of inflammatory mediators
	Decreases capillary permeability to prevent inflammatory edema
	Depresses phagocytosis by white blood cells to reduce the release of inflammatory mediators
	Suppresses the immune response
	Causes atrophy of lymphoid tissue
	Decreases eosinophils
	Decreases antibody formation
	Decreases the development of cell-mediated immunity
	Reduces fever
	Inhibits fibroblast activity
Psychic effect	Tends to contribute to emotional stability
Permissive effect	Facilitates the response of the tissues to humoral and neural influences, such as that of the catecholamines, during trauma and extreme stress

tical hormones have displayed behavior ranging from mildly aberrant to psychotic.

Antiinflammatory Effects. Large quantities of cortisol are required for an effective antiinflammatory action. This is achieved by the administration of pharmacologic doses of synthetic cortisol. The increased cortisol blocks inflammation at an early stage by decreasing capillary permeability and stabilizing the lysosomal membranes so that inflammatory mediators are not released. Cortisol suppresses the immune response by reducing humoral and cell-mediated immunity. With this lessened inflammatory response comes a reduction in fever. During the healing phase, cortisol suppresses fibroblast activity and thereby lessens scar formation. Cortisol also inhibits prostaglandin synthesis, which may account in large part for its antiinflammatory actions.

SUPPRESSION OF ADRENAL FUNCTION

A highly significant aspect of long-term therapy with pharmacologic preparations of the adrenal cortical hormones is adrenal insufficiency on withdrawal of the drugs. The deficiency is due to suppression of the HPA system. Chronic suppression causes atrophy of the entire system, and abrupt withdrawal of drugs can cause acute adrenal insufficiency. Furthermore, recovery to a state of normal adrenal function may be prolonged, requiring up to 12 months.

TESTS OF ADRENAL FUNCTION

There are a number of diagnostic tests by which adrenal cortical function and the HPA may be evaluated. Blood levels of cortisol, aldosterone, and ACTH can be measured using radioimmunoassay methods. A 24-hour urine specimen measures the excretion of 17-ketosteroids, 17-ketogenic steroids, and 17-hydroxycorticosteroids. These metabolic end-products of the adrenal hormones and the male androgens provide information about alterations in the biosynthesis of the adrenal cortical hormones. Suppression and stimulation tests afford a means of assessing the state of the HPA feedback system. For example, a test dose of ACTH may be given to assess the response of the adrenal cortex to pituitary stimulation. Similarly, administration of dexamethasone (a synthetic glucocorticoid drug) provides a means of measuring negative feedback suppression of ACTH. Adrenal tumors and ectopic ACTH-producing tumors are generally unresponsive to ACTH suppression by dexamethasone. Metyrapone (Metopirone) blocks the final step in cortisol synthesis, producing 11-dehydroxycortisol, which does not inhibit ACTH.

This test measures the ability of the pituitary to release ACTH.

CONGENITAL ADRENAL HYPERPLASIA (ADRENOGENITAL SYNDROME)

Congenital adrenal hyperplasia (CAH) describes a congenital disorder caused by an autosomal recessive trait in which a deficiency exists in any of the five enzymes necessary for the synthesis of cortisol. A common characteristic of all types is a defect in the synthesis of cortisol that results in increased levels of ACTH and adrenal hyperplasia. The increased levels of ACTH overstimulate the pathways for production of adrenal androgens. Mineralocorticoids may be produced in excessive or insufficient amounts, depending on the precise enzyme deficiency. Both males and females are affected. Males are seldom diagnosed at birth, unless they have enlarged genitalia or lose salt and manifest adrenal crisis; in female infants, an increase in androgens is responsible for creating the virilization syndrome of ambiguous genitalia with an enlarged clitoris, fused labia, and urogenital sinus (Fig. 45-10). In both males and females, other secondary sex characteristics are normal, and fertility is unaffected if appropriate therapy is instituted.

The two most common enzyme deficiencies are the 21-hydroxylase and 11-β-hydroxylase deficien-

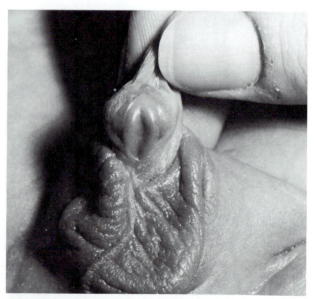

FIG. 45-10. Female infant with congenital adrenal hyperplasia demonstrating virilization of the genitalia. Note the enlarged clitoris and the fused labia, which resembles a scrotal sac. (Hurwitz, L. S. [1980]. Nursing implications of selected endocrine disorders. *Nursing Clinics of North America, 15*[3], 528. Reprinted with permission)

cies. The clinical manifestations of both deficiencies are largely determined by the functional properties of the steroid intermediates and the completeness of the block in the cortisol pathway.

A spectrum of 21-hydroxylase deficiency states exists, ranging from simple virilizing CAH to a complete salt-losing enzyme deficiency. Simple virilizing CAH impairs the synthesis of cortisol, and steroid synthesis is shunted to androgen production. People with these deficiencies usually produce sufficient aldosterone or aldosterone intermediates to prevent signs and symptoms of mineralocorticoid deficiency. The salt-losing form is accompanied by deficient production of aldosterone and its intermediates. This results in fluid and electrolyte disorders after the fifth day of life, including hyponatremia, hyperkalemia, vomiting, dehydration, and shock.

The 11-β-hydroxylase deficiency is rare and manifests a spectrum of clinical severity. There is not only excessive androgen production but also impaired conversion of 11-deoxycorticosterone to corticosterone. The overproduction of 11-deoxycorticosterone, which has mineralocorticoid activity, is responsible for the hypertension that accompanies this deficiency.

Diagnosis of adrenogenital syndrome depends on the precise biochemical evaluation of metabolites in the cortisol pathway as well as on clinical signs and symptoms. Medical treatment of adrenogenital syndrome includes oral or parenteral cortisol replacement. Fludrocortisone acetate, a mineralocorticoid, may also be given to children who are salt losers. Depending on the degree of virilization, reconstructive surgery during the first 2 years of life is indicated to reduce the size of the clitoris, separate the labia, and exteriorize the vagina. Surgery has provided excellent results and does not impair sexual function.

ADRENAL INSUFFICIENCY

There are two forms of adrenal insufficiency: primary and secondary. Primary adrenal insufficiency, or Addison's disease, is due to the destruction of the adrenal gland. Secondary adrenal insufficiency is due to a disorder of the HPA system.

PRIMARY ADRENAL INSUFFICIENCY (ADDISON'S DISEASE)

In 1855, Thomas Addison, an English physician, provided the first detailed clinical description of primary adrenal insufficiency. Addison's disease is a relatively rare disorder in which all the layers of the adrenal cortex are destroyed. Autoimmune destruction is the most common cause of Addison's disease

in the United States. Tuberculosis is an infrequent cause in the United States but common where tuberculosis is more prevalent. Rare causes include metastatic carcinoma, fungal infection (particularly histoplasmosis), cytomegalovirus (mostly in people with acquired immunodeficiency syndrome [AIDS]), amyloid disease, and hemochromatosis. Bilateral adrenal hemorrhage may occur in people taking anticoagulants, during open heart surgery, and during birth or major trauma. The use of the term *Addison's disease* is reserved for adrenal insufficiency due to adrenocortical disease in which adrenocortical hormones are deficient and ACTH levels are elevated because of feedback stimulation.

Addison's disease, like insulin-dependent diabetes mellitus, is a chronic metabolic disorder that requires lifetime hormone replacement therapy. The adrenal cortex has a large reserve capacity, and the manifestations of adrenal insufficiency do not usually become apparent until about 90% of the gland has been destroyed.[10] These manifestations are primarily related to (1) mineralocorticoid deficiency, (2) glucocorticoid deficiency, and (3) hyperpigmentation resulting from elevated ACTH levels. Although lack of the adrenal androgens exerts few effects in men because the testes produce these hormones, women will have sparse axillary and pubic hair. The manifestations of adrenal insufficiency are summarized in Table 45-3.

Mineralocorticoid deficiency causes increased urinary losses of sodium, chloride, and water along with decreased excretion of potassium. The result is hyponatremia, loss of extracellular fluid, decreased cardiac output, and hyperkalemia. There may be an abnormal appetite for salt. Orthostatic hypotension is common. Dehydration, weakness, and fatigue are often present as early symptoms. If loss of sodium and water is extreme, cardiovascular collapse and shock ensue. Because of a lack of glucocorticoids, the person with Addison's disease has poor tolerance to stress. This deficiency causes hypoglycemia, lethargy, weakness, fever, and gastrointestinal symptoms such as anorexia, nausea, vomiting, and weight loss. Hyperpigmentation results from elevated levels of ACTH. The skin looks bronzed or suntanned in both exposed and unexposed areas, and the normal creases and pressure points tend to become especially dark. The gums and oral mucous membranes may become bluish black. This hyperpigmentation becomes more pronounced during periods of stress. The amino acid sequence of ACTH is strikingly similar to that of melanocyte-stimulating hormone (MSH); thus, hyperpigmentation is seen in about 98% of people with Addison's disease and is helpful in distinguishing the primary and secondary forms of adrenal insufficiency.

TABLE 45-3. MANIFESTATIONS OF ADRENAL CORTICAL INSUFFICIENCY AND EXCESS

PARAMETER	ADRENAL CORTICAL INSUFFICIENCY	GLUCOCORTICOID EXCESS
Electrolytes	Hyponatremia* Hyperkalemia*	Hypokalemia
Fluids	Dehydration* (elevated BUN, others)	Edema
Blood pressure	Hypotension* Shock* Orthostatic hypotension	Hypertension
Musculoskeletal	Muscle weakness* Fatigue*	Muscle wasting Fatigue
Hair and skin	Skin pigmentation	Easy bruisability Hirsutism, acne, and striae (abdomen and thighs)
Inflammatory response	Low resistance to trauma, infection, and stress	Decrease in eosinophils Lymphocytopenia
Gastrointestinal	Nausea, vomiting* Abdominal pain*	Possible gastrointestinal bleeding
Glucose metabolism	Hypoglycemia*	Impaired glucose tolerance Glycosuria Elevated blood sugar
Emotional	Depression and irritability	Emotional lability to psychosis
Other	Menstrual irregularity Decreased axillary and pubic hair in women	Oligomenorrhea Impotence in the male Centripetal obesity (moon face and buf- falo hump)

* Present in acute adrenal insufficiency.

SECONDARY ADRENAL INSUFFICIENCY

Secondary adrenal insufficiency can occur as the result of hypopituitarism or because the pituitary gland has been surgically removed. However, a far more common cause than either of these is the rapid withdrawal of glucocorticoids that have been administered therapeutically. These drugs suppress the HPA system, with resulting adrenal cortical atrophy and lack of cortisol. It is important to note that this suppression continues long after drug therapy has been discontinued and could be critical during periods of stress or when surgery is performed.

ACUTE ADRENAL CRISIS

Acute adrenal crisis is a life-threatening situation. If Addison's disease is the underlying problem, exposure to even a minor illness or stress can precipitate nausea, vomiting, muscular weakness, hypotension, dehydration, and vascular collapse. The onset of adrenal crisis may be sudden, or it may progress over a period of several days. The symptoms may also occur suddenly in children with salt-losing forms of the adrenogenital syndrome. Massive bilateral adrenal hemorrhage causes an acute fulminating form of adrenal insufficiency. Hemorrhage can be caused by meningococcal septicemia (called *Waterhouse-Friderichsen syndrome*), adrenal trauma, anticoagulant therapy, adrenal vein thrombosis, or adrenal metastases.

Adrenal insufficiency is treated with hormone replacement therapy that includes a combination of glucocorticoids and mineralocorticoids. In acute adrenal insufficiency, cortisol is given intravenously followed by rapid infusion of saline and glucose. The day-to-day regulation of the chronic phase of Addison's disease is usually accomplished with oral cortisol, and higher doses are given during periods of stress. Because these people with the disorder are likely to have episodes of hyponatremia and hypoglycemia, they need to have a regular schedule for meals and exercise.

GLUCOCORTICOID HORMONE EXCESS (CUSHING'S SYNDROME)

The term *Cushing's syndrome* refers to the manifestations of hypercortisolism due to any cause. Three important forms of Cushing's syndrome result from excess glucocorticoid production by the body. One is a *pituitary form*, which results from excessive production of ACTH by a tumor of the pituitary gland; it accounts for about two thirds of the disease cases, and because this form of the disease was the one originally described by Cushing, it is called Cushing's disease. The second form is the *adrenal form*, caused by an adrenal tumor (benign or malignant). The third form is *ectopic* Cushing's, due to a nonpituitary ACTH-secreting tumor. Certain extrapituitary malignant tumors such as small cell carcinoma of the lung may secrete ACTH or, more rarely, CRF and produce severe Cushing's syndrome. Cushing's syndrome can also result from long-term therapy with one of the potent pharmacologic preparations of glucocorticoids (*iatrogenic Cushing's syndrome*).

The major manifestations of Cushing's syndrome represent an exaggeration of the many actions of cortisol (see Table 45-3). Altered fat metabolism causes a peculiar deposition of fat characterized by a protruding abdomen; subclavicular fat pads or "buffalo hump" on the back; and a round, plethoric "moon face." There is muscle weakness, and the extremities are thin because of protein breakdown and muscle wasting. In advanced cases, the skin over the forearms and legs becomes thin, having the appearance of parchment. Purple striae or stretch marks, from stretching of the catabolically weakened skin and subcutaneous tissues, are distributed on the breast, thighs, and abdomen. Osteoporosis may develop due to destruction of bone proteins and alterations in calcium metabolism, resulting in back pain, compression fractures of the vertebrae, and rib fractures. As calcium is mobilized from bone, renal calculi may develop. Derangements in glucose metabolism are found in some 90% of patients, with clinically overt diabetes mellitus occurring in about 20%.[10] The glucocorticoids possess mineralocorticoid properties; this causes hypokalemia as a result of excessive potassium excretion and hypertension resulting from sodium retention. Inflammatory and immune responses are inhibited, resulting in increased susceptibility to infection. Cortisol increases gastric acid secretion, and this may provoke gastric ulceration and bleeding. An accompanying increase in androgen levels causes hirsutism, mild acne, and menstrual irregularities in women. Excess levels of the glucocorticoids may give rise to extreme emotional lability, ranging from mild euphoria and absence of normal fatigue to grossly psychotic behavior.

Diagnosis of Cushing's syndrome depends on the finding of elevated plasma levels of cortisol. One of the prominent features of Cushing's syndrome is loss of the diurnal pattern of cortisol secretion. Therefore, cortisol determinations are often made on three blood samples: one taken in the morning, one in late afternoon or early evening, and a third drawn the following morning after a midnight dose of dexamethasone. Measurement of plasma ACTH, 24-hour urinary 17-ketosteroids, 17-ketogenic steroids, and 17-hydroxycorticosteroids, and suppression or stimulation tests of the HPA system are often made. Skull x-ray films and intravenous pyelograms, which outline the shadows of the kidneys and adrenal glands, may be done. CT scans afford a means for locating adrenal or pituitary tumors.

Untreated, Cushing's syndrome produces serious morbidity and even death. The treatment method, whether by surgery, irradiation, or pharmacologic, is largely determined by the cause of the hypercortisolism. The goal of treatment for Cushing's syndrome is to remove or correct the source of hypercortisolism without causing any permanent pituitary or adrenal damage.[13] A transsphenoidal removal of a pituitary adenoma or a hemihypophysectomy is the preferred method of treatment for Cushing's disease. This allows for removal of the tumor rather than the entire pituitary gland. After successful removal, the person must take replacement glucocorticoid therapy for 6 to 12 months. Patients may also receive pituitary irradiation, but the cure rate is only about 25% and remissions require up to 6 months. An adrenalectomy (unilateral or bilateral) may be done in the case of adrenal adenoma. When possible, ectopic ACTH-producing tumors are removed. Pharmacologic agents that block steroid synthesis (ketoconazole, metyrapone, and aminoglutethimide) may used to treat people with ectopic tumors that cannot be resected.

In summary, the adrenal cortex produces three types of hormones: mineralocorticoids, glucocorticoids, and adrenal sex hormones. The mineralocorticoids along with the renin–angiotensin mechanism aid in controlling body levels of sodium and potassium. The glucocorticoids have antiinflammatory actions and aid in regulating glucose, protein, and fat metabolism during periods of stress. These hormones are under the control of the hypothalamic–pituitary–adrenal (HPA) system. The adrenal sex hormones exert little effect on the day-to-day control of body function, but probably contribute to the development of body hair in women. The adrenal genital syndrome describes a genetic defect in the cortisol pathway resulting from a deficiency of one of the enzymes needed for its synthesis. Depending on the enzyme involved, the disorder causes virilization of female infants and, in some instances, fluid and electrolyte disturbances because of impaired mineralocorticoid synthesis. Chronic adrenal insufficiency is called Addison's disease. It can be caused by destruction of the adrenal gland or by dysfunction of the HPA system. Adrenal insufficiency requires replacement therapy with cortical hormones. Acute adrenal insufficiency is a life-threatening situation. Cushing's syndrome exists when the glucocorticoid level is abnormally high. This syndrome may be a result of pharmacologic doses of cortisol, a pituitary or adrenal tumor, or an ectopic tumor that produces ACTH. The clinical manifestations of Cushing's syndrome reflect the very high level of cortisol that is present.

■ REFERENCES

1. Guyton, A. (1991). *Medical physiology* (8th ed., pp. 822–824, 835, 843). Philadelphia: W.B. Saunders.
2. Ganong, W.F. (1991). *Medical physiology* (15th ed., pp. 378–383). Norwalk, CT: Appleton Lange.
3. Findling, J.W., & Tyrell, B.J. (1991). Anterior pituitary. In F.S. Greenspan (Ed.). *Basic and clinical endocrinology* (3rd ed., pp. 84–86, 121, 133–146, 166, 200–202). Norwalk, CT: Appleton Lange.
4. Wheeler, M.D., & Styne, D.M. (1990). Diagnosis and management of precocious puberty. *Pediatric Clinics of North America, 37,* 1255–1271.
5. Melmed, S. (1990). Acromegaly. *New England Journal of Medicine, 322,* 966–977.
6. Glorieux, J., Dussault, J.H., Morissette, J., et al. (1985). Follow-up at ages 5 and 7 years on mental development in children with hypothyroidism detected in the Quebec Screening Program. *Journal of Pediatrics, 107,* 913.
7. New England Congenital Hypothyroid Collaborative. (1985). Neonatal hypothyroid screening: Status of patients at 6 years of age. *Journal of Pediatrics, 107,* 915.
8. Klein, A.H., Meltzer, S., Kenney, F., et al. (1972). Improved prognosis in congenital hypothyroidism treated before age three months. *Journal of Pediatrics, 81,* 912.
9. Guters, A. (1992). Congenital hypothyroidism. *Pediatric Annals, 31,* 17–28.
10. Cotran, R.S., Kumar, V., & Robbins, S.L. (1989). *Pathologic basis of disease* (4th ed., pp. 1220–1221, 1252, 1254). Philadelphia: W.B. Saunders.
11. Gavin, L.A. (1990). Thyroid crisis. *Medical Clinics of North America, 75,* 179–193.
12. McEwan, B.S. (1978). Influences of the adrenocortical hormone on pituitary and brain function. *Monographs on Endocrinology, 12,* 467.
13. Gumowski, J., Proch, M., & Kessler, C.A. (1992). Endocrinopathies of hyperfunction: Cushing's syndrome and hyperaldosteronism. *AACN Clinical Issues in Critical Care Nursing, 3,* 331–347.

■ BIBLIOGRAPHY

Aron, D.C. (1987). Cushing's syndrome: Current concepts in diagnosis and treatment. *Comprehensive Therapy, 13,* 37–44.

Bartuska, D.G. (1991). Thyroid disease in the elderly. *Hospital Practice, 26*(12A), 85102.

Biglieri, E.G. (1989). ACTH effects on aldosterone, cortisol, and other steroids. *Hospital Practice, 24*(1A), 145–164.

Cara, J.F., & Johanson, A.J. (1990). Growth hormone for short stature not due to classic growth hormone deficiency. *Pediatric Clinics of North America, 37,* 1229–1253.

Cutler, G.B., & Laue, L. (1990). Congenital adrenal hyperplasia due to 21-hydroxylase deficiency. *New England Journal of Medicine, 323,* 1806–1813.

Foley, T.P. (1992). Thyrotoxicosis in childhood. *Pediatric Annals, 21,* 43–49.

Gavin, L.A. (1988). The diagnostic dilemmas of hyperthyroxinemia and hypothyroxinemia. *Advances in Internal Medicine, 33,* 185.

Hurwitz, L.S. (1980). Nursing implications of selected pediatric endocrine disorders. *Nursing Clinics of North America, 15*(3):525.

Kay, T.B., & Crapo, L. (1990). The Cushing's syndrome: An update on diagnostic tests. *Annals of Internal Medicine, 112,* 434.

Lee, L.M. (1992). Adrenocortical insufficiency: A medical emergency. *AACN Clinical Issues in Critical Care Nursing, 3,* 319–330.

Levy, E.G. (1991). Thyroid disease in the elderly. *Medical Clinics of North America, 75,* 151–167.

Orth, D.N. (1991). Differential diagnosis of Cushing's syndrome. *New England Journal of Medicine, 325,* 957–959.

Sawin, C.T. (1991). Thyroid dysfunction in older persons. *Advances in Internal Medicine, 37,* 223–249.

Singer, P.A. (1991). Thyroiditis. *Medical Clinics of North America, 75,* 61–77.

Small, R.C. (1992). Metabolic and anatomic thyroid emergencies: A review. *Critical Care Medicine, 20,* 276–291.

Spittle, L. (1992). Diagnoses in opposition: Thyroid storm and myxedema coma. *AACN Clinical Issues in Critical Care Nursing, 3,* 300–308.

Utiger, F.D. (1991). The pathogenesis of autoimmune thyroid disease. *New England Journal of Medicine, 325,* 278–279.

Wass, J.A.H., Laws, E.R., Jr., Randall, R.V., immune thyroid disease. *New England Journal of Medicine, 325,* 278–279.

Zimmerman, D., & Gan-Gaisano, M. (1990). Hyperthyroidism in children and adolescents. *Pediatric Clinics of North America, 37,* 1273–1297.

CHAPTER 46

DIABETES MELLITUS

CAROL MATTSON PORTH
LINDA S. HURWITZ

■ OBJECTIVES

After you have studied this chapter, you should be able to meet the following objectives:

■ Describe the actions of insulin with reference to glucose, fat, and protein metabolism.

■ Explain what is meant by a counterregulatory hormone and describe the actions of glucagon, epinephrine, growth hormone, and the adrenocortical hormones in regulation of blood glucose levels.

■ List the distinguishing characteristics of insulin-dependent diabetes mellitus (IDDM) and non–insulin-dependent diabetes mellitus (NIDDM), other types of diabetes, and gestational diabetes mellitus.

■ Explain why IDDM predisposes to the development of ketoacidosis, whereas NIDDM does not.

■ Describe the altered physiologic functioning underlying three "polys" that characterize diabetes mellitus.

■ Describe measures used in the treatment of an insulin reaction.

■ Compare blood glucose regulation during exercise in people without diabetes and those with IDDM, and relate this to the increased risk for development of hypoglycemia in a person with IDDM.

■ List five principles for diet management in people with diabetes.

■ State the actions of the oral hypoglycemic agents in terms of the lowering of blood glucose.

■ Name and describe the three types (according to duration of action) of insulin.

■ Describe the clinical manifestations of diabetic ketoacidosis and their physiologic significance.

■ Describe the clinical condition resulting from the nonketotic hyperosmolar state.

■ Describe the clinical manifestations of insulin-induced hypoglycemia and state how these might differ in elderly people.

Carol Mattson Porth: PATHOPHYSIOLOGY: CONCEPTS OF
ALTERED HEALTH STATES, 4th ed. © 1994, 1990, 1986, 1982
J.B. Lippincott Company

927

■ Describe and compare the Somogyi effect and the dawn phenomenon.
■ Cite a common characteristic of tissues that are affected by the chronic complications of diabetes.
■ Describe alterations in physiologic function that accompany diabetic peripheral neuropathies.
■ Describe the pathology underlying diabetic retinopathy.

■ Cite the relation between diabetes mellitus and the occurrence of macrovascular complications.
■ Describe the causes of foot ulcers in people with diabetes mellitus.
■ Explain the relation between diabetes mellitus and infection.

Diabetes mellitus is a chronic alteration in health that affects more than 12 million people in the United States. The disease affects people in all age groups and from all walks of life. The acute complications of diabetes are the most common causes of medical emergencies resulting from metabolic disease. Diabetes is the leading risk factor in coronary heart disease, stroke, and peripheral vascular disease, and it is the leading cause of blindness and end-stage renal disease.

HORMONAL CONTROL OF BLOOD GLUCOSE

The body uses glucose, fatty acids, and other substrates as fuel to satisfy its energy needs. Although the respiratory and circulatory systems combine efforts to furnish the body with oxygen needed for metabolic purposes, it is the liver, in concert with the pancreatic hormones insulin and glucagon, that controls the body's fuel supply. The secretion of both insulin and glucagon is regulated by blood glucose levels. Insulin is released in response to an increase in blood glucose, and glucagon, in response to a decrease in blood glucose. Both insulin and glucagon are transported from the pancreas through the portal circulation to the liver where they exert an almost instantaneous effect on blood glucose levels.

Glucose is an optional fuel for tissues such as muscle, adipose tissue, and the liver, which can use fatty acids and other fuel substrates for energy. When glucose is not needed for energy it is either stored as glycogen or converted into fat. When the cells (primarily the liver and skeletal muscle cells) approach saturation with glycogen, the additional glucose is converted into fatty acids, and then stored as triglycerides in fat cells. When blood glucose levels fall below normal, glycogen is broken down (*glycogenolysis*). However, only liver glycogen stores can be released into the blood stream to raise blood glucose levels. Skeletal muscle lacks the enzyme glucose 6-phosphatase that allows glucose to leave the cell, thus limiting the use of its glycogen stores to the

muscle cell. When body stores of glucose decrease below normal, the liver synthesizes additional glucose (*glucogenesis*) from amino acids and the glycerol portion of fat. Glucose metabolism is discussed more fully in Chapter 43.

In contrast to muscle, liver, and other body tissues, the brain and nervous system relies almost exclusively on glucose for its energy needs. Because the brain can neither synthesize nor store more than a few minutes' supply of glucose, normal cerebral function requires a continuous supply from the circulation. Severe and prolonged hypoglycemia can cause brain death, and even moderate hypoglycemia can result in substantial brain dysfunction.[1] The body maintains a system of *counterregulatory mechanisms* to counteract hypoglycemia-producing situations and thus ensure brain function and survival. The physiologic mechanisms that prevent or correct hypoglycemia include the actions of the counterregulatory hormones: glucagon, the catecholamines, growth hormone, and the glucocorticoids.

INSULIN

Insulin is produced by the pancreatic β cells in the islets of Langerhans. The active form of the hormone is composed of two polypeptide chains—an A chain and a B chain (Fig. 46-1). The chains emerge with the appropriate linkage required for biologic activity from a single chain called *proinsulin*. In converting proinsulin to insulin, enzymes in the β cell cleave proinsulin at specific sites to form two substances, active *insulin* and a *C-peptide* chain (the link that served to join the A and B chains before they were separated), which has no biologic activity. Both active insulin and the inactive C-peptide chain are released simultaneously from the β cell (Fig. 46-2). The C-peptide chains can be measured, and this measurement can be used to study β-cell activity. For example, injected insulin in a person with mature-onset diabetes would provide few, if any, C-peptide chains, whereas insulin secreted by the β cells would be accompanied by secretion of C-peptide chains.

Insulin secreted by the β cells enters the portal

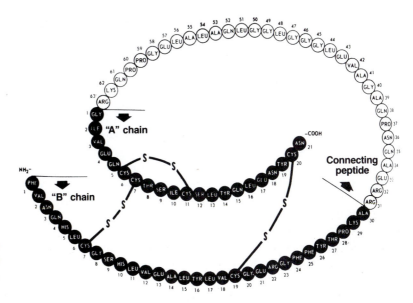

FIG. 46-1. Amino acid sequence of porcine proinsulin showing the A chain, B chain, and C peptide link. (Shaw, W. N., & Change, R. E. [1968]. *Diabetes, 17*[12], 738.)

circulation and travels directly to the liver where about 50% is either utilized or degraded. Once it has been released into the general circulation, insulin has a half-life of about 15 minutes. This is because circulating insulin is rapidly bound to peripheral tissues or destroyed by the liver or kidneys.

The actions of insulin are three-fold: (1) it provides for glucose storage, (2) it prevents fat and glycogen breakdown, and (3) it inhibits gluconeogenesis and increases protein synthesis. Although several hormones are known to increase blood glucose, insulin is the only hormone known to have a direct effect in lowering blood glucose. The actions of insulin are summarized in Chart 46-1.

Insulin lowers blood glucose by facilitating its transport into skeletal muscle and adipose tissue. Although liver cells do not require insulin for glucose transport, a rise in insulin levels does cause an increase in the hepatic uptake of glucose and its conversion to glycogen. Insulin also decreases the breakdown of glycogen both within the liver and in muscle tissue. Fat is the most efficient form of fuel storage. It

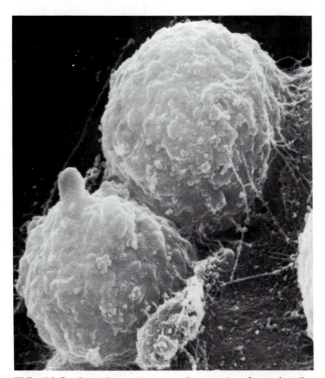

FIG. 46-2. Scanning electron micrograph of an insulin-secreting β cell from the islets of Langerhans in the pancreas. (Courtesy of Kenneth Siegesmund, Ph.D., Anatomy Department, Medical College of Wisconsin, Milwaukee, WI.)

CHART 46-1: ACTIONS OF INSULIN ON GLUCOSE, FATS, AND PROTEIN

Glucose

Increases glucose transport into skeletal muscle and adipose tissue
Increases glycogen synthesis
Decreases gluconeogenesis

Fats

Increases glucose transport into fat cells
Increases fatty acid transport into adipose cells
Increases triglyceride synthesis

Proteins

Increases active transport of amino acids into cells
Increases protein synthesis by accelerating translation of RNA by ribosomes and increased transcription of DNA in the nucleus to form increased amounts of RNA
Decreases protein breakdown by enhancing the use of glucose and fatty acids as a fuel source

provides 9 kcal/g of stored substrate in contrast to the 4 kcal/g provided by carbohydrates and proteins. Insulin acts to promote fat storage by increasing the transport of glucose into fat cells and by both facilitating triglyceride synthesis from glucose within fat cells and inhibiting the intracellular breakdown of stored triglycerides. In relation to body proteins, insulin both inhibits protein breakdown and increases protein synthesis by increasing the active transport of amino acids into body cells. Insulin also inhibits gluconeogenesis or the building of glucose from new sources, mainly amino acids. When sufficient glucose and insulin are present, protein breakdown is minimal because the body is able to use glucose and fatty acids as a fuel source. In children and adolescents, insulin is needed for normal growth and development.

Insulin release is regulated by blood glucose levels, increasing as blood glucose levels rise and decreasing when blood glucose levels decline. Serum insulin levels begin to rise within minutes after a meal, reach a peak in about 30 minutes, and then return to baseline levels within 3 hours. Between periods of food intake, insulin levels remain low and sources of stored glucose and amino acids are mobilized to supply the energy needs of glucose-dependent tissues. The glucose tolerance test, described later in this chapter, uses a glucose challenge as an indirect measure of the body's ability to secrete insulin and remove glucose from the blood.

GLUCAGON

Glucagon, a small protein molecule produced by the pancreatic α cells of the islets of Langerhans, maintains blood glucose between meals and during periods of fasting. Like insulin, glucagon travels by way of the portal vein to the liver where it exerts its main action. In contrast to insulin, glucagon secretion is inhibited by glucose.

The actions of glucagon are opposite to those of insulin. Glucagon stimulates glycogenolysis and gluconeogenesis, increases lipolysis and the output of ketones by the liver, and enhances the uptake of amino acids by the liver. The actions of glucagon are summarized in Chart 46-2.

It has been suggested that abnormalities in glucagon secretion contribute to the elevation of blood glucose levels observed in diabetes mellitus. Unger has suggested that it is the ratio of insulin to glucagon, rather than the absolute amount of either hormone, that determines blood glucose levels.[2] According to theory, glucagon secretion is unopposed in a person with diabetes because of the lack of insulin, which therefore leads to increased production of glucose by the liver.

CHART 46-2: ACTIONS OF GLUCAGON ON GLUCOSE, FATS, AND PROTEINS

Glucose
Promotes the breakdown of glycogen into glucose-phosphate
Increases gluconeogenesis

Fats
Enhances lipolysis in adipose tissue, liberating glycerol for use in gluconeogenesis

Proteins
Increases breakdown of proteins into amino acids for use in gluconeogenesis
Increases transport of amino acids in hepatic cells
Increases conversion of amino acids into glucose precursors

CATECHOLAMINES

The catecholamines, epinephrine and norepinephrine, help to maintain blood glucose levels during periods of stress. The actions of epinephrine are summarized in Chart 46-3. Epinephrine inhibits insulin release and promotes glycogenolysis by stimulating the conversion of muscle and liver glycogen to glucose. Muscle glycogen cannot be released into the blood; nevertheless, the mobilization of these stores for muscle use conserves blood glucose for use by other tissues such as the brain and the nervous system. During periods of exercise and other types of stress, epinephrine inhibits insulin release from the β cells and thereby decreases the movement of glucose into muscle cells. The catecholamines also increase lipase activity and thereby cause increased mobilization of fatty acids; this also serves to conserve glucose. The blood glucose–elevating effect of epinephrine is an important homeostatic mechanism in hypoglycemia.

GROWTH HORMONE

Growth hormone has many specific metabolic effects. It increases protein synthesis in all cells of the body, mobilizes fatty acids from adipose tissue, and

---

CHART 46-3: ACTIONS OF EPINEPHRINE ON METABOLISM

Mobilizes glycogen stores
Decreases movement of glucose into body cells
Inhibits insulin release from β cells
Mobilizes fatty acids from adipose tissue

antagonizes the effects of insulin. Growth hormone produces a decrease in both cellular uptake and utilization of glucose, thereby producing an increase in blood glucose, sometimes to as high as 50% to 100% of normal.[3] In turn, this increase in blood glucose increases the stimulus for insulin secretion by the β cells. The secretion of growth hormone normally is inhibited by insulin and increased levels of blood glucose. During periods of fasting, when both blood glucose levels and insulin secretion fall, growth hormone levels increase. Exercise, such as running and cycling, and various stresses, including anesthesia, fever, and trauma, produce an increase in growth hormone levels.

A chronic hypersecretion of growth hormone, as occurs in acromegaly (see Chapter 45), can lead to glucose intolerance and the development of diabetes mellitus. In people who already have diabetes, moderate elevations in growth hormone levels that occur during periods of stress and periods of growth in children can produce the entire spectrum of metabolic abnormalities associated with poor regulation, despite optimized insulin treatment.

GLUCOCORTICOID HORMONES

The glucocorticoid hormones exhibit an important effect in increasing blood glucose. They are synthesized in the adrenal cortex along with other corticosteroid hormones. There are several steroid hormones with glucocorticoid activity; the most important of these is cortisol, which accounts for about 95% of all glucocorticoid activity.[3]

The glucocorticoid hormones are critical to survival during periods of fasting and starvation. They stimulate gluconeogenesis by the liver, sometimes producing a 6- to 10-fold increase in hepatic glucose production. These hormones also cause a moderate decrease in tissue utilization of glucose. In predisposed people, the prolonged elevation of glucocorticoid hormones can lead to hyperglycemia and the development of diabetes mellitus. In people with diabetes, even transient increases in cortisol can complicate control.

Cortisol levels increase during periods of stress, such as that produced by infection, pain, trauma, surgery, prolonged and strenuous exercise, and acute anxiety. Hypoglycemia is a potent stimulus for cortisol secretion. The control of cortisol secretion is discussed in Chapter 45.

In summary, energy metabolism is controlled by a number of hormones, including insulin, glucagon, epinephrine, growth hormone, and the glucocorticoids. Of these hormones, only insulin has the effect of lowering blood glucose. Insulin's blood glucose–lowering action results from its ability to increase the transport of glucose into body cells and decrease hepatic production and release of glucose into the bloodstream. Other hormones—glucagon, epinephrine, growth hormone, and the glucocorticoids—serve to maintain or increase blood glucose and are referred to as counterregulatory hormones. Glucagon and epinephrine promote glycogenolysis. Glucagon and the glucocorticoids increase gluconeogenesis. Growth hormone decreases the peripheral utilization of glucose. Whereas insulin has the effect of decreasing lipolysis and the utilization of fats as a fuel source, both glucagon and epinephrine increase fat utilization.

■ DIABETES MELLITUS

The term *diabetes mellitus* means "the running through of sugar." Reports of the disorder can be traced back to the 1st century A.D. when Aretaeus the Cappadocian described the disorder as a chronic affection characterized by intense thirst and voluminous honey-sweet urine—"the melting down of flesh into urine."[4] It was the discovery of insulin by Banting and Best in 1921 that transformed the once-fatal disease into a chronic health problem.

Diabetes is a disorder of carbohydrate, protein, and fat metabolism resulting from an imbalance between insulin availability and insulin need. It can represent an absolute insulin deficiency, the impaired release of insulin by the pancreatic β cells, the presence of inadequate or defective insulin receptors, or the production of insulin that is inactive or destroyed before it can carry out its action. A person with uncontrolled diabetes is unable to transport glucose into fat and muscle cells; as a result, the body cells are starved and the breakdown of fat and protein is increased.

CLASSIFICATION AND ETIOLOGY

Although diabetes mellitus is clearly a disorder of insulin availability, it is probably not a single disease. A classification system that divides diabetes into insulin-dependent and non–insulin-dependent forms was developed by an international workshop sponsored by the National Diabetes Data Group of the National Institutes of Health (Table 46-1).[5] Included in the classification system is a category for gestational diabetes (diabetes that develops during pregnancy), impaired glucose tolerance (abnormal glucose tolerance test without other signs of diabetes), and a secondary form of diabetes caused by other conditions (*e.g.*, Cushing's syndrome).

TYPE I INSULIN-DEPENDENT DIABETES MELLITUS

Type I or insulin-dependent diabetes mellitus (IDDM) is characterized by an absolute insulin defi-

TABLE 46-1. CLASSIFICATION OF DIABETES AND GLUCOSE INTOLERANCE STATES

CLASSIFICATION	FORMER TERMINOLOGY	CHARACTERISTICS
Diabetes Mellitus (DM)		
Type I		
Insulin-dependent diabetes mellitus (IDDM)	Juvenile-onset diabetes	People in this subclass are dependent on injected insulin
		Ketosis prone
Type II		
Non–insulin-dependent diabetes mellitus (NIDDM)	Adult-onset, maturity-onset diabetes	People in this subclass are not insulin-dependent, but they may use insulin
1. Nonobese NIDDM		Not ketosis prone
2. Obese NIDDM (60%–90%)		Frequently obese
Other types		
Pancreatic disease	Secondary diabetes	Presence of diabetes and associated condition
Hormonal		
Drug- or chemical-induced insulin receptor abnormalities		
Certain genetic defects		
Other types		
Impaired Glucose Tolerance (IGT)		
Nonobese IGT	Asymptomatic, chemical, subclinical, borderline, latent diabetes	Based on nondiagnostic fasting glucose levels and glucose tolerance test between normal and diabetic
Obese IGT		
IGT associated with other conditions, including (1) pancreatic disease, (2) hormonal, (3) drug or chemical, (4) insulin-receptor abnormalities, or (5) genetic syndromes		
Gestational Diabetes Mellitus (GDM)	Gestational diabetes	Glucose intolerance that developed during pregnancy
		Increased risk of perinatal complications
		Increased risk of developing diabetes within 5–10 years after parturition

(Adapted from National Diabetes Data Group. [1979]. Classification and diagnosis of diabetes mellitus and other categories of glucose intolerance. *Diabetes, 28,* 1042. Reprinted with permission of the American Diabetic Association)

ciency state. In the United States and Europe, about 10% to 20% of people with diabetes have IDDM.[6] This type of diabetes, formerly called juvenile diabetes, occurs more commonly in young people but can occur at any age. IDDM is a catabolic disorder characterized by an elevation in blood glucose and a breakdown of both body fats and proteins. One of the actions of insulin is the inhibition of lipolysis (fat breakdown) and the release of free fatty acids from fat cells. In the absence of insulin, ketosis develops when these fatty acids are released from fat cells and converted to ketones in the liver. Because of their absolute lack of insulin, people with type I diabetes mellitus are particularly prone to develop keto-acidosis. All people with IDDM require exogenous insulin replacement to reverse the catabolic state, control blood glucose levels, and prevent ketosis.

It has been suggested that IDDM results from

a genetic predisposition (diabetogenic genes), a hypothetical triggering event that involves an environmental agent that serves to incite an immune response, and immunologically mediated β cell destruction.[7,8] Much recent evidence has focused on the inherited major histocompatibility complex (MHC) genes that code the human leukocyte antigens (HLA) found on the surface of body cells (see Chapter 13). There is a strong association between certain HLA antigens (DR3 and DR4) in Caucasians coded by these immune response genes and IDDM. Thus, it appears that what is inherited as part of the HLA genotype in IDDM is a susceptibility to an abnormal immune response that affects β cells. Islet cell antibodies have been found in as many as 60% to 95% of newly diagnosed people with IDDM and in people who later develop the disease.[7,8] In addition to the MHC genes, an insulin gene relating β-cell replication and function has been identified on chromosome 11.

Environmental agents that have been associated with altered pancreatic β-cell function include viruses and chemical toxins. Mumps, congenital rubella, and the coxsackievirus have been associated with IDDM. Among the suspected chemical toxins are the nitrosamines, which are sometimes found in smoked and cured meats. The nitrosamines are related to streptozocin, which is used to induce diabetes in experimental animals, and to the rat poison Vacor, which can produce diabetes when ingested by humans.

The fact that IDDM is thought to result from an interaction between genetic and environmental factors has led to research into methods directed at prevention and early control of the disease. These methods include the identification of genetically susceptible people and early intervention in newly diagnosed people with IDDM. After the diagnosis of IDDM, there often is a short period of β-cell regeneration, sometimes called the *honeymoon period*, during which symptoms of diabetes disappear and insulin injections are not needed. Immune interventions designed to interrupt the destruction of β cells during the so-called honeymoon period are being investigated with hopes of finding a way to prevent complete and irreversible β-cell failure.

TYPE II NON–INSULIN-DEPENDENT DIABETES MELLITUS

Non–insulin-dependent diabetes mellitus (NIDDM), formerly known as maturity-onset diabetes, describes a condition of fasting hyperglycemia that occurs despite the availability of insulin. NIDDM is a nonketotic form of diabetes, it is not associated with HLA markers or inset-cell antibodies, and people with the disease usually are not dependent on insulin to sustain life. Most people with NIDDM are older and overweight and have fewer problems with control than do people with IDDM. Insulin levels in people with NIDDM usually are sufficient to prevent lipolysis and the development of ketosis but are inadequate to lower blood glucose by effecting the transport of glucose into fat cells. The metabolic abnormalities that contribute to the hyperglycemia that occurs in NIDDM include impaired insulin secretion, peripheral insulin resistance, and increased hepatic glucose production. Two subgroups of NIDDM are distinguished by the presence or absence of obesity.

Most people with NIDDM (about 80%) are overweight.[9] The type of obesity as well as the presence of obesity are important considerations in the development of NIDDM. Research has shown that people with upper-body obesity are at greater risk for developing NIDDM than people with lower-body obesity (see Chapter 43).[9, 10] Obese people have been shown to have increased resistance to the action of insulin and impaired suppression of glucose production by the liver, resulting in both hyperglycemia and hyperinsulinemia (Fig. 46-3). The increased insulin resistance has been attributed to either a decreased number of insulin receptors in the peripheral adipose tissues or the impairment of insulin receptor function. In addition to insulin resistance, there is an impairment of insulin release from β cells in response to glucose. Insulin resistance and β-cell function usually improve with weight loss, to the extent that many people with NIDDM can be managed with a weight-reduction program and exercise.

A second type of NIDDM occurs in nonobese people. These people have an absent or blunted early insulin response to glucose. Included in this subgroup are younger people with a strongly positive family history that suggests autosomal dominant transmission. Most people with the nonobese type of NIDDM respond well to dietary therapy or to the oral antidiabetic agents.

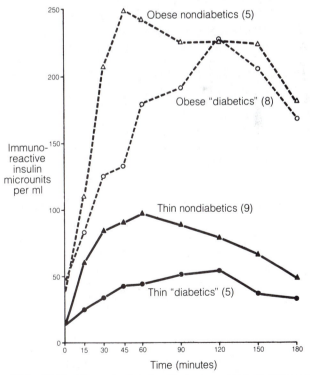

FIG. 46-3. Mean absolute insulin responses in both thin and obese patients with diabetes during a 3-hour (100-g) oral glucose tolerance curve. (Bagdade, J. D., Biermann, E. L., & Porter, D. [1967]. The significance of basal insulin levels in evaluation of the insulin response to glucose in diabetic and nondiabetic subjects. *Journal of Clinical Investigation (New York)*, 46(10), 1553.)

OTHER TYPES

The category labeled *other types* of diabetes, formerly known as secondary diabetes, describes diabetes that is associated with certain other conditions and syndromes. Such diabetes can occur secondary to pancreatic disease or the removal of pancreatic tissue; endocrine diseases, such as acromegaly; Cushing's syndrome; or pheochromocytoma. Endocrine disorders that produce hyperglycemia do so by either increasing the hepatic production of glucose or decreasing the cellular utilization of glucose.

Several diuretics—thiazides, furosemide, and ethacrynic acid—elevate blood glucose. These diuretics increase potassium loss, which is thought to impair insulin release. Other drugs known to cause hyperglycemia are diazoxide, glucocorticoids, levodopa, oral contraceptives, sympathomimetics, phenothiazines, phenytoin, and total parenteral nutrition (hyperalimentation). Drug-related increases in blood glucose usually are reversed once the drug has been discontinued.

IMPAIRED GLUCOSE TOLERANCE

The diagnosis *impaired glucose tolerance* describes a person with plasma glucose levels that range between those considered normal and those considered diabetic. Calorie restriction and weight reduction are important for overweight people in this class.

GESTATIONAL DIABETES

Gestational diabetes refers to glucose intolerance of varying degrees that occurs during pregnancy. It most frequently is seen in women with a family history of diabetes, glycosuria, a history of stillbirth or spontaneous abortion, the presence of fetal anomalies in previous pregnancy, a previous large or heavy-for-date baby, obesity in the mother, advanced maternal age, or five or more pregnancies. The presence of more than one of these risk factors is particularly indicative of increased risk. All pregnant women, however, should be screened for glucose intolerance because selective screening based on history and other attributes have been shown to be inadequate.[11] The Clinical Practice Recommendations of the American Diabetes Association suggest that all pregnant women who have not been identified as having glucose intolerance before the 24th week have a screening load glucose intolerance test between the 24th and 28th weeks of pregnancy. This test consists of 50 g of glucose given without regard for the last meal and followed in 1 hour by a venous blood sample for glucose.[11]

Diagnosis and careful medical management are essential because women with gestational diabetes are at higher risk for complications of pregnancy, mortality, and fetal abnormalities. Fetal abnormalities include macrosomia (large body size), hypoglycemia, hypocalcemia, polycythemia, and hyperbilirubinemia.

Treatment of gestational diabetes includes close observation of mother and fetus. Maternal fasting and postprandial blood glucose levels should be measured regularly. Fetal surveillance depends on the degree of risk for the fetus. The frequency of growth measurements and determinations of fetal distress depends on available technology and gestational age. All women with gestational diabetes mellitus require nutritional guidance. If dietary management alone does not achieve a fasting blood glucose level equal to or less than 105 mg/dL or a 2-hour postprandial blood glucose equal to or less than 120 mg/dL, insulin therapy with highly purified non-beef or human insulin may be indicated. Oral antidiabetic agents are teratogenic and not recommended in pregnancy. Self-monitoring of blood glucose levels is essential because urine glucose monitoring in pregnancy is not acceptable practice.

Women with gestational diabetes are at increased risk of developing diabetes 5 to 10 years after delivery. Women in whom gestational diabetes is diagnosed should be followed post partum to detect diabetes early in its course. It is recommended that they be evaluated during their first postpartum visit with a 2-hour oral glucose tolerance test with a 75-g glucose load.[11]

MANIFESTATIONS

Diabetes mellitus may have a rapid or an insidious onset. In IDDM, signs and symptoms often are acute and of sudden origin. On the other hand, NIDDM often develops more insidiously; its presence may be detected during a routine medical examination or when a patient seeks medical care for other reasons.

The most commonly identified signs and symptoms of diabetes are referred to as the three "polys"—*polyuria* (excessive urination), *polydipsia* (excessive thirst), and *polyphagia* (excessive hunger). These three symptoms are closely related to the hyperglycemia and glycosuria present in diabetes. Glucose is a small, osmotically active molecule. When blood glucose levels are sufficiently elevated, the amount of glucose filtered by the glomeruli of the kidney exceeds the amount that can be reabsorbed by the renal tubules; this results in glycosuria accompanied by large losses of water in the urine. Thirst results from intracellular dehydration that occurs as blood glucose levels rise and water is pulled out of body cells, including those in the thirst center. Cellular dehydration also causes dryness of the mouth. This early symptom may be easily overlooked in NIDDM, in which there is a gradual increase in blood glucose without accompanying signs of ketoacidosis. Polyphagia usually is not present in people with NIDDM. In IDDM, it probably results from cellular starvation and the depletion of cellular stores of carbohydrates, fats, and proteins.

Weight loss despite normal or increased appetite is a common occurrence in a person with uncontrolled IDDM. The cause of weight loss is two-fold. First, loss of body fluids results from osmotic diuresis. Vomiting may exaggerate the fluid loss in ketoacidosis. Second, body tissue is lost because the lack of insulin forces the body to use its fat stores and cellular proteins as sources of energy. In terms of weight loss, there often is a marked difference between NIDDM and IDDM. Weight loss is a frequent phenomenon in people with uncontrolled IDDM, whereas many people with uncomplicated NIDDM have problems with obesity.

Other signs and symptoms of hyperglycemia include recurrent blurred vision, fatigue, paresthesias, and skin infections. In NIDDM, these often are the symptoms that prompt a person to seek medical treatment. Blurred vision develops as the lens and retina are exposed to hyperosmolar fluids. Lowered plasma volume produces weakness and fatigue. Paresthesias reflect a temporary dysfunction of the peripheral sensory nerves. Chronic skin infections are common in NIDDM. Both hyperglycemia and glycosuria favor the growth of yeast organisms. Pruritus and vulvovaginitis resulting from candidal infections are common initial complaints in women with diabetes.

DIAGNOSIS AND MANAGEMENT

The diagnosis of diabetes mellitus is based on fasting blood glucose levels or the results of a glucose challenge test. Capillary blood glucose and self-monitoring of blood glucose can be performed by persons with diabetes to manage their disease. Glycosylated hemoglobin is used to determine metabolic control in people with chronic hyperglycemia. The treatment plan for diabetes usually involves diet, antidiabetic agents, and exercise. Weight loss and dietary management may be sufficient to control blood glucose levels in people with NIDDM.

BLOOD TESTS

Fasting Blood Glucose Test. The fasting blood glucose test measures glucose levels after food has been withheld for 8 to 12 hours. If the fasting plasma glucose level is higher than 140 mg/dL on more than one occasion, further evaluation with a standardized oral glucose tolerance test may be indicated.[12]

Glucose Tolerance Test. The oral glucose tolerance test is an important screening test for diabetes. The test measures the body's ability to store glucose by removing it from the blood. Using blood glucose levels, the test measures the response to a given amount of concentrated glucose at selected intervals, usually 30 minutes, 1 hour, 90 minutes, 2 hours, and 3 hours. Urine glucose may also be measured at these times. Insulin levels as well as proinsulin and C peptide levels may also be measured at these intervals. In people with normal glucose tolerance, blood glucose levels return to normal within 2 to 3 hours after ingestion of a glucose load, in which case it can be assumed that sufficient insulin is present to allow glucose to leave the blood and enter body cells. Because a person with diabetes lacks the ability to respond to an increase in blood glucose by releasing adequate insulin to facilitate storage, blood glucose levels not only rise above those observed in normal people but remain elevated for longer periods (Fig. 46-4). The glucose tolerance test is a useful diagnostic measure for detecting subclinical forms of diabetes—the stage of the disease in which the fasting blood glucose may still be normal and other obvious signs of diabetes are not yet detectable. A variation of the glucose tolerance test is the cortisone glucose tolerance test. The administration of cortisone challenges the body's ability to metabolize glucose. Another form of the glucose tolerance test is used for screening purposes; this form of the test involves sampling blood 2 hours after a glucose challenge.

Capillary Blood Tests and Self-Monitoring of Blood Glucose Levels. Technologic advances have provided the means for monitoring blood glucose

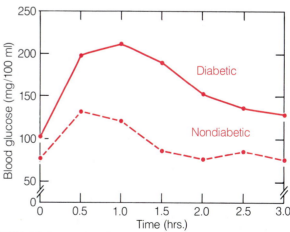

FIG. 46-4. *Results of a glucose tolerance test for people with and without diabetes. Blood samples usually are taken at 30-minute intervals after ingestion of a glucose solution containing 1.75 g of glucose per kilogram of body weight. The test may be modified for use as a screening tool.*

levels by using a drop of capillary blood. This method has not only provided health professionals with a rapid and economical method for monitoring blood glucose but also given people with diabetes a means of maintaining near-normal blood glucose levels through self-monitoring of blood glucose levels. These methods use a drop of capillary blood obtained by pricking the finger with a special needle or small lancet. Small trigger devices make use of the lancet virtually painless. The drop of capillary blood is placed on a reagent strip, and glucose levels are determined either electronically, using a glucose meter, or visually, using a color chart.

Glycosylated Hemoglobin. This test measures the amount of glycosylated hemoglobin (hemoglobin into which glucose has been incorporated) present in the blood. Hemoglobin normally does not contain glucose when it is released from the bone marrow. During its 120-day life span in the red blood cell, hemoglobin normally becomes glycosylated to form glycohemoglobins A_{1a} and A_{1b} (2% to 4%) and A_{1c} (4% to 6%). In uncontrolled diabetes there is an increase in hemoglobin A_{1c}. In diabetes with hyperglycemia, there is an increase in hemoglobin A_{1c}. A hemoglobin A_{1c} value of 11% to 15% indicates poor control of blood glucose over time. Because glucose entry into the red blood cell is not insulin-dependent, the rate at which glucose becomes attached to the hemoglobin molecule depends on blood glucose. Glycosylation is essentially irreversible; hence, the level of glycosylated hemoglobin present in the blood provides an index of blood glucose levels over the previous 2 months or more.

URINE TESTS

The ease, accuracy, and convenience of self blood glucose monitoring techniques have made urine testing obsolete for most people with diabetes. Urine tests only reflect blood glucose levels; they are influenced by such factors as the renal threshold for glucose, fluid intake and urine concentration, urine testing methodologies, and some drugs. Because of these factors, the American Diabetes Association recommends that all people who use insulin should self-monitor their blood, not urine, glucose.[13] Unlike glucose tests, urine ketone determinations remain an important part of monitoring diabetic control, particularly in people with IDDM who are at risk for developing ketoacidosis.

DIETARY MANAGEMENT

Diet therapy usually is prescribed to meet the specific needs of each person with diabetes. Goals and principles of diet therapy differ between type I and type II diabetes as well as between lean and obese people.

A task force of the American Diabetes Association met in 1986 to develop nutritional recommendations and principles for people with diabetes mellitus. These recommendations are similar to those of the American Heart Association, the American Cancer Society, the Nutritional Committee for Recommendations for Children with Diabetes of the American Academy of Pediatrics, and the 1985 U.S. Dietary Guidelines.[14] The task force recommended that (1) calories should be prescribed to achieve and maintain a desirable weight with additional allocation of calories to provide for growth and metabolic needs in children and pregnant or lactating women; (2) carbohydrates should be liberalized, ideally up to 55% to 65% of the total calories, and individualized, with the amount depending on blood glucose, lipid levels, and individual eating patterns; (3) the recommended dietary allowance for protein of 0.8 g/kg of body weight for adults should be used and modified if needed; and (4) total fat should constitute less than 30% of the diet and cholesterol should be less than 300 mg/d.

In an obese person with type II diabetes, the principles of diet therapy are different. Dietary interventions are directed toward weight reduction, improvement in blood glucose and lipid levels, and consistency in day-to-day nutrient intake. These interventions include (1) well-balanced and nutritious meals, (2) control of calories for weight loss and achievement of ideal body weight, (3) control of monosaccharides in the diet, and (4) distribution of carbohydrate, protein, and fat according to individual desires and need for weight management.

Several methods of dietary control can be used. One method is the free diet, which essentially allows a person to eat in a method that is satisfying but avoids concentrated sugars. A complete diet history should be taken before this method is suggested. The free diet may be acceptable for people who have already established therapeutic eating habits. A second method involves weighing food. This method is difficult for many people but may be useful for those who are having difficulty in portion control.

The third and most frequently prescribed meal plan is the exchange system.[15] In this system, foods are divided into six categories. Each food in a particular category (in the amount designated) has an equivalent amount of carbohydrate, protein, and fat. The six exchange categories are milk, meats, fruits, breads or grains, vegetables, and fats. The foods within each category are interchangeable in the prescribed amounts. For example, in the fruit list, one half cup of orange juice can be exchanged for one quarter cup of grape juice or one half a grapefruit. In the meat group, one egg can be exchanged for 1 oz of cheese or 1 oz of chicken. Fats are included, based on whether the meat choices are lean, medium, or high in fat content. Polyunsaturated fats are encouraged to avoid problems with hyperlipidemia. The exchange system is easy to learn and provides a highly nutritious well-balanced diet.

Current evidence suggests that high-fiber, complex-carbohydrate diets prevent large fluctuations in blood glucose levels, thereby providing better glucose control. For some people with diabetes, pasta provides better glucose control than potatoes; rice may provide better control than bread. These concepts are particularly important during pregnancy, in which the goal is to maintain glucose levels between 60 and 120 mg/dL. Even mild hyperglycemia has been shown to be detrimental to the fetus; increased episodes of hyperglycemia have been shown to cause significant increases in congenital anomalies. The recommendation that pregnant women with diabetes avoid monosaccharides and include high-fiber complex carbohydrates in their diets is widely accepted. In some instances, milk and other complex carbohydrate sources are used to treat hypoglycemia for the primary purpose of avoiding counterregulatory responses.

In addition to improved glycemic response, other benefits of fiber may include lowering of low-density lipoprotein cholesterol and total cholesterol and improving the satiety of a meal. The best fiber to achieve this is the soluble-fiber variety of foods that include legumes, oat bran, barley, and fruits. The insoluble variety, which is most effective for relief of constipation, includes wheat bran and whole grains.

Two thirds of adults who have diabetes also have hypertension. For this reason, reducing daily sodium intake is desirable. The American Heart Association and the American Diabetes Association suggest a daily intake of 1000 mg/1000 kcal, not to exceed 3000 mg. This can be achieved by choosing foods naturally low in sodium and by modifying cooking habits to use less salt. Given the complications and risks presented to people with diabetes, the low-sodium diet may be useful in preventing complications.

Sucrose (common table sugar) should be limited not only because of its glycemic response, but because its long-term effects coupled with increased lipid levels may lead to cardiovascular disease. In addition, sucrose is considered an empty-calorie food. Moderate use of an alternative low-calorie sweetener by people with diabetes is acceptable. Excessive use of any food is not without adverse effects.

The American Diabetes Association provides literature with more detailed information on diet therapy and patient education. Included is the method of calculating individual meal plans. Nutritionists are valuable resources to the nurse, physician, and patient and should be included in diet management.

EXERCISE

The benefits of exercise include cardiovascular fitness and psychological well-being. In addition, many people with NIDDM benefit from a decrease in body fat, better weight control, and improvement in insulin sensitivity. The resulting improvement in glucose tolerance may free them from the use of antidiabetic drugs. Exercise is so important in diabetes management that a planned program of regular exercise usually is considered an integral part of the therapeutic regimen for every person with diabetes.

In a person without diabetes, the uptake of glucose into the exercising muscle increases 7- to 20-fold during short-term exercise and blood levels of glucose are maintained by an adrenergically induced decrease in insulin release from β cells and an increased breakdown of liver glycogen stores mediated by counterregulatory hormones. When exercise is prolonged for more than 2 hours, the exercising muscles obtain the greater amount of their energy from fatty acids, and glucose release from the liver is derived from gluconeogenesis.

In a person with IDDM, the beneficial effects of exercise are accompanied by an increased risk of hypoglycemia. Although muscle uptake of glucose increases significantly, the ability to maintain blood levels of glucose is hampered by failure to suppress the absorption of injected insulin and activate the counterregulatory mechanisms that maintain blood glucose. Not only is there an inability to suppress insulin levels, but insulin absorption may increase. This increased absorption is more pronounced when insulin is injected into the subcutaneous tissue of the exercised muscle, but it occurs even when insulin is injected into other body areas. Even after exercise ceases, the lowering effect on blood glucose levels continues.

In some people with IDDM, the symptoms of hypoglycemia occur many hours after cessation of exercise. This may be because subsequent insulin doses (in people using multiple daily insulin injections) are not adjusted to accommodate the exercise-induced decrease in blood glucose. The cause of hypoglycemia in people who do not administer a subsequent insulin dose is unclear. It may be related to the fact that the liver and skeletal muscles increase their uptake of glucose after exercise as a means of replenishing their glycogen stores or that the liver and skeletal muscles are more sensitive to insulin during this time. People with IDDM should be aware that delayed hypoglycemia may occur after exercise and that there may be a need to alter their insulin dose, their carbohydrate intake, or both.

Although of benefit to people with diabetes, exercise must be weighed on the risk–benefit scale. For those with complications, vigorous exercise can be harmful and can cause eye hemorrhage as well as other problems. For people with IDDM who exercise during periods of poor control (when blood glucose is elevated and ketonemia is present), blood glucose and ketone levels rise to even higher levels. This is because the stress of exercise is superimposed on preexisting insulin deficiency and increased counter-regulatory hormone activity.

Because most sporadic exercise has only transient benefits, a regular exercise or training program is the most beneficial. It is not only better for cardiovascular conditioning but also can maintain a muscle–fat ratio that enhances peripheral insulin receptivity.

ANTIDIABETIC AGENTS

There are two forms of antidiabetic agents—oral sulfonylureas and injectable insulin.

Sulfonylureas. The sulfonylureas were discovered accidentally in 1942 when scientists noted that one of the sulfonamide drugs being developed at the time caused hypoglycemia. These drugs reduce blood glucose by stimulating the release of insulin from β cells in the pancreas and increasing the sensitivity of peripheral tissues to insulin. This means that these agents are effective only when some residual β-cell function remains. They are used in the treatment of NIDDM and cannot be substituted for insulin in people with IDDM, who have an absolute insulin deficiency. Slight modifications in the basic structure of the members of this drug group produce agents that have similar qualitative actions but markedly different potency. The sulfonylureas are traditionally grouped into two generations. The first generation of drugs includes tolbutamide, acetohexamide, tolazamide, and chlorpropamide. The second generation of drugs (*e.g.*, glyburide and glipizide)

that have emerged are considerably more potent that the earlier drugs. These preparations differ in dosage and duration of action (Table 46-2). Because the sulfonylureas increase the rate at which glucose is removed from the blood, it is important to recognize that they can cause hypoglycemic reactions. This problem is more common in elderly people with impaired hepatic and renal function who are taking the longer-acting sulfonylureas.[16]

Insulin. Insulin-dependent diabetes mellitus requires treatment with insulin. Insulin is destroyed in the gastrointestinal tract and must be administered by injection. All insulin is measured in units, the international unit of insulin being defined as the amount of insulin required to lower the blood glucose of a fasting 2-kg rabbit from 145 mg to 120 mg/dL of blood. Most types of insulin are available in U100 (units per milliliter) strength. Insulin preparations are categorized according to onset, peak, and duration of action. There are three principal types of insulin: (1) short-acting, for rapid onset of action; (2) intermediate-acting; and (3) long acting (Table 46-3). Insulin regimens that call for two or three daily injections of regular insulin or regular mixed with intermediate-acting insulin are the most common. These regimens provide a blood glucose level that is within a more normal physiologic range than that provided by the once-a-day injection.

Over the past several decades, many pharmaceutical companies have entered the insulin-manufacturing market. After much research, human insulin has become available, providing an alternative to previous forms of insulin that were obtained from bovine (beef) and porcine (pork) sources. The manufacture of human insulin uses recombinant DNA or a modification of pork insulin. Beef insulin differs from human insulin by three amino acids, whereas pork insulin differs by only one amino acid. Many people

TABLE 46-2. SULFONYLUREA PREPARATIONS: HALF-LIFE AND DURATION OF ACTION		
SULFONYLUREA PREPARATIONS	**HALF-LIFE (HR)**	**DURATION OF ACTION (HR)**
First Generation		
Tolbutamide (Orinase)	4–6	6–12
Tolazamide (Tolinase)	7	10–14
Acetohexamide (Dymelor)	5–7	12–14
Chlorpropamide (Diabinese)	36	Up to 60
Second Generation		
Glyburide (Diabeta, Micronase)	10	24
Glipizide (Glucotrol)	4	≤24

TABLE 46-3. INSULIN: ACTIVITY PEAK AND DURATION OF ACTION

TYPE OF PREPARATION	ACTIVITY PEAK (H)	DURATION (H)
Rapid-Acting		
Insulin injection (regular)	2–4	5–7
Prompt insulin zinc suspension (eg, Semi-lente)	2–8	12–16
Intermediate-Acting		
Isophane insulin suspension (NPH)	6–12	18–24
Insulin zinc suspension (Lente)	6–12	18–24
Long-Acting		
Protamine zinc insulin suspension (PZI)	16–18	24–36
Extended insulin zinc suspension (Ultra-lente)	16–18	24–36

(From information in Gilman, A.G., Rall, T.W., Nies, A.S., et al. [Eds.] [1990]. *Goodman and Gilman's The pharmacological basis of therapeutics* (8th ed., p. 1476). New York: Pergamon.)

with diabetes develop antibodies to beef and pork insulin. Recent improvements in the purification techniques for insulin extracted from animal pancreas have made it possible to reduce or eliminate many of the contaminants that were capable of inciting antibody formation. The use of human insulin or purified pork insulins is indicated when insulin of conventional purity and containing beef species has been associated with allergy, immune resistance, or lipoatrophy at the site of injection. A change from pork or beef to human insulin should be carefully monitored because hypoglycemia can occur from an increased receptivity to the human insulin.

Two intensive treatment regimens—multiple daily injections and continuous subcutaneous infusion of insulin (CSII)–have been developed that closely simulate the normal pattern of insulin secretion by the body.[17] With each method, a basal insulin level is maintained and bolus doses of regular insulin are delivered before meals. The choice of management is determined by the patient.

Multiple Daily Injections. In multiple-daily-injection programs, the basal insulin requirements are met by long-acting insulin (ultralente) administered before breakfast or by intermediate-acting insulin (lente or NPH) administered at bedtime.[17] The development of convenient injection devices (*e.g.*, pen injector) has made it easier for people with diabetes to comply with the multiple doses of regular insulin that are administered before meals.

Continuous Subcutaneous Insulin Infusion. With the CSII method, the basal insulin requirements are met by subcutaneous infusion whose dose can be varied to accommodate diurnal variations. The CSII technique involves the insertion of a small needle into the subcutaneous tissue of the abdomen. Tubing from the needle is connected to a syringe set into a small infusion pump worn on a belt or in a jacket pocket. The computer-operated pump then delivers a set basal amount of insulin. In addition to the basal amount delivered by the pump, a bolus amount of insulin may be delivered when needed by pushing a button. Self blood glucose monitoring is a necessity when using this method of management. Each basal and bolus dose is determined individually and programmed into the infusion pump computer. Only those people who are highly motivated to do frequent blood glucose tests and to make daily insulin adjustments are candidates for this method of injection. Although the pump's safety has been proven, strict attention must be paid to signs of hypoglycemia. People with diabetes who do not sense hypoglycemia or whose counterregulatory response is impaired are not candidates for the CSII technique. Ketotic episodes caused by pump failure and infections at the needle site are possible complications.

PANCREAS TRANSPLANTATION

Pancreas transplantation is being performed with increased frequency and success rate for the treatment of diabetes. When successful, pancreas transplants can restore carbohydrate metabolism to normal or nearly normal. By the end of 1990, 3216 pancreatic transplantations had been recorded in the International Pancreas Transplantation Registry. Between 1987 and 1990, the 1- and 3-year survival rates were 91% and 80%, respectively, and the graft survival rates (with total freedom from insulin therapy) were 72% and 57%, respectively.[18]

The indications for pancreas transplantation are early nephropathy, progressive retinopathy, neuropathy, and extreme difficulty with diabetic management. People with pancreas transplants require immunosuppression, usually a combination of cyclosporine, azathioprine, and prednisone, to prevent transplant rejection. The procedure often is done on people who need a kidney transplant and require immunosuppression for that purpose.[18]

As with kidney transplantation, pancreas transplantation is not a life-saving procedure. It does, however, afford the potential for significantly improving the quality of life. The most serious problems are the requirement for immunosuppression and the need for diagnosis and treatment of rejection.

ACUTE COMPLICATIONS

The three major acute complications of diabetes are ketoacidosis, hyperosmolar hyperglycemic nonketotic (HHNK) coma, and hypoglycemia.

DIABETIC KETOACIDOSIS

Ketoacidosis occurs when ketone production by the liver exceeds cellular utilization and renal excretion. In people with IDDM, the lack of insulin leads to mobilization of fatty acids and subsequent increase in ketone production.

Compared with an insulin reaction (to be discussed), diabetic ketoacidosis usually is slower in onset and recovery is more prolonged. There typically is a history of 1 or 2 days of polyuria, polydipsia, nausea, vomiting, and marked fatigue with eventual stupor that can progress to coma. Abdominal pain and even tenderness may be present in the absence of abdominal disease. Hypotension and tachycardia may be present because of a decrease in blood volume. Blood glucose levels are elevated (ranging from 250 mg/dL to greater than 1000 mg/dL), and urine glucose is greater than 2% to 5%. Plasma pH and bicarbonate are decreased, and serum or urine tests for ketones are positive. Serum potassium levels may be normal or elevated, despite total potassium depletion resulting from protracted polyuria and vomiting. The signs and symptoms of ketoacidosis are summarized in Chart 46-4.

There are two major metabolic derangements in diabetic ketoacidosis, *hyperglycemia* and *metabolic acidosis*. Hyperglycemia leads to osmotic diuresis, dehydration, and a critical loss of electrolytes. Metabolic acidosis is caused by the excess ketoacids that require buffering by the bicarbonate ion; this leads to a marked decrease in serum bicarbonate levels. The breath has a characteristic fruity smell because of

CHART 46-4: SIGNS AND SYMPTOMS OF DIABETIC KETOACIDOSIS

Onset 1 to 24 hours
Laboratory findings
   Blood glucose greater than 250 mg/dL
   Ketonemia and presence of ketones in the urine
   Decreased plasma pH (less than 7.3) and bicarbonate (less than 15 mEq/L)
Dehydration caused by hyperglycemia
   Warm, dry skin
   Dry mucous membranes
   Tachycardia
   Weak, thready pulse
   Acute weight loss
   Hypotension
Ketoacidosis
   Anorexia, nausea, and vomiting
   Odor of ketones on the breath
   Depression of the central nervous system
      Lethargy and fatigue
      Stupor
      Coma
   Abdominal pain
Compensatory responses
   Rapid, deep respirations (Kussmaul's respiration)

the presence of the volatile ketoacids. A number of the signs and symptoms that occur in diabetic ketoacidosis are related to compensatory mechanisms. The heart rate increases as the body compensates for a decrease in blood volume, and the rate and depth of respiration increase (Kussmaul's respiration) as the body attempts to prevent further decreases in pH. Metabolic acidosis is discussed further is Chapter 30.

Diabetic ketoacidosis most frequently is seen in a person with IDDM. It can occur at the onset of the disease, often before the disease has been diagnosed. For example, a mother may bring a child into the hospital with reports of lethargy, vomiting, and abdominal pain, unaware that the child has diabetes. Stress increases the release of gluconeogenic hormones and predisposes the person to the development of ketoacidosis. Consequently, the development of ketoacidosis often is preceded by physical or emotional stress—for example, infection, pregnancy, or extreme anxiety.

The treatment of diabetic ketoacidosis focuses on correcting the fluid and electrolyte imbalances and returning the blood pH to normal. This usually is accomplished through the administration of insulin and intravenous fluid and electrolyte replacement solutions. Because insulin resistance accompanies severe acidosis, low-dose insulin therapy is used. An initial loading dose of regular insulin often is given intravenously, followed by continuous low-dose infusion. Frequent monitoring of laboratory tests of blood glucose and serum electrolytes is used as a guide for fluid and electrolyte replacement. It is important to replace fluid and electrolytes and correct *p*H before bringing the blood glucose to a normal level. Too rapid a drop in blood glucose may cause hypoglycemic symptoms and cerebral edema. A sudden change in the osmolality of extracellular fluid occurs when blood glucose is lowered rapidly, and this can cause cerebral edema. Serum potassium levels often fall as acidosis is corrected and extracellular potassium moves into the intracellular compartment; at this time, it may be necessary to add potassium to the intravenous infusion. Identification and treatment of the underlying cause, such as infection, are also important.

HYPEROSMOLAR HYPERGLYCEMIC NONKETOTIC COMA

Hyperosmolar hyperglycemic nonketotic (HHNK) coma is characterized by plasma osmolarity of 300 mosm/L or more, blood glucose in excess of 600 mg/dL of blood, the absence of ketoacidosis, and depression of the sensorium.[12]

HHNK coma may occur in various conditions, including NIDDM, acute pancreatitis, severe infection, myocardial infarction, and treatment with oral or parenteral nutrition solutions. It is seen most frequently in persons with NIDDM. Two factors appear to contribute to the hyperglycemia that precipitates the condition: an increased resistance to the effects of insulin and an excessive carbohydrate intake.

In hyperosmolar states, the increased serum osmolarity has the effect of pulling water out of body cells, including brain cells. The most prominent manifestations are dehydration, neurologic signs and symptoms, polyuria, and thirst (Chart 46-5). The neurologic signs include grand mal seizures, hemiparesis, Babinski's reflexes, aphasia, muscle fasciculations, hyperthermia, hemianopia, nystagmus, and visual hallucinations. The onset of HHNK coma often is insidious, and because it occurs most frequently in older people, it may be mistaken for a stroke.

The treatment of HHNK coma requires judicious medical observation and care. This is because water moves back into brain cells during treatment, posing a threat of cerebral edema. Extensive potassium losses that have also occurred during the diuretic phase of the disorder require correction. Because of the problems encountered in the treatment and the serious nature of the disease conditions that cause HHNK coma, the prognosis for this disorder is less favorable than that for ketoacidosis; the mortality rate has been reported to be 40% to 70%.[19]

CHART 46-5: SIGNS AND SYMPTOMS OF HYPEROSMOLAR COMA

Onset insidious; 24 hours to 2 weeks
Laboratory findings
    Blood glucose greater than 600 mg/dL
    Serum osmolarity 300 mOsm/L or greater
Severe dehydration
    Dry skin and mucous membranes
    Extreme thirst
Neurologic manifestations
    Depressed sensorium lethargy to coma
    Neurologic deficits
        Positive Babinski's sign
        Paresis or paralysis
        Sensory impairment
        Hyperthermia
        Hemianopia
Seizures

HYPOGLYCEMIA

Hypoglycemia, or an insulin reaction, usually occurs in people with IDDM. It occurs when blood glucose falls below 50 mg/dL of blood and is characterized by sudden onset and rapid progression (Chart 46-6). The signs and symptoms of hypoglycemia can be divided into two categories: those caused by altered cerebral function and those related to activation of the autonomic nervous system. Because the brain relies on blood glucose as its main energy source, hypoglycemia produces behaviors related to altered cerebral function. Headache, difficulty in problem

---

CHART 46-6: SIGNS AND SYMPTOMS OF INSULIN REACTION

Onset sudden
Laboratory findings
    Blood glucose less than 50 mg/dL
Impaired cerebral function (caused by decreased glucose availability for brain metabolism)
    Feeling of vagueness
    Headache
    Difficulty in problem solving
    Slurred speech
    Impaired motor function
    Change in emotional behavior
    Seizures
    Coma
Autonomic nervous system responses
    Hunger
    Anxiety
    Hypotension
    Sweating
    Vasoconstriction of skin vessels (skin is pale and cool)
    Tachycardia

solving, disturbed or altered behavior, coma, and seizures are common. At the onset of the hypoglycemic episode, activation of the parasympathetic nervous system often causes hunger. The initial parasympathetic response is followed by activation of the sympathetic nervous system; this causes anxiety, tachycardia, sweating, and constriction of the skin vessels (the skin is cool and clammy). Although different people respond in different ways to an insulin reaction, each person usually has the same individual pattern of response during each insulin reaction. For this reason, it is helpful if this response pattern can be identified during the early stages of treatment in the person with IDDM.

There is a wide variation in the manifestation of signs and symptoms; that is, not every person with diabetes manifests all or even most of the symptoms. The signs and symptoms of hypoglycemia are more variable in children and in elderly people. Elderly people may not display the typical autonomic responses associated with hypoglycemia but frequently develop signs of impaired function of the central nervous system, including mental confusion. Some medications, such as β-adrenergic blocking drugs, interfere with the symptomatic response normally seen in hypoglycemia.

Many factors precipitate an insulin reaction in a person with IDDM, including error in insulin dose, failure to eat, increased exercise, decreased insulin need after removal of a stress situation, and a change in insulin site. Alcohol decreases liver gluconeogenesis, and a person with diabetes needs to be cautioned about its potential for causing hypoglycemia, especially if it is consumed in large amounts or on an empty stomach.

The most effective treatment of an insulin reaction is the immediate ingestion of a concentrated carbohydrate source, such as sugar, honey, candy, or orange juice. Alternative methods for increasing blood glucose may be required when the person having the reaction is unconscious or unable to swallow. Glucagon may be given intravenously, intramuscularly, or subcutaneously. The liver contains only a limited amount of glycogen (about 75 g); glucagon is ineffective in people whose glycogen stores have been depleted. It is recommended, therefore, that glucagon be given only once and not repeated. Repeating the dose may cause vomiting, which will worsen the situation. A small amount of honey or glucose gel (available in most pharmacies) can be inserted into the buccal pouch (under the tongue) when swallowing is impaired. Monosaccharides such as glucose or fructose, which can be absorbed directly into the bloodstream, work best for this purpose. It is important not to overtreat hypoglycemia so as to cause hyperglycemia. Treatment usually con-

sists of an initial administration of about 10 g of glucose, which can be repeated as necessary. Complex carbohydrates may be administered once the acute reaction has been controlled (see the section on diabetic diet). In gestational diabetes, milk is recommended to treat hypoglycemia. This use of a complex carbohydrate prevents rebound hyperglycemia, which can be harmful to the fetus. In situations of severe, life-threatening hypoglycemia, it may be necessary to administer glucose (20 to 50 mL of a 50% solution) intravenously.

SOMOGYI EFFECT AND DAWN PHENOMENON

The *Somogyi effect* describes a cycle of insulin-induced posthypoglycemic episodes. In 1924, Joslin and his associates noted that hypoglycemia was associated with alternate episodes of hyperglycemia.[20] It was not until 1959 that Somogyi presented the results of his 20 years of studies, which confirmed the observation that "hypoglycemia begets hyperglycemia."[21] In a person with diabetes, insulin-induced hypoglycemia produces a compensatory increase in blood levels of catecholamines, glucagon, cortisol, and growth hormone. These counterregulatory hormones cause blood glucose to become elevated and produce some degree of insulin resistance. A vicious circle begins when the increase in blood glucose and insulin resistance are treated with larger insulin doses. The hypoglycemic episode often occurs during the night or at a time when it is not recognized, rendering the diagnosis of the phenomenon more difficult. Figure 46-5 shows the events that occur with the Somogyi effect.

Research suggests that even rather mild insulin-associated hypoglycemia, which may be asymptomatic, can cause hyperglycemia in IDDM through the recruitment of counterregulatory mechanisms, although the insulin action does not wane. A concomitant waning of the effect of insulin (end of the duration of action), when it occurs, exacerbates post-

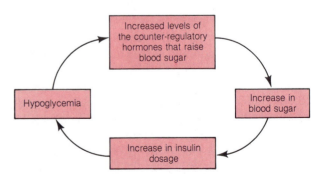

FIG. 46-5. Cycle of events that occur with the Somogyi phenomenon.

hypoglycemic hyperglycemia and accelerates its development. It has been suggested that these research findings may explain the labile nature of the disease in some people with diabetes. Measures to prevent hypoglycemia and the subsequent activation of counterregulatory mechanisms include a redistribution of dietary carbohydrates and an alteration in insulin dose or method of administration.[22]

The *dawn phenomenon* is characterized by increased levels of fasting blood glucose or insulin requirements or both between 5 and 9 A.M. in the absence of antecedent hypoglycemia. It occurs in people with IDDM or NIDDM. It has been suggested that a change in the normal circadian rhythm for glucose tolerance, which usually is higher during the later part of the morning, is altered in people with diabetes.[23] Growth hormone has been suggested as a possible factor. When the dawn phenomenon occurs alone, it may produce only mild hyperglycemia, but when it is combined with the Somogyi effect, it may produce profound hyperglycemia.[12]

CHRONIC COMPLICATIONS

The chronic complications of diabetes include neuropathies, disorders of the microcirculation (nephropathies and retinopathies), macrovascular complications, and foot ulcers. Interestingly, these disorders occur in the insulin-independent tissues of the body—those tissues that do not require insulin for glucose entry into the cell. This probably means that intracellular glucose concentrations in many of these tissues approach or equal those in the blood.

THEORIES OF PATHOGENESIS

The interest among researchers in explaining the causes and development of chronic lesions in a person with diabetes has led to a number of theories. Several of these theories have been summarized to prepare the reader for understanding specific chronic complications.

Polyol Pathway. A polyol is an organic compound that contains three or more hydroxyl groups. The polyol pathway refers to the intracellular mechanisms responsible for changing the number of hydroxyl units on a glucose. In the sorbitol pathway, glucose is transformed first to sorbitol and then to fructose. Although glucose is readily converted to sorbitol, the rate at which sorbitol can be converted to fructose and then metabolized is limited. Sorbitol is osmotically active, and it has been hypothesized that the presence of excess intracellular amounts may alter cell function in those tissues that use this pathway

(*e.g.*, lens, kidneys, nerves, and blood vessels). In the lens, for example, the osmotic effects of sorbitol cause swelling and opacity. Increased sorbitol is also associated with a decrease in myoinositol and reduced adenosinetriphosphatase activity. The reduction of these compounds may be responsible for the peripheral neuropathies caused by Schwann cells.

Formation of Abnormal Glycoproteins. Glycoproteins, or what might be termed glucose proteins, are normal components of the basement membrane in smaller blood vessels and capillaries. It has been suggested that the increased intracellular concentration of glucose associated with uncontrolled blood glucose levels in diabetes favors the formation of abnormal glycoproteins. These abnormal glycoproteins are thought to produce structural defects in the basement membrane of the microcirculation and to contribute to eye, kidney, and vascular complications.

Problems with Tissue Oxygenation. Proponents of the tissue oxygenation theories suggest that many of the chronic complications of diabetes arise because of a decrease in oxygen delivery in the small vessels of the microcirculation. Among the factors believed to contribute to this inadequate oxygen delivery is a defect in red blood cell function that interferes with the release of oxygen from the hemoglobin molecule. In support of this theory is the finding of a two- to three-fold increase in glycosylated hemoglobin (HbA_{1c}) in some people with diabetes. In glycosylated hemoglobin, a glycoprotein is substituted for valine in the β chain, causing a high affinity for oxygen. There is a reported decline in red blood cell 2,3-diphosphoglycerate (2,3-DPG) during the acidotic and recovery phases of diabetic ketoacidosis. The glycolytic intermediate 2,3-DPG reduces the hemoglobin affinity for oxygen. Both an increase in glycosylated hemoglobin and a decrease in 2,3-DPG increase the hemoglobin's affinity for oxygen, and less oxygen is released for tissue use.

PERIPHERAL NEUROPATHIES

Although the incidence of peripheral neuropathies is known to be high among people with diabetes, it is difficult to document exactly how many are affected by these disorders. This is because of the diversity in clinical manifestations and because the condition often is far advanced before it is recognized.

Two types of pathologic changes have been observed in connection with diabetic peripheral neuropathies. The first is a thickening of the walls of the nutrient vessels that supply the nerve, leading to the assumption that vessel ischemia plays a major role in the development of these neural changes. The second and more recent finding has been a segmental demyelinization process that affects the Schwann cell. This demyelinization process is accompanied by a slowing of nerve conduction. Research on the sorbitol pathway suggests that the formation and accumulation of sorbitol or the reduction of myoinositol within Schwann cells may lead to injury and impair nerve conduction.

It appears that the diabetic peripheral neuropathies are not a single entity. The clinical manifestations of these disorders vary with the location of the lesion. Although there are several methods for classifying the diabetic peripheral neuropathies, a simplified system divides them into somatic and autonomic disturbances (Chart 46-7).

In addition to the discomforts associated with the loss of sensory or motor function, lesions in either the somatic or the peripheral nervous system predispose a person with diabetes to other complications. The loss of feeling, touch, and position sense increases the risk of falling. Impairment of temperature and pain sensation increases the risk of serious burns and injuries to the feet. Defects in vasomotor reflexes can lead to dizziness and syncope when the person moves from the supine to the standing position. In-

complete emptying of the bladder because of impaired innervation predisposes the person to urinary stasis and bladder infection and increases the risk of renal complications (see Chapter 32).

In the male, disruption of sensory and autonomic nervous system function can cause impotence. Diabetes is the leading physiologic cause of impotence, and it occurs in both IDDM and NIDDM. Of the 5 million men with diabetes in the United States, 30% to 60% suffer from impotence.[24]

NEPHROPATHIES

Diabetic nephropathy is the most common cause of end-stage kidney disease. By far, the most common kidney lesions in people with diabetes are those that affect the glomeruli. Diabetes affects the arterioles as well, causing arteriolar sclerosis; it also increases the susceptibility to pyelonephritis and papillary sclerosis. The term diabetic nephropathy is used to describe the combination of lesions that occur concurrently in the diabetic kidney. In the United States, 33% of all people who enter renal replacement therapy (see Chapter 33) have diabetes.[25]

Not all people with diabetes develop clinically significant nephropathy; for this reason, attention is focusing on risk factors for the development of this complication. Among the suggested risk factors are genetic and familial predisposition, kidney and glomerular enlargement, poor glycemic control, and capillary and systemic hypertension.[26] Diabetic nephropathy occurs in family clusters, suggesting a family predisposition, although this does not rule out the possibility of environmental factors shared by siblings.[27] Kidney enlargement, nephron hypertrophy, and hyperfiltration occur early in the disease, suggesting increased work of the kidneys in reabsorbing excessive amounts of glucose. Evidence suggests that strict glycemic control can reverse or prevent these phenomena. Hypertension places increased stress on the arteriolar and capillary structures of the kidneys.

Various glomerular changes may be present in diabetic nephropathy, including capillary basement membrane thickening, diffuse glomerular sclerosis, and nodular glomerulosclerosis. Changes in the capillary basement membrane take the form of thickening of basement membranes along the length of the glomeruli. Diffuse glomerulosclerosis consists of thickening of both the basement membrane and the mesangial matrix. It is found in most people with diabetes of more than 10 years' duration.[28] Nodular glomerulosclerosis, also called intercapillary glomerulosclerosis or *Kimmelstiel-Wilson disease*, is a form of glomerulosclerosis that involves the development of nodular lesions in the glomerular capillary of

---

CHART 46-7: CLASSIFICATION OF DIABETIC PERIPHERAL NEUROPATHIES

Somatic

Polyneuropathies (bilateral sensory)
  Paresthesias, including numbness and tingling
  Impaired pain, temperature, light touch, two-point discrimination, and vibratory sensation
  Decreased ankle and knee-jerk reflexes
Mononeuropathies
  Involvement of a mixed nerve trunk that includes loss of sensation, pain, and motor weakness
Amyotrophy
  Associated with muscle weakness, wasting, and severe pain of muscles in the pelvic girdle and thigh

Autonomic

Impaired vasomotor function
  Postural hypotension
Impaired gastrointestinal function
  Gastric atony
  Diarrhea, often postprandial and nocturnal
Impaired genitourinary function
  Paralytic bladder
  Incomplete voiding
  Impotence
  Retrograde ejaculation
Cranial nerve involvement
  Extraocular nerve paralysis
  Impaired pupillary responses
  Impaired special senses

the kidneys, causing impaired blood flow with progressive loss of kidney function and, eventually, renal failure. Nodular glomerulosclerosis is thought to occur only in people with diabetes. This syndrome is encountered in 10% to 35% of people with diabetes and is a major cause of morbidity and mortality.[28] Changes in the basement membrane in diffuse glomerulosclerosis and Kimmelstiel-Wilson syndrome allow plasma proteins to escape in the urine, causing proteinuria, the development of hypoproteinemia (decreased levels of plasma proteins), and edema. Glomerular disorders of the kidneys are further discussed in Chapter 32.

RETINOPATHIES

Diabetes is the leading cause of acquired blindness in the United States. Although a person with diabetes is at increased risk for developing cataracts and glaucoma, retinopathy is the most common pattern of eye disease. Diabetic retinopathy is characterized by abnormal retinal vascular permeability, microaneurysm formation, neovascularization and associated hemorrhage, scarring, and retinal detachment (see Chapter 52). By 20 years after the onset of diabetes, nearly all people with IDDM and more than 60% of people with NIDDM have some degree of retinopathy. Diabetic retinopathy is estimated to be the most frequent cause of new blindness among Americans aged 20 to 74.[29]

Because of the risk of retinopathy, it is important that people with diabetes have regular eye examinations. People with IDDM should have an initial examination for retinopathy shortly after the diagnosis of diabetes is made. The recommendation for follow-up examinations is based on the type of examination that was done and the findings of that examination. People with persistently elevated glucose levels or proteinuria should be examined yearly.[30] Women who are planning a pregnancy should be counseled on the risk of development or progression of diabetic retinopathy. Women with diabetes who become pregnant should be followed closely throughout their pregnancy. This does not apply to women who develop gestational diabetes because such women are not at risk for developing diabetic retinopathy.[30]

People with macular edema, moderate to severe nonproliferative retinopathy, or any proliferative retinopathy should receive the care of an ophthalmologist. Methods used in the treatment of diabetic retinopathy include the destruction and scarring of the proliferative lesions with laser photocoagulation. The diabetic retinopathy study demonstrated that photocoagulation may delay or prevent visual loss in more than 50% of eyes with proliferative retinopathy.[31]

MACROVASCULAR COMPLICATIONS

Diabetes mellitus is a major risk factor for coronary artery disease, cerebrovascular disease, and peripheral vascular disease. The prevalence of these macrovascular complications is increased two- to four-fold in people with diabetes.[32]

Multiple risk factors for macrovascular disease frequently are found in people with diabetes, including obesity, hypertension, hyperglycemia, hyperinsulinemia, hyperlipidemia, altered platelet function, and elevated fibrinogen levels. The prevalence of coronary artery disease, stroke, and peripheral vascular disease is substantially increased in people with diabetes, even in the absence of these risk factors. Furthermore, there appear to be differences between NIDDM and IDDM in terms of duration of disease and the development of macrovascular disease. In people with NIDDM, the known duration of the disease does not seem to exert a major effect on the occurrence of macrovascular disease. In IDDM, however, both the attained age and the duration of diabetes appear to be correlated with macrovascular disease.[32] The reason for these discrepancies remains unknown.

DIABETIC FOOT ULCERS

Foot problems are common among people with diabetes and may become severe enough to cause ulceration, infection, and, eventually, a need for amputation. Foot problems have been reported as the most common complication leading to hospitalization among people with diabetes. In a controlled study of 854 outpatients with diabetes followed in a general medical clinic, foot problems accounted for 16% of hospital admissions over a 2-year period and 23% of total hospital days.[33] More than one half of all nontraumatic amputations of lower extremities in the United States are reported among people with diabetic foot problems.[34]

In people with diabetes, lesions of the feet represent the effects of both neuropathy and vascular insufficiency. About 60% to 70% of people with diabetic foot ulcers have neuropathy without vascular disease, 15% to 20% have vascular disease, and 15% to 20% have both neuropathy and vascular disease.[35]

People with sensory neuropathies have impaired pain sensation and often are unaware of the constant trauma to the feet caused by poorly fitting shoes, improper weight bearing, hard objects or pebbles in the shoes, or infections such as athlete's foot. Neuropathy prevents people from detecting pain; therefore, they are unable to adjust their gait to avoid walking on an area where pressure is causing trauma and necrosis. Common sites of trauma are the back of the heel, the plantar metatarsal area, or the great toe, where weight is borne during walking. Motor neuropathy with weakness of the intrinsic muscles of the foot may result in increased weight bearing over the metatarsal heads. Because of the constant risk of foot problems, it is important that people with diabetes wear shoes that have been fitted correctly and inspect their feet daily, looking for blisters, open sores, and fungal infection (athlete's foot) between the toes. If their eyesight is poor, a family member should do this for them. In the event a lesion is detected, prompt medical attention is needed to prevent serious complications. Smoking should be avoided because it causes vasoconstriction and contributes to vascular disease. Because cold produces vasoconstriction, appropriate foot coverings should be used to keep the feet warm and dry. Toenails should be cut straight across to prevent ingrown toenails. The toenails often are thickened and deformed, requiring the services of a podiatrist.

INFECTIONS

Although not specifically an acute or a chronic complication, infections are common concerns of a person with diabetes. Certain types of infections occur with increased frequency in people with diabetes: soft tissue infections of the extremities, osteomyelitis, urinary tract infections and pyelonephritis, candidal infections of the skin and mucous surfaces, and tuberculosis. Controversy exists over whether infections are more frequent in people with diabetes or whether infections seem more prevalent because they often are more serious in people with diabetes.

There are several known causes for the suboptimal response to infection in a person with diabetes. One is the presence of chronic complications, such as vascular disease and neuropathies; the other is the presence of hyperglycemia and altered neutrophil function. Sensory deficits may cause a person with diabetes to ignore minor trauma and infection, and vascular disease may impair circulation and delivery of blood cells and other substances needed to produce an adequate inflammatory response and effect healing. Pyelonephritis and urinary tract infections are relatively common in a person with diabetes, and it has been suggested that these infections may bear some relation to the presence of a neurogenic bladder or nephrosclerotic changes in the kidneys. Hyperglycemia and glycosuria may influence the growth of microorganisms and increase the severity of the infection. Diabetes and elevated blood glucose levels may also impair host defenses such as the function of neutrophils and immune cells.

In summary, diabetes mellitus is a disorder of carbohydrate, protein, and fat metabolism resulting from an imbalance between insulin availability and insulin need. The disease can be classified as insulin-dependent (IDDM), in which there is an absolute insulin deficiency, or non–insulin-dependent (NIDDM), in which there is a lack of insulin availability or effectiveness. The cause of IDDM and NIDDM is unknown. Other types of diabetes include secondary forms of carbohydrate intolerance, which occur secondary to some other condition, such as pancreatic disorders, which destroy β cells, or endocrine diseases such as Cushing's syndrome, which cause increased production of glucose by the liver and decreased utilization of glucose by the tissues. Gestational diabetes develops during pregnancy, and although glucose tolerance often returns to normal after childbirth, it indicates increased risk of developing diabetes.

The diagnosis of diabetes mellitus is based on clinical signs of the disease, fasting blood glucose levels, and the glucose tolerance test. In people with IDDM, self-monitoring provides a means of maintaining near-normal blood glucose levels through frequent testing of blood glucose and adjustment of insulin dosage. Glycosylation involves the irreversible attachment of glucose to the hemoglobin molecule; the measurement of glycosylated hemoglobin provides an index of blood glucose levels over several months. The treatment of diabetes includes diet, exercise, and, in many cases, the use of an antidiabetic agent. Dietary management focuses on maintaining a well-balanced diet, controlling calories to achieve and maintain an optimum weight, and regulating the distribution of carbohydrates, proteins, and fats. Two types of antidiabetic agents are used in the management of diabetes: injectable insulin and oral sulfonylurea drugs. Type I diabetes requires treatment with injectable insulin. The sulfonylurea agents increase insulin release from the β cells in the pancreas and increase the sensitivity of the peripheral tissues to insulin. These drugs require a functioning pancreas and may be used in the treatment of NIDDM. The benefits of exercise include cardiovascular fitness and psychological well-being. In addition, many people with NIDDM benefit from a decrease in body fat, better weight control, and an improvement in insulin sensitivity. In people with IDDM, the benefits of exercise are accompanied by a risk of hypoglycemia.

The metabolic disturbances associated with diabetes affect almost every body system. The acute complications of diabetes include diabetic ketoacidosis, HHNK coma, and hypoglycemia. The chronic complications of diabetes affect the non–insulin-dependent tissues, including the retina, blood vessels, kidneys, peripheral nervous system, and feet.

■ REFERENCES

1. Cryor, P.E., & Gerich, J.E. (1985). Glucose counter-regulation, hypoglycemia, and intensive insulin therapy in diabetes mellitus. *New England Journal of Medicine, 313,* 232.
2. Unger, R.H. (1985). The essential role of glucagon in pathogenesis of diabetes mellitus. *Lancet, 1,* 14.
3. Guyton, A. (1986). *Medical physiology* (7th ed., pp. 888, 910). Philadelphia: W.B. Saunders.
4. Waif, S.O. (Ed.). (1980). *Diabetes mellitus.* Indianapolis: Eli Lilly.

5. National Diabetes Data Group. (1979). Classification and diagnosis of diabetes mellitus and other categories of glucose intolerance. *Diabetes, 28,* 1039.

6. Karam, J.H., Solber, P.R., & Forsham, P.H. (1991). Pancreatic hormones and diabetes mellitus. In F.S. Greenspan (Ed.). *Basic clinical endocrinology* (3rd ed., pp. 592–650). E. Norwalk, CT: Appleton Lange.

7. Eisenbarth, G.S. (1986). Type I diabetes mellitus: A chronic autoimmune disease. *New England Journal of Medicine, 314,* 1360.

8. Skyler, J.S., & Rabinovitch, A. (1987), Etiology and pathogenesis of insulin dependent diabetes mellitus. *Pediatric Annals, 16,* 682.

9. Tuomilehto, J., & Wolf, E. (1987). Primary prevention of diabetes. *Diabetes Care, 10,* 238.

10. Karam, J.H. (1988). Therapeutic dilemmas in type II diabetes mellitus—improving and maintaining B-cell and insulin sensitivity. *Western Journal of Medicine, 148,* 685.

11. American Diabetes Association. (1991). Gestational diabetes mellitus (position paper). *Diabetes Care, 14* (Suppl. 2), 5–6.

12. Karam, J.H. (1993). Diabetes mellitus and hypoglycemia. In L. M. Tierney, S.J. McPhee, M.A. Papadakis, et al. (Eds.). *Current medical diagnosis and treatment.* E. Norwalk, CT: Appleton Lange.

13. American Diabetes Association. (1992). Urine glucose and ketone determinations (position paper). *Diabetes Care, 15*(Suppl. 2), 38–39.

14. American Diabetes Association. (1992). Nutritional recommendations and principles for individuals with diabetes mellitus. *Diabetes Care, 17*(Suppl. 2), 21–28.

15. American Diabetes Association and American Dietetic Association. (1986). *Exchange lists for meal planning.* New York and Chicago: ADA/ADA.

16. Gilman, A.G., Rall, T.W., Nies, A.S., et al. (Eds.) (1990). *Goodman and Gilman's The pharmacological basis of therapeutics* (8th ed., pp. 1484–1487). New York: Permagon Press.

17. Zinman, B. (1989). The physiologic replacement of insulin. *New England Journal of Medicine, 321,* 363–370.

18. Robertson, R.P. (1992). Pancreatic and islet cell transplantation for diabetes–cures or curiosities. *New England Journal of Medicine, 327,* 1861–1868.

19. Kitabachi, A.E., & Rumbak, M. (1989). The management of diabetic emergencies. *Hospital Practice, 24*(6A), 129–159.

20. Joslin, E.P., Gray, H., & Root, H.L. (1924). Insulin in hospital and home. *Journal of Metabolic Research, 2,* 651.

21. Somogyi, M. (1957). Exacerbation of diabetes in excess insulin action. *American Journal of Medicine, 26,* 169.

22. Bolli, G.B., Gotterman, I.S., & Campbell, P.J. (1984). Glucose counterregulation and waning of insulin in the Somogyi phenomenon (posthypoglycemic hyperglycemia). *New England Journal of Medicine, 311,* 1214.

23. Bolli, G.B., & Gerich, J.E. (1984). The Dawn phenomenon—a common occurrence in both non-insulin and insulin dependent diabetes mellitus. *New England Journal of Medicine, 310,* 746–750.

24. Carlin, B.W. (1988). Impotence and diabetes. *Metabolism, 37,* 19.

25. Viberti, G., Yip-Messent, J., & Morocutti, A. (1992). Diabetic nephropathy. *Diabetes Care, 15,* 1216–1222.

26. Hostetter, T.H. (1992). Diabetic nephropathy. *Diabetes Care, 15,* 1205–1211.

27. Sequist, E.R., Goetz, F.C., Rich, S., et al. (1989). Familial clustering of diabetic kidney disease. *New England Journal of Medicine, 320,* 1161–1165.

28. Kumar, V., Cotran, R.S., & Robbins, S.L. (1992). *Basic pathology* (5th ed., pp. 576–577). Philadelphia: W.B. Saunders.

29. Singer, D.E., Nathan, D.M., Fogel, H.A., et al. (1992). Screening for diabetic retinopathy. *Annals of Internal Medicine, 116,* 660–671.

30. American Academy of Ophthalmology. (1992). Screening for diabetes retinopathy (Guidelines of the American College of Physicians, American Diabetes Association). *Diabetes Care, 15*(Suppl. 2), P16–P18.

31. Browner, W.S. (1986). Preventable complications of diabetes mellitus. *Western Journal of Medicine, 145,* 701.

32. American Diabetes Association. (1992). Role of cardiovascular risk factors in prevention and treatment of macrovascular disease in diabetes (consensus statement). *Diabetes Care, 15*(Suppl. 2), 68–74.

33. Smith, D., Weinberger, M., & Katz, B. (1987). A controlled trial to increase office visits and reduce hospitalizations of diabetic patients. *Journal of General Internal Medicine, 2,* 232–238.

34. Reiber, G.E. (1992). Diabetes foot care. *Diabetes Care, 15*(Suppl. 1), 29–31.

35. Grunfeld, C. (1991). Diabetic foot ulcers: Etiology, treatment, and prevention. *Advances in Internal Medicine, 37,* 103–133.

■ **BIBLIOGRAPHY**

American Diabetes Association. (1992). Diabetes neuropathy (position statement). *Patient Care, 15,* 62–67.

American Diabetes Association. (1992). Proceedings of a Consensus Development Conference on Standarization Measures in Diabetic Neuropathy. *Diabetes Care, 15*(Suppl. 3), 1080–1083.

Ashbury, A.K. (1988). Understanding diabetic neuropathy. *New England Journal of Medicine, 319,* 577.

Atkinson, M., & Maclaren, N.K. (1990). What causes diabetes. *Scientific American, 263,* (1), 62–71.

Colwell, J.A. (1991). Oral treatment of diabetes mellitus: The contribution of gliclazide. *American Journal of Medicine, 90*(Suppl. 6A), 6A-1S-7S.

Dinneen, S., Gerich, J., & Rizza, R. (1992). Carbohydrate metabolism in non-insulin-dependent diabetes mellitus. *New England Journal of Medicine, 327,* 707–713.

Donahue, R.P., & Orchard, T.J. (1992). Diabetes mellitus and macrovascular complications. *Diabetes Care, 15*(9), 1141–1160.

Duckworth, W.C. (1991). Intensive management of type II diabetes. *Hospital Practice, 26*(5), 65–85.

Galloway, J.A., Hooper, J.A., Spradlin, T.C., et al. (1992). Biosynthesis of human insulin (review). *Diabetes Care, 15,* 666–692.

Gluck, S.L., & Klahr, S. (1991). Enlarging our view of the diabetic kidney. *New England Journal of Medicine, 324,* 1662–1664.

Groop, L.C. (1992). Sulfonylureas in NIDDM. *Patient Care, 15,* 737–753.

Horton, E.S. (1991). Exercise and decreased risk of

NIDDM. *New England Journal of Medicine, 325,* 196–197.

Kahn, S.E., Schwartz, R.S., Porte, D., et al. (1991). The glucose intolerance of aging: Implications for intervention. *Hospital Practice, 26*(4), 29–38.

Kitabachi, A.E., & Rumbar, M. (1989). The management of diabetic emergencies. *Hospital Practice, 24*(6A), 129–160.

Porte, D., & Kahn, S. (1991). Mechanisms of hyperglycemia in type II diabetes mellitus: Therapeutic implications for sulfonylurea treatment—an update.

American Journal of Medicine, 90(Suppl. 6A), 8S–14S.

Robertson, P. (1991). Pancreas transplantation in humans with diabetes mellitus. *Diabetes, 40,* 1085–1089.

Siperstein, M.D. (1992). Diabetic ketoacidosis and hyperosmolar coma. *Endocrinology and Metabolism Clinics of North America, 21,* 415.

Viberti, G., Yip-Messent, J., & Morocutti, A. (1992). Diabetic nephropathy. *Diabetes Care, 15,* 1216–1222.

Watkins, P.J. (1990). Diabetic autonomic neuropathy. *New England Journal of Medicine, 322,* 1078.

ALTERATIONS IN NEUROMUSCULAR FUNCTION

CHAPTER 47

ORGANIZATION AND CONTROL OF NEURAL FUNCTION

EDWARD W. CARROLL
ROBIN L. CURTIS

Introductory Concepts
Hierarchy of Control
Terminology
Central and Peripheral
Nervous Systems
Development and Organization
of the Nervous System
Embryologic Development

Soma and Viscera
Segmental Organization
of the Nervous System
Cell Columns
Longitudinal Tracts
Nervous Tissue Cells
Neurons

Supporting Cells
Metabolic Requirements
Nerve Cell Communication
Impulse Generation
and Conduction
Synaptic Transmission
Messenger Molecules

■ OBJECTIVES

After you have studied this chapter, you should be able to meet the following objectives:

■ State the difference between the central nervous system (CNS) and the peripheral nervous system (PNS).

■ Cite the significance of the hierarchy of control levels of the CNS.

■ Use the segmental approach to explain the development of the nervous system and the organization of the postembryonic nervous system.

■ Explain the difference between the viscera and the soma of a body segment.

■ State the origin and destination of nerve fibers contained in the dorsal and ventral roots.

■ Define *ganglia, cell column*, and *tract*.

■ State the type of structures that are innervated by general somatic afferent, general visceral afferent, special somatic afferent, general visceral efferent, pharyngeal efferent, and general somatic efferent neurons.

■ State the function of association neurons in the nervous system.

■ Name and describe the anatomy of the three parts of a neuron.

■ State the function of the supporting cells of the nervous system.

■ Describe the interaction of the presynaptic and postsynaptic terminals.

■ Explain the occurrence of both spatial and temporal summation.

■ Briefly describe how neurotransmitters are synthesized, stored, released, and inactivated.

■ Describe current thinking on how alterations in neurotransmitter release or action can alter body function.

Carol Mattson Porth: PATHOPHYSIOLOGY: CONCEPTS OF
ALTERED HEALTH STATES, 4th ed. © 1994, 1990, 1986, 1982
J.B. Lippincott Company

The nervous system, in coordination with the endocrine system, provides the means by which cell and tissue functions are integrated into a solitary, surviving organism. It controls skeletal muscle movement and helps to regulate cardiac and visceral smooth muscle activity. The nervous system makes possible the reception, integration, and perception of sensory information; it provides for memory and problem solving; and it facilitates adjustment to an ever-changing external environment. No part of the nervous system functions separately from other parts, and in the human, who is a thinking and feeling creature, the effects of emotion can exert a strong influence on both neural and hormonal control of body function. On the other hand, alterations in both neural and endocrine function (particularly at the biochemical level) can exert a strong influence on psychological behavior. This chapter is divided into three parts: the development and organization of the nervous system, nervous tissue cells, and neuronal communication.

■ DEVELOPMENT AND ORGANIZATION OF THE NERVOUS SYSTEM

The development of the nervous system can be traced far back into evolutionary history. In the course of its development, newer functional features and greater complexity resulted from the modification and enlargement of more primitive structures. In a moving organism, rapid reaction to environmental danger, to potential food sources, or to a sexual partner was required for the survival of the species. Thus, the front, or rostral, end of the central nervous system became specialized as a means of sensing the external environment and controlling reactions to it. In time, the ancient organization, which is largely retained in the spinal cord segments, was expanded in the forward segments of the nervous system. Of these, the most forward segments have undergone the most radical modification and have developed into the forebrain: the diencephalon and the cerebral hemispheres. The dominance of the front end of the central nervous system is reflected in a hierarchy of control levels—brain stem over spinal cord, forebrain over brain stem. Because the newer functions were added onto the outside of older functional systems and because the newer functions became concentrated at the rostral end of the nervous system, they are much more vulnerable to injury. These three principles—(1) no part of the nervous system functions independently of the other parts, (2) newer systems control older systems, and (3) the newer systems are more vulnerable to injury—form a basis

for understanding many of the manifestations that occur when the nervous system suffers injury or disease.

EMBRYONIC DEVELOPMENT

The nervous system appears very early in embryonic development. The early development of the nervous system is essential because it has a strong inducing influence that directs the development and organization of many other body systems, including the axial skeleton, skeletal muscles, and sensory organs such as the eyes and ears. Later, during the last trimester, the nervous system begins its second major function as a communication and integrative system.

During the second week of development, there are two layers of embryonic tissue, the endoderm and ectoderm. At the beginning of the third week, the ectoderm begins to invaginate and migrate between the two layers, forming a third layer called the *mesoderm* (Fig. 47-1). The mesoderm along the midline of the embryo rostral to the primitive pit forms a specialized rod of embryonic tissue called the *notocord*.

The notochord and adjacent mesoderm provides the necessary induction signal for the overlying ectoderm to differentiate and form the thickened neural plate: the primordium of the nervous system. The neural plate develops an axial groove (the neural groove) which sinks into the underlying mesoderm, its walls fusing across the top, forming a hollow ectodermal tube called the *neural tube*. The process, which is called *closure*, occurs during the later third and fourth weeks of gestation and is vital to the survival of the embryo. The neural tube will develop into the central nervous system (CNS). The notochord becomes the foundation around which the vertebral column ultimately develops. The surface ectoderm separates from the neural tube and fuses over the top to become the outer layer of skin. Closure begins at the cervical and high thoracic levels and zippers both rostrally toward the cephalic end of the embryo and caudally toward the posterior end. The last locations for completion of closure are at the rostral-most end of the brain (anterior neuropore, 25 days) and at the lumbosacral region (posterior neuropore, 27 days).

As the neural tube closes, ectodermal cells called *neural crest cells* migrate away from the dorsal surface of the forming neural tube and are progenitors of the neurons and supporting cells of the peripheral nervous system (see Fig. 47-1). Some of these cells gather into clumps or ganglia at the sides of each spinal cord segment (*dorsal root ganglia*) and most brain segments (*cranial ganglia*). Neurons of these ganglia become the afferent or sensory neurons of

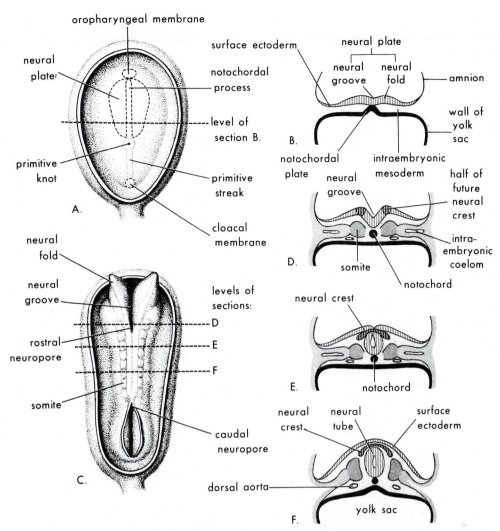

FIG. 47-1. Diagram showing formation of the neural crest and folding of the neural tube. (**A**). Dorsal view of an embryo of about 18 days, exposed by removing the amnion. (**B**) Transverse section of this embryo showing the neural plate and early development of the neural groove. The developing notochord is also shown. (**C**) Dorsal view of an embryo of about 22 days. The neural folds have fused opposite the somites but are widely spread out at both ends of the embryo. The rostal and caudal neuropores are indicated. (**D, E, F**) Transverse sections of this embryo at the levels shown in **C**, illustrating formation of the neural tube and its detachment from the surface ectoderm. Note that some neuroectodermal cells are not included in the neural tube but remain between it and the surface ectoderm as the neural crest. These cells first appear as paired columns on the dorsolateral aspect of the neural tube, but they soon become broken up into a series of segmented masses. (Moore, K. L. [1993]. *The developing human.* Philadelphia: W.B. Saunders)

the peripheral nervous system (PNS). Other neural crest cells become the pigment cells of the skin or contribute to the formation of the meninges, many of the structures of the face, and the peripheral ganglion cells of the autonomic nervous system. The latter include cells of the adrenal medulla.

The neural tube, which becomes the CNS, has a very early and critical role in inducing and organizing cell migration and differentiation of the neural crest, which in turn forms the PNS and contributes to many structures of the head and meninges. Further, the neural tube induces closure of the axial skeleton and induces the formation of special sensory organs. During later fetal life and thereafter, the nervous system provides communication, signal processing, integrative, and memory functions by means of electrochemical and chemical secretory functions of neurons. Both the early induction and later lifelong communication functions of the nervous system are at the center of the integrity, survival, and individuality of each person.

CLOSURE DEFECTS

If closure of the neural tube does not occur at any point, normal CNS development does not occur. Closure defects also prevent development of the protective skeletal and skin structures. Closure defects can occur over any area of the neural tube. The most common are in the area of the posterior neuropore and the anterior neuropore. Closure defects of the posterior neuropore result in a condition called *spinal bifida*.

Complete closure of the anterior neuropore is essential to subsequent normal brain and skull development. Failure to close results in severe developmental defects of the brain and cranium, a condition called *anencephaly*. This defect involves the forebrain and leaves the newborn with only brain stem reflexes. There is also an absence of the surrounding cranial vault (acrania) and scalp. It is a common malformation, occurring about once in every 1000 live births, and occurs four times more frequently in females than males. The condition is incompatible with long-term survival, and most babies die within several days of birth. Many factors have been implicated as a cause of anencephaly. There is a familial incidence, suggesting a genetic component. During the first trimester of pregnancy, environmental factors can increase the incidence of such neural closure defects. A significant correlation with exposure to x-rays has been established. Recent evidence suggests that increased frequency of closure defects may be related to increases in environmental temperature (fever, hot tubs, saunas)[1] as well as decreased levels of folic acid.[2] Anencephaly can serve as a cause of other developmental defects. For instance, the normal fetus swallows amniotic fluid and excretes it through the kidneys. Because the anencephalic fetus lacks the neural development for swallowing, anencephalic pregnancies are often associated with excess amniotic fluid (polyhydramnios).

THE CENTRAL AND PERIPHERAL NERVOUS SYSTEMS

The nervous system can be divided into two parts—the central nervous system (CNS) and the peripheral nervous system (PNS). The CNS consists of the brain and spinal cord, which is located within the pro-

tected confines of the axial skeleton (cranium and spinal column). The PNS is located outside these structures. The basic design of the nervous system provides for the concentration of computational and control functions within the CNS. In this design, the PNS functions as an input–output system for relaying input to the CNS and for transmitting output messages that control effector organs, such as muscles and glands.

The functioning cells of the nervous system are called *neurons*. Neurons have branching cytoplasm-filled processes, the dendrites and the axons, which project from the cell body and are unique to the nervous system. The axonal processes are particularly designed for rapid communication with other neurons and the many body structures that are innervated by the nervous system. Afferent, or sensory, neurons transmit information from the PNS to the CNS. Efferent, or motor neurons, carry information away from the CNS. Interspersed between the afferent and efferent neurons is a network of interconnecting neurons that serve to modulate and control the body's response to changes in the internal and external environments. These interconnecting networks facilitate the establishment of response patterns and allow for storage of information on which learning and memory are based. Complex neural networks provide the means for subjective experiences, such as perception and emotion. These also provide for intelligence, judgment, and anticipation of events.

TERMINOLOGY

One aspect of understanding the nervous system has to do with orientation of the nervous system in relation to the body. Structures that are located toward the front of the body are described as being in an *anterior* or *ventral* position; those that are located toward the back are *posterior* or *dorsal*. The term *superior* indicates upper; *inferior* indicates lower. The term *cephalic*, which also means head end, is sometimes used to indicate a superior position and *caudal*, an inferior position. Another important term is the Latin word *rostrum* (beak), which refers to the front end in the embryo and to the region of the nose and mouth in postembryonic life. Other terms that are used to describe the position of nervous system structures are *medial*, which means near the middle, and *lateral*, which means toward the side or furthest from the middle. A *proximal* structure is one that is located nearest the trunk, and a *distal* structure is one that is located furthest from the trunk. An *afferent* nerve fiber is one that conveys information toward the

CNS, and an *efferent* nerve fiber is one that conveys information away from the CNS.

THE SOMA AND VISCERA

On cross section, the body is organized into a soma and a viscera (Fig. 47-2). The soma, or body wall, includes all of the structures derived from the embryonic ectoderm, such as the epidermis of the skin and the CNS. The mesodermal connective tissues of the soma include the dermis of the skin, skeletal muscle, bone, and the outer lining of the body cavity (parietal pleura and peritoneum). For the nervous system, all of the more internal structures constitute the *viscera*, including the great vessels derived from the intermediate mesoderm, the urinary system, and the gonadal structures. The viscera also includes the inner lining of the body cavities, such as the visceral pleura and peritoneum, and the mesodermal tissues that surround the entoderm-lined gut and its derivative organs (lungs, liver, and pancreas).

Each body segment receives a bilaterally symmetric segmental nerve, which lies in the soma and provides afferent innervation of the skin, muscles, bones, meninges of the CNS, and the somatic lining of body cavities. It also provides efferent innervation of the skeletal muscle, smooth muscle, and glands of the soma. Branches from the segmental nerve supply the visceral organs of the body, providing both afferent and efferent functions through the autonomic nerves, including control of smooth and cardiac muscle as well as the glands of the visceral organs.

SEGMENTAL ORGANIZATION OF THE NERVOUS SYSTEM

Throughout life, the organization of the nervous system retains many patterns that were established during early embryonic life. It is this early pattern of organization that is presented as a framework for understanding the nervous system.

In the process of development, the basic organizational pattern of the body is that of a longitudinal series of segments, each repeating the same fundamental pattern (Fig. 47-3). Although the early muscular, skeletal, vascular, and excretory systems and the nerves that supply these somatic and visceral structures have the same segmental pattern, it is the nervous system that most clearly retains this organization in the adult. The CNS and its associated peripheral nerves are thus made up of 43 or so segments, 33 of which form the spinal cord and spinal nerves, and 10, the brain and its cranial nerves (Fig. 47-4).

Each segment of the CNS is accompanied by two pairs (one member of a pair on each side) of bundled

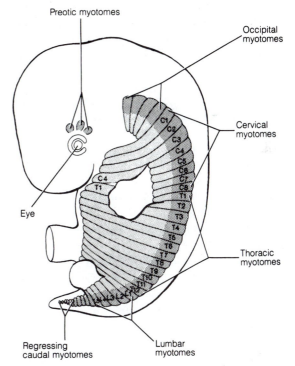

FIG. 47-3. The developing muscular system in a 6-week-old embryo. The segmental muscle masses, or myotomes, which give rise to most skeletal muscles, reflect the basic segmental organization of the body and head. Efferent cranial nerves innervating the myotomes of the head are as follows: preotic myotomes (nerves III, IV, and VI) and the occipital myotomes (XII). (Moore, K. L. [1977]. *The developing human* [2nd ed., p. 317]. Philadelphia: W.B. Saunders)

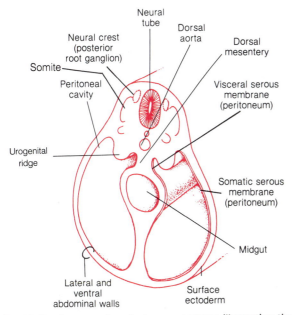

FIG. 47-2. Cross section of a human embryo, illustrating the development of the somatic and visceral structures.

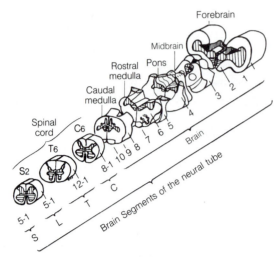

FIG. 47-4. The adult human central nervous system. The dorsal (*vertical hatching*) and ventral (*horizontal hatching*) horns of the gray matter are surrounded by the white matter that contains the longitudinal tracts. Numbers indicate segmental divisions of the neural tube. (Adapted from Elliott, H. C. [1969]. *Neuroanatomy.* Philadelphia: J.B. Lippincott)

nerve fibers, or *roots*: a ventral pair and a dorsal pair. The paired dorsal roots interconnect a pair of *dorsal root ganglia* and their corresponding CNS segment. These ganglia contain the afferent nerve cell bodies, each of which has two axon-like processes—one that ends in a peripheral receptor and another that enters the central neural segment. The axon-like process that enters the central neural segment communicates with a neuron called an *input association (IA)* neuron. Somatic afferents transmit information from the soma to somatic IA neurons, and visceral afferents transmit information from the viscera to visceral IA neurons. The paired ventral roots of each segment are bundles of axons that provide efferent (motor) output to effector sites such as muscle and glandular cells of the body segment.

On cross section, the hollow embryonic neural tube can be divided into a central canal, or ventricle, that contains the cerebrospinal fluid (CSF) and the wall of the tube. The latter develops into an inner gray cellular portion, which contains nerve cell bodies, and an outer white matter portion, which contains tract systems of the CNS that are made up of nerve cell processes. The dorsal half of the gray matter is called the *dorsal horn*. It contains sensory IA neurons that receive afferent information from the dorsal roots. The ventral portion, or *ventral horn*, contains efferent neurons that communicate by way of the ventral roots with effector cells of the body segment. Many of the CNS neurons develop axons that grow longitudinally as tract systems that intercommunicate between neighboring and distal segments of the neural tube.

CELL COLUMNS

The complexity of the organizational structure of the nervous system is somewhat simplified by a pattern in which PNS and CNS neurons are repeated as parallel cell columns running lengthwise along the nervous system. In this organizational pattern, afferent neurons, dorsal horn cells, and ventral horn cells are organized as a series of 11 cell columns. A box of 22 colored beverage straws (a set of 11 straws on each side of the midline) can be used as an analogy to represent the cell columns. In this model, each lateral half of the nervous system (right and left sides) is represented in mirror fashion by one set of 11 colored straws. If these straws were cut crosswise (equivalent to a transverse section through the nervous system) at several places along their length, the spatial relationship among the different colored straws would be repeated in each section (Fig. 47-5).

The cell columns on each side can be further grouped according to their location in the PNS and CNS: four in the dorsal root ganglia that contain sensory neurons, four in the dorsal horn that contain the sensory IA neurons, and three in the ventral horn that contain motor neurons. Each column of dorsal root ganglia projects to its particular column of IA neurons in the dorsal horn. The IA neurons distribute afferent information to local reflex circuitry and more rostral and elaborate segments of the CNS. The ventral roots contain both output association (OA) neurons and lower motor neurons (LMNs). The lower motor neurons provide the final circuitry for organizing efferent nerve activity. The efferent neurons send their axons into the body to innervate skeletal, smooth, or cardiac muscle, and glandular cells.

Between the input association neurons and the output association neurons are networks of small internuncial neurons, which are arranged in complex circuits. The internuncial neurons provide the discreteness, appropriateness, and intelligence of responses to stimuli. Most of the billions of CNS cells in the spinal cord and brain gray matter are internuncial neurons.

The effectiveness of a CNS-mediated response to changing environmental conditions depends on the functional integrity of the neurons and effector cells in a particular sequence called a *reflex*. A reflex is a highly predictable relationship between a stimulus and a response. It is mediated by the transmission of receptor-derived action potentials in the afferent neurons that stimulate activity in a network of CNS association neurons of the dorsal or ventral gray matter leading to action potentials in efferent neurons. These efferents, in turn, stimulate effector responses

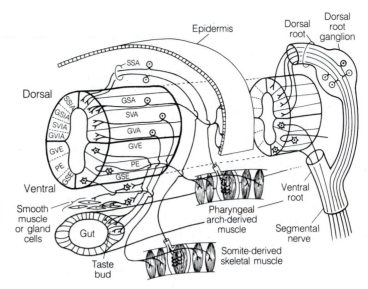

FIG. 47-5. Cell columns of the central nervous system. The columns in the dorsal horn contain input association neurons: special sensory (SSIA), general sensory (GSIA), special visceral (SVIA), and general visceral (GVIA). The ventral horn contains the efferent neurons: the general visceral efferent (GVE), pharyngeal efferent (PE), and general somite efferent (GSE).

in structures such as skeletal, smooth, or cardiac muscle and glands. The activity of these effectors constitutes the reflex response.

There are four columns of afferent (sensory) neurons in the dorsal root ganglia that directly innervate four corresponding columns of input association neurons in the dorsal horn. These columns are categorized as special and general afferents: *special somatic afferent, general somatic afferent, general visceral afferent,* and *special visceral afferent.*

Special somatic afferent (SSA) fibers are concerned with internal sensory information such as joint and tendon sensation (proprioception). The general somatic afferents (GSA) innervate the skin and other somatic structures; they respond to stimuli such as those that produce pressure or pain. The general somatic afferent IA column cells relay the sensory information to protective and other reflex circuits and also project the information to the forebrain where it is perceived as painful, warm, cold, and so on. The special somatic afferent IA column cells relay their information to local reflexes concerned with posture and movement. These neurons also relay information to the cerebellum, contributing to coordination of movement, and to the forebrain, contributing to experience. Afferents innervating the labyrinth and derived auditory end organs of the inner ear also belong to the special soma category.

General visceral afferent (GVA) neurons innervate visceral structures such as the gastrointestinal tract and urinary bladder; they project to the general visceral IA column, which relays to vital reflex circuits and sends information to the forebrain regarding visceral sensations of stomach fullness, bladder pressure, sexual experience, and others. Special visceral afferent (SVA) cells innervate specialized gut-related receptors, such as the taste buds and receptors of the olfactory mucosa. Their central processes

communicate with special sensory input association column neurons that project to reflex circuits to produce salivation, chewing, swallowing, and other responses. The forebrain projection fibers from these association cells provide for the sensations of taste (gustation) and smell (olfaction).

The ventral horn contains three separate longitudinal cell columns: *general visceral efferent, pharyngeal efferent,* and *general somite efferent.* Each of these cell columns contain both OA and efferent neurons. The OA neurons coordinate and integrate the function of the efferent lower motor neuron (LMN) cells of its column.

General visceral efferent (GVE) neurons transmit the efferent output of the autonomic nervous system and are called *preganglionic neurons.* The GVE are structurally and functionally divided into the sympathetic and parasympathetic nervous system, and their axons project through the segmental ventral roots to innervate smooth and cardiac muscle and glandular cells of the body, most of which are in the viscera. In the viscera three additional neural crest–derived cell columns are present on each side of the body. These become the postganglionic neurons of the autonomic nervous system. For the sympathetic nervous system, the columns are the paravertebral or sympathetic chain ganglia and the prevertebral series of ganglia (*e.g.,* celiac ganglia). For the parasympathetic system, these become the enteric plexus in the wall of the gut-derived organs (discussed in Chapter 49).

Pharyngeal efferent (PE) neurons innervate the branchial arch skeletal muscles: the muscles of mastication, facial expression, head turning, and muscles of the pharynx and larynx. The general somite efferent (GSE) column neurons supply the somite-derived muscles of the body and head, which include the skeletal muscles of the body, limbs, tongue, and

TABLE 47-1. THE SEGMENTAL NERVES AND THEIR COMPONENTS

SEGMENT	NERVE	COMPONENT	INNERVATION	FUNCTION
1. Forebrain				
	I. Olfactory	SVA	Receptors in olfactory mucosa	Reflexes, olfaction (smell)
2.	II. Optic nerve		Optic nerve and retina (part of brain system, not a peripheral nerve)	
3. Midbrain				
	V. Trigeminal (V₁) ophthalmic division			
		SSA	Muscles: upper face: forehead upper lid: frontal and ethmoid sinuses	Facial expression, proprioception
		GSA	Skin, subcutaneous tissue; conjunctiva; frontal/ethmoid sinuses	Somesthesia Reflexes (blink)
	III. Oculomotor	GVE	Iris spincter: ciliary muscle	Pupillary constriction Accommodation
		GSE	Extrinsic eye muscles	Eye movement, lid movement
4. Pons				
	V. Trigeminal (V₂) maxillary division			
		SSA	Muscles: facial expression	Proprioception
		GSA	Skin, oral mucosa, upper teeth, hard palate, maxillary sinus	Reflexes (sneeze) Somesthesia
	V. Trigeminal (V₃) mandibular division			
		SSA	Lower jaw, muscles: mastication	Proprioception, jaw jerk
		GSA	Skin, mucosa, teeth, anterior ²/₃ tongue	Reflexes, somesthesia
		PE	Muscles: mastication, tensor tympani, tensor veli palantini	Mastication: speech Protects ear from loud sound Tenses soft palate
	IV. Trochlear	GSE	Extrinsic eye muscle	Moves eye down and in
5. Caudal Pons				
	VIII. Vestibular, cochlear			
		SSA	Vestibular end organs Organ of Corti	Reflexes: sense of head position Reflexes: hearing
	VII. Facial nerve, intermedius portion			
		GSA	External auditory meatus	Somesthesia
		GVA	Nasopharynx	Gag reflex: sensation
		SVA	Taste buds anterior ²/₃ tongue	Reflexes: gustation (taste)
		GVE	Nasopharynx; lacrimal, sublingual, and submandibular glands	Mucous secretion Reflexes (lacrimation and salivation)
	Facial nerve	PE	Muscles: facial expression, stapedius	Facial expression Protects ear from loud sounds
	VI. Abducens			
		GSE	Extrinsic eye muscle	Lateral eye deviation
6. Middle Medulla				
	IX. Glossopharyngeal			
		SSA	Stylopharyngeus muscle	Proprioception
		GSA	Posterior external meatus	Somesthesia
		SVA	Taste buds posterior ¹/₃ tongue	Gustation (taste)
		GVA	Oral pharynx	Gag reflex: sensation
		GVE	Parotid gland: pharyngeal mucosa	Salivary reflex: mucous secretion
		PE	Stylopharyngeus	Assists swallowing

(Continued)

TABLE 47-1. THE SEGMENTAL NERVES AND THEIR COMPONENTS (CONTINUED)

SEGMENT NERVE	COMPONENT	INNERVATION	FUNCTION
7,8,9,10. Caudal Medulla			
X. Vagus			
	SSA	Muscles: pharynx, larynx	Proprioception
	GSA	Posterior surface pinna	Somesthesia
	SVA	Taste buds, pharynx, larynx	Reflexes, gustation
	GVA	Visceral organs (esophagus to mid-transverse colon, liver, pancreas, heart, lungs)	Reflexes, sensation
	GVE	Visceral organs as above	Parasympathetic efferent
	PE	Muscles pharynx, larynx	Swallowing, phonation, emesis
XIII. Hypoglossal			
	GSE	Muscles of tongue	Tongue movement, reflexes
Spinal Segments			
C1–C4 Upper Cervical			
XI. Spinal assessory Spinal nerves	PE	Sternocleidomastoid, trapazius	Head, shoulder movement
	SSA	Muscles of neck	Proprioception, DTRs
	GSA	Neck, back of head	Somesthesia
	GSE	Neck muscles	Head, shoulder movement
C5–C8 Lower Cervical			
	SSA	Upper limb muscles	Proprioception, DTRs
	GSA	Upper limbs	Reflexes, somesthesia
	GSE	Upper limb muscles	Movement, posture
T1–L2 Thoracic, Upper Lumbar			
	SSA	Trunk, abdominal wall muscles	Proprioception
	GSA	Trunk, abdominal wall	Reflexes, somesthesia
	GVA	All of viscera	Reflexes and sensation
	GVE	All of viscera	Sympathetic reflexes, vasomotor control, sweating, piloerection
	GSE	Trunk, abdominal wall, back muscles	Movement, posture, respiration
L2–S1 Lower Lumbar, Upper Sacral			
	SSA	Lower limb muscles	Proprioception, DTRs
	GSA	Lower trunk, limbs, back	Reflexes, somesthesia
	GSE	Trunk, lower limbs, back muscles	Movement, posture
S2–S4 Lower Sacral			
	SSA	Pelvic, perineal muscles	Proprioception
	GSA	Pelvis, genitalia	Reflexes, somesthesia
	GVA	Hindgut, bladder, uterus	Reflexes, sensation
	GVE	Hindgut, visceral organs	Visceral reflexes, defecation, urination, erection
S5–Co2 Lower Sacral, Coccygeal			
	SSA	Perineal muscles	Proprioception
	GSA	Lower sacrum, anus	Reflexes, somesthesia
	GSE	Perineal muscles	Reflexes, posture

extrinsic eye muscles. These efferent neurons transmit the commands of the CNS to peripheral effectors—the skeletal muscles. Thus they are the "final common path neurons" in the sequence leading to motor activity. They are often called lower motor neurons (LMNs) because they are under the control of higher levels of the CNS, including precise control by upper motor neurons (UMNs).

With rare exceptions, peripheral nerves, including the cranial nerves, contain afferent and efferent neuronal processes of more than one of four afferent and three efferent cell columns. This provides the basis for assessing the function of any peripheral nerve. The functional components of each end of the cranial nerves and of spinal nerve roots are presented in Table 47-1.

LONGITUDINAL TRACTS

The gray matter of the cell columns in the CNS is surrounded by bundles of myelinated axons (white matter) and unmyelinated axons that travel longitudinally along the length of the neural axis. This white matter can be divided into three layers—an inner, a middle, and an outer layer (Fig. 47-6). The inner, or *archi*, layer contains short fibers that project for a maximum of about five segments before reentering the gray matter. The middle, or *paleo*, layer projects six or more segments. Both the archi and the paleo layer fibers have many branches, or *collaterals*, that enter the gray matter of intervening segments. The outer, or *neo*, layer contains large-diameter axons that can travel the entire length of the nervous system (Table 47-2). The term *suprasegmental* refers to higher levels of the CNS, such as the brain stem and cerebrum and structures above a given CNS segment. Both paleo- and neo-level fibers have suprasegmental projections.

The longitudinal layers are arranged in bundles, or fiber tracts, which contain axons that have the same destination, origin, and function. These longitudinal tracts are named systematically to reflect their origin and destination, the site of origin being named first and the site of destination second. For example, the *spinothalamic tract* originates in the *spinal* cord and terminates in the *thalamus*. The *corticospinal* tract originates in the cerebral *cortex* and ends in the *spinal* cord.

Inner Layer. The inner layer of white matter contains the axons of neurons of the gray matter that interconnect with neighboring segments of the nervous system. The axons of this layer permit the pool of motor neurons of several segments to work together as a functional unit. They also allow the afferent neurons of one segment to trigger reflexes that activate motor units in neighboring as well as the same segments. In terms of evolution, this is the oldest of the three layers; thus, it is sometimes referred to as the archi-level layer. It is the first of the longitudinal layers to become functional, and it appears to be limited to reflex types of movements. Reflex movements of the fetus (quickening) that begin during the fifth month of intrauterine life involve the inner archi-level layer.

The inner layer of the white matter differs from the other two layers in one important aspect. Many neurons in the embryonic gray matter migrate out into this layer, resulting in a rich mixture of neurons and local fibers called the *reticular formation*. The circuitry of most reflexes is contained in the reticular formation. In the brain stem, the reticular formation becomes quite large and contains major portions of vital reflexes, such as those controlling respiration, cardiovascular function, swallowing, and vomiting, to mention a few.

A functional system called the *reticular activation system* (RAS) operates in the lateral portions of the reticular formation of the medulla, pons, and especially the midbrain. The convergence of information from all sensory modalities, including those of the somesthetic, auditory, visual, and visceral afferent nerves, bombards the neurons of this system. The RAS has both descending and ascending portions. The descending portion communicates with all spinal segmental levels through paleo-level reticulospinal tracts and serves to facilitate many of the cord-level reflexes. For example, it speeds up reaction time and stabilizes postural reflexes. The ascending portion, sometimes called the *centroencephalic system*, accelerates brain activity, particularly thalamic and cortical activity. This is reflected by the appearance of awake brain-wave patterns. Thus, sudden stimuli result not only in protective and attentive postures but also in increased awareness.

Middle Layer. The middle layer of the white matter contains most of the major fiber tract systems required for sensation and movement. It contains the ascending spinoreticular and spinothalamic tracts. This system consists of larger-diameter and longer suprasegmental fibers, which ascend to the brain stem and are largely functional at birth. In terms of evolutionary development, these tracts are quite old; therefore, this layer is sometimes called the paleo layer. It facilitates many of the primitive functions, such as the "auditory startle reflex," which occurs in response to loud noises. This reflex consists of turning the head and body toward the sound, dilating the pupils of the eyes, catching of the breath, and quickening of the pulse.

Outer Layer. The outer layer of the tract systems is the newest of the three layers in terms of evolutionary development; hence, it is sometimes called the neo layer. It becomes functional at about the second year of life, and it includes the pathways needed for bladder training. Myelination of the neo-layer suprasegmental tracts, which include many of those required for the most delicate coordination and skill, is not complete until sometime around the fifth year of life. This includes the development of tracts needed for fine manipulative skills, such as the finger–thumb coordination required for the use of many tools and the toe movements needed for acrobatics. Being the newest to evolve and being on the outside of the brain and spinal cord, these tracts are the most vulnerable to injury. When these outer tracts are damaged, the paleo and archi tracts often remain

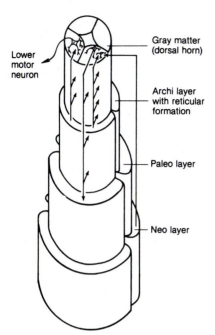

FIG. 47-6. The three concentric subdivisions of the tract systems of the white matter. Migration of neurons into the archi layer converts it into the reticular formation of the white matter.

Labels in figure:
- Lower motor neuron
- Gray matter (dorsal horn)
- Archi layer with reticular formation
- Paleo layer
- Neo layer

functional, and rehabilitation methods can result in quite effective use of the older systems. Delicacy and refinement may be lost, but basic function remains. For example, a very important outer system (or neo-system), the corticospinal system, permits the fine manipulative control required for writing. If this is lost, paleo-level systems remaining intact permit the grasping and holding of objects. Thus, the hand can still be used to perform its basic functions.

Collateral Communication Pathways. Axons in the archi and paleo layers characteristically possess many collateral branches, which move into the gray cell columns or synapse with the reticular formation as the axon passes each succeeding CNS segment.

Should a major axon be destroyed at some point along its course, these collaterals provide multi-synaptic alternative pathways that bypass the local damage. Neo-level tracts do not possess these collaterals but are instead highly discrete as to the target neurons with which they communicate. Because of their discreteness, damage to the neo tracts causes permanent loss of function. Damage to the archi or paleo systems, on the other hand, is usually followed by slow return of function, presumably through the use of these collateral connections. For example, the surgical sectioning of pathways carrying pain impulses (spinothalamic paleo-level tracts) can be used for temporary relief of intractable pain. The pain experience usually returns after some weeks or months. When it does return, it is often poorly localized and sometimes more unpleasant than it was initially. Consequently, this surgical procedure, which is called a tractotomy, is usually reserved for persons who are not expected to survive for longer than a few months.

In summary, the nervous system can be divided into two parts: the central nervous system (CNS) and the peripheral nevous system (PNS). The CNS develops from the ectoderm of the early embryo by formation of a hollow tube that closes and sinks below the surface of its longitudinal axis. The cavity of the tube forms the ventricles of the brain and spinal canal, and the side wall develops to form the brain stem and spinal cord. The brain stem and spinal cord are subdivided into the dorsal horn, which contains neurons that receive and process incoming or afferent information, and the ventral horn, which contains efferent motor neurons that handle the final stages of output processing.

The segmental pattern of early embryonic development is retained in the fully developed nervous system. Each one of the 43 or more body segments is interconnected to corresponding CNS or neural tube segments by segmental afferent and efferent neurons. Afferent neuronal processes enter the CNS by way of the dorsal root ganglia and the dorsal roots. Afferent neurons of the dorsal root ganglia are of four types: general

TABLE 47-2. CHARACTERISTICS OF THE CONCENTRIC SUBDIVISIONS OF THE LONGITUDINAL TRACTS IN THE WHITE MATTER OF THE CENTRAL NERVOUS SYSTEM

CHARACTERISTICS	ARCHI-LEVEL TRACTS	PALEO-LEVEL TRACTS	NEO-LEVEL TRACTS
Segmental span	Intersegmental (less than five segments)	Suprasegmental (five or more segments)	Suprasegmental
Number of synapses	Multisynaptic	Multisynaptic but fewer than archi-level tracts	Monosynaptic with target structures
Conduction velocity	Very slow	Fast	Fastest
Examples of functional systems	Flexor withdrawal reflex circuitry	Spinothalamic tracts	Corticospinal tracts

somatic afferent, special somatic afferent, general visceral afferent, and special visceral afferent. These afferent neurons synapse with their appropriate input association neurons in the cell columns of the dorsal horn (*e.g.*, general somatic afferents synapse with neurons in the general somatic afferent IA cell column). Efferent fibers from motoneurons in the ventral horn exit the CNS in the ventral roots. General somatic efferent neurons are LMNs that innervate somite-derived skeletal muscles, and general visceral efferent neurons are preganglionic fibers that synapse with postganglionic fibers that innervate visceral structures. This pattern of afferent and efferent neurons, which is generally repeated in each segment of the body, forms parallel cell columns running lengthwise through the CNS and PNS.

Longitudinal communication between CNS segments is provided by neurons that send the axons into nearby segments by means of the innermost layer of the white matter, the ancient archi-level system of fibers. These cells provide for coordination between neighboring segments. Neurons have invaded this layer, and the mix of these cells and axons, called the reticular formation, is the location of much of the important reflex circuitry of the spinal cord and the brain stem. Paleo-level tracts, which are located outside this layer, provide the longitudinal communication between more distant segments of the nervous system; this layer includes most of the important ascending and descending tracts. The recently evolved neo-level systems, which become functional during infancy and childhood, travel at the outside of the white matter and provide the means for very delicate and discriminative function. The outside position of the neo tracts, as well as their lack of collateral and redundant pathways, makes them the most vulnerable to injury.

■ NERVOUS TISSUE CELLS

Nervous tissue contains two types of cells—neurons and supporting cells. The neurons are the functional cells of the nervous system. Neurons exhibit membrane excitability and conductivity and secrete neurotransmitters and hormones, such as epinephrine and antidiuretic hormone. The *supporting cells*, such as Schwann cells in the PNS and the glial cells in the CNS, function to *protect* the nervous system and *supply* metabolic support for the neurons.

NEURONS

To understand the brain and nervous system, it is necessary to understand how neurons are constructed, how they work, and how they communicate with one another. The human brain consists of several trillion cells, each of which must communicate with several thousand others. The average nerve cell ranges in size from 0.02 mm to 0.04 mm, and a synaptic cleft no more than 0.001 mm.[3]

Neurons have three distinct parts—the cell body and its cytoplasm-filled processes, the dendrites, and the axons (Fig. 47-7). These processes form the functional connections, or synapses, with other nerve cells, with receptor cells, or with effector cells.

The *cell body*, or *soma*, contains a large, vesicular nucleus, one or more distinct nucleoli, and a well-developed rough endoplasmic reticulum. The nucleus has the same DNA code content that is present in other cells of the body. The nucleoli, which are composed of both DNA and RNA, are associated with protein synthesis. There are large masses of ribosomes, which are prominent in many neurons. These acidic RNA masses, which are involved in protein synthesis, stain as dark *Nissl* bodies with basic histologic stains (see Fig. 47-7).

The *dendrites* (treelike) are multiple, branched extensions of the nerve cell body; they are the main source through which neurons receive information and conduct information *toward* the cell body. The dendrites and cell body are studded with synaptic terminals from axons and dendrites of other neurons (Fig. 47-8).

The *axon* is a long efferent process that projects from the cell body and carries impulses away from the cell. There is usually only one axon to a nerve cell. Most axons undergo multiple branching, resulting in many axonal terminals. The cytoplasm of the cell body extends to fill both the dendrites and the axon (see Fig. 47-7B). There are no Nissl bodies in the *axon hillock*, which is the point where the axon leaves the cell body. The proteins and other materials that are used by the axon are synthesized in the cell body and then flow down the axon through its cytoplasm.

The cell body of the neuron is equipped for a high level of metabolic activity. This is necessary because the cell body must synthesize the cytoplasmic and membrane constituents required to maintain the function of the axon and its terminals. Some of these axons extend for a distance of 1 to 1.5 m and have a volume that is sometimes 200 to 500 times greater than the cell body itself. Two axonal transport systems, one slow and one rapid, move molecules from the cell body through the cytoplasm of the axon to its terminals. Replacement and nutrient molecules are slowly forced out of the cell body and down the axon as they are synthesized, moving at the rate of about 1 mm/day. Other molecules, such as some of the neurosecretory granules or their precursors, are conveyed by a rapid energy-dependent active transport system, moving at the rate of about 400 mm/day. In many instances, membrane-bound vesicles containing neurosecretory granules (neurotransmitters, neuromodulators, or neurohormones) are moved to the axon synaptic terminals by the active transport process. For example, rapid axonal transport carries antidiuretic hormones and oxytocin from hypothalamic neurons through their axons to the poste-

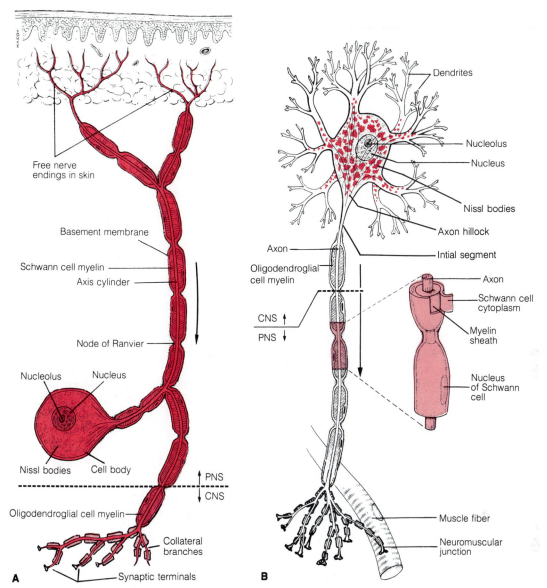

FIG. 47-7. **(A)** A typical afferent neuron that carries information from surface receptors (in this case, the skin) to the central nervous system (CNS). The cell body and axons are in the peripheral nervous system (PNS), whereas the central axon penetrates into the CNS wherein myelin is provided by oligodendroglial cells. **(B)** Myelinated efferent neuron with axon entering the PNS to innervate skeletal muscle cells. (Chaffee, E. E., & Lytle, I. M. [1980]. *Basic physiology and anatomy* [4th ed.]. Philadelphia: J.B. Lippincott)

rior pituitary, where the hormones are released into the blood. A reverse rapid axonal transport system serves to move materials including target cell messenger molecules from axonal terminals back to the cell body.

SUPPORTING CELLS

Supporting cells of the nervous system, Schwann cells of the PNS and the several types of glial cells of the CNS, provide the neurons with protection and metabolic support. The supporting cells segregate the neurons into isolated metabolic compartments, which are required for normal neural function. Together with the tightly joined endothelial cells of the capillaries in the CNS, these supporting cells may contribute to what is called the blood–brain barrier. This term is used to emphasize the impermeability of the nervous system to large and potentially harmful molecules. In addition, the many-layered myelin wrappings of Schwann cells of the PNS and the oligodendroglia of the CNS provide the myelin sheath seg-

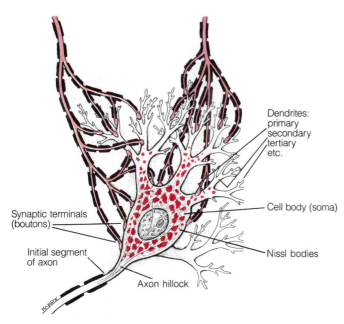

FIG. 47-8. Synaptic terminals in contact with the dendrites and cell body of an efferent neuron. (Chaffee, E. E., & Lytle, I. M. [1980]. *Basic physiology and anatomy* [4th ed.]. Philadelphia: J.B. Lippincott)

ments that serve to increase the velocity of nerve impulse conduction in axons having larger diameters.

Normally, the nerve cell bodies in the PNS are collected into *ganglia*, such as the dorsal root and autonomic ganglia. Each of the cell bodies and processes of the peripheral nerves is surrounded, or enclosed, in cellular sheaths of supporting cells. The cells that surround the ganglion cells are called *satellite cells*. The satellite cells secrete a basement membrane that apparently protects the cell body from the diffusion of large molecules. Collagen, secreted by fibroblasts, protects the axon from mechanical forces. Thus, in the PNS, all parts of a neuron and its supporting cells are surrounded by a covering called the *endoneurial sheath*, which is made up of a continuous basement membrane surrounded by layers of collagen. The presence of the endoneurial sheath is essential to the regeneration of peripheral axons. This sheath provides a collagenous tube through which a regenerating axon can again reach its former target. Finally, the entire ganglion is protected by a heavy collagenous layer, which also surrounds the large bundles of neural processes in the PNS, called the epineurial sheath.

The processes of the larger nerves, the axons of both the afferent and efferent neurons, are surrounded by the cell membrane and cytoplasm of Schwann cells, which are close relatives of the satellite cells. The Schwann cell surrounds the nerve process and then wraps itself around it many times in jelly-roll fashion (Fig. 47-9). Schwann cells line up along the neuronal process, and each of these cells, in turn, forms its own discrete myelin segment. The end of each myelin segment attaches to the cell membrane of the axon by means of sealed junctions. Successive Schwann cells are separated by short extracellular fluid gaps called the *nodes of Ranvier*, where

the myelin is missing (Fig. 47-10). The nodes of Ranvier serve to increase nerve conduction by allowing the impulse to jump from node to node in a process called *saltatory conduction*. In this way, the impulse can travel more rapidly through the extracellular fluid than it could if it were required to move system-

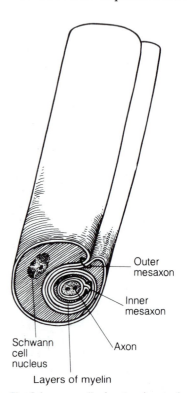

FIG. 47-9. The Schwann cell migrates down a larger axon to a bare region, settles down, and encloses the axon in a fold of its plasma membrane. It then rotates around and around, wrapping the axon in many layers of plasma membrane, with most of the Schwann cell cytoplasm squeezed out. The resultant thick, multiple-layered coating around the axon is called myelin.

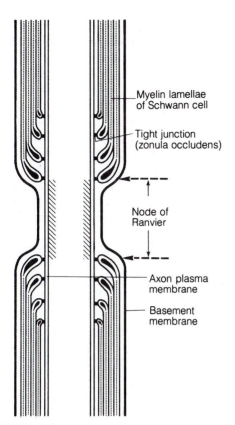

FIG. 47-10. Schematic drawing of a longitudinal section through a node of a myelinated axon of the PNS. Sealed junctions between myelin lamellae of the Schwann cell and the axon plasma membrane seal in the intracellular fluids within the internodal region. Extracellular fluids of the PNS communicate directly with the bare axon at the node. In the CNS, there is no basement membrane in the internode and nodal regions.

atically along the entire nerve process. This increased conduction velocity greatly reduces reaction time, or time between the application of a stimulus and the subsequent motor response. The short reaction time that occurs when there is a rapid conduction velocity is of particular importance in peripheral nerves with long distances (sometimes 1–2 m) for conduction between the CNS and distal effector organs.

In addition to its role in increasing conduction velocity, the myelin sheath aids in nourishing the neuronal process. Because there are essentially no glycogen stores within the cytoplasm of the neuron, the major source of energy is derived from the supporting cells, in this case the myelin sheath, or from the vascular system at the nodes of Ranvier. In some pathologic conditions, such as multiple sclerosis in the CNS and Guillain–Barré syndrome in the PNS, the myelin may degenerate or be destroyed, leaving a section of bare axonal process, which eventually dies unless remyelinization takes place. Thus, the metabolic intervention of the supporting cells is essential for the long-term survival of the neuron and its processes.

Each of the end-to-end series of Schwann cells is enclosed within a continuous tube of basement membrane, which is surrounded by a multilayered, collagen-rich *endoneurial tube* (Fig. 47-11). These endoneurial tubes are bundled together with blood vessels and lymphatics into nerve *fascicles*, which are surrounded by a collagenous *perineurial sheath*. Usually, several fascicles are further surrounded by the heavy, protective *epineurial sheath* of the peripheral nerve. The protective layers that surround the pe-

FIG. 47-11. Schematic representation of a nerve and a reflex arc. In this example, the sensory stimulus starts in the skin and passes into the spinal cord via the dorsal root ganglion. The sensory stimulus then activates one or more interneurons, which in turn activate an LMN innervating skeletal muscle. Examples of the operation of this reflex are withdrawal of the finger from a hot surface. (Slightly modified, redrawn from Ham, A. W. [1969]. *Histology* [6th ed.]. Philadelphia: J.B. Lippincott. From Junqueira, L. C., Carneiro, J., Kelly, R. O. [1992]. *Basic histology* (7th ed.). Norwalk, CT: Appleton & Lange)

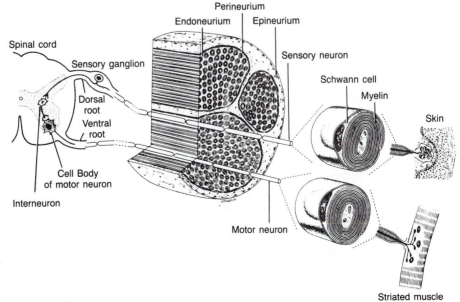

ripheral nerve processes are continuous with the connective tissue capsule of the sensory endings and the connective tissue that surrounds the effector structures, such as the skeletal muscle cell. Centrally, the connective tissue layers continue along the dorsal and ventral roots of the nerve and fuse with the meninges that surround the spinal cord and brain. The endoneurial tube does not penetrate the CNS. The absence of these tubular collagenous structures is thought to be a major factor in the less effective axonal regeneration that occurs within the CNS compared with the PNS.

The supporting cells of the CNS consist of the oligodendroglia, astroglia, microglia, and the ependymal cells. The *oligodendroglial cells* form the myelin for the CNS. Instead of forming a myelin covering for a single axon, these cells reach out with several processes, each wrapping around and forming a multi-layered myelin segment around several different axons (Fig. 47-12). The coverings of the nerve axons in the CNS also function in speeding the velocity of nerve conduction in a manner similar to that of the peripheral myelinated fibers. Myelin has a high lipid content, which gives it a whitish color; thus, the name *white matter* is given to the masses of myelinated fibers of the spinal cord and brain.

A second type of glial cell, the *astroglia*, is particularly prominent in the gray matter, or more central portion of the brain. These large cells have many processes, some reaching to the surface of the capillaries, others reaching to the surface of the nerve cells, and still others filling most of the intercellular space of the CNS (see Fig. 47-12B). The astrocytic linkage between the blood vessels and the neurons may provide a transport mechanism for the exchange of oxygen, carbon dioxide, and metabolites. They also have an important role in sequestering cations such as calcium and potassium from the intercellular fluid. The astrocytes are capable of filling their cytoplasm with microfibrils (fibrous astrocytes), and masses of these cells form the special type of scar tissue called *gliosis* that develops in the CNS when brain tissue is destroyed.

A third type of glial cell, the *microglia*, is a phagocytic cell that is available for cleaning up debris following cellular damage, infection, or cell death. The *ependymal* cells form the lining of the neural tube cavity, the ventricular system. In some areas, these cells combine with a rich vascular network to form the choroid plexus where production of the cerebrospinal fluid (CSF) takes place (see Fig. 47-12C,D).

METABOLIC REQUIREMENTS

Nervous tissue has a high need for metabolic energy. Although the brain amounts to only 2% of the body's weight, it consumes 20% of its oxygen. Despite this

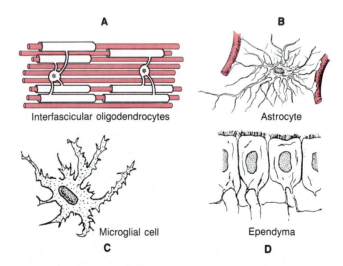

FIG. 47-12. Neuroglial cells of the central nervous system (CNS). **(A)** Oligodendrocyte providing myelin segments for several axons in the CNS. **(B)** Protoplasmic astrocyte of gray matter with prolific, long, highly branched processes that occupy most of the interneural spaces. Most of these processes end in terminal expansions on the walls of capillaries, called perivascular feet. **(C)** Microglial cell. **(D)** Cuboidal ependymal cells lining the CNS ventricles and central canal. Cilia on the apical surface move the cerebrospinal fluid (CSF) and may also secrete CSF into the ventricle. **(B, C, D,** Barr, M.L. [1988]. *The human nervous system: An anatomical viewpoint.* [5th ed., p. 28]. Philadelphia: J.B. Lippincott)

high need, the brain cannot store oxygen nor can it engage in anaerobic metabolism. An interruption in the blood or oxygen supply to the brain leads to clinically observable signs and symptoms. In the absence of oxygen, brain cells continue to function for about 10 seconds. Unconsciousness occurs almost simultaneously when cardiac arrest occurs, and the death of brain cells begins within 4 to 6 minutes. Interruption of blood flow also leads to the accumulation of metabolic by-products that are toxic to neural tissue.

Glucose is the major fuel source for the nervous system, yet the nervous system has no provisions for storing glucose. Unlike muscle cells, the nervous system has no glycogen stores and must rely on glucose from the blood or the glycogen stores of supporting glial cells. Persons receiving insulin for diabetes may experience signs of neural dysfunction and unconsciousness (insulin reaction or shock) when blood glucose drops as a result of an insulin excess (see Chapter 46).

In summary, nervous tissue is composed of two types of cells, neurons and supporting cells. Neurons are composed of three parts: a cell body, which controls cell activity; the dendrites, which conduct information toward the cell body; and the axon, which carries impulses from the cell body. The supporting cells consist of Schwann cells of the PNS and the glial cells of the CNS. The supporting cells protect and provide metabolic support for the neurons and aid in segregating them into isolated compartments, which is necessary for normal neuronal function. The function of the nervous system demands a high amount of metabolic energy. Glucose is the major fuel for the nervous system. Although the brain constitutes only 2% of body weight, it consumes 20% of its oxygen supply. In general, neurons exemplify the principle that the more specialized the function of a cell type, the less its ability to regenerate.

■ NERVE CELL COMMUNICATION

Neurons are classified as excitable tissue. This means that they are able to initiate and conduct electrical impulses. Basic to an understanding of nerve function is an appreciation of the events that occur during the excitation and initiation of an action potential in a nerve or muscle cell (see Chapter 1). The discussion in this chapter focuses on action potentials that occur in axons; many of the same types of phenomena occur in other types of excitable tissue, such as muscle.

IMPULSE GENERATION AND CONDUCTION

An impulse, or action potential, represents the lateral, or lengthwise, movement of electrical charge along the axon membrane. This phenomenon is based on the rapid flow, sometimes called *conductance*, of charged ions through the membrane in a progressive manner. In excitable tissue, ions such as sodium, potassium, chloride, and calcium carry the electrical charges that are involved in the initiation and transmission of such impulses.

During the depolarization process, the neuronal membrane becomes selectively permeable to the sodium ion, and the rapid inflow of sodium ions produces local currents that travel through the adjacent cell membrane. This, in turn, causes the sodium channels in this part of the membrane to open. These channels have a characteristic *threshold* potential. When this threshold potential is reached, gatelike structures in the membrane open widely in an all-or-none manner (see Chapter 1). Under ordinary circumstances the threshold stimulus is sufficient to open large numbers of these channels, triggering massive depolarization of the membrane—the action potential. In unmyelinated axons, the action potential depolarizes the surface ahead of itself and thus moves along the axon. Conduction in myelinated fibers follows a similar pattern, but because of the high resistance in the myelinated segments, the current flow jumps from node to node (saltatory conduction) as was described earlier. This is a more rapid process, and myelinated axons conduct up to 50 times faster than unmyelinated fibers.

SYNAPTIC TRANSMISSION

Neurons communicate with neighboring neurons or other target cells by one of two methods: ionic passage between cells (*electrical synapse*) or neurosecretion (*chemical synapse*). The function of neurons can be closely linked by opposition of their cell membranes in a *gap junction* where submicroscopic channels between the cells permit the passage of sodium and potassium ions, with the result that an action potential can pass directly and quickly from one cell to another. Gap junctions can communicate in either direction. Thus they may couple the two cells into a close functional relationship in circuits where this is required.

The more common mechanism by which neurons communicate with other neurons or target cells is the chemical synapse. These involve special presynaptic and postsynaptic membrane structures. The synaptic cleft separates the pre- and postsynaptic membranes. The presynaptic terminal secretes one, and often several, chemical messenger molecules (neurotransmitters, neuromodulators, and trophic factors) into the synaptic cleft. The most rapid acting of these neuromediators, the neurotransmitters, diffuse into and unite with receptors on the postsynaptic membrane, and this causes either excitation or inhibition of the postsynaptic neuron by producing hypopolarization or hyperpolarization of the postsynaptic membrane, respectively (Fig. 47-13). *Hyopolarization* increases the excitability of the postsynaptic neuron by bringing the membrane potential closer to threshold potential so that a smaller stimulus is needed to cause the neuron to fire. Such a synapse is termed *excitatory*. *Hyperpolarization* has the opposite effect—it decreases the likelihood that an action potential will be generated and has an *inhibitory* effect. Thus synapses fall into two main classes: excitatory or inhibitory, depending on the type of receptors that are present on the postsynaptic membrane.

Chemical synapses are the slowest component in progressive communication through a sequence of neurons such as in a spinal reflex. In contrast to the conduction of electrical action potentials, each successive event at the chemical synapse—transmitter secretion, diffusion across the synaptic cleft, and interaction with postsynaptic receptors and generation of a subsequent action potential in the postsynaptic neuron—consumes time. On the average, conduction across a chemical synapse requires approximately 0.3 milliseconds. In addition, the chemical synapse serves as a valve, permitting only one-way communication.

A neuron's cell body and dendrites are covered by thousands of synapses, any or many of which can be active at any moment in time. Because of this rich synaptic capability, each neuron resembles a little integrator in which there are many circuits of neurons that interact with one another. It is the complexity of these interactions that gives the system its intelligence in terms of the subtle integrations involved in producing behavioral responses, and that makes the prediction of stimulus–response relationships somewhat hazardous in the absence of a millisecond-to-millisecond knowledge of the excitatory and inhibitory activity that takes place on the surfaces of each neuron in a functional circuit. With billions of these little integrators capable of becoming involved in such a response, it is amazing that predictions are possible at all. It is even more astounding that the basic microcircuitry involved in the nervous system is reproduced reliably during the development of each new organism.

There are several types of synapses. Axonic terminals of an afferent neuron can develop in close apposition to the dendrites (*axodendritic synapse*), to the cell body (*axosomatic synapse*), or to the axon (*axoaxonic synapse*) of a CNS neuron. The mechanism of communication between the *presynaptic* axonic terminal and the *postsynaptic* neuron is similar in all three types of synapses. In all three, the action potential sweeps into the axonic terminals of the afferent neuron and triggers rapid secretion of neurotransmitter molecules from the axonic, or presynaptic, surface. Conversion of action potentials into secretion is called *coupling*, and, although it is not completely understood, it is believed that the release of calcium ions is involved.

Many CNS neurons possess thousands of synapses on their dendritic or somatic surfaces. The combination of the neurotransmitter with the receptor sites can produce either excitation or inhibition. When the combination of a neurotransmitter with a receptor site causes partial depolarization of the postsynaptic membrane, it is called an *excitatory postsynaptic potential* (*EPSP*). In other synapses, the combination of a transmitter with a receptor site is inhibitory in the sense that the combination of the transmitter with the receptor site causes the local nerve membrane to become hyperpolarized and less excitable. Then it is called an *inhibitory postsynaptic potential* (*IPSP*).

An action potential does not begin in the membrane adjacent to the synapse. Instead it begins in the *initial segment* of the axon, just before the first myelin segment, at which point the axon is more excitable than the rest of the neuron. The local currents resulting from any one EPSP (sometimes called a *generator potential*) are usually insufficient to pass threshold and cause depolarization of the axon's initial segment. However, if several EPSPs occur simultaneously, the area of depolarization can become large enough and the currents at the initial segment can become strong enough to exceed the threshold potential and initiate a conducted action potential. This summation of depolarized areas is called *spatial summation*. The EPSPs can also summate and cause

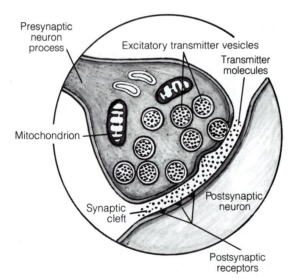

FIG. 47-13. Synapse, showing the pre- and postsynaptic neuronal surface. (Chaffee, E. E., & Lytle, I. M. [1980]. *Basic physiology and anatomy* [4th ed.]. Philadelphia: J.B. Lippincott)

Presynaptic neuron process

Excitatory transmitter vesicles

Transmitter molecules

Mitochondrion

Synaptic cleft

Postsynaptic neuron

Postsynaptic receptors

an action potential if they come in close temporal (time) relation to one another. This temporal aspect of the occurrence of two or more EPSPs is called *temporal summation*.

IPSPs can also undergo spatial and temporal summation with each other and with EPSPs, reducing the effectiveness of the latter by a roughly algebraic summation. If the sum of EPSPs and IPSPs keeps the depolarization at the initial segment below threshold levels, the generation of an action potential does not occur.

The spatial and temporal summation required in the distribution and timing of synaptic activity serves as a sensitive and very complicated switch requiring just the right combination of incoming activity before the cell releases its own message in the form of the action potential. The frequency of action potentials in the axon, on the other hand, is an all-or-none language (digital language), which can vary only as to the presence or absence of such impulses and their frequency. Action potentials permit rapid communication over distances, but it is the rich capacity for integration of excitatory and inhibitory synaptic bombardment of the soma and dendrites that gives the neuron, and thus the nervous system, the capability for complexity, memory, and intelligence.

MESSENGER MOLECULES

Neurotransmitters are the chemical messenger molecules of the nervous system. The process of neurotransmission involves the synthesis, storage, and release of a neurotransmitter; the reaction of the neurotransmitter with a receptor; and termination of the receptor action. The recent development of new research methods, including staining techniques and the use of radiolabeled antibodies, has allowed scientists to study and gain answers in each of these areas.

Both the nervous system and the endocrine system use chemicals as messengers. As more information is obtained about the chemical messengers of both systems, the distinction between the nervous system and the endocrine system becomes somewhat blurred. Many neurons, such as those in the adrenal medulla, secrete transmitters that are released into the bloodstream, and it has been found that other neurons possess receptor sites for hormones. On the other hand, many hormones have turned out to be neurotransmitters. Vasopressin, a peptide hormone that is released from the posterior pituitary gland, is also a neurotransmitter for nerve cells in the hypothalamus. Today, more than a dozen of these cell-to-cell messengers are known to be capable of relaying signals in either the nervous system or the endocrine system.[4]

Neurotransmitters usually are synthesized in the cytoplasm of the axon terminal. The synthesis of transmitters may require one or more enzyme-catalyzed steps (one for acetylcholine and three for norepinephrine). The various types of neurons are limited in terms of the type of transmitter they can synthesize by their enzyme systems. The suffix *-ergic* and the name of the transmitter produced is often used to classify neurons. Accordingly, a dopaminergic neuron is one that produces dopamine. After synthesis, the transmitter molecules are stored in the axon terminal in tiny membrane-bound sacs called *synaptic vesicles*. There may be thousands of vesicles in a single terminal, each containing 10,000 to 100,000 molecules of transmitter. The vesicle protects transmitters from enzyme destruction within the nerve terminal.

The arrival of an impulse at a nerve terminal causes a large number of transmitter molecules to be released into the synaptic space. Neurotransmitters exert their actions through specific proteins, called *receptors*, embedded in the postsynaptic membrane. These receptors are tailored precisely to match the size and shape of the transmitter. In each case, the interaction between a transmitter and receptor results in a specific physiologic response. The action of a transmitter is determined by the type of receptor to which it binds. For example, acetylcholine is excitatory when it is released at a myoneural junction and inhibitory when it is released at the sinoatrial node in the heart. Receptors are named according to the type of neurotransmitter with which they interact. For example, the term *cholinergic receptor* is used to indicate a receptor that binds acetylcholine. Some neurotransmitters act as modulators of neural action rather than initiators.

Rapid removal of a transmitter, once it has exerted its effects on the postsynaptic membrane, is necessary to maintain precise control of neural transmission. A transmitter that has been released can undergo one of three fates. It can be broken down into inactive substances by enzymes, it can be taken back up into the presynaptic neuron in a process called *reuptake*, or it can diffuse away into the intercellular fluid until its concentration is too low to influence postsynaptic excitability. Acetylcholine, for example, is rapidly broken down by acetylcholinesterase into acetic acid and choline, with the choline being taken back into the presynaptic neuron for reuse in acetylcholine synthesis. The catecholamines, on the other hand, are largely taken back into the neuron in an unchanged form for reuse. The catecholamines can also be degraded by enzymes in the synaptic space or by enzymes that are present in the nerve terminals.

Neurotransmitters tend to be small molecules

that incorporate a positively charged nitrogen atom; they include amino acids, peptides, and monoamines. Amino acids are the building blocks of proteins and are present in body fluids. Peptides are low-molecular molecules that yield two or more amino acids on hydrolysis. They include substance P, vasopressin, endorphins, and the enkephalins. Monoamines are an amine molecule containing one amino group (NH_2). Serotonin, dopamine, norepinephrine, and epinephrine are monoamines that are synthesized from amino acids. Fortunately, the nervous system is protected by the blood–brain barrier from circulating amino acids and other molecules that could act in an unregulated manner as neurotransmitters (see Chapter 51).

There is still much to be learned about the role of certain amino acids and peptides as neurotransmitters. For example, several amino acids (glutamic acid and aspartic acid) appear to exert powerful excitatory effects on synaptic transmission. Glycine, another amino acid, is known to have strong inhibitory effects. One of the most common inhibitory transmitters is gamma-aminobutyric acid (GABA). This amino acid is unique in that it is synthesized almost exclusively in the brain and spinal cord. It has been established that almost one-third of all synapses use GABA.[4] With the inclusion of amino acids as neurotransmitters comes the puzzling aspect that the same amino acid can function as both a neurotransmitter and a building block for protein synthesis.

It was not until the mid 1970s that it became known that peptides could act as neurotransmitters.[5] Some of the newest and most exciting of the neuropeptides are the endorphins, enkephalins, and substance P, which appear to be involved in pain sensation. The endorphins and enkephalins, which have been described as the body's own morphine, undoubtedly contribute to a decrease in pain perception and a feeling of well-being (see Chapter 48). Substance P, a chain of 11 amino acids, is present in a number of neuronal pathways in the brain and primary sensory fibers in the PNS. Because it excites spinal neurons that respond to painful stimuli, it has been suggested that substance P is involved in transmitting painful information from the periphery to the CNS.[6]

The actions of most neurotransmitters are localized in specific clusters of neurons with axons that project to highly specific brain regions. As more is learned about the locations and mechanisms of action of the various neurotransmitters, it becomes increasingly apparent that many disease conditions have their origin in altered neurotransmitter responses. In some cases, there is evidence of degeneration or dysfunction of the neurons producing the neurotransmitters; in others, there is an apparent alteration in the postsynaptic response to the neurotransmitter. For example, the neurons containing dopamine are concentrated in regions of the midbrain known as the *substantia nigra* and *ventral tegmentum*. Many of these dopamine-containing neurons project their axons to areas of the forebrain that are thought to be involved in regulation of emotional behavior. Other dopamine fibers terminate in regions near the middle of the brain called the *corpus striatum*; these fibers seem to play an essential role in the performance of complex motor movements. Degeneration of the dopamine fibers in this area of the brain leads to the tremor and rigidity that are characteristic of Parkinson's disease. Some forms of mental illness, such as schizophrenia, are thought to involve abnormal release or responses to neurotransmitters in the brain. Pharmacologic methods of supplying neurotransmitters (as in Parkinson's disease) or modifying their actions (as in the case of psychoactive drugs) are used to treat some of these disorders. Undoubtedly, more specific treatment methods will become available as more is learned about the transmission of neural information.

Other classes of messenger molecules are often secreted by axon terminals in addition to or instead of neurotransmitters. Neuromodulator molecules apparently react with postsynaptic receptors to produce slower and longer-lasting changes in membrane excitability. This has the effect of making the action of the faster-acting neurotransmitter molecules more or less effective. Some of the peptide molecules may fall into the modulator category. Neurohumoral mediators reach the target cell through the blood stream and produce an even slower action than the neuromodulators. Neurotrophic factors are required to maintain the long-term survival of the postsynaptic cell and are secreted by axon terminals independent of an action potential. Examples include LMN-to-muscle cell trophic factors and neuron-to-neuron trophic factors in sequential chains of CNS sensory systems. Trophic factors from the target cell that can enter the axon terminal and are essential to the long-term survival of the presynaptic neuron have also been demonstrated. Target cell-to-neuron trophic factors probably have great significance in establishment of specific neural connections during normal embryonic development.

In summary, neurons, which are able to generate and conduct impulses, are classified as excitable tissue. Neurotransmitters are chemical messengers that serve to control neural function; they selectively cause either excitation or inhibition of action potentials. A synapse is a one-way communication link between neurons; it has both presynaptic and postsynaptic components. Neurotransmitters released from the presynaptic terminals of one neuron diffuse across the synaptic cleft and unite with receptors in the postsynaptic surface of another neuron as a means of communicating information between the two neurons. Thus, a neuron integrates ongoing synaptic activity, resulting in the production or nonproduction of an action potential. Once initiated, an action potential travels rapidly along the cell's axon to trigger transmitter release for synaptic communication with the next neuron in the circuit. This combination of integration of excitatory and inhibitory synaptic activity and rapid communication of impulses permits the complex functioning that is characteristic of the nervous system. Axon terminals often secrete other messenger molecules in addition to or instead of neurotransmitters. These have slower and longer-lasting postsynaptic effects and include neuromodulators, neurohormones, and neurotrophic factors. Target cells also secrete trophic factors required for the long-term survival of the innervating neuron.

■ REFERENCES

1. Milunsky, A., Ulcickas, M., Rothman, K.J., et al. (1992). Maternal heat exposure and neural tube defects. *Journal of the American Medical Association, 268*, 882–885.
2. Palca, J. (1992). Folic acid: Agencies split on nutrition advice. *Science, 257*, 1857.
3. National Institutes of Health, National Institute on Communicative Disorders and Stroke. (1979). *Report on convulsive and neuromuscular disorders to the National Advisory Neurological and Communicative Disorders and Stroke Council* (p. 103). Washington, DC: US Department of Health, Education, and Welfare, Public Health Service, NIH Publication No. 79–1913.
4. Bloom, F.E. (1981). Neuropeptides. *Scientific American, 245*(10), 148.
5. Iverson, L.L. (1979). The chemistry of the brain. *Scientific American, 241*(9), 134.
6. Snyder, S.H. (1985). The molecular basis for communication between cells. *Scientific American, 253*(4), 132.

■ BIBLIOGRAPHY

Aoki, C., & Siekevitz, P. (1988). Plasticity in brain development. *Scientific American, 259*(6), 56.

FitzGerald, M.J.T. (1985). *Neuroanatomy: Basic and applied.* Philadelphia: Bailliere Tindall.

Ganong, W.F. (1991). *Review of medical physiology* (15th ed.). Norwalk, CT: Appleton & Lange.

Junqueira, L.C., Carniro, J., & Long, J.A. (1986). *Basic histology* (5th ed., Chaps. 9, 10). Los Altos, CA: Lange.

Kalil, R.E. (1989). Synapse formation in the developing brain. *Scientific American, 261*(6), 76.

Kimelberg, H.K., & Norenberg, M.D. (1989). Astrocytes. *Scientific American, 260*(4), 66.

Moore, K.L. (1982). *The developing human* (3rd ed., Chap. 18). Philadelphia: W.B. Saunders.

Sadler, T.W. (1991). *Langman's medical embryology* (6th ed., Chap. 20). Baltimore: Williams & Wilkins.

Shatz, C.J. (1992). The developing brain. *Scientific American, 267*(3), 60.

Stevens, S. (1979). The neuron. *Scientific American, 241*(9), 54.

Telford, I.R., & Bridgeman, C.F. (1990). *Introduction to functional histology* (Chaps. 11, 12). New York: Harper & Row.

Wurtman, R.J. (1982). Nutrients that modify brain behavior. *Scientific American, 246*(4), 50.

CHAPTER 48

SOMATOSENSORY FUNCTION AND PAIN

SHEILA M. CURTIS
ROBIN L. CURTIS

■ OBJECTIVES

After you have studied this chapter, you should be able to meet the following objectives:

■ Name the three somatosensory modalities.

■ Define *proprioception* and *kinesthesia*.

■ Trace the pathway of an impulse that originates in a somatosensory receptor.

■ State the significance of the dermatomes in a neurologic examination.

■ Contrast the role of rapid-adapting and slow-adapting afferents in maintaining posture.

■ Compare the discriminative pathway with the anterolateral pathway, and explain the clinical usefulness of this distinction.

■ Describe the sensory homunculus in the cerebral cortex.

■ Differentiate between the specificity and pattern theories of pain.

■ Explain the gate control theory of pain.

■ Describe the function of nociceptors in response to pain information.

■ State the difference between the A-delta and C-fiber neurons in the transmission of pain information.

■ Trace the transmission of pain signals with reference to the neospinothalamic, paleospinothalamic, and reticulospinal pathways.

■ Describe the function of endogenous analgesic mechanisms as they relate to transmission of pain information.

■ Differentiate acute pain from chronic pain.

■ Describe the mechanisms of referred pain, and list the common sites of referral for cardiac and other types of visceral pain.

■ Compare pain threshold and pain tolerance.

■ Cite common physiologic manifestations of pain.

■ State how the pain response may differ in children and elderly people.

Carol Mattson Porth: PATHOPHYSIOLOGY: CONCEPTS OF ALTERED HEALTH STATES, 4th ed. © 1994, 1990, 1986, 1982 J.B. Lippincott Company

■ Define *hypesthesia, hyperesthesia, hyperalgesia, dysesthesia, paresthesias, anesthesia, hyperpathia, analgesia,* and *hypoalgesia.*

■ Describe three methods for assessing pain.

■ State the mechanisms whereby nonnarcotic and narcotic analgesic, tricyclic antidepressant, and anticonvulsive drugs relieve pain.

■ Describe the proposed mechanisms of pain relief associated with the use of heat, cold, and transcutaneous electrical nerve stimulation.

■ Compare the methods used in acupuncture and acupressure.

■ Explain the advantage of intravenously versus intramuscularly administered opioid drugs for relief of pain in children.

■ Differentiate between the causes of tension-type headaches and migraine headaches and their treatments.

■ Cite the most common cause of temporomandibular joint pain.

■ Describe the cause and characteristics of trigeminal neuralgia and postherpetic neuralgia.

■ Cite a possible mechanism of phantom limb pain.

Sensory mechanisms provide a continuous stream of information about the seeming realities of the person, the outside world, and the interactions between the two. The term *somesthesia* (body + sensation) describes a person's awareness of his or her body. The somatosensory component of the nervous system provides an awareness of body sensations such as touch, temperature, and limb position, which are different from the special senses such as vision, hearing, smell, and taste. This chapter is divided into two parts: the first describes the organization and control of somatosensory function and the second focuses on pain as a somatosensory modality.

■ ORGANIZATION AND CONTROL OF SOMATOSENSORY FUNCTION

Somatosensory experience can be divided into *modalities*, a term used for qualitative, subjective distinctions between sensations such as *touch, heat,* and *pain.* Such experiences require the function of both sensory receptors and forebrain structures in the thalamus and cerebral cortex. The sensory receptors for somatosensory function consist of discrete nerve endings in the skin and other body tissues. Between 2 and 3 million sensory neurons deliver a steady stream of encoded action potentials that represent the status of their sensory endings. Only a small proportion of this information reaches awareness; most provides input essential for a myriad of reflex and automatic mechanisms that keep us alive and manage our functioning.

Somesthesia can be subdivided with reference to the location of the sensory nerve endings. Cutaneous modalities include touch (tactile) and the more complex sensations of itch and tickle; temperature (warm to hot and cool to cold); and pain, including the bright, sharp type and the dull, stinging, burning, aching type. In deeper structures of the body wall

and the limbs, afferent nerve endings supply the deep connective tissues, joint capsules, ligaments, muscles, tendons, periosteum of bone, and blood vessel walls. Some of these sensory endings provide the basis for the coordination of movement and contribute to the experience of body, head, and limb position (*proprioception*) and movement (*kinesthesia*). When stimulated at a frequency high enough to be associated with tissue damage, these afferents also send a message that is interpreted as pain.

SOMESTHETIC INNERVATION PATTERNS

The somesthetic innervation of the body, including the head, retains a basic segmental organizational pattern that was established during embryonic development. Thirty-three spinal (segmental) nerves provide sensory and motor innervation of the body wall, the limbs, and the viscera (see Chapter 47). Sensory input to each spinal cord segment is provided by afferent sensory neurons with cell bodies in the dorsal root ganglia. A *sensory unit* consists of a dorsal root ganglion neuron, its peripheral branch innervating a small region of the periphery, and its central axon, which synapses with a dorsal horn association neuron. The many distal endings of the peripheral branch are receptive endings, tuned to specific forms of physical or chemical energy. Less commonly, the peripheral branch terminals innervate specialized receptor cells that are themselves sensitive to specific physical (*e.g.,* baroreceptors) or chemical (*e.g.,* chemoreceptors) agents. The peripheral branches of the general soma afferent (GSA) neurons divide repeatedly as they supply the skin, fascial sheets, muscles, tendons, joint capsules, periosteum, marrow cavities, and parietal lining of the body cavities. Action potentials that originate from any of the numerous receptive endings of an afferent neuron are conducted toward and into the central nervous system (CNS) through the peripheral branch, dorsal root, and central axon into the spinal cord association cell columns. The afferent neuron, in a sense, cannot distinguish among information coming from its various peripheral terminals. If the applied stimulus results in an action potential in any terminal branch, the impulse is transmitted to the dorsal horn association cells in the CNS.

PERIPHERAL DISTRIBUTION OF THE GENERAL SOMA AFFERENT NEURONS (DERMATOMES)

Each segment of the body, with few exceptions, contains a pair of dorsal root ganglia. The general soma afferent neurons that innervate the body wall, or soma, of that segment are located within these gan-

glia. Between 30,000 and 50,000 afferent neuron cell bodies reside in each of the paired dorsal root ganglia of each segment; their central axons project to the corresponding spinal segment through the dorsal roots.[1] The segmental innervation of head segments follows the same pattern by means of cranial nerves.

The region of the body wall that is supplied by a single pair of dorsal root ganglia is called a *dermatome*. These dorsal root ganglion–innervated strips occur in a regular sequence moving upward from the second coccygeal segment through the cervical segments, reflecting the basic segmental organization of the body and the nervous system (Fig. 48-1). Neighboring dermatomes overlap one another sufficiently that a loss of one dorsal root or root ganglion results in reduced but not total loss of sensory innervation of a dermatome. Maps have been prepared that are helpful in detecting the level and extent of sensory defects resulting from segmental nerve and spinal cord damage.

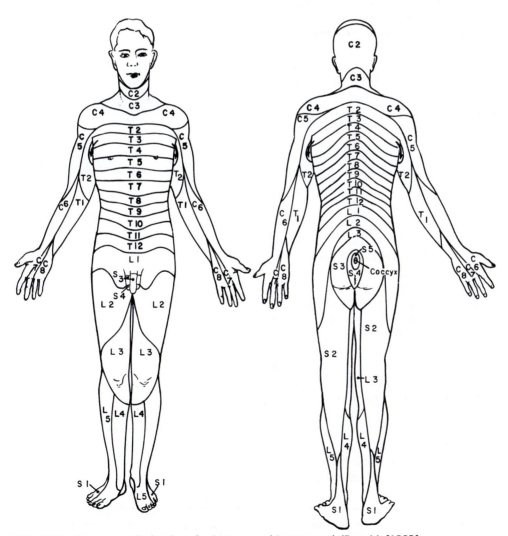

FIG. 48-1. Cutaneous distribution of spinal nerves (dermatomes). (Barr, M. [1993]. *The human nervous system.* New York: Harper & Row.)

In the peripheral nervous system, fusion between neighboring spinal nerves results in an overlapping of sensory innervation from neighboring dermatomes. This overlapping system provides a built-in protection, so that damage to one or two adjacent dorsal roots does not result in a complete loss of sensory input from those segments. Partial loss of sensory innervation results in reduced discrete localization within a sensory field.

CENTRAL DISTRIBUTION OF SENSORY INPUT

Sensory systems are organized as a serial succession of neurons consisting of (1) first-order (primary) afferent neurons, which transmit sensory information from the periphery; (2) second-order (secondary) CNS association neurons, which communicate with various reflex networks and sensory pathways that travel directly to the thalamus; and (3) third-order (tertiary) neurons, which relay information from the thalamus to the cerebral cortex.[2] Many interneurons process and modify the sensory information at the level of the second- and third-order neurons, and myriads more participate before coordinated and appropriate learned-movement responses occur. The number of participating neurons increases exponentially from the primary through the secondary and the secondary through the tertiary levels. By providing multiple parallel projections along with mechanisms for filtering, amplifying, and modulating information, this expansion of the number of participating neurons serves as a safety feature.

FIRST-ORDER NEURONS

Sensory input from primary neuron receptors is distributed to one or more dorsal horn input association cell columns, each of which has a characteristic pattern of central projection. For instance, afferent neuron axons relaying light touch information project to the general somatic input association (GSIA) neuron column (see Chapter 47). Afferent axons conveying muscle or tendon stretch information project to both the GSIA and a special association column that relays to the cerebellum, the special somatic input association (SSIA) column. The function of these input association column neurons is to relay afferent signals to (1) local reflex circuits, providing rapid, lower motoneuron responses; (2) more rostral parts of the reflex hierarchy, permitting more complex, organized response patterns; (3) the reticular activating system, contributing to general wakefulness of forebrain systems; and (4) the thalamus, where sensation and perceptive functions begin.

SECOND-ORDER NEURONS

One function of the second-order association cells is to relay afferent information into reflex circuits. If a skin receptor on the finger, which responds to increased temperature, is stimulated by skin contact with a hot object, a series of events takes place (Fig. 48-2). First, the heat produces local changes in the receptors that are converted to action potentials. The action potentials are then transmitted through the peripheral nerve to the cell body in the dorsal root ganglion and from there through its axon into the spinal cord segment. In the spinal cord segment, association neurons can trigger an action potential in a lower motoneuron, resulting in skeletal muscle contraction and movement of the skin surface away from the stimulus. This protective reflex is called the *withdrawal reflex*.

General somesthetic input association (GSIA) column neurons of the dorsal horn distribute the afferent signals to different reflex circuits: pain and temperature to the withdrawal circuit and deep pressure to a stepping reflex circuit. All the somesthetic input signals are projected by other association neurons to higher levels of the nervous system as necessary input for more complex reflex patterns. The same information that triggered the spinal cord withdrawal reflex is projected by spinoreticular fibers to other reflexes at the brain stem level, where the circuitry for catching the breath, a sudden rise in heart rate, and other responses such as vocalization occur. At a higher level of control, for instance, projections of the spinoreticular fibers to midbrain circuits allow the regaining of position when balance is lost. This illustrates the concept of the *hierarchy of reflexes* in which the same afferent information contributes to more and more complex reaction patterns, each at a progressively more rostral location in the CNS that controls the various components organized at lower levels.

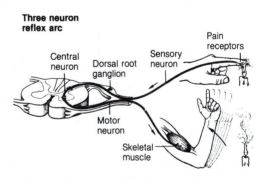

FIG. 48-2. Withdrawal reflex. (Adapted from Chaffee, E E., & Lytle, I. M. [1980]. *Basic physiology and anatomy* [4th ed., p. 240]. Philadelphia: J.B. Lippincott.)

THIRD-ORDER NEURONS

Some second-order neurons project across the midline of the CNS and ascend to the forebrain to innervate the thalamus. The third-order neurons of the somesthetic system are the thalamic nuclei. Input to the contralateral thalamus (*i.e.*, on the side opposite the stimuli) can be distributed to the lateral or intermediate nuclei. The lateral nuclei project to the sensory cortex where meaning and the perceptive aspects of somesthetic experience are integrated. The intermediate nuclei project to the limbic system where many of the emotional aspects of sensation are mediated. The intermediate nuclei are also capable of contributing a crude, poorly localizable sensation from the opposite side of the body. For instance, the thalamus, in the absence of the cortex, provides an awareness of pain, but it has no meaning.

STIMULUS DISCRIMINATION

Discrimination of the location of a somesthetic stimulus is called *acuity* and is based on the sensory field within a dermatome innervated by an afferent neuron. High acuity (*i.e.*, the ability to make fine discriminations of location) requires a high density of innervation by afferent neurons. For example, acuity is high on the thumb, but lower on the back of the hand. High acuity also requires a projection system through the nervous system to the forebrain that preserves distinctions between activity in neighboring sensory fields.

Receptors or receptive endings of primary afferent neurons differ as to the intensity at which they begin to fire. This afferent threshold usually is lower than the stimulus threshold required for first brain-level subjective sensation threshold. For instance, when a single hair on the back of the hand is bent more and more, some bending occurs before action potentials appear in the primary (tactile) sensory neuron (afferent threshold). The hair must be bent further and the sensory action potentials must increase in frequency before a person is able to reliably detect the bending of the hair (subjective sensation threshold). For highly developed discriminative systems, under ideal conditions, these thresholds may correspond closely. Many factors, such as attention and emotion, can greatly elevate the subjective threshold. Once the subjective threshold is reached, the intensity of the experienced sensation is based on the rate of impulse generation in the afferent neuron, such that gradations in stimulus intensity are discriminated proportional to the logarithm of stimulus strength. This means that once the subjective threshold has been reached, greater changes in stimulus strength are needed for discrimination. This is known as the *Weber-Fechner principle*. For example, once the subjective threshold has been reached, a person could have difficulty detecting a 1-g increase in weight when holding 30 g or a 10-g increase in weight when holding 300 g (in each case, the ratio of change [logarithm] remains about 1 to 30).[3] This relationship holds true for all sensory systems, including the somesthetic system, and is based on characteristics of the receptor endings.

Some afferent neurons maintain a more or less steady rate of firing to a continuous stimulus. This is true for afferents from muscles, tendons, and joints, where continuous feedback information is necessary for maintaining posture. These slow-adapting afferent neurons contrast with rapid-adapting afferent neurons, which signal only the onset, sudden change, and conclusion of a stimulus. Rapid-adapting afferent neurons are required to signal moving, brief, or vibrating stimuli.

SENSORY MODALITY

The qualitative aspects of different types of stimuli are based on the differential sensitivity of primary sensory neuron peripheral terminals to different forms of physical and chemical energy. Receptive endings of different afferent neurons are particularly sensitive to a specific form of energy. They can initiate action potentials to many forms of energy at high energy levels, but they usually are especially "tuned" or differentially sensitive to low levels of a particular energy class. For instance, a receptive ending may be particularly sensitive to a small increase in local skin temperature. Stimulating the ending with electric current or strong pressure can also result in action potentials. The amount of energy required, however, is much less for temperature change. Increases in the action potential rate in the "warm" afferent, when the information reaches the thalamus and cerebral cortex, is experienced as the sensation "warm" and at higher levels of action potentials as "hot." Other afferent sensory terminals are most sensitive to slight indentations of the skin, and their signals are subjectively interpreted as "touch." Cool versus warm, sharp versus dull pain, delicate touch versus deep pressure, and joint movement versus joint position are all based on different populations of afferent neurons or on central integration of simultaneous input from several differently tuned afferents. For example, the sensation of itch results from a combination of high activity in pain- and touch-sensitive afferents, and the sensation of tickle requires a gentle moving tactile stimulus over cool skin.

When this tuned aspect of different primary afferents reaches the forebrain and subjective experience, the qualitative differences between warm and touch are called *sensory modalities*. These are based on the separate relays of primary, secondary, and tertiary neurons of the receptor-detected information to the thalamus and cortex. But the experience of a modality, such as cold versus warm, is uniquely subjective. The projection pathways for modalities differ considerably in (1) the location of secondary and tertiary neurons and (2) the precision with which the sensory information is transmitted to the forebrain.

ASCENDING PATHWAYS

Different somesthetic afferents transmit signals related to delicate vibratory or fine tactile stimuli. Other afferents transmit signals from less sensitive pain or temperature receptors. For all classes of somesthetic afferents, the input association cell columns in the dorsal horn of the spinal cord are the source of secondary or association axons that project through spinoreticular tract systems to the reticular activating system of the brain stem. The spinoreticular projections provide the basis for increased wakefulness or awareness after strong somatesthetic stimulation and for the generalized startle reaction that occurs with sudden and intense somesthetic stimuli. The responses of the reticular activating system include postural as well as autonomic nervous system responses, such as a rise in blood pressure and heart rate, dilation of the pupils, and the pale, moist skin that results from constriction of the cutaneous blood vessels and activation of sweat glands. In addition, the sensory association cell columns relay afferent information to the forebrain, where sensation and perception occur.

The somesthetic cell columns also send afferent information to the forebrain of the opposite (contralateral) side, where sensation and perception occur. Two parallel pathways, the *dorsal column discriminative* and the *anterolateral (spinothalamic)* pathways, reach the thalamic level of sensation, each taking a different route through the CNS. These pathways differ in the location of the secondary GSIA nucleus neurons and in the level of the CNS at which the information is projected across the midline to the contralateral thalamus and cortex. The discriminative pathway provides for rapid transmission of information relating fine touch and pressure, vibration, and position sense. The anterolateral system provides for slower transmission of pain, thermal sensations, crude touch and pressure, and tickle and itch sensations.

DISCRIMINATIVE PATHWAY

The rapid-transmission discriminative pathway to the thalamus and cerebral cortex involves branches of

primary afferent axons that travel up the ipsilateral dorsal columns of the spinal cord white matter and synapse with highly evolved somesthetic input association neurons in the medulla. Second-order neurons provide a further large-diameter projection through the brain stem without collateral branches (Fig. 48-3). This discriminative pathway transmits accurate localization and delicate intensity discriminative information to the opposite side of the brain. There, third-order neurons relay information to the primary somesthetic cerebral cortex. Sensory information arriving at the thalamus by this route is discretely localizable and delicately analyzable in terms of intensity grades. This pathway is highly dependent on parietal cortical function and has little projection into the intermediate thalamic nuclei. This is the only pathway taken by sensations of joint movement (kinesthesia), body position (proprioception), vibration, and delicate, discriminative touch, such as is required to differentiate correctly between touching skin at two neighboring points (two-point discrimination) versus only at one point.

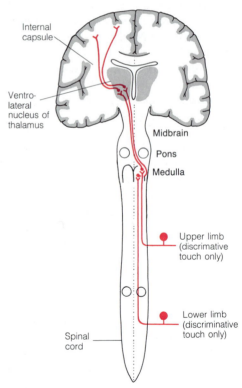

FIG. 48-3. Discriminative pathway. This pathway is an ascending system for rapid transmission of sensations that relate joint movement (kinesthesis), body position (proprioception), vibration, and delicate touch. Primary afferents travel up the dorsal columns of the spinal cord white matter and synapse with somesthetic input association neurons in the medulla. Secondary neurons project through the brain stem to the thalamus and synapse with tertiary neurons, which relay the information to the primary somesthetic cortex on the opposite side of the brain.

The discriminative pathway uses only three neurons to transmit information from a sensory receptor to the somesthetic strip of parietal cerebral cortex of the opposite side: (1) the primary sensory neuron that projects its central axon to the dorsal column nuclei; (2) the dorsal column neuron that sends its axon through a rapid conducting tract, the *medial lemniscus*, that crosses at the base of the medulla and travels to the thalamus on the opposite side of the brain where basic sensation begins; and (3) the thalamic neuron that projects its axon to the primary sensory cortex, site of discriminative sensation.

SOMATOSENSORY CORTEX

The somatosensory cortex is located in the parietal lobe, which lies behind the central sulcus and above the lateral sulcus (Fig. 48-4). The strip of parietal cortex that borders the central sulcus is called the *primary sensory cortex* because it receives primary sensory information by way of direct projections from the lateral nuclei of the thalamus. A distorted map of the body and head surface, called a *homunculus*, reflects the density of cortical neurons devoted to sensory input from afferents in corresponding periphery areas. As depicted in Figure 48-5, much more cortical surface is devoted to areas of the body such as the thumb, forefinger, lips, and tongue, where fine touch and pressure are essential for function. The cortical area devoted to body surface area correlates with the density of afferent innervation in that area.

Parallel to and just behind the primary somatosensory cortex (toward the occipital cortex) lie the parietal association areas, which are required to transform the raw material of sensation into meaningful learned perception. Most of the *perceptive* aspects of body sensation, or somesthesia, require the function of this parietal association cortex. Thalamic association nuclei are also involved. The perceptive aspect, or meaningfulness, of a stimulus pattern in-

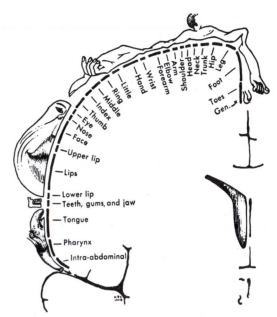

FIG. 48-5. Homunculus, as determined by stimulation studies on the human cortex during surgery. (Penfield, E., & Rasmussen, T. [1955]. *The cerebral cortex of man.* New York: Macmillan. Copyright © by Macmillan Publishing Co., Inc., renewed 1978 by Theodore Rasmussen)

volves the integration of present sensation with past learning. For instance, your past learning plus present tactile sensation give you the perception of sitting on a soft chair rather than on a hard bicycle seat. One of the important functions of the discriminative pathway is to integrate the input from multiple receptors. The sense of shape and size of an object in the absence of visualization, called *stereognosis*, is based on precise afferent information from muscle, tendon, and joint receptors. A screwdriver has a different shape from a knife, not only in the texture of its parts (tactile sensibility) but also in its shape based on the relative position of the fingers as they are moved over the object (proprioception). This complex, interpretive perception requires not only that the discriminative system must be functioning optimally but also that higher-order parietal association cortex processing and prior learning must have occurred.

If the discriminative somesthetic pathway is functional but the parietal associational cortex has become discretely damaged, the person can correctly describe the object but does not recognize that it is indeed a screwdriver. This deficit is called *astereognosis*. If the somesthetic but not the parietal association cortex is irritated by a growing tumor or meningeal scar tissue, hallucinations of a "strange tingling sensation" or of "something moving over the skin" are experienced. These usually are unpleasant and without meaning. This abnormal neural firing may cause an "aura" (sensory seizure), which can then progress to a generalized tonic-clonic seizure.

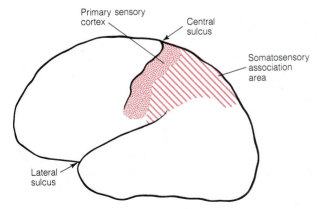

FIG. 48-4. Primary somatosensory and association somatosensory cortex.

Cortical lesions from cerebrovascular accidents or growing tumors usually destroy large areas, affecting both the somatosensory and the parietal association cortex. Damage to the somatosensory cortex on the nondominant (usually right) side of the brain can produce a condition called the *hemi-inattention syndrome* in which the entire left side of the body is ignored as if it does not exist as part of the self (see Chapter 51). This syndrome is less evident after lesions of the same region on the dominant side.

ANTEROLATERAL PATHWAY

The anterolateral, or spinothalamic, pathway consists of bilateral multisynaptic slow-conducting tracts that transmit sensory signals that do not require discrete localization of signal source or discrimination of fine gradations in intensity (Fig. 48-6). This slow-conducting system is also called the *paleospinothalamic tract*, indicating that it is phylogenetically older than

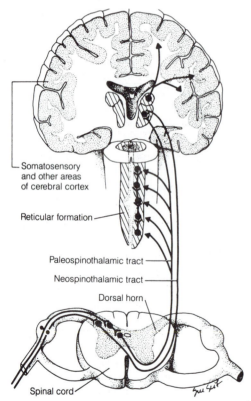

FIG. 48-6. Neospinothalamic and paleospinothalamic subdivisions of the anterolateral sensory pathway. The neospinothalamic tract runs to the thalamic nuclei and has fibers that project to the somatosensory cortex. The paleospinothalamic tract sends collaterals to the reticular formation and other structures, from which further fibers project to the thalamus. These fibers influence the hypothalamus and the limbic system as well as the cerebral cortex. (Rodman, M. J., & Smith, D. W. [1979]. *Pharmacology and drug therapy in nursing* [2nd ed., p. 263]. Philadelphia: J.B. Lippincott.)

Labels in figure:
Somatosensory and other areas of cerebral cortex
Reticular formation
Paleospinothalamic tract
Neospinothalamic tract
Dorsal horn
Spinal cord

the neospinothalamic discriminative system. The anterolateral fibers originate in the dorsal horns where the dorsal root neurons enter the spinal cord; they cross in the anterior commissure, within the few segments of origin, to the opposite anterolateral white column where they ascend upward toward the brain. The anterolateral system carries the sensations of crude touch, temperature, and pain.

The anterolateral pathway also projects into the intermediate nuclei of the thalamus, which have close connections with the limbic cortical systems. This circuitry that gives touch its affective or emotional aspects (*e.g.*, the particular unpleasantness of heavy pressure and the peculiar pleasantness of the tickling and gentle rubbing of the skin). The anterolateral pathway is multisynaptic and, therefore, slow and crudely graded.

Tactile Sensation. In addition to the discriminative pathway, tactile sensibility uses a primitive and crude alternative relay to the thalamus. The afferent axons that carry tactile information up the dorsal columns have many branches or collaterals, and some of these synapse in the dorsal horn near the level of dorsal root entry. After several synapses, axons are projected up *both sides* of the anterolateral aspect of the spinal cord to the thalamus. From there, some projections travel to the somesthetic cortex, especially of the side opposite the stimulus. Few fibers travel all the way to the thalamus. Most synapse on reticular formation neurons, which send their axons on toward the thalamus. Because of these multiple routes, total destruction of the pathway seldom occurs. The lateral nuclei of the thalamus that receive this information are capable of contributing a crude, poorly localized sensation from the opposite side of the body.

The only time this crude alternative system becomes essential is when the discriminative pathway is damaged. Then, despite projection to the somesthetic cortex of anterolateral system information, only a poorly localizable, high-threshold sense of touch remains. Such people lose all kinesthesia, proprioception, and two-point discrimination. They can detect touch stimuli to one versus the other hand, but more force must be delivered to the skin.

Thermal Sensation. Dorsal root ganglion afferents with receptive endings in the skin for warm-hot or cool-cold send their central axons into the segmental dorsal horn of the spinal cord. Cranial nerves that innervate the face and inside of the mouth send their axons to equivalent nuclei of the brain stem. Thermal information is projected to the forebrain through the multisynaptic, slow-conducting anterolateral *paleospinothalamic* system of the *opposite side*.

Thalamic and cortical somesthetic regions for temperature are mixed with those for tactile sensibility. Connections through the medial thalamus into the limbic system are associated with the high emotional content of thermal sensation. The ascending information for temperature sensation does not use the discriminative path.

Conduction of thermal information through peripheral nerves is quite slow compared with the rapid tactile afferents. If a person places a foot in a tub of hot water, the tactile sensation of the water on the skin occurs well in advance of the burning sensation. The anterolateral thermal projection system is also quite slow compared with the discriminative tactile pathway. Thus, the foot has been withdrawn from the hot water by the withdrawal reflex well before the excessive heat is perceived by centers in the forebrain. Local anesthetic agents block the small-diameter afferents that carry thermal sensory information before they block the large-diameter axons that carry discriminative touch information. Absence of thermal sensitivity (athermia) resulting from partial peripheral nerve block or from damage to the anterolateral system is not experienced as a loss of hot and cold sensations. The affected area does not become numb until all tactile information has been blocked from reaching the thalamus and cortex.

CLINICAL ASSESSMENT OF SOMESTHETIC FUNCTION

Clinically, neurologic assessment of somesthetic function can be done by testing the integrity of spinal segmental nerves. A pinpoint pressed against the skin of the sole that results in a withdrawal reflex and a complaint of pain confirms the functional integrity of the afferent terminals in the skin, the entire pathway through the peripheral nerves of the foot, leg, and thigh to the sacral (S1) dorsal root ganglion, and through the dorsal root into the spinal cord segment. It confirms that the somesthetic input association cells receiving this information are functioning and that the reflex circuitry of the cord segments (L5 to S2) is functioning. Further, the lower motoneurons of the L4 to S1 ventral horn can be considered operational, and their axons through the ventral roots, the mixed peripheral nerve, and the muscle nerve to the muscles producing the withdrawal response can be considered intact and functional. The communication between the lower motoneuron and the muscle cells is functional, and these muscles have normal responsiveness and strength. Testing is done at each segmental level, or dermatome, moving upward along the body and neck from coccygeal segments through the high cervical levels to test the functional integrity of all the spinal nerves. Similar dermatomes cover the

face and scalp, and these, although innervated by cranial segmental nerves, are tested in the same manner.

The observation of a normal withdrawal reflex rules out peripheral nerve disease, disorders of the dorsal root and ganglion, diseases of the myoneural junction, and severe muscle diseases. Normal reflex function also indicates that many major descending CNS tract systems are functioning within normal limits. If the person reports the pinprick sensation and accurately identifies its location, then many ascending systems through much of the spinal cord and brain are also functioning normally, as are basic intellect and speech mechanisms.

The integrity of the discriminative dorsal column–medial lemniscus versus the anterolateral tactile pathways is tested with the person's eyes closed by gently brushing the skin with a wisp of cotton, touching an area with two versus one pin points, touching corresponding parts of the body on each side simultaneously or in random sequence, and passively bending the person's finger one way and then another in random order. If only the anterolateral pathway is functional, the tactile threshold is markedly elevated, two-point discrimination and proprioception are missing, and the patient has difficulty discriminating which side of the body received stimulation.

In summary, the somatosensory component of the nervous system provides an awareness of body sensations such as touch, temperature, and pain. Afferent neurons of the dorsal root ganglia innervate a corresponding segment of the body as general soma afferent (somesthetic) neurons. A sensory unit consists of a single dorsal root ganglion afferent neuron, its terminals in a small region of the periphery, and its central axon that terminates on dorsal horn association neurons. The soma innervated by somesthetic afferent neurons of one set of dorsal root ganglia is called a dermatome. By means of a multisynaptic circuit, pressure stimuli sufficiently strong to cause tissue damage trigger a highly predictable withdrawal reflex by activating a lower motoneuron–innervated skeletal muscle contraction. Somesthetic afferents transmit the discriminative sensations of vibration and delicate touch as well as the cruder sensations of pain and temperature.

The tactile system can be considered the basic somesthetic system. Loss of temperature or pain sensitivity leaves the person with no awareness of deficiency; if the tactile system is lost, total anesthesia (numbness) of the involved body part results. The tactile system uses two anatomically separated pathways to relay touch information to the opposite side of the forebrain: the dorsal column discriminative pathway and the anterolateral pathway. Both pathways cross to the opposite side of the nervous system. The discriminative pathway crosses at the base of the medulla, and the anterolateral pathway crosses within the first few segments of entering the cord. Normal delicate touch, vibration, position, and movement sensations use the discriminative, two-neuron pathway to reach the thalamus where tertiary relay occurs to the primary somesthetic strip of parietal cortex. The anterolateral pathway consists of bilateral multisynaptic slow-conducting tracts that preserve crude tactile sensation even when there is considerable damage to the spinal cord. In contrast to the tactile system, temperature sensations of warm-hot and cool-cold result from skin thermal afferents, which project to the thalamus and cortex only through the anterolateral system of the opposite side. Testing of the ipsilateral dorsal column (discriminate touch) system or the contralateral temperature projection systems permits diagnostic analysis of the level and extent of damage in spinal cord lesions.

■ PAIN

Pain is a complex and personal phenomenon. It involves not only anatomic structures and physiologic behaviors but psychological, social, cultural, and cognitive factors as well. Pain can be a prepotent or overwhelming experience, often disruptive to customary behavior, and when severe it demands and directs all of one's attention.

Pain probably is the most common symptom that motivates a person to seek professional help. Indeed, it sends those who suffer to the physician's office more often, and with greater speed, than any other symptom. Its location, radiation, duration, and severity give important clues to its etiology. Despite its unpleasantness, pain can serve a useful purpose because it warns of impending tissue injury, motivating the person to seek relief. For example, an inflamed appendix could progress in severity, rupture, and even cause death were it not for the warning afforded by the pain. Pain can be an indication of depression or dependency. It may also be used for secondary gain, either consciously or unconsciously.

DEFINITIONS AND THEORIES

What is pain? What is its purpose? Is it of any use? Does it help or harm? Scientific disciplines have attempted to answer these and other questions about pain. The many definitions of pain flowing from these efforts serve to highlight its complex nature. Despite intense interest and research, the puzzle of pain persists; we still have much to learn about this common and human experience.

Historically, pain often has been looked on as a punishment or a means of atonement. The term itself—Greek *poine;* Latin *poena;* French *peine*—means punishment. Some Western cultures have viewed pain as something to be avoided at all costs. Aristotle regarded pain as the antithesis of pleasure, whereas Freud discussed the pleasure principle in relation to the avoidance of pain. It is impossible to really separate the pain sensation from emotion because the sensation itself is only part—and perhaps not even the main part—of the total pain experience. Responses to pain are patterned according to the norms of a person's cultural group. Zborowski, in his studies of Italian and Jewish women, found that both groups had low levels of pain tolerance and complained loudly when in pain. Interestingly, this behavior occurred for different reasons. The Italian women were relatively satisfied once their pain was relieved, whereas the Jewish women pursued the matter further, demanding to know its meaning.[4]

Sternbach described pain as "an abstract concept that refers to (1) a personal, private sensation of hurt; (2) a harmful stimulus which signals current and impending tissue damage; (3) a pattern of responses which operate to protect the organism from harm."[5] Useful as this definition is, it fails to describe all facets of the experience called pain.

Margo McCaffery, a nurse in private practice with more than 25 years of experience in the management of pain, has provided one of the most clinically useful definitions to date. She states: "Pain is whatever the experiencing person says it is, existing whenever he says it does."[6] Clinically, there are advantages to this definition. It is broad enough to cover the client's expression of pain, verbal or nonverbal, but perhaps more important, it indicates that the client is believed, which is critical to developing the trust relationship so important in managing pain. Merskey believes that if pain is accepted as a psychological phenomenon with physiologic correlates rather than vice versa, some clinical problems can be prevented. For example, the patient will not be considered a malingerer or liar if no objective cause for the pain can be found.[7]

NOCICEPTION

Scientifically, pain has been viewed within the context of nociception. *Nociception* is associated with tissue damage (Latin *nocere,* to injure). Researchers have used the withdrawal reflex (*e.g.,* withdrawal of the hand away from a nociceptive stimulus) to describe nociceptive stimuli. Such stimuli include pressure from a sharp object, strong electric current to the skin, or application of heat or cold (about 10°C above or below skin temperature). Nociceptive stimuli are those that occur at or close to an intensity that causes tissue damage; therefore, they can be objectively defined. This does not imply that pain is experienced whenever noxious stimuli activate nociceptors. Pain occurs when nociceptive stimuli are perceived as painful. In addition to triggering withdrawal reflexes, nociceptive stimuli are actively avoided and function as negative reinforcers for learning.

PAIN THEORIES

Traditionally, two theories have been offered to explain the physiologic basis for painful experience. The first, the *specificity theory*, regards pain as a separate sensory modality evoked by the activity of specific receptors that transmit information to pain centers or regions in the forebrain where pain is experienced. The second theory includes a group of theories collectively referred to as *pattern theory*. It proposes that pain receptors share endings or pathways with other sensory modalities but that different patterns of activity (spatial or temporal) of the same neurons can be used to signal painful and nonpainful stimuli. For example, light touch applied to the skin would produce the sensation of touch through low-frequency firing of the receptor; intense pressure would produce pain through high-frequency firing of the same receptor. Both theories focus on the neurophysiologic basis of pain, and both probably apply. Specific nociceptive afferents have been identified. In addition, almost all afferents, if driven at a very high frequency, can be experienced as painful. What these theories fail to address are the motivational, cognitive, cultural, and affective components of pain.

The *gate control theory* originally proposed by Melzack and Wall in 1965 was a modification of the specificity theory to meet the challenges proposed by the pattern theories. This theory postulated the presence of neural gating mechanisms at the segmental spinal level to account for interactions between pain and other sensory modalities.[8] The original gate control theory proposed a spinal cord level network of transmitting (t) or projection cells and internuncial neurons that can inhibit the t cells to form a segmental level gating mechanism that can block projection of pain information to the brain.

According to the gate control theory, the internuncial neurons involved in the gating mechanism are activated by large-diameter, faster-propagating fibers that carry touch (tactile) information. Thus, the simultaneous firing of the large-diameter touch fibers can block the transmission of impulses from the small-diameter myelinated and unmyelinated pain fibers. Pain therapists have long known that pain intensity can be temporarily reduced during active tactile stimulation. For example, repeated sweeping of a soft-bristled brush on the skin (brushing) over or near a painful area may result in pain reduction for several minutes to several hours.

Pain modulation is now known to be a much more complex phenomenon than that proposed by the original gate control theory. Tactile information is transmitted by small- as well as large-diameter fibers. Also, major interactions between sensory modalities, including the gating phenomenon, occur at several levels of the CNS rostral to the input segment. Perhaps the most puzzling aspect of locally applied stimuli, such as brushing, that can block the experience of pain is the relatively long-lasting effects (minutes, hours) of such treatments. This prolonged effect has been difficult to explain on the basis of specificity theories, including the gate control theory. Other extremely important factors include endogenous opioids and their receptors at both the segmental and the brain stem level, descending feedback modulation, altered sensitivity, learning, and culture. Despite this, the Melzack and Wall theory has served a useful purpose. It excited interest in pain and stimulated research and clinical activity related to the pain-modulating systems.

PAIN MECHANISMS AND RESPONSES

The mechanisms of pain are many and complex. There are (1) primary sensory peripheral nerve fibers and their receptive endings that monitor the stimuli for pain; (2) the spinal cord circuitry that processes pain information; (3) the pathways that project pain information to the brain; (4) the thalamus and cortex that integrate and modulate pain; and finally, (5) the subjective reaction to pain.

PAIN RECEPTORS AND MEDIATORS

Receptors that have pain as their lowest-intensity threshold stimulus are known as nociceptors, or pain receptors. Structurally, the receptive endings of the peripheral pain fibers are free nerve endings. These receptive endings are widely distributed in the skin, dental pulp, some internal organs, periosteum, and meninges. Considerable controversy remains regarding the production of pain by the overstimulation of other receptors, such as those for temperature and pressure.

The available evidence seems to support the idea that cellular destruction leads to the release of pain-producing substances. Bradykinin (a peptide) is one of the most potent examples; experimentally, it causes pain when extremely low doses are injected intraarterially or intraperitoneally. It is broken down relatively rapidly and, therefore, may be involved primarily in acute pain. Prostaglandins increase sensitivity of pain receptors by enhancing bradykinin's pain-provoking effect.[9] Other substances implicated in producing pain are histamine, potassium, serotonin, leukotrienes, acetylcholine, adenosine triphosphate, and substance P. These chemical mediators are effective in producing nociceptive reflexes and the experience of pain by (1) activating peripheral receptors of nociceptors, (2) sensitizing peripheral endings of nociceptors, or (3) stimulating the release of pain-producing substances.[10] The effectiveness of these compounds in provoking nociceptive reflexes and the experience of pain suggests that pain afferents are, at least in part, chemoreceptors.[11]

SPINAL CORD CIRCUITRY AND PATHWAYS

The peripheral branches of the afferent fibers that transmit pain information to the spinal cord form two subpopulations: small unmyelinated types of fibers referred to as *C fibers* and small myelinated fibers called *A-delta fibers*. The C fibers are the smallest of all peripheral fibers; they transmit impulses at the rate of 0.5 to 2.0 m per second. The A-delta fibers have considerably greater conduction velocities, transmitting impulses at a rate of 5 to 30 m per second.

The axons of the C fiber and A-delta neurons travel through the dorsal root to the white matter of the dorsal lateral spinal cord where they bifurcate and ascend or descend one or two segments, projecting collaterals into the dorsal horn association columns of these segments. Activated circuits of the association columns communicate with four categories of circuitry: (1) the segmental level withdrawal reflex, (2) the reticular activating system, (3) the forebrain limbic system, and (4) the thalamus and cortex. The local cord level withdrawal reflex is designed to remove endangered tissue from a damaging stimulus.

From the dorsal horn, axons of association projection neurons cross through the anterior commissure to the opposite side and ascend upward in a pathway called the *anterolateral sensory pathway* to the brain. There are three subdivisions in the anterolateral pathway: the neospinothalamic, paleospinothalamic, and spinoreticular systems (see Fig. 48-6).

The fibers in the *neospinothalamic tract* are mainly associated with the spatial and temporal aspects of sharp, bright, or fast pain. The A-delta afferent fibers project, after a single spinal level synapse, through the moderately rapid neospinothalamic pathway to the thalamus. Projections of this system to the contralateral parietal somesthetic area probably provide the precise location of first pain (bright, sharp, stabbing pain).

The *paleospinothalamic tract* is a slower-conducting multisynaptic tract concerned with the diffuse, dull, aching, and unpleasant pain that travels through the small unmyelinated C fibers. This system also ascends in the contralateral anterolateral pathway to terminate in several thalamic regions, including the intralaminar nuclei, which project to the limbic cortex, and is associated with the emotional aspects of pain.

The *spinoreticular system* projects primarily bilaterally to the reticular formation of the brain stem. This system, in conjunction with the collaterals of the paleospinothalamic system, facilitates avoidance reflexes at all levels. It also contributes to an increase in the electroencephalographic activity associated with alertness and indirectly influences hypothalamic functions associated with sudden alertness, such as increased heart rate and blood pressure. This may explain the tremendous arousal effects of certain pain stimuli. Further projections of these systems send information to the mesencephalic periaqueductal gray and hypothalamus.

BRAIN CENTERS AND PAIN PERCEPTION

The basic sensation of hurtfulness, or pain, occurs at the level of the thalamus. In the neospinothalamic system, interconnections between the lateral thalamus and the somatosensory cortex are necessary to add precision and discrimination to the pain sensation. Association areas of the parietal cortex are essential to the perception, or learned meaningfulness, of the pain experience. For example, if a mosquito bites a person's index finger on the left hand and only the thalamus is functional, the person will complain of pain somewhere on the hand. With the primary sensory cortex functional, the person can localize the pain to the precise area on the index finger. The association cortex, on the other hand, is necessary to interpret the buzzing and the sensation that preceded the pain as being related to a mosquito bite. The paleospinothalamic system projects diffusely from the intralaminar nuclei of the thalamus to large areas of the limbic cortex. These connections are probably associated with the hurtfulness as well as the mood-altering and attention-narrowing effect of pain.

PAIN THRESHOLD, TOLERANCE, AND REACTION

Reactions to pain are affected by pain threshold and tolerance. Although the terms often are used interchangeably, pain threshold and pain tolerance are not the same entity. Pain threshold is more closely associated with nociceptive (*i.e.*, tissue-damaging) stimuli. Pain tolerance relates more to the total pain experience; it is defined as the maximum intensity or duration of pain that a person is willing to endure—the point beyond which the person wants something done about the pain. Tolerance is not necessarily indicative of the severity of pain. Psychological, familial, cultural, and environmental factors significantly influence the intensity of pain a person is willing to tolerate. Separation and identification of the role of each of these two aspects of pain continue to pose fundamental problems for the pain management team as well as for pain researchers.

Physical reactions to pain may be manifested by biting the lips, clenching the teeth, and facial expressions such as frowning and wrinkling the brows. Protective body movements can be both involuntary and voluntary. The previously mentioned withdrawal reaction, which moves the body part away from the pain source, is involuntary. Voluntary movements, such as changes in posture and relaxation exercises, often relieve discomfort.

ENDOGENOUS ANALGESIC MECHANISMS

One of the exciting advances in understanding pain is the elucidation of neuroanatomic pathways that arise in the midbrain and brain stem, descend to the spinal cord, and function in the modulation of ascending pain impulses. One such pathway begins in an area of the midbrain called the *periaqueductal gray (PAG)* region. Soon after the introduction of the gate control theory, it was found that focal stimulation of the midbrain PAG regions produced a state of analgesia. The resultant analgesia lasted for many hours and was sufficient to permit abdominal surgery, although levels of consciousness and reactions to auditory and visual stimuli remained unaffected. A few years later, opiate receptors were found to be highly concentrated in this and other regions of the CNS where electrical stimulation produced analgesia. Because of these findings, the PAG area of the midbrain often is referred to as the *endogenous analgesia center*.

Recent studies have shown that the PAG area receives input from widespread areas of the CNS, including the cerebral cortex, hypothalamus, brain stem reticular formation, and spinal cord by way of the paleospinothalamic and neospinothalamic tracts. This region is intimately connected to the limbic system, which is associated with emotional experience. The neurons of the PAG area have axons that descend into the nucleus raphe magnus (NRM) in the rostral medulla. The axons of these NRM neurons project to the dorsal horn of the spinal cord where they terminate in the same layers as the entering primary pain fibers (Fig. 48-7). Stimulation of the medullary nuclei is thought to inhibit pain transmission by dorsal horn projection neurons.[11] There is also evidence of noradrenergic neurons that can inhibit transmission of pain impulses at the level of the spinal cord. Studies indicate that the rostral pons has noradrenergic neurons with axons that project to the medullary nuclei and to the dorsal horn cells of the spinal cord.[12] The discovery that norepinephrine can block pain transmission had led to studies directed at the combined administration of narcotics and clonidine (a central-acting α-adrenergic agonist) for pain relief.

The *opioids* are morphine-like substances that are manufactured in many regions of the CNS, including the pituitary gland. The discovery of morphine receptors led to a search for natural body substances capable of interacting with these receptors. The natural ligands (binding molecules) for these opiate receptors are the endogenous opioid peptides (the endorphins and enkephalins), which were discovered in 1975. New therapeutic approaches to the treatment of pain were envisioned when it was discovered that these peptides exert inhibitory modulation of pain transmission and that the release of endogenous opioids after CNS stimulation correlated with patient reports of pain relief. Endorphins are found primarily in the amygdala, limbic system, hypothalamic-pituitary axis, and other brain stem structures. The enkephalins are found primarily in short interneurons in the PAG of the midbrain, limbic system, basal ganglia, hypothalamus, and spinal cord dorsal horn. These morphine-like substances mimic the peripheral and central effects of morphine and the central effects of other opiate drugs.

Since the discovery of the opioids, other neuromodulators for pain have been identified. Serotonin has been identified as a neuromodulator in the NRM medullary nuclei that project to the spinal cord. It has been shown that tricyclic antidepressant compounds, such as amitriptyline, have analgesic properties independent of their antidepressant effects. These drugs, which enhance the effects of serotonin by blocking its presynaptic uptake, have been found to be effective in the management of certain types of chronic pain.[13, 14] Neurons that secrete substance P, another neuropeptide, are widely distributed throughout the nervous system. Considerable research data support the role of substance P as a transmitter substance used by unmyelinated C-fiber afferents related to nociception and slow pain.[15] There is evidence that enkephalins and other opioid peptides modulate pain at the spinal level by inhibiting the release of substance P.

TYPES OF PAIN

The types of pain can be classified into four categories according to (1) source, (2) fast versus slow pain, (3) referral, and (4) duration (acute versus chronic).

Source. The sources of pain commonly are divided into four general categories: (1) cutaneous, (2) deep somatic, (3) visceral, and (4) functional or psychogenic.

Cutaneous pain arises from superficial structures, such as the skin and subcutaneous tissues. A paper cut on the finger is an example of easily localized superficial, or cutaneous, pain. It is a sharp, bright pain with a burning quality and may be either abrupt

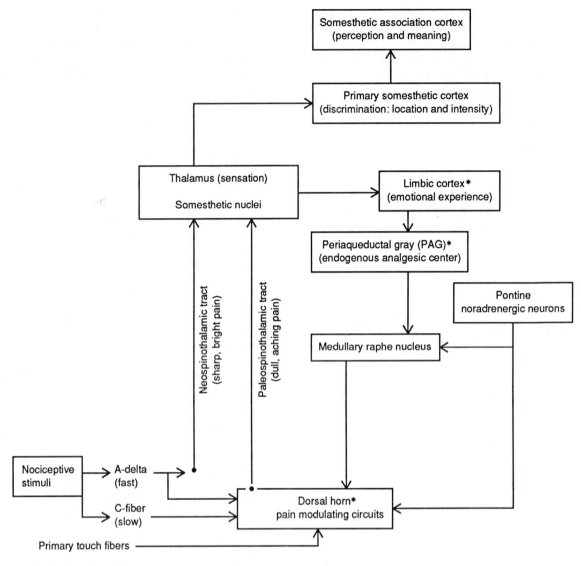

FIG. 48-7. *Primary pain pathways. The transmission of incoming nociceptive impulses is modulated by dorsal horn circuitry that receives inhibitory input from peripheral touch receptors and from descending pathways that involve the periaqueductal endogenous analgesic center in the midbrain, pontine noradrenergic neurons, and the raphe nucleus in the medulla.*

or slow in onset. It can be localized accurately and may be distributed along the dermatomes. Because there is an overlap of nerve fiber distribution between the dermatomes, the boundaries of pain frequently are not as clear-cut as the dermatomal diagrams indicate.

Deep somatic pain originates in deep body structures, such as the periosteum, muscles, tendons, joints, and blood vessels. This pain is more diffuse than cutaneous pain. Various stimuli, such as strong pressure exerted on bone, ischemia to a muscle, and tissue damage, can produce deep somatic pain. This is the type of pain one experiences from a sprained

ankle. Radiation of pain from the original site of injury can occur. For example, damage to a nerve root can cause a person to experience pain radiating along its fiber distribution.

Visceral, or *splanchnic*, pain has its origin in the visceral organs. Common examples of visceral pain are renal colic, pain caused by cholecystitis, pain associated with acute appendicitis, and ulcer pain. Although the viscera are diffusely and richly innervated, cutting or burning of viscera, as opposed to similar noxious stimuli applied to cutaneous or superficial structures, is unlikely to cause pain. Instead, strong abnormal contractions of the gastrointestinal system, distention, or ischemia affecting the walls of the viscera can induce severe pain. Anyone who has suffered from either severe gastrointestinal distress or ureteral colic can readily attest to the misery involved. We are most accustomed to thinking of visceral pain as emanating from the abdominal cavity. It tends to be diffuse, especially in early stages.

Visceral pain is transmitted by small unmyelinated pain fibers that travel with the axons of the autonomic nervous system and project to visceral input association neurons of the cord or brain stem. Besides sending projections to the forebrain, these input association neurons also project through the paleospinal and spinoreticular pathways into visceral reflex circuits. Consequently, visceral pain typically is accompanied by autonomic responses such as nausea, vomiting, sweating, pallor, and, possibly, shock. Ascending pathways resulting in the experience of visceral pain have three different overlapping general visceral afferent (GVA) sources: (1) pharynx through lower esophagus via cranial nerves IX and X, (2) stomach through mid-transverse colon via T1–L2, and (3) below the mid-transverse colon via S2–S4. The peripheral GVA pathways involved travel with the parasympathetic distribution for the upper and lower viscera and with the sympathetic distribution for the intervening viscera.

Pain from the viscera may be localized only with difficulty. There are several explanations for this. First, innervation of visceral organs is poorly represented at the forebrain (perception) levels. A second possible explanation is that the brain does not easily learn to localize sensations that originate in organs that are only imprecisely visualized. For example, a cut on the third finger of the right hand can be readily seen, identified, and localized, whereas an inflamed internal organ can be localized only vaguely. A third explanation is that sensory information from thoracic and abdominal viscera can travel by two pathways to the CNS. The first route is called the *visceral*, or *true visceral*, *pathway*. According to this hypothesis, the pain information travels with the fibers of the autonomic nervous system that enter the spinal cord in only the T1 to T12 and S1 to S4 segments. Therefore, the pain is felt at a site on the surface of the body distant to the pain locus.

The second route, the parietal pathway, which is somatic, usually is not considered a pathway for visceral pain but may be the pain route with inflammation of the parietal pleura, pericardium, and peritoneum. Sensations that travel along this pathway can be localized directly over the affected part; a common example is pain in the right lower quadrant associated with an inflamed appendix.

Pain may have a known or unknown physical cause. Unlike organic or somatogenic pain, which

originates in the body, or soma, *functional*, or *psychogenic*, *pain* (*i.e.*, pain of unknown physical cause) is attributed to the psyche or emotions. In both situations, the physical sensation of pain is the same. The person may be unaware that the origin of the pain is emotional and may experience it as if the pain were truly originating from an organic disorder. People with pain usually experience both its physical and its emotional aspects. It is difficult to conceive of pain as being either purely organic or purely functional. McCaffery's statement that "pain is whatever the experiencing person says it is and exists whenever he says it does" is particularly applicable here.[6] Because all pain appears to have both mental and physical components, McCaffery and others recommend that all pain be considered real pain experienced by real people.

Fast Pain Versus Slow Pain. Two qualitatively different types of pain can be readily appreciated— fast pain and slow pain. Fast pain is a short, well-localized sensation; it starts and stops abruptly when the stimulus is instituted or stopped. Examples are a pinprick or strong pinch. Fast pain has its origin in the free nerve endings of myelinated A-delta axons located in the skin that respond to strong mechanical pressure and high temperature. It is associated with the withdrawal reflex and with the sensation of bright, sharp pain experience. Slow pain is experienced as a throbbing, burning, or aching sensation. It has its origin in the free nerve endings of the very slow conducting unmyelinated C fibers. The slow-pain receptors have chemoreceptor properties and respond to compounds liberated as a result of tissue damage from excessive mechanical, chemical, and cold or hot stimuli. These two fiber-conduction groups of afferents partially explain the two components of pain. The farther the stimulus is from the brain, the more time separates the fast and slow components.

Referred Pain. Referred pain is that pain perceived at a site different from its point of origin but innervated by the same spinal segment. It is hypothesized that visceral and somatic afferent neurons converge on the same dorsal horn projection neurons. For this reason, it can be difficult for the brain to correctly identify the original source of pain. Pain that originates in the abdominal or thoracic viscera is diffuse and poorly localized and often perceived at a site far removed from the affected area. For example, the pain associated with myocardial infarction commonly is referred to the left arm, neck, and chest.

Referred pain may arise alone or concurrent with pain located at the origin of the noxious stimuli. Although the term *referred* usually is applied to pain that originates in the viscera and is experienced as if originating from the body wall, it may also be applied to pain that arises from somatic structures. An example would be pain referred to the chest wall caused by nociceptive stimulation of the peripheral portion of the diaphragm, which receives somatic (somesthetic) innervation from the intercostal nerves.

An understanding of pain reference is of great value in diagnosing illness because afferent neurons from visceral or deep somatic tissue enter the spinal cord at the same level as those from the cutaneous areas to which the pain is referred (Fig. 48-8).

The sites of referred pain are determined during the development of the organ systems in the embryo. Let us say that a person has peritonitis but complains

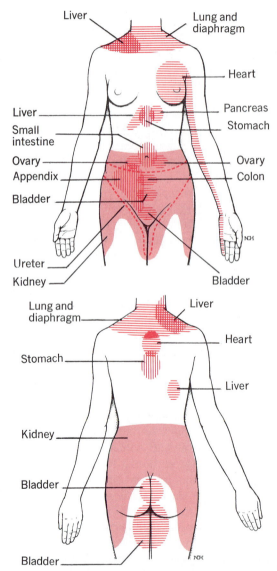

FIG. 48-8. Areas of referred pain. (**Top**) Anterior view. (**Bottom**) Posterior view. (Chaffee, E. E., & Lytle, I. M. [1980]. *Basic physiology and anatomy* [4th ed., p. 266]. Philadelphia: J.B. Lippincott.)

of pain in the shoulder. Internally, there is irritation or inflammation of the central diaphragm. In the embryo, the diaphragm originates in the neck, and its central portion is innervated by the phrenic nerve, which enters the cord at the level of the third to fifth cervical segment (C3 to C5). As the fetus develops, the diaphragm descends to its adult position between the thoracic and abdominal cavities, innervated by the phrenic nerve. Therefore, fibers that enter the spinal cord at the C3 to C5 level carry information from the neck area as well as from the diaphragm, and the diaphragmatic pain is interpreted by the forebrain as originating in the shoulder or neck area.

Although the *visceral* pleura, pericardium, and peritoneum are said to be relatively free of pain fibers, the *parietal* pleura, pericardium, and peritoneum do react to nociceptive stimuli. Visceral inflammation can involve parietal and somatic structures, and this in turn may give rise to diffuse local or referred pain. For example, irritation of the parietal peritoneum resulting from appendicitis typically gives rise to pain directly over the inflamed area in the lower right quadrant. Also, such stimuli can evoke pain referred to the umbilical area.

Muscle spasm, or *guarding*, occurs when somatic structures are involved. Guarding is a protective-reflex rigidity; its purpose is to protect the affected body parts (*e.g.*, an abscessed appendix or a sprained muscle). This protective guarding may give rise to pain of muscle ischemia, causing both local and referred pain.

Acute Versus Chronic Pain. Pain can also be classified according to duration and characterized as acute or chronic. The pain research of the past 25 to 30 years has emphasized the importance of differentiating acute pain from chronic pain and dealing with them separately. This is because they differ from each other not only temporally but also in cause, mechanisms, pathophysiology, and function and because the diagnosis of and therapy for each are distinctive (Table 48-1).[16]

Acute pain is defined as pain of less than 6 months' duration. It consists of unpleasant sensory, perceptual, and emotional components with associated somatic, autonomic, psychological, and behavioral responses. Acute pain is caused by noxious, or tissue-damaging, stimuli; its purpose is to serve as a protective, or warning, system. Besides alerting the person to the existence of actual or impending tissue damage, it prompts a search for professional help. The pain's location, intensity, duration, and radiation as well as those factors that aggravate or relieve it are essential diagnostic clues. Unlike chronic pain, it is rare for acute pain to be due to pain of unknown origin or to psychological factors alone. Acute pain

TABLE 48-1. CHARACTERISTICS OF ACUTE AND CHRONIC PAIN

CHARACTERISTIC	ACUTE PAIN	CHRONIC PAIN
Onset	Recent	Continuous or intermittent
Duration	Short duration	6 mo or more
Autonomic responses	Consistent with sympathetic fight or flight response*	Absence of autonomic responses
	Increased heart rate	
	Increased stroke volume	
	Increased blood pressure	
	Increased pupillary dilation	
	Increased muscle tension	
	Decreased gut motility	
	Decreased salivary flow (dry mouth)	
Psychological component	Associated anxiety	Increased irritability
		Associated depression
		Somatic preoccupation
		Withdrawal from outside interests
		Decreased strength of relationships
Other types of response		Decreased sleep
		Decreased libido
		Appetite changes

Responses are approximately proportional to intensity of the stimulus.

commonly is accompanied by anxiety, which usually disappears when the pain is relieved. The likelihood of acute pain progressing to chronic pain is decreased by appropriate treatment.

Chronic pain has classically been defined as pain of 6 months' duration or longer. In practice, this time frame varies, and the differences between acute and chronic pain are more than temporal. The International Association for the Study of Pain defines chronic pain as that which persists beyond the expected normal time of healing.[16, 17] The pain may be continuous (*e.g.*, arthritis) or intermittent (*e.g.*, angina or intermittent claudication). Unlike acute pain, persistent chronic pain usually serves no useful function. To the contrary, it imposes physiologic, psychological, family, and economic stresses and may exhaust a person's resources. In contrast to acute pain, psychological and environmental influences may play an important role in the development of behaviors associated with chronic pain. Chronic pain often is associated with depression and despair rather than anxiety. Amazingly, this depression commonly is relieved spontaneously when the pain is removed.

People suffering chronic pain may not exhibit the somatic, autonomic, or affective behaviors associated with acute pain. One reason for this is that the stress response cannot be maintained for long periods. Also, certain behaviors viewed as acceptable in patients with severe but short-lived pain are not expected or considered appropriate in the chronic situation. With chronic pain, it is important to heed the person's own description of the pain because the expected psychophysiologic responses may or may not be present.

One proposed classification of chronic pain divides affected people into two broad groups according to life expectancy (brief versus normal). This classification assumes clinical importance primarily if a decision must be reached concerning long-term use of narcotics for pain relief.

RESPONSES TO PAIN

The responses to pain are both physiologic and psychosocial.

Physiologic responses to pain involve activation of the sympathetic nervous system, which evokes the fight-or-flight reaction, with catecholamine release from the adrenal medulla. What happens is this: as blood is shifted from nonvital to vital parts of the body, the vessels of the skin and abdominal viscera (spleen, kidneys, and intestine) constrict, whereas those of the heart, skeletal muscles, lungs, and brain dilate. The face becomes pallid and the pupils dilate. Respiratory and heart rates and the strength of cardiac contraction increase. Muscle tension rises and energy stores are mobilized to supply the body with glucose. A relative decline in parasympathetic activity may result in loss of appetite, nausea, and vomiting. Gastrointestinal motility and digestive gland secretion also diminish. After a period of time, a parasympathetic rebound response occurs, and the heart rate, blood pressure, and respiratory rate may fall below the prepain level. This is likely when pain is intense but of short duration.

Pain that persists or is repetitive results in adaptive responses, with observable decreases in sympathetic activity. Pain receptors show little, if any, adaptation. On the contrary, reactions to long-term pain are centrally mediated. With time, physiologic and psychological coping mechanisms evolve, but these behavioral responses do not necessarily indicate pain relief. The person may merely be too fatigued to respond.

Psychosocial reactions to pain are deeply influenced by the same factors that affect pain tolerance, including past experiences with pain. A verbally competent person may be able to accurately describe the location, duration, and intensity of the pain as well as his or her ability or willingness to tolerate it. A change in the tone of voice may be as revealing as the words spoken. Previous personal and family experiences with certain diseases, such as cancer, can significantly affect the degree of fear, anxiety, and depression associated with pain and, consequently, the person's reaction to it.

Pain that necessitates absence from work probably is of greater importance to one who is paid an hourly wage than to one who has ample health insurance and sick time available.

Vocalizations comprise a group of responses such as crying, groaning, grunting, and gasping. Their frequency, loudness, and duration can assume greater significance in situations where the person is either too young or too confused to be verbally competent. These manifestations are particularly important in young children and elderly people.

Cultural and environmental factors may also play a role in pain perception. For example, a person who values stoicism is unlikely to cry out in public when subjected to painful stimuli, whereas this may be an accepted response for someone of another culture.

Pain can provide reassurance. In one study, the members of a group of men matched as to injuries gave very different responses, depending on the cir-cumstances of their wounding.[18] Trauma inflicted on the battlefield evoked denial of pain and refusal of medication; the same types of injuries inflicted on civilians evoked complaints of pain and requests for pain relief. These striking differences have been attributed to the emotional state at the time of injury as well as to the significance each person attached to the injuries. For the soldier, being wounded may have afforded a face-saving escape from unpleasant, life-threatening situations. It meant being transported to a relatively safe environment, perhaps even home. But a civilian with the same type of injury may have felt that life-style as well as income was threatened.

ALTERATIONS IN PAIN SENSITIVITY AND PERCEPTION

Sensitivity to pain varies among people as well as in the same person under different conditions and in different parts of the body. Irritation, mild hypoxia, and mild compression of a peripheral nerve often result in hyperexcitability of the sensory nerve fibers or cell bodies. This is experienced as unpleasant hypersensitivity (*hyperesthesia*) or increased painfulness (*hyperalgesia*). Possible causes of increased sensitivity to noxious stimuli include (1) a decrease in threshold of nociceptors or (2) an increase in pain produced by suprathreshold stimuli. Primary hyperalgesia occurs at the site of injury. Secondary hyperalgesia occurs in nearby uninjured tissue.[10, 16]

Spontaneous, unpleasant sensations called *paresthesias* occur with more severe irritation (*e.g.*, the pins-and-needles sensation that follows temporary compression of a peripheral nerve). The general term *dysesthesia* is given to distortions (usually unpleasant) of somesthetic sensation that typically accompany partial loss of sensory innervation. *Hyperpathia* is a syndrome in which the sensory threshold is raised, but when it is reached, continued stimulation, especially if repetitive, results in a prolonged and unpleasant experience. This pain can be explosive and radiates through a peripheral nerve distribution. It is associated with pathologic changes in peripheral nerves, such as localized hypoxia. More severe pathology can result in reduced or lost tactile (*hypesthesia, anesthesia*), temperature (*hypothermia, athermia*), and pain sensation (*hypalgesia*). *Analgesia* is the absence of pain on noxious stimulation or the relief of pain without loss of consciousness.

The inability to sense pain may result in trauma, infection, and even loss of a body part or parts. Inherited insensitivity to pain may take the form of congenital indifference or congenital insensitivity to pain. In the former, transmission of nerve impulses appears normal but appreciation of painful stimuli at higher levels appears to be absent. In the latter, a peripheral nerve defect apparently exists such that transmission of painful nerve impulses does not result in perception of pain. Whatever the cause, people who lack the ability to perceive pain are at constant risk of tissue damage because pain is not serving its protective function.

Allodynia (Greek *allo*, other, and *odynia*, painful) is the term used for the puzzling phenomenon of pain that follows a nonnoxious stimulus to apparently normal skin. This term is intended to refer to instances in which otherwise normal tissues may be abnormally innervated or may be referral sites for other loci that give rise to pain with nonnoxious stimuli.[17] It may be that an area is hypersensitive because of inflammation or another cause, and a normally subthreshold stimulus is sufficient to trigger the sensation of pain. This response is thought to be chemically mediated, possibly the result of tissue damage in the surrounding area.

Trigger points that are fired off by light tactile stimulation to a highly localized point on the skin or mucous membrane can repeatedly produce immediate intense pain at that site or elsewhere. *Myofascial trigger points* are foci of exquisite tenderness found in many muscles and can be responsible for pain projected to sites remote from the points of tenderness. Trigger points are widely distributed in the back of the head and neck and in the lumbar and thoracic regions. These trigger points cause reproducible myofascial pain syndromes in specific muscles. According to recent reports, these pain syndromes are the major source of pain in clients at chronic pain treatment centers. One report indicated that 85% of 233 consecutive admissions to one comprehensive pain center were assigned a primary organic diagnosis of myofascial pain syndrome.[19] The diagnosis of myofascial pain frequently is overlooked and, as a consequence, inadequately treated.

MANAGEMENT OF PAIN

In 1992, the Clinical Practice Guidelines for Acute Pain Management were released.[20] They were developed by a multidisciplinary expert group under the sponsorship of the Agency for Health Care Policy and Research (AHCPR), Public Health Service, U.S. Department of Health and Human Services. The guidelines, which focus on postoperative pain, emphasize the need for (1) a collaborative, interdisciplinary approach to pain control, which includes members of the health care team and input from the patient and the patient's family when appropriate; (2) an individualized proactive pain control plan developed preoperatively by patients and practitioners (because

pain is easier to prevent than to bring under control once it has begun); (3) assessment and frequent reassessment of the patient's plan; (4) use of both drug and nondrug therapies to control or prevent pain; and (5) a formal, institutional approach to management of acute pain, with clear lines of responsibility.

ASSESSMENT OF PAIN

The relief and management of pain require careful assessment to consider the cause of the pain, evaluate its severity, and determine the type of pain that is present. As with other disease states, it is preferable to eliminate the cause rather than treat the symptoms. A careful history often provides information about triggering factors (injury, infection, or disease) and site of nociception (peripheral receptor or visceral organ). Observation of facial expression and posture may provide additional information about the severity and accompanying responses to pain. For example, alterations in normal posture, such as limping, may increase the spread of pain to neighboring myotomes with progressive complaints, such as stiffness and soreness, that are worsened by activity or cold. The AHCPR pain guidelines emphasize that the "the single most reliable indicator of the existence and intensity of acute pain—and any resultant affective discomfort or distress—is the patient's self report."[20]

Unlike many other bodily responses, such as temperature and blood pressure, the degree or severity of pain cannot be measured objectively. To overcome this problem, various methods have been developed for quantifying the severity of pain in a given person. Among the methods used for pain measurement are (1) numerical value and visual analog scales, (2) verbal descriptor scales, (3) physiologic and behavioral measures, and (4) multidimensional measures, such as the two-component scale and the McGill Pain Questionnaire.[21] Because of the personal nature of pain, most pain instruments are more useful in evaluating individual versus group responses to pain.

The *numeric value* and *visual analog scales* ask a person to give a numeric value to his or her pain, with 0 representing no pain and 10 representing the most intense pain imaginable. The visual analog scale uses a straight line, often 10 cm in length, which represents a continuum of pain intensity. The person is asked to choose a point on the continuum that represents his or her present state of pain intensity. *Verbal descriptor scales* consist of three to five numerically ranked choices of words such as none, slight, mild, moderate, and severe. The word that is chosen is used to determine the intensity of pain on an ordinal scale.

The *physiologic and behavioral measures* incorporate the observation of physiologic and behavorial variables into the pain assessment tool. For example, Hanken and McDowell designed a multidimensional rating scale that uses six variables to measure pain: (1) attention directed toward the pain, (2) anxiety, (3) verbal statement of the degree of pain, (4) skeletal muscle response, (5) characteristics of the respirations, and (6) amount of perspiration.[22] Johnson and Rice developed an instrument that measures two components of pain experience: the physical sensation component and the reactive component.[23] The physical sensation of pain was rated on a scale of 0 to 100, and the distress caused by the pain was rated on a scale labeled slightly distressing, mildly distressing, moderately distressing, and just bearable.

The McGill Pain Questionnaire (Fig. 48-9) measures both the physiologic and the psychological dimensions of pain.[24, 25] The instrument is divided into four parts. The first part uses a drawing of the body on which the person indicates the location of pain. The second part uses a list of 20 words to describe the sensory, affective, evaluative, and other qualities of pain, with the selected words being given a numeric score (*e.g.*, words implying the least pain are assigned a value of 1 and next a value of 2, and so on). The third part asks the person to select words such as brief, momentary, and constant to describe the pattern of pain. The fourth part of the instrument evaluates the present pain intensity on a scale of 0 to 5.

TREATMENT OF PAIN

The treatment of pain may use a number of methods, including cognitive-behavioral interventions, pharmacologic treatment, intermittent or continuous neural blockade, physical agents such as heat and cold, spinal analgesia, electroanalgesia, and surgical interventions. A multidisciplinary approach often is used. The decision about which approach should be tried is based on the duration, characteristics, cause, and mechanisms of pain, if known; the age and social responsibilities of the person; the prognosis; any previous therapy; patient preference; and psychological considerations.

COGNITIVE-BEHAVIORAL

Cognitive-behavioral interventions include relaxation, distraction and imagery, and biofeedback. If the person is having surgery, these techniques can be taught preoperatively.

Relaxation. Relaxation is one of the most evaluated cognitive-behavioral approaches to pain relief.[20]

The relaxation methods need not be complex. Relatively simple strategies, such as brief jaw relaxation procedures, have been successful in decreasing self-reported pain and analgesic use.

Distraction and Imagery. Distraction (*i.e.*, focusing one's attention on stimuli other than painful stimuli) is used to make pain more tolerable but usually does not eliminate it.[5] It could be considered a type of sensory shielding whereby attention to pain is sacrificed for attention to objective or physical stimuli that are already present or easily obtained. Examples are counting, repeating phrases or poems, engaging in activities that require concentration, such as projects, activities, work, conversation, describing slides or pictures, and rhythmic breathing. Television, adventure movies, music, and humor can also provide diversion. It is a mistake to assume that a person who appears to be able to cope with pain by the use of distraction does not have pain. The person should not be punished for his or her efforts by having appropriate medications withheld.[5]

Imagery consists of using one's imagination to develop a mental picture—a visual image. In pain management, therapeutic guided imagery (goal-directed imaging) is used. It can be used in conjunction with relaxation techniques, biofeedback, and other management methods to develop sensory images that can decrease the perceived intensity of pain. It can also be used to lessen anxiety and reduce muscle tension.

Biofeedback. Biofeedback is used to provide feedback to a person concerning the current status of some body function (*e.g.*, finger temperature, temporal artery pulsation, blood pressure, or muscle tension). It is a process of learning designed to make the person aware of certain of his or her own body functions for the purpose of modifying these functions at a conscious level. Interest in this treatment modality rose with the possibility of using biofeedback in the management of migraine and tension headaches or for other pain that had a muscle tension component.

HEAT AND COLD

Both heat and cold are used in the treatment of pain. Each temperature modality has its advantages and advocates. The type of thermal modality used depends on the type of pain being treated and, in many cases, personal preference.

Heat. Historically, heat has proved to be a useful method for relieving pain. Some of the earliest sources of therapeutic heat were heated stones,

McGill Pain Questionnaire

Patient's Name _____ Date _____ Time _____ am/pm

PRI: S_____ A_____ E_____ M_____ PRI(T)_____ PPI_____
    (1–10)   (11–15)   (16)   (17–20)   (1–20)

1 FLICKERING QUIVERING PULSING THROBBING BEATING POUNDING	11 TIRING EXHAUSTING
2 JUMPING FLASHING SHOOTING	12 SICKENING SUFFOCATING
3 PRICKING BORING DRILLING STABBING LANCINATING	13 FEARFUL FRIGHTFUL TERRIFYING
4 SHARP CUTTING LACERATING	14 PUNISHING GRUELLING CRUEL VICIOUS KILLING
5 PINCHING PRESSING GNAWING CRAMPING CRUSHING	15 WRETCHED BLINDING
6 TUGGING PULLING WRENCHING	16 ANNOYING TROUBLESOME MISERABLE INTENSE UNBEARABLE
7 HOT BURNING SCALDING SEARING	17 SPREADING RADIATING PENETRATING PIERCING
8 TINGLING ITCHY SMARTING STINGING	18 TIGHT NUMB DRAWING SQUEEZING TEARING
9 DULL SORE HURTING ACHING HEAVY	19 COOL COLD FREEZING
10 TENDER TAUT RASPING SPLITTING	20 NAGGING NAUSEATING AGONIZING DREADFUL TORTURING

BRIEF MOMENTARY TRANSIENT	RHYTHMIC PERIODIC INTERMITTENT	CONTINUOUS STEADY CONSTANT

E = EXTERNAL
I = INTERNAL

PPI
0 NO PAIN
1 MILD
2 DISCOMFORTING
3 DISTRESSING
4 HORRIBLE
5 EXCRUCIATING

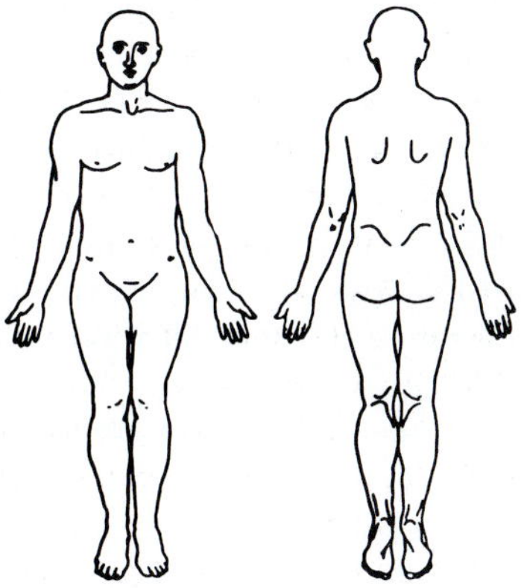

COMMENTS:

FIG. 48-9. McGill pain questionnaire. The pain rating index (PRI) is the sum of rank values for the 20 words: S, sensory; A, affective; E, evaluative; M, miscellaneous; PRI(T), total; PPI, present pain intensity. (Cousins, M. J., & Bridenbaugh, P. O. [1988]. *Neural blockade in clinical anesthesia and management of pain* [2nd ed., p. 853]. Philadelphia: J.B. Lippincott.)

sand, oils, and water or simply the radiant heat from the sun or a fire.[26] Currently, application is achieved through a number of methods, such as immersion in hot water, hot packs, electrically heated pads, infrared rays, and shortwave diathermy.

Care must be taken not to use excessive heat. When excessive heat is used, the heat itself becomes a noxious stimulus, which results in the perception of pain. More important, this can be regarded as a warning signal of impending tissue damage and an indication that removal of the heat source is essential to avoid a burn.

Heat dilates blood vessels and increases local blood flow; it can also influence the transmission of pain impulses and it increases collagen extensibility.[27] Overall, an increase in local circulation can reduce the level of nociceptive stimulation by reducing local ischemia caused by muscle spasm or tension, it can increase the removal of metabolites and inflammatory mediators that act as nociceptive stimuli, and it can help to reduce swelling and relieve pressure on local nociceptive endings. Heat is carried to the posterior horn of the spinal cord in the large-diameter myelinated fibers and may exert its effect by "closing the pain gate" to the predominantly small-diameter fibers.[26] It may also produce the release of endogenous opioids through placebo-type mechanisms. Limitation in the range of movement often is the result of muscle shortening. Heat alters the collagen fibers in ligaments, tendons, and joint structures so that they are more easily extended and can be stretched further before the nociceptive endings are stimulated. Thus, heat often is applied before therapy aimed at stretching joint structures and increasing range of motion.

Cold. Like heat, the application of cold may produce a dramatic reduction in the level of pain that some people perceive. Ice is the major source of cold application to the body. When placed on the skin, heat is conducted to the ice-exposed surface from the deeper tissues; as a result, there is a rapid cooling of the superficial tissues of up to 15°C within 2 to 5 minutes.[27] The deeper tissues are not cooled as much and take longer to cool; it can take up to 20 minutes to develop a temperature drop of 5°C—longer if there is a thick subcutaneous fat layer.

Cold exerts its effect on pain through both circulatory and neural mechanisms. The initial response to local application of cold is sudden local vasoconstriction. This initial vasoconstriction is followed by alternating periods of vasodilatation and vasoconstriction during which the body "hunts" for its normal level of blood flow to prevent local tissue damage. This gives rise to the so-called *Lewis hunting reaction* whereby the circulation to the cooled area

undergoes alternating periods of pallor caused by ischemia and flushing caused by hyperemia.[28] The vasoconstriction is caused by local stimulation of sympathetic fibers and direct cooling of blood vessels and the hyperemia, by local autoregulatory mechanisms. In situations of acute injury, cold is used to produce vasoconstriction and prevent extravasation of blood into the tissues; pain relief results from decreased swelling and decreased stimulation of nociceptive endings. The vasodilatation that follows can be useful in removing substances that stimulate nociceptive endings.

Cold can also have a marked and dramatic effect on chronic pain that results from muscle spasm that causes an accumulation of metabolites within the muscle. For example, the severe pain of joint inflammation suffered by people with rheumatoid arthritis often is appreciably reduced with the application of ice. In terms of pain modulation, cold may reduce afferent activity reaching the posterior horn of the spinal cord by way of large-diameter fibers and thereby influence the closing of the pain gate. The application of ice can be considered a noxious stimulus and, as such, may influence the release of endogenous opioids from the PAG area.

STIMULATION-INDUCED ANALGESIA

Chapman has called the early 1970s the "stimulation-induced analgesia" period of investigation.[29] Electrical stimulation, which includes transcutaneous electrical nerve stimulation (TENS) and electrical acupuncture, may gradually increase the pain threshold to almost double.[30] Stimulation-induced analgesia is one of the oldest known methods of pain relief. Historical references to the use of electricity to decrease or control pain date back to A.D. 46 when a Roman physician, Scribonius Largus, described how the stimulus from an electric eel was able to provide pain relief for headache and gout.[30]

Transcutaneous Electrical Nerve Stimulation. TENS refers to the transmission of electrical energy across the surface of the skin to the peripheral nerve fibers. TENS units have been developed that are convenient, easily transported, and relatively economical to use. Most are about the size of a transistor radio or cigarette package. These battery-operated units deliver a measurable amount of current to a target site.

The system usually consists of three parts: a pair of electrodes, lead wires, and a stimulator. The electrical stimulation is delivered in a pulsed waveform that can be varied in terms of pulse amplitude, width, and rate. The type of stimulation used varies with the type of pain being treated. Electrode placement is determined by the physiologic pathways and an understanding of the pain mechanisms involved. They may be placed on either side of a painful area, over an affected dermatome, over an affected peripheral nerve where it is most superficial, or over a nerve trunk. For example, the electrodes commonly are placed medial and lateral to the incision when treating postoperative pain.

There is probably no one explanation for the physiologic effects of TENS. Each specific type of stimulator may have different sites of action and, thus, may be explained by more than one theory.[31] The gate control theory has been proposed as one possible mechanism.[32] According to this theory, pain information is transmitted by small-diameter A-delta and C fibers. Large-diameter afferent A fibers, as well as small-diameter fibers, carry tactile information mediating touch, pressure, and kinesthesia. Transcutaneous electrical nerve stimulators function on the basis of differentially firing off impulses in the large fibers that carry nonpainful information. According to the gate control theory, increased activity in these large fibers closes the gate to block or modulate transmission of painful information to the forebrain. A second possible explanation is that the high-frequency stimulation (50 to 60 Hz) produced by some units simply acts as a counterirritant.[33] A third possible explanation is that stimulators that produce strong rhythmic contractions may act through the release of endogenous analgesics such as the endorphins and enkephalins.[34] A fourth, and probably the best, explanation for quick analgesia with brief, intense stimulation, is that of a conduction block.[35] TENS has the advantage that it is noninvasive, easily regulated by the person or health professional, and effective in some forms of acute and chronic pain. Its use can be taught preoperatively, affording a reduction in both hospital days and postoperative analgesic medication.

Acupuncture. The practice of acupuncture consists of achieving a therapeutic effect by introducing needles into specific points on the surface of the body. Charts are available that describe the points used to relieve pain at certain anatomic sites. Sometimes palpation is used. It usually is useful to stimulate points that are not normally painful but that become so when symptoms are present. The practice of acupuncture dates back thousands of years to ancient China when the stimulation was achieved by using needles made of bone, stone, or bamboo. Interest in acupuncture peaked in the 1970s as communication between the Eastern and Western medical communities became established and reports of complete surgical analgesia by use of acupuncture alone reached the Western world. Later findings indicated

that complete analgesia is unlikely. The Chinese are practicing electroacupuncture, in which electrical impulses are passed through the needles. Heat may also be applied to the needles, resulting in heat penetration to the depth of the needle. Various theories of how acupuncture achieves analgesia have been proposed, including the gate control theory and stimulation of endogenous opioid release. Pain relief from acupuncture and electroacupuncture has been shown to be reversible by the morphine antagonist naloxone.[36]

Acupressure is the means of stimulating acupressure points without using needles. It is particularly popular in Japan, where it is called *Shiatsu* (*shi* meaning finger and *atsu* meaning pressure).[31] Pressure may be applied with a finger, thumb, or any blunt instrument. Many techniques are used, including massaging in a circular motion for 3 to 5 minutes, pressing inward toward the center of the body and releasing three times, or vibrating the point with fingertip pressure.

PHARMACOLOGIC TREATMENT

The use of drugs to control pain is only one aspect of the overall program for pain relief. These agents have been used for many years to relieve pain of short duration, enabling the person to achieve mobility—for example, after surgery, when exercises such as coughing and deep breathing may be required.

An analgesic drug is defined as a medication that acts on the nervous system to decrease or eliminate pain without inducing loss of consciousness. Analgesic drugs have no powerful curative effects. They are categorized as narcotic or nonnarcotic, addictive or nonaddictive, prescriptive or over-the-counter, strong or weak, and peripherally or centrally acting. The ideal analgesic would be potent but nonaddicting and would produce few adverse effects. It would be effective but would not alter the state of awareness. Tolerance would not occur. Finally, it would be inexpensive.

Nonnarcotic Oral Analgesics. Aspirin, or acetylsalicylic acid, is an example of a nonnarcotic, nonaddictive, over-the-counter analgesic drug. Aspirin acts both centrally and peripherally to block the transmission of pain impulses. It also has antipyretic and antiinflammatory properties, and, like steroids, it is known to inhibit prostaglandins, which make the nerves more sensitive to chemicals such as bradykinin. It does produce the well-known adverse effect of bleeding owing to local and systemic effects. Locally, it causes irritation of the gastrointestinal tract; systemically, it causes prolonged bleeding time by inhibiting platelet aggregation. The latter effect may last for several days, so regular daily doses should be avoided for at least 1 week before surgery. Severe liver disease, vitamin K deficiency, hypoprothrombinemia, or any type of bleeding disorder, like hemophilia, can be a contraindication to the use of aspirin in some people.

Acetaminophen may be an effective alternative to aspirin in some people. Although equivalent to aspirin as an effective analgesic and antipyretic agent, it differs by its lack of antiinflammatory properties. It lacks platelet-inhibiting properties and does not cause gastric bleeding. The drug can cause liver damage. Children under age 5 appear to be less susceptible to this hepatotoxicity. Because there is controversy regarding prolonged use or large doses, the drug should be used with caution.

Another group of drugs with aspirin-like properties are the nonsteroidal antiinflammatory drugs (NSAIDs). The NSAIDs include ibuprofen (Motrin, Rufen), naproxen (Anaprox, Naprosyn), fenoprofen (Nalfon), and indomethacin (Indocin). These drugs act mainly through the inhibition of prostaglandin synthesis. They decrease the sensitivity of blood vessels to bradykinin and histamine, affect lymphokine production from T lymphocytes, reverse vasodilatation, and decrease the release of inflammatory mediators from granulocytes, mast cells, and basophils. To varying degrees, all the NSAIDs are inhibitors of prothrombin synthesis; all are analgesic, antiinflammatory, and antipyretic; and all inhibit platelet aggregation. They are all gastric irritants but to a lesser extent than aspirin. Nephrotoxicity has also been observed. In addition to their use in rheumatoid and osteoarthritis, the NSAIDs (ibuprofen and naproxen) have proved useful in primary dysmenorrhea.

Narcotic Analgesics. The term *narcotic*, or *opioid*, is used to refer to a group of drugs, natural or synthetic, with morphine-like actions. The older term *opiate* was used to designate drugs derived from opium—morphine, codeine, and many other semisynthetic congeners of morphine. The pain-relieving (analgesic) and psychopharmacolgic properties of morphine have been known for centuries. The discovery that the brain contains its own (endogenous) analgesic, morphine-like chemicals, which comprise a group of peptides known as endorphins, is recent. Three distinct families of opioid peptides have been identified thus far: *enkephalins*, *endorphins*, and *dynorphins*. Each family of opioid peptides is derived from a genetically distinct precursor molecule (*e.g.*, proenkephalin, proendorphin, and prodynorphin). Each of these precursors contains a number of biologically active peptides, both opioid and nonopioid. The precursor molecules are found not only in the CNS but also in blood and various other tissues.

The opioids exert their action through opioid receptors. There is reasonably firm evidence of three major categories of opioid receptors in the CNS, designated mu (μ), kappa (κ), and delta (δ); in addition, two subtypes of each category have been identified tentatively.[37] These receptors are particularly concentrated in areas of the brain where the enkephalins have also been located. Inferences have been drawn from data that attempt to relate pharmacologic effects of opioid drugs to interactions with a particular type of receptor. For example, analgesia is thought to involve mu receptors (largely at supraspinal sites) and kappa receptors (principally within the spinal cord). The function of delta receptors is more speculative. Both endogenous and exogenous opioids bind to these receptors; some may interact at variable extent with all three types of receptors and act as an agonist, partial agonist, or antagonist at each.[37] There is evidence that morphine and other morphine-like opioid agonists produce analgesia primarily through interaction with mu-opioid receptors. Other consequences of mu receptor activation include respiratory depression, miosis, reduced gastrointestinal motility, and feelings of well-being (euphoria). Two types of mu receptors have been identified, based on their affinities for agonists: mu_1 (higher affinity), thought to mediate supraspinal analgesia, and mu_2 (lower affinity), thought to mediate respiratory depression and gastrointestinal actions among others.[37] As more information becomes available regarding the opioids and their receptors, it seems likely that pain medications can be developed that act selectively at certain receptor sites, thus providing more effective pain control while producing fewer adverse effects and affording less danger of addiction. For example, it might be possible to develop opioid drugs that produce effective analgesia but not undesirable adverse effects, such as respiratory depression.

The term *tolerance* implies a decreased responsiveness to a drug that occurs with continued administration. The development of tolerance and physical dependence with repeated use is a characteristic of opioid drugs, and the potential for developing psychological dependence on the drugs is one of the major limitations to their clinical use. There are three classes of narcotic drugs: agonists, antagonists, and opioids with mixed actions.[37] The latter group includes the agonist-antagonists that appear to be agonists at some receptors and antagonists at others. The morphine-like agonists bind to discrete opioid receptors and cause analgesia. They include morphine, hydromorphone (Dilaudid), methadone (Dolophine), levorphanol (Levo-Dromoran), oxymorphone (Numorphan), heroin, meperidine (Demerol), and codeine. The narcotic antagonists, such as naloxone (Narcan), are drugs that bind to opioid receptors but block the action of morphine-like agonists and do not have analgesic properties of their own. Naloxone can reverse the effects of morphine immediately and frequently is used in the treatment of narcotic overdose. The mixed agonist-antagonist drugs produce analgesia in nontolerant people but produce withdrawal in people who are tolerant to morphine-like drugs. The mixed agonist-antagonist drugs include pentazocine (Talwin), nalbuphine (Nubain), and butorphanol (Stadol). All the agonist opioid drugs can produce significant respiratory depression by inhibiting brain stem respiratory mechanisms, and all can suppress the cough reflex. Another adverse effect common to narcotic analgesics is constipation. Tolerance develops to the respiratory depression and cough suppression but not to the constipation. The agonist-antagonist drugs usually produce sedation in addition to analgesia when given in therapeutic doses. Severe respiratory depression may be less common with agonist-antagonist analgesics than with pure agonist drugs.

The narcotics are indicated for relief of pain that cannot be relieved with less effective agents, such as the nonnarcotic analgesic drugs. When used for temporary relief of severe pain, such as that occurring postoperatively, there is much evidence that narcotics given routinely before the pain becomes extreme are far more effective than those administered in a sporadic manner; patients seem to require fewer doses and are better able to resume regular activities earlier. Narcotics are also used for treatment of pain in people with limited life expectancy. Because there often is undue concern about the possibility of addiction, many chronic pain sufferers with a short life expectancy receive inadequate pain relief. Most pain experts agree that it is appropriate to provide the level of narcotic necessary to relieve the severe, intractable pain of people whose life expectancy is limited. Oral medications are preferable to injection; tolerance usually is minimal after a few weeks. Addiction is not considered a problem in cancer patients.[38]

In people with cancer pain, morphine remains the most useful strong narcotic. The World Health Organization has recommended that oral morphine be part of the essential drug list and made available throughout the world as the drug of choice.[39] Oral forms of morphine are well absorbed from the gastrointestinal tract and have a half-life of about 2.5 hours and a duration of action of 4 to 6 hours. Liquid forms of the drug usually are given at 4-hour intervals to maintain an adequate blood level for analgesia, while minimizing the potential for toxic side effects.[40] A controlled-release tablet form of the drug, morphine sulfate pentahydrate (MS Contin), is available. The controlled-release tablets are designed to maintain a steady level of analgesia over a 12-hour period, allowing the patient to have long periods of rest and sleep through the night.

A recently developed approach to opioid administration is the use of continuous infusion pumps. Infusion pumps can be used to deliver narcotics by way of the subcutaneous or intravenous route on a continuous or demand basis.[41, 42] Continuous subcutaneous narcotic infusion can be accomplished using a portable infusion pump attached to a small butterfly needle inserted into the subcutaneous tissues. Continuous intravenous infusion of narcotics is also used, but this method presents problems with adjusting the infusion rate to meet changing dose requirements. An alternate approach, patient-controlled analgesia (PCA), has proved effective for relieving postoperative pain and for pain management in people with cancer.[41] This system consists of a microprocessor-controlled infusion pump that delivers the opioid drug through an intravenous cannula. A pushbutton on the system enables patients to deliver their own narcotic dose as needed. A lock-out system, which prevents overdosing, is programmed into the system.

The administration of narcotics into the intrathecal or epidural spaces for the relief of acute and chronic pain has gained popularity in clinical practice.[43] The procedure requires the introduction of a catheter into the epidural or intrathecal space by an anesthesiologist or other physician trained in the technique. With this method, every precaution must be taken that no drugs or solutions are given that could damage the spinal cord. This method offers the advantage of providing effective analgesia while minimizing the central depressant effects common to systemic narcotic administration.[37] The intrathecal or epidural administration route is particularly effective in patients who have had surgery and in whom respiratory function is already compromised (*e.g.,* chest trauma, respiratory insufficiency, or obesity). The procedure is also used for chronic pain such as that associated with cancer or long-term debilitating diseases. This type of pain control is based on the finding of opioid receptors in the cell bodies of the primary afferent neurons in the dorsal root ganglia and in the dorsal horn cells of the spinal cord that are involved in pain transmission.

Tricyclic Antidepressants. The fact that the pain-suppression system has nonendorphin synapses raises the possibility that potent centrally acting nonopiate drugs may be useful in relieving pain. Serotonin has been shown to play an important role in producing analgesia. The tricyclic antidepressant drugs that block the removal of serotonin from the synaptic cleft (imipramine, amitriptyline, and doxepin) have been shown to produce pain relief in some people. The drugs are particularly useful in some chronic painful conditions, such as postherpetic neuralgia.

Anticonvulsant Drugs. Certain anticonvulsant drugs, such as carbamazepine (Tegretol) and phenytoin (Dilantin), have specific analgesic effects that are effective in some pain conditions. These drugs, which suppress spontaneous neuronal firing, are particularly useful in the management of pain that occurs after nerve injury.

Placebo Response. An interesting phenomenon that deserves comment is the placebo response (Latin, "I will please"). The definition of a placebo can include the use of any treatment strategy that produces a positive placebo response. This positive reaction occurs because of the person's belief that the treatment will be effective, rather than because of any specific or therapeutic properties of the placebo itself. For example, a *positive placebo reactor* might report pain relief after the administration of a medication believed to be an analgesic when in fact it was composed of an inert substance.

At one time, placebo reactors were thought to have psychogenic or functional pain that was more imaginary than real. Newer research indicates that most people are, to a greater or lesser degree, placebo reactors. In fact, numerous studies have shown that a minimum of 20% to 40% of those with objective physical stimuli for pain consistently report pain relief from a placebo.

Placebos are not recommended as a test to determine if pain is imaginary or real, mild or severe, nor are they recommended as a means of assessing other physiologic or psychological reactions, such as changes in blood pressure, respiratory rate, heart rate, gastrointestinal activity, and temperature.

SURGICAL INTERVENTION

Surgery for severe intractable pain of either peripheral or central origin has met with some success. It can be used to remove the cause or block the transmission of pain. People with phantom limb pain, severe neuralgia, inoperable cancer of certain types, or causalgia sometimes suffer so intensively that they consider suicide as their only means of escape. In these extreme cases, surgery may be the only remaining treatment that seems to offer relief from the agony. Surgical methods to relieve pain usually are considered a last resort because damage to nerve cell bodies is irreversible. In addition, a penalty is paid because of the damage to other systems, predisposing the patient to other problems. Although severed

axons may regenerate, full recovery is highly unlikely. After a few weeks or months, the pain often returns and may be more disturbing than the condition for which the surgery was done. Regenerating nerve fibers may give rise to dysesthesias (extremely uncomfortable sensations); but if survival time is short, surgery may be warranted. In some cases, such as removal of a tumor pressing on nerve fibers or removal of an inflamed appendix, pain is completely relieved.

Surgery to block the transmission of pain signals along peripheral or central pathways may be successful. Peripherally, nerve section (neurotomy) or section of a dorsal root ganglion (rhizotomy) is not uncommon; some success has been reported for this type of surgery, particularly in trigeminal neuralgia.

At the spinal cord level, cordotomy (severing of the anterolateral quadrant of the cord) and tractotomy (interruption of the lateral spinothalamic tract) may require deep incisions into the cord to give adequate relief. With such deep incision, bladder function may be affected. The success of these types of surgery depends on the source of pain and the cord level involved. Electrical stimulation or pharmacologic agents, or both, often are used either to determine the appropriate surgical site or to eliminate the need for surgery.

Hypophysectomy, the removal of the pituitary gland, has an interesting history. It was done originally in efforts to prevent metastasis in certain hormone-dependent cancers, including some breast cancers. It was found, rather unexpectedly, that the pain often was immediately and totally relieved. It is now most likely to be used to relieve intractable pain caused by disseminated cancer of the prostate or breast that cannot be controlled by morphine or more localized means. The mechanism of pain relief is not yet understood. It is particularly mysterious because the pituitary is a rich source of endogenous opioids.

INTERDISCIPLINARY APPROACH

The Clinical Practice Guidelines for Acute Pain Management: Operative and Medical Procedures and Trauma emphasize the need for a collaborative, interdisciplinary approach to pain control, including members of the health care team and input from the patient and the patient's family, when appropriate.[20]

The interdisciplinary approach to complex chronic pain was introduced more than 30 years ago. Today, a number of pain clinics have been established. This team approach uses the knowledge and expertise of many health professionals to diagnose and manage complex types of pain. Besides being useful clinically, the team approach is effective in both teaching and collaborative research. The acute pain model assumes an objective cause that can be treated and diminished or eliminated within a short time, but the most perplexing difficulties are those relating to chronic pain. This approach has demonstrated its value in addressing many of the chronic pain problems from the physical, physiologic, and psychosocial aspects simultaneously.

PAIN MANAGEMENT IN CHILDREN

Pain is multidimensional, and each person is affected differently. When the problems of pain are addressed, elderly people and children may require special attention compared with young or middle-aged adults.

One startling finding has been that children, unlike adults, often are permitted to suffer intense postoperative pain even when pain medication has been ordered and is available. One of the problems rests with the administration of fixed doses of opioid, ordered to be given as needed by the intramuscular route.[44] Although children are less able to articulate their needs than adults, pain medications often are ordered on an as-needed basis; when they are given, it is by the instrument most feared by children—a syringe and needle. Other factors that contribute to inadequate pain treatment in children include the incorrect belief that children do not feel pain or, if they do, do not remember it and a lack of specific knowledge about the assessment, physiology, pathology, and treatment of pain in children. Unfounded concerns about addiction and adverse effects, such as excess sedation and respiratory depression, contribute to the undertreatment of children.[44]

Circumcision, heel-lancing, and other noxious stimuli to preterm and full-term neonates result in physiologic changes. These include cardiorespiratory effects, such as marked increases in heart rate and blood pressure; large changes in transcutaneous partial pressure of oxygen; and increased palmar sweating. Hormonal and metabolic changes include increased plasma renin activity and increased plasma levels of epinephrine, norepinephrine, and cortisol. Marked hormonal changes associated with surgery under light anesthesia result in severe stress reactions and increased postoperative morbidity and mortality. Evidence is now mounting that the use of anesthetics for surgery in the neonate is not only recommended as effective but as necessary to prevent pathologic stress reactions.

In their well-referenced paper, Anand and Hickey discuss their own work and a number of other studies related to pain and its control in the neonate.[45] The same authors identify behavioral changes indicative of pain in neonates subjected to circumcision without anesthesia. They warn that the persistence of certain of these responses implies a greater capacity for memory than commonly is assumed. They suggest that memory of these experiences associated with pain and stress may disrupt normal adaptation of the neonate.

Pain in the human fetus and neonate presents special problems because it often is assumed that they suffer less intensely, or not at all, because of the immaturity of their nervous systems. Considerable research evidence suggests that by late gestation, pain pathways, cortical and subcortical pain centers, and neurochemical systems associated with pain transmission and modulation are developed and functional.[46] As with systems associated with pain perception in the adult, the neuropeptides and endogenous opioid systems also seem to be involved in the neonate. Endogenous opioids are released by the human fetus at birth and in response to fetal and neonatal distress.[47] β-Endorphin plasma concentrations increase with difficult births, and evidence suggests that birth asphyxia may be a potent stimulus to the release of these endogenous opioids.[48]

In children, complex relationships may occur between previous threats or experiences with pain and their current response. Like adults, children appear better able to cope with pain when they are informed about what is happening to them and helped to develop appropriate coping strategies. Doll play, various sensory inputs, films, and videotapes may help them cope. Distraction, hypnosis, guided-relaxation imagery, and other techniques can be used effectively, depending on the child's age. Children who have an inaccurate understanding of what is happening to them may develop fantasies of mutilation, become extremely anxious, and doubt their ability to cope. Realistic reassurance measures that promote their sense of control and coping abilities are recommended. The child's developmental level, position in the family, and understanding of what happened or is happening and why are only a few of the variables that need study. Allowing parents to be with the child can be a great comfort.

The Acute Pain Management Guideline Panel recommends that children receive systemic opioids by the intravenous, epidural, oral, or transmucosal route.[20] This is because intramuscular injections are painful and frightening to the child; many children would rather have pain than a "shot." Continuous intravenous infusions avoid fluctuating blood levels that occur with oral and intramuscular administration. The regular assessment of vital signs and level of consciousness is necessary when parenteral opioids are used for treating pain. Because of the wide interindividual and intraindividual variations in response to opioids, some children have adverse reactions despite the careful tritration of dose and intervals.[20]

PAIN MANAGEMENT IN ELDERLY PEOPLE

The literature regarding pain in elderly people is sparse, and more studies are needed. Several aspects require particular attention.[49] Many elderly people receive inappropriate doses of medications because of tissue changes resulting from the normal aging process. Abrupt hospitalization may cause disorientation, decreased exercise, loss of control over one's life, inability to express pain, and regression. Depression and fear of death may also cause special problems. Degenerative changes can result in intermittent or continuous chronic pain. These problems must be considered when dealing with pain in elderly people.

In summary, pain is an elusive and complex phenomenon; it is a symptom common to many illnesses. Pain is a highly individualized experience that is shaped by a person's culture and previous life experiences, and, thus, it is difficult to measure. Traditionally, there have been two principal theories of pain; specificity and pattern theories. Scientifically, pain is viewed within the context of nociception. Nociceptors are receptive nerve endings that respond to noxious stimuli. Neither theory accounts for the motivational, cognitive, cultural, and affective components of pain. Pain can be classified according to source, duration, objective signs, and areas of referral. Reactions to pain, which are affected by pain threshold, pain tolerance, and age factors, are manifested through physical reactions, physiologic responses, and psychosocial reactions. Referred pain is pain that is perceived at a site different from its point of origin but innervated by the same spinal segment.

Pain may occur with or without an adequate stimulus, or it may be absent in the presence of an adequate stimulus—either of which describes a pain disorder. There may be analgesia (lack of pain without loss of consciousness), hyperalgesia (increased sensitivity to pain), hypalgesia (decreased sensitivity to pain), or hyperpathia (an unpleasant and prolonged response to pain).

Pain can be either acute or chronic; the latter is particularly difficult to manage. Controversy continues as to whether chronic pain should be viewed as a physiologic phenomenon with psychological correlates or as a psychological phenomenon with physiologic correlates. A growing body of data suggest that the latter definition may eliminate many of the chronic pain management problems.

Treatment modalities include the use of physiologic and behavioral measures, heat and cold, stimulation-induced analgesic methods, and pharmacologic agents singly or in combination. It is becoming apparent that even with chronic pain, the most effective approach is early treatment or even prevention. Once pain is present, the greatest success in the management of problems related to assessment and appropriate effective treatment is achieved with the use of an interdisciplinary approach. Pain management in both children and elderly people requires special consideration.

■ SPECIAL TYPES OF PAIN

HEADACHE

Headache is discussed here because it is a type of pain that is recognized almost universally. Although headache is extremely common, its cause frequently is not known. There are many types of headache, the most common of which are tension-type (muscle contraction) headache and migraine headache. Hypertension as well as traction on intracranial pain-sensitive structures by tumors, subdural hemorrhages, or the weight of the brain after cerebrospinal fluid removal can also induce headaches. Depression can result in headache and is a frequently overlooked cause in children and adolescents.[50] Other causes of headaches include systemic infections with fever, seizure disorders, and hypoxic conditions, such as cyanotic heart disease and severe asthma. Physicians estimate that at least 20% of the complaints they receive are related to headache.[51] Bille's study revealed that 40% of children have experienced headache by age 7 and 75%, by age 15.[52]

Although it is difficult to classify and define diseases, the field of pain related to headache presents particular problems. The absence of laboratory tests, which could serve as diagnostic criteria for any of the primary headache forms, reflects the paucity of physiologic data available. There are typical and pure forms of headache, but transitional forms also occur, and these cause confusion. Over time a person may have more than one form of headache, and those they have may undergo not only quantitative but also qualitative changes. Therefore, a new system has been developed that classifies headaches, rather than people. A person may have more than one form of headache; however, each particular headache can fit only one set of diagnostic criteria.

Until 1988, most headache classifications were derived from a 1962 publication of the Ad Hoc Committee on the Classification of Headache.[53] In 1988, the first edition of The Classification and Diagnostic Criteria for Headache Disorders, Cranial Neuralgias, and Facial Pain, prepared by the Headache Classification Committee of the International Headache Society, was published, along with ten general rules considered essential to the correct use of this new system.[54] The new classification system is constructed in an hierarchical manner with up to four digits, and there are operational diagnostic criteria for all headache disorders. Routine diagnoses are expected at the one- or two-digit level. Diagnoses to the fourth digit are expected at specialized diagnostic and treatment centers. Although the primary purpose for development of this classification system was research, the operational diagnostic criteria are expected to influence the diagnosis and treatment of headaches. The chosen criteria for a particular diagnosis represent a compromise between sensitivity and specificity and are expected to help clarify some of the problems of the 1962 classification system. The major classifications of the new system are given in Chart 48-1. Subclassifications to the second digit are included for migraine and tension-type headaches because these are the two most commonly encountered types of headaches in clinical practice.

TENSION-TYPE HEADACHE

Under the new classification system, the various muscle contraction and psychogenic headaches are called tension-type headaches. The most common form of headache in adults and adolescents is the tension headache resulting from sustained contraction of the muscles of the neck and scalp. Contraction of these muscles causes pressure on nerves in the

CHART 48-1: CLASSIFICATION AND DIAGNOSTIC CRITERIA FOR HEADACHE DISORDERS, CRANIAL NEURALGIAS, AND FACIAL PAIN

1. Migraine
   1.1 Migraine without aura
   1.2 Migraine with aura
   1.3 Ophthalmoplegic migraine
   1.4 Retinal migraine
   1.5 Childhood periodic syndromes that may be precursors to or associated with migraine
   1.6 Complications with migraine
   1.7 Migrainous disorder not fulfilling above criteria
2. Tension-type headache
   2.1 Episodic tension-type headache
   2.2 Chronic tension-type headache
   2.3 Headache of the tension-type not fulfilling the above criteria
3. Cluster headache and chronic paroxysmal hemicrania
4. Miscellaneous headaches unassociated with structural lesion
5. Headache associated with head trauma
6. Headache associated with vascular disorders
7. Headache associated with nonvascular intracranial disorders
8. Headache associated with substances or their withdrawal
9. Headache associated with noncephalic infection
10. Headache associated with metabolic disorder
11. Headache or facial pain associated with disorder of cranium, neck, eyes, ears, nose, sinuses, teeth, mouth or other facial or cranial structures
12. Cranial neuralgias, nerve trunk pain, and deafferentation pain
13. Headache not classifiable

(Adapted from Oleson, J. [1988]. Classification and diagnostic criteria for headache disorders, cranial neuralgias and facial pain. *Cephalgia, 8*(Suppl 7):13–19.)

area, and it can also constrict blood vessels at the base of the neck. When these mechanisms increase pressure, waste products (*e.g.*, lactic acid) also accumulate, causing more pain. The usual source of this tensing of muscles is an unconscious reaction to stress. Any activity that requires the head to be held in one position, such as typing, repairing jewelry, or using a microscope, can cause muscle contraction headache. Even sleeping in a cold room or with the neck in an inappropriate or strained position can cause a tension headache.

Prevention and treatment are best approached by identifying and removing precipitating factors. This can include such measures as sleeping in a warm room, wearing a scarf to avoid muscle spasms when exposed to the cold, and using a small pillow under the neck for sleeping. Proper eye care, light, and posture during reading as well as frequently exercising the neck and shoulders should lower the incidence of muscle spasms. Sleep, deep relaxation exercises, and massage of sore or tense muscles can help to decrease or eliminate painful headaches. Biofeedback (to be discussed) may be used in the treatment of tension headache. The use of medication often can be decreased or eliminated by successfully using one or more of the above alternative approaches to pain relief.

MIGRAINE HEADACHE

Migraine headache affects between 12 million and 16 million Americans. It occurs in all age groups, even infants. Incidence according to sex is equal in young children, but in adolescents and adults, it occurs three times more frequently in females than in males.[55, 56] In some cases, it can be associated with certain days in the menstrual cycle. The disorder is characterized by paroxysmal attacks of intense head pain. Throbbing unilateral pain, photophobia, anorexia, and nausea with vomiting frequently accompany these headaches. Such neurologic deficits as hemiparesis and hemisensory defects may be noted with vasoconstriction followed by vasodilatation, or normal blood flow followed by hyperemia.

In contrast to the 1962 headache classification system,[53] which included migraine headaches in the vascular headache classification, the 1988 system has added a separate classification for migraine headaches.[54] This is in accord with recent research findings that have demonstrated a probable neurogenic cause to this type of headache.

The two major types of migraine are called *migraine without aura* (formerly referred to as common migraine) and *migraine with aura* (formerly called classic or classical migraine). An aura is a complex of focal neurologic symptoms that initiates or accompanies a migraine headache attack. About 85% of people with migraine do not have an aura.[55] Prodromal symptoms of migraine without aura may precede the headache by 1 or 2 days or by several hours. These symptoms differ from an aura, which precedes the headache by no more than 60 minutes. The prodramata may consist of one or more alterations that affect mood (depression or euphoria), consciousness (drowsiness or alertness), or energy (sluggishness or increased energy). Autonomic manifestations such as yawning or unusual hunger may occur. Any of these symptoms may follow the headache as well as precede it. The headache itself usually develops gradually. The initial, relatively mild headache becomes moderate or severe with pulsating and throbbing qualities and usually is one-sided. Nausea with or without vomiting and hypersensitivity to light, noise, and odors are the most common associated phenomena.

The aura of migraine typically begins 20 to 30 minutes before the headache itself and disappears soon after the headache begins.[56] Alterations in sensory or motor function can occur. A typical visual aura can consist of flashing lights, blind spots, double vision, or hallucinations. These symptoms are consistent with foci of cerebral ischemia and, therefore, changes in oxygen availability. Pain receptors are sensitive to this diminution in oxygen.

The old concept that vasospasm causes the aura of migraine or the vasodilation has largely been discarded. It is now thought that the aura represents a spreading depression of neuronal activity in the cerebral cortex; the decreased blood flow is thought to represent the decreased metabolism rather than the ischemia of vasospasm.[57] It is also thought that the pain of the migraine headache is related, not to the dilated blood vessels, but to their increased permeability and the exudation of polypeptides. In recent years, it has been shown that substance P and other polypeptides are released by the perivascular nerve endings. It is thought that these polypeptides play an important role in initiating the headache. These observations are consistent with current theory, which attributes migraine headaches to dysfunctional vascular endothelial cells.[58]

Migraine headache sufferers are advised to moderate caffeine intake and avoid large fluctuations in estrogen levels by eliminating oral contraceptives and postmenopausal hormones. Reducing psychological and environmental stresses can also decrease the precipitation of attacks. Dietary changes include avoiding tyramine-containing foods, cured meats, and monosodium glutamate (Chart 48-2). Smoke-filled rooms and hypoglycemia, whether early-morning or fast-induced, can increase migraine attacks.

When dietary and life-style changes and non-

CHART 48-2: FOODS THAT CAUSE MIGRAINE HEADACHE

Tyramine-Containing Foods

Red wine
Strong or aged cheese
Smoked herring
Chicken livers
Canned figs
Broad bean pods

Sodium Nitrate–Containing Cured Meats

Bacon
Hot dogs
Salami

Fruits

Avocados
Bananas
Citrus fruits

Dairy Products

Yogurt
Sour cream

Baked Goods

Fresh bread
Coffee cake
Doughnuts

Other

Monosodium glutamate
Chocolate
Nuts, peanut butter
Fermented, pickled, and marinated foods
Onions

pharmacologic approaches, such as biofeedback and relaxation techniques, fail to achieve relief, medications may be necessary. The goal is prevention because it is much more effective than treatment. The drugs most commonly used in the migraine prophylaxis are β-adrenergic blocking drugs (e.g., propranolol, nadolol). Tricyclic antidepressant drugs have central analgesic effects apart from their antidepressant effects and can be highly useful in migraine prophylaxis. Calcium-channel blocking drugs, particularly verapamil and diltiazem, are also used in migraine prophylaxis. Other drugs used are monoamine oxidase inhibitors, platelet antagonists, and steroidal and nonsteroidal antiinflammatory drugs.

Administration of ergotamine tartrate at the onset of symptoms is effective in most cases, including adults, adolescents, and children over age 10. This drug should not be used in pregnancy because of its oxytocic effect.

Serotonin (5-hydroxytryptamine) is thought to play a central role in the pathogenesis of migraine.[58] Its metabolism is abnormal in people with migraine, and intravenous administration of 5-hydroxytryptamine can alleviate migraine attacks. Antimigraine drugs share the ability to activate 5-hydroxytryptamine receptors. The drug sumatriptan, a selective agonist of 5-hydroxytryptamine, has recently been shown to be effective in the treatment of acute migraine.[59]

TEMPOROMANDIBULAR JOINT PAIN

Temporomandibular joint (TMJ) syndrome is one of the major causes of headaches. It usually is caused by an imbalance in the joint movement because of poor bite, bruxism (teeth grinding), or joint problems such as inflammation, trauma, and degenerative changes. The pain is almost always referred. Headache associated with this syndrome is common in both adults and children and can cause chronic pain problems. Treatment of TMJ pain is aimed at correcting the problem, and in some cases, this may be difficult.

CAUSALGIA

Causalgia is an extremely painful condition that follows sudden and violent deformation of peripheral nerves. This problem often is initiated in combat because of nerve damage by high-velocity missiles (*e.g.*, bullets or metal fragments). The nerve typically is damaged but not severed. The classic syndrome was described by Mitchell in 1864 for men sustaining gunshot wounds to the extremities.[60] The median and sciatic nerves most commonly are affected. The pain is characteristically burning and can be elicited with the slightest movement or touch to the affected area. It is excruciating, and even clothing or puffs of air are sufficient to set it off in severe cases. It can be exacerbated by emotional upsets or any increased peripheral sympathetic nerve stimulation. Sympathetic components are part of all variations of causalgia. These are characterized by vascular and trophic (nutritive) changes to the skin, soft tissue, and bone. Reflex sympathetic dystrophy is a disorder of the sympathetic nervous system characterized by rubor or pallor, sweating or dryness, edema, pain, or skin atrophy (see Chapter 49).

Treatment by sympathetic blockade usually is successful and may be the reason this condition is considered a dysautonomia (*i.e.*, a dysfunction of the autonomic nervous system). In some cases, prolonged cooling and intravenous administration of guanethedine into the affected limb (with venous outflow blocked for several minutes) has been shown to alleviate the pain for days or longer.[17] Electrical stimulation of the large myelinated fibers that inner-

vate the area from which the pain arises is also effective. Controversy remains regarding the mechanisms involved in these pain-relief measures. The long-term use of narcotics is discouraged because of the danger of addiction. Effective treatment is imperative to prevent invalidism and, in severe cases, suicide.

NEURALGIA

Neuralgia is characterized by severe, brief, often repetitive attacks of lightning-like or throbbing pain. It occurs along the distribution of a spinal or cranial nerve and usually is precipitated by stimulation of the cutaneous region supplied by that nerve.

TRIGEMINAL NEURALGIA

Trigeminal neuralgia, or *tic douloureux*, is one of the most common and severe neuralgias. It is manifested by facial tics or grimaces and characterized by stabbing, paroxysmal attacks of pain that usually are limited to the unilateral sensory distribution of one or more branches of the trigeminal nerve, most often the maxillary division. Victims describe the pain as excruciating. It may be triggered by light touch, eating, swallowing, shaving, talking, chewing gum, washing the face, or sneezing or have no apparent cause. Stimulation of small-diameter afferent fibers is more effective in provoking attacks than cold, warm, or noxious stimuli. Abnormalities of facial sensation are not likely between attacks. Neurologic deficits are rare, as they are in neuralgias of cranial nerves VII, IX, and X.

Carbamazepine (Tegretol), which is a tricyclic compound, may be used to control the pain of trigeminal neuralgia and may delay or eliminate the need for surgery. Surgical release of vessels, dural structures, or scar tissue surrounding the semilunar ganglion or root in the middle cranial fossa often eliminates the symptoms. If not, destruction or blocking peripheral branches or central root of cranial nerve V produces loss of all sensation, including pain. A more satisfactory treatment is section of the descending spinal tract of nerve V in the brain stem. This may be effective because it removes background inflow of impulses on which spontaneous attacks depend. Dissociation of facial sensation occurs, in that pain and temperature disappear, but there is only a slight decrease in tactile activity. This neurosurgical procedure provides evidence that the nucleus caudalis of the trigeminal complex is necessary for the transmission of facial pain. Considerable controversy remains regarding the pathophysiology of trigeminal neuralgia.

POSTHERPETIC NEURALGIA

The pain associated with postherpetic neuralgia (herpes zoster, or shingles) follows recovery from an infection of the dorsal root ganglia and corresponding areas of innervation by the herpes zoster virus (see Chapter 11). Postherpetic neuralgia most often affects the thoracic spinal nerves. The ophthalmic division of the trigeminal nerve, which innervates the upper face and eye, is the cranial nerve most often affected.

Herpes zoster is caused by the same herpes virus that causes varicella (chickenpox) and is thought to represent a localized recurrent infection by the varicella virus that has remained latent in the dorsal root ganglia since the initial attack of chickenpox. Reactivation of viral replication is associated with a decline in immunity, such as that which occurs with aging. During the acute attack of herpes zoster, the reactivated virus travels centrifugally from the ganglia to the skin of the corresponding dermatomes, causing a localized vesicular eruption and hyperpathia (abnormally exaggerated subjective response to pain). In the acute infection, proportionately more of the large nerve fibers are destroyed. Regenerated fibers appear to have smaller diameters. Older patients have pain, dysesthesia, and hyperesthesia after the acute phase; these are increased by minor stimuli. Because there is a relative loss of large fibers with age, elderly people are particularly prone to suffering because of the shift in the proportion of large- to small-diameter nerve fibers.

Postherpetic neuralgia is extremely distressing and most efficaciously treated early (*i.e.*, in the first 3 months), before the condition becomes established. High doses of systemic corticosteroids and oral acyclovir (a drug that inhibits herpesvirus DNA replication) may reduce the incidence of postherpetic neuralgia when used early in the disease.[61] A tricyclic antidepressant drug, such as amitriptyline, may be used for pain relief. Regional nerve blockade (stellate ganglion, epidural, local infiltration, or peripheral nerve) has been used with limited success.

PHANTOM LIMB PAIN

Phantom limb pain, a type of neurologic pain, follows amputation of a limb or part of a limb. At first, it is characterized by sensations of tingling, heat and cold, or heaviness. The pain that follows is burning, shooting, or crushing. It may disappear spontaneously or persist for many years. The basic mechanisms involved remain controversial. One theory is that abnormal sensory input secondary to limb amputation or trauma alters the pattern of information processing in the CNS. A closed self-exciting neuro-

nal loop in the posterior horn of the spinal cord is postulated to send impulses to the brain, resulting in pain. Even the slightest irritation to the amputated limb area can initiate this cycle. In some people, neuromas form near the regenerating end of a nerve. It is known that when a peripheral nerve is cut, the scar tissue that forms becomes a barrier to regenerating outgrowth of the axon. The growing axon often becomes trapped in the scar tissue, forming a tangled growth (neuroma) of small-diameter axons, including both primary nociceptive afferents and sympathetic efferents.

These afferents show increased sensitivity to innocuous mechanical stimuli and to sympathetic activity and circulating catecholamines. The absence of the inhibitory effects of the large-diameter fibers may contribute to the pain problem.

Treatment has been accomplished by the use of sympathetic blocks, transcutaneous electrical nerve stimulation of the large myelinated afferents innervating the area, hypnosis and relaxation training. Controversy continues as to the precise mechanisms responsible for the usefulness of these methods. Many of the complications of limb amputation can be alleviated by immediate fitting of a prosthesis and conscientious stump care. Stump care includes bandaging to support the remaining muscles, protect the soft tissues, and prevent the formation of edematous fluids. Care must be taken to prevent infection. After the amputation wound has healed, the stump must be shrunk and shaped into a conical form to permit the correct fitting of a prosthesis. This is done by the proper application of elastic bandages or devices. The reader is referred to a specialty text for more complete information on stump care.

In summary, pain and pain disorders are universal experiences. Headache is so common that it is experienced by 75% of the population by age 15. There are many types of headache, the most common of which are tension-type (muscle contraction) headache and migraine headache. In 1988, the first edition of The Classification and Diagnostic Criteria for Headache Disorders, Cranial Neuralgias, and Facial Pain, prepared by the Headache Classification Committee of the International Headache Society, was published, along with 10 general rules considered essential to the correct use of this new system. TMJ syndrome is one of the major causes of headaches. It usually is caused by an imbalance in the joint movement because of poor bite, teeth grinding, or joint problems such as inflammation, trauma, and degenerative changes.

Causalgia is an extremely painful condition that follows sudden and violent deformation of peripheral nerves. Neuralgia is characterized by severe, brief, often repetitiously occurring attacks of lightning-like or throbbing pain that occurs along the distribution of a spinal or cranial nerve and usually is precipitated by stimulation of the cutaneous region supplied by that nerve. Trigeminal neuralgia, or *tic douloureux*, is one of the most common and severe neuralgias. It is manifested by facial tics or grimaces. Postherpetic neuralgia or shingles is caused by an infection of the dorsal root ganglia and corresponding areas of innervation by the herpes zoster virus. Phantom limb pain, a neurologic pain, follows amputation of a limb or part of a limb.

■ REFERENCES

1. Bkinkov, S.M. (1968). *The human brain in figures and tables* (p. 57). New York: Plenum Press.
2. Martin, J.H., & Jessell, T.M. (1991). Anatomic substrates for somatic sensation. In E.R. Kandel & J.H. Schwartz (Eds.). *Principles of neuroscience* (3rd ed., pp. 353–366). New York: Elsevier.
3. Guyton, A. (1991). *Textbook of medical physiology* (8th ed., p. 515). Philadelphia: W.B. Saunders.
4. Zborowski, M. (1952). Cultural components in response to pain. *Journal of Social Issues, 8,* 16.
5. Sternbach, R. (Ed.). (1978). *The psychology of pain*. New York: Raven Press.
6. McCaffery, M., & Beebe, A. (1989). *Pain: Clinical manual for nursing practice*. St. Louis: C.V. Mosby.
7. Merskey, H. (1978). Pain and personality. In R.A. Sternbach (Ed.). *The psychology of pain* (pp. 123–124). New York: Raven Press.
8. Melzack, R., & Wall, P.D. (1965). Pain mechanisms: A new theory. *Science, 150,* 971.
9. Ottoson, D. (1983). *Physiology of the nervous system* (pp. 462–463). New York: Oxford University Press.
10. Kelley, D.D., & Jessell, T.M. (1991). Pain and analgesia. In E.R. Kandel & J.H. Schwartz (Eds.) *Principles of neuroscience* (3rd ed., pp. 385–399). New York: Elsevier.
11. Cooper, J.R., Bloom, F.E., & Roth, R.H. (1991). *The biochemical basis of neuropharmacology* (6th ed., p. 263). New York: Oxford University Press.
12. Basabaum, A.I. (1987). Cytochemical studies of the neural circuitry underlying pain and pain control. *Acta Neurochirurgica (Wien), 38*(Suppl.), 5.
13. Payne, R.P. (1987). Anatomy, physiology, and neuropharmacology of cancer pain. *Medical Clinics of North America, 71*(2), 153.
14. Fields, H.L., Heinricher, M.M., & Mason P. (1991). Neurotransmitters in nociceptive modulatory circuits. *Review of Neuroscience, 14,* 219.
15. Saria, A. (1987). The role of substance P and other neuropeptides in transmission of pain. *Acta Neurochirurgica (Wien), 38*(Suppl.), 33.
16. Grichnick, K., & Ferrante, F.M. (1991). The difference between acute and chronic pain. *Mount Sinai Journal of Medicine, 58,* 217–220.
17. Fields, H.L. (1987). *Pain* (pp. 121–122, 141, 1123, 1161). New York: McGraw-Hill.
18. Beecher, H.K. (1956). Nature of significance of wound to pain experienced. *Journal of the American Medical Association, 161,* 1609.
19. Fishbain, A.A., Goldberg, M., Meagher, B.R., et al. (1986). Male and female chronic pain patients categorized by DSM-III psychiatric diagnostic criteria. *Pain, 26,* 181.
20. Acute Pain Management Guideline Panel. (1992, Feb.). *Acute pain management: Operative or medical procedures and trauma* (AHCPR Pub. No. 92-0032). Rockville, MD: Agency for Health Care Policy and Research, Public Health Service, U.S. Department of Health and Human Services.
21. McGuire, D.B. (1984). The measurement of clinical pain. *Nursing Research, 33,* 152.
22. Hanken, A., & McDowell, W. (1964). Development of a rating scale to measure pain. In M. Newton, W. Hunt, W. McDowell, et al. (Eds.). *A study of nurse action in relief of pain.* Columbus: Ohio State University School of Nursing.
23. Johnson, J.E., & Rice, V.H. (1974). Sensory and distress components of pain: Implications for the study of clinical pain. *Nursing Research, 23,* 203.
24. McGuire, D.B. (1984). Assessment of pain in cancer patients using the McGill Pain Questionnaire. *Oncology Nursing Forum, 11*(6), 32.
25. Melzack, R. (1975). The McGill Pain Questionnaire: Major properties and scoring methods. *Pain, 22,* 1.
26. Licht, S. (1984). History of therapeutic heat and cold. In J.F. Lehman (Ed.). *Therapeutic heat and cold* (3rd ed.). Baltimore: Williams & Wilkins.
27. Nigel, P.P. (1988). Heat and cold. In P.E. Wells, V. Frampton, & D. Bowsher (Eds.). *Pain management in physical therapy* (pp. 169–180). E. Norwalk, CT: Appleton & Lange.
28. Keating, W. (1961). Cold vasodilatation after adrenalin. *Journal of Physiology, 159,* 101.
29. Chapman, C.R. (1979). Contribution of research on acupuncture and transcutaneous electrical stimulation to the understanding of pain mechanisms and pain relief. In F. Roland, J. Beers, & E.G. Bassett (Eds.). *Mechanisms of pain and analgesic compounds* (pp. 7–183). New York: Raven Press.
30. Hymes, A. (1984). A review of the historical area of electricity. In J.S. Mannheimer & G.N. Lampe (Eds.). *Clinical transcutaneous electrical stimulation* (p. 1). Philadelphia: F.A. Davis.
31. Michel, T.H. (Ed.). (1985). *International perspectives in physical therapy* (pp. 96–97, 129–130). Edinburgh: Churchill Livingstone.
32. Wolf, S.L. (1984). Neurophysiologic mechanisms of pain modulation: Relevance to TENS. In J.S. Mannheimer & G.N. Lampe (Eds.). *Clinical transcutaneous electrical stimulation* (p. 41). Philadelphia: F.A. Davis.
33. Anderson, S.A. (1979). Pain control by sensory stimulation. In J.J. Bonica (Ed.). *Advances in pain research and therapy* (p. 569). New York: Raven Press.
34. Sjolund, B.H., Terenius, L., & Erickson, M.B.E. (1977). Increased cerebrospinal fluid levels of endorphin after electroacupuncture. *Acta Physiologica Scandinavica, 100,* 382.
35. Ignelzi, R.J., & Nyquist, J.K. (1979). Excitability changes in peripheral nerve fibers after repetitive electrical stimulation: Implications for pain modulation. *Journal of Neurosurgery, 51,* 824.
36. Sherman, J.E., & Liebeskind, J.C. (1980). An endorphinergic centrifugal substrate of pain modulation: Recent findings, current concepts and complexities. In J.J. Bonica (Ed.). *Pain.* New York: Raven Press.
37. Jaffe, J.H., & Martin, W.R. (1990). Opioid analgesics and antagonists. In A.G. Gilman, L.S. Goodman, T.W. Rall, et al. (Eds.). *Goodman and Gilman's The pharmacological basis of therapeutics* (8th ed., pp. 485–497). New York: Macmillan.
38. Melzak, R. (1990). The tragedy of needless pain. *Scientific American, 262*(2), 2–8.
39. Swerdlow, M., & Stjernward, J. (1982). Cancer pain relief—an urgent problem. *World Health Forum, 3,* 325–330.
40. Foley, K.M., & Inturrisi, C.E. (1987). Analgesic therapy in cancer pain: Principles and practice. *Medical Clinics of North America, 71,* 207.
41. Fields, H.L., & Levine, J.D. (1984). Pain—mechanisms and management. *Western Journal of Medicine, 141,* 347.
42. Dennis, E.M.P. (1984). An ambulatory infusion pump

for pain control: A nursing approach to home care. *Cancer Nursing, 7,* 309.

43. Lieb, R.A., & Hurtig, J.B. (1985). Epidural and intrathecal narcotics for pain management. *Heart and Lung, 14,* 164.

44. Haberkern, C.M., Tyler, D.C., & Krane, E.J. (1991). Postoperative pain management in children. *Mount Sinai Journal of Medicine (NY), 58,* 247–255.

45. Anand, K.J.S., & Hickey, P.R. (1987). Pain and its effects in the human neonate and fetus. *New England Journal of Medicine, 317*(21), 1321.

46. Gilles, F.J., Shankle, W., & Dooling, E.C. (1983). Myelinated tracts: Growth patterns. In F.H. Gilles, A. Leviton, & E.C. Dooling (Eds.). *The developing human brain: Growth and epidemiologic neuropathology* (pp. 117–183). Boston: John Wright.

47. Gautray, J.P., Jolivet, A., Vielh, J.P., et al. (1977). Presence of immunoassayable *b*-endorphin in human amnionic fluid: Elevation in cases of fetal distress. *American Journal of Obstetrics and Gynecology, 129,* 211.

48. Puolakka, J., Kauppila, A., Leppaluoto, J., et al. (1982). Elevated beta-endorphin immunoreactivity in umbilical cord blood after complicated delivery. *Acta Obstetricia et Gynecologica Scandinavica, 61,* 513.

49. Wachter-Shikora, N.L. (1983). The elderly patient in pain and the acute care setting. *Nursing Clinics of North America, 18*(2), 395.

50. Rothner, A.D. (1991). Headaches in adolescents: Diagnosis and management. *Medical Clinics of North America, 73*(3), 653–660.

51. Diamond, S. (1983). In A.P. Kahn (Ed.). *Headaches* (p. 4). Chicago: Contemporary Books.

52. Bille, B. (1962). Migraine in school children. *Acta Paediatrica Scandinavica, 51*(Suppl. 136), 1.

53. Friedman, A.P. (Chair). (1962). Ad Hoc Committee on the Classification of Headache: Classification of headache. *Archives of Neurology, 6,* 173–176.

54. Olesen, J. (Chair). (1988). Headache Classification Committee of the International Headache Society. The classification and diagnostic criteria for headache disorders, cranial neuralgias, and facial pain. *Cephalalgia, 8*(Suppl. 7), 1–96.

55. Stewart, W.F., Lipton, R.B., Celentano, D.D., et al. (1992). Prevalence of migraine headache in the United States. *Journal of the American Medical Association, 267,* 64–69.

56. Linet, M.S., Stewart, W.F., Celentano, D.D., et al. (1989). An epidemiological study of headaches among adolescents and young adults. *Journal of the American Medical Association, 261,* 2211–2216.

57. Solomon, S. (1991). Migraine: Current approaches to diagnosis and management. *Hospital Practice, 26*(4A), 141–160.

58. Appenzeller, O. (1991). Pathogenesis of migraine. *Medical Clinics of North America, 75*(3), 763–789.

59. The Subcutaneous Sumatriptan International Study Group. (1991). Treatment of migraine headache with sumatriptan. *New England Journal of Medicine, 325,* 316–321.

60. Hitchcocke, K.E. (1986). Current views on the role of neurosurgery for pain relief. In M. Swerdlow (Ed.). *The therapy of pain* (2nd ed., p. 187). Norwell, MA: MTP Press.

61. Goldstein, S.M., & Odom, R.B. (1992). Skin and appendages. In S.A. Schroeder, L.M. Tierney, S.J. McPhee, et al. (Eds.). *Current medical diagnosis and treatment* (pp. 84–85). E. Norwalk, CT: Appleton & Lange.

■ BIBLIOGRAPHY

Bonica, J.J. (1991). History of pain concepts and pain therapy. *Mount Sinai Journal of Medicine (NY), 58,* 191–202.

Diamond, S. (1991). Migraine headaches. *Medical Clinics of North America, 75,* 545–565.

Eland, J.M., & Coy, J.A. (1990). Assessing pain in the critically ill child. *Focus on Critical Care (AACN), 17,* 469–479.

Grunau, R.V.E., & Craig, K. (1987). Pain expression in neonates: Facial action and cry. *Pain, 28,* 395–410.

Kahn, C.H., & Warfield, C.A. (1989). Orofacial pain. *Hospital Practice, 24*(2A), 247–271.

Katz, J., & Melzak, R. (1987). Referred sensations in chronic pain. *Pain, 28,* 51–59.

Koren, G., Butt, W., Chinyanga, H., et al. (1985). Postoperative morphine infusion in newborn infants: Assessment of disposition characteristics and safety. *Journal of Pediatrics, 107,* 963–967.

McCrory, L.B. (1991). A review of the second international symposium on pediatric pain. *Pediatric Nursing, 17,* 366–370.

Melzak, R. (1992 April). Phantom limbs. *Scientific American, 264,* 120–129.

Nation, E.M., & Warfield, C.A. (1989). Pain in the elderly. *Hospital Practice, 24*(7A), 113–118.

Page, G.G., & Halvorson, M. (1991). Pediatric nurses: The assessment and control of pain in preverbal infants. *Journal of Pediatric Nursing, 6,* 99–106.

Payan, D.G. (1989). Substance P: A modulator of neuroendocrine-immune function. *Hospital Practice, 24*(2A), 67–80.

Procacci, P., Zoppi, M., & Maresca, M. (1986). Clinical approach to visceral sensation. *Progress in Brain Research, 67,* 21–28.

Richlin, D.M. (1991). Nonnarcotic analgesics and tricyclic antidepressants for the treatment of chronic nonmalignant pain. *Mount Sinai Journal of Medicine (NY), 58,* 221–228.

Sorkin, L.S. (1991). Nociceptive transmission within the spinal cord. *Mount Sinai Journal of Medicine (NY), 58,* 208–215.

Tarbell, S.E., Cohen, T., & Marsh, J.L. (1992). The toddler-preschooler postoperative pain scale: An observational scale for measuring postoperative pain in children aged 1–5. Preliminary report. *Pain, 51,* 273–280.

Von Korff, M., Ormel, J., Keefe, F.J., et al. (1992). Grading the severity of chronic pain. *Pain, 51,* 133–149.

Wall, P.D. (1992). The placebo effect: An unpopular topic. *Pain, 51,* 1–3.

Wild, L., & Coyne, C. (1992). Epidural analgesia: The basics and beyond. *American Journal of Nursing, 92,* 26–36.

Woolsey, R.M. (1986). Chronic pain following spinal cord injury. *Journal of the American Paraplegia Society, 9*(3–4), 39–41.

Young, P.A. (1986). The anatomy of the spinal cord pain paths: A review. *Journal of the American Paraplegia Society, 9*(3–4), 28–38.

CHAPTER 49

NORMAL AND ALTERED AUTONOMIC NERVOUS SYSTEM FUNCTION

CAROL MATTSON PORTH
ROBIN L. CURTIS

◼ OBJECTIVES

After you have studied this chapter, you should be able to meet the following objectives:

◼ Compare the sensory and motor components of the autonomic nervous system (ANS) with those of the somatic nervous system.

◼ Describe major sources of afferent input to the ANS.

◼ Compare the characteristics of central nervous system outflow, general effector functions, and neurotransmission for the sympathetic and parasympathetic nervous systems.

◼ Describe the synthesis, reuptake, and metabolism of catecholamines.

◼ Describe the synthesis and metabolism of acetylcholine.

◼ Differentiate the main locations of α_1-, α_2-, β_1-, and β_2-receptors.

◼ Differentiate the locations of muscarinic and nicotinic receptors.

◼ Compare the general features of effector function produced by interruption of somatic motor neuron and an autonomic motor neuron.

◼ State the effect of interruption of ANS innervation on the eye and vision; skin and thermal regulation; circulatory system and control of blood flow and blood pressure; gastrointestinal system and gastrointestinal function; metabolic functions; and sexual function.

◼ State the pathology associated with a pheochromocytoma.

◼ List the possible manifestations of autonomic peripheral neuropathies.

◼ Describe the condition called progressive autonomic failure.

◼ Describe at least three diagnostic methods of assessing autonomic function.

Carol Mattson Porth: PATHOPHYSIOLOGY: CONCEPTS OF ALTERED HEALTH STATES, 4th ed. © 1994, 1990, 1986, 1982 J.B. Lippincott Company

The ability to maintain homeostasis and perform the activities of daily living in an ever-changing physical environment is largely vested in the autonomic nervous system (ANS). The ANS functions at the subconscious level and is involved in regulating, adjusting, and coordinating vital visceral functions such as blood pressure and blood flow, body temperature, respiration, digestion, metabolism, and elimination. Common synonyms for the ANS are the *involuntary nervous system* and *vegetative nervous system*. The ANS is strongly affected by emotional influences and is involved in many of the expressive aspects of behavior. Blushing, pallor, palpitations of the heart, clammy hands, and dry mouth are several emotional expressions that are mediated through the ANS. Of recent interest has been the use of biofeedback and relaxation exercises for modifying the subconscious functions of the ANS.

For purposes of organization, this chapter has been divided into two parts: (1) the organization and control of ANS function and (2) disorders of ANS function. Additional content on ANS function as it relates to specific alterations in body function is integrated into other chapters of the book.

■ ORGANIZATION AND CONTROL OF AUTONOMIC NERVOUS SYSTEM FUNCTION

The nervous system can be conceptually divided into the somatic and autonomic nervous systems. The somatic nervous system, with its sensory and motor components, provides contact with the external world and regulation of behaviors directed toward interacting with the external environment. The ANS functions by responding to stimuli from within the body and by maintaining the constancy of the internal environment. Although the nervous system can be conceptually divided, the distinction between the somatic and the autonomic nervous system becomes blurred when the higher levels of integrated responses are considered. Indeed, almost all somatic reflexes have a visceral component and vice versa. For example, the response to cold stimulates contraction of the piloerector skin muscles (goose bumps) by way of the ANS and contraction of the voluntary muscles (shivering), which is controlled by the somatic nervous system. Exposure to a bright light produces avoidance movements (somatic) as well as constriction of the pupils (ANS).

As with the somatic nervous system, the ANS is represented in both the central nervous system (CNS) and the peripheral nervous system (PNS). Traditionally, the ANS has been defined as a general efferent system that innervates visceral organs. The efferent outflow from the ANS is divided between its two divisions—the sympathetic nervous system and the parasympathetic nervous system. The afferent input to the ANS is provided by visceral afferent neurons, generally not considered to be part of the ANS.

The functions of the sympathetic nervous system include maintaining body temperature and adjusting blood flow and blood pressure to meet the changing needs of the body that occur with activities of daily living, such as moving from the supine to the standing position. The sympathoadrenal system can also discharge as a unit when there is a critical threat to the integrity of the person—the fight-or-flight response. During a stress situation, the heart rate accelerates; blood pressure rises; blood sugar increases; the bronchioles and pupils dilate; sphincters of the stomach, intestine, and internal urethra constrict; and the rate of secretion of exocrine glands that are involved in digestion diminishes. Emergency situations often require vasoconstriction and shunting of blood away from the skin and gastrointestinal tract to the skeletal muscles and brain, a mechanism that provides for a reduction in blood flow if a wound should occur and preservation of vital functions needed for survival. Sympathetic function often is summarized as catabolic in that its actions predominate during periods of pronounced energy expenditure, such as when survival is threatened.

In contrast to the sympathetic nervous system, the functions of the parasympathetic nervous system are concerned with conservation of energy, resource replenishment and storage (anabolism), and maintenance of organ function during periods of minimal activity. The parasympathetic nervous system slows heart rate, stimulates gastrointestinal function and related glandular secretion, promotes bowel and bladder elimination, and contracts the pupil, protecting the retina from excessive light during periods when visual function is not vital to survival.

The two divisions of the ANS are viewed as having opposite and antagonistic actions (*i.e.,* if one activates, the other inhibits a function). Exceptions are functions, such as sweating and regulation of arteriolar blood vessel diameter, that are controlled by a single division of the ANS, in this case the sympathetic nervous system. Both the sympathetic and the parasympathetic nervous system are continually active. The effect of this continual or basal (baseline) activity is referred to as *tone*. The tone of an effector organ or system can be increased or decreased and usually is regulated by a single division of the ANS. For example, vascular smooth muscle tone is controlled by the sympathetic nervous system. Increased sympathetic activity produces local vasoconstriction due to increased vascular smooth muscle tone, and decreased activity results in vaso-dilatation due to decreased tone. In structures such as the sinoatrial (SA) node and atrioventricular (AV) node of the heart, which are innervated by both divisions of the ANS, one division predominates in controlling tone. In this case, the tonically active parasympathetic nervous system exerts a constraining or braking effect on heart rate, and when parasympathetic outflow is withdrawn, similar to releasing a brake, heart rate increases. The increase in heart rate that occurs with vagal withdrawal can be further augmented by sympathetic stimulation. Table 49-1 describes the responses of effector organs to sympathetic and parasympathetic impulses.

VISCERAL AFFERENT PATHWAYS

Sensory information from the viscera is conveyed to the CNS by way of visceral afferent fibers. Both the parasympathetic and sympathetic peripheral nerves have fibers that carry visceral afferent and sensation information (about 80% of vagal fibers are sensory afferent fibers that supply the heart, lungs, and other viscera). The general visceral afferent fibers are involved in the mediation of vasomotor, respiratory, and viscerosomatic reflexes and interrelated visceral activities, such as gastrointestinal functioning and bladder emptying. In addition, they carry information concerning visceral sensations such as discomfort and pain.

The receptors of the *general visceral afferent* neurons monitor conditions of the internal environment, such as the chemical composition of body fluids and the pressure and stretch of internal organs. Some visceral afferents terminate in specialized chemoreceptors, such as those of the carotid and aortic bodies that monitor blood pH, oxygen (P_{O_2}), and carbon dioxide (P_{CO_2}). The pressure-sensitive baroreceptor endings in the carotid sinus and aorta sense changes in blood pressure. General visceral afferent receptors in the mucosal, smooth muscle, and connective tissue of the gastrointestinal tract monitor smooth muscle stretch and changes in the composition of the gastrointestinal contents. Distention of the bowel can stimulate increased motility, and the presence of microbial growth products can stimulate sensory receptors and cause diarrhea. The pharynx, trachea, bronchi, and lungs are richly innervated by visceral afferent endings. These endings provide the afferent input for the sneezing and cough reflexes.

Some general visceral afferent fibers join sympathetic nerves, such as the splanchnic nerves, whereas others from the same viscera travel in parasympathetic nerves, such as the vagus and the pelvic nerves. The cell bodies for the visceral afferents are located in the ganglia of the facial (VII), glossopharyngeal (IX), and vagus (X) cranial nerves; the thoracic and upper lumbar dorsal root ganglia; and the dorsal root ganglia of sacral levels 2, 3, and 4. The central axons of the afferent neurons enter the dorsal horn gray matter or its equivalent in the brain stem and synapse with association neurons (interneurons) of the same or neighboring segments. The association neurons use multisynaptic pathways that project to (1) local reflex circuits, (2) centers in the brain stem that contribute to the hierarchic control mechanisms of visceral reflexes, and (3) the thalamus and other higher centers where visceral sensations are perceived and integrated into cognitive and emotional responses. Spinal interneurons frequently receive convergent input from both somatic and visceral efferent fibers. These convergent pathways are thought to contribute to the referred pain that occurs with visceral pathology such as the referred pain in the left arm that commonly occurs with myocardial infarction.

General visceral afferent neurons monitor visceral sensations such as feelings of hunger, fullness of the bladder and rectum, sensations that originate in the sexual organs during coitus, and visceral pain.[1] Visceral afferent information reaches the sensation level in an area of the thalamus that has projections to a small area of the parietal sensory cortex. Visceral pain, which is discussed in Chapter 48, can arise from a common visceral sensation. For example, fullness of the bladder is perceived as the need to micturate. If it is inconvenient to empty the bladder, the sensation becomes stronger and more unpleasant. During severe urinary retention, as occurs with outflow obstruction, the sensation becomes exceedingly painful. At the point when visceral sensations become unpleasant and painful, autonomic effector responses often manifest themselves. Distention of the gut to the point that the sensation of nausea occurs typically is accompanied by increased heart rate and sweating. Because the intermediate thalamic nuclei that receive visceral signals communicate with the limbic system, visceral sensation can have a strong emotional component. For example, sensations of fullness, pressure, and visceral pain and those associated with deep structure stimulation during voiding, defecation, and sexual activity can have strong emotional components.

AUTONOMIC EFFERENT PATHWAYS

The afferent outflow of both divisions of the ANS follow a two-neuron pathway. The first motoneuron, called the *preganglionic neuron*, lies in a motor cell

TABLE 49-1. RESPONSES OF EFFECTOR ORGANS TO AUTONOMIC NERVE IMPULSES

EFFECTOR ORGANS	ADRENERGIC IMPULSES		CHOLINERGIC IMPULSES
	Receptor Type	Responses	Responses
Eye			
Radial muscle, iris	α_1	Contraction (mydriasis) + +	—
Sphincter muscle, iris		—	Contraction (miosis) + + +
Ciliary muscle	β_2	Relaxation for far vision +	Contraction for near vision + + +
Heart			
SA node	β_1	Increase in heart rate + +	Decrease in heart rate; vagal arrest + + +
Atria	β_1	Increase in contractility and conduction velocity + +	Decrease in contractility, and shortened action potential duration + +
AV node	β_1	Increase in automaticity and conduction velocity + +	Decrease in conduction velocity; AV block + + +
His–Purkinje system	β_1	Increase in automaticity and conduction velocity + + +	Little effect
Ventricles	β_1	Increase in contractility, conduction velocity, automaticity, and rate of idioventricular pacemakers + + +	Slight decrease in contractility claimed by some
Arterioles			
Coronary	$\alpha_1\alpha_2;\beta_2$	Constriction +; dilatation[2] + +	Constriction +
Skin and mucosa	α_1, α_2	Constriction + + +	Dilatation[3]
Skeletal muscle	$\alpha; \beta_2$	Constriction + +; dilatation[2,4] + +	Dilatation[5] +
Cerebral	α_1	Constriction (slight)	Dilatation[3]
Pulmonary	$\alpha_1; \beta_2$	Constriction +; dilatation[2]	Dilatation[3]
Abdominal viscera	$\alpha_1; \beta_2$	Constriction + + +; dilatation[4] +	—
Salivary glands	α_1, α_2	Constriction + + +	Dilatation + +
Renal	$\alpha_1, \alpha_2, \beta_1, \beta_2$	Constriction + + +; dilatation[4] +	—
Veins (Systemic)	$\alpha_1; \beta_2$	Constriction + +; dilatation + +	—
Lung			
Tracheal and bronchial muscle	β_2	Relaxation +	Contraction + +
Bronchial glands	$\alpha_1; \beta_2$	Decreased secretion; increased secretion	Stimulation + + +
Stomach			
Motility and tone	$\alpha_1, \alpha_2; \beta_2$	Decreased (usually)[6] +	Increase + + +
Sphincters	α_1	Contraction (usually) +	Relaxation (usually) +
Secretion		Inhibition (?)	Stimulation + + +
Intestine			
Motility and tone	$\alpha_1, \alpha_2; \beta_1, \beta_2$	Decrease[6] +	Increase + + +
Sphincters	α_1	Contraction (usually) +	Relaxation (usually) +
Secretion	α_2	Inhibition	Stimulation + +
Gallbladder and Ducts	β_2	Relaxation +	Contraction +
Kidney			
Renin secretion	$\alpha_1; \beta_1$	Decrease +; increase + +	—
Urinary Bladder			
Detrusor	β_2	Relaxation (usually) +	Contraction + + +
Trigone and sphincter	α_1	Contraction + +	Relaxation + +

(Continued)

TABLE 49-1. RESPONSES OF EFFECTOR ORGANS TO AUTONOMIC NERVE IMPULSES (Continued)

EFFECTOR ORGANS	ADRENERGIC IMPULSES		CHOLINERGIC IMPULSES
	Receptor Type	Responses	Responses
Ureter			
Motility and tone	α_1	Increase	Increase (?)
Uterus	α_1; β_2	Pregnant: contraction (α_1); relaxation (β_2). Nonpregnant: relaxation (β_2)	Variable[7]
Sex Organs, Male	α_1	Ejaculation + + +	Erection + + +
Skin			
Pilomotor muscles	α_1	Contraction + +	—
Sweat glands	α_1	Localized secretion[8] +	Generalized secretion + + +
Spleen Capsule	α_1; β_2	Contraction + + +; relaxation +	—
Adrenal Medulla		—	Secretion of epinephrine and norepinephrine (nicotinic effect)
Skeletal Muscle	β_2	Increased contractility; glycogenolysis; K^+ uptake	—
Liver	α; β_2	Glycogenolysis and gluconeogenesis[9] + + +	—
Pancreas			
Acini	α	Decreased secretion +	Secretion + +
Islets (β cells)	α_2	Decreased secretion + + +	—
	β_2	Increased secretion +	—
Fat Cells	α; β_1 (β_3)	Lipolysis[9] + + +	—
Salivary Glands	α_1	Potassium and water secretion +	Potassium and water secretion + + +
	β	Amylase secretion +	
Lacrimal Glands	α	Secretion +	Secretion + + +
Nasopharyngeal Glands		—	Secretion + + +
Pineal Gland	β	Melatonin synthesis	—
Posterior Pituitary	β_1	Antidiuretic hormone secretion	—

Responses are designated 1+ to 3+ to provide an approximate indication of the importance of adrenergic and cholinergic nerve activity in the control of the various organs and functions listed. A dash signifies no known functional innervation.

[1] Heart also contains α_1 and β_2 receptors, but they are less important for physiologic responses.

[2] Dilatation predominates in situ due to metabolic autoregulatory phenomena.

[3] Cholinergic vasodilatation at these sites is of questionable physiologic significance.

[4] Over the usual concentration range of physiologically released, circulating epinephrine, β-receptor response (vasodilatation) predominates in blood vessels of skeletal muscle and liver; α-receptor response (vasoconstriction), in blood vessels of other abdominal viscera. The renal and mesenteric vessels also contain specific dopaminergic receptors, activation of which causes dilatation.

[5] Sympathetic cholinergic system causes vasodilatation in skeletal muscle, but this is not involved in most physiologic responses.

[6] It has been proposed that adrenergic fibers terminate at inhibitory β-receptors on smooth muscle fibers, and at inhibitory α receptors on parasympathetic cholinergic (excitatory) ganglion cells of Auerbach's plexus.

[7] Depends on stage of menstrual cycle, amount of circulating estrogen and progesterone, and other factors.

[8] Palms and some other sites ("adrenergic sweating").

[9] There is significant variation among species in the type of receptor that mediates certain metabolic responses; α and β responses have not been determined in humans. A β_3 receptor has been cloned and may mediate responses in fat cells in some species.

(From Gilman, A. G., Rall, T. W., Nies, A. S., & Taylor, P. [1990]. *Goodman and Gilman's pharmacologic basis of therapeutics* [8th ed., pp. 89, 90]. New York: Pergamon Press.)

column in the ventral horn of the spinal cord or its equivalent location in the brain stem and is located within the CNS. The second motoneuron, called the *postganglionic neuron*, synapses with a preganglionic neuron in an autonomic ganglion and is located in the PNS. The two divisions of the ANS differ in terms of location of preganglionic cell bodies, relative length of preganglionic fibers, general function, nature of peripheral responses, and preganglionic and postganglionic neuromediators (Table 49-2). This two-neuron outflow pathway and the interneurons in the autonomic ganglia that add further modulation to ANS function are features distinctly different from the arrangement in somatic motor innervation.

TABLE 49-2. CHARACTERISTICS OF THE SYMPATHETIC AND PARASYMPATHETIC NERVOUS SYSTEMS

CHARACTERISTIC	SYMPATHETIC OUTFLOW	PARASYMPATHETIC OUTFLOW
Location of preganglionic cell bodies	Thoracic 1–12, lumbar 1 and 2	Cranial nerves: III, VII (intermedius), IX, X; sacral segments 2, 3, and 4
Relative length of preganglionic fibers	Short—to paravertebral chain of ganglia or to aortic prevertebral of ganglia	Long—to ganglion cells near or in the innervated organ
General function	Catabolic—mobilizes resources in anticipation of challenge for survival (preparation for "fight-or-flight" response)	Anabolic—concerned with conservation, renewal, and storage of resources
Nature of peripheral response	Generalized	Localized
Transmitter between preganglionic terminals and postganglionic neurons	Acetylcholine (ACh)	ACh
Transmitter of postganglionic neuron	ACh (sweat glands and skeletal muscle vasodilator fibers); norepinephrine (NE) (most synapses); NE and epinephrine (secreted by adrenal gland)	ACh

Most visceral organs are innervated by both sympathetic and parasympathetic fibers. Exceptions are structures, such as blood vessels and sweat glands, that have input from only one division of the ANS. The fibers of the sympathetic nervous system are distributed to effectors throughout the body, and as a result, sympathetic actions are more diffuse than those of the parasympathetic nervous system, in which there is a more localized distribution of fibers. The preganglionic fibers of the sympathetic nervous system may traverse a considerable distance and pass through several ganglia before finally synapsing with postganglionic neurons, and their terminals make contact with a large number of postganglionic fibers. In some ganglia, the ratio of preganglionic to postganglionic cells may be 1:20; because of this, the effects of sympathetic stimulation are diffuse.[2] In addition, there is considerable overlap, so that one ganglion may be supplied by several preganglionic fibers. In contrast to the sympathetic nervous system, the parasympathetic nervous system has its postganglionic neurons located very near or within the organ of innervation, and the ratio of preganglionic to postganglionic communication often is 1:1, so that its effects are much more circumscribed.[2]

SYMPATHETIC NERVOUS SYSTEM

The preganglionic fibers of the sympathetic nervous system are in the thoracic and upper lumbar segments of the spinal cord, and this part of the ANS is also called the *thoracolumbar division*. These preganglionic neurons, which are located primarily in the ventral horn intermediolateral cell columns, are largely myelinated and relatively short. The postganglionic neurons of the sympathetic nervous system are located in either the paravertebral ganglia of the sympathetic chains that lie on either side of the vertebral column or in prevertebral sympathetic ganglia, such as the celiac ganglia (Fig. 49-1). In addition to postganglionic efferent neurons, the sympathetic ganglia contain neurons of the internuncial, short-axon type, similar to those associated with complex circuitry in the brain and spinal cord. Many of these appear to inhibit, whereas others modulate preganglionic to postganglionic transmission. The full significance of these modulating circuits remains under investigation.

The axons of the preganglionic neurons leave the spinal cord by way of the ventral root of the spinal nerve and travel by way of nerve branches called *white rami* to the paravertebral ganglia (Fig. 49-2). Within the sympathetic chain of ganglia, preganglionic fibers may synapse with neurons of the ganglion it enters; pass up or down the chain and synapse with one or more ganglia; or pass through the chain and move outward through a splanchnic nerve to terminate in one of the prevertebral ganglia (celiac, superior mesenteric, or inferior mesenteric) that are scattered along the dorsal aorta and its branches. Preganglionic fibers from the thoracic segments of the cord pass upward to form the cervical chain interconnecting the inferior, middle, and superior cervical

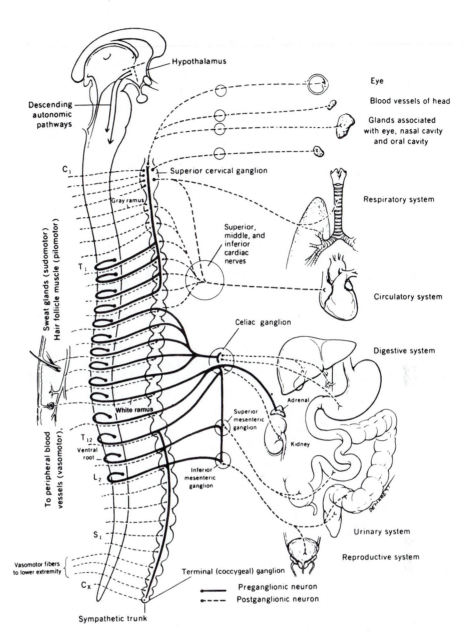

FIG. 49-1. Diagrammatic representation of the sympathetic division of the autonomic nervous system. (Noback, C. R., & Demarest, R. J. [1977]. *The nervous system—introduction and review* [2nd ed.]. New York: McGraw-Hill.)

sympathetic ganglia with the rest of the sympathetic chain at lower levels. Postganglionic sympathetic axons of the cervical and lower lumbosacral chain ganglia spread further through nerve plexuses along continuations of the great arteries. Thus, cranial structures, particularly blood vessels, are innervated by the spread of postganglionic axons along the external and internal and carotid arteries into the face and the cranial cavity. The sympathetic fibers from T1 pass up the sympathetic chain into the head; those from T2 pass into the neck; those from T1 to T5, to the heart: those from T3, T4, T5, and T6, to the thoracic viscera; those from T7, T8, T9, T10, and T11, to the abdominal viscera; and those from T12, L1, L2, and L3, to the kidneys and pelvic organs.[3] Many of the preganglionic fibers from the fifth to the last tho-

racolumbar segment pass through the paravertebral ganglia to continue as the splanchnic nerves. Most of these fibers do not synapse until they reach the celiac ganglion; others pass to the adrenal medulla. The adrenal medulla, which is part of the sympathetic nervous system, contains postganglionic sympathetic neurons that secrete sympathetic neurotransmitters directly into the bloodstream.

Some of the postganglionic fibers from the paravertebral ganglia reenter the segmental nerve through unmyelinated branches called *gray rami* and are then distributed to all parts of the body wall in the spinal nerve branches. These fibers innervate the sweat glands, piloerector muscles of the hair follicles, the blood vessels of the skin and skeletal muscles, and the CNS itself.

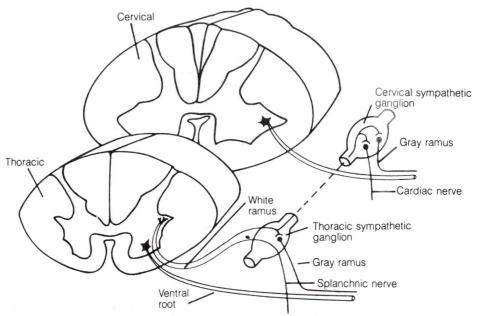

FIG. 49-2. Autonomic elements of the spinal nerves. In the thoracolumbar region, each ventral nerve root carries a contingent of efferent sympathetic fibers. These pass to the neighboring sympathetic trunk as a white ramus. Some of the fibers synapse in ganglia of corresponding levels, whereas others emerge from the trunk without synapsing. Fibers emerge from the ganglia to pass to plexuses or to rejoin the nerves as gray rami passing to peripheral or meningeal structures. In the cervical and sacral regions, the ventral roots give off no white rami. Fibers from other levels synapse in the ganglia, however, and secondary fibers pass off as gray rami to join the nerve trunks. (Elliott, H. C. [1969]. *Neuroanatomy.* Philadelphia: J.B. Lippincott.)

PARASYMPATHETIC NERVOUS SYSTEM

The preganglionic fibers of the parasympathetic nervous system, also referred to as the *craniosacral division* of the ANS, originate in the brain stem cranial nerves and sacral segments of the spinal cord (Fig. 49-3). The central regions of origin are the midbrain, pons, medulla oblongata, and sacral part of the spinal cord. The midbrain outflow passes through the oculomotor (III) cranial nerve to the ciliary ganglia that lies in the orbit behind the eye; it supplies the pupillary sphincter muscle of the eye and the ciliary muscles that control lens thickness for accommodation. Pontine outflow comes from preganglionic fibers of the facial (VII) nerve, which synapse in the submandibular ganglia, supplying the submandibular and sublingual glands, and the pterygopalatine ganglia, supplying the lacrimal and nasal glands. The medullary outflow develops from cranial nerves VII, IX, and X. Fibers in the glossopharyngeal (IX) nerve synapse in the otic ganglia, which supply the parotid salivary glands. About 75% of parasympathetic efferent fibers are carried in the vagus (X) nerve. The vagus nerve provides parasympathetic innervation for the heart, trachea and lungs, esophagus, stomach, small intestine and proximal half of the colon, liver, gallbladder, pancreas, kidneys, and upper portions of the ureters.

The sacral preganglionic axons leave the S2 to S4 segmental nerves by gathering into the pelvic nerves, also called the *nervi erigentes*. The pelvic nerves leave the sacral plexus on each side of the cord and distribute their peripheral fibers to the bladder, uterus, urethra, prostate, distal portion of the transverse colon, descending colon, and rectum. The sacral parasympathetic fibers also supply the external genitalia to facilitate sexual function.

With the exception of cranial nerves III, VII, and IX that synapse in discrete ganglia, the long parasympathetic preganglionic fibers pass uninterrupted to short postganglionic fibers located in the organ wall. In the walls of these organs, postganglionic neurons send axons to smooth muscle and glandular cells that modulate their functions.

The gastrointestinal tract has its own intrinsic network of ganglionic cells located between the smooth muscle layers, called the *enteric* (intramural) *plexus*, that controls local peristaltic movements. This network of parasympathetic postganglionic neurons and interneurons runs from the upper portion of the esophagus to the internal anal sphincter. Local afferent sensory neurons respond to mechanical and chemical stimuli and communicate these influences

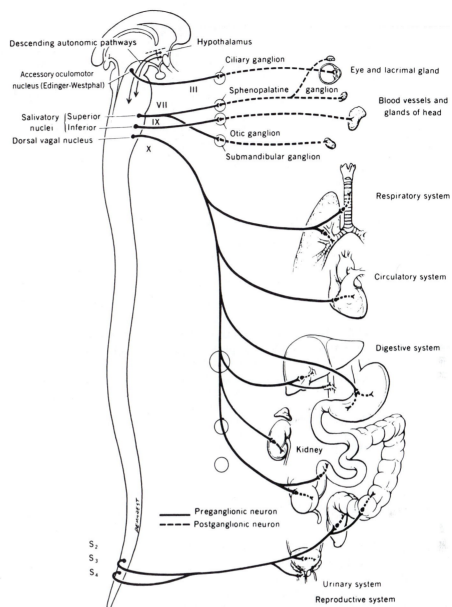

FIG. 49-3. Diagrammatic representation of the parasympathetic division of the autonomic nervous system. (Noback, C. R., & Demarest, R. J. [1977]. *The nervous system—introduction and review* [2nd ed.]. New York: McGraw-Hill.)

to motor fibers in the enteric plexus. The number of neurons in the enteric neural network (10^8) is so large that it approximates that of the spinal cord.[4] This enteric nervous system is thought to be capable of independent function without control from CNS fibers.[4] The CNS has a modulating role, by way of preganglionic innervation of the plexus, converting local peristalsis to longer distance movements, thereby speeding the transit of intestinal contents.

CENTRAL INTEGRATIVE PATHWAYS

Local reflex circuits that interrelate visceral afferent and autonomic efferent activity are integrated into a hierarchic control system in the spinal cord and brain stem. Progressively greater complexity in the re-

sponses and greater precision in their control occur at each higher level of the nervous system. As mentioned earlier, most visceral reflexes contain contributions from the lower motoneurons that innervate skeletal muscles as part of their response patterns. The distinction between purely visceral and somatic reflex hierarchies becomes less and less meaningful at the higher levels of hierarchic control and behavioral integration.

For most autonomic-mediated functions, the hypothalamus serves as the major control center. The hypothalamus, which has connections with the cerebral cortex, limbic system, and pituitary gland, is in a prime position to receive, integrate, and transmit information to other areas of the nervous system. The neurons concerned with thermoregulation, thirst, and feeding behaviors are found in the hypothalamus. The hypothalamus is also the site for integrating neuroendocrine function. Hypothalamic releasing and inhibiting hormones control the secretion of anterior pituitary hormones (thyroid-stimulating hormone, adrenocorticotropic hormone, growth hormone, luteinizing hormone, follicle-stimulating hormone, and prolactin). The supraoptic nuclei of the hypothalamus are involved in water metabolism through synthesis of antidiuretic hormone (ADH) and its release from the posterior pituitary gland (see Chapter 29). Oxytocin, which causes contraction of the pregnant uterus and milk let-down during breastfeeding, is synthesized in the hypothalamus and released from the posterior pituitary gland in a manner similar to that of ADH.

The organization of many life-support reflexes occurs in the reticular formation of the medulla and pons. These areas of reflex circuitry, often called *centers*, produce complex combinations of autonomic and somatic efferent functions required for the respiration, gag, cough, sneeze, swallow, and vomit reflexes as well as the more purely autonomic control of the cardiovascular system. At the hypothalamic level, these reflexes are integrated into more general response patterns, such as rage, defensive behavior, eating, drinking, voiding, and sexual function. Forebrain and especially limbic system control of these behaviors involves inhibiting or facilitating release of the response patterns according to social pressures during general emotion-provoking situations.

Reflex adjustments of cardiovascular and respiratory function occur at the level of the brain stem. A prominent example is the carotid sinus baroreflex. Increased blood pressure in the carotid sinus increases the discharge from afferent fibers that travel by way of the ninth cranial nerve to cardiovascular centers in the brain stem. These centers increase the activity of descending efferent vagal fibers that slow heart rate, while inhibiting sympathetic fibers that increase heart rate and blood vessel tone. One of the striking features of ANS function is the rapidity and intensity with which it can change visceral function. Within 3 to 5 seconds, it can increase heart rate to about twice its resting level. Bronchial smooth muscle tone is largely controlled by way of parasympathetic fibers carried in the vagus nerve. These nerves produce mild to moderate constriction of the bronchioles (see Chapter 27).

Other important ANS reflexes are located at the level of the spinal cord. As with other spinal reflexes, these reflexes are modulated by input from higher centers. When there is loss of communication between the higher centers and the spinal reflexes, as occurs in spinal cord injury, these reflexes function in an unregulated manner (see Chapter 50). There is uncontrolled sweating, vasomotor instability, and reflex bowel and bladder function.

NEUROTRANSMISSION

The generation and transmission of impulses in the ANS occur in the same manner as transmission in other neurons (see Chapter 47). There are self-propagating action potentials with transmission across synapses and other tissue junctions by way of neurohumoral transmitters. The somatic motoneurons that innervate skeletal muscles divide into many branches, with each branch innervating a single muscle fiber; this is in contrast to the distribution of postganglionic fibers of the ANS, which form a diffuse neural plexus at the site of innervation. The membranes of the cells of many smooth muscle fibers are connected by conductive protoplasmic bridges, called *gap junctions*, that permit rapid conduction of impulses through whole sheets of smooth muscle, often in repeating waves of contraction. Thus, autonomic neurotransmitters released near a limited portion of these fibers provide a modulating function extending to a large number of effector cells. The muscle layers of the gut and the bladder wall are examples. In some instances, isolated smooth muscle cells are individually innervated by the ANS; the piloerector cells that elevate the hair on the skin during cold exposure are an example.

The main neurotransmitters of the autonomic nervous system are acetylcholine and the catecholamines epinephrine and norepinephrine. Acetylcholine is released at all the sites of preganglionic transmission in the autonomic ganglia of both sympathetic and parasympathetic nerve fibers and at the sites of postganglionic transmission in parasympathetic nerve endings. It is also released at sympathetic nerve endings that innervate the sweat glands and cholinergic vasodilator fibers found in skeletal muscle. Norepinephrine is released at most sympathetic nerve endings. The adrenal medulla, which is a modified prevertebral sympathetic ganglion, produces epinephrine along with small fractions of norepinephrine. Dopamine, which is an intermediate compound in the synthesis of norepinephrine, also acts as a neurotransmitter. It is the principal inhibitory transmitter of internuncial neurons in the sympathetic ganglia. It also has vasodilator effects on renal, splanchnic, and coronary blood vessels when given intravenously and sometimes is used in the treatment of shock (see Chapter 25).

ACETYLCHOLINE AND CHOLINERGIC RECEPTORS

Acetylcholine is synthesized in the terminal endings of cholinergic fibers from choline and acetylcoenzyme A (acetyl-CoA) through the catalytic action of the enzyme acetyltransferase. Once acetylcholine is secreted by the cholinergic nerve endings, it is rapidly broken down by the enzyme acetylcholinesterase. The choline molecule is transported back into the nerve ending where it is used again in the synthesis of acetylcholine. Receptors that respond to acetylcholine are called *cholinergic receptors*. There are two types of cholinergic receptors: muscarinic and nicotinic. Muscarinic receptors are present on the innervational targets of postganglionic fibers, particularly those of the parasympathetic nervous system. Nicotinic receptors are found in autonomic ganglia and the end plates of skeletal muscle. Acetylcholine has excitatory effects on both muscarinic and nicotinic receptors; yet in the heart and lower esophageal sphincter, it has an inhibitory effect.

The drug atropine is an antimuscarinic or muscarinic cholinergic-blocking drug that prevents the action of acetylcholine at both excitatory and inhibitory muscarinic receptor sites. Because it is a muscarinic-blocking drug, it exerts little effect at nicotinic receptor sites.

CATECHOLAMINES AND ADRENERGIC RECEPTORS

The catecholamines, which include norepinephrine, epinephrine, and dopamine, are synthesized in the axoplasm of sympathetic nerve terminal endings from the amino acid tyrosine (Fig. 49-4). In the process of catecholamine synthesis, tyrosine is hydroxylated (has a hydroxyl group added) to form DOPA, DOPA is decarboxylated (has a carboxyl group removed) to form dopamine, and dopamine is hydroxylated to form norepinephrine. In the adrenal gland, an additional step occurs during which norepinephrine is methylated (a methyl group is added) to form epinephrine. Epinephrine is also called *adrenalin*, and sympathetic neurons, *adrenergic* neurons. Each of the steps in neurotransmitter synthesis requires a different enzyme, and the type of neurotransmitter that is produced depends on the type of enzymes that are available in a nerve terminal. For example, the postganglionic sympathetic neurons that supply blood vessels synthesize norepinephrine, whereas postganglionic neurons in the adrenal medulla produce both epinephrine and norepinephrine. Epinephrine accounts for about 80% of the catecholamines released from the adrenal gland. The synthesis of epinephrine by the adrenal medulla is influenced by the glucocorticoid secretion from the adrenal cortex. These hormones are transported by way of an intraadrenal vascular network from the adrenal cortex to the adrenal medulla where they cause the sympathetic neurons to increase their production of epinephrine by way of increased enzyme activity.[2] Thus, any stress situation sufficient to evoke increased levels of glucocorticoids also increases epinephrine levels.

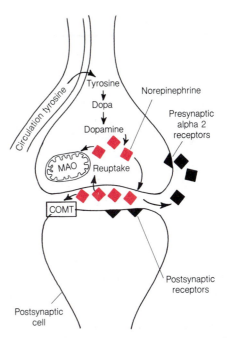

FIG. 49-4. Synthesis, reuptake, and metabolism of norepinephrine. Presynaptic α_2-receptors control norepinephrine release in the central nervous system.

As the catecholamines are synthesized, they are stored in vesicles. The final step of norepinephrine synthesis occurs in these vesicles. During an action potential, the neurotransmitter molecules are released from the storage vesicles. The storage vesicles not only provide a means for concentrated storage of the catecholamines but also protect them from the cytoplasmic enzymes that degrade the neurotransmitter.

In addition to neuronal synthesis, there is a second major mechanism for replenishment of norepinephrine in sympathetic nerve terminals. This mechanism consists of the active recapture or reuptake of the released neurotransmitter into the nerve terminal. From 50% to 80% of the norepinephrine that is released during an action potential is removed from the synaptic area by an active reuptake process.[3] This process not only terminates the action of the neurotransmitter but also allows it to be reused by the neuron. The remainder of the released catecholamines either diffuse into the surrounding tissue fluids or are degraded by two special enzymes: catechol-O-methyltransferase (COMT), which is diffusely present in all tissues, and monoamine oxidase (MAO), which is found in the nerve endings themselves.[3] Some drugs, such as the tricyclic antidepressants, are thought to increase the level of catecholamines at the site of nerve endings in the brain by blocking the reuptake process. Others, such as the MAO inhibitors, decrease the enzymatic degradation of the neurotransmitters and, thus, increase their levels.

The catecholamines can cause either excitation or inhibition of smooth muscle contraction, depending on the site, dose, and type of receptor present. Norepinephrine has potent excitatory activity and low inhibitory activity. Epinephrine is potent as both an excitatory agent and an inhibitory agent. The excitatory or inhibitory responses of organs to neurotransmitters are mediated by interaction with special structures in the cell membrane called *receptors*. The receptors in sympathetic neurons are called *adrenergic receptors*. In 1948, Ahlquist proposed the terms alpha (α) and beta (β) for the receptor sites where catecholamines produce their excitatory (α) and inhibitory (β) effects.[5]

In vascular smooth muscle, excitation of α-receptors causes vasoconstriction, and excitation of β-receptors causes vasodilatation. Both endogenous and exogenously administered norepinephrine produce marked vasoconstriction of the blood vessels in the skin, kidneys, and splanchnic circulation that are supplied with α-receptors. β-Receptors are most prevalent in the heart, blood vessels of skeletal muscle, and bronchioles. Blood vessels in skeletal muscle have both α- and β-receptors. In these vessels, high levels of norepinephrine produce vasoconstriction; low levels produce vasodilatation. The low levels are thought to have a diluting effect on norepinephrine levels in the arteries of these blood vessels so that the beta effect predominates.[6] In vessels with few receptors, such as those that supply the brain, norepinephrine has little effect.

α-Receptors have been further subdivided into α$_1$- and α$_2$-receptors, and β-adrenergic receptors, into β$_1$- and β$_2$-receptors. β$_1$-receptors are found primarily in the heart and can be selectively blocked by β$_1$-receptor blockers. β$_2$-Receptors are found in the bronchioles and in other sites that have β-mediated functions. α$_1$-Receptors are found primarily in postsynaptic effector sites; they mediate responses in vascular smooth muscle. α$_2$-Receptors are mainly located presynaptically and can inhibit the release of norepinephrine from sympathetic nerve terminals. α$_2$-Receptors are abundant in the CNS and are thought to influence the central control of blood pressure. Table 49-1 lists the receptor type and effector responses of the various organs that are innervated by the ANS.

The various classes of adrenergic receptors provide a mechanism by which the same adrenergic neurotransmitter can have many discretely different effects on differing effector cells. This mechanism also permits neurotransmitters carried in the bloodstream, whether from neuroendocrine secretion by the adrenal gland or from subcutaneously or intravenously administered drugs, to produce the same effects.

The catecholamines that are produced and released from sympathetic nerve endings are referred to as *endogenous neuromediators*. Sympathetic nerve activity can also be mediated by exogenous forms of these neurotransmitters that reach the nerve endings and their receptors by way of the bloodstream after being injected or inhaled. Drugs that are not catecholamines but that mimic their effects are said to have *sympathomimetic* actions. Many of these drugs can be given orally. Other drugs can selectively block the receptor sites on the neurons and temporarily prevent the neurotransmitter from exerting its action.

In summary, the ANS regulates, adjusts, and coordinates the visceral functions of the body. The ANS, which is divided into the sympathetic and parasympathetic systems, is an efferent system. It receives its afferent input from visceral afferent neurons. The ANS has both CNS and PNS components. The outflow of both the sympathetic and the parasympathetic nervous system follows a two-neuron pathway, which consists of a preganglionic neuron located within the CNS and a postganglionic neuron located outside the CNS. Sympathetic fibers leave the CNS at the thoracolumbar level, and the parasympathetic fibers leave at the craniosacral level. In general, the sympathetic and parasympathetic nervous systems have opposing effects on visceral function—if one excites, the other inhibits. The hypothalamus serves as the major control center for most ANS functions; local reflex circuits that interrelate visceral afferent and autonomic efferent activity are integrated in a hierarchic control system in the spinal cord and brain stem.

The main neurotransmitters for the ANS are acetylcholine and the catecholamines epinephrine and norepinephrine. Acetylcholine is the transmitter for all preganglionic neurons, for postganglionic parasympathetic neurons, and for selected postganglionic sympathetic neurons. The catecholamines are the neurotransmitters for most postganglionic sympathetic neurons. The neurotransmitters exert their target action through specialized cell surface receptors—cholinergic receptors that bind acetylcholine and adrenergic receptors that bind the catecholamines. The cholinergic receptors are divided into nicotinic and muscarinic receptors, and the adrenergic receptors are divided into α- and β-receptors.

■ ALTERATIONS IN ANS FUNCTION

Disorders of ANS function seldom occur as a separate disease. Because the control of the internal environment is vested in the ANS, most conditions that threaten the physiologic or psychological integrity of a person are accompanied by changes in ANS function.

The manifestations of altered ANS function are quite different from disorders of the somatic nervous system. When motoneurons are interrupted, the skeletal muscles they innervate are paralyzed. In contrast, the smooth muscle and other tissues that are innervated by the ANS usually have some level of spontaneous activity, and it is the control over this spontaneous activity that is lost when ANS innervation is disrupted. For example, the heart continues to beat when all innervation from the ANS is removed. This has been repeatedly demonstrated in heart transplantation procedures in which the cardiac innervation is severed. Likewise, the peristaltic movement of the gastrointestinal tract continues, despite the loss of ANS innervation in spinal cord injury, although modified so that transit time may become altered.

ORGAN AND SYSTEM DYSFUNCTION

Disorders of the ANS can be manifested as dysfunction of a single body organ or system or as a dysfunction of multiple organ systems. Disturbances in function of a single organ system can result from disorders of either central or peripheral ANS function. These disorders may occur singly or as a symptom of an accompanying disease condition.

VISION

Three functions of the eye are controlled by the ANS: pupil size, lens thickness, and lacrimation or tearing. Sympathetic activity causes pupil dilatation by contraction of the radial muscle of the iris. This enhances visual acuity by increasing the amount of light that enters the eye. The parasympathetic nervous system controls the circular muscles of the iris and causes pupil constriction; it is reflexly stimulated when excess light enters the eye.

Adjustment of lens thickness, used for focusing on near objects (called *accommodation*), is controlled almost entirely by the parasympathetic division of the ANS. At rest, the lens normally is held in a flattened shape by the tension (from the sclera) on its radial suspensory ligaments. Thus, the resting eye is in focus for distant objects (see Chapter 52). Parasympathetic excitation results in contraction of the ciliary muscle; this releases the tension and allows the lens to assume a more convex or thickened shape, which brings near objects into focus. Sometimes atropine, a cholinergic blocking drug, is used to facilitate thorough inspection of the retina and optic disk during an ophthalmoscopic eye examination. When instilled into the conjunctival sac, the drug diffuses into the iris and ciliary body and blocks signal transmission at parasympathetic synapses with a resultant paralysis of lens accommodation and pupillary enlargement. Homatropine, which is less potent and has a shorter duration of action than atropine, usually is used.

Tearing or lacrimation is controlled by the parasympathetic nervous system; it is increased with lo-

cal irritation and reflex stimulation. Emotional reactions that involve crying are undoubtedly mediated by way of input from the cortex and limbic systems.

Horner's Syndrome. Horner's syndrome is a disorder of sympathetic function that causes a drooping of the upper eyelid (ptosis), backward displacement of the eye into the orbit (enophthalmos), a fixed and constricted pupil (miosis), and generalized vascular dilatation (erythematosus) and loss of sweating (anhidrosis) over the affected half of the face. Postganglionic neurons of the superior cervical ganglion follow the internal carotid artery and then the ophthalmic artery into the orbit to innervate the blood vessels of the face, the dilator muscles of the iris, and the tarsal muscles of the eyelid. Horner's syndrome usually is caused by damage to the sympathetic chain, the superior cervical ganglion, or the internal carotid artery. The most common causes are mediastinal tumors, particularly bronchiogenic carcinoma, Hodgkin's disease, and metastatic tumors. Other causes are surgical or accidental trauma to the neck and CNS conditions, such as occlusion of the posterior inferior cerebellar artery and multiple sclerosis. Hemisection or transection of the cervical spine interrupts descending control of sympathetic outflow, causing ipsilateral (hemisection) or bilateral (transection) Horner's syndrome. This is called *central Horner's syndrome.*

Tonic Pupil (Adie's Syndrome). Tonic pupil is characterized by a pupil that is initially larger than normal and responds poorly to light. The disorder results from damage to the ciliary ganglion that contains the parasympathetic postganglionic fibers and aberrant regeneration of its nerve fibers. The affected pupil usually remains larger than normal for 2 to 6 months and then becomes smaller than the normal one.[7] The reduction in pupil size is thought to be caused by an aberrant regeneration process in which fibers that normally control accommodation grow to innervate the affected pupillary sphincter muscles. The neuronal drive associated with normal ciliary function then constricts the pupil by way of the aberrant nerves to give a small pupil. The initial changes in accommodation resolve as the ciliary fibers regenerate.

Argyll Robertson Pupil. In the condition called Argyll Robertson pupil, the pupil does not respond to light but is capable of accommodation. The condition usually is bilateral and characterized by small (1 to 2 mm) and irregular-shaped pupils. The pupils do not dilate to atropine. In the past, the most common cause of the Argyll Robertson pupil was CNS syphilis. At present, other causes include diabetes mellitus, degenerative disorders, and tumors of the midbrain. The sites of the CNS lesion usually are not known.

SKIN AND THERMAL REGULATION

The sweat glands of the skin, the piloerector muscles, and the skin blood vessels are all controlled by the sympathetic nervous system. All these mechanisms are involved in temperature regulation (see Chapter 10). Contraction of the pilomotor muscles causes "goose bumps" when the skin is exposed to a cold environment. This slightly reduces the surface area for heat loss. It also elevates the hair, trapping more air and, thus, reducing heat loss. In humans with delicate hairs on their bodies, this ancient reflex is not effective. Skin blood flow regulates the conduction of heat from internal body structures to the skin, where heat can be released into the external environment. Skin blood vessels dilate when there is a need to dissipate body heat and constrict when there is a need to conserve body heat. Skin blood flow also decreases when there is a need to divert blood flow to vital centers, such as occurs with circulatory shock.

Unlike most sympathetically innervated organs, the sweat glands have cholinergic rather than adrenergic receptors. The fact that sweat glands have cholinergic receptors allows them to be active during fever and exposure to hot weather when sympathetic outflow to skin vessels is reduced as a means of maintaining vasodilatation. The sweat glands and skin vessels are also innervated by separate efferent neurons; thus, the two functions are sorted out by CNS mechanisms as well.

Sweating disorders may take the form of increased sweating above normal to a given stimulus (hyperhidrosis) or absent or decreased sweating (anhidrosis).

Hyperhidrosis, particularly of the hands and feet, can be a social embarrassment and can occur without pathology. It commonly is associated with emotional reactions. It can also be caused by endocrine disorders such as hyperthyroidism, acromegaly, or pheochromocytoma (to be discussed). Recurring and transient periods of hyperhidrosis accompanied by vasomotor instability typically accompany hormonal changes that occur during menopause. Localized cutaneous areas of sweating may occur after injury to a peripheral nerve that carries both afferent and efferent fibers. It often is accompanied by severe pain (causalgia) along the course of the nerve (discussed in Chapter 48). It is most common after injury to the median or sciatic nerves. Sweating may occur as part of an isolated spinal cord reflex that is provoked by bladder distention or other sensory stimuli in people with spinal cord transection.

Anhidrosis can result from impaired sympathetic innervation of sweat glands, degeneration of sweat glands, or decreased sensitivity of the sweat glands to acetylcholine. Many people with diabetic neuropathy that involves sympathetic pathways show signs of anhidrosis over the lower extremities and trunk. There may be hyperhidrosis of the face and neck and drenching nocturnal sweats independent of a hypoglycemic event.[8] Another unusual feature of diabetic neuropathy is severe facial sweating at mealtimes. The presence of abnormal sweating patterns in diabetes should suggest the possibility of peripheral neuropathy and should be considered when sweating is used as an indicator of a hypoglycemic event.

Impairment of sweating and vasodilatation occurs in people with cervical cord injuries. Such people may become vulnerable to the effects of environmental heat and to hyperpyrexia during infection.

Sweating may be impaired in elderly people because of degenerative changes in the sweat glands and changes in sweat gland sensitivity to acetylcholine. A reduction in sweating capability is thought to be one of the factors that contribute to the increased incidence of heatstroke in elderly people during a heat wave.[8]

CIRCULATORY FUNCTION

The heart is innervated by both divisions of the ANS. The sympathetic nervous system innervates both the SA and the AV node as well as the ventricles; it increases both heart rate and force of ventricular contraction. The parasympathetic innervation of the heart, by way of the vagus, is largely restricted to the SA and AV nodes; its effect is to slow heart rate. The resistance of the peripheral blood vessels, which is a major determinant of blood pressure and flow, is largely controlled by the sympathetic nervous system. Most blood vessels, especially those of the abdominal viscera and skin, constrict when there is increased sympathetic activity. These blood vessels normally constrict and divert the flow of blood to the vital organs, such as the heart and brain, during times of need.

The cardiovascular system assumes a pivotal role in homeostasis by adjusting the blood supply to the various organs in relation to need. The circulation to the brain and other vital centers is largely controlled by autonomically mediated circulatory reflexes that match pressure and flow to the needs of the individual tissue beds. When going from the supine to the standing position, for example, cerebral blood flow is protected by the baroreceptor reflex. This reflex incorporates pressure-sensitive receptors in the carotid sinus and aorta, cardiovascular regulatory centers in the brain stem, and autonomic effector responses that alter heart rate and total peripheral resistance to meet the changing demands of the circulatory system and to maintain blood flow to vital centers. Volume receptors control total blood volume and are the circulatory system's protection against inadequate filling of the vascular compartment. Disorders of circulatory function occur when the autonomic reflexes that control cardiovascular function are exaggerated, deficient, or inappropriate. They include such disorders as cardiac dysrhythmias and abnormal blood pressure responses to normal activities of daily living.

Orthostatic hypotension (see Chapter 20) represents an abnormal drop in blood pressure that occurs with assumption of the upright position. It may result from an impaired vasoconstrictor response and peripheral pooling of blood with a temporary lack of blood flow to the brain.

Fainting or syncope refers to a transient loss of consciousness resulting from inadequate cerebral blood flow. It usually is preceded by sweating, pallor, blurred vision, dizziness, and nausea. Fainting may have an abrupt onset, with an initial increase in sympathetic activity leading to increased heart rate and vascular resistance. The initial sympathetic response is brief and followed by a sudden drop in heart rate, a decrease in vascular resistance, a profound fall in blood pressure and cerebral blood flow, and loss of consciousness.[9] Fainting is more common in people who are in the upright position, and assumption of the supine position during a faint usually results in a return of consciousness. Factors that predispose to fainting include a reduction in venous return to the heart resulting from orthostatic or postural stress, blood loss, or an increased intrathoracic pressure because of performance of Valsalva's maneuver.[10] The risk of syncope is increased in a hot environment because of vasodilatation and loss of extracellular fluid volume caused by sweating. Emotional fainting can occur as the result of reduced vasoconstrictor outflow and increased vasodilator outflow from CNS centers that influence blood vessel tone. Most healthy people can precipitate presyncopal conditions, particularly in hot weather, when they hyperventilate and produce cerebral vasoconstriction secondary to decreased cerebral carbon dioxide levels. Assumption of the standing position or standing without moving the legs to promote venous return contributes to the presyncopal condition.[9] Immobility and prolonged bed rest lead to a decrease in vascular volume and deconditioning of vascular smooth muscle and the skeletal muscle pumps that return blood to the heart. Thus, dizziness and the potential for fainting are common after immobility or bed rest.

Micturition syncope can occur immediately after bladder emptying. Loss of consciousness is abrupt, and recovery is rapid and complete. A full bladder causes vasoconstriction, a condition that does not usually produce hypertension because it is counteracted by the baroreceptor reflex. It has been suggested that syncope occurs when the constricted vessels suddenly dilate. It is more common in males than in females, probably because the standing position contributes to pooling of blood in the extremities. The reflex effects of bladder distention on circulation are much more pronounced in paraplegic people with cord injuries above T6.

The baroreceptor reflex is less efficient in many elderly people, and this may contribute to syncope and falls.[11, 12] This is particularly true when multiple stresses are placed on the circulation. These stresses include sudden assumption of the standing position from either the seated or supine position, vasodilatation caused by a warm room or bed, a full bladder, use of medications that impair autonomic function, and decreased vascular volume because of inadequate fluid intake or the use of diuretics. Orthostatic hypotension is further discussed in Chapter 21.

Postprandial hypotension is a decrease in blood pressure that occurs after a meal. Insulin release has a depressant effect on baroreflex function.[13] Consequently, the consumption of a meal that is high in carbohydrate content, with the subsequent release of insulin, has the potential for producing a postprandial decrease in blood pressure. This aspect of autonomic function has many practical implications for people who already have disorders of ANS function, such as elderly people and people who have had a stroke. Several studies have shown a significant reduction of postprandial blood pressure in elderly people.[13–15] In people who have had a stroke, autoregulation of the cerebral vessels in the affected area is lost; slight orthostatic falls in blood pressure after carbohydrate ingestion have the potential of further compromising blood flow to the area. Therefore, ingestion of small, low-carbohydrate meals and afterward avoidance of positions that produce orthostatic hypotension are suggested as a means of minimizing brain ischemia.

PHEOCHROMOCYTOMA

A pheochromocytoma is a tumor of chromaffin tissue (tissue that contains sympathetic nerve cells that stain with chromium salts) found in the adrenal medulla; it can arise in other sites, however, where there is chromaffin tissue, such as the sympathetic ganglia. Although only 0.1% to 0.2% of people with hypertension have an underlying pheochromocytoma, the disorder can cause lethal hypertensive crises; 8% to 10% of the tumors are malignant.[16]

Like adrenal medullary cells, the tumor cells of a pheochromocytoma produce and secrete the cate-cholamines epinephrine and norepinephrine. Thus, the hypertension is the result of massive release of these catecholamines. Their release often is paroxys-mal, occurring several times a month to several times a day and lasting for 1 minute to several hours. The most frequent symptoms, in addition to hyperten-sion, are headache, sweating, and tachycardia. Ner-vousness, tremor, pallor of the face, weakness, fatigue, and weight loss occur less frequently. Marked variability in blood pressure between epi-sodes is typical. Several tests are available to differen-tiate this type of hypertension from other types. One of the most commonly used diagnostic methods is the determination of 24-hour levels of urinary cate-cholamines and their metabolites, including vanillyl-mandelic acid. Once the presence of a pheochromo-cytoma has been established, the tumor needs to be located. Computed tomographic scans may be used for this purpose. Surgical removal of operable tumors is curative.[16]

GASTROINTESTINAL FUNCTION

Normal digestive function requires both digestive secretions and motility. The parasympathetic ner-vous system has the major control of the salivary gland activity. The sympathetic nervous system con-trols blood flow in the mouth and related structures, including the salivary glands. Its effect on salivation is probably indirect, by way of vasoconstriction of the salivary gland arterioles, resulting in reduced extra-cellular fluid delivery and, thus, increasing the vis-cosity of the salivary secretions, experienced as a dry mouth. The muscarinic anticholinergic drug atropine blocks parasympathetic activity and, thus, produces a dry mouth. If the parasympathetic innervation of the salivary gland is interrupted, the gland ceases to secrete saliva. If only one gland is affected, a dry mouth may not pose a problem and swallowing may not be affected.

The gastrointestinal tract has its own set of nerves known as the intramural, or enteric, plexus. Both sympathetic and parasympathetic stimulation can affect gastrointestinal tract motility (see Chapter 40). Parasympathetic activity increases the activity of the gastrointestinal tract, and sympathetic activity decreases the activity. Alterations in intramural plexus function can result in problems with swallow-ing or movement of food through the gastrointes-tinal tract.

Achalasia. Achalasia (cardiospasm) involves a failure of relaxation of the lower esophagus and is thought to result from abnormal parasympathetic innervation. In advanced cases, there is absence or degeneration of the ganglion cells in the intramural plexus. The main symptom is difficulty swallowing, with weight loss and vomiting occurring in some people.

Hirschsprung's Disease. Hirschsprung's disease, also called *congenital megacolon*, is a congenital ab-sence of many autonomic ganglion cells from the intramural plexus of the colon. The ganglia are defi-cient from the anorectal junction, in most cases from the rectum, and sometimes from sections of the sig-moid colon.[17] Constipation is present from birth. There is a delay in the initial passing of meconium; the rectum usually is empty and the rest of the colon is distended. Vomiting typically follows. In some cases, there are alternating periods of obstruction and sudden passage of diarrheal stools. Complica-tions include fluid and electrolyte disturbances and perforation of the distended bowel. The treatment for this condition is surgical resection of the affected portion of the colon.

METABOLIC FUNCTION

Sympathetic stimulation also has metabolic func-tions: it inhibits insulin release from β cells in the pancreas, it increases glucose release from the liver, and it increases lipolysis. All these functions result in increased availability of blood glucose or its lipid precursors, which supports increased skeletal mus-cle and brain function required during the fight-or-flight reaction. The hypothalamus is thought to play an important role in appetite, satiety, and hunger. There is increasing evidence that the ANS contrib-utes to feeding patterns and weight gain. In animal studies, for example, decreased sympathetic activity leads to excess energy storage in fat cells by means of decreased lipolysis (fat breakdown) and increased lipogenesis (fat generation).[18] Studies have shown an association between the percentage of body fat and responses to tests of ANS function.[19]

SEXUAL FUNCTION

In the male, sexual function requires erection and emission-ejaculation. Erection involves vascular en-gorgement of the spongelike erectile tissue in the corpora cavernosa and corpora spongiosum that re-sults from arterial dilatation and venous constriction. This is primarily a parasympathetic function and re-quires sacral outflow by way of the pelvic nerves.

Parasympathetic impulses, in addition to promoting erection, cause the urethral glands and the bulbourethral glands to secrete mucus. This mucus flows through the urethra and aids in lubrication. Emission consists of expulsion of semen into the posterior urethra and reflex closure of the internal sphincter of the bladder to prevent reflux of secretions into the bladder. Both expulsion of semen into the posterior urethra and closure of the internal sphincter depend on sympathetic impulses that leave the cord at the lower thoracic and upper lumbar regions. The afferent neurons that trigger emission run in the pudendal and pelvic nerves to the sacral cord and with the sympathetic fibers to the thoracolumbar cord. Ejection of semen from the anterior urethra (ejaculation) depends on the rhythmic contractions of the bulbocavernous and ischiocavernous muscles supplied by the somatic pudendal nerve. The entire period of emission and ejaculation is called the male orgasm.

Both erection and emission-ejaculation are largely reflex in nature. Erection can occur despite partial or complete lesions above the level of the sacral cord. Afferent impulses resulting from stimulation of the genitalia or perineum are transmitted through the pudendal nerve to the sacral cord, and efferent parasympathetic impulses from the same segments reach the corpora cavernosa and spongiosum, leading to vasodilation and congestion. In some cases, persistent erection (priapism) may occur. For emission-ejaculation to occur, the lower thoracic and upper lumbar sympathetic connections must be intact.

Impotence (failure of erection) can result from any disorder that affects sacral parasympathetic function, including injury, polyneuropathy, and multiple sclerosis. Emission-ejaculation can be inhibited by drugs that act directly on the sympathetic nervous system (*e.g.*, antihypertensive drugs and many tranquilizers). Impotence and problems with emission-ejaculation may occur in men who suffer from diabetic autonomic neuropathy. Ejection of semen from the urethra is controlled by the somatic pudendal nerve and does not occur in men with lower motor neuron lesions of this nerve.

Fertility may also be impaired in men with partial loss of ANS function caused by lesions of the spinal cord above the lumbar or sacral segments. Even if they are able to ejaculate, sperm counts show few motile sperms in the ejaculate. The cause of the decreased sperm count is unknown, but it is thought that impairment of temperature regulation in the scrotum may be a contributing factor.

In women, disorders of ANS function interfere with orgasm. This occurs with lesions of the cauda equina and spinal cord. There is no evidence that ovulation or menstruation is affected. Delivery of a baby can occur after spinal cord transection or interruption of sympathetic nerve supply. After spinal cord transection, labor may occur without the mother knowing that labor has begun and may be accompanied by autonomic hyperreflexia.

DISORDERS OF PERIPHERAL ANS FUNCTION

Disorders of the peripheral autonomic nervous system may occur in isolation, as in acute and subacute autonomic neuropathies, or in association with a generalized peripheral neuropathy, as in Guillain-Barré syndrome (see Chapter 50). The peripheral neuropathies most likely to cause severe ANS dysfunction are those in which small myelinated and unmyelinated fibers are damaged in baroreflex afferents, the afferents to the heart, and the afferent pathways to the mesenteric blood vessels.[20]

Autonomic neuropathy is common in diabetes mellitus, and clinical features include impaired sweating, postural hypotension, impaired control of heart rate, diarrhea, impaired esophageal and gastric motility, impotence, and sphincter and pupillary disturbances of the eye. Long-term alcohol abuse can lead to alcohol-induced neuropathy. Degeneration of both the vagus and the sympathetic neurons occur in severe cases. Disturbances of esophageal motility in chronic alcoholics with peripheral neuropathies may be a manifestation of damage to the vagus nerve. Peripheral neuropathies with associated autonomic manifestations may result from the toxic effects of exposure to heavy metals such as thallium as well as exposure to arsenic, organic solvent, and other chemicals. Other disease conditions that can affect the peripheral ANS are chronic renal failure, rheumatoid arthritis, systemic lupus erythematosus, and mixed connective tissue disorders.

DENERVATION HYPERSENSITIVITY

When autonomically innervated smooth muscle is deprived of its innervation, it becomes extremely sensitive to its neurotransmitters. During the first week or so after sympathetic or parasympathetic nerve injury, the innervated organ becomes more and more sensitive to circulating neurotransmitters. This is called *denervation hypersensitivity*. The mechanisms of the hypersensitivity are not completely understood. The number of receptors on the postsynaptic membrane are increased when acetylcholine or norepinephrine are no longer released from the neuron. This is called *upregulation* and is caused by genetic mechanisms that are responsible for replacing the receptors. The increased number of receptors produces an increased response to neurotransmitters that circulate in the blood—whether they are from endogenous sources, such as the adrenal gland, or from exogenous sources, such as medications.

DISORDERS OF CENTRAL ANS FUNCTION

The most common pathologies of disturbed autonomic function of CNS origin are degeneration of the intermediolateral cell columns (progressive autonomic failure) or diseases that cause damage to the descending pathways that synapse with the intermediolateral column cells (spinal cord tumors, cerebrovascular accidents, brain stem tumors, multiple sclerosis, and Parkinson's disease).[20]

PROGRESSIVE AUTONOMIC FAILURE

A condition called progressive autonomic failure is a degenerative disorder of CNS and PNS autonomic neurons. It can occur as a primary disorder (idiopathic autonomic insufficiency) or as a secondary disorder associated with other diseases, such as Parkinson's disease and Wernicke's encephalopathy (see Chapter 54), spinal cord injury (see Chapter 50), and stroke (see Chapter 51).

Idiopathic autonomic insufficiency is a disorder of unknown cause. The condition is more common in males than in females and usually strikes during middle age. The disorder may occur as an uncomplicated progressive autonomic failure, or it may be complicated by parkinsonian features or multisystem atrophy. In males, impotence is an early symptom, and manifestations of sphincter disturbances, such as urinary hesitancy, urgency, and incontinence, are common. Loss of sweating ability is characteristic. These early signs, which may go unrecognized, are followed by orthostatic hypotension—a hallmark of the disorder. Postural hypotension may be manifested by dizziness and weakness after standing or walking. There may be sudden drop attacks, but more often there is a gradual fading of consciousness over 30 seconds or so while the person is walking or standing. A neck ache radiating to the occipital region of the skull and shoulders often precedes the actual loss of consciousness. Sometimes there are transient visual disturbances, scotomata, position hallucinations, or tunnel vision.[21] The visual disturbances may be particularly troubling when the person is standing or walking. Symptoms typically are worse in the morning, after meals, and in hot weather or other conditions that predispose to an unfavorable redistribution of blood volume. People treated with bed rest for hypotension may develop persistent recumbent hypertension, mainly caused by loss of baroreflex function.[22]

The prognosis is better for people with uncomplicated idiopathic autonomic insufficiency; in these people, postural hypotension, impairment of sweating, and disturbances of heart rate and blood pressure may be the only manifestations. In people in whom the condition is complicated by parkinsonian features, there is facial immobility, bradykinesia, tremor, and rigidity. Multisystem failure (sometimes called Shy-Drager syndrome) is characterized by progressive pyramidal, bulbar, extrapyramidal, and cerebellar deterioration; iris atrophy; Horner's syndrome; and other ocular disturbances. There may also be a laryngeal stridor during sleep, sudden inspiratory gasps, sleep apnea, and cluster breathing as well as other disturbances of respiration. The presence of parkinsonian features or multisystem atrophy is associated with a much poorer outcome, with death occurring in 4 to 8 years.[20]

The most troubling aspect of progressive autonomic failure is orthostatic hypotension. Treatment measures, including drug therapy, are used to increase blood volume, vasomotor tone, or both.[22] Treatment is complicated by the fact that the supine position produces hypertension. Elevation of the head of the bed at night usually is advocated for this reason.[22] Tights, a tightly fitting elastic support garment that compresses the vessels in the legs and lower abdomen, may be used to control symptoms by decreasing the amount of blood that can be pooled in the abdomen and legs. In severe cases, antigravity suits may be used. These support devices are restricting and uncomfortable, particularly in hot weather. The mineralocorticoid drug 9-a fluorocortisol and sodium chloride may be used to increase blood volume. Oral sympathomimetic drugs (*e.g.*, ephedrine, phenylephrine) may be prescribed for people with severe symptoms. β-Adrenergic blocking drugs have been used to prevent possible β-agonist–induced vasodilatation. Caffeine has a pressor effect and may be useful in preventing postprandial decreases in blood pressure.

DIAGNOSTIC METHODS

The integrity and function of the ANS usually are assessed through the use of tests that stress selected autonomic reflexes. These tests include the blood pressure and heart rate response to a change in posture (tilt test or free standing), respiration (respiratory sinus arrhythmia), isometric (handgrip) exercise, Valsalva test, cold pressor test, and mental stress. Plasma catecholamines and catecholamine metabolites in the urine can be measured. Pupillary innervation can be assessed using various autonomic drugs. These tests are summarized in Table 49-3.

In summary, disorders of the ANS can affect a single organ or system and can result in diseases that affect either central or peripheral ANS function. The visceral structures that are innervated by the ANS usually have some level of spontaneous activity, and it is modulation of this spontaneous activity that is lost when ANS function is interrupted. Alterations in ANS function can alter the ability of the eye to control pupil size, lens focus, accommodation, and tearing; the function of the sweat glands, piloerector muscles, and blood vessels of the skin; the ability of the circulatory system to maintain blood flow and blood pressure; the motility and release of digestive secretion by the gastrointestinal tract; the control of metabolic functions; and sexual functioning. Disorders of the peripheral ANS may occur in isolation as acute or subacute neuropathies or in association with generalized peripheral neuropathies. Autonomic neuropathy is common in diabetes mellitus. Progressive autonomic failure describes a degenerative disorder of the central and peripheral ANS.

TABLE 49-3. TESTS OF AUTONOMIC NERVOUS SYSTEM (ANS) FUNCTION

TEST	NORMAL RESPONSE	PART OF THE ANS TESTED
Graded postural stress (a tilt table is used; heart rate and blood pressure are monitored)	Fall in pulse pressure (decrease in systolic and increase in diastolic pressures) and increased heart rate at high levels of tilt	Sympathetic vasoconstriction at low levels of tilt; arterial baroreceptors at high levels tilt
Heart rate to standing	Increase in heart rate to about 15th beat with slowing to about 30th beat; then stabilizes	Baroreflex afferents; parasympathetic withdrawal of the vagal heart rate response (immediate); peripheral sympathetic vasoconstriction (stabilization of heart rate)
Isometric handgrip (a handgrip device is used; contraction is maintained at a given percentage of maximum contraction for 5 min)	Increase in systolic and diastolic pressure	Input from central CNS command and metabolic or mechanical changes in contracting muscle; sympathetic vasoconstrictor response
Valsalva test (done by blowing into a mouthpiece for 15 s; heart rate is monitored during and immediately after the strain). Intra-arterial blood pressure may also be monitored	Rise in phase II (end of strain) and phase IV slowing (5–20 s post strain) of heart rate	Baroreflex afferents; sympathetic increase in heart rate and vasoconstriction; vagal slowing of heart rate
Respiratory sinus arrhythmia—heart rate variation with respiration (heart rate is measured during normal or forced breathing and the difference between inspiratory and expiratory rate calculated)	Heart rate increases during inspiration and decreases during expiration	Pulmonary receptors in the lung; vagal efferent control of heart rate
Cold pressor test (hand immersed in cold or ice water for 1 to 2 min)	Increase in blood pressure	Afferent pain and temperature receptors; sympathetic vasoconstrictor response
Emotional stress (mental arithmetic, loud noise, confusing instructions for task, and so forth)	Increase in blood pressure; decrease in skin blood flow	Input from the cortex; sympathetic vasomotor response
Sweat tests (done by applying radiant heat to body)	Sweat is detected with chemicals that change color when wet	Pattern of sweating can be observed. Postganglionic lesions can be distinguished from preganglionic lesions with iontophoresis or injection of a cholinergic drug into the skin
Pupillary innervation (instillation of adrenergic or cholinergic drugs into the conjunctival sac)	Appropriate constriction or dilatation	Postganglionic control of autonomic innervation of pupil

■ REFERENCES

1. Procacci, P., Zoppi, M., & Maresca, M. (1986). Clinical approach to visceral sensation. *Progress in Brain Research, 67,* 21.
2. Gilman, A.G., Rall, T.W., Nies, A.S., et al. (1990). *Goodman and Gilman's pharmacological basis of therapeutics* (8th ed., p. 87). New York: Pergamon.
3. Guyton, A. (1991). *Medical physiology* (8th ed., pp. 668, 670). Philadelphia: W.B. Saunders.
4. Appenzeller, O. (1990). *The autonomic nervous system* (4th ed., p. 368). New York: Elsevier.
5. Ahlquist, R.P. (1948). A study of the adrenotropic receptors. *American Journal of Physiology, 153,* 586.
6. Schmitt, R.F., & Thews, G. (1983). *Human physiology* (p. 115). New York: Springer-Verlag.
7. Smith, S.A. (1988). Pupillary function in autonomic failure. In R. Bannister (Ed.). *Autonomic failure* (2nd ed., pp. 396–397). New York: Oxford Medical Publications.
8. Collins, K.J. (1988). Autonomic control of sweat glands and disorders of sweating. In R. Bannister (Ed.). *Autonomic failure* (2nd ed., pp. 748–765). New York: Oxford Medical Publications.
9. Porth, C.J., Bamrah, V.S., Tristani, F.E., et al. (1984). The Valsalva maneuver: Mechanisms and clinical implications. *Heart and Lung, 13,* 507.
10. Hainsworth, R. (1988). Fainting. In R. Bannister (Ed.). *Autonomic failure* (2nd ed., pp. 142–158). New York: Oxford Medical Publications.
11. Weiner, W.J., Nora, L.M., & Glantz, R.H. (1984). Elderly inpatients: Postural reflex impairment. *Neurology, 34,* 945.
12. Smith, S.A., & Fasler, J.J. (1983). Age-related changes in autonomic function: Relationship with postural hypotension. *Age and Ageing, 12,* 206.
13. Lipsitz, L.A., & Fullerton, K.J. (1986). Postprandial blood pressure reduction in healthy elderly. *Journal of the American Geriatrics Society, 34,* 267.
14. Fagan, T.C., Conrad, K.A., Mar, J.H., et al. (1986). Effects of meals on hemodynamics: Implications for antihypertensive drug studies. *Clinical Pharmacology and Therapeutics, 39,* 255.
15. deMey, C., Enterling, D., & Brendel, E. (1987). Postprandial changes in supine and erect heart rate, systemic blood pressure and renin activity in normal subjects. *European Journal of Pharmacology, 32,* 471.
16. Bravo, E.L., & Gifford, R.W. (1984). Pheochromocytoma: Diagnosis, localization, and management. *New England Journal of Medicine, 311*(20), 1298.
17. Robbins, S.L., & Kumar, V. (1987). *Basic pathology* (p. 540). Philadelphia: W.B. Saunders.
18. Bray, G.A., & York, D.A. (1979). Hypothalamic and genetic obesity in experimental animals: An autonomic and endocrine hypothesis. *Physiological Reviews, 59,* 719.
19. Peterson, H.R., Rothchild, M., & Weinber, C.R. (1988). Body fat and activity of the autonomic nervous system. *New England Journal of Medicine, 318*(17), 1077.
20. McLeod, J.G., & Tuck, R.R. (1987). Disorders of the autonomic nervous system: Part I. Pathology and clinical features. *Annals of Neurology, 21,* 419.
21. Bannister, R. (1988). Autonomic failure: Symptoms. In R. Bannister (Ed.). *Autonomic failure* (2nd ed., pp. 267–288). New York: Oxford Medical Publications.
22. McLeod, J.G., & Tuck, R.R. (1987). Disorders of the autonomic nervous system: Part II. Investigation and treatment. *Annals of Neurology, 21,* 519.

■ BIBLIOGRAPHY

Bradshaw, M.J., & Edwards, R.T.M. (1986). Postural hypotension—pathophysiology and management. *Quarterly Journal of Medicine, 60,* 643.

Bray, G.A. (1986). Autonomic and endocrine factors in the regulation of energy balance. *Federation Proceedings, 45*(5), 1404.

Kaijser, L., & Sachs, C. (1985). Autonomic cardiovascular responses in old age. *Clinical Physiology, 5,* 347.

Onrot, J., Goldberg, M.R., Biagioni, I., et al. (1985). Hemodynamic and humoral effects of caffeine in autonomic failure. *New England Journal of Medicine, 313,* 549.

Onrot, J., Goldberg, M.R., Hollister, A.S., et al. (1986). Management of chronic orthostatic hypotension. *American Journal of Medicine, 80,* 454.

Wallin, B.G., & Stjernberg, L. (1984). Sympathetic activity in man after spinal cord injury. *Brain, 107,* 183.

Warfield, C.A. (1984). The sympathetic dystrophies. *Hospital Practice, 19*(5), 52c.

ALTERATIONS IN MOTOR FUNCTION

ROBIN L. CURTIS
SYLVIA EICHNER MCDONALD

■ OBJECTIVES

After you have studied this chapter, you should be able to meet the following objectives:

■ Trace a voluntary muscle movement from its initiation in the supplementary motor cortex, through the basal ganglia, cerebellum, brain stem circuits, spinal cord circuits, to the lower motoneuron (LMN) and myoneural junction, and state the contribution of each of these neural components.

■ Define the function of the following muscle types: *extensors, flexors, adductors, abductors, rotators, agonists, antagonists,* and *synergists.*

■ Describe the longitudinal and transverse organization of the spinal cord.

■ Define *motor unit* and explain why this is the smallest unit of motor function.

■ Compare the myotatic, reverse myotactic, and flexor-withdrawal reflexes.

■ State the contributions of the primary motor cortex, the premotor area, and the supplementary motor cortex to motor function.

■ Describe the functions of the pyramidal versus extra-pyramidal systems.

■ Describe the pathology associated with Duchenne muscular dystrophy.

■ Relate the clinical manifestations of myasthenia gravis to its etiology.

■ Trace the steps in regeneration of an injured peripheral nerve.

■ Describe the manifestation of peripheral nerve root injury due to a prolapsed intervertebral disk.

■ Compare the cause and manifestations of peripheral mononeuropathies with peripheral polyneuropathies.

■ Define *paresis, paralysis, monoparesis, hemiparesis, diparesis, paraparesis,* and *quadriparesis* or *tetraplegia.*

■ Compare the manifestations of upper motoneuron (UMN) and lower motoneuron (LMN) injury.

Carol Mattson Porth: PATHOPHYSIOLOGY: CONCEPTS OF
ALTERED HEALTH STATES, 4th ed. © 1994, 1990, 1986, 1982
J.B. Lippincott Company

1027

■ State the pathology associated with amyotrophic lateral sclerosis (ALS)

■ Describe the function of the cerebellum in motor function and relate it to the cerebellar ataxia and tremor.

■ State the alterations in motor control that occur with chorea, athetosis, hemiballismus, and tremor.

■ Briefly state the mechanisms of neural injury in spinal cord injury (SCI).

■ Describe the classification of SCI in terms of tetraplegia and paraplegia and complete and incomplete injuries.

■ Describe the alterations in ventilation/communication, autonomic nervous system function, sensorimotor integrity, bowel and bladder function, and sexual functioning that occur following SCI.

■ Use the concepts of health stabilization, life-style modification, and community integration to explain the continuum of care for a person with SCI.

Effective motor function requires not only that muscles move but also that the mechanics of their movement be programmed in a manner that provides for smooth and coordinated movement. In some cases, purposeless and disruptive movements can be almost as disabling as the relative or complete absence of movement. This chapter is organized into four sections: control of motor function, alterations in function of the neuromuscular unit, alterations in pyramidal versus extrapyramidal function, and spinal cord injury. Although motor function relies on continuous input from sensory neurons, the focus of this chapter is on the efferent output that controls movement. Spinal cord injury is presented as an example of a condition that affects multiple motor systems.

■ CONTROL OF MOTOR FUNCTION

Movement begins *in utero* at about 21 weeks' gestation with the quickening of the fetus, and the capability for some coordinated movement is present at birth. Maturation of the spinal cord and brain circuitry during the first year or two of life allows the child to defy the force of gravity and learn to sit, then stand, and in rapid sequence master the skills of walking, running, jumping, and climbing.

Motor function, whether it involves walking, running, or precise finger movements, requires both movement and maintenance of posture. Posture can be described as the active muscular resistance to the displacement of the body or its parts by gravity or other applied forces.[1] The two functions are intricately related, and it is virtually impossible to successfully perform one without the other. Purposeful movement of the hands and feet is accomplished only by first placing the body and the arm or leg in a stable posture and appropriate position.

The structures that control posture and movement are located throughout the neuromuscular system. The system consists of the neuromuscular unit, which includes the motoneurons, the myoneural junction, and the muscle fibers; the spinal cord, which contains the basic reflex circuitry for posture and movement; the descending pathways from the brain stem circuits, the cerebellum, basal ganglia, and the motor cortex (Fig. 50-1). Delicate, skillful, intentional movement of distal and especially flexor muscles of the limbs and the speech apparatus is initiated and controlled from the frontal motor regions of cerebral cortex. These areas receive information from the somesthetic thalamus and cortex, and, indirectly, from the cerebellum and basal ganglia. Planning a movement sequence to accomplish a precise goal, such as moving a body part to a precise point in three-dimensional space, involves higher-order functions of the prefrontal cortex. This plan is translated into a "model" of the sequential component actions, a learned function performed by the premotor cortex. The model is activated (initiated) via the supplemental motor cortex, and precise control of distal muscle participation requires the primary motor cortex. Descending axons from the motor cortex project to the brain stem or spinal cord; there they indirectly or, in special instances, directly innervate lower motoneurons (LMNs) that supply the muscle fibers. The inherited as well as the learned repertoire of basic movement sequences providing axial and proximal positioning and support required by the model is governed by the basal ganglia, which control the brain stem reticular formation as well as influence the primary motor cortex. Continuous sensory feedback from the involved muscles as well as from all sensory systems are matched against the model and adjustments for errors in timing or in sequence are continuously relayed from the cerebellum, the basal ganglia, and the primary sensory cortex back to the motor cortex. The

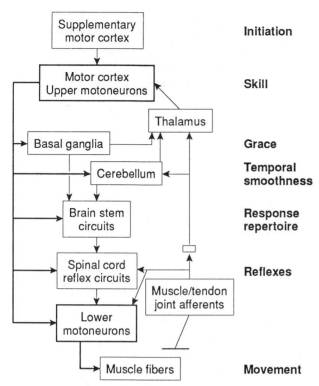

Supplementary motor cortex	**Initiation**
Motor cortex Upper motoneurons	**Skill**
Thalamus	
Basal ganglia	**Grace**
Cerebellum	**Temporal smoothness**
Brain stem circuits	**Response repertoire**
Spinal cord reflex circuits	**Reflexes**
Muscle/tendon joint afferents	
Lower motoneurons	
Muscle fibers	**Movement**

FIG. 50-1. Diagram of neural pathways for control of motor function.

programmed model, continuously corrected and adjusted, progresses until the precise goal is accomplished. The efficiency of the entire motor system depends on optimally facilitated motor units on a background of stretch reflex and vestibular system input to maintain stable postural support. Motor function involves both parallel functioning and ongoing interactive communication between these functions. A highly skilled movement is beautiful to behold, but because of the necessary complexity of its control, it can be easily damaged or distorted.

FUNCTIONAL ORGANIZATION OF MOTOR FUNCTION

Skeletal muscle is composed of muscle cells, or fibers, which contain the interacting actin and myosin filaments that generate the contractile force required for movement (see Chapter 1). In terms of function, muscles can be classified as *extensors*, muscles that increase the angle of a joint, or *flexors*, muscles that decrease the angle of a joint. In the legs, groups of extensor muscles work together to resist gravity and function to maintain the upright posture and provide locomotion power. In general, flexor muscle groups assist gravity, participate in withdrawal reflexes, and provide the more delicate aspects of manipulation. Other muscle groups act roughly in pairs: *adductors*

versus *abductors*, which move a part toward or away from the midline of the body, and *rotators*, which work in pairs to rotate a part of the limb, the trunk, or the head around each part's longitudinal axis. Many muscles participate in more than one of these functions. Coordinated movement requires the action of two or more muscle groups—*agonists*, which promote a movement; *antagonists*, which oppose it; and *synergists*, which assist the agonist muscles by stabilizing a joint or contributing additional force to the movement. Some simple types of movement require only a burst of energy from an agonist muscle group. Other types of movements, such as self-terminated actions, require a smooth sequence of movements: agonist, antagonist, and, finally, co-contraction of agonist and antagonist to stop and stabilize the end of the movement. Agonist and antagonist contractions are programmed by higher brain centers to fit the situation. Simple movements are programmed before they start so that the movement proceeds from start to finish without modification. Self-terminated movements are more complex; they are programmed to start and are then modified as they proceed.

THE NEUROMUSCULAR UNIT

The neurons that control motor function are referred to as *motoneurons* or sometimes as *alpha motoneurons*. A motor unit consists of one motoneuron and the group of muscle fibers it innervates within a muscle. All muscles contain thousands of muscle fibers and are innervated by many—often many hundred—motor units. The alpha motoneurons supplying a motor unit are located in the ventral horn of the spinal cord and are called lower motoneurons (LMNs). The synapse between an LMN and the muscle fibers of a motor unit is called the *neuromuscular junction*. The motor unit functions as a single unit. If an action potential is generated in the LMN, then, by way of the neuromuscular junction, all the muscle cells in the motor unit will fire simultaneously. Upper motoneurons (UMNs), which exert control over LMNs, project from the motor strip in the cerebral cortex to the ventral horn and are fully contained within the CNS.

Axons of the LMNs exit the spinal cord at each segment to innervate skeletal muscle cells, including those of the limbs, back, abdomen, and chest. Each LMN undergoes multiple branching, making it possible for a single LMN to innervate from 10 to 2000 muscle cells. In general, large muscles—those containing hundreds and thousands of muscle cells and providing gross motor movement—have large motor units. This is in sharp contrast to those that control the hand, tongue, and eye movements in which the motor units are small and permit very discrete control.

THE SPINAL CORD

All of the basic circuitry needed for movement is contained in the spinal cord and brain stem. Although the basic interneural reflex circuitry of the spinal cord is anatomically fixed, the mode of function is governed to a great extent by descending input from higher centers.

In the adult, the spinal cord is located in the upper two thirds of the spinal canal of the vertebral column (Fig. 50-2). It extends from the foramen magnum at the base of the skull to a cone-shaped termination, the conus medullaris, which is usually located at the level of the first or second lumbar vertebra in the adult. From this point, the dorsal and ventral roots angle downward from the cord, forming what is called the *cauda equina*, or horse's tail. The filum terminale, which is composed of nonneural tissues and the *pia mater*, continues caudally and attaches to the second sacral vertebra.

The location of the spinal cord in relation to the vertebral column results in a disparity between the positions of each succeeding cord segment and the exit of its dorsal and ventral nerve roots through the corresponding intervertebral foramina (Fig. 50-3). This disparity becomes more pronounced at the more caudal levels. The arachnoid and its enclosed

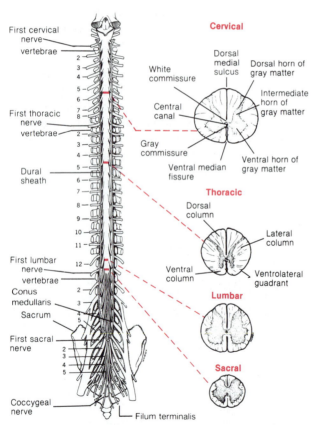

FIG. 50-2. The spinal cord within the vertebral canal. The spinal canal and meninges have been opened. The spinal nerves and vertebrae are numbered on the *left.* Cross (transverse) sections with regional variations in gray matter and increasing proportions of white matter as the cord is ascended appear on the *right.* (Modified from Chaffee, E.E., & Lytle, I.M. [1980]. *Basic physiology and anatomy* [4th ed.]. Philadelphia: J.B. Lippincott)

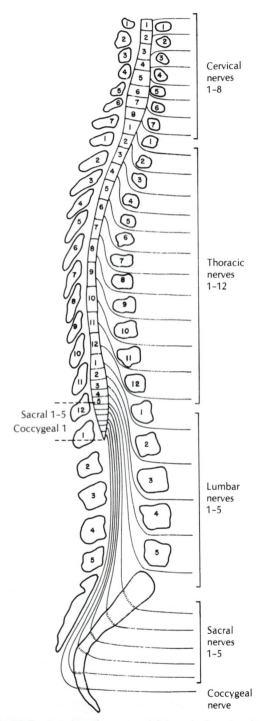

FIG. 50-3. Relation of segments of the spinal cord and spinal nerves to the vertebral column. (Barr, M.L., & Kiernan, J.A. [1988]. *The human nervous system: An anatomical viewpoint* [5th ed., p. 65]. Philadelphia: J.B. Lippincott)

subarachnoid space, which is filled with cerebrospinal fluid (CSF), do not close down on the filum terminale until they reach the second sacral vertebra. This results in the formation of a pocket of CSF, the dural *cisterna spinalis*, which extends from about the second lumbar vertebra to the second sacral vertebra. Because there is an abundant supply of spinal fluid and the spinal cord does not extend this far, the area is often used for sampling the CSF. A procedure called a spinal tap, or puncture, can be done by inserting a special type of needle into the dural sac at the level of L3 and L4. The spinal roots, which are covered with pia mater, are in relatively little danger of trauma from the needle used for this purpose.

Longitudinal Organization. The peripheral nerves that carry information to and from the spinal cord are called spinal nerves. There are 32 or more pairs of spinal nerves (8 cervical, 12 thoracic, 5 lumbar, 5 sacral, and 2 or more coccygeal); each pair is named for the segment of the spinal cord from which it exits. Because the first cervical (C1) spinal nerve exits the spinal cord just above the first cervical vertebra, the nerve is given the number of the bony vertebra just below it. The numbering was changed for all lower levels, however. Thus, an extra cervical nerve, the C8 nerve, exits above the T1 vertebra, and each subsequent nerve is numbered for the vertebra just above its point of exit (see Fig. 50-3).

Segmental Spinal Nerves. Each spinal cord segment communicates with its corresponding body segment through the paired segmental spinal nerves. Each spinal nerve, along with blood vessels that supply the spinal cord, enters the spinal canal through an intervertebral foramen where it divides into two branches, or roots, one of which enters the dorsolateral surface of the cord (the dorsal root), carrying the axons of afferent neurons into the CNS. The other leaves the ventrolateral surface of the cord (the ventral root), carrying the axons of efferent neurons into the periphery (Fig. 50-4). These two roots fuse at the intervertebral foramen, forming the mixed spinal nerve—mixed because it has both afferent and efferent axons.

After emerging from the vertebral column, the mixed spinal nerve divides into two branches: a small dorsal primary ramus and a larger ventral primary ramus (Fig. 50-5). The thoracic and upper lumbar spinal nerves also give rise to a third branch (the ramus communicans) that contains sympathetic axons supplying the blood vessels, the genitourinary system, and the gastrointestinal system. The dorsal ramus contains sensory fibers from the skin and motor fibers to muscles of the back. The anterior primary ramus contains motor fibers that innervate the skel-

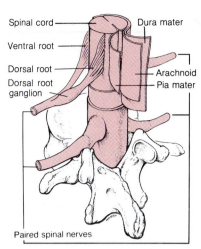

FIG. 50-4. Spinal cord and meninges. (Chaffe, E.E., & Lytle, I.M. [1980]. *Basic physiology and anatomy* [4th ed., p. 234]. Philadelphia: J.B. Lippincott)

etal muscles of the anterior body wall and the legs and arms.

The spinal nerves do not go directly to skin and muscle fibers; instead, they form complicated nerve networks called *plexuses*. A plexus is a site of intermixing nerve branches. A number of spinal nerves enter a plexus and interconnect with other spinal nerves before exiting from the plexus. The nerves that emerge from a plexus form smaller and smaller branches that supply the skin and muscles of the various parts of the body. There are four plexuses of the peripheral nervous system: the cervical plexus, the brachial plexus, the lumbar plexus, and the sacral plexus (Fig. 50-6).

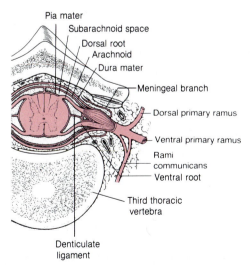

FIG. 50-5. Cross-section of vertebral column at the level of the third thoracic vertebra, showing the meninges, the spinal cord, and the origin of a spinal nerve and its branches or rami. (Modified from Chaffee, E.E., & Lytle, I.M. [1980]. *Basic physiology and anatomy* [4th ed., p. 235]. Philadelphia: J.B. Lippincott)

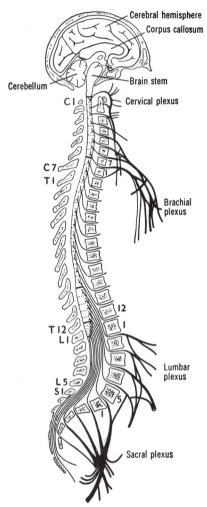

FIG. 50-6. Drawing of the brain and cord *in situ*. The brain is shown in the median plane. Although not illustrated, the first cervical vertebra articulates with the base of the skull. The letters along the vertebral column indicate cervical, thoracic, lumbar, and sacral. Note that the cord ends at the upper border of the second lumbar vertebra. (Gardner, E. [1975]. *Fundamentals of neurology* [2nd ed., p. 35]. Philadelphia: W.B. Saunders)

Transverse Organization. The spinal cord is oval or rounded on transverse section. The internal gray matter has the appearance of a butterfly or letter H (see Fig. 50-5). Some of the neurons that make up the gray matter of the cord have processes or axons that leave the cord, enter the peripheral nerves, and supply tissues such as autonomic ganglia or skeletal muscles. Other neurons in the gray portion of the cord are concerned with input or reflex mechanisms and are called *internuncial neurons* or *interneurons* (see Chapter 47). The white matter of the cord that surrounds the gray matter contains nerve fiber tracts or descending axons that transmit information between segments of the cord or from higher levels of the CNS, such as the brain stem or cerebrum.

The extensions of the gray matter that form the letter H are called the horns. Those that extend posteriorly are called the *dorsal horns*; those that extend anteriorly are called the *ventral horns*. The dorsal horns contain input association neurons that receive afferent impulses through the dorsal roots and other interconnecting neurons. The ventral horns contain output association neurons and the efferent LMNs that leave the cord by way of the ventral roots.

The spinal cord contains many small internuncial neurons that surround the efferent motoneurons and synapse with the cell body or dendrites of the efferent cells. Action potentials of these internuncial neurons exert either excitatory or inhibitory effects on the LMN, and, if the sum of the action potentials passes threshold, LMN action potentials are triggered. Although some CNS systems communicate directly with the LMN, almost all LMN activity is controlled by systems communicating through excitatory or inhibitory internuncial neurons. These internuncial neurons represent the final stage of communication between elaborate CNS neuronal circuits and transmission of information to the skeletal muscle cells of the motor unit. A central portion of the cord, which connects the dorsal and ventral horns and surrounds the central canal, is called the *intermediate gray matter*. In the thoracic area, the small, slender projections that emerge from the intermediate gray matter are called the *intermediolateral columns of the horns*. These columns contain the visceral output association neurons and the efferent neurons of the sympathetic nervous system.

The amount of gray matter present in the cord is largely determined by the amount of tissue innervated by a given segment of the cord (see Fig. 50-2). Larger amounts of gray matter are present in the lower lumbar and upper sacral segments, which supply the lower extremities, and in cervical segment 5 to thoracic segment 1, which supply the upper limbs. The volume of white matter in the spinal cord also increases progressively toward the brain because more and more ascending fibers are added and because the number of descending axons is greater.

SPINAL REFLEXES

A reflex provides a highly reliable relationship between a stimulus and a motor response. Its anatomic basis consists of an afferent neuron, the connection or synapse with CNS neurons that communicate with the effector neuron, and the effector neuron that innervates a muscle or organ. Reflexes are essentially "wired in" to the CNS in that normally they are always ready to function; with training, most reflexes can be modulated to become parts of more complicated movements. A reflex may involve neurons within a single cord segment (segmental reflexes), several or many segments (intersegmental reflexes), or structures in the brain (suprasegmental reflexes). Two important types of spinal motor reflexes are discussed in this chapter: the myotatic reflex and the withdrawal reflex. Autonomic reflexes, which control visceral function, are discussed in Chapter 49.

Myotatic Reflex. Specialized sensory nerve terminals in skeletal muscles, in their tendons and connective tissue sheaths, and in joints relay information on tension in these structures to the CNS. This information, which drives postural reflex mechanisms, is also relayed to the thalamus and the sensory cortex and is experienced as *proprioception* (sense of the body, itself). Two of these sensory mechanisms are very important: (1) muscle spindle receptors and (2) Golgi tendon organs.

Essentially all skeletal muscles contain large numbers of specialized stretch receptor apparatus called *muscle spindles* (Fig. 50-7). These consist of a group of specialized, miniature, thin skeletal muscle fibers (intrafusal fibers) within a connective tissue capsule attached to the connective tissues surrounding the muscle fibers (extrafusal muscle fibers) of a skeletal muscle. Endings of large-diameter afferent neurons (Group Ia) wind in helical fashion around the central region of each of the intrafusal muscle fibers in a spindle; these are "skinniness" receptors. If a skeletal muscle is stretched, the muscle fibers, the spindle, and the intrafusal muscle fibers inside the spindle are stretched and therefore become more slender. Increased slenderness of the intrafusal fibers results in an increased firing rate of the Ia nerve fiber that is proportional to the degree of spindle stretch and therefore extrafusal muscle stretch.

Axons of Ia spindle afferent neurons enter the spinal cord through the dorsal root and have several branches, including one that terminates mainly in the segment of entry and one that ascends the dorsal col-

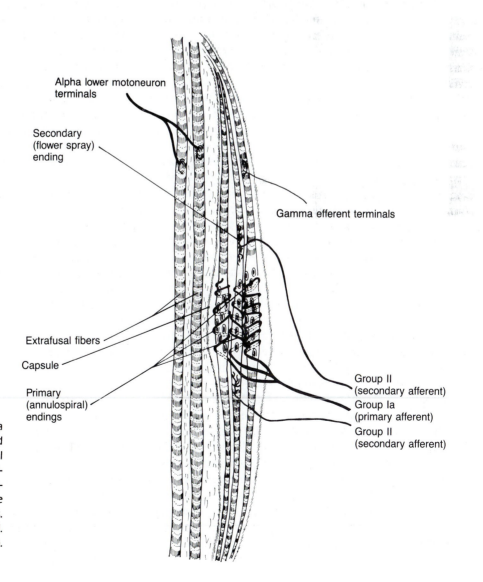

Alpha lower motoneuron terminals

Secondary (flower spray) ending

Gamma efferent terminals

Extrafusal fibers

Capsule

Primary (annulospiral) endings

Group II (secondary afferent)
Group Ia (primary afferent)
Group II (secondary afferent)

FIG. 50-7. Schematic diagram of a muscle spindle showing afferent and efferent innervation of intrafusal muscle fibers and the efferent innervation of neighboring extrafusal muscle fibers. The diameter of the muscle spindle is expanded to show details. (Modified from Cormack, D.H. [1987]. *Ham's histology* [9th ed., p. 408]. Philadelphia: J.B. Lippincott)

umn of the cord to the medulla of the brain stem. The *segmental branch* makes a connection, among several others, that passes directly to the anterior gray matter of the cord and establishes monosynaptic contact with each of the LMNs that have motor units in the muscle containing the spindle source of input. This single synapse or monosynaptic connection is the only known instance of direct afferent-to-efferent neuron reflex in the nervous system.

When a muscle begins to be lengthened, the spindle is stretched; this causes the afferent spindle fibers to increase their rate of firing and produce an opposing muscle contraction through monosynaptic contact with the LMNs that supply the muscle. Another segmental branch of the same Ia neuron's central axon innervates an internuncial neuron, which is, in turn, inhibitory to motor units of antagonistic muscles. Inhibition of these muscle units assists further in opposing muscle stretch. If the extrafusal muscle fibers of a muscle contract and shorten, stretch on the spindle intrafusal muscle fibers is reduced, the Ia firing frequency is reduced, and the Ia is no longer sensitive to minor changes in muscle length. Branches of the Ia axon ascend the spinal cord, sending collateral branches into the dorsal horn of the adjacent segments influencing reflex function at each level. The intersegmental reflexes are particularly important in coordinating hand, neck, and limb movements. The ascending fibers ultimately provide information about muscle length to the cerebellum and cerebral cortex. Descending motor systems can also inhibit or modulate the reflex, making the muscle available for use as a part of programmed movement.

The role of Ia and other classes of muscle spindle afferents is to inform the CNS of the status of muscle length. When a skeletal muscle lengthens or shortens against tension, a mechanism needs to be available for readjustments such that sensory feedback from a muscle remains sensitive to the moment-to-moment status of muscle stretch even while change in muscle length is occurring. The spindle apparatus is adjustable; this is accomplished by a special class of LMNs, the *gamma* LMNs or *gamma* efferents. Their cell bodies also are in the ventral horn, and their axons innervate the tiny intrafusal muscle fibers inside the spindle. This contrasts with alpha LMNs, which control extrafusal muscle contraction that produces muscle force and joint movement. By increasing or decreasing the length of the spindle muscle fibers, gamma LMNs directly affect Ia afferent activity. If the extrafusal muscle fibers of a muscle contract and shorten, stretch on the spindle intrafusal muscle fibers is reduced, the Ia firing frequency is reduced, and the Ia is no longer sensitive to minor changes in muscle length. Central control of gamma LMN activ-

ity can readjust the spindle fiber length and return spindle afferent sensitivity to the momentary contractional situation of the muscle.

Control of intrafusal muscle fiber length provides the CNS with a means of varying the Ia afferent firing rate, thereby controlling the level of stretch reflex activity and, thus, muscle tone. When a muscle is supporting body weight, the stretch reflex operates continuously, producing a continuous *resistance to passive stretch* or continuous *muscle tone*. All muscles possess the stretch reflex mechanism, and, with practice, the excitability of the stretch reflex in a muscle can be estimated by assessing the "floppiness" of a relaxed muscle. If the stretch reflex is not operating within normal limits, this usually indicates that the reflex pathway has suffered damage or that the excitability of the ventral horn LMN pool of the muscle is abnormal. *Hypotonia* (reduced excitability of the stretch reflex) can be due to reduced function in descending facilitatory systems or to damage to the muscle stretch afferent–motor unit circuit. Hypotonia can range from postural weakness to total flaccid paralysis. *Hypertonia* can result from excessive descending facilitation or to changes in segmental circuitry, such as occurs some weeks after an UMN lesion (spasticity) or following damage to the portions of the basal ganglia (rigidity). Under these conditions of greatly increased stiffness (resistance to passive stretch), movement becomes difficult (paresis) or impossible.

A high level of stretch reflex–produced muscle tone in both the agonist and the antagonist muscles around a joint results in a fixed, stable situation. Central control over the gamma LMN mechanism permits increases or decreases in muscle tone in anticipation of changes in the muscle force required to oppose ongoing conditions, such as when weight is about to be lifted. In addition, the gamma LMNs contribute to centrally programmed movements by raising the sensitivity of the stretch reflex in antagonistic muscles and thereby reducing opposition to the oncoming joint movement. Without this programmed adjustability of the stretch reflex, any movement is immediately opposed and prevented. All reflex and learned movement patterns involve programmed control of gamma efferents, resulting in continuous readjustments of stretch reflex sensitivity in agonists, antagonists, and synergists as the movement progresses.

Inverse Myotatic Reflex. The inverse myotatic reflex, most prominent in antigravity muscles, reduces the strength of alpha LMN–driven muscle contraction when the force generated by the muscle threatens the integrity of the muscle or tendon. This protective reflex, which involves two or more synapses in its path, has a very high threshold and activates inhibitory interneurons in the ventral horn that decrease the firing rate of alpha LMNs. Muscle spindle afferents other than the Ia, the Golgi tendon organ afferent, and nociceptive afferents from the connective tissue of the homonymous (same) muscle and tendon drive this high-threshold, protective reflex. The inverse myotatic reflex also has a contralateral component. If, for example, the inverse myotatic reflex produces relaxation of the quadriceps in one leg, the cross-component would produce contraction in the quadriceps of the other leg. The inverse myotatic reflex provides postural stability to ambulatory movements. For example, when the inverse myotatic reflex produces relaxation of antigravity muscles (with flexion) of one leg as we walk, the cross-component produces contraction and extension of the opposite leg.

In persons with spastic paralysis (to be discussed), the inverse myotatic reflex becomes hyperactive and produces what is called the *clasp-knife reaction*. If one were to flex passively the lower limb of such a person at the knee, increasing resistance would be encountered. This resistance would continue to increase until, at some point, it would abruptly cease and the leg could then be passively flexed. Similar signs are seen in spastic upper limbs.

Withdrawal Reflex. Spinal level reflexes provide the "bricks" that are used by higher brain centers to build complex motor movements. Other than the myotatic reflex, most spinal reflexes are entirely polysynaptic and require several segments of the spinal cord to function at a more complex organizational level. They involve automatic integration of many muscle groups into the response, modifying local stretch reflex excitability in the process. The *withdrawal reflex* (sometimes called the flexor-withdrawal reflex) is stimulated by any tissue-threatening or -damaging stimulus and quickly moves the body part away from the offending stimulus (usually by flexing a limb part). When the sole of the foot receives firm pressure stimulation, the *extensor-thrust* reflex pattern results in forceful extension, providing stable body support in basic standing patterns. Alternate *stepping* between opposite limbs during walking and running also involves all four limbs and the entire length of the spinal cord. This is retained as the swinging of the arms in normal human walking and running. Other spinal level reflexes include reflex relaxation of the external anal and urethral sphincters during defecation and urination and coordinated contraction of intercostal, diaphragmatic, back, and shoulder muscles during the inspiratory part of the

respiratory cycle. Intact neuronal circuitry and normal-range excitability of these reflexes are required for brain stem and forebrain motor control to operate properly.

THE BRAIN STEM

Normally one does not have to think about controlling the muscle activity that allows one to stand erect despite the force of gravity. Instead, input from brain stem structures automatically influences reflex mechanisms of the spinal cord and allows maintenance of body posture, pacing of steps, and recovery of posture when balance is disrupted.

The anatomic components of the brain stem are the medulla, pons, and midbrain (Fig. 50-8). At its caudal end, the brain stem is continuous with the spinal cord; at its rostral end, it is continuous with the diencephalon that is bounded by the cerebral hemispheres. The motor centers of the brain stem are the red nucleus, lateral vestibular nucleus, superior colliculus, and certain parts of the reticular formation.

The brain stem centers are located between the higher motor centers and the spinal cord and form part of the descending control systems that influence the motor component of spinal cord and cranial nerve reflexes. The lateral vestibular nucleus gives rise to an uncrossed tract, which projects to the ventral horn of the spinal cord; it is excitatory to extensor motor neurons and inhibits flexor neurons. For example, when the head and body begin to tilt to one side, the tilt is opposed by vestibular reflex contraction of the neck flexors of the opposite side and of limb extensor muscles of the same side, maintaining a stable head and body posture. Input from the labyrinth (see Chapter 53) is concerned with bending, rotation, and linear acceleration or deceleration.

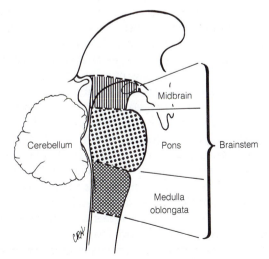

FIG. 50-8. Brain stem structures.

The reticular formation in the pons and medulla gives rise to two reticulospinal tracts: (1) the medullary fibers, which excite flexor neurons and inhibit extensor motoneurons, and (2) the pontine fibers, which excite extensors and inhibit flexors. Interplay between these descending tract systems modifies the excitability of spinal reflexes to produce complex motor movements, such as coordination of walking and running movements, and righting reflexes, which maintain or reestablish body and head positions. Many fundamental automatic movement patterns are provided by the brain stem's reticular formation circuitry, including respiratory movements, sneezing and coughing, and chewing and swallowing. The brain stem also contains circuitry for coordination of autonomic and somatic motor functions, such as shivering and vomiting. Damage to brain stem motor areas often results in death because of the fundamental importance of these life-sustaining responses.

THE CEREBELLUM

The cerebellum is located in the posterior fossa of the cranium superior to the pons (see Fig. 50-8). It is separated from the cerebral hemispheres by a fold of dura mater, the tentorium cerebelli. The cerebellum consists of a small unpaired median portion, called the *vermis*, and two large lateral masses, the cerebellar hemispheres. In contrast to the brain stem with its external white matter and internal gray nuclei, the cerebellum, like the cerebrum, has an outer cortex of gray matter and a core of white matter. A series of nuclei are embedded deep in the white matter. Axons from cells of the cortex and association fibers of the nuclei connect cortex-to-cortex communication, cortex-to-nuclei communication, and vice versa. Projection fibers from the nuclei relay information to many regions, particularly to the motor cortex by means of a thalamic relay.

The synergistic (temporal smoothing) functions of the cerebellum participate in all movement of limbs, trunk, head, larynx, and eyes, whether the movement is part of a voluntary movement or of a highly learned semiautomatic or automatic movement. During highly skilled movements, the motor cortex sends signals to the cerebellum, informing it about the movement that is to be performed. The cerebellum makes continuous adjustments, resulting in smoothness of movement, particularly during delicate maneuvers. Highly skillful movement requires extensive motor training, and there is considerable evidence that many of these learned movement patterns involve cerebellar circuits.

The cerebellum receives sensory input from the vestibular system, eyes, ears, skin, muscles, joints, and tendons that monitor movement. It is the main central target for proprioceptive information. The sensory input from a given area of the body arrives at the same area in the cerebellum as input from the motor cortex that controls the motor units in that body area. In this way, the cerebellum is able to assess continuously the status of each body part—position, rate of movement, and forces such as gravity that are opposing movement. The cerebellum compares what is actually happening with what is intended to happen; it then transmits appropriate corrective signals back to the motor system, instructing it to increase or decrease the activity of certain muscle groups and regulating their contractions so that smooth and accurate movements are performed.

One of the functions of the cerebellum is the dampening of muscle movement. All body movements are basically pendular (swinging to and fro). As movement begins, momentum develops and must be overcome before movement can be stopped. Because of momentum, all movements have a tendency to overshoot if they are not dampened. In the intact cerebellum, automatic signals stop movement precisely at the intended point. In providing for this type of control, the cerebellum predicts the future position of moving parts of the body; the rapidity with which the limb is moving, as well as the projected time for the course of movement, is detected from incoming proprioceptive signals. This allows the cerebellum to inhibit agonist muscles and excite antagonist muscles when movement approaches the intended target.

THE BASAL GANGLIA

The basal ganglia are the several large masses of neurons that lie on either side of the thalamus and surround the internal capsule. The term *corpus striatum* (striped body) is sometimes used interchangeably with basal ganglia. The major components of the basal ganglia are the caudate (tailed) nucleus, the putamen, and the globus pallidus (pale body). The globus pallidus and putamen make up the lentiform nucleus. As with the motor cortex, the nuclei on the left side control movement on the right side of the body, and vice versa. Circuits interconnecting the premotor cortex and supplementary motor cortex, the basal ganglia, and parts of the thalamus provide associated movements that accompany highly skilled behaviors. The basal ganglia provide gracefulness to the performance as well as the supportive background for highly skilled movements. Intact and functional basal ganglia provide the swinging of the arms during walking and running and the follow-through movements that accompany throwing a ball or swinging a club. Parkinson's disease, Huntington's chorea, some forms of cerebral palsy, among other dysfunctions involving the basal ganglia, result in a frequent or continuous release of abnormal postural or axial and proximal movement patterns. If damage to the basal ganglia is localized to one side, the movements are of the opposite side of the body. These automatic movement patterns stop only in sleep, but in some conditions the movements are so violent that getting to sleep becomes difficult.

THE MOTOR CORTEX

The motor cortex is located in the posterior part of the frontal lobe. It consists of the primary, premotor, and supplementary motor cortex. The primary motor cortex (area 4) is located on the rostral surface and adjacent portions of the central sulcus (see Fig. 51-6). The premotor area (area 6) lies immediately rostral to the primary motor cortex. The neurons in the primary motor cortex are arranged in a somatotopic array or distorted map of the body (motor homunculus [Fig. 50-9]). The distorted body map represents the neurons that control voluntary movement of a particular body part. The body parts that require the greatest dexterity have the greatest cortical areas devoted to them. Over one-half of the primary motor cortex is concerned with controlling the muscles of the hands and muscles of speech.[2] The supplementary motor cortex is found in the part of area 6 that lies on the medial surface of the hemisphere.

The primary motor cortex is very thick. It contains many layers of pyramid-shaped output neurons that project to the cortex of the opposite side, to the premotor cortex, to the somesthetic strip of the parietal cortex that is located on the other side of the central sulcus, to the basal ganglia, and to the thalamus on the same side of the brain. The large pyramidal cells located in the fifth layer project to the brain stem and spinal cord. These UMNs send their axons through the subcortical white matter and the internal capsule to the deep surface of the brain stem, through the ventral bulge of the pons, to the ventral surface of the medulla where they form a ridge or pyramid. At the junction between the medulla and cervical spinal cord, 80% or more of the UMN axons cross the midline (decussate) to form the lateral *corticospinal tract* or pyramidal tract in the lateral white matter of the spinal cord. This tract extends throughout the spinal cord, with roughly 50% of its fibers terminating in the cervical segments, 20% in the thoracic segments, and 30% in the lumbosacral segments.[3] Most of the remaining uncrossed fibers travel down the ventral column of the cord, mainly to cervical levels, where they cross and innervate contralateral LMNs.

The premotor area sends some fibers into the corticospinal tract but mainly innervates the primary motor strip. A movement pattern to accomplish a particular objective, such as throwing a ball or picking up a fork, is planned by the prefrontal association cortex and associated thalamic nuclei. The "model" for the movement pattern includes both the muscle contractional sequences for complex distal manipulation as well as the larger preparative and supportive actions of whole limbs and limb girdles. It involves the function of the premotor cortex (areas 6 and 8) just anterior to the primary motor cortex and its projections to the primary motor cortex. The primary motor cortex, often called the *motor strip*, controls discrete muscle sequences and is the first level of descending control for precise movements. Discrete lesions within the most posterior part of the primary motor cortex result in profound weakness in specific distal flexor muscle groups and permanent inability to perform delicate manipulative motor patterns on the opposite side of the body or face. Lesions restricted to the more anterior part of the motor strip result in weakness of larger limb and girdle muscles.

On the medial surface of the hemisphere in the premotor region, a *supplementary motor region* contains representation of all parts of the body. The supplementary cortex is intimately involved in the initiation of planned, delicate, skillful movement. Bilateral lesions result in long-lasting loss (akinesia) of movements involving both hands or both feet and can result in long-term loss of speech (mutism).

Monosynaptic innervation of LMNs by UMNs of

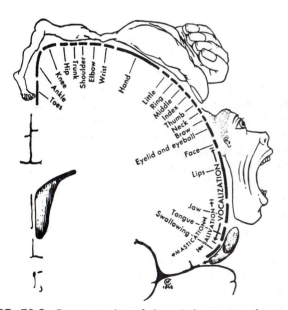

FIG. 50-9. Representation of the relative extent of motor cortical area 4 devoted to muscles of the various body regions. Medial surface is at the left, lateral fissure is at the right, with pharyngeal and laryngeal muscle representation extending toward the insula. (Penfield, E., & Rasmussen, T. [1968]. *The cerebral cortex in man: A clinical study of localization of function.* New York: Macmillan)

the primary motor cortex only occurs for the most distal muscles involved with delicate manipulative skills (*e.g.*, those of the hands and fingers, tongue, mouth, and pharynx). For LMNs of other muscles, the connection is multisynaptic and less discrete. As the UMN axons pass along their long pathways, collateral branches move out and innervate regions of the basal ganglia, the thalamus, the brain stem, and nuclei that project into the cerebellum. The cerebellum matches the temporal smoothness aspect of the "model" with the ongoing movement against proprioceptive feedback from the actual movement and sends error signals back to the thalamus and motor cortex for corrective modifications of the ongoing movement. Similarly, sensory feedback to the basal ganglia results in error-correcting feedback for supportive and background aspects of the movement and sensory cortex for somesthetic based error correction. Ongoing error correction becomes less and less important for well-learned movements, which can proceed without sensory feedback.

THE PYRAMIDAL VERSUS EXTRAPYRAMIDAL SYSTEMS

By convention, motor tracts are classified as belonging to one of two motor systems: pyramidal and extrapyramidal systems. The so-called pyramidal system consists of the motor pathways originating in the motor cortex and terminating in the brain stem (corticobulbar fibers) and the spinal cord (corticospinal fibers). The corticospinal fibers traverse the ventral surface of the medulla in a bundle called the *pyramid* before decussating (crossing to the opposite side) at the medulla–spinal cord junction—hence the name *pyramidal system*. The cortex and basal ganglia also project to the brain stem reticular formation, and reticulospinal systems provide an ancient pathway to LMNs of proximal and extensor muscles. These fibers do not decussate in the pyramids—hence the name *extrapyramidal*. The pyramidal and extrapyramidal systems have different effects on muscle tone. The pyramidal system is largely excitatory; it provides control of delicate muscle movement. The extrapyramidal system provides the more crude, background supportive movement patterns. In terms of actual function, the pyramidal and extrapyramidal systems do not function independently of each other. The concept of two separate systems is helpful, however, in understanding motor function. Following severe damage to the pyramidal system, the crude movements and (under heightened emotional conditions) crude, slurred speech that can still occur are due to extrapyramidal function. Table 50-1 summarizes the characteristics of the pyramidal and extrapyramidal motor systems.

In summary, motor function involves the neuromuscular unit, spinal cord circuitry, brain stem neurons, the cerebellum, the basal ganglia, and the motor cortex. A motor unit consists of one LMN and the group of muscle fibers it innervates within the muscle. Stretch receptors provide muscle tone by means of the stretch reflex. The basic reflex circuitry controlling muscle function is located in the spinal cord. Brain stem circuits contribute basic movement patterns, the cerebellum provides temporal smoothness to movement, and the basal ganglia provides gracefulness. Upper motoneurons, which provide delicate control over LMNs, project from the motor strip in the cerebral cortex to the ventral horn. The UMNs in the motor cortex send their axons through the subcortical white matter, internal capsule, and the deep surface of the brain stem, to the ventral surface to the opposite side of the medulla, where they form a pyramid before crossing the midline to form the lateral corticospinal tract in the spinal cord. A skillful movement pattern is planned in the prefrontal cortex; a sequential model is organized in the premotor cortex, initiated via the supplementary motor cortex and carried out by the primary motor cortex. The basal ganglia and cerebellum provide ongoing support functions contributing gracefulness and temporal smoothness to the ongoing movement. If the UMN system is severely damaged, delicate and skillful movement is lost but crude movement still can be made using extrapyramidal systems.

■ DISORDERS OF NEUROMUSCULAR FUNCTION

SKELETAL MUSCLE DISORDERS

Disorders of skeletal muscle groups involve both atrophy and dystrophy. *Atrophy* describes a shrinkage, death, or disappearance of muscle cells secondary to some type of nerve injury or disease. *Muscular dystrophy* is a primary disorder of muscle tissue and is characterized by a defect in the muscle fibers.

MUSCLE ATROPHY

Maintenance of muscle strength requires relatively frequent movements against resistance. Reduced use results in muscle atrophy, which is characterized by a reduction in the diameter of the muscle fibers due to a loss of protein filaments. When a normally innervated muscle is not used for long periods of time, the muscle cells shrink in diameter, and although the muscle cells do not die, they become weakened. This is called *disuse atrophy* and occurs with conditions such as immobilization and chronic illness.

The most extreme examples of muscle atrophy, however, are found in disorders that deprive muscles of their innervation. This is called *denervation atrophy*. During early embryonic development, outgrowing skeletal nerves innervate partially mature muscle cells. If the developing muscle cells are not innervated, they will not mature and will eventually die. In the

TABLE 50-1. CHARACTERISTICS OF PYRAMIDAL AND EXTRAPYRAMIDAL MOTOR CONTROL

FEATURE	PYRAMIDAL	EXTRAPYRAMIDAL	PERIPHERAL
Nomenclature	(1) Voluntary motor pathway (2) Upper motor neuron (UMN) pathway (3) Corticospinal pathway	(1) Involuntary motor pathway (2) Extracorticospinal	(1) Final common pathway (2) Lower motor neuron (LMN) pathway
Location	From the Betz cells of the frontal lobe motor strip to the anterior horn cell of the spinal cord	Motor cortex with projections into basal ganglia, and communication with the reticular formation	From the ventral horn cells of the spinal cord to the neuromuscular junction
Function	Initiates and transmits impulses for highly skilled voluntary movement to spinal cord	(1) Inhibits muscle tone throughout the body (2) Initiates and regulates associated or background movement patterns	Transmits impulses from the spinal cord to skeletal muscles
Disruption	Muscle weakness; loss of fine manipulative skills; hyperactive reflexes and spastic paralysis on the contralateral side—hemiplegia	Muscle rigidity and incoordination Loss of discrete movement Abnormal postures and automatic movements	Hypoactive reflexes and paresis or flaccid paralysis, usually monoplegia. Destruction results in denervation atrophy followed by muscle cell degeneration and muscle wasting
Extent of damage	Small amount of damage in important area (*e.g.,* internal capsule) causes extensive decrease in function	If part of basal ganglia is left intact, gross postural and ''fixed'' movements can still be performed; widespread damage leads to muscle rigidity throughout the body	Extensive damage (several levels) before function is significantly decreased

process of innervation, randomly contracting muscle cells become enslaved by the innervating neurons; from then on, the muscle cell contracts only when stimulated by that particular neuron. If the LMN dies or its axon is destroyed, the skeletal muscle cell is again free of neural domination. When this happens, it begins to have temporary spontaneous contractions (called *fibrillations*) of its own. It also begins to lose its contractile proteins and, if not reinnervated, will degenerate after several months.

If a peripheral motor neuron is crushed and its endoneurial tube remains intact, regenerating axons can grow down the connective tissue tube to reinnervate the muscle cell. If the nerve is cut, however, scar tissue between the cut ends of the endoneurial tube reduces the likelihood of axonic reinnervation by the original axon, and muscle cell loss is likely to occur. If some intact LMN axons remain within the muscle, nearby denervated muscle cells apparently emit what is called a *trophic signal*, probably a chemical messenger, that signals intact axons to sprout and send outgrowing collaterals into the denervated area and recapture control of some of the denervated muscle fibers. The degree of axonic regeneration that occurs

after injury to an LMN depends on the amount of scar tissue that develops at the site of injury and how quickly reinnervation occurs. If reinnervation occurs after the muscle cell has degenerated, no recovery is possible. Thus, peripheral nerve section usually results in some loss of muscle cell function, which is experienced as weakness. Collateral sprout reinnervation results in enlarged motor units and, therefore, a reduction in the discreteness of muscle control following recovery.

MUSCULAR DYSTROPHY

Muscular dystrophy is a term applied to a number of genetic disorders that produce progressive deterioration of skeletal muscles because of mixed muscle cell hypertrophy, atrophy, and necrosis. They are primary diseases of muscle tissue and probably do not involve the nervous system. As the muscle undergoes necrosis, fat and connective tissue replace the muscle fibers, which increases muscle size and results in muscle weakness. The increase in muscle size resulting from connective tissue infiltration is called *pseudohypertrophy*. The muscle weakness is insidious in onset but continually progressive, varying with the type of disorder.

The most common form of the disease is Duchenne's muscular dystrophy, which has an incidence of about 3 per 100,000. Duchenne's muscular dystrophy is inherited as a recessive single gene defect on the X chromosome and, hence, is transmitted from the mother to her male offspring. A spontaneous (mutation) form may occur in females. Another form of dystrophy, Becker's muscular dystrophy, is similarly X-linked but has its onset later in childhood or adolescence and has a slower course. In Duchenne's muscular dystrophy, the postural muscles of the hip and shoulder are affected first; the child usually performs normally until around 3 years of age when frequent falling begins to occur. Wheelchairs are usually needed at a mean age of 9.5 years.[4] Death due to respiratory and cardiac muscle involvement usually occurs in young adulthood. About 70% of deaths result from respiratory causes alone.[4] Observation of the child's voluntary movement and a complete family history provide important diagnostic data for the disease. Muscle biopsy, which shows fat in the muscle tissues, electromyograms, and serum levels of the enzyme creatine phosphokinase (CPK), which leaks out of damaged muscle fibers, can be used to confirm the diagnosis. Gene probes are being developed that can be used for carrier detection and prenatal diagnosis.[5]

To date, there is no cure for any of the muscular dystrophies. Although there have been exciting research advances toward identifying the gene and gene product involved in Duchenne's muscular dystrophy,[6, 7] new cases continue to occur. Imbalances between agonist and antagonist muscles lead to abnormal postures and the development of contractures and joint immobility. Management of the disease is directed toward maintaining ambulation and preventing deformities. Passive stretching, correct or counter posturing, and splints help to prevent deformities. Precautions should be taken to avoid respiratory infections.

DISORDERS OF THE MYONEURAL JUNCTION

The transmission of impulses at the myoneural junction is mediated by the release of the neurotransmitter *acetylcholine* (ACh) from the axon terminals. Acetylcholine binds to specific receptors in the end-plate region of the muscle fiber surface to cause muscle contraction. Studies suggest that there are over a million binding sites per motor end-plate.[1]

Acetylcholine is active in the myoneural junction for only a brief period of time, during which an action potential is generated in the innervated muscle cell. Some of the transmitter diffuses out of the synapse, and the remaining transmitter is rapidly inactivated by an enzyme called *acetylcholinesterase*. This enzyme splits the ACh molecule into choline and acetic acid. The choline is transported back into the nerve terminal and reused in the synthesis of acetylcholine. The rapid inactivation of acetylcholine at the myoneural junction allows for repeated muscle contractions and, thus, gradations of contractile force.

A number of drugs and agents can alter neuromuscular function by changing the release, inactivation, or receptor binding of ACh. Curare acts on the postjunctional membrane of the motor end-plate to prevent the depolarizing effect of the neurotransmitter. Blocking of neuromuscular transmission by curare-type drugs is used during many types of surgical procedures to facilitate relaxation of involved musculature. Physostigmine and neostigmine inhibit acetycholinesterase and allow acetylcholine released from the motoneuron to accumulate. These drugs are used in the treatment of myasthenia gravis (to be discussed). Toxins from the botulism organism produce paralysis by blocking acetylcholine release. Spores from the botulism organism may be found in soil-grown foods that are not cooked at temperatures of at least 100°C in home-canning procedures. The organophosphates (*e.g.*, malathion and parathion) that are used in some insecticides bind acetylcholinesterase. They produce excessive and prolonged ACh action with depolarization block of cholinergic receptors, including those of the myoneural junction. Other organophosphate compounds were developed as nerve gases during World War I with similar and, if absorbed in high concentrations, lethal effects due to loss of respiratory muscle function.

MYASTHENIA GRAVIS

Myasthenia gravis is a disorder of transmission at the myoneural junction that affects communication between the motoneuron and the innervated muscle cell. The prevalence of myasthenia gravis is 4 to 6 per 100,000.[8] The disease is about three times more common in women than men; it may occur at any age, but the peak incidence of onset is between 20 and 30 years of age. A small second peak occurs in later life and affects men more often than women. The disorder appears transiently and lasts for days to weeks in about 10% of infants born to mothers with myasthenia gravis.

Myasthenia gravis is thought to result from a decrease in ACh receptor sites at the myoneural junction that leads to decreased muscle function. Evidence indicates that the reduction in ACh receptors results from an autoimmune response.[8] Autoantibodies binding to acetylcholine receptors are found in most persons with the disease. This receptor antibody is thought to cause receptor degradation and inhibition of receptor synthesis. The exact mechanism that triggers the autoimmune response is unknown but is thought to be related to abnormal T-lymphocyte characteristics. About 15% to 40% of persons with myasthenia gravis also have thymic abnormalities, either a thyoma (thymus tumor) or thymic hyperplasia (increased thymus weight due to increased number of thymus cells).[9]

The primary clinical manifestations of myasthenia are weakness of the eye muscles, with ptosis (drooping of the upper eyelids) and diplopia (double vision) caused by weakness of the extraocular muscles. Neuromuscular and eyelid weakness can be checked following instructions to have a person firmly close his or her eyes. Normally eyelashes are not seen with firm eye closure. In persons with myasthenia gravis, the eyelid muscles are weakened and the eyelashes often remain visible.[10] Extraocular muscle weakness can be tested by having the person maintain an upward gaze for 2 to 3 minutes while observations for eye muscle fatigue are made.

The clinical course varies. The disease may progress from ocular muscle weakness to generalized weakness, including respiratory weakness. Chewing and swallowing may be difficult, and persons with the disease often choose to eat soft puddings and cereals rather than meats and hard fruit. Masticatory weakness can be checked by having the person repetitively open and close the jaw against resistance.[10] Weakness in limb movement is usually more pronounced in proximal than in distal parts of the extremity, so that climbing stairs and lifting objects are difficult. As the disease progresses, the muscles of the lower face are affected, causing speech impairment. When this happens, the person often supports the chin with one hand to assist in speaking. In most people, symptoms are least evident when arising in the morning but grow worse with effort and as the day proceeds. General muscle weakness can be assessed by having the person continuously maintain a position, such as holding the arms overhead or extending the fingers.

Cranial nerve weakness and progressive muscle fatigue after exertion without sensory symptoms, changes in consciousness, or autonomic dysfunction are early signs of myasthenia gravis. Because the disease is relatively uncommon, it frequently goes undiagnosed until generalized weakness occurs. The diagnosis is based on the Tensilon (edrophonium chloride) test, during which edrophonium, a short-acting acetylcholinesterase inhibitor, is administered intravenously. The drug has the effect of decreasing the breakdown of ACh at the myoneural junction by

the enzyme acetylcholinesterase. When weakness is due to myasthenia gravis, a dramatic transitory improvement in muscle function occurs. Another diagnostic method is to assay the titer of ACh receptor antibodies circulating in the blood.

A recent advance in diagnostic methods for myasthenia gravis is the single-fiber electromyography, which is available in many medical centers. The technique involves recording the action potential from two or more muscle fibers within a muscle unit. This method can diagnose myasthenia gravis in most cases.

Treatment methods include use of pharmacologic agents, management of myasthenic crisis, thymectomy, and plasmapheresis. Pharmacologic treatment with anticholinesterase drugs inhibits the hydrolysis of ACh at the myoneural junction by acetylcholinesterase. Pyridostigmine (Mestinon) and neostigmine (Prostigmin) are the drugs of choice. Corticosteroid drugs, which suppress the immune response, are used in cases of a poor response to anticholinesterase drugs and thymectomy. Immunosuppressant drugs may also be used, often in combination with plasmapheresis.

Thymectomy, or surgical removal of the thymus, may be performed as a treatment for myasthenia gravis. Because the mechanism whereby surgery exerts its effect is unknown, the treatment is controversial. Currently, thymectomy is performed in persons with thymoma regardless of age and in persons 50 to 60 years of age or older with recent onset of moderate disease. Plasmapheresis, a procedure in which the plasma with the IgG immunoglobulin fraction is separated and removed from the person's blood, is a recent treatment method yielding variable results. Usually six to eight treatments are needed to bring about a transient improvement.

Persons with myasthenia gravis may develop a sudden exacerbation of symptoms and weakness known as *myasthenic crisis*. This usually occurs during a period of stress, such as infection, emotional upset, pregnancy, alcohol ingestion, cold, or following surgery. Many times, no primary cause can be identified. However, myasthenic crisis resulting from the need for more medication is virtually indistinguishable from cholinergic crisis resulting from too much medication. In the case of too much medication, cholinergic crisis is often accompanied by nausea, vomiting, pallor, sweating, salivation, colic, diarrhea, miosis, or bradycardia due to the muscarinic effects of the anticholinesterase drugs. Whatever the cause, prompt medical treatment is needed. To determine whether the crisis was precipitated by the disease process or by cholinergic drugs, the Tensilon test is used. If the crisis is myasthenic, the symptoms will improve. Provision for respiratory support should be available in either case.

PERIPHERAL NERVE DISORDERS

The peripheral nervous system (PNS) consists of the motor and sensory nerves of the cranial and spinal nerves, the peripheral parts of the autonomic nervous system, and peripheral ganglia. A peripheral neuropathy is any primary disorder of the peripheral nerves. The result is usually muscle weakness, with or without atrophy, or sensory changes, or both. The disorder can involve a single nerve (mononeuropathy) or multiple nerves (polyneuropathy).

Unlike the tracts of the CNS, peripheral nerves are fairly strong and resilient. This is because they contain a series of connective tissue sheaths that enclose their nerve fibers.[12] An outer fibrous sheath called the *epineurium* surrounds the moderate to large-sized nerves; inside, a sheath called the *perineurium* invests each bundle of nerve fibers; within each bundle, a delicate sheath of connective tissue known as the *endoneurium* surrounds each individual nerve fiber (see Chapter 47, Fig. 47-11). Small peripheral nerves lack the epineurial covering. Within its endoneurial sheath, each nerve fiber is invested by a segmented sheath of Schwann's cells. The Schwann's cells produce the myelin sheath that surrounds the peripheral nerves. Each Schwann's cell, however, can only myelinate one segment of a single axon so that myelination of an entire axon requires the participation of a long line of these cells.[11]

PERIPHERAL NERVE INJURY

Neurons exemplify the general principle that the more specialized the function of a cell type, the less able it is to regenerate. For most neurons, cell division ceases by the time of birth; from then on the cell body of a neuron is unable to divide and replace itself. Although the entire neuron cannot be replaced, it is often possible for the dendritic and axon cell processes to regenerate as long as the cell body remains viable.

When a peripheral nerve is destroyed by a crushing force or by a cut that penetrates the nerve, the portion of the nerve fiber that is separated from the cell body rapidly undergoes degenerative changes, while the central stump and cell body of the nerve are often able to survive (Fig. 50-10). Because the cell body synthesizes the material required for nourishing and maintaining the axon, it is likely that the loss of these materials results in the degeneration of the separated portion of the nerve fibers.

Following injury, the Schwann cells that are distal to the site of damage are also able to survive, but their myelin degenerates in a process called *Wallerian degeneration*. The Schwann cells assist other phagocy-

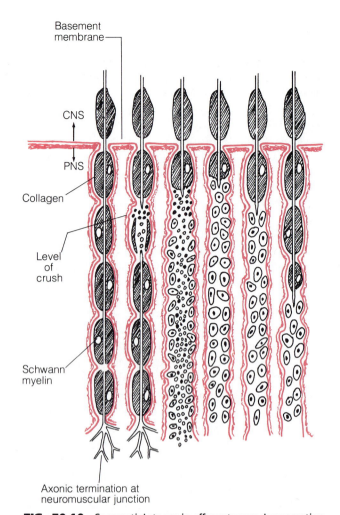

FIG. 50-10. Sequential stages in efferent axon degeneration and regeneration within its endoneurial tube, following peripheral nerve crush injury.

tic cells in the area in the cleanup of the debris caused by the degenerating axon and myelin. As they remove the debris, the Schwann cells multiply and fill the empty endoneurial tube. At this point nothing further happens unless a regenerating nerve fiber penetrates into the endoneurial tube, in which case the Schwann cells reform the myelin segments around the fiber.

Meanwhile, the cell body of the neuron responds to the loss of part of its nerve fiber by shifting into a phase of greatly increased protein and lipid synthesis. It does this by dispersing the masses of ribosomes, which stain as Nissl granules. They cease to be stainable and disappear in a process called *chromatolysis*. In the process, the nucleus moves away from the axonal side of the cell body as if displaced by the active synthetic apparatus of the cells. These changes reach their height within about 10 days of injury and continue until regrowth of the nerve fiber ceases.

In the process of regeneration, the injured nerve

fiber develops one or more new branches from the proximal nerve stump, which grow into the developing scar tissue. If a crushing injury has occurred and the endoneurial tube is intact through the trauma area, the outgrowing fiber will grow back down this tube to the structure that was originally innervated by the neuron. However, if the injury involves the severing of an axon, then the outgrowing branch must come in contact with its original endoneurial tube if it is to be reunited with its original target structure. The rate of outgrowth of regenerating nerve fibers is about 1 mm to 2 mm per day, so that the recovery of conduction to a target structure depends not only on regrowth into the appropriate endoneurial tube but also on the distance involved. It can take weeks or months for the regrowing fiber to reach the end organ and communicative function to be reestablished. Further time is required for the Schwann cells to form new myelin segments and for the axon to recover its original diameter and conduction velocity.

The successful regeneration of a nerve fiber in the PNS depends on many factors. If a nerve fiber is destroyed relatively close to the neuronal cell body, the chances are that the nerve cell will die, and if it does it will not be replaced. If a crushing type of injury has occurred, partial or often full recovery of function occurs. A cutting-type trauma to a nerve is an entirely different matter. Connective scar tissue forms rapidly at the wound site, and only the most rapidly regenerating axonal branches are able to get through to the intact distal endoneurial tubes. A number of scar-inhibiting agents have been used in an effort to reduce this hazard but have met with only moderate success. In another attempt to improve nerve regeneration, various types of tubular implants have been placed to fill longer gaps in the endoneurial tube.

Perhaps the most difficult problem is the alignment of the proximal and distal endoneurial tubes so that regenerating fiber can return down its former tube and innervate its former organ. This problem is similar to realigning a large telephone cable that has been cut so that all the wires are reconnected exactly as before the separation. Microscopic alignment of the cut edges during microsurgical repair results in improved success. An efferent nerve fiber that formerly innervated a skeletal muscle will regrow down an endoneurial tube formerly occupied by an afferent fiber and reach the former sensory area; then its cell body will eventually die. A sensory fiber that grows down an endoneurial tube that connects with a skeletal muscle fiber will undergo the same fate. If, however, these fibers grow down endoneurial tubes that innervate the appropriate type of target organ, reinnervation and function may return, even though the fibers have changed places. Under the best of conditions, a 10% regeneration to the appropriate organ is considered a success once a peripheral nerve has been severed. Even so, considerable function will return with that amount of innervation.

PERIPHERAL NERVE ROOT INJURY: PROLAPSED INTERVERTEBRAL DISK

The intervertebral disk is considered the most critical component of the load-bearing structures of the spinal column. The structural components of the disk make it capable of absorbing shock and changing shape while allowing movement.[12] The intervertebral disk can become dysfunctional owing to trauma or the effects of aging. This results in movement between the articulating vertebral segments and the loss of the elastic properties of the disk itself. With aging or dysfunction, the nucleus pulposus (inner portion of the disk) can be squeezed out of place and herniate through the annulus fibrosus (outer portion of the disk), a condition referred to as a herniated or prolapsed disk (Fig. 50-11). When this happens, the nucleus pulposus usually moves laterally or dorsally, causing irritation or crushing of a nerve root or the spinal cord. This irritation causes spontaneous firing of the sensory afferents and severe pain is experienced—local pain due to injured tissue and pain referred to the area of dermatomal distribution of the spinal nerve root. Crushing damage to the dorsal roots results in reduction or loss of sensation, and crushing of the ventral roots produces muscle weakness. The signs and symptoms of a prolapsed disk

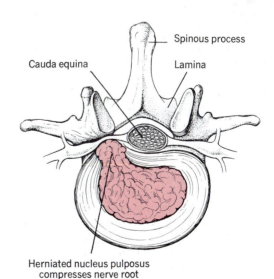

FIG. 50-11. A prolapsed (herniated) intervertebral disk. The soft central portion of the disk is protruding into the vertebral canal, where it exerts pressure on a spinal nerve root. (Chaffee, E.E., & Lytle, I.M. [1980]. *Basic physiology and anatomy* [4th ed., p. 103]. Philadelphia: J.B. Lippincott)

are localized to the area of the body innervated by the nerve roots.

The level at which a prolapsed disk occurs is important. Usually it occurs at the lower levels of the lumbar spine, where both the mass being supported and the bending of the vertebral column are greatest. When the injury occurs in this area, only the cauda equina will be irritated or crushed. Because these elongated dorsal and ventral roots contain endoneurial tubes of connective tissue, regeneration of the nerve fibers is likely. However, several weeks or months are required for full recovery to occur because of the distance to the innervated muscle or skin of the lower limbs. A prolapsed disk pressing into the spinal canal at higher levels can destroy the ventral white matter or can completely transect the cord. Here regeneration is unlikely, and the paralysis and anesthesia of the caudal body regions may be permanent.

MONONEUROPATHIES

Mononeuropathies are usually caused by localized conditions, such as trauma, compression, or infections, that affect a single spinal nerve, plexus, or peripheral nerve trunk. Fractured bones may lacerate or compress nerves; excessively tight tourniquets may injure nerves directly or produce ischemic injury; and infections such as herpes zoster may affect a single segmental afferent nerve distribution. Recovery of nerve function is usually complete following compression lesions and incomplete or faulty following nerve transection.

Carpal Tunnel Syndrome. Carpal tunnel syndrome is an example of a compression-type mononeuropathy that is relatively common. It is caused by compression of the median nerve as it travels with the flexor tendons through a canal made by the carpal bones and transverse carpal ligament. The condition can be caused by a variety of conditions that produce either a reduction in the capacity of the carpal tunnel (bony or ligament changes) or an increase in the volume of the tunnel contents (*e.g.*, inflammation of the tendons, synovial swelling, or tumors).[12] Carpal tunnel syndrome can be a feature of many systemic diseases, such as rheumatoid arthritis, hyperthyroidism, acromegaly, and diabetes mellitus. The condition can result from wrist injury; it can occur during pregnancy and use of birth control drugs; and it is seen in persons with repetitive use of the wrist (flexion–extension movements and stress associated with pinching and gripping motions). One cause of carpal tunnel syndrome is the hand motions used by supermarket checkers.[13, 14]

Carpal tunnel syndrome is characterized by pain, paresthesia, and numbness of the thumb and first two-and-a-half digits of the hand; pain in the wrist and hand, both worsening at night; atrophy of the abductor pollicis muscle; and weakness in precision grip. All of these abnormalities may contribute to clumsiness of fine motor activity. Diagnosis is usually based on hypoesthesia confined to median nerve distribution, a positive Tinel's sign, and a positive Phalen's sign. Tinel's sign denotes the development of a tingling sensation radiating into the palm of the hand that is elicited by light percussion over the median nerve at the wrist. The Phalen test is performed by having the person hold the wrist in complete flexion for about a minute; if numbness and paresthesia along the median nerve are reproduced or exaggerated, the test is considered to be positive. Electromyography and nerve conduction studies are often done to confirm the diagnosis and rule out other causes of the disorder. Treatment includes rest and splinting; splints may be confined to nighttime use. In patients in whom splinting is ineffective, corticosteroids may be injected into the carpal tunnel to reduce inflammation and swelling. Surgical intervention consists of operative division of the volar carpal ligaments as a means of relieving pressure on the medial nerve.

POLYNEUROPATHIES

Polyneuropathies lead to symmetric sensory, motor, or mixed sensorimotor deficits. The condition is characterized by demyelination or axonal degeneration of peripheral nerves. Typically, the longest axons are involved first, with symptoms beginning in the distal part of the extremities. If the autonomic nervous system is involved, there may be postural hypotension, constipation, and impotence. Polyneuropathies can result from immune mechanisms (Guillain-Barré syndrome), toxic agents (arsenic polyneuropathy, lead polyneuropathy, alcoholic polyneuropathy), and metabolic diseases (diabetes mellitus and uremia). Different causes tend to affect axons of different diameters and to affect sensory, motor, or autonomic neurons to different degrees.

Guillain-Barré Syndrome. Guillain-Barré syndrome is an acute and subacute polyneuropathy. The manifestations of the disease involve an infiltration of mononuclear cells around the capillaries of the peripheral neurons, edema of the endoneurial compartment, and demyelination of ventral spinal roots. The annual incidence of Guillain-Barré syndrome ranges from 0.6 to 1.9 cases per 100,000 population. About 85% of persons with the disease achieve a spontaneous recovery.

The cause of Guillain-Barré syndrome is unknown. About two-thirds of cases follow a viral infection, usually mundane but including HIV, cytomegalovirus, or Epstein-Barr virus with hepatitis or infectious mononucleosis. A widely studied outbreak of the disorder followed the swine flu vaccination program of 1976–77. It has been suggested that an altered immune response to peripheral nerve antigens contributes to the development of the disorder.

The disorder is characterized by progressive ascending muscle weakness of the limbs, producing a symmetric flaccid paralysis. Symptoms of paresthesia and numbness often accompany the loss of motor function. The rate of disease progression varies, and there may be disproportionate involvement of either the upper or lower extremities. Paralysis may progress to involve the respiratory muscles; about 20% of persons with the disorder require ventilatory assistance.[15] Autonomic nervous system involvement that causes postural hypotension, arrhythmias, facial flushing, abnormalities of sweating, and urinary retention is common.

Guillain-Barré syndrome is usually a medical emergency. There may be a rapid development of ventilatory failure and autonomic disturbances that threaten circulatory function. Treatment includes support of vital functions and prevention of complications such as skin breakdown and thrombophlebitis. Recent clinical trials have shown the effectiveness of plasmapheresis in decreasing morbidity and shortening the course of the disease. Treatment is most effective if initiated early in the course of the disease. Intravenous immunoglobulin therapy has also proved effective.[16]

ALTERATIONS IN CNS CONTROL OF MUSCLE TONE AND MOTOR MOVEMENT

Disorders of motor function include weakness and paralysis, which result from lesions in the voluntary motor pathways, including the UMNs of the corticospinal and corticobulbar tracts and the LMNs that leave the CNS and travel by way of the peripheral nerve to the muscle. Muscle tone, which is a necessary component of muscle movement, is a function of the muscle spindle (myotatic) system and the extrapyramidal system, which monitors and buffers input to the LMNs by way of the UMNs.

Alterations in Muscle Tone. Disorders of skeletal muscle tone are characteristic of many nervous system pathologies. Any interruption of the myotatic reflex circuit by peripheral nerve injury, disease of the neuromuscular junction and of skeletal muscle fibers, damage to the corticospinal system, or injury to the spinal cord or spinal nerve root results in

disturbance of muscle tone. As explained earlier in this chapter, muscle tone is defined as resistance to passive movement around a joint. It may be described as less than normal (*hypotonia*), absent (*flaccidity*), or excessive (*hypertonia, rigidity, spasticity,* or *tetany*). The latter three terms are extremes of hypertonia that include other distinguishing features.

Clinically, muscle tone is evaluated by asking a person to relax while supporting the limb except at the joint being investigated; the distal part of the extremity is then moved passively around the joint. Normally there is mild resistance to movement. A method for assessing muscle stretch excitability is to tap the tendon of a muscle briskly with a reflex hammer, which is normally immediately followed by a sudden contraction or *muscle jerk* (Fig. 50-12). Here the stretch reflex has been "tricked" by the sudden tug on the tendon. A synchronous burst of Ia nerve activity from the many spindles in the muscle results in essentially simultaneous firing of a large number of LMN units. The stretch reflex is tricked into responding as if the muscle has been suddenly stretched. These muscle jerk reflexes are called *deep tendon reflexes* (DTRs). They are usually checked at the wrists, elbows, knees, and Achilles tendons.

The DTRs can provide a great amount of information in a brief period of time. A normal-range DTR indicates that (1) the afferent peripheral process in the peripheral muscle and nerves is normal; (2) the dorsal root ganglion function is normal; (3) the dorsal root function is normal; and (4) the dorsal, intermediate, and ventral horns are functioning appropriately, as are the ventral root and lower motor neuron cell body and axon. It also means that (5) the neuromuscular synapse is functioning normally; (6) the muscle fibers are capable of normal contraction; and (7) suprasegmental input is normal. Using this method of assessment, it is possible to test the function of many spinal nerves and spinal cord segments and some of the cranial nerves and brain stem segments in a short time. If abnormality of excitability is detected, further tests are required to determine the nature and location of the pathologic process.

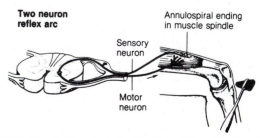

FIG. 50-12. Testing the stretch reflex with a reflex hammer. (Adapted from Chaffee, E.E., & Lytle, I.M. [1980]. *Basic physiology and anatomy* [4th ed., p. 240]. Philadelphia: J.B. Lippincott)

Paresis and Paralysis. The word *plegia* is Greek for a blow, stroke, or paralysis. Terms used to describe the extent and anatomic location of motor damage are *paralysis*, meaning loss of movement, and *paresis*, meaning weakness or incomplete loss of muscle function. *Monoparesis* or *monoplegia* results from the destruction of pyramidal innervation of one limb; *hemiparesis or hemiplegia*, of both limbs on one side; *diparesis/diplegia* or *paraparesis/paraplegia*, of both upper or lower limbs; and *quadriparesis/quadriplegia* (tetraparesis/tetraplegia), of all four limbs. Paresis or paralysis can be further categorized by upper motor neuron origin or lower motor neuron origin.

UPPER MOTONEURON LESIONS

A UMN lesion can involve the motor cortex, the internal capsule, other brain structures through which the corticospinal tract descends, or the spinal cord. When the lesion is above the level of the pyramids at the caudal end of the brain stem, paralysis will affect structures on the opposite side of the body. In UMN disorders involving injury to the T12 level or above, there is an immediate profound weakness and loss of fine, skilled, voluntary limb movement, reduced bowel and bladder control, and diminished sexual functioning, followed by an exaggeration of muscle tone. With UMN lesions, the LMN spinal reflexes remain intact while communication and control from higher brain centers are lost. Descending excitatory influences via the pyramidal system and some descending inhibitory influences from other cortical regions are lost, resulting in a net immediate weakness accompanying a loss of delicate control. After several weeks, this becomes converted to hypertonicity or spastic paralysis (mechanism to be discussed later). The spasticity is often greatest in the flexor muscles of the upper limbs and extensor muscles of the lower limbs. Sometimes a lesion of the pyramidal tract is not severe enough to cause total paralysis but produces a relatively minor degree of weakness. In this case, the finer and more skilled movements are most severely impaired. Spasticity is manifested by increased resistance to passive movement of a joint in which the initial strong resistance to movement quickly fades away.

Clonus is rhythmic, repeated contraction in response to the sudden stretch of a muscle that has been maintained by gentle pressure. It is seen in hypertonia associated with UMN lesions. It is caused by an oscillating stimulation of the muscle spindles that occurs when the spindle fibers are activated by an initial muscle stretch. This results in reflex contraction of the muscle and unloading of the spindle fibers with decreased afferent activity. The reduced spindle fiber activity causes the muscle to relax, which again causes the spindle fiber to be stretched, and the cycle starts over.

UMN Lesions Associated with Stroke. Damage to the corticospinal system is a common component of stroke because the system passes through much of the internal capsule, a common target of cerebrovascular accidents. Also, it is a very long tract system and therefore is vulnerable at many locations. Further, damage to the system has profound consequences to functions that are uniquely human—fine manipulative skills of the fingers and of the speech apparatus. Severe damage to the fibers controlling digital manipulation results in profound and permanent weakness of the small hand muscles, with total loss of finger–thumb opposition and independent control of individual fingers. The hand can still be moved as a whole, and crude grasping and holding of items return after a recovery period. If the lower limb is affected, other signs of corticospinal damage include the loss of certain superficial abdominal reflexes and the appearance of a dorsiflexion (especially of the big toe) and splaying of the toes on stimulation of the sole of the foot, called *Babinski's sign*.

During the third through eighth week after corticospinal damage, muscle tone gradually increases and eventually reaches an excessive level, accompanied by other signs of hyperactive stretch reflexes such as clonus and exaggerated DTRs. The resultant *spastic paralysis* in the upper limb is selective for the in-rotators of the shoulder, flexors of the elbow, supinators of the forearm, and flexors of the fingers. Motor units in these muscles are particularly innervated by the UMNs. As a result, the classic spastic posture for the upper limb is a very stiffly held, flexed forearm rotated against the chest, with the fingers curled tightly over the thumb and hand turned upward. Spasticity of the lower limb particularly affects the adductor extensors of the hip and extensors of the knee, so that the gait of a fully developed spastic leg is stiff-legged with no movement at the knee and with the foot adducted (toes turned in toward the midline).

There are two major theories as to the cause of this slowly developing but permanent spasticity. The older theory is that the pyramidal tract also contains fibers delivering inhibition to the segmental stretch reflexes. With interruption of the pyramidal tract, this inhibition is lost and extremely hyperactive muscle tone results.[19] A more recent theory suggests that the loss of UMN synapses on spinal segmental neurons is followed by outgrowth or plastic replacement of the denuded synapses by the segmental stretch afferents.[20] This would result in greatly increased facilitory power of the stretch reflexes. The only LMNs affected would be those that before were directly or indirectly innervated by UMNs. This theory recognizes the malleability of CNS synaptic relationships, which has been well demonstrated during maturation[21] and in other adult CNS systems.[22] At present no decisive data support either theory, and both mechanisms may contribute. The slow onset of spasticity favors the plasticity or outgrowth theory, however.

In spite of various exercise and movement routines, the loss of strength and of fine manipulative movement apparently cannot be prevented. Attempts to slow and prevent the gradually developing spasticity have had some success, giving promise that at least this crippling aspect of corticospinal damage eventually might be preventable. Stroke is discussed further in Chapter 51.

LOWER MOTONEURON LESIONS

In contrast to UMN lesions in which the spinal reflexes remain intact, LMN disorders disrupt communication between the muscle and all neural input from spinal cord reflexes, including the stretch reflex, which maintains muscle tone.

Infection or irritation of the cell body of the LMN or its axon can lead to hyperexcitability, which causes spontaneous contractions of the muscle units. These can be observed as a twitching and squirming on the muscle surface, a condition called *fasciculations*. Toxic agents, such as the tetanus toxin (*Clostridium tetani*), produce extreme hyperexcitability of the LMN, which results in continuous firing at maximum rate. The resultant sustained contraction of the muscles is called *tetany*. Tetany of muscles on both sides of a joint produces immobility or tetanic paralysis. When the poliomyelitis virus attacks an LMN, it first irritates the LMN, causing fasciculations to occur. These fasciculations are often followed by neuronal death. Weakness and severe muscle wasting of denervation atrophy results. If muscles are totally denervated, total weakness, called *flaccid paralysis*, occurs.

With complete LMN lesions, the muscles of the limbs, bowel, bladder, and genital areas become atonic, and it is impossible to elicit contraction by stretching the tendons. One of the outstanding features of lower motoneuron lesions is the profound development of muscle atrophy. Damage to the LMNs with or without spinal cord damage may be called *peripheral nerve injury* and may occur at any level of the spinal cord (*e.g.*, C7 peripheral nerve injury will lead to LMN hand weakness only). All segments below the level of injury that have intact LMNs will manifest UMN signs. Usually injury to the spinal cord at the T12 level or below results in LMN injury and flaccid paralysis to all areas below the level of injury. This is because the spinal cord ends at the T12–L1 level of the vertebral column, and from this level the spinal roots of the LMNs continue caudally within the spinal canal.

AMYOTROPHIC LATERAL SCLEROSIS

Amyotrophic lateral sclerosis (ALS), also known as *Lou Gehrig's disease* after the famous New York Yankee baseball player, is a devastating neurologic disorder that selectively affects motor function. There are about 5000 new cases of ALS in the United States each year. ALS is primarily a disorder of middle life, affecting persons between the ages of 40 and 60 years, with men developing the disease nearly twice as often as women. Persons who develop the disease in childhood or early adulthood probably have an inherited form of the disorder. The disease typically follows a progressive course, with a mean survival of 2 to 5 years from the onset of symptoms. At present, the cause of ALS is unknown. Interest has focused on searching for an immunologic or autoimmune factor in the pathogenesis of the disease.

The disease can affect both the UMNs (large pyramidal and Betz cells) contained in the cerebral cortex and the cell bodies of the LMNs contained in the brain stem and anterior horn cells of the spinal cord.[17] The fact that the disease is more extensive in the distal parts of the affected tracts in the lower spinal cord, rather than the proximal parts, suggests that affected neurons first undergo degeneration at their distal terminals and the disease proceeds in a centripedal direction until ultimately the parent nerve cell dies.[18] A remarkable feature of the disease is that the entire sensory system, the regulatory mechanisms of control and coordination of movement, and the intellect remain intact. The neurons controlling ocular motility as well as the parasympathetic neurons in the sacral spinal cord are also spared.

The death of LMNs leads to denervation with subsequent shrinkage of musculature and muscle fiber atrophy. It is this fiber atrophy, termed *amyotrophy*, which appears in the common name of the disease. The loss of nerve fibers in lateral columns of the white matter of the spinal cord, along with fibrillary gliosis, imparts a firmness or sclerosis to this CNS tissue; the term *lateral sclerosis* in the name of the disorder designates these changes.

Symptomatology may be referable to either UMN or LMN involvement. Upper motoneuron symptoms include weakness, spasticity or stiffness, and impaired fine motor control. Dysphagia (difficulty swallowing), dysarthria (impaired articulation of speech), and dysphonia (difficulty speaking) may be due to either brain stem LMN involvement or to dysfunction of UMNs descending to the brain stem. Symptoms of destruction of lower motoneurons include fasciculations, weakness, muscle atrophy, and hyporeflexia. Muscle cramps involving the distal legs are often an early symptom. The most common clinical presentation is slowly progressive weakness and atrophy in the distal muscles of one upper extremity. This is followed by regional spread of clinical weakness, reflecting involvement of neighborhood areas of the spinal cord. Eventually there is involvement of both UMNs and LMNs affecting multiple limbs and the head. In the more advanced stages, the muscles of the palate, pharynx, tongue, neck, and shoulders become involved, causing impairment of chewing, swallowing, and speech. Dysphagia with recurrent aspiration and weakness of the respiratory muscles produce the most significant acute complications of the disease. Death usually results from involvement of cranial and respiratory musculature.

Currently, there is no treatment that has influence on the progress of the pathologic changes that occur with the disease. Rehabilitation measures assist persons with the disorder to manage their disability, and respiratory and nutritional support allow persons with the disorder to survive longer than would otherwise be the case.

ALTERATIONS IN MOVEMENT COORDINATION

Increased muscle tone or uncoordinated muscle movements are usually due to disorders of the extrapyramidal system. The extrapyramidal system arises from the motor cortex and is routed indirectly through the brain, with projections to the basal ganglia and the brain stem reticular formation. From the reticular formation, the extrapyramidal system projects to LMNs. The extrapyramidal system is usually considered a functional rather than an anatomic unit because of its many projections. In contrast with the direct route of the corticospinal or pyramidal tract, the extrapyramidal system reaches the spinal cord only after many detours and indirect routing.

DISORDERS OF CEREBELLAR FUNCTION

The functions of the cerebellum, or "little brain," are essential for smooth, coordinated, skillful movement. The cerebellum influences both voluntary and automatic aspects of movement. It does not initiate activity, but it is responsible for the temporal smoothness of correlated muscle action throughout the body.

The signs of cerebellar dysfunction can be grouped into three classes: vestibulo-cerebellar, cerebellar ataxia or decomposition of movement, and cerebellar tremor. These disorders occur on the side of cerebellar damage, whether by congenital defect, cerebrovascular accident, or growing tumor. The abnormality of movement occurs whether the eyes are open or closed. Thus, visual monitoring of movement cannot compensate for cerebellar defects.

Damage to the part of the cerebellum associated with the vestibular system leads to difficulty or inability to maintain a steady posture of the trunk, which normally requires constant readjusting movements. This is seen as an unsteadiness of the trunk, called *trunkal ataxia*, and it can be so severe that standing is not possible. The ability to fix the eyes on a target can also be affected. Constant conjugate readjustment of eye position (*nystagmus*) results, making reading extremely difficult, especially when the eyes are deviated toward the side of cerebellar damage.

Cerebellar ataxia and tremor are different aspects of defects in the smooth, continuously correcting functions. Cerebellar dystaxia or (if severe) ataxia includes a *decomposition of movement*: each succeeding component of a complex movement occurs separately instead of being blended into a smoothly proceeding action. Because ethanol specifically affects cerebellar function, persons who are inebriated often walk with a staggering and unsteady gait. Rapid alternating movements such as supination–pronation–supination of the hands is jerky and performed slowly (dysdiadochokinesia). Reaching to touch a target breaks down into small sequential components, each going too far, followed by overcorrection. The finger moves jerkily toward the target, misses, corrects in the other direction, and misses again until finally the target is reached. This is called *over-and-under reaching*; the general term is *dysmetria*.

Cerebellar tremor is a rhythmic back-and-forth movement of a finger or toe that worsens as the target is approached. The tremor results from the inability of the damaged cerebellar system to maintain ongoing fixation of a body part and to make smooth, continuous corrections in the trajectory of the movement; overcorrection occurs, first in one direction and then the other. Often the tremor of an arm or leg can be detected during the beginning of an intended movement; thus, the common term for cerebellar tremor is *intention tremor*. Cerebellar function as it relates to tremor can be assessed by asking the person to touch one heel to the opposite knee, to gently move the toes along the back of the opposite shin, or to move the hand so as to touch the nose with a finger.

Cerebellar function can also affect the motor skills of chewing and swallowing (dysphagia) and of speech (dysarthria). Normal speech requires smooth control of respiratory muscles and highly coordinated control of the laryngeal, lip, and tongue muscles. Cerebellar dysarthria is characterized by slow, slurred speech of continuously varying loudness. Rehabilitative efforts directed by speech therapists include learning to slow the rate of speech and to compensate as much as possible through the use of less-affected muscles.

DISORDERS OF THE BASAL GANGLIA

Disorders of the basal ganglia comprise a complex group of motor disturbances characterized by involuntary movements, alterations in muscle tone, and disturbances in body posture. The basal ganglia contribute *gracefulness* to cortically initiated and controlled, skilled movements. The basal ganglia receive indirect input from the cerebellum and from all sensory systems, including vision, and direct input from the motor cortex. The basal ganglia appear to organize the basic movement patterns into more complex patterns and to *release* them when commanded by the motor cortex. Many aspects of movement of the trunk, shoulder or hip girdles, and proximal parts of the limbs are automatic (*e.g.,* the swinging of the arms during walking and running or the follow-through of a throwing movement). The coordination and precision with which these movements are performed can be improved through learning and practice. Not everyone, however, can become an accomplished ballerina or gymnast. The basic repertoire of these fundamental complex movement patterns is built into brain stem circuitry that is under gene control, and individual differences limit the extent to which learning and practice can enhance their accomplishment.

The globus pallidus is the site where basic movement patterns are generated. It is normally under constant inhibition by the caudate, putamen, and subthalamic nuclei. This inhibition is removed (*disinhibited*) by the motor cortex when a particular motor sequence is required as a part of a skilled sequence. Damage to this area of the basal ganglia results in extremely reduced movement (bradykinesia or hypokinesia). There is a loss of the automatic movements of the opposite side of the body, such as swinging of the arms when walking. The affected limbs can be passively placed in any position, even a very unusual one, and that position may be held for long periods. On the other hand, if the globus pallidus is functionally intact and inhibitory control by caudate, putamen, or subthalamic nuclei is removed, constant movements (*hyperkinesia*) result. These movements, which include tremor, hemiballismus, chorea, and athetosis, cannot be intentionally controlled and thus are called *involuntary movements.*

Tremor is an involuntary, alternating, rhythmic contraction of opposing muscle groups. It is usually fairly uniform in frequency and amplitude. Tremor of extrapyramidal origin is usually increased during rest and diminished during voluntary activities. *The parkinsonian syndrome* (see Chapter 54) results in hypokinesis—tremor of body parts when they are not being used for skillful purposes. Certain tremors are considered physiologic; they are transient and occur with unusual experiences in normal people. They may be related to fatigue, emotional stress, or environmental conditions, such as shivering that occurs with cold exposure. Toxic tremors are produced by endogenous toxic states such as thyrotoxicosis.

The term *ballismus* originated from a Greek word meaning *to jump around. Hemiballismus* involves a constant, violent flinging movement of one arm or leg that may occur in elderly persons as the result of a small stroke that involves the subthalamic nucleus on the opposite side of the body. The movements may disappear only during deep sleep, but falling asleep with this continuous violent movement can be most difficult.

The caudate and putamen are inhibitory to movements that are driven by the globus pallidus. Localized damage to these structures can result in slow, twisting, wormlike movements of the face, leg, arm, or wrist and fingers, as if using a screwdriver. These movements, called *athetoid,* result from continuous and prolonged contraction of both agonist and antagonist muscle groups. They are normal, smooth, useful movements except that they occur continuously in nonrhythmic, often irregular sequence.

Choreiform movements, which are quick and jerky but also coordinated and graceful, involve the face, tongue, swallowing muscles, and distal arm or leg. Choreiform movements are accentuated by movement and environmental stimulation; they often interfere with normal voluntary activities. The lesions causing the movements are principally located in the caudate and lentiform nuclei (*e.g.,* globus pallidus or putamen). The word *chorea* originates from the Greek word meaning *to dance.* There may be grimacing movements of the face, raising of the eyebrows, rolling of the eyes, and curling, protrusion, and withdrawal of the tongue. In the limbs the movements are largely peripheral; there may be *piano-playing* flexion, extension movements of the fingers, and elevations and depressions of the shoulders. The limb movements disappear during sleep. Movements of the face or limbs may occur alone or, more commonly, in combination.

Sydenham's chorea, sometimes called St. Vitus' dance, can occur in children during rheumatic fever. It is usually a self-limited disorder and leaves no permanent signs. *Huntington's chorea* is a hereditary (autosomal dominant) disease of sometimes late onset, appearing in middle maturity. It is a chronic and progressive degenerative disorder involving the basal ganglia, with progressive widespread destruction in the cerebral cortex. After onset, the chorea and an accompanying mental deterioration progress toward death over a period of about 15 years. The condition appears to be at least partially caused by a progressive loss of the inhibitory GABA-ergic neurons and small acetylcholine neurons in the caudate and putamen (see Chapter 54).

The term *dystonia* refers to the abnormal maintenance of a posture resulting from a twisting, turning movement that involves the limbs, neck, or trunk. In some disorders of movement, simultaneous opposing movements can result in paralysis or nonmovement. Long-sustained simultaneous hypertonia across a joint can result in degenerative changes and permanent fixation in unusual postures. *Spasmodic torticollis*, the most common type of dystonia, affects the muscles of the neck and shoulder. The condition, which is caused by bilateral and simultaneous contraction of the neck and shoulder muscles, results in the unilateral head turning or head extension, sometimes limiting rotation. Elevations of the shoulder often accompany the spasmodic movements of the head and neck. Eventually, immobility of the cervical vertebrae can lead to degenerative fixation in the twisted posture. Torsional spasm involving the trunk can also occur.

The "extrapyramidal" signs in all of these conditions intensify during highly emotional situations. When skilled movement is required, such as attempting to get out of a bus, make change, or write, the defect apparently can be partially overridden by motor cortical function. For instance, if a mildly affected person with parkinsonian syndrome is carrying an open newspaper and attending to something else, arm and hand tremor can be severe; the moment the person begins to read, the tremor decreases or is lost. However, persons with movement disorders are very self-conscious, and if people stare the emotional aspect often results in an intensification of the tremor.

In summary, disorders of motor function can result from altered function of the skeletal muscles, the myoneural junction, the peripheral nerves or peripheral nerve roots, or CNS-controlled UMN and LMN activity, as well as from the loss of coordinated movement due to disorders of the cerebellum and basal ganglia.

Disorders of the neuromuscular unit include muscular dystrophy, myasthenia gravis, and peripheral nerve disorders. Muscular dystrophy is a term used to describe a number of disorders that produce progressive deterioration of skeletal muscle. The disease usually affects children. One form, Duchenne's muscular dystrophy, is inherited as a sex-linked trait and transmitted by the mother to her offspring. Myasthenia gravis is a disorder of the myoneural junction, most likely resulting from a deficiency of functional acetylcholine receptors, which causes weakness of the skeletal muscles. Because the disease affects the myoneural junction, there is no loss of sensory function. Disorders of peripheral nerves include mononeuropathies and polyneuropathies. Mononeuropathies involve a single spinal nerve, plexus, or peripheral nerve trunk. Carpal tunnel syndrome, a mononeuropathy, is caused by compression of the medial nerve that passes through the carpal tunnel in the wrist. Polyneuropathies produce symmetric sensory, motor, and mixed sensorimotor deficits. A number of conditions, including immune mechanisms, toxic agents, and metabolic disorders, are implicated as causative agents in polyneuropathies. Guillain-Barré syndrome is a subacute polyneuropathy of uncertain etiology. It causes progressive ascending motor, sensory, and autonomic nervous system manifestations.

Alterations in CNS control of muscle tone and movement result from lesions of voluntary UMN pathways of the corticobulbar and corticospinal tracts and the LMN of the peripheral nerves. Muscle tone is maintained through the combined function of the muscle spindle system and the extrapyramidal system that monitors and buffers UMN innervation of the LMNs. Hypotonia is a condition of less than normal muscle tone, and hypertonia or spasticity is a condition of excessive tone. Paresis refers to weakness in muscle function, and paralysis refers to a loss of muscle movement. UMN lesions produce spastic paralysis, and LMN lesions produce flaccid paralysis. Damage to the UMNs of the corticospinal and corticobulbar tracts is a common component of stroke.

Alterations in coordination of muscle movements and abnormal muscle movements result from disorders of the cerebellum and basal ganglia. The function of the cerebellum is essential for smooth, coordinated movements. Cerebellar disorders include vestibulo-cerebellar dysfunction, cerebellar ataxia, and cerebellar tremor. The basal ganglia supply the aspect of gracefulness to muscle movement. Disorders of the basal ganglia are characterized by involuntary movements, alterations in muscle tone, and disturbances in posture. These disorders include tremor, hemiballismus, chorea, and athetosis.

■ SPINAL CORD INJURY

Despite the protective mechanisms built in during the development of the CNS, spinal cord injury (SCI) continues to occur. Currently, estimates of the national population of people living with SCI vary from 200,000 to 500,000. Nationally, there are an additional 8000 to 10,000 new spine injuries that result in paralysis each year. The most frequent cause of SCI is motor vehicle accidents, followed by falls, violence (which is increasing in numbers), sports injuries, and other types of injuries, which include attempted suicide and occupational injuries. Of sports-related injuries, 66% are due to diving.[23]

The average age for SCI is between 16 years and 30 years, with 19 years being the most frequent age. As age increases, the etiology of injury changes, with falls becoming the most frequent cause. Males sustain SCI at a rate four times higher than that of females. Alcohol and drugs have been cited as contributing factors in an increasing number of cases.

THE SPINAL COLUMN

The spinal column, which is located in the posterior midline of the body, begins at the base of the skull and ends at the coccyx or "tailbone." There are 32 or 33 individual and fused vertebral bodies, or vertebrae, that make up the spinal column: 7 cervical, 12 thoracic, 5 lumbar, 5 fused sacral, and 3 or 4 fused coccygeal vertebrae. Each vertebra in the vertebral column, with the exception of the first cervical vertebra, shares common characteristics (*e.g.*, each consists of an anterior portion, or body, and a posterior portion, called the *vertebral* or *neural arch*; Fig. 50-13). The vertebral arch or posterior elements are composed of two pedicles, two laminae, a spinous process, two transverse processes, and four articular processes known as *facets*. The transverse foramen within the transverse processes of cervical vertebrae forms a passageway for the vertebral artery, vertebral vein, and a sympathetic nerve plexus, all supplying the brain stem and meninges of the posterior fossa.

The design of the vertebra is to provide bony support and protection for the spinal segmental nerves by forming an intervertebral foraminae and for the spinal cord by forming the spinal canal. The size and function of the vertebrae are directly related to their specific location in the spinal column. Generally, vertebral bodies increase in size to bear additional weight as they descend along the spinal column. The width of the spinal canal varies at different levels also. The atlas (C1) and the axis (C2) are smaller than the rest of the vertebrae and are formed in a manner that allows for flexion, extension, and rotation of the head. The intermediate-sized thoracic vertebrae are heart-shaped and limited in movement, making the thoracic spine, especially the lower levels, more rigid. They also possess tubercles for rib attachment. Each vertebra articulates with the next above and below by means of articular processes called *facets* that function as sliding synovial joints. These provide some support as well as major limitation of movement. They also can be a frequent source of back pain. The design of the lumbar spine allows for powerful flexion and some extension; the lumbar vertebrae are large and heavy to accommodate the attachment of lower limb muscles.

The presence of the fibrocartilaginous disks and strong bands of fibers known as ligaments assists the vertebral column in supporting and protecting the spinal cord. The intervertebral disks contain a firm, gelatinous structure called the *nucleus pulposus*, surrounded by a layer of fibrocartilage called the *anulus*

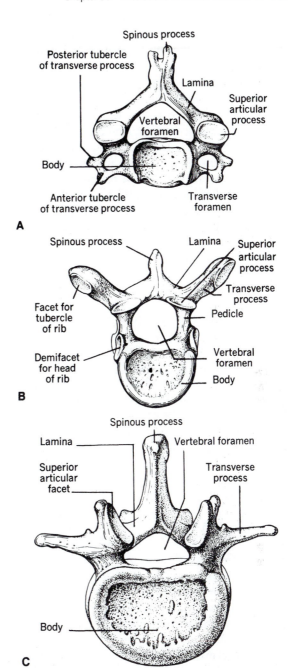

FIG. 50-13. Views of three types of vertebrae. (**A**) Fourth cervical vertebra, superior aspect; (**B**) sixth thoracic vertebra, superior aspect; (**C**) third lumbar vertebra, superior aspect. (Chaffee, E.E., & Greisheimer, E.M. [1974]. *Basic physiology and anatomy*. Philadelphia: J.B. Lippincott)

fibrosus. The intervertebral disks, along with the facet joints, carry all of the compressive loading to which the trunk of the body is subjected. The vertebrae and intervertebral disks are held in place by the ligaments. Two major longitudinal ligaments extend from the axis (C2) to the sacrum on the anterior and posterior surfaces of the vertebral bodies and disks. These ligaments have many different functions: they allow adequate motion and maintenance of alignment between vertebrae, protect the spinal cord by limiting motions with well-defined limits, share with the muscles in providing stability to the spine within its defined range of motion, and protect the spinal cord in traumatic situations with high loads and fast speeds.[24] Other fibrous connective tissue ligaments that attach at various sites between the parts of neighboring vertebrae also support and limit movement of the spinal column, thereby protecting the spinal cord. Additional stabilizing forces are the rib cage, the superficial and deep-trunk muscles, and the normal curvature of the spine, which is anteriorly convex at the cervical and lumbar regions and posteriorly convex in the thoracic and sacral levels.

SPINAL CORD BLOOD SUPPLY

The blood flow to the spinal cord is supplied by three sources: the anterior spinal artery, which provides the main blood supply for the anterior two-thirds of the spinal cord; the posterior spinal arteries, which provide the main blood supply for the posterior one-third of the cord; and the radicular arteries, which bring arterial blood into the spinal cord and supply the outer circumference of the cord at various levels. Interruption of blood flow to the cord can cause permanent damage.

MECHANISMS OF INJURY

VERTEBRAL COLUMN INJURY

Injuries to the vertebral column include fractures, dislocations, and subluxations. A fracture can occur at any part of the bony vertebrae, causing fragmentation of the bone. It most often involves the pedicle, lamina, or processes (facets). Dislocation/subluxation (partial dislocation) injury causes the vertebral bodies to become displaced, with one overriding another to prevent correct alignment of the verebral column. The extent of injury to the vertebral column caused by motion or trauma is related to (1) the amount and direction of motion and (2) the rate of application of force causing the motion. Most injuries result from some combination of a compression force and bending movement.

Damage to the ligaments and/or bony vertebrae may make the spine unstable. In an unstable spine, further unguarded movement of the spinal column could result in compression or overstretching of neural tissue, whereas in a stable spine, further movement of the spinal column will not impinge on the spinal cord. Most traumatic injuries to the spinal column render it unstable, warranting precautionary measures such as immobilization with collars and

backboards and limiting the movement of persons at risk or with known SCI.

Flexion injuries occur when there is forward bending of the spinal column that exceeds the limits of normal movement. Typical flexion injuries result, for example, when the head is struck from behind, such as in a fall with the back of the head as the point of impact. *Extension injuries* occur when there is excessive forced bending (hyperextension) of the spine backward. A typical extension injury involves a fall in which the chin or face is the point of impact, causing hyperextension of the neck. Injuries of flexion and extension occur more commonly in the cervical spine (C4 to C6) than in any other area. Limitations imposed by the ribs, spinous processes, and joint capsules in the thoracic and lumbar spine make this area less flexible and less susceptible to flexion and extension injuries than the cervical spine. The exact location of increased stiffness and inflexibility may vary among individuals and may range from T11 to L1. Therefore, this area is more subject to mechanical failure and accounts for a high number of spine injuries in the thoracolumbar junction.

A *compression injury* causing the vertebral bones to shatter, squash, or even burst occurs when there is spinal loading from a high-velocity blow to the top of the head or by landing forcefully on the feet (Fig. 50-14). This typically occurs at the cervical level (*e.g.,* diving injuries) or in the thoracolumbar area (*e.g.,* falling from a distance and landing on the feet). Compression injuries may occur when the vertebrae are weakened owing to conditions such as osteoporosis and cancer with bone metastasis.

Axial rotation injuries can produce highly unstable injuries. Maximal axial rotation occurs in the cervical region, especially between C1 and C2 and at the lumbosacral joint. *Coupling* of vertebral motions is common in injury when two or more individual motions occur (*e.g.,* lateral bending and axial rotation). The motion being produced by the external force is termed the main motion, and all the accompanying motions are considered coupled motions. *Penetrating injuries* occur with or without spinal column damage as direct trauma to the cord. The most frequent penetrating injuries are caused by gunshot or knife wounds.

SPINAL CORD INJURY

The pathophysiology of SCI can be divided into two types—primary and secondary. The primary neurologic injury occurs at the time of mechanical injury and is irreversible. It is characterized by small hemorrhages in the gray matter of the cord, followed by edematous changes in the white matter leading to necrosis of neural tissue. This type of pathology results from the forces of compression, stretch, and

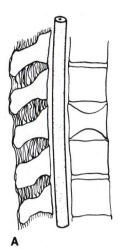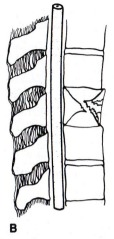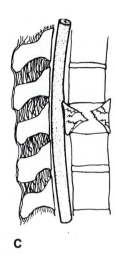

A   **B**   **C**

FIG. 50-14. Progressive degrees of compression fracture. (**A**) Severe compression fracture showing the biconcave profile produced by the adjacent discs. (**B**) A more severe degree of fracture. A vertical fracture has joined the deformed, concave endplates. The anterior body fragment is comminuted and displaced anteriorly. (**C**) A more severe degree of compression fracture. The posterior body fragment is now comminuted and displaced posteriorly into the spinal canal. Neural damage may occur. The neural arch is intact. This spine is stable. (Rockwood, C.A., & Green, D.P. [1977]. *Fractures.* Philadelphia: J.B. Lippincott)

shear associated with fracture or compression of the spinal vertebrae, dislocation of vertebrae (flexion, extension, subluxation), and jarring of the cord within the spinal canal (contusions). Lacerations occur when there is cutting or tearing of the spinal cord. This causes injury to nerve tissue with associated bleeding and edema. Penetrating injuries produce lacerations and direct trauma to the cord and may occur with or without spinal column damage. The most frequent penetrating injuries are caused by gunshot or knife wounds.

Secondary injuries follow the primary injury and promote the spread of injury. Although there is considerable debate about the pathogenesis of secondary injuries, the end result is a progression in neurologic damage. Following SCI, several mechanisms of pathology occur: (1) vascular pathology, (2) neuronal pathology that leads to loss of reflexes below the level of injury, and (3) release of vasoactive agents and cellular enzymes. Vascular pathology (*e.g.*, vessel trauma and hemorrhage) can lead to ischemia, increased vascular permeability, and edema. Blood flow to the spinal cord may be further compromised by spinal shock that results from a loss of neural reflexes below the level of injury. The release of vasoactive substances (norepinephrine, seratonin, dopamine, and histamine) from the wound tissue can cause vasospasm and impede blood flow in the microcirculation, thereby producing further necrosis of blood vessels and neurons. The release of proteolytic and lipolytic enzymes from injured cells causes delayed swelling and necrosis in the spinal cord.

As in spine trauma, the greater the magnitude of force applied to the spinal cord, the greater the associated damage. There may also be some areas of hemorrhage (and injury) rostral and caudal to the site of impact. For this reason the severity of bony injury or radiographic findings may not always correspond with the extent of neurologic damage. Also, the location of bony injury may not coincide with the clinical findings of motor and sensory deficits (*e.g.*, C6 compression fracture with motor and sensory level of functioning at C7, C4, or C5).

CLASSIFICATION AND TYPES OF INJURY

Recently, the American Spinal Injury Association (ASIA) published *Standards for Neurological and Functional Classification of Spinal Cord Injury.*[25] According to the ASIA, tetraplegia (preferred to "quadriplegia") refers to impairment or loss of motor and/or sensory function in the cervical segments of the cord due to damage of neural elements within the spinal canal. Tetraplegia results in impairment of function in the arms, trunk, legs, and pelvic organs. It does not include peripheral nerve injuries. *Paraplegia*, according to the ASIA, refers to impairment or loss of motor and/or sensory function in the thoracic, lumbar, or sacral (not cervical) segments of the spinal cord, secondary to damage of neural elements within the spinal canal. With paraplegia, arm functioning is spared but, depending on the level of injury, functioning of the trunk, leg, and pelvic organ may be involved. Paraplegia also refers to conus medullaris and cauda equina injuries but not to injury to peripheral nerves outside the spinal canal.

Further definitions describe the extent of neurologic damage as complete or incomplete injuries. An *incomplete* SCI is present if partial preservation of sensory/or motor function is found below the neurologic level of injury and includes the lowest sacral segment (*e.g.*, sparing of S2-S4 innervation of myocutaneous and deep anal sensation and rectal sphincter control). Therefore, the necessary test of motor function is the voluntary contraction of the anal sphincter upon digital exam. A *complete* injury refers to the absence of sensory and motor function, which includes the lowest sacral segment. The myotome and dermatome charts (see Chapter 48, Fig. 48-1) show skeletal muscle and sensory areas of skin innervated by specific spinal cord segments.

The level and extent of injury to the spinal cord can be determined by the presenting clinical symptoms, which reflect the predominant area of the cord that is involved. Complete cord injuries can result from severance of the cord, disruption of nerve fibers although they remain intact, or interruption of blood supply to that segment resulting in complete destruction of neural tissue and UMN and LMN paralysis. However, complete severance of the cord is rarely seen. Incomplete injuries may present in a variety of patterns but can be organized into certain patterns or "syndromes," which occur more frequently and reflect the predominant area of the cord that is involved.

A condition called *central cord syndrome* occurs when injury is predominantly in the central gray or white matter of the cord. Because the corticospinal tract fibers are organized with those controlling the arms being located more centrally and those controlling the legs located more laterally, some external axonal transmission remains intact. Therefore, motor function of the upper extremities is affected but the lower extremities may not be affected or may be affected to a lesser degree, with some sparing of sacral sensation. Bowel, bladder, and sexual functions are usually affected to varying degrees and may parellel the degree of lower extremity involvemnt. This syndrome occurs almost exclusively in the cervical cord, rendering the lesion a UMN with spastic paralysis. Central cord damage is more frequent in elderly persons with narrowing or stenotic changes in the spinal canal related to arthritis. It may also occur in persons with congenital stenosis. As in any incomplete injury, prognosis for return of function is more likely than in complete injury.

Anterior artery or *anterior cord syndrome* is usually caused by damage due to infarction of the ante-rior spinal artery resulting in damage to the anterior two-thirds of the cord. The deficits result in loss of motor function provided by the corticospinal tracts, as well as loss of pain and temperature sensation caused by damage to the lateral spinothalamic tracts. The posterior one-third of the cord is relatively unaffected, preserving position, vibration, and touch sense.

A condition called *Brown-Sequard syndrome* results from damage to a hemisection of the anterior and posterior cord. The effect is a loss of voluntary motor function from the corticospinal tract and proprioception from the ipsilateral side of the body and contralateral loss of pain and temperature from the lateral spinothalamic tracts for all levels below the lesion.

Conus medullaris syndrome involves damage to the conus medullaris or the sacral cord (conus) and lumbar nerve roots with the neural canal at the L1 vertebral level. Functional deficits resulting from this type of injury usually result in LMN or flaccid bowel, bladder, and sexual function. Motor function in the legs and feet may be impaired without significant sensory impairment. Damage below the L2 vertebra level usually results in LMN and sensory neuron damage known as *cauda equina syndrome*. Functional deficits present as varying patterns of asymmetric flaccid paralysis, sensory impairment, and pain.

ALTERATIONS IN FUNCTION

Alterations in body function that result from spinal cord injury depend on the level of injury and the amount of cord involvement. Both functional abilities and spinal reflex activity are affected. The physical problems discussed in this chapter are those associated with ventilation/communication, autonomic regulation, sensorimotor integrity, bowel and bladder function, and sexual function. Because of the variations that occur with incomplete injuries, the discussion related to physical problems focuses on complete (total motor and sensory) spinal cord injuries.

FUNCTIONAL ABILITIES

Functional abilities following SCI cover varying degrees of sensorimotor loss and altered reflex activity based on the level of cord injury and extent of cord damage. Table 50-2 summarizes the functional abilities by level of injury. Motor function in cervical injuries ranges in levels from complete dependence to independence with or without assistive devices in activities of mobility and self care. The functional levels of cervical injury relate to C5, C6, C7, and C8 innervation. At the C5 level deltoid and biceps func-

TABLE 50-2. FUNCTIONAL ABILITIES BY LEVEL OF CORD INJURY

INJURY LEVEL	SEGMENTAL SENSORIMOTOR FUNCTION	DRESSING, EATING	ELIMINATION	MOBILITY*
C1	Little or no sensation or control of head and neck. No diaphragm control. Requires continuous ventilation	Dependent	Dependent	Limited. Voice or sip-N-puff controlled electric wheelchair
C2 to C3	Head and neck sensation; some neck control. Independent of mechanical ventilation for short periods	Dependent	Dependent	Same as for C1
C4	Good head and neck sensation and motor control; some shoulder elevation; diaphragm movement	Dependent; may be able to eat with adaptive sling	Dependent	Limited to voice, mouth, head, chin, or shoulder-controlled electric chair
C5	Full head and neck control; shoulder strength; elbow flexion	Independent with assistance	Maximal assistance	Electric or modified manual wheel chair, needs transfer assistance
C6	Fully innervated shoulder; wrist extension or dorsiflexion	Independent and/or with minimal assistance	Independent and/or with minimal assistance	Independent in transfers and wheel chair independently
C7 to C8	Full elbow extension; wrist plantar flexion; some finger control	Independent	Independent	Independent; manual wheelchair
T1 to T5	Full hand and finger control; use of intercostal and thoracic muscles	Independent	Independent	Independent; manual wheelchair
T6 to T10	Abdominal muscle control, partial to good balance with trunk muscles	Independent	Independent	Independent; manual wheelchair
T11 to L5	Hip flexors, hip abductors (L1–3); knee extension (L2–4); knee flexion and ankle dorsiflexion (L4–5)	Independent	Independent	Short distance to full ambulation with assistance
S1 to S5	Full leg, foot and ankle control; innervation of perineal muscles for bowel, bladder, and sexual function (S2–4)	Independent	Normal to impaired bowel and bladder function	Ambulate independently with or without assistance

*Assistance refers to adaptive equipment, set up, or physical assistance.

tion is spared, allowing full head, neck, and diaphragm control with good shoulder strength and full elbow flexion. At the C6 level wrist dorsiflexion by the way of wrist extensors is functional, allowing for *tenodesis*, which is the natural bending inward and flexion of the fingers when the wrist is extended and bent backward. Tenodesis is a key movement because it can be used to pick up objects when finger movement is absent. A functional C7 injury allows full elbow flexion and extension, wrist plantar flexion, and some finger control. At the C8 level finger flexion is added. Thoracic cord injuries (T1 to T12) allow for full upper-extremity control with limited to full control of inter-costal and trunk muscles and balance. Injury at the T1 level allows for full fine motor control of the fingers. Because of the lack of specific functional indicators at the thoracic levels, the level of injury is usually determined by sensory level testing. Functional capacity in the L1 through L5 nerve innervations allows for hip flexors, hip abductors (L1 to L3), movement of the knees (L2 to L5), and ankle dorsiflexion (L4 to L5). Sacral (S1 to S5) innervation allows for full leg, foot, and ankle control, as well as innervation of perineal musculature for bowel, bladder, and sexual function.

SPINAL REFLEX ACTIVITY

Altered spinal reflex activity in SCI is essentially determined by UMN and LMN lesions. UMNs, which are fully contained within the CNS, are generally affected by any injury at the T12 level or above. This results in spastic paralysis of the affected skeletal muscle groups and muscles that control bowel, bladder, and sexual functions. LMN injuries generally occur with injuries below T12 and result from damage to the peripheral nerves that exit each segment of the spinal cord. The LMN injuries cause flaccid paralysis of involved skeletal muscle groups and muscles that control bowel, bladder, and sexual function. However, injuries near the T12 level may result in mixed UMN/LMN deficits (*e.g.*, spastic paralysis of the bowel and bladder with flaccid muscle tone).

Spinal shock or *neurogenic shock* is the term used to describe the state of areflexia that occurs following cord injury. It involves the motor pathways, and the manifestations are flaccid paralysis and lack of tendon reflexes and autonomic function, regardless of whether the level of lesion will eventually produce spastic (UMN) or flaccid (LMN) paralysis. The basic mechanisms accounting for the transient spinal shock are unknown. Spinal shock may last for minutes, hours, days, or weeks, after which isolated spinal cord activity returns. Usually, if reflex function returns by the time the person reaches the hospital, the neuromuscular changes are reversible. This kind of reversible spinal shock may occur in football-type injuries in which jarring of the spinal cord within the canal produces a concussion-like phenomenon in which there is temporary loss of movement and reflexes followed by full recovery within days. In persons in whom paralysis or weakness persists, hypotension and bradycardia may become critical, but manageable, problems. Generally, the higher the level of cord injury, the greater the effect. This aspect of spinal shock will be discussed under autonomic nervous system function.

VENTILATION/COMMUNICATION

Ventilation requires movement of both the expiratory and inspiratory muscles, all of which receive innervation from the spinal cord. The main muscle of ventilation, the diaphragm, is innervated by segments C3 to C5. The intercostal muscles, located between the ribs, are innervated by spinal segments T1 through T7. These muscles function in elevating the rib cage and are needed for coughing and deep breathing. The major muscles of expiration are the abdominal muscles, which receive their innervation from levels T6 to T12. By forcing the abdominal viscera against the diaphragm, the muscles exert pressure on the diaphragm and return the thoracic cage to its resting position. Coughing and deep breathing, which are vital to the removal of mucus and foreign particles from the respiratory tract, are facilitated by the elevation of the rib cage and expansion of the anteroposterior and lateral dimensions of the chest wall, followed by strong respiratory and abdominal muscle contraction forcing air out of the lungs.

Although the ability to inhale and exhale may be preserved at various levels of spinal cord injury, functional deficits in ventilation are most apparent in the quality of the breathing cycle and the ability to oxygenate tissues, give off carbon dioxide, and mobilize secretions. Cord injuries involving C1 to C3 result in lack of respiratory effort and will require assisted ventilation. Although C3 to C5 injury allows for partial or full diaphragmatic function, ventilation will be diminished due to loss of intercostal muscle function, resulting in shallow breaths and a weak cough. Below C5 level, as less intercostal and abdominal musculature is affected, the ability to take a deep breath and cough is less impaired. Maintenance therapy consists of muscle training to strengthen existing muscles for endurance and mobilizing secretions.

With assisted ventilation, whether continuous or intermittent, ensuring adequate communication of needs is also essential. There are several ways of ensuring this communication with the use of verbal or nonverbal communication systems. Verbal approaches may consist of fenestrated tracheal tubes to provide air flow and vibration of the vocal cords, talking tracheostomy tubes, diaphragmatic pacing, electrolarynx-type devices, and mechanical ventilation with an air leak. Nonverbal communication techniques include boards or cards displaying the person's most frequently used words, computerized scanning programs, and mouth-stick control devices.

AUTONOMIC NERVOUS SYSTEM DYSFUNCTION

Spinal cord injury not only interrupts the function of the somatic nerves that control skeletal muscle function but also interrupts visceral afferent input and autonomic outflow from below the site of injury. This affects parasympathetic outflow from the sacral segments of the spinal cord and sympathetic outflow from the thoracic and lumbar segments. Following SCI, the spinal reflex circuits are largely isolated from the rest of the CNS. Afferent somatic and visceral sensory input that enters the spinal cord through intact segmental nerves is unaffected. Similarly, the efferent outflow from intact reflex centers below the site of injury is largely unaffected. However, the transmission of ascending sensory input to higher centers and descending motor control output from higher centers is blocked at the site of injury. Thus, what are lacking are the regulation and integration of reflex function from higher autonomic and motor control control centers in the brain and brain stem. Interruption of autonomic outflow results in continued function above the level of injury, whereas the spinal and autonomic reflexes below the level of injury are uncontrolled.

The autonomic regulation of circulatory function and thermoregulation present the most severe problems in SCI. The higher the level of injury and the greater the body surface area affected, the more profound the effects on circulation and thermoregulation. Persons with injury at the T6 level or above experience problems in regulating vasomotor tone; those with injuries below the T6 level usually have sufficient sympathetic function to maintain adequate vasomotor function. The level of injury and its corresponding problems may vary among persons and situations, and some dysfunctional effects may be seen at levels below T6. With lower lumbar and sacral injuries, sympathetic function remains essentially unaltered (see Chapter 49).

Spinal Shock. In persons in whom high-level paraplegia or tetraplegia persists beyond the first few hours or days after injury, hypotension and bradycardia may be critical, but manageable, problems. Circulatory function is impaired owing to a loss of sympathetic control of heart rate, peripheral vascular resistance, and lack of muscle tone in paralyzed limbs, resulting in sluggish circulating blood flow and venous return. The resulting bradycardia and hypotension can usually be managed with slow fluid resuscitation and body positioning that facilitates venous return. Spinal shock and true hemorrhagic shock (hypotension and tachycardia) must be differentiated and treated accordingly. Spinal shock is usually self-limiting; the return of reflexes in UMN lesions usually occurs in a caudal–rostral direction, with the first returning reflexes being those in the sacral area (rectal sphincter contraction), followed by those of the lumbar area (the lower extremities). However, bradycardia and hypotension may persist and become asymptomatic normal parameters. The length of time that it takes to adjust to the altered circulatory status is variable and may be as long as a year.

Vasovagal Response. The vagus (X) nerve normally exerts a continuous inhibitory effect on heart rate. Vagal stimulation that causes marked bradycardia by way of an intact cervical branches of the vagus nerve is called the vasovagal response. Visceral afferent input to the vagal centers in the brain stem of persons with tetraplegia or high-level paraplegia can produce marked bradycardia when unchecked by a dysfunctional sympathetic nervous system. Severe bradycardia and even asystole can result when the vasovagal response is elicited by deep endotracheal suctioning or rapid position change. Preventive measures, such as hyperoxygenation before, during, and after suctioning, are advised. Rapid position changes should be avoided or anticipated, and anticholinergic drugs should be immediately available to counteract severe episodes of bradycardia.

Autonomic Dysreflexia. The terms *autonomic dysreflexia* or *autonomic hyperreflexia* refer to an acute episode of exaggerated sympathetic reflex responses that occurs in persons with SCI. It is usually characterized by severe hypertension ranging as high as 300/160 mmHg, bradycardia, and headache ranging from dull to severe and pounding.[25] Below the level of injury the reflex response stimulates major sympathetic outflow tracts, resulting in vasospasm, hypertension, skin pallor, and gooseflesh that represents the piloerector response. Continued hypertension produces a baroreflex-mediated vagal slowing of heart rate to bradycardia levels. Above the level of the lesion the sympathetic vasomotor response results in arterial vasodilatation, headache, flushed skin, nasal stuffiness, profuse sweating, and anxiety.

Autonomic dysreflexia results when an exaggerated response from the sympathetic nervous system occurs due to lack of control from higher centers. This exaggerated response is usually caused by visceral stimuli, which normally cause pain or discomfort in the abdominopelvic region. Persons with injuries at the T6 level or below usually have sufficient sympathetic outflow to control visceral reflexes. In persons with T6 injuries and above, the aortic and carotid baroreceptors and afferent input to the cardiovascular centers in the brain stem, as well as the parasympathetic cranial outflow that controls heart rate, remain intact. The sympathetic outflow controlling peripheral vascular resistance is through the thoracic spinal nerves innervating preganglionic neurons in the sypathetic chain, the axons of the latter reentering the spinal nerves through the gray rami. This outflow becomes nonfunctional below the level of injury; when stimulated, the sympathetic reflexes that regulate peripheral vascular resistance function in an unregulated manner, causing rapid vasoconstriction and severe hypertension. As blood pressure rises, the uncoordinated baroreflex response produces a slowing of heart rate, resulting in severe hypertension accompanied by a reflex-mediated bradycardia.

The stimuli initiating the dysreflexic response include visceral distention (full bladder or rectum), stimulation of pain receptors (such as occurs with pressure, ingrown toenails, dressing changes, and diagnostic or operative procedures), and visceral contractions, such as ejaculation, bladder spasms, or uterine contractions. In approximately 80% of cases, the dysreflexic response results from a full bladder.[26]

Autonomic dysreflexia is a clinical emergency, and without prompt and adequate treatment, convulsions, loss of consciousness, and even death can occur. The major components of treatment include monitoring blood pressure while removing or correcting the initiating cause or stimulus. The person should be placed in an upright position, and all support hose or binders should be removed to promote venous pooling of blood and reduce venous return, thereby decreasing blood pressure. If the stimuli have been removed or the stimuli cannot be identified and the upright position established but the blood pressure remains elevated, drugs that block autonomic function are administered. Persons should be monitored for several hours after the dysreflexic event.

Postural Hypotension. Postural or orthostatic hypotension usually occurs in persons with T4 to T6 injuries and above, related to the interruption of sympathetic innervation to blood vessels in the extremities and abdomen. Pooling of blood, along with gravitational forces, impairs venous return to the heart, and there is a subsequent decrease in cardiac output when the person is placed in an upright position. This usually occurs when the person is placed in the seated position in bed or transferred from the bed to the wheelchair. The signs of orthostatic hypotension include dizziness, pallor, excessive sweating above the level of the lesion, complaints of blurred vision, and possibly fainting. Because of the disruption in

autonomic function at the time of injury, the blood pressure and heart rate may already be low but asymptomatic. Postural hypotension is usually prevented by slow changes in position and devices to promote venous return.

Body Temperature Regulation. The sympathetic nervous system is influential in maintaining temperature homeostasis. The central mechanisms for thermoregulation are located in the hypothalamus. In response to cold, the hypothalamus stimulates vasoconstrictor responses in peripheral blood vessels, particularly those of the skin. This results in decreased loss of body heat to the external environment, thereby maintaining heated circulation to vital internal organs. Increased heat production results from increased metabolism, voluntary activity, or shivering. Shivering can almost double the heat production of the body. In order to reduce heat, hypothalamic-stimulated mechanisms produce vasodilatation of skin blood vessels to dissipate heat and sweating to increase evaporative heat losses.

Following SCI, the communication between the thermoregulatory centers in the hypothalamus and the sympathetic effector responses below the level of injury are disrupted—the ability to control blood vessel responses that conserve or dissipate heat is lost, as are the abilities to sweat and shiver. The higher the level of injury, the greater the disturbance in thermoregulation. In tetraplegia and high paraplegia, there are few defenses against changes in the environmental temperature, and body temperature tends to assume the temperature of the external environment, a condition known as *poikilothermy*. Persons with lower-level injuries will have varying degrees of thermoregulation. Disturbances in thermoregulation are chronic and may cause continual loss of body heat. Treatment consists of education in the adjustment of clothing and awareness of how environmental temperatures affect the person's ability to accommodate these changes.

EDEMA

Edema following SCI is related to decreased peripheral vascular resistance, areflexia or decreased tone in paralyzed limbs, and immobility that causes increased venous pressure and abnormal pooling of blood in the abdomen, lower limbs, and upper extremities. Orthostatic or dependent edema in dependent body parts is usually relieved by positioning to overcome gravitational forces or compression devices (such as support stockings and binders) that encourage venous return.

DEEP VEIN THROMBOSIS

Deep vein thrombosis (DVT), as a complication of SCI, occurs in 14% to 100% of persons with SCI, depending on the method of diagnosis.[27] Although it is seen more frequently in the postacute phase of SCI, it often has its origin during the events surrounding the initial injury. Impairment of vasomotor tone, initial loss of muscle tone, trauma to the vein wall, hypercoagulability, and immobility predispose to sluggish venous blood flow and the risk of DVT. Prevention includes measures to prevent venous pooling of blood, especially in the paralyzed limbs (*e.g.*, range of motion and vascular compression devices) and assessment of the risk and presence of DVT beginning immediately after injury.

SENSORIMOTOR INTEGRITY

Following the period of spinal shock, isolated spinal reflex activity and muscle tone that is not under the control of higher centers returns in an UMN injury. This may result in hypertonia and spasticity of skeletal muscles below the level of injury, where the normal communication pathways to higher centers for voluntary motor control have been interrupted by the spinal cord lesion. These spastic movements are involuntary versus voluntary, a distinction that needs to be explained to both the person with SCI and his or her family members. Spastic movements in flexor and extensor patterns, which occur below the level of injury, can be tonic (sustained tone) or clonic (intermittent) and are usually heightened initially after injury, reaching a peak and then becoming stable in about 2 years, with exacerbations due to medical conditions.

These movements occur in most spinal injuries above the T12 level in which the reflex arc is preserved. In T12 or below injuries, the reflex response itself is damaged at the cord or spinal nerve level, preventing spasticity. Spasticity in and of itself is not detrimental to the person with SCI and may even facilitate maintenance of muscle tone to prevent muscle wasting, improve venous return, and aid in mobility. Spasms become detrimental, however, when they impair safety and the ability to make functional gains in mobility and activities of daily living, such as feeding, dressing, and toileting, as well as vocational and avocational interests. Spasms may also cause trauma to bones and tissues, leading to joint contractures and skin breakdown.

The stimuli for reflex muscle spasms arise from somatic and visceral afferent pathways that enter the cord below the level of injury. The most common of these stimuli are muscle stretching, bladder infec-

tions or stones, fistulas, bowel distention or impaction, pressure areas or irritation of the skin, and infections. Because the stimuli that precipitate spasms vary from person to person, careful assessment needs to be done to identify the factors that precipitate spasm in each person. Passive range-of-motion exercises to stretch spastic muscles should be done twice a day, avoiding stimuli that elicit spasm. Antispasmodic medications may be warranted and need to be carefully monitored for effectiveness.

Skin. The entire surface of the skin is innervated by cranial or spinal nerves organized into dermatomes showing cutaneous distribution. The central and autonomic nervous systems also play a vital role in skin function. Impulses from the peripheral nervous system carry sensory information to the brain and receive information for motor control and reflex activity at each dermatome. The autonomic nervous system, through control of vasomotor and sweat gland activity, influences the health of the skin by providing adequate circulation, excretion of body fluids, and temperature regulation. The lack of sensory warning mechanisms and voluntary motor ability below the level of injury, coupled with circulatory changes, places the person with SCI major risk for disruption of skin integrity. Significant factors associated with disruption of skin integrity are pressure, shearing forces, and localized trauma and skin irritation. Relieving pressure, allowing adequate circulation to the skin, and inspecting skin are primary ways of maintaining skin integrity. Of all the complications following SCI, skin breakdown is the most preventable.

Pain. Pain following SCI is a diverse and unpredictable experience that, for some people, can be severe.[28, 29] Initially, pain arises from soft tissues such as the skin, muscles, and joint structures, as well as from fractures and dislocations of bony elements. With healing and/or decompression of neurologic tissue, much of the pain associated with the injury resolves. For many people, however, chronic pain syndromes develop.[28] About 90% of persons will have delayed pain following SCI; about 40% of these will have increasing pain contributing to disability.[28] Chronic pain is more common among persons with paraplegia than in those with tetraplegia.[29] There are four types of pain syndromes following SCI: mechanical, radicular, visceral, and central.[29, 30] Mechanical or fracture pain usually occurs at the level of injury related to soft tissue damage, most commonly from damaged facet joints or spinal fracture. It is dull and aching, often aggravated by movement. Radicular (spinal nerve root) pain presents as an aching or shooting type of pain that radiates into a more or less well-defined nerve root distribution affecting the arm, leg, or trunk. Although the pain occurs in its severest form in incomplete SCI lesions, it is also seen in transected cauda equina lesions. The cause of radicular pain in SCI is obscure but may result from compression or injury of nerve roots by a herniated nucleus pulposus, a fracture fragment, or a dislocated veretebra or from neuronal hyperexcitability due to local ischemia. Visceral pain involves a poorly localized, burning discomfort of the abdomen and pelvis. It is often related to some intra-abdominal event such as bladder distention or urinary tract infection. It is thought that the etiology of visceral pain may be similar to that of central pain. Central pain is a diffuse, burning sensation that is experienced in body parts below the level of injury and is aggravated by touch, movement, and visceral distention. The mechanism of central pain is possibly an abnormal firing of deafferented input association or projection neurons. Because this type of pain has resulted from loss of normal input, it is often called *deafferentation pain*.

The management of pain syndrome in a person with SCI begins with assessment measures to determine the type of pain that is present and, if possible, the underlying mechanisms. Transcutaneous electrical nerve stimulation (TENS) and the tricyclic antidepressant drugs (*e.g.*, amitriptyline, doxepin, and imipramine) have proved useful in treating central pain.[30] Mechanical pain is often treated with nonsteroidal anti-inflammatory drugs (NSAID) and physical therapy.[30] Anticonvulsant drugs (carbamazepine and phenytoin) are often effective in relieving radicular pain.[30] The mechanisms of drug action and specifics of chronic pain management are discussed in Chapter 48.

BOWEL AND BLADDER FUNCTION

Among the most devastating consequences of spinal cord injury is the loss of bowel and bladder function. Loss of these functions are apparent immediately after injury and require a great deal of time, expense, materials, and human energy for management. Micturition, or the act of voiding, can be described as the sequence of events involving sensory input that occurs with bladder filling, activation of the spinal reflex voiding center, stimulation and provision of cerebral control, and progression and termination of actual voiding.[31] Although the anatomy and function of the kidneys or production of urine is not greatly altered following SCI, almost all persons with SCI experience some loss of bladder function. Therefore, management must be directed toward functional improvement of the voiding problem itself.

The neural control of bladder function is supplied by sympathetic nerve fibers that allow for relaxation of the detrusor muscle during bladder filling (T1 to L2), parasympathetic nerve fibers that supply the reflex voiding center (S2 to S4), the motoneurons that travel in the pelvic nerve and supply the external urethral sphincter (S2 to S4), and the micturition center in the brain stem (see Chapter 34). The micturition center coordinates the activity of the detrusor muscle and the external sphincter by way of input from ascending spinal pathways and descending pathways from higher voluntary control centers in the cortex. Following resolution of spinal shock, which renders the bladder areflexic, bladder dysfunction is manifested by disruption of neural pathways between the bladder and the reflex voiding center (lower motoneuron lesion) or between the reflex voiding center and higher brain centers for communication and coordinated sphincter control (upper motoneuron lesion). Persons with UMN or spastic bladders lack awareness of bladder filling (storage) and voluntary control of voiding (evacuation). In LMN or flaccid bladder dysfunction, lack of awareness of bladder filling and lack of bladder tone render the person unable to void voluntarily or involuntarily. Of specific importance to optimal bladder function is the storage and evacuation of urine under low pressure to prevent damage to the bladder and urethra and, more importantly, to the kidneys.

Normally, the low-pressure urine storage mechanism is achieved through sympathetic inhibition of detrusor muscle contractile activity coordinated with increased urethral closing pressure until the reflex voiding threshold is reached. At threshold, the stretched detrusor muscle elicits a parasympathetic response, inducing urethral smooth muscle relaxation along with balanced bladder contraction until complete emptying is achieved. After SCI, involuntary voiding reflexes (UMN) may be elicited during filling along with higher-level external sphincter response, which may lead to incontinence and prevent full emptying of the bladder. These reflexes usually occur at high volumes. In LMN injury, there is no bladder function other than storage or external sphincter response, leading to retention with overflow and leakage of urine. This loss of control of bladder emptying not only influences the quality of a person's life but also carries with it a lifetime threat of severe renal problems.

The principal goals of bladder management are to provide low-pressure drainage to the urinary bladder and to prevent complications with consideration for the person's physical life-style, potential for cooperation, and support from family and community. Management techniques for neurogenic bladder dysfunctions consist of methods of continuous or intermittent drainage, external collection, and manual techniques (*e.g.*, Credé's maneuver, Valsalva's maneuver, or bladder tapping).

Bowel elimination in SCI is also a coordinated effort involving the intrinsic nerve supply (intramural plexus) to the large intestine, autonomic nervous system, and, like voiding, CNS innervation. Intrinsic control of the bowel is supplied by networks of nerve fibers in the bowel wall (enteric plexus) that respond to fecal distention with increased peristalsis. Parasympathetic innervation from the vagus nerve and the S2 to S4 cord segments, or the defecation reflex center, affects the colon, rectum, and internal and external sphincters. Sympathetic innervation from T6 through L3 segments affects the same area. Parasympathetic effects are seen in increased motility and peristalsis, relaxed sphincter tone, increased gastrointestinal secretions, and maintenance of smooth muscle tone, whereas sympathetic activity provides the antagonistic control to the parasympathetic effects as well as vasomotor control.

Defecation is controlled by communications between the brain, the defecation center (S2 to S4), and the external anal sphincter. After SCI, UMN damage can occur when injury to the cord is sustained above the S2 to S4 cord segments. The person acquires spastic functioning of the defecation reflex with involuntary control of the external sphincter. Lower motoneuron injury occurs with damage to the cord at the defecation reflex center or between the S2 to S4 segments and the external sphincters. This causes flaccid functioning of the defecation reflex and loss of anal sphincter tone. Even though intrinsic contractile responses are intact, without the defecation reflex peristaltic movements are ineffective in evacuating stool.

The goal of bowel management following SCI is to establish complete evacuations, which minimize incontinence and complications and afford dignity and independence to the person. The principal methods of bowel management include measures such as a high-fluid and high-fiber diet, mobility at the highest level that is possible, medications, consistent timing of evacuation, privacy and positioning, and techniques such as digital stimulation and Valsalva's maneuver.

SEXUAL FUNCTION

Although the physical act of sex itself may change with SCI, the ability to enjoy a sexual and caring relationship with another person remains and often takes on greater importance than before the injury.

Spinal cord injury at any level abolishes communication pathways between the genital and higher centers. Erotic and emotional feelings and thoughts, however, may still be experienced in areas above the level of injury, especially when the mouth and neck are stimulated. Extragenital circulatory, musculoskeletal, and respiratory responses such as increased heart rate, breathing, and muscle tone that are mediated by centers above the level of injury may occur.

Sexual function, as in bladder and bowel control, is mediated by the S2 to S4 segments of the spinal cord. The genital sexual response in SCI, which is manifested by an erection in men and vaginal lubrication in women, may be initiated by mental or touch stimuli depending on the level of injury. The T11 to L2 cord segments have been identified as the mental-stimuli sexual response area where autonomic nerve pathways in communication with the cortex leave the cord and innervate the genitalia. The S2 to S4 cord segments have been identified as the sexual-touch reflex center. In an injury at T10 or above (UMN lesion), reflex sexual response to genital touch may occur freely. However, a sexual response to mental stimuli (T11 to L2) will not occur, owing to the spinal lesion blocking the communication pathway. In an injury at T12 or below (LMN), the sexual reflex center may be damaged and there may be no response to touch. Therefore, cord damage below the T12 segment may result in sexual arousal by mental stimuli. For persons with lesions between L2 to S1, sexual response to mental or touch stimuli may occur. Aids for men with erectile dysfunction include medications, vacuum devices, and penile implants. In women, water-soluble lubricants assist with vaginal lubrication. The severity of injury is not the most important determining factor in the outcome of sexual well-being. Satisfaction is most often the result of good sexual communication and shared intimacy and is independent of orgasm.

In men, lack of erectile ability or inability to experience penile sensations or orgasm is not a reliable indicator of fertility, which should be evaluated by an expert. In women, fertility is parallel to menses; usually it is delayed 3 months to 5 months after injury. There are hazards to pregnancy, labor, and birth control devices relative to SCI that require knowledgeable health care providers, but they need not be prohibitive.

TREATMENT AND MANAGEMENT STRATEGIES

CONTINUUM OF CARE

Prevention of SCI is of paramount importance. In the meantime, the major questions revolve around the optimal care for persons who sustain SCI. The issues relate to the methods of management that allow for the best chance of preserving neurologic function and preventing complications. In general, adequate immobilization immediately following injury is a necessary and effective treatment. It is now known that the cord suffers not only the immediate physical effects of trauma but also from secondary pathologic processes such as ischemia and edema, as discussed earlier. The use of steroid therapy has been reported in the literature since 1972, suggesting that there may be some benefit to SCI patients if given promptly after injury. More recently, Bracken and colleagues conducted a double blind study in ten centers, using a structured protocol for methylprednisolone use, that demonstrated some improvement in neurologic status.[31] There is evidence that the drug stabilizes the membranes of injured cells; this may decrease edema as well as ischemia in the injured spinal cord axon.

Early surgical treatment of the spine aims at internal skeletal stabilization so that early mobilization and rehabilitation can occur. Other research involves functional electrical stimulation to reactivate paralyzed systems and nerve regeneration and tissue-bridge implants to provide support for regenerating CNS axons across a damaged area. Until a cure is found, prevention in the form of health promotion, early diagnosis, and prompt intervention and rehabilitation to prevent further complications and restore optimal functioning is essential.

The spinal cord continuum of care begins at the moment of injury and ensues throughout the life span. Although it is not in the scope of this text to address the psychosocial issues surrounding SCI, one cannot deal with the physical problems without encountering the emotional and behavioral effects. Some aspects of SCI may be predictable; however, there are many factors that influence the outcome.

One approach to life with SCI may be with rela-

tion to concepts of health stabilization or restoration of physical function, life-style modification or integration of physical deficits with premorbid life-style and postinjury status, and community integration or independent functioning and socialization in the community (Table 50-3). Rather than stages, or phases, of recovery and rehabilitation in SCI, it may be thought of as a perpetual cycle that the person enters and reenters at any point along the life span. As aspects of one area change, so do the others in response to the needs of the person in establishing a mind-and-body wellness equilibrium. Health stabilization concerns surround the restoration of physical function, whether due to acute or chronic changes, as well as the psychosocial mechanisms necessary to deal with the situation on a short-term basis. Life-style modification deals with incorporating the changes in physical function with developmental tasks and cognitive exploration of beliefs and values regarding health, wellness, disability, self, and others. Community integration focuses on applying life-style modifications for independent living in realistic situations. The impact of physical disability in unstructured and unpredictable situations provides the ultimate challenge in socialization and independent functioning.

In summary, SCI is a disabling neurologic condition most commonly caused by motor vehicle accidents, falls, and sports injuries. It occurs most frequently in males and persons under 30 years of age. SCI is caused by abnormal motion or trauma to the spinal column; it includes injuries caused by excessive forward flexion and lateral bending, rotation, and extension of the spinal column. Dysfunctions of the nervous system following SCI cover varying degrees of sensorimotor loss and altered reflex activity, based on the level of injury and extent of cord damage. Dependent on the level of injury, the physical prob-

TABLE 50-3. THE SPINAL CORD CONTINUUM OF CARE

HEALTH STABILIZATION	LIFE-STYLE MODIFICATION	COMMUNITY INTEGRATION
Ventilation/communication function	Self care	Physical barriers
Autonomic nervous system regulation	Mobility	Equipment needs
Bowel and bladder control		Home care availability
Sensorimotor integrity		Professional health-care availability
Psychosocial impact	Psychosocial barriers	Psychosocial balance
	Developmental/cognitive level	Community re-entry
	Values/beliefs	Support systems
	Self concept/sexuality	Role adjustment
	Client/family education	

lems of SCI include spinal shock; ventilation/communication problems; autonomic nervous system dysfunction that predisposes to the vasovagal response, autonomic hyperreflexia, impaired body temperature regulation, and postural hypotension; impaired muscle pump and venous innervation leading to edema of dependent areas of the body and risk of deep vein thrombosis; altered sensorimotor integrity that contributes to uncontrolled muscle spasms, altered pain responses, and threat to skin integrity; alterations in bowel and bladder elimination; and impaired sexual function. The treatment of SCI involves a continuum of care that begins at the moment of injury and ensues throughout the life span. SCI research focuses on prevention of injury, preservation of neurologic function, and prevention of complications. The continuum of care incorporates health stabilization or restoration of physical function, life-style modification or integration of physical deficits with premorbid life-style and postinjury status, and community integration or independent functioning and socialization in the community.

■ REFERENCES

1. Berne, R.M., & Levy, M.N. (1988). *Physiology* (2nd ed., pp. 51, 244). St. Louis: C.V. Mosby.
2. Guyton, A. (1991). *Medical physiology* (8th ed., p. 602). Philadelphia: W.B. Saunders.
3. Noback, C.R., & Demarest, R.J. (1981). *The human nervous system* (3rd ed., p. 197). New York: McGraw-Hill.
4. Smith, P.E.M., Calverley, P.M.A., Edwards, R.H.T., et al. (1987). Practical problems in the respiratory care of patients with muscular dystrophy. *New England Journal of Medicine, 316,* 1197.
5. Bartlett, R.J., Pericak-Vance, M.A., Koh, J., et al. (1988). Duchenne muscular dystrophy: High frequency of deletions. *Neurology, 38,* 1.
6. Slater, C.R. (1987). The missing link in DMD? *Nature, 330,* 693.
7. Webster, C., Silberstein, L., Hays, A.R., et al. (1988). Fast muscle fibers are preferentially affected in Duchenne muscular dystrophy. *Cell, 52,* 503.
8. LaPate, G., & Pestronk, A. (1993). Autoimmune myasthenia gravis. *Hospital Practice, 28*(1A), 109.
9. Cotran, R.S., Kumar, V., & Robbins, S.L. (1989). *Robbins' pathologic basis of disease* (4th ed., pp. 1366–1367). Philadelphia: W.B. Saunders.
10. Sellman, M.S., & Mayer, R.F. (1985). Weakness and "tiredness": When to suspect myasthenia gravis. *Geriatrics, 40*(1), 92.
11. Cormack, D.H. (1987). *Ham's histology* (9th ed., pp. 335, 373–374). Philadelphia: J.B. Lippincott.
12. Hodgkins, M.L., & Grady, D. (1988). Carpal tunnel syndrome. *Western Journal of Medicine, 148,* 217.
13. Margolis, W., & Krause, J.F. (1987). The prevalence of carpal tunnel syndrome in female supermarket checkers. *Journal of Occupational Medicine, 29,* 953.
14. Barnhardt, S., & Rosinstock, L. (1987). Carpal tunnel in grocery checkers. *Western Journal of Medicine, 147,* 37.
15. Ferner, R., Barnet, M., & Hughes, R.A.C. (1987). Management of Guillain-Barré syndrome. *British Hospital Medicine, 2,* 525.
16. Ropper, A.H. (1992). The Guillain-Barre syndrome. *New England Journal of Medicine, 326,* 1130.
17. Pascuzz, R.M. (1988). Amyotrophic lateral sclerosis. *Indiana Medicine, 81,* 607.
18. Beal, M.F., Richardson, E.P., & Martin, J.B. (1991). Degenerative disease of the nervous system. In J. Wilson, E. Braunwald, & K.J. Isselbacher (Eds.). *Harrison's principles of internal medicine* (12th ed., pp. 2072–2074). New York: McGraw-Hill.
19. Magoun, H.W., & Rhines, R. (1946). An inhibitory mechanism in the bulbar reticular formation. *Journal of Neurophysiology, 9,* 165.
20. McCouch, G.P., Austin, G.M., Liu, C.-N., et al. (1958). Sprouting as a cause of spasticity. *Journal of Neurophysiology, 21,* 205.
21. Mariani, J., & Delhaye-Bouchaud, N. (1987). Elimination of functional synapses during development of the nervous system. *News in Psychological Sciences, 2,* 93.
22. Lund, R.D. (1978). *Development and plasticity of the brain.* New York: Oxford University Press.
23. National Spinal Cord Injury Statistical Center. (1987). *Spinal cord injury fact sheet.* Birmingham: University of Alabama.
24. White, A.A., & Panjabl, M.M. (1990). *Clinical biomechanics of the spine* (2nd ed.). Philadelphia: J.B. Lippincott.
25. American Spinal Injury Association. (1992). *Standards of neurological and functional classification of spinal cord injury.* Chicago: American Spinal Cord Injury Association.
26. Chui, L., & Bhatt, K. (1983). Autonomic dysreflexia. *Rehabilitation Nursing, March–April,* 16.
27. Myllynen, P., Kammonen, F., Rokkanen, P., et al. (1985). Deep venous thrombosis and pulmonary embolism in patients with acute spinal cord injury: A comparison with nonparalyzed patients immobilized due to spinal fractures. *Journal of Trauma, 21,* 541.
28. Zejdlik, C.P. (1992). *Management of spinal cord injury* (2nd ed., pp. 594–601). Boston: Jones and Bartlett.
29. Woolsey, R.M. (1986). Chronic pain following spinal cord injury. *Paraplegia, 19*(3 & 4), 27.
30. Farkash, A.E., & Portenoy, R.K. (1986). The pharmacologic management of chronic pain in the paraplegic patient. *Paraplegia, 19*(3 & 4), 41.
31. Bracken, M.B., Shepard, M.J., Collins, W.F., et al. (1990). A randomized, controlled trial of methylprednisolone or naloxone in the treatment of acute spinal cord injury. *New England Journal of Medicine, 332*(20), 1405.

■ BIBLIOGRAPHY

Alonso, R.J., & Mancall, E.L. (1991). The clinical management of spasticity. *Seminars in Neurology, 11,* 215.

Chipps, E. (1991). Myasthenia gravis: The patient in crisis. *Critical Care Nursing, 11*(7), 18.

Coon, W.W., Horsh, J., & Rubin, L.J. (1987). Preventing deep venous thrombosis. *Patient Care, February 15,* 82.

Ducker, T.B. (1990). Treatment of spinal cord injury. *New England Journal of Medicine, 322,* 1459.

Gilman, S. (1992). Advances in neurology (Parts 1 and 2). *New England Journal of Medicine, 326,* 1608.

Hughes, J.T. (1991). Neuropathology of the spinal cord. *Neurologic Clinics, 9,* 551.

Hughes, R.A.C. (1992). The management of Guillain-Barre syndrome. *Hospital Practice, 27,* 107.

Koller, W.C. (1990). Evaluation of tremor disorders. *Hospital Practice, 25*(5A), 23.

Meyer, P.R., Cybulski, G.R., Rusin, J.J., et al. (1991). Spinal cord injury. *Neurologic Clinics, 9,* 626.

Oaks, D.D., Wilmot, C.B., Hall, K.M., et al. (1990). Benefits of early admission to a comprehensive trauma center for spinal cord injury. *Archives of Physical Medicine and Rehabilitation, 71,* 637.

Richmond, T.S. (1990). Spinal cord injury. *Nursing Clinics of North America, 25,* 57.

Schoenen, J. (1991). Clinical anatomy of the spinal cord. *Neurologic Clinics, 9,* 503–533.

Sipsky, M.L. (1991). The impact of spinal cord injury on female sexuality, menstruation and pregnancy: A review of literature. *Journal of the American Paraplegia Society, 14*(3), 40.

Sipsky, M.L., & Alexander, C.J. (1991). Infertility following spinal cord injury: Current methods of treatment. *SCI Psychosocial Process,* Special Edition—Sexuality and Disability, 45.

Young, R.R. (1989). Treatment of spastic paresis. *New England Journal of Medicine, 920,* 1553.

CHAPTER 51

DISORDERS OF BRAIN FUNCTION

SHEILA M. CURTIS
PATRICK WALSH
ROBIN L. CURTIS

■ OBJECTIVES

After you have studied this chapter, you should be able to meet the following objectives:

■ Describe the organization of the brain on the basis of embryonic development.

■ Cite the origin and function of the cranial nerves.

■ Describe the location of the frontal, parietal, temporal, occipital, and limbic lobes of the cerebral cortex, and state their general classes of function.

■ State the characteristics of the dominant and non-dominant hemispheres of the brain.

■ Contrast and compare the blood–brain and CSF–brain barriers.

■ State the contribution of the internal carotid arteries, the vertebral arteries, and the circle of Willis to the cerebral circulation.

■ Explain autoregulation of cerebral blood flow.

■ Differentiate between cerebral hypoxia and cerebral ischemia.

■ Compare the concepts of focal and global ischemia.

■ Define *cerebrovascular occlusive disease* and compare the characteristics of transient ischemic attacks and stroke.

■ Define auditory-receptive aphasia, visual-receptive aphasia, Wernicke's aphasia, anomic aphasia, conduction aphasia, expressive aphasia, sensory agnosia, motor speech apraxia, and fluent and nonfluent aphasia.

■ Describe the characteristics of the denial or hemi-inattention syndrome.

■ State the complications associated with subarachnoid hemorrhage.

■ Describe the alterations in cerebral vasculature that occur with arteriovenous malformations.

Carol Mattson Porth: PATHOPHYSIOLOGY: CONCEPTS OF
ALTERED HEALTH STATES, 4th ed. © 1994, 1990, 1986, 1982
J.B. Lippincott Company

- ■ Describe the compensatory mechanisms used to prevent large changes in intracranial pressure (ICP) from occurring when there are changes in brain, blood, and CSF volume.
- ■ Compare the causes of communicating and non-communicating hydrocephalus.
- ■ Differentiate between cytotoxic, vasogenic, and interstitial cerebral edema.
- ■ Describe the postural changes that occur with decorticate and decerebrate rigidity.
- ■ Compare the symptoms of concussion with those of contusion.
- ■ Differentiate among location, manifestations, and morbidity associated with epidural, subdural, and intracerebral hematoma.

- ■ Compare the pathology of meningitis and encephalitis.
- ■ State a definition of consciousness.
- ■ Trace rostral-caudal progression of consciousness, pupillary changes, respiration, and motor function resulting from dysfunction of the diencephalon, midbrain, pons, and medulla.
- ■ State two criteria for diagnosis of brain death.
- ■ Explain the difference between the terms *seizure activity* and *seizure* or *epileptic syndrome*.
- ■ Compare the manifestations of simple partial seizures and complex partial seizures and those of absence seizures and tonic-clonic seizures.

The brain is protected from external forces by the rigid confines of the skull and the cushioning afforded by the cerebrospinal fluid (CSF). The metabolic stability required by its electrically active cells is maintained by a number of regulator mechanisms, including the blood–brain barrier and autoregulatory mechanisms that insure its blood supply. Nonetheless, the brain remains remarkably vulnerable to injury by ischemia, trauma, tumors, degenerative processes, and metabolic derangements.

The content in this chapter has been organized into six sections: (1) brain structure and function, (2) alterations in cerebral blood flow, (3) increased intracranial pressure, (4) head injury and infection, (5) altered levels of consciousness, and (6) seizure disorders.

■ BRAIN STRUCTURE AND FUNCTION

The brain is the center for meaningful activity. It provides us with a conscious awareness of our surroundings and the ability to feel, hear, see, taste, and smell; to direct and plan our movements; to speak to the people we come in contact with; and to remember previous experience and use that memory as a basis for decision making.

DEVELOPMENT OF THE BRAIN

In the process of development, the more rostral part of the embryonic neural tube—approximately 10 segments—undergoes extensive modification and enlargement to form the brain (Fig. 51-1). In the early embryo, three swellings, or primary vesicles, de-

velop, subdividing these 10 segments into the prosencephalon (forebrain), which contains the first two segments; the mesencephalon, or midbrain, which develops from segment 3; and the rhombencephalon, or hindbrain, which develops from segments 4 to 10 (Fig. 51-2). The 10 brain segments represent modifications of the spinal cord level neural tube and are often called, collectively, *the brain stem*. The brain stem does not include later developed outgrowths—the cerebral hemispheres, the optic nerve and retina, and the cerebellum.

The central canal of the prosencephalon develops two pairs of lateral outpouchings that carry the neural tube with them: (1) the optic cup, which becomes the optic nerve and retina, and (2) the telencephalic vesicles, which become the olfactory bulbs and the cerebral hemispheres. The central canal of the neural tube extends into the cerebral hemispheres as enlarged CSF–filled cavities, the first and second (lateral) ventricles. The remaining neural tube of these three segments is called the *diencephalon*; it develops into the thalamus and hypothalamus. The neurohypophysis (posterior pituitary) grows as a midline ventral outgrowth at the junctions of segments 1 and 2. A dorsal outgrowth, the pineal body, develops between segments 2 and 3, the diencephalic–mesencephalic junction.

The ventral half of the neural tube gray matter, the basal lamina, becomes the output-oriented ventral horn of the spinal cord and brain stem, including the hypothalamus. Most of the brain, as seen grossly, represents tremendous enlargements, outpouchings, outgrowths, and cortex formation derived from the alar lamina, which in the spinal cord is the source of the dorsal horns.

Both the central and peripheral nervous systems differentiate very early in embryonic life and hold a

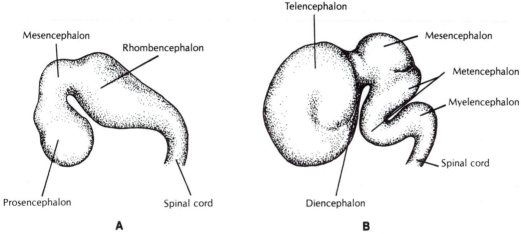

FIG. 51-1. **(A)** Primary brain vesicles (fifth week). **(B)** Secondary brain vesicles (seventh week). The diencephalon is partly hidden by the expanding telencephalon, which develops into the cerebral hemispheres. (Barr, M. L., & Kiernan, J. A. [1988]. *The human nervous system: An anatomical viewpoint* [5th ed., p. 5]. Philadelphia: J.B. Lippincott)

critical position in providing a necessary stimulus for differentiation of many other body tissues, particularly the skeletal muscles. By the end of the third month of gestation, the gross structure of the brain and spinal cord is established. The remaining period of intrauterine growth involves increases in numbers of both neurons and glial cells to a final neural-to-glial ratio of about 1:20. The synaptic relationships that develop during this period provide the basic circuitry required for subsequent mature neural function. Axon outgrowth of the major tract systems and the myelination of most of these occur during this vulnerable period. A phenomenal increase in brain weight occurs during the last 3- to 5-month period of intrauterine life. At birth, the average brain weighs about 300 g, approximately 12.5% of total body weight. During postuterine life, brain growth continues but at a decreasing rate, while body growth continues at an increasing rate. As a result, the adult human brain weight (1450–1500 g in the male, and 1200–1300 g in the female) is about five times that of the brain at birth and yet is only about 2.4% of total body weight. Maximum brain weight is reached between ages 20 and 29 and is then followed by a gradual decrease in weight with advancing years.

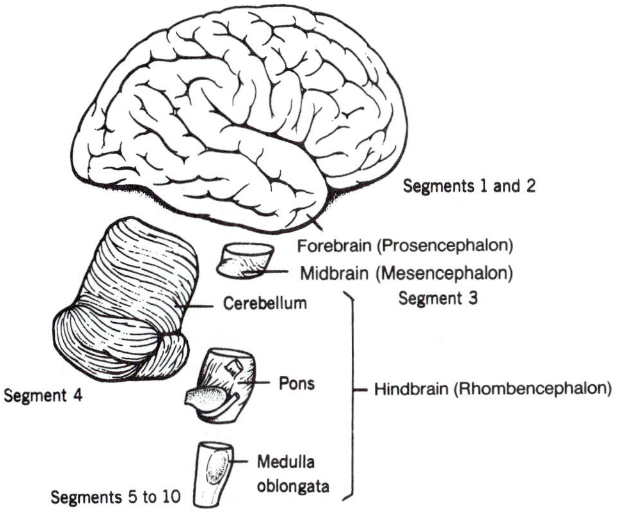

During the latter two-thirds of intrauterine life, the cerebral cortex increases its volume relative to that of deeper structures; this is achieved by a greatly increased surface area, which occurs with increasing development of the number and depth of infoldings. The adult cerebral cortex, with its many gyri (ridges) and infoldings, or sulci (grooves), is equivalent to an area of about 160,000 mm^2 and contains about 16.5 billion neurons.[1] The cerebellar cortex also undergoes a tremendous increase in area during the latter half of embryonic life and infancy, achieving an area of 84,000 mm^2, again with the development of many deep sulci and narrow gyri. The cerebellar cortex of the adult contains approximately 100 billion neurons.

The third neural tube segment, which forms the midbrain, retains its basic spinal segment–like organization. Segment 4 of the rhombencephalon becomes much enlarged and flattened laterally, giving the fourth ventricle its rhomboid shape. This segment, called the *metencephalon* or pons, also grows up and over the fourth ventricle to form much of the cerebellum. The pons and cerebellum retain important functional interrelationships in the adult.

The remaining segments, 5 through 10, become

FIG. 51-2. The segments of the forebrain, midbrain and hindbrain. (Modified from Chaffee, E. E., & Lytle, I.M. [1980]. *Basic physiology and anatomy* [4th ed., p. 203]. Philadelphia: J.B. Lippincott)

the medulla oblongata, with the widened fourth ventricle narrowing to form a central canal, which continues through the spinal cord segments. The most rostral segment (5) of the medulla fuses with the pons and is often called the caudal pons. It also contributes to the caudal part of the cerebellum. The junction of segment 10 of the brain stem with the cervical spinal segments occurs at the foramen magnum, the large opening in the skull through which the neural tube passes.

Each of these brain segments, except for segment 2, retains some portion of the basic segmental organization of the nervous system. The evolutionary development of the brain is reflected in the cranial and upper cervical paired segmental nerves. This reflects the prototype or original pattern: a segmented neural tube, each segment of which has multiple paired branches containing a grouping of particular component axons. One segment would have paired branches to body muscles and another set of visceral structures, and so on. The classic pattern of the spinal nerve organization, which consists of a pair of dorsal and a pair of ventral roots, is a more recent evolutionary development that has not occurred in the cranial nerves. Consequently, the cranial nerves, which are arbitrarily numbered 1 through 12, retain the ancient pattern with more than one cranial nerve branching from a single segment. The truly segmental nerve pattern of the cranial nerves is further clouded by the loss of all branches from segment 2 and most of the branches from segment 1. It should be noted that the second cranial nerve, the optic nerve, is not a segmental nerve branch. Rather, it is a brain tract connecting the retina (modified brain) with the first forebrain segment from which it developed.

HINDBRAIN

The hindbrain (medulla and pons) is a distorted, enlarged, and elaborated version of the spinal cord. It contains the neuronal circuits required for the basic breathing, eating, and locomotive functions required for survival. It is surrounded on the outside by the long tract systems that interconnect the forebrain with lower parts of the CNS (see Fig. 51-1).

MEDULLA

The medulla oblongata represents the caudal five segments of the brain part of the neural tube; thus, the cranial nerve branches entering and leaving it have similar functions, as do the spinal segmental nerves. The ventral horn area in the medulla is quite small, but the dorsal horn is enlarged, processing a great amount of the information pouring through the cranial nerves. The segmental peripheral nerve components of the medulla can be divided into those that leave the neural tube ventromedially (hypoglossal and abducens cranial nerves) and those that exit dorsolaterally (vagus, spinal accessory, glossopharyngeal, and vestibulocochlear cranial nerves). Because the signs and symptoms of pathology reflect the spatial segregation of brain stem components, neurologic syndromes resulting from trauma, tumors, aneurysms, and cerebrovascular accidents are often classified as ventral or dorsolateral syndromes.

The lower motoneurons (LMNs) of the lower segments of the medulla supply the extrinsic and intrinsic muscles of the tongue by means of the *hypoglossal (XII) cranial nerve*. Damage to the hypoglossal nerve results in partial or total denervation and, therefore, weakness or paralysis of tongue muscles. When the tongue is protruded, it deviates toward the damaged and therefore weak side because of the greater protrusion strength on the normal side. The axons of the hypoglossal nerve leave the medulla adjacent to two long, longitudinal ridges along the medial undersurface of the medulla called the *pyramids*. The pyramids contain the corticospinal axons that provide for fine manipulative control for the spinal LMNs. Lesions of the ventral surface of the caudal medulla result in the syndrome of *alternating hypoglossal hemiplegia*, characterized by signs of ipsilateral (same side) denervation of the tongue and contralateral (opposite side) weakness or paralysis of both the upper and lower extremities.

The *vagus nerve (X)* has both afferent (sensory) and efferent (motor) fibers that innervate the gastrointestinal tract (from the laryngeal pharynx to the midtransverse colon), the heart, and the lungs; the pharyngeal taste buds (special visceral afferents) and muscles of the pharynx and larynx. The fibers carried in the vagus are responsible for both afferent and efferent innervation of these structures. Therefore, initiation of many essential reflexes and normal functions depend on intact vagal innervation. For example, 80% of the fibers of the vagus are afferents, some of which are involved in initiated vomiting and hiccup reflexes and in ongoing feedback during swallowing and speech. The unilateral loss of vagal function can result in slowed gastrointestinal motility, a permanently husky voice, and deviation of the uvula away from the damaged side. Bilateral loss of vagal function can seriously damage reflex maintenance of cardiovascular and respiratory reflexes. Swallowing may become difficult, and in some cases paralysis of laryngeal structures causes life-threatening airway obstruction.

The sternocleidomastoid, a powerful head-turning muscle, and the trapezius muscle, which elevates the shoulders, are innervated by cranial nerve XI, the *spinal assessory* (*XI*) cranial nerve with LMNs in the upper four cervical spinal segments. Lateral rootlets from these segmental levels combine and enter the cranial cavity through the foramen magnum and then exit through the jugular foramen with cranial nerves (IX) and (X). Loss of spinal accessory nerve function results in drooping of the shoulder on the damaged side and weakness when turning the head to the opposite side.

The dorsolateral *glossopharyngeal nerve*, cranial nerve IX, contains the same components as the vagus nerve but for a more rostral segment of the gastrointestinal tract and the pharynx. This nerve provides the special sensory innervation of the taste buds of the oral pharynx and the back of the tongue; the afferent innervation of the oral pharynx and the baroreceptors of the carotid sinus; the efferent innervation of the otic ganglion, which controls the salivary function of the parotid gland; and the efferent innervation of the stylopharyngeal muscle of the pharynx. This cranial nerve is seldom damaged, but when it is, anesthesia of the ipsilateral oral pharynx and dry mouth due to reduced salivation develop.

The *vestibulocochlear* cranial nerve (VIII), formerly called the auditory nerve, is attached laterally at the junction of the medulla oblongata and the pons. It consists of two distinct fiber divisions, both of which are sensory: (1) the cochlear division, which arises from cell bodies in the cochlea in the inner ear and transmits impulses related to the sense of hearing, and (2) the vestibular division, which arises from two ganglia that innervate cell bodies in utricle, saccule, and semicircular canals and transmits impulses related to head position and movement of the body through space. Injury to the cochlear division results in tinnitus or nerve deafness versus conduction deafness; injury to the vestibular division leads to vertigo, nystagmus, and some postural instability (see Chapter 53).

In the most rostral segment of the medulla, LMNs send their axons out ventrally on either side of the pyramids and then forward into the orbit through the *abducens* (VI) cranial nerve to innervate the lateral rectus muscle of the eye. As the name indicates, the abducens nerve abducts the eye (lateral and outward rotation); peripheral damage to them results medial strabismus, which is a weakness or loss of eye abduction (see Chapter 52).

The facial cranial nerve (VII) and its intermediate component (the intermedius) contain both afferent and efferent components. The intermedius nerve innervates the nasopharynx and taste buds of the palate, the forward two-thirds of the tongue, the submandibular and sublingual salivary glands, the lacrimal glands, and mucous membranes of the nose and roof of the mouth. Loss of this branch of the facial nerve can lead to eye dryness with risk of corneal scarring and blindness. The LMNs of the facial nerve innervate muscles that control facial expression, such as wrinkling of the brow and smiling. Unilateral loss of facial nerve function results in flaccid paralysis of the muscles of one-half of the head, a condition called *Bell's palsy*. The facial nerve passes through a bony tunnel behind the middle ear cavity. Bell's palsy has been attributed to inflammatory reactions involving the facial nerve in or near this bony tunnel. Because such injuries result from pressure caused by edematous tissue, the integrity of the endoneurial tube is retained, and regeneration with full recovery of all muscles generally occurs within a period of several months.

PONS

The pons, or bridge, develops from the fourth neural tube segment. The central canal of the spinal cord, which remains small but is greatly enlarged in the pons and rostral medulla, forms the fourth ventricle (Fig. 51-3). An enlarged area on the ventral surface of the pons contains the pontine nuclei, which receive information from all parts of the cerebral cortex. The axons of these neurons form a massive bundle that swings around the lateral side of the fourth ventricle to enter the cerebellum. The reticular formation of the pons is large and contains the circuitry for masticating food and manipulating the jaws during speech. The trigeminal (V) and facial (VII) cranial nerves have their origin in the pons.

The *trigeminal* cranial nerve (V), which has both sensory and motor subdivisions, exits the brain stem laterally on the forward surface of the pons. The trigeminal is the main sensory nerve conveying the modalities of pain, temperature, touch, and proprioception to the superficial and deep regions of the face. The regions innervated include the skin of the anterior scalp and face, the conjunctiva and orbit, the meninges, the paranasal sinuses, and the mouth, including the teeth and the anterior two-thirds of the tongue. The LMNs of the trigeminal nerve innervate skeletal muscles involved with mastication and also contribute to swallowing and speech, movements of the soft palate, and tension of the tympanic membrane. The latter apparently has a protective reflex function, dampening movement of the middle ear ossicles during high-intensity sound.

CEREBELLUM

The cerebellum, or "little brain," is located above the fourth ventricle. Similar to a complicated computer system, the cerebellum serves to interrelate visual,

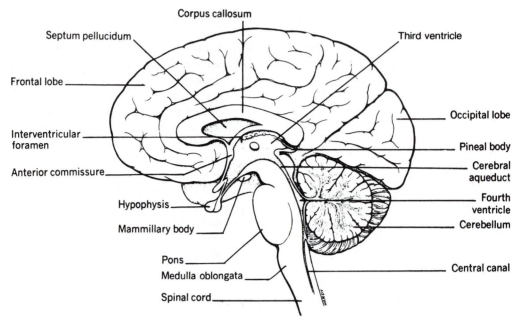

FIG. 51-3. Midsagittal section of the brain. (Chaffee, E. E., & Lytle, I. M. [1980]. *Basic physiology and anatomy* [4th ed., p. 214]. Philadelphia: J.B. Lippincott)

auditory, somesthetic, and vestibular information with ongoing motor activity so that highly skilled movement can be smoothly performed. Functions of the cerebellum are discussed in Chapter 50.

MIDBRAIN

The midbrain develops from the third segment of the neural tube, and its organization is similar to that of a spinal segment. The central canal is reestablished as the cerebral aqueduct, interconnecting the fourth ventricle with the third ventricle (see Fig. 51-3). The oculomotor (III) and trochlear (IV) cranial nerves are located in the midbrain.

Massive fiber bundles of the cerebral peduncles pass from the forebrain to the pons along the ventral surface of the midbrain. On the dorsal surface, four "little hills," the superior and inferior colliculi, are areas of cortical formation. The inferior colliculus is involved in directional turning and, to some extent, in experiencing the direction of sound sources. The superior colliculus is an essential part of the reflex mechanisms that control eye movements when the visual environment is being surveyed.

The central gray matter contains the LMNs that innervate most of the skeletal muscles that move the optic globe about and raise the eyelids. These axons leave the midbrain through the *oculomotor (III)* cranial nerve. This nerve also contains axons that control pupillary constriction and ciliary muscle focusing of the lens. Damage to the ventrally exiting cranial

nerve III and to the adjacent cerebral peduncle, which includes the corticospinal axon system on one side, results in paralysis of eye movement combined with contralateral hemiplegia (discussed in Chapter 52).

A small, compact group of cells in the ventral part of the central gray matter contains the LMNs that innervate the superior oblique eye muscles that move the upper part of the eye downward and toward the nose when the eye is adducted, or turned inward. These axons emerge dorsolaterally and caudally as the *trochlear (IV)* cranial nerve and decussate (cross over) in the medulla before exiting the brain stem. Lesions involving the trochlear cranial nerve are unusual. The diplopia, or double vision, resulting from such lesions affects downward gaze to the opposite side. Walking downstairs becomes particularly difficult. The trochlear nerve–innervated superior oblique muscle has as its major function intorsion of the optic globe; to avoid diplopia, the person usually carries the head tilted to the side of damage.

FOREBRAIN

The forebrain is the most rostral part of the brain; it consists of the telencephalon or "end-brain," and the diencephalon or "between-brain." The diencephalon forms the core of the forebrain, and the telencephalon forms the cerebral hemispheres.

DIENCEPHALON

The two most forward brain segments form an enlarged dorsal horn–ventral structure with a narrow, deep, enlarged central canal—the third ventricle—separating the two sides. This region is called the *diencephalon*. The dorsal horn part of the diencephalon is the thalamus and subthalamus, and the ventral horn part is the hypothalamus (Fig. 51-4).

The thalamus consists of two large, egg-shaped masses, one on either side of the third ventricle. The thalamus is divided into several major parts, and each part is divided into distinct nuclei, which are the major relay stations for information going to and from the cerebral cortex. All sensory pathways, except those for smell, have direct projections to thalamic nuclei, which in turn convey the information to restricted areas of the sensory cortex. The coordination and integration of peripheral sensory stimuli occur within the thalamus, and there is some crude interpretation of highly emotion-laden auditory experiences that not only occur but can be remembered. A person can come out of a deep coma and remember a considerable amount of what was said at the bedside. The thalamus also plays a role in relaying critical information regarding motor activities to and from selected areas of the motor cortex. Two neuronal circuits that are significant in this regard are (1) the pathway from the cerebral cortex to the pons and cerebellum and then, by way of the thalamus, back to the motor cortex, and (2) the feed-back circuit that travels from the cortex to the basal ganglia, then to the thalamus, and from the thalamus back to the cortex. Through its connections with the ascending reticular activating system, the thalamus processes neural influences that are basic to cortical excitatory rhythms (those recorded on the electroencephalogram) that are essential to sleep–wakefulness cycles and to the process of attending to stimuli. In addition to their cortical connections, the thalamic nuclei have connections with each other and with neighboring nonthalamic brain structures such as the limbic system. Through their connections with the limbic system, some thalamic nuclei are involved in the relationship between stimuli and their emotional responses. The subthalamus contains movement control systems related to the basal ganglia (see Chapters 50 and 54). The *optic (II) nerve* and retina are outgrowths of the diencephalon from the region of the optic chiasm. The structure and function of the optic nerve are presented in Chapter 52.

The ventral horn portion of the diencephalon is the hypothalamus, which borders the third ventricle and includes a ventral extension, the neurohypophysis (posterior pituitary). The hypothalamus is the area of master-level integration of homeostatic control of the body's internal environment. Maintenance of blood gas concentration, water balance, food consumption, and major aspects of endocrine and autonomic nervous system control require hypothalamic function.

The internal capsule is a broad band of projection fibers that lies between the thalamus medially and the basal ganglia laterally (see Fig. 51-4). The internal capsule contains all of the fibers that interconnect the cerebral cortex with deeper structures, including the basal ganglia, thalamus, midbrain, pons, medulla, and spinal cord.

CEREBRAL HEMISPHERES

The two cerebral hemispheres are lateral outgrowths of the diencephalon. The cerebral hemispheres contain the lateral ventricles (ventricles I and II), which are interconnected with the third ventricle of the diencephalon by a small opening called the interventricular foramen (of Monro). Axons of the *olfactory cranial (I) nerve* terminate in the most ancient portion of the cerebrum—the olfactory bulb, where initial processing of olfactory information occurs. Projection axons from the olfactory bulb relay through the olfactory tracts to the thalamus and to other parts of the cerebral cortex, where both olfactory-related reflexes and olfactory experience occur.

The corpus callosum is a massive commissure, or bridge, of myelinated axons interconnecting the cerebral cortex of the two sides of the brain. Two

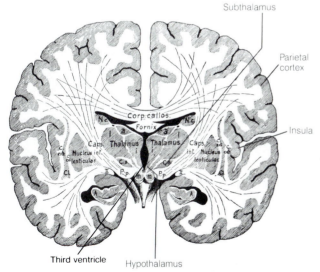

FIG. 51-4. Frontal section of the brain passing through the third ventricle, showing the thalamus, subthalamus, hypothalamus, internal capsule (*caps int.*), external capsule (*c. ext.*), corpus callosum (*corp. callos.*), basal ganglia (caudate nucleus [*c.s.*], lenticular nucleus), insula, and parietal cortex. (Modified from Villiger, E., & Addison, W. H. F. [Eds.]. [1931]. *Brain and spinal cord.* Philadelphia: J.B. Lippincott)

smaller commissures, the anterior and posterior commissures, connect the two sides of the more specialized regions of the cerebrum and diencephalon.

A section through the cerebral hemispheres will reveal the surface of the cerebral cortex, a subcortical layer of white matter made up of masses of myelinated axons, and deep masses of gray matter: the basal ganglia that border the lateral ventricle. The *basal ganglia* comprise the comma-shaped caudal nucleus, the shield-shaped putamen, and the globus pallidus. The basal ganglia supply axial and proximal unlearned and learned postures and movements, which enhance and add gracefulness to UMN-controlled fine manipulative movements. These background movement functions, called "associated movements," provide, for example, the swinging of the arms during walking or the set-up and follow-through during the swinging of a baseball bat. The structure and function of basal ganglia are further described in Chapters 50 and 54.

The surfaces of the hemispheres are lateral (side), medial (area between the two sides of the brain), and basal (ventral). The cerebral cortex exposed to view laterally is the recently evolved layered cortex. The surface of the hemispheres contains many ridges and grooves. The ridge between two grooves is called a *gyrus*, and the groove is called a *sulcus* or *fissure*. The cerebral cortex is arbitrarily divided into lobes named after the bones that cover them: the frontal, parietal, temporal, and occipital lobes (Fig. 51-5).

Frontal Lobe. The frontal lobe extends from the frontal pole to the central sulcus (fissure) and is separated from the temporal lobe by the lateral sulcus. The frontal lobe can be subdivided rostrally into the frontal pole and laterally into the superior, middle, and inferior gyri, which continue on the undersur-

face over the eyes as the orbital cortex. These areas are associated with the medial thalamic nuclei, which is also related to the limbic system. In general terms, the prefrontal cortex appears to be involved in anticipation and prediction of consequences of behavior. This "future-oriented" region is particularly depressed by many drugs, including alcohol.

The precentral gyrus (area 4), adjacent to the central sulcus, is the primary motor cortex (Fig. 51-6). The frontal cortex just rostral to the precentral gyrus is called the *premotor* or *motor association cortex* (areas 8, 6). This area is involved in the organization of more complex, learned movement patterns, and damage results in dyspraxia or apraxia. Such patients can manipulate a screwdriver, for instance, but cannot use it to loosen a screw. Both the primary and the association motor cortex are interconnected with lateral thalamic nuclei through which they receive feedback information from the basal ganglia and cerebellum.

Parietal Lobe. The parietal lobe of the cerebrum lies behind the central sulcus (the post-central gyrus) and above the lateral sulcus. The strip of cortex bordering the central sulcus is called the primary somatosensory cortex (areas 3, 1, 2) because it receives very discrete sensory information from the lateral nuclei of the thalamus (see Fig. 51-6). Just behind the primary sensory cortex is a region of somesthetic association cortex (areas 5, 7), which is interconnected with thalamic nuclei and with the primary sensory cortex. This region is necessary to appreciate perception or meaningfulness of sensory information. The somesthetic functions of the sensory cortex are discussed in Chapter 48.

Temporal Lobe. The temporal lobe lies below the lateral sulcus and merges with the parietal and occipital lobes (see Fig. 51-5). It has a polar region and

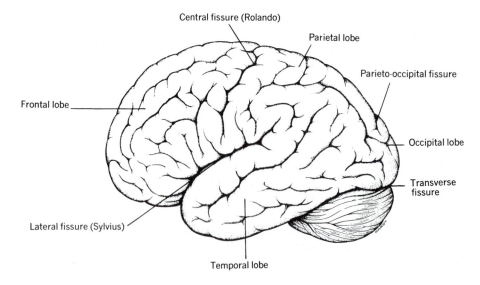

FIG. 51-5. Lateral aspect of the left cerebral and cerebellar hemispheres.

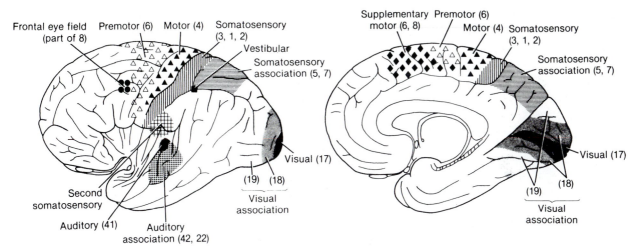

FIG. 51-6. Motor and sensory areas of the cerebral cortex. The lateral view (**left**) of the left (dominant) side is drawn as though the lateral sulcus had been pried open, exposing the insula. The diagram on the **right** represents the areas in a brain that has been sectioned in the median plane. (Reproduced by permission from Nolte, J. [1981]. *The human brain.* St. Louis: C.V. Mosby)

three primary gyri: superior, middle, and inferior. It is separated from the limbic areas on the ventral surface by the collateral or rhinal sulcus. The primary auditory cortex (area 41) involves the part of the superior temporal gyrus that extends into the lateral sulcus (see Fig. 51-6). This area is particularly important for fine discrimination from sound entering the opposite ear. It receives auditory input projections by way of the inferior colliculus of the midbrain and a ventral-lateral thalamic nucleus. The more exposed part of the superior temporal gyrus involves the auditory association or perception area (area 22). The gnostic aspects of hearing (*e.g.,* the meaning of a certain sound pattern) require the function of this area. The remaining portion of the temporal cortex has a less well-defined function but is apparently important in long-term memory recall. Irritation or stimulation can result in vivid hallucinations of long-past events. These higher-order temporal and parietal cortical regions are interconnected with a large, recently evolved dorsal lateral thalamic nuclear complex.

The cortices of the frontal, parietal, and temporal lobes surrounding the older cortex of the *insula,* located deep in the lateral fissure, represent the most recently evolved parts of the cerebral cortex. These areas contain primary and association functions for motor control and somesthesias for the lips and tongue and for audition; thus, they are particularly involved in speech mechanisms.

Occipital Lobe. The occipital lobe is located posterior to the temporal and parietal lobes and is only arbitrarily separated from them. The medial surface of the occipital lobe contains a deep sulcus

extending from the limbic lobe to the occipital pole, the *calcarine sulcus,* which contains the primary visual cortex (area 17). Stimulation of this cortex causes the experience of bright lights (phosphenes) in the visual field. Just superior and inferior and extending onto the lateral side of the occipital pole is the association cortex for vision (areas 18 and 19). This area is closely connected with the primary visual cortex and with complex nuclei of the thalamus. The integrity of the association cortex is required for gnostic visual function—the meaningfulness of visual experience.

The neocortical areas of the parietal lobe, between the somesthetic and the visual cortices, have a function in interrelating the texture, or "feel," of an object with its visual image. Between the auditory and visual association areas, the parieto-occipital region is necessary for interrelating the sound and image of an object or person.

Limbic System. The medial aspect of the cerebrum is organized as three concentric bands of cortex, the limbic system, which surround the interconnection between the lateral and third ventricle (the interventricular foramen). The innermost band just above and below the cut surface of the corpus callosum is folded out of sight but is an ancient, three-layered cortex ending as the hippocampus in the temporal lobe. Just outside the folded area is a band of transitional cortex, which includes the cingulate and the parahippocampal gyri (Fig. 51-7). This limbic lobe has reciprocal connections with the medial nuclei and the intralaminar nuclei of the thalamus, with the deep nuclei of the cerebrum (amygdaloid nuclei, septal nuclei) and with the hypothalamus. In general, this region of the brain is involved in emotional

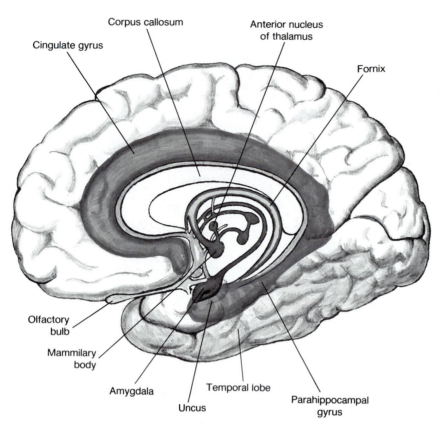

Cingulate gyrus

Corpus callosum

Anterior nucleus of thalamus

Fornix

Olfactory bulb

Mammillary body

Amygdala

Uncus

Temporal lobe

Parahippocampal gyrus

FIG. 51-7. The limbic system. This includes the limbic cortex (cingulate gyrus, parahippocampal gyrus, uncus) and associated subcortical structures (thalamus, hypothalamus, amygdala). (Chaffee, E. E., & Lytle, I. M. [1980]. *Basic physiology and anatomy* [4th ed., p. 211]. Philadelphia: J.B. Lippincott)

experience and in the control of emotion-related behavior. Stimulation of specific areas in this system can lead to feelings of dread, high anxiety, or exquisite pleasure.

Cerebral Dominance. Cerebral dominance refers to the fact that control of certain learned forms of behavior is exerted primarily by one of the two cerebral hemispheres. Handedness, perception of language, performance of speech, and appreciation of spatial relationships are primarily expressions of one or the other hemispheres.[2] By convention, speech is usually used to designate the dominant hemisphere. The dominant hemisphere has a major role in verbal and analytic abilities; the nondominant hemisphere has a lesser role in these functions and a major role in nonverbal and spatial abilities. In most persons, even left-handed persons, the left hemisphere is the dominant hemisphere for speech. Although it is assumed that the dominance of speech and handedness are assigned to the same hemisphere, this is not always the case. In clinical practice, communication dominance is a determinant of cerebral dominance. It may be tested, in special cases, by the use of the WADA test in which barbiturate is injected via the carotid artery to a single hemisphere and neurologic status is assessed. It should be noted that there is substantial overlap; therefore, the concept of strict lateralization may not be appropriate other than in primary sensory areas.

The interhemispheric communication pathways are largely undeveloped at birth. The communication between the two hemispheres increases with age and is fairly well developed by the second or third year of life. Cerebral dominance probably develops gradually throughout childhood. This explains why a child with an injury to the normally dominant hemisphere can be trained to become left-handed and proficient in speech, whereas an older person with similar deficits finds such learning difficult or impossible.

MENINGES

Inside the skull and vertebral column, the brain and spinal cord are loosely suspended and protected by several connective tissue sheaths called the *meninges* (Fig. 51-8). The surfaces of the spinal cord, brain, and segmental nerves are covered with a delicate connective tissue layer called the *pia mater* (delicate mother). The surface blood vessels and those that penetrate the brain and spinal cord are encased in this protective tissue layer. A second very delicate, nonvascular, and waterproof layer, called the *arachnoid* because of its spider-web appearance, encloses the entire CNS (Fig. 51-9). The CSF is contained within the subarachnoid space. Immediately outside the arachnoid is a continuous sheath of strong connective tissue, the *dura mater* (tough mother), which provides the major protection for the brain and spinal cord carried

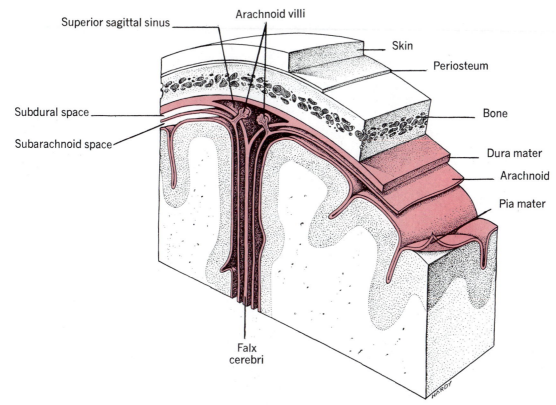

FIG. 51-8. The cranial meninges. Arachnoid villi, shown within the superior sagittal sinus, are one site of cerebrospinal fluid absorption into the blood. (Chaffee, E. E., & Lytle, I. M. [1980]. *Basic physiology and anatomy* [4th ed.]. Philadelphia: J.B. Lippincott)

within it. The cranial dura often splits into two layers, and the outer layer serves as the periosteum of the inner surface of the skull.

The inner layer of the dura forms two folds. The first, a longitudinal fold called the *falx cerebri*, separates the cerebral hemispheres and fuses with a second transverse fold called the *tentorium cerebelli* (Fig.

51-10). The latter acts as a hammock, supporting the occipital lobes above the cerebellum. The tentorium forms a tough septum, which divides the cranial cavity into the anterior and middle fossae and contains the cerebral hemispheres and a posterior fossa, which lies inferior to it and contains the brain stem and cerebellum. The tentorium attaches to the pe-

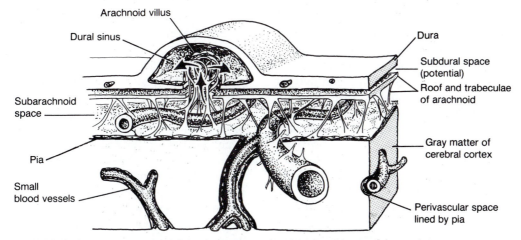

FIG. 51-9. Schematic diagram of the three connective tissue membranes (pia, arachnoid, and dura) constituting the meninges of the central nervous system. Cerebrospinal fluid is resorbed by way of the arachnoid villi projecting into the dural sinuses, as indicated by *arrows*. (After Weed; from Cormack, D. H. [1987]. *Ham's histology* [9th ed., p. 367]. Philadelphia: J.B. Lippincott)

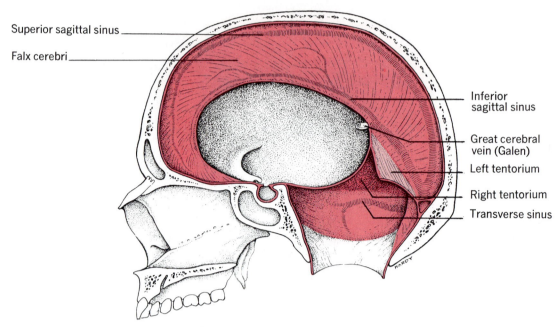

Superior sagittal sinus

Falx cerebri

Inferior sagittal sinus

Great cerebral vein (Galen)

Left tentorium

Right tentorium

Transverse sinus

FIG. 51-10. Cranial dura mater. The skull is open to show the falx cerebri and the right and left portions of the tentorium cerebelli, as well as some of the cranial venous sinuses. (Chaffee, E. E., & Lytle, I. M. [1980]. *Basic physiology and anatomy* [4th ed., p. 219]. Philadelphia: J.B. Lippincott)

trous portion of the temporal bone and the dorsum sellae of the cranial floor, with a semicircular gap, or *incisura*, formed at the midline to permit the midbrain to pass forward from the posterior fossa. The resultant compartmentalization of the cranial cavity is the basis for the commonly used terms *supratentorial*— above the tentorium—and *infratentorial*—below the tentorium. The cerebral hemispheres and the diencephalon are supratentorial structures, and the pons, cerebellum, and medulla are infratentorial. The strong folds of the inner dura, the tentorium and falx cerebri, normally support and protect the brain, which floats in the CSF within the enclosed space. During extreme trauma, however, the sharp edges of these folds can damage the brain. Space-occupying lesions such as enlarging tumors or hematomas can squeeze the brain against these edges or through the small openings of the tentorium, the incisura (herniation). As a result, brain tissue can be compressed, contused, or destroyed, often with permanent deficits (to be discussed).

VENTRICULAR SYSTEM AND CEREBROSPINAL FLUID

The ventricular system is a series of CSF-filled cavities within the brain (Fig. 51-11). The lining of the ventricles and central canal of the spinal cord, called the *ependymal lining*, undergoes great expansion in the roof of the lateral, third and fourth ventricles,

with multiple foldings called the choroid plexuses, which are the source of 90% of the CSF. The other 10% is produced by the remainder of the ependymal lining of the ventricles and central canal of the spinal cord. The choroid plexuses total only 2 to 3 g of tissues, or approximately 0.25% of the brain weight. The surface of the choroid epithelium facing the CSF contains many microvilli, from which about 800 mL of CSF are secreted each day. The total volume in the ventricular system is only about 150 mL, meaning that the CSF is completely replaced several times a day. The CSF is a closed system, and there is a net flow back and forth in the cerebral aqueduct that reflects the pulsatile nature of the arterial blood pressure.

The CSF is an ultrafiltrate of blood plasma composed of 99% water, with other constituents very close to that of the brain extracellular fluid (Table 51-1). The functions of the CSF are twofold: (1) it provides a supporting and protective fluid within which float the brain and spinal cord, and (2) it provides a relatively constant ionic environment that serves as a medium for diffusion of nutrients, electrolytes, and metabolic products between the extracellular fluid surrounding CNS neurons and glia. Filling the ventricles, the CSF supports the mass of the brain. Because it fills the subarachnoid space surrounding the CNS, physical force delivered to the cranial or spinal skeleton is to some extent diffused and cushioned.

The CSF produced in the ventricles must exit

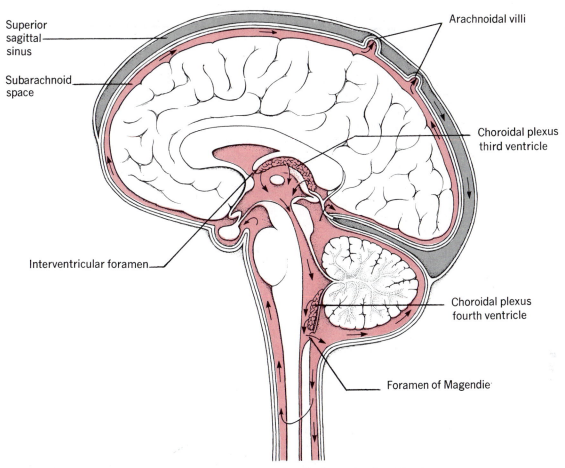

FIG. 51-11. The flow of cerebrospinal fluid from the time of its formation from blood in the choroid plexuses until its return to the blood in the superior sagittal sinus. (Note: Plexuses in the lateral ventricles are not illustrated.) (Chaffee, E. E., & Lytle, I. M. [1980]. *Basic physiology and anatomy* [4th ed., p. 221]. Philadelphia: J.B. Lippincott)

through the interventricular foramen, the third ventricle, the cerebral aqueduct, and the fourth ventricle to escape from the neural tube. Three other openings, or *foramina*, allow the CSF to pass into the subarachnoid space. Two of these, the *foramina of Luschka*, are located at the lateral corners of the fourth

ventricle. The third, the medial *foramen of Magendie*, is located in the midline at the caudal end of the fourth ventricle (see Fig. 51-11). About 30% of the CSF passes down into the subarachnoid space that surrounds the spinal cord, mainly on its dorsal surface, and moves back up to the cranial cavity along its ventral surface.

Reabsorption of CSF into the vascular system occurs along the sides of the superior sagittal sinus in the anterior and middle fossa. To reach this area, the CSF must pass along the sides and ventral surface of the medulla and pons and then through the tentorial incisura or opening that surrounds the midbrain. Some of the CSF exits the posterior fossa ventrally, along the sides of the basilar artery rostrally and through a CSF cistern between the midbrain peduncles (basilar cistern). The major part of the flow continues along the sides of the hypothalamus to the region of the optic chiasma and then laterally and superiorly along the lateral fissure and over the parietal cortex to the superior sagittal sinus region. Here the waterproof arachnoid has protuberances, the

TABLE 51-1. COMPOSITION OF CEREBROSPINAL FLUID COMPARED WITH PLASMA

SUBSTANCE	PLASMA	CEREBROSPINAL FLUID
Protein mg/dL	7500.00	20.00
Na$^+$ mEq/L	145.00	141.00
CL$^-$ mEq/L	101.00	124.00
K$^+$ mEq/L	4.50	2.90
HCO$^-$ mEq/L	25.00	24.00
pH	7.4	7.32
Glucose mg/dL	92.00	61.00

arachnoid villi, which penetrate the inner dura and venous walls of the superior sagittal sinus.

The reabsorption of CSF into the vascular system occurs by way of a pressure gradient. The normal CSF pressure is about 150 mm H_2O. The microstructures of the arachnoid villi are such that if the CSF pressure falls below approximately 50 mm H_2O, the passageways collapse and reverse flow is blocked. The arachnoid villi, therefore, function as one-way valves, permitting CSF outflow into the blood but not allowing blood to pass into the arachnoid spaces.

BLOOD–BRAIN AND CSF–BRAIN BARRIERS

Maintenance of a chemically stable environment is essential to the function of the brain. Elsewhere in the body, the extracellular fluid concentrations of hormones, amino acids, pH, and ions such as potassium undergo small fluctuations during daily activities such as eating and exercising. If the brain were to undergo such fluctuations, the result would be uncontrolled neural activity, because some substances such as amino acids act as neurotransmitters and ions such as potassium influence the threshold for neural firing. Two barriers, the blood–brain barrier and the CSF–brain barrier, provide the means for maintaining the stable chemical environment of the brain. Only water, carbon dioxide, and oxygen enter the brain with relative ease; the transport of other substances between the brain and the blood is slow. The site of the barrier is the endothelial cells of the cerebral capillaries in the blood–brain barrier and the choroid epithelium in the CSF–brain barrier.

BLOOD–BRAIN BARRIER

The blood–brain barrier depends on the unique characteristics of the brain capillaries. The endothelial cells of brain capillaries are joined by continuous tight junctions. In addition to the endothelial cell junctions, the brain capillaries are almost completely surrounded by processes of supporting cells of the brain, called astrocytes. The blood–brain barrier permits passage of essential substances while excluding unwanted materials. Reverse transport systems remove materials from the brain. Large molecules such as proteins and peptides are largely excluded from crossing the blood–brain barrier. Acute cerebral lesions, such as trauma and infection, increase the permeability of the blood–brain barrier and alter brain concentrations of proteins, water, and electrolytes.

The blood–brain barrier prevents many drugs from entering the brain. Most highly water-soluble compounds are excluded from the brain, whereas those that are lipid soluble cross the lipid layers of the blood–brain barrier with ease. Some drugs, such as the antibiotic chloramphenicol, are highly lipid soluble and, therefore, enter the brain readily. Other medications have a low solubility in lipids and enter the brain slowly, if at all. Alcohol, nicotine, and heroin are very lipid soluble and rapidly enter the brain. Some substances that enter the capillary endothelium are converted by metabolic processes to a chemical form incapable of moving into the brain.

The cerebral capillaries are much more permeable at birth than in adulthood, and the blood–brain barrier develops during the early years of life. In severely jaundiced infants, bilirubin can cross the immature blood–brain barrier, producing kernicterus and brain damage (see Chapter 18). In adults the mature blood–brain barrier prevents bilirubin from entering the brain, and the nervous system is not affected.

CSF–BRAIN BARRIER

The ependymal lining cells of the choroid plexus are linked together by tight junctions, forming a blood–CSF barrier to diffusion of many molecules from the blood plasma of choroid plexus capillaries to the CSF. Water is transported through the choroid epithelial cells by osmosis. Oxygen and carbon dioxide move into the CSF by diffusion, resulting in partial pressures roughly equal to those of plasma. Both the high sodium and low potassium contents of the CSF are actively regulated and kept relatively constant. Lipids and nonpeptide hormones diffuse through the barrier rather easily, but most large molecules, such as proteins, peptides, many antibiotics, and other medications, do not normally get through. The choroid epithelium uses energy (ATP) to actively secrete many components into the CSF, including proteins; sodium ions; a number of micronutrients such as vitamins C, B_6 (pyridoxine), and folates; and ribonucleosides and deoxyribonucleosides. Because the resultant CSF has a relatively high sodium content, the negatively charged chloride and bicarbonate diffuse into the CSF along an ionic gradient. The choroid also generates bicarbonate from carbon dioxide that is present in the blood. The generation of bicarbonate is important to the regulation of the pH of the CSF. Mechanisms exist that facilitate the transport of other molecules such as glucose without energy expenditure. Ammonia, a toxic metabolite of neuronal activity, is converted to glutamine by astrocytes. Glutamine moves by facilitated diffusion through the choroid epithelium into the plasma. This exemplifies a major function of the CSF, that of providing a means of removal of toxic waste products from the CNS. Since the brain and spinal cord have no lymphatic channels, the CSF serves this function.

There are several specific areas of the brain where the blood–CSF barrier does not exist. One area is at the caudal end of the fourth ventricle (area postrema) where specialized receptors for the carbon dioxide level of the CSF influence respiratory function. Another area consists of the walls of the third ventricle, which permit hypothalamic neurons to monitor blood glucose levels reflected in CSF glucose levels. This mechanism permits hypothalamic centers to respond to these blood glucose levels, contributing to hunger and eating behaviors.

In summary, in the process of development, the most rostral part of the embryonic neural tube develops to form the brain. The brain can be divided into three parts: the hindbrain, midbrain, and forebrain. The hindbrain, consisting of the medulla oblongata and pons, contains the neuronal circuits required for eating, breathing, and locomotive functions required for survival. Cranial nerves XII, XI, X, IX, VIII, VII, VI, and V are located in the hindbrain. The midbrain contains cranial nerves III and IV. The forebrain is the most rostral part of the brain; it consists of the diencephalon and the telencephalon. The dorsal horn part of the diencephalon is the thalamus and subthalamus, and the ventral horn part is the hypothalamus. The cerebral hemispheres are the lateral outgrowths of the diencephalon. Although there may be considerable overlap, one of the hemispheres is the more dominant hemisphere; it has a major role in verbal and analytic abilities. The less dominant hemisphere has a major role in nonverbal and spatial abilities.

The cerebral hemispheres are arbitrarily divided into lobes—the frontal, parietal, temporal, and occipital lobes—named after the bones of the skull that cover them. The premotor area and primary motor cortex are located in the frontal lobe; the primary sensory cortex and somesthetic association area in the parietal cortex; the primary auditory cortex and the auditory association area, in the temporal lobe; and the primary and association visual cortex, in the occipital cortex. The limbic system, which is involved in emotional experience, is located in the medial aspect of the cerebrum. These cortical areas are reciprocally interconnected with underlying thalamic nuclei via the internal capsule. Thalamic involvement is essential for normal forebrain function. The brain is enclosed and protected by the pia mater, arachnoid, and dura mater. The protective CSF in which the brain and spinal cord float isolates them from minor and moderate trauma. The CSF is secreted into the ventricles, circulates through the ventricular system, passes outside to surround the brain, and is reabsorbed into the venous system through the arachnoid villi. The CSF–brain barrier and the blood–brain barrier protect the brain from substances in the blood that would disrupt brain function.

■ ALTERATIONS IN CEREBRAL BLOOD FLOW

CEREBRAL CIRCULATION

The blood flow to the brain is supplied by the two internal carotid arteries (anteriorly) and the vertebral arteries (posteriorly) (Fig. 51-12).

The internal carotid artery, a terminal branch of the common carotid artery, branches into several arteries: the ophthalmic, posterior communicating, anterior cerebral, and middle cerebral arteries (Fig. 51-13). Most of the arterial blood within the internal carotid arteries is distributed by way of the anterior and middle cerebral arteries.

The anterior cerebral arteries supply the medial surface of the cerebrum and the anterior half of the thalamus, the corpus striatum, part of the corpus callosum, and the internal capsule.

The middle cerebral artery passes laterally, supplying the insula, and then emerges on the lateral cortical surface, supplying the inferior frontal gyrus, the motor and premotor frontal cortex concerned with delicate face and hand control. It is the major vascular source for the primary and association somesthetic cortex for the face and hand and the superior temporal gyrus with the primary and association auditory cortex. It also is a major source of blood supply for the genu and the posterior limb of the internal capsule and much of the basal ganglia. The middle cerebral artery is, functionally, a continuation of the internal carotid; emboli of the internal carotid most frequently become lodged in branches of the middle cerebral artery. Consequences of ischemia of these areas may be most devastating, resulting in damage to the fine manipulative skills of the face or upper limb and to both receptive and expressive communication functions. Occlusion of the local branches of the artery result in more restricted deficits.

The two vertebral arteries arise from the subclavian arteries and enter the foramina in the transverse spinal processes at the level of the sixth cervical spine and continue upward through the foramina of the upper six vertebrae; they wind behind the atlas and enter the skull through the foramen magnum and unite to form the basilar artery. Branches of the basilar and vertebral arteries supply the medulla, pons, cerebellum, midbrain, and caudal part of the diencephalon. The basilar artery terminates in the two posterior cerebral arteries which supply the remaining occipital and inferior regions of the temporal cortex.

The posterior communicating arteries connect the vertebrobasilar and internal carotid systems completing the circle of Willis at the base of the brain. This anastomosis of arteries may provide continued circulation should blood flow through one of the main vessels be disrupted. Without collateral circulation, cessation of blood flow in the cerebral arteries may result in neural damage because the metabolic needs of the electrically active cells of the brain can no longer be met. The vertebrobasilar arteries supply the basic life support reflexes; the internal carotid arteries support higher order functions. Interruption of blood flow in the carotid arteries may result in coma and death.

The cerebral blood is drained by two sets of veins

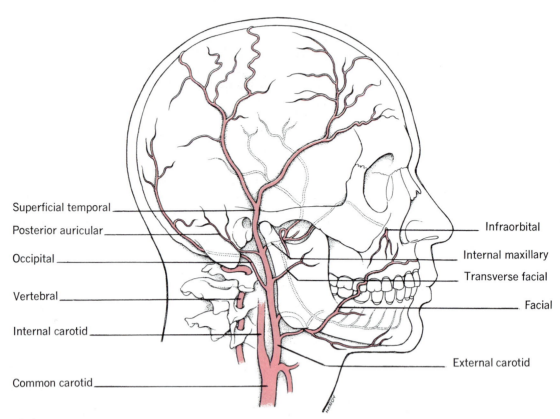

Superficial temporal

Posterior auricular

Occipital

Vertebral

Internal carotid

Common carotid

Infraorbital

Internal maxillary

Transverse facial

Facial

External carotid

FIG. 51-12. Branches of the right external carotid artery. The internal carotid artery ascends to the base of the brain. The right vertebral artery is also shown as it ascends through the transverse foramina of the cervical vertebrae. (Chaffee, E. E., & Lytle, I. M. [1980]. *Basic physiology and anatomy* [4th ed., p. 338]. Philadelphia: J.B. Lippincott)

that empty into the dural venous sinuses: the deep (great) cerebral venous system and the superficial venous system. The deep system is well protected, in contrast to the superficial cerebral veins, which travel through the pia mater on the surface of the cerebral cortex. These superficial vessels connect directly to the sagittal sinuses within the falx cerebri by way of bridging veins. They travel through the CSF-filled subarachnoid space, penetrate the arachnoid and then the dura to reach the dural venous sinuses. This system of sinuses returns blood to the heart primarily by way of the internal jugular veins. Alternate routes

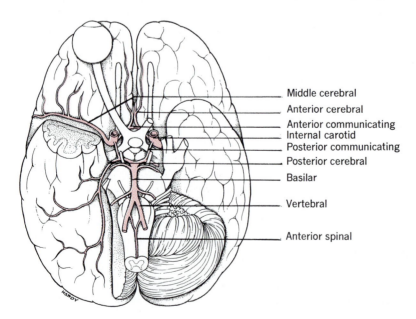

Middle cerebral

Anterior cerebral

Anterior communicating

Internal carotid

Posterior communicating

Posterior cerebral

Basilar

Vertebral

Anterior spinal

FIG. 51-13. The circle of Willis as seen at the base of a brain removed from the skull. (Chaffee, E. E., & Lytle, I. M. [1980]. *Basic physiology and anatomy* [4th ed., p. 852]. Philadelphia: J.B. Lippincott)

for venous flow also exist; for example, venous blood may exit through the emissary veins that pass through the skull and through veins that traverse various foramina to empty into extracranial veins.

The intracranial venous system has no valves. Thus, the direction of flow depends on gravity or the pressure in the venous sinuses relative to that in the extracranial veins. Increases in intrathoracic pressure, such as occur with coughing or performance of Valsalva's maneuver, produce a rise in central venous pressure that is reflected back into the internal jugular veins and to the dural sinuses. This produces a brief rise in intracranial pressure.

REGULATION OF CEREBRAL BLOOD FLOW

The blood flow to the brain is maintained at about 750 mL/min, or one-sixth of the resting cardiac output. The regulation of blood flow to the brain is largely controlled by autoregulatory or local mechanisms that respond to the metabolic needs of the brain. Cerebral autoregulation has been classically defined as the ability of the brain to maintain constant cerebral blood flow despite changes in systemic arterial pressure. The autoregulation (self-regulation) of cerebral blood flow is very efficient within a mean arterial blood pressure range of about 60 mmHg to 140 mmHg. If blood pressure falls below 60 mmHg, cerebral blood flow becomes severely compromised; if it rises above the upper limit of autoregulation, blood flow rises rapidly and causes overstretching of the cerebral vessels. In persons with hypertension, this autoregulatory range shifts to a higher level. More recently, cerebral autoregulation has been further defined to describe the ability of local areas of the cerebral cortex to adjust their blood flow dependent upon metabolic needs. Athough total cerebral blood flow remains relatively stable throughout marked changes in cardiac output and arterial blood pressure, regional blood flow may change markedly owing to local changes in metabolism.

At least three different metabolic factors have been shown to affect cerebral blood flow: (1) carbon dioxide concentration, (2) hydrogen ion concentration, and (3) oxygen concentration. Increased carbon dioxide and hydrogen ion concentration produce an increase in cerebral blood flow, whereas decreased oxygen concentration increases blood flow. Carbon dioxide, by way of the hydrogen ion, provides a potent stimulus for control of cerebral blood flow—a doubling of the carbon dioxide pressure (PCO_2) in the blood results in a doubling of cerebral blood flow. Other substances that alter the pH of the brain produce similar changes in cerebral blood flow. Because increased hydrogen ion concentration greatly de-

presses neural activity, it is fortunate that blood flow increases to wash the hydrogen ions and other acidic materials away from the brain tissue.[3] Profound extracellular acidosis also induces vasomotor paralysis, in which case cerebral blood flow may depend entirely on systemic arterial blood pressure.

The deep cerebral blood vessels appear to be completely controlled by autoregulation, whereas the superficial and major cerebral blood vessels are innervated by the sympathetic nervous system. Under normal physiologic conditions, however, the sympathetic nervous system exerts little effect on superficial cerebral blood flow. This is because local regulatory mechanisms are so powerful that they compensate almost entirely for the effects of sympathetic stimulation. However, when there is a failure of local mechanisms, sympathetic control of cerebral blood pressure becomes very important. For example, when the arterial pressure rises to very high levels, the sympathetic nervous system constricts the large and intermediate-sized superficial blood vessels as a possible means of protecting the smaller, more easily damaged vessels. Also, sympathetic reflexes are believed to provide one possible cause of vasospasm in the intermediate and large arteries in some types of brain damage, such as that caused by rupture of a cerebral aneurysm.

HYPOXIC AND ISCHEMIC INJURY

The energy requirements of the brain are provided mainly by adenosine triphosphate (ATP); the ability of the cerebral circulation to deliver oxygen in sufficiently high concentrations to facilitate metabolism of glucose and generate ATP is essential to brain function. Although the brain makes up only 2% of the body weight, it receives one-sixth of the resting cardiac output and accounts for 20% of the oxygen consumption.[4] It follows that deprivation of oxygen or blood flow can have a deleterious effect on brain structures. By definition, *hypoxic hypoxia* denotes a deprivation of oxygen with maintained blood flow; *ischemic hypoxia* denotes a situation of hypoxia due to greatly reduced or interrupted blood flow. Hypoxia is usually seen in conditions such as exposure to reduced atmospheric pressure, carbon monoxide poisoning, severe anemia, and failure to oxygenate the blood. Because hypoxia indicates decreased oxygen levels at the tissue level, it produces a generalized depressant effect on the brain.

The cellular pathophysiologies of hypoxia and ischemia are quite different, and the brain tends to have a very different sensitivity to the two conditions. Contrary to popular belief, hypoxia is fairly well tolerated, particularly in situations of chronic hypoxia. Neurons are capable of substantial anaerobic metabolism and are fairly tolerant of pure hypoxia; it commonly produces euphoria, listlessness, drowsiness, and impaired problem solving. Unconsciousness and convulsions may occur when hypoxia is sudden and severe. However, the effects of severe hypoxia (anoxia) on brain function are seldom seen because the condition rapidly leads to cardiac arrest and ischemia.[4]

Ischemia can be *focal*, as in stroke, or *global*, as in cardiac arrest. Persons with global ischemia have no collateral circulation during the ischemic event. In contrast, collateral circulation may provide low levels of blood flow during focal ischemia. The residual perfusion may provide sufficient substrates to maintain a low level of metabolic activity, thereby preserving membrane integrity. At the same time, the delivery of glucose under anaerobic conditions may result in additional lactic acid production and worsening of lactic acidosis.[5]

POSTISCHEMIC HYPOPERFUSION

Although the threshold for ischemic neuronal injury is unknown, there is a period of time during which neurons can survive if blood flow is reestablished. Unfortunately, brain injury may not be reversible if the duration of ischemia is such that the threshold of injury has been reached. Even after circulation has been reestablished, damage to blood vessels and changes in blood flow can prevent return of adequate tissue perfusion. This period of postischemic hypoperfusion is thought to be associated with mechanisms such as desaturation of venous blood, capillary and venular clotting, and sludging of blood, called particulate flow.[5] Because of sludging, blood viscosity increases and there is increased resistance to blood flow. There is also experimental evidence of immediate vasomotor paralysis of surface conducting blood vessels due to extracellular acidosis, followed by ischemic vasoconstriction due to secondary vasospasm. The term secondary vasospasm is used to distinguish ischemic vasoconstriction from that induced by subarachnoid hemorrhage.[5] The vasoconstriction may be due to calcium influx, increased extracellular potassium, or release of endogenous vasoconstrictors such as norepinephrine.

Hypermetabolism due to increased circulating catecholamines has been implicated as a contributing factor in postischemic hypoperfusion. Catecholamine release results in an increased cerebral metabolic rate and increased need for all energy-producing substrates, which the damaged brain is unable to maintain. Treatment is aimed at providing oxygen to the troubled brain and decreasing the metabolic rate through the use of barbiturates.[6] However, the beneficial effects of barbiturates are minimal un-

less administered before the anticipated ischemia (*e.g.*, before neurosurgery).[5]

Another area of recent interest in postischemic injury is free oxygen radicals that are liberated from partially damaged tissue or from blood once blood flow has been restored. Free radicals are highly reactive chemical species that combine with and injure cerebrovascular endothelium; they also impair the vessel's ability to respond to carbon dioxide by increasing blood flow.

Under abnormal conditions such as ischemia and acidosis, brain trauma results from *cytotoxic edema*, causing neuronal cell damage or possible death. If blood flow in the brain falls to abnormally low levels, cellular hypoxia results in reduced energy (ATP) production and depletion of energy stores. Low energy production, in turn, reduces the function of the membrane ion pumps. Altered membrane permeability results, leading to increased extracellular concentrations of potassium and plasma membrane hypopolarization. Further, low blood flow results in inadequate removal of anaerobic metabolic end-products such as lactic acid, producing extracellular acidosis. The altered osmotic conditions result in water entry and cell swelling. Depending on the nature of the insult, such cellular edema can occur in the vascular endothelium or smooth muscle cells, astrocytes, the myelin-forming processes of oligodentrocytes, or neurons. If blood flow is reduced to low levels for extended periods or to extremely low levels for a few minutes, cellular edema can cause the cell membrane to rupture, resulting in escape of intracellular contents into the surrounding extracellular fluid. This leads to damage of neighboring cells.

Cytotoxic edema is a slowly progressing process. When neurons are involved in this cytopathic process, presynaptic as well as postsynaptic elements become hypopolarized. Presynaptic hypolarization opens voltage-gated calcium channels, producing increased levels of free intracellular calcium and release of neurotransmitters. In addition to increased transmitter release, the gradually falling membrane potential brings both pre- and post-synaptic neurons into the threshold range, resulting in electrical hyperactivity; this continues until there is insufficient energy for recovery to the threshold potential, at which time the cells fall into electrical silence. This progression suggests possible mechanisms of seizure generation, loss of neuronal funtion, and eventual cell death.

Ischemic Neurotoxicity. The cells most vulnerable to ischemia are neurons, which suffer first reversible and then irreversible damage. Some types of neurons, notably those in the hypothalamus and cerebral cortex, including the hippocampus, are particularly vulnerable to ischemia and are often the first to be damaged. Some of these neurons have been clearly implicated in memory functions. The reason for this selective vulnerability is still somewhat unclear, but attention has focused on the role of excitatory neurotransmitters called excitotoxins.

CNS neurons can be divided into two major categories: (1) macroneurons, which number in the thousands and (2) microneurons, which make up the overwhelming majority of the many billions of CNS neurons. Macroneurons are large cells with long axons that leave the local network of intercommunicating neurons to send action potentials to other regions of the nervous system at distances of centimeters to meters (*e.g.*, UMNs that communicate with LMNs that control leg movement). In contrast, microneurons are very small cells that are intimately involved in local circuitry. Their axons transmit action potentials to other members of the same local network.

Macroneurons synapse on the postsynaptic excitatory receptors of the microneurons. Many macroneurons use amino acids, primarily glutamate and aspartate, as excitatory transmitters in their communication with microneurons. The excitatory transmitters exert many of their effects through receptor-mediated membrane channels. Glutamate channels are large, complex proteins that bridge the plasma membrane and contain a central pore or channel that, when open, permits ions to diffuse across the cell membrane. One subtype of glutamate receptor opens a large-diameter calcium channel, which permits calcium and sodium to enter the cell and allows potassium to exit, resulting in prolonged (seconds) action potentials. The particular subtype, called the glutamate N-methyl-D-asparate (NMDA) receptor, has several other important roles in CNS function. The open calcium channel results in increased free intracellular calcium, and this initiates a multistep process of protein (including enzyme) synthesis. Among the proteins that may be synthesized are additional membrane NMDA receptors. This suggests a possible mechanism for long-term change in synaptic function, such as may be involved in long-term memory.

The microneurons of the hypothalamus and the cerebral cortex, including the hippocampus, are particularly vulnerable to low energy supply conditions. These neurons bear large numbers of NMDA receptors and are particularly vulnerable to a special and possible pathologic process called the *calcium cytotoxic cascade*. Calcium has a critical role in normal cellular functions as a second messenger, a metabolic regulator, and an effector in neurotransmitter release. Activation of this NMDA receptor–mediated cascade not only causes cellular edema but also a major increase in intracellular free calcium. Increased intracellular calcium facilitates the release and activa-

tion of degradative enzymes, including proteases, lipases, and endonucleases. The proteases attack cellular structures including membranes, endonucleases damage protein synthesis, and lipases damage membranes and create free radicals. This cascade leads to cell death at blood flow rates that are somewhat higher than those inducing cytotoxic edema in other neurons. As a result of this mechanism, many of the small interneurons that make up essential parts of complex control and memory functions of the brain are selectively damaged, even if the rest of the CNS survives the insult. This may account for the long-term effects of brain insult, which frequently include subtle and not-so-subtle reductions in cognitive and memory functions.

Research currently is being directed toward a means of attenuating or preventing the calcium cascade. Considerable success has been achieved by (1) blocking the synthesis or release of excitatory amino acid transmitters; (2) blocking the NMDA receptors; (3) stabilizing the membrane potential to prevent initiation of the calcium cascade, using lidocaine and certain barbiturates; (4) specifically blocking certain intracellular proteases, endonucleases, and lipases that are known to be cytotoxic; and (5) increasing scavenging of oxygen free radicals.[7-9]

Global Ischemia. Global ischemia occurs when blood flow is inadequate to meet the metabolic needs of the entire brain. The result is a spectrum of neurologic disorders. Unconsciousness occurs within seconds of severe global ischemia—that resulting from complete cessation of blood flow, as in cardiac arrest, or with marked decrease in blood flow, as in serious cardiac dysrhythmias. If circulation is restored immediately, consciousness will be quickly regained. However, if blood flow is not promptly restored, severe pathologic changes take place. Energy sources, glucose and glycogen, are exhausted in 2 to 3 minutes and cellular adenosine triphosphate (ATP) in 4 to 5 minutes. When ischemia is sufficiently severe or prolonged, infarction or death of all cellular elements of the brain occurs.

An exception to the time frame above is the circumstance of cold-water drowning in which a person, especially a child, is submerged in cold water for longer than 10 minutes.[10] Hypothermia develops and causes a reduction in the cerebral metabolic requirements for oxygen; it subsequently serves as a protective mechanism for the neurons. In such a case, recovery can be rapid and remarkable. Resuscitation efforts should not be discontinued prematurely.

The neurologic deficits that result from global ischemia vary widely. If the period of no flow/low flow is minimal, there is usually minimal neurologic damage. When the period is prolonged, the early neurologic picture may be that of fixed and dilated pupils, abnormal motor posturing, and coma.[11] Gradual improvement in neurologic status may occur, although cognitive defects usually persist and can prevent a return to preischemic functioning level.

With less profound global ischemia (*e.g.*, hypotension) the damage is concentrated in the anatomically vulnerable border zones (called *watershed zones*) between territories provided by major arteries of the cerebral cortex, cerebellum, basal ganglia, and spinal cord. It is most severe in the border areas supplied by the middle, anterior, and posterior cerebral arteries. This is because the watershed zones (*i.e.*, territories of the brain where the distal branches of these vessels abut against one another) form extremely vulnerable areas in terms of ischemia. These territories receive less blood with profound lowering of blood flow, such as in severe hypotension, predisposing to infarction (death) of brain tissues.

There are three types of watershed infarctions that appear between vascular territories: (1) superficial infarction, (2) deep infarction, and (3) infarction located at the angular gyrus. Superficial watershed infarctions are located between the anterior and middle cerebral artery territories and between the middle and posterior cerebral artery territories. Deep infarction develops between cortical and deep penetrating branch territories, usually between the insula and putamen. Angular gyrus infarctions develop in the adjacent territories of the anterior, middle, and posterior cerebral arteries. After severe hypotension, areas of the cortex that are supplied by the major cerebral arteries may regain function upon recovery of adequate blood flow; however, infarctions may occur in the watershed boundary strips, resulting in severe neurologic deficits.[12]

In extreme ischemia, there is a central core of dead or dying cells, surrounded by an ischemic area of minimally surviving cells called the penumbra (halo). The cells of the penumbra receive marginal blood flow; thus, their metabolic activities are altered. Whether the cells of a pneumbra continue to survive depends on the successful return of adequate circulation, the volume of toxic products released by the neighboring dying cells, cerebral edema, and alterations in local blood flow. If the toxic products of dead tissue result in cell death in the penumbra, the core of tissue enlarges and the volume of surrounding tissue at risk increases.

CEREBROVASCULAR OCCLUSIVE DISEASE

Cerebrovascular occlusive disease is a heterogeneous disorder involving a variety of vascular pathologies that can cause focal ischemia and infarction of brain cells. The process (1) may involve obstruction within a cerebral vessel as occurs in atherosclerosis; (2) may originate remotely, as when an embolus from the heart lodges in an intracerebral vessel; or (3) may result from a ruptured vessel in the intracerebral tissue. The terms *cerebrovascular accident* (CVA) and *stroke* are often used to designate the acute neurologic deficits that these processes produce. In the United States stroke remains the third leading cause of death, despite a general decline in incidence over the past 35 years. This decline cannot be traced to a single factor, but it is probably due to early identification and treatment of risk factors such as hypertension.

Various methods have been used to classify cerebrovascular occlusive disease. One classification system, largely defined by results from brain-imaging and vascular studies, identifies six major subtypes: (1) atherosclerotic large-artery disease, (2) nonatherosclotic large-artery disease, (3) penetrating artery disease, (4) cardioembolism, (5) stroke of undetermined origin, and (6) miscellaneous causes (*e.g.*, sickle cell or migraine-related). The fifth group was included because the use of sophisticated technology (computed tomography [CT] scans, magnetic resonance imaging [MRI], echocardiogram, carotid and transcranial Doppler ultrasound, and cerebral angiography) demonstrated normal vascular studies in a large percentage of persons with ischemic stroke. The reported incidence of large-artery stroke is 16%; cardioembolism, 19%; penetrating artery disease, 27%; and stroke of undetermined origin, 40%.[13]

Among the reported risk factors for stroke are age, race, lipid abnormalities, hypertension, diabetes mellitus, elevated fibrinogen levels, sickle cell disease, polycythemia, moderate to increased levels of alcohol use, use of tobacco, amphetamines, cocaine, and other chemicals, diet, obesity, sedentary lifestyle, previous ischemic episodes, and heart disease.[14] Alcohol can contribute to stroke by several mechanisms: (1) induction of cardiac arrhythmias and defects in ventricular wall motion that lead to cerebral embolism, (2) induction of hypertension, (3) enhancement of blood coagulation disorders, and (4) reduction of cerebral blood flow.[15]

Another factor that is credited with increased risk of cerebrovascular occlusive disease is use of oral contraceptives. With the exception of selected subgroups that demonstrate additional risk factors, the increased risk may be slight. However, the overall prevalence is significant owing to frequency of use. Analysis of data regarding use of estrogen in postmenopausal women remains controversial.

A recent cause of stroke has been cocaine. Cardiovascular events begin soon after cocaine use and include increased blood pressure, heart rate, body temperature, and metabolic rate. Cocaine also causes vasospasm and enhances the platelet response. The reported ages of persons with cocaine stroke have ranged from newborn (maternal cocaine use) to 48 years of age. Both ischemic and hemorrhagic strokes have been reported. The mechanisms of cocaine-related stroke vary. In some persons, stroke was associated with hemorrhage from aneurysms or arteriovenous malformations; in other cases, it was associated with thrombotic lesions.[16–18]

Elimination or control of certain risk factors for stroke (*e.g.*, use of tobacco, control of blood lipids, and hypertension) offers the best opportunity to prevent cerebral ischemia due to cerebral atherosclerosis. Early detection and treatment affords significant advantages over waiting until a serious event has occurred.

TRANSIENT ISCHEMIC ATTACKS

Transient ischemic attacks (TIAs) are focal ischemic cerebral neurologic deficits that last for less than 24 hours (usually less than 1–2 hours). The causes of TIAs are multiple and include atherosclerotic disease of cerebral vessels and emboli. TIAs are important because they may provide warning of impending stroke. Diagnosis may permit surgical or medical intervention and, thus, prevent extensive damage. Overall, the risk of stroke varies. There is about a 20% risk of stroke within 1 month of a first classic carotid TIA; that risk falls to and remains at about 5% annually after the first 6 months. This risk is reduced to about 2.5% with the best medical care available.[19]

The signs and symptoms of TIA depend on the cerebral vessel that is involved. There is often numbness and mild weakness of contralateral body structures. The forearm, hand, and angle of the mouth are commonly affected areas with middle cerebral involvement. Brief global aphasia may occur in transient ischemia of the left hemisphere. There may be transient visual disturbances such as graying-out, blurring, or fogging of vision if the posterior cerebral artery is affected.

Treatment of TIA depends on the type and location of the ischemia-producing lesion. After numerous studies, it is now generally accepted that a small daily dose of aspirin results in reduction in the frequency of stroke after TIA.[20] It has been shown that other platelet antiaggregates (sulfinpyrazone or dipyridamole) are no more effective than aspirin. Anticoagulants, such as warfarin, may be appropriate in certain situations but do increase the risk of hemorrhage. In some cases, ischemia may be due to focal loss of cerebral autoregulation, and blood flow to the area of the brain involved can be particularly sensitive to any rise or fall in blood pressure. Dehydration and relative hypotension should be avoided.

In persons with hypertension, the judicious use of medication to lower blood pressure may be indicated. However, care must be taken to avoid rapid decreases in blood pressure or hypotensive episodes.[21] Surgical treatment using endarterectomy (arterial surgery to remove atherosclerotic plaque) may be done for persons with ulcerative carotid lesions. A procedure called an *extracranial–intracranial bypass operation* involves redirecting blood flow from an artery in the scalp, through the cranium, and into the arteries that supply the brain. Usually the superficial temporal artery is anastomosed with the middle cerebral artery. This procedure remains controversial and may be used in a small number of persons who fail to gain relief from other therapeutic measures.[22, 23]

Subclavian Steal. Subclavian steal is a phenomenon in which there is transient cerebral ischemia as blood flows in a reverse direction from the vertebral artery into the vessels of the arm, stealing blood from the basilar artery and the circle of Willis. This usually occurs when the arm is exercised and the subclavian artery becomes occluded near its origin. The result is transient cerebral ischemia due to vertebrobasilar insufficiency as blood is siphoned or "stolen" from the vertebrobasilar circulation and circle of Willis.[24]

Symptoms of the disorder include dizziness, lightheadedness, and syncope; the radial pulse is absent or diminished; and there is usually a 20-mmHg or more difference in blood pressure between the affected and unaffected arms. Although relatively rare—accounting for only 4% of all cerebrovascular diseases and 17% of extracranial carotid disorders—subclavian steal should be considered when there are complaints of dizziness and lightheadedness, especially if accompanied by blood pressure differences between the two upper extremities. With the vascular surgery that is now available to redirect blood flow, the prognosis for recovery is excellent.

STROKES

Strokes are characterized by local areas of cerebral infarction. Almost all cerebral infarctions are caused by local vessel occlusion, although they can occur without obstruction, as in the border zone infarctions, or when there is reduction of perfusion pressure combined with severe atherosclerotic disease. Most occlusive strokes are caused by thrombi or emboli. Other types of stroke include lacunar infarcts and intracerebral hemorrhage.

In contrast to a transient ischemic attack, stroke is characterized by a neurologic deficit that persists for at least 24 hours. A neurologic deficit that continues to progress or worsen over a period of 1 or 2 days is called a *stroke-in-evolution*. A *completed stroke* describes the condition in which there has been maximum neurologic deficit, the person's condition has stabilized or is improving, and there is residual neurologic damage. Recovery may take place over days, weeks, or months and may be only partial.

Thrombotic and Embolic Strokes. Thrombi are the most common cause of stroke. Thrombi usually occur in atherosclerotic blood vessels. In the cerebral circulation, altherosclerotic plaques are found most commonly at arterial bifurcations. Common sites of plaque formation include larger vessels of the brain, notably the origin of the internal carotid or vertebral arteries, and junctions of the basilar and vertebral arteries. In most cases only one region supplied by a single cerebral artery is affected. Atherosclerotic thrombosis may occur gradually over several days, during which the CNS symptomatology may plateau and then deteriorate further. Usually, thrombotic strokes are seen in older people and are frequently accompanied by evidence of arteriosclerotic heart disease. Thrombotic strokes are not associated with activity and may occur in a person at rest. Consciousness may or may not be lost, and improvement may be rapid.

An embolic stroke is caused by a moving blood clot. It usually affects the smaller cerebral vessels, often at bifurcations. The most frequent site of embolic strokes is the middle cerebral artery distribution, probably because it offers the path of least resistance. Although most cerebral emboli originate in a thrombus in the left heart, they may also originate in an atherosclerotic plaque in the carotid arteries. The embolus travels quickly to the brain and becomes lodged in a small artery through which it cannot pass. Therefore, embolic stroke usually has a sudden onset with immediate maximum deficit.

Various cardiac conditions predispose to formation of emboli that produce embolic stroke, including rheumatic heart disease, atrial fibrillation, recent myocardial infarction, ventricular aneurysm, and bacterial endocarditis. Recent advances in the diagnosis and treatment of heart disease can be expected to alter favorably the incidence of embolic stroke.

Lacunar Infarcts. Lacunar infarcts are small (1.5–2.0 cm) to very small (3–4 mm) lesions located in the deeper subcortical parts of the brain or in the brain stem. They are found in the territory of single deep penetrating arteries supplying the internal capsule, basal ganglia, or brain stem. They result from occlusion of the smaller branches of large cerebral arteries—commonly the middle cerebral and posterior cerebral, and less commonly the anterior cerebral, vertebral, or basilar arteries. In the process of healing, lacunar infarcts leave behind small cavities,

or lacunae. Six basic causes of lacunar infarcts have been proposed: (1) embolism, (2) hypertension, (3) small-vessel occlusive disease, (4) hematologic abnormalities, (5) small intracerebral hemorrhages, and (6) vasospasm. Because of their size and location, lacunar infarcts do not usually cause profound deficits such as aphasia or apractic agnosia of the minor hemisphere. Instead, they often produce syndromes such as pure motor hemiplegia, pure sensory hemiplegia, and dysarthria.

Intracerebral Hemorrhage. The most frequently fatal stroke is rupture of an intracerebral blood vessel. With rupture of an intracerebral vessel, hemorrhage into the brain parenchyma occurs, resulting in edema, compression of the brain contents, or spasm of the adjacent blood vessels. The most common predisposing factor is hypertension. Other causes of hemorrhage are aneurysms, trauma, erosion of the vessels by tumors, arteriovenous malformations, and blood dyscrasias (aneurysmal subarachnoid hemorrhage and arteriovenous malformations are discussed at the end of this section). A cerebral hemorrhage occurs suddenly, usually when the person is active. Vomiting occurs very frequently at the onset, and headache is invariably present. Focal symptoms depend on which vessel is involved. Even a small hemorrhage into the internal capsule results in contralateral hemiplegia, with initial flaccidity progressing to spasticity. A large hemorrhage and resultant edema exert great pressure on the brain substance, and the clinical course progresses rapidly to coma and frequently to death.

CLINICAL MANIFESTATIONS OF STROKE

The specific manifestations of stroke are determined by the cerebral artery that is affected, the area of brain tissue that is supplied by that vessel, and the adequacy of the collateral circulation (Table 51-2). The manifestations may include loss of consciousness, cognitive and motor disorders, specific motor and/or sensory impairment, aphasia, and hemi-inattention syndrome. When the patient regains consciousness, deficits in higher-order function become evident. Certain classic syndromes are expected, but in the clinical situation they frequently overlap one another.

Motor Deficits. Initially following a stroke affecting the corticospinal tract (*e.g.*, the motor cortex, posterior limb of the internal capsule, or medullary pyramids), there is profound weakness on the contralateral side. It is characterized by a decrease or absence of normal muscle tone, immediate loss of fine manipulative skills, and a tendency of the af-

TABLE 51-2. SIGNS AND SYMPTOMS OF STROKE BY INVOLVED CEREBRAL ARTERY

CEREBRAL ARTERY	BRAIN AREA INVOLVED	SIGNS AND SYMPTOMS*
Anterior cerebral	Infarction of the medial aspect of one frontal lobe if lesion is distal to communicating artery; bilateral frontal infarction if flow in other anterior cerebral artery is inadequate	Paralysis of contralateral foot or leg; impaired gait; paresis contralateral arm; contralateral sensory loss over toes, foot, and leg; problems making decisions or performing acts voluntarily; lack of spontaneity, easily distracted; slowness of thought; aphasia dependent on the hemisphere involved; urinary incontinence; cognitive and affective disorders
Middle cerebral	Massive infarction of most of lateral hemisphere and deeper structures of frontal, parietal, and temporal lobes; internal capsule; basal ganglia	Contralateral hemiplegia (face and arm); contralateral sensory impairment; aphasia; homonymous heminanopsia; altered consciousness (confusion to coma); inability to turn eyes toward paralyzed side; denial of paralyzed side or limb (hemi-inattention); possible acalculia, alexia, finger agnosia and left–right confusion; vasomotor paresis and instability
Posterior cerebral	Occipital lobe; anterior and medial portion of temporal lobe	Homonymous hemianopia and other visual defects such as color blindness, loss of central vision, and visual hallucinations; memory deficits, perseveration (repeated performance of same verbal or motor response)
	Thalamus involvement	Loss of all sensory modalities; spontaneous pain; intentional tremor; mild hemiparesis; aphasia
	Cerebral peduncle involvement	Oculomotor nerve palsy with contralateral hemiplegia
Basilar and vertebral	Cerebellum and brain stem	Visual disturbances such as diplopia, dystaxia, vertigo, dysphagia, dysphonia

* Dependent on hemisphere involved and adequacy of collaterals.

fected limbs to move as a whole. A small corticospinal lesion may be indicated by clumsiness in carrying out fine movements of the fingers (*e.g.*, buttoning or sewing) rather than obvious weakness. There is a tendency toward foot drop, outward rotation of the leg, and dependent edema in the affected extremities. Putting the extremities through passive range-of-motion exercises helps to maintain joint function and prevent edema, shoulder subluxation (incomplete dislocation), and muscle contractures. The smooth sequential movement of the exercises may also help to reestablish motor patterns.

When the corticospinal tract has been affected, tone gradually returns after a few weeks, and then spasticity usually begins to replace initial flaccidity within 6 to 8 weeks. Spasticity involves an increase in the tone of affected muscles and, generally, an element of weakness. Owing to the distribution of muscle hypertonia with spasticity, the flexor muscles are usually more strongly affected in the upper extremities and the extensor muscles more strongly affected in the lower extremities. Various mechanisms, including disinhibition of segmental and suprasegmental reflexes and reorganization of segmental circuitry, appear to contribute to spasticity. As a result, altered limb posture may be manifested by shoulder adduction, forearm pronation, finger flexion, and knee and hip extension.[25] If no voluntary movement or movement on command appears within a few months, function will probably not return to that extremity. Passive range-of-motion exercises should be continued, and positioning should be directed toward keeping all the joints in functional position. Motor deficits associated with stroke are discussed further in Chapter 50.

Aphasia. Aphasia is a general term that encompasses varying degrees of inability to comprehend, integrate, and express language. It is most accurately described as a disorder of language abilities rather than a speech disorder. The most common cause is a vascular lesion in the distribution of the middle cerebral artery of the dominant hemisphere—that is, the hemisphere responsible for mediation of language. (The left hemisphere is dominant in about 95% of right-handed and 70% of left-handed people.) The cerebral hemispheres usually function similarly in controlling opposite sides of the body. However, some functions, such as body language, are controlled by the dominant hemisphere but also require the simultaneous action of both hemispheres. Language dominance by one hemisphere does not occur before 1 to 2 years of age. Because the other hemisphere appears to take over, unilateral lesions between the ages of 4 and 12 years usually result in only transient language disorders.[26]

Communication is a complex process by which ideas and feelings are exchanged; it is accomplished by means of various behavioral patterns, gestures, expressions, and symbols. Communication involves memory, reasoning, and emotions, as well as speech and language.[27] Two key aspects of communication are language and speech. *Language* involves higher-order integrative functions of the forebrain. It is used to communicate thoughts and feelings through the use of symbolic formulations, such as words or numbers, and information is transmitted either vocally or graphically. *Speech*, on the other hand, involves the mechanical act of articulating language, the "motor act" of verbal expression.[27] Speech depends upon the functional integrity of the peripheral musculature involved and its control by UMNs and LMNs.

Disorders of language can be caused by perceptual and integrative abnormalities or disturbances of higher-level communication skills. Disorders of speech can be caused by motor deficits of the lips, tongue, palate, or pharynx (dysarthria, anarthria) or by problems secondary to disease of the larynx or its nerve supply (dysphonia, aphonia). A person with a speech problem such as dysarthria may demonstrate an inability to articulate while retaining language ability.

Disorders of language and speech generally fall into two categories: (1) disturbances of the central processing mechanisms of language, which result in aphasia (or, more accurately, dysphasia, since the disturbance is seldom complete), and (2) dysarthria (anarthria). Dysarthria may present as a disturbance of articulation mechanisms of speech production; dysphonia is a disorder of volume, quality, or pitch of the voice. Aphasia may be localized above the tentorium, whereas dysphonia may be localized at other levels as well.

Two categories are usually used when describing aphasia: (1) receptive (sensory, fluent, posterior) and (2) expressive (motor, nonfluent, and frontal). Lesions of the posterior temporal or lower parietal lobe (areas 22 or 39) are associated with receptive aphasia lesions. Expressive aphasia is associated with lesions of Broca's area of the dominant frontal lobe (areas 44 and 45) and with abnormal programming of the motor function of language (motor speech ataxia).

Receptive Aphasia. Receptive or sensory aphasia is the inability to comprehend spoken (Wernicke's aphasia) and, often, written words. Thus, two major forms may be distinguished: (1) auditory-receptive aphasia and (2) visual-receptive aphasia. In *auditory-receptive aphasia*, auditory acuity remains intact but the person is unable to understand the spoken word. In *visual-receptive aphasia*, understanding of written language is impaired (dyslexia, alexia). *Alexia* may occur with visual object agnosia—that is, difficulty in recognizing or naming objects (anomia) or colors (color anomia). Sometimes the ability to read numbers is retained, although the person is unable to read letters or words.[2]

One of the most common characteristics of aphasia is distorted spontaneous or conversational speech. This has been classified as (1) fluent (many words) and (2) nonfluent (few words). Receptive aphasia has been classified as *fluent* aphasia. The term fluent refers to the characteristics of the speech generated, not to its content or the ability of the person to comprehend what is being said. Fluent speech requires little or no effort, is articulate, and is of increased quantity. There are three categories of fluent aphasia: Wernicke's, anomic, and conductive aphasia. *Wernicke's aphasia* is characterized by an inability to comprehend speech, not only that of others but also of oneself. Sometimes Wernicke's aphasia is also used to include reading and writing. *Anomic aphasia* is speech that is nearly normal except for difficulty the person has in selecting words. *Conductive aphasia* (disconnection syndrome) is inappropriate word use in the presence of good comprehension; it is due to destruction of the fiber system under the insula that connects Wernicke's and Broca's areas.

Expressive Aphasia. Expressive or *motor aphasia* is the inability to translate thoughts or ideas into meaningful speech or writing. The person with expressive aphasia may be able, with difficulty, to utter two or three words, especially those with an emotional overlay. Automatic speech appears to be intact, and social phrases are easier to articulate. Although comprehension may be intact, some words are omitted or inappropriate words are substituted (*e.g.*, "weathery winter"). Use of neologisms (invented words) or paraphrasic errors result in telegraphic speech. The sentences produced are meaningless, although the person believes them to be correct and appropriate.

Expressive aphasia has been classified as *non-fluent aphasia*. Speech production is limited and often poorly articulated. If Broca's area or the precentral gyrus of the dominant frontal lobe is affected, automatic speech appears to be intact, but neologisms, paraphasic errors, and cursing are common. The person seems to be aware of communication problems but is unable to correct them. This often leads to frustration, anger, and depression.

Receptive and Expressive Aphasia. The person with receptive aphasia demonstrates a *sensory agnosia*, whereas a person with expressive aphasia demonstrates a *motor speech apraxia*. Some persons manifest elements of both expressive and receptive aphasia; these disorders are called *mixed aphasias*. When all language ability is lost (both expressive and receptive), the aphasia is said to be total or global. Most aphasias are partial, and a thorough speech evaluation is needed to determine the type and extent of language disorder as well as appropriate therapy.

Unilateral Neglect or Hemi-inattention. Because of an inability to analyze and interpret incoming sensory information due to the disruptive lesion of the brain and the internal production of abnormal signals, a high percentage of persons with stroke have a form of denial of illness and a denial of one half of their own body and environment on that side of the body (hemi-inattention).[2, 27] Importantly, such persons are unaware of the deficit. For example, a person with left hemiplegia may raise the right arm when asked, but when asked to raise the left arm, respond by saying, "I just did." Spatial orientation is often impaired, and there is difficulty in localizing stimuli, their own limbs, and objects in space. Affected persons may totally disregard stimuli coming from the involved side of the body, even though they can see and hear them. The affected side of the body may go unattended and ungroomed (hemi- or unilateral neglect). Frequently a person will wash or shave the unaffected but not the affected side of the body. When asked to draw a picture of themselves, these persons often draw a person with only one arm and leg. The condition is more common in persons with strokes that affect the nondominant side of the brain—usually the right hemisphere, which is more involved with spatial orientation, body image, and inductive modes of reasoning.

DIAGNOSIS AND TREATMENT

Accurate diagnosis of stroke is based on a complete history and thorough physical and neurologic ex-

amination. A careful history, including TIAs, their rapidity of onset and focal symptoms, as well as those of any other diseases that may be present, will help to determine the type of stroke that is involved. CT scans and MRI have also become important tools in diagnosing stroke and in differentiating cerebral hemorrhage and intracranial lesions that mimic stroke. MRI provides a sensitive study of brain parenchymal tissue for evidence of ischemic injury. Arteriography may be used to demonstrate the site of the vascular abnormality and afford visualization of most intracranial vascular areas. Magnetic resonance angiography (MRA) has improved the reliability of noninvasive techniques and provides a sensitive screening test for large-vessel occlusive disease. Two other types of imaging, positron emission tomography (PET) and single-photon emission computed tomography (SPECT), are used to study the distribution of blood flow and metabolic activity of the brain. Both methods involve the detection of photons emitted from radionuclides. The radionuclides used for these two tests are very short-lived (minutes), and they emit radioactive energy as they move through the circulation. The use of PET makes it possible to define the location and size of strokes by providing data on cerebral blood flow and volume as well as brain cell metabolism. SPECT provides metabolic and flow-related information, without the cost and complexity of regular PET scanning. The introduction of several Doppler ultrasound techniques has facilitated the noninvasive evaluation of cerebral circulation. Emitted signals may be uninterrupted (continuous-wave Doppler) or intermittent (pulsed-Doppler). The flow characteristics of all vessels within the depth of field is demonstrated on the continuous-wave Doppler; the pulsed-wave Doppler samples flow at any depth. Use of these methods has increased due to low cost, ease of application, safety features, continuous technical advances, improved imaging quality, and increased reliability.[12, 28]

The treatment of stroke is largely symptomatic. The main goals are prevention of complications and treatment of any underlying disease. The chief consideration is to maintain oxygenation of brain tissue, and the possibility exists that a rapid fall in blood pressure could compromise blood flow and oxygenation, particularly in persons with ischemic pathology. Athough hypertension may be implicated in stroke, controversy exists over the safety of dramatically lowering blood pressure after stroke. There is also debate over the use of anticoagulants as a means of preventing further occlusion. Anticoagulants represent a double-edged sword because they could precipitate hemorrhage or cause continued bleeding in persons with stroke due to intracerebral hemorrhage. Surgical attempts at restoring blood supply to the brain focus on removing clots or plaque from afferent arteries, reconstructing vessels, and bypassing occluded vessels.

Symptomatic treatment is aimed at preventing complications and promoting the fullest possible recovery of function. During the acute phase, proper positioning and range-of-motion exercises are essential. Early rehabilitation efforts include all members of the rehabilitation team—physician, nurse, speech therapist, physical therapist, and occupational therapist—and the family.

ANEURYSMAL SUBARACHNOID HEMORRHAGE

Aneurysmal subarachnoid hemorrhage represents bleeding into the subarachnoid space, caused by a ruptured cerebral aneurysm. Bleeding into the subarachnoid space can extend well beyond the site of origin, flooding the basal cistern, ventricles, and spinal subarachnoid space. Aneurysmal subarachnoid hemorrhages are seen most frequently between the ages of 35 to 65 and seldom in children.[29] The mortality and morbidity of aneurysmal subarachnoid hemorrhage are high. About 50% of persons who suffer from the hemorrhage die within 3 months, and half of the survivors have serious disability.[30]

An aneurysm is a bulge at the site of localized weakness in the muscular wall of an arterial vessel. Most cerebral aneurysms are small saccular aneurysms called *berry aneurysms*. They are most often found at bifurcations and other junctions of vessels of the circle of Willis, with about 85% located anteriorly. The posterior ventrobasilar system is the site in the remaining 15% of cases. In 20% to 30% of cases, berry aneurysms are multiple. There is angiographic evidence that these aneurysms enlarge with time and produce weakening of the vessel wall, often to the extent that only a thin fibrous vessel wall remains. The likelihood of rupture increases with an increase in aneurysm size. Large aneurysms may also cause chronic headache, neurologic deficits, or both. For example, giant aneurysms of the internal carotid artery may cause persistent headache and ptosis because of pressure on the third cranial nerve. On the other hand, small aneurysms may go unnoticed; intact aneurysms are frequently found at autopsy as an incidental finding.[4]

Two theories regarding the pathogenesis of aneurysm formation have been proposed. One proposes a developmental defect in the vessel wall; the other proposes degeneration of the vessel wall due to conditions such as atherosclerosis and hypertension and fragile vessel walls due to connective tissue disease and situations of abnormal blood flow.[31, 32]

The onset of subarachnoid aneurysmal rupture is often heralded by a sudden and severe headache, described as "the worst headache of my life." Other manifestations of subarachnoid hemorrhage include signs of meningeal irritation such as nuchal rigidity (neck stiffness) and photophobia; cranial nerve deficits, especially cranial nerve II, III, VI, and sometimes IV (diplopia and blurred vision); stroke syndrome; loss of consciousness; increased intracranial pressure; and pituitary dysfunction. Bleeding into the subarachnoid space causes meningeal irritation or a chemical meningitis, resulting in signs of headache and nuchal rigidity. Occasionally nausea and vomiting will accompany the presenting symptoms. In other cases, there may be no focal neurologic findings. If bleeding is severe, headache may be accompanied by collapse and loss of consciousness. Depending on the course of the bleeding, the headache subsides slowly over a matter of days. Hypertension is a frequent finding and may be the result of the hemorrhage. Cardiac dysrhythmias and noncardiac edema result from massive release of catecholamines triggered by the subarachnoid hemorrhage.

The deficits that can result as complications of aneurysm rupture make this entity a major health problem. These complications include rebleeding, vasospasm with cerebral ischemia, hydrocephalus, hypothalamic dysfunction, and seizure activity. Rebleeding and vasospasm are the most severe and most difficult to treat. Rebleeding carries the same mortality risk as the initial hemorrhage and may result in further and usually catastrophic neurologic deficits.

Vasospasm is a dreaded complication of aneurysmal bleeding. The condition is difficult to treat and is associated with a high incidence of morbidity and mortality. Although the description of aneurysm-associated vasospasm is relatively uniform, its proposed mechanisms are controversial.[31, 32] Usually the condition develops 3 to 10 days (peak, 7 days) after aneurysm rupture and involves a focal narrowing of the cerebral artery or arteries that can be visualized on arteriography. Clinically, there is a gradual deterioration in neurologic status as blood supply to the brain in the region of the spasm is decreased; this can usually be differentiated from the rapid deterioration seen in rebleeding. Vasospasm can often be predicted by the amount of blood seen in the basal cistern on CT scan. Vasospasm is treated by attempting to maintain adequate cerebral perfusion pressure by use of vasopressors or increased intravascular volume to increase or maintain vessel patency, or both. There is a risk of rebleeding from this therapy; early surgery reduces this risk. Endovascular techniques, including balloon dilatation, have been developed to mechanically treat narrowed arterial segments. Elevation of blood pressure before the occlusion of the aneurysm may increase the risk of rebleeding.

Various pharmacologic regimens to treat vasospasm have been proposed. The calcium channel-blocking drug nimopidine has been proposed to effect an improvement in neurologic outcomes after subarachnoid hemorrhage, although angiographic evidence of vasodilation has not been demonstrated. Improved microcirculatory flow and direct neuronal protection are two mechanisms of action proposed to explain the positive outcomes observed.[5, 21]

Another complication of aneurysm rupture is the development of hydrocephalus. It is thought to result from obstruction of the arachnoid villi of the CSF system, which are responsible for reabsorption of CSF. The lysis of blood in the subarachnoid space causes the protein content of the CSF to increase, thereby preventing diffusion of CSF across the arachnoid villi, plugging the system and resulting in hydrocephalus. Occasionally, hydrocephalus can be medically managed by the use of osmotic diuretics, but if neurologic deterioration is significant, surgical placement of a shunt or drain may be indicated. Hydrocephalus is diagnosed by serial CT scans, increasing size of the ventricles, and clinical signs of increased intracranial pressure (to be discussed).

The diagnosis of subarachnoid hemorrhage is made by clinical presentation, CT, MRI, lumbar puncture, and arteriogram. Within the first 48 hours, CT will demonstrate the presence of blood in the subarachnoid space in about 75% to 85% of cases.[29, 34, 35] Lumbar puncture may show blood in the CSF. However, there is risk of rebleeding and brain herniation with lumbar puncture. CT will show blood in the basilar cistern and around the cerebral convexities. Arteriography is the definitive diagnostic tool for establishing the presence and location of the aneurysm. This procedure involves the injection of a contrast medium into an artery so that the vessel can be visualized using fluoroscopic or x-ray methods and defects, such as vasospasm, can be detected. In 5% to 10% of cases, angiography fails to identify an etiology. In these cases, repetition of the study is considered 7 to 10 days after the hemorrhage.

The course of treatment after aneurysm rupture depends on the extent of neurologic deficit. Persons with less severe deficits (with or without headache and no neurologic deficits) may undergo cerebral arteriography and early surgery, usually within 24 to 72 hours. A procedure involving craniotomy and *clipping* is often used. In this procedure, a specially designed metal clip is inserted and tightened around the neck of the aneurysm. This procedure offers protection from rebleeding and may permit removal of the hematoma. Some persons with subarachnoid hemorrhage are managed medically for 10 days or more in an attempt to improve their clinical status before surgery. Endovascular techniques have been developed to treat selected aneurysms.

ARTERIOVENOUS MALFORMATIONS

Arteriovenous (AV) malformations are congenital abnormal communications between arterial and venous channels that result from failure in development of the capillary network in the embryonic brain and spinal cord (Fig. 51-14). As the child's brain grows,

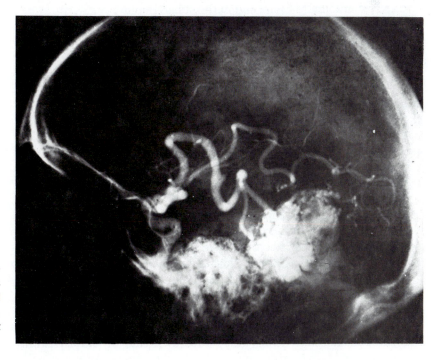

FIG. 51-14. Arteriovenous malformations consist of dilated arterial and venous channels with the apex pointing toward the lateral ventricle. (Smith, R. R. [1980]. *Essentials of neurosurgery.* Philadelphia: J.B. Lippincott)

the malformation acquires additional arterial contributions that enlarge to form a tangled collection of thin-walled vessels that shunt blood directly from the arterial to the venous circulation. About 90% of AV malformations are in the cerebral hemispheres, half being superficial and the other half buried more deeply. Within the brain, the malformations are often separated by gliotic tissue in which there is evidence of repeated bleeding.[4] The hemodynamic effects of arteriovenous malformations are twofold.[30] First, blood is shunted from the high-pressure arterial system to the low-pressure venous system without the buffering advantage of the capillary network. As a result the draining venous channels are exposed to high levels of pressure, predisposing to rupture and hemorrhage. Second is the effect of impaired perfusion on the cerebral tissue adjacent to the AV malformation. The elevated arterial and venous pressures and lack of a capillary circulation impair cerebral perfusion by producing a high-flow situation that diverts blood away from the surrounding tissue. Clinically, this is evidenced by slowly progressive neurologic deficits. The diversion of blood to the AV malformation has been referred to as a vascular "steal" phenomenon.[4]

The major clinical manifestations of AV malformations are hemorrhage, seizures, headache, and progressive neurologic deficits. AV malformations are the third most common cause of intracranial bleeding after aneurysm and spontaneous intracerebral hemorrhage.[36] Bleeding from the malformations is most frequent between ages 10 and 30 and is rare after age 60, with males being affected more often than females.[4] In about 65% of cases, bleeding occurs both into brain tissue and in the subarachnoid space; in about 25% of cases it is confined to the subarachnoid space; and in the remainder, it occurs only in brain tissue. Seizures occur as an initial symptom between 20% and 50% of the time. Headaches are often severe, and persons with the disorder may describe them as being throbbing, synchronous with their heart beat. Other less common symptoms include visual symptoms (diplopia and hemianopia), hemiparesis, mental deterioration, and speech deficits. Definitive diagnosis is often obtained through cerebral angiography.

Treatment methods include surgical excision, embolization, radiation therapy, and laser (Nd:YAG) therapy. Because of the nature of the malformation, each of these methods is accompanied by some risk of complications. If the AV malformation is accessible, surgical excision is usually the treatment of choice. Embolization, which is performed on large AV malformations, is accomplished by insertion of a catheter into the carotid or vertebral circulation to allow a substance such as Silastic spheres, Gelfoam, or metallic pellets to form emboli and gradually oblit-erate blood flow in the malformation. Radiation therapy may be recommended when the lesion is incompletely removed or when the lesion is considered inoperable. When the radiation beam is directed into the malformation, it causes a thickening of its vascular elements. The ND:YAG laser, which is still considered experimental, permits photocoagulation of the malformation.

In summary, blood flow to the brain is supplied by the two internal carotid arteries and the two vertebral arteries and drained by two sets of veins: the deep cerebral venous system and the superficial venous system. Deprivation of oxygen (hypoxic hypoxia) or blood flow (ischemic hypoxia) can have deleterious effects on the brain structures. Ischemia can be *focal*, as in stroke, or *global*, as in cardiac arrest. Neurons of the hypothalamus and the cerebral cortex, including the hippocampus, are particularly vulnerable to hypoxia and ischemia. These neurons bear large numbers of special glutamine NMDA receptors and are particularly vulnerable to a proposed pathologic mechanism called the *calcium cytotoxic cascade*. Global ischemia occurs when blood flow is inadequate to meet the metabolic needs of the brain, as in cardiac arrest. The most serious effect of global ischemia occurs in brain tissues supplied by the most distal branches of the cerebral arteries, in territories called *watershed zones*. These territories receive less blood with profound lowering of blood flow, such as in severe hypotension, predisposing to infarction of brain tissues.

Cerebral vascular accident, or stroke, results in abrupt onset of neurologic deficits and is caused by a focal vascular occlusion. It is the third leading cause of death in the United States and a major cause of disability. Uncontrolled hypertension is a significant risk factor for the development of stroke. Stroke can result from hemorrhage, embolus, or thrombus. The effects of stroke depend on the location of the blood vessel that is involved and can include motor, sensory, and speech manifestations. Treatment is directed toward prevention and rehabilitation and involves the combined efforts of the members of the rehabilitation team, the patient, and the family. A subarachnoid hemorrhage involves bleeding into the subarachnoid space. Most subarachnoid hemorrhages are the result of a ruptured cerebral aneurysm. Fifty percent of people with subarachnoid hemorrhage do not survive the initial hemorrhage. Presenting symptoms include headache, nuchal rigidity, photophobia, and nausea. Complications include rebleeding, vasospasm, and hydrocephalus. Arteriovenous malformations are congenital abnormal communications between arterial and venous channels that result from failure in development of the capillary network in the embryonic brain and spinal cord. The vessels in AV malformations may enlarge to form a space-occupying lesion, become weak and predisposed to bleeding, and divert blood away from other parts of the brain; they can cause brain hemorrhage, seizures, headache, and other neurologic deficits.

ALTERATIONS IN CEREBRAL VOLUMES AND PRESSURES

Intracranial pressure (ICP) is the pressure within the cranial cavity. The standard measurement is that pressure within the lateral ventricles. The cranial cavity contains: (1) blood (about 10%), (2) brain tissue (about 80%), and (3) CSF (about 5% to 10%), within the rigid confines of a nonexpandable skull. Each of these three volumes contributes to the ICP, which normally is maintained within a range of 0 mmHg to 15 mmHg. The volumes of each of these components can vary slightly without causing marked changes in intracranial pressure, because small increases in the volume of one component can be compensated for by a decrease in the volume of one or both of the other two components. This is termed the *Monro-Kellie hypothesis*. Normal fluctuations in ICP occur with respiratory movements and activities of daily living such as straining, coughing, and sneezing.

Abnormal variation in intracranial volume with subsequent changes in ICP can be caused by a volume change in any of the three intracranial components. For example, an increase in tissue volume can result from a brain tumor, brain edema, or bleeding into brain tissue. An increase in blood volume develops when there is vasodilatation of cerebral vessels or obstruction of venous outflow. Excess production, decreased absorption, or obstructed circulation of CSF affords the potential for an increase in the CSF component. When the change in volume is due to a brain tumor, it tends to occur slowly and is usually localized to the immediate area, whereas the increase resulting from head injury usually develops rapidly.

According to the modified Monro-Kellie hypothesis, reciprocal compensation occurs between the three intracranial compartments.[25, 37] Of the three intracranial volumes, tissue volume is relatively restricted in ability to undergo change; CSF and blood volume are the most able to compensate for changes in ICP. Initial increases in ICP are buffered by both a

translocation of CSF to the spinal subarachnoid space and an increased reabsorption of CSF. The rate of CSF production by the choroid plexuses of the third and fourth ventricles is relatively constant. However, the rate of reabsorption and removal is controlled by the pressure difference between the CSF in the subarachnoid space and the blood in the dural sinuses. Because changes in ICP produce an increase in CSF pressures without increasing dural sinus pressures, reabsorption of CSF is increased. Intracranial blood volume is determined by the cerebral blood flow, the resistance of the cerebral blood vessels to flow, and the cerebral perfusion pressure. The cerebral vascular resistance refers to the resistance across the blood vessels in the brain; it increases with vessel constriction and decreases with vessel dilatation. As explained earlier, increases in P_{CO_2} produce vasodilatation of cerebral blood vessels and rapid and significant changes in cerebral blood flow.

The impact of increases in blood, brain tissue, or CSF volumes on ICP varies among individuals and depends on the amount of increase that occurs, the effectiveness of compensatory mechanisms, and the compliance of brain tissue. Compliance represents the ratio of change in volume to the resulting change in pressure (compliance = change in volume/change in pressure). The effect of intracranial volume changes (horizontal axis) on ICP changes (vertical axis) are depicted in Figure 51-15.[31] The shape of the curve demonstrates effects of intracranial volume changes on ICP. The ICP remains constant from point A to point B when volume is added to the intracranial space. Because the compensatory mechanisms are adequate, compliance is high in this area of the curve and there is little change in ICP. From points B to C

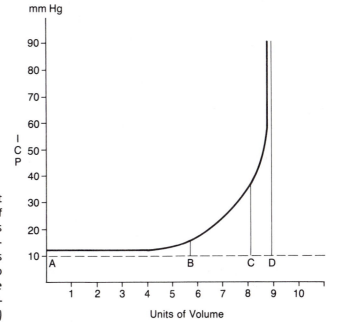

FIG. 51-15. Pressure–volume curve. From point A to just before B, the ICP remains constant although there is addition of volume (compliance is high). At point B, even though the ICP is within normal limits, compliance begins to change, as evidenced by the slight rise in ICP. From points B to C, the ICP rises with an increase in volume (low compliance). From points C to D, ICP rises significantly with each minute increase in volume (compliance is lost). (Hickey, J. [1992]. *Neurological and neurosurgical nursing* [3rd ed., p. 250]. Philadelphia: J.B. Lippincott)

the compensatory mechanisms become less efficient; compliance decreases and ICP begins to rise. At points C to D, the compensatory mechanisms have been exceeded such that even small changes in volume produce large changes in ICP.

The cerebral perfusion pressure (CPP) is the difference between the mean arterial blood pressure (MABP) and the intracranial pressure (CPP = MABP − ICP). The cerebral perfusion pressure is determined by the pressure gradient between the internal carotid artery and the subarachnoid veins, which in turn reflect cerebral vascular resistance and cerebral blood flow. Both the MABP and ICP are frequently monitored in persons with brain conditions that increase ICP and impair brain perfusion. Normal CPP ranges from 70 mmHg to 100 mmHg. Brain ischemia develops at levels below 60 mmHg to 70 mm Hg.[31] When the pressure in the cranial cavity approaches or exceeds the mean systemic arterial pressure, tissue perfusion becomes inadequate, cellular hypoxia results, and, if maintained, neuronal death may occur. The highly specialized cortical neurons are the most sensitive to oxygen deficit; therefore, a decrease in the level of consciousness is one of the earliest and most reliable signs of increased ICP. The increasing cellular hypoxia leads to general neurologic deterioration. The level of consciousness may deteriorate on a continuum from alertness through coma or unresponsiveness. The deteriorating levels of consciousness are described behaviorally.

One of the late reflexes seen with marked increase in ICP is the CNS ischemic response, which is triggered by ischemia of the vasomotor center in the brain stem. Neurons in the vasomotor center respond directly to ischemia by producing a marked increase in mean arterial blood pressure, sometimes to levels as high as 270 mmHg, accompanied by a widening of the pulse pressure and a reflex slowing of the heart rate. This triad of signs, sometimes called the *Cushing reflex* (or response), is an important but late indicator of increased ICP. It results from a severely increased ICP that compromises the blood flow to the brain stem. If the increase in blood pressure initiated by the CNS ischemic reflex is greater than the pressure surrounding the compressed vessels, blood flow will be reestablished. The ischemic reaction is a last-ditch effort by the nervous system to maintain the cerebral circulation.

MANIFESTATIONS AND ASSESSMENT METHODS

Changes in ICP can be assessed through direct or indirect methods. *Direct* methods for continuous monitoring of ICP have been developed over the past 3 decades and are available in many acute care settings. Sophisticated bedside equipment for direct monitoring of ICP can provide continuous information about volume–pressure relationships, cerebral compliance, pulse pressure waves, and cerebral perfusion pressure. These parameters can be measured by direct placement of monitoring devices in the ventricles, subarachnoid, subdural, or epidural space, or in the parenchyma of the brain. The intraventricular method is considered the gold standard for ICP monitoring.

Indirect methods used to estimate fluctuations in ICP are assessment of physiologic parameters such as blood pressure, heart rate, pupillary response, and alterations in levels of consciousness. Other indirect methods include radiologic studies such as CT and MRI. CT scans detect changes in the position of brain structures and provide indirect evidence of ICP changes. The introduction of CT scanning to emergency neurologic care has had a significant impact on the speed of diagnosis of neurologic injury. MRI will also indicate shifting of brain structures. The technique uses a magnetic field to align atomic nuclei along their axis of rotation. When the magnetic field is discontinued, the atoms emit energy as they return to their original position. By using special tomographic computing techniques a tissue image can be obtained. MRI has been useful in degenerative neurologic disease and detection of small brain tumors. It is not useful in an emergency because all metal objects must be removed from the scanning area—a difficult task with intravenous fluids, traction, and ventilator equipment.

HYDROCEPHALUS

One form of increased volume in the cranial cavity is hydrocephalus, which is defined as an abnormal increase in CSF volume within any part or all of the ventricular system. The three causes of hydrocephalus are decreased absorption, overproduction of CSF, and obstruction of CSF circulation. Decreased absorption can result from a block in the CSF pathway to the arachnoid villi or a failure of the villi to transfer the CSF to the venous system. An obstruction to CSF flow can be caused by congenital malformations, infections, or tumors encroaching on the ventricular system. This is sometimes called *noncommunicating* or *obstructive hydrocephalus* because CSF flow is prevented from exiting the ventricular system. Impaired transfer of CSF through the subarachnoid space to or through the villi to the venous system is sometimes called *communicating* or *malabsorption hydrocephalus*. Communicating hydrocephalus can occur if too few villi are formed, if postinfective (meningitis) scarring occludes them, or if the villi become obstructed with fragments of blood or infectious debris. Adenomas of the choroid plexus can cause an overproduction of CSF. This form of hydrocephalus is much less common than that resulting from decreased absorption of CSF.

The signs of ICP elevation associated with hydrocephalus depend on the type of hydrocephalus, the age of onset, and the extent of pressure rise. When hydrocephalus occurs in infants and small children before the sutures of the skull have fused, head enlargement with bulging fontanels is a prominent manifestation. Head enlargement does not occur in adults, and increases in ICP depend on whether the condition developed rapidly or slowly. Acute hydrocephalus is usually manifested by increased ICP. Slowly developing hydrocephalus is less apt to produce an increase in ICP but may produce deficits such as progressive dementia and gait changes. CT scans are used to diagnose all types of hydrocephalus. The usual treatment is a shunting procedure, which provides an alternative route for return of CSF to the circulation.

CEREBRAL EDEMA

Cerebral edema, or brain swelling, is an increase in tissue volume secondary to abnormal fluid accumulation. There are three types of brain edema: vasogenic, cytotoxic, and interstitial.[25, 38] *Vasogenic edema* results from an increase in the extracellular fluid that surrounds brain cells. *Cytotoxic edema* involves the actual swelling of brain cells themselves. *Interstitial edema* is associated with an increase in sodium and water content of the periventricular white matter. Brain edema may or may not produce an increase in intracranial pressure. The impact of brain edema depends on the brain's compensatory mechanisms and the extent of the swelling.

Vasogenic edema occurs in conditions such as tumors, prolonged ischemia, hemorrhage, brain injury, and infectious processes (*e.g.*, meningitis) that impair function of the blood–brain barrier and allow transfer of water and protein into the interstitial space. When brain injury occurs, the blood–brain barrier is disrupted and increased permeability occurs. Although increased permeability has been attributed to a defect in endothelial cell tight junctions, more recent evidence indicates a more important factor may be increased vesicular transport across the endothelial cell.[25] Vasogenic edema occurs primarily in the white matter of the brain, possibly because the white matter is more compliant than the gray matter

and offers less resistance to flow. Vasogenic edema can displace a cerebral hemisphere and can be responsible for various types of herniation. The functional manifestations of vasogenic edema include focal neurologic deficits, disturbances in consciousness, and severe intracranial hypertension.

Cytotoxic (cellular) edema involves an increase in fluid within the intracellular space, chiefly the gray matter, although the white matter may be involved. Cytotoxic edema results from hypo-osmotic states such as water intoxication or severe ischemia that impairs the function of the sodium–potassium membrane pump.[25, 38] This causes rapid accumulation of sodium within the cell, followed by water moving along the osmotic gradient. Major changes in cerebral function, such as stupor and coma, may occur with cytotoxic edema. The edema associated with ischemia may be severe enough to produce cerebral infarction with necrosis of brain tissue.

Interstitial edema involves movement of the CSF across the ventricular wall so there is increased water and sodium in the periventricular white matter due to transependymal passage of CSF.[38] It is most commonly seen in noncommunicating or obstructive hydrocephalus.

Arterial occlusion usually produces both vasogenic and cytotoxic edema. Although edema is viewed as a pathologic process, it does not necessarily disrupt brain function unless it results in an increase in ICP. The localized edema surrounding a brain tumor often responds to corticosteroid therapy (*e.g.*, dexamethasone), but use of these drugs in other situations is controversial. The mechanism of action of the corticosteroids in treatment of cerebral edema is unknown, but in therapeutic doses they seem to stabilize cell membranes and scavenge free radicals. Osmotic diuretics (*e.g.*, mannitol) may be useful in the acute phase of vasogenic and cytotoxic edema when hypoosmolarity is present.

BRAIN HERNIATION

Brain herniation is the displacement of brain tissue under the tough dural folds of the falx cerebri or through the notch or incisura of the tentorium cerebelli. A rising ICP created by increased volume causes displacement of the cerebral tissue toward a more compliant area. There are different types of herniation syndromes, based on the area of the brain that has herniated and the structure under which it has been pushed (Fig. 51-16). They are commonly divided into two broad categories, supratentorial and infratentorial, according to whether they are located above or below the tentorium.

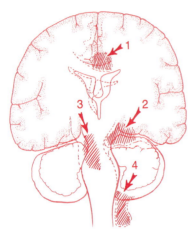

FIG. 51-16. Brain herniations: *1*, cingulate or across the falx; *2*, uncal or lateral; *3*, central or transtentorial; and *4*, infratentorial.

SUPRATENTORIAL HERNIATION

There are three major patterns of supratentorial herniation: (1) cingulate or under the falx, (2) uncal or lateral, and (3) central or transtentorial. Each herniation syndrome has distinguishing features in the early phases, but as forced downward displacement on the pons and medulla continues, clinical signs become similar. Any of the supratentorial herniation syndromes can compress vascular and CSF flow, which can further complicate the neurologic manifestations of brain lesions. Downward displacement of the brain in any of the supratentorial herniation syndromes can cause brain stem herniation, in which the medulla herniates into the foramen magnum. Death is immediate due to medullary compression.

Cingulate Herniation. Cingulate (subfalcial) herniation involves the displacement of the cingulate gyrus and hemisphere beneath the sharp edge of the falx cerebri to the opposite side of the cranial vault. Displacement beneath the falx can cause compression of the local blood supply and parenchymal brain tissue, leading to ischemia and edema, which further increase ICP levels. Little is known about the specific signs and symptoms that would facilitate recognition of cingulate herniation.

Central or Transtentorial Herniation. Central or transtentorial herniation involves the downward displacement of the cerebral hemispheres, basal ganglia, diencephalon, and midbrain through the tentorial incisura. The diencephalon may be compressed tightly against the mibrain with such force that edema and hemorrhage result. It may or may not be associated with uncal herniation. In the early diencephalic stage, central herniation is manifested by a clouding of consciousness with bilaterally small pu-

pils (about 2 mm in diameter) with a full range of constriction, and motor responses to pain that are purposeful or semipurposeful (localizing) and often asymmetric. The clouding of consciousness is due to pressure on the reticular activating system (RAS) in the upper midbrain. As herniation progresses to the late diencephalic stage, painful stimulation results in decorticate posturing, possibly asymmetric, and there is a waxing and waning of respirations with periods of apnea (Cheyne-Stokes respirations). With midbrain involvement, the pupils are fixed and midsize (about 5 mm in diameter), reflex adduction of the eyes and upward gaze are impaired due to cranial nerve III involvement, and pain elicits decerebrate posturing (Fig. 51-17). Respirations change from Cheyne-Stokes breathing to neurogenic hyperventilation in which the frequency of ventilation may exceed 40 breaths per minute because of uninhibited stimulation of both the inspiratory and expiratory centers. Progression to involve the pons and medulla also produces fixed, midsized pupils, but with loss of reflex abduction as well as adduction of the eyes, and absence of a motor response or only leg flexion upon painful stimulation.

Uncal Herniation. Uncal herniation occurs when a lateral mass pushes the brain tissue centrally and forces the medial aspect of the temporal lobe, which contains the uncus and hippocampal gyrus, under the edge of the tentorial incisura into the posterior fossa. The diencephalon and midbrain are compressed and displaced to the opposite side in uncal herniations. Cranial nerve III (oculomotor) and the posterior cerebral artery are frequently caught between the uncus and the tentorium. The oculomotor nerve controls pupillary constriction; the entrapment of this nerve results in ipsilateral pupillary dilatation, which is usually an early sign of uncal herniation. Consciousness may be unimpaired at first because the RAS has not yet been affected. Deterioration, however, may proceed rather rapidly—making it important to recognize the distinguishing early features of lateral herniations. As both central and lateral herniations progress, there are changes in motor strength and coordination of voluntary movements because of compression of the descending motor pathways. It is not unusual for initial changes in motor function to occur on the side of the lesion, owing to compression of the contralateral cerebral peduncle. This is important because it may result in false localizing signs of hemiparesis on the same side as the affected cranial nerve III, rather than on the opposite side. As the condition progresses, bilateral positive Babinski responses as well as respiratory changes (*e.g.*, Cheyne-Stokes, ataxic patterns) occur. Decorticate and decerebrate posturing may develop

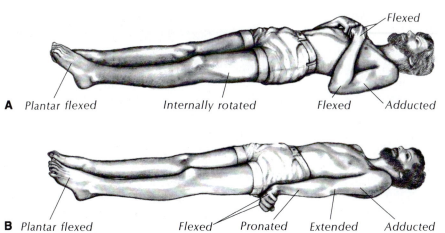

A Plantar flexed   Internally rotated   Flexed   Adducted

B Plantar flexed   Flexed   Pronated   Extended   Adducted

FIG. 51-17. Abnormal rigidity. (**A**) Decorticate rigidity. In decorticate rigidity, the upper arms are held tightly to the sides, with elbows, wrists, and fingers flexed. The legs are extended and internally rotated. The feet are plantar flexed. This posture implies a destructive lesion of the corticospinal tracts within or very near the cerebral hemispheres. When rigidity is unilateral, this is the posture of chronic spastic hemiplegia. (**B**) Decerebrate rigidity. In decerebrate rigidity, the jaws are clenched and the neck extended. The arms are adducted and stiffly extended at the elbows, with forearms pronated, wrists and fingers flexed. The legs are stiffly extended at the knees, with the feet plantar flexed. Decerebration is caused by a lesion in the diencephalon, midbrain, or pons, although severe metabolic disorders, such as hypoxia or hypoglycemia, may also produce it. (From Bates, B. [1991]. *Guide to physical examination* [5th ed.]. Philadelphia: J.B. Lippincott)

(Fig. 51-17), followed by dilated, fixed pupils, flaccidity, and respiratory arrest.

INFRATENTORIAL HERNIATION

Infratentorial herniation results from increased pressure in the infratentorial compartment. It often progresses rapidly and can cause death because it is likely to involve the lower brain stem centers that control vital cardiopulmonary functions. Herniation may occur either superiorly (upward) through the tentorial incisura or inferiorly (downward) through the foramen magnum.

Upward displacement of brain tissue can cause blockage of the aqueduct of Sylvius and lead to hydrocephalus and coma. Downward displacement of the midbrain through the tentorial notch or the cerebellar tonsils through the foramen magnum can interfere with medullary functioning and cause cardiac or respiratory arrest. In cases of preexisting increased ICP, herniation may occur when pressure is released from below, such as in a lumbar puncture.

If the CSF pathway is blocked and fluid cannot leave the ventricles, the volume will expand, as will the downward displacement through the tentorial notch. The expanding volume will cause all function at a given level to cease as destruction progresses in a rostral–caudal direction. The result of this displacement is brain stem ischemia and hemorrhage extending from the diencephalon to the pons. If the lesion expands rapidly, displacement and obstruction occur quickly, leading to irreversible infarction and hemorrhage.

In summary, the contents of the cranial cavity consist of brain tissue, blood, and CSF. The collective volumes of these three intracranial components determine intracranial pressure (ICP). A variation in volume of any of these three components can cause ICP to rise, affecting cerebral function. Compensatory mechanisms protect the brain from small variations in the volume of any of these three components. Large variations, however, exceed the compensatory mechanisms of the CNS and may lead to ischemia, brain herniation, and death. Among the causes of elevated ICP are hydrocephalus and head injury. Hydrocephalus represents an abnormal increase in CSF volume within a part or all of the ventricular system. It is caused by overproduction of CSF or obstruction of its flow through the ventricular system. Brain edema represents an increase in tissue volume secondary to abnormal fluid accumulation. There are three types of brain edema: vasogenic, which results from an increase in extracellular fluid; cytotoxic, which involves the actual swelling of brain cells; and interstitial, which involves increased fluid in the periventricular white matter. Brain herniation is the displacement of brain tissue under the tough dural folds of the falx cerebri or past the incisura or notch of the tentorium cerebelli. Brain herniation is commonly divided into two broad categories, supratentorial and infratentorial, based on location of the herniation.

■ BRAIN INJURY AND INFECTION

The brain is enclosed within the protective confines of the rigid, bony skull. Although the skull affords protection for the tissues of the CNS, it may provide the potential for development of traumatic brain injuries. This is because the skull cannot expand to accommodate the increase in volume that occurs when there is swelling or bleeding within the confines of the skull. The bony structures themselves can cause injury to the nervous system. Fractures of the skull can compress sections of the nervous system, or they can splinter and cause penetrating wounds.

One potential serious type of direct injury is skull fracture. Skull fractures can be divided into four groups: simple, comminuted, depressed, and basilar. A *simple* or *linear* skull fracture is a break in the continuity of bone. A comminuted skull fracture refers to a splintered or multiple fracture line. When bone fragments impinge on brain tissue, the fracture is said to be *depressed*. A fracture of the bones that form the base of the skull is called a *basilar* skull fracture.

Usually radiologic examination is needed to confirm the presence and extent of a skull fracture. This is important because of the possible damage to the underlying tissues. The ethmoid cribiform plate through which the olfactory fibers enter the skull represents the most fragile portion of the neurocranium and can be shattered by basal skull fractures. A frequent complication of basilar skull fractures is leakage of CSF from the nose (rhinorrhea) or ear (otorrhea); this occurs because of the proximity of the base of the skull to the nose and ear. This break in protection of the brain becomes a potential source of infection of the meninges or of brain substance. There may be lacerations to the vessels of the dura, with resultant intracranial bleeding. Damage to the cranial nerves (I, II, III, VI, VII, VIII) may also result from basilar skull fractures if the fracture is in the vicinity of the foramina from which the cranial nerves exit the skull.

The effects of traumatic brain injuries can be divided into two categories: (1) primary or direct injury, in which damage is due to impact, and (2) secondary injury, in which damage results from the subsequent brain swelling, intracranial hematomas, infection, cerebral hypoxia, and ischemia. Because secondary injuries follow rapidly, usually within hours of direct injury, it is often difficult to distinguish them from the damage done by the primary injury. The distinction between primary or direct and secondary injuries is crucial, however, because the main objective of treatment is to prevent or minimize secondary brain injury.

Even if there is no break in the skull, a blow to the head can cause severe and diffuse brain damage. Such closed injury can be classified as (1) focal or diffuse and (2) mild, moderate, or severe. Focal injuries include contusion, laceration or hemorrhage. Diffuse injuries include concussion, contusion, diffuse axonal injury (formerly known as shearing lesion [Fig. 51-18]), and hypoxic brain injury.

In mild head injury, there may be momentary loss of consciousness without demonstrable neurologic symptoms or residual damage, except for possible residual amnesia. Microscopic changes can usually be detected in the neurons and glia within hours of injury. *Concussion* is defined as a momentary interruption of brain function with or without loss of consciousness. Although recovery usually takes place within 24 hours, mild symptoms, such as headache, irritability, insomnia, and poor concentration and memory, may persist for months. This is known as the *postconcussion syndrome*. Because these complaints are vague and subjective, they are sometimes regarded as being of psychological origin. An organic basis for the postconcussion symptoms is suspected. Postconcussion syndrome can have a significant effect on activities of daily living and return to employment. Persons with postconcussion syndrome may need retraining for severe disabilities.

Moderate head injury is characterized by a longer period of unconsciousness and may be associated with neurologic manifestations, such as hemiparesis, aphasia, and cranial nerve palsy. In this type of injury, small hemorrhages and some swelling of brain tissue may occur. Frequently, a *contusion* or bruising of brain tissue is visualized on CT scan.

In severe head injury, there may be cerebral contusion and tearing and shearing of brain structures. It is often accompanied by neurologic deficits such as hemiplegia. Severe head injuries often occur with injury to other parts of the body, such as the extremities, chest, and abdomen. Extravasation of blood may occur; if the contusion is severe, the blood may accumulate, as a result of intracranial bleeding. Similarly, when laceration of the brain directly under the area of injury occurs, especially if the skull is fractured, hemorrhage may be sufficiently extensive to form a hematoma. Contusions of the cerebral cortex are often distributed along the rough, irregular inner surface of the skull and are more likely to affect the frontal or temporal lobes, resulting in cognitive and motor deficits.

Although the skull and CSF provide protection for the brain, they can also contribute to trauma of this nature. A form of brain injury that can cause concussion or contusion due to bouncing of the brain within the enclosed confines of the rigid skull is called a *coup/contrecoup injury*. In this mechanism of injury, the brain is thrown against the same side of

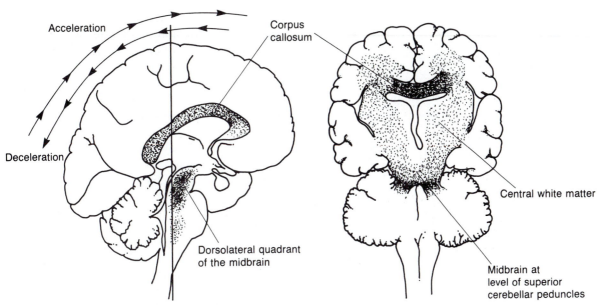

FIG. 51-18. Diffuse axonal injury. Diffuse axonal injury results from acceleration–deceleration and shearing force on the brain. Depending on the severity of the injury, the areas of the brain most often affected are the corpus callosum, the dorsolateral area of the midbrain, and the parasagittal white matter. (Hickey, J. [1992]. *Neurological and neurosurgical nursing* [3rd ed., p. 362]. Philadelphia: J.B. Lippincott)

the skull (coup) in one continuous motion, which causes damage immediately below the site of impact (see Fig. 51-18). The brain then rebounds and strikes the opposite side of the skull (contrecoup), which causes injury in regions opposite the side of impact. This occurs because the brain is suspended in the CSF, whereas the brain stem is stable. As the brain strikes the rough surface of the cranial vault, brain tissue, blood vessels, nerve tracts, and other structures are bruised and torn.

Persons with this type of injury can remain minimally responsive to their environment and have a normal CT scan. They may develop a chronic vegetative state characterized by sleep–wake cycles and alertness but no cognitive awareness of self and environment. This state may be caused by torquing motion on the brain stem disrupting the tracts of the reticular activating system and causing widely scattered shearing of axons. This shearing lesion, which can only be visualized microscopically, is called diffuse axonal injury and is related to high-speed acceleration-deceleration injuries, such as those seen after automobile accidents (see Fig. 51-18). This injury causes widespread damage to axons in the brain. Although neurons do not regenerate, nearby undamaged axons will sprout and grow into new and usually inappropriate connections.

Coma, decerebration, and initially low ICP are clinically common, and mortality is extremely high. Hypoxic injury occurs if neurons are deprived of adequate oxygenation beyond their particular threshold. Any sudden loss of oxygen supply to the brain, including cardiac arrest, can cause hypoxic brain injury. Clinical signs and symptoms depend on the brain area(s) affected and the duration of oxygen deprivation. Clinically, varying degrees of ICP and outcomes ranging from mild to severe deficits can be seen.

The significance of secondary injuries depends on the extent of damage caused by the primary injury. Certain secondary injuries have been discussed, such as increased ICP, cerebral edema, and brain herniation. In addition, hematoma can result from shearing of a blood vessel, which also causes contusion. Intracerebral hematomas can be caused by trauma and can result in increased ICP, which may proceed to herniation of cranial contents through the tentorial notch.

EPIDURAL HEMATOMA

Epidural hematomas are usually caused by a blow to the head that fractures the skull. An epidural (extradural) hematoma is one that develops between the inner table of the bones of the skull and the dura (Fig. 51-19). It is usually due to a tear in a meningeal artery, most often the middle meningeal, which is located under the thin temporal bone. Because bleed-

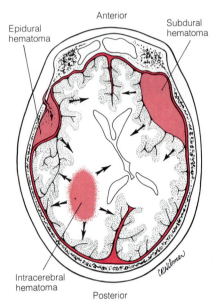

FIG. 51-19. Location of epidural, subdural, and intracerebral hematomas.

ing is arterial in origin, rapid compression of the brain occurs. Epidural hematoma is more common in a young person because the dura is not so firmly attached to the skull surface as it is in an older person; as a consequence, the dura can be easily stripped away from the inner surface of the skull, allowing the hematoma to form.

Typically, a person with an epidural hematoma presents with the following picture: a history of head injury, a brief period of unconsciousness followed by a lucid period in which consciousness is regained, followed by rapid progression to unconsciousness. The lucid interval is not always present, but when it is, it is of great diagnostic value. With rapidly developing unconsciousness, there are focal symptoms related to the area of the brain involved. These symptoms can include ipsilateral pupil dilatation and contralateral hemiparesis. If the hematoma is not removed, the condition may progress, leading to increased ICP, tentorial herniation, and finally death.

SUBDURAL HEMATOMA

A subdural hematoma (Fig. 51-19) develops in the area between the dura and the arachnoid (subdural space) and is usually the result of a tear in the small bridging veins that connect veins on the surface of the cortex to dural sinuses. The bridging veins pass from the pial vessels, through the CSF-filled subarachnoid space, penetrate the arachnoid and the

dura, and finally empty into the intradural sinuses. These veins are readily snapped in head injury when the brain moves suddenly in relation to the cranium. Bleeding can occur between the dura and arachnoid (subdural hematoma) or into the CSF-filled subarachnoid space (subarachnoid hematoma). A subdural hematoma develops more slowly than an epidural hematoma because the tear is in the venous system, whereas epidural hematomas are arterial.

Subdural hematomas are classified as (1) acute, (2) subacute, and (3) chronic. This classification system is based on the approximate time intervals before the appearance of symptoms. Symptoms of acute hematoma are seen within 24 hours of the injury, whereas subacute hematoma does not produce symptoms until 2 to 10 days following injury. Symptoms of chronic subdural hematoma may not arise until several weeks after the injury. These classifications are based partially on pathologic considerations.

Acute subdural hematomas may progress rapidly and carry a high mortality rate. Associated symptoms may progress rapidly because of severe cranial injury and increased ICP. The high mortality rate has been associated with uncontrolled ICP increase, loss of consciousness, decerebrate posturing, and delay in surgical removal of the hematoma.[40] The clinical picture is similar to that of epidural hematoma except that there is usually no lucid interval. In subacute hematoma, there may be a period of improvement in the level of consciousness and neurologic symptoms, only to be followed by deterioration if the hematoma is not removed.

Symptoms of chronic subdural hematoma develop weeks after a head injury—so much later, in fact, that the person may not remember having had a head injury. This is especially true of older persons with fragile vessels and whose brain has shrunk away from the dura. Seepage of blood into the subdural space may occur very slowly. Because the blood in the subdural space is not absorbed, vascular granulation tissue forms from which additional bleeding may occur. Within this encapsulated area, the cells are slowly lysed and a fluid with a high osmotic pressure is formed. This creates an osmotic gradient with fluid from the surrounding subarachnoid space being pulled into the area; as a result of this and additional bleeding, the mass increases in size, exerting pressure on the cranial contents. In some instances the clinical picture is less defined, the most prominent symptom is a decreasing level of consciousness indicated by drowsiness, confusion, and apathy. Headache is also almost invariably present. Morbidity and mortality are higher with subdural hematoma than with epidural and intracerebral hematoma.

INTRACEREBRAL HEMATOMA

Intracerebral hematoma can also result from head injury. This type of bleeding occurs in the brain tissue itself (Fig. 51-19). Blood often leaks into the CSF, causing the same problems as a bridging vein bleed, only the phenomenon is more rapid because of the arterial origin. The severe motion that the brain undergoes can cause bleeding within brain tissue, or a contusion can coalesce into a hematoma. Intracerebral hematoma occurs more frequently in older people and alcoholics, whose brain vessels are more friable. Intracerebral hematomas can occur in any lobe of the brain but are seen most frequently in the frontal or temporal lobes. There can be one hematoma or many.

The signs and symptoms produced by an intracerebral hematoma depend on its size and location within the brain. Signs of increased ICP can be manifested if the hematoma is large and encroaches on vital structures. A hematoma in the temporal lobe can be dangerous because of the potential for lateral herniation.

Treatment of an intracerebral hematoma can be medical or surgical. For a patient with a large hematoma and a rapidly deteriorating neurologic condition, surgery to evacuate the clot is generally indicated. Surgery may not be needed in someone who is neurologically stable despite neurologic deficits; in this case, the hematoma may resolve much like a contusion.

INFECTIONS

Infections of the CNS may be classified according to the structure involved: the meninges—meningitis; the brain parenchyma—encephalitis; the spinal cord—myelitis; the brain and spinal cord—encephalomyelitis. They may also be classified by the type of invading organism: bacterial, viral, or other. In general, the pathogens enter the CNS through the bloodstream by crossing the blood–brain barrier or by direct invasion through skull fracture, a bullet hole, or, more rarely, contamination during surgery or lumbar puncture.

MENINGITIS

Meningitis is an infection of the pia mater, the arachnoid, and the CSF-filled subarachnoid space. Inflammation spreads rapidly since CSF circulates around the brain and spinal cord. Usually the inflammation is caused by an infection, but chemical meningitis may also occur. There are two types of acute infectious meningitis: acute pyogenic meningitis (usually bacterial) and acute lymphocytic (generally viral) meningitis.[4]

In the United States the incidence of bacterial meningitis is approximately 3 to 10 cases per 100,000, of which two-thirds are children under 5 years of age. The most common pyogenic infectious agents are *Hemophilus influenzae, Neisseria meningitidis* (the meningococcus), *Streptococcus pneumoniae,* and *Escherichia coli.* Under the age of 5, the most common agent of infection is *H. influenzae* sero type b; above that age, infection with *S. pneumoniae* is most frequent. The meningococcus can be carried asymptomatically in the throat and nasopharynx and has its highest incidence in children and young adults. Epidemics occur in settings such as the military, where recruits must reside in close contact after recent exposure to one another.[41, 42] The very young and the very old are at most risk for pneumococcus meningitis. Meningitis due to *E. coli* occurs most often in the neonate, especially if there is a neural tube defect. Risk factors associated with contracting meningitis include head trauma with basilar skull fractures, otitis media, sinusitis or mastoiditis, neurosurgery, dermal sinus tracts, systemic sepsis, or an immunocompromised host.

The most common symptoms of acute pyogenic meningitis are fever and chills; headache; back, abdominal, and extremity pains; and nausea and vomiting. Nuchal rigidity and photophobia are often present. Two assessment techniques can help determine whether or not meningeal irritation is present. Kernig's sign is resistance to extension of the leg while the patient is lying with the hip flexed at a right angle. Brudzinski's sign is seen when flexion of the neck results in flexion of the hip and knee. These postures are caused by stretching of the inflamed meninges from the lumbar level to the head. Stretching of the inflamed meninges is extremely painful, hence the resistance to stretching. A petechial rash is found in most persons with meningococcal meningitis. These petechiae may vary from pinhead size to large ecchymoses or even areas of skin gangrene that slough if the person survives. Other types of meningitis may also produce a petechial rash. Persons infected with *H. influenzae* and pneumococcus may present with difficulty in arousal and seizures, whereas those with the meningococcus may present with delirium or coma.[41] Lumbar puncture (spinal tap) yields a cloudy and purulent CSF under increased pressure. The CSF typically contains large numbers of neutrophils (polymorphonuclear white blood cells) (up to 90,000 per mm³), increased protein content, and reduced sugar content. Bacteria can be seen on smear and can be easily cultured with appropriate media.

Arthritis, cranial nerve damage (especially the eighth nerve, with resulting deafness), and hydrocephalus may occur as complications of pyogenic meningitis. As the pathogens enter the subarachnoid space they cause inflammation, characterized by a cloudy, purulent exudate. Thrombophlebitis of the bridging veins and dural sinuses may develop, followed by congestion and infarction in the surrounding tissues. Ultimately, the meninges thicken and adhesions form. These adhesions may impinge on the cranial nerves, giving rise to cranial nerve palsies, or may impair the outflow of CSF, causing hydrocephalus.

The bacteria responsible for meningitis must overcome sequential host defense mechanisms to invade and replicate in the CSF. Host response to the particular pathogen appears largely responsible for the signs and symptoms of clinical meningitis. The organisms that initiate the host response in meningitis demonstrate an affinity for the nervous system (neurotropism). They colonize and invade the nasopharyngeal mucosa, survive intravascularly, penetrate the damaged blood–brain barrier, and survive within the CSF. The least understood step in this process has been the molecular mechanism by which these organisms penetrate the blood–brain barrier.[43–46]

In the pathophysiology of bacterial meningitis, the bacterial organisms replicate and undergo lysis in the CSF, releasing endotoxins or cell wall fragments. These substances initiate the release of inflammatory mediators (cytokines), which set the stage for a complex but coordinated sequence of events by which activated neutrophils bind to cerebral endothelial cells of the blood–brain barrier, damage these cells by the release of toxic oxygen products (free radicals), and increase movement of fluid across the capillary wall. Experimental evidence strongly suggests that inflammatory mediators released into the CSF induce inflammation and impair the blood–brain barrier to the extent that pathogens, neutrophils, and albumin cross the endothelial cell wall into the CNS. The development of brain edema, hydrocephalus, or increased cerebral blood flow can increase ICP.[43–46]

Factors responsible for the severity of meningitis include (1) virulence factors of the pathogen, (2) host factors, (3) brain edema, and (4) permanent neurologic damage. Brain edema can be induced by any agent that causes meningitis and can be vasogenic, due to increased permeability of the blood–brain barrier; cytotoxic, due to fragments of the infecting organisms; or interstitial, due to resistance to CSF outflow.[43]

Although antibiotic therapy was introduced approximately 50 years ago, morbidity and mortality remain high for bacterial meningitis. In fact, mortality due to *S. pneumoniae* remains between 20% and 30%, and neurologic sequelae such as deafness affect half of the survivors. This has important implications for the growth and development of children.[43, 44] Recent elucidation of some of the pathophysiologic molecular mechanisms involved in meningitis has stimulated the investigation of increasingly effective approaches to therapy.[44–46]

Rapidly acting antibiotic bacterical therapy is essential. However, high concentration of bacterial fragments (*e.g., H. influenzae* lipopolysaccharide or *S. pneumoniae* cell wall fragments) have the potential for exacerbating both the abnormalities of the blood–brain barrier (*i.e.,* impaired cerebral microvascular endothelium) and the inflammatory process within the CNS. Adjunctive corticosteroid therapy, especially that given before antibiotic therapy, has been shown to reduce inflammation and decrease the neurologic sequelae.[46] More clinical investigations are needed to study these and other adjunctive agents such as nonsteroidal anti-inflammatory drugs, phosphodiesterase inhibitors, and monoclonal antibodies, which show promise of decreasing the morbidity and mortality rates due to bacterial meningitis.[44, 45]

Viral meningitis presents in much the same way as bacterial meningitis, but the course is less severe and the CSF findings are markedly different—there are lymphocytes in the fluid rather than polymorphonuclear cells, the protein is only moderately elevated, and the sugar content is usually normal. The acute viral meningitides are self-limiting and usually require only symptomatic treatment. Viral meningitis can be caused by many different viruses including mumps, coxsackie, Epstein-Barr virus, and herpes simplex type II. In many cases, the virus cannot be identified.

CSF analysis will confirm or rule out meningitis and will often identify the organism. Other observations should include (1) the presence of infection, (2) alterations in behavior or level of consciousness, and (3) neurologic symptoms. Treatment depends on the etiologic agent. In bacterial meningitis, prompt therapy is essential to prevent death and minimize serious sequelae. Persons who have been exposed to someone with meningococcal meningitis should be treated prophylactically.

ENCEPHALITIS

Generalized infection of the parenchyma of the brain or spinal cord is almost always caused by a virus but may also be caused by bacteria, fungi, and other organisms. Other less frequent causes of encephalitis are toxic substances such as ingested lead and vaccines for measles, mumps, and rabies, which cause postvaccination encephalitis. Encephalitis due to the human immunodeficiency virus (HIV) is discussed in Chapter 15.

The pathologic picture of encephalitis includes local necrotizing hemorrhage, which ultimately becomes generalized, with prominent edema. There is progressive degeneration of nerve cell bodies. The histologic picture, although rather general, demonstrates some specific characteristics; for example, the poliovirus selectively destroys the cells of the anterior horn of the spinal cord.

Encephalitis, like meningitis, is characterized by fever, headache, and nuchal rigidity. In addition, a wide range of neurologic disturbances are present, such as lethargy, disorientation, seizures, dysphagias, focal paralysis, delirium, and coma. The nervous system is subject to invasion by many viruses, such as arbovirus, poliovirus, and rabies virus. The mode of transmission may be the bite of a mosquito (arbovirus) or rabid animal (rabies virus) or ingestion (poliovirus). A common cause of encephalitis in the United States is herpes simplex virus. Diagnosis of encephalitis is made by clinical history and presenting symptoms, in addition to the traditional CSF studies.

In summary, although the skull and the CSF provide protection for the brain, they can also contribute to brain injury through compression and bone splinters that occur with skull fracture and contrecoup injuries. Head injuries may be due to either penetration or impact, each type affecting the brain and supporting structures in different ways. Head injuries can be classified as direct, resulting from the immediate effects of injury, skull fracture, concussion, or contusion, or as secondary, resulting from edema or hemorrhage and infection. Secondary injury may result from epidural, subdural, or intracerebral hematoma formation. Infections of the CNS may be classified according to the structures involved (meningitis, encephalitis) or the type of organism causing the infection. The damage caused by infection may predispose to hydrocephalus, seizures, and other neurologic abnormalities.

■ ALTERED LEVELS OF CONSCIOUSNESS AND BRAIN DEATH

Consciousness is a condition in which the individual is fully responsive to stimuli and demonstrates awareness of the environment. Arousal from sleep, wakefulness, and the ability to respond to stimuli rely on an intact reticular activating system (RAS) in the brain stem. Cognition and the ability to respond to the environment rely on an intact forebrain, cerebral cortex, and thalamus. Therefore, altered forms of consciousness can result from dysfunction or inter-

ruption along the pathways of the reticular activating system (RAS).

The RAS is a diffuse, primitive system of interlacing nerve cells and fibers, driven by input from all sensory systems. It is composed of an intrinsically active core reticular facilitatory area, located in the reticular formation of the upper lateral medulla, and all of the pons, midbrain, and diencephalon, plus its ascending RAS and descending RAS projections. The ascending RAS projects upward to the diencephalon and cerebral cortex, and the descending RAS projects downward to the LMNs of the spinal cord influencing postural muscle tone.

The RAS has two positive feedback loops. The first projects to the cerebral cortex and back to the reticular formation. The second projects to the peripheral muscles and back to the reticular formation. Thus once the RAS becomes activated, feedback impulses from both the cerebral cortex and the periphery maintain excitation. Unless inhibitory signals are received by the RAS, continuous nerve impulses will be transmitted upward to the diencephalon and cortex and downward to the spinal cord. Stimuli such as a loud noise or stamping of the feet will induce further activation of the cerebral cortex (EEG arousal) and increased muscle tone. After prolonged wakefulness, the neurons in the RAS become less excitable. When this happens, neuronal mechanisms give way to lower-level functioning and sleep.

ROSTRAL–CAUDAL PROGRESSION OF COMA

A person's level of consciousness can vary due to the extent of injury, medical stability, fever, and pain-producing stimuli.

Deterioration of brain function usually follows a rostral to caudal progression, which is observed as the brain initially compensates for the injury and subsequently decompensates with the loss of autoregulation and cerebral perfusion if the mass effect progresses (Table 51-3). The hemispheres are most susceptible to damage; thus, the most frequent sign of brain dysfunction is altered level of consciousness and change in behavior. As brain structures in the diencephalon, midbrain, pons, and medulla are affected sequentially; additional motor and pupillary signs become evident. Signs of hemodynamic and respiratory instability are the last to appear because their regulatory centers are located low in the medulla.

Disruptions affecting the diencephalon, midbrain, pons, and medulla usually cause a predictable pattern of change in level of consciousness. The highest level of consciousness is seen in an alert person

TABLE 51-3. ROSTRAL–CAUDAL PROGRESSION OF COMA

AREA INVOLVED	LEVELS OF CONSCIOUSNESS	PUPILS	MUSCLE TONE	RESPIRATION
Diencephalon (thalamus/hypo-thalamus)	Decreased concentration, agitation, dullness, lethargy Requires continuous stimulation to arouse	Respond to light briskly Full range of eye movements only on "doll's head" maneuver or caloric test	Some purposeful movement in response to pain; combative movement Decorticate	Yawning and sighing → Cheyne-Stokes
Midbrain	Stupor → coma	Midposition fixed (MPF), nystagmus with caloric test	Decerebrate	Neurogenic hyper-ventilation
Pons	Coma	MPF	Decerebrate	Apneustic
Medulla	Coma	MPF	Flaccid	Atactic

(Courtesy of Mary Wierenga, R.N., Ph.D., School of Nursing, University of Wisconsin-Milwaukee)

who is oriented to person, place, and time and is totally aware of the surroundings. The first symptoms of diminution in level of consciousness are decreased concentration, agitation, dullness, and lethargy. With further deterioration, the person becomes more difficult to arouse and may respond only to vigorous shaking. Early respiratory changes include yawning and sighing with progression to Cheyne-Stokes breathing. These signs are indicative of bilateral hemisphere damage with danger of tentorial herniation. If the vertebrobasilar arterial blood supply to occipital and inferior temporal cortex remains intact, the eyes may follow a bright moving target (smooth pursuit movements). The pupils may respond briskly to light (a subcortical function), but the ability to visually search the environment is lost, and the eyes stare straight ahead. The full range of conjugate eye movements is seen only when the head is passively rotated (unless contraindicated by neck injury) and eyes compensate by retaining a stationary fixation point (oculocephalic reflex or "doll's eyes" phenomenon) or when the caloric test (injection of warm or cold water in the external ear canal) is done to elicit vestibular driven nystagmus (see Chapter 53). There is some nonpurposeful as well as purposeful movement in response to pain. As coma progresses, the brain stem facilitory area of the RAS becomes more active as fewer descending signals from the cortex and basal ganglia are received. This results in decorticate posturing with forceful adduction of the upper arms, flexion of the elbows, wrists, and fingers, and extension and internal rotation of the legs (see Fig. 51-17).

With progression continuing in a rostral–caudal direction, the midbrain becomes involved. Respirations change from Cheyne-Stokes breathing to neu-

rogenic hyperventilation in which the frequency of ventilation may exceed 40 breaths per minute because of uninhibited stimulation of both the inspiratory and expiratory centers. The pupils become nonreactive and fixed in midposition as parasympathetic (pupillary constriction [cranial nerve III]) and sympathetic (pupillary dilation [descending reticulospinal]) control is compromised. Nystagmus can still be elicited by the caloric test. Muscle hypertonia produces decerebrate posturing in which arms are adducted, rigidly extended, and pronated, wrist and fingers are flexed, and legs are rigidly extended.

As coma advances to involve the pons, the pupils remain in midposition and fixed and the decerebrate posturing continues. Breathing comes apneustic, with sighs evident in midinspiration and with prolonged inspiration and expiration because of excessive stimulation of the respiratory center.

With medullary involvement, the pupils remain fixed in midposition. Respiration become ataxic (i.e., totally uncoordinated and irregular). Apnea may occur because of the loss of responsiveness to carbon dioxide stimulation. Complete ventilatory assistance should be considered for any person with ataxic breathing. With loss of the vestibular system input (a major source of RAS stimulation), as well as loss of most of the descending reticular facilitatory system, hypertonia gives way to reduced muscle tone approaching flaccidity.

In progressive brain deterioration, the patient's neurologic capabilities appear to fall off in stepwise fashion. Similarly, as neurologic function returns, there appears to be stepwise progress to higher levels of consciousness. An assessment tool called the *Glasgow Coma Scale* is often used to describe levels of coma. This scale uses three aspects of neurologic

TABLE 51-4. THE GLASGOW COMA SCALE*

Eye Opening (E)	
Spontaneous	4
To call	3
To pain	2
None	1
Motor Response (M)	
Obeys commands	6
Localizes pain	5
Normal flexion (withdrawal)	4
Abnormal flexion (decorticate)	3
Extension (decerebrate)	2
None (flaccid)	1
Verbal Response (V)	
Oriented	5
Confused conversation	4
Inappropriate words	3
Incomprehensible sounds	2
None	1

*GSC Score = E + M + V. Best possible score = 15; worst possible score = 3.

function—eye-opening, verbal, and motor response—to arrive at a numeric score that represents the level of coma (Table 51-4).[47, 48]

BRAIN DEATH

With advances in scientific knowledge and technology that have provided the means for artificially maintaining ventilatory and circulatory function, the definition of death has had to be reexamined. In 1968, criteria for irreversible coma were published by a Harvard Medical School Ad Hoc Committee,[49] but advances in recent years, including the development of effective artificial cardiopulmonary support for brain-injured persons, led to the need for reevaluation of the determination of death.

The definitive criteria for brain death currently followed in the United States were proposed in 1981 by the President's Commission for the Study of Ethical Problems in Medicine and Biomedical and Behavioral Research.[50] According to these criteria, a diagnosis of death requires both cessation of all brain functions, including the brain stem, and irreversibility. The bases for demonstrating brain death are the absence of brain stem reflexes, absence of cortical activity, and demonstration of irreversibility of the state.[50, 51]

Clinical examination must disclose at least the absence of responsiveness, and respiratory effort. Medical circumstances may require use of confirmatory tests. In the United States, the electroencephalogram (EEG) is one test used to establish brain death. At least a 6-hour period following all cessation of brain activity as indicated by the EEG is usually required to confirm brain inactivity. Longer periods of observation of absent brain activity are required in cases of drug overdose (e.g., barbiturates and other CNS depressants), drug toxicity (e.g., neuromuscular blocking drugs or aminoglycoside antibiotics), neuromuscular diseases (e.g., myasthenia gravis) hypothermia, or shock.

Diagnostic tests that determine the functional conduction of impulses in the brain include the brain stem auditory-evoked response (BAER) and the somatosensory-evoked response (SSER). Recently these evoked responses have been used in determining the prognosis in brain injury and brain death.[52] With these tests, a waveform is produced when (1) an auditory stimulus is presented through earphones and transmitted to pathways of the auditory system in the brain stem, or (2) electrical stimulation of the median or peroneal nerve is transmitted by ascending pathways of the CNS somatosensory system. Computer impulse averaging produces waveforms that are repeatable, much like an electrocardiogram. Normal waveforms indicate normal impulse conduction in the brain stem (BAER) and cortex (SSER). When neurologic injury occurs, the waveform is altered and damage can be localized but not pinpointed.

Brain stem reflexes that are assessed include pupillary reaction to light, corneal reflexes, the gag/swallowing reflex, and the oculovestibular reflex. Adequate testing for apnea is very important. An acceptable method is ventilation with pure oxygen or an oxygen-and-carbon-dioxide mixture for 10 minutes before withdrawal from the ventilator, followed by passive flow of oxygen. This method allows blood levels of carbon dioxide to rise without hazardously lowering the oxygen content of the blood. If respiratory reflexes are intact, the hypercarbia that develops should stimulate ventilatory effort within 30 seconds when the carbon dioxide tension (P_{CO_2}) is greater than 60 mmHg. A 10-minute period of apnea is usually sufficient to attain this level of P_{CO_2}. Spontaneous breathing efforts indicate that the brain stem is functioning.

Irreversibility implies that brain death cannot be reversed. Some conditions, such as drug and metabolic intoxication, can cause cessation of brain functions that are reversible even when they produce clinical cessation of brain functions and EEG silence. This needs to be ruled out before declaring that a person is brain dead. The brains of infants and small children have increased resistance to damage and may recover substantial function after exhibiting unresponsiveness. Therefore, particular caution needs to be used when applying neurologic criteria to determine death in children younger than 5 years.[50]

In summary, consciousness is a state of awareness of self and environment. It exists on two continua: a normal continuum of wakefulness and sleep and a pathologic continuum of wakefulness and coma. Consciousness depends on the normal functioning of the reticular activating system. Coma can be metabolic or structural (supratentorial or tentorial) in origin. It may follow a rostral—caudal progression, with characteristic changes in levels of consciousness, pupillary response, muscle tone, and respiratory activity occurring as the diencephalon through the medulla are affected.

The definitive criteria for brain death currently followed in the United States were proposed in 1981 by the President's Commission for the Study of Ethical Problems in Medicine and Biomedical and Behavioral Research. According to these criteria, a diagnosis of death requires both cessation of all brain functions, including the brain stem, and irreversibility.

■ SEIZURE DISORDERS

Seizures (sometimes called convulsions) are paroxysmal motor, sensory, or cognitive manifestations of spontaneous, abnormally synchronous discharge of collections or ensembles of CNS neurons. This uncontrolled neuronal activity causes signs and symptoms that vary based on location of the involved area or focus, the surrounding neurons, and their connections to other parts of the brain. These signs and symptoms can include strange sensations and perceptions (hallucinations), unusual or repetitive muscle movements, autonomic visceral activity, and the onset of a confusional state or loss of consciousness. The neuronal hyperexcitability that results in a seizure occurs irrespective of the discrete functions of individual neurons; however, its manifestations depend on the particular population of nerve cells involved.

It has been estimated that between 1.5 and 1.65 million persons in the United States are subject to recurrent seizures. Seizure activity is the most common disorder encountered in pediatric neurology; among adults, its incidence is exceeded only by cerebrovascular disorders.[52, 53] Age of onset can be a clue to the type or cause of seizure. When there is no known cause, seizures may be due to vulnerability of the developing nervous system to seizure activity. In most persons, the onset of a first seizure episode occurs before 20 years of age. After 20 years of age, seizure is most often due to structural change, trauma, tumor, or stroke.

A seizure is not a disease but a symptom of an underlying CNS dysfunction. Seizures may occur during almost any serious illness or injury affecting the brain, including infections, tumors, drug abuse, vascular lesions, congenital deformities, and brain injury.

Clinically, seizures may be categorized as (1) provoked (secondary or acute symptomatic) and (2) unprovoked (primary or idiopathic). Provoked or symptomatic seizures include febrile seizures, precipitated by systemic metabolic conditions, and seizures that follow a primary insult to the CNS. Unprovoked or idiopathic seizures are those in which no identifiable cause can be determined.

Multiple episodes or frequent recurrences of apparently unprovoked seizures are considered a seizure disorder or epilepsy (the less preferred term). These persons are evaluated to determine and, if possible, treat the underlying dysfunction. In these cases, anticonvulsant therapy may be prescribed in an attempt to keep seizure activity under control.[54]

The most common subgroup of seizures under the category of provoked seizures is that of febrile seizures in children—those associated with a high fever (usually a temperature over 104°F). In the United States, 2% to 5% of children will experience a febrile seizure before the age of 5 years. Of these, approximately 30% will have one recurrence, and only one-half of those will have yet another recurrence. Since the risks of treatment (*e.g.*, side effects of medications used to control seizures) often exceed the benefits, anticonvulsant medications may be avoided in these cases.[55]

Seizures precipitated by systemic or metabolic disturbances and by primary CNS insult also fall into the category of provoked seizures. Transient systemic metabolic disturbances that may precipitate seizures include electrolyte imbalances, hypoglycemia, hypoxia, and alkalosis. Toxemia of pregnancy, water intoxication, uremia, and CNS infections such as meningitis may also precipitate a seizure. The rapid withdrawal of sedative-hypnotic drugs, such as alcohol or barbiturates, is another cause of seizures. Approximately 5% to 10% of those who suffer a CNS insult such as occurs with cerebral bleeding, edema, or neuronal damage will experience a seizure at the time. Treatment of the precipitating cause of these seizures often results in their disappearance. Long-term prophylactic treatment with anticonvulsant medications remains controversial in these situations.[56]

Many theories have been proposed to explain the initiation of the abnormal brain activity that occurs with seizures. Seizures may be caused by alterations in cell membrane permeability or distribution of ions across the neuronal cell membranes. Another cause may be decreased inhibition of cortical or thalamic neuron activity or structural changes such as glial scarring that alter the excitability of neurons. Neurotransmitter imbalances such as an acetylcholine excess or a deficiency of gamma aminobutyric acid (GABA), an inhibitory neurotransmitter, have been proposed as a cause.[57]

Everyone has a seizure threshold, which, when exceeded, can result in seizure activity. Whether seizure activity occurs depends on the individual's seizure threshold and the extent to which it has been altered by pathologic processes. Some individuals have a low seizure threshold and thus are more likely to experience seizures, even in response to benign stimuli. The role of genetic or familial predisposition to seizures and *interictal* (between seizures) alterations in electroencephalogram (EEG) tracings remains under active investigation. The incidence of certain types of seizure activity is statistically higher in families with a genetic predisposition toward cerebral dysrhythmia; however, evidence of cerebral dysrhythmia is not invariably associated with clinical manifestations of a primary seizure disorder.

SEIZURE/EPILEPSY SYNDROMES

The terms *seizure disorder* or *epilepsy syndromes* are often used interchangeably, although most clinicians prefer seizure disorder because of the negative connotations still associated with the term epilepsy. A seizure disorder can be defined as a syndrome in which there is a tendency to have recurrent, paroxysmal seizure activity without evidence of reversible metabolic cause. It is a chronic condition for which long-term medication may be appropriate.[54, 58]

CLASSIFICATION

Although a knowledge of the etiology is important, seizure management is usually directed toward identifying the seizure type and controlling seizure occurrence. In 1969, a classification system was developed by the International League Against Epilepsy. This system, which was prompted by the need for more accurate diagnosis and quantification of seizure activity for use with new and more specific types of medications, combined clinical and EEG manifestations to describe seizure activity.[59] A revision of the original classification was proposed in 1981 that allows for description of seizure progression, which helped to improve the accuracy of diagnosis (Chart 51-1).[60] As technology advances, the knowledge of medications, and their effects on the various types of seizures is increased. Therefore, the classification system is considered a dynamic one and will continue to need refinement.

Currently, there are two classification systems in use. The first is based on seizure type, and the second on the concept of seizure disorders or epilepsy syndromes. The International Classification of Epileptic Seizures is based on seizure type and symptoms during the seizure (*i.e.*, during the ictal period)

CHART 51-1: CLASSIFICATION OF EPILEPTIC SEIZURES

Partial Seizures

Simple partial seizures (no impairment of consciousness)
    With motor symptoms
    With sensory symptoms
    With autonomic signs
    With psychic symptoms
Complex partial seizures (impairment of consciousness)
    Simple partial onset followed by impaired consciousness
    Impairment of consciousness at onset
Partial seizures evolving to secondarily generalized seizures
    Simple partial leading to generalized seizures
    Complex partial leading to generalized seizures

Unclassified Seizures

    Classification not possible due to inadequate or incomplete data

Generalized Seizures

Absence seizures (typical or atypical)
Atonic seizures
Myoclonic seizures
Clonic seizures
Tonic
Tonic-clonic seizures

(Adapted from Commission on Classification and Terminology of the International League Against Epilepsy [1981]. *Epilepsia, 22,* 489)

---

and EEG patterns during and between seizures (*i.e.*, during ictal and interictal periods). It divides seizures into two broad categories: (1) partial seizures, in which the seizure begins in a specific or focal area of one cerebral hemisphere, and (2) generalized seizures, which involve virtually simultaneous onset in both cerebral hemispheres.[60]

Partial Seizures. Partial or focal seizures are the most common type of seizures among newly diagnosed cases in all age groups over 10 years of age. Partial seizures can be subdivided into three major groups: (1) simple partial (consciousness is not impaired), (2) complex partial (impairment of consciousness), and (3) secondarily generalized partial seizures. These categories are primarily based on current neurophysiologic theories related to seizure propagation and the extent of involvement of the brain's hemispheres.

Simple Partial Seizures. Simple partial seizures usually involve only one hemisphere and are not accompanied by loss of consciousness or responsiveness.

These seizures have also been referred to as elementary partial seizures, partial seizures with elementary symptomatology, or focal seizures. The 1981 Commission on Classification and Terminology of the International League Against Epilepsy classified simple partial seizures according to (1) motor signs, (2) sensory symptoms, (3) autonomic manifestations, and (4) psychic symptoms. The observed clinical signs and symptoms depend on the area of the brain where the abnormal neuronal discharge is taking place. If the motor area of the brain is involved, the earliest symptom is motor movement corresponding to the location of onset on the contralateral side of the body. The motor movement may remain localized or may spread to other cortical areas with sequential involvement of body parts in a characteristic "march," formerly known as a Jacksonian march or seizure. If the sensory portion of the brain is involved, there may be no observable clinical manifestations. Sensory symptoms correlating with the location of seizure activity on the contralateral side of the brain may involve somatic sensory disturbance (*e.g.*, tingling or crawling sensations) or special sensory disturbance (visual, auditory, gustatory, or olfactory phenomena). When abnormal cortical discharge stimulates the autonomic nervous system, flushing, tachycardia, diaphoresis, hypotension or hypertension, or pupillary changes may be evident.

The term *prodrome* or *aura* has traditionally meant a sensory warning sign of impending seizure activity or the onset of seizure that affected persons could describe because they were conscious. It is now thought that the aura itself is part of the seizure. Because consciousness is maintained and only a small portion of the brain is involved, an aura is regarded as a simple partial seizure. Simple partial seizures may progress to complex partial seizures or generalized tonic-clonic seizures that result in unconsciousness. Therefore, the aura in simple partial seizure may, in fact, be a warning sign of impending complex partial seizures.

Complex Partial Seizures. Complex partial seizures involve impairment of consciousness and often arise from the temporal lobe. The seizure begins in a localized area but may rapidly progress to both hemispheres. These seizures formerly were referred to as temporal lobe seizures or psychomotor seizures. Complex partial seizures are often accompanied by automatisms—repetitive, nonpurposeful activity such as lip-smacking, grimacing, or patting or continual rubbing of clothing. Confusion during the postictal (following a seizure) state is common. Hallucinations and illusionary experiences such as *déjà vu* (familiarity with unfamiliar events or environments) or *jamais vu* (unfamiliarity with a known environ-

ment) have been reported. There may be overwhelming fear, uncontrolled forced thinking or flood of ideas, and feelings of detachment and depersonalization. A person with partial seizures is sometimes misunderstood and believed to require hospitalization for a psychiatric disorder.

Secondarily Generalized Partial Seizures. During these seizures, the ictal neuronal discharge spreads, involving deeper structures of the brain, such as the thalamus or the reticular formation. Discharges spread to both hemispheres, resulting in progression to tonic-clonic seizure activity. These seizures may start as simple or complex partial seizures. The aura, or peculiar sensation(s) that precedes the seizure, is usually the result of partial seizure activity.

Generalized Seizures. Generalized onset seizures are the most common type in young children. These seizures are classified as primary or generalized when clinical signs and symptoms, as well as supporting EEG changes, indicate involvement of both hemispheres. The clinical symptoms include unconsciousness and involve varying bilateral degrees of symmetric motor responses without evidence of localization to one hemisphere. These seizures are divided into four broad categories: (1) absence seizures (typical and atypical), (2) atonic (akinetic) seizures, (3) myoclonic seizures, and (4) major motor (formerly grand mal) seizures (characterized by tonic, clonic, or tonic-clonic activity).[54]

Although *typical absence seizures* have been characterized by a blank stare, motionlessness, and unresponsiveness, motion occurs in about 90% of absence seizures. This motion takes the form of automatisms such as lip-smacking; mild clonic motion, usually in the eyelids; increased or decreased postural tone; and autonomic phenomena. There is often a brief loss of contact with the environment. The seizure usually lasts only a few seconds, and then the person is able to resume normal activity immediately. The manifestations are often so subtle that they may pass unnoticed. *Atypical absence seizures* are similar to typical absence seizures except for greater alterations in tone and less abrupt onset and cessation. In practice, it is difficult to distinguish between typical and atypical absence seizures without benefit of supporting EEG findings. However, it is important for the clinician to distinguish between complex partial and absence seizures because the drugs of choice are different. Medications that are effective for partial seizures may increase the frequency of absence seizures.[54] Absence seizures typically occur only in children and either cease in adulthood or evolve to generalized major motor seizures, especially if the absence seizures occurred early in childhood. The risk/benefit decision is in favor of treating these seizures. However, since absence seizures are often outgrown in 1 to 2 years, medication may be discontinued at that time.

In *akinetic* or *atonic seizures*, there is a sudden split-second loss of muscle tone leading to slackening of the jaw, drooping of a limb, or falling to the ground. These seizures are also known as *drop attacks*.

Brief, involuntary muscle contractions induced by stimuli of cerebral origin are called *myoclonic seizures*. A myoclonic seizure involves bilateral jerking of muscles, either generalized or confined to the face, trunk, or one or more extremities. *Tonic seizures* are characterized by a rigid, violent contraction of the muscles fixing the limbs in a strained position. *Clonic seizures* consist of repeated contractions and relaxations of the major muscle groups.

The *tonic-clonic seizure*, formerly called a *grand mal seizure*, is the most common major motor seizure. Frequently the person has a vague warning (probably a simple partial seizure) and experiences a sharp tonic contraction of the muscles with extension of the extremities and immediate loss of consciousness. Incontinence of bladder and bowels is common. Cyanosis may occur from contraction of airway and respiratory muscles. The tonic phase is followed by the clonic phase, which involves rhythmic, bilateral contraction and relaxation of the extremities. At the end of the clonic phase, the person may remain unconscious for a period of time. This is termed the *postictal phase*. The tonic-clonic phases last approximately 60 to 90 seconds.

It is likely that the prevalence of primary tonic-clonic seizures has been overestimated. Most tonic-clonic seizures are probably secondarily generalized partial seizures or perhaps less dramatic seizures such as absence seizures. Generalized tonic-clonic seizures can develop within 7 to 48 hours of reducing or eliminating ethanol intake in alcohol-dependent persons.[61]

Unclassified Seizures. Unclassified seizures are those seizures that cannot be placed in one of the above categories. These seizures are observed in the neonatal and infancy period of life. Determination of whether the seizure is focal or generalized is not possible. Unclassified seizures are difficult to control with medication.

DIAGNOSIS AND TREATMENT

The diagnosis of a seizure disorder is based on a thorough history and neurologic examination, including a full description of the seizure. The physical examination helps rule out any metabolic disease that could precipitate seizures. Skull x-rays and CT or MRI scans are used to identify structural defects. One of the most useful diagnostic tests is the electroencephalogram, which is used to record changes in the brain's electrical activity. It is used to support the clinical diagnosis of epilepsy, to provide a guide for prognosis, and to assist in classifying the seizure disorder.

The first rule of treatment is to protect the person from injury during a seizure; the next is to treat any underlying disease. Persons with a seizure disorder or epilepsy syndrome should be advised to avoid situations that could be dangerous or life-threatening if seizures should occur. Treatment of the underlying disorder may reduce the frequency or eliminate the occurrence of seizures. Once the underlying disease is treated, the aim of treatment is to bring the seizures under control with the least possible disruption in life-style and minimum side effects from medication. With proper drug management, 65% to 90% of persons with a seizure disorder can obtain good seizure control.[62, 63] During the last 25 years, the therapy for epilepsy has changed dramatically owing to the improved classification system, the ability to measure serum anticonvulsant levels, and the availability of potent new anticonvulsant drugs.

Anticonvulsant Medications. Whenever possible, a single drug should be used in seizure therapy. This eliminates drug interactions and additive side effects. Among the drugs used in treatment of seizures are carbamazepine, phenytoin, ethosuximide, valproate, phenobarbital, primidone, and clonazepam.[62, 63] Carbamazepine and phenytoin are the drugs of choice in partial seizures. They are also used for tonic-clonic seizures secondary to partial seizures. Ethosuximide is the drug of choice for absence seizures but is not effective for tonic-clonic seizures progressed from partial seizures. Valproate is helpful for people with many of the minor motor seizures and tonic-clonic seizures. Valproate and ethosuximide can be used together. Phenobarbital is used for tonic-clonic seizures, as is primidone. In addition, primidone is prescribed for simple and complex partial seizures. Absence and myoclonic seizures can be treated with clonazepam. Atonic seizures are highly resistant to therapy.

Determining the proper dose of the anticonvulsant drug(s) is often a long and tedious process, which can become very frustrating to the person with a seizure disorder or epilepsy syndrome. Consistency in taking the medication is essential. Anticonvulsant drugs should never be discontinued abruptly; rather, the dose should be decreased slowly to prevent seizure recurrence. The most frequent cause of recurrent seizures is patient noncompliance with drug regimens.[62, 63] Ongoing education and support are extremely important in the management of seizures. The psychosocial implications of a diagnosis of a seizure disorder or epilepsy syndrome continue to have a large impact on those affected with the disorder.

The neurologist and primary care physician must work together when a person on anticonvulsant medication(s) becomes ill and must take additional medications. Some drugs act synergistically, and others interfere with the actions of anticonvulsant medications. Therefore, this situation needs to be carefully monitored to avoid overmedication or interference with successful seizure control.

Other Therapy. Although surgical therapy has limited use in the treatment of seizure disorders, surgical removal of a single isolated cortical lesion is sometimes indicated if a single lesion can be identified and removed leaving minimal neurologic deficit and seizures have not been controlled with adequate trials of anticonvulsant drugs. Corpus callosum section, another procedure used in the treatment of intractable seizures, involves sectioning or separating the fibers of the corpus callosum to prevent spread of a unilateral seizure to the contralateral cerebral hemisphere. Indications for this type of surgery include drop attacks with secondary generalization that occur several times a week and cause repeated injury despite adequate drug levels. The number of persons who can benefit from this type of surgical procedure is small.

STATUS EPILEPTICUS

Seizures that do not stop spontaneously or occur in succession without recovery are called *status epilepticus*. There are as many types of status epilepticus as there are types of seizures. Tonic-clonic status epilepticus is a medical emergency and, if not promptly treated, may lead to respiratory failure and death.

The main cause of status epilepticus in persons with chronic seizure disorders is noncompliance with medication therapy, and in a person with no history of a seizure disorder or epilepsy syndrome it is neurologic or systemic disease. If status epilepticus is due to neurologic or systemic disease, the cause needs to be identified and treated immediately because the seizures will probably not respond until the underlying cause has been corrected. When status epilepticus is the result of discontinuing medication, the drug regimen should be reinstituted as soon as possible. The prognosis is related to the underlying cause more than to the seizures themselves.

In summary, seizures are caused by spontaneous, uncontrolled, paroxysmal, abnormally synchronized, transitory discharges from cortical centers. Seizures may occur as a reversible symptom of another disease condition or as a recurrent condition called a seizure or epilepsy syndrome. Seizures are classified as partial or generalized seizures. Partial seizures have evidence of local onset, beginning in one hemisphere. They include simple partial seizures, in which consciousness is not lost, and complex partial partial seizures, which begin in one hemisphere but progress to involve both and in which consciousness is lost. Generalized seizures involve both hemispheres and include unconsciousness and rapidly occurring, widespread, bilaterally symmetric motor responses. They include absence (typical and atypical), atonic (akinetic), myotonic, and major motor seizures. Control of seizures is the primary goal of treatment and is accomplished with anticonvulsant medications. Anticonvulsant medications interact with one another and need to be monitored closely when more than one drug is used.

■ REFERENCES

1. Blinkov, S.M., & Glezer, I.I. (1968). *The human brain in figures and tables* (p. 201). New York: Basic Books.
2. Walsh, K. (1987). *Neuropsychology: A clinical approach* (2nd ed.). New York: Churchill Livingstone.
3. Guyton, A. (1991). *Textbook of medical physiology* (8th ed., p. 679). Philadelphia: W.B. Saunders.
4. Cotran, R.S., Kumar, V., & Robbins, S.L. (1989). *Robbins' pathologic basis of disease* (4th ed., pp. 347–343, 1388–1397, 1402–1408). Philadelphia: W.B. Saunders.
5. Meyer, F.B. (1992). Brain metabolism, blood flow, and ischemic thresholds. In I.A. Awad (Ed.). *Neurosurgical topics: Cerebrovascular occlusive disease and brain ischemia* (pp. 1–24). Cleveland: AANS.
6. Hunter, C. (1987). Cardiopulmonary cerebral resuscitation: Nursing interventions. *Critical Care Nursing, 7*(3), 46.
7. Feurerstein, G., Hunter, J., & Barone, F.C. (1992). Calcium blockers and neuroprotection. In P.J. Marangos, & H. Lal (Eds.). *Advances in neuroprotection: Emerging strategies in neuroprotection* (p. 129). Boston: Birkhauser.
8. Sauer, D., Massiu, L., Allegrini, P.R., Amacker, H., Schmutz, M., & Fagg, G.E. (1992). Excitotoxicity, cerebral ischemia, and neuroprotection by competitive NMDA receptor antagonists. In P.J. Marangos, & H. Lal (Eds.). *Advances in neuroprotection: Emerging strategies in neuroprotection* (pp. 93–105). Boston: Birkhauser.
9. Meldrum, B. (1992). Excitatory amino acids and neuroprotection. In P.J. Marangos, & H. Lal (Eds.). *Advances in neuroprotection: Emerging strategies in neuroprotection* (p. 106). Boston: Birkhauser.
10. Martin, T.G. (1986). Drowning and near drowning. *Hospital Medicine, 22*(7), 53.
11. Neatherlin, J.S., & Brillhardt, B. (1988). Glasgow coma scores in the patient post cardiopulmonary resuscitation. *Journal of Neurosciences Nursing, 20*(2), 104.
12. Zabramski, J.M., & Anson, J.A. (1992). Diagnostic evaluation of ischemic cerebrovascular disease. In I.A. Awad (Ed.). *Neurosurgical topics: Cerebrovascular occlusive disease and brain ischemia* (pp. 73–101). Cleveland: AANS.
13. Chimowitz, M.L. (1992). Clinical spectrum and natural history of cerebrovascular occlusive disease. In I.A. Awad (Ed.). *Neurosurgical topics: Cerebrovascular occlusive disease and brain ischemia* (pp. 59–71). Cleveland: AANS.

14. Dempsey, F.J., & Moore, R.W. (1992). Risk factor modification and medical therapy in stroke prevention. In I.A. Awad (Ed.). *Neurosurgical topics: Cerebrovascular occlusive disease and brain ischemia* (pp. 117–134). Cleveland: AANS.

15. Gorelick, P.B. (1987). Alcohol and stroke. *Current Concepts in Cerebrovascular Disorders, 21*(5), 21.

16. Levine, S.R., & Welch, K.M.A. (1987). Cocaine and stroke. *Current Concepts in Cerebrovascular Disorders, 22*(5), 25.

17. Levine, S.R., & Welch, K.M.A. (1988). The neurologic impact of cocaine abuse. *Emergency Medicine, 20,* 99.

18. Wojack, J.C., & Flamm, E.S. (1987). Intracranial hemorrhage and cocaine abuse. *Stroke, 18,* 712.

19. Loftus, C.M. (1992). Indications for surgery in extracranial carotid disease. In I.A. Awad (Ed.). *Neurosurgical topics: Cerebrovascular occlusive disease and brain ischemia* (pp. 155–165). Cleveland: AANS.

20. Grotta, J.C. (1987). Current medical and surgical therapy for cerebrovascular accident. *New England Journal of Medicine, 317*(24), 1505.

21. Davis, S. (1992). Medical management of acute brain ischemia. In I.A. Awad (Ed.). *Neurosurgical topics: Cerebrovascular occlusive disease and brain ischemia* (pp. 135–154). Cleveland: AANS.

22. The EC/IC Bypass Study Group. (1985). Failure of extracranial-intracranial arterial bypass to reduce the risk of ischemic stroke: Results of an international randomized trial. *New England Journal of Medicine, 313,* 1191.

23. Awad, I.A. (1992). Extracranial-intracranial bypass surgery: Current indictions and techniques. In I.A. Awad (Ed.). *Neurosurgical topics: Cerebrovascular occlusive disease and brain ischemia* (pp. 215–230). Cleveland: AANS.

24. Diaz, F.G. (1992). Vertebrobasilar occlusive disease. In I.A. Awad (Ed.). *Neurosurgical topics: Cerebrovascular occlusive disease and brain ischemia* (pp. 213–214). Cleveland: AANS.

25. Adams, R.D., & Victor, M. (1993). *Principles of neurology* (5th ed., pp. 541, 542, 556–559, 652, 653, 669–748). New York: McGraw-Hill.

26. Daube, J.R., Reagan, T.J., Sandok, B.A., & Westmoreland, B.F. (1986). *Neurosciences: An approach to anatomy, pathology, and physiology by system and levels* (2nd ed., pp. 394–395). Rochester, MN: Mayo Clinic.

27. Bronstein, K.S., Popovich, J.M., & Stewart-Amidei, C. (1991). *Promoting stroke recovery: A research-based approach for nurses* (p. 200). St. Louis: C.V. Mosby.

28. Fayad, P.B., & Brass, L.M. (1992). Doppler ultrasonography in occlusive cerebrovascular disease. In I.A. Awad (Ed.). *Cerebrovascular occlusive disease and brain ischemia* (pp. 103–116). Cleveland: AANS.

29. Cook, H.A. (1900). Aneurysmal subarachnoid hemorrhage: Neurosurgical frontiers and nursing challenges. *AACN Clinical Issues in Critical Care, 2,* 665.

30. Biller, J., Godersky, J.C., & Adams, H.P. (1988). Management of aneurysmal subarachnoid hemorrhage. *Stroke, 19,* 1300.

31. Hickey, J.V. (1992). *Neurological and neurosurgical nursing* (3rd ed., pp. 541–556).

32. Stehbens, W.E. (1989). Etiology of intracerebral berry aneurysms. *Journal of Neurosurgery, 70,* 823–831.

33. Mitchel, S.K., & Yates, R.R. (1986). Cerebral vasospasm: Theoretical causes, medical management, and nursing implications. *Journal of Neurosciences Nursing, 18,* 315.

34. Welty, T.E., & Horner, T.G. (1990). Pathophysiology and treatment of subarachnoid hemorrhage. *Clinical Pharmacology, 9,* 35–39.

35. McDonald, E. (1989). Aneurysmal subarachnoid hemorrhage. *Journal of Neurosciences Nursing, 21,* 313–321.

36. McNair, N. (1988). Arteriovenous malformations. *Critical Care Nurse, 8*(4), 35–40.

37. Vos, H.R. (1993). Making headway with intracranial hypertension. *American Journal of Nursing, 93*(2), 28–35.

38. Rowland, L.P., Fink, M.E., & Rubin, L. (1991). Cerebrospinal fluid: Blood–brain barrier, brain edema, and hydrocephalus. In E.R. Kandel, J.H. Schwartz, & T.M. Jessell. *Principles of neural science* (3rd ed., pp. 1050–1060). New York: Elsevier.

39. Kelly, D.D. (1991). Disorders of sleep and consciousness. In E.R. Kandel, J.H. Schwartz, & T.M. Jessell. *Principles of neural science* (3rd ed., pp. 805–819). New York: Elsevier.

40. Cotman, C.W., & Nieto-Sampedro, M. (1985). Progress in facilitating the recovery of function after central nervous system trauma. *Annals of the New York Academy of Science, 457,* 83.

41. Benenson, A.S. (Ed.). (1990). *Control of communicable diseases in man* (15th ed., pp. 279–286). Washington, D.C.: APHA.

42. McLean, D.M., & Smith, J.A. (1991). *Medical microbiology synopsis* (pp. 67, 70–71, 89–90). Philadelphia: Lea and Febriger.

43. Davis, B.D. Dulbecco, R., Eisen, H.N. & Ginsberg, H.S. (1990). *Microbiology* (4th ed., pp. 615–619). Philadelphia: J.B. Lippincott.

44. Quagliarello, V., & Scheld, M. (1992). Bacterial meningitis: Pathogenesis, pathophysiology, and progress. *New England Journal of Medicine, 327,* 864.

45. Saez-Llorens, X., & McCracken, G.H. (1991). Mediators of meningitis: Therapeutic implications. *Hospital Practice, 26*(1A), 68.

46. Odio, C.M., Faingelzight, I., Paris, M., et al. (1991). The beneficial effects of early dexamethasone administration in infants and children with bacterial meningitis. *New England Journal of Medicine, 324,* 1525.

47. Ingersoll, G.L., & Leyden, D.B. (1987). The Glasgow Coma Scale for patients with head injuries. *Critical Care Nursing, 7*(5), 26.

48. Knight, R.L. (1986). The Glasgow Coma Scale: Ten years later. *Critical Care Nursing, 6*(3), 65.

49. Beecher, H.K. (1968). A definition of irreversible coma: Report of the Ad Hoc Committee of the Harvard Medical School to examine the definition of brain death. *Journal of the American Medical Association, 237,* 337.

50. President's Commission for the Study of Ethical Problems in Medicine and Biomedical and Behavioral Research. (1981). Guidelines for determination of death. *Neurology, 32,* 395.

51. Bernat, J.L., Culver, C.M., & Gert, B. (1981). On the definition of death. *Annals of Internal Medicine, 94,* 389.

52. Martin, J.H. (1991). The collective electrical behavior of cortical neurons: The electroencephalogram and the mechanisms of epilepsy. In E.R. Kandel, J.H. Schwartz, & T.M. Jessell. *Principles of neural science* (3rd ed., p. 785). New York: Elsevier.

53. Hauser, W.A., & Annegers, J.E. (1989). Epidemiologic measurements for the determination of genetic risks. In G. Beck-Mannagetta, V.E. Anderson, H. Doose, & D. Janz (Eds.). *The genetics of the epilepsies* (pp. 7–12). New York: Springer-Verlag.

54. Hauser, W.A. (1991). Classification of seizures and epilepsy. In R.P. Lesser (Ed.). *Diagnosis and management*

of seizure disorders (pp. 1–19). New York: Demos Publications.

55. Freeman, J.M. (1992). What have we learned from febrile seizures? *Pediatric Annals, 21*(6), 355–361.

56. Tempkin, N., et al. (1990). A randomized double blind study of phenytoin for the prevention of posttraumatic seizures. *New England Journal of Medicine, 323.*

57. Lothman, E.W., & Collins, R.C. (1984). Seizures. In A.L. Pearlman, & R.C. Collins (Eds.). *Neurological pathophysiology* (3rd ed., pp. 229–249). New York: Oxford Univrsity Press.

58. Hauser, W.A., & Hesdorffer, D.D. (1990). *Epilepsy: Frequency, causes, and consequences.* New York: Demos.

59. Gastault, H. (1970). Clinical and encephalographic classification of epileptic seizures. *Epilepsia, 11,* 102.

60. Commission on Classification and Terminology of the International League Against Epilepsy. (1981). Proposal for revised clinical and electroencephalographic classification of epileptic seizures. *Epilepsia, 22,* 489–501.

61. Messing, R.O., & Diamond, I. (1993). Molecular biology of alcohol dependence. In R.N. Rosenberg, S.B. Prusiner, S. DiMauro, R.L. Barchi, & L.M. Kunkel (Eds.). *The molecular and genetic basis of neurological disease* (pp. 129–142). Boston: Butterworth-Heinemann.

62. Faingold, C.L. & Fromm, G.H. (1992). *Drugs for control of epilepsy: Actions on neuronal networks involved in seizure disorders.* Boca Raton: CRC Press.

63. Lesser, R.P. (Ed.). (1991). *Diagnosis and management of seizure disorders.* New York: Demos Publications.

■ BIBLIOGRAPHY

Bates, D. (1991). Defining prognosis in coma. *Journal of Neurology, Neurosurgery and Psychiatry, 54,* 309.

Berg, A.T., & Shinnar, S. (1991). The risk of seizure recurrence following a first unprovoked seizure. *Neurology, 41,* 965.

Davis, M., & Lucatorto, M. (1992). The false localizing signs of increased intracranial pressure. *Journal of Neurosciences Nursing, 24,* 24550.

Feldmann, E., & Wilterdink, J. (1991). The symptoms of transient cerebral ischemic attacks. *Seminars in Neurology, 11,* 135.

Furlan, A.J. (1992). Transient ischemic attacks: Recognition and management: *Heart Disease and Stroke, 1*(1), 33.

Gold, D.J., & Mahre, M. (1993). Endovascular therapy of neurovascular malformations. *Journal of Neurosurgical Nursing, 25,* 38.

Lehman, L.B. (1990). Intracranial pressure monitoring and treatment: A contemporary view. *Annals of Emergency Medicine, 19,* 295.

Leonard, A.D., & Newburg, S.M. (1992). Cardioembolic stroke. *Journal of Neurosciences Nursing, 24,* 69.

Manifold, S.L. (1990). Aneurysmal SAH: Cerebral vasospasm and early repair. *Critical Care Nursing, 10,* 62.

Pellock, J.M. (1990). The classification of childhood seizures and epilepsy syndromes. *Neurologic Clinics, 8,* 619.

Pellock, J.M., & Willmore, L.J. (1991). A rationale guide to routine blood monitoring in patients receiving antiepileptic drugs. *Neurology, 41,* 961.

Rosen, M.J., & Daughton, S. (1990). Cerebral perfusion pressure management in head injury. *Journal of Trauma, 30,* 933.

Scheinberg, P. (1991). The biologic basis for the treatment of acute stroke. *Neurology, 41,* 1867.

Scheurer, M.I., & Pedley, T.A. (1990). The evaluations and treatment of seizures. *New England Journal of Medicine, 323,* 1468.

Segatore, M., & Way, C. (1992). The Glasgow coma scale: Time for change. *Heart and Lung, 92,* 548.

Snead, O.C. (1988). Epilepsy in children: A practical approach. *Seminars in Neurology, 8*(1), 24.

Solomon, D.H., & Hart, R.G. (1993). Advances in stroke management. *Emergency Medicine, 25*(3), 25.

CHAPTER 52

ALTERATIONS IN VISION

SHEILA M. CURTIS
EDWARD W. CARROLL

■ OBJECTIVES

After you have studied this chapter, you should be able to meet the following objectives:

■ Differentiate between exophthalmos and proptosis.
■ Cite the differences in marginal blepharitis, a hordeolum, and a chalazion.
■ Compare symptoms associated with the red eye caused by conjunctivitis, corneal irritation, and acute glaucoma.
■ List at least four causes of dry eye.
■ Describe the appearance of corneal edema.
■ List the symptoms of keratitis.
■ Explain the mechanism of pupillary constriction and dilation.
■ Compare closed-angle and open-angle glaucoma.
■ Define *refraction* and *accommodation* and describe the changes that occur with myopia, hyperopia, and presbyopia.
■ Describe the visual changes that occur with cataract.
■ Describe the function of the retina and its photoreceptors.

■ State the cause of color blindness.
■ Relate the phagocytic function of the retinal pigment epithelium to the development of retinitis pigmentosa.
■ Explain how prematurity and oxygen administration interact in producing retinopathy of prematurity.
■ Describe the function of the macula and fovea and state the visual changes that occur with macular degeneration.
■ Describe the pathogenesis of background and proliferative diabetic retinopathy and their mechanisms of visual impairment.
■ Explain the pathology and visual changes associated with macular degeneration.
■ Discuss the cause of retinal detachment.
■ Trace the pathways of the nasal and temporal retina from the optic nerve to the primary visual cortex.
■ Define *scotoma* and discuss its significance.

Carol Mattson Porth: PATHOPHYSIOLOGY: CONCEPTS OF
ALTERED HEALTH STATES, 4th ed. © 1994, 1990, 1986, 1982
J.B. Lippincott Company

1113

■ Explain the mechanism of pupillary constriction and dilation.

■ Define *smooth pursuit, saccadic, vestibular, vergence,* and *tremor eye movements.*

■ Explain the difference between paralytic and nonparalytic strabismus.

■ Explain the need for early diagnosis and treatment of strabismus in infants and small children.

■ Define *amblyopia* and explain its pathogenesis.

Nearly 11.5 million people in the United States—1 in every 19—suffer from some degree of visual impairment. Of these, 12% are unable to see well enough to read ordinary newsprint, even with the aid of glasses, and another 4% are classified as legally blind.[18] More than 50% of blind people are over age 65, and the majority of these are over 85 years of age. Alterations in vision can result from disorders of the eyeball and supporting structures, increased intraocular pressure, optics and lens function, vitreous and retinal function, visual pathways and cortical function, and eye movements.

■ THE EYE AND SUPPORTING STRUCTURES

The optic globe, or eyeball, is a remarkably mobile, nearly spherical structure contained within a pyramid-like cavity of the skull called the *orbit* (Fig. 52-1). The eyeball consists of three layers: an outer supporting fibrous layer (sclera), a vascular layer (uveal tract), and a neural layer (retina). The interior is filled with transparent media (the aqueous and vitreous humors), which allow the penetration and transmission of light to photoreceptors in the retina. The exposed surface of the eye is protected by the eyelid, a skin flap that provides a means for shutting out most light. Tears bathe its surface, preventing friction between the eye and the lid, maintaining the hydration of the cornea, and protecting the eye from irritation by foreign objects. Two eyes on the same horizontal plane, with extraocular muscles for directional rotation of the eyeball, provide different images of the same objects and depth perception.

DISORDERS OF THE ORBIT

The orbit is a pyramid-shaped cavity with walls formed by the union of seven cranial and facial bones: the frontal, maxillary, zygomatic, lacrimal, sphenoid, ethmoid, and palatine bones (Fig. 52-2). The superior surface of the maxillary bone forms the main floor of the orbit. The maxillary, lacrimal, and eth-

moid bones form the medial wall of the orbit. The lateral wall of the orbit is triangular in shape; it is formed anteriorly by zygomatic bone and posteriorly by the sphenoid bone. It forms the thickest part of the orbit, particularly at the orbital margin where the wall is most apt to be exposed to trauma. The apex of the orbital pyramid, located in the posterior medial part of the orbit, is pierced by an opening called the *optic foramen*, through which the optic nerve, ophthalmic artery, and sympathetic nerves from the carotid plexus pass. A larger opening, the superior orbital fissure, permits passage of branches of cranial nerves III, IV, V (ophthalmic division), and VI. These nerves provide motor innervation of the extrinsic and intrinsic eye muscles and sensory innervation of the orbit and its contents. The eyeball occupies only the anterior one fifth of the orbit; the remainder is filled with muscles, nerves, the lacrimal gland, and adipose tissue that supports the normal position of the optic globe. A layer of fascia known as Tenon's capsule surrounds the globe of the eye from the cornea to the posterior segment and separates the eye from the orbital fat.

Because the walls of the orbit are rigid, any space-occupying lesion results in protrusion of the eyeball, a condition called *exophthalmos*. Exophthalmos may be caused by swelling or trauma of orbital tissues, tumors of the orbit, or forward displacement of the eye due to endocrine disorders of pituitary or hypothalamic origin. It is commonly seen in people with a form of hyperthyroidism called *Graves' disease* (see Chapter 45). When the eyelid also protrudes, the condition is known as *proptosis*. The condition causes a delay in lid closure (lid lag) and, in severe cases, an inability of the lids to close completely, resulting in exposure and drying of the cornea. Because the optic nerve has sufficient length within the orbit, protrusion greater than 5 mm is required before nerve damage occurs.

Enophthalmos, or deeply sunken eyes, may be an individual characteristic, but it also occurs with severe loss of orbital fat during malnutrition and starvation. Severe developmental defects during the first month of fetal life can result in the absence of one or both optic globes (*anophthalmos*), and growth defects

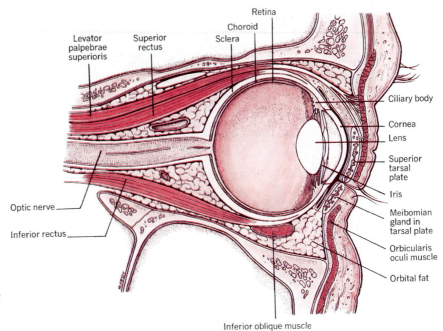

FIG. 52-1. The eye and its appendages, lateral view. (Chaffee, E. E., & Lytle, I. M. [1980]. *Basic anatomy and physiology* (4th ed.). Philadelphia: J.B. Lippincott)

during the last 3 months of gestation can result in abnormally small eyes (*microphthalmos*).

DISORDERS OF THE EYELIDS

The eyelids are called the *palpebrae*, and the oval space between the upper and lower lids is the *palpebral fissure*. The angle where the upper and lower lids meet is referred to as a *canthus*; the lateral canthus is the outer, or temporal, angle and the medial canthus is the inner, or nasal, angle (Fig. 52-3). A line through the lateral and medial canthi defines the angle of the palpebral fissure and is usually horizontal. In children with Down's syndrome, this line slants upward laterally, giving the child a Mongolian appearance (see Chapter 4). A fold of skin, the *epicanthic fold*, covers the medial canthus and is characteristic of the Asian race as well as people with certain chromosomal abnormalities.

In each lid, a tarsus, or plate of dense connective tissue, gives the lid its shape (see Fig. 52-1). Each tarsus contains modified sebaceous glands (meibomian glands), the ducts of which open onto the eyelid margins. The sebaceous secretions enable airtight closure of the lids and prevent rapid evaporation of tears.

Entropion and Ectropion. Normally the edges of the eyelids are in such a position that the palpebral conjunctiva that lines the eyelids is not exposed and the eyelashes do not rub against the cornea. Turning in of the lid is called *entropion*. It is usually caused by scarring of the palpebral conjunctiva or degeneration of the fascial attachments to the lower lid that occurs with aging. Turning inward of the eyelashes causes corneal irritation. *Ectropion* refers to eversion of the lower lid. The condition is usually bilateral and caused by relaxation of the orbicularis oculi muscle because of seventh nerve weakness or the aging process. Ectropion causes tearing and ocular irritation and may lead to inflammation of the cornea. Both entropion and ectropion can be treated surgically. Electrocautery penetration of the lid conjunctiva can also be used to treat mild forms of ectropion. Contrac-

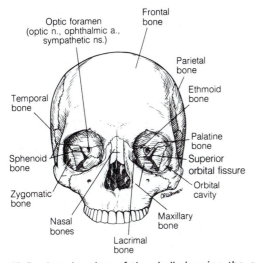

FIG. 52-2. Anterior view of the skull showing the orbital cavity and optic foramen that form an opening for the optic nerve, blood vessels (*e.g.,* ophthalmic artery), and sympathetic nerves that supply the eye.

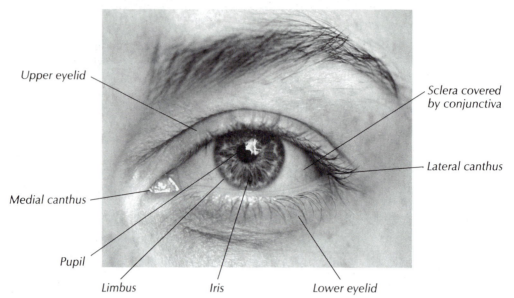

Upper eyelid

Sclera covered by conjunctiva

Lateral canthus

Medial canthus

Pupil

Limbus   Iris   Lower eyelid

FIG. 52-3. Left eye. (Bates, B. [1991]. *A guide to physical examination and history taking* [5th ed.]. Philadelphia: J.B. Lippincott)

tion of the scar tissue that follows tends to draw the lid up to its normal position.

Eyelid Inflammation. Blepharitis, or inflammation of the eyelid margins, is a common disorder of the eyelid margins. There are two main types: seborrheic and staphylococcal. The seborrheic form is usually associated with seborrhea (dandruff) of the scalp or brows. Staphylococcal blepharitis may be due to *Staphylococcus aureus*, in which case it is often ulcerative.[2] The chief symptoms are irritation, burning, redness, and itching of the eyelid margins. Treatment includes careful cleansing with a wet applicator or clean washcloth to remove the scales. A nonirritating baby shampoo can be used. When the disorder is associated with a microbial infection, an antibiotic ointment is prescribed.

A *hordeolum* (*sty*) is caused by infection of the sebaceous glands of the eyelid and can be either internal or external. The main symptoms are pain, redness, and swelling. The treatment is similar to that for abscesses in other parts of the body: heat in the form of warm compresses is applied, and antibiotic ointment may be used. Incision or expression of the infectious contents of the abscess may be necessary. A *chalazion* is a small nodule that is formed due to fatty degeneration of a hordeolum. It is treated by surgical excision.

Eyelid Weakness. The two striated muscles that provide movement of the eyelids are the levator palpebrae superioris and the orbicularis oculi, which is a circular ring of muscle that surrounds the eye. The levator palpebrae, which is innervated by the oculomotor (III) cranial nerve, raises the upper lid. The orbicularis oculi, which is supplied by the facial (VII) cranial nerve, closes the lid. The palpebral portion of this muscle is used for gentle closure, and the orbital portion is used for forcible closure of the lids.

Drooping of the eye lid is called *ptosis*. It can result from weakness of the levator muscle that elevates the upper lid in conjunction with the unopposed action of orbicularis oculi that forcefully close the palpebral fissure. Weakness of the orbicularis oculi causes not ptosis, but an open eyelid. Neurologic causes of eyelid weakness include damage to the innervating cranial nerves or to the nerves' central nuclei in the midbrain and the caudal pons.

The facial (VII) cranial nerve reaches the orbicularis oculi after exiting the skull under the parotid gland and traveling deep to the skin across the face. Thus, trauma to the zygomatic and buccal branches of the facial nerve with a resultant ptosis is relatively common. Weakness of the orbicularis oculi is tested by placement of the examiner's fingers on the muscular sphincter ring while the eye is open and then asking the person to close the eye. Movement of the eyelid is also affected in a condition called *Bell's palsy*, which involves paralysis of muscles on one side of the face because of a lesion of the facial nerve or its nucleus in the caudal pons.

Damage to the oculomotor nerve is much less common than damage to the facial nerve because the oculomotor nerve is protected by the skull throughout its path. However, ptosis resulting from third cranial nerve injury can occur in midbrain stroke and basal skull fractures and from tumors located deep in the orbit or in the cavernous sinus.

DISORDERS OF THE CONJUNCTIVA

The conjunctiva is a thin layer of mucous membrane that lines the inner surface of both eyelids and covers the optic globe to the junction of the cornea and sclera (Fig. 52-4). The portion of the conjunctiva that lines the eyelids is called the *palpebral conjunctiva*, and the part that covers the eyeball is called the *bulbar conjunctiva*. When the eyes are closed, the conjunctiva lines the closed conjunctival sac. The conjunctiva is extremely sensitive to irritation and inflammation. The lining of the upper lid is innervated by the ophthalmic division of the trigeminal (V_1) cranial nerve and that of the lower lid, by the maxillary division of the same nerve.

CONJUNCTIVITIS

Conjunctivitis, or inflammation of the conjunctiva (also called redeye or pinkeye) is one of the most common forms of eye disease. It varies in severity from mild hyperemia with tearing (hay fever conjunctivitis) to a severe necrotizing process (membranous conjunctivitis). Conjunctivitis may result from infection, allergens, chemical agents, physical irritants, or radiant energy. Infections may extend from areas adjacent to the conjunctiva or may be bloodborne, such as in measles or chickenpox.

The main symptoms of conjunctivitis are redness of the eye, which is most obvious peripherally; ocular discomfort or foreign body sensation; a gritty or burning sensation; and tearing. Severe pain suggests corneal rather than conjunctival disease. Itching is common in allergic conditions. A discharge, or exudate, may be present with all types of conjunctivitis and may cause transient blurring of vision. It is usually watery when the conjunctivitis is caused by allergy, foreign body, or viral infection and mucopurulent in the presence of bacterial or fungal infection. A characteristic of many forms of conjunctivitis is papillary hypertrophy. This occurs because the palpebral conjunctiva is bound to the tarsus by fine fibrils. As a result, inflammation that develops between the fibrils causes the conjunctiva to be elevated in mounds called *papillae*. When the papillae are small, the conjunctiva has a smooth, velvety appearance. A red papillary conjunctivitis suggests bacterial or chlamydial conjunctivitis. In allergic conjunctivitis, the papillae often become flat-topped, polygonal, and milky in color and have a cobblestone appearance. Edema of the conjunctiva is called *chemosis*.

Allergic Conjunctivitis. Allergic conjunctivitis (hay fever) is a common disorder associated with exposure to allergens such as pollen. It causes bilateral tearing, itching, and redness of the eyes. The treatment includes the use of cold compresses, antihistamines, and vasoconstrictor eyedrops. The local application of corticosteroids may be used on a short-term basis.

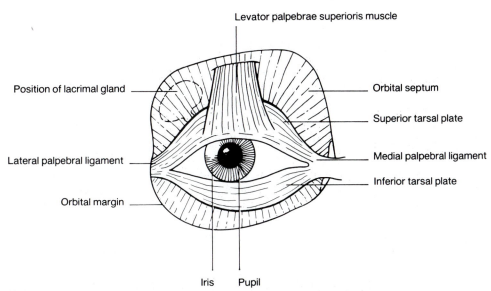

FIG. 52-4. *Right orbit (anterior view showing superficial structures). (Akesson, E. J., Loeb, J. A., & Wilson-Pauwels, L. [1990]. Thompson's core textbook of anatomy [2nd ed., p. 351]. Philadelphia: J.B. Lippincott)*

Bacterial Conjunctivitis. Common agents of bacterial conjunctivitis are *Streptococcus pneumoniae*, *Staphylococcus aureus*, *Neisseria gonorrhoeae*, *Neisseria meningitidis*, and *Hemophilus influenzae*. All of these organisms produce a copious purulent discharge. The eyelids are sticky, and there may be excoriation of the lid margins. Treatment may include local application of antibiotics. The disease is usually self-limiting, lasting about 10 to 14 days if untreated. Scrupulous personal hygiene and prompt adequate treatment of infected people and their contacts are effective.

Viral Conjunctivitis. Etiologic agents of viral conjunctivitis include adenoviruses, herpesviruses, and enteroviruses.[3] Adenovirus type 3 is usually associated with pharyngitis, fever, and malaise. It causes generalized hyperemia, copious tearing, and minimal exudate. Children are affected more often than adults. Contaminated swimming pools due to inadequate chlorination are common sources of infection. Adenoviruses types 4 and 7 are associated with acute respiratory disease of military recruits. Adenovirus type 8 epidemics are associated with inadequate sterilization of ophthalmic equipment. There is no specific treatment for this type of viral conjunctivitis; it usually lasts 7 to 14 days. Preventive measures include scrupulous personal hygiene such as avoiding shared use of eyedroppers, eye makeup, goggles, and towels.[4]

Herpes simplex virus conjunctivitis is characterized by unilateral infection, irritation, mucoid discharge, pain, and mild photophobia. Herpetic vesicles may develop on the eyelids and lid margins. Although the infection is usually caused by the type 1 herpes virus, it can also be caused by the type 2 virus. It is often associated with herpes simplex virus keratitis, in which the cornea shows discrete epithelial lesions. Topical application of acyclovir or idoxuridine provides prompt relief.[5] Local corticosteroid preparations increase the activity of the herpes simplex virus, apparently by enhancing the destructive effect of collagenase on the collagen of the cornea. Therefore, the use of these medications should be avoided in people suspected of having herpes simplex conjunctivitis or keratitis.

Chlamydial Conjunctivitis. Inclusion conjunctivitis is usually a benign suppurative conjunctivitis transmitted by the type of *Chlamydia trachomatis* that causes venereal infections (see Chapter 39). It is spread by contaminated genital secretions and occurs in newborns of mothers having *C. trachomatis* birth canal infections. It can also be contracted through swimming in unchlorinated pools. The incubation period varies from 5 to 12 days, and the disease may last for several months if untreated. The infection is usually treated with systemic erythromycin and topical tetracycline ointment.

A more serious form of infection is caused by a different type of *C. trachomatis*. This form of chlamydial infection not only affects the conjunctiva, but also causes ulceration and scarring of the cornea. It is the leading cause of preventable blindness in the world. Although the agent is widespread, it is seen mostly in dry and sandy regions and among poor people and nomads.[8] In the United States, the infection is largely confined to the American Indians of the Southwest. It is transmitted by direct human contact, contaminated particles (fomites), and flies.

Diagnosis. The diagnosis of conjunctivitis is based on history, physical examination, and microscopic and culture studies to identify the cause. Because a red eye may be the sign of several eye conditions, it is important to differentiate between redness caused by conjunctivitis and that caused by more serious eye disorders such as corneal lesions and acute glaucoma. In contrast to corneal lesions and acute glaucoma, conjunctivitis produces injection (enlargement and redness) of the peripheral conjunctival blood vessels rather than those radiating around the corneal limbus; causes mild discomfort rather than moderate to severe discomfort associated with corneal lesions or the severe and deep pain associated with acute glaucoma; does not affect vision, except for blurring due to discharge; does not cause pupil dilation as compared with acute glaucoma; and does not produce changes in the appearance of the cornea (the clarity of the cornea may be changed in corneal injury, depending on the cause, and is steamy or cloudy in acute glaucoma). Infectious forms of conjunctivitis are often bilateral and involve other family members. Unilateral disease suggests irritant sources, such as foreign bodies or chemical irritation.

DISORDERS OF THE LACRIMAL APPARATUS

The lacrimal gland is the source of the serous secretions called tears. This gland lies in the orbit, superior and lateral to the eyeball (Fig. 52-5). Approximately 12 small ducts connect the tear gland to the superior conjunctival fornix. Tears, which contain about 98% water, 1.5% sodium chloride, and the antibacterial enzyme lysozyme, are essential to the maintenance of vision because of their lubricant and possibly antibacterial properties. Lubrication between the two layers of conjunctiva permits comfortable eye and lid movement.

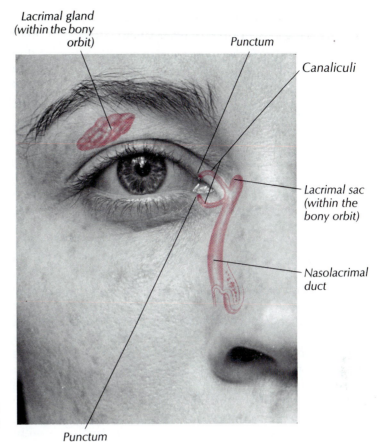

Lacrimal gland (within the bony orbit)

Punctum

Canaliculi

Lacrimal sac (within the bony orbit)

Nasolacrimal duct

Punctum

FIG. 52-5. Lacrimal apparatus. (Bates, B. [1991]. *A guide to physical examination and history taking* [5th ed., p. 157]. Philadelphia: J.B. Lippincott)

A reddish elevation, the lacrimal caruncle, is in the medial canthus. Minute openings, the lacrimal puncta, in the edge of the lids just above and below the caruncle, are the entrances of the superior and inferior canaliculi, which permit entrance of tears into the lacrimal sac and nasolacrimal duct (tear duct). The nasolacrimal duct empties into the nasal cavity.

Dry Eyes. The thin layer of tears that covers the cornea is essential in preventing drying and damage of the outer layer of the cornea. Tear film is from glands in the eyelid as well as the lacrimal gland. The tear film is composed of three layers: (1) the superficial lipid layer, derived from the meibomian glands and thought to retard evaporation of the aqueous layer; (2) the aqueous layer, secreted by the lacrimal glands; and (3) the mucinous layer that overlies the cornea and epithelial cells.[2] Because the epithelial cell membranes are relatively hydrophobic and cannot be wetted by aqueous solutions alone, the mucinous layer plays an essential role in wetting these surfaces. Periodic blinking of the eyes is needed to maintain a continuous tear film over the ocular surface. Disruption of any of the tear film components or of the blinking action of the eyelids can lead to the breakup of the tear film and dry spots on the cornea.

A number of conditions cause reduced function of the lacrimal glands. With aging, the lacrimal glands tend to diminish their secretion, and, as a result, many older people awaken from a night's sleep with highly irritated eyes. Dry eyes also result from loss of reflex lacrimal gland secretion due to congenital defects, infection, irradiation, damage to the parasympathetic innervation of the gland, and medications such as antihistamines, β-adrenergic blocking drugs, and anticholinergic drugs (atropine and scopolamine). The wearing of contact lenses tends to contribute to eye dryness through decreased blinking.

Sjögren's syndrome is a systemic disorder in which there is lymphocytic and plasma cell infiltration of the lacrimal and parotid glands. The disorder is associated with diminished salivary and lacrimal secretions (sicca complex), resulting in keratoconjunctivitis sicca and xerostomia (dry mouth). The syndrome occurs mainly in women near menopause and is often associated with connective tissue disorders such as rheumatoid arthritis.

People with dry eyes complain of dry or gritty sensation in the eye, burning, itching, inability to produce tears, photosensitivity, redness, pain, and difficulty in moving the eyelids. Dry eyes and the absence of tears can cause keratinization of the cornea and conjunctival epithelium. In severe cases, corneal ulcerations can occur. Consequent corneal scarring can cause blindness.

The treatment of dry eyes includes frequent instillation of artificial tear solutions into the conjunctival sac. More prolonged duration of action can be obtained from drop preparations containing methylcellulose (*e.g.*, Isopto Plain) or polyvinyl alcohol (*e.g.*, Liquifilm Tears or Hypo Tears) or by using petrolatum ointment (Lacri-Lube). These artificial tear preparations are generally safe and without side effects. However, the preservatives necessary to maintain their sterility are potentially allergenic.

Dacryocystitis. Dacryocystitis is an infection of the lacrimal sac. It occurs most often in infants or in people over 40 years of age. It is usually unilateral and most often occurs secondary to obstruction of the nasolacrimal duct. Often the cause of the obstruction is unknown, although there may be a history of severe trauma to the midface. The symptoms include tearing and discharge, pain, swelling, and tenderness. The treatment includes application of heat (warm compresses) and antibiotic therapy. In chronic forms of the disorder, surgical repair of the tear duct may be necessary. In infants, dacryocystitis is usually due to failure of the nasolacrimal ducts to open spon-

taneously before birth. When one of the ducts fails to open, a secondary dacryocystitis may develop. These infants are usually treated with gentle massage of the tear sac, instillation of antibiotic drops into the conjunctival sac, and, if that fails, probing of the tear duct.

DISORDERS OF THE SCLERA, CORNEA, AND UVEAL TRACT

DISORDERS OF THE SCLERA

The outer layer of the eyeball consists of a tough, opaque, white fibrous layer called the sclera (Fig. 52-6). Its strong yet elastic properties maintain the shape of the globe. The sclera is homologous to the dermis of the facial skin and is continuous except for a number of tiny holes at the optic disk, the lamina cribrosa sclerae through which the optic nerve axons exit the retina. The sclera is continuous with the extension of the cranial dura mater that surrounds and protects the optic nerve. In an inherited collagen disease known as *osteogenesis imperfecta* (see Chapter 57), the sclera is thin, and the pigmented choroid shows through, providing a bluish cast to the sclera. Subconjunctival hemorrhage frequently is associated with even light trauma to the head or optic globe. In

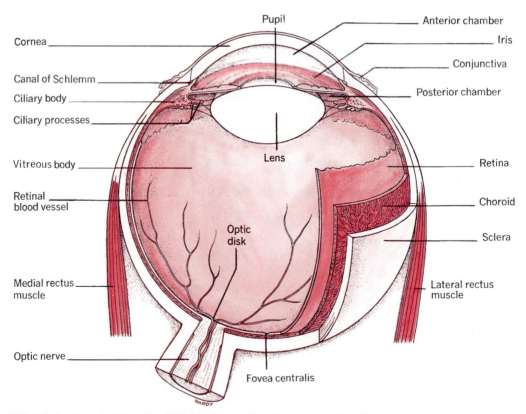

FIG. 52-6. Transverse section of the eyeball. (Chaffee, E. E., & Lytle, I. M. [1980]. *Basic physiology and anatomy* [4th ed., p. 775]. Philadelphia: J.B. Lippincott)

jaundice, the sclera appears yellow because of staining from excessive levels of circulating bilirubin.

DISORDERS OF THE CORNEA

At the anterior part of the eyeball, the scleral structure becomes the transparent cornea. The point at which the cornea joins the sclera is called the *limbus* (see Fig. 52-3). Because light passes from air into the liquid and solid transparent media of the eye at the corneal surface, the major part of refraction (bending) of light rays and focusing of vision occurs at this point. The cornea has three layers: (1) an extremely thin outer epithelial layer, which is continuous with the ocular conjunctiva; (2) a middle stromal layer called the *substantia propria;* and (3) an inner endothelial layer, which lies adjacent to the aqueous humor of the anterior chamber. The thick substantia propria constitutes 90% of the cornea; its anterior condensation (Bowman's membrane) is attached to the basement membrane of the epithelial layer. Descemet's membrane, the basement membrane of the endothelium, separates the endothelium from the stromal layer. The substantia propria is composed of regularly arranged collagen bundles embedded in a mucopolysaccharide matrix. The regular organization of the collagen fibers, which makes the substantia propria transparent, is necessary for light transmission. Hydration within a limited range is necessary to maintain the spacing of the collagen fibers and transparency.

The cornea is avascular and derives its nutrient and oxygen supply by means of diffusion from blood vessels of the adjacent sclera, from the aqueous humor at its deep surface, and from tears. The corneal epithelium is heavily innervated by sensory neurons. Epithelial damage causes discomfort that ranges from a foreign body sensation and burning of the eyes to severe stabbing or knifelike incapacitating pain. Reflex lacrimation is common.

Trauma that causes abrasions of the cornea can be extremely painful, but, if minor, the abrasions usually heal in a few days. The epithelial layer is capable of regeneration, and small defects heal without scarring. If the stroma is damaged, healing occurs more slowly and the danger of infection is increased. Injuries to Bowman's membrane and the stromal layer heal with scar formation and permanent opacification. Opacities of the cornea impair the transmission of light. A minor scar can severely distort vision because it disturbs the refractive surface.

The integrity of both the epithelium and the endothelium is necessary to maintain the cornea in its relatively dehydrated state. Damage to either structure leads to edema and loss of transparency. Among the causes of corneal edema are prolonged and uninterrupted wearing of hard contact lenses, which can deprive the epithelium of oxygen, disrupting its integrity. The edema disappears spontaneously when the cornea comes in contact with the atmosphere. Corneal edema also occurs when there is a sudden rise in intraocular pressure. If intraocular pressure rises rapidly above 50 mmHg, as in acute glaucoma, subendothelial edema develops. With corneal edema, the cornea appears dull, uneven, and hazy. A decrease in visual acuity and iridescent vision (rainbows around lights) occur. Iridescent vision results from epithelial and subepithelial edema, which splits white light into its component parts with blue in the center and red on the outside.

Abnormal Corneal Deposits. The cornea is frequently the site of deposition of abnormal metabolic products. In hypercalcemia, calcium salts can precipitate within the cornea, producing a cloudy band keratopathy. Cystine crystals are deposited in cystinosis, cholesterol esters in hypercholesterolemia, and a golden ring of copper in hepatolenticular degeneration due to Wilson's disease (called a Kayser-Fleischer ring). Pharmacologic agents, such as chloroquine, can result in crystal deposits in the cornea.

Arcus Senilis. Arcus senilis is an extremely common, bilateral, benign corneal degeneration that may occur at any age, but is more common in the elderly. It consists of a grayish white infiltrate, about 2 mm in width, that occurs at the periphery of the cornea. It represents an extracellular lipid infiltration and is commonly associated with hyperlipidemia. Arcus senilis does produce visual symptoms, and there is no treatment for the disorder.

Keratitis. Keratitis refers to inflammation of the cornea. It can be caused by infections, hypersensitivity reactions, ischemia, defects in tearing, trauma, and interruption in sensory innervation, such as occurs with local anesthesia. Scar tissue formation due to keratitis is the leading cause of blindness and impaired vision throughout the world. Most of this vision loss is preventable if the condition is diagnosed early and appropriate treatment is instituted.

Keratitis can be divided into two types: ulcerative, in which part of the epithelium, stroma, or both are destroyed, and nonulcerative, in which all the layers of the epithelium are affected by the inflammation but the epithelium remains intact. Causes of ulcerative keratitis include infectious agents such as those causing conjunctivitis (*e.g.*, *Staphylococcus*, *Pneumococcus*, and *Chlamydia*), exposure trauma, and misuse of contact lenses. Herpes simplex is a common cause of ulcerative keratitis. Exposure trauma may be due to deformities of the lid, paralysis of the lid muscles, or severe exophthalmos. Mooren's ulcer is a chronic, painful, indolent ulcer that occurs in the absence of infection. It is usually seen in older people and may affect both eyes.

Nonulcerative keratitis is associated with a number of diseases, including syphilis, tuberculosis, and lupus erythematosus. It may also result from a viral infection entering through a small defect in the cornea.

Symptoms of keratitis include photophobia, discomfort, and lacrimation. The discomfort may range from foreign body sensation to severe pain. Defective vision results from the changes in transparency and curvature of the cornea that occur. If ulceration is present, it stains green when a drop of fluorescein dye is instilled. Generally, peripheral involvement of the cornea is related to the same disorders that affect the conjunctiva (discussed earlier).

Herpes simplex virus (HSV) keratitis is the most common cause of corneal ulceration in the United States. Most cases are due to HSV type 1 infections. However, in neonatal infections acquired during passage through the birth canal, about 80% are due to HSV type 2.[7] The disease can occur as a primary or recurrent infection. Primary infections cause follicular conjunctivitis and blepharitis, characterized by a round cobblestone pattern of avascular lesions. Epithelial keratitis may develop. After the initial primary infection, the virus remains in the trigeminal ganglion and possibly in the cornea without causing signs of infection.

Recurrent infection may be precipitated by various poorly understood stress-related factors that reactivate the virus. Involvement is usually unilateral. The first symptoms are irritation, photophobia, and tearing. There may be some reduction in vision when the lesion affects the central part of the cornea. Because corneal anesthesia occurs early in the disease, the symptoms may be minimal and, therefore, the person may delay seeking medical care. There is often a history of fever blisters or other herpetic infection, but corneal lesions may be the only sign of recurrent herpes infection. Most typically the corneal lesion involves the epithelium and has a typical branching pattern. These epithelial lesions heal without scarring. Topical antiviral agents such as trifluridine (Viroptic) drops, idoxuridine (Herplex, stoxil) drops, or vidarabine (arabinofuranosyl adenine, ara-A, adenine arabinoside) ointment are used to promote healing.[7] Corticosteroid drugs increase viral replication and should not be used. Lesions that involve the stromal layer of the cornea produce increasingly severe corneal opacities. They are thought to have an immune rather than an infectious cause. Stromal keratitis may be treated with topically applied corticosteroids to suppress the immune response.

Corneal Transplantation. Advances in ophthalmologic surgery permit corneal transplantation using a cadaver cornea. Unlike kidney or heart transplantation procedures, which are associated with considerable risk of rejection of the transplanted organ, the use of cadaver corneas entails minimal danger of rejection, because this tissue is not exposed to the vascular and, therefore, immunologic defense system. Instead, the success of this type of transplantation operation depends on the prevention of scar tissue formation, which would limit the transparency of the transplanted cornea.

DISORDERS OF THE UVEAL TRACT

The middle vascular layer, or uveal tract, of the eye includes the choroid, the ciliary body, and the iris (see Fig. 52-6). The uveal tract is an incomplete ball with gaps at the pupil and at the optic disk, where it is continuous with the arachnoid and pial layers surrounding the optic nerve. The choroid is rich in dispersed melanocytes, which function to prevent the diffusion of light through the wall of the optic globe. The pigment of these cells absorbs light within the eyeball and light that penetrates the retina. The light absorptive function prevents the scattering of light and is important for visual acuity, particularly with high background illumination levels.

The ciliary body is an anterior continuation of the choroid layer. It has both smooth muscle and secretory functions. Its smooth muscle function contributes to alteration in lens shape, and its secretory function contributes to production of aqueous humor.

The iris is an adjustable diaphragm that permits alteration in pupil size and in the amount of light entering the eye. The pupillary diameter can be varied from approximately 2 to 8 mm. The posterior surface of the iris is formed by a two-layer epithelium continuous with those layers covering the ciliary body. The anterior layer contains the dilator, or radial, muscles of the iris (Fig. 52-7). Just anterior to these muscles is the loose, highly vascular connective tissue stroma. Embedded in this layer are concentric rings of smooth muscle cells that compose the sphincter muscle of the pupil. The anteriormost layer of the iris forms a highly irregular anterior surface and contains many fibroblasts and melanocytes. Eye color differences result from the density of the pigment. The amount of pigment decreases from dark brown eyes through shades of brown and gray to blue.

Several mutations affect the pigment of the uveal tract, including albinism. Albinism is a genetic (autosomal recessive trait) deficiency of tyrosinase, which is necessary for the synthesis of melanin by the

FIG. 52-7. Schematic construction of the ciliary body and angle recess in humans. Anteriorly the area is covered by the cornea and posteriorly by the sclera, which contains the canal of Schlemm. The termination of the corneal endothelium is marked by the line of Schwalbe. The ciliary muscle consists of longitudinal fibers, which are mainly parallel to the sclera; radial fibers, which are intermediate; and a circular muscle, which is most internal. The corneal-scleral trabecula provide a filtering area between the anterior chamber angle and the canal of Schlemm. (Redrawn from Von Mollendorf, W., & Bargmann, W. [Eds.]. [1964]. *Handbuch der mikroskopischen Anatomie des Menschen.* Berlin: Springer-Verlag, 1964. From Newell, F. W. [1982]. *Ophthalmology: Principles and concepts* [5th ed.]. St. Louis: C.V. Mosby)

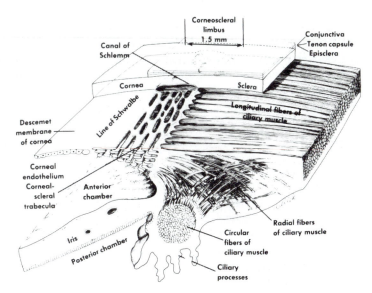

melanocytes. Classic albinism is termed tyrosine-negative albinism, and the affected person has white hair, pink skin, and light blue eyes. In these people, excessive light penetrates the unpigmented iris and, to some extent, the anterior sclera and unpigmented choroid. Their photoreceptors are flooded with excess light, and visual acuity is markedly reduced. In addition, excess stimulation of the photoreceptors at normal or high illumination levels is experienced as painful (photophobia). Tyrosine-positive albinism results from a genetic defect in which a reduced but variable amount of tyrosine is synthesized by the pigment cells. Hair and skin color vary among these people. Reduced choroid and iris pigment results in variable acuity and photophobic abnormalities. A third type of hereditary defect involves the absence of pigment in the choroid and iris with normal pigmentation elsewhere. This is called ocular albinism and results from a chromosomal abnormality of the X chromosome. Other hereditary syndromes include reduced or absent choroid and iris pigment, as in phenylketonuria. People with tyrosine-negative albinism or ocular albinism usually have continuous back-and-forth excursion eye movements (physiologic nystagmus), which makes reading difficult.

Uveitis. Inflammation of the entire uveal tract is termed *uveitis*. One of the serious consequences of the condition can be the involvement of the underlying retina. Parasitic invasion of the choroid can result in local atrophic changes that usually involve the retina; examples include toxoplasmosis and histoplasmosis. Sarcoid deposition in the form of small nodules results in irregularities of the underlying retinal surface.

In summary, the optic globe, or eyeball, is protected posteriorly by the bony structures of the orbit and anteriorly by the eyelids. It is continuously bathed by a protective layer of tears. Protrusion of the eyes is called exophthalmos, and the condition of deeply sunken eyes is called enophthalmos. The eyelids are called the palpebrae. Marginal blepharitis is the most common disorder of the eyelids. It is commonly caused by a staphylococcal infection or seborrhea (dandruff). The term *ptosis* refers to a drooping of the upper lid. It can be caused by injury to the facial (VII) or oculomotor (III) cranial nerves or fibers of the sympathetic nervous system.

The conjunctiva lines the inner surface of the eyelids and covers the optic globe to the junction of the cornea and sclera. Conjunctivitis (also called redeye or pinkeye) is a common eye disorder. It is important to differentiate between redness caused by conjunctivitis and that caused by more serious eye disorders, such as acute glaucoma or corneal lesions. Tears protect the cornea from drying and irritation. Impaired tear production or conditions that prevent blinking and the spread of tears produce drying of the eyes and predispose them to corneal irritation and injury. Trauma or disease that involves the stromal layer of the cornea heals with scar formation and permanent opacification. These opacities interfere with the transmission of light and may impair vision. The uveal tract is the middle vascular layer of the eye. It contains melanocytes that prevent diffusion of light through the wall of the optic globe. Inflammation of the uveal tract (uveitis) can affect visual acuity; albinism, an inherited pigment defect, can cause photophobia.

■ ANTERIOR AND POSTERIOR CHAMBERS AND CONTROL OF INTRAOCULAR PRESSURE

The fluid-filled anterior and posterior chambers of the anterior segment of the eye are divided by the iris and the closely adjacent lens into the posterior and anterior chambers, the pupil forming the only passageway between the two chambers (Fig. 52-8). The posterior chamber, which is the smaller chamber, lies posterior to the iris and anterior to the lens. The gel-like vitreous humor fills the remaining space within the cavity of the globe.

The transparent aqueous humor, which fills the space between the cornea and lens, is secreted by the ciliary epithelium in the posterior chamber. The secreted aqueous humor flows slowly through the thin passageway between the lens and the iris and is reabsorbed by a specialized region at the iridocorneal angle. At the iridocorneal angle, the aqueous humor normally passes through a porous trabeculated region of the sclera (see Fig. 52-7) that permits entry into a circular venous ring called *Schlemm's canal* and from there into the anterior ciliary veins. The anterior ciliary veins continue into the choroid and enter the ophthalmic veins at the back of the eye.

The aqueous humor helps to maintain the intraocular pressure and metabolism of the lens and posterior cornea. The interior pressure of the eye must exceed atmospheric pressure to prevent the eyeball from collapsing. In addition, the aqueous humor serves a nutritive function for the lens and the posterior surface of the cornea. It contains a low protein concentration and a high concentration of ascorbic acid, glucose, and amino acids. It also mediates the exchange of respiratory gases.

The hydrostatic pressure of the aqueous humor results from a balance of several factors: (1) the rate of secretion, (2) the resistance to flow through the narrow opening between the lens and iris at the entrance into the anterior chamber, and (3) the resistance to resorption at the trabeculated region of the sclera at the iridocorneal angle. Normally the rate of aqueous production is equal to the rate of aqueous outflow, so that the intraocular pressure is maintained within a normal range of 9 to 21 mmHg. However, data suggest that the value is closer to 12 ± 1 mmHg in young healthy adults during daylight hours. The mean value increases by approximately 1 mmHg per decade after 40 years of age.[8] Abnormalities in the balance between these factors lead to increased intraocular pressure, a disease complex called *glaucoma*. The sustained increase in intraocular pressure that occurs with glaucoma leads to a gradual loss of peripheral vision (Fig. 52-9), followed by loss of central vision.

Intraocular Pressure Measurements. Intraocular pressure can be estimated by direct palpation or measured indirectly by means of a tonometer. Direct palpation, by gentle use of the examiner's index fingers on each upper tarsal plate, is not quantitative but can indicate whether the eye is soft or hard. For indirect measurement, two types of tonometers in current use are contact tonometers, such as the Goldmann applanation tonometer, which is placed on the anesthetized eye, and a noncontact tonometer, which uses an air pulse. Applanation tonometry is the most accurate clinically applicable method to measure the intraocular pressure. It functions by flattening the curvature of the cornea to a degree dependent on the pressure applied and the resistance of the cornea to deformation. As long as the cornea is structurally intact, its resistance to deformation varies directly with intraocular pressure. The noncontact (air puff) tonometer is not as accurate as the applanation tonometer. It does not require eye drops since no instrument touches the eye. Another familiar method, Schiøtz tonometry, requires only a handheld instrument—the Schiøtz contact tonometer. It is less accurate than applanation tonometry but is useful for screening.

Ophthalmoscopy. Increased intraocular pressure causes damage to optic nerve structures (optic disk) that can be recognized on ophthalmoscopic examination. The normal optic disk has a centrally placed depression called the *optic cup*. With progressive atrophy of axons caused by increased intraocular pressure, pallor of the optic disk develops, and the size and depth of the optic cup increase. Because changes in the optic cup precede the visual field loss, regular ophthalmoscopic examination is important for detecting eye changes that occur with increased intraocular pressure.

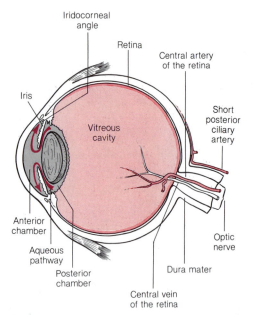

FIG. 52-8. Anterior and posterior chambers of the eye. *Arrows* indicate the pathway of aqueous flow.

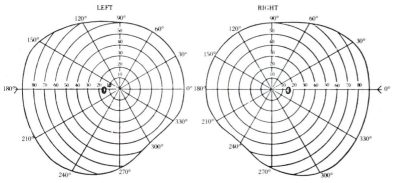

THE FIELD OF VISION (peripheral vision) with both eyes is 180° recorded on these charts.

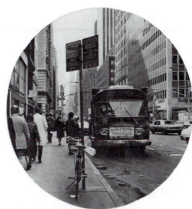

NORMAL VISION A person with normal or 20/20 vision sees this street scene.

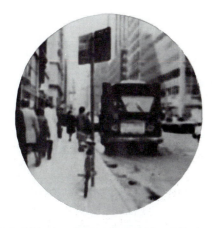

CATARACT diminished acuity from an opacity of the lens. The field of vision is unaffected. There is no scotoma, but the person has an overall haziness of the view, particularly in glaring light conditions.

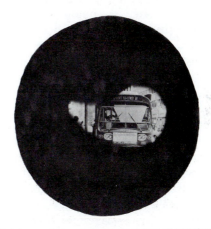

GLAUCOMA Advanced glaucoma involves loss of peripheral vision but the individual still retains most of his central vision.

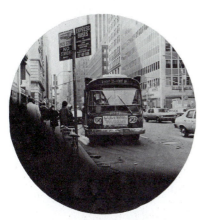

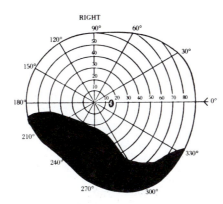

RETINAL DETACHMENT shown here in the active stage. There are many causes for detachment, but the hole or tear allows fluid to lift the retina from its normal position. This elevated retina causes a field or vision defect, seen as a dark shadow in the peripheral field. It may be above, or below as illustrated.

FIG. 52-9. Photographs representing the eye diseases, done as if the camera were the right eye. The accompanying visual-field chart showing the area of visual loss also represents the right eye. (Photo courtesy The Lighthouse, The New York Association for the Blind)

GLAUCOMA

Glaucoma includes a group of conditions that cause a rise in intraocular pressure. If left untreated, the pressure may increase sufficiently to cause ischemia and degeneration of the optic nerve; this leads to progressive blindness. Glaucoma is a major contributor to the incidence of more than 500,000 legally blind people in the United States. It accounts for 13% of all cases of blindness and affects about 2% of people over 40 years of age.[6] It is the second leading cause of irreversible blindness in the United States and the most common etiology among African Americans. Although the latter have been reported to have an incidence six times that of whites, they are only twice as likely to receive appropriate surgical intervention.[9] The condition is often asymptomatic, and a significant loss of peripheral vision may occur before medical attention is sought, emphasizing the need for routine screening measurement of intraocular pressure in people over age 40.

TYPES OF GLAUCOMA

The secretion of aqueous humor is an active process that continues regardless of the pressure in the secreted fluid. The secretory activity of the ciliary epithelium requires the enzyme carbonic anhydrase. Rarely is increased intraocular pressure due to the overproduction of aqueous humor; instead, it usually results from interference with outflow anywhere along the outflow pathway (pupil, trabecular meshwork, or Schlemm's canal). Congenital deformities of the trabecular meshwork, clogging of the meshwork with cellular debris from various intraocular pathologies, and adhesions of the peripheral iris to the trabecular meshwork can all result in increased intraocular pressure. As intraocular pressure rises because of impaired outflow, Schlemm's canal is compressed, causing a further reduction in aqueous outflow.

Glaucoma is commonly classified as (1) closed-angle (narrow-angle) or (2) open-angle (wide-angle) glaucoma depending on the location of the compromised aqueous humor circulation and resorption. Glaucoma may occur as a congenital or an acquired condition, and it may present as a primary or secondary disorder. Primary glaucoma occurs without evidence of preexisting ocular or systemic disease. Secondary glaucoma can result from inflammatory processes that affect the eye, tumors or blood cells from trauma-produced hemorrhage that obstruct the outflow of aqueous humor, or hemorrhage caused by trauma.

Congenital (Infantile) Glaucoma. Congenital glaucoma is caused by a disorder in which the ante-rior chamber retains its fetal configuration, with the trabecular meshwork attached to the root of the iris, or is covered with a membrane. The earliest symptoms are excessive lacrimation and photophobia. Affected infants tend to be fussy, have poor eating habits, and rub their eyes frequently. Diffuse edema of the cornea is usually present, giving the eye a grayish-white appearance. Chronic elevation of the intraocular pressure before the age of 3 years causes enlargement of the entire globe (buphthalmos). Early surgical treatment is necessary to prevent blindness.

Closed-Angle Glaucoma. In closed-angle (narrow-angle) glaucoma, the anterior chamber is narrow, and outflow becomes impaired when the iris thickens as the result of pupil dilation (Fig. 52-10). As the iris thickens, it restricts the circulation pathway between the base of the iris and the sclera, reducing or eliminating access to the angle where aqueous reabsorption occurs. Approximately 5% to 10% of all cases of glaucoma fall into this category.

The symptoms of closed-angle glaucoma are related to sudden intermittent increases in intraocular pressure. These occur after prolonged periods in the dark, emotional upset, and other conditions that cause extensive and prolonged pupil dilation. Administration of pharmacologic agents such as atropine, which cause pupillary dilation (mydriasis), can also precipitate an acute episode of increased intraocular pressure in people with the potential for closed-angle glaucoma. Attacks of increased intraocular pressure are manifested by ocular pain and blurred or iridescent vision caused by corneal edema. The pupil may be enlarged and fixed. The symptoms

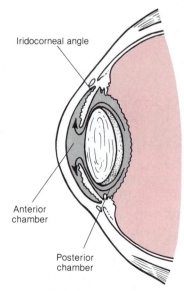

Iridocorneal angle

Anterior chamber

Posterior chamber

FIG. 52-10. Narrow anterior chamber and iridocorneal angle in closed-angle (narrow-angle) glaucoma.

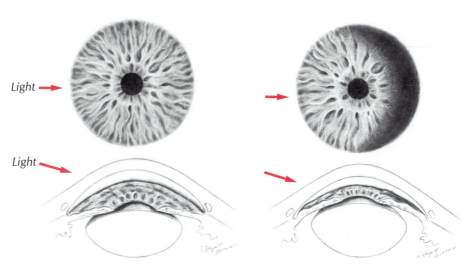

FIG. 52-11. Transillumination of the iris. In the eye with a normal anterior chamber, the iris is evenly illuminated by light shining obliquely into the anterior chamber. In the eye with a narrow anterior chamber, the iris is unevenly illuminated and shadowed. (Bates, B. [1991]. *A guide to physical examination and history taking* [5th ed.]. Philadelphia: J.B. Lippincott)

are often spontaneously relieved by sleep and conditions that promote pupillary constriction. With repeated or prolonged attacks, the eye becomes reddened, and edema of the cornea may develop, giving the eye a hazy appearance. A unilateral, often excruciating, headache is common. Nausea and vomiting may be present, causing the headache to be confused with migraine.

Closed-angle glaucoma usually occurs as the result of an inherited anatomic defect that causes a shallow anterior chamber. This defect is exaggerated by the anterior displacement of the peripheral iris that occurs in older people because of the increase in lens size that occurs with aging. Some people with a congenitally narrow anterior chamber never develop symptoms, and others develop symptoms only when they are elderly. Because of the dangers of vision loss, people with narrow anterior chambers should be warned about the significance of blurred vision, halos, and ocular pain should these symptoms occur. Sometimes decreased visual acuity and an unreactive pupil may be the only cue to closed angle glaucoma in the elderly.

The depth of the anterior chamber can be evaluated by transillumination or by a technique called *gonioscopy*. Gonioscopy uses a special contact lens and either mirrors or prisms so that the angle of the anterior chamber can be seen and measured. The transillumination method requires only a penlight. The light source is held at the temporal side of the eye and directed horizontally across the iris. In persons with a normal-sized anterior chamber, the light passes through the chamber to illuminate both halves of the iris. In contrast, in persons with a narrow anterior chamber, only the half of the iris adjacent to the light source is illuminated (Fig. 52-11).

The treatment of closed-angle glaucoma is primarily surgical. It involves creating an opening between the anterior and posterior chambers by either removing part of the iris (peripheral iridectomy) or cutting a window through the base of the iris (iridectomy). The anatomic abnormalities responsible for closed-angle glaucoma are usually bilateral, but progression may not be symmetric.

Open-Angle Glaucoma. With open-angle glaucoma, an abnormal increase in intraocular pressure occurs in the absence of an obstruction between the trabecular meshwork and the anterior chamber. Instead, it usually occurs because of an abnormality of the trabecular meshwork that impairs the flow of aqueous humor between the anterior chamber and Schlemm's canal. Open-angle glaucoma tends to manifest after age 35 and is the most common type of glaucoma, accounting for approximately 90% of all cases. The condition is usually asymptomatic and chronic, causing progressive loss of visual field unless it is appropriately treated. Because it is usually asymptomatic, routine screening tonometry is the best means of detecting the disorder. In some people, the use of moderate amounts of topical corticosteroid medications can cause an increase in intraocular pressure. Sensitive people may also sustain an increase in intraocular pressure with the use of systemic corticosteroid drugs.

In contrast to closed-angle glaucoma, which can be treated surgically, open-angle glaucoma is usually treated medically. Five classes of antiglaucoma drugs used in the treatment of glaucoma: β-adrenergic blockers, adrenergic agonists, parasympathomimetics, carbonic anhydrase inhibitors, and hyperosmolar agents.[10] All but the carbonic anhydrase inhibitors and hyperosmolar agents are given topically (*i.e.*, instilled as eyedrops). Beta blockers (timolol, betaxolol, levobunolol, and metipranolol) are the drugs of first choice for lowering intraocular pressure. These drugs, which are administered topically as eyedrops, can have significant absorption and related side effects, particularly in the elderly. The adrenergic agonists (epinephrine and dipivefrin) lower ocular pressure by decreasing aqueous humor production and increasing outflow from the anterior chamber. These drugs produce mydriasis (pupillary dilation), and many people become sensitive to the drugs over time, developing a red eye that persists until the treatment is discontinued. The parasympathomimetic drugs directly (pilocarpine) or indirectly (echothiophate iodide, physostigmine, and demecarium bromide) cause contraction of the ciliary muscle, which through its scleral attachment alters the shape of the trabecular meshwork and allows the aqueous to drain more freely. Both drugs cause contraction of the iris sphincter muscle, which causes pupillary miosis.

Carbonic anhydrase inhibitors (acetazolamide, methazolamide, and dichlorphenamide) reduce the secretion of aqueous humor by the ciliary epithelium. These drugs, which must be administered orally, have considerable side effects and are usually reserved for people whose elevated intraocular pressure cannot be controlled by topical therapy.[10] The hyperosmolar agents are administered systemically; the most commonly used are glycerin (taken by mouth) and 20% mannitol (administered intravenously). These drugs, which lower intraocular pressure by creating an osmotic gradient between the vitreous humor and the blood so that water is temporarily drawn from the vitreous humor, are only used when there is a need to lower intraocular pressure rapidly.[10]

When a reduction in intraocular pressure cannot be maintained through pharmacologic methods, surgical treatment may become necessary. Until recently, the main surgical treatment for open-angle glaucoma was a filtering procedure in which an opening is created between the anterior chamber and the subconjunctival space. A new argon or neodymium-YAG laser technique, in which multiple spots are applied 360 degrees around the trabecular meshwork, has been developed.[2] The microburns resulting from the laser treatment scar rather than penetrate the trabecular meshwork, a process that is thought to enlarge the outflow channels by increasing the tension exerted on the trabecular meshwork. Cryotherapy, diathermy, and high-frequency ultrasound may be used in some cases to destroy the ciliary epithelium and reduce aqueous humor production.

In summary, glaucoma is one of the leading causes of blindness in the United States. It is characterized by conditions that cause an increase in intraocular pressure, which, if untreated, can lead to atrophy of the optic disk and progressive blindness. The aqueous humor is formed by the ciliary epithelium in the posterior chamber and flows through the pupil to the angle formed by the cornea and the iris. Here it filters through the trabecular meshwork and enters Schlemm's canal for return to the venous circulation. Glaucoma results from the impeded outflow of aqueous humor from the anterior chamber of the eye. There are two major forms of glaucoma: closed-angle and open-angle. Closed-angle glaucoma is caused by a narrow anterior chamber and blockage of the outflow channels at the angle formed by the iris and the cornea. This occurs when the iris becomes thickened during pupillary dilation. In open-angle glaucoma, microscopic obstruction of the trabecular meshwork occurs. Open-angle glaucoma is usually asymptomatic, and considerable loss of the visual field often occurs before medical treatment is sought. Routine screening tonometry provides the means for early detection of glaucoma before vision loss has occurred.

■ OPTICS AND LENS FUNCTION

The function of the eye is to transform light energy into nerve signals that can be transmitted to the brain for interpretation. Optically, the eye is similar to a camera. It contains a lens system that inverts the image, an aperture for controlling light exposure (the pupil), and a retina that corresponds to the film.

The lens is an avascular transparent biconvex body, whose posterior side is more convex than the anterior side. It measures about 9 to 10 mm in the transverse diameter and about 4 mm in the anteroposterior diameter. A thin, homogeneous, and highly elastic carbohydrate-containing lens capsule is attached to the surrounding ciliary body by delicate suspensory radial ligaments called *zonules*, which hold the lens in place (Fig. 52-12). In providing for a change in lens shape, the tough and elastic sclera acts as a bow, and the zonule and lens capsule act as the bow string. Thus, the lens capsule is normally under tension, and the lens is flattened. Some

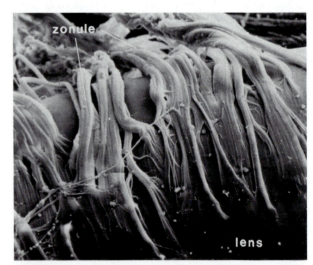

FIG. 52-12. Scanning micrograph of a portion of the zonule, attached to the periphery of the lens, from a monkey's eye. Note the large bundles of fibers attached to the capsule of the lens below. (Courtesy of P. Basu. From Ham, A. W., & Cormack, D. H. [1979]. *Histology* [8th ed.]. Philadelphia: J.B. Lippincott)

of the smooth muscle fibers of the ciliary body are oriented parallel to the scleral surface and insert more anteriorly at the sclera–cornea junction. Many of the fibers are oriented radially as a sphincter around the eyeball. Contraction of the muscle fibers of the ciliary body results in a bending-in of the anterior sclera, relieving the tension on the zonules and thus on the lens capsule. Under these conditions, the rather elastic lens assumes a nearly spherical shape. Altering the normally flat lens shape to a more spherical shape increases the focusing power of the lens and has the effect of bringing the focused image of a near object forward to the retinal surface.

REFRACTION AND ACCOMMODATION

When light passes from one medium to another, its velocity is either decreased or increased, and the direction of light movement is changed. The bending of light at an angulated surface is called *refraction*. When light rays pass through the center of a lens, their direction is not changed; however, rays passing laterally through a lens are bent (Fig. 52-13). Usually, the refractive power of a lens is described as the distance (in meters) from its surface, at which the rays come into focus (focal length), or as the reciprocal of this distance (diopters). For example, a lens that brings an object into focus at 0.5 m has a refractive power of 2 diopters (1.0/0.5 = 2.0). With a fixed power lens, the closer an object is to the lens, the further behind the lens the focus point will be. The closer the object, the stronger, as well as the more perfect, the focusing system must be.

In the eye, the major refraction of light begins at the convex corneal surface. Further refraction occurs as light moves from the posterior corneal surface to the aqueous humor, from the aqueous humor to the anterior lens surface, and from the posterior lens surface to the vitreous humor. In the eye, the focusing surface, the retina, is at a fixed distance from the lens; thus, adjustability in the refractive power of the lens is needed to keep the image of close objects in sharp focus on the retina. This is called *accommodation*. The adjustable lens shape and the adjustable pupillary opening must be under the control of a feedback system that makes these adjustments while evaluating image sharpness. All of this is accomplished by accommodation and pupillary reflexes under the control of the visual acuity centers in the primary visual and association cortex. These areas provide feedback control for modifying lens shape and, therefore, of visual clarity.

When a refractive defect of the corneal surface does not permit the formation of a sharp image, the

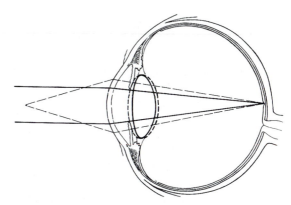

FIG. 52-13. Accommodation. The *solid lines* represent rays of light from a distant object, and the *dotted lines* represent rays from a near object. The lens is flatter for the former, more convex for the latter. In each case the rays of light are brought to a focus on the retina. (Chaffee, E. E., & Lytle, I. M. [1980]. *Basic physiology and anatomy* [4th ed.]. Philadelphia: J.B. Lippincott)

accommodative reflex continues the unsuccessful attempts of ciliary muscle contraction to alter the lens shape. The discomfort or pain associated with continuous muscle contraction is experienced as eye strain.

DISORDERS OF REFRACTION

A perfectly shaped optic globe and cornea result in optimal visual acuity (emmetropia), that is, a sharp image in focus at all points on the retinal surface in the posterior part, or fundus, of the eye. Unfortunately, individual differences in the formation and growth of the eyeball and cornea frequently result in inappropriate image focal formation. If the optic globe is too short for distant vision, the image is focused posterior to (in back of) the retina. This is called *hyperopia* or *farsightedness* (Fig. 52-14). In such cases, the accommodative changes of the lens cannot bring near objects into focus. This type of defect is corrected by appropriate biconvex lenses. If the eyeball is too long for near vision, an infinitely distant target is focused anterior to (in front of) the retina. This condition is called *myopia* or *nearsightedness* (see Fig. 52-14). It can be corrected with an appropriate biconcave lens. Radial keratotomy, a form of refractive corneal surgery, can be performed to correct the defect. This surgical procedure involves the use of radial incisions to alter the corneal curvature. Nonuniform curvature of the horizontal plane, in contrast with the vertical plane, of the refractive transparent media, usually of the cornea, is called *astigmatism* and must be corrected by a compensatory lens. Spherical aberration involves a cornea with a nonspherical surface. Lens correction can be made for this defect as well.

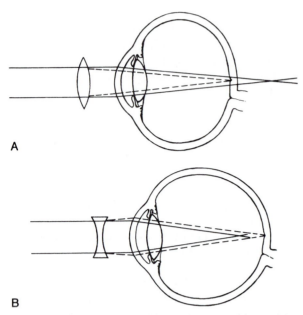

FIG. 52-14. (**A**) Hyperopia corrected by a biconvex lens, as shown by the *dotted lines.* (**B**) Myopia corrected by a biconcave lens, shown by the *dotted lines.* (Chaffee, E. E., & Lytle, I. M. [1980]. *Basic physiology and anatomy* [4th ed.]. Philadelphia: J.B. Lippincott)

DISORDERS OF ACCOMMODATION

Accommodation is the process whereby a clear image is maintained as the gaze is shifted from a far to a near object. It requires convergence of the eyes, pupillary constriction, and thickening of the lens through contraction of the ciliary muscle. Accommodation is under the control of the parasympathetic portion of the oculomotor (III) cranial nerve. The cell bodies of this nerve are contained in the oculomotor nuclear complex located in the midbrain, and its preganglionic axons synapse with postganglionic neurons of the ciliary ganglion in the orbit. The postganglionic axons enter the back of the eye and travel in the choroid layer to the ciliary muscle fibers. Visual function must be present to evaluate and adjust the clarity of the image. Thus, accommodation depends on the functional integrity of the entire visual system, including the forebrain and midbrain circuitry. Accommodation does not occur during sleep. An absolutely blind person cannot accommodate, nor can a person in coma.

Paralysis of the ciliary muscle, and thus of accommodation, is called *cycloplegia.* Pharmacologic paralysis is sometimes necessary to facilitate ophthalmoscopic examination of the fundus of the eye, especially in small children who are unable to hold a steady fixation during the examination. The lens shape is totally under the control of the pretectal region and the parasympathetic pathway by way of the oculomotor nerve to the ciliary muscle. Accommodation is lost with the destruction of this pathway.

The lens consists of transparent fibers arranged in concentric layers, of which the external layers are the newest and softest. There is no loss of lens fibers with aging. Instead, additional fibers are added to the outermost portion of the lens. As the lens ages, it thickens and its fibers become less elastic, so that the range of focus or accommodation is diminished to the point where reading glasses become necessary for near vision. This is called *presbyopia.*

CATARACTS

A cataract is a lens opacity that interferes with the transmission of light to the retina. It has been estimated that 5 million to 10 million people in the United States are visually disabled because of cataracts.[1] Cataracts are the most common cause of age-related visual loss in the world; they are found in about 50% of people 65 to 74 years old and in 70% of those over age 75.

The chief symptom of cataracts is a gradual decline in visual acuity (see Fig. 52-9). Vision for far and near objects decreases. Dilation of the pupil in dim light improves vision. With nuclear cataracts (those involving the lens nucleus), the refractive power of the anterior segment often increases to produce an acquired myopia. Thus, people with hyperopia may experience a "second sight" or improved reading acuity until increasing opacity reduces acuity. Central lens opacities may divide the visual axis and cause an optical defect in which two or more blurred images are seen. On ophthalmoscopic examination, cataracts may appear as a gross opacity filling the pupillary aperture or as an opacity silhouetted against the red background of the fundus.

A number of factors contribute to the development of cataracts, including genetic defects, environmental and metabolic influences, viruses, injury, and aging.[2] Both long-term exposure to sunlight (UVB radiation) and heavy smoking are associated with increased risk of cataract formation.[11] Although there is no accepted method of classification, most cataracts can be described as congenital, senile, traumatic, or secondary to systemic or ocular disease.

Congenital Cataract. A congenital cataract is one that is present at birth. Among the causes of congenital cataracts are genetic defects, toxic environmental agents, and viruses such as rubella. Maternal rubella during the first trimester can cause congenital cataract. Exposure of the embryo to ionizing radiation levels as low as 50 rads, such as occurs during barium enema or fluoroscopy, can induce congenital cataract. Cataracts and other developmental defects of the ocular apparatus depend both on the total dose and the embryonic stage at the time of exposure. During the last trimester of fetal life, genetically or environmentally influenced malformation of the superficial lens fibers can occur. Most congenital cataracts are not progressive and are not dense enough to cause significant visual impairment. However, if the cataracts are bilateral, and significant opacity is present, lens extraction should be done on one eye by age 2 months to permit the development of vision and prevent nystagmus. If the surgery is successful, the other eye should be done soon after.

Traumatic Cataract. Traumatic cataracts are most often caused by foreign body injury to the lens or blunt trauma to the eye. Foreign body injury that interrupts the lens capsule allows aqueous and vitreous humor to enter the lens and initiate cataract formation. Other causes of traumatic cataract are overexposure to heat (glassblower's cataract) or to ionizing radiation. The radiation dose necessary to cause a cataract varies with the amount and type of energy; younger lenses are most vulnerable.

Senile Cataract. Cataract is the most common cause of age-related vision loss in the world. With normal aging, both the nucleus and the cortex of the lens enlarge as new fibers are formed in the cortical zones of the lens. In the nucleus, the old fibers become more compressed and dehydrated. In addition, metabolic changes occur. Lens proteins become more insoluble, and concentrations of calcium, sodium, potassium, and phosphate increase. During the early stages of cataract formation, a yellow pigment and vacuoles accumulate in the lens fibers. Unfolding of protein molecules, cross-linking of sulfhydryl groups, and conversion of soluble to insoluble proteins lead to the loss of lens transparency. The onset is gradual, and increasingly blurred vision and visual distortion are the only symptoms.

Cataracts Due to Metabolic and Toxic Agents. Disorders of carbohydrate metabolism are the most common metabolic causes of cataract. Normally, glucose enters lens cells by diffusion and is reduced to sorbitol (an alcohol) by the intracellular enzyme aldose reductase. Sorbitol diffuses out of the lens fibers slowly, creating an osmotic gradient for the entry of water. In uncontrolled diabetes mellitus, the entry of water into the lens fibers accelerates with increased production of osmotically active sorbitol. The lens fibers swell and change their refractive properties, causing myopic changes and blurring of vision. The condition is slowly reversible unless it is longstand-

ing, in which case lens fiber destruction and permanent cataracts occur. The sugar galactose exerts the same effect in people with galactosemia.

Cataracts can result from a number of drugs. Dinitrophenol, a drug widely used for weight reduction during the 1930s; triparanol; chlorpromazine; and the adrenocorticosteroid drugs have all been implicated as causative agents in cataract formation. Busulfan, a cancer treatment drug, has been clearly linked to cataract formation. Frequent examination of lens transparency should accompany the use of these and any other substances with cataract-forming effects.

Treatment. There is no medical treatment for cataract. Surgery is the only treatment for correcting cataract-related vision loss. Surgery involves lens extraction and intraocular lens implantation, or the lens can be removed and the person fitted with contact lenses or occasionally with glasses. The American Academy of Ophthalmology has established the standard for when cataract surgery should be performed as the "best corrected" visual acuity of 20/50 or worse in the affected eye.[12] However, surgery may still be indicated when a person's best corrected acuity is 20/40 or better, if there is disabling glare or work-related disability, or if the cataract threatens to cause other eye problems, such as secondary glaucoma or uveitis. Surgery is commonly performed on an outpatient basis and with the use of local anesthesia. The absence of the lens is called *aphakia;* the eye with an implanted lens is described as being *pseudophakic.*

In summary, the refractive properties of the eye depend on the size and shape of the eyeball and the cornea and on the focusing abilities of the lens. In terms of visual function, refraction refers to the ability to focus an image on the retina. Errors in refraction occur when the visual image is not focused on the retina because of individual differences in the size or shape of the eyeball or cornea. In hyperopia, or farsightedness, the image falls in back of the retina. In myopia, or nearsightedness, the image falls in front of the retina. Because the focusing power of the eyeball and cornea is fixed, it is the lens that provides the means for the focusing of near images on the retina. The lens is a transparent and avascular biconvex structure suspended behind the iris and between the anterior chamber and the vitreous body that aids in visual focus. It is enclosed in an elastic capsule and attached to the ciliary body suspensory ligament. When the ciliary muscle contracts, the ligament relaxes and the lens becomes more nearly spherical, enabling the eye to focus on objects that are nearer to the eye. Relaxation of the ciliary muscle allows the eye to focus on distant objects. This mechanism is called accommodation and is controlled by the autonomic nervous system. Stimulation of the parasympathetic nervous system contracts the ciliary muscle and increases refractive power. With aging, the lens thickens and loses its ability to focus on near objects, a condition called *presbyopia*.

A cataract is a lens opacity. It can occur as the result of congenital influences, metabolic disturbances, infection, injury, and aging. The most common type of cataract is the senile cataract that occurs with aging. The treatment for a totally opaque or mature cataract is surgical extraction. An intraocular lens implant may be inserted during the surgical procedure to replace the lens that has been removed; otherwise, thick convex lenses or contact lenses are used to compensate for the loss of lens function.

■ THE VITREOUS AND RETINA

The posterior segment, which constitutes five sixths of the eyeball, contains the transparent vitreous humor and the neural retina. It is this interior part of the posterior chamber, called the *fundus*, that is visualized through the pupil with an ophthalmoscope.

DISORDERS OF THE VITREOUS

The vitreous humor is a colorless, structureless gel that fills the posterior segment of the eye. It consists of about 99% water, some salts, glycoproteins, and dispersed collagen fibrils. The vitreous is attached to the ciliary body and the peripheral retina in the region of the ora serrata and to the periphery of the optic disk.

The vitreous is a biologic gel. Disease, aging, and injury can disturb the factors that maintain water in suspension, causing liquefaction to occur. With the loss of gel structure, fine fibers, membranes, and cellular debris develop. When this occurs, floaters (images) can often be noticed as these substances move within the vitreous cavity during head movement. In disease, blood vessels may grow from the surface of the retina or optic disk onto the posterior surface of the vitreous, and blood may fill the vitreous cavity.

In a procedure called a *vitrectomy*, the removal and replacement of the vitreous with a balanced saline solution can restore sight in some people with vitreous opacities resulting from hemorrhage or vitreoretinal membrane formations that cause legal blindness. In this procedure, a small probe with a cutting tip is used to remove the opaque vitreous and membranes. The procedure is difficult and requires complex instrumentation. It is of no value if the retina is not functional.

DISORDERS OF THE RETINA

The function of the retina is to receive visual images, partially analyze them, and transmit this modified information to the brain. Disorders of the retina and

its function include (1) congenital photoreceptor abnormalities such as color blindness, (2) disturbances in blood vessels such as vascular retinopathies with hemorrhage and the development of opacities, (3) separation of the pigment and sensory layers of the retina (retinal detachment), (4) derangements of the pigment epithelium (retinitis pigmentosa), and (5) abnormalities of Bruch's membrane and choroid (macular degeneration). The retina has no pain fibers; therefore, most diseases of the retina are painless and do not cause redness of the eye.

The retina is composed of two parts: an outer pigmented layer and an inner neural layer. The neural retina covers the inner aspect of the posterior two thirds of the eyeball. Posteriorly, the retina is continuous with the optic nerve; anteriorly, the neural retina ends a short distance behind the ciliary body in a wavy border called the *ora serrata*.

The single pigment layer is separated from the vascular portion of the choroid by a thin layer of elastic tissue (Bruch's membrane), which contains collagen fibrils in its superficial and deep portions. The cells of the pigmented layer receive their nourishment by diffusion from the choroid vessels. Its tight junctions (and those of the retinal blood vessels) provide the blood–retina barrier. The neural retina is composed of three layers of neurons: a posterior layer of photoreceptors, a middle layer of bipolar cells, and an inner layer of ganglion cells that communicate with the photoreceptors. A superficial marginal layer contains the axons of the ganglion cells as they collect and leave the eye by way of the optic nerve (Fig. 52-15). These fibers lie adjacent to the vitreous humor. The interneurons, the horizontal and amacrine cells, have cell bodies in the bipolar layer, and they play an important role in modulating retinal function. Light must pass through the transparent inner layers of the sensory retina before it reaches the photoreceptors.

PHOTORECEPTORS

There are two types of photoreceptors: rods, capable of black–white discrimination, and cones, capable of color discrimination. Both types of photoreceptors are thin, elongated, mitochondria-filled cells with a single highly modified cilium (Fig. 52-16). The cilium has a short base, or inner segment, and a highly modified outer segment. The plasma membrane of the outer segment is highly folded to form membranous disks (rods) or conical shapes (cones) containing visual pigment. These disks are continuously synthesized at the base of the outer segment and shed at the distal end. The discarded membranes are phagocytized by the retinal pigment cells. If this phagocytosis is disrupted, as in retinitis pigmentosa, the sensory retina degenerates.

Rods. Photoreception involves the transduction of light energy into an altered ionic membrane potential of the rod cell. Light passing through the eye penetrates the nearly transparent neural elements to produce decomposition of the photochemical substance (visual pigment) called *rhodopsin* in the outer segment of the rod. Light that is not trapped by a rhodopsin molecule is absorbed by either the retinal pigment melanin or the more superficial choroid melanin. Rhodopsin consists of a protein (opsin) and a vitamin A-derived pigment called *retinal pigment*. During light stimulation, rhodopsin is broken down into its component parts (opsin and retinal), and retinal is converted into vitamin A. The reconstitution of rhodopsin occurs during total darkness; vitamin A is transformed into retinal, and then opsin and retinal combine to form rhodopsin. Because there are considerable stores of vitamin A in the retinal pigment cells and in the liver, a vitamin A deficiency must exist for weeks or months to have an impact on the photoreceptive process. Reduced sensitivity to light, a symptom of vitamin A deficiency, first affects night vision and is quickly reversed by injection or ingestion of the vitamin.

A pattern of light on the retina falls on a massive array of photoreceptors. These photoreceptors communicate with bipolar and other interneurons before action potentials in ganglion cells relay the message to the brain. For rods, this microcircuitry involves the convergence of signals from many rods on a single ganglion cell. This arrangement maximizes spatial summation and the detection of stimulated (light versus dark) receptors. Rod-based vision is partic-

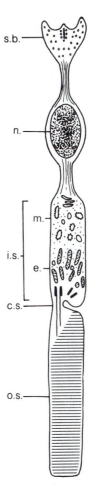

FIG. 52-16. Retinal rod, showing its component parts and the distribution of its organelles. Its outer segment (*o.s.*) contains the disks. The connecting structure between the outer and inner segments is labeled *c.s.* The inner segment is labeled *i.s.* In the outermost part of this there is a basal body, from which a modified cilium extends into the inner part of the outer segment. The inner segment is described as consisting of two parts, the ellipsoid portion (*e*) and the myoid portion (*m*). The former contains abundant mitochondria. The myoid portion contains rER, free ribosomes, and Golgi saccules. Farther in, the cell is constricted until it bulges to surround the nucleus (*n*). It then narrows again and ends in an expansion called the synaptic body (*s.b.*) because here the photoreceptor synapses with other nerve cells. (Courtesy of R. Young. From Ham, A. W., & Cormack, D. H. [1979]. *Histology* [8th ed.]. Philadelphia: J.B. Lippincott)

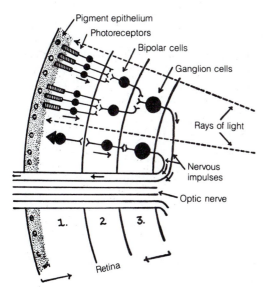

FIG. 52-15. Basic arrangement of the three orders of neurons in the nervous portion of the retina. Note that light rays and nerve impulses travel in opposite directions through the retina. (Ham, A. W., & Cormack, D. H. [1979]. *Histology* [8th ed.]. Philadelphia: J.B. Lippincott)

ularly sensitive to detecting light, and especially moving light stimuli at the expense of clear pattern discrimination. Thus, rod vision is particularly adapted for night and low-level illumination.

Dark adaptation is the process by which rod sensitivity increases to the optimum level. This requires approximately 4 hours in total or near-total darkness and involves only rod receptor (black-and-white) vision. During daylight, or high-intensity bombardment, the concentration of vitamin A increases and the concentration of the photopigment retinal decreases. During dark adaptation, increased synthesis of retinal from vitamin A results in a higher concentration of rhodopsin available to capture the light energy.

Cones and Color Sensitivity. Cone receptors that are selectively sensitive to different wavelengths of light provide the basis for color vision. Three types of cones, or cone-color systems, respond to the more blue, green, and red portions of the visible electromagnetic spectrum. This selectivity is due to the presence of one of three color-sensitive molecules to which the photochemical substance (visual pigment) is bound. The decomposition and reconstitution of the cone visual pigments are believed to be similar to that of the rods. The color a person senses depends on which set of cones or combination of sets of cones is stimulated in a given image.

Cones do not have the dark adaptation of rods. Consequently, the dark-adapted eye is a rod receptor eye with only black–gray–white experience (*scotopic vision*). The light-adapted eye (*photopic vision*) adds the capacity for color discrimination. Rhodopsin has its maximum sensitivity in the blue–green region of the spectrum. If red lenses are worn in daylight, only the red cones (and green cones to some extent) are in use; the rods (and blue cones) are essentially in the dark, and dark-adaptation proceeds. This method is used by military and night-duty airport control tower personnel to allow adaptation to take place before they go on duty in the dark.

Color Blindness. Color blindness is a misnomer for a condition in which people appear to confuse, mismatch, or experience reduced acuity for color discrimination. Such people are often unaware of their defect until challenged by problems resulting from difficulties in discriminating a red from a green traffic light or mismatches of colors in an art class. Most often the result of genetic factors, the deficit can result from defective function of one or more of the three color-cone mechanisms.[13] The deficiency is usually partial but can be complete. Rarely are two of the color mechanisms missing. When this does occur, usually red and green are missing. Extremely rare are people with no color mechanisms. For such people, the world is experienced entirely as black, gray, and white.

The genetically color-blind person has never experienced the full range of normal color vision and is unaware of what he or she is missing. Color discrimination is necessary for everyday living, and color-blind people, knowingly or unknowingly, make color discriminations based on other criteria, such as brightness or position. For example, the red light of a traffic signal is always the upper light, and the green

is the lower light. The color-blind person gets into trouble when brightness differences are minimal and discrimination must be based on hue and saturation qualities.

The genes responsible for color blindness affect receptor mechanisms rather than central acuity. The gene for red and green mechanisms is sex-linked (on the X chromosomes), resulting in a much higher incidence among males of red, green, or red-green color blindness. The gene affecting the blue mechanism is autosomal. Acquired color defects are more complex but tend to follow a general rule: disease of the more peripheral retina affects blue discrimination, and disease of the more central retina affects red and green discrimination. This is because there are no blue cones in the central fovea. Clinically, a defective color vision may be the only after effect of optic neuritis.

The simplest test for color discrimination defects employs pseudoisochromatic plates (*e.g.,* Ishihara plates) that use numbers or letters buried in a matrix of colored dots. These plates are arranged so that common color-blindness defects result in misreading of the number or letter. Proper testing conditions require good lighting and the use of a control plate interpretable by the most color-blind people, to eliminate inability to read as a confounding factor.

Retinitis Pigmentosa. Retinitis pigmentosa is a group of hereditary diseases that cause slow degenerative changes in the retinal receptors. In the United States, the incidence for all types of retinitis pigmentosa is 1 in 3500 and the carrier state may be 1 in 80. Slow destruction of the rods occurs, progressing from the peripheral to the central regions of the retina. Based on research with animal models, one probable mechanism of the disorder is a defect in phagocytic mechanisms of the pigment cells that cause membrane debris to accumulate and destroy the photoreceptors. The destruction results in dark lines and areas in which the pigment of the retinal pigment layer is unmasked by receptor loss. Night blindness, the first symptom of the disorder, often begins in early youth, with gross visual handicap occurring in the middle or advanced years. There is no effective treatment for this group of hereditary eye disorders.

MACULA AND FOVEA

A small area (approximately 1.5 mm in diameter) near the center of the retina, called the *macula*, is especially capable of acute and detailed vision. This area is composed entirely of cones. In the central portion of the macula, the *fovea centralis*, the blood vessels and innermost layers are displaced to one side instead of resting on top of the cones. This allows light to pass unimpeded to the cones without passing through several layers of retina. The density of cones drops off rapidly away from the fovea. There are no rods in the fovea, but their density increases as the cones decrease in density toward the periphery of the retina. Many cones are connected on a one-to-one basis with ganglion cells. In addition, retinal microcircuitry for cones emphasizes the detection of edges. This type of circuitry favors high acuity. A concentration of acuity favoring cones at the fovea supports the use of this part of the retina for fine analysis of focused central vision.

MACULAR DEGENERATION

Macular degeneration is characterized by destructive changes of the yellow pigmented area surrounding the central fovea (the macula) resulting from vascular disorders. It is the leading cause of blindness in people over 75 and of new blindness among people over age 65 years.[1] Although rare, macular degeneration can occur as a hereditary condition in young people and sometimes in adults.

Macular degeneration is characterized by the loss of central vision, usually in both eyes. The person may find it difficult to see at long distances (*e.g.*, in driving), do close work (*e.g.*, reading), see faces clearly, or distinguish colors. However, the person may not be severely incapacitated because the peripheral retinal function usually remains intact. With the help of low-vision aids, people can usually continue their normal activities.

There are two types of age-related macular degeneration: an atrophic nonexudative or "dry" form and an exudative or "wet" form.[14] The atrophic form is characterized by a gradual progressive bilateral vision loss due to atrophy and degeneration of the rod and cone photoreceptors. The exudative form is characterized by a formation of a neovascular (new blood vessel) membrane that separates the pigmented epithelium from the neuroretina. These new blood vessels have weaker walls than normal and are prone to leakage. This combination allows the leakage of serous or hemorrhagic into the subretinal space, causing separation of the pigmented epithelium from the neurosensory retina. Over time, the subretinal hemorrhages organize to form scar tissue. When this happens, retinal tissue death and loss of all visual function in the corresponding macular area occurs. Although about 80% to 85% of people with age-related macular degeneration have the atrophic form, 80% to 85% of severe vision loss can be ascribed to the exudative form.[15]

Although there is no treatment for the dry form of macular degeneration, argon laser photocoagula-tion may be useful in treating the wet form.[16] People with macular degeneration should be reassured that loss of central vision does not progress to loss of peripheral vision; most people can maintain their independence assisted by low vision aids.

RETINAL BLOOD SUPPLY

The blood supply for the retina is derived from two sources: the choriocapillaries of the choroid and the branches of the central retinal artery. The nutritional needs of the retina, including oxygen supply to the pigment cells and rods and cones, involve diffusion from blood vessels in the choroid. Because the choriocapillaries provide the only blood supply for the fovea centralis, detachment of this part of the sensory retina from the pigment epithelium causes irreparable visual loss. The bipolar, horizontal, amacrine, and ganglion cells, as well as the ganglion cell axons that gather at the disk, are supplied by branches of the retinal artery. The central artery of the retina is a branch of the ophthalmic artery. It enters the globe through the optic disk. Branches of the artery radiate over the entire retina, except for the central fovea, which is surrounded but is not crossed by arterial branches. The retinal veins follow a distribution parallel to the arterial branches and bring venous blood to the central vein of the retina, which exits the back of the eye through the optic disk. Funduscopic examination of the eye with an ophthalmoscope provides an opportunity to examine the retinal blood vessels as well as other aspects of the retina (Fig. 52-17). Because the retina is an extension of the brain and the blood vessels are, to a considerable extent, representative of brain blood vessels, the ophthalmoscopic examination of the fundus of the eye provides an opportunity for the study and diagnosis of metabolic and vascular diseases of the brain, as well as pathologic processes that are specific to the retina.

The functioning of the retina, like that of other cellular portions of the CNS, is highly dependent on an oxygen supply from the vascular system. One of the earliest signs of decreased perfusion pressure in the head region is a graying-out or blackout of vision, which usually precedes loss of consciousness. This can occur during large increases in intrathoracic pressure, which interferes with the return of venous blood to the heart (such as occurs with straining during defecation), with systemic hypotension, and often during sudden postural movements under conditions of decreased vascular adaptability.

Ischemia of the retina occurs under general circulatory collapse. If a person survives cardiopulmonary arrest, for instance, permanent decreased visual acuity can occur as a result of edema and the ischemic death of retinal neurons. This is followed by primary

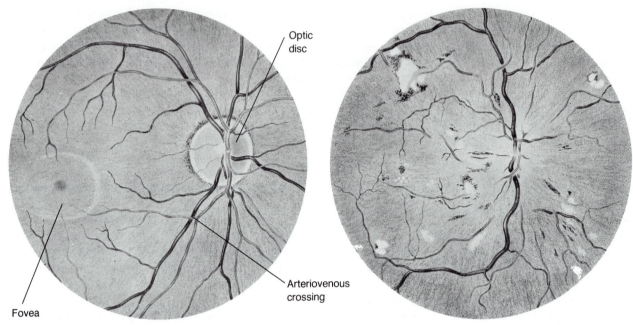

FIG. 52-17. Fundus of the eye as seen in retinal examination with an ophthalmoscope: (**left**) normal fundus; (**right**) pathologic fundus. The macula is not evident, but one can see flame-shaped hemorrhages and interrupted arteriovenous crossings. (Chaffee, E. E., & Lytle, I. M. [1980]. *Basic physiology and anatomy* [4th ed.]. Philadelphia: J.B. Lippincott)

optic nerve atrophy proportional to the extent of ganglionic cell death. The ophthalmic artery, the source of the central artery of the retina, takes its origin from the internal carotid artery. Intermittent retinal ischemia can accompany internal carotid or common carotid stenosis. In addition to ipsilateral intermittent blindness, contralateral hemiplegia or sensory deficits may accompany the episodes, depending on the competency of the circle of Willis in providing the brain with alternative arterial support. Treatment with anticoagulants or surgical endarterectomy may provide relief. Arteritis of the ophthalmic and central artery occurs more frequently in aged people; if severe, it can result in occlusive disease and permanent visual deficits.

Papilledema. The central retinal artery enters the eye through the optic *papilla* in the center of the optic nerve. The central vein of the retina follows the same path. The entrance and exit of the central artery and veins of the retina through the tough scleral tissue at the optic papilla can be compromised by any condition causing persistent increased intracranial pressure. The most common of these conditions are cerebral tumors, subdural hematomas, hydrocephalus, and malignant hypertension. The thin-walled, low-pressure veins are the first to collapse, with the consequent backup and slowing of arterial blood flow. Under these conditions, capillary permeability increases, and leakage of fluid results in

edema of the optic papilla, called papilledema. The interior surface of the papilla is normally cup-shaped and can be evaluated through an ophthalmoscope. With papilledema, sometimes called *choked disk*, the optic cup is distorted by protrusion into the interior of the eye. Because this sign does not occur until the intracranial pressure is significantly elevated, compression damage to the optic nerve fibers passing through the lamina cribrosa may have begun. Thus, as a warning sign, papilledema occurs quite late. Unresolved papilledema results in the destruction of the optic nerve axons and blindness.

Retinal Artery Occlusion. Complete occlusion of the central artery of the retina results in sudden unilateral blindness (anopsia). This is an uncommon disorder of older people and is most often due to embolism or atherosclerosis. Because the retina has a dual blood supply, the survival of retinal structures is possible if blood flow can be reestablished within 90 minutes.[2] If blood flow is not restored, the infarcted retina swells and opacifies. Because the receptors of the central fovea are supplied with blood from the choroid, they survive. A cherry-red spot (healthy fovea) is seen surrounded by the pale white opacified retina. Although the nerve fibers of the optic disks are adequately supplied by the choroid, the disk becomes pale because of the death of the optic fibers (optic atrophy) after the death of their ganglionic cells.

Occlusions of branches of the central artery, called branch arterial occlusions, are essentially retinal strokes. These occur mainly as a result of emboli and local infarction in the neural retina. The opacification that follows is often slowly resolved, and retinal transparency is restored. Local blind spots (scotomas) occur, however, because of the destruction of local elements of the retina. Loss of the axons of destroyed ganglion cells results in some optic nerve atrophy.

Central Retinal Vein Occlusion. Occlusion of the central retinal vein results in venous dilation, stasis, and reduced flow through the retinal veins. It is usually monocular and causes rapid deterioration of visual acuity. Superficial and deep hemorrhages throughout the retina follow, because of the increased capillary wall fragility resulting from the decreased venous outflow as well as lack of arterial inflow.

Among the causes of central retinal vein obstruction are hypertension, diabetes mellitus, and conditions such as sickle cell anemia, which slow the venous blood flow. The reduction in blood flow results in neovascularization with fibrovascular invasion of the space between the retina and the vitreous humor. In addition to obstructing normal visual function, the new vessels are fragile and prone to hemorrhage. Escaped blood may fill the space between the retina and vitreous, producing the appearance of a sudden veil over the visual field. The blood can find its way into the aqueous humor (hemorrhagic glaucoma). Photocoagulation of the spreading new blood vessels with high-intensity light or laser beam is used to prevent blindness and eye pain. As the hemorrhage is resolved, degenerating blood products can produce contraction of the vitreous and formation of fibrous tissue within it, causing tears and detachment of the retina.

Much more common are local vein occlusions with regional and focal capillary microhemorrhages that produce the same but more restricted pathologic effects. These microhemorrhages result in the formation of rings of yellow exudate composed of lipid and lipoprotein blood-breakdown products. Microhemorrhages deep in the neural retina are somewhat restricted by the vertical organization of the neural elements and result in dot hemorrhages. Microhemorrhages in the layer of ganglionic cell axon bundles result in cotton-wool spots.

VASCULAR RETINOPATHIES

Vascular disorders of the retina result in microaneurysms, neovascularization, hemorrhage, and formation of retinal opacities. *Microaneurysms* are outpouchings of the retinal vasculature. On ophthalmoscopic examination, they appear as minute unchanging red dots associated with blood vessels. They tend to leak plasma and are often surrounded by edema, which gives the retina a hazy appearance. Microaneurysms can be identified with certainty using fluorescein angiography (the fluorescein dye is injected intravenously and the retinal vessels are subsequently photographed using a special ophthalmoscope and fundus camera). The microaneurysms may bleed. Areas of hemorrhage and edema tend to clear spontaneously; however, they reduce visual acuity if they encroach on the macula and cause degeneration before they are absorbed.

Neovascularization involves the formation of new blood vessels. They can develop from the choriocapillaries, extending between the pigment layer and the sensory layer, or from the retinal veins, extending between the sensory retina and the vitreous cavity and sometimes into the vitreous. These new blood vessels are fragile, leak protein, and tend to bleed. Neovascularization occurs in a number of conditions that impair retinal circulation, including stasis because of hyperviscosity of blood or decreased flow, vascular occlusion, sickle cell disease, sarcoidosis, diabetes mellitus, and retinopathy of prematurity (retrolental fibroplasia). The cause of new blood vessel formation is uncertain. The stimulus is presumably a diffusible factor that is released during impaired perfusion or oxygenation of retinal tissue. The vitreous humor is thought to contain a substance that normally inhibits neovascularization, and this factor is apparently suppressed under conditions in which the new blood vessels invade the vitreous cavity.

Hemorrhage can be preretinal, intraretinal, or subretinal. Preretinal hemorrhages occur between the retina and the vitreous. These hemorrhages tend to be large because the blood vessels are only loosely restricted; they may be associated with a subarachnoid or subdural hemorrhage and are usually regarded as a serious manifestation of the disorder. They usually reabsorb without complications unless they penetrate into the vitreous. Intraretinal hemorrhages occur because of abnormalities of the retinal vessels, diseases of the blood, increased pressure within the retinal vessels, or vitreous traction on the vessel. Systemic causes include diabetes mellitus, hypertension, and blood dyscrasias. Subretinal hemorrhages are those that develop between the choroid and pigment layer of the retina. A common cause of subretinal hemorrhage is neovascularization. Photocoagulation may be used to treat microaneurysms and neovascularization.

Light normally passes through the transparent inner portions of the sensory retina before reaching the photoreceptors. *Opacities* such as hemorrhages, exudate, cotton-wool patches, edema, and tissue proliferation produce a localized loss of transparency that can be observed with the use of an ophthalmoscope. *Exudates* are opacities resulting from inflammatory processes. The development of exudates often results in the destruction of the underlying retinal pigment and choroid layer. *Deposits* are localized opacities consisting of lipid-laden macrophages or accumulated cellular debris. *Cotton-wool patches* are retinal opacities with hazy, irregular outlines. They occur in the nerve fiber layer and contain cell organelles. Cotton-wool patches are associated with retinal trauma, severe anemia, papilledema, and diabetic retinopathy.

Retinopathy of Prematurity. Retinopathy of prematurity, previously called *retrolental fibroplasia*, is a potentially blinding abnormal proliferation of retinal blood vessels that is unique to the preterm infant. The improved survival rates of low-weight premature infants during the past several decades has resulted in an increased incidence of retinopathy of prematurity.[17] The survival rate for infants weighing 500 to 750 g at birth is approaching 60%, and, for those weighing 751 to 1000 g, it is approaching 90%.[18]

The immature retina has two blood supplies, the choroidal and the inner retinal vessels. The choroidal blood vessels, which lie on the outside of the retina, develop early and are the sole supplier of nourishment for the immature retina. Vascularization of the inner retina begins during the 16th week of gestation as the retinal vessels grow and advance outward in a 360-degree circle from the optic nerve; they reach the ora serrata at the nasal periphery by 32 weeks, and the temporal periphery by around the 40th week of gestation.[19] Retinopathy of prematurity develops at the site of these newly forming retinal vessels. Normally, these vessels develop under hypoxic conditions that exist in utero. Unfortunately, most premature babies require some supplemental oxygen to sustain extrauterine life. When confronted with the hyperoxic conditions that occur when a baby is born prematurely, these immature vessels constrict and obliterate. After cessation of oxygen therapy, the blood vessels that were not obliterated begin to proliferate and grow rapidly in an attempt to reestablish and complete the vascularization of the inner retina. This area of rapid vascular growth usually forms an abrupt, rather than a gradual, junction between the vascular and avascular retina; the vessels are often abnormal and weak and can grow into the vitreous body, where they may cause leakage of fluid or hemorrhage with resultant formation of scar tissue. As the scar tissue shrinks, it can exert traction on the retina, causing retinal detachment and permanent loss of vision.

The more premature the infant, the greater the risk of retinopathy developing. The incidence of retinopathy of prematurity in infants weighing 500 to 750 g is almost 100% with severe disease developing in about 30% of these infants; the incidence of retinopathy in those weighing 751 to 1000 g is almost 80% with severe disease occurring in about 10% of infants.[18]

In 1984, the Committee for the Classification of Retinopathy of Prematurity developed an international system for classification that divides the retina into three zones (360-degree circles spaced between the optic nerve and the ora serrata) and characterizes the extent of involvement by the number of clock hours involved.[20] The system includes four stages of retinopathy. In *stage I disease*, a flat white line of demarcation has developed, separating the vascularized retina from the undeveloped avascular retina. In *stage II disease*, the line of demarcation has height and width; it extends out of the plane of the retina into the vitreous. In *stage III disease*, extraretinal proliferation of vascular tissue is present along the ridge of the demarcation line and may extend into the vitreous. A plus (+) is added to the stage (*e.g.*, III+ retinopathy of prematurity) when the retinal vasculature posterior to the ridge becomes enlarged, dilated, and tortuous. *Stage IV* disease is characterized by detachment of the retina. Retinal detachment results in blindness, therefore, treatment should be initiated before stage IV disease.

It has been recommended that all infants born less than 1251 g have an ophthalmic examination at 4 to 6 weeks of life. If no disease or stage I or II disease is detected, repeat ophthalmic exams should be scheduled according to the infant's level of risk until the retina is completely vascularized.[21] In many cases of stage I and II disease, partial or complete regression may occur in one or both eyes. Infants having stage III+ disease in zones I or II in five contiguous or eight cumulative clock hours (threshold retinopathy of prematurity) should be treated promptly because rapid progression to stage IV disease is possible.

Treatment consists of cryotherapy to the vascular portion of the retina. During cryotherapy, the trained ophthalmologist or ocular surgeon places the cryoprobe on the outside of the eye to produce transcleral freezing and destruction of the abnormal vessels. Cryotherapy has been shown to reduce the risk of unfavorable outcome due to retinopathy of prematurity by 50%.[21] Because the incidence of myopia and astigmatism is greater among children treated with cryotherapy, infants requiring treatment should be closely followed by an ophthalmologist.

Diabetic Retinopathy. Diabetic retinopathy is the third leading cause of new blindness, for all ages, in the United States. It ranks first as the cause of new blindness in people between the ages of 20 and 74 years, with 12% of all new cases of blindness caused by diabetes.[22] The risk of blindness for the nation's 12 million diabetics is 25 times that of the general population.

Diabetic retinopathy can be divided into two types: (1) background and (2) proliferative (Fig. 52-18). Background retinopathy is confined to the retina. It involves thickening of the retinal capillary walls and microaneurysm formation. Ruptured capillaries cause small intraretinal hemorrhages, and microinfarcts may cause cotton-wool exudates. A sensation of glare (because of the scattering of light) is a common complaint. The most common cause of decreased vision in people with background retinopathy is macular edema. It represents fluid accumulation within the retina stemming from a breakdown in the blood–retina barrier.

Proliferative diabetic retinopathy represents a more severe retinal change than background retinopathy. It is characterized by formation of new fragile blood vessels (neovascularization) at the disk and elsewhere in the retina. These vessels grow in front of the retina along the posterior surface of the vitreous or into the vitreous. They threaten vision in two ways. First, because they are abnormal, they tend to bleed easily, causing leakage of blood into the vitreous cavity, with subsequent decrease in visual acuity. Second, the blood vessels attach firmly to the retinal surface and posterior surface of the vitreous, such that normal movement of the vitreous may exert a pull on the retina, causing retinal detachment and progressive blindness. Early proliferative diabetic retinopathy is likely to be asymptomatic so it is important that it be identified early, before bleeding occurs and obscures the view of the fundus or leads to fibrosis and retinal attachment.

The American Academy of Ophthalmology has published suggested guidelines for the management and follow-up of people with diabetic retinopathy.[23] These recommendations suggest that the first retinal examination for people whose diabetes was diagnosed before age 30 can be safely delayed until 5 years after diagnosis. For older people, the first retinal examination should be performed at the time of initial diagnosis. After the initial eye examination, every person with diabetes should have regular ocular follow-ups, at least once a year and more frequently if warranted by the severity of the retinopathy. The ocular examination by the ophthalmologist should include acuity measurements, slit-lamp biomicroscopy, and direct and indirect ophthalmoscopy of the retina through fully dilated pupils. When indicated, color fundus photographs and fluorescein angiograms should be done.

There is growing evidence to suggest that careful control of blood sugars in people with diabetes mellitus may retard the onset and progression of retinopathy. Photocoagulation provides the only major direct treatment modality for the neovascularization that leads to microhemorrhage. It destroys not only the proliferating vessels, but also the ischemic retina, and therefore reduces the stimulus for further

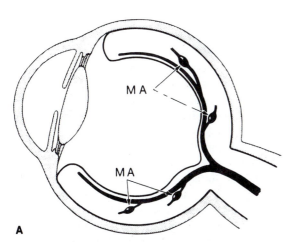
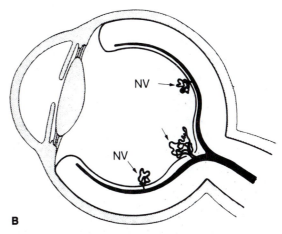

A **B**

FIG. 52-18. Nonproliferative and proliferative lesions in retinopathy of the person with diabetes. (**A**) Background retinopathy in which the abnormal blood vessels are contained in the retina. The microaneurysms (MA) are shown schematically within the retina. (**B**) Proliferative retinopathy in which neovascularization or new vessel (NV) formation occurs and breaks through the surface of the retina, growing into the vitreous cavity. (Copyright 1978 by the American Diabetes Association, Inc. Reprinted from Diabetes Forecast by permission)

neovascularization. Vitrectomy has proved effective in removing vitreous hemorrhage and severing vitreoretinal membranes that develop.

Hypertensive Retinopathy. Longstanding systemic hypertension results in the compensatory thickening of arteriolar walls, which effectively reduces capillary perfusion pressure. Ordinarily, retinal blood vessels are transparent and are seen as a red line; in venules, the red cells resemble a string of boxcars. On ophthalmoscopy, arteries appear paler than veins because they have thicker walls. The thickened arterioles in chronic hypertension become opaque and have a copperwiring appearance. Edema, microaneurysms, intraretinal hemorrhages, exudates, and cotton-wool spots are all observed. Malignant hypertension involves swelling of the optic disk as a result of the local edema produced by escaped fluid. If the condition is permitted to progress long enough, serious visual deficits result.

Sudden increases in blood pressure do not permit the protective thickening of arteriolar walls, and hemorrhage is likely to occur. Trauma to the optic globe or the head, sudden high blood pressure in eclampsia, and some types of renal disease are characteristically accompanied by edema of the retina and optic disk as well as an increased likelihood of hemorrhage.

Atherosclerosis of Retinal Vessels. In atherosclerosis, the lumen of the arterioles becomes narrowed. As a result, the retinal arteries become tortuous and narrowed. At sites where the arteries cross and compress veins, the red cell column of the vein appears distended. Exudate accumulates on arteriolar walls as plaque or cytoid bodies. Deep and superficial hemorrhages are common. Atheromatous plaques of the central artery are associated with danger of stasis, thrombi of the central veins, and occlusion.

RETINAL DETACHMENT

Retinal detachment involves the separation of the sensory retina from the pigment epithelium (Fig. 52-19). It occurs when traction on the inner sensory layer or a tear in this layer allows fluid, usually vitreous, to accumulate between the two layers. Retinal detachment that occurs secondary to breaks in the sensory layer of the retina is termed *rhegmatogenous detachment* (*rhegma* in Greek meaning "rent" or "hole"). The vitreous is normally adherent to the retina at the optic disk, macula, and periphery of the retina. When the vitreous shrinks, it separates from the retina at the posterior pole of the eye (posterior vitreous detachment), but at the periphery the vitreous pulls on the attached retina, which can lead to

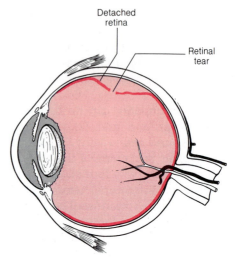

FIG. 52-19. Detached retina.

tearing of the retina. Sometimes flashing lights (photopsias) are experienced when this occurs. Vitreous fluid can enter the tear and contribute to further the separation of the retina from its overlying pigment layer. Myopia and aphakia are two of the most common predisposing factors. Detachment may also occur secondary to the presence of exudates that separate the two retinal layers. Exudative detachment may occur secondary to intraocular inflammations, intraocular tumors, or certain systemic diseases. Inflammatory processes include posterior scleritis, uveitis, or parasitic invasion.

Detachment of the neural retina from the retinal pigment layer (retinal detachment) separates the receptors from their major blood supply, the choroid. If detachment continues for some time, permanent destruction and therefore blindness of that part of the retina occur. The bipolar and ganglion cells survive because their blood supply, by way of the retinal arteries, remains intact. Without receptors, however, there is no visual function.

The primary symptom of retinal detachment is loss of vision. There is no pain. Because the process begins in the periphery and spreads circumferentially and posteriorly, initial visual disturbances may involve only one quadrant of the visual field. Large peripheral detachments may be present without involvement of the macula, so that visual acuity remains unaffected. The tendency, however, is for detachments to enlarge until all of the retina is detached.

Diagnosis is based on the ophthalmoscopic appearance of the retina. Treatment is aimed at closing retinal tears and reattaching the retina. Small tears may be closed using cryotherapy (freezing), diathermy (heat), or photocoagulation (laser). Rhegmatogenous detachment usually requires surgical treatment. Scleral buckling is the primary surgical procedure performed to reattach the retina. The procedure requires careful location of the retinal break and treatment with diathermy, cryotherapy, or laser to produce chorioretinal adhesions that seal the retinal tears so that the vitreous can no longer leak into the subretinal space. With scleral buckling, a piece of silicone (the buckle) is sutured and infolded into the sclera, physically indenting the sclera so it comes in contact with the separated pigment and retinal layers. Pneumatic retinopexy involves the intraocular injection of an expandable gas instead of a piece of silicone to form the indentation. An overall reattachment rate of 90% is reported; however, the visual results depend on the preoperative status of macula.[12]

Tests of Retinal Function. The diagnosis of retinal disease is based on history, tests of visual acuity, refraction, visual field tests, color vision tests, and often fluorescein angiography. Electroretinography (ERG) can be used to measure the electrical activity of the retina in response to a flash of light. The recorded ERG represents the difference in electrical potential between an electrode placed in a corneal contact lens and one placed on the forehead. The test can be used to evaluate retinal function in people with an opaque lens or vitreous body. The electro-oculogram (EOG) records the electrical potentials between the front of the eye and the retina in the back of the eye. It is recorded from two electrodes, one placed above and the other lateral to the eye. The EOG measures eye movement and is frequently used in sleep studies.

In summary, the retina covers the inner aspect of the posterior two thirds of the eyeball and is continuous with the optic nerve. It contains the neural receptors for vision, and it is here that light energy of different frequencies and intensities is converted to graded local potentials, which are converted to action potentials and transmitted to visual centers in the brain. The retina is composed of an outer pigmented layer, which prevents the scattering of light stimuli and contains the enzymes for the synthesis of visual pigments. There are two types of photoreceptors: rods, capable of black-and-white discrimination, and cones, capable of color discrimination. Both rods and cones contain visual pigments. With exposure to light energy within a particular frequency, the visual pigment decomposes, causing nerve excitation. There is a maximal density of cones in an area of the posterior retina called the macula. Macular degeneration, a leading cause of blindness in the elderly, results from destructive changes in the macula. The rods, which sense maximal spatial relationships, have their highest density toward the periphery of the eye. The photoreceptors normally shed portions of their outer segments. These segments are phagocytized by cells in the pigment epithelium. Failure of phagocytosis, as occurs in one form of retinitis pigmentosa, results in degeneration of the pigment layer and blindness.

*The retina receives its blood from two sources: the cho-*riocapillaries, which supply the pigment layer and the outer portion of the sensory retina adjacent to the choroid, and the branches of the retinal artery, which supply the inner half of the retina. The retinal blood vessels are normally apparent through the ophthalmoscope. Disorders of retinal vessels can result from a number of local and systemic disorders, including retinopathy of prematurity, diabetes mellitus, and hypertension. They cause vision loss through changes that result in hemorrhage, the production of opacities, and separation of the pigment epithelium and sensory retina. Retinal detachment involves separation of the sensory receptors from their blood supply; it causes blindness unless reattachment is promptly accomplished.*

■ NEURAL PATHWAYS AND CORTICAL CENTERS

Full visual function requires normally developed brain-related functions of photoreception, visual sensation and perception, and pupillary reflex. These functions depend on the integrity of all visual pathways including the retinal circuitry and the pathway from the optic nerve.

OPTIC PATHWAYS

Visual information is carried to the brain by the axons of the retinal ganglion cells forming the optic nerve. Surrounded by pia mater, cerebrospinal fluid, arachnoid, and dura mater, the optic nerve represents an outgrowth of the brain rather than a peripheral nerve. The optic nerve extends from the back of the optic globe through the orbit and the optic foramen, into the middle fossa, and on to the optic chiasm at the base of the brain—a distance of 40 to 50 mm in the adult (Fig. 52-20). Axons from the nasal half of the retina remain medial and those from the temporal retina remain lateral in the optic nerve.

The two optic nerves meet and fuse at the optic chiasm, located on the ventral and most rostral end of the brain stem, just in front of the infundibular stalk and pituitary gland. In the chiasm, axons from the nasal retina of the opposite side and axons from the temporal retina on the same side are organized to form the optic tracts. Thus, one optic tract contains fibers from both eyes that transmit information from the same visual field. The fibers of the optic tracts move laterally around the cerebral peduncles to synapse in the lateral geniculate nucleus (LGN) of the thalamus. Axons from these neurons in the LGN form the optic radiations to the primary visual cortex in the calcarine area of the occipital lobe. The LGN receives input from the visual cortex, oculomotor centers in the brain stem, and the brain stem reticular formation. It is thought to modify the pattern and

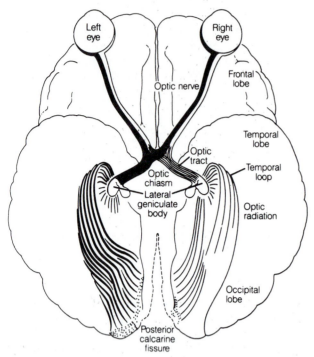

FIG. 52-20. Optic pathways. All of the nasal fibers of the right and left eye decussate (cross) at the optic chiasm. (Newell, F. W. [1982]. *Ophthalmology: Principles and concepts* [5th ed.]. St. Louis: C.V. Mosby)

strength of the retinal input. The pattern for information transmission that was established in the optic tract is retained in the optic radiations. For example, the axons from the right visual field, represented by the nasal retina of the right eye and the left temporal retina of the left eye, are united at the chiasm and continue through the left optic tract and left optic radiation to the left visual cortex, where visual experi-

ence is first perceived. The left primary visual cortex thus receives two representations of the right visual field. The left LGN and the left primary visual cortex retain physical separation of information from the left and right representations of the right visual field. At the cortical level, interaction between these slightly disparate representations occurs and provides the basis for the sensation of depth in the near visual field.

VISUAL CORTEX

The primary visual cortex (area 17) is located in the calcarine fissure of the occipital lobe. It is at this level that visual sensation is first experienced (Fig. 52-21). The immediately neighboring associational visual cortex (areas 18 and 19), together with their thalamic nuclei, must be functional for added meaningfulness of visual perception. This higher-order aspect of the visual experience depends on previous learning.

Approximately 1 million retinal ganglion cell axons pass through the optic nerve and tract to reach the LGN in the thalamus, and more than 100 million arising from geniculate neuron axons provide the input to the billions of neurons in the visual cortex. Here the spatial representation of the visual field is retained in a distorted retinal map. The proportion of cells of the LGN and of the primary visual area devoted to analysis of the central visual field is greatly expanded, compared with that of the peripheral retina. From 80% to 90% of the cellular mass and area of the primary visual cortex is concerned with central vision. This accounts for the greatly increased visual acuity of central vision, not only at the retina but also at all levels of the visual pathway.

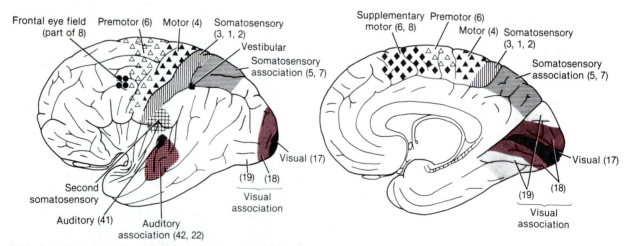

FIG. 52-21. Lateral view of the cortex with the lateral sulcus pried open to expose the insula (**left**) and medial view of the cortex (**right**), illustrating the location of the visual, visual association, auditory, and auditory association areas. (Nolte, J. [1981]. *The human brain* [p. 271]. St. Louis: C.V. Mosby. Reproduced with permission)

Circuitry in both the primary visual cortex and the associational visual areas is extremely discrete with respect to the location of retinal stimulation. For example, specific neurons respond to the moving edge of a particular inclination, specific colors, or familiar shapes.

This fine-grained organization of the visual cortex with functionally separate and multiple representations of the same visual field provides the major basis for visual sensation and perception. Because of this discrete circuitry, lesions of the visual cortex must be large to be detected clinically.

A flash of light delivered to the retina evokes potentials that can be measured and recorded by placing electrodes on the scalp over the occipital lobes. The waves of the evoked potentials, called pattern-reversed-evoked potentials or visual-evoked potentials, have proven to be a useful tool for clinical evaluation of the functional integrity of the successive levels of the visual pathway.

VISUAL FIELDS

The visual field refers to that area that is visible during fixation of vision in one direction. Because the visual system is organized with reference to the visual fields rather than to direct measures of neural function, the terminology for normal and abnormal visual characteristics is usually based on visual field orientation.

Most of the visual field is binocular, or seen by both eyes. This binocular field is subdivided into central and peripheral portions. The central portion provides high visual acuity and corresponds to the field focused on the central fovea; the peripheral and surrounding portion provides the capacity to detect objects, particularly moving objects. Beyond the visual field shared by both eyes, the left lateral periphery of the visual field is seen exclusively by the left nasal retina, and the right peripheral field is seen by the right nasal retina.

As with a camera, the simple lens system of the eye inverts the image of the external world on each retina. The right and left sides of the visual field are also reversed. The right binocular visual field is seen by the left retinal halves of each eye: the nasal half of the right eye and the temporal half of the left eye.

Once the level of the retina is reached, the nervous system plays a consistent game. The upper half of the visual field is received by the lower half of the retinas of both eyes, and the representations of this upper half of the field are carried in the lower half of each optic nerve to synapse in the lower half of the LGN of each side of the brain. Neurons in this part of the LGN send their axons through the inferior half of the optic radiation, which loops into the temporal lobe to the lower half of the primary visual cortex on each side of the brain.

Because of the lateral separation of the two eyes, the visual field as viewed by the two eyes results in a slightly different view of the world by each eye, called *binocular disparity*. Disparity between the laterally displaced images seen by the two eyes provides a powerful source of three-dimensional depth perception for objects within a distance of 30 m. Beyond that distance, the difference in the two images becomes insignificant, and depth perception is based on other cues such as the superimposition of the image of near objects over that of far objects, or the relatively faster movement of near objects than of far objects.

VISUAL FIELD DEFECTS

Visual field defects occur as a result of damage to the visual pathways or the visual cortex. Visual field testing or perimetry is used to identify defects and determine the location of lesions. The periphery of the opposite visual field is represented on the medial surface and in the depths of a deep medial calcarine sulcus of the occipital cortex (area 17). The central, high acuity part of the visual half field extends somewhat over the occipital pole. The visual association cortex surrounds the primary cortex on the superior, lateral, and inferior occipital lobe. This area is required for complex analysis and learned meaningfulness of visual stimuli.

Retinal Defects. All of us possess a hole, or *scotoma*, in our visual field of which we are unaware. Because the optic disc, where the optic nerve fibers exit the retina, does not contain photoreceptors, a corresponding location in the visual field constitutes a blind spot. Local retinal damage caused by small vascular lesions (retinal stroke) and other localized pathology can produce additional blind spots. As with the normal blind spot, people are not usually aware of the existence of scotomata in their visual fields unless they encounter problems seeing objects in certain restricted parts of the visual field.

Absences near or in the center of the bilateral visual field can be annoying and even disastrous. Although the hole is not recognized as such, the person finds that a part of a printed page appears or disappears depending on where the fixation point is held. Most people learn to position their eyes so as to use the remaining central foveal vision for high-acuity tasks. Defects in the peripheral visual field, including the monocular peripheral fields, are less annoying but potentially more dangerous. Often the person is unaware of the defect and, when walking or driving an automobile, does not see cars or bicyclists until their image reaches the functional visual field—sometimes too late to avert an accident. With careful education, a person can learn to shift the gaze constantly in such a way as to obtain visual coverage of important parts of the visual field. If the damage is at the retinal or optic nerve level, only the monocular field of the damaged eye becomes a problem. A lesion affecting the central foveal vision of one eye can result in complaints of eye strain during reading and other close work, because only one eye is really being used. Localized damage to the optic tracts, LGN, optic radiation, or primary visual cortex affects corresponding parts of the visual fields of both eyes.

Disorders of the Optic Pathways. The visual pathway extends from the front to the back of the head. It is much like a telephone line between distant points in that damage at any point along the pathway results in functional defects (Fig. 52-22). Among the disorders that can interrupt the visual pathway are vascular lesions, trauma, and tumors. For example, normal visual system function depends on vascular adequacy in the ophthalmic artery and its branches; the central artery of the retina; the anterior and middle cerebral arteries, which supply the intracranial optic nerve, chiasm, and optic tracts; and the posterior cerebral artery, which supplies the lateral geniculate, optic radiation, and visual cortex. In turn, adequacy of the posterior cerebral artery function depends on that of the vertebral and basilar arteries that supply the brain stem. Vascular insufficiency in any one of these arterial systems can seriously affect vision. Examination of the visual system function is

of particular diagnostic use because lesions at various points along the pathway have characteristic symptoms that assist in the localization of pathology.

Visual field defects of each eye and of the two eyes together are useful in localizing lesions affecting the system. Blindness in one eye is termed *anopia*. If half of the visual field for one eye is lost, the defect is termed *hemianopia;* loss of a quarter field is called *quadrantanopia.* Enlarging pituitary tumors can produce longitudinal damage through the optic chiasm with loss of the medial fibers of the optic nerve representing both nasal retinas and thus, both temporal visual half-fields. Loss of the temporal or peripheral visual fields on both sides results in a narrow binocular field, commonly called *tunnel vision.* The loss of different half-fields in the two eyes is called a *heteronymous* loss, and the abnormality is called *heteronymous hemianopia.* Destruction of one or both lateral halves of the chiasm is not uncommon with multiple aneurysms of the circle of Willis. Here the function of the left or both temporal retinas occurs, and the nasal fields of the left or of both eyes are lost. The loss of the nasal fields of both eyes is called *bitemporal heteronymous anopia.* With both eyes open, the person with bilateral defects still has the full binocular visual field.

Loss of the optic tract, lateral geniculate, full optic radiation, or complete visual cortex on one side results in loss of the corresponding visual half-fields in each eye. *Homonymous* means the same for both eyes. In left-side lesions, the right visual field is lost for each eye and is called *complete right homonymous hemianopia.* Partial injury to the left optic tract, LGN, or optic radiation can result in the loss of a quarter of

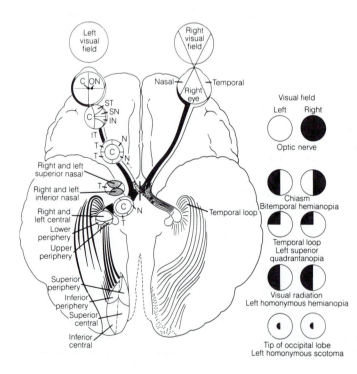

FIG. 52-22. Typical visual field defects that occur with damage to different regions of the optic pathways. Visual fields are diagrammed to reflect the source of the light that stimulates the retina. *C* = central, *ON* = optic nerve, *ST* = superior temporal, *IT* = inferior temporal, *SN* = superior nasal, *IN* = inferior nasal, *T* = temporal, *N* = nasal. Light from the temporal side stimulates the nasal portion of the retina, light from above stimulates the lower portion, and so on. Thus, the visual field defect caused by a lesion affecting fibers arising from the nasal half of the retina is diagrammed as a temporal field defect. (Newell, F. W. [1982]. *Ophthalmology: Principles and concepts* [5th ed.]. St. Louis: C.V. Mosby)

the visual field, again the same for both eyes. This is called *homonymous quadrantanopia* and, depending on the lesion, it can involve the upper (superior) or lower (inferior) fields. Because the optic radiation fibers for the superior quarter of the visual field traverse the temporal lobe, superior quadrantanopia is more common. The LGN, optic radiation, and visual cortex all receive their major blood supply from the posterior cerebral artery; thus, unilateral occlusion of this artery results in complete loss of the opposite field (homonymous hemianopia). Bilateral occlusion of these arteries results in total cortical blindness.

Disorders of the Visual Cortex. Discrete damage in the binocular portion of the primary visual cortex can also result in scotomas in the corresponding visual fields. If the visual loss is in the central high-acuity part of the field, severe loss of visual acuity and pattern discrimination occurs. The central, high-acuity portion of the visual field is located at the occipital pole. This region can be momentarily compressed against the occipital bone (contrecoup) after severe trauma to the frontal part of the cranium. Mechanical trauma to the cortex results in firing of neurons, experienced as flashes of light or "seeing stars." Destruction of the polar visual cortex causes severe loss of visual acuity and pattern discrimination. Such damage is permanent and cannot be corrected with lenses.

The bilateral loss of the entire primary visual cortex, called *cortical blindness,* eliminates all visual experience. Some suggestion remains that crude analysis of visual stimulation exists on reflex levels. Eye-orienting and head-orienting responses to bright moving lights, pupillary reflexes, and blinking at sudden bright light are retained even though vision has been lost. Extensive damage to the visual association cortex (areas 18, 19) that surrounds an intact primary visual cortex results in a loss of the learned meaningfulness of visual images (visual agnosia). The patient can see the patterns of color, shapes, and movement, but can no longer recognize formerly meaningful stimuli. Familiar objects can be described but not named or reacted to meaningfully. However, if other sensory modalities (hearing and touch) can be applied, full recognition occurs. Thus, this disorder represents a problem of recognition rather than intellect.

Testing of Visual Fields. Crude testing of the binocular visual field and the visual field of each individual eye (monocular vision) can be accomplished without specialized equipment. In the confrontation method, the examiner stands or sits 2 to 3 feet in front of the person to be tested and instructs the person to focus on an object such as a penlight with one eye closed. The object is moved from the center toward the periphery of the person's visual field and from the periphery toward the center, and the person is instructed to report the presence or absence of the object. By moving the object through the vertical, horizontal, and oblique aspects of the visual field, a crude estimate can be made of the visual field. If the test object is kept midway between the examiner and the person being tested, the examiner can close the corresponding eye and compare the person's monocular vision with his or her own. Large field defects can be estimated by the confrontation method, and it may be the only way for testing young children and uncooperative adults. Rapidly presenting the examiner's fingers toward the eyes and observing for a reflex blink to the threat is sometimes the only way to detect a visual field deficit in someone with decreased consciousness.

Accurate determination of the presence, size, and shape of smaller holes, or scotomata, in the visual field of a particular eye can be demonstrated by the ophthalmologist only through the use of a method known as *perimetry.* This is done by having the person look with one eye toward a central spot directly in front of the eye while the head is stabilized by a chin rest or bite board. A small dot of light or a colored object is moved back and forth in all areas of the visual field. The person reports whether or not the stimulus is visible and, if a colored stimulus is used, what the perceived color is. A hemispherical support is used to control and standardize the movement of the test object, and a plot of radial coordinates of the visual field is made. Perimetry provides a means of determining alterations from normal and, with repeated testing, a way of following the progress of the disease or treatment.

PUPILLARY REFLEXES

The pupillary reflex, which controls the size of the pupillary opening, is controlled by the autonomic nervous system. The sphincter muscle that produces pupillary constriction is innervated by postganglionic parasympathetic neurons of the ciliary ganglion and other scattered ganglion cells between the scleral and choroid layers (Fig. 52-23). The oculomotor (III) cranial nerve nucleus, located in the midbrain, provides the preganglionic innervation for these parasympathetic axons. Innervation for the dilator muscle is derived from thoracic sympathetic preganglionic neurons that send axons along the sympathetic chain to innervate the postganglionic neurons in the superior cervical ganglion. The postganglionic neurons send axons along the internal carotid and ophthalmic arteries to the posterior surface of the optic globe.

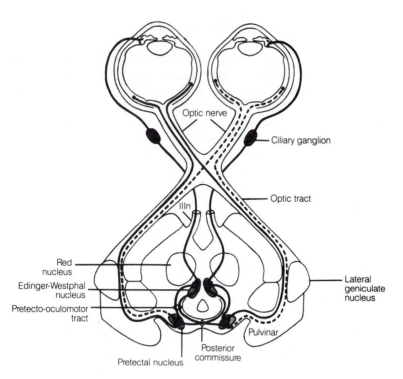

FIG. 52-23. Diagram of the path of the pupillary light reflex. (Reproduced with permission from Walsh, F. B., & Hoyt, W. F. [1969]. *Clinical neuro-ophthalmology* [3rd ed., vol. 1]. Baltimore: Williams & Wilkins)

These axons travel between the scleral and choroid layers to reach the dilator muscles of the iris. The pupillary reflex is controlled by a region in the midbrain called the *pretectum*. The pretectal areas on each side of the brain are interconnected, accounting for the binocular aspect of the light reflex. These areas project axons to nuclei of the midbrain called the *Edinger-Westphal nuclei*. These nuclei contain the parasympathetic preganglionic neurons, which innervate the ciliary ganglion and thus control the sphincters of the iris. Midbrain level evaluation with feedback control provides an automatic brightness control mechanism. The functional importance of this reflex mechanism is its rapidity, compared with the slow light and dark-adaptive retinal mechanism.

Normal function of the pupillary reflex mechanism is tested by shining a penlight into one eye of the person being tested. To avoid accommodation, the person is asked to stare into the distance. A rapid constriction of the pupil exposed to light should occur (direct light reflex, or direct pupillary reflex). Because the reflex is normally bilateral, the contralateral pupil should also constrict (consensual light reflex, or consensual pupillary reflex). Reflex pupillary dilation occurs more quickly in lightly pigmented eyes than in more darkly pigmented eyes. By shining the light first into one eye and then into the other eye and noting the response of both pupils, considerable information can be gathered about the function of the central nervous system (CNS) circuitry.

The circuitry of the light reflex is partially separated from the main visual pathway. This is illustrated by the fact that the pupillary reflex remains unaffected when lesions to the optic radiations or the visual cortex occur. The cortically blind person retains direct and consensual light reflexes. The light reflex also functions under light anesthetic levels and is used to evaluate the depth of anesthesia. When the reflex is lost, the anesthesia level is approaching that which depresses the respiratory reflexes as well.

Careful attention to inappropriate or unequal pupil diameters is diagnostically important. The integrity of the dual control of pupillary diameter is somewhat vulnerable to trauma, tumor enlargement, or vascular disease. Damage to the oculomotor nucleus or nerve not only eliminates innervation of many of the extraocular muscles and the levator muscle of the upper lid but also results in permanent pupillary dilation (*mydriasis*) in the affected eye. People with mydriasis experience discomfort in normal or brightly lit environments because of loss of pupillary constriction in the affected eye.

Lesions affecting (1) descending brain control of sympathetic outflow that passes through the cervical spinal cord, (2) ascending sympathetic preganglionic axons of the sympathetic ganglia, or (3) sympathetic postganglionic axonal plexus in the wall of the carotid artery can interrupt the sympathetic control of the iris dilator muscle, resulting in permanent pupillary constriction (*miosis*). Tumors of the orbit that compress structures behind the eye can eliminate all pupillary reflexes, usually before destroying the optic nerve.

The function of the sympathetic and parasym

pathetic control of the iris (and pupillary size) is differentially affected by many pharmacologic agents. Bilateral pupillary constriction is characteristic of opiate usage. Pupillary dilation results when topical parasympathetic blocking agents such as atropine or homatropine are applied and sympathetic pupillodilatory function is left unopposed. These medications are used by ophthalmologists to facilitate the examination of the transparent media and fundus of the eye. Miotic drugs such as pilocarpine have the opposite effect, facilitating aqueous humor circulation.

In summary, visual information is carried to the brain by axons of the retinal ganglion cells forming the optic nerve. The two optic nerves meet and fuse in the optic chiasm. The axons of each nasal retina cross in the chiasm and join the uncrossed fibers of the temporal retina of the opposite eye in the optic tract. From the optic chiasm, the crossed fibers of the nasal retina of one eye and the uncrossed temporal fibers of the other eye pass to the LGN and then to the primary visual cortex, which is located in the calcarine fissure of the occipital lobe. Damage to the visual pathways or visual cortex leads to visual field defects that can be identified through visual field testing or perimetry and used to determine the lesion's location. Damage to the visual association cortex can result in seeing an object, but with loss of learned recognition (visual agnosia).

The pupillary reflex, which controls the size of the pupil, is controlled by the autonomic nervous system. The parasympathetic nervous system controls pupillary constriction, and the sympathetic nervous system controls pupillary dilation.

■ EYE MOVEMENTS

Normal vision depends on the coordinated action of the entire visual system as well as a number of central control systems. It is through these mechanisms that an object is simultaneously imaged on the fovea of both eyes and perceived as a single image. Strabismus and amblyopia are two disorders that affect this highly integrated system.

EXTRINSIC EYE MUSCLES

Each eyeball can rotate around its vertical axis (lateral or medial rotation in which the pupil moves away from or toward the nose), its horizontal left–right axis (vertical elevation or depression in which the pupil moves up or down), and its longitudinal horizontal axis (in which the top of the pupil moves toward [intorsion] or away from [extorsion] the nose). *Conjugate movements* are those in which the optical axes of the two eyes are kept parallel, sharing the same visual field. *Gaze* refers to the act of looking steadily in one direction.

Six extrinsic muscles (four rectus and two oblique muscles) control the movement of each eye (Fig. 52-24). The four rectus muscles are named according to where they insert into the sclera on the medial, lateral, inferior, and superior surfaces of the eye. The two oblique muscles insert on the lateral posterior

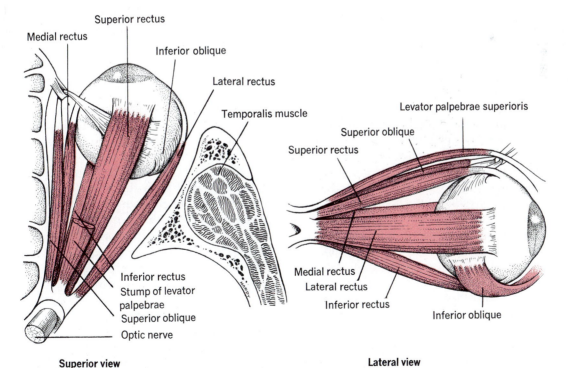

FIG. 52-24. Extrinsic muscles of the right eye: (**left**) viewed from above within the orbital cavity; (**right**) lateral view. (Chaffee, E. E., & Lytle, I. M. [1980]. *Basic anatomy and physiology* [4th ed.]. Philadelphia: J.B. Lippincott)

quadrant of the eyeball: the superior oblique on the upper surface and the inferior oblique on the lower. Each of the three sets of muscles in each eye is reciprocally innervated so that one muscle relaxes when the other contracts. The medial and lateral recti contract reciprocally to move the eye from side to side; the superior and inferior recti contract to move the eye up and down. The oblique muscles rotate the eye around its optic axis. Although the origins and insertions of the extrinsic eye muscles would seem to make their role in eye movement predictable, their function is somewhat complex. This is because the muscles insert into a rotatable eyeball.

Inserting approximately on the horizontal plane, the antagonistic medial and lateral recti rotate the eye medially (adduction) or laterally (abduction). When the optical axes of the two eyes are parallel, these muscles provide horizontal conjugate (paired) gaze. Convergence (moving toward a common point) and divergence (moving away from a common point) of the optical axes of the eyes result from the differential contraction of the recti muscles accompanied by coordinated inhibition of the antagonistic muscles. The phrase *being yoked together* is often used to describe such direct antagonism between eye muscles.

The actions of the superior and inferior recti are more complex. Their predominant action is the elevation and depression of the eyeball, usually a conjugate movement. Because of their medial orbit origin, both muscles contribute to medial rotation. In addition, each contributes to some extent to intorsion (superior rectus) and extorsion (inferior rectus).

Major functions of the oblique muscles are extorsion (the inferior oblique pulls the inferior surface of the eyeball medially) and intorsion (the superior oblique pulls the superior surface of the eyeball medially) of the optic globe. These muscles function as antagonists for rotation around the longitudinal axis of the eye. Because of its insertion position posterior to the equator of the eyeball, the superior oblique pulls the upward-pointed eye downward, assisting the function of the inferior rectus. The inferior oblique, similarly, pulls upward a downward-pointed eye, assisting the superior rectus. When the eye is strongly medially deviated, the oblique muscles function almost entirely as elevator and depressor muscles.

The extraocular muscles are innervated by three cranial nerves: the trochlear (IV) innervates the superior oblique, the abducens (VI) innervates the lateral rectus, and the oculomotor (III) innervates the remaining four muscles. The medial longitudinal fasciculus (MLF) connects the nuclei of these cranial nerves. This important tract system transmits impulses that coordinate conjugate movements of the

eye. Eye movements are further influenced by input from control centers in the frontal cortex (frontal premotor area), the visual association area, and the superior colliculus, a midbrain optic reflex center that is concerned with eye movements. Strong signals are also transmitted into the oculomotor system from the vestibular nuclei by way of the MLF (to be discussed later).

EYE MOVEMENTS AND GAZE

Eye movements can be categorized into five classes of movement: smooth pursuit, saccadic, vestibular, vergence, and tremor. Smooth pursuit (object following), saccadic (position correcting), and vestibular (nystagmus) movements involve conjugate coordination. *Vergence* (divergence and convergence) movements involve coordinated movements of the eyes in opposite directions. A *tremor* refers to involuntary rhythmic oscillatory (quivering) movements. Small-range optical tremor is a normal and useful independent function of each eye. Eye movements are important motor capabilities that are integrated into vestibular, auditory, and visual reflex and learned functions.

Smooth Pursuit Movements. Smooth pursuit movements are tracking movements that serve to maintain an object at a fixed point in the center of the visual fields of both eyes. The object may be moving and the eyes following it, or the object may be stationary and the head of the observer moving. Voluntary pursuit movements are tested by asking the person to follow a finger or another object as it is moved smoothly through the visual field. Successful conjugate tracking requires a functional optic system communicating to the superior colliculus and to the primary visual cortex. The communication from the primary visual cortex to the superior colliculus must also be functional.

Normal eye posture is a conjugate gaze directed straight forward with the head held in a forward-looking posture. Smooth pursuit movements normally begin from this position. In fact, holding a strongly deviated gaze becomes tiring within about 30 seconds, and most people make head and body rotation adjustments to bring the eyes to a central position within that time period.

Saccadic Movements. Saccadic eye movements are sudden, jerky conjugate movements that quickly change the fixation point. During reading, the fixation pattern involves a focus on a word or short series of words and then a sudden jump of the eyes to a new fixation point on the next word or phrase. These shifts in fixation points are saccadic movements. The neural circuitry that makes coordinated saccadic movements possible remains under study, but certain areas of the midbrain reticular formation are essential for these movements. Saccadic movements are quick readjustments of the binocular fixation point that must occur to accomplish a change in fixation. This readjustment occurs while searching the visual environment. Changes in fixation point must be accomplished quickly to provide the person with a new, stable part of the visual field on which to focus. No sensation of blur is experienced during the period of rapid eye movement, although the mechanism by which the blurred vision is eliminated is not understood.

The visual startle reaction in which the eyes are quickly turned in the direction of a sudden and intense visual stimulus entering the periphery of the visual field, is saccadic movement initiated by the optic system. This reflex occurs in the absence of the cortical portion of the visual system (cortical blindness). The auditory startle reaction (startle reflex) involves rapid saccadic movements in the direction of a sudden auditory stimulus. It is present in the neonate and in people with impaired cortical auditory apparatus.

The frontal eye fields of the premotor cortex are of critical importance for voluntary saccadic movements such as reading. If this frontal premotor area is not functional, a person can describe objects in the visual field but cannot voluntarily search the visual environment.

Vergence Movements. Convergence of the optical axes of the two eyes is an automatic aspect of changing binocular fixation from a distant to a close fixation point. This readjustment of the position of each eye in relation to the other accompanies changes in ciliary muscle activity that affect the lens shape and pupillary dilation that exposes more of the lens refractive surface. All of these adjustments function to permit a closer and sharper binocular retinal image and are included in the function of accommodation. Convergence can occur smoothly as a pursuitlike, continuous adjustment when a moving object approaches the observer. Convergence can also occur as a saccadic movement when fixation is changed from a distant to a near object, or vice versa. Divergence occurs when a fixated object recedes in the visual field. The convergence–divergence aspect of accommodation requires a functional visual cortex and intact projection to the pretectal area and to the parasympathetic efferent neurons of the oculomotor nerve. A region of the midbrain reticular formation near the oculomotor nuclei must also be functional for convergence to occur. Master control is by the depth perception mechanism of the occipital visual association cortex. Voluntary convergence is achieved by altering the fixation point to one close to the eyes, requiring participation of the frontal eye fields.

Optic Tremor. Without special equipment, the fine continuous tremor of each eye is difficult to detect. This tremor is attributed to the inequality in the number of motor units active in opposing extraocular muscles at any moment. Because of the great amplification factor between minute shifts in eye position relative to the large shifts in a distant fixation point, one might expect eye tremor to be a serious impediment to acuity. Yet, the visual system functions rapidly enough to keep up with these minute shifts in fixation; if the tremor were eliminated, the visual image would quickly fade away through adaptation of the individual cone receptors. The function of the tremor is to keep the retinal image moving over the receptor array so that it is constantly encountering recovered or unadapted receptors.

Horizontal Gaze. Lateral conjugate gaze is accomplished through a reflex mechanism involving the medulla, pons, and midbrain, which contain the sixth, fourth, and third cranial nerve nuclei. Lateral rotation of an eye results from the increased activity of the sixth-nerve-innervated lateral rectus muscle accompanied by the corresponding reduced activity of the third-nerve-innervated medial rectus muscle. Synergists of the medial rectus, the third-nerve-innervated superior and inferior recti, also must be inhibited. Communication between the sixth nerve and third nerve nuclei must be rapid and precise. Conjugate (bilateral) side-to-side eye movement involves lateral rotation of one eye and medial rotation of the other. This requires close coordination between the sixth nerve nucleus of one side and the third nerve nucleus of the other. Further, smooth movement in conjugate gaze requires continuous variation in the contractional tone in synergists as well as in opposing eye muscles throughout the full range of dual eye rotation.

Reflex coordination of lateral gaze involves a longitudinal tract system of the brain stem, the medial longitudinal fasciculus (MLF), that interconnects the lower motor neurons of the sixth and third cranial nerves. A region in the reticular formation near the sixth nerve nucleus, called the pontine gaze center, controls this highly coordinated reflex mechanism.

Destruction of the lateral gaze control region on one side results in ipsilateral gaze palsy (*i.e.*, there is lateral gaze to the contralateral side but not to the affected side). Interruption of the MLF on one side between the sixth and third nerve nuclei, called internuclear ophthalmoplegia which occurs in multiple sclerosis, results in abnormality of the contralateral lateral gaze: the eye on the affected side fails to adduct (cranial nerve III) when the contralateral eye abducts (cranial nerve VI). Bilateral destruction of the MLF results in loss of adduction during lateral gaze to either side. A visual target moving smoothly in the horizontal plane is followed by this conjugate gaze mechanism through the intervention of the superior colliculus, which communicates directly with this gaze center through tectobulbar fibers. Conjugate following of a bright, smoothly moving target occurs automatically, even in the absence of a functional visual cortex. In deep coma, for instance, the presence of visual following indicates that the brain stem, including the midbrain, remains functional. Voluntary control of conjugate following of a horizontally moving object in the visual field requires the function of the primary and associational visual cortices that project axons to the superior colliculus.

When a lateral conjugate following movement exceeds the range of eye rotation, head rotation is often added. The MLF extends down to cervical spinal levels. Descending control from the horizontal gaze center by way of this tract is exerted on the spinal accessory and other cervical-level lower motoneurons. By this means the powerful head-turning muscles, the sternocleidomastoid, and other cervical muscles are smoothly brought into play. The major function of the MLF is the coordination circuitry of the lateral gaze mechanism.

Vertical Gaze. Vertical gaze, or the upward and downward rotation of an eye, involves four extraocular muscles. The third-nerve-innervated superior rectus and inferior oblique work in concert to rotate the eye upward with coordinated inhibition of the inferior rectus (III) cranial nerve and superior oblique (IV) cranial nerve. Conjugate vertical gaze, upward or downward, with parallel optical axes of the two eyes is coordinated by a vertical gaze center located in the midbrain deep to the rostral end of the MLF. Communication between this center and the innervational nuclei does not use the MLF. Instead, another major longitudinal tract system, the central tegmental fasciculus (CTF), provides longitudinal communication.

Torsional Conjugate Eye Movements. Conjugate twisting, or torsion, of the two eyes occurs when the head is tipped to one side. Exact, appropriate countertorsion of the two eyes serves to preserve a stable visual field in spite of minor head movements. A torsion gaze center, or control region, in the reticular formation of the brain stem has yet to be clearly localized.

Conjugate gaze control is extremely precise, and the central circuits providing this capability are complex. The superior colliculus, the midbrain vertical and medullary horizontal gaze centers, and the cerebellum, which add temporal smoothness to these coordinated movements, are all involved.

DISORDERS OF EYE MOVEMENT

STRABISMUS

Strabismus, or squint, refers to any abnormality of eye coordination or alignment that results in loss of binocular vision. When images from the same spots in visual space do not fall on corresponding points of the two retinas, diplopia or double vision occurs. In standard terminology, the disorders of eye movement are described according to the direction of movement. *Esotropia* refers to medial deviation, *exotropia* refers to lateral deviation, *hypertropia* refers to upward deviation, *hypotropia* refers to downward deviation, and *cyclotropia* refers to torsional deviation. The term *concomitance* refers to equal deviation in all directions of gaze. A nonconcomitant strabismus is one that varies with the direction of gaze. Strabismus may be divided into (1) paralytic (nonconcomitant) forms, in which there is weakness or paralysis of one or more of the extraocular muscles, or (2) nonparalytic (concomitant), in which there is no primary muscle impairment. Strabismus is termed *intermittent*, or *periodic*, when there are periods in which the eyes are parallel. It is *monocular* when the same eye always deviates and the fellow eye fixates.

Paralytic Strabismus. Paralytic strabismus results from paresis (weakness) or plegia (paralysis) of one or more of the extraocular muscles. When the normal eye fixates, the affected eye is in the position of primary deviation. In the case of esotropia, there is weakness of one of the lateral rectus muscles, usually the result of weakness of the abducens (VI) cranial nerve. When the affected eye fixates, the unaffected eye is in a position of secondary deviation. The secondary deviation of the unaffected eye is greater than the primary deviation of the affected eye. This is because the affected eye requires an excess of innervational impulse to maintain fixation; the excess impulses also are distributed to the unaffected eye (Hering's law of equal innervation), causing overaction of its muscles.[2]

Paralytic strabismus is uncommon in children but accounts for nearly all cases of adult strabismus; it can be caused by a number of conditions. Paralytic strabismus is most commonly seen in adults who have had cerebral vascular accidents and may also occur as the first sign of a tumor or inflammatory condition involving the CNS. One type of muscular dystrophy exerts its effects on the extraocular muscles. Initially eye movements in all directions are weak, with later progression to bilateral optic immobility. Weakness of eye movement and lid elevation is often the first evidence of myasthenia gravis. The pathway of the oculomotor (III), trochlear (IV), and abducens (VI) cranial nerves through the cavernous sinus and the back of the orbit make them vulnerable to basal skull fracture and tumors of the cavernous sinus (cavernous sinus syndrome) or orbit (orbital syndrome). In infants, paralytic strabismus can be caused by birth injuries affecting either the extraocular muscles or the cranial nerves supplying these muscles. It can also result from congenital anomalies of the muscles. In general, paralytic strabismus in an adult with previously normal binocular vision causes diplopia (double vision). This does not occur in people who have never developed binocular vision.

Nonparalytic Strabismus. In nonparalytic strabismus, there is no extraocular muscle weakness or paralysis, and the angle of deviation is always the same in all fields of gaze. With persistent deviation, secondary abnormalities may develop because of overaction or underaction of the muscles in some fields of gaze. Nonparalytic esotropia is the most common type of strabismus. The disorder may be accommodative, nonaccommodative, or a combination of the two. Accommodative strabismus is caused by disorders such as uncorrected hyperopia, in which the esotropia occurs with accommodation. The onset of this type of esotropia characteristically occurs between 18 months and 4 years of age (because accommodation is not well developed until that time). The disorder is most often monocular but may be alternating. About 50% of the cases of esotropia fall into this category. The causes of nonaccommodative strabismus are obscure. The disorder may be related to faulty muscle insertion, fascial abnormalities, or faulty innervation. There is evidence that idiopathic strabismus may have a genetic basis; siblings may have similar disorders.

Diagnosis and Treatment. Examination by a qualified practitioner is indicated in any infant whose eyes are not aligned at all times during waking hours after 3 months of age.[2] Diagnostic measures emphasize two major areas: (1) ocular deviation due to altered extrinsic muscle function and (2) visual acuity. Rapid assessment of extraocular muscle function is accomplished by three methods. First, in a somewhat darkened room and with the child staring straight ahead, a penlight is pointed at the midpoint between the two eyes, and a bright dot of reflected light can be seen on the cornea of each eye. With normal eye alignment, the reflected light should appear at the same spot on the cornea of each eye. Nonparallelism of the two eyes indicates muscle imbalance because of weakness or paralysis of the deviant eye. Second, the child is asked to follow the movement of a small object (a pencil point or lighted penlight) as it is moved through the extremes of what are called the six cardinal positions of gaze. In extreme lateral gaze, normal subjects can show a few quick beats of a jerky or nystagmoid movement (to be discussed). Nystagmoid movement is abnormal if it is prolonged or present in any other eye posture. The third method (called the cover–uncover test) eliminates binocular fusion as a factor in maintaining parallelism between the eyes and is used to determine which eye is used for fixation. The child's attention is directed toward a fixation object such as a small picture or tongue blade. A light should not be used because it may not stimulate accommodation. If a mild weakness is present, the eye with blocked vision drifts into a resting position, the extent of which depends on the relative strength of the muscles. The eye should snap back when the card is removed. The test is always done for both near and far fixation. Visual acuity is evaluated to obtain a comparison of the two eyes. An illiterate E chart (or similar test chart) can be used for young children.

Treatment of strabismus is directed toward the development of normal visual acuity, the correction of the deviation, and superimposition of the retinal images to provide binocular vision. Both nonsurgical and surgical methods can be used. In children, early treatment is important; the ideal age to begin is 6 months. Nonsurgical treatment includes occlusive patching, pleoptics, and prism glasses. Because prolonged occlusive patching leads to loss of useful vision in the covered eye, patching is alternated between the affected and unaffected eyes. This improves the vision in the affected eye without sacrificing vision in the unaffected eye. Prism glasses compensate for an abnormal alignment of an optic globe. Long-acting miotics in weak strengths (echothiophate iodide solution, Phospholine, or isoflurophate ointment, Floropryl) may be used in treating accommodative esotropia. In young children, these drugs can be used instead of glasses. They act by altering the accommodative convergence relationship in a favorable manner so that fusion is maintained despite accommodation. Miosis also allows for clearer vision with less accommodation in both near and far vision. Surgical procedures may be used to strengthen a muscle or weaken a muscle by altering its length or attachment site.

AMBLYOPIA

Amblyopia describes a condition of diminished vision (uncorrectable by lenses) in which no detectable organic lesion of the eye is present. This condition is sometimes referred to as *lazy eye*. It is caused by visual deprivation (conditions such as cataracts) or abnormal binocular interactions (strabismus or anisometropia) during visual immaturity. Normal development of the thalamic and cortical circuitry necessary for binocular visual perception requires simultaneous binocular use of each fovea during a critical period of time early in life (0 to 5 years). In infants with unilateral cataracts that are dense, central, and larger than 2 mm in diameter, this time is before 2 months of age.[2] In conditions causing abnormal binocular interactions, one image is suppressed to provide clearer vision. In esotropia, vision of the deviated eye is suppressed to prevent diplopia. A similar situation exists in anisometropia in which the refractive indexes of the two eyes are different. Although the eyes are correctly aligned, they are unable to focus together and the image of one eye is suppressed. In experimental animals, monocular deprivation results in reduced synaptic density in the LGN and the primary visual cortical areas that process input from the affected eye or eyes.[24]

The reversibility of amblyopia depends on the maturity of the visual system at the time of onset and the duration of the abnormal experience. If esotropia is involved, some people will alternate eyes and not experience diplopia. With late-adolescent or adult onset, this habit pattern must be unlearned after correction.

Peripheral vision is less affected than central foveal vision in amblyopia. Suppression becomes more evident with high illumination and high contrast. It is as if the affected eye did not possess central vision and the person learns to fixate with the nonfoveal retina. If bilateral congenital blindness or near blindness (*e.g.*, cataracts) occurs and remains uncorrected during infancy and early childhood, the person remains without pattern vision and has only overall field brightness and color discrimination. This is essentially bilateral amblyopia.

Treatment. The treatment of children with the potential for developing amblyopia must be instituted well before the age of 6 to avoid the suppression phenomenon. Surgery for congenital cataracts and ptosis should be done early. Severe refractive errors should be corrected. In strabismus, alternately blocking vision in one eye and then the other forces the child to use both eyes for form discrimination. The duration of occlusion of vision in the good eye must be short (2 to 5 hours per day) and closely monitored,

or deprivation amblyopia can develop in the good eye as well.[27] Although amblyopia is not likely to occur after the age of 8 or 9, plasticity in central circuitry is evident even in adulthood. For example, after refractive correction for longstanding astigmatism in adults, visual acuity improves slowly, requiring several months to reach normal levels.

In summary, normal vision depends on coordinated movement of the two eyes. Eye movements depend on the action of six extraocular muscles (four recti and two oblique) and their cranial (III, IV, and VI) nerve innervation. Conjugate eye movements are those in which the optical axes of the two eyes are kept parallel, sharing the same visual field. There are five types of eye movements: smooth pursuit (tracking movements), saccadic (positional correcting), vestibular (nystagmus), vergence (divergence and convergence), and tremor (fine movements). Lateral gaze is used in viewing lateral objects. It involves the coordinated movements of the extraocular muscles and their cranial nerve nuclei, the MLF tract of the brain stem, and the pontine lateral gaze center. Unilateral destruction of the pontine gaze center results in ipsilateral gaze paralysis. Vertical gaze facilitates looking upward and downward. It is controlled by the action of the extraocular muscles and their cranial nerve nuclei, the central tegmental fasciculus pathway, and the midbrain vertical gaze center.

Disorders of eye movements include strabismus and amblyopia. Strabismus refers to abnormalities in the coordination of eye movements with loss of binocular eye alignment. This inability to focus a visual image on corresponding parts of the two retinas results in diplopia. Esotropia refers to medial deviation, exotropia refers to lateral deviation, hypertropia refers to upward deviation, hypotropia refers to downward deviation, and cyclotropia refers to torsional deviation. Paralytic strabismus is caused by weakness or paralysis of the extraocular muscles. Nonparalytic strabismus results from the inappropriate length or insertion of the extraocular muscles or from accommodation disorders. Amblyopia (lazy eye) is a condition of diminished vision that cannot be corrected by lenses and one in which no detectable organic lesion in the eye can be observed. It results from inadequately developed CNS circuitry due to visual deprivation (cataracts) or abnormal binocular interactions (strabismus or anisometropia) during the period of visual immaturity.

■ REFERENCES

1. National Society to Prevent Blindness. (1980). *Vision problems in the U.S.* New York.
2. Vaughan, D.G., Ashbury, T., & Riordan-Eva, P. (1992). *General ophthalmology* (13th ed., pp. 79, 90–91, 169–170, 200–201, 225, 233). Norwalk, CT: Appleton Lange.
3. Benenson, A.S. (Ed.). (1990). *Control of communicable disease in man* (15th ed., pp. 103–104, 442). Washington, DC: APHA.
4. McLean, D.M., & Smith, J.A. (1991). *Medical microbiology synopsis* (p. 164). Philadelphia: Lea & Febiger.
5. Davis, B.R., Dulbecco, H.N., Eisen, H.S., et al. (1990).

Microbiology (4th ed., pp. 926–927). Philadelphia: J.B. Lippincott.

6. Cotran, R.S., Kumar, V., & Robbins, S.L. (1989). *Robbins' pathologic basis of disease* (4th ed., p. 327, 1466). Philadelphia: W.B. Saunders.

7. Bienfang, D.C., Kelly, L.D., Nicholson, D.H., et al. (1990). Ophthalmology. *New England Journal of Medicine, 323,* 956–967.

8. Javitt, J.C., McBean, A.M., Nicholson, G.A., et al. (1991). Underestimation of glaucoma among Black Americans. *New England Journal of Medicine, 325,* 1418–1422.

9. Martin, X.D. (1992). Normal intraocular pressure in man. *Ophthalmologicia, 205,* 57–63.

10. Capino, D.G., & Leibowitz, H.M. (1990). Glaucoma screening, diagnosis and therapy. *Hospital Practice, 25(5),* 73–91.

11. West, S.K. (1991). Who develops cataracts. *Archives of Ophthalmology, 109,* 196–198.

12. Quality of Care Committee—Anterior Segment Panel. (1989). *Cataract in the otherwise healthy eye.* San Francisco: American Academy of Ophthalmology.

13. Kandel, E.R., Schwartz, J.H., & Jessell, T.M. (1991). *Principles of neural science* (3rd ed., pp. 467–469). New York: Elsevier.

14. Capino, D.G., & Leibowitz, H.M. (1988). Age-related macular degeneration. *Hospital Practice, 22(3A),* 23–42.

15. Woods, S. (1992). Macular degeneration. *Nursing Clinics of North America, 27,* 761–755.

16. Macular Photocoagulation Study Group. (1991). Argon laser photocoagulation for neovascular maculopathy. *Archives of Ophthalmology, 109,* 1109–1114.

17. Valinine, R.H., Jackson, J.C., Kalina, R.E., et al. (1989). Increased survival of low birth weight infants: Impact on the incidence of retinopathy of prematurity. *Pediatrics, 84,* 442–445.

18. Kretzer, F.L., & Hittner, H.M. (1988). Retinopathy of prematurity: Clinical implications of retinal development. *Archives of Disease in Childhood, 63,* 1151–1167.

19. Shapiro, C. (1986). Retrolental fibroplasia: What we know and what we don't know. *Neonatal Network, 4(6),* 33–45.

20. The Committee for the Classification of Retinopathy of Prematurity. (1984). An international classification of retinopathy of prematurity. *Archives of Ophthalmology, 102,* 1130–1134.

21. Cryotherapy for Retinopathy of Prematurity Cooperative Group. (1988). Multicenter trial of cryotherapy for retinopathy of prematurity: Preliminary results. *Pediatrics, 81,* 697–706.

22. Al, E. (1992). Current management of diabetic retinopathy. *Western Journal of Medicine, 157,* 67–70.

23. American Academy of Ophthalmology Quality of Care Committee Retina Panel. (1989). *Preferred practice pattern: Diabetic retinopathy* (pp. 1–28). San Francisco: American Academy of Ophthalmology.

24. Wong-Riley, M.T.T., & Carroll, E.W. (1984). The effect of impulse blockage on cytochrome oxidate activity in the monkey visual system. *Nature, 307,* 262–264.

■ BIBLIOGRAPHY

Baylor, D.A. (1987). How photoreceptors respond to light. *Scientific American, 256(4),* 40.

Boyd-Monk, H. (1990). Assessing acquired ocular disease. *Nursing Clinics of North America, 25,* 811–822.

Dasbach, E.J., Fryback, D.G., Newcomb, P.A., et al. (1991). Cost effectiveness of strategies for detecting diabetes retinopathy. *Medical Care, 29,* 20–39.

Endres, W., & Shin, Y.S. (1990). Cataract and metabolic disease. *Journal of Inherited Metabolic Disease, 13,* 509–516.

Fulton, A. (1992). Screening preschool children to detect visual and ocular disorders. *Archives of Ophthalmology, 110,* 1553–1554.

Krachmer, J.H., & Palay, D.A. (1991). Corneal disease. *New England Journal of Medicine, 325,* 1804–1806.

Lerman, S. (1988). Ocular phototoxicity. *New England Journal of Medicine, 319,* 1475.

Liesengang, T.J. (1991). Diagnosis and therapy of herpes zoster ophthalmicus. *Ophthalmology, 98,* 1216–1229.

Limberg, M.B. (1991). A review of bacterial keratitis and bacterial conjunctivitis. *American Journal of Ophthalmology, 112,* 2S–9S.

Merimee, T.J. (1990). Diabetic retinopathy: A synthesis of perspectives. *New England Journal of Medicine, 322,* 978–987.

Phelps, D.L. (1989). Retinopathy of prematurity. *New England Journal of Medicine, 326,* 1078–1080.

Ramachandran, V.S. (1992). Blind spots. *Scientific American, 266(5),* 86–91.

Ruehl, C.A., & Schremp, P.S. (1992). Nursing care of the cataract patient: Today's outpatient approach. *Nursing Clinics of North America, 27,* 727–743.

Schmitt, C., & Hockwin, O. (1990). The mechanisms of cataract formation. *Journal of Inherited Metabolic Disease, 13,* 501–508.

Seddon, J.M. (1991). The differential burden of blindness in the United States. *New England Journal of Medicine, 325,* 1440–1442.

Shingleton, B.J. (1991). Eye injuries. *New England Journal of Medicine, 325,* 40814.

Smith, S.C. (1992). Diabetic retinopathy. *Nursing Clinics of North America, 27,* 745–759.

Tiesisch, J.M., Sommer, A., Witt, K., et al. (1990). Blindness and visual impairment in an American urban population. *Archives of Ophthalmology, 108,* 286–290.

Vader, L.A. (1992). Vision and vision loss. *Nursing Clinics of North America, 27,* 705–714.

ALTERATIONS IN HEARING AND VESTIBULAR FUNCTION

ROBIN L. CURTIS
CAROL MATTSON PORTH

■ OBJECTIVES

After you have studied this chapter, you should be able to meet the following objectives:

■ List the structures of the external, middle, and inner ear and cite their function.

■ Cite the impact of damage to Wernicke's area in the brain.

■ Describe the symptoms of impacted cerumen.

■ Relate the functions of the eustachian tube to the development of otitis media.

■ Explain why infants and young children are more prone to develop otitis media.

■ List three common symptoms of otitis media.

■ Describe the disease process that occurs with otosclerosis and relate this to the hearing loss that occurs.

■ Differentiate between conductive and sensorineural hearing loss.

■ List at least three drug groups that have potential ototoxicity.

■ Explain the function of the vestibular system.

■ Describe normal nystagmus eye movements.

■ List the symptoms of motion sickness.

■ Describe the pathology associated with Meniere's disease.

Carol Mattson Porth: PATHOPHYSIOLOGY: CONCEPTS OF
ALTERED HEALTH STATES, 4th ed. © 1994, 1990, 1986, 1982
J.B. Lippincott Company

The ears are paired organs that are responsible for hearing and the maintenance of equilibrium and effective posture (vestibular function). The ear consists of an external ear, a middle, and an inner ear. The external and middle ear functions are capturing, transmitting, and amplifying sound. The inner ear contains the receptive organs that are selectively stimulated by either sound waves (hearing) or head position and motion (vestibular function).

■ HEARING

Hearing is a specialized sense that provides the ability to perceive vibration of sound waves. The compression waves that produce sound have both frequency and intensity. *Frequency* indicates the rate of change with time (cycles per second [cps] or hertz [Hz]). Most people cannot hear compression waves that have a frequency higher than 20,000 Hz. Waves of higher frequency are called ultrasonic waves, meaning that they are above the audible range. In the audible frequency range, the subjective experience correlated with sonic frequency is the pitch of a sound. Waves below 20 to 30 Hz are experienced as a rattle or drum beat rather than a tone. The ear is most sensitive to waves in the frequency range of 1000 to 3000 Hz. Wave intensity is represented by either amplitude or units of sound pressure. By convention, the *intensity* (in power units, or ergs per square centimeter) of a sound is expressed as the ratio of intensities between the sound and a reference value. A 10-fold increase in sound pressure is called a *bel*, after Alexander Graham Bell. This representation often is too crude to be of use; the most often used unit is the decibel (db), or one tenth of a bel. In the normal sonic environment, about 1 db of increased intensity (loudness) can be detected. The region of audible speech sounds falls between 42 and 70 db.

AUDITORY SYSTEM

The ear receives sound waves, distinguishes their frequency, translates this information into nerve impulses, and transmits them to the central nervous system (CNS). The auditory system can be divided into five parts: the external ear, the middle ear, the inner ear, auditory brain stem pathways, and the primary and associational auditory cortex of the brain's temporal lobe.

EXTERNAL EAR

The external ear is called the *pinna*, or *auricle*. It is supported by elastic cartilage and shaped like a funnel. The funnel shape concentrates high-frequency sound entering from the lateral-forward direction into the *external acoustic meatus*, or *ear canal* (Fig. 53-1). The shape also helps to prevent front–back confusion of sound sources. The anterior portion of the pinna and the external ear canal are innervated by branches of the mandibular division of the trigeminal (V) cranial nerve. The posterior portions, including the back of the external ear as well as the posterior wall of the ear canal, are innervated by auricular branches of the facial (VII), glossopharyngeal (IX), and vagus (X) cranial nerves. Because of the vagal innervation, the insertion of a speculum or an otoscope into the external ear canal can stimulate coughing or vomiting reflexes, particularly in young children.

The external ear canal extends from the auricle to the tympanic membrane, or eardrum. Its outer two thirds is supported by elastic cartilage, and its inner one third by the tympanic bone. It is somewhat S-shaped and acts as a resonator, amplifying frequencies around 3500 Hz. A thin layer of skin containing fine hairs, sebaceous glands, and ceruminous glands lines the ear canal. The ceruminous glands secrete cerumen, or earwax, which has certain antimicrobial properties and is thought to serve a protective function.

TYMPANIC MEMBRANE

The tympanic membrane (or eardrum), which separates the external ear from the middle ear, has three layers: (1) an outer layer of thin skin continuous with the lining of the external acoustic meatus, (2) a middle layer of tough collagenous fibers mixed with fibrocytes and some elastic fibers, and (3) an inner epithelial layer continuous with the lining of the middle ear. It is attached in a manner that allows it to vibrate freely when audible sound waves enter the external auditory canal. When viewed through an otoscope, the tympanic membrane appears as a shallow, almost circular cone pointing inward toward its apex, the umbo (Fig. 53-2). The landmarks include the lightened stripe over the handle of the malleus; the umbo at the end of the handle; the pars tensa, which constitutes most of the drum; and the pars flaccida, the small area above the malleus attachment. Light usually is reflected from the pars tensa at about the 4 o'clock position. The tympanic membrane is semitransparent, and a small whitish cord, which traverses the middle ear from back to front, can be seen just under its upper edge. This is the corda tympani, a branch of the intermedius component of the facial (VII) cranial nerve.

MIDDLE EAR
AND EUSTACHIAN TUBE

The middle ear is a tiny cavity, roughly the shape of a red blood cell set on edge, located in the petrous

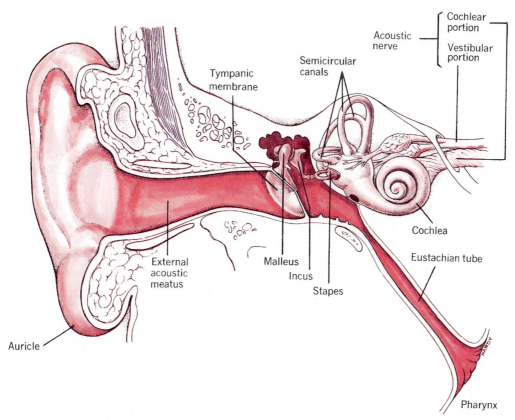

FIG. 53-1. External, middle, and internal subdivisions of the ear. (Chaffee, E. E., & Lytle, I. M. [1980]. *Basic physiology and anatomy* [4th ed.]. Philadelphia: J.B. Lippincott)

(stony) temporal bone. Its lateral wall is formed by the tympanic membrane, and its medial wall is formed by the bone dividing the middle and inner ear. Two tissue-covered openings in the medial wall, the oval and the round windows, provide for the transmission of sound waves between the air-filled middle ear and the fluid-filled inner ear. Posteriorly, the middle ear is continuous with small air pockets in the temporal bone called *mastoid air spaces* or *cells* (Fig. 53-3). In early life these air spaces are filled with

hematopoietic tissue. Replacement of hematopoietic tissue with air sacs begins during the 3rd year of life and is completed at puberty.

Auditory Tube. There is a gap in the bone between the anterior and medial walls for a canal, called the *eustachian tube*, or *auditory tube*, which connects with the nasopharynx (see Fig. 53-3). The middle ear is filled with the air that reaches it from the nasopharynx by way of the auditory tube; it is lined

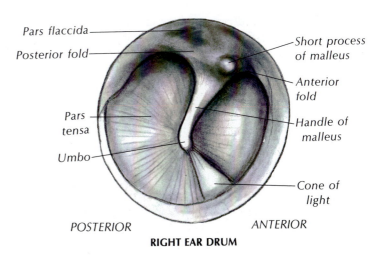

FIG. 53-2. Right eardrum. (Bates, B. [1991]. *A guide to physical examination* [5th ed.]. Philadelphia: J.B. Lippincott)

Pars flaccida

Posterior fold

Pars tensa

Umbo

Short process of malleus

Anterior fold

Handle of malleus

Cone of light

POSTERIOR   ANTERIOR

RIGHT EAR DRUM

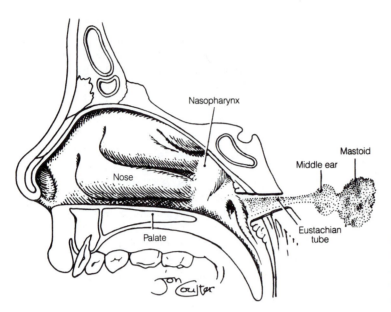

FIG. 53-3. Nasopharynx—eustachian tube—mastoid air cell system. (Bluestone, C. D. [1981]. Recent advances in pathogenesis, diagnosis, and management of otitis media. *Pediatric Clinics of North America, 28*(4), 36. Reproduced with permission)

with a mucous membrane that is continuous with the pharynx and mastoid air cells. Infections from the nasopharynx can travel from the nasopharynx along the mucous membrane of the auditory tube to the middle ear, causing otitis media. Near the opening of the auditory tube, the columnar epithelial lining changes to the pseudostratified cilated-columnar surface of the pharynx, which contains occasional mucus-secreting cells. Hypertrophy of the mucus-secreting cells contributes to the mucoid secretions that develop during certain types of otitis media.

The auditory tube, which connects the middle ear with the nasopharynx, serves three basic functions: (1) ventilation of the middle ear, along with equalization of middle ear and ambient pressures; (2) protection of the middle ear from unwanted nasopharyngeal sound waves and secretions; and (3) drainage of middle ear secretions into the nasopharynx.[1] The nasopharyngeal entrance to the auditory tube, which usually is closed, is opened by the action of the tensor veli palatini muscles (Fig. 53-4). Stimulation occurs as part of the swallowing and yawning reflexes and provides the mechanism for equalizing the pressure of the middle ear with that of the atmosphere. This equalization ensures that the pressures on both sides of the tympanic membrane are the same, so that sound transmission is not reduced and rupture does not result from sudden changes in external pressure, such as occurs during plane travel.

Ossicles. Three tiny bones, the auditory ossicles, are suspended from the roof of the middle ear cavity and connect the tympanic membrane with the oval window (see Fig. 53-1). They are connected by synovial joints and are covered with the epithelial lining of the cavity. The *malleus* (hammer) has its

handle firmly fixed to the upper half of the tympanic membrane. The head of the malleus articulates with the *incus* (anvil), which, in turn, articulates with the *stapes* (stirrup), which is inserted and sealed into the oval window by an annular ligament. The ossicles are arranged so that their lever movements transmit vibrations from the tympanic membrane to the oval window and from there to the fluid in the inner ear. It is the piston-like action of the stapes footplate that sets up compression waves in the inner ear fluid. Air and liquid offer different degrees of impedance (resistance) to the transmission of sound waves. Therefore, the bones of the middle ear serve as impedance-

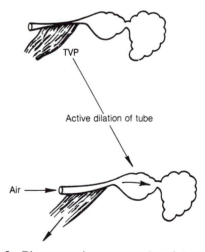

FIG. 53-4. Diagrammatic representation of physiologic pressure regulation of the middle ear by the active opening of the eustachian tube by the tensor veli palatini muscle (TVP). An alternative mechanism is by gradient-activated opening of the eustachian tube. (Bluestone, C. D. [1981]. Recent advances in the pathogenesis, diagnosis, and management of otitis media. *Pediatric Clinics of North America, 28*(4), 727. Reproduced with permission)

matching devices between the low impedance of the air and the high impedance of the cochlear fluid. This matching is accomplished by (1) concentrating the pressure from the large area of the tympanic membrane (43 to 55 mm^2) to the small area of the oval window (about 3 mm^2) and (2) amplifying the air-transmitted sound waves into the force required to set up compression waves in the fluid of the inner ear. The latter is accomplished by the ossicular lever system, which increases the pressures from the tympanic membrane to the oval window.

Two tiny skeletal muscles, the *tensor tympani* and the *stapedius*, insert into the ossicles. The tensor tympani is positioned in the roof of the auditory tube and inserts on the base of the malleus handle. The functional role of this muscle is in dispute. The stapedius muscle alters the movement of the stapes, reducing the displacement of fluid in the inner ear. Reflex contraction of this muscle by means of the facial nerve, the stapedial reflex, provides a protective mechanism for the delicate inner ear structures when high-intensity sound occurs.

INNER EAR

The inner ear contains a labyrinth or system of intercommunicating channels and the receptors for hearing and position sense. The outer bony wall of the inner ear, the bony labyrinth, encloses a thin-walled, membranous duct system, the membranous labyrinth (Fig. 53-5). Two separate fluids are found in the inner ear. A fluid called the *perilymph* (*periotic fluid*) separates the bony labyrinth from the membranous labyrinth, and one called the *endolymph* (*otic fluid*) fills

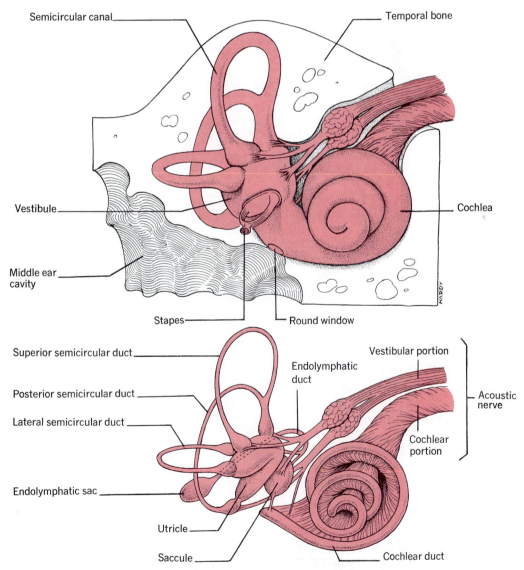

FIG. 53-5. (**Top**) Diagram of the bony labyrinth; (**bottom**) membranous labyrinth as seen when removed from the bony labyrinth. (Chaffee, E. E., & Lytle, I. M. [1980]. *Basic physiology and anatomy* [4th ed.]. Philadelphia: J.B. Lippincott)

the membranous labyrinth. The bony labyrinth is divided into three compartments: the cochlea, the vestibule, and the semicircular canals. The cochlea, which contains the auditory receptors, is a bony tube shaped like a snail shell that winds around a central bone column called the modiolus. The utricle, saccule, and semicircular canals contain the receptors for head position sense and are discussed later in the chapter. The entire bony labyrinth occupies a volume with a diameter less than the size of a dime.

The membranous cochlear duct is a triangular-shaped structure that stretches across the cochlear canal, separating it into two parallel tubes, each containing perilymph: the scala vestibuli and the scala tympani (Fig. 53-6). One side of the cochlear duct, the basilar membrane, stretches under tension lat-

erally from the modiolus to an elastic spiral ligament. The second side, the vestibular membrane (Reissner's membrane), is a delicate double layer of squamous epithelial cells. The third side consists of a well-vascularized epithelium, the stria vascularis, which is the source of endolymph. The cochlear duct separates the scala vestibuli and the scala tympani from the base of the cochlea throughout its two and one half spiral turns to its apex. An opening at the apex, called the helicotrema, permits fluid waves to move between the two scalae. Sound waves, delivered by the stapes footplate to the perilymph, travel throughout the fluid of the inner ear, including up the scala vestibuli, to the apex of the cochlea. The fluid pressure wave results in compensatory displacements of the round window, compressing the air of the middle

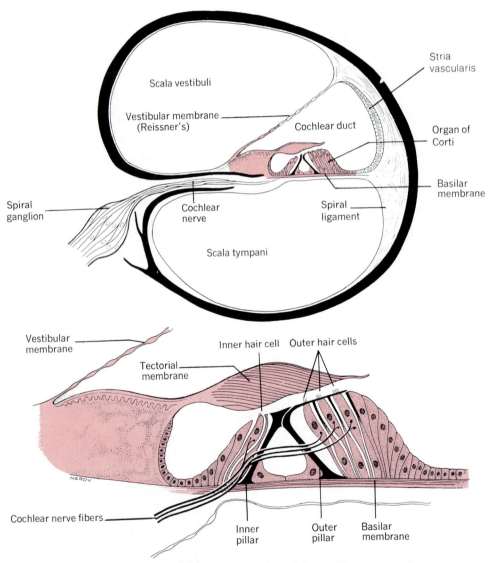

FIG. 53-6. (**Top**) Portion of cochlea. Note the relation of the cochlear duct to the scalae, vestibuli, and tympani. (**Bottom**) Spiral organ of Corti has been removed from the cochlear duct and greatly enlarged. (Chaffee, E. E., & Lytle, I. M. [1980]. *Basic physiology and anatomy* [4th ed.]. Philadelphia: J.B. Lippincott)

ear cavity and auditory canal. The basilar membrane becomes progressively more massive from base to distal apex and, thus, resonates to higher frequencies near the base and lower frequencies toward the apex as the fluid pressure wave travels up the cochlear spiral. This "tuned" aspect of the basilar membrane results in increased amplitude of displacement at the resonant locations, responding to a particular sound frequency and greater firing of cochlear neurons innervating this region. This mechanism provides the major basis for the discrimination of sound frequency.

Perched on the basilar membrane and extending along its entire length is an elaborate arrangement of columnar epithelium called the organ of Corti. Continuous rows of hair cells separated into inner and outer rows can be found within the cell arrangement. The cells have hairlike cilia that protrude through openings in an overlying supporting reticular membrane into the endolymph of the cochlear duct. A gelatinous mass, the tectorial membrane, extends from the medial side of the duct to enclose the cilia of the outer hair cells. Vibrations of the organ of Corti cause the hairs to be bent against the less flexible tectorial membrane. Each hair cell is supplied by a nerve fiber, some by more than one. It is the bending of the hair fibers that transform (transduce) sound

energy, which thus far has been mechanical, into membrane potential changes, transmitter release, and stimulation of nerve endings. It is generally agreed that the inner rows of hair cells, transducing different frequencies, are arranged sequentially with those transducing the higher tones located on the lower (basal) end of the cochlear duct and those transducing lower tones located near its apex. Thus, selective destruction of hair cells in a particular segment of the cochlea can lead to hearing loss of particular tones. The outer rows of hair cells appear to provide the signals on which the experience of sound loudness is based.

NEURAL PATHWAYS

Afferent fibers from the organ of Corti have their cell bodies in the spiral ganglion in the central portion of the cochlea. Nerve fibers from the spiral ganglion (vestibulocochlear, or auditory, nerve [VIII]) travel to the cochlear nuclei located in the pons (Fig. 53-7). Many of the secondary nerve fibers from the cochlear nuclei pass to the opposite side of the pons. These secondary fibers may project to cell groups called the trapezoid, the superior olivary nucleus, or rostrally toward the inferior colliculus of the midbrain. Ipsilateral projections and interconnections between the

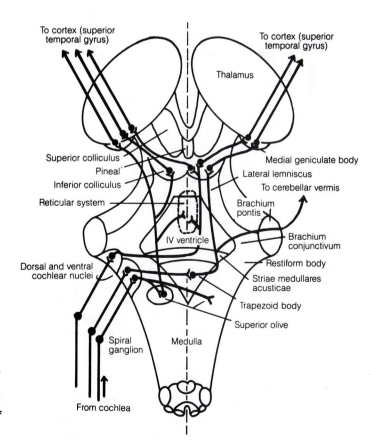

FIG. 53-7. Simplified diagram of main auditory pathways superimposed on a dorsal view of the brain stem. Cerebellum and cerebral cortex removed. (Reproduced with permission from Ganong, W. [1975]. *Review of medical physiology* [7th ed.]. Los Altos, CA: Lange)

nuclei of the two sides occur throughout the central auditory system. Consequently, impulses from either ear are transmitted through the auditory pathways to both sides of the brain stem.

A number of reflexes, initiated by sound stimuli, are integrated in the central auditory pathways. The superior olivary nucleus is involved in basic auditory reflexes, including the stapedial and tensor tympani reflexes. A comparison of impulses from the two sides, which provides the basis for spatial localization of a sound source, occurs at the level of the inferior colliculus. Superior colliculus function is required for auditory startle reflexes, which include rapid saccadic eye movements and turning of the head and body toward the sound source. The superior olivary nucleus, which has extensive connections with the brain stem respiratory and cardiovascular centers, integrates the heart rate, blood pressure, and respiratory changes that occur with the auditory startle reflex.

From the inferior colliculus, the auditory pathway passes to the medial geniculate nucleus of the thalamus, where all the fibers synapse. Considerable evidence supports the capability of this level of organization to provide crude auditory experience, including crude tone and intensity discrimination as well as the directionality of a sound source. From the medial geniculate nucleus, the auditory tract spreads by way of the auditory radiation to the primary auditory cortex (area 41) located mainly in the superior temporal gyrus and insula (see Chapter 52, Fig. 52-21). This area and its corresponding higher-order thalamic nucleus are required for high-acuity loudness discrimination and for precise discrimination of pitch. The auditory association cortex (areas 42 and 22) borders the primary cortex on the superior temporal gyrus. This area and its associated high-order thalamic nuclei are necessary for auditory gnosis or the meaningfulness of sound to occur. Past experience, as well as precise analysis of momentary auditory information, is integrated during this process.

DISORDERS OF AUDITORY FUNCTION

Hearing loss may be the most common physical disability suffered by people in the United States. More than 13 million people in the United States have some hearing impairment. Of these people, 6 million are seriously handicapped and more than 1.7 million are deaf.[2]

ALTERATIONS IN EXTERNAL EAR FUNCTION

The external ear conducts sound waves to the tympanic membrane. The function of the external ear is disturbed when sound transmission is obstructed by excessive amounts of accumulated cerumen or inflammation of the external ear (otitis externa).

Impacted Cerumen. Although the cerumen (earwax) produced by the glands of the ear canal normally dries up and leaves the ear, it can accumulate, causing narrowing of the canal. Repeated unskilled attempts to remove the wax may pack it more deeply into the ear canal. Impacted earwax usually produces no symptoms until the canal becomes completely occluded, at which point a feeling of fullness, deafness, tinnitus (ringing in the ears), or coughing because of vagal stimulation develops.

In most cases, impacted cerumen can be relieved with detergent ear drops. A few drops of baby shampoo, baby oil, or hydrogen peroxide can be instilled into the ear for several days to soften the wax. Commercial products are available and effective. If necessary, the wax is then removed using suction or a large syringe to produce a water stream.

Otitis Externa. Otitis externa may vary in severity from a mild eczematoid dermatitis to severe cellulitis. It can be caused by infectious agents or materials contained in earphones or earrings (contact dermatitis). Most infections of the external ear are bacterial, with occasional secondary infection by fungi. Predisposing factors include moisture in the ear canal after swimming (swimmer's ear) or bathing, trauma resulting from scratching or attempts to clean the ear, and allergic dermatitis. External otitis commonly is accompanied by redness, scaliness, narrowing of the canal because of swelling, itching, and pain. Inflammation of the pinna or canal makes movement of the auricle painful. There may be watery or purulent drainage and intermittent deafness. Treatment methods include the use of topical antibiotic ointments, eardrops, and topical corticosteroids to reduce inflammation.

ALTERATIONS IN MIDDLE EAR FUNCTION

Otitis Media. Otitis media, or inflammation of the middle ear, may occur in any age group, although children are most commonly affected; it is the most common diagnosis made by physicians who care for children. Otitis media can be acute, subacute, or chronic. It may or may not be infectious in origin and may or may not be associated with effusion (collection of fluid and exudate). Infants and young children are at highest risk for developing it, the peak prevalence occurring between 6 and 36 months. There are two reasons for the increased risk in infants and young children: (1) the auditory tube is shorter, more horizontal, and wider in this age group than in older children and adults; and (2) infection can spread more easily through the canal of the infant who spends most of the day lying in bed. Bottle-fed babies have a higher incidence of otitis media than breastfed babies, probably because bottle-fed babies are held in a more horizontal position during feeding, and swallowing while in the horizontal position facilitates the reflux of milk into the middle ear. Breastfeeding also provides for the transfer of protective maternal antibodies to the infant. The incidence of otitis media is higher among children with craniofacial anomalies (cleft palate and Down syndrome), Alaskan natives (Inuits [Eskimos]), and Native Americans.

Abnormalities of the auditory tube are important factors in the pathogenesis of middle ear infections. Two major types of auditory tube dysfunction contribute to otitis media: obstruction and abnormal patency (Fig. 53-8). Obstruction can be either mechanical or functional. Functional obstruction results from the persistent collapse of the auditory tube because of a lack of tubal stiffness or an abnormal muscular opening mechanism. It is common in infants and young children because the amount and stiffness of the cartilage supporting the auditory tube are less than in older children and adults. Also, age-related changes in the craniofacial base render the muscle responsible for opening the auditory tube less efficient in this age group. Mechanical obstruction can be either intrinsic or extrinsic, the most common obstruction being caused by intrinsic swelling resulting from upper respiratory tract infection or allergy. Extrinsic obstruction can result from the enlargement

of adenoid tissue or a tumor. With obstruction, air in the middle ear is absorbed, causing a negative pressure and the transudation of serous fluid into the middle ear.

The abnormally patent auditory tube either does not close or does not close completely. In children, air and secretions may be pumped into the auditory tube during nose blowing and crying. Organisms or foreign material from the nasopharynx incite an inflammatory response (see Chapter 13) with exudate, leukocytosis, and hypertrophy of the mucous glands in the eustachian tube and mucous membrane lining the middle ear.

Acute Otitis Media. Acute otitis media is characterized by either a suppurative (purulent or pus-containing) or serous (serum-type) exudate. Most cases of otitis media follow an upper respiratory tract infection that has been present for several days. *Streptococcus pneumoniae* and *Haemophilus influenzae* are the most frequently isolated organisms.

Acute suppurative otitis media is characterized by otalgia (earache), fever (up to 104°F), and hearing loss. There may be rhinorrhea, vomiting, and diarrhea. Pain usually increases as purulent exudate accumulates behind the tympanic membrane. An infant may cry and rub the infected ear, and an older child will complain of sharp or severe pain in the ear. If the tympanic membrane ruptures because of excessive pressure, the pain is relieved and a purulent drainage is present in the external ear canal.

Acute serous otitis media may also occur after a viral disease, with an allergy, or after sudden changes in atmospheric pressure. If air cannot pass back through the auditory tube on descent during an airplane flight, hearing loss and discomfort develop. This most commonly occurs in those who travel while suffering from an upper respiratory tract infection. Yawning, swallowing, and chewing gum seem to facilitate the opening of the auditory tube, which equalizes air in the middle ear. Signs of acute serous otitis media include conductive hearing loss, eardrum retraction, and fluid level or air bubbles visible through the tympanic membrane.

Recurrent Otitis Media. Recurrent otitis media can occur as an acute episode of otitis media along with almost every respiratory tract infection. Most children with recurrent otitis media respond well to treatment and have fewer recurrences with advancing age. Some children have persistent middle ear effusion with superimposed recurrent episodes of acute otitis media.

Chronic Otitis Media. Otitis media that persists beyond 3 months is considered chronic.[3] Chronic otitis media can occur with or without effusion.

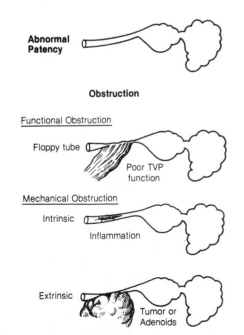

FIG. 53-8. Pathophysiology of the eustachian tube. (Bluestone, C. D. [1981]. Recent advances in the pathogenesis, diagnosis, and management of otitis media. *Pediatric Clinics of North America, 28*(4), 737. Reproduced with permission)

Chronic suppurative otitis media is most common in those who have suffered ear problems during early childhood. With the chronic infection, permanent perforation of the tympanic membrane often occurs. Ear ossicles may be destroyed, and chronic changes can occur in the mucosal lining of the middle ear. The chronic condition frequently is exacerbated by upper respiratory tract infections.

Diagnosis and Treatment. Diagnosis of otitis media often is made by otoscopic examination of the tympanic membrane. A bulging, lusterless membrane with subsequent obliteration of the bony landmarks and cone of light are observed. Gentle movement of the pinna can help to distinguish otitis media from otitis externa. This maneuver does not produce pain in purulent otitis media but causes severe discomfort in otitis externa. A culture of middle ear effusion fluid is used for verifying the presence of a microorganism and identifying its type. A needle can be inserted through the inferior part of the tympanic membrane to obtain a specimen of effusion fluid, or a culture can be made of the drainage present in the external ear canal when the tympanic membrane has perforated.

The use of the pneumatic otoscope permits the introduction of air into the canal for the purpose of determining tympanic membrane flexibility. The movement of this membrane is decreased in some cases of acute otitis media and absent in chronic middle ear infection. Tympanometry is an important advance in the identification of middle ear disease. A tympanogram is obtained by inserting a small probe into the external auditory canal; a tone of fixed characteristics is then presented through the probe, and the mobility of the tympanic membrane is measured electronically while the external canal pressure is artificially varied.

The treatment of otitis media includes the use of appropriate antibiotic therapy. Additional supportive therapy, including analgesics, antipyretics, and local heat, may be indicated. A myringotomy (surgical incision of the tympanic membrane) may be done to relieve pressure on the membrane, reduce pain and hearing loss, and prevent the ragged opening that can follow spontaneous rupture of the tympanic membrane. The use of antihistamines and decongestants is controversial. They usually are of most benefit to children with serous otitis media of an allergic origin.

Pressure-equalization tubes may be used in the treatment of children with recurrent or chronic otitis media. Insertion of the tubes is one of the most commonly performed surgical procedures in the United States; the long-term benefits are controversial. Indications for tube insertion include the persistence of middle ear fluid for 3 or more months per episode, the presence of speech-language delay, and conductive hearing loss of 20 db or more.[4] Placement of the tubes usually is performed under general anesthesia. The ears of children with the tubes must be kept out of water. Spontaneous extrusion of the tubes usually occurs after 5½ to 7 months.[5,6] The adverse effects include recurrent otorrhea, persistent perforation, scarring and atrophy of the tympanic membrane, and cholesteatoma.

Complications. Complications of otitis media are not common, but they can follow inadequate treatment. The most common are those associated with the aural (ear) cavity and surrounding temporal bone. Intracranial complications are rare but are the most serious.

One of the most common complications of otitis media is persistent conductive hearing loss. Fluid may be present in the middle ear for weeks or months after an acute bout of otitis media. This may impair hearing and affect the child's learning of language skills. Hearing loss that is associated with fluid collection usually resolves when the effusion clears. Permanent hearing loss may occur as the result of damage to the tympanic membrane or other middle ear structures.

Perforation of the tympanic membrane occurs most often after acute otitis media; although it usually heals spontaneously, tympanoplasty may be necessary.

Adhesive otitis media involves an abnormal healing reaction to an inflamed middle ear. It produces irreversible thickening of the mucous membranes and may cause impaired movement of the ossicles and, possibly, conductive hearing loss. Tympanosclerosis involves the formation of whitish plaques and nodular deposits on the submucosal surface of the tympanic membrane with possible adherence of the ossicles and conductive hearing loss.

A cholesteatoma is a saclike mass containing a silvery white debris of keratin, which is shed by the squamous epithelial lining of the tympanic membrane. As the lining of the epithelium sheds and desquamates, the lesion expands and erodes the surrounding tissues. The lesion, which is associated with chronic middle ear infection, is insidiously progressive, and erosion may involve the temporal bone, causing intracranial complications. The treatment involves microsurgical techniques to remove the cholesteatomatous material.

The mastoid antrum and air cells constitute a portion of the temporal bone and may become inflamed as an extension of an acute or chronic otitis media. Because of the use of antibiotics, acute mastoiditis (a complication of acute otitis media) is unusual. If it does occur, there is necrosis of the mastoid process and destruction of the bony intercellular matrix, which are visible by radiologic examination. Mastoid tenderness and drainage of exudate through a perforated tympanic membrane can occur. Chronic mastoiditis can develop as the result of chronic middle ear infection. The usefulness of antibiotics for this condition is limited. Mastoid or middle ear surgery, along with other medical treatment, may be indicated.

Intracranial complications, although rare, can develop if the infection spreads through vascular channels, by direct extension, or through preformed pathways such as the round window. These complications are seen more often with chronic suppurative otitis media and mastoiditis. They include meningitis, focal encephalitis, brain abscess, lateral sinus thrombophlebitis or thrombosis, labyrinthitis, and facial nerve paralysis. Any child who develops persistent headache, tinnitus, stiff neck, or visual or other neurologic symptoms should be investigated for possible intracranial complications.

Otosclerosis. Otosclerosis is a familial, autosomal dominant disorder that causes conductive deafness, sensorineural hearing loss, and tinnitus. It is a disorder of the otic capsule, which becomes the petrous part of the temporal bone that surrounds the inner ear. Otosclerosis may begin at any time in life but usually does not appear until after puberty, most frequently between ages 20 and 30. There is an increase in the disease process during pregnancy.

In otosclerosis, the disease process begins with resorption of bone in one or more foci. During active bone resorption, the bone structure appears spongy and softer than normal (osteospongiosis). The resorbed bone is replaced by an overgrowth of new, hard sclerotic bone. The process is slowly progressive, involving more areas of the temporal bone, especially in front of and posterior to the stapes footplate. As it invades the footplate, the pathologic bone increasingly immobilizes the stapes, reducing the transmission of sound. Pressure of otosclerotic bone on inner ear structures or the eighth nerve may contribute to the development of tinnitus, sensorineural hearing loss, and vertigo.

The symptoms of otosclerosis involve an insidious hearing loss. Initially, one is unable to hear a whisper or someone speaking at a distance. In the earliest stages, the bone conduction by which the person's own voice is heard remains relatively unaffected. Therefore, the person's own voice sounds unusually loud and the sound of chewing becomes intensified. Because of bone conduction, most of these people can hear fairly well on the telephone,

which provides an amplified signal. Also, many are able to hear better in a noisy environment, probably because the masking effect of background noise causes people to speak louder.

The treatment of otosclerosis can be either medical or surgical. A carefully selected, well-fitting hearing aid may allow a person with conductive deafness to lead a normal life. Sodium fluoride has been used in the medical treatment of osteospongiosis. Because much of the conductive hearing loss associated with otosclerosis is due to stapedial fixation, the surgical treatment involves stapedectomy with stapedial reconstruction using either the patient's own stapes or a stapedial prosthesis. The argon laser beam may be used in the surgical procedure.

ABNORMALITIES OF CENTRAL AUDITORY PATHWAYS

The auditory pathways in the brain involve intercommunication between the two sides of the brain at many levels. As a result, strokes, tumors, abscesses, and other focal abnormalities seldom produce more than a mild reduction in auditory acuity on the side opposite the lesion. When it comes to the intelligibility of auditory language, lateral dominance becomes important. On the dominant side, usually the left side, the more medial and dorsal portion of the associational auditory cortex is of crucial importance. This area is called *Wernicke's area*, and damage here is associated with auditory receptive aphasia (an agnosia of speech). People with damage to this area of the brain can speak intelligibly and read normally but are unable to understand the meaning of major aspects of audible speech.

Irritative foci that affect the auditory radiation or the primary auditory cortex can produce roaring or clicking sounds, which appear to come from the auditory environment of the opposite side (auditory hallucinations). Focal seizures that originate in or near the auditory cortex often are immediately preceded by the perception of ringing or other sounds preceded by a prodrome (aura). Damage to the auditory association cortex, especially if bilateral, results in deficiencies of sound recognition and memory (auditory agnosia). If the damage is in the dominant hemisphere, speech recognition can be affected (sensory aphasia).

HEARING LOSS

There are many causes of hearing loss or deafness. Most fit into the categories of conductive, sensorineural (perceptive), or mixed deficiencies that involve a combination of conductive and sensorineural function deficiencies of the same ear.

CONDUCTIVE HEARING LOSS

Conductive hearing deficit occurs with external ear or middle ear disorders such as impacted cerumen, perforation of the tympanic membrane, fluid or pus in the middle ear, and ossicle fusion. A partial hearing loss can occur if sonic stimuli are not adequately transmitted to the inner ear through the external acoustic meatus (auditory canal), tympanic membrane, middle ear, and chain of ossicles.

SENSORINEURAL HEARING LOSS

Sensorineural, or perceptive, hearing loss occurs with disorders that affect the inner ear, auditory nerve, or auditory pathways of the brain. With this type of deafness, sound waves are conducted to the inner ear, but abnormalities of the cochlear apparatus or auditory nerve decrease or distort the transfer of information to the brain. Tinnitus or ringing of the ears accompanies cochlear nerve irritation. Abnormal function resulting from damage or malformation of the central auditory pathways and circuitry is included in this category. Sensorineural hearing loss may be congenital as a result of birth trauma, maternal rubella, or malformations of the inner ear. Trauma to the inner ear, vascular disorders with hemorrhage, or thrombosis of vessels that supply the middle ear can also cause sensorineural deafness. Other causes of sensorineural deafness are infections and drugs.

Environmentally induced deafness can occur through direct exposure to excessively intense sound, as in the workplace or at a concert. This type of deafness was once called "boilermaker's deafness" because of the intense reverberating sound to which riveters were exposed when putting together boiler tanks. Sustained or repeated exposure to noise pollution at sound intensities greater than 100 to 120 db can cause corresponding mechanical damage to the organ of Corti on the tuned basilar membrane. If damage is severe, permanent sensorineural deafness to the offending sound frequencies results. Thus, the wearing of earplugs or ear protection is important under many industrial conditions and for musicians and music listeners exposed to high sound amplification. Noise pollution often is characterized by high-intensity sounds of a specific frequency that cause corresponding damage to the organ of Corti.

Deafness or some degree of hearing impairment is the most common serious complication of bacterial meningitis in infants and children. It has been reported that sensorineural deafness complicates bacterial meningitis in 10% of cases and is most likely to follow *Streptococcus pneumoniae* meningitis.[7]

Drugs that damage inner ear structures are labeled ototoxic. Vestibular symptoms of ototoxicity include light-headedness, giddiness, and dizziness; if severe, cochlear symptoms can consist of tinnitus or hearing loss. The hearing loss is sensorineural and may be bilateral or unilateral, transient or permanent. Several classes of drugs have been identified as having ototoxic potentials: aminoglycoside antibiotics and other basic antibiotics with similar ototoxic potential, antimalarial drugs, loop diuretics, and salicylates. In addition to these drug groups, many other drug groups have been implicated in causing ototoxicity. The risk of ototoxicity depends on the total dose of the drug and its concentration in the bloodstream. The risk is increased in people with impaired kidney functioning and in those previously or currently treated with another potentially ototoxic drug. Table 53-1 lists drugs with the potential for producing ototoxicity.

OLD-AGE HEARING LOSS

Hearing loss is a common disability in elderly people. About 23% of people between ages 65 and 75 and 40% of the population over age 75 are affected.[8] This contrasts with other sensory losses in the aged that tend to reach a plateau in functional deficit. High-frequency sounds are affected more than low-frequency sounds because both high and low frequencies distort the base of the basilar membrane, whereas only low frequencies affect the distal (apical) region. Through the years, permanent mechanical damage to the organ of Corti is more likely near the base of cochlea where the high sonic frequencies are discriminated. Men are affected earlier and experience a greater loss than women. Some people also experience phonetic regression, or word discrimination loss, which interferes with normal communication.

DIAGNOSIS

Hearing loss may be estimated by having the person report soft whispered, normal spoken, or shouted words. A ticking watch may also be used, but this only tests the higher frequencies.

The *audiogram* is an important method of analyzing a person's hearing. It is done by an audiologist and requires highly specialized sound production and control equipment. Pure tones of controlled intensity are delivered, usually to one ear at a time, and the minimum intensity needed for hearing to be experienced is plotted as a function of frequency.

Tuning forks are used to differentiate conductive and sensorineural hearing loss. A 512-Hz or higher frequency tuning fork is used because frequencies below this level elicit a tactile response. The *Weber test* evaluates conductive hearing loss by lateralization of sound. It is done by placing the lightly vibrating

TABLE 53-1. MAJOR OTOTOXIC DRUGS		
DRUG	**AUDITORY FUNCTION**	**VESTIBULAR FUNCTION**
Aminoglycoside Antibiotics		
Amikacin	+	0
Gentamicin	+	+
Kanamycin	+	+
Neomycin	+	+
Streptomycin	+	+
Tobramycin	+	+
Other Antibiotics		
Colistin (topical middle ear)	0	+
Erythromycin (intravenous)	+*	0
Minocycline	0	+
Polymyxin B (topical middle ear)	0	+
Vancomycin	+	0
Antimalarial Drugs		
Chloroquine and quinine	+*	0
Loop Diuretics		
Ethacrynic acid	+	+
Furosemide	+*	0
Bumetanide	+*	0
Salicylate (aspirin)	+*	0
Cisplatin	+	0

* Effects are rarely permanent.
+, yes; 0, no.

tuning fork on the forehead or vertex of the head. In persons with conductive losses, the sound is louder on the side with the hearing loss, whereas in persons with sensorineural loss, it radiates to the side with the better hearing. The *Rinne test* compares air and bone conduction. The test is done by alternately placing the tuning fork on the mastoid bone and in front of the ear canal. In conductive losses, bone conduction exceeds air conduction; in sensorineural losses, the opposite occurs.

The *brain stem–evoked response* (BSER) is a noninvasive method that permits functional evaluation of certain defined parts of the central auditory pathways. Scalp electrodes and high-gain amplifiers are required to produce a record of the electrical wave activity elicited during repeated acoustic stimulations of either or both ears. With this method, certain of the early waves that come from discrete portions of the pons and midbrain auditory pathways can be correlated with specific sensorineural abnormalities.

TREATMENT

Conduction deafness can be corrected through the use of electrical amplification methods (hearing aids). Hearing aids deliver sound stimuli directly to the skull bones with sufficient added power to, in turn, directly vibrate the inner ear apparatus. This method bypasses the middle ear conduction apparatus. Amplification is of no assistance with sensorineural hearing loss. With sensorineural deficit, a hearing aid serves only to increase the intensity of a signal experienced as distorted. In mixed hearing loss, amplification can provide improvement only for the conduction problems that are part of the syndrome. Although most standard tests for auditory acuity use pure tone stimuli, intelligibility of sound stimuli is not necessarily correlated with pure tone loss. Damage to the important communicative function of auditory language produces a social isolation that is potentially damaging to a person's mental attitude and motivation for rehabilitation.

Surgically implantable cochlear prostheses for the profoundly deaf have been developed. A number of auditory prostheses have been produced that use electrodes implanted outside or within the cochlea or in the modiolus. A cochlear prosthesis does not provide normal hearing; rather, it provides perception of background noises. For example, the cochlear prosthesis allows a person to hear footsteps and become aware that someone is speaking, so that lipreading can be used. It also allows for recognition of protective sounds, such as an automobile approaching, a fire alarm, and the opening and closing of doors.

Improvements now permit at least some speech recognition in some instances.[9] The method has promise except for those few pathologic conditions in which total labyrinthine destruction or total cochlear nerve degeneration has occurred.

Unlike visual deficiency, which can lead to amblyopia and visual impairment, unilateral conduction deafness in early childhood, if corrected in later years, apparently does not lead to differential use of only the unaffected ear for speech perception.[10, 11] Also, damage to the central auditory pathways or auditory cortex on one side of the brain in childhood does not result in serious impairment in hearing and speech perception.[12, 13] In the adolescent or adult, damage to the auditory association cortex on the speech dominant side (usually the left side) can result in serious difficulties in speech perception called *receptive aphasia*.

In summary, hearing is a specialized sense whose external stimulus is the vibration of sound waves. The ear receives the sound waves, distinguishes their frequencies, translates this information into nerve impulses, and transmits these to the CNS. The auditory system consists of the external ear, middle ear, inner ear, auditory pathways, and central auditory cortex. Among the disorders of the auditory system are infections of the external and middle ear, otosclerosis, and conduction and sensorineural deafness. Otitis externa is an inflammatory process of the external ear. The middle ear is a tiny air-filled cavity located in the temporal bone. The auditory tube connects the middle ear to the nasopharynx and allows for equalization of pressure between the middle ear and the atmosphere. Infections can travel from the nasopharynx to the middle ear along the auditory tube, causing otitis media, or inflammation of the middle ear. The auditory tube is shorter and more horizontal in infants and young children, and infections of the middle ear are a common problem in these age groups. Otitis media can be acute, subacute, or chronic. The most common form, acute suppurative otitis media, usually follows an upper respiratory tract infection. It is characterized by otalgia, fever, and hearing loss. The effusion that accompanies otitis media can persist for weeks or months, interfering with hearing and impairing speech development. Otosclerosis is a familial disorder of the otic capsule. It causes bone resorption followed by excessive replacement with sclerotic bone. The disorder eventually causes immobilization of the stapes and conduction deafness. Deafness, or hearing loss, can develop as the result of a number of auditory disorders. It can be conductive, sensorineural, or mixed. Conduction deafness occurs when transmission of sound waves from the external to the inner ear is impaired. Sensorineural deafness can involve cochlear structures of the inner ear or the neural pathways that transmit auditory stimuli.

■ VESTIBULAR FUNCTION

The vestibular receptive organs, which are located in the inner ear, and their CNS connections contribute to the reflex activity necessary for effective posture and movement in a physical world governed by momentum and a gravitational field. Because the vestibular apparatus is part of the inner ear and, thus, located in the head, it is head motion and acceleration that are sensed. The vestibular system serves two general and related functions: (1) it maintains and assists recovery of stable body and head position through control of postural reflexes and (2) it maintains a stable visual field despite marked changes in head position.

VESTIBULAR SYSTEM

The peripheral apparatus of the vestibular system lies embedded in the petrous portion of the temporal bone, adjacent to and continuous with the cochlea of the auditory system. All the vestibular structures are contained in bony canals called the bony labyrinth. A membranous labyrinth that has the same shape as the bony labyrinth is fitted into the bony canals. The area immediately surrounding the membranous labyrinth is filled with perilymph, in which the membranous labyrinth floats. The composition of perilymph is similar to that of cerebrospinal fluid (CSF), and a tubular perilymphatic duct connects the perilymph fluid with the CSF in the subarachnoid space of the posterior fossa. The membranous labyrinth is filled with endolymph. A small-diameter tubular extension, the endolymphatic sac, connects this system with the subdural space near the jugular foramen, providing an exit for the slowly circulating endolymph into the lymphatic system. The endolymph has a high potassium concentration and is similar to intracellular fluid.

The vestibular apparatus is divided into five prominent divisions: three semicircular ducts, a utricle, and a saccule (see Fig. 53-5). The receptors of these structures are differentiated into the angular acceleration–deceleration receptors of the semicircular canals and the linear acceleration–deceleration and static gravitational receptors of the utricle and saccule. The utricle and saccule are two widened membranous sacs within the bony vestibule. The utricle connects the ends of each semicircular duct. The saccule communicates with the utricle through a small duct and with the cochlear duct of the auditory apparatus through the ductus reuniens.

Small patches of tall columnar hair-like ciliated epithelial cells are located in the floor of the utricle (utricular macula), in the side wall of the saccule (saccular macula), at the base of each semicircular duct (cristae), and along the floor of the cochlear duct (organ of Corti; see Fig. 53-6). Each hair cell has several microvilli and one true cilium called a kinocilium. Ganglion cells, homologous with dorsal root ganglion cells, form three afferent ganglia: the superior vestibular ganglion, which innervates the hair cells of the utricular macula and the cristae of the superior and horizontal semicircular ducts; the inferior vestibular ganglion, which innervates the saccular macula and the cristae of the inferior semicircular duct; and the spiral (or acoustic) ganglion, which innervates the cochlear duct. The central axons of these ganglion cells become the superior and inferior vestibular nerves and the cochlear auditory nerve. They often are collectively called the *eighth cranial nerve,* and they enter the side of the nearby medullary–pontine junction of the brain stem. The axons of the vestibular nerves terminate in the four vestibular nuclei (superior, lateral, medial, and inferior vestibular nuclei).

SEMICIRCULAR DUCTS

The three semicircular ducts, each about two thirds of a circle, are arranged at right angles to one another, with the horizontal duct tilted at about 12 degrees above the normal horizontal plane of the head (see Fig. 53-5). The horizontal ducts of the two sides of the head are in the same plane and the superior duct of one side is parallel with the inferior duct of the other side. At the junction of each semicircular duct and the utricle, an enlargement of each semicircular duct, called an *ampulla,* contains the hair cell sensory surface raised into a crest, or crista, at right angles to the duct. The stereocilia of each hair cell extend into a flexible gelatinous mass, the cupula, which essentially closes off fluid flow through the semicircular ducts. When the head begins to rotate around the axis of a semicircular duct (*i.e.,* undergoes angular acceleration), the momentum of the endolymph causes an increase in pressure to be applied to one side of the cupula. This is similar to the lagging behind of the water in a glass that is suddenly rotated, except that the endolymph cannot flow past the cupula and instead applies a differential pressure to its two sides, bending it and the cilia of the hair cells. This results in a reduced membrane potential across the hair cell plasma membrane when the hair is bent toward the microvilli and an increased membrane potential when the hair cell is bent in the opposite direction. Impulses from the cristae are transmitted by the vestibular part of the vestibulocochlear (VIII) cranial nerve to the vestibular nuclei of the caudal pons.

Maximal stimulation of the afferents of a semicircular duct results when rotation of the head occurs exactly in the plane of the membranous duct. Because of the orientation of the three semicircular ducts, angular accelerations of the head result in action potentials in at least one and usually more than one of the vestibular nerve branches to the three

cristae. If the angular acceleration reduces to a steady angular velocity, friction between the endolymph and the duct wall gradually results in first a reduction of pressure and then a loss of differential pressure on the two sides of the cupula—a form of sensory adaptation. On the sudden reduction or cessation of head rotation, the momentum of the endolymph applies pressure on the cupula from the opposite direction. Thus, the semicircular duct system provides a mechanism for signaling to the CNS the direction and rate of accelerations and decelerations in head rotation.

UTRICLE AND SACCULE

The hair cell surface (macula) of the utricle is oriented approximately in the horizontal plane. The macula of the saccule is oriented in the vertical plane. In both instances, the stereocilia of the hair cells extend into a gelatinous mass within the endolymph. Myriad microscopic crystals of calcium carbonate and calcium phosphate, called *otoliths,* are embedded in this gelatinous material, adding considerably to its total mass. The gelatinous mass with its otoliths is called the otolithic membrane. When the head is tilted, the gelatinous mass shifts its position because of the pull of the gravitational field, bending the stereocilia of the macular hair cells. Although each hair cell becomes hyperpolarized or hypopolarized, depending on the direction in which the cilia are bending, the hair cells are oriented in all directions, making these sense organs sensitive to static or changing head position in relation to the gravitational field. The central connections from the maculae provide the mechanism by which head, body, and eye postural adjustments occur in response to tilting the head and by which a stable visual fixation point ("optic grasp" of the visual field), as well as postural support of a stable head position, is maintained. Projections to the forebrain provide the basis for sensations of head tilt away from the horizontal plane.

In addition to this rather static tilt reception function, the utricle and saccule provide the organism with linear acceleration and deceleration reception. When the head is accelerated in a linear manner, such as the initial or terminal phase of an elevator ride or during automobile acceleration or deceleration, differential movement between the head and the otolithic membranes provides the basis for reflex compensatory bracing of neck, trunk, and limbs. The utricle and saccule also provide the input data on which the air-righting reflexes are based. A cat dropped from an upside-down position lands on its feet and does so even if blindfolded. Most vestibular reflexes, including air-righting, are functional at birth. If a neonate is supported in the prone position and the support is momentarily (and with great care) removed, the trunk is extended and all four limbs are extended as falling begins. In the supine position, the trunk is flexed and the limbs are flexed as the fall progresses. On the other hand, the head-on-body vestibular reflexes of the infant are not sufficiently operational during the first 6 weeks or so after birth to maintain head posture. This is why the neonate's head must be supported when the neonate is lifted in the supine position.

CENTRAL NERVOUS SYSTEM CONNECTIONS

The nerve fibers from the vestibular receptors travel in the vestibular portion of the vestibulocochlear (VIII) cranial nerve (see Fig. 53-7) to the superior, medial, lateral, and inferior vestibular nuclei located at the junction of the medulla and pons. In addition, some of the afferent fibers travel to the ipsilateral cerebellar cortex and a deep cerebellar nucleus called the *fastigial nucleus*. The part of the cerebellum that receives vestibular input is called the *archicerebellum*, or the *flocculonodular lobe*. On the output side, cells in the fastigial nucleus that receive afferent terminals and terminals from cortical neurons send their axons back to the vestibular nuclei of the same and opposite sides of the brain stem.

A fiber tract called the *medial longitudinal fasciculus* (MLF) extends from the midbrain to the upper part of the spinal cord; it lies close to the medial plane and interconnects the vestibular nuclei with motor nuclei, particularly those of cranial nerves III, IV, VI, and XI. In addition to complex internal circuitry, neurons from the vestibular nuclei project into the nearby reticular formation and provide powerful control on postural reflexes of the eyes, head, body, and limbs. Projections occur to the pons lateral gaze control center, to the vertical and torsional gaze control regions, to the sixth cranial nerve nuclei, to the MLF, to the fourth and third nerve nuclei, and to cervical-level lower motoneurons innervating the sternocleidomastoid and other neck muscles that control head turning and posture. The MLF projections primarily control horizontal or lateral turning and conjugate gaze. In addition, extensive projections into and through the reticular formation follow the central tegmental fasciculus pathway that controls the vertical and rotatory (torsion) gaze reflexes.

EYE MOVEMENT REFLEXES

Vestibular control of conjugate eye posture can be understood in terms of complex reflex bilateral (conjugate) eye movements that preserve eye fixation on stable objects in the visual field. The term *nystagmus* is used to describe vestibular-controlled eye move-ments that occur in response to angular and rotational movements of the head. As one begins to sway or fall, such visual stability is essential to successful recovery attempts. Thus, as the body and head begin rotation, the eyes in a conjugate manner move in exactly the opposite direction, maintaining the previous fixation point. This is called the slow phase of nystagmus. If the rotation continues beyond the range of lateral eye movement, a quick (rapid phase of nystagmus) conjugate eye correction (saccadic return) occurs as if to obtain a new stable fixation point, and then the slow phase continues again. This nystagmus pattern continues as long as angular acceleration continues. When a steady rotational velocity is reached, compensatory nystagmus movements gradually wane as the disparity between the movement of endolymph and the semicircular duct wall is lost, as the pressure on the two sides of the cupula is equalized.

Clinically, the direction of this nystagmus pattern is named for the fast, or saccadic, phase. The reflex circuitry is in precise control of motor units in the nuclei that innervate the extrinsic muscles of the eye by way of cranial nerves III, IV, and VI. In fact, the precision of nystagmus movements is as great in people whose eyes are closed and in the congenitally blind as it is in normal-sighted people. If the eyes are not allowed to move, or if stimulation is strong, the head also moves in a nystagmoid manner as a result of vestibular control of the sternocleidomastoid muscles by cranial nerve XI.

Vestibular-driven nystagmus can occur in any plane. Beginning rotation of the head around a transverse axis in a head-over-heels manner is accompanied by compensatory nystagmus, which has its slow, smooth-pursuit phase in the upward direction and its fast phase in the direction of rotation. Starting rotation around the frontal–occipital axis (*i.e.*, head tilting to the side) is accompanied by compensatory slow-phase torsion eye movements, twisting in the direction opposite to the rotation. The saccadic phase is in the direction of body rotation. In each instance, nystagmus can be understood in terms of repeated attempts to grasp stable fixed visual fields as the head rotates, with a quick correction to a new, stable fixation point.

Nystagmus can be classified in terms of the direction of eye movement: horizontal, vertical, rotatory, or mixed. Nystagmus derived from a sense organ or vestibular nerve is of the slow phase–fast phase or jerky type described previously. Nystagmus resulting from CNS pathology usually has equal slow and fast rates in each direction, called pendular nystagmus.

If the visual environment is rotated or appears to rotate past a person with a normally functioning visual system, even though the head remains in a fixed position, a fixation point is selected and a smooth pursuit movement rotates the eyes to the limit of the binocular field. At this point, a saccadic correction quickly moves the eyes back to a new fixation point, and the pursuit occurs again. This visually induced, or optokinetic, nystagmus and the associated sensation of movement are experienced when a moving object such as a car or train moves past the visual field. The phenomenon demonstrates the ability of visual stimuli to overpower the vestibular end organs' signals that the head is indeed stable in relation to gravitational and inertial forces.

THALAMIC AND CORTICAL PROJECTIONS

Some of the neurons of the vestibular nuclei project their axons rostrally to the ventrolateral nuclei of the thalamus. In addition to the intrathalamic circuitry, thalamic projections go to the primary vestibular cortex near the somesthetic area of the parietal lobe. These thalamic and cortical projections provide the basis for the subjective experiences of position in space, rotation, and vertigo that accompany the onset or sudden cessation of head rotation. During such episodes, nystagmus is observed.

Severe damage to the forebrain or to the brain stem rostral to the pons often results in loss of rostral control of these static vestibular reflexes. If the patient's head is moved from side to side or up and down, the eyes retain a stable fixation point. Thus, the eyes move in conjugate gaze, much as those of a doll with counterweighted eyes. This phenomenon, called doll's head phenomenon, demonstrates the always-present vestibular static reflexes without forebrain interference or suppression. If doll's head phenomenon is present, brain stem function at the level of the pons is considered intact (in a comatose person). These static vestibular reflexes are to be contrasted with rapid or dynamic vestibular reflexes (nystagmus and the linear acceleration–deceleration reflexes).

POSTURAL REFLEXES

Sudden changes in balance or orientation, such as falling to the right or left or backward or forward, result in powerful reflexes needed to maintain equilibrium and posture.

The descending portion of the MLF, essentially a medial vestibulospinal tract, continues at least into thoracic cord levels and provides vestibular control of the muscle tone of axial muscles, including the dorsal back muscles. A rapid-conducting lateral vestibulo-

spinal tract descends the spinal cord to provide powerful vestibular control of the lower motoneurons of the upper and lower limbs. As the head begins to tip (*i.e.*, rotate) on the neck or as part of general body tipping, the vestibular system activates the appropriate extensor muscles of the neck, trunk, and limbs, opposing the direction of the tilt. These powerful reflex adjustments in muscle tone assist in maintaining stable head and, therefore, body postural support during static posture and during passive or active movement.

All the vestibular nuclei receive input from the cerebellum as well as the vestibular nerve. The cerebellar connections of the vestibular system are necessary for adjustments of temporally smooth, coordinated movements to ongoing head movement, tilt, or angular acceleration. For instance, accurate grasping can occur during a fall, indicating cerebellar adjustments based on vestibular information during the performance of a smooth, accurate movement.

Vestibular reflexes are quite powerful, and considerable learning is required to inhibit or greatly modify them, as is necessary for acrobatic pilots, divers, and gymnasts. Dancers and skaters who engage in rapid spinning movements also learn to use or at least partially inhibit these reflexes.

ALTERATIONS IN VESTIBULAR FUNCTION

Disorders of vestibular function are characterized by a condition called *vertigo*, in which a hallucination of motion occurs; that is, either the person is stationary and the environment is in motion (objective vertigo), or the person is in motion and the environment is stationary (subjective vertigo). Vertigo should be differentiated from dizziness, which is characterized by light-headedness, fainting, and unsteadiness. Abnormal nystagmus, tinnitus, and hearing loss are other common manifestations of vestibular dysfunction, as are autonomic manifestations such as perspiration, nausea, and vomiting. Disorders of vestibular function can be either peripheral (involving the labyrinth) or central (involving the vestibular connections).

Spontaneous nystagmus that occurs without head movement or visual stimuli is always pathologic. It seems to appear more readily and more severely when fatigue is present and, to some extent, can be influenced by psychological factors. Nystagmus derived from the CNS, in contrast with peripheral end organ or eighth cranial nerve sources, seldom is accompanied by vertigo. If present, the vertigo is of mild intensity.

DISORDERS OF PERIPHERAL VESTIBULAR FUNCTION

Motion Sickness. One of the most common alterations of vestibular function is motion sickness. It is caused by repeated rhythmic stimulation of the vestibular system, such as is encountered in car, air, or boat travel. Vertigo, malaise, nausea, and vomiting are the principal symptoms. Autonomic signs, including lowered blood pressure, tachycardia, and excessive sweating, may occur. Anti–motion sickness drugs may be used to ameliorate these symptoms. Motion sickness usually decreases in severity with repeated exposure.

Vestibular System Injury or Irritation. The inner ear is vulnerable to injury caused by fracture of the petrous portion of the temporal bones; infection of nearby structures, including the middle ear and meninges; and blood-borne toxins and infections. Damage to the vestibular system can occur as an adverse effect of certain drugs or from allergic reactions to foods. The aminoglycosides (*e.g.,* streptomycin and gentamicin) have a specific toxic affinity for the vestibular portion of the inner ear. Alcohol can cause transient episodes of vertigo.

Severe irritation or damage of the vestibular end organs or nerves results in severe balance disorders reflected by instability of posture, dystaxia, and falling accompanied by vertigo. With irritation, falling is away from the affected side; with destruction, it is toward the affected side. Adaptation to asymmetric stimulation occurs within a few days, after which the signs and symptoms diminish and eventually are lost. After recovery, there usually is a slightly reduced acuity for tilt, and the person walks with a somewhat broadened base to improve postural stability. The neurologic basis for this adaptation to unilateral loss of vestibular input is not understood. After adaptation to the loss of vestibular input from one side, the loss of function of the opposite vestibular apparatus produces signs and symptoms identical to those resulting from unilateral rather than bilateral loss. Within weeks, adaptation is again sufficient for locomotion and even driving a car. Such a person relies heavily on visual and proprioceptive input and has severe orientational difficulty in the dark, particularly when traversing uneven terrain.

Meniere's Disease. A disorder of peripheral vestibular function, Meniere's disease is caused by an overaccumulation of endolymph, also called endolymphatic hydrops. It is characterized by fluctuating episodes of tinnitus, feelings of ear fullness, and violent rotary vertigo that often renders the person unable to sit or walk. There is a need to lie quietly with the head fixed in a comfortable position, avoiding all head movements that aggravate the vertigo. Symptoms referable to the autonomic nervous system, including pallor, sweating, nausea, and vomiting, usually are present. The more severe the attack, the more prominent the autonomic manifestations. A fluctuating hearing loss occurs, and initially, there is a return to normal after the episode subsides. As the disease progresses, it becomes more severe and permanent. Meniere's disease usually is unilateral, and because the sense of hearing is bilateral, many people with the disorder are not aware of the full extent of their hearing loss.

A number of conditions, such as allergy, adrenal–pituitary insufficiency, trauma, and hypothyroidism, can cause Meniere's disease. The most common form of the disease is an idiopathic form thought to be caused by a single viral injury to the fluid transport system of the inner ear. An area of recent interest has been the investigation of the relation between immune disorders and Meniere's disease.

Methods used in the diagnosis of Meniere's disease include audiograms, vestibular testing by electronystagmography, and petrous pyramid x-rays. The administration of hyperosmolar substances, such as glycerin and urea, often produces acute temporary hearing improvement in people with Meniere's disease and sometimes is used as a diagnostic measure of endolymphatic hydrops. The diuretic furosemide may also be used for this purpose.

The treatment of Meniere's disease can be either medical or surgical. Medical treatment consists primarily of sedation (*e.g.,* diazepam [Valium]) and diuretic therapy (hydrochlorothiazide or hydrochlorothiazide with triamterene [Dyazide]).[14] A low-sodium diet is recommended in addition to these medications. The steroid hormone prednisone may be used to maintain satisfactory hearing and resolve dizziness. Streptomycin therapy has been used for ablation of the vestibular system.[14]

Vestibular rehabilitation, a relatively new treatment modality for peripheral vestibular disorders, has met with considerable success.[15, 16] It commonly is done by physical therapists and uses a home exercise program that incorporates habituation exercises, balance retraining exercises, and a general conditioning program.[16] The habituation exercises take advantage of physiologic fatigue of the neurovegetative response to repetitive movement or positional stimulation and are done to decrease motion-provoked dizziness, light-headedness, and unsteadiness. The exercises are selected to provoke the vestibular symptoms. The person moves quickly into the position that causes symptoms, holds the position until the symptoms subside (fatigue of the neurovegetative response), relaxes, and then repeats the exercise for a prescribed number of times. The exercises usually are repeated twice daily. The habituation effect is characterized by decreased sensitivity and duration of symptoms. It may occur in as quickly as 2 weeks or take as long as 6 months.[16] Balance retraining exercises consist of activities directed toward improving individual components of balance that may be abnormal. General conditioning exercises, a vital part of the rehabilitation process, are individualized to the person's preferences and life-style. They should consist of motion-oriented activity that the person is interested in and should be done on a regular basis (*e.g.*, four to five times per week).[16]

Surgical methods include (1) the creation of an endolymphatic shunt in which excess endolymph from the inner ear is diverted into either the subarachnoid space or the mastoid and (2) vestibular nerve section. Advances in vestibular nerve section have facilitated the monitoring of seventh and eighth nerve potentials. These methods are used to prevent hearing damage.[14]

DISORDERS OF CENTRAL VESTIBULAR FUNCTION

Abnormal nystagmus and vertigo can occur as a result of CNS pathology. Compression of the vestibular nuclei by cerebellar tumors invading the fourth ventricle results in progressively severe signs and symptoms. In addition to abnormal nystagmus and vertigo, vomiting and broad-base and dystaxic gait become progressively more evident. Some drugs (*e.g.*, anticonvulsants) can also cause abnormal nystagmus. Centrally derived nystagmus usually has equal excursion in both directions (pendular). In contrast to peripherally generated nystagmus, CNS-derived nystagmus is relatively constant rather than episodic, can occur in any direction rather than being primarily in the horizontal or torsional (rotatory) dimensions, often changes direction through time, and cannot be suppressed by visual fixation. Repeated induction of nystagmus results in rapid diminution or "fatigue" of the reflex with peripheral abnormalities, but fatigue is not characteristic of central lesions. Congenital and lifelong nystagmus abnormalities are not uncommon and occur as part of a number of hereditary syndromes. Nystagmus can also accompany other motor defects in cerebral palsy and degenerative syndromes such as multiple sclerosis. Abnormal nystagmus can make reading and other tasks that require precise eye positional control difficult.

DIAGNOSTIC METHODS

Diagnosis of vestibular disorders is based on a description of the symptoms, a history of trauma or exposure to agents that are destructive to vestibular structures, and physical examination. Tests of eye movements (nystagmus) and muscle control of balance and equilibrium often are used. Current tests of vestibular function focus on the horizontal semicircular reflex because it is the easiest reflex to stimulate (rotationally and calorically) and record using electronystagmography.

Electronystagmography. Electronystagmography (ENG) is a precise and objective diagnostic method of evaluating nystagmus eye movements. Electrodes are placed lateral to the outer canthus of each eye and above and below each eye. A ground electrode is placed on the forehead. With ENG the velocity, frequency, and amplitude of spontaneous or induced nystagus and the changes in these measurements brought by a loss of fixation, either with the eyes open or closed, can be quantified. The advantages of ENG are that it is easily administered, noninvasive, does not interfere with vision, and does not require head restraint.[17]

Caloric Stimulation. Caloric testing involves positioning the head at a 30-degree angle and irrigating the external auditory canal with either warm (40°C) or cold (25°C) water. The resulting changes in temperature, as conducted through the petrous portion of the temporal bone, set up convection currents in the otic fluid that mimic the effects of angular acceleration. With the head positioned at 30 degrees, the endolymph is induced primarily in the horizontal semicircular canals. When cold water is used, there is initial conjugate eye movement (lasting 30 to 120 seconds) toward the ear being irrigated if the oculovestibular reflex is intact.[18] This movement is controlled by the brain stem and represents the slow component of nystagmus. The fast component (occurring within 20 to 30 seconds) follows, moving the eyes back toward the opposite side. Eye movements can be monitored by ENG. An advantage of the caloric stimulation method is the ability to test the vestibular apparatus on one side at a time.

Rotational Tests. Rotational testing involves rotation using a rotatable chair or motor-driven platform. Unlike caloric testing, rotational testing depends only on the inner ear and is unrelated to conditions of the external ear or temporal bone. A major disadvantage of the method is that both ears are tested simultaneously.

Motor-driven platforms can be precisely controlled and multiple graded stimuli can be delivered in a relatively short period of time. For rotational testing, the person is seated in a chair mounted on the motor-driven platform. Testing is usually performed in the dark without visual influence and with selected light stimuli. Eye movements are monitored using ENG.

A rotatable chair (Bárány chair), much like a barber's chair, can be used for assessing postrotational vestibular reflexes. The person is strapped into the chair with the head positioned so that the plane of one pair of semicircular ducts is in the horizontal plane (plane of rotation); each of the three primary planes of the ducts is tested, in turn. The person is rotated until a steady rate of rotation is achieved. The chair is suddenly stopped, and the ensuing postrotational reflex nystagmus and the compensatory movements of the body and limbs are observed.

Romberg Test. The Romberg test is used to demonstrate disorders of static vestibular function. The person being tested is requested to stand with feet together and arms extended forward so that the degree of sway and arm stability can be noted. The person is then asked to close his or her eyes. When visual clues are removed, postural stability is based on proprioceptive sensation from the joints, muscles, and tendons and from static vestibular reception. Deficiency in vestibular static input is indicated by greatly increased sway and a tendency for the arms to drift toward the side of deficiency.

If vestibular input is severely deficient, the subject falls toward the deficient side. Care must be taken because defects of proprioceptive projection to the forebrain also result in some arm drift and postural instability toward the deficient side. Only if two-point discrimination and vibratory sensation from the lower and upper limbs are bilaterally normal can the deficiency be attributed to the vestibular system.

ANTIVERTIGO DRUGS

Among the methods used to treat vertigo are the antivertigo or anti–motion sickness drugs. Drugs used in the treatment of vertigo include anticholinergic drugs (scopolamine, atropine), monoaminergic drugs (amphetamine, ephedrine), and antihistamines (meclizine [Antivert], cyclizine [Marezine], dimenhydrinate [Dramamine], and promethazine [Phenergan]). Animal studies have documented that drugs with anticholinergic or monoaminergic activity diminish the excitability of neurons in the vestibular nucleus. Although the antihistamines have long been used in treating vertigo, little is known about their mechanism of action. Most of these drugs have some anticholinergic activity, and some also enhance sympathetic activity by blocking the reuptake of monoamines at the synaptic nerve terminals. A transdermal scopolamine preparation (Transderm-V) is available for use in treating motion sickness. The medication is prepared on a slow-release micro-porous polypropylene membrane contained in a patch that can be placed behind the ear. A small dose of the drug is released slowly and absorbed over a 3-day period. This method of drug delivery has proved effective in preventing motion sickness with minimal adverse effects. To be effective, the patch must be in place for several hours before exposure to motion.

In summary, the vestibular system plays an essential role in the equilibrium sense, which is closely integrated with the visual and proprioceptive (position) senses. The receptors for the vestibular system, which are located in the semicircular ducts of the inner ear, respond to changes in linear and angular acceleration of the head. The vestibular nerve fibers travel in the vestibulocochlear (VIII) cranial nerve to the vestibular nuclei located at the junction of the medulla and pons. Some of the fibers pass through the nuclei to the cerebellum. The cerebellar connections are necessary for temporally smooth, coordinated movements during ongoing head movements, tilt, and angular acceleration. The vestibular nuclei also connect with the nuclei of the oculomotor (III), trochlear (IV), and abducens (VI) cranial nerves. Vestibular control of conjugate eye movements serves to preserve eye fixation on stable objects in the visual field during head movement. The term nystagmus is used to describe vestibular-controlled eye movements that occur in response to angular and rotational movements of the head. Neurons of the vestibular nuclei also project to the thalamus, to the temporal cortex, and to the somatesthetic area of the parietal cortex. The thalamic and cortical projections provide the basis for the subjective experiences of position in space and of rotation and vertigo.

Disorders of the vestibular system include motion sickness and Meniere's disease. Meniere's disease, which is caused by an overaccumulation of endolymph, is characterized by severe disabling episodes of tinnitus, feelings of ear fullness, and violent rotary vertigo. The diagnosis of vestibular disorders is based on a description of the symptoms, a history of trauma or exposure to agents destructive to vestibular structures, and tests of eye movements (nystagmus) and muscle control of balance and equilibrium. Among the methods used in the treatment of vertigo that accompanies vestibular disorders are the antivertigo, or anti–motion sickness, drugs. These drugs act by diminishing the excitability of neurons in the vestibular nucleus.

■ REFERENCES

1. Bluestone, C.D. (1982). Otitis media in children: To treat or not to treat. *New England Journal of Medicine, 306,* 1399.
2. Meyerhoff, W.L., & Carter, J.B. (1984). *Diagnosis and management of hearing loss* (p. 1). Philadelphia: W.B. Saunders.
3. Senturia, B.H., Bluestone, C.D., Paradise, J.L., et al. (1980). Report of the Ad Hoc Committee on Definition and Classification of Otitis Media and Otitis Media with Effusion. *Annals of Otolaryngology, 89*(Suppl), 3.

4. Barfold, C., & Roborg, J. (1980). Secretory otitis media: Long-term observations after treatment with grommets. *Archives of Otolaryngology, 106,* 553.

5. Al-Sheikhle, A.R.J. (1980). Secretory otitis media in children. (A retrospective study of 249). *Journal of Laryngology and Otology, 94,* 1117.

6. Heald, M.M., Matkin, N.D., & Merideth, K.E. (1990). Pressure-equalization (PE) tubes in treatment of otitis media: National survey of otolaryngologists. *Laryngology—Head and Neck Surgery, 102,* 334–338.

7. Dodge, P.R., Hallowell, D., Feigin, R.D., et al.(1984). Prospective evaluation of hearing impairment as a sequela of acute bacterial meningitis. *New England Journal of Medicine, 311,* 879.

8. Gates, G.A. (Chairperson). (1989). Invitational Geriatric Otorhinolaryngology Workshop: Presbycusis. *Otolaryngology—Head and Neck Surgery, 100,* 266–271.

9. Dawson, P.W., Blamey, P.J., Rowland, L.C., et al.(1992). Cochlear implants in children, adolescents, and prelinguistically deafened adults: Speech perception. *Journal of Speech and Hearing Research, 35,* 401–417.

10. Bess, F.H., & Tharp, A.M. (1986). Case history data on unilaterally hearing-impaired children. *Ear and Hearing, 7,* 14–19.

11. Martin, D.S. (Ed.). (1991). *Advances in cognition, education and deafness.* Washington, DC: Gallaudet University Press.

12. Feldman, H.M., Holland, A.L., Kemp, S.S., et al. (1992). Language development after unilateral brain injury. *Brain and Language, 42,* 89–102.

13. Bishop, D.V.M. (1992). The underlying nature of specific language impairment. *Journal of Child Psychology and Psychiatry and Allied Disciplines, 33,* 3–66.

14. Dickins, J.R.E., & Graham, S.S. (1990). Meniere's disease–1983–1989. *American Journal of Otolaryngology, 11,* 51–65.

15. Horak, F.B., Jones-Rycewicz, C., Black, F.W., et al. (1992). Effects of vestibular rehabilitation on dizziness and imbalance. *Otolaryngology—Head and Neck Surgery, 106,* 175–180.

16. Smith-Whellock, M., Shepard, N.T., & Telian, S.A. (1991). Physical therapy program for vestibular rehabilitation. *American Journal of Otology, 12,* 218–225.

17. Baloh, R.W. (1989). Modern vestibular function testing. *Western Journal of Medicine, 150,* 59–67.

18. Hickey, J.V. (1992). *Neurological and neurosurgical nursing* (3rd ed., p. 109). Philadelphia: J.B. Lippincott.

■ BIBLIOGRAPHY

Bluestone, C.D. (1989). Modern management of otitis media. *Pediatric Clinics of North America, 36,* 1371–1387.

Bluestone, C.D., Fria, T.J., Arjona, S.K., et al. (1986). Controversies in screening for middle ear disease and hearing loss in children. *Pediatrics, 77,* 57.

Brackemann, D.E. (1990). Surgical treatment of vertigo. *Journal of Laryngology and Otology, 164,* 849–859.

Callahan, C.W., & Lazoritz, S. (1988). Otitis media and language development. *American Family Practice, 37,* 186.

Croteau, N., Pless, B., & Infante-Rivard, C. (1990). Trends in medical visits and surgery for otitis media among children. *American Journal of Diseases in Children, 144,* 535–536.

Fireman, P. (1987). Newer concepts in otitis media. *Hospital Practice, 22*(11A), 85.

Fireman, P. (1988). Otitis media and its relationship to allergy. *Pediatric Clinics of North America, 35,* 1075–1091.

Giebink, G.S. (1992). Otitis media update: Pathogenesis and treatment. *Annals of Otology, Rhinology, and Laryngology, 101,* 21–23.

Langman, A.W., Jackler, R.K., & Sooy, F.A. (1991). Stapedectomy: Long-term hearing results. *Laryngoscope, 101,* 810–814.

Mohr, D. (1986). The syndrome of paroxysmal positional vertigo—a review. *Western Journal of Medicine, 145,* 645.

Mulrow, C.D. (1991). Screening for hearing impairment in the elderly. *Hospital Practice, 26,* 79–86.

Paradise, J.L. (1987). On classifying otitis media as suppurative or nonsuppurative, with a suggested clinical schema. *Journal of Pediatrics, 111,* 948.

Paradise, J.L. (1992). Antimicrobial prophylaxis for recurrent otitis media. *Annals of Otolaryngology, 101,* 33–36.

Sade, J., & Luntz, M. (1991). Adenodectomy in otitis media. *Annals of Otology, Rhinology, and Laryngology, 100,* 226–231.

Stringer, S.P., & Meyerhoff, W.L. (1990). Diagnosis, causes, and management of vertigo. *Comprehensive Therapy, 16*(3), 34–41.

Swan, I.R. (1989). The Rinne tuning fork test. *Hospital Practice, 24,* 99–102.

CHAPTER 54

DEGENERATIVE, DEMYELINATING, AND NEOPLASTIC DISORDERS OF THE NERVOUS SYSTEM

■ OBJECTIVES

After you have studied this chapter, you should be able to meet the following objectives:

■ State the criteria for a diagnosis of dementia.
■ Compare the etiologies associated with Alzheimer's disease, multi-infarct dementia, Pick's disease, Creutzfeldt-Jakob disease, Wernicke-Korsakoff syndrome, and Huntington's disease.
■ Describe the changes in brain tissue that occur with Alzheimer's disease.
■ Explain how a diagnosis of Alzheimer's disease is arrived at.
■ Use the three stages of Alzheimer's disease to describe its progress.
■ Compare the causes of the primary and secondary forms of parkinsonism.

■ Explain the symptoms of Parkinson's disease with reference to the extrapyramidal system.
■ Differentiate between the actions of anticholinergic drugs and dopamine agonists in controlling the symptoms of Parkinson's disease.
■ Explain the significance of demyelinization and plaque formation in multiple sclerosis.
■ Describe the manifestations of multiple sclerosis.
■ List the major categories of brain tumors.
■ Interpret the meaning of benign and malignant as they relate to brain tumors.
■ Describe the general manifestations of brain tumors.
■ List the methods used in diagnosis of brain tumors.

There are several types of nervous system disorders that produce progressive deterioration of function. These include degenerative brain disorders, such as dementia and parkinsonism, and demyelinating diseases, such as multiple sclerosis. Brain tumors are neoplasms that arise from central nervous system (CNS) tissues or as metastases from tumors outside the CNS. Although some brain tumors are successfully treated, many produce progressive destruction of brain tissue.

Carol Mattson Porth: PATHOPHYSIOLOGY: CONCEPTS OF ALTERED HEALTH STATES, 4th ed. © 1994, 1990, 1986, 1982 J.B. Lippincott Company

■ DEGENERATIVE BRAIN DISORDERS

Degenerative brain disorders are diseases that selectively affect one or more functional systems of neurons while leaving others intact. They generally produce symmetric and progressive involvement of the CNS, affect similar areas of the brain, and produce similar clinical syndromes.[1] Thus, degenerative disorders affecting the cortex tend to produce dementias; those affecting the basal ganglia produce extrapyramidal movement disorders.

DEMENTIAS

Dementia is a syndrome of intellectual deterioration severe enough to interfere with occupational or social performance. It involves disturbances in memory, language use, perception, and motor skills and in the ability to learn necessary skills, solve problems, think abstractly, and make judgments. Chart 54-1 describes the characteristics of dementia as presented in the *Diagnostic and statistical manual for mental disorders* (DSM-III-R).[2] Depression is the most common treatable illness that may masquerade as dementia and needs to be ruled out when a diagnosis of dementia is considered (see Chapter 7 for a discussion of delirium and depression in the elderly). This is important because cognitive functioning usually returns to baseline levels when depression is treated. Dementia can be caused by any disorder that permanently damages large association areas of the cerebral hemispheres, including Alzheimer's disease, multi-infarct dementia, Pick's disease, Creutzfeldt-Jakob disease, Wernicke-Korsakoff syndrome, and Huntington's chorea.

ALZHEIMER'S DISEASE

Dementia of the Alzheimer's type occurs in middle or late life and accounts for 50% to 70% of all cases of dementia. The disorder affects 2 to 4 million Americans and may be the fourth leading cause of death in the United States.[3] The risk of developing Alzheimer's disease increases with age. Approximately 4% of persons over age 65 years have Alzheimer's disease; by age 80, prevalence reaches 20%. As the elderly population in the United States continues to increase, the number of persons with Alzheimer's-type dementia can also be expected to increase.

Pathophysiology. Alzheimer's disease is characterized by cortical atrophy and loss of neurons, particularly in the frontal and temporal lobes. With significant atrophy, there is ventricular enlargement

---

CHART 54-1: DIAGNOSTIC CRITERIA FOR DEMENTIA

A. Demonstrable evidence of impairment in short-term and long-term memory. Impairment of short-term memory (inability to learn new information) may be indicated by inability to remember three objects after 5 minutes. Long-term memory impairment (inability to remember information that was known in the past) may be indicated by inability to remember personal information (*e.g.*, what happened yesterday, place, occupation) or facts of common knowledge (*e.g.*, past presidents, well-known dates).

B. At least one of the following:
   (1) Impairment in abstract thinking, as indicated by inability to find similarities and differences between related words, difficulty in defining words and concepts, and other similar tasks
   (2) Impaired judgment, as indicated by inability to make reasonable plans to deal with interpersonal, family, and job-related problems and issues
   (3) Other disturbances of higher cortical function, such as aphasia (disorder of language), apraxia (inability to carry out motor activities despite intact comprehension and motor function), agnosia (failure to recognize and identify objects despite intact sensory function), and "constructual difficulty" (*e.g.*, inability to copy three-dimensional figures, assemble blocks, or arrange sticks in specific designs)
   (4) Personality change (*i.e.*, alteration or accentuation of premorbid traits)

C. The disturbance in A and B significantly interferes with work or usual social activities or relationship with others.

D. The disturbance does not occur exclusively during the course of delirium.

(American Psychiatric Association. [1987]. *Diagnostic and statistical manual of mental disorders* [3rd ed., revised]. Washington, DC: American Psychiatric Association. Reprinted with permission)

(hydrocephalus) secondary to the loss of brain tissue. The major microscopic features of Alzheimer's disease are the presence of neurofibrillary tangles and senile plaques. The neurofibrillary tangles, found within the cytoplasm of abnormal neurons, consist of fibrous proteins wound around one another in a helical fashion. These tangles are resistant to chemical or enzymatic breakdown, and so they persist in brain tissue long after the neuron in which they arose has died and disappeared. The senile plaques are patches or flat areas composed of clusters of degenerating nerve terminals arranged around a central core of β-amyloid peptide. The β peptide is a fragment of a much larger β-amyloid precursor protein (βAPP), the normal function and source of which is still unknown. Formation of the β peptide appears to represent one of several possible cleavage patterns of BAPP.[1] Also characteristic of Alzheimer's disease is the accumulation of amyloid deposits in the cerebral and meningeal microvessels. The amyloid is the same as that found in the plaque core.

The basic pathogenic defect in Alzheimer's disease remains unclear, although much of the current research has focused on the βAPP. The gene for this protein is located on the long arm of chromosome 21, just distal to the genetic defect on the same chromosome that underlies at least some cases of familial (autosomal dominant) Alzheimer's disease. Interestingly, persons with Down syndrome (trisomy 21) develop the pathologic changes of Alzheimer's disease and comparable decline in cognitive functioning at a relatively young age. Virtually all persons with Down syndrome who survive past the age of 50 develop the full-blown pathologic features of Alzheimer's disease.[4]

It is important to recognize that some plaques and tangles can be found in the brains of older persons who do not show cognitive impairment. It is appears that it is the number and distribution of the plaques and tangles that contribute to the intellectual deterioration that occurs in persons with Alzheimer's disease. The plaques and tangles are found throughout the neocortex (with relative sparing of the primary sensory cortex) and in the hippocampus and amygdala.[1] The hippocampus is crucial to information processing, acquisition of new memories, and retrieval of old memories. The development of neurofibrillary tangles in the endorhinal cortex and superior portion of the hippocampal gyrus interferes with cortical input and output, thereby isolating the hippocampus from the remainder of the cortex and rendering it functionless.[5]

Neurochemically, Alzheimer's disease has been associated with a decrease in the level of choline acetyltransferase activity in the cortex and hippocampus. This enzyme is required for the synthesis of acetylcholine, a neurotransmitter that is associated with memory. The reduction in choline acetyltransferase is quantitatively related to the numbers of neuritic plaques and severity of dementia. Evidence supporting the role of acetylcholine in Alzheimer's disease comes from studies using scopolamine, a drug that blocks acetylcholine receptors. Memory deficits similar to those found in normal elderly persons have been induced in healthy young persons through the administration of scopolamine.[6] Furthermore, these deficits were reversed by administering physostigmine, a drug that prevents acetylcholine breakdown and thereby enhances its action. Unfortunately, attempts to increase brain levels of acetylcholine or its precursors in persons with Alzheimer's disease have been unsuccessful. Initial trials using

choline and lecithin, the precursors of acetylcholine, have failed to demonstrate any improvement in memory. Physostigmine has produced some improvement in a few patients. However, the drug has limited usefulness because of its potentially toxic side effects and short half-life (about 2 hours).[7]

Manifestations. Alzheimer's-type dementia follows an insidious and progressive course. Major symptoms include loss of memory, disorientation, impaired abstract thinking and impulse control, and changes in personality and affect.[8] Three stages of Alzheimer's dementia have been identified, each characterized by progressive degenerative changes (Chart 54-2).

The *first stage*, which may last for 2 to 4 years, is characterized by a subjective memory deficit that is often difficult to differentiate from the normal forgetfulness that occurs in the elderly. Whereas most elderly forget unimportant events and details, persons with Alzheimer's disease randomly forget both important and unimportant details. They forget where things are placed, get lost easily, and have trouble remembering appointments. Both recent and remote memory are affected. Mild changes in personality, such as a flat affect, lack of spontaneity, and loss of a previous sense of humor, occur during this stage.

As the disease progresses, the person with Alz-

CHART 54-2: STAGES OF ALZHEIMER'S DISEASE

Stage 1

Memory loss
Lack of spontaneity
Subtle personality changes
Disorientation to time and date

Stage 2

Impaired cognition and abstract thinking
Restlessness and agitation
Wandering, "sundown"
Inability to carry out activities of daily living
Impaired judgment
Inappropriate social behavior
Lack of insight, abstract thinking
Repetitive behavior
Voracious appetite

Stage 3

Emaciation—indifference to food
Inability to communicate
Urinary and fecal incontinence
Seizures

(Matteson, M. A., & McConnell, E. S. [1988]. *Gerontological nursing* [p. 251]. Philadelphia: J.B. Lippincott)

heimer's disease enters the *second* or *confusional stage* of dementia. This stage may last several years and is marked by a more global impairment of cognitive functioning. During this stage there are changes in higher cortical functioning needed for language, spatial relationships, and problem solving. Depression may occur in persons who are aware of their deficits. There is extreme confusion, disorientation, lack of insight, and inability to carry out the activities of daily living. Personal hygiene is neglected and language becomes impaired due to difficulty in remembering and retrieving words. Wandering, especially in the late afternoon or early evening, becomes a problem. The *sundown syndrome*, which is characterized by confusion, restlessness, agitation, and wandering, may become a daily occurrence late in the afternoon. Some persons may become hostile and abusive toward family members. Persons who enter this stage can no longer live alone and should be assisted in making decisions about supervised placement, whether with family or friends or in a community-based facility.

Stage 3 is the *terminal stage*. It is usually relatively short (1 to 2 years) in comparison with the other stages, but has been known to last for as long as 10 years.[9] The person becomes incontinent, apathetic, and unable to recognize family or friends. It is usually during this stage that the sufferer is institutionalized.

Diagnosis and Treatment. Alzheimer's disease is essentially a diagnosis of exclusion. There are no peripheral biochemical markers or tests for the disease. The diagnosis can be confirmed only by microscopic examination of tissue obtained from a cerebral biopsy or at autopsy. At present the diagnosis is based on clinical findings. Criteria for the clinical diagnosis of Alzheimer's disease have been established by a work group under the auspices of the Department of Health and Human Services Task Force on Alzheimer's Disease.[9] The diagnosis requires the presence of dementia established by clinical examination and documented by results of a Mini-Mental State Exam, Blessed Dementia Test, or similar examination that yield evidence of deficits in two or more areas of cognition and progressive worsening of memory or other cognitive functions. Brain imaging, either computed tomography (CT) scan or magnetic resonance imaging (MRI), is done to rule out other brain disease. Metabolic screening should be done for known reversible causes of dementia such as vitamin B_{12} deficiency, thyroid dysfunction, and electrolyte imbalance. A diagnostic accuracy of 80% can be achieved on the basis of clinical examination alone, and laboratory tests to exclude other disorders increase the accuracy to 90%.[7]

There is no specific treatment for Alzheimer's dementia. Drugs are used primarily to control depression, agitation, and sleep disorders. Two major goals of care are maintaining the person's socialization and providing support for the family. Validation therapy can be used to encourage persons with dementia to express their feelings.[10] Reminiscence group therapy has been found useful in maintaining socialization and establishing group relationships. Self-help groups that provide support for family and friends have become available, with support from the Alzheimer's Disease and Related Disorders Association. Day-care and respite centers are available in many areas to provide relief for caregivers.

MULTI-INFARCT DEMENTIA

Multi-infarct dementia is associated with cerebral vascular disease that does not result directly from atherosclerosis but rather from infarction due to multiple emboli that disseminate throughout the brain. About 20% to 25% of dementias are vascular in origin, and the incidence is closely associated with hypertension.[8] Other contributing factors are arrhythmias, myocardial infarction, peripheral vascular disease, diabetes mellitus, and smoking. The usual onset is between the ages of 55 and 70 years. The disease differs from Alzheimer's in its presentation and tissue pathology. The onset may be gradual or abrupt, and there may be focal neurologic symptoms related to local areas of infarction.

PICK'S DISEASE

Pick's disease is a rare form of dementia characterized by atrophy of the frontal, temporal, and parietal lobes of the brain. The neurons in the affected areas contain cytoplasmic inclusions called Pick bodies.

The average age at onset of Pick's disease is 54 years. The disease is more common in women than men. Behavioral manifestations may be noted earlier than memory deficits, taking the form of a striking absence of concern and care, a loss of initiative, echolalia (automatic repetition of anything said to the person), hypotonia, and incontinence. The course of the disease is relentless, with death ensuing within 2 to 10 years. The immediate cause of death generally is infection.

CREUTZFELDT-JAKOB DISEASE

Creutzfeldt-Jakob disease is a rare, transmissible form of dementia, thought to be caused by an infective protein agent called a *prion*. The pathogen is resistant to chemical and physical methods commonly used for sterilizing medical and surgical equipment. The disease has reportedly been transmitted through corneal transplants and human growth hormone obtained from cadavers. The National Hormone and Pituitary Program halted the distribution of human-pituitary hormone in 1985 after reports that three young persons who had received the hormone had died of Creutzfeldt-Jakob disease.[11] Because of the uncertainty and dangers surrounding the transmission of Creutzfeldt-Jakob disease, it is recommended that persons who received human-derived growth hormone refrain from blood, tissue, or organ donation.[12]

Creutzfeldt-Jakob disease causes degeneration of the pyramidal and extrapyramidal systems and is most readily distinguished by its rapid course. Affected persons are usually demented within 6 months of onset. The disease is uniformly fatal, with death often occurring within months, although occasional persons may survive for several years.[1] The early symptoms consist of abnormalities in personality and visual/spatial coordination. Extreme dementia and myoclonus follow as the disease progresses.

WERNICKE-KORSAKOFF SYNDROME

Wernicke-Korsakoff syndrome is due to chronic alcoholism. Wernicke's disease is characterized by weakness and paralysis of the extraocular muscles, nystagmus, ataxia, and confusion. Signs of peripheral neuropathy may be present. The person has an unsteady gait and complains of diplopia. There may be signs attributable to alcohol withdrawal—delirium, confusion, hallucinations, and others. It is generally agreed that this disorder is caused by a deficiency of thiamine (vitamin B_1), and many of the symptoms are reversed when nutrition is improved with supplemental thiamine.

The Korsakoff component of the syndrome involves severe impairment of recent memory. There is often difficulty in dealing with abstractions, and the person's capacity to learn is defective. Confabulation (the recitation of imaginary experiences to fill in gaps in memory) is probably the most distinctive feature of the disease. Polyneuritis is also common. Unlike Wernicke's disease, Korsakoff's psychosis does not improve significantly with treatment.

HUNTINGTON'S DISEASE

Huntington's disease is a rare hereditary disorder characterized by chronic progressive chorea, psychological changes, and dementia. Although the disease is inherited as an autosomal dominant disorder,

symptoms do not usually develop until after 30 years of age.[13] By the time the disease has been diagnosed, the person has often passed the gene on to his or her children.

Huntington's disease produces localized death of brain cells. The first and most severely affected neurons are the caudate nucleus and putamen of the basal ganglia. The neurochemical changes that occur with the disease are complex. The neurotransmitter gamma-aminobutyric acid (GABA) is an inhibitory neurotransmitter in the basal ganglia. Postmortem studies have shown a decrease of GABA and GABA receptors in the basal ganglia of persons dying of Huntington's disease. It has also been shown that the levels of acetylcholine, an excitatory neurotransmitter in the basal ganglia, are reduced in persons with Huntington's disease. At the same time, the dopaminergic pathway of the nigrostrital system, which is affected in parkinsonism (discussed later in this chapter), is preserved in Huntington's disease, suggesting that an imbalance in dopamine and acetylcholine may contribute to manifestations of the disease.

Depression and personality changes are the most common early psychological manifestations; memory loss is often accompanied by impulsive behavior, moodiness, antisocial behavior, and a tendency to emotional outbursts.[13] Other early signs of the disease are lack of initiative, loss of spontaneity, and inability to concentrate. Fidgetiness or restlessness may represent early signs of dyskinesia, followed by choreiform and some dystonic posturing (see Chapter 50). Eventually, progressive rigidity and akinesia (rather than chorea) develop in association with dementia.

There is no cure for Huntington's disease. The treatment is largely symptomatic. Drugs may be used to treat the dyskinesias and behavioral disturbances.

In recent years the study of the genetics of Huntington's disease has led to the discovery that the gene for the disease is located on chromosome 4.[13] The discovery of a marker probe for the gene locus has raised the possibility of predictive testing for the disease. The testing procedure requires obtaining DNA samples from the person at risk and several relatives to determine which member of the gene pair travels with the marker probe for the Huntington's gene in a particular family. DNA for determining the genotype can be obtained from the blood of a consenting person, from amniotic fluid, or from frozen brain tissue from a diseased person.[13] Presymptomatic testing raises many ethical questions, including that of providing a person with knowledge that he or she is carrying a gene that will eventually lead to prolonged physical and mental deterioration.

PARKINSON'S DISEASE AND PARKINSONISM

Parkinsonism is a degenerative disorder of basal ganglia function that results in variable combinations of slowness of movement (bradykinesia), increased muscle tonus (rigidity), tremor, and impaired automatic postural responses. About 500,000 to 1 million persons in the United States are affected by Parkinson's disease. Onset is most common at about 55 years, with the highest prevalence in the eighth decade.[14]

The basal ganglia, a group of deep cerebral nuclei, include the caudate nucleus, the globus pallidus, the subthalamic nucleus, and the substantia nigra. The putamen and globus pallidus are collectively termed the lentiform nucleus; the combination of the lentiform nucleus and caudate nucleus is designated the corpus striatum. The basic circuitry of the basal ganglia consists of three interacting neuronal loops (Fig. 54-1).[15] One loop is a corticocortical loop that passes from the premotor supplementary areas of the cerebral cortex, through the caudate and putamen, the internal segment of the globus pallidus, and the thalamus, and then back to the primary motor cortex and portions of supplementary and premotor cortex associated with the primary motor cortex. A second loop projects from the caudate and putamen to the external segment of globus pallidus,

then to the subthalamic nucleus, and finally to the internal segment of the globus pallidus. A third loop, the nigrostriatal pathway, connects the substantia nigra with the caudate and putamen. Normally, the pigmented neurons in the substantia nigra produce and store the neurotransmitter dopamine, which is subsequently transported via the nigrostriatal fibers to receptors in the corpus striatum. It is assumed that this pathway is inhibitory to the striatal neurons that communicate with the motor cortex via the thalamic nuclei. The striatum also contains many cholinergic interneurons that functionally oppose the dopaminergic input.

The movement disorders associated with parkinsonism result primarily from a defect in the nigrostriatal pathway. Destruction of neurons in the substantia nigra causes this tract to degenerate, and as a result the dopamine that is normally delivered to the striatum is markedly decreased. Loss of approximately 80% of the pigmented neurons in the substantia nigra, leading to an 80% depletion of striatal dopamine, is required for the appearance of clinical parkinsonism. The neurons that secrete acetylcholine remain functional, however, and in the absence of dopamine become overactive, thus contributing to the motor symptoms that are characteristic of parkinsonism.

ETIOLOGY

The alterations in motor function that characterize parkinsonism are seen in many different toxic and disease states. The most common form of parkinsonism is idiopathic Parkinson's disease (paralysis agitans), named after James Parkinson, who first described the disorder in 1817. In idiopathic parkinsonism, dopamine depletion is due to degeneration of the dopamine nigrostriatal system. It usually begins after age 50 years; most cases are diagnosed in the sixth and seventh decade of life. Parkinsonism can also develop as a postencephalitic syndrome, as a side effect of therapy with antipsychotic drugs that block dopamine receptors, as a toxic reaction to a chemical agent, or as an outcome of severe carbon monoxide poisoning. Symptoms of parkinsonism may also accompany conditions such as cerebral vascular disease, neoplasms, or degenerative neurologic diseases that structurally damage the nigrostriatal pathway.

Postencephalitic parkinsonism was a particular problem in the 1930s and 1940s, as a result of an outbreak of lethargic encephalitis (sleeping sickness) that occurred in 1914 to 1918.[16] Drug-induced parkinsonism can follow the taking of antipsychotic drugs in high doses (*e.g.*, phenothiazines and butyrophenones). These drugs block dopamine receptors

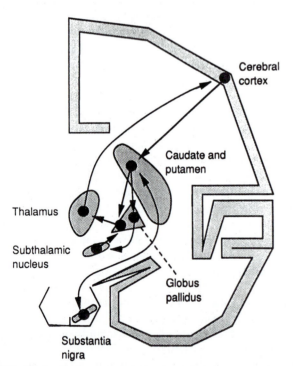

FIG. 54-1. Basic neuronal circuitry of the basal ganglia. (Greenberg, D. A., Aminoff, M. J., & Simon, R. P. [1993]. *Clinical neurology* [3rd ed., p. 208]. Norwalk, CT: Appleton-Lange)

Cerebral cortex

Caudate and putamen

Thalamus

Subthalamic nucleus

Globus pallidus

Substantia nigra

and dopamine output by the cells of the substantia nigra. Of recent interest was the development of parkinsonism in a group of individuals who had attempted to make a narcotic drug and instead synthesized a compound called *MPTP* (1-methyl-4-phenyl-1,2,3,6-tetrahydropyridine).[17–19] This compound selectively destroys the dopaminergic neurons of the substantia nigra. This incident has led to investigations into the role of toxins, both those that are produced by the body as a part of metabolic processes and those that enter the body from outside sources, in the pathogenesis of Parkinson's disease.

MANIFESTATIONS

Parkinson's disease often begins insidiously with slowness of movement, weakness, and tremor. Tremor of the distal segments of the limbs is an early symptom; it usually is unilateral, occurs at rest but disappears with movement, and involves a rhythmic alternating flexion and contraction of the muscles that produces the appearance of pill-rolling movements. The tremor is gradually followed by rigidity, which is most evident on passive joint movement, and involves jerky, cogwheel-type movements that require considerable energy to perform. Flexion contractions may occur as a result of the rigidity. In addition, there is slowness in initiating (bradykinesia) movements and difficulty in sudden unexpected stopping of voluntary movements and loss of unconscious associative movements. People with Parkinson's disease have difficulty initiating walking and difficulty turning. While walking, they may freeze in place and feel as if their feet are glued to the floor, especially when moving through a doorway or preparing to turn. When they walk, they lean forward with their head bent and take small, shuffling steps without swinging their arms, tend to move faster and faster, and stop only with difficulty. Loss of postural reflexes make the person prone to fall, often backwards.

As the disease progresses, the facial expression becomes stiff and masklike. There is loss of eye-blinking and failure to express emotion. There is rigidity of the tongue, palate, and throat muscles; the person may drool because of difficulty in moving the saliva to the back of the mouth and swallowing it. The speech is slow, monotonous, without modulation, and poorly articulated.

Because the basal ganglia also influence the autonomic nervous system, persons with Parkinson's disease often have excessive and uncontrolled sweating, sebaceous secretion, and salivation. Autonomic symptoms such as constipation, urinary incontinence, and lacrimation may also be present.

Dementia is an important feature associated with Parkinson's disease. It occurs in approximately 40% of persons with the disease and seems to occur independent of drug therapy.[20] The mental state of some persons with Parkinson's disease may be indistinguishable from that seen in Alzheimer's disease.[21] It has been suggested that many of the brain changes in both diseases may be due to degeneration of acetylcholine-containing neurons in a region of the brain called the *nucleus basalis of Maynert*, which is the main source of cholinergic innervation of the cerebral cortex.[22] Persons with Parkinson's disease also have other neurochemical disturbances that might account for some of the features of dementia.

There are several stages in the progression of Parkinson's disease. The symptoms are usually noted first on one side of the body and progress to bilateral involvement, with early postural changes beginning 1 to 2 years after onset. The tremor often begins in one or both hands and then becomes generalized. Postural changes and gait disturbances continue to become more pronounced until the person has significant disability and requires constant care.

TREATMENT

The treatment of parkinsonism consists of education regarding the nature of the disorder, drug therapy, and general supportive measures to provide emotional support and encouragement to continue as much physical activity as possible. Physical therapy and speech therapy are often helpful. The quality of life can often be improved by the provision of simple aids to activities of daily living, such as rails placed in strategic parts of the home and special silverware with large handles.

Drug Therapy. Drug treatment is usually reserved until disability mandates its use. Antiparkinson drugs act in one of two ways: (1) to increase the functional ability of the underactive dopaminergic system, or (2) to reduce the excessive influence of excitatory cholinergic neurons. The first type of drugs includes levodopa and Sinemet, amantadine (Symmetrel), and bromocriptine (Parlodel). Dopamine does not cross the blood–brain barrier. Administration of levodopa, a precursor of dopamine that does cross the blood–brain barrier, has yielded significant improvement in clinical symptoms of Parkinson's disease. The second type of drugs is the anticholinergic drugs. Because dopamine transmission is disrupted in Parkinson's disease, there is a preponderance of cholinergic activity, which is decreased with anticholinergic drugs.

Drugs That Increase Dopamine. Dopamine does not cross the blood–brain barrier. The evidence of decreased dopamine levels in the striatum in Parkinson's disease led to the administration of large doses of L-dopa (L-dihydroxyphenylalanine) or the synthetic compound levodopa, which is absorbed from the intestinal tract, crosses the blood-brain barrier, and is converted to dopamine by centrally acting dopa decarboxylase. Unfortunately, only a small percentage (1% to 3%) of administered levodopa actually enters the brain unaltered; the rest is metabolized outside the brain, predominantly by decarboxylation to dopamine, which cannot cross the blood–brain barrier. This means that large doses of levodopa are needed when the drug is used alone, and this leads to many side effects. However, when levodopa is given in combination with a dopa decarboxylase inhibitor (carbidopa) that does not cross the blood–brain barrier, the peripheral metabolism of levodopa is reduced, plasma levels of levodopa are higher, plasma half-life is longer, more levodopa is available for the entry into the brain, and a smaller dose is needed.

Sinemet is a preparation containing levodopa and carbidopa. Individuals are started on very small doses of Sinemet, and the dose is gradually increased until therapeutic levels are reached. Some of the side effects of levodopa may be relatively mild when the drug is given in combination with carbidopa to reduce its extracerebral metabolism. Side effects such as nausea and vomiting, cardiac dysrhythmias, and postural hypotension are considerably reduced when Sinemet is used. Dyskinesias occur in about 80% of persons receiving levodopa for long periods and appears to be dose related.[22] Other adverse effects of levodopa include depression, restlessness, somnolence, confusion, hallucinations, nightmares, changes in mood, and other changes in behavior or personality that occur later in the course of treatment and become more common with time. Dyskinesias and behavioral side effects are more common in persons receiving levodopa in combination with carbidopa rather than levodopa alone, presumably because higher levels are reached in the brain.

A later complication of levodopa treatment is the "on-off phenomenon," in which frequent abrupt and unpredictable fluctuations in motor performance occur during the day.[22] These fluctuations include periods of dyskinesias (the "on" response) and periods of marked bradykinesia (the "off" response). Some fluctuations are due to the timing of drug administration, in which the on response coincides with peak drug levels and the off response with low drug levels.[23]

Amantadine (Symmetrel) was introduced as an antiviral agent for prophylaxis of A_2 influenza and was unexpectedly found to cause symptomatic improvement of persons with parkinsonism. Although the exact mechanism of action remains to be elucidated, it may augment release of dopamine from the remaining intact dopaminergic terminals in the nigrostriatal pathway of persons with Parkinson's disease. It is used to treat persons with mild symptoms but no disability.

Bromocriptine (Parlodel) acts directly to stimulate dopamine receptors. It is used as adjunctive therapy in Parkinson's disease. It is often used for persons who have become refractory to L-dopa or have developed an on-off phenomenon.

Selegiline (also called Eldepryl or deprenyl) is a monamine oxidase B inhibitor and thereby inhibits the metabolic breakdown of dopamine. Selegiline may be used as adjunctive treatment to reduce mild on-off fluctuations in responsiveness of persons who are receiving levodopa. Some clinical studies suggest that selegiline may be used early in parkinsonism to delay the progression of the disease.

Anticholinergic Drugs. Anticholinergic drugs are more helpful in alleviating tremor and rigidity than bradykinesia. Treatment is started with a small dose of one preparation, and the dose is increased until benefit occurs or side effects develop. If treatment is ineffective, the drug is gradually withdrawn and another preparation tried. Ethopropazine (Parsidol) is probably the most helpful drug in this group for relieving tremor.[24] Other anticholinergic drugs are benztropine (Cogentin), biperiden (Akineton), chlorphenoxamine (Phenoxene), Orphenadrine (Disipal, Norflex), procyclidine (Kemadrin), and trihexyphenidyl (Artane).[24] The anticholinergic drugs lessen the tremors and rigidity and afford some improvement of function. However, their potency seems to decrease over time, and increasing the dosage merely increases side effects such as blurred vision, dry mouth, bowel and bladder problems, and some mental changes.

Surgery. Thalamotomy is generally reserved for the patient who is relatively young and has predominantly unilateral tremor and rigidity that fails to respond to medication.

Autologous (self) adrenal medullary tissue[25, 26] or fetal brain tissue[27] has been surgically implanted into the caudate nucleus in the belief that the transplanted tissue will connect with host cells, producing dopamine, and stimulate receptors, thus correcting the defect responsible for the disease. Results of this research have been contradictory, and this approach is highly controversial.

In summary, degenerative diseases are disorders that selectively affect one or more functional systems of neurons while leaving others intact. Dementia is a degenerative syndrome in which intellectual deterioration is severe enough to interfere with occupational and social performance. Dementia can be caused by any disorder that permanently damages large association areas of the cerebral hemispheres, including Alzheimer's disease, multi-infarct dementia, Pick's disease, Creutzfeldt-Jakob disease, and Huntington's disease. Multi-infarct dementia is associated with vascular disease, and Pick's disease with atrophy of the frontal and temporal lobes. Creutzfeldt-Jakob disease is a rare transmissible form of dementia. Wernicke-Korsakoff syndrome is due to chronic alcoholism. Huntington's disease is a rare hereditary disorder characterized by chronic progressive chorea, psychological change, and dementia. By far the most common cause of dementia (50% to 70%) is Alzheimer's disease. The condition is a major health problem among the elderly. It is characterized by cortical atrophy and loss of neurons, the presence of neuritic plaques, granulovacuolar degeneration, and cerebrovascular amyloid. The disease follows an insidious and progressive course that begins with memory impairment and terminates in inability to recognize family or friends and loss of bodily functions. The particular tragedy of Alzheimer's disease and other related dementias is that they dissolve the mind and rob the victim of humanity. Simultaneously, these disorders devastate the lives of spouses and other family members, who must endure an insidious loss of the person and the relationship.

Parkinson's disease is a disorder of the basal ganglia that results in variable combinations of bradykinesia, rigidity, tremor, and impaired automatic postural responses to position and movement. The striatal structures of the basal ganglia modulate the excitatory input that travels from the thalamus to the motor cortex, particularly the premotor cortex and supplementary motor cortex. Parkinsonism is characterized by a defect in the nigrostriatal pathway and a resultant decrease in dopamine levels in the striatum. The striatum also contains many cholinergic interneurons that normally oppose the dopaminergic input. In the absence of dopamine, these neurons become overactive, causing the motor symptoms that are characteristic of parkinsonism. Treatment consists of medications to increase brain dopamine levels or to decrease acetylcholine with anticholinergic agents.

■ DEMYELINATING DISEASES

The loss of myelin sheaths with relative preservation of the demyelinated nerve axons is characteristic of a group of neurologic disorders called *demyelinating diseases*. The most common of these is multiple sclerosis.

In the central nervous system (CNS), myelin is formed by the oligodendrocytes, chiefly those lying between the nerve fibers and the white matter. This function is equivalent to that of the Schwann cells in the peripheral nervous system (see Chapter 46). The properties of the myelin sheath—high electrical resistance and low capacitance—permit it to function as an electrical insulator. Small uninsulated junctures, called the *nodes of Ranvier*, exist between the cells of the myelin sheath. Impulses jump from node to node, thus speeding conduction of impulses and reducing the metabolic work required to maintain the ionic gradients necessary for neural conduction.

The process of myelination of the CNS begins early in the fourth month of fetal life. It is incomplete at birth, and some fibers continue to become myelinated during the first year of life.[28] The total amount of myelin increases from birth to maturity. Although myelin is relatively stable, there is continual removal and replacement of individual components. Studies indicate that the myelin formed early in life is the most stable and that newly formed myelin is more easily broken down and replaced.[29] There are two major myelin proteins, proteolipid protein and basic protein, that are incorporated in the myelin sheath and are involved in the replacement process. Myelin enzymes, capable of degrading myelin proteins, have been identified. These enzymes may be involved in normal catabolic processes and could have a role in some forms of demyelination.[29]

Demyelinated nerve fibers display a variety of conduction abnormalities ranging from decreased conduction velocity to conduction blocks. In the demyelinated fiber, conduction velocity is decreased so that the threshold for excitation is reached very slowly or not at all.[30]

MULTIPLE SCLEROSIS

Multiple sclerosis is a major cause of neurologic disability among young and middle-aged adults. The disease is rarely diagnosed in persons under age 15 or over 55 years, with a peak incidence of onset around the age of 30.[31] Estimates of the total number of cases of multiple sclerosis in the United States range from 123,000 to 250,000. In approximately 60% of the cases, the disease is characterized by exacerbations and remissions over many years from several different sites in the CNS. Initially, there is normal or near-normal neurologic function between exacerbations. As the disease progresses, there is less improvement between exacerbations and increasing neurologic dysfunction.

PATHOPHYSIOLOGY

Multiple sclerosis is characterized by demyelination in the white matter of the brain (usually periventricular), brain stem, or spinal cord. Sharp-edged demyelinated patches, ranging from 1 mm to 4 cm, are macroscopically visible throughout the white matter of the central nervous system.[32] These lesions, which represent the end result of acute myelin breakdown, are called *plaques*. Oligodendrocytes are decreased in number and may be absent, especially in older lesions. The sequence of myelin breakdown is not well understood, although it is known that the lesions contain small amounts of myelin basic proteins, increased amounts of proteolytic enzymes, macrophages, lymphocytes, and plasma cells. Acute, subacute, and chronic sclerotic lesions are scattered throughout the CNS.

The recent use of MRI has shown that the lesions of multiple sclerosis may occur in two stages: a first stage that involves the sequential development of small inflammatory lesions, and a second stage during which the lesions extend and consolidate and during which both demyelination and gliosis (scar tissue development) occur.[33] It is not known whether the inflammatory process, present during the first stage, is directed against the myelin or against the oligodendrocytes. Remyelination of the nervous system was considered to be impossible until a few years ago. Recent evidence has shown that remyelination can occur in the CNS if the process that initiated the demyelination is halted before the oligodendrocyte dies.[29]

ETIOLOGY

The cause of multiple sclerosis remains unknown. Geographic distribution and migration studies suggest an environmental influence. The disease is more prevalent in the colder northern latitudes; it is more common in the northern Atlantic states, the Great Lakes region, and the Pacific Northwest than in the southern parts of the United States. Other high-incidence areas include northern Europe, Great Britain, southern Australia, and New Zealand. Migration studies have shown that persons who move from a high-risk area tend to retain the risk of their birthplace if they move after age 15 or adopt the risk of their new home if they migrate as children.[1]

There is also a family tendency in some cases of multiple sclerosis, suggesting a genetic influence on susceptibility. However, studies of monozygotic twins have found that the second twin develops the disease only in 30% of cases, suggesting that an exogenous or environmental trigger such as an infectious agent is required to produce the disease.[30] There is also a strong association between multiple sclerosis and certain HLA antigens (see Chapter 13).[1]

Many believe that the disease has an immunologic basis, but this has not been confirmed. The demyelination process in multiple sclerosis is marked by prominent lymphocytic invasion in the lesion. Both T_4 helper cells and T_8 suppressor cells are present. In some persons, a sharp decline in the suppressor T-cell population in the blood accompanies exacerbations of the disease.[1]

MANIFESTATIONS AND CLINICAL COURSE

The interruption of neural conduction in the demyelinated nerves is manifested by a variety of symptoms, depending on the location and duration of the lesion.

Areas commonly affected by multiple sclerosis are the optic chiasm, optic nerves, brain stem, cerebellum, the corticospinal tracts, and posterior cell columns of the spinal cord. Typically, an otherwise healthy person suffers an acute or subacute episode of paresthesias, optic neuritis (visual clouding or loss of vision in part of the visual field with pain on movement of the globe), diplopia, or paralysis. Paresthesias are evidenced as numbness and tingling on the face or involved extremities. Lhermitte's symptom is an electric-shock–like tingling down the back and onto the legs that is produced by flexion of the neck. Other common symptoms are abnormal gait, bladder dysfunction, vertigo, nystagmus, and speech disturbance. The symptoms are usually painless, last for several days to weeks, and then completely or partially resolve. After a period of normal or relatively normal function, new symptoms appear. Psychological manifestations, such as mood swings, may represent a reaction to the nature of the disease or, more likely, involvement of the white matter of the cerebral cortex. Depression, euphoria, inattentiveness, apathy, forgetfulness, and loss of memory may occur.

Small increases in body temperature can temporarily worsen existing neurologic deficits in persons with multiple sclerosis by producing a block of impulse conduction in demyelinated nerve fibers. This observation forms the basis for the hot bath test, which is sometimes used to aid in the diagnosis of multiple sclerosis.[34] The test is performed by having the person recline in a whirlpool or hot bath. The water level is adjusted so that both axillae are submerged, and the temperature of the water is raised to 110°F while neurologic function is monitored. If new neurologic deficits are observed, the test is terminated and the water is cooled to reverse the conduction block and its attendant symptoms. Prolonged neurologic sequelae have been observed in persons with multiple sclerosis following unintentional exposure to high environmental temperatures such as those encountered in a hot tub or while sunbathing.[35, 36]

A small percentage of people develop an acute form of multiple sclerosis that progresses rapidly with incomplete remissions of short duration. This form of multiple sclerosis can be fatal within a few months or years. There is also a benign form of the disease that has a few mild exacerbations followed by complete recovery. In the benign form, a person remains relatively asymptomatic without neurologic dysfunction for many years. There may also be a subclinical form of the disease, since demyelination has been observed in asymptomatic persons on autopsy.[32] Because of the varied clinical courses of multiple sclerosis, persons in whom the disease is recently diagnosed have some justification for optimism.

DIAGNOSIS

The diagnosis of multiple sclerosis is difficult because there is no specific laboratory test for the disease, manifestations are variable, and there may be lengthy delays between the first appearance of symptoms and recurrence. A definite diagnosis of multiple sclerosis requires evidence of two attacks and clinical findings consistent with two separate lesions or clinical evidence of one lesion and paraclinical (*e.g.*, MRI or CT scans) evidence of a second lesion.[37] The attacks must each last a minimum of 24 hours, be separated by a period of at least 1 month, and be unexplained by other mechanisms.[37]

Although no laboratory test can be used to diagnose multiple sclerosis, examination of the cerebrospinal fluid (CSF) is helpful. A large percentage of patients with multiple sclerosis have elevated IgG levels, and some have oligoclonal patterns (discrete electrophoretic bands) even with normal IgG levels. There may also be a mild increase in total protein or lymphocytes in the CSF. These tests can be altered in a variety of inflammatory neurologic disorders and are not specific for multiple sclerosis.

Recently, electrophysiologic evaluations (evoked potential studies) and CT scans have aided in the identification and documentation of lesions, but they still do not provide information about the cause of the lesions. MRI studies can detect the multiplicity of lesions even when CT scans are normal. A computer-assisted method of MRI has been developed that measures lesion size. Many new areas of myelin abnormality are asymptomatic. Serial MRI studies can be done to detect asymptomatic lesions, monitor the progress of existing lesions, and evaluate the effectiveness of treatment.

TREATMENT

The variety of symptoms, unpredictable course, and lack of specific diagnostic methods have made the evaluation and treatment of multiple sclerosis difficult. Persons who are minimally affected by the disorder require no specific treatment. The person should be encouraged to live as healthy a life-style as possible, including good nutrition and adequate rest and relaxation. Physical therapy may help maintain muscle tone. Every effort should be made to avoid excessive fatigue, physical deterioration, emotional stress, and extremes of environmental temperature, which may precipitate exacerbation of the disease.

Adrenocorticotropin (ACTH) and corticosteroids can be used to shorten the duration of an acute attack. Long-term administration does not, however, appear to alter the course of the disease and may have harmful side effects. Several studies have indicated that intensive immunosuppressive therapy with intravenous cyclophosphamide may help arrest the chronic progressive course of active multiple sclerosis. Plasmapheresis has proved beneficial in some cases.

The primary treatment of multiple sclerosis is symptomatic. Pharmacologic treatment may include (1) dantrolene (Dantrium), baclofen (Lioresal), or diazepam (Valium) for spasticity; (2) cholinergic drugs for bladder problems; and (3) antidepressant drugs for depression.

Two substances, copolymer 1 and β-interferon, are currently undergoing extensive clinical testing. Both agents have shown some benefits in persons with multiple sclerosis that follows a course of remissions and exacerbations rather than steady progress. Copolymer 1 (COP 1) is a synthetic polypeptide simulating parts of the myelin basic protein. Its mechanism of action is still uncertain. β-Interferon, a lymphokine that acts as an immune enhancer, has recently been released for use in treatment of persons with multiple sclerosis.

In summary, multiple sclerosis is an example of a demyelinating disease in which there is a slowly progressive breakdown of myelin and formation of plaques but sparing of the axis cylinder of the neuron. The cause of multiple sclerosis remains unknown. Geographic distributions and migration studies suggest an environmental influence. Interruption of neural conduction in multiple sclerosis is manifested by a variety of disabling signs and symptoms that depend on the neurons that are affected. The most common symptoms are paresthesias, optic neuritis, and motor weakness. The disease is usually characterized by exacerbations and remissions. Initially, near-normal function returns between exacerbations. The variety of symptoms, course of the disease, and lack of specific diagnostic tests make diagnosis and treatment of the disease difficult. At present treatment is largely symptomatic.

■ BRAIN TUMORS

Brain tumors account for 2% of all cancer deaths. The American Cancer Society reports that there are over 16,900 new cases and over 11,800 deaths from brain and CNS cancers each year.[38] Another 17,000 to 18,000 patients (18% of all cancer patients) develop metastases to the brain from other sites. More adults die each year of brain tumors than of Hodgkin's disease or multiple sclerosis.[39] In children, brain tumors are second only to leukemia as a cause of death from cancer and kill about 1600 children and young adults annually.

Brain tumors can be divided into three types: (1) primary intracranial tumors of central nervous system tissue (neurons and neuroglia), (2) primary intracranial tumors that originate within the skull cavity but are not derived from the brain parenchyma itself (*e.g.*, meninges, pituitary gland, pineal gland), and (3) metastatic tumors. Primary intracranial neoplasms of central nervous system origin can be classified according to site of origin and histologic type (Chart 54-3).

"Benign" versus "malignant" has its own meaning when it relates to brain tumors. In most neoplasms, the term *malignant* is used to describe the lack of cell differentiation, the invasive nature of the tumor, and its ability to metastasize. In the brain, however, even a well-differentiated and histologically benign tumor may grow and cause death because of its location.

Collectively, the neoplasms of astrocyte origin are the most common type of primary brain tumor in the adult. Astocytomas fall into three clinicopathologic groups: (1) astrocytomas, including glioblastoma multiforme, (2) brain stem glioma, and (3) pilocyte astrocytoma.[1] Astrocytomas of the cerebral hemispheres are commonly divided into three grades of increasing pathologic anaplasia and rapidity of progression: astrocytoma, anaplastic astrocytoma, and glioblastoma multiforme (see Chapter 5 for a discussion of cell differentiation and anaplasia). Together these tumors account for 80% to 90% of all neuroglial tumors in adults. They are most frequent in middle age, with the anaplastic astrocytomas having a peak incidence in the sixth decade. *Glioblastoma multiforme* is commonly used as a synonym for highly malignant forms of astrocytoma, namely, grades III and IV. Astrocytomas have a marked tendency to become more anaplastic with time, so that a tumor beginning as an astrocyoma may develop into a glioblastoma. Brain stem gliomas occur in the first 2 decades of life and make up about 20% of brain tumors in this age group.[1] Pilocytic astrocytomas are distinguished from other astrocytomas by their cellular appearance and their benign behavior. Typically, they occur in children and young adults and are usually located in the cerebellum, but can also be found in the floor and walls of the third ventricle, the optic chiasm and nerves, and occasionally in the cerebral hemispheres. Oligodendrogliomas comprise about 5% of glial tumors; they are most common in middle life and are found in the cerebral hemispheres.[1] Ependymomas are derived from the single layer of epithelium that lines the ventricles and spinal canal. Although they can occur at any age, they are most likely to occur in the first 2 decades of life and most frequently affect the fourth ventricle; they constitute 5% to 10% of brain tumors in this age group.[1] The spinal cord is the most common site for ependymomas in middle life.

Medulloblastomas, which consist of primitive, undifferentiated neuronal cells, make up 30% of primary brain tumors in children.[1]

Meningiomas develop from the meningothelial cells of the arachnoid and are thus outside the brain. They comprise about 20% of primary brain tumors and generally have their onset in the middle or later years of life.[1] Meningiomas are slow-growing, well-circumscribed, and often highly vascular tumors. They are usually benign, and complete removal is possible if the tumor does not involve vital structures. Pituitary adenomas comprise 12% to 14% of brain tumors; they are usually nonmalignant.[1]

Craniopharyngiomas are composed of cells derived from the embryonic notochord and are tumors of children and young adults. They commonly occur in the midline of the nervous system and are highly invasive, making surgical removal difficult or impossible.

ETIOLOGY

The cause of brain tumors is unknown. Although a number of chemical and viral agents can cause brain tumors in laboratory animals, there is no evidence that these agents cause brain cancer in humans. Cranial irradiation and exposure to some chemicals may lead to an increased incidence of both astrocytomas and meningiomas. There may also be a hereditary factor; 16% of persons with primary brain tumors have a family history of cancer. Childhood tumors are considered to be developmental in origin.

CHART 54-3: TYPES OF BRAIN TUMORS

Primary Parenchymal Tumors

Tumors of the neuroglia
  Astrocytoma
    Glioblastoma multiforme
    Brain stem glioma
    Pilocyte astrocytoma
  Oligodendrocytes
    Oligodendroglioma
  Ependymal cells
    Ependymona
  Mixed gliomas

Tumors of Neural Cells

Neuroblastoma
Ganglion cell tumors
Tumors of primative cells
  Medulloblastoma

Primary Nonparenchymal Tumors

Meningioma and tumors of related tissue
Pineal tumors
Pituitary tumors
Developmental tumors
  Hemangioblastoma and tumors of blood vessel origin
  Craniopharyngiomas

Metastatic Tumors

MANIFESTATIONS

Intracranial tumors give rise to focal disturbances in brain function and increased intracranial pressure. Focal disturbances occur because of brain compression, tumor infiltration, disturbances in blood flow, and brain edema. Alterations in brain function due to focal lesions, increased intracranial pressure, and cerebral edema are discussed in Chapter 51.

Tumors may be located intra-axially (within brain tissue) or extra-axially (outside brain tissue). Disturbances in brain function are generally greatest with fast-growing, infiltrative, intra-axial tumors because of compression, infiltration, and necrosis of brain tissue. Extra-axial tumors, such as meningiomas, may reach a large size without producing signs and symptoms. Cysts may form within tumors and contribute to brain compression. Cerebral edema develops around brain tumors, is usually of the vasogenic type, and is characterized by increased brain water and expanded extracellular fluid. The edema is thought to result from increased permeability of tumor capillary endothelial cells.

Because the volume of the intracranial cavity is fixed, brain tumors cause generalized intracranial pressure when they reach sufficient size. Tumors can obstruct the flow of cerebrospinal fluid in the ventricular cavities and produce hydrocephalic dilatation of the proximal ventricles and atrophy of the cerebral hemispheres. Complete compensation of ventricular volumes can occur with very-slow-growing tumors, but with rapidly growing tumors increased intracranial pressure becomes an early sign. Depending on the location of the tumor, brain displacement and herniation of the uncus or cerebellum may occur (see Chapter 51).

The clinical manifestations of brain tumors depend on the size and location of the tumor. General signs and symptoms include headache, nausea and vomiting, mental changes, papilledema and visual disturbances (diplopia), alterations in sensory and motor function, and seizures.

The brain itself is insensitive to pain. The headache that accompanies brain tumors results from compression or distortion of pain-sensitive dural or vascular structures. It may be felt on the same side of the head as the tumor but is more commonly diffuse in nature. In the early stages, the headache, which is caused by irritation, compression, and traction on the dural sinuses or blood vessels, is mild and occurs in the morning when the person awakens. It usually disappears when the person has been up for a short time. The headache becomes more constant as the tumor enlarges and is often worsened by coughing, bending, or sudden movements of the head.

Vomiting occurs with or without preceding nausea and is a common symptom of increased intracranial pressure and brain stem compression. Direct stimulation of the vomiting center, which is located in the medulla, may contribute to the vomiting that occurs with brain tumors. The vomiting is often projectile in nature. Vomiting due to a brain tumor is usually unrelated to meals and is often, but not always, associated with headache.

Papilledema (edema of the optic disk) results from increased intracranial pressure and obstruction of the cerebrospinal fluid pathways. It is associated with decreased visual acuity, diplopia, and deficits in the visual fields. Visual defects associated with papilledema are often the reason that persons with brain tumor seek medical care.

Personality and mental changes are common with brain tumors. Persons are often irritable initially and later become quiet and apathetic. They may become forgetful, seem preoccupied, and appear to be psychologically depressed. Because of the mental changes, a psychiatric consultation may be sought before a diagnosis of brain tumor is made.

Focal signs and symptoms are determined by the location of the tumor. Tumors arising in the frontal lobe may grow to large size, produce an increase in intracranial pressure, and cause signs of generalized brain dysfunction before focal signs are present. On the other hand, tumors that impinge on the visual system cause visual loss or visual field defects long before generalized signs develop. Certain areas of the brain have a relatively low threshold for seizure activity; tumors arising in relatively silent areas of the brain may produce focal epileptogenic discharges. Temporal lobe tumors often produce seizures as their first symptom. Hallucinations of smell or hearing, as well as déjà vu phenomena, are common focal manifestations of temporal lobe tumors. Brain stem tumors commonly produce upper and lower motor neuron signs, such as weakness of facial muscles and ocular palsies that occur with or without involvement of sensory or long motor tracts. Cerebellar tumors often cause ataxia of gait.

DIAGNOSIS AND TREATMENT

Diagnostic procedures for brain tumor include physical and neurologic examinations, visual field and funduscopic examination, CT scans and MRI, skull x-rays, technetium pertechnetate brain scans, electroencephalography, and cerebral angiography. Physical examination is used to assess motor and sensory function. Since the visual pathways travel through many areas of the cerebral lobes, detection of visual field defects can provide information about the location of tumors. A funduscopic examination is done to determine the presence of papilledema. CT scans have become the screening procedure of choice for diagnosing and localizing brain tumors as well as other intracranial masses. MRI scans may be diagnostic when a clinically suspected tumor is not detected by CT scanning. Skull x-rays are used to detect calcified areas within a neoplasm or erosion of skull structures due to tumors. Brain tumors tend to disrupt the blood–brain barrier; as a result, the uptake of the radioactive isotope used in a brain scan is increased within a tumor. About 75% of persons with a brain tumor have an abnormal electroencephalogram; in some cases, the results of the test can be used to localize the tumor. Cerebral angiography can be used to locate a tumor and visualize its vascular supply, information that is important when planning surgery.

The three general methods for treatment of brain tumors are surgery, radiation, and chemotherapy.[40] Surgery is part of the intial management of virtually all brain tumors; it establishes the diagnosis and allows for tumor removal in many cases. The development of microsurgical neuroanatomy, the operating microscope, the fusion of imaging systems with resection techniques, advanced stereotactic and ultrasound technology, and intraoperative monitoring of evoked potentials have all served to improve the effectivenss of surgical resection.[40] However, removal may be limited by the location of the tumor and its invasiveness. Stereotactic surgery uses three-dimensional coordinates and CT and MRI to localize a brain lesion precisely. Ultrasound technology has been used for both localizing and removing tumors. The ultrasonic aspirator, which combines a vibrating head with suction, permits atraumatic removal of tumors from cranial nerves and important cortical areas. Intraoperative monitoring of evoked potentials is an important adjunct to some types of surgery. For example, evoked potentials can be used to monitor auditory, visual, speech, or motor responses during surgery done under local anesthesia.

Most malignant brain tumors respond to external irradiation. Radiation can increase longevity and, at times, can allay symptoms when tumors recur. The treatment dose depends on the tumor's histologic type and radioresponsiveness and on the anatomic site and the level of tolerance of the surrounding tissue. Radiation therapy is now being avoided in children younger than 2 years of age because of the long-term effects, which include developmental delay, panhypopituitarism, and secondary tumors.[40]

The use of chemotherapy for brain tumors is somewhat limited by the blood-brain barrier. Chemotherapeutic agents can be administered intravenously, intra-arterially, intrathecally (into the spinal canal), or intraventricularly. The intravenous route is the one used most often. For malignant gliomas in adults, the nitrosoureas (carmustine or lomustine), cisplatin, and procarbazine have been most effective. Methotrexate is used in the treatment of medulloblastomas. Other agents are being tested. Chemotherapy is now the initial treatment for many childhood brain tumors. Currently, the most useful drugs for childhood brain tumors are vincristine, cisplatin, procarbazine, and methotrexate.

The most recent promising area of improved delivery of chemotherapeutic agents is through the use of biodegradable anhydrous wafers impregnated with the drug and implanted into the tumor at the time of surgery. These wafers are constructed so that they release the drug over a period of many months.[41]

In summary, brain tumors account for 2% of all cancer deaths and are the second most common type of cancer in children. Brain tumors can arise primarily from intracranial structures; in addition, tumors from other parts of the body often metastasize to the brain. Primary brain tumors can arise from any structure within the cranial cavity. Most begin in brain tissue, but the pituitary, the pineal region, and the meninges are also sites of tumor development. Brain tumors give rise to focal disturbances in brain function and increased intracranial pressure. Focal disturbances result from brain compression, tumor infiltration, disturbances in blood flow, and cerebral edema. The clinical manifestations of brain tumor depend on the size and location of the tumor. General signs and symptoms include headache, nausea and vomiting, mental changes, papilledema and visual disturbances, alterations in motor and sensory function, and seizures. Diagnostic tests include physical examination, visual field testing and funduscopic examination, CT scans, MRI studies, skull x-rays, brain scans, electroencephalography, and cerebral angiography. Treatment includes surgery, radiation, and chemotherapy.

■ REFERENCES

1. Robbins, S.L., & Kumar, V. (1992). *Basic pathology* (5th ed., pp. 712–713, 720–725, 725–727, 729–731). Philadelphia: W.B. Saunders.
2. American Psychiatric Association. (1987). *Diagnostic and statistical manual of mental disorders* (3rd ed., revised). Washington, DC: American Psychiatric Association.
3. Kwentus, J.A., Hart, R., Lingon, W., et al. (1986). Alzheimer's disease. *American Journal of Medicine*, 81, 91–95.
4. Karlinsky, H. (1986). Alzheimer's disease in Down's syndrome. *Journal of the American Geriatrics Society*, 34, 728.
5. Hyman, B.T., Van Hoesen, G.W., Kromer, I., et al. (1986). Understanding the memory loss in Alzheimer's disease. *American Journal of Alzheimer's Care and Related Disorders*, 1, 18.
6. Hasan, M.K., & Baker, D.J. (1987). Alzheimer's disease: Recent advances. *West Virginia Medical Journal*, 83, 427–429.

7. Katzman, R. (1986). Alzheimer's disease. *New England Journal of Medicine, 314*, 964–973.
8. Matteson, M.A., & McConnell, E.S. (1988). *Gerontological nursing* (pp. 249–254). Philadelphia: J.B. Lippincott.
9. McKhann, G., Drachman, D., Folstein, M., et al. (1984). Clinical diagnosis of Alzheimer's disease: Report of the NINCDS-ADRDA Work Group under the Auspices of the Department of Health and Human Services Task Force on Alzheimer's Disease. *Neurology, 34*, 939–944.
10. Babino, L. (1988). Conceptual analysis of validation therapy. *International Journal of Aging and Human Development, 26*, 161–168.
11. Brown, P., Gajdusek, C., Gibbs, C.J., et al. (1985). Potential epidemic of Creutzfeldt-Jakob disease from human growth hormone therapy. *New England Journal of Medicine, 313*, 728–731.
12. Rappaport, E.B. (1987). Iatrogenic Creutzfeldt-Jakob disease. *Neurology, 37*, 1520–1521.
13. Martin, J.B. (1987). Huntington's disease: Pathogenesis and management. *New England Journal of Medicine, 315*, 1267–1276.
14. Goetz, C.G., Jankovic, J., & Paulson, G.W. (1992). Update on Parkinson's disease. *Patient Care, March 30*, 172–208.
15. Greenberg, D.A., Aminoff, M.J., & Simon, R.P. (1993). *Clinical neurology* (2nd ed., pp. 208–209). Norwalk, CT: Appleton Lange.
16. Cotran, R.S., Kumar, V., & Robbins, S.L. (1989). *Pathologic basis of disease* (4th ed., pp. 1430–1431). Philadelphia: W.B. Saunders.
17. Ballard, P.A., Tetrud, J.W., & Langston, J.W. (1985). Permanent human parkinsonism due to 1-methyl-4-phenyl-1,2,3,6-tetrahydropydrine (MPTP): Seven cases. *Neurology, 35*, 949–956.
18. Langston, J.W. (1987). MPTP: Insights into the etiology of Parkinson's disease. *European Neurology, 26* (Suppl. 1), 2–10.
19. Lewin, R. (1985). Parkinson's disease: An environmental cause? *Science, 229*, 257–258.
20. Cummings, T. (1988). The dementia of Parkinson's disease. *European Neurology, 28* (Suppl. 1), 15–23.
21. Hakim, A.M., & Mathieson, G. (1979). Dementia in Parkinson disease: A neuropathologic study. *Neurology, 29*, 1209–1214.
22. Nutt, J.G., Woodward, W.R., & Hammerstad, J.P. (1984). The "on-off" phenomenon in Parkinson's disease. *New England Journal of Medicine, 310*, 483–488.
23. Katzung, B.G. (1992). *Basic and clinical pharmacology* (pp. 383–391). Norwalk, CT: Appleton & Lange.
24. Aminoff, M.J. (1993). Nervous system. In S.A. Schroeder, M.A. Krupp, & L.M. Tierney (Eds.). *Current medical diagnosis and treatment* pp. 757–758). Norwalk, CT: Appleton & Lange.
25. Backlund, E.O., Granberg, P.O., Hamberger, B., et al. (1985). Transplantation of adrenal medullary tissue to striatum in parkinsonism. *Journal of Neurosurgery, 62*, 169–173.
26. Merz, B. (1987). Adrenal-to-brain transplants improve the prognosis for Parkinson's disease. *Journal of the American Medical Association, 257*, 2691–2692.
27. Fahn, S. (1992). Fetal-tissue implants in Parkinson's disease. *New England Journal of Medicine, 327*, 1589–1590.
28. Cormack, D.H. (1987). *Ham's histology* (9th ed., pp. 344–345). Philadelphia: J.B. Lippincott.
29. Norton, W.T. (1984). Recent advances in myelin biochemistry. *Annals of the New York Academy of Sciences, 70*, 5–10.
30. Gonzalez-Scarano, F., Spellman, R.S., & Nathanson, N. (1986). Epidemiology. In W.E. McDonald, & D.H. Silberg (Eds.). *Multiple sclerosis* (pp. 37–55). Boston: Butterworth.
31. Waxman, S.G. (1982). Membranes, myelin and the pathophysiology of multiple sclerosis. *New England Journal of Medicine, 306*, 1529.
32. McFarlin, D.E., & McFarland, H.F. (1982). Multiple sclerosis. *New England Journal of Medicine, 307*, 1183–1188.
33. Paty, D.W. (1987). Multiple sclerosis: Assessment of disease progression and effects of treatment. *Canadian Journal of Neurology, 14*, 518.
34. Davis, F.A. (1984). The hot tub test in multiple sclerosis. In D.W. Poser, L. Scheinber, W.I. McDonald, & G.C. Ebers (Eds.). *The diagnosis of multiple sclerosis* (pp. 44–48). New York: Thieme-Stratton.
35. Berger, J.R., & Sheremata, W.A. (1983). Persistent neurological deficit precipitated by hot bath test in multiple sclerosis. *Journal of the American Medical Association, 249*, 171.
36. Berger, J.R., & Sheremata, W.A. (1985). Letter to the editor. *Journal of the American Medical Association, 253*, 203.
37. Poser, C., Paty, D., Scheinber, L., et al. (1983). New diagnostic criteria for multiple sclerosis. *Annals of Neurology, 13*, 227.
38. American Cancer Society. (1992). *Cancer facts and figures—1992.* New York: American Cancer Society.
39. Black, P.M. (1991). Brain tumors (second of two parts). *New England Journal of Medicine, 324*, 1555–1564.
40. Black, P.M. (1991). Brain tumors (first of two parts). *New England Journal of Medicine, 324*, 1471–1476.
41. Ransohoff, J., Koslow, M., & Cooper, P.R. (1991). Cancer of the central nervous system and pituitary. In A.I. Hollieb, D.J. Fink, & G.P. Murphy (Eds.). *American Cancer Society textbook of clinical oncology* (pp. 229–237). Atlanta: American Cancer Society.

▪ BIBLIOGRAPHY

Consensus Conference. (1987). Differentiating diagnosis of dementing diseases. *Journal of the American Medical Association, 258*, 3411–3416.

Danielczyk, W. (1992). Mental disorders in Parkinson's disease. *Journal of Neural Transmission [Supplementum], 38*, 115–127.

Delgado, J.M., & Billo, J.M. (1988). Care of the patient with Parkinson's disease: Surgical and nursing interventions. *Journal of Neuroscience Nursing, 20*, 142.

Growdon, J.H. (1992). Treatment for Alzheimer's disease? *New England Journal of Medicine, 327*, 1306–1308.

Jenner, P. (1992). What process causes nigral cell death in Parkinson's disease? *Neurologic Clinics, 10*, 387–403.

Jenner, P., Schapira, A.H.V., & Maraden, D.C. (1992). New insights into the cause of Parkinson's disease. *Neurology, 42*, 2241–2250.

Katzman, R. (1991). Alzheimer disease: Basic and clinical advances. *Journal of the American Geriatric Society, 39*, 516–525.

Korczyn, A.D. (1991). The clinical differential diagnosis of dementia: Concepts and methodology. *Psychiatric Clinics of North America, 14,* 237–249.

McDonald, W.I. (1993). The dynamics of multiple sclerosis: The Charcot Lecture. *Journal of Neurology, 240,* 28–36.

Morris, J.C., & Rubin, E.H. (1991). Clinical diagnosis and course of Alzheimer's disease. *Psychiatric Clinics of North America, 14,* 223–235.

Przuntek, H. (1992). Early diagnosis of Parkinson's disease. *Journal of Neural Transmission [Supplementum], 38,* 105–114.

Ransmayr, G., Kunig, G., & Gerstenbrand, F. (1992). Modern therapy of Parkinson's disease. *Journal of Neural Transmission [Supplementum], 38,* 129–140.

Tanner, C.M. (1992). Epidemiology of Parkinson's disease. *Neurologic Clinics, 10,* 317–329.

Treves, T. (1991). Epidemiology of Alzheimer's disease. *Psychiatric Clinics of North America, 14,* 251–249.

Weinshenker, B.G., & Nelson, R. (1990). The Second Canadian Conference on Multiple Sclerosis. *Canadian Journal of Neurological Sciences, 17,* 53–60.

ALTERATIONS IN SKELETAL SUPPORT AND MOVEMENT

CHAPTER 55

STRUCTURE AND FUNCTION OF THE SKELETAL SYSTEM

Characteristics of Skeletal Tissue
Bone
Cartilage

Tendons and Ligaments
Joints and Articulations
Synarthroses

Diarthroses
Bursae
Intraarticular Menisci

■ OBJECTIVES

After you have studied this chapter, you should be able to meet the following objectives:

- List the common components of bone, cartilage, and the dense connective tissue of ligaments and tendons.
- Compare the properties of the intercellular collagen and elastic fibers of skeletal tissue.
- Name and state the function of the four types of bone cells.
- Draw a long bone, and label the diaphysis, epiphysis, and metaphysis.
- State the location and function of the periosteum and the endosteum.
- Compare bone and cartilage in terms of their structure and function.
- Cite the characteristics and name at least one location of elastic cartilage, hyaline cartilage, and fibrocartilage.

- Define a *tendon* and a *ligament*.
- State the difference between synarthrodial and diarthrodial joints.
- Describe the articular structures of a diarthrodial joint.
- Describe the source of blood supply to a diarthrodial joint.
- Explain why pain is often experienced in all the joints of an extremity when only a single joint is affected by a disease process.
- Describe the structure and function of a bursa.
- Explain the pathology associated with a torn meniscus of the knee.

Without the skeletal system, movement in the external environment would not be possible. The bones of the skeletal system serve as a framework for the attachment of muscles, tendons, and ligaments. The skeletal system protects and maintains soft tissues in their proper position, provides stability for the body, and maintains the body's shape. The bones act as a storage reservoir for calcium, and the central cavity of some bones contains the hematopoietic connective tissue in which blood cells are formed.

The skeletal system consists of the axial and appendicular skeleton. The axial skeleton, which is composed of the bones of the skull, thorax, and vertebral column, forms the axis of the body. The appen-

Carol Mattson Porth: PATHOPHYSIOLOGY: CONCEPTS OF ALTERED HEALTH STATES, 4th ed. © 1994, 1990, 1986, 1982 J.B. Lippincott Company

dicular skeleton consists of the bones of the upper and lower extremities, including the shoulder and hip. For our purposes, the skeletal system is considered to include the bones and cartilage of the axial and appendicular skeleton as well as the connective tissue structures (ligaments and tendons) that connect the bones and join muscles to bone.

CHARACTERISTICS OF SKELETAL TISSUE

The tissues found in bones, cartilage, tendons, and ligaments have many things in common. Each of these connective tissue types consists of living cells, nonliving intercellular protein fibers, and an amorphous, or shapeless, ground substance. The tissue cells are responsible for secreting and maintaining the intercellular substances in which they are housed. These substances provide the structural characteristics of the tissue. For example, the intercellular matrix of bone is impregnated with calcium salts, providing the hardness that is characteristic of this tissue.

Two main types of intercellular fibers are found in skeletal tissue: collagenous and elastic. Collagen is an inelastic and insoluble fibrous protein. Because of its molecular configuration, collagen has great tensile strength; the breaking point of collagenous fibers found in human tendons is reached with a force of several hundred kilograms per square centimeter. Fresh collagen is colorless, and tissues that contain large numbers of collagenous fibers generally appear white. The collagen fibers in tendons and ligaments give these structures their white color. Elastin is the major component of elastic fibers that allows them to stretch several times their length and rapidly return to their original shape when the tension is released. Ligaments and structures that must undergo repeated stretching contain a high proportion of elastic fibers.

BONE

Bone is connective tissue in which the intercellular matrix has been impregnated with inorganic calcium salts so that it has great tensile and compressible strength but is light enough to be moved by coordinated muscle contractions. The intercellular matrix is composed of two types of substances—organic matter and inorganic salts. The organic matter, including bone cells, blood vessels, and nerves, constitutes about one third of the dry weight of bone; the inorganic salts make up the other two thirds.

The organic matter consists primarily of collagen fibers embedded in an amorphous ground substance.

The inorganic matter consists of hydroxyapatite, an insoluble macrocrystalline structure of calcium phosphate salts, and small amounts of calcium carbonate and calcium fluoride. Bone may also take up lead and other heavy metals, thereby removing these toxic substances from the circulation. This can be viewed as a protective mechanism. The antibiotic tetracycline drugs are readily bound to calcium deposited in newly formed bones and teeth. When tetracycline is given during pregnancy, it can be deposited in the teeth of the fetus, causing discoloration and deformity. Similar changes can occur if the drug is given for long periods to children under 6 years of age.

TYPES OF BONE

There are two types of mature bones, cancellous and compact bone (Fig. 55-1). Both types are formed in layers and are therefore called lamellar bone. Cancellous, or spongy, bone is found in the interior of bones and is composed of trabeculae, or spicules, of bone, which form a latticelike pattern. These latticelike structures are lined with osteogenic cells and filled with either red or yellow bone marrow. Cancellous bone is relatively light, yet its structure is such

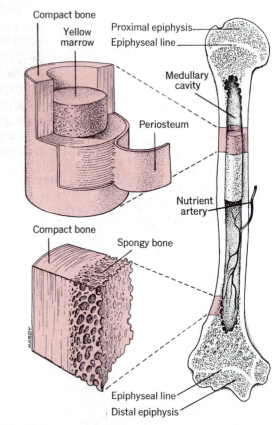

FIG. 55-1. A long bone shown in longitudinal section. (Chaffee, E. E., & Lytle, I. M. [1980]. *Basic physiology and anatomy* [4th ed.]. Philadelphia: J.B. Lippincott)

that it has considerable tensile strength and weight-bearing properties. Compact (cortical) bone has a densely packed calcified intercellular matrix that makes it more rigid than cancellous bone. The relative quantity of compact and cancellous bone varies in different types of bones throughout the body and in different parts of the same bone, depending on the need for strength and lightness. Compact bone is the major component of tubular bones. It is also found along the lines of stress on long bones and forms an outer protective shell on other bones.

BONE CELLS

Four types of bone cells participate in the formation and maintenance of bone tissue: (1) osteogenic cells, (2) osteoblasts, (3) osteocytes, and (4) osteoclasts (Table 55-1).

Osteogenic Cells. The undifferentiated osteogenic cells are found in the periosteum, endosteum, and epiphyseal plate of growing bone. These cells differentiate into osteoblasts and are active during normal growth; they may also be activated in adult life during healing of fractures and other injuries. Osteogenic cells also participate in the continual replacement of worn-out bone tissue.

Osteoblasts. The osteoblasts, or bone-building cells, are responsible for the formation of the bone

matrix. Bone formation occurs in two stages: ossification and calcification. Ossification involves the formation of osteoid, or prebone. Calcification of bone involves the deposition of calcium salts in the osteoid tissue. The osteoblasts synthesize collagen and other proteins that make up osteoid tissue. They also participate in the calcification process of the osteoid tissue, probably by controlling the availability of calcium and phosphate. Osteoblasts secrete the enzyme alkaline phosphatase, which is thought to act locally in bone tissue to raise calcium and phosphate levels to the point at which precipitation occurs. The activity of the osteoblasts undoubtedly contributes to the rise in serum levels of alkaline phosphatase that follows bone injury and fractures.

Osteocytes. The osteocytes are mature bone cells that are actively involved in maintaining the bony matrix. Death of the osteocytes results in the resorption of this matrix. The osteocytes lie in a small lake filled with extracellular fluid, called a *lacuna*, and are surrounded by a calcified intercellular matrix. Extracellular fluid-filled passageways permeate the calcified matrix and connect with the lacunae of adjacent osteocytes. These passageways are called *canaliculi*. Because diffusion does not occur through the calcified matrix of bone, the canaliculi serve as communicating channels for the exchange of nutrients and metabolites between the osteocytes and the blood vessels on the surface of the bone layer.

The osteocytes, together with their intercellular matrix, are arranged in layers, or lamellae. In compact bone, 4 to 20 lamellae are arranged concentrically around a central haversian canal, which runs essentially parallel to the long axis of the bone. Each of these units is called a *haversian system*, or *osteon*. The haversian canals contain blood vessels that carry nutrients and wastes to and from the canaliculi (Fig. 55-2). The blood vessels from the periosteum enter the bone through tiny openings called *Volkmann's canals* and connect with the haversian systems. Cancellous bone is also composed of lamellae, but its trabeculae are usually not penetrated by blood vessels. Instead, the bone cells of cancellous bone are nourished by diffusion from the endosteal surface through canaliculi, which interconnect their lacunae and extend to the bone surface.

Osteoclasts. Osteoclasts are bone cells that function in the resorption of bone, removing both the mineral content and the organic matrix. Unlike the osteoblasts, which originate in osteogenic cells, the osteoclasts are formed by the fusion of blood-derived monocytes. Although the mechanism of osteoclast formation and activation remains elusive, it is known that parathyroid hormone increases the number and

TABLE 55-1. FUNCTION OF BONE CELLS

TYPE OF BONE CELL	FUNCTION
Osteogenic cells	Undifferentiated cells that differentiate into osteoblasts. They are found in the periosteum, endosteum, and epiphyseal growth plate of growing bones.
Osteoblasts	Bone-building cells that synthesize and secrete the organic matrix of bone. Osteoblasts also participate in the calcification of the organic matrix.
Osteocytes	Mature bone cells that function in the maintenance of bone matrix. Osteocytes also play an active role in releasing calcium into the blood.
Osteoclasts	Bone cells responsible for the resorption of bone matrix and the release of calcium and phosphate from bone.

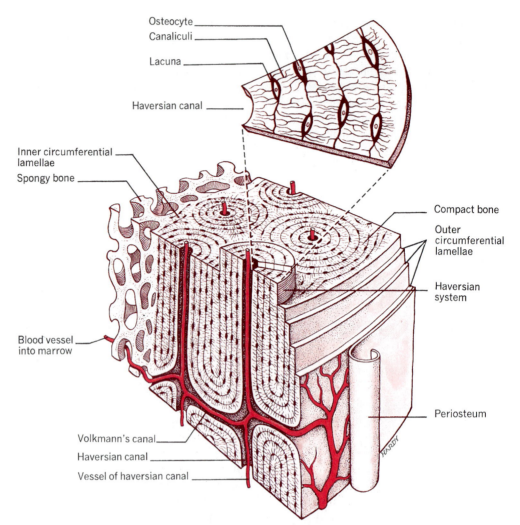

FIG. 55-2. Haversian systems as seen in a wedge of compact bone tissue. The periosteum has been peeled back to show a blood vessel entering one of Volkmann's canals. (**Upper right**) Osteocytes lying within lacunae; canaliculi permit interstitial fluid to reach each lacuna. (Chaffee, E. E., & Lytle, I. M. [1980]. *Basic physiology and anatomy* [4th ed.]. Philadelphia: J.B. Lippincott)

resorptive function of the osteoclasts. Calcitonin, on the other hand, is thought to reduce the number and resorptive function of the osteoclasts. The mechanism whereby osteoclasts exert their resorptive effect on bone is also unclear. These cells may secrete an acid that removes calcium from the bone matrix, thus releasing the collagenic fibers for digestion by either osteoclasts or mononuclear cells.

CLASSIFICATION OF BONES

Bones are classified, on the basis of their shape, as (1) long, (2) short, (3) flat, and (4) irregular. Long bones are found in the upper and lower extremities. Short bones are irregularly shaped bones located in the ankle and the wrist. Except for their surface, which is compact bone, these bones are spongy throughout. Flat bones are composed of a layer of spongy bone

between two layers of compact bone. They are found in areas such as the skull and rib cage, where extensive protection of underlying structures is needed or, as in the scapula, where a broad surface for muscle attachment must be provided. Irregular bones, because of their shapes, cannot be classified in any of the previous groups. This group includes such bones as the vertebrae and the bones of the jaw.

A typical long bone has a shaft, or diaphysis, and two ends, called epiphyses. Long bones are usually narrow in the midportion and broad at the ends so that the weight they bear can be distributed over a wider surface. The shaft of a long bone is formed mainly of compact bone roughly hollowed out to form a marrow-filled medullary canal. The ends of long bones are covered with articular cartilage that rests on a bony plate, the subchondral bone.

In growing bones, the part of the bone shaft that

funnels out as it approaches the epiphysis is called the metaphysis (Fig. 55-3). It is composed of bony trabeculae that have cores of cartilage. In the child, the epiphysis is separated from the metaphysis by the cartilaginous growth plate. After puberty, the metaphysis and epiphysis merge, and the growth plate is obliterated.

BONE MARROW

Bone marrow occupies the medullary cavities of the long bones throughout the skeleton and the cavities of cancellous bone in the vertebrae, ribs, sternum, and flat bones of the pelvis. The cellular composition of the bone marrow varies with both age and skeletal location. Red bone marrow contains developing red blood cells and is the site of blood cell formation. Yellow bone marrow is composed largely of adipose cells. At birth, nearly all of the marrow is red and hematopoietically active. As the need for red blood cell production decreases during postnatal growth, red marrow is gradually replaced with yellow bone marrow in most of the bones. In the adult, red marrow persists in the vertebrae, ribs, sternum, and ilia.

PERIOSTEUM AND ENDOSTEUM

Bones are covered, except at their articular ends, by a membrane called the periosteum (see Fig. 55-1). The periosteum has an outer fibrous layer and an inner layer that contains the osteogenic cells needed for

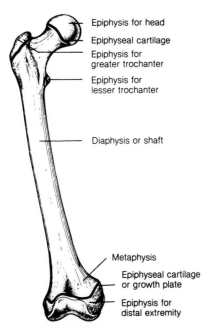

Epiphysis for head
Epiphyseal cartilage
Epiphysis for greater trochanter
Epiphysis for lesser trochanter

Diaphysis or shaft

Metaphysis
Epiphyseal cartilage or growth plate
Epiphysis for distal extremity

FIG. 55-3. A femur, showing epiphyseal cartilages for the head, metaphysis, trochanters, and distal end of the bone. (Adapted from Chaffee, E. E., & Lytle, I. M. [1980]. *Basic physiology and anatomy* [4th ed.]. Philadelphia: J.B. Lippincott)

bone growth and development. The periosteum contains blood vessels and acts as an anchorage point for vessels as they enter and leave the bone. The endosteum is the membrane that lines the spaces of spongy bone, the marrow cavities, and the haversian canals of compact bone. It is composed mainly of osteogenic cells. These osteogenic cells contribute to the growth and remodeling of bone and are necessary for one repair.

CARTILAGE

Cartilage is a firm but flexible type of connective tissue consisting of cells and intercellular fibers embedded in an amorphous gel-like material. It has a smooth and resilient surface and a weight-bearing capacity exceeded only by that of bone.

Cartilage is essential for growth both before and after birth. It is able to undergo rapid growth while maintaining a considerable degree of stiffness. In the embryo, most of the axial and appendicular skeleton is formed first as a cartilage model and is replaced by bone. In postnatal life, cartilage continues to play an essential role in the growth of long bones and persists as articular cartilage in the adult.

There are three types of cartilage: elastic cartilage, hyaline cartilage, and fibrocartilage. *Elastic cartilage* contains some elastin in its intercellular substance. It is found in areas, such as the ear, where some flexibility is important. Pure cartilage is called *hyaline cartilage* (from the Greek, meaning glass) and is pearly white. It is the type of cartilage seen on the articulating ends of fresh soup bones found in the supermarket. *Fibrocartilage* has characteristics that are intermediate between dense connective tissue and hyaline cartilage. It is found in the intervertebral disks, in areas where tendons are connected to bone, and in the symphysis pubis.

Hyaline cartilage is the most abundant type of cartilage. It forms much of the cartilage of the fetal skeleton. In the adult, hyaline cartilage forms the costal cartilages, which join the ribs to the sternum and vertebrae, many of the cartilages of the respiratory tract, the articular cartilages, and the epiphyseal plates.

Cartilage cells, which are called *chondrocytes*, are located in lacunae. These lacunae are surrounded by an uncalcified gel-like intercellular matrix of collagen fibers and ground substance. Cartilage is devoid of blood vessels and nerves. The free surfaces of most hyaline cartilage, with the exception of articular cartilage, is covered by a layer of fibrous connective tissue called the *perichondrium*.

It has been estimated that about 65% to 80% of the wet weight of cartilage is water held in its gel structure. Because cartilage has no blood vessels, this tissue fluid allows for the diffusion of gases, nutrients, and wastes between the chondrocytes and blood vessels outside the cartilage. Diffusion cannot take place if the cartilage matrix becomes impregnated with calcium salts. Therefore, cartilage dies if it becomes calcified.

TENDONS AND LIGAMENTS

In the skeletal system, tendons and ligaments are dense connective tissue structures that connect muscles and bones. Tendons connect muscles to bone, and ligaments connect the movable bones of joints. Tendons can appear as cordlike structures or as flattened sheets, called aponeuroses, such as in the abdominal muscles.

The dense connective tissue found in tendons and ligaments has a limited blood supply and is composed largely of intercellular bundles of collagen fibers arranged in the same direction and plane. This type of connective tissue provides great tensile strength and can withstand tremendous pulls in the direction of fiber alignment. At the sites where tendons or ligaments are inserted into cartilage or bone, a gradual transition from pure dense connective tissue to either bone or cartilage occurs. In cartilage this transitional tissue is called fibrocartilage.

Tendons that might rub against bone or other friction-generating surfaces are enclosed in double-layered sheaths. An outer connective tissue tube is attached to the structures surrounding the tendon, and an inner sheath encloses the tendon and is attached to it. The space between the inner and outer sheath is filled with a fluid similar to synovial fluid.

In summary, skeletal tissue includes bone, cartilage, ligaments, and tendons. These skeletal structures are composed of similar tissue types; each has living cells and nonliving intercellular fibers and ground substance that is secreted by the cells. The characteristics of the various skeletal tissue types are determined by the intercellular matrix. In bone, this matrix is impregnated with calcium salts to provide hardness and strength. There are four types of bone cells: osteocytes, or mature bone cells; osteoblasts, or bone-building cells; osteoclasts, which function in bone resorption; and osteogenic cells, which differentiate into osteoblasts. A typical long bone has a shaft, or diaphysis, and two ends called epiphyses. Densely packed compact bone forms the outer shell of a bone, and latticelike cancellous bone forms the interior. Cartilage is a firm, flexible type of skeletal tissue that is essential for growth both before and after birth. There are three types of cartilage: elastic, hyaline, and fibrocartilage. Hyaline cartilage, which is the most abundant type, forms the costal cartilages that join the ribs to the sternum and vertebrae, many of the cartilages of the respiratory tract, and the articular cartilages. Tendons and ligaments are dense connective skeletal tissue that connect muscles and bones. Tendons connect muscles to bones and ligaments connect the movable bones of joints.

■ JOINTS AND ARTICULATIONS

Articulations, or joints, are areas where two or more bones meet. The term *arthro* is the affix used to designate a joint. For example, *arthrology* is the study of joints and *arthroplasty* is the repair of a joint. There are two classes of joints, based on movement and the presence of a joint cavity: synarthroses and diarthroses.

SYNARTHROSES

Synarthroses are joints that lack a joint cavity and move little or not at all. There are three types of synarthroses: synostoses, synchondroses, and syndesmoses. *Synostoses* are nonmovable joints in which the surfaces of the bones are joined by dense connective tissue or bone. The bones of the skull are joined by synostoses; they are joined by dense connective tissue in children and young adults and by bone in older people. *Synchondroses* are joints in which bones are connected by hyaline cartilage and have limited motion. The ribs are attached to the sternum by this type of joint. *Syndesmoses* permit a certain amount of movement; they are separated by a fibrous disk and joined by interosseous ligaments. The symphysis pubis of the pelvis and the bodies of the vertebrae that are joined by intervertebral disks are examples of syndesmoses.

DIARTHROSES

Diarthrodial joints (synovial joints) are freely movable joints. Most joints in the body are of this type. Although they are classified as freely movable, their movement actually ranges from almost none (sacro-iliac joint) to simple hinge movement (interphalangeal joint), to movement in many planes (shoulder or hip joint). The bony surfaces of these joints are covered with thin layers of articular cartilage, and the cartilaginous surfaces of these joints slide past each other during movement. As discussed in Chapter 58, diarthrodial joints are the joints most frequently affected by rheumatic disorders.

In a diarthrodial joint, the articulating ends of the bones are not connected directly but are indirectly linked by a strong fibrous capsule (joint capsule) that surrounds the joint and is continuous with the periosteum (Fig. 55-4). This capsule supports the joint and helps to hold the bones in place. Additional support may be provided by ligaments that extend between the bones of the joint.

The joint capsule consists of two layers: an outer fibrous layer and an inner membrane, the synovium.

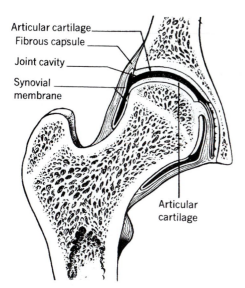

FIG. 55-4. Diarthrodial joint, showing the articular cartilage, fibrous joint capsule, joint cavity, and synovial membrane. (Chaffee, E. E., & Lytle, I. M. *Basic physiology and anatomy* [4th ed.]. Philadelphia: J.B. Lippincott)

The synovium surrounds the tendons that pass through the joints as well as the free margins of other intraarticular structures such as ligaments and menisci. The synovium forms folds that surround the margins of articulations but do not cover the weight-bearing articular cartilage. These folds permit stretching of the synovium so that movement can occur without tissue damage.

The synovium secretes a slippery synovial fluid with the consistency of egg white. This fluid acts as a lubricant and facilitates the movement of the articulating surfaces of the joint. Normal synovial fluid is clear or pale yellow, does not clot, and contains fewer than 100 cells/mm^3. The cells are predominantly mononuclear cells derived from the synovium. The composition of the synovial fluid is altered in many inflammatory and pathologic joint disorders. Aspiration and examination of the synovial fluid play an important role in the diagnosis of joint diseases.

The articular cartilage is an example of hyaline cartilage and is unique in that its free surface is not covered with perichondrium. It has only a peripheral rim of perichondrium, and calcification of the portion of cartilage abutting the bone may limit or preclude diffusion from blood vessels supplying the subchondral bone. Articular cartilage is apparently nourished by the diffusion of substances contained in the synovial fluid bathing the cartilage. Regeneration of most cartilage is slow; it is accomplished primarily by growth that requires the activity of perichondrium cells. In articular cartilage, which has no perichondrium, superficial injuries heal slowly.

BLOOD SUPPLY

The blood supply to a joint arises from blood vessels that enter the subchondral bone at or near the attachment of the joint capsule and form an arterial circle around the joint. The synovial membrane has a rich blood supply, and constituents of plasma diffuse rapidly between these vessels and the joint cavity. Because many of the capillaries are near the surface of the synovium, blood may escape into the synovial fluid after relatively minor injuries. Healing and repair of the synovial membrane are usually rapid and complete. This is important because synovial tissue is injured in many surgical procedures that involve the joint.

INNERVATION

The nerve supply to joints is provided by the same nerve trunks that supply the muscles that move the joints. These nerve trunks also supply the skin over the joints. As a rule, each joint of an extremity is innervated by all the peripheral nerves that cross the articulation; this accounts for the referral of pain from one joint to another. For example, hip pain may be perceived as pain in the knee.

The tendons and ligaments of the joint capsule are sensitive to position and movement, particularly stretching and twisting. These structures are supplied by the large sensory nerve fibers that form proprioceptor endings (see Chapter 50). The proprioceptors function reflexively to adjust the tension of the muscles that support the joint and are particularly important in maintaining muscular support for the joint. For example, when a weight is lifted, there is a proprioceptor-mediated reflex contraction and relaxation of appropriate muscle groups to support the joint and protect the joint capsule and other joint structures. Loss of proprioception and reflex control of muscular support leads to destructive changes in the joint.

The synovial membrane is innervated only by autonomic fibers that control blood flow. It is relatively free of pain fibers, as is evidenced by the fact that surgical procedures on the joint are often done under local anesthesia. The joint capsule and the ligaments have pain receptors; these receptors are more easily stimulated by stretching and twisting than other joint structures. Pain arising from the capsule tends to be diffuse and poorly localized.

BURSAE

In some diarthrotic joints, the synovial membrane forms closed sacs that are not part of the joint. These sacs, called *bursae*, contain synovial fluid. Their purpose is to prevent friction on a tendon. Bursae are present in areas where pressure is exerted because of

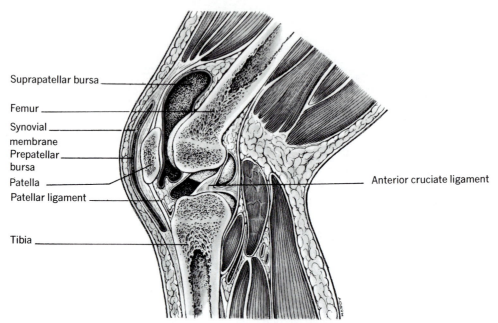

FIG. 55-5. Sagittal section of knee joint, showing prepatellar and suprapatellar bursae. (Chaffee, E. E., & Lytle, I. M. [1980]. *Basic physiology and anatomy* [4th ed.]. Philadelphia: J.B. Lippincott)

close approximation of joint structures (Fig. 55-5). Such conditions occur when tendons are deflected over bone or where skin must move freely over bony tissue. Bursae may become injured or inflamed, causing discomfort, swelling, and limitation in movement of the involved area. A bunion is an inflamed bursa of the metatarsophalangeal joint of the great toe.

INTRAARTICULAR MENISCI

Intraarticular menisci are fibrocartilage structures that develop from portions of the articular disk that occupied the space between articular cartilage surfaces during fetal development. Menisci may extend partway through the joint and have a free inner border (as at the lateral and medial articular surfaces of the knee), or they may extend through the joint, separating it into two separate cavities (as in the sternoclavicular joint). The menisci of the knee joint may be torn as the result of an injury. The detached portion may interfere with joint motion and cause recurring pain and locking or giving way of the joint. When this happens, the injured structure is often removed surgically. After removal, a new structure sometimes grows in from the fibrous capsule of the joint. The new meniscus is almost a complete duplicate of the old except that it is made up of dense connective tissue rather than the fibrocartilage of the original structure.

In summary, articulations, or joints, are areas where two or more bones meet. Synarthroses are joints in which bones are joined together by fibrous tissue, cartilage, or bone; they lack a joint cavity and move little or no movement. Diarthrodial or synovial joints are freely movable. The surfaces of the articulating ends of bones in diarthrodial joints are covered with a thin layer of articular cartilage and they are enclosed in a fibrous joint capsule. The joint capsule consists of two layers: an outer fibrous layer and an inner membrane, the synovium. A slippery fluid called the synovial fluid, which is secreted by the synovium and is present in the joint capsule, acts as a lubricant and facilitates movement of the joint's articulating surfaces. Bursae, which are closed sacs containing synovial fluid, prevent friction in areas where tendons are deflected over bone or where skin must move freely over bony tissue. Menisci are fibrocartilaginous structures that develop from portions of the articular disk that occupied the space between the articular cartilage during fetal development. The menisci may have a free inner border, or they may extend through the joint, separating it into two cavities. The menisci in the knee joint may be torn as a result of injury.

■ BIBLIOGRAPHY

Bloom, W., & Faucett, D.W. (1975). *A textbook of histology.* Philadelphia: W.B. Saunders.

Cormack, D.H. (1987). *Ham's histology* (9th ed., pp. 234–338). Philadelphia: J.B. Lippincott.

Junqueira, L.C., Carneiro, J., & Long, J.A. (1986). *Basic histology* (pp. 140–165). Los Altos, CA: Lange Medical Publications.

C H A P T E R 5 6

ALTERATIONS IN SKELETAL FUNCTION: TRAUMA AND INFECTION

KATHLEEN E. GUNTA

Injury and Trauma of
Musculoskeletal Structures
Soft Tissue Injury
Strains and Sprains
Dislocations

Chondromalacia
Loose Bodies
Fractures
Bone Infections
Iatrogenic Bone Infections

Osteomyelitis
Treatment
Tuberculosis

■ OBJECTIVES

After you have studied this chapter, you should be able to meet the following objectives:

■ Describe the physical agents responsible for soft tissue trauma.
■ Name the three types of soft tissue injuries.
■ Compare muscle strains and ligamentous sprains.
■ Describe the healing process of soft tissue injuries.
■ Differentiate between open and closed fractures.
■ List the signs and symptoms of a fracture.
■ Describe the fracture healing process.
■ Relate individual and local factors to the healing process in bone.

■ Explain the importance of immobilization for fracture healing.
■ Explain why muscle and joint function should be maintained during fracture healing.
■ Differentiate between the early complications of fractures and later complications of fracture healing.
■ Explain the implications of bone infection.
■ Describe how an acute form of osteomyelitis becomes chronic.

The musculoskeletal system includes the bones, joints, and muscles of the body together with associated structures such as ligaments and tendons. This system, which constitutes more than 70% of the body, is subject to a large number of disorders. These disorders affect people in all age groups and walks of life, causing pain, disability, and deformity. The discussion in this chapter focuses on trauma and infections of skeletal structures.

■ INJURY AND TRAUMA OF MUSCULOSKELETAL STRUCTURES

Trauma, which commonly includes injury to musculoskeletal structures, is the third leading cause of death in the United States. A broad spectrum of injuries result from numerous physical forces. Injuries to the musculoskeletal system include blunt tis-

Carol Mattson Porth: PATHOPHYSIOLOGY: CONCEPTS OF
ALTERED HEALTH STATES, 4th ed. © 1994, 1990, 1986, 1982
J.B. Lippincott Company

sue trauma, disruption of tendons and ligaments, and fractures of bony structures.

Many of the external physical agents that cause injury to the musculoskeletal system are typical of a particular environmental setting, activity, or age group. Trauma resulting from high-speed motor accidents is ranked as the number one killer of adults under the age of 35. Motorcycle accidents are especially common in young men, with fractures of the distal tibia, midshaft femur, and radius occurring most often.

Trauma in children is usually the result of an accident. Bicycle-related injuries account for more than 50,000 emergency room visits annually, the majority being in the 5- to 14-year-old age group.[1]

Elderly people are at particular risk for injuries caused by falls. Impaired hearing and sight, dizziness, and unsteadiness of gait contribute to falls in the older person. These falls are often compounded by osteoporosis, or bone atrophy, which makes fractures more likely. Fractures of the vertebrae, proximal humerus, and hip are particularly common in this age group.

SOFT TISSUE INJURY

Most skeletal injuries are accompanied by soft tissue injuries. These injuries include contusions, hematomas, and lacerations. They are discussed here because of their association with skeletal injuries.

A *contusion* is an injury to soft tissue that results from direct trauma and is usually caused by striking a body part against a hard object. With a contusion, the skin overlying the injury remains intact. Initially, the area becomes ecchymotic (black and blue) because of local hemorrhage; later, the discoloration gradually changes to brown and then to yellow as the blood is reabsorbed.

A large area of local hemorrhage is called a *hematoma* (blood tumor). Hematomas cause pain as blood accumulates and exerts pressure on nerve endings. The pain increases with movement or when pressure is applied to the area. The pain and swelling of a hematoma take longer to subside than that accompanying a contusion. A hematoma may become infected because of bacterial growth. Unlike a contusion, which does not drain, a hematoma may eventually split the skin because of increased pressures and subsequently produce drainage.

The treatment for both a contusion and a hematoma consists of elevating the affected part and applying cold for the first 24 hours to reduce the bleeding into the area. A hematoma may need to be aspirated. After the first 24 hours, heat or cold should be applied intermittently for periods of 20 minutes at a time.

A *laceration* is an injury in which the skin is torn or its continuity is disrupted. The seriousness of a laceration depends on the size and depth of the wound and on whether there is contamination from the object that caused the injury. Puncture wounds from nails or rusted material may result in the growth of toxic bacteria, leading to gas gangrene or tetanus.

Lacerations are usually treated by wound closure, which is done once the area is sufficiently cleansed; the closed wound is covered with a sterile dressing. It is important to minimize contamination of the wound and to control bleeding. Contaminated wounds and open fractures are copiously irrigated and debrided, and the skin is usually left open to heal to prevent the development of an anaerobic infection or a sinus tract.

STRAINS AND SPRAINS

Tendons and ligaments, which connect bones and muscles, can be severed by cutting injuries or damaged by forcible twisting or stretching. A *strain* is a stretching injury to a muscle or a musculotendinous unit caused by mechanical overloading. This type of injury may result from either an unusual muscle contraction or an excessive forcible stretch. Although there is usually no external evidence of a specific injury, pain, stiffness, and swelling are present. The most common sites for muscle strain are the lower back and the cervical region of the spine. The elbow and the shoulder are also supported by musculotendinous units that are subject to strains. Foot strain is associated with the weight-bearing stresses of the feet; it may be caused by inadequate muscular and ligamentous support, overweight, or excessive exercise such as standing, walking, or running.

A *sprain*, which involves the ligamentous structures surrounding the joint, resembles a strain, but the pain and swelling subside more slowly (Fig. 56-1). It is usually caused by abnormal or excessive movement of the joint. With a sprain, the ligaments may be incompletely torn or, as in a severe sprain, completely torn or ruptured. The signs of sprain are pain, rapid swelling, heat, disability, discoloration, and limitation of function. Any joint may be sprained, but the ankle joint is most commonly involved. Most ankle sprains occur when the foot is turned inward under a person, forcing the ankle into inversion beyond the structural limits. Other common sites of sprain are the knee (the collateral ligament and anterior cruciate ligament) and elbow (on the ulnar side). As with a strain, the soft tissue injury that occurs with a sprain is not evident on x-ray. Occasionally, however, a chip of bone is evident when the entire ligament, including part of its bony attachment, has been ruptured or torn from the bone.

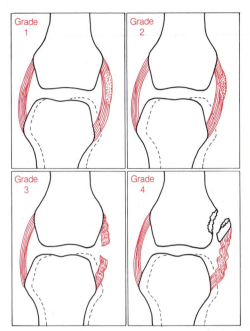

FIG. 56-1. Degrees of sprain on the medial side of the right knee: grade 1, mild sprain of the medial collateral ligament; grade 2, moderate sprain with hematoma formation; grade 3, severe sprain with total disruption of the ligament; and grade 4, severe sprain with avulsion of the medial femoral condyle at the insertion of the medial collateral ligament. (Adapted from Spickler, L. L. [1983]. Knee injuries of the athlete. *Orthopedic Nursing*, 2(5), 12–13)

A tear of the meniscus can be associated with a sprained knee (see Chapter 55). Meniscus tears can be described by their appearance (such as parrot-beak and bucket handle) or their location (such as posterior horn or anterior horn). Meniscus injury commonly occurs as the result of a rotational injury from a sudden or sharp pivot or a direct blow to the knee as in hockey, basketball, or football. The injured knee is edematous and painful especially with hyper-flexion and hyperextension. A loose fragment may cause knee instability and locking. Diagnosis is made by arthroscopy.

Healing of the dense connective tissues in tendons and ligaments is similar to that of other soft tissues. If properly treated, injuries usually heal with the restoration of the original tensile strength. Repair is accomplished by fibroblasts from the inner tendon sheath or, if the tendon has no sheath, from the loose connective tissue that surrounds the tendon. Capillaries infiltrate the injured area during the initial healing process and supply the fibroblasts with the materials they need to produce large amounts of collagen. Formation of the long collagen bundles begins within 4 to 5 days, and, although tensile strength increases steadily thereafter, it is not sufficient to permit strong tendon pulls for 4 to 5 weeks.[2] During the first 3 weeks, there is a danger that muscle con-

traction will pull the injured ends apart; should this occur, the tendon will heal in the lengthened position. There is also a danger that adhesions will develop in areas where tendons pass through fibrous channels, such as in the distal palm of the hands, rendering the tendon useless.

The treatment of muscle strains and ligamentous sprains is similar in several ways. For an injured extremity, elevation of the part followed by local application of cold may be sufficient. Compression, accomplished through the use of adhesive wraps or a removable splint, helps reduce swelling and provides support. A cast is applied for severe sprains, especially those severe enough to warrant surgical repair. Immobilization for a muscle strain is continued until the pain and swelling have subsided. In a sprain, the affected joint is immobilized for several weeks. Immobilization may be followed by graded active exercises. Early diagnosis, treatment, and rehabilitation are essential in preventing chronic ligamentous instability.

In the lumbar and cervical spine regions, muscle strains are more common than sprains. For these strains, treatment usually consists of bedrest, traction, application of heat, and massage. Cold should be used during the first 24 hours to reduce pain and swelling of the affected area. Exercises, correct posture, and good body mechanics help to reduce the risk of reinjury. Mechanical low back pain is becoming increasingly common in the adolescent athlete. Overuse, especially hyperextension of the lumbar spine in such sports as track, wrestling, gymnastics, and diving, can tear the muscles, fascia, and ligaments. Chronic low back pain may indicate a stress fracture. Fractures near the top and bottom surface of the vertebrae can occur when the growing lumbar spine is overstressed, causing the disks to push into the bone. Early detection and treatment are important to prevent complications and prevent disability.

Rotator cuff injury occurs in one or more of the four muscles that lie deep in the shoulder bridging the glenohumeral joint. It is caused by excessive usage, a direct blow or stretch injury usually involving throwing or swinging as with baseball pitchers or tennis players. Rotator cuff tendinitis, also known as *shoulder impingement syndrome*, is also common, especially in swimmers. Many physical examination maneuvers are used to define shoulder pathology. The history and mechanism of injury are important. In addition to standard x-rays, an arthogram, computed tomography (CT) scan, or magnetic resonance imaging (MRI) scan may be done. Arthroscopic examination under anesthesia is done for diagnostic as well as operative arthroscopy to repair severe tears. A period of rest is followed by a customized exercise and rehabilitation program to improve strength, flexibility, and endurance. The rotator cuff is not unlike other muscle groups of the body in that its risk of injury increases when asked to perform a high stress function in an unconditioned state.

DISLOCATIONS

Dislocation of a joint is the loss of articulation of the bone ends within the joint capsule caused by displacement or separation of the bone end from its position in the joint. It usually follows a severe trauma that disrupts the holding ligaments. Dislocations are seen most often in the shoulder and acromioclavicular joints. A *subluxation* is a partial dislocation in which the bone ends within the joint are still in partial contact with each other.

Dislocations can be congenital, traumatic, or pathologic. Congenital dislocations occur in the hip and knee. Traumatic dislocations occur after falls, blows, or rotational injuries. For example, car accidents often cause dislocations of the hip and accompanying acetabular fractures because the direction of impact. This is true of both people wearing seatbelts and those who are unrestrained. In the shoulder and patella, dislocations may become recurrent, especially in athletes. They recur with the same motion but require less and less force each time. Pathologic dislocation in the hip is a late complication of infection, rheumatoid arthritis, paralysis, and neuromuscular diseases. Dislocations of the phalangeal joints are not serious and are usually reduced by manipulation. Less common sites of dislocation, seen mainly in young adults, are the wrist and midtarsal region. They are usually the result of violent force.

Diagnosis of a dislocation is made by physical examination and confirmed by x-ray. The symptoms are pain, deformity, and limited movement. With recurrent dislocations, the person often senses the impending dislocation and may have a look of apprehension when range of joint motion is tested.

The treatment depends on the site, mechanism of injury, and associated injuries such as fractures. Dislocations that do not reduce spontaneously usually require manipulation or surgical repair. Various surgical procedures can also be used to prevent redislocation of the patella, shoulder, or acromioclavicular joints. Immobilization is necessary for several weeks after reduction of a dislocation; this allows for healing of the joint structures. In dislocations affecting the knee, alternatives to surgery are isometric quadriceps-strengthening exercises and a temporary brace. Surgical procedures, such as joint replacement, may be necessary in certain pathologic dislocations.

Recurrent subluxation and dislocation of the patella are common injuries in young adults. They account for about 10% of all athletic injuries and are more common in females. Sports such as skiing or tennis may cause stress on the patella. These sports involve external rotation of the foot and lower leg with knee flexion, a position that exerts rotational stresses on the knee. There is often a sensation of the patella "popping out" when the dislocation occurs. Other complaints include the knee giving out, swelling, crepitus, stiffness, and loss of range of motion. Congenital knee variations are predisposing factors. Treatment can be difficult, but nonsurgical methods are used first. They include immobilization with the knee extended, bracing, administration of salicylates, and isometric quadriceps-strengthening exercises. Surgical intervention is often necessary.

CHONDROMALACIA

Chondromalacia, or softening of the articular cartilage, is seen most commonly on the undersurface of the patella and occurs most frequently in young adults. It can be the result of recurrent subluxation of the patella or overuse in strenuous athletic activities. Patients with this disorder typically complain of pain, particularly when climbing stairs or sitting with the knees bent. Occasionally there is weakness of the knee. The treatment consists of rest, isometric exercises, and application of ice after exercise. Part of the patella may be surgically removed in severe cases. In less severe cases, the soft portion is shaved, using a saw inserted through an arthroscope.

LOOSE BODIES

Loose bodies are small pieces of bone or cartilage inside the joint. These can be the result of trauma to the joint or may occur when cartilage has worn away from the articular surface, causing a part of the surface bone to die. When this happens, a piece of bone separates and becomes free-floating. The symptoms are painful catching and locking of the joint. Loose bodies are commonly seen in the knee, elbow, hip, and ankle. The loose body repeatedly gets caught in the crevice of a joint, pinching the underlying healthy cartilage; unless the loose body is removed, it may cause osteoarthritis and restricted movement. The treatment consists of removal using operative arthroscopy.

FRACTURES

Normal bone can withstand considerable compression and shearing forces and, to a lesser extent, tension forces. A fracture is any break in the continuity of bone that occurs when more stress is placed on the bone than it is able to absorb. Grouped according to their etiology, fractures can be divided into three major categories: (1) fractures caused by sudden injury, (2) fatigue or stress fractures, and (3) pathologic fractures. The most common fractures are those resulting from sudden injury. The force causing the fracture may be direct, such as a fall or blow, or indirect, such as a massive muscle contraction or trauma transmitted along the bone. For example, the head of the radius or clavicle can be fractured by the indirect forces that result from falling on an outstretched hand. A fatigue, or stress, fracture results from repeated wear on a bone. Overuse injuries of the lower extremities, especially posterior medial tibial pain is one of the most common symptoms that physically active people experience. Stress fractures in the tibia may be confused with "shin splints" (a nonspecific term for pain in the lower leg from overuse in walking and running) because they frequently don't appear on x-ray until 2 weeks after the onset of symptoms.

A pathologic fracture occurs in bones that are already weakened by disease or tumors. Fractures of this type may occur spontaneously with little or no stress. The underlying disease state can be local, as with infections, cysts, or tumors, or it can be generalized, as in osteoporosis, Paget's disease, or disseminated tumors.

CLASSIFICATION

Fractures are usually classified according to (1) type, (2) location, and (3) direction of the fracture line (Fig. 56-2).

Types. The type of fracture is determined by its communication with the external environment, the degree of break in continuity of the bone, and the character of the fracture pieces. A fracture can be classified as either open or closed. When the bone fragments have broken through the skin, the fracture is called an *open* or *compound* fracture. Open fractures are often complicated by infection, osteomyelitis, delayed union, or nonunion. In a *closed* fracture there is no communication with the outside skin.

The degree of a fracture is described in terms of a partial or complete break in the continuity of bone. A *greenstick* fracture, which is seen in children, is an example of a partial break in bone continuity and resembles the kind seen when a young sapling is broken. This kind of break occurs because children's bones, especially until about age 10, are more resilient than the bones of adults.

A fracture is also described by the character of the fracture pieces. A *comminuted* fracture has more than two pieces. A *compression* fracture, such as oc-

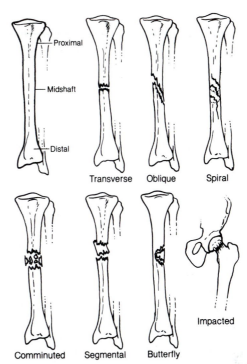

FIG. 56-2. Classification of fractures. Fractures are classified according to location (proximal, midshaft, or distal), the direction of fracture line (transverse, oblique, spiral), and type (comminuted, segmental, butterfly, or impacted).

curs in the vertebral body, involves two bones that are crushed or squeezed together. A fracture is called *impacted* when the fracture fragments are wedged together. This type usually occurs in the humerus and is often less serious and generally treated without surgery.

Pattern. The direction of the trauma or mechanism of injury produces a certain configuration or pattern of fracture. *Reduction* is the restoration of a fractured bone to its normal anatomic position. The pattern of a fracture indicates the nature of the trauma and provides information about the easiest method for reduction. Transverse fractures are caused by simple angulatory forces. A spiral fracture results from a twisting motion, or torque. A transverse fracture is not likely to become displaced or lose its position after it is reduced. On the other hand, spiral, oblique, and comminuted fractures are often unstable and may change position after reduction.

Location. A long bone is divided into three parts: proximal, midshaft, and distal (see Fig. 56-2). A fracture of the long bone is described in relation to its position in the bone. Other descriptions are used when the fracture affects the head or neck of a bone, involves a joint, or is near a prominence such as a condyle or malleolus.

Signs and Symptoms. The signs and symptoms of a fracture include pain, tenderness at the site of bone disruption, swelling, loss of function, deformity of the affected part, and abnormal mobility. The deformity varies according to the type of force applied, the area of the bone involved, the type of fracture produced, and the strength and balance of the surrounding muscles. In long bones, three types of deformities—angulation, shortening, and rotation—are seen. Severely angulated fracture fragments may be felt at the fracture site and often push up against the soft tissue to cause a tenting effect on the skin. Bending forces and unequal muscle pulls cause angulation. Shortening of the extremity occurs as the bone fragments slide and override each other because of the pull of the muscles on the long axis of the extremity (Fig. 56-3). Rotational deformity occurs when the fracture fragments rotate out of their normal longitudinal axis; this can result from rotational strain produced by the fracture or unequal pull by the muscles that are attached to the fracture fragments. A crepitus or grating sound may be heard as the bone fragments rub against each other. In the case of an open fracture, there is bleeding from the wound where the bone protrudes. Blood loss from a pelvic fracture or multiple long bone fractures can cause hypovolemic shock in a trauma victim (see Chapter 25).

Shortly after the fracture has occurred, nerve function at the fracture site may be temporarily lost. The area may become numb, and the surrounding muscles may become flaccid. This condition has been termed *local shock*. During this period, which may last for a few minutes to half an hour, fractured bones may be reduced with little or no pain. After this brief period, pain sensation returns, and with it muscle spasms and contractions of the surrounding muscles.

HEALING

Bone healing occurs in a manner similar to soft tissue healing. It is, however, a more complex process and takes longer. Although the exact mechanisms of bone healing are open to controversy, five stages of the healing process have been identified: (1) hematoma formation, (2) cellular proliferation, (3) callus formation, (4) ossification, and (5) consolidation and re-

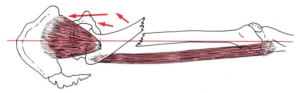

FIG. 56-3. Displacement and overriding of fracture fragments of a long bone (femur) caused by severe muscle spasm.

modeling (Fig. 56-4). The degree of response during each of these stages is in direct proportion to the extent of trauma.

Hematoma Formation. Hematoma formation occurs during the first 48 to 72 hours after fracture. It develops as blood from torn vessels in the bone fragments and surrounding soft tissue leaks between and around the fragments of the fractured bone. As a result of hematoma formation, clotting factors remain in the injured area to initiate the formation of a fibrin meshwork, which serves as a framework for the ingrowth of fibroblasts and new capillary buds. Granulation tissue, the result of fibroblasts and new capillaries, gradually invades and replaces the clot. When a large hematoma develops, healing is delayed because macrophages, platelets, oxygen, and nutrients for callus formation are prevented from entering the area.

Cellular Proliferation. Three layers of bone structure are involved in the cellular proliferation that occurs during bone healing after a fracture: the periosteum or outer covering of the bone; the endosteum or inner covering; and the medullary canal, which contains the bone marrow. During this process, the osteoblasts, or bone-forming cells, multiply

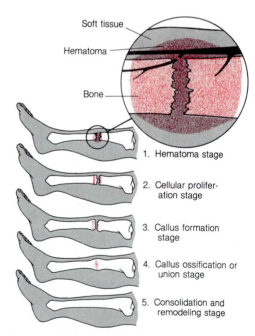

1. Hematoma stage

2. Cellular proliferation stage

3. Callus formation stage

4. Callus ossification or union stage

5. Consolidation and remodeling stage

FIG. 56-4. Healing of a fracture. During hematoma formation (*1*), a locally formed clot serves as a fibrin meshwork for subsequent cellular invasion. Cellular proliferation (*2*) involves the invasion of the hematoma area by fibroblastic and endothelial cells. During callus formation (*3*), osteoblasts enter the area and produce the osteoid matrix. Callus formation is followed by union (*4*). The remodeling of the healed fracture is the last stage of the healing process (*5*).

and differentiate into a fibrocartilaginous callus. The fibrocartilaginous callus is softer and more flexible than callus. Cellular proliferation begins distal to the fracture, where there is a greater supply of blood. After a few days, a fibrocartilage "collar" becomes evident around the fracture site. The collar edges on either side of the fracture eventually unite to form a bridge, which connects the bone fragments.

Callus Formation. During the early stage of callus formation, the fracture becomes "sticky" as osteoblasts continue to move in and through the fibrin bridge to help keep it firm. Cartilage forms at the level of the fracture, where there is less circulation. In areas of the bone with muscle insertion, periosteal circulation is better, bringing in the nutrients necessary to bridge the callus. The bone calcifies as mineral salts are deposited. This stage occurs in 3 to 4 weeks.

Ossification. Ossification involves the final laying down of bone. This is the stage at which the fracture has been bridged and the fracture fragments are firmly united. Mature bone replaces the callus, and the excess callus is gradually resorbed by the osteoclasts (cells that resorb bone). The fracture site feels firm and immovable and appears united on x-ray. At this point, it is safe to remove the cast.

Remodeling. Remodeling involves resorption of the excess bony callus that develops within the marrow space and encircling the external aspect of the fracture site. The remodeling process is directed by mechanical stress and direction of weight bearing. It continues according to Wolff's law—bone responds to mechanical stress by becoming thicker and stronger in relation to its function.

Healing Time. Healing time depends on the site of the fracture, the condition of the fracture fragments, hematoma formation, and other local and host factors. In general, fractures of long bones, displaced fractures, and fractures with less surface area heal slower. Function usually returns within 6 months after union is complete. However, return to complete function may take longer.

Factors Affecting Healing. The factors that influence bone healing are local factors and those specific to the patient. Local factors include (1) the nature of the injury or the severity of the trauma, including fracture displacement and edema; (2) the degree of bridge formation that develops during bone healing; (3) the amount of bone loss (*e.g.*, it may be too great for the healing to bridge the gap); (4) the type of bone that is injured (*e.g.*, cancellous bone heals faster than

cortical bone); (5) the degree of immobilization that is achieved (movement disrupts the fibrin bridge and cartilage forms instead of bone); (6) local infection, which retards or prevents healing; (7) local malignancy, which must be treated before healing can proceed; (8) bone necrosis, which prevents blood flow into the fracture site; and (9) intraarticular fractures (those through a joint), which may heal more slowly and may eventually produce arthritis. Individual factors that may delay bone healing are the patient's age, current medications, debilitating diseases, such as diabetes and rheumatoid arthritis, local stress around the fracture site, circulatory problems, coagulation disorders, and poor nutrition.

DIAGNOSIS AND TREATMENT

A *splint* is a device for immobilizing the movable fragments of a fracture. When a fracture is suspected, the injured part should always be splinted before it is moved. This is essential for preventing further injury.

Diagnosis is the first step in the care of fractures and is based on history and physical manifestations. X-ray examination is used to confirm the diagnosis and direct the treatment. The ease of diagnosis varies with the location and severity of the fracture. In the trauma patient, the presence of other more serious injuries may make diagnosis more difficult. A thorough history includes the mechanism, time, and place of the injury, first recognition of symptoms, and any treatment initiated. A complete history is important because a delay in seeking treatment or weight bearing on a fracture may have caused further injury or displacement of the fracture.

Treatment of fractures depends on the general condition of the patient, the presence of associated injuries, the location of the fracture, its displacement, and whether the fracture is open or closed. There are three objectives for treatment of fractures: (1) reduction of the fracture, (2) immobilization, and (3) preservation and restoration of the function of the injured part.

Reduction. Reduction of a fracture is directed toward replacing the bone fragments to as near a normal anatomic position as possible. This can be accomplished by closed manipulation or surgical (open) reduction. Closed manipulation uses methods such as manual pressure and traction. Fractures are held in reduction by external or internal fixation devices. Surgical reduction involves the use of various types of hardware to accomplish internal fixation of the fracture fragments (Fig. 56-5). Primary closure of crush injuries in the extremities is delayed until tissue viability is determined. The wound is first

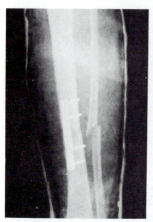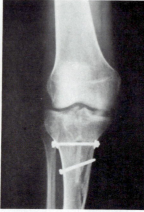

FIG. 56-5. (**Left**) Internal fixation of the tibia with compression plate. (**Right**) Internal fixation of an intraarticular fracture of the upper tibia with a screw and bolt. (Farrell, J. [1986]. *Illustrated guide to orthopedic nursing* [3rd ed.]. Philadelphia: J.B. Lippincott)

debrided and immobilized with an external fixation device. Reconstruction is done later using cancellous bone grafts, microvascular composite tissue grafts, or by way of tissue regeneration with distraction devices.[3]

Immobilization. Immobilization prevents movement of the injured parts and is the single most important element in obtaining union of the fracture fragments. Immobilization can be accomplished through the use of external devices, such as splints, casts, external fixation devices, or traction, or by means of internal fixation devices inserted during surgical reduction of the fracture.

Splints are made from many different materials. Metal splints or air splints may be used during transport to a health care facility as a temporary measure until the fracture has been reduced and another form of immobilization instituted. Plaster of Paris splints, which are molded to fit the extremity, work well. Splinting should be done if there is any suspicion of a fracture because motion of the fracture site can cause pain, bleeding, more soft tissue damage, and nerve or blood vessel compression. If the fracture has sharp fragments, movement can cause perforation of the skin and conversion of a closed fracture into an open one. When a splint is applied to an extremity, it should extend from the joint above the fracture site to the joint below it.

Casts (plaster or synthetic material) are commonly used to immobilize fractures of the extremities. They are often applied with a joint in partial flexion to prevent rotation of the fracture fragments. Without this flexion, the extremity, which is essentially a cylinder, tends to rotate within the cylindrical structure of the cast.

The application of a cast brings the risk of impaired circulation to the extremity because of blood vessel compression. A cast applied shortly after a fracture may not be large enough to accommodate the swelling that inevitably occurs in the hours that follow. Therefore, after a cast is applied, the peripheral circulation must be observed carefully until this danger has passed. Should the circulation become inadequate, the parts that are exposed at the distal end of the cast (*e.g.*, the toes with a leg cast and the fingers with an arm cast) usually become cold and cyanotic or pale. An increase in pain may occur initially, followed by paresthesia (tingling or abnormal sensation) or anesthesia as the sensory neurons that supply the area are affected. There is a decrease in the amplitude or absence of the pulse in areas where the arteries can be palpated. Capillary refill time, which is assessed by applying pressure to the fingernail and observing the rate of blood return, is prolonged to greater than 3 seconds. This condition demands immediate measures, such as splitting the cast, to restore the circulation and prevent permanent damage to the extremity. A casted extremity should always be elevated above the level of the heart for the first 24 hours to minimize swelling.

A brace may be used after a cast is removed or instead of a cast, as with a tibial stress fracture.

With *external fixation devices*, pins or screws are inserted directly into the bone above and below the fracture site. They are secured to a metal frame and adjusted to align the fracture. This method of treatment is used primarily for open fractures, infections such as osteomyelitis and septic joints, unstable closed fractures, and limb lengthening.

Limb-lengthening devices are being used for traumatic losses of bone and soft tissue. Limb-lengthening systems, such as the Ilizarov external fixator (Fig. 56-6) are used to lengthen or widen bones, correct angular or rotational defects, or immobilize fractures.[4] The apparatus is applied with a surgical technique called a corticotomy (a percutaneous osteotomy that preserves the periosteal and endosteal tissues). A circular external apparatus is attached to bone by tensioned Kirschner wires. The corticotomy site is gradually distracted or pulled apart, about 1 mm per day, until the desired length is achieved. The continuous distraction activates regeneration of bone, soft tissue, nerves, and blood vessels. New bone forms (osteogenesis) in the distraction gap. This newly formed bone can fill defects (posttraumatic or after resection for osteomyelitis), consolidate nonunions, regenerate bone in limb lengthening, correct deformities, and eliminate the need for bone grafting. This apparatus is left on until the desired length is achieved and consolidation is complete.

Another method for achieving immobility and

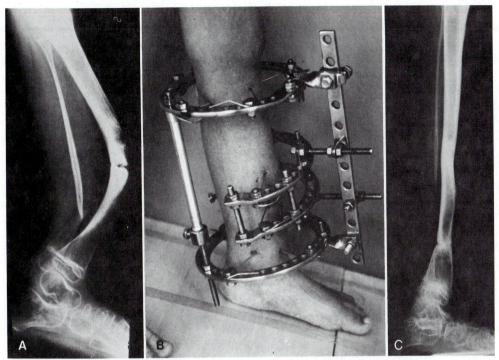

FIG. 56-6. Ilizarov device used to treat a tibial fracture with anterolateral bow and medullary sclerosis: before (**A**), with Ilizarov device in place (**B**), and three-year follow-up lateral roentgenograph (**C**). (Paley, D., Catagni, M., Argnani, F. et al. [1992]. Treatment of congenital pseudoarthrosis of the tibia using Ilizarov technique. *Clinical Orthopedics and Related Research, 280,* 84)

maintaining reduction is *traction.* Traction is a pulling force applied to an extremity or part of the body while a counterforce, or countertraction, pulls in the opposite direction. Countertraction is usually exerted by the body's weight on the bed. Traction is used to maintain alignment of the fracture fragments and reduce muscle spasm.

Effective traction prevents movement of the fracture site. Fractures caused by trauma are associated with muscle injury and spasm. These muscle contractions cause overriding and displacement of the bone fragments, particularly when the fractures affect long bones. The five goals of traction therapy are to (1) correct and maintain the skeletal alignment of either entire bones or joints; (2) reduce pressure on a joint surface; (3) correct, lessen, or prevent deformities such as contractures and dislocations; (4) decrease muscle spasm; and (5) immobilize a part to promote healing. Traction may be used as a temporary measure before surgery or as a primary treatment method.

There are three types of traction: manual traction, skin traction, and skeletal traction. *Manual traction* consists of a steady, firm pull that is exerted by the hands. It is a temporary measure used to manipulate a fracture during closed reduction, for support of a neck injury during transport when cervical-spine

fracture is suspected, or for reduction of a dislocated joint. *Skin traction* is a pulling force applied to the skin and soft tissue. It is accomplished by strips of adhesive, flannel, or foam secured to the injured part.

Skeletal traction is a pulling force applied directly to the bone. Pins, wires, or tongs are inserted through the skin and subcutaneous tissue into the bone distal to the fracture site. Muscles, tendons, arteries, and nerves are identified during the insertion process so that they are not penetrated. Pins are not inserted into joints or open areas. Skeletal traction provides an excellent pull. It can be used for long periods and with large amounts of weight. It is commonly used for fractures of the femur, the humerus, and the cervical spine (Crutchfield tongs applied to the skull). Skeletal traction is also used in maintaining alignment of fractures that are casted and in certain types of reconstructive foot surgery. Pin tract infection is a complication of skeletal traction. Pin insertion sites should be inspected daily for redness, drainage, and shifting of the traction device. Larger pins need to be cleansed daily with hydrogen peroxide or an antibiotic solution.

Preservation and Restoration of Function. During the period of immobilization required for fracture healing, the preservation and restoration of function of muscles and joints are an ongoing process in the unaffected as well as the affected extremities. Exercises designed to preserve function, maintain muscle strength, and reduce joint stiffness should be started early. Active range of motion, in which the person moves the extremity, is done on unaffected extremities; and isometric, or muscle-tensing, exercises are done on the affected extremities. In some instances, an electrical muscle stimulator is applied directly to the skin to stimulate isometric muscle contraction as a means of preventing disuse atrophy. After the fracture has healed, a program of physical therapy may be necessary. However, the most important factor in restoring function is the person's own active exercises.

Muscles tend to atrophy during immobilization because of lack of use. Joints stiffen as muscles and tendons contract and shorten. The degree of muscle atrophy and joint stiffness depends on several factors. In adults, the degree of atrophy and muscle stiffness are directly related to the length of immobilization, with longer periods of immobility resulting in greater stiffness. Children have a natural tendency to move on their own, and this movement maintains muscle and joint function. Therefore, they usually have less atrophy and recover sooner once the source of immobilization has been removed. Associated soft tissue injury, infection, and preexisting joint disease increase the risk of stiffness. Although limbs are immobilized in a functional position, casts are removed as soon as fracture healing has taken place.

COMPLICATIONS

The complications of fractures can be divided into two groups: (1) early complications associated with loss of skeletal continuity, injury from bone fragments, pressure due to swelling and hemorrhage, or development of fat emboli, and (2) complications associated with fracture healing. The early complications of fractures depend on the severity of the fracture and the area of the body that is involved. For example, bone fragments from a skull fracture may cause injury to brain tissue, or multiple rib fractures may lead to a flail chest and respiratory insufficiency. With flail chest, the chest wall on the fractured side becomes so unstable that it may move in the opposite direction as the patient breathes (*i.e.*, in during inspiration and out during expiration).

Compartment Syndrome. Compartment syndrome is the result of increased pressure within a limited anatomic space that compromises circulation and threatens the viability and function of the nerves and muscle within a closed compartment (see Chapter 20). It can be acute or chronic. Acute compartment

syndrome can occur after a fracture or crushing injury when excessive swelling around the site of injury results in increased pressure (30 mmHg or more) within a closed compartment. This increase in pressure occurs because fascia, which covers and separates muscles, is inelastic and unable to compensate for the extreme swelling.

The condition causes severe pain because of passive stretching of soft tissue and skin. Nerve compression may cause changes in sensation (paresthesias such as burning or tingling or loss of sensation), diminished reflexes, and eventually loss of motor function. Compression of blood vessels may cause muscle ischemia and loss of function. Muscles and nerves may be permanently damaged if the pressure is not relieved. In contrast to ischemia caused by a tight bandage or cast, in the compartment syndrome the peripheral pulses are often normal. The compartment syndrome is more common with crushing injuries, in closed fractures, and when external compression of a limb produces a tourniquet effect. The most common sites are the four compartments of the lower leg (deep posterior, superficial posterior, lateral, and anterior compartments) and the dorsal and volar compartments of the forearm.

Treatment is directed at reducing the compression of blood vessels and nerves. Constrictive dressings and casts are loosened. Intracompartmental pressure is often monitored, either with needle injection or continuous measurements. A fasciotomy, or transection of the fascia that is restricting the muscle compartment, may be required when the pressure in the area rises above 30 mmHg, which is roughly equal to the perfusion pressure in the capillary beds. Irreversible nerve and muscle damage can be avoided if the fasciotomy is done within 24 hours of the onset of clinical symptoms for compartment pressures of 40 mmHg or less.[5]

Fat Emboli. Fat emboli result from the presence of intracellular fat globules in the lung parenchyma and peripheral circulation after a long-bone fracture or other major trauma. There are two theories about the origin of fat emboli. One theory is that fat globules are released from the bone marrow or subcutaneous tissue at the fracture site into the venous system through torn veins.[6] The second theory postulates that the fat emboli develop intravascularly secondary to an alteration in lipid stability caused by increased release of tissue lipases, catecholamines, glucagon, or other steroid hormones in response to the stress of injury.[7] Fat emboli may also be caused by exogenous sources of fat, such as blood transfusions, intravenous fat emulsions, or bone marrow transplantation.

Fat embolism syndrome (FES) describes a respiratory deficiency state caused by decreased alveolar diffusion of oxygen due to fat embolism. Three degrees of severity are seen: subclinical, overt clinical, and fulminating. Although the subclinical and overt clinical forms of FES respond well to treatment, the fulminating form is often fatal. There are three possible outcomes when fat emboli enter the pulmonary circulation: (1) small emboli can mold to vessel caliber, pass through the lung, and enter the systemic circulation, where they are either trapped in the tissues or eliminated through the kidney; (2) the fat particles can be broken down by alveolar cells and eliminated through sputum; and (3) there can be local lipolysis with release of free fatty acid.[8] Free fatty acids cause direct injury to the alveolar capillary membrane, which leads to hemorrhagic interstitial pneumonitis with disruption of surfactant production and development of the adult respiratory distress syndrome. In addition, the fat globules become coated with platelets, causing thrombocytopenia. Serotonin released by the sequestered platelets causes bronchospasm and vasodilatation.

Clinically, the incidence of fat embolization is related to fractures of bones containing the most marrow (*i.e.*, long bones and the bones of the pelvis). Initial symptoms begin to develop within a few hours to 3 to 4 days after injury and do not appear beyond 1 week after the injury. The first symptoms include a subtle change in behavior and signs of disorientation due to the presence of emboli in the cerebral circulation combined with respiratory depression. There may be complaints of substernal chest pain and dyspnea accompanied by tachycardia and a low-grade fever. Diaphoresis, pallor, and cyanosis become evident as respiratory function deteriorates. A petechial rash that does not blanch with pressure often occurs 2 to 3 days after the injury. This rash is usually found on the anterior chest, axillae, neck, and shoulders. It may also appear on the soft palate and conjunctiva. The rash is thought to be related to embolization of the skin capillaries or thrombocytopenia.

An important part of the treatment of fat emboli is early diagnosis. Arterial blood gases should be assayed immediately after recognition of clinical manifestations. In a person suspected of having FES, a sustained arterial oxygen tension (Po_2) of less than 60 mmHg, an arterial carbon dioxide tension (Pco_2) of more than 55 mmHg, or a blood pH of less than 7.3 is diagnostic.[9] Treatment is directed toward correcting hypoxemia and maintaining adequate fluid balance. Mechanical ventilation may be required. Corticosteroid drugs are administered to decrease the inflammatory response of lung tissues, decrease the edema, stabilize the lipid membranes to reduce lipolysis, and combat the bronchospasm. Corticosteroids are also given prophylactically to high-risk peo-

ple. The only preventive approach to FES is early stabilization of the fracture.

Impaired Healing. *Union* of a fracture has occurred when the fracture is solid enough to withstand normal stresses and it is clinically and radiologically safe to remove the external fixation. In children, fractures generally heal within 4 to 6 weeks; in adolescents, they heal within 6 to 8 weeks; and, in adults, they heal within 10 to 18 weeks.

Delayed union is the failure of a fracture to unite within the normal time period (*e.g.*, 20 weeks for a fracture of the tibia or femur in an adult). The treatment for delayed union consists in determining and correcting the cause of the delay. *Malunion* is healing with deformity, angulation, or rotation that is visible on x-ray. It is usually treated by surgery. *Nonunion* is failure to produce union and cessation of the processes of bone repair. It is characterized by mobility of the fracture site and pain on weight bearing. Muscle atrophy and loss of range of motion may also be present. Nonunion is usually established 6 to 12 months after the time of the fracture. The complications of fracture healing are summarized in Table 56-1.

Treatment methods for impaired bone healing include surgical interventions including bone grafts, bracing, external fixation, or electrical stimulation of the bone ends. Electrical stimulation is thought to stimulate the osteoblasts to lay down a network of bone. Three types of commercial bone growth stimulators are available: a noninvasive model, which is placed outside the cast; a seminoninvasive model, in which pins are inserted around the fracture site; and a totally implantable type, in which a cathode coil is wound around the bone at the fracture site and is operated by a battery pack implanted under the skin. Figure 56-7 depicts a noninvasive type of electrical stimulator. The Ilizarov method of circular external fixation is being used with increasing frequency to treat nonunions, especially those that are infected.

In summary, many external physical agents can cause trauma to the musculoskeletal system. There are particular factors that can place a person at greater risk for injury. Some soft tissue injuries such as contusions, hematomas, and lacerations are relatively minor and easily treated. Muscle strains and ligamentous sprains are caused by mechanical overload on the connective tissue. They heal more slowly than the minor soft tissue injuries and require some degree of immobilization. Healing of soft tissue begins within 4 to 5 days of the injury and is primarily the function of fibroblasts, which produce collagen. Joint dislocation is caused by trauma to the supporting structures. Repeated trauma to the joint can cause articular softening (chondromalacia) or the separation of small pieces of bone or cartilage, called loose bodies, within the joint.

Fractures occur when more stress is placed on a bone than

TABLE 56-1. COMPLICATIONS OF FRACTURE HEALING

COMPLICATION	MANIFESTATIONS	CONTRIBUTING FACTORS
Delayed union	Failure of fracture to heal within predicted time as determined by x-ray	Large displaced fracture Inadequate immobilization Large hematoma Infection at fracture site Excessive loss of bone Inadequate circulation
Malunion	Deformity at fracture site Deformity or angulation on x-ray	Inadequate reduction Malalignment of fracture at time of immobilization
Nonunion	Failure of bone to heal before the process of bone repair stops Evidence on x-ray Motion at fracture site Pain on weight bearing	Inadequate reduction Mobility at fracture site Severe trauma Bone fragment separation Soft tissue between bone fragments Infection Extensive loss of bone Inadequate circulation Malignancy Bone necrosis Noncompliance with restrictions

the bone can absorb. The nature of the stress determines the type of fracture and the character of the resulting bone fragments. Healing of fractures is a complex process that takes place in five stages: hematoma formation, cellular proliferation, callus formation, ossification, and consolidation and remodeling. For satisfactory healing to take place, the affected bone has to be reduced and immobilized. This is accomplished by either a surgically implanted internal fixation device or devices such as splints, casts, or traction or external fixation apparatus. The complications associated with fractures can occur early when damage to soft tissue, blood vessels, and nerves is present or later when the healing process is interrupted. Local factors related to the healing environment and the person's general physical condition affect the healing process.

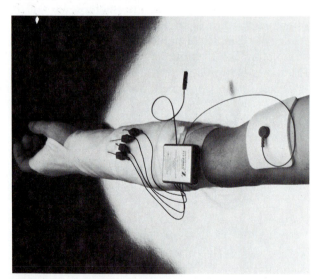

FIG. 56-7. One type of electrical stimulator used in the treatment of nonunion. (Courtesy of Zimmer, Inc., Warsaw, IN; Farrell, J. [1986]. *Illustrated guide to orthopedic nursing* [3rd ed.]. Philadelphia: J.B. Lippincott)

■ BONE INFECTIONS

Bone infections are difficult to treat and eradicate. Their effects can be devastating; they can cause pain, disability, and deformity. Chronic bone infections may drain for years because of a sinus tract. This occurs when a passageway develops from an abscess or cavity within the bone to an opening through the skin.

IATROGENIC BONE INFECTIONS

Iatrogenic bone infections are those inadvertently brought about by surgery or other treatment. These infections include complications of pin tract infection in skeletal traction, sepsis (infected) joints in joint replacement surgery, and wound infection after any surgery. Measures to prevent these infections include: (1) preparation of the skin to reduce bacterial growth before surgery or insertion of traction devices or wires; (2) strict operating room protocols, including disinfection of the operative site and a wide surrounding field with draping to prevent egress of the patient's and operating room personnel's flora into the area; (3) prophylactic use of antibiotics including topical wound irrigation; and (4) maintenance of sterile technique after surgery when working with drainage tubes and dressing changes. Because of the danger of infection, orthopedic wounds are kept covered with a sterile dressing until they are closed.

OSTEOMYELITIS

Osteomyelitis represents an acute or chronic pyogenic infection of the bone. The term *osteo* refers to bone and *myelo* refers to the marrow cavity, both of which are involved in this disease. Osteomyelitis can be caused by hematogenous (through the bloodstream) seeding, direct extension, or direct contamination of an open fracture or wound. In most cases, *Staphylococcus aureus* is the infecting organism.[10]

The most common cause of osteomyelitis is the direct contamination of bone from an open wound. It may be the result of an open fracture, a gunshot wound, or a puncture wound. Inadequate irrigation or debridement, introduction of foreign material into the wound, and extensive tissue injury increase the bone's susceptibility to infection. If the infection is not sufficiently treated, the acute infection may become chronic. Osteomyelitis may also occur as a complication of surgery, such as in the sternum after open heart surgery or in extremities after bone allograft or total joint replacement.

ACUTE HEMATOGENOUS OSTEOMYELITIS

Acute hematogenous osteomyelitis is almost always limited to those under 21 years of age. It affects, in order of frequency, the femur, tibia, humerus, and radius.[10] The condition usually manifests as an acute febrile systemic illness of 48 hours or less duration accompanied by the signs of local bone involvement. Although the incidence of the acute form of osteomyelitis has declined, there is an apparent increase in the subacute form.[11] Subacute osteomyelitis has an insidious onset in which symptoms are typically present for 2 weeks or more before diagnosis. The infection generally begins in the metaphysis of the bone where the nutrient artery channels terminate and the blood flow is sluggish. Because of the bone's rigid structure, there is little room for swelling, and the pus that forms finds its way to the surface of the bone to form a subperiosteal abscess. The blood sup-

ply to the bone may become obstructed by septic thrombi, in which case the ischemic bone becomes necrotic. It separates from the viable surrounding bone to form a fragment of bone known as a sequestrum (Fig. 56-8).

In children, acute hematogenous osteomyelitis is usually preceded by staphylococcal or streptococcal infections of the skin, sinuses, teeth, or middle ear. There is a history of trauma in one third of the cases; the trauma apparently reduces the bone's ability to respond to infection. Intravenous drug users are at risk for infections with *Streptococcus* and *Pseudomonas*.

The signs and symptoms of acute hematogenous osteomyelitis are those of bacteremia accompanied by symptoms referable to the site of the bone lesion. There is often pain on movement of the affected extremity, loss of movement, and local tenderness followed by heat and swelling. X-ray studies may appear normal initially, but they show evidence of periosteal elevation and increased osteoclastic activity once an abscess has formed. Changes are evident on a bone scan 10 to 14 days before any radiographic changes are seen.

In the adult, hematogenous osteomyelitis usually affects the axial skeleton and the irregular bones in the wrist and ankle. It is most common in debilitated patients and in those with a history of chronic skin infections, chronic urinary tract infections, and intravenous drug use.

The treatment of acute osteomyelitis begins with identification of the causative organism through blood cultures, aspiration cultures, and Gram's stain. Antibiotics are first given intravenously and then orally. The amount of rest needed by the affected limb and pain control measures used are based on symptomatology. Debridement and surgical drainage may also be necessary.

CHRONIC OSTEOMYELITIS

Chronic osteomyelitis has long been recognized as a disease. The incidence, however, has decreased in the last century because of improvements in surgical techniques and antibiotic therapy. Chronic osteomyelitis includes all inflammatory processes in the bone, excluding those in rheumatic diseases, that are caused by microorganisms. It may be the result of delayed or inadequate treatment of acute hematogenous osteomyelitis or osteomyelitis caused by direct contamination of bone. Acute osteomyelitis is considered to have become chronic when either the infection persists beyond 6 to 8 weeks or when the acute process has been adequately treated and is expected to resolve. Chronic osteomyelitis can persist for years; it may appear spontaneously, after a

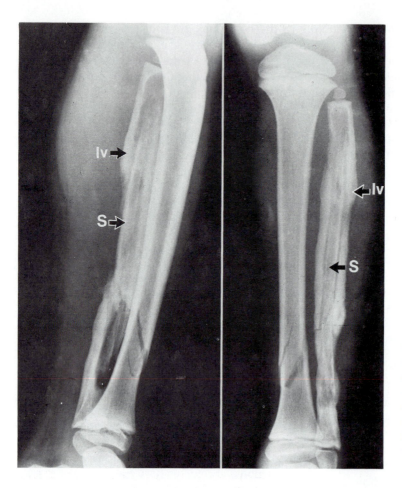

FIG. 56-8. Hematogenous osteomyelitis of the fibula of 3 months' duration. The entire shaft has been deprived of its blood supply and has become a sequestrum (*S*) surrounded by new immature bone, involucrum (*Iv*). Pathologic fractures are present in the lower tibia and fibula. (Wilson, F. C. [1980]. *The musculoskeletal system: Basic processes and disorders* [2nd ed., p. 150]. Philadelphia: J.B. Lippincott)

minor trauma, or when resistance is lowered. The hallmark feature of chronic osteomyelitis is the presence of infected dead bone, a sequestrum, that has separated from the living bone. A sheath of new bone, called the involucrum, forms around the dead bone. Radiologic techniques such as x-rays, bone scans, and sinograms are used to identify the infected site. Chronic osteomyelitis or infection around a total joint prosthesis can be difficult to diagnose because the classic signs of infection are not apparent and the blood leukocyte count may not be elevated. A subclinical infection may be present for years. Bone scans are used in conjunction with bone biopsy for a definitive diagnosis.

TREATMENT

The treatment of bone infections begins with wound cultures to identify the microorganism and its sensitivity to antibiotic therapy. This is followed by surgery to remove foreign bodies (*e.g.*, metal plates or screws) or sequestra and by long-term antibiotic therapy. Wounds may be left open and packed or closed with a continuous wound-irrigation system being left in place for several days to several weeks after surgery. The irrigation system consists of an antibiotic or sodium chloride solution that is flushed directly into the site of the infection and suctioned out by means of a closed drainage system. Immobilization of the affected part is usually necessary, with restriction of weight bearing on a lower extremity. External fixation devices are used.

Methicillin-resistant *Staphylococcus aureus* (MRSA) has become increasingly common, especially in people with total joint replacements, those treated in intensive care units or trauma centers, residents of long-term care facilities, and patients with indwelling catheters and intravascular devices.[12] The Ilizarov method has been used in Russia for osteomyelitis since 1951.[13] With this method, chronic refractory osteomyelitis can frequently be cured because the mass regeneration of new bone within the focus of infection serves as a highly vascularized bone graft.[14]

Hyperbaric Oxygenation. Chronic refractory osteomyelitis that has been resistant to other forms of treatment may be treated with hyperbaric oxygenation. Hyperbaric oxygenation, which is the intermittent, short-term administration of 100% oxygen at a pressure above normal atmospheric pressure, increases tissue oxygenation and vascularity and reduces edema by releasing pressure on the capillary bed. The improvement in local vascularity enhances bone and soft tissue healing and produces a bactericidal effect by facilitating the host's leukocyte defense response and augmenting the action of antibiotic therapy. The increased oxygen also creates a favorable environment for the removal of bony debris and remnants of the infectious process by osteoclasts. Hyperbaric oxygenation is known to increase the rate of granulation tissue formation but has not been proved effective in all forms of osteomyelitis. It is thought to be best used for anaerobic infections. Not all hospitals and medical centers have facilities for hyperbaric oxygenation treatment.

TUBERCULOSIS

Tuberculosis can spread from one part of the body, such as the lungs or occasionally the lymph nodes, to the bones and joints. It is caused by *Mycobacterium tuberculosis*. The disease is localized and progressively destructive. In about 50% of cases it affects the vertebrae, but it is also frequently seen in the hip and knee. The disease is characterized by bone destruction and abscess formation. Local symptoms include pain, immobility, and muscle atrophy; joint swelling, mild fever, and leukocytosis may also be present. Diagnosis is confirmed by a positive culture. The most important part of the treatment is antituberculosis drug therapy. Because of improved methods to prevent and treat tuberculosis, its incidence had diminished in recent decades. However, the incidence is on the rise again: in 1986, there was an increase of 2.5%, the first substantial rise since 1952.[15] Unfortunately, however, the diagnosis of tuberculosis in the bones and joints may still be missed.

In summary, bone infections occur because of either the direct or indirect invasion of the skeletal circulation by microorganisms, most commonly the bacterium Staphylococcus aureus. *Osteomyelitis, or infection of the bone and marrow, can be an acute or chronic disease. Acute osteomyelitis is seen most often as a result of the direct contamination of bone by a foreign object. Chronic osteomyelitis is a long-term process that can recur spontaneously at any time throughout a person's life. The incidence of all types of bone infection has been dramatically reduced since the advent of antibiotic therapy.*

■ REFERENCES

1. Centers for Disease Control. (1987). Bicycle-related injuries: Data from the National Electronic Injury Surveillance System. *MMWR. Morbidity and Mortality Weekly Report, 36,* 269.
2. Wright, P.H., & Brashear, H.R. (1980). The local response to trauma. In F.C. Wilson (Ed.). *The musculoskeletal system: Basic processes and disorders* (2nd ed., p. 264). Philadelphia: J.B. Lippincott.
3. Martini, Z., & Castaman, E. (1987). Tissue regeneration in the reconstruction of lost bone and soft tissue in the limbs: A preliminary report. *British Journal of Plastic Surgery, 40,* 142.
4. Paley, D., Catagni, M., Argnani, F., et al. (1992). Treatment of congenital pseudoarthrosis of the tibia using Ilizarov technique. *Clinical Orthopaedics and Related Research, 280,* 81.
5. Rorabeck, C.H. (1984). The treatment of compartment syndromes of the leg. *Journal of Bone and Joint Surgery, 66(B),* 93.
6. Oh, W.H., & Mital, M.A. (1976). Fat embolism: Current concepts of pathogenesis, diagnosis, and treatment. *Orthopedic Clinics of North America, 9,* 767.
7. Maylan, J.A., & Evenson, M.A. (1979). Diagnosis and treatment of fat embolism. *Annual Review of Medicine, 28,* 885.
8. Oldman, G.L., & Weise, W. (1979). Fat embolism. *Arizona Medicine, 36,* 885.
9. Lindeque, B.G.P., Schoeman, H.S., Dommisse, G.F., et al. (1987). Fat embolism and the fat embolism syndrome. *Journal of Bone and Joint Surgery, 1,* 128.
10. Robbins, S.L., & Cotran, R.S. (1984). *Pathologic basis of disease.* Philadelphia: W.B. Saunders.
11. Jones, N.S., Anderson, D.J., & Stiles, P.J. (1987). Osteomyelitis in a general hospital. *Journal of Bone and Joint Surgery 69(B),* 779.
12. Bitar, C.M., Mayahll, C.G., Lamb, V.A., et al. (1987). Outbreak due to methicillin-and-rifampin resistant *Staphylococcus aureus.* Epidemiology and eradication of the resistant strain from the hospital. *Infection Control, 8(1),* 15.
13. Ilizarov, G.A., & Ledyaev, V.I. (1992). The replacement of long tubular bone defects by lengthening distraction osteotomy of one of the fragments. *Clinical Orthopaedics and Related Research, 280,* 7.
14. Green, S.A. (1991). Osteomyelitis: The Ilizarov perspective. *Orthopedic Clinics of North America, 22(3),* 515.
15. Tuberculosis, final data—United States, 1986. (1988). *Morbidity and Mortality Weekly Report, 36,* 817.

■ BIBLIOGRAPHY

Anderson, P.A., Rivara, F.P., Maier, R.V., et al. (1991). The epidemiology of seatbelt-associated injuries. *Journal of Trauma, 31(1),* 60.

Aronson, D.D., Singer, R.M., & Higgins, R.F. (1987). Skeletal traction for fractures of the femoral shaft in children. *Journal of Bone and Joint Surgery, 69(A),* 1435.

Barden, R.M., & Sinkora, G.L. (1991). Bone stimulators for fusions and fractures. *Nursing Clinics of North America, 26(3),* 89.

Calhoun, J.H., Cobos, J.A., & Mader, J.T. (1991). Does hyperbaric oxygen have a place in treatment of osteomyelitis. *Orthopedic Clinics of North America, 22,* 467.

Cattaneo, R., Catagni, M., & Johnson, E.E. (1992). The treatment of infected nonunions and segmental defects of the tibia by means of Ilizarov. *Clinical Orthopedics, 280,* 143.

Dirschl, D.R., & Wilson, F.C. (1991). Topical antibiotic irrigation in prophylaxis of operative wound infections in orthopedic surgery. *Orthopedic Clinics of North America, 22,* 419.

Folcik, M.A. (1991). Meniscal injuries. *Nursing Clinics of North America, 26*(1), 181.

Gamron, R.B. (1988). Taking the pressure off compartment syndrome. *American Journal of Nursing, 88*, 1076.

Merritt, K. (1988). Factors increasing the risk of infection in patients with open fracture. *Journal of Trauma, 28*, 823.

Newman, K.D., Bowman, L.M., Eichelberger, M.R., et al. (1990). The lap belt complex: Intestinal and lumbar- spine injury in children. *Journal of Trauma, 30*(9), 1133.

Sly, D.A. (1991). Orthopedic complication: Compartment syndrome, fat embolization syndrome, and venous thromboembolism. *Nursing Clinics of North America, 26*(1), 113.

Whitelaw, G.P., Wetzler, M.J., Levy, A.S., et al. (1991). A pneumatic leg brace for the treatment of tibial stress fracture. *Clinical Orthopaedics and Related Research, 270*, 301.

CHAPTER 57

ALTERATIONS IN SKELETAL FUNCTION: CONGENITAL DISORDERS, METABOLIC BONE DISEASE, AND NEOPLASMS

KATHLEEN E. GUNTA

■ OBJECTIVES

After you have studied this chapter, you should be able to meet the following objectives:

■ Describe the function of the epiphysis in skeletal growth.

■ Explain how an infant's limbs differ from those of an adult.

■ Define *femoral anteversion*.

■ Differentiate between toeing-in and internal tibial torsion.

■ Define *genu varum* and *genu valgum*.

■ Identify two childhood diseases that are classified as osteochondroses.

■ Describe the pathology of Legg–Calvé–Perthes disease.

■ List the symptoms of Osgood–Schlatter disease.

■ Explain why it is important to treat a slipped capital femoral epiphyseal as soon as it is diagnosed.

■ List the cardinal signs of scoliosis that serve as a basis for school screening programs.

■ Describe the physical appearance of an infant with congenital dislocation of the hip.

■ Explain the treatment for a newborn with clubfoot.

■ List the problems that occur because of defective tissue synthesis in osteogenesis imperfecta.

■ Name the three factors responsible for maintaining the equilibrium of bone tissue.

■ Compare structural remodeling of bone with internal remodeling.

■ Cite the functions of parathyroid hormone, vitamin D, and calcitonin in bone metabolism.

■ Trace the activation of vitamin D in the body.

■ List three factors that contribute to the development of osteoporosis.

■ Describe the action of fluoride in the treatment of osteoporosis.

■ Describe the primary features of osteoporotic bone.

Carol Mattson Porth: PATHOPHYSIOLOGY: CONCEPTS OF
ALTERED HEALTH STATES, 4th ed. © 1994, 1990, 1986, 1982
J.B. Lippincott Company

- Cite the sex, race, and age groups of people most frequently affected by osteoporosis.
- Contrast osteomalacia, rickets, and osteoporosis.
- Relate vitamin D deficiency to the inadequate mineralization of bone that occurs in osteomalacia and rickets.
- List the clinical manifestations of Paget's disease.
- Differentiate between the properties of benign and malignant bone tumors.

- Name the three major symptoms of bone cancer.
- Contrast osteogenic sarcoma and chondrosarcoma.
- List the primary sites of tumors that frequently metastasize to the bone.
- State the three primary goals for treatment of metastatic bone disease.

During childhood, skeletal structures grow in both length and diameter and sustain a large increase in bone mass. The term *modeling* refers to the formation of the macroscopic skeleton, which ceases at maturity (age 18 to 20 years). Bone remodeling functions to replace existing bone and occurs in both children and adults. It involves both resorption and formation of bone. With aging, bone resorption and formation are no longer perfectly coupled, and there is loss of bone. Alterations in musculoskeletal structure and function may develop as a result of normal growth and developmental processes or as a result of impairment of skeletal development due to hereditary or congenital influences. Other skeletal disorders can occur later in life as a result of metabolic disorders or neoplastic growth.

■ ALTERATIONS IN SKELETAL GROWTH AND DEVELOPMENT

BONE GROWTH AND REMODELING

EMBRYONIC DEVELOPMENT

The skeletal system develops from the mesoderm, the thin middle layer of embryonic tissue, by two different ossification processes: endochondral or intramembranous ossification. Endochondral ossification involves ossification of a cartilaginous bone model. Intramembranous ossification occurs where there is no preexisting cartilage model. In the skull, it involves ossification of the loose layer of mesenchymal tissue that fills the space between the brain and the skin.

Development of the vertebrae of the axial skeleton begins at about the fourth week in the embryo; during the ninth week, ossification begins with the appearance of ossification centers in the lower thoracic and upper lumbar vertebrae. The limb buds of the appendicular skeleton make their appearance late

in the fourth week. The hand pads are present on day 33, and the finger rays are evident on day 41 of embryonic development.[1]

BONE GROWTH IN CHILDHOOD

During the first two decades of life, the skeleton undergoes general overall growth. The long bones of the skeleton, which grow at a relatively rapid rate, are provided with a specialized structure called the epiphyseal growth plate. As long bones grow in length, the deeper layers of cartilage cells in the growth plate multiply and enlarge, pushing the articular cartilage further away from the metaphysis and diaphysis of the bone. As this happens, the mature and enlarged cartilage cells at the metaphyseal end of the plate become metabolically inactive and are replaced by bone cells (Fig. 57-1). This process allows bone growth to proceed without changing the shape of the bone or causing disruption of the articular cartilage. The cells in the growth plate stop dividing at puberty, at which time the epiphysis and metaphysis fuse.

A number of factors can influence the growth of cells in the epiphyseal growth plate. Epiphyseal separation can occur in children as the result of accidents. The separation usually occurs in the zone of the mature enlarged cartilage cells, which is the weakest part of the growth plate. The blood vessels that nourish the epiphysis, which pass through the growth plate, are ruptured when the growth plate separates. This can cause cessation of growth and a shortened extremity.

The growth plate is also sensitive to nutritional and metabolic changes. Scurvy (vitamin C deficiency) impairs the formation of the organic matrix of bone, causing slowing of growth at the epiphyseal plate and cessation of diaphyseal growth. In rickets (vitamin D deficiency) calcification of the newly developed bone on the metaphyseal side of the growth plate is impaired. Thyroid and growth hormones are both required for normal growth. Alterations in these

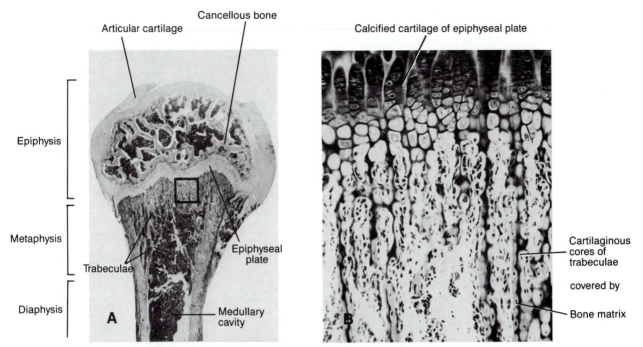

FIG. 57-1. (**A**) Low-power photomicrograph of one end of a growing long bone (rat). Osteogenesis has spread from the epiphyseal center of ossification so that only the articular cartilage above and the epiphyseal disk below remain cartilaginous. On the diaphyseal side of the epiphyseal plate (disk), metaphyseal trabeculae extend down into the diaphysis. (**B**) Medium-power photomicrograph of the area indicated in **A**, showing trabeculae on the diaphyseal side of the epiphyseal plate (disk). These have cores of calcified cartilage on which bone has been deposited. The cartilaginous cores of the trabeculae were formerly partitions between columns of chondrocytes in the epiphyseal plate (disk). (Cormack, D. H. [1987]. *Ham's histology* [9th ed., p. 299]. Philadelphia: J.B. Lippincott)

and other hormones can affect growth (see Chapter 45).

Growth in the diameter of bones occurs by oppositional growth of new bone on the surface of existing bone along with an accompanying resorption of bone on the endosteal surface; in this manner the shape of the bone is maintained. As a bone grows in diameter, concentric rings are added to the bone surface, much as rings are added to a tree trunk: these rings form the lamellar structure of mature bone. Osteocytes, which develop from osteoblasts, become buried in the rings. Haversian channels form as periosteal vessels running along the long axis become surrounded by bone.

ALTERATIONS DURING NORMAL GROWTH PERIODS

Infants and children undergo changes in muscle tone and joint motion during growth and development. These changes usually cause few problems and are corrected during normal growth processes. The normal folded position of the fetus in utero causes physiologic flexion contractures of the hips and a froglike appearance of the lower extremities. The hips are externally rotated and the patellae point outward, whereas the feet appear to point forward because of the internal pulling force of the tibiae. During the first year of life the lower extremities begin to straighten out in preparation for walking. Internal and external rotation become equal, and the hips extend. Flexion contractures of the shoulders, elbows, and knees are also commonly seen in newborns, but they should disappear by 3 months of age.[2]

All infants and toddlers have lax ligaments that become tighter with age and assumption of the weight-bearing posture. The hypermobility that accompanies joint laxity along with torsional, or twisting, forces exerted on the limbs during growth are responsible for a number of variants seen in young children. Torsional forces caused by intrauterine positions or sleeping and sitting patterns twist the growing bones and can produce the deformities seen with growth and development.

FEMORAL ANTEVERSION

Femoral anteversion (internal femoral torsion) is a normal variant commonly seen during the first 6 years of life, especially in 3- and 4-year-old girls. Hip rotation in both flexion and extension can be measured with computed tomography (CT). Internal rotation of the hips exceeds external rotation by 30 degrees or more. It is related to the increased ligamentous laxity of the anterior capsule of the hip: this joint does not provide the stable pressure needed to correct the approximately 50 degrees of anteversion present at birth. Children are most comfortable sitting in the "M" position, with the hips between the heels. When the child stands, the knees turn in whereas the feet appear to point straight ahead; when the child walks, both knees and toes point in. Children with this problem are encouraged to sit in the so-called Indian chief or "W" position. If left untreated, the tibiae compensate by becoming externally rotated so that by 8 to 12 years of age the knees may turn in but the feet no longer do. A derotational osteotomy may be done in severe cases (*e.g.*, with excessive anteversion) if the hip is in excess of 50 degrees or if there is a functional disability.

TOEING-IN

Toeing-in (metatarsus abductus) is the most common congenital foot deformity. It occurs in approximately 1 per 1000 births, affecting boys and girls equally. It can be caused by torsion in the feet, lower legs, or entire leg. Toeing-in due to adduction of the forefoot (congenital metatarsus adductus) is usually the result of the fetal position maintained in utero. It may occur in one foot or both. A supple deformity can be passively manipulated into a straight position and requires no treatment. Treatment consisting of serial long leg casting or an orthosis that pushes the metatarsals (not the hindfoot) into abduction is usually required in a fixed deformity (*i.e.*, one in which the forefoot cannot be passively manipulated into a straight position).

TOEING-OUT

Toeing-out is a common problem in children caused by external femoral torsion. This occurs when the femur can be externally rotated to about 90 degrees but internally rotated only to a neutral position or slightly beyond. When a child habitually sleeps in the prone position, the femoral torsion persists and an external tibial torsion may also develop. If external tibial torsion is present, the feet point lateral to the midline of the medial plane. External tibial torsion rarely causes toeing-out: it only intensifies the condition. Toeing-out usually corrects itself as the child becomes proficient in walking. Occasionally a night splint is used. Both toeing-in and toeing-out are less noticeable when the child is running or barefoot. Overcorrection of a flexible foot can cause flatfoot deformity. A rigid deformity that is untreated can cause pain and improper footwear fitting.

INTERNAL TIBIAL TORSION

Internal tibial torsion (bowing of the tibia) is a rotation of the tibia that makes the feet appear to turn inward. It is present at birth and fails to correct itself if children either sleep on their knees with the feet turned in or sit on in-turned feet. In 80% of cases, it resolves by the time the child is 18 months of age.[3] In the other 20% of cases, the Denis Browne splint (a bar to which shoes are attached) may be used to put the feet into mild external rotation while the child is sleeping. This treatment stimulates the proximal growth plate of the tibia to grow in a spiral fashion and correct the defect. Surgery may be necessary if tibial torsion persists beyond age 3, but only if the condition is severe and significantly interferes with walking and running.

GENU VARUM AND GENU VALGUM

Genu varum (bowlegs) is an outward bowing of the knees greater than 1 inch when the medial malleoli of the ankles are touching. Most infants and toddlers have some bowing of their legs up to age 2. If there is a large separation between the knees (*i.e.*, greater than 15 degrees) after age 2, the child may require bracing. The child should also be evaluated for diseases such as rickets or tibia vara (Blount's disease).

Genu valgum (knock-knees) is a deformity in which there is decreased space between the knees. The medial malleoli in the ankles cannot be brought in contact with each other when the knees are touching. It is seen most frequently in children between the ages of 2 and 6 years and should resolve by ages 7 to 10 years. The condition is usually the result of lax medial collateral ligaments of the knee and may be exacerbated by sitting in the "M" position. Genu valgum can be ignored up to age 7, unless it is more than 15 degrees, unilateral, or associated with short stature. It usually resolves spontaneously and rarely requires treatment. If either genu varum or genu valgum persists and is uncorrected, osteoarthritis may develop in adulthood as a result of abnormal intraarticular stress. Genu varum can cause gait awkwardness and increased risk of sprains and fractures. In addition, uncorrected genu valgum may cause subluxation and recurrent dislocation of the patella with a predisposition to chondromalacia and joint pain and fatigue.

FLATFOOT

Flatfoot is a deformity characterized by the absence of the longitudinal arch of the foot. Infants normally have a wider and fatter foot than adults. The fat pads that are normally accentuated by pliable muscles create an illusion of fullness often mistaken for flatfeet. Until the longitudinal arch develops at age 2 to 3 years, all children have flatfeet. The true criterion for flatfoot (pes planus) is that the head of the talus points medially and downward, so that the heel is everted and the forefoot must be inverted (toed in) for the metatarsal heads to be planted equally on the ground. Weight bearing may cause pain in the longitudinal arch and up the leg.

There are two types of flatfeet—supple and rigid. Supple flatfeet are always bilateral, occur more often in African-American people, and tend to be familial.[3] In supple flatfeet, the arch disappears only with weight bearing. The rigid flatfoot is fixed with no apparent arch in any position. It is seen in conjunction with neuromuscular diseases and juvenile rheumatoid arthritis.

In the adult, treatment of flatfeet is conservative and aimed at relieving fatigue, pain, and tenderness. Supportive well-fitting shoes with arch supports may be helpful and prevent ligaments from becoming overstretched. Women may complain of pain in the forefoot when wearing poorly fitting high heels. Surgery may be done in cases of severe and persistent symptoms.

JUVENILE OSTEOCHONDROSES

The term *juvenile osteochondroses* is used to describe a group of children's diseases in which one or more growth ossification centers undergo a period of degeneration, necrosis, or inactivity that is followed by regeneration and usually deformity. The osteochondroses are separated into two groups according to their etiologies. The first group consists of the true osteonecrotic osteochondroses, so called because the diseases are caused by localized osteonecrosis of an apophyseal or epiphyseal center (Legg–Calvé–Perthes disease, Freiberg's infarction, Panner's disease, and Kienböck's disease). The second group of juvenile osteochondroses are caused by abnormalities of endochondral ossification, due either to a genetically determined normal variation or to trauma (Osgood–Schlatter disease, Blount's disease, Sever's disease, and Scheuermann's disease). The discussion in this section focuses on Legg–Calvé–Perthes disease from the first group and Osgood–Schlatter disease from the second group.

LEGG–CALVÉ–PERTHES DISEASE

Legg–Calvé–Perthes disease (coxa plana) is an osteonecrotic disease of the proximal femoral (capital) epiphysis, which is the growth center for the head of the femur. It occurs in 1 out of 1200 children, affecting primarily those between ages 3 and 12 years with a peak age of 6 years.[4] It occurs primarily in boys and is much more common in whites than African Americans. Although no definite genetic pattern has been established, it occasionally affects more than one family member. The incidence for siblings developing the disease is 1 in 25.[5]

The cause of Legg–Calvé–Perthes disease is unknown. The disorder is usually insidious in onset and occurs in otherwise healthy children. It may, however, be associated with acute trauma. The children usually affected have a shorter stature. Undernutrition has been suggested as a causative factor. When girls are affected, they usually have a poorer prognosis than boys because they are skeletally more mature. This means that they would have a shorter period for growth and remodeling than boys of the same age. Although both legs can be affected, in 85% of the cases only one leg is involved.[5]

The primary pathologic feature of Legg–Calvé–Perthes disease is an avascular necrosis of the bone and marrow involving the epiphyseal growth center in the femoral head. The disorder may be confined to part of the epiphysis, or it may involve the entire epiphysis. In severe cases, there is a disturbance in the growth pattern that leads to a broad, short femoral neck. The necrosis is followed by slow absorption of the dead bone over 2 to 3 years. Although the necrotic trabeculae are eventually replaced by healthy new bone, the epiphysis rarely regains its normal shape. The process occurs in four predictable stages, each with its distinctive radiologic characteristics:

1. The incipient or synovitis stage is characterized by synovial inflammation and increased joint fluid. This stage usually lasts 1 to 3 weeks.

2. During the aseptic or avascular stage, the ossification center becomes necrotic. This stage may last from several months to a year. Damage to the femoral head is determined by the degree of necrosis that occurs during this stage.

3. The regenerative or revascularization stage involves the resorption of the necrotic bone. This stage lasts 1 to 3 years, during which the necrotic bone is gradually replaced by new immature bone cells and the contour of the bone is remodeled.

4. The healed or residual stage is characterized by the formation and replacement of immature bone

cells by normal bone cells. Remodeling of the femoral head continues throughout the growing years but is ultimately determined by the amount of collapse that has occurred during the avascular stage.

Legg–Calvé–Perthes disease has an insidious onset with a prolonged course. The main symptoms are pain in the groin, thigh, or knee and difficulty in walking. The child may have a painless limp with limited abduction and internal rotation, and a flexion contracture of the affected hip. The age of onset is important because young children have a greater capability for remodeling of the femoral head and acetabulum, and thus less flattening of the femoral head occurs. Early diagnosis is important and is based on correlating physical symptoms with x-ray findings that are related to the stage of the disease.

The goal of treatment is to reduce deformity and preserve the integrity of the femoral head. Both conservative and surgical interventions are used in the treatment of Legg–Calvé–Perthes disease. Children under 4 years of age with little or no involvement of the femoral head may require only periodic observation. In all other children, some intervention is needed to relieve the force of weight bearing, the muscular tension, and subluxation of the femoral head. It is important to maintain the femur in a well-seated position in the concave acetabulum to prevent deformity. This is done by keeping the hip in abduction and mild internal rotation.

The initial treatment usually involves bedrest with Russell or Buck's traction (see Chapter 55) or with a device to keep the legs separated in abduction with mild internal rotation (*e.g.*, hip spica cast or abduction brace). Once the inflammatory stage has subsided (usually several weeks), the child is allowed up but is not permitted to bear weight on the femoral head. The child walks with crutches and may be required to wear a brace, splint, or walking cast.

Surgery may be done to contain the femoral head within the acetabulum. This treatment is usually reserved for children older than 6 years who at the time of diagnosis have more serious involvement of the femoral head. Several sources indicate that the best surgical results are obtained when surgery is done early, before the epiphysis becomes necrotic.[6, 7]

OSGOOD–SCHLATTER DISEASE

Osgood–Schlatter disease is a partial separation of the tibial tuberosity caused by sudden or continued strain on the patellar tendon during growth. It occurs most frequently in boys between the ages of 10 and 16 years.[8] The disorder is characterized by pain in the front of the knee associated with inflammation and thickening of the patellar tendon. An ossification center of growing cartilage forms within the tibial tubercle, making it susceptible to the pull of the quadriceps muscle. A partial avulsion or tearing of the tubercle is the result of extraordinary stress placed on the knee during a critical growth period. Follow-up studies have indicated that the disorder may really be a mechanical tendonitis with partial avulsion of the tibial tubercle.[8]

With Osgood–Schlatter disease, pain is usually associated with specific activities such as kneeling, running, bicycle riding, or stair climbing. The symptoms are self-limiting; although they may recur during adolescence, they usually resolve after closure of the tibial growth plate. In some cases, limitations on activity, braces, and even a plaster cast to immobilize the knee may be necessary to relieve the pain. The objective of treatment is to release tension on the quadriceps to permit revascularization and reossification of the tibial tubercle. Surgery may be indicated to excise painful bony fragments from the patellar tendon. Occasionally minor symptoms or an increased prominence of the tibial tubercle may continue into adulthood.

SLIPPED CAPITAL FEMORAL EPIPHYSIS

Normally, the proximal femoral epiphysis unites with the neck of the femur between ages 16 and 19 years. Before this time (10 to 17 years in girls and 13 to 16 years in boys), the femoral head may slip from its normal position directly at the head of the femur and become displaced medially and posteriorly.[8] This produces an adduction, lateral rotation, and extension deformity. About 1 in 50,000 children suffer a slipped capital femoral epiphysis.[5] It is the most common disorder of the hip in adolescents.

The etiology of slipped capital femoral epiphysis is obscure, but it may be related to the child's susceptibility to stress on the femoral neck as a result of genetics or abnormal structure. Boys are affected twice as often as girls, and in 50% of cases the condition is bilateral.[8] Affected children are often overweight with poorly developed secondary sex characteristics or, in some instances, are extremely tall and thin. In many cases there is a history of rapid skeletal growth preceding displacement of the epiphysis. It may also be affected by an inflammatory autoimmune process, excess levels of growth hormone, or nutritional deficiencies.

There are often complaints of referred knee pain in children with the condition, accompanied by reports of difficulty walking, fatigue, and stiffness. The diagnosis is confirmed by x-ray studies in which the degree of slipping can be determined on a lateral view. Early treatment is imperative to prevent life-long crippling. Avoidance of weight bearing on the femur and bedrest are essential parts of the treatment. Traction or gentle manipulation under anesthesia is used to reduce the slip. Surgical insertion of pins to keep the femoral neck and head of the femur aligned is a common method of treatment for children with moderate or severe slips. Crutches are used for several months after surgical correction to prevent full weight bearing until the growth plate is sealed by the bony union. Long-term prognosis depends on the amount of displacement that occurs. Complications include avascular necrosis, leg shortening, malunion, and problems with the internal fixation.

SCOLIOSIS

Scoliosis is a lateral deviation of the spinal column that may or may not include rotation or deformity of the vertebrae. It has been estimated that over 1 million Americans have a significant degree of scoliosis.[9] It is most commonly seen during adolescence and is eight times more frequent in girls than boys. An increase in joint laxity, which causes excessive joint motion and is more common in girls, has been associated with development of idiopathic scoliosis.[10]

Scoliosis can develop as the result of another disease condition or it can occur without known cause. Idiopathic scoliosis, or scoliosis of unknown cause, accounts for 75% to 80% of the total number of cases of the disorder and affects between 2% and 8% of the population in the United States.[11] The other 20% to 25% of cases are caused by over 50 different etiologies, including poliomyelitis, congenital hemivertebrae, neurofibromatosis, and cerebral palsy. Family history is positive for scoliosis in about 30% of the cases.[12]

Scoliosis is classified as either postural or structural. With postural scoliosis there is a small curve that corrects with bending. It can be corrected with passive and active exercises. Structural scoliosis does not correct with bending. It is a fixed deformity classified into three categories based on etiology: (1) idiopathic, (2) congenital, and (3) neuromuscular.

Idiopathic scoliosis is a structural spinal curvature for which no etiology has been established. It occurs primarily in infants of the United Kingdom and Europe during the first 3 years of life. Its usual effect on males is a curve in the thoracic area that is convex and to the left. Juvenile idiopathic scoliosis occurs in children between 5 and 6 years of age and is rare. Adolescent idiopathic scoliosis that begins at about 10 years

of age is the most common type of scoliosis; it is more common and progressive in girls.[13] Although the curve may be present in any area of the spine, the most common curve is a right thoracic curve, which produces a rib prominence on the convex side and hypokyphosis from rotation of the vertebral column around its long axis as the spine begins to curve.

Congenital scoliosis is caused by disturbances in vertebral development during the third to fifth week of embryologic development.[14] There are structural anomalies in the vertebrae that can cause a severe curvature. The child may have other anomalies and neurologic complications if the spine is involved.

Neuromuscular scoliosis develops from neuropathic or myopathic diseases. Neuropathic scoliosis is seen with cerebral palsy and poliomyelitis. There is often a long C-shaped curve from the cervical to the sacral region. In cerebral palsy there may be severe deformity that makes treatment difficult. Myopathic neuromuscular scoliosis develops with muscular dystrophy and is usually not severe.

Scoliosis is usually first noted because of the deformity it causes. A high shoulder, prominent hip, or projecting scapula may be noticed by a parent or in a school screening program. In girls, difficulty in hemming or fitting a dress may call attention to the deformity. Pain is present in severe cases, usually in the lumbar region. The pain may be caused by pressure on the ribs or the crest of the ilium. There may be shortness of breath as a result of diminished chest expansion and gastrointestinal disturbances from crowding of the abdominal organs. Adults with less severe deformity may experience mild backache. If scoliosis is left untreated, the curve may progress to a point where cardiopulmonary function is compromised and there is a risk of neurologic complications. New surgical techniques are available to successfully treat adults with undetected or progressive scoliosis.[15, 16]

Early diagnosis of scoliosis is important in prevention of severe spinal deformity. The cardinal signs of scoliosis are: (1) uneven shoulders or iliac crest, (2) prominent scapula on the convex side of the curve, (3) malalignment of spinous processes, (4) asymmetry of the flanks, (5) asymmetry of the thoracic cage, and (6) rib hump or paraspinal muscle prominence when bending forward (Fig. 57-2). School screening programs are an excellent method for early detection of scoliosis in adolescents. Screening should be done yearly in the fifth through tenth grades. School nurses and teachers can be trained to perform the examination. Both boys and girls should be screened. Students are examined from the front, back, and sides while standing and bending with arms both at the sides and out in front with palms

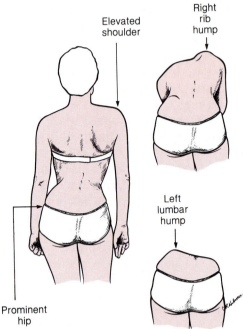

Elevated shoulder

Right rib hump

Left lumbar hump

Prominent hip

FIG. 57-2. Scoliosis. Abnormalities to be determined at initial screening examination. (Gore, D. R., Passehl, R., Sepic, S., & Dalton, A. [1981]. Scoliosis screening: Results of a community project. *Pediatrics, 67*[2]. Copyright 1981 by the American Academy of Pediatrics)

touching. A scoliometer should be used at the apex of curvature to quantify a prominence (a scoliometer reading of greater than 10 degrees requires physician referral).[13]

Diagnosis is made by physical examination and confirmed by radiography. The curve is measured by determining the amount of lateral deviation present on x-ray films and is labeled right or left for the convex portion of the curve. Several different methods are used.

The treatment of scoliosis depends on the sever-ity of the deformity. A conservative approach includes periodic assessment and either an exercise program or some form of external bracing. An exercise program is designed to promote the maximum degree of correction possible based on the degree of flexibility present at the time of diagnosis. The pelvic tilt exercise is an example of an exercise done both with and without a brace.

A brace is used to control the progression of the curvature during growth and also provides some correction. The most commonly used brace is the Milwaukee brace, which was developed by Blount and Schmitt in 1945 (Fig. 57-3). This was the first brace to provide some degree of active correction. It is the treatment of choice for curvatures of 40 degrees or less in adolescents with idiopathic scoliosis. The decision to use the brace has to be an individual one, with consideration being given to the likelihood of progression to 40 degrees or more and the cosmetic impact on the person. Lateral pads apply pressure to the apex of the curve (*i.e.*, the point most deviated from the vertical axis) on the convex side. The brace is usually prescribed for 23 hours per day, with removal permitted only for hygienic purposes. In reality, however, few adolescents comply with this program. Compliance is higher in younger children, with most high-school-age children wearing their braces only 9 to 12 hours per day. Because of the high noncompliance in the full-time programs, part-time programs have been initiated with 16 hours or less of prescribed brace-wear for curvatures of less than 35 degrees.[17] In this program, the adolescent does not have to wear the brace to school.

Exercises are done during the time out of the brace and when the brace is on. Good skin care is essential to prevent breakdown under the brace. It is important for health care professionals to work with the adolescent to ensure compliance with the treat-

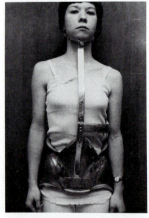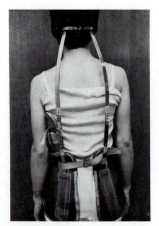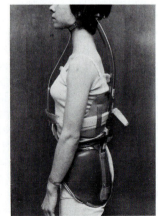

FIG. 57-3. The Milwaukee brace as seen from front, back, and side. (Farrell, J. [1986]. *Illustrated guide to orthopedic nursing* [3rd ed., p. 172]. Philadelphia: J.B. Lippincott)

ment program. This is particularly important because the brace may present an additional stress to an already threatened body image. Lateral electrical surface stimulation may be used for progressive curves between 20 and 35 degrees in a growing child to prevent progression of the curvature. There are conflicting data regarding its efficacy, and it is ineffective in the mature person.[13]

Surgical intervention with instrumentation and spinal fusion is done in severe cases—when the curvature has progressed to 40 degrees or beyond at the time of diagnosis or when curves of a lesser degree are compounded with imbalance or rotation of the vertebrae. Several methods of instrumentation are used, including: Harrington rod instrumentation and posterior spinal fusion, Dwyer (or Zielke) instrumentation and anterior spinal fusion, segmental (Luque) spinal instrumentation and posterior spinal fusion, or Cotrel–Dubousset bilateral segmental fixation.

With the Harrington rod instrumentation and posterior spinal fusion, a distraction rod is attached to the posterior aspect of the spinal column on the concave side of the curvature. A second, more flexible rod, may be used to compress the convex side. The Drummond or Wisconsin technique includes wires placed through the base of the spinous process and around the Harrington rod to provide multiple points of fixation. With the anterior instrumentation method, a wire cable (Dwyer) or steel rod (Zielke) is threaded through screw and staple units inserted directly into the vertebral body as a means of exerting tension on the convex side of the curve. The spine is fused anteriorly. This is usually followed several weeks later by a posterior fusion done for added correction and stability. A Dwyer or Zielke instrumentation procedure is difficult because the anterior fusion requires a transthoracic and retroperitoneal approach (through the rib cage and pulmonary cavity). With the segmental instrumentation method, a posterior fusion is used along with the Luque instrumentation. Wire loops are attached to the laminae as a means of securing rods to both sides of the spine. This provides a rigid internal fixation at the level of each vertebra. Cotrel–Dubousset instrumentation consists of two gnarled rods linked together with various hooks and transverse fixation rods that provide a three-dimensional correction of the curve and rotational stability. The system is used to treat a variety of spinal problems, including scoliosis, kyphosis, fractures, and tumors. Despite great advances in spinal surgery, no one method seems to be the best for all cases. The Cotrel–Dubousset instrumentation procedure has gained popularity because it is a rigid system of immobilization that provides three-dimensional correction and preserves or improves sagittal

contours (thoracic kyphosis and lumbar lordosis). It does not require postoperative immobilization and allows for resumption of their normal activities within a short time.

Patients who have had a Harrington rod inserted or a Dwyer procedure performed are immobilized in a body cast or Milwaukee brace. Traction may be used initially, applied directly to the Milwaukee brace. A CircOlectric bed, Stryker frame, or Foster frame may be used to assist with turning. Patients with a Harrington rod or Dwyer instrumentation require a longer period of postoperative bedrest than those who had the segmental (Luque) spinal instrumentation procedure. The Cotrel–Dubousset instrumentation system necessitates a shorter period of immobilization after surgery. A brace is not required except for adults or adolescents with neuromuscular disease.

HEREDITARY AND CONGENITAL DEFORMITIES

Congenital deformities are abnormalities that are present at birth. They can be caused by hereditary influences or by disturbances in embryonic development. They range in severity from mild limb deformities, which are relatively common, to major limb malformations, which are relatively rare. There may be a simple webbing of the fingers or toes (syndactyly) or the presence of an extra digit (polydactyly). Joint contractures and dislocations produce more severe deformity, as does the absence of entire bones, joints, or limbs. An epidemic of limb deformities occurred from 1957 to 1962 as a result of maternal ingestion of thalidomide. This drug was withdrawn from the market in 1961.

Congenital deformities are caused by many factors, some as yet unknown. These factors include genetic influences, external agents that injure the fetus (*e.g.*, radiation, alcohol, medications, and viruses), and in utero environmental factors. As discussed in Chapter 4, the fourth to the seventh week of gestation is the most vulnerable period for development of limb deformities.

CONGENITAL DISLOCATION OF THE HIP

Congenital dislocation of the hip is seen in 1.6 out of every 1000 live births. It occurs most frequently in first-born children and is six times more common in female than in male infants.[14] It is thought that the instability of the hip is a consequence of laxity of the ligaments, which is genetically determined, and displacement is the result of environmental factors such as fetal position or breech delivery.[14]

In a child with congenital dislocation of the hip, the head of the femur is located outside of the acetabulum. In less severe cases, the hip joint may be either unstable or subluxed, so that the joint surfaces are separated and there is a partial dislocation.

Normal development of the hip requires that a normal positional relationship should exist between the femoral head and the acetabulum. If this relationship is not maintained, there may be a delay in the maturation, size, and development of both the femoral head and the acetabulum. Early diagnosis of congenital hip dislocation is important because treatment is easiest and most effective if begun during the first 6 months of life. Repeated dislocation causes damage to both the femoral head and the acetabulum. Clinical examinations to detect dislocation of the hip should be done at birth and every several months during the first year of life. If the femoral head can be displaced by the examiner, it is considered dislocatable.

Several examination techniques are used to screen for congenital hip dislocation. In infants, signs of dislocation include asymmetry of the hip or gluteal folds, shortening of the thigh so that one knee (on the affected side) is higher than the other, and limited abduction of the affected hip (Fig. 57-4). The asymmetry of gluteal folds is not definitive but indicates the need for further evaluation. A specific examination involves an attempt to manually dislocate and reduce the abnormal hip while the infant is in the supine position with both knees flexed. With gentle downward pressure being applied to the knees, the knee and thigh are manually abducted as an upward and medial pressure is applied to the proximal thigh. In infants with the disorder, the initial downward pressure on the knee produces a dislocation of the hip, which is followed by a palpable or audible click (Ortolani's sign) as the hip is reduced and moves back into the acetabulum. In an older child, instability of the hip may produce a delay in standing or walking and eventually a characteristic waddling gait. When the thumbs are placed over the anterior iliac crest and the hands are placed over the lateral pelvis in examination, the levels of the thumbs are not even; in addition, the child is unable to elevate the opposite side of the pelvis (positive Trendelenburg's test). Diagnosis is confirmed by radiography.

The treatment of congenital hip dislocation is begun as soon as the diagnosis has been made. The best results are obtained if the treatment is begun before changes in the hip structure (*e.g.*, 2 to 3 months) prevent it from being reduced by gentle manipulation or abduction devices. Infants with dislocatable hips due to anatomic changes and toddlers who may lack development of the acetabular socket require

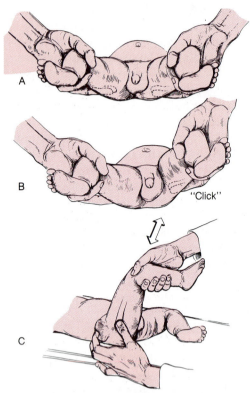

FIG. 57-4. Congenital dislocation of the hip. (**A**) In the newborn, both hips can be equally flexed, abducted, and externally rotated without producing a "click." (**B**) A diagnosis of a congenital dislocation of the hip may be confirmed by Ortolani's "click" test. The involved hip cannot be abducted as far as the opposite one, and there is a "click" as the hip reduces. (**C**) Telescoping of the femur to aid in the diagnosis of a congenitally dislocated hip. (*Hoppenfeld's physical examination of the spine and extremities.* [1976]. New York: Appleton-Century-Crofts)

more aggressive treatment such as open reduction and joint reconstruction. Treatment at any age includes reduction of the dislocation and immobilization of the legs in an abducted position. The most serious complication of any treatment is avascular necrosis of the femoral head as a result of the forced abduction. With children under 3 years of age, gentle traction is used when reduction cannot be easily obtained. This treatment is followed by several months of immobilization in a hip spica cast, plaster splints, or an abduction splint such as a Frejka pillow or Pavlik harness. The harness allows the child more mobility as the leg is slowly and gently brought into abduction. Failure to use the harness correctly can result in a need for surgery. Older children or adults with unreduced congenital dislocation of the hip may require hip surgery because of damage to the articulating surface of the joint. These people have considerable problems after surgery because of their soft tissue contractures.

CONGENITAL CLUBFOOT

Congenital clubfoot can affect one or both feet. Like congenital dislocation of hip, its occurrence follows a multifactorial inheritance pattern. The condition has an incidence of 1 per every 1000 live births and occurs twice as often in males as in females.[18] The chance that a sibling will have the defect is 3%, and the chance that the offspring of an affected person will have the disorder is 8% to 11%.

In forefoot adduction, which accounts for about 95% of cases, the foot is plantar flexed and inverted.[23] This is the so-called equinovarus type where the foot resembles a horse's hoof (Fig. 57-5). The other 5% of cases are of the calcaneovalgus type (reverse clubfoot) in which the foot is dorsiflexed and everted. The reverse clubfoot can occur as an isolated condition or in association with multiple congenital defects.

At birth, the feet of many infants assume one of these two positions, but they can be passively overcorrected or brought back into the opposite position. If the foot cannot be overcorrected, some type of correction may be necessary. Although the exact cause of clubfoot is unknown, three theories are generally accepted: (1) an anomalous development occurs during the first trimester of pregnancy, (2) the leg fails to rotate inward and move from the equinovarus position at about the third month, or (3) the soft tissues in the foot do not mature and lengthen. Clubfoot is seen in association with chromosomal abnormalities and may occur in association with other congenital syndromes that are transmitted by mendelian inheritance (see Chapter 4). However, it is most commonly idiopathic and found in a normal infant in whom no genetic or chromosomal abnormality or other extrinsic cause can be found.[19]

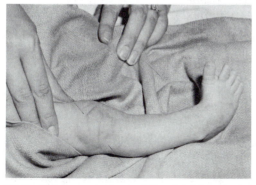

FIG. 57-5. Talipes equinovarus deformity. Note the internal tibial torsion. (Turek, S. L. [1984]. *Orthopaedics: Principles and their application* [4th ed.]. Philadelphia: J.B. Lippincott)

Clubfoot varies in severity from a mild deformity to one in which the foot is completely inverted. The treatment is begun as soon as the diagnosis is made. When treatment is initiated during the first few weeks of life, a nonoperative procedure is effective within a short period. Serial manipulations and casting are used to gently correct each component in the forefoot varus, the hindfoot varus, and the equinus. The treatment is continued until the foot is in a normal position with full correction evident clinically and on x-ray studies. Surgery may be required for severe deformities or when nonoperative treatment methods are unsuccessful. An external distractor such as the Ilizarov external fixator may be used to correct the deformity of a relapsed or neglected clubfoot.

OSTEOGENESIS IMPERFECTA

Osteogenesis imperfecta is a hereditary disease characterized by defective synthesis of connective tissue, including bone matrix. It is perhaps the most common hereditary bone disease, with an occurrence rate of approximately 1 in 20,000 births.[20] Although it is usually transmitted as an autosomal dominant trait, a distinct form of the disorder with multiple lethal defects is thought to be inherited as an autosomal recessive trait.[21]

The disorder is characterized by thin and poorly developed bones that are prone to multiple fractures. These children have short limbs and a soft, thin cranium with bifrontal prominences that give a triangular appearance to the face. Other problems associated with defective connective tissue synthesis include short stature, thin skin, blue or gray sclera, abnormal tooth development, hypotonic muscles, loose-jointedness, scoliosis, and a tendency for hernia formation. Hearing loss is common in adults with this disorder because of otosclerosis of the middle and inner ear.

The most serious defects occur when the disorder is inherited as a recessive trait. Severely affected fetuses have multiple intrauterine fractures, and bowing and shortening of the extremities. Many of these babies are stillborn or die during infancy. Less severe affliction occurs when the disorder is inherited as a dominant trait. The skeletal system is not so weakened, and fractures often do not appear until the child becomes active and starts to walk, or even later in childhood. These fractures heal rapidly, but with a poor-quality callus. In some cases, parents may be suspected of child abuse when the child is admitted to the health care facility with multiple fractures.

There is no known medical treatment for correction of the defective collagen synthesis that is characteristic of osteogenesis imperfecta. Instead, treatment modalities focus on preventing and treating fractures. Precise alignment is necessary to prevent deformities. Nonunion is common, especially with repeated fractures at a progressively deforming site. Surgical intervention is often needed to correct deformities (internal fixation of long bones may be done with an intramedullary rod that "grows" with the child), stabilize fractures, remove hardware devices after a nonunion, and occasionally amputate the site of a failed bone graft.

In summary, skeletal disorders can be due to congenital or hereditary influences or to factors that occur during normal periods of skeletal growth and development. Newborn infants undergo normal changes in muscle tone and joint motion, causing conditions such as femoral anteversion and toeing-in. Many of these conditions are corrected as skeletal growth and development take place. Other childhood skeletal disorders, such as the osteochondroses, slipped capital femoral epiphysis, and scoliosis, are not corrected by the growth process. These disorders are progressive, can cause permanent disability, and require treatment. Disorders such as congenital dislocation of the hip and congenital clubfoot are present at birth. Both of these disorders are best treated during infancy. Regular examinations during the first year of life are recommended as a means of achieving early diagnosis of such disorders. Osteogenesis imperfecta is a rare autosomal hereditary disorder characterized by defective synthesis of connective tissue, including bone matrix. It results in poorly developed bones that fracture easily.

■ METABOLIC BONE DISEASE

The process of bone resorption and formation is continuous throughout life. This process is called bone remodeling. There are two types of bone remodeling: structural and internal remodeling.[22] Structural remodeling involves deposition of new bone on the outer aspect of the shaft at the same time that bone is resorbed from the inner aspect of the shaft. It occurs during growth and results in a bone having adult form and shape. Internal remodeling involves the replacement of bone. In the adult skeleton, remodeling involves formation of new packets of bone on trabecular surfaces and is important in replacing existing bone. Internal remodeling involves a coupled sequence of bone cell activity (Fig. 57-6). The sequence is activated by one of many stimuli, including the actions of parathyroid hormone. It begins with osteoclastic resorption of existing bone, during which both the organic and the inorganic components are removed. The sequence proceeds to the formation of new bone by osteoblasts. In the adult, the length of one sequence (bone resorption and formation) is about 4 months. Ideally, the replaced bone should equal the absorbed bone. If it does not, there is a net loss of bone. In the elderly, for example, bone

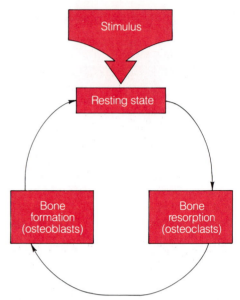

FIG. 57-6. Coupled sequence of bone resorption and formation.

resorption and formation are no longer perfectly coupled, and bone mass is lost.

The three major influences on the equilibrium of bone tissue are: (1) mechanical stress, which helps stimulate osteoblastic activity and formation of the organic matrix; (2) calcium and phosphate levels in the extracellular fluid; and (3) hormones and local factors, which influence bone resorption and formation. Mechanical stress stimulates osteoblastic activity and formation of organic matrix. It is important in preventing bone atrophy and in healing fractures. Bone serves as a storage site for extracellular calcium and phosphate ions. Consequently, alterations in the extracellular levels of these ions affect their deposition in bone (see Chapter 29).

HORMONAL CONTROL OF BONE FORMATION AND METABOLISM

The process of bone formation and mineral metabolism is complex. It involves the interplay between the action of parathyroid hormone, calcitonin, and vitamin D. Other hormones, such as cortisol, growth hormone, thyroid hormone, and the sex hormones, also influence bone formation either directly or indirectly. The actions of parathyroid hormone, calcitonin, and vitamin D are summarized in Table 57-1.

PARATHYROID HORMONE

Parathyroid hormone (PTH) is one of the important regulators of calcium and phosphate levels in the blood. The hormone is secreted by the parathyroid

TABLE 57-1. ACTIONS OF PARATHYROID HORMONE, CALCITONIN, AND VITAMIN D

ACTIONS	PARATHYROID HORMONE	CALCITONIN	VITAMIN D
Intestinal absorption of calcium	Increases indirectly through increased activation of vitamin D	Probably not affected	Increases
Intestinal absorption of phosphate	Increases	Probably not affected	Increases
Renal excretion of calcium	Decreases	Increases	Probably increases but less effect than PTH
Renal excretion of phosphate	Increases	Increases	Increases
Bone resorption	Increases	Decreases	1,25 $(OH)_2D_3$ increases
Bone formation	Decreases	Uncertain	24,25 $(OH)_2D_3$ increases(?)
Serum calcium levels	Produces a prompt increase	Decreases with pharmacologic doses	No effect
Serum phosphate levels	Prevents an increase	Decreases with pharmacologic doses	No effect

glands, which are located on the posterior outer surface of the thyroid gland.

PTH acts to prevent serum calcium levels from falling below and serum phosphate levels from rising above normal physiologic concentrations. The secretion of PTH is regulated by negative feedback according to serum calcium levels. PTH, which is released from the parathyroid gland in response to a decrease in plasma calcium, acts to restore the concentration of the calcium ion to just above the normal set point. This, in turn, inhibits further secretion of the hormone. Other factors, such as serum phosphate and arterial blood *p*H, indirectly influence parathyroid secretion by altering the amount of calcium that is complexed to phosphate or bound to albumin.

PTH functions to maintain serum calcium levels by initiating (1) release of calcium from bone, (2) conservation of calcium by the kidney, (3) enhanced intestinal absorption of calcium through activation of vitamin D, and (4) reduction of serum phosphate levels (Fig. 57-7). PTH also increases the movement of calcium and phosphate from bone into the extracellular fluid. Calcium is immediately released from the canaliculi and bone cells; a more prolonged release of calcium and phosphate is mediated by increased osteoclast activity. In the kidney, PTH stimulates tubular reabsorption of calcium while reducing the reabsorption of phosphate. The latter effect ensures that increased release of phosphate from bone during mobilization of calcium does not produce an elevation in serum phosphate levels. PTH increases intestinal absorption of calcium because of its ability to stimulate production of 1,25-dihydroxyvitamin D_3 by the kidney.

CALCITONIN

Whereas PTH acts to increase blood calcium levels, the hormone calcitonin acts to lower blood calcium levels. Calcitonin (sometimes called thyrocalcitonin) is secreted by the parafollicular, or C, cells of the thyroid gland.

Calcitonin inhibits the release of calcium from bone into the extracellular fluid. It is thought to act by causing calcium to become sequestered in bone cells

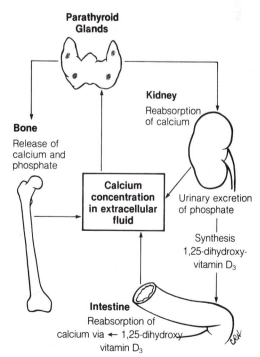

FIG. 57-7. Regulation and actions of parathyroid hormone.

and by inhibiting osteoclast activity. Calcitonin also reduces the renal tubular reabsorption of calcium and phosphate; the decrease in serum calcium level that follows administration of pharmacologic doses of calcitonin may be related to this action.[23]

The major stimulus for calcitonin synthesis and release is a rise in serum calcium. The actual role of calcitonin in the overall mineral homeostasis is unclear. There are no clearly definable syndromes of calcitonin deficiency or excess, which suggests that calcitonin does not directly alter calcium metabolism. It has been suggested that the physiologic actions of calcitonin are related to the postprandial handling and processing of dietary calcium.[23] This theory proposes that after meals calcitonin maintains parathyroid secretion at a time when it normally would be reduced by calcium entering the blood from the digestive tract. Although excess or deficiency states associated with alterations in physiologic levels of calcitonin have not been observed, it has been shown that pharmacologic doses of the hormone reduce osteoclastic activity. Because of this action, calcitonin has proved effective in the treatment of Paget's disease. The hormone is also used to reduce serum calcium levels during hypercalcemic crises.

VITAMIN D

Vitamin D and its metabolites are not vitamins but steroid hormones. There are two forms of vitamin D: vitamin D_2 (ergocalciferol) and vitamin D_3 (cholecalciferol). The two forms differ by the presence of a double bond, yet have identical biologic activity. The term *vitamin D* is used to indicate both forms.

Vitamin D has little or no activity until it has been metabolized to compounds that mediate its activity. Figure 57-8 depicts sources of vitamin D and pathways for activation. The first step of the activation process occurs in the liver, where vitamin D is hydroxylated to form the metabolite 25-hydroxyvitamin D_3 (25-OH D_3). From the liver, 25-OH D_3 is transported to the kidneys, where it undergoes conversion to either 1,25-dihydroxyvitamin D_3 [1,25-$(OH)_2D_3$] or 24,25-dihydroxyvitamin D_3 [24,25-$(OH)_2D_3$]. Other metabolites of vitamin D have been and are still being discovered.

There are two sources of vitamin D: intestinal absorption and skin production. Intestinal absorption occurs mainly in the jejunum and includes both vitamin D_2 and vitamin D_3. The most important dietary sources of vitamin D are fish, liver, and irradiated milk. Because vitamin D is fat-soluble, its absorption is mediated by bile salts and occurs by means of the lymphatic vessels. In the skin, ultraviolet radiation from sunlight spontaneously converts 7-dehydrocholesterol previtamin D_3 to vitamin D_3.

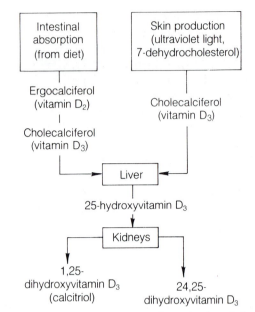

FIG. 57-8. *Sources and pathway for activation of vitamin D.*

A circulating vitamin D–binding protein provides a mechanism to remove vitamin D from the skin and make it available to the rest of the body. With adequate exposure to sunlight, the amount of vitamin D that can be produced by the skin is usually sufficient to meet physiologic requirements. The importance of sunlight exposure is evidenced by population studies that report lower vitamin D levels in countries, such as England, that have less sunlight than the United States.[24] Elderly people who are either housebound or institutionalized frequently have low vitamin D levels.[25] The deficiency often goes undetected until there are problems such as pseudofractures or electrolyte imbalances. Seasonal variations in vitamin D levels probably reflect changes in sunlight exposure.

The most potent of the vitamin D metabolites is 1,25-$(OH)_2D_3$. This metabolite increases intestinal absorption of calcium and resorption of calcium and phosphate from bone. Bone resorption by the osteoclasts is increased and bone formation by the osteoblasts is decreased; there is also an increase in acid phosphatase and a decrease in alkaline phosphatase. Both intestinal absorption and bone resorption increase the amount of calcium and phosphorus available to the mineralizing surface of the bone. The role of 24,25-$(OH)_2D_3$ is less clear. There is increasing evidence that 24,25-$(OH)_2D_3$, in conjunction with 1,25-$(OH)_2D_3$, may be involved in normal bone mineralization.[26]

The regulation of vitamin D activity is influenced by several hormones. PTH and prolactin stimulate 1,25-$(OH)_2D_3$ production by the kidney. States of hyperparathyroidism are associated with increased levels of 1,25-$(OH)_2D_3$, whereas hypoparathyroidism leads to lowered levels of this metabolite. Prolactin may have an ancillary role in regulating vitamin D metabolism during pregnancy and lactation. Calcitonin inhibits $1,25\text{-}(OH)_2D_3$ production by the kidney. In addition to hormonal influences, changes in the concentration of ions such as calcium, phosphate, hydrogen, and potassium exert an effect on both $1,25\text{-}(OH)_2D_3$ and $24,25\text{-}(OH)_2D_3$ production. Under conditions of deprivation of phosphate and calcium, $1,25\text{-}(OH)_2D_3$ levels are increased, whereas hyperphosphatemia and hypercalcemia decrease the levels of metabolite.

DISORDERS OF BONE METABOLISM

OSTEOPENIA

Osteopenia is a condition that is common to all metabolic bone diseases. It is characterized by a reduction in bone mass greater than expected for age, race, or sex, and it occurs because of a decrease in bone formation, inadequate bone mineralization, or excessive bone deossification. Osteopenia is not a diagnosis but a term used to describe an apparent lack of bone on x-ray studies. The major causes of osteopenia are osteoporosis, osteomalacia, malignancies such as multiple myeloma, and endocrine disorders such as hyperparathyroidism and hyperthyroidism.

OSTEOPOROSIS

Osteoporosis is a disorder in which the rate of bone resorption is greater than the rate of bone formation. There are parallel losses of both the organic matrix and mineral content of the bone. The total composition of bone remains the same: there is just too little of it. Osteoporotic bone is brittle and fragile, and it fractures easily. Osteoporosis can occur as the result of an endocrine disorder or malignancy but is most often associated with the aging process. Loss of bone mass begins at about age 25. After age 40, the rate of bone loss is approximately 0.5% per year, and it increases to about 1% per year or more in menopausal women.[27] An estimated 25 million Americans are affected with osteoporosis. This include over 50% of women over 45 years of age and 90% of women over 75 years of age.[28] It has been estimated that osteoporosis affects about 14 million women in the United States. Overall, up to 85% of the female population develop osteoporosis.[28] Age-related bone losses in men are seen 15 to 20 years later than in women and occur at a slower rate.[29] It has also been shown that bone mass positively correlates with the amount of skin pigmentation; whites have the least amount of bone mass and African Americans have the most.[29]

Although osteoporosis is uncommon among African-American women, many cases are seen among postmenopausal women with brown and yellow skin. One of the reasons for the increased risk in postmenopausal women of white or Asian descent may be that their original bone mass is less and therefore the losses associated with aging affect them sooner.

With osteoporosis, changes occur in both the diaphysis and the metaphysis. The diameter of the bone enlarges with age, causing the outer supporting cortex to become thinner. In severe osteoporosis, the bones begin to resemble the fragile structure of a fine china vase. There is loss of trabeculae from cancellous bone and thinning of the cortex to such an extent that minimal stress causes fractures. The changes that occur with osteoporosis have been explained by two distinct disease processes affecting women both early and late in life.[30] The first type is caused by early postmenopausal estrogen deficiency and is manifested by loss of trabecular bone with predisposition to fractures of the vertebrae and distal radius. The second type is caused by a calcium deficiency and is a slower process in which both cortical and trabecular bone are lost. Hip fractures, which are seen later in life, result from the second type. The heterogeneity of pathogenic mechanisms and presentations makes it difficult to generalize about osteoporosis.

The development of osteoporosis involves many factors. It is related to hormone levels, physical fitness, and general nutrition (Table 57-2). It is thought that an indirect action of estrogen is the suppression of bone resorption. This action is reduced after menopause. Exercise helps to prevent involutional bone loss and may serve to prevent or delay the progression of osteoporosis.[30, 31] Poor nutrition or an age-related decrease in intestinal absorption of calcium because of deficient activation of vitamin D may contribute to osteoporosis, particularly in the elderly. People with endocrine disorders such as hyperthyroidism, hyperparathyroidism, Cushing's syndrome, or diabetes mellitus are at high risk for developing osteoporosis. The prolonged use of medications that increase calcium excretion, such as aluminum-containing antacids, corticosteroids, and anticonvulsants, is also associated with bone loss.[32] Other factors found to be associated with osteoporosis are a diet high in protein, cigarette smoking, alcohol ingestion, and a family history of osteoporosis.[33]

Osteoporosis is rare in children. When it does occur, it is related to causes such as the excess corticosteroid levels associated with Cushing's syndrome, colon disease, prolonged immobility, or osteogenesis imperfecta. The cardinal features occur at the onset or just before puberty and may include pain in the back and extremities and multiple fractures. There is radiologic evidence of osteoporotic new bone. Idiopathic juvenile osteoporosis, which is more common in children, resembles rickets.

The true etiology of osteoporosis is unknown, but most data suggest that the primary problem is an acceleration of bone resorption. The serum alkaline phosphatase level, a measure of osteoblastic activity, is increased slightly.[29] There may also be a lower level of calcitonin and a decreased response to a calcium stimulus.[27] Decreases in sex hormone levels, which seem to act as an intermediate to prevent bone loss, in both men and women are somehow important in the pathogenesis of osteoporosis. In postmenopausal women, these changes can be reversed by estrogen therapy. There is some evidence that osteoporosis is caused, at least in part, by abnormalities in local factors, such as prostaglandins, interleukins, and growth factors, that influence bone cell function.[31] Further study is needed, particularly because local factors cannot be measured directly but have to be identified with in vitro organ-culture methods and tissues from laboratory animals.

The first clinical manifestations of osteoporosis are pain accompanied by skeletal fractures—a vertebral compression fracture or fractures of the hip, pelvis, humerus, or any other bone. Estimates are

that 25% to 30% of all white women in the United States will experience an osteoporosis-related fracture.[32] Unfortunately, fractures represent an end stage of the disease. Women who present with fractures are much more likely to suffer another fracture than are women of the same age without osteoporosis. Wedging and collapse of vertebrae causes a loss of height in the vertebral column and kyphosis, a condition commonly referred to as dowager's hump. Usually, there is no generalized bone tenderness. When pain occurs, it is related to fractures.

The initial diagnosis of osteoporosis is often made on the basis of standard x-ray studies when a woman presents with a fracture. However, radiologic evidence of decreased bone density is nonspecific. Bone loss is apparent on standard x-ray studies only when there is a 30% or greater loss in bone mass. A CT scan is the most accurate indicator of early bone loss in the spine, but it is expensive and involves exposure to high radiation doses. Dual-photon absorptiometry of the spine and hip and single-photon absorptiometry of the wrist can detect bone losses of only 1% to 2%. The latter are used as an inexpensive diagnostic tool in osteoporosis screening programs.

In all cases of osteoporosis, clinical examination and x-ray findings must be considered in conjunction with various blood chemistry levels. Assays of calcium, phosphorus, and alkaline phosphatase levels and protein electrophoresis should be done before treatment is started. These levels may all be within the normal range in postmenopausal osteoporosis, with only a slight rise in serum calcium and phosphate reflecting the increased bone destruction. Unfortunately, the only measure of bone density and calcium level is through bone biopsy. This is usually reserved for people who do not respond to treatment.

Prevention and early detection of osteoporosis is essential to the prevention of the deformities and fractures associated with its presence. It is important to identify people in high-risk groups so treatment can be begun early. Postmenopausal women of small stature or lean body mass, those with sedentary lifestyles, those whose calcium intake is poor, and those suffering from diseases that demineralize bone are at greatest risk. Regular exercise and adequate calcium intake are important factors in preventing osteoporosis. Studies have indicated that premenopausal women need over 1000 mg and postmenopausal women 1500 mg of calcium daily.[8] This means that adults should drink three to four glasses of milk daily or substitute other foods that are high in calcium. Unfortunately, the average American diet only provides about 600 mg.[8]

The efficacy of treatment methods for osteoporosis is questionable. A combination of fluoride, calcium, and vitamin D is most often used. Increas-

TABLE 57-2. RISK FACTORS ASSOCIATED WITH OSTEOPOROSIS

Personal
  Advanced age
  Female
  Caucasian (fair, thin skin)
  Small bone structure
  Postmenopausal
  Family history
Lifestyle
  Sedentary
  Calcium deficiency (long-term)
  High-protein diet
  Excessive alcohol intake
  Excessive caffeine intake
  Smoking
Drug- and Disease-Related
  Aluminum-containing antacids
  Anticonvulsants
  Corticosteroids
  Heparin
  Diabetes mellitus
  Chronic obstructive lung disease
  Gastrectomy
  Malignancy
  Hyperparathyroidism
  Rheumatoid arthritis

ing calcium intake enhances peak bone mass and reduces bone loss and is best done before menopause. Calcium supplements such as calcium carbonate are readily available. The popular 500-mg tablet provides 200 mg of elemental calcium and 20% of the recommended daily requirement. The usual dose is 500 mg taken three times a day with meals to avoid gastric upset. A daily intake of 400 IU of vitamin D is recommended.[8] Administration of fluoride does lead to widespread formation of new bone, but the quality of the bone is still questionable. Because the new bone is laid down on existing bone, the treatment must be started while there is still adequate bone onto which the fluoride bone can be built. Calcitonin can be used to increase osteoblast activity. It has some effect on bone pain but is only available by injection. There is evidence that deficient activation of vitamin D may be an important factor in the impaired intestinal absorption of calcium in the elderly. On the basis of this evidence, 1,25-dihydroxyvitamin D_3 is being studied as a treatment for osteoporosis.[34]

The use of estrogen therapy in postmenopausal women in the United States is relatively common and is becoming less controversial. Several studies have shown a reduction in postmenopausal bone loss in women using estrogen therapy, particularly those treated within the first 3 years of menopause.[31] Studies have indicated that administering estrogen to older women, at least up to age 74 years, may prevent hip fractures.[35] However, there is strong evidence that women who have not undergone a hysterectomy are at increased risk for developing endometrial cancer when taking estrogens.[30, 36] This risk appears to be related to the length of treatment, dose, and concomitant use of progestins. Further research is needed to determine the ideal dose and duration of estrogen therapy needed to prevent loss of bone mass.

People with osteoporosis have many special needs. In treating fractures, it is important to minimize immobility. Surgical intervention is done for stable fracture fixation that allows early restoration of mobility and function. This means early weight bearing in the lower extremities. Walking and swimming are encouraged. Unsafe conditions that predispose people to falls and fractures should be corrected or avoided.

OSTEOMALACIA AND RICKETS

In contrast to osteoporosis, which causes a loss of total bone mass and results in brittle bones, osteomalacia and rickets produce a softening of the bones and do not involve the loss of bone matrix. About 60% of bone is mineral content, about 30% is organic matrix, and the rest is living bone cells. Both the organic matrix and the inorganic mineral salts are needed for normal bone consistency. As an example, if the inorganic mineral salts are removed from fresh bone (dilute nitric acid removes them), the organic matrix that remains still resembles a bone, but it is so flexible that it can be tied in a knot. On the other hand, when a bone is placed over a hot flame, the organic material is destroyed and the bone becomes brittle.

Osteomalacia. Osteomalacia is a generalized bone condition in which inadequate mineralization of bone matrix results from a calcium or phosphate deficiency (or both). It is sometimes referred to as the adult form of rickets.

There are two main causes of osteomalacia: (1) insufficient calcium absorption from the intestine because of either a lack of calcium or resistance to the action of vitamin D and (2) increased renal phosphorus losses. As discussed previously, vitamin D is a fat-soluble vitamin that is either absorbed intact through the intestine or produced in the skin as a result of ultraviolet irradiation. Vitamin D that is absorbed from the intestine or synthesized in the skin is inactive. Vitamin D is activated in a two-step process that begins in the liver and is completed in the kidney. Vitamin D deficiency is most commonly due to reduced vitamin D absorption as a result of biliary tract or intestinal diseases that impair fat and fat-soluble vitamin absorption. Lack of vitamin D in the diet is rare in the United States because many foods are fortified with the vitamin. Anticonvulsant medications, such as phenobarbital and phenytoin, induce hepatic hydroxylases that accelerate breakdown of the active forms of vitamin D. The long-term use of antacids, such as aluminum hydroxide, that bind dietary forms of phosphate and prevent their absorption is another cause of phosphate deficiency. Longstanding primary hyperparathyroidism causes hypophosphatemia, which can lead to rickets in children and osteomalacia in adults. A form of osteomalacia called renal rickets occurs in persons with chronic renal failure. It is caused by the inability of the kidney to activate vitamin D and excrete phosphate and is accompanied by hyperparathyroidism, increased bone turnover, and increased bone resorption. Another form of osteomalacia is due to renal tubular defects that cause excessive phosphorus losses. This form of osteomalacia is commonly referred to as vitamin D–resistant rickets and is often a familial disorder. It is inherited as an x-linked dominant gene, being passed by mothers to half of all their children and by fathers to their daughters only. This form of osteomalacia affects boys more severely than girls.

The incidence of osteomalacia is high among the

elderly because of diets deficient in both calcium and vitamin D and is often compounded by intestinal malabsorption problems that accompany aging. Osteomalacia is often seen in cultures in which the diet is deficient in vitamin D, such as in northern China, Japan, and northern India. Women in these areas have a higher incidence of the disorder than men because of the combined effects of pregnancy, lactation, and more indoor confinement. Osteomalacia is occasionally seen in strict vegetarians; people who have had a gastrectomy; and those on long-term anticonvulsant, tranquilizer, sedative, muscle relaxant, or diuretic drugs. There is also a greater incidence of osteomalacia in colder regions of the world, particularly during the winter months, probably because of lessened exposure to sunlight.

The clinical manifestations of osteomalacia are bone pain, tenderness, and fractures as the disease progresses. In severe cases, muscle weakness is often an early sign. The cause of muscle weakness is unclear. The combined effects of gravity, muscle weakness, and bone softening contribute to the development of deformities. There may be a dorsal kyphosis in the spine, rib deformities, a heart-shaped pelvis, and marked bowing of the tibiae and femurs. Osteomalacia predisposes a person to pathologic fractures in the weakened areas, especially in the distal radius and proximal femur. In contrast to osteoporosis, it is not a significant cause of hip fractures. There may be delayed healing and poor retention of internal fixation devices.

Osteomalacia is usually accompanied by a compensatory hyperparathyroidism stimulated by low serum calcium levels. Parathyroid hormone reduces renal absorption of phosphate and removes calcium from the bone. Thus, calcium levels are only slightly reduced in osteomalacia.

Diagnostic measures are directed toward identifying osteomalacia and establishing its cause. Diagnostic methods include x-ray studies, laboratory work-up, bone scan, and bone biopsy. X-ray findings typical of osteomalacia are the development of transverse lines or pseudofractures called Looser's zones. These are apparently caused by pulsations of the major arteries where they cross the bone.[21] A bone biopsy may be done to confirm the diagnosis of osteomalacia in a person with nonspecific osteopenia who shows no improvement after treatment with exercise, vitamin D, and calcium.

The treatment of osteomalacia is directed at the underlying cause. If the problem is nutritional, restoring adequate amounts of calcium and vitamin D to the diet may be sufficient. The elderly with intestinal malabsorption may also benefit from vitamin D. The least expensive and most effective long-term treatment is a diet rich in vitamin D (fish, dairy products, and margarine) along with careful exposure to the midday sun. Vitamin D is specific for adult osteomalacia and vitamin D–resistant rickets, but large doses are usually needed to overcome the resistance to its calcium absorption action and to prevent renal loss of phosphate. The biologically active form of vitamin D, calcitriol, is available for use in the treatment of osteomalacia resistant to vitamin D (e.g., osteomalacia resulting from chronic liver disease and kidney failure). If osteomalacia is due to malabsorption, the treatment is directed toward correcting the primary disease condition. For example, adequate replacement of pancreatic enzymes is of paramount importance in pancreatic insufficiency. In renal tubular disorders, the treatment is directed at the altered renal physiology.

Rickets. Vitamin D deficiency rickets, seen in children, is called infantile or nutritional rickets. It is a disturbance in the formation of bone in the growing skeleton and affects the epiphyseal plate as well as the bones of the immature child. It is characterized by softened and deformed bones caused by failure of the organic matrix of bone to calcify normally. Rickets occurs primarily in underdeveloped areas of the world and in urban areas where pigmented ethnic groups have migrated from sunny to cloudy climates. It is seen most often in infants from 6 to 24 months of age.

Nutritional rickets is caused by either a lack of vitamin D in the diet or malabsorption diseases. Inadequate amounts of calcium and phosphorus in the diet also play a part in the development of rickets. The bony changes are a result of inadequate absorption of calcium.

The pathology of rickets is the same as that of osteomalacia seen in adults. Because rickets affects children during periods of active growth, however, the structural changes seen in the bone are somewhat different. Bones become deformed; ossification at epiphyseal plates is delayed and disordered. This results in widening of the epiphyseal cartilage plate. Any new bone that does grow is unmineralized.

The symptoms of rickets are usually noted between 6 months and 3 years. There is usually stunting of growth with height sometimes far below the normal range. Weight is often not affected so that the children, many of whom present with a protruding abdomen (rachitic potbelly), have been described as presuming a Buhddalike appearance when sitting. Early symptoms are lethargy and muscle weakness, which may be accompanied by convulsions or tetany related to hypocalcemia. Irritability is common. In severe cases, children lose their skin pigment, develop flabby subcutaneous tissue, and have poorly developed musculature. The ends of long bones and ribs are enlarged. The thorax may be abnormally shaped with prominent rib cartilage (rachitic rosary). The legs exhibit either bowlegged (varus) or knock-kneed (valgus) deformities. The skull is enlarged and soft, and closure of the fontanels is delayed. The child is slow to develop teeth and may have difficulty standing.

Rickets is treated with a balanced diet sufficient in calcium, phosphorus, and vitamin D. Exposure to sunshine is also important, especially for premature infants and those on artificial milk feedings. Supplemental vitamin D in excess of normal requirements is given for several months. Maintaining good posture, positioning, and bracing in older children are used to prevent deformities. Once the disease is controlled, deformities may have to be surgically corrected as the child grows.

PAGET'S DISEASE (OSTEITIS DEFORMANS)

Paget's disease is discussed separately because it is not a true metabolic disease. It is a progressive skeletal disorder that involves excessive bone destruction and repair and is characterized by increasing structural changes of the long bones, spine, pelvis, and cranium. The disease affects about 3% of the population over age 40 and 10% of those over age 70.[37] It is rarely diagnosed before age 40. In children, hyperostosis corticalis deformans juvenilis (a rare inherited disorder), hyperphosphatemia, and diseases that cause diaphyseal stenosis may mimic Paget's disease and are sometimes referred to as juvenile Paget's disease. The etiology of Paget's disease is unknown. One theory proposes that it may be caused by a virus with osteoclastic capability that has remained dormant for some years.[38]

The disease usually begins insidiously and progresses slowly over many years. An initial osteolytic phase is followed by an osteoblastic sclerotic phase. During the initial osteolytic phase, abnormal osteoclasts proliferate. Bone resorption occurs so rapidly that new bone formation cannot keep up, and the bone is replaced by fibrous tissue. The bones actually increase in size and thickness because of accelerated bone resorption followed by abnormal regeneration. Irregular bone formation results in sclerotic and osteoblastic lesions. The result is a thick layer of coarse bone with a rough and pitted outer surface that has the appearance of pumice. Histologically, the Paget's lesions show increased vascularity and bone marrow fibrosis with intense cellular activity. The bone has a somewhat mosaic pattern caused by areas of density outlined by heavy blue lines, called cement lines.

The disease varies in severity and may be present long before it is clinically detected. The clinical manifestations of Paget's disease depend on the specific area involved. About 20% of those people with the disorder are totally asymptomatic, and the disease is discovered accidentally.[38] Involvement of the skull causes headaches, intermittent tinnitus, vertigo, and eventual hearing loss. In the spine, collapse of the anterior vertebrae causes kyphosis of the thoracic spine. The femur and tibia become bowed. Softening of the femoral neck can cause coxa vara (reduced angle of the femoral neck). Coxa vara, in combination with softening of the sacral and iliac bones, causes a waddling gait. When the lesion affects only one bone, it may cause only mild pain and stiffness. Progressive deossification weakens and distorts the bone structure. The deossification process begins along the inner cortical surfaces and continues until the substance of the bone disappears. Pathologic fractures may occur, especially in the bones subjected to the greatest stress (*e.g.*, the upper femur, lower spine, and pelvic bones). These fractures often heal poorly, with excessive and poorly distributed callus.

Other manifestations of Paget's disease include nerve palsy syndromes from lesions in the upper extremities, mental deterioration, and cardiovascular disease. Cardiovascular disease is the most serious complication and is listed as the most common cause of death in advanced generalized Paget's disease. It is caused by vasodilation of the vessels in the skin and subcutaneous tissues overlying the affected bones. When one third to one half of the skeleton is affected, the increased blood flow may lead to high-output cardiac failure.[38] Ventilatory capacity may be limited by rib and spine involvement.

Sarcoma occurs in about 7% of people with Paget's disease, with a slight predominance in men.[39] One fifth of all osteogenic sarcomas in people 50 years or older originate in people with Paget's disease.[40] The bones most often affected, in order of frequency, are the femur, pelvis, humerus, and tibia. There appears to be a close histopathogenic relationship between Paget's disease and the associated sarcoma.[41] The fact that the cellular activity seen in sarcoma (*e.g.*, these tumors have a large number of osteoclasts and atypical osteoblasts) seems to be an exaggeration of the remodeling process of Paget's disease gives credence to the theory that both diseases have a viral origin.[38]

Diagnosis of Paget's disease is based on characteristic bone deformities and x-ray changes. Elevated levels of serum alkaline phosphatase and urinary hydroxyproline support the diagnosis, and continued surveillance of these levels may be used to monitor the effectiveness of treatment. Bone scans are used to detect the rapid bone turnover indicative of active disease and to monitor the response to treatment. The scan cannot identify bone activity due to malignant lesions. Bone biopsy may be done to differentiate the lesion from osteomyelitis or a primary or metastatic bone tumor.

The treatment of Paget's disease is based on the degree of pain and the extent of the disease. Pain can be reduced with either nonsteroidal or other anti-inflammatory agents. Suppressive agents such as calcitonin, mithramycin, and diphosphate compounds are used to manage pain and prevent further spread of the disease and neurologic defects. Calcitonin and etidronate disodium (a phosphate compound) decrease bone resorption. Mithramycin is a cytotoxic agent that causes osteoclasts to reduce their resorption of bone. Because this drug is toxic, it is reserved for resistant cases. Decreases in serum alkaline phosphatase and urinary hydroxyproline levels and radiologically evident improvement indicate response to treatment. However, symptomatic improvement is usually considered the best measure of success.

In summary, in addition to its structural function, the skeleton is a homeostatic organ. Metabolic bone diseases such as osteoporosis, osteomalacia, rickets, and Paget's disease are the result of a disruption in the equilibrium of bone formation and resorption. Osteoporosis, which is the most common of the metabolic bone diseases, occurs when the rate of resorption is greater than that of bone formation. It is seen frequently in postmenopausal women and is the major cause of fractures in people over 45 years of age. Osteomalacia and rickets are caused by inadequate mineralization of bone matrix, primarily because of a deficiency of vitamin D. Paget's disease results from excessive osteoclastic activity and is characterized by the formation of poor-quality bone. The success rate of the various drugs and hormones that are used to treat metabolic bone diseases varies. Further research is needed to clarify the etiology, pathology, and treatment of these diseases.

■ NEOPLASMS

Neoplasms in the skeletal system are usually referred to as bone tumors. Primary malignant tumors of the bone are uncommon, constituting about 1% of all cancers.[40] Metastatic disease of the bone, however, is relatively common. Primary bone tumors may arise from any of the skeletal components, including osseous bone tissue, cartilage, and bone marrow. The discussion in this section focuses on primary benign and malignant bone tumors of osseous or cartilaginous origin and metastatic bone disease. Tumors of bone marrow origin (leukemia and multiple myeloma) are discussed in Chapter 16.

Like other types of neoplasms, bone tumors may be either benign or malignant. The benign types, such as osteochondromas and giant cell tumors, tend to grow rather slowly and usually do not destroy the supporting or surrounding tissue or spread to other parts of the body. Malignant tumors, such as osteosarcoma and Ewing's sarcoma, grow rapidly and can spread to other parts of the body through the bloodstream or lymphatics. Specific types of bone tumors affect different age groups. Adolescents have the highest incidence, with a rate of 3 cases per 100,000. In children less than 15 years of age, only 3.2% of all malignancies are primary bone tumors.[40] The two major forms of bone cancer in children and young adults are osteogenic sarcoma and Ewing's sarcoma. It is unusual for either condition to be seen after age 25. The incidence of bone tumors declines in young adults to a rate of 0.3 per 100,000 between the ages of 30 and 35 years and slowly begins to rise until the incidence at age 60 equals that at adolescence.[40] The classification of benign and malignant bone tumors is described in Table 57-3.

CHARACTERISTICS OF BONE TUMORS

There are three major symptoms of bone tumors: pain, presence of a mass, and impairment of function (Chart 57-1).[42] Pain is a feature common to almost all malignant tumors but may or may not be present in benign tumors. For example, a benign bone cyst is usually asymptomatic until a fracture occurs. Pain that persists at night and is not relieved by rest is suggestive of malignancy. A mass or hard lump may be the first sign of a bone tumor. A malignant tumor is suspected when a painful mass exists that is enlarging or eroding the cortex of the bone. The ease of discovery of a mass depends on the location of the tumor: A small lump arising on the surface of the tibia is easy to detect, whereas a tumor that is deep in the medial portion of the thigh may grow to a considerable size before it is noticed. Both benign and malignant tumors may cause the bone to erode to the point where it cannot withstand the strain of ordinary use. In such cases, even a small amount of bone stress or trauma precipitates a pathologic fracture. A tumor may produce pressure on a peripheral nerve causing decreased sensation, numbness, a limp, or limitation of movement.

BENIGN NEOPLASMS

Benign bone tumors usually are found to be limited to the confines of the bone, have well-demarcated edges, and are surrounded by a thin rim of sclerotic bone. The four most common types of benign bone tumors are (1) osteoma, (2) chondroma, (3) osteochondroma, and (4) giant cell tumor.

An *osteoma* is a small bony tumor found on the

TABLE 57-3. CLASSIFICATION OF PRIMARY BONE NEOPLASMS

TISSUE TYPE	BENIGN NEOPLASM	MALIGNANT NEOPLASM
Bone	Osteoid osteoma	Osteosarcoma
	Benign osteoblastoma	Parosteal osteogenic
	Osteoma	sarcoma
Cartilage	Osteochondroma	Chondrosarcoma
	Chondroma	
	Chondroblastoma	
	Chondromyxoid fibroma	
Bone marrow		Multiple myeloma
		Reticulum cell sarcoma
Uncertain	Giant cell tumor	Ewing's sarcoma
	Fibrous histiocytoma	Malignant giant cell tumor
		Malignant fibrous histiocytoma
		Adamantinoma

surface of a long bone, flat bone, or the skull. It is usually composed of hard, compact (ivory osteoma) or spongy (cancellous) bone. It may be either excised or left alone.

A *chondroma* is a tumor composed of cartilage. It either grows outward from the bone (ecchondroma) or within the bone (enchondroma). These tumors may become large and are especially common in the hands and feet. At times a chondroma may persist for many years and then take on the attributes of a malignant chondrosarcoma. A chondroma is usually not treated unless it becomes unsightly or uncomfortable.

An *osteochondroma* is the most common form of benign tumor in the skeletal system. It grows only during periods of skeletal growth, originating in the epiphyseal cartilage plate and growing out of the

bone like a mushroom. An osteochondroma is composed of both cartilage and bone and usually occurs singly but may affect several bones in a condition called multiple exostoses. Malignant changes are rare, and excision of the tumor is done only when necessary.

A *giant cell tumor*, or osteoclastoma, is an aggressive tumor of multinucleated cells that often behaves like a malignant tumor, metastasizing through the bloodstream and recurring locally after excision. It occurs most often in young adults, predominantly female, and is most commonly found in the knee, wrist, or shoulder. The tumor begins in the metaphyseal region, grows into the epiphysis, and may extend into the joint surface. Pathologic fractures are common because the tumor destroys the bone substance. Clinically, pain may occur at the tumor site, with gradually increasing swelling. X-rays show destruction of the bone with expansion of the cortex.

The treatment of giant cell tumors depends on their location. If the affected bone can be eliminated without loss of function, such as the clavicle or fibula, the entire bone or part of it may be removed. When the tumor is near a major joint, such as the knee or shoulder, a local excision is done. Irradiation may be used in an attempt to prevent recurrence of the tumor.

MALIGNANT BONE TUMORS

In contrast to benign tumors, malignant tumors tend to be ill-defined, lack sharp borders, and extend beyond the confines of the bone, showing that it has destroyed the cortex. Malignant bone tumors are rare

CHART 57-1: SYMPTOMS OF BONE CANCER

■ Bone pain in an adult or child that comes on slowly but lasts for as long as a week, is constant or intermittent, and may be worse at night.

■ Unexplained swelling or lump of the arms, legs, thigh, or other bone that is firm and slightly tender and may be felt through the skin. It may interfere with normal movement and can cause the bone to break.

These symptoms are not sure signs of cancer. They may also be caused by other, less serious problems. Only a physician can tell for sure.

(Adapted from *What you need to know about cancers of the bone.* [1990]. U.S. Dept of Health and Human Services, NIH Publication No. 90-1571)

before age 10, have their peak incidence in the teen years, and have a high mortality rate. In addition, there is much morbidity and trauma from the often mutilating surgical excision.

The diagnosis of bone tumors includes both radiologic staging and biopsy. Radiographs (x-rays) give the most general diagnostic information, such as malignant versus benign and primary versus metastatic. The x-ray demonstrates the region of bone involvement, extent of destruction, and amount of reactive bone formed. Radioisotope scans are used to estimate the local intramedullary extent of the tumor and screen for other skeletal areas of involvement. CT scans further aid diagnosis and anatomic localization and can identify small pulmonary metastasis not seen by conventional x-ray. Magnetic resonance imaging (MRI) is the most accurate method of evaluating the intramedullary extent of bone tumor and can demarcate the soft structures in relation to neurovascular structures without the use of a contrast media. It is best used in conjunction with a CT scan.[43] A biopsy is also done because the definitive treatment of most bone tumors is based on pathologic interpretation of the biopsy specimen. A bone biopsy can be performed by means of a large needle or open surgical methods.

The treatment of malignant bone tumors primarily involves surgical removal of the tumor with either amputation of the limb or wide resection of the tumor and surrounding tissue. Radiation therapy is used as a definitive and adjuvant treatment to slow the progression of the cancer, decrease bone pain, and prevent pathologic fractures. A pathologic fracture spreads the tumor cells through formation of a hematoma. Because high-grade bone and soft tissue sarcomas produce clinically undetectable metastases called micrometastases, immunotherapy, irradiation, and chemotherapy are often used in combination as adjuvant therapy. Chemotherapy is the most effective modality for controlling metastases. Extremely aggressive drug combinations have been developed, particularly in the pediatric and young adult age groups. Many advances have been made in the limb salvage and reconstructive surgical procedures being used as an alternative to limb amputation. They are more often used in younger people in an attempt to increase their functioning and mobility. The tumor must have minimal soft tissue involvement and no involvement of major blood vessels.

OSTEOGENIC SARCOMA

Osteogenic sarcoma is the seventh most common cancer in children and males are affected 1.5 to 2 times more often than females.[40] The tumor most commonly affects adolescents, with peak incidence occurring during the period of maximum growth. The primary tumor is most often located at the anatomic sites associated with maximum growth velocity—the distal femur, proximal tibia, and proximal humerus. People affected with osteogenic sarcoma are usually tall and are found to have a high plasma level of somatomedin. Bone tumors in the elderly, often with Paget's disease, are more common in the humerus, pelvis, and proximal femur.

Osteogenic sarcoma is a malignant tumor of mesenchymal cells, characterized by the direct formation of osteoid or immature bone by malignant osteoblasts. These cells synthesize thin, wispy, and purposeless fragment of bone. Osteogenic sarcomas are aggressive tumors that grow rapidly; they are often eccentrically placed in the bone and move from the metaphysis of the bone out to the periosteum, with subsequent spread to adjacent soft tissues.

The causes of osteogenic sarcoma are unknown. The correlation of age and location of most of the tumors with the period of maximum growth suggests some relation to increased osteoblastic activity. Paget's disease, which is linked to osteosarcoma in the adult, is also associated with increased osteoblastic activity. Also, radiation from either an internal source, such as the radioactive pharmaceutical technetium used in bone scans, or an external source, such as x-rays, has also been associated with osteosarcoma.

The primary clinical feature of osteosarcoma is severe pain in the affected bone, usually of sudden onset. There is a wide variation in the hardness of osteogenic tumors. Osteosarcoma usually begins as a firm white or reddish mass and later becomes softer with a viscous interior. Swelling is often present over the area. The skin overlying the tumor may be shiny and stretched, with prominent superficial veins. The range of motion of the adjacent joint may be restricted. Even though this type of tumor extends through the medullary cavity, there is usually no evidence on x-ray images.

Sarcomas infrequently metastasize to the lymph nodes because the cells are unable to grow within the node. Nodal metastases usually occur only in the late course of disseminated disease. Most often the tumor cells exit the primary tumor through the venous end of the capillary, and early metastasis to the lung is common. Lung metastases, even if massive, are usually relatively asymptomatic. The prognosis in osteosarcoma depends on the aggressiveness of the disease, radiologic features, presence or absence of pathologic fracture, size of the tumor, rapidity of tumor growth, and sex of the person. There is some suggestion that females have a better survival rate than males.[42]

Chemotherapy, using various drug combinations, is the most effective treatment for metastatic osteosarcoma. The treatment for sarcomas is a combination of surgery, chemotherapy, and radiation therapy used preoperatively or postoperatively. In the past, treatment usually entailed amputation above the level of the tumor. Limb salvage surgical procedures, using a metal prosthesis or cadaver allografts, are becoming a more viable alternative. Studies have shown that limb salvage surgery has no adverse effects on the long-term survival of people with osteosarcoma. The success of limb salvage appears to depend on the use of a wide surgical margin and use of adjuvant chemotherapy.[46] The increasing success of limb-salvage surgery is due to improved radiographic imaging studies and effective use of adjuvant therapy, including chemotherapy and irradiation.[47] Microscopic examination has shown that tumor filaments may extend 1 to 3 inches or more beyond the cortical bone.[45] Advanced imaging techniques and the use of angiography assist the surgeon in determining the best type of definitive surgery. Successful limb conservation has been achieved in a limited population with a technique involving en bloc resection (removal of the tumor and a portion of uninvolved soft tissue), extracorporeal irradiation, and reimplantation of the irradiated bone.[48] Irradiation is used for inoperable tumor, such as in the mandible, maxilla, or pelvis. Pulmonary irradiation is being used with increasing success to treat pulmonary metastases in children under age 12. The use of immunotherapy, including interferon, is still in the experimental stage, as it is with other types of cancers.

CHONDROSARCOMA

Chondrosarcoma, a malignant tumor of cartilage that can develop either within the medullary cavity or peripherally, is the second most common form of malignant bone tumor. It occurs primarily in middle or later life, slightly more often in males. The tumor arises from points of muscle attachment to bone, particularly the knee, shoulder, hip, and pelvis. About 10% of all chondrosarcomas arise from underlying benign lesions.[41]

Chondrosarcomas are slow-growing, metastasize late, and are often painless. They can remain hidden in an area like the pelvis for a long time. This type of tumor, like many primary malignancies, tends to destroy bone and extend into the soft tissues beyond the confines of the bone of origin. Chondrosarcomas mainly affect the bones of the trunk, pelvis, or proximal femur and rarely develop in the distal portion of a bone. Often irregular flecks and ringlets of calcification are a prominent radiographic finding. Early diagnosis is important because chondrosarcoma responds well to early radical surgical excision.

It is generally resistant to radiation therapy and available chemotherapeutic agents.

EWING'S SARCOMA

Ewing's sarcoma is the third most common type of primary bone tumor and is highly malignant. It is frequently seen in males under 30 years of age, with the incidence being highest in the second decade of life.[40] Ewing's tumor arises from immature bone marrow cells and causes bone destruction from within. It usually occurs in the shaft of long bones or any portion of the pelvis.

Manifestations of Ewing's tumor include pain, tenderness, fever, and leukocytosis. Pathologic fractures are common because of bone destruction. Immediate combination chemotherapy is the first treatment of Ewing's sarcoma.[44] Wide resection of the tumor is done if the nerves and blood vessels are free of disease. Most protocols use several courses of intensive chemotherapy before surgery and continue it for a year after surgery. Ewing's sarcoma is more radiosensitive than most bone tumors, but there is risk of a secondary radiation-induced osteosarcoma. It may be necessary to increase the intensity of the treatment with total body irradiation, autologous bone marrow transplantation, and administration of growth factors.[44]

METASTATIC BONE DISEASE

Skeletal metastases are the most common malignancy of osseous tissue, accounting for 60% to 65% of all skeletal tumors.[49] Metastatic lesions are seen most often in the spine and pelvis and are less common in anatomic sites that are further removed from the trunk of the body. Tumors that frequently spread to the skeletal system are those of the breast, lung, prostate, kidney, and thyroid, although any cancer can ultimately involve the skeleton. More than 80% of bone metastases are due to primary lesions in the breast, lung, or prostate.[50] The incidence of metastatic bone disease is highest in people over 40 years of age. In 90% of cases, there are several bony metastases, with or without metastatic spread to other organs.[49] Because of the effectiveness of current cancer treatment modalities, cancer patients are living longer, so that the incidence of clinically apparent skeletal involvement appears to be increasing in the long run. These skeletal metastases cause great pain, increase the risk of fractures, and increase the disability of the cancer patient.

Metastasis to the bone frequently occurs without involving other organs. This is because the blood flow in the veins of the skeletal system is sluggish. These are thin-walled valveless veins, and there are many storage sites along the way. The pattern of metastasis is often related to the specific vascular pathway involved (*e.g.*, metastases to the shoulder girdle and pelvis occur when prostatic cancers invade the vertebral vein system). If metastasis is limited to the skeletal system, without other major organ involvement, a person can live for many years. Death is usually a consequence of metastasis to vital organs rather than a consequence of the primary tumor.

The major symptom of bone metastasis is pain with evidence of an impending pathologic fracture. Pain is caused by either stretching of the periosteum of the involved bone or by nerve entrapment, as in the nerve roots of the spinal cord by the vertebral body. X-ray examinations are used along with CT or bone scans to detect, diagnose, and localize metastatic bone lesions. About one third of people with skeletal metastases have positive bone scans without radiologic findings, and about 28% have metastatic lesions on x-ray studies with a negative bone scan.[51] Arteriography, using radiopaque contrast media, may be helpful in outlining the tumor margins. Serum levels of alkaline phosphatase and calcium are often elevated in people with metastatic bone disease. A bone biopsy usually is done when there is a question regarding the diagnosis or treatment.

The primary goals in treatment of metastatic bone disease are to prevent pathologic fractures and to promote survival with maximum functioning to help the patient maintain as much mobility and pain control as possible. Treatment methods include surgery, chemotherapy, and irradiation. The discovery of new and more effective drugs along with the use of combination protocols has increased the effectiveness of chemotherapy in treating metastatic bone disease secondary to tumors of the breast, prostate, and lung.[52] Radiation therapy is primarily used as a palliative treatment to alleviate pain and prevent pathologic fractures. Localized radiation therapy provides partial or complete pain relief and prevention of fractures in about 73% to 96% of people with metastases to weight-bearing bones.[50]

Pathologic fractures occur in about 10% to 15% of people with metastatic bone disease. The affected bone appears to be eaten away on x-ray images and, in severe cases, crumbles on impact, much like dried toast. Many pathologic fractures occur in the femur, humerus, and vertebrae. In the femur, fractures occur because the proximal aspect of the bone is under great mechanical stress. Lesions may be treated prophylactically with surgery and radiation therapy to prevent pathologic fractures. Flexible intramedullary rods, such as an Enders rod, may be used to stabilize long bones when lytic lesions involve 30% or more of the bone or are longer than 3 cm and in non-weight–bearing bones (humerus, ulna, and radius) when lesions involve 50% or more of the bone or are longer

than 5 cm.[50] When a pathologic fracture has occurred, bracing, intramedullary nailing of the femur and spine stabilization may be done. Because adequate fixation is often difficult in diseased bone cement (methyl methacrylate) is often used with internal fixation devices to stabilize the bone. The selection of a treatment modality for either prevention or treatment of pathologic fractures depends on the severity of the lesion, the degree of pain, and the life expectancy of the patient. The goal is to give people flexibility, mobility, and pain relief. Surgeons employ a certain degree of aggressiveness in treating metastatic lesions so that patients can function as normally as possible.

In summary, bone tumors, like any other type of neoplasms, may be either benign or malignant. Benign bone tumors grow slowly and usually do not destroy the surrounding tissues. Malignant tumors can be either primary or metastatic. Primary bone tumors are relatively rare, grow rapidly, metastasize to the lungs and other parts of the body through the bloodstream, and have a high mortality rate. Metastatic bone tumors are usually multiple, originating primarily from cancers of the breast, lung, and prostate. The incidence of metastatic bone disease is probably increasing because the improved treatment methods enable people with cancer to live longer. Advances in chemotherapy, radiation therapy, and surgical procedures have substantially increased the survival and cure rates for many types of bone cancers. A primary goal in metastatic bone disease is the prevention of pathologic fractures.

■ REFERENCES

1. Moore, K.L. (1983). *Before we are born* (pp. 2–3). Philadelphia: W.B. Saunders.
2. Hopper, W.C. (1983). Genetics in orthopedics. *Orthopedic Nursing, 1,* 38.
3. DeAngles, C. (1984). *Pediatric primary care* (pp. 289, 292). Boston: Little, Brown.
4. *Core curriculum for orthopedic nursing* (p. 125). (1986). Pitman, NJ: National Association of Orthopedic Nurses.
5. Renshaw, T.S. (1986). *Pediatric orthopedics* (pp. 77, 83). Philadelphia: W.B. Saunders.
6. Axer, A., Gershuni, D.H., Hendel, D., Mirovski, Y., et al. (1980, July-August). Indications for femoral osteotomy in Legge Calvé Perthes disease. *Clinical Orthopaedics and Related Research, 150,* 78.
7. Jani, L.F.H., & Dick, W. (1980). Results of three different types of therapeutic groups in Perthes disease. *Clinical Orthopaedics and Related Research, 150*(4), 88.
8. Rodman, G.P., & Shumacker, H.R. (Ed.). (1988). *Primer on rheumatic disorders* (9th ed., pp. 243, 245, 277). Atlanta: Arthritis Foundation.
9. Harrel, J., & Meehan, P.L. (1977). School screening in spinal deformity. *Orthopedic Nursing Association Journal, 6,* 201.
10. Binns, M. (1988). Joint laxity in idiopathic adolescent scoliosis. *Journal of Bone and Joint Surgery, 70*(B), 420.
11. Harrington, P.R. (1977, July-August). The etiology of idiopathic scoliosis. *Clinical Orthopaedics and Related Research, 126,* 17.

12. Bunnell, W.P. (1988, April). The natural history of idiopathic scoliosis. *Clinical Orthopaedics and Related Research, 229,* 20.

13. Salmon, S.W., Mooney, N.E., & Verdisco, L.A. (Eds.). (1991). *Core curriculum for orthopedic nursing* (2nd ed., pp. 359–361). Pitman, NJ: Anthony J Jannetti IM.

14. Holt deToledo, C. (1979). The patient with scoliosis: The defect, the classification, and detection. *American Journal of Nursing, 79,* 1588.

15. Bradford, D.S. (1988). Adult scoliosis: Current concepts of treatment. *Clinical Orthopaedics and Related Research, 229,* 70.

16. Drummond, D.S. (1991). A perspective on recent trends in scoliosis correction. *Clinical Orthopaedics and Related Research, 264,* 90.

17. Kehl, D.K., Morrissy, R.T. (1988). Brace treatment in adolescent scoliosis: An update on concepts and techniques. *Clinical Orthopaedics and Related Research, 229,* 34.

18. Hooker, C.W., & Greene, W.B. (1983). Congenital malformations. In F.C. Wilson (Ed.). *The musculoskeletal system* (2nd ed., p. 27). Philadelphia: J.B. Lippincott.

19. Cowell, H., & Wein, B. (1980). Current concepts review: Genetic aspects of clubfoot. *Journal of Bone and Joint Surgery, 62-A,* 1381.

20. Tachdjian, M.O. (1990). *Pediatric orthopedics.* Philadelphia: W.B. Saunders.

21. Cotran, R.S., Kumar, V., & Robbins, S.L. (1989). *Pathologic basis of disease* (4th ed., pp. 441, 1318). Philadelphia: W.B. Saunders.

22. Cormack, D.H. (1987). *Ham's histology* (9th ed., p. 305). Philadelphia: J.B. Lippincott.

23. Talmadge, R.V., Grubb, S.A., & VanderWeil, C.J. (1983). Physiologic processes in bone. In F. C. Wilson (Ed.), *The musculoskeletal system* (2nd ed.). Philadelphia: JB Lippincott.

24. Stamp, T.C.B., & Round, J.M. (1974). Seasonal changes in human plasma levels of 25-dihydroxyvitamin D. *Nature, 247,* 563.

25. Anderson, M.E.K., & Conley, D.M. (1987). Let the sun shine in. *Geriatric Nursing, 8,* 174.

26. Bickle, D.D. (1982). The vitamin D endocrine system. *Annals of Internal Medicine, 27,* 45.

27. Raisz, L.G. (1982). Osteoporosis. *Journal of the American Geriatric Society, 30,* 127.

28. American Academy of Orthopaedic Surgeons. (1988). *Osteoporosis.* Park Ridge, IL: American Academy of Orthopedic Surgeons.

29. Gordon, G.S., & Vaughn, C. (1980). Osteoporosis: Early detection, prevention, and treatment. *Consultant, 25,* 64.

30. Riggs, B.L. (1987). Pathogenesis of osteoporosis. *American Journal of Obstetrics and Gynecology, 156,* 1342.

31. Raisz, L.G. (1988). Local and systemic factors in the pathogenesis of osteoporosis. *New England Journal of Medicine, 318,* 818.

32. Notelovitz, M., & Ware, M. (1988). *Stand tall: The informed woman's guide to osteoporosis.* Gainesville, FL: Triad.

33. Spencer, H. (1982). Osteoporosis: Goals of therapy. *Hospital Practice, 3,* 131.

34. Slovik, D.M., Adams, J.S, Neer, R.M., et al. (1981). Deficient production of 1,25 dihydroxyvitamin D in elderly osteoporotic patients. *New England Journal of Medicine, 305,* 372.

35. Kiel, D.P., Felson, D.T., Anderson, J.J., et al. (1987). Hip fracture and the use of estrogens in postmenopausal women: The Framingham Study. *New England Journal of Medicine, 317,* 1169.

36. Weinerman, S.A., & Bockman, R.S. (1990). Medical therapy for osteoporosis. *Orthopedic Clinics of North America, 21*(1), 109.

37. Aroncheck, J.M., & Haddad, J.G. (1983). Paget's disease. *Orthopedic Clinics of North America, 14,* 3.

38. Wallach, S. (1982). Treatment of Paget's disease. *Advances in Internal Medicine 27,* 1.

39. Schajowicz, F., Arauyo, E.S., & Berenstein, M. (1983). Sarcoma complicating Paget's disease of bone. *Journal of Bone and Joint Surgery, 65*(B), 299.

40. Rubin, R. (Ed.). (1983). *Clinical oncology: A multidisciplinary approach* (pp. 296–306). New York: American Cancer Society.

41. Dahlin, D.C. (1978). *Bone tumors: General aspects and data on 6,221 cases* (3rd ed.). Springfield, IL: Charles C Thomas.

42. *What you need to know about cancers of the bone.* (1990). U.S. Department of Health and Human Services. NIH Publication No 90-1571.

43. Heare, T.C., Enneking, W.F., & Heare, M.H. (1989). Staging techniques and biopsy of bone tumors. *Orthopedic Clinics of North America, 20,* 273.

44. Mankin, H.J., Willett, C.G., & Harmon, D.C. (1991). Malignant tumors of the bone. In A.I. Holleb, D.J. Fink, & G.P. Murphy (Eds.). *American Cancer Society textbook of clinical oncology* (pp. 355–358). Atlanta: American Cancer Society.

45. Brashear, H.R. (1980). Tumors and tumorlike conditions of bone. In F.C. Wilson (Ed.). *The musculoskeletal system* (2nd ed., p. 158). Philadelphia: J.B. Lippincott.

46. Simon, M.A. (1987). Limb salvage for osteosarcoma. *Journal of Bone and Joint Surgery, 70*(A), 307.

47. Springfield, D.S. (1991). Introduction to limb-salvage surgery for sarcoma. *Orthopedic Clinics of North America, 22,* 1.

48. Uyttendaele, D., DeSchyver, A., & Claessen, H. (1988). Limb conservations in primary bone tumors by resection, extracorporeal irradiation and re-implantation. *Journal of Bone and Joint Surgery, 70*(B):348.

49. Sherry, H.S., Levy, R.N., & Siffert, R.S. (1982). Metastatic disease of bone in orthopedic surgery. *Clinical Orthopaedics and Related Research, 169,* 44.

50. Mauch, P.M., & Drew, M.A. (1985). Treatment of metastatic cancer to bone. In V.T. DeVita, S. Hellman, & S.A. Rosenberg (Eds.). *Cancer: Principles of practice of oncology* (2nd ed., pp. 2132, 2133, 2135). Philadelphia: J.B. Lippincott.

51. Bhardwaj, S., & Holland, J.F. (1982). Chemotherapy of metastatic cancer in bone. *Clinical Orthopaedics and Related Research 169,* 28.

52. Schocker, J.D., & Brady, L.W. (1982). Radiation therapy for bone metastasis. *Clinical Orthopaedics and Related Research 169,* 38.

■ BIBLIOGRAPHY

Abramowicz, M. (Ed.). (1987). Prevention and treatment of postmenopausal osteoporosis. *Medical Letter, 29*(746), 75.

Birch, J.C., Herrig, J.H., Roach, J.W., et al. (1988). Cotrel–Dubousset instrumentation in idiopathic scoliosis. *Clinical Orthopaedics and Related Research, 228,* 25.

Christodouloy, A.G., Prince, H.G., & Webb, J.K., et al. (1987). Adolescent idiopathic thoracic scoliosis: A prospective trial with and without bracing during postoperative care. *Journal of Bone and Joint Surgery, 69*(1), 13.

Corbett, D. (1988). Information needs of parents of a child with Pavlik harness. *Orthopedic Nursing, 7*(2), 20.

Cornell, C.N. (1990). Management of fractures in patients with osteoporosis. *Orthopedic Clinics of North America, 21*(11), 125.

Einhorn, T.A., & Levine, B. (1990). Nutrition and bone. *Orthopedic Clinics of North America, 21*(1), 43.

Gelberman, R.H., Cohen, M.S., Desai, S.S., et al. (1987). Femoral anteversion: A clinical assessment of idiopathic intoeing gait in children. *Journal of Bone and Joint Surgery, 69*(B), 75.

Gerther, J.M., & Root, L. (1990). Osteogenesis imperfecta. *Orthopedic Clinics of North America, 21*(1), 151.

Habermann, E.T., & Lopez, R.A. (1989). Metastatic disease of bone and treatment of pathologic fractures. *Orthopedic Clinics of North America, 20*(3), 469.

Jaffe, N. (1989). Chemotherapy for malignant bone tumors. *Orthopedic Clinics of North America, 20*(3), 487.

Kaplan, F.S., Soffer, S.R., Fallon, M.D., et al. (1988). Osteomalacia as a very late manifestation of primary hyperparathyroidism. *Clinical Orthopaedics and Related Research 228*, 26.

Klein, M.J., Kehan, S., & Lewis, M.M. (1989). Osteosarcoma: Clinical and pathological considerations. *Orthopedic Clinics of North America, 30*(3), 327.

Liscum, B. (1992). Osteoporosis: The silent disease. *Orthopedic Nursing, 11*(4), 21.

Mankin, H.J. (1990). Rickets, osteomalacia, and renal distrophy: An update. *Orthopedic Clinics of North America, 21*(1), 81.

McKibbin, B., Freedman, L., Howard, C., et al. (1988). The management of congenital dislocation of the hip in the newborn. *Journal of Bone and Joint Surgery, 70*(B), 423.

O'Connor, M.I., & Pritchard, D.J. (1991). Ewing's sarcoma: Prognostic factors, disease control, and the re-emerging role of surgical treatment. *Clinical Orthopaedics and Related Research, 262*, 78.

Renshaw, T.S. (1988). Screening school children for scoliosis. *Clinical Orthopaedics and Related Research, 229*, 26.

Rinsky, L.A. (1992). Advances in management of idiopathic scoliosis. *Hospital Practice, 27*(4), 49.

Rodts, M.F. (1987). Surgical intervention for adult scoliosis. *Orthopedic Nursing, 6*(6), 11.

Shane, E. (1988). Osteoporosis. *Contemporary Issues in Endocrinology and Metabolism, 5*, 151.

Thomas, I.H., Cole, W.G., & Waters, K.D. (1987). Function after partial pelvic resection of Ewing's sarcoma. *Journal of Bone and Joint Surgery, 69*(B), 271.

Winter, R.B. (1986). Adolescent idiopathic scoliosis. *New England Journal of Medicine, 314*, 1379.

CHAPTER 58

ALTERATIONS IN SKELETAL FUNCTION: RHEUMATIC DISORDERS

JANICE SMITH PIGG
DEBRA ANN BANCROFT

**Systemic Autoimmune
Rheumatic Diseases**
Rheumatoid Arthritis
Systemic Lupus Erythematosus
Systemic Sclerosis
Polymyositis and
Dermatomyositis
**Arthritis Associated
with Spondylitis**
Ankylosing Spondylitis
Reactive Arthritis

Psoriatic Arthritis
Enteropathic Arthritis
Degenerative Joint Disease
Osteoarthritis
**Metabolic Diseases Associated
with Rheumatic States**
Crystal-Induced Arthropathies
Gout
Calcium Crystal Deposition
Disease

**Rheumatic Diseases
in Children and the Elderly**
Rheumatic Diseases in Children
Rheumatic Diseases in the
Elderly

■ OBJECTIVES

After you have studied this chapter, you should be able to meet the following objectives:

■ Describe the pathologic changes that may be found in the joint of a person with rheumatoid arthritis.
■ List the extraarticular manifestations of rheumatoid arthritis.
■ Describe the immunologic process that occurs in systemic lupus erythematosus.
■ List four major organ systems that may be involved in systemic lupus erythematosus.
■ Cite the primary features of ankylosing spondylitis.
■ Describe how the site of inflammation differs in spondyloarthropathies from that in rheumatoid arthritis.
■ Compare rheumatoid arthritis and osteoarthritis in terms of joint involvement, level of inflammation, and local and systemic manifestations.

■ Describe the pathologic joint changes associated with osteoarthritis.
■ Cite the common features in the management of rheumatoid arthritis, systemic lupus erythematosus, osteoarthritis, and ankylosing spondylitis.
■ Differentiate between the type of crystals found in the joint in acute gout and pseudogout.
■ State two mechanisms of hyperuricemia.
■ List three types of juvenile rheumatoid arthritis and differentiate among their major characteristics.
■ Name one rheumatic disease that by definition affects only the elderly population.

Carol Mattson Porth: PATHOPHYSIOLOGY: CONCEPTS OF
ALTERED HEALTH STATES, 4th ed. © 1994, 1990, 1986, 1982
J.B. Lippincott Company

Arthritis, literally inflammation of the joint, is a generic term used for rheumatic disorders characterized by inflammatory and degenerative joint changes. More than 100 diverse rheumatic diseases exist, ranging from localized self-limiting conditions to those that are systemic autoimmune processes. One person in every seven is affected.[1] Arthritis affects people in all age groups and is the second leading cause of disability in the United States.[2] The disabling effects may be manifested in an individual's personal, professional, and social activities.

Some forms of arthritis may develop as a primary joint disorder, whereas other forms may occur as a secondary disorder resulting from another disease condition. A review of Chart 58-1, providing a classification of the rheumatic diseases, demonstrates this distinction. Not yet included in this 1988 classification, but being reported in the literature, are the frequent joint complaints in people who are positive for human immunodeficiency virus (HIV).[3] The common use of the term *arthritis* oversimplifies the nature of the varied disease processes, the difficulty in distinguishing (diagnosing) one form of arthritis or rheumatic disease from another, and the complexity of treatment of these generally chronic conditions.

The content in this chapter focuses on: (1) systemic autoimmune rheumatic disease, (2) arthritis associated with spondylitis, (3) degenerative joint disease, (4) metabolic diseases associated with arthritis, (5) rheumatic disease in children and the elderly. A review of normal joint structures is presented in Chapter 55.

■ SYSTEMIC AUTOIMMUNE RHEUMATIC DISEASES

Systemic autoimmune diseases are a group of chronic disorders that are characterized by diffuse inflammatory vascular lesions and degenerative changes in connective tissue. These disorders share similar clinical features and may affect the same organs. Rheumatoid arthritis (RA), systemic lupus erythematosus (SLE), polymyalgia rheumatica, temporal arteritis, and juvenile arthritis and dermatomyositis, which share an autoimmune systemic pathology are discussed.

RHEUMATOID ARTHRITIS

Rheumatoid arthritis is a systemic inflammatory disease that affects 0.3% to 1.5% of the population, women being affected two to three times more frequently than men.[1] Although the disease occurs in all age groups, its prevalence increases with age. The peak incidence in women is between ages 40 and 60 with onset at age 30 to 50.

Although the cause of RA remains somewhat mysterious, there is evidence that immunologic events may play an important role (see Chapters 13 and 14). About 70% to 80% of those with the disease have a substance called the *rheumatoid factor* (RF), an antibody directed against an autologous (self-produced) IgG antibody, in their blood.[4]

Why the body would begin to produce antibodies against its own IgG cannot be answered. It is possible that an infectious agent, such as a virus, could alter the immunoglobulin so that it is recognized as foreign. Another possibility is that genetic predisposition plays a role in the development of the response. A large number of people (60%) with RA have been found to have the histocompatibility antigen, human lymphocyte antigen (HLA), HLA-DR4.[1] HLA-DR4 may not only play a role in identifying susceptibility to RA but is also related to the severity of the disease.

PATHOLOGIC CHANGES

RF has been found not only in the blood, but also in the synovial fluid and synovial membrane of affected people. In fact, it has been shown that much of the RF is produced by lymphocytes present in the inflammatory infiltrate of the synovial tissue.[5] To explain the destructive changes that occur in RA, it has been suggested that the RF reacts with IgG or other types of antibodies to form immune complexes. These immune complexes activate the complement system, which, in turn, initiates the inflammatory reaction. Polymorphonuclear leukocytes, monocytes, and lymphocytes are attracted to the area. These cells phagocytize the immune complexes and, in the process, release lysosomal enzymes capable of causing destructive changes in the joint cartilage. The inflammatory response that follows attracts additional lymphocytes and plasma cells, setting into motion a chain of events that perpetuates the condition. As the inflammatory process advances, the synovial cells and the subsynovial tissue undergo a reactive hyperplasia. Vasodilation and increased blood flow cause warmth and redness. Swelling results from the increased capillary permeability that accompanies the inflammatory process.

Characteristic of RA is the development of an extensive network of new blood vessels in the synovial membrane, which contributes to the advancement of the rheumatoid synovitis. This destructive vascular granulation tissue, which is called *pannus*, extends from the synovium to involve the articular cartilage (Fig. 58-1). The inflammatory cells found in the pannus have a destructive effect on the adjacent

CHART 58-1: CLASSIFICATION OF THE RHEUMATIC DISEASES

I. Diffuse connective tissue diseases
  A. Rheumatoid arthritis
  B. Juvenile arthritis
    1. Systemic onset (Still's disease)
    2. Polyarticular onset
    3. Pauciarticular onset
  C. Systemic lupus erythematosus
  D. Systemic sclerosis
  E. Polymyositis/dermatomyositis
  F. Necrotizing vasculitis and other vasculopathies
    1. Polyarteritis nodosa group (includes hepatitis B–associated arteritis and Churg–Strauss allergic granulomatosis)
    2. Hypersensitivity vasculitis (includes Schönlein-Henoch purpura)
    3. Wegener's granulomatosis
    4. Giant cell arteritis (temporal arteritis, Takayasu's arteritis)
    5. Mucocutaneous lymph node syndrome (Kawasaki disease)
    6. Behçet's disease
    7. Cryoglobulinemia
    8. Juvenile dermatomyositis
  G. Sjögren's syndrome
  H. Overlap syndromes (includes undifferentiated and mixed connective tissue disease)
  I. Others (includes polymyalgia rheumatica, panniculitis (Weber–Christian disease), erythema nodosum, relapsing polychondritis, diffuse fasciitis with eosinophilia, adult onset Still's disease and others)

II. Arthritis associated with spondylitis
  A. Ankylosing spondylitis
  B. Reactive arthritis (Reiter's syndrome)
  C. Psoriatic arthritis
  D. Arthritis associated with chronic inflammatory bowel disease

III. Degenerative joint disease (osteoarthritis, osteoarthrosis)
  A. Primary (includes erosive osteoarthritis)
  B. Secondary

IV. Arthritis, tenosynovitis, and bursitis associated with infectious agents
  A. Direct
    1. Bacterial (staphylococci, gonococci, mycobacteria, spirochetes, and others)
    2. Viral, including hepatitis
    3. Fungal
    4. Parasitic
    5. Unknown, suspected (Whipple's disease)
  B. Indirect (reactive)
    1. Bacterial (includes acute rheumatic fever, intestinal bypass, postdysenteric—*Shigella*, *Yersinia*)
    2. Viral (hepatitis B)

V. Metabolic and endocrine diseases associated with rheumatic states
  A. Crystal-induced conditions
    1. Monosodium urate (gout)
    2. Calcium pyrophosphate dihydrate (pseudogout, chondrocalcinosis)
    3. Apatite and other basic calcium phosphates
    4. Oxalate
  B. Biochemical abnormalities
    1. Amyloidosis
    2. Vitamin C deficiency (scurvy)
    3. Specific enzyme deficiency states (includes Fabry's, Farber's, and others)
    4. Hyperlipoproteinemias (types II, IIa, IV, and others)
    5. Mucopolysaccharidoses
    6. Hemoglobinopathies (SS disease and others)
    7. True connective tissue disorders (Ehlers-Danlos, Marfan's osteogenesis imperfecta, and pseudoxanthoma elasticum)
    8. Hemochromatosis
    9. Wilson's disease (hepatolenticular degeneration)
    10. Ochronosis (alkaptonuria)
    11. Gaucher's disease
    12. Others
  C. Endocrine diseases
    1. Diabetes mellitus
    2. Acromegaly
    3. Hyperparathyroidism
    4. Thyroid disease (hyperthyroidism, hypothyroidism, thyroiditis)
  D. Immunodeficiency diseases (primary immunodeficiency, acquired immunodeficiency syndrome [AIDS])
  E. Other hereditary disorders
    1. Arthrogryposis multiplex congenita
    2. Hypermobility syndromes
    3. Myositis ossificans progressiva

VI. Neoplasms
  A. Primary (*e.g.*, synovioma, synoviosarcoma)
  B. Metastasis
  C. Multiple myeloma
  D. Leukemia and lymphoma
  E. Villonodular synovitis
  F. Osteochondromatosis
  G. Others

VII. Neuropathic disorders
  A. Charcot's joints
  B. Compression neuropathies
    1. Peripheral entrapment (carpal tunnel syndrome and others)
    2. Radiculopathy
    3. Spinal stenosis
  C. Reflex sympathetic dystrophy
  D. Others

VIII. Bone, periosteal, and cartilage disorders associated with articular manifestations
  A. Osteoporosis
    1. Generalized
    2. Localized (regional and transient)

(Continued)

CHART 58-1: CLASSIFICATION OF THE RHEUMATIC DISEASES (continued)

B. Osteomalacia
C. Hypertrophic osteoarthropathy
D. Diffuse idiopathic skeletal hyperostosis (includes ankylosing vertebral hyperostosis—Forrestier's disease)
E. Osteitis
   1. Generalized (osteitis deformans—Paget's disease of bone)
   2. Localized (osteitis condensans ilii; osteitis pubis)
F. Osteonecrosis
G. Osteochondritis (osteochondritis dissecans)
H. Bone and joint dysplasias
I. Slipped capital femoral epiphysis
J. Costochondritis (includes Tietze's syndrome)
K. Osteolysis and chondrolysis
L. Osteomyelitis
IX. Nonarticular rheumatism
   A. Myofascial pain syndromes
      1. Generalized (fibrositis, fibromyalgia)
      2. Regional
   B. Low back pain and intervertebral disk disorders
   C. Tendinitis (tenosynovitis) and/or bursitis
      1. Subacromial/subdeltoid bursitis
      2. Bicipital tendinitis, tenosynovitis
      3. Olecranon bursitis
      4. Epicondylitis, medial or laterial humeral
      5. DeQuervain tenosynovitis
      6. Adhesive capsulitis of the shoulder (frozen shoulder)
      7. Trigger finger
      8. Others

D. Ganglion cysts
E. Faciitis
F. Chronic ligament and muscle strain
G. Vasomotor disorders
   1. Erythromelalgia
   2. Raynaud's disease or phenomenon
H. Miscellaneous pain syndromes (includes weather sensitivity, psychogenic rheumatism)
X. Miscellaneous disorders
   A. Disorders frequently associated with arthritis
      1. Trauma (the result of direct trauma)
      2. Internal derangement of joints
      3. Pancreatic disease
      4. Sarcoidosis
      5. Palindromic rheumatism
      6. Intermittent hydrarthrosis
      7. Erythema nodosum
      8. Hemophilia
   B. Other conditions
      1. Multicentric reticulohistiocytosis (nodular panniculitis)
      2. Familial Mediterranean fever
      3. Goodpasture's syndrome
      4. Chronic active hepatitis
      5. Drug-induced rheumatic syndromes
      6. Dialysis-associated syndromes
      7. Foreign body synovitis
      8. Acne and hyradenitis suppurativa
      9. Pustulosis palmaris et plantaris
      10. Sweet's syndrome
      11. Others

(*Primer on the rheumatic diseases* [9th ed.]. [1988]. Atlanta: Arthritis Foundation)

cartilage and bone. Eventually, the pannus develops between the joint margins, leading to reduced joint motion and the possibility of eventual ankylosis. With the progression of the disease, joint inflammation and the resulting structural changes can lead to joint instability, muscle atrophy from disuse, stretching of the ligaments, and involvement of the tendons and muscles. The effect of the pathologic changes in the joint is related to the disease activity, which can change at any time. The destructive changes are irreversible.

CLINICAL MANIFESTATIONS

RA is often associated with extraarticular as well as articular manifestations. The disease, which is characterized by exacerbations and remissions, may involve only a few joints for brief durations or it may be relentlessly progressive and debilitating. About 3% of people with the disease have a progressive, unremitting form of RA that does not respond to aggressive therapy.[6]

Joint Manifestations. RA usually has an insidious onset marked by systemic manifestations such as fatigue, anorexia, weight loss, and generalized aching and stiffness. Joint involvement is usually symmetric and polyarticular. Any diarthrodial joint can be involved. The person may complain of joint pain and stiffness that lasts 30 minutes and frequently for several hours. The limitation of joint motion that occurs early in the disease is usually due to pain; later, it is due to fibrosis. The most frequently affected joints initially are the fingers, hands, wrists, knees, and feet. Later, other diarthrodial joints may become involved. Spinal involvement is usually limited to the cervical region. In the hands, there is usually bilateral and symmetric involvement of the proximal interphalangeal (PIP) and metacarpophalangeal (MCP) joints in the early stages of RA; the distal interphalangeal (DIP) joints are rarely affected. The fingers often take on a spindle-shaped appearance because of inflammation of the PIP joints (Fig. 58-2).

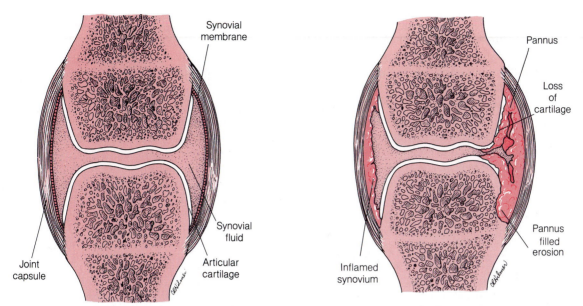

FIG. 58-1. (**Left**) Normal joint structures. (**Right**) Joint changes in rheumatoid arthritis. The left side denotes early changes occurring within the synovium, and the right side shows progressive disease that leads to erosion and the formation of pannus.

Progressive joint destruction may lead to subluxation and instability as well as limitation in movement. Swelling and thickening of the synovium can result in stretching the joint capsule and ligaments. When this occurs, muscle and tendon imbalance develop, and mechanical forces applied to the joints through daily activities produce joint deformities. In the MCP joints, the extensor tendons can slip to the ulnar side of the metacarpal head, causing ulnar deviation of the finger. Subluxation of the MCP joints

may develop when this deformity is present. Hyperextension of the PIP joint and partial flexion of the DIP joint is called a *swan neck deformity*. Once this condition becomes fixed, severe loss of function occurs, because the person can no longer make a fist. When flexion of the PIP joint with hyperextension of the DIP joint occurs, it is called a *boutonnière deformity*.

The knee is one of the most commonly affected joints and is responsible for much of the disability associated with the disease.[7] Active synovitis may be

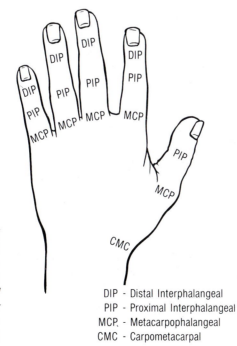

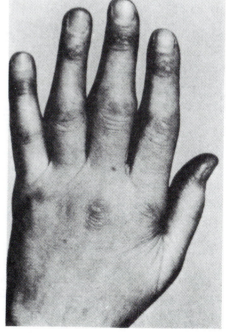

FIG. 58-2. (**Left**) Diagram of the joints of the hand. (**Right**) Early rheumatoid arthritis—spindling of the fingers. (Photograph reprinted from the *Revised clinical slide collection on the rheumatic diseases.* [1972]. Used by permission of the Arthritis Foundation)

DIP - Distal Interphalangeal
PIP - Proximal Interphalangeal
MCP - Metacarpophalangeal
CMC - Carpometacarpal

apparent as visible swelling that obliterates the normal contour over the medial and lateral aspects of the patella. The bulge sign, which involves milking fluid from the lateral to the medial side of the patella, may be used to determine the presence of excess fluid when it is not visible. Joint contractures, instability, and valgus (knock-knee) deformity are further manifestations that can occur. There is often severe quadriceps atrophy, which contributes to disability. A *Baker's cyst* may occur behind the knee. This is caused by enlargement of the bursa and usually does not cause symptoms unless the cyst ruptures, in which case symptoms mimicking thrombophlebitis appear.

Disease activity can limit flexion and extension of the ankle, which can create difficulty in walking. Involvement of the metatarsophalangeal joints can cause subluxation, hallux valgus, and cock-up toe deformities.

Neck discomfort is common. In rare cases, longstanding disease can lead to neurologic complications. Dislocation of the first cervical vertebra and subluxation of the odontoid process of the second vertebra into the foramen magnum is an uncommon but potentially fatal complication.

Extraarticular Manifestations. Although characteristically a joint disease, RA can affect a number of other tissues. Extraarticular manifestations probably occur with a fair degree of frequency but are usually mild enough to cause few problems. They are thought to be caused by circulating immune complexes and most likely to be present in people with a positive RF assay.

Because RA is a systemic disease, it may be accompanied by the previously mentioned complaints of fatigue, weakness, anorexia, weight loss, and low-grade fever when the disease is active. The erythrocyte sedimentation rate (ESR), which is commonly elevated during inflammatory processes, has been found to correlate with the amount of disease activity.[1] Anemia associated with a low serum iron level or low iron-binding capacity is common.[1] This anemia is generally resistant to iron therapy.

Rheumatoid nodules are granulomatous lesions that develop around small blood vessels. The nodules may be tender or nontender, movable or immovable. The size is variable. Typically they are found over pressure points such as the extensor surfaces of the ulna. The nodules may remain unless surgically removed, or they may resolve spontaneously.

Vasculitis is an uncommon manifestation of RA seen in people with a long history of active arthritis and high titers of RF. It is possible that some people have vasculitis that remains silent. Vasculitis is caused by the inflammatory process affecting the small and medium-sized arterioles. Manifestations

include ischemic areas in the nail fold and digital pulp that appear as brown spots. Ulcerations may occur in the lower extremities, particularly around the malleolar areas. In some cases, neuropathy may be the only symptom of vasculitis. The visceral organs, such as the heart, lungs, and gastrointestinal (GI) tract, may also be affected.

Other extraarticular manifestations include eye lesions such as episcleritis and scleritis, hematologic abnormalities, pulmonary disease, cardiac complications, infection, and Felty's syndrome (leukopenia with or without splenomegaly).

DIAGNOSIS AND TREATMENT

The diagnosis of RA is based on history, physical examination, and laboratory tests. Information should be elicited regarding the duration of symptoms, systemic manifestations, stiffness, and family history. The diagnostic criteria developed by the American Rheumatism Association are used in establishing the diagnosis (Chart 58-2). At least four of the criteria must be present to make a diagnosis of RA.

In the early stages, the disease is often difficult to diagnose. On physical examination, the affected joints show signs of inflammation, swelling, tenderness, and possibly warmth and reduced motion. The joints have a soft, spongy feeling because of the synovial thickening and inflammation. Body movements may be guarded to prevent pain. Changes in joint structure are usually not visible early in the disease.

RF may be used as a diagnostic test, but is incon-

CHART 58-2. PROPOSED 1987 REVISED AMERICAN RHEUMATISM ASSOCIATION CRITERIA FOR RHEUMATOID ARTHRITIS

Four or more of the following conditions must be present to establish a diagnosis of rheumatoid arthritis:
1. Morning stiffness for at least 1 hour and present for at least 6 weeks.
2. Swelling of three or more joints for at least 6 weeks.
3. Swelling of wrist, metacarpophalangeal or proximal interphalangeal joints for 6 or more weeks.
4. Symmetric joint swelling.
5. Hand roentgenogram changes typical of rheumatoid arthritis that must include erosions or unequivocal bony decalcification.
6. Rheumatoid nodules.
7. Serum rheumatoid factor found present by a method that is positive in less than 5% of normals.

(*Primer on the rheumatic diseases* [9th ed.]. [1988]. Atlanta: Arthritis Foundation. Used with the permission of the Arthritis Foundation)

clusive[8] because 1% to 5% of healthy people have RF.[1] The presence of RF seems to be more common with advancing age. A person can have RA without RF being present. Radiologic findings are not diagnostic in RA because joint erosions are often not seen on radiographic images in the early stages of the disorder.

Synovial fluid analysis can be helpful in the diagnostic process. The fluid has a cloudy appearance because the white blood cell count is elevated as a result of inflammation, whereas the complement components of the synovial fluid are depressed.

The treatment goals for a person with RA are to reduce pain, minimize stiffness and swelling, maintain mobility, and become an informed health care consumer. The treatment plan includes education about the disease and its treatment, rest, therapeutic exercises, and medications. Because of the chronicity of the disease and the need for continuous long-term adherence to the prescribed treatment modalities, it is important that the treatment be integrated with the person's lifestyle.

Basic education is fundamental in removing misconceptions. Both the person with arthritis and the general population need to know that although arthritis cannot be cured, much can be done to control its progress. Fear of being crippled is a major concern that should be addressed so the disease can be perceived realistically. All aspects of the treatment require that the person with arthritis accept responsibility for the health care program. Family members should be included in education programs; their support in integrating prescribed treatment regimens is important. Because many unproven remedies for arthritis are offered, patients need information on how to assess the validity of the available treatments. The Arthritis Foundation provides information and community services to people with arthritis and their families.

Both physical and emotional rest are important aspects of care. Physical rest reduces joint stress. Rest should include total body rest of 8 to 10 hours at night and one to two naps or rest periods during the day. Rest of specific joints is recommended to relieve pain. For example, sitting reduces the weight on an inflamed knee, and the use of lightweight splints reduces undue movement of the hand or wrist. Emotional rest is also important. Some people find that discomfort increases with emotional stress; with emotional rest, muscles relax and discomfort is reduced.

Although rest is essential, therapeutic exercises are important in maintaining joint motion and muscle strength. Range of motion exercises involve the active and passive movement of joints. Isometric (muscle tensing) exercises may be used to strengthen muscles. These exercises are frequently taught by a physical therapist and performed daily at home.

There is also a need to emphasize the difference between normal activity and therapeutic exercise. One of the most striking changes in the treatment of RA is the addition of aerobic exercises to the regimen of selected patients. Before this, it was felt that exercising patients with inflammatory arthritis would cause undue stress and strain on the joints and increase joint inflammation. Studies have shown that although people with RA have generally low levels of physical fitness, they can benefit from individualized exercise programs without experiencing joint damage or flares of the disease.[9]

Instruction in the safe use of heat and cold modalities to relieve discomfort and in the use of relaxation techniques is also important. Proper posture, positioning, body mechanics, and the use of supportive shoes can provide further comfort. Patients often need information about the principles of joint protection and work simplification. Some need assistive devices to reduce pain and improve their ability to perform activities of daily living.

Strategies to aid in symptom control also involve regulating activity by pacing, establishing priorities, and setting realistic goals. Support groups and group education experiences benefit some people. The home and work environments should be assessed, and interventions should be incorporated as the situation warrants.

Salicylates and their derivatives are often selected as the first medication of choice in treatment of RA. The dose required for treatment is within a range that reduces inflammation. The analgesic dose of aspirin is often less than the dose required to suppress inflammation, and people should be instructed that the antiinflammatory dose needs to be maintained to control symptoms. The exact mechanism of aspirin's action is not completely understood, but it is known to inhibit prostaglandin synthesis. Enteric-coated and buffered forms of aspirin are available and are sometimes better tolerated in people who are prone to GI side effects. Tinnitus and decreased hearing are common side effects that resolve when the medication dosage is reduced or discontinued. Sometimes other aspirin preparations are better tolerated, such as salsalate, choline magnesium trisalicylate, and diflunisal.[1] If the person cannot tolerate or does not receive benefit from aspirin, other nonsteroidal antiinflammatory drugs (NSAID) may be tried.

A slow-acting (or disease-modifying) drug may be added to the medication regimen to induce remission of the disease if it is not responding to the NSAIDs or other conservative therapy. The exact mechanism of action for the slow-acting medications such as gold compounds, hydroxychloroquine, penicillamine, methotrexate, azathioprine, and sulfasalazine is unknown, however, they do suppress the signs and symptoms of joint inflammation over periods of time. Their beneficial effects do not usually become evident until after 3 to 6 months of therapy.

Corticosteroid drugs may be used to reduce discomfort. To avoid long-term side effects, they are only used in specific situations for short-term therapy at a low dose level. They may be used for unremitting disease with extraarticular manifestations. This medication does not modify the disease, so it is unable to prevent joint destruction. Intraarticular corticosteroid injections can provide rapid relief of acute or subacute inflammatory synovitis (after infection is ruled out) in a few joints. They should not be repeated more than a few times a year.

Immunosuppressant drugs, such as azathioprine, cyclophosphamide, chlorambucil, and methotrexate have the potential for modifying the disease process in RA. Only azathioprine and methotrexate have U.S. Food and Drug Administration (FDA) approval for treatment of arthritis. Sulfasalazine, also not approved for treatment of RA, is an antibacterial antiinflammatory compound. Plasmapheresis, leukopheresis, lymphapheresis, thoracic-duct drainage, chemical or local radiation synovectomy, and total body irradiation are procedures considered experimental. More recent research and experimental treatments are in the area of immunobiologics. The new treatments focus on deleting only the destructive cells in the immune system rather than suppressing all of the immune system cells, which occurs with such drugs as methotrexate and azathioprine. These new treatments may hold promise for the future.

Surgery may be a part of the treatment of RA. Synovectomy may be indicated to reduce pain and joint damage when synovitis does not respond to medical treatment. The most common soft tissue surgery is tenosynovectomy (repair of damaged tendons) of the hand to release nerve entrapments. Total joint replacements may be indicated to reduce pain and increase motion.

Although the course of RA is unpredictable, the past 20 years have brought more effective treatment for the disease. Sufferers are being diagnosed and treated earlier. Criteria have been developed for remission in RA (Chart 58-3).

SYSTEMIC LUPUS ERYTHEMATOSUS

Systemic lupus erythematosus is a chronic inflammatory disease that ranges in severity from mild to potentially fatal. It is characterized by the formation of autoantibodies and immune complexes that can affect virtually any organ system including the musculoskeletal system. It is a major rheumatic disease

---

CHART 58-3: PROPOSED CRITERIA FOR CLINICAL REMISSION IN RHEUMATOID ARTHRITIS

Five or more of the following requirements must be fulfilled for at least 2 consecutive months:
1. Duration of morning stiffness not exceeding 15 minutes.
2. No fatigue.
3. No joint pain (by history).
4. No joint tenderness or pain on motion.
5. No soft tissue swelling in joints or tendon sheaths.
6. Erythrocyte sedimentation rate (Westergren method) less than 30 mm/h for a female or 20 mm/h for a male.

(*Primer on rheumatic diseases* [9th ed.]. [1988]. Atlanta: Arthritis Foundation. Used with permission of the Arthritis Foundation)

---

with a prevalence of about 1 in 2000, with approximately 500,000 people in the United States being afflicted with this disease. There is a female predominance, 9:1 over men, and closer to 30:1 during the childbearing years. SLE is more common in African Americans and Asians than whites, and the incidence in some families is higher.

The etiology of lupus is unknown. However, there is evidence the disease results from an autoimmune disorder brought about by a combination of factors that may include genetic, hormonal, and environmental factors.[10] Genetic studies suggest a genetic predisposition as evidenced by the occurrence of familial cases of lupus, especially among identical twins. In addition, the increased incidence in African Americans versus whites suggests genetic factors. As many as four genes may be involved in the expression of lupus in humans. HLA genes may be important in that certain HLA genes encode proteins that are keys to immune recognition and play a part in the development of SLE.[11]

Studies also suggest that an imbalance in sex hormone levels may play a role in the development of the disease, especially because the disease is so prevalent in women. Androgens appear to protect, whereas estrogens seem to favor the development of SLE. It has been suggested that an imbalance in sex hormone levels may lead to a heightened helper T cell and weakened suppressor T cell immune response that could lead to the development of autoantibodies.[1]

Possible environmental triggers include ultraviolet light, chemicals (hydralazine, hair dyes, drugs), some foods, and possibly infectious agents.[10] Ultraviolet (UV) light, specifically UVB associated with exposure to the sun or unshielded fluorescent bulbs, may trigger an exacerbation. Photosensitivity is present in approximately one third of lupus patients.

Pathologic Process. People with lupus appear to have increased production of both self and nonself antigens and B-cell hyperreactivity. The basis for the B-cell hyperreactivity could result from several mechanisms. In theory, excessive helper T-cell function or defective suppressor T-cell function could alter the B-cell response (see Chapter 13).

The pathologic process likely begins with the activation of polyclonal B-cells, causing exaggerated production of autoantibodies. The autoantibodies team up with corresponding antigens to form immune complexes (see Chapter 14). When there is a disorder of immune regulation, as in lupus, these immune complexes build up and are deposited in vascular and tissue surfaces, triggering an inflammatory response and ultimately causing local tissue injury. Some autoantibodies that have been identified in lupus are antinuclear antibodies (ANA), including anti-DNA. Other antibodies may be produced against various cells, including red cell surface antigens, platelets, coagulation factors, and other antibodies. Autoantibodies against red blood cells can lead to anemia, and those against platelets to thrombocytopenia.

CLINICAL MANIFESTATIONS

SLE can manifest in a variety of ways. The disease has been called the *great imitator* because it has the capacity for affecting so many different body systems. It can affect the musculoskeletal system, the skin, the pericardium, the lungs, the kidney, the central nervous system (CNS), and the red blood cells and platelets. The onset may be acute or insidious, and the course of the disease is characterized by exacerbations and remissions.

Arthralgias and arthritis are among the most commonly occurring early symptoms of SLE, and approximately 90% of all patients with lupus complain of joint pain at some point during the course of their disease.[1] The polyarthritis of lupus initially can be confused with other forms of arthritis, especially RA, because of the symmetric arthropathy. However, on radiologic examination, there is rarely articular destruction. Ligaments, tendons, and the joint capsule may be involved, causing varied deformities in approximately 30% of patients. Flexion contractures, hyperextension of the interphalangeal joint, and subluxation of the carpometacarpal joint contribute to the deformity and subsequent loss of function in the hands. Other musculoskeletal man-

ifestations of lupus include tenosynovitis, tendon rupture of the intrapatellar and Achilles tendon, and avascular necrosis (frequently of the femoral head). Besides the musculoskeletal system, SLE can affect other major organ systems, including the skin, heart, lungs, GI system, kidneys, CNS, lymph and vascular systems.

Skin manifestations can be of many different types and may be classified as acute, subacute, or chronic. The acute skin lesions comprise the classic malar or "butterfly" rash on the nose and cheeks (Fig. 58-3). This rash is seen in SLE and may also be associated with other skin lesions, such as hives, livedo reticularis (reticular-cyanotic discoloration of the skin, often precipitated by cold), and fingertip lesions such as periungual erythema, nail fold infarcts, and splinter hemorrhages. Hair loss is common. Mucous membrane lesions tend to occur during periods of exacerbation. Sun sensitivity may occur in lupus even after mild sun exposure.

Discoid lupus (chronic cutaneous) involves plaque-like lesions on the head, scalp, and neck. These lesions first appear as red, swollen patches of skin, and later there can be scarring, depigmenta-

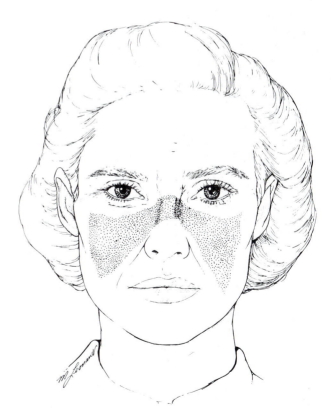

FIG. 58-3. The butterfly (malar) rash of systemic lupus erythematosus. (Smeltzer, S. C., & Bare, B. C. [1992]. *Brunner & Suddarth's textbook of medical-surgical nursing* [7th ed.]. Philadelphia: J.B. Lippincott)

tion, and plugging of hair follicles. Ninety percent of patients with discoid lupus have disease that only involves the skin.

Subacute cutaneous lupus (SCLE) is a less severe form of lupus. The skin lesions in this condition may resemble psoriasis. These lesions are found in sun-exposed areas such as the face, chest, upper back, and arms. Patients with SCLE may have mild systemic problems, which are usually limited to joint and muscle pains. There is a low incidence of lupus nephritis in SCLE.

Renal involvement in SLE occurs in about 50% of patients. Several forms of glomerulonephritis may occur including mesangial, focal proliferative, diffuse proliferative, and membranous (see Chapter 32). Interstitial nephritis may also occur. Nephrotic syndrome causes proteinuria with resultant edema in the legs, abdomen, and around the eyes. Renal failure may or may not be preceded by nephrotic syndrome. Kidney biopsy is the best determinant of renal damage and the extent of treatment needed.

Pulmonary involvement in SLE occurs in 40% to 50% of patients and is manifested primarily by pleural effusions or pleuritis. Less frequently occurring pulmonary problems include acute pneumonitis, pulmonary hemorrhage, chronic interstitial lung disease, and pulmonary embolism.

Pericarditis is the most common of the cardiac manifestations occurring in up to 30% to 40% of lupus patients and is often accompanied by pleural effusions. Myocarditis can be seen in up to 25% of patients. Congenital heart block can occur in infants of mothers with lupus who have a specific type of ANA (anti-Ro) in their serum. Secondary heart disease is also a problem in lupus. Hypertension may be associated with lupus nephritis and long-term corticosteroid use. Ischemic heart disease can occur in older patients with longer duration lupus. Infective carditis is rare but can occur with valvular lesions.[12]

The CNS may also be involved in 30% to 75% of lupus patients. SLE can cause damage in several ways: vasculitis may impede blood flow, causing strokes or hemorrhage; the immune system may produce antineuronal antibodies, which attack nerve cells; and lupus anticoagulants or anticariolipin antibodies may indirectly cause blood clots in the brain. Seizures can occur and with increased frequency when renal failure is present. Psychiatric symptoms may vary, including psychosis, depression, unnatural euphoria, dementia (decreased cognitive functioning), confusion, and altered consciousness. More research is being done on the role of psychological factors triggering the onset of lupus.

Hemolytic disorders may involve hemolytic anemia, leukopenia, lymphopenia, or thrombocytope-

nia. Lymphadenopathy may also occur in 50% of all lupus patients.[13]

DIAGNOSIS AND TREATMENT

The diagnosis of lupus can be complicated and difficult. The American College of Rheumatology has defined eleven criteria to be considered in the diagnosis of lupus, but these are intended for use in clinical trials rather than individual diagnosis.[14] Diagnosis is based on a complete history and physical examination, as well as analysis of the blood work. No single test can diagnose lupus in all patients.

The most common laboratory test performed is the immunofluorescence test for ANA. Ninety-five percent of untreated lupus patients have a high ANA level. The ANA test is not specific for lupus, though, and positive ANA results may be found in healthy people or may be associated with other disorders. The anti-DNA antibody test is more specific for the diagnosis of lupus.[15] Other serum testing may reveal moderate to severe anemia, thrombocytopenia, and leukocytosis or leukopenia. Additional immunologic tests may be done to give support to the diagnosis or to differentiate SLE from other connective tissue diseases.

Treatment of lupus focuses on managing both the acute and chronic symptoms of the disease. Patient–physician communication and trust are the basis for long-term disease management. Patients are the best source of information about the pattern of their own disease activity. Teamwork can reduce the need for unnecessary hospitalization, testing, expense, and anxiety.

The goals of treatment include preventing progressive loss of organ function, reducing the possibility of exacerbations, minimizing disability from the disease process, and preventing complications from medication therapy.[16]

Treatment with medications may be as simple as a drug to reduce inflammation, such as an NSAID. NSAIDs can control fever, arthritis, and mild pleuritis. An antimalarial drug may be the next medication considered to treat cutaneous and musculoskeletal manifestations of lupus. Adrenal corticosteroids are used to treat more significant symptoms of SLE, such as renal and CNS disorders. High-dose corticosteroid treatment is used for acute symptoms, and the drug is tapered to the lowest therapeutic dose as soon as possible to minimize the adverse effects. Immunosuppressive drugs are used in cases of severe disease. Cyclophosphamide, under closely monitored circumstances, has been found to be beneficial in the treatment of lupus nephritis.

SYSTEMIC SCLEROSIS

Systemic sclerosis, sometimes prefixed by the term progressive, is sometimes called *scleroderma*. In this disorder, the skin is thickened through fibrosis with an accompanying fixation to the subdermal structures, including the sheaths or fascia covering tendons and muscles. Clinical manifestations include muscular atrophy, pain, edema, calcification, and arthrodesis. The condition is systemic and may involve the CNS, lungs, esophagus, heart, duodenum, and kidneys. African Americans and women are more susceptible to this disease than white men. The etiology of this rare disorder, although characterized by proliferative vascular changes, is not well understood. A variant of systemic sclerosis is the *CREST* syndrome. This acronym represents the manifestations of *calcinosis, Raynaud's phenomenon, esophageal dysmotility, sclerodactyly* (localized scleroderma of the fingers), and *telangiectasia*.

POLYMYOSITIS AND DERMATOMYOSITIS

Polymyositis and dermatomyositis are chronic inflammatory myopathies. The pathogenesis is multifactorial and includes cellular and humoral immune mechanisms.[17] Systemic manifestations are common, and cardiac and pulmonary complications often adversely affect the outcome. These conditions are characterized by symmetric proximal muscle weakness and occasional muscle pain and tenderness.

In summary, RA is a systemic inflammatory disorder that affects 0.3% to 1.5% of the population. Women are affected more frequently than men. This form of arthritis, the cause of which is unknown, has a chronic course and is usually characterized by remissions and exacerbations. Joint involvement is symmetric and begins with inflammatory changes in the synovial membrane. As joint inflammation progresses, structural changes can occur, leading to joint instability. Systemic manifestations include weakness, anorexia, weight loss, and low-grade fever. Some extraarticular features include rheumatoid nodules, vasculitis, and Sjögren's syndrome. The treatment goals include reducing pain, stiffness, and swelling, maintaining mobility, and assisting the person to become an informed health care consumer.

SLE is a chronic autoimmune disorder that affects multiple body systems. There is no known cause of lupus, however, the disease may result from an immunoregulatory disturbance brought about by a combination of factors that may involve genetic, hormonal, and environmental triggers. Some drugs have been shown to induce lupus, especially in the elderly. There is an exaggerated production of autoantibodies, which team up with antigens to produce an immune complex. The buildup of immune complexes causes an inflammatory response in affected tissues. Treatment focuses on preventing loss of organ function, controlling inflammation, and minimizing complications of medication therapy.

■ ARTHRITIS ASSOCIATED WITH SPONDYLITIS

The spondlyoarthropathies are disorders of the axial skeleton. Inflammation of the axial skeleton develops at sites where ligament inserts into bone rather than the synovium. It frequently involves the sacroiliac joints. Sometimes a person with spondyloarthropathy also has inflammation and involvement of the peripheral joints, in which case, the signs and symptoms overlap with other inflammatory types of arthritis (*e.g.*, RA). However, the disorders differ from RA in that there is an absence of the RF factor; hence, they are often referred to as *seronegative spondyloarthropathies*.

The seronegative spondyloarthropathies include ankylosing spondylitis, juvenile ankylosing spondylitis, reactive arthritis (Reiter's syndrome), psoriatic arthritis, and enteropathic (inflammatory bowel disease) arthritis. There is also clinical evidence of overlap between the various seronegative spondyloarthropathies.

ANKYLOSING SPONDYLITIS

Ankylosing spondylitis is an inflammatory disease of the axial skeleton, including the sacroiliac joints, intervertebral disk spaces, and the apophyseal and costovertebral articulations. Bilateral sacroiliitis is a primary feature of the disease. Occasionally, large synovial joints may be involved, usually the hips, knees, and shoulders. Small peripheral joints are usually not affected.

This disorder is more common than was once believed; it probably affects about 1% to 2% of the population, which is comparable to the prevalence of RA.[18] At one time the disease was thought to occur 4 to 10 times more frequently in men than in women. It appears that the prevalence in women is probably the same or only slightly less than in men, but the disease is not usually as severe in women.[19] Although ankylosing spondylitis can occur in people of any age, it is usually diagnosed in the second or third decade of life. The disease is seen frequently in North American native Americans and is rarely seen in African Americans and Asians.[20]

Ankylosing spondylitis may cause fibrosis, calcification, and ossification of joints with progression to ankylosis. The disease generally brings to mind an image of a person with a rigid bamboolike spine.

Fortunately, however, few people develop a progressive disease pattern that leads to this outcome. The disease spectrum ranges from an asymptomatic sacroiliitis to a progressive disease that can affect many body systems. When a progressive disease pattern does develop, it is usually in men.

PATHOLOGIC CHANGES

The basic pathogenesis of ankylosing spondylitis is unknown. However, the presence of mononuclear cells in acutely involved tissue suggests an immune response. HLA-B27 remains one of the best-known examples of an association between a disease and a hereditary marker. Although about 90% of people with ankylosing spondylitis possess the HLA-B27 antigen, HLA-B27 is also present in about 8% of the normal population.[21] Several theories have been advanced to account for the association between HLA-B27 and ankylosing spondylitis. One possibility is that the gene that determines the HLA-B27 antigen may be linked to other genes that determine pathologic autoimmune phenomena or that lead to increased susceptibility to infections or environmental agents. A second theory has to do with molecular mimicry. The general idea is that an autoimmune reaction to an antigenic determinant site in the host's tissues may occur as a consequence of an immunologic response to an identical or closely related antigen of a foreign agent (usually infectious).

CLINICAL MANIFESTATIONS

The person with ankylosing spondylitis typically complains of low back pain, which may be persistent or intermittent. The pain, worse when resting, particularly when lying in bed, may initially be blamed on muscle strain or spasm from physical activity. Lumbosacral pain may also be present, with discomfort in the buttocks and hip areas. Sometimes pain can radiate to the thigh in a manner similar to that of sciatic pain. Although the pain is usually in the lower back, some people may complain of pain at a higher vertebral level as an initial symptom. Prolonged stiffness is present in the morning and after periods of rest. Mild activity helps reduce pain and stiffness. It is understandable that sleep patterns are frequently interrupted because of these manifestations. Walking or exercise may be needed to provide the comfort needed to return to sleep. Muscle spasm may also contribute to discomfort.

Loss of motion in the spinal column is characteristic of the disease. The severity and duration of disease activity influence the degree of mobility. Motion can be lost in anterior or lateral flexion, extension, and rotation of the spinal column. Loss of lumbar lordosis occurs as the disease progresses, and this is followed by kyphosis of the thoracic spine and extension of the neck. A spine fused in the flexed position is the end result in severe ankylosing spondylitis. A kyphotic spine makes it difficult for the patient to look ahead and to maintain balance while walking.

Some form of peripheral arthritis occurs in 20% to 30% of people with ankylosing spondylitis.[20] Women seem to have peripheral joint disease more frequently than men. Involvement is usually asymmetric and affects hip, shoulder, and knee joints. Hip pain can be a major cause of disability. The lower the age at onset, the greater the likelihood of progression to total hip replacement.[1]

Systemic features of weight loss, fever, and fatigue may be apparent. Uveitis develops in up to 25% of those affected by ankylosing spondylitis.[1] Osteoporosis can occur, especially in the spine, which contributes to the risk of spinal fracture. Fusion of the costovertebral joints can lead to reduced lung volume.

Complications of ankylosing spondylitis, although infrequent, include fractures in ankylosed areas of the spine, atlantoaxial subluxation (the atlas is the first cervical vertebra and articulates above with the occipital bone and below with the axis), spinal cord compression, aortic regurgitation, apical fibrosis of the lung, amyloidosis, and cauda equina syndrome with bowel and bladder dysfunction. The complications are more likely in longstanding disease.

The disease process varies considerably among individuals. Exacerbations and remissions are common; their unpredictability can create uncertainty in planning daily activities as well as future goals and expectations. Fortunately, most of those affected are able to lead productive lives.

The prognosis in ankylosing spondylitis is generally good. The first decade of disease predicts the remainder. Severe disease usually occurs early and is marked by peripheral arthritis, especially of the hip. Mortality is low (6%), and significant disability occurs in less than 20% of people with the disorder.

DIAGNOSIS AND TREATMENT

The early and precise diagnosis of ankylosing spondylitis is closely related to a favorable prognosis. Early recognition allows for implementation of a conservative and usually effective treatment program on a lifelong basis. The diagnosis of ankylosing spondylitis is based on history, physical examination, and x-ray examination. Several methods are available to assess mobility and detect sacroiliitis. These methods include pressure on the sacroiliac joints with the person in a forward bending position to elicit pain and muscle spasm, measurement of the distance between the tips of fingers and the floor in a bent over position with straight knees, and the modified Schöber's test in which contralateral flexion of the back is measured. Although these measures alone do not provide a diagnosis of ankylosing spondylitis or other spondyloarthropathies, they can provide useful measurements for monitoring the disease status. Chest expansion may be used as an indirect indicator of thoracic involvement, which usually occurs late in the disease. Measurements are taken at the fourth intercostal space. Normally the chest expands by 4 to 5 cm with inspiration. This measurement is more difficult to obtain in women and less specific in older people with a normal decrease in expansion, smokers, or those with emphysema.

Laboratory findings frequently include an elevated ESR. A mild normocytic normochromic anemia may also be present. HLA typing is not diagnostic of the disease and should not be used as a routine screening procedure.

Radiologic evaluations help differentiate sacroiliitis from other diseases. In early disease, x-ray images may be normal. Vertebrae are normally concave on the anterior border. In ankylosing spondylitis the vertebrae take on a squared appearance (Fig. 58-4). Spinal changes usually follow a progressive ascending pattern up the spine.

Treatment is directed at controlling pain and maintaining mobility by suppressing inflammation. Instruction should address proper posture and positioning. This includes sleeping in a supine position on a firm mattress using one small pillow or no pillow. Sleeping in extension may reduce the possibility of flexion contractures. A bed board may be used to supply additional firmness. Therapeutic exercises are important to assist in maintaining motion in peripheral joints and in the spine. Muscle-strengthening exercises for extensor muscle groups are also prescribed. Heat applications or a shower or bath may be beneficial before exercise to improve ease of movement. These strategies can also be used in the morning or at bedtime to reduce stiffness and pain. Immobilizing joints is not recommended.

Maintaining ideal weight reduces the stress on weight-bearing joints. Smoking should be discouraged because it can exacerbate respiratory problems. Swimming is an excellent general conditioning exercise that avoids joint stress and enhances muscle tone. Occupational counseling or job evaluation may be warranted because of postural abnormalities.

Aspirin or NSAIDs are used to reduce inflammation, which, in turn, helps to control pain and reduce muscle spasm. Phenylbutazone is highly effective, but its use should be limited to people with severe disease in whom other agents have failed because of

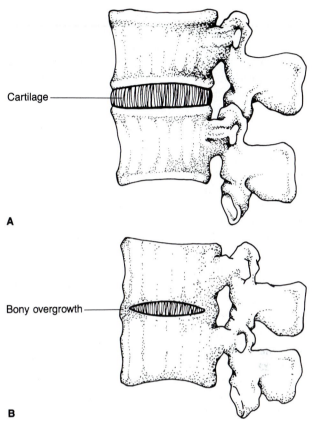

A

B

FIG. 58-4. The bony overgrowth (**B**) of the vertebra characteristic of ankylosing spondylitis is evident when compared with normal vertebra (**A**).

potential bone marrow suppression in long-term usage.[20]

Most peripheral joint pain and limitations of motion occur in the hip. Total hip replacement surgery helps reduce pain and increase mobility. Anesthesia can be problematic for people with cervical rigidity or with reduced chest expansion. These factors need to be weighed before surgery is considered.

REACTIVE ARTHRITIS

Reactive arthritis, including Reiter's syndrome, is a seronegative arthritis in which an infective trigger mechanism (sexually transmitted or enteric infection) is suspected. The reactive arthropathies may be defined as a sterile inflammatory arthropathy distant in time and place from the initial inciting infective process. It can occur after *Shigella-, Salmonella-, Campylobacter-,* or *Yersinia*-associated diarrhea or sexually transmitted *Ureaplasma* or *Chlamydia* infections (the gonococcus produces direct infection of the joint and is not a cause of reactive arthritis). Reactive arthritis has been observed in people with acquired immunodeficiency syndrome (AIDS).[21] Urethritis is ordinarily the first feature of the disease; conjunctivitis and arthritis, typically of the lower extremities, usually follow. Not all people exhibit this triad of features; some people may have only one or two of them. In addition to urethritis, other mucocutaneous manifestations may be present, including mouth ulcerations, balanitis circinata, and skin rashes. Low back pain is common. Spinal radiologic changes are similar to ankylosing spondylitis but may be more asymptomatic. Reactive arthritis may follow a self-limited course; it may involve recurrent episodes of arthritis, or, in a small number of cases, it may follow a continuous unremitting course. The treatment is largely symptomatic. NSAIDs are used in treating the arthritic symptoms. Although the disease is precipitated by an infection, there is no evidence that antibiotic therapy alters the course of the disease.

PSORIATIC ARTHRITIS

Psoriatic arthritis is a seronegative inflammatory arthropathy that affects 5% to 7% of people with cutaneous psoriasis. Psoriatic lesions precede or appear concomitantly with joint lesions in about 85% of cases.[22] At least 20% of those with psoriatic arthritis have an elevated serum uric acid. The abnormally elevated serum uric acid is caused by the rapid skin turnover of psoriasis, the breakdown of nucleic acid, and the metabolism to uric acid value. This finding may lead to misdiagnosis of gout.[23] Psoriatic arthritis tends to be slowly progressive. For clinical purposes, it is useful to recognize two major groups of patients: those with axial and those with peripheral psoriatic arthritis. Asymmetric oligoarthritis occurs most commonly (60% to 70%).[22] When fingers or toes are involved, there is diffuse swelling or *sausaging*. Often, affected joints are surprisingly functional and only minimally symptomatic.

ENTEROPATHIC ARTHRITIS

Spondyloarthritis is also associated with inflammatory bowel diseases such as Crohn's disease, regional enteritis, and ulcerative colitis in about 15% of the cases. When arthritis is present, it has usually developed before the bowel disease, especially in Crohn's disease. Knees are most frequently involved (75%), followed by ankles and wrists. Sacroiliitis occurs in approximately 10% of people with inflammatory bowel disease. In this form of arthritis, the activity of the bowel disease is not related to the activity of the arthritis.

In summary, spondyloarthropathies affect the axial skeleton. Inflammation develops at sites where ligaments insert into bone. Ankylosing spondylitis is considered a prototype of this classification category. Bilateral sacroiliitis is the primary feature of ankylosing spondylitis. The disease spectrum ranges from asymptomatic sacroiliitis to a progressive disorder affecting many body systems. The etiology remains unknown; however, a strong association between HLA-B27 antigen and ankylosing spondylitis has been identified. Loss of motion in the spinal column is characteristic of the disease. Peripheral arthritis may occur in some people. Other forms of spondyloarthritis include reactive arthritis and spondyloarthritis associated with inflammatory bowel disease. Although there are overlapping features of each of the spondyloarthropathies (Table 58-1), clinical distinction is important to identify etiologic differences and determine the specific treatment.

■ DEGENERATIVE JOINT DISEASE

OSTEOARTHRITIS

Osteoarthritis, also referred to as *degenerative joint disease* or *osteoarthrosis*, is the most familiar form of arthritis. It is a chronic condition of unknown etiol-

TABLE 58-1. COMPARISON OF THE SPONDYLOARTHROPATHIES

CHARACTERISTIC	ANKYLOSING SPONDYLITIS	REITER'S DISEASE	PSORIATIC ARTHRITIS	INFLAMMATORY BOWEL DISEASE
Age at onset	Young adult	Young to middle age	Any age	Any age
Type of onset	Gradual	Sudden	Variable	Gradual
Sacroiliitis	>95%	20%	20%	10%
Peripheral joint involvement	25%	90%	All (about 5% to 7% of those patients with psoriasis)	Occasional
HLA-B27 (in whites)	>90%	75%	<50%	<50%
Eye involvement	25% to 30%	Common	Occasional	Occasional

(Adapted from Arnett, F.C., Khan, M.A., & Willkens, R.F. [1989]. A new look at ankylosing spondylitis. *Patient Care, 23* [19], 82–101)

ogy that can lead to loss of mobility and chronic pain, often causing significant disability, especially when the involved joints are critical to the performance of daily activities.

One third of all adults in the United States have x-ray evidence of osteoarthritis of the hand, foot, knee, or hip. The incidence of osteoarthritis increases with age until by the late fifties or early sixties, more than 60% and possible as great as 85% of the population probably have some degree of cartilage abnormality in many of their major joints.[24] However, only 15% to 25% of this number experience significant symptoms, discrediting the hypothesis that symptomatic osteoarthritis is an inevitable result of aging.[25] Even in patients with clinically apparent (by radiologic evidence of narrowed joint space) osteoarthritis, progressive age does not necessarily imply increases in pain or disability.

The joint changes associated with osteoarthritis are progressive loss of articular cartilage and an associated synovitis that is secondary. These changes are accompanied by joint pain, stiffness, limitation of motion, and possibly joint instability and deformity. Although there may be periods when mild inflammation is present, it is not the severe destructive type seen in the inflammatory forms of rheumatic diseases such as RA.

Osteoarthritis may occur as a primary idiopathic or a secondary disorder although this distinction is not always clear. Idiopathic osteoarthritis of the hip may reflect subtle developmental defects or as a sequela of diseases of childhood because these conditions produce joint incongruity and increase impact loading.[26] Primary osteoarthritis occurs without an obvious reason and is the most common form. There is a genetic predisposition to some forms of osteoarthritis, such as Heberden's nodes, which affect the DIP joints of the hand. Studies also implicate immunologic factors in the perpetuation and acceleration of the osteoarthritic change.[27]

The secondary form of the disease develops because of some identifiable reason. For example, osteoarthritis can occur secondary to joint instability caused by injury to a knee ligament or a meniscus cartilage tear. Other joint disorders such as RA, damage from metabolic alterations of the cartilage, and crystal deposition may also cause secondary osteoarthritis. Repetitive use or abuse of the joint related to occupation or sports may contribute to the development of osteoarthritis. The anecdotal evidence for association of osteoarthritis with injury, both acute and chronic, is strong. The response to mechanical trauma may be influenced by genetics, endocrine, psychological and cultural factors as well as the aging process. The ability of articular cartilage to withstand fatigue testing (*i.e.*, to resist fracture with the applica-

tion of repetitive low-magnitude loads) diminishes progressively with age.

The relationship between obesity and the development of osteoarthritis is still controversial, but obesity has been associated with osteoarthritis of the knee in women, probably as a result of additional mechanical stress.[28] Excess fat may have a direct metabolic effect on cartilage, over and above the effects of excess joint stress.

Two primary prevention efforts for osteoarthritis are (1) reduction of excessive weight to decrease the incidence of osteoarthritis of the knee and (2) efforts to reduce the rate of accidental injuries to decrease site-specific osteoarthritis.[29]

PATHOLOGIC CHANGES

Osteoarthritis is a disorder of the articular cartilage and subchondral bone (bony plate that supports the articular cartilage) of diarthroidal joints (Fig. 58-5). A balance between mechanical stress and the ability of the joint tissues to resist that stress exists in the diarthrodial joints. Osteoarthritis represents a deterioration (degeneration) of the articular cartilage caused by a physiologic imbalance between the stress applied to the joint tissues and the ability of the joint tissues to withstand the stress. Either the articular cartilage and underlying bone are normal but excessive loads applied to the joints causes the tissues to fail, or a physiologic reasonable load is applied to the joint but the articular cartilage or bone is defective.

Articular cartilage plays two essential mechani-

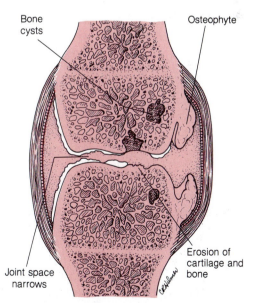

FIG. 58-5. Joint changes in osteoarthritis. The left side denotes early changes and joint space narrowing with cartilage breakdown. The right side shows more severe disease progression with lost cartilage and osteophyte formation.

cal roles in joint physiology. First, the articular cartilage serves as a remarkably smooth bearing surface. In combination with synovial fluid, the articular cartilage provides extremely low friction during movement. Second, the cartilage also transmits load down to the bone, dissipating the mechanical stress. The subchondral bone serves to protect the overlying articular cartilage, providing it with a pliable bed and absorbing energy.

Cartilage is a specialized type of connective tissue. As with other types of tissue, it consists of cells (the chondrocytes) nested in an extracellular matrix. In articular cartilage, the extracellular matrix is composed of water, proteoglycans, collagen, and ground substance. The proteoglycans, which are large macromolecules made up of disaccharides and amino acids, afford elasticity and stiffness, permitting articular cartilage to resist compression. The ground substance constitutes a highly hydrated semisolid gel. Collagen molecules consist of polypeptide chains that form long fibrous strands. They provide form and tensile strength. The primary function of the collagen fibers is to provide a rigid scaffold to support the chondrocytes and ground substance of cartilage. The hydrated proteoglycan molecules, because of their macromolecular size and charge, are entrapped within the collagen meshwork of the extracellular matrix. Because of the inextensibility of the collagen fibers, the proteoglycans are prevented from expanding to their maximum size. This confers a high osmotic pressure within the tissue.

Under physiologic conditions of impact loading, the joint is protected with both passive and active mechanisms. Passive mechanisms include fracture and deformation of the subchondral bone. Deformation is essential for maximizing the contact area and for minimizing the stress. A progressive increase in the number of microfractures in subchondral bone may be detrimental to normal joint function because the remodeled trabeculae may be stiffer than normal and less effective as shock absorbers. Under such circumstances, the subchondral bone cannot deform normally with load. The increased incongruity of joint surfaces that occurs normally with loading is diminished, and stress is concentrated at contact areas on the articular cartilage (Fig. 58-6).

Under conditions of repeated movement, articular cartilage is highly resistant to wear. But repetitive impact loading rapidly leads to joint failure, hence the high prevalence of osteoarthritis specific to vocational or avocational sites (*i.e.,* shoulders and elbows of baseball pitchers, ankles of ballet dancers, knees of basketball players). Although this process is occurring in the cartilage, changes are also taking place in the underlying subchondral bone. The subchondral bone plate thickens and can become eburnated (like

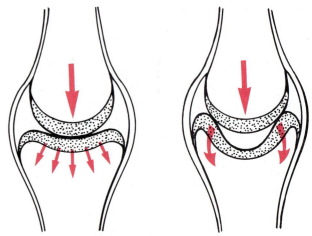

FIG. 58-6. (Left) A joint normally undergoes deformation of the articular cartilage and the subchondral bone when carrying a load. This maximizes the contact area and spreads the force of the load. **(Right)** If the joint does not deform with a load, the stresses are concentrated and the joint breaks down. (Redrawn from Brandt, K. D., & Radin, E. [1987]. The physiology of articular stress: Osteoarthroses. *Hospital Practice* [January 15], 111)

an ivorylike mass). Sclerosis, or formation of new bone and cysts, usually occurs in the juxtaarticular bone (the bone near the joint). New bone that forms at the joint margins is called an *osteophyte (spur)*.

To further understand the pathology of osteoarthritis, the lubrication of the joint must be considered. Under high loads, lubrication depends on a film of interstitial fluid squeezed out of the cartilage after compression of the opposing surfaces of the joint. The greater the load is, the better the lubrication. With depletion of proteoglycans from the cartilage matrix in osteoarthritis, the mechanisms that normally operate under high loads to produce a pressurized lubricating squeeze film may be impaired. Attempts to devise artificial lubricants have been unsuccessful because they impede the flow of interstitial fluid into and out of the cartilage surface.

Mild synovitis may occur in osteoarthritis. This inflammation represents a reactive process and is more likely to be seen in advanced disease. The synovitis may be related to the release of free cartilage proteoglycan from the deteriorating articular cartilage. Immunologic factors may also be involved. Calcium pyrophosphate and apatite crystals are common in osteoarthritic knee effusions.[1]

Immobilization is another factor that can produce degenerative changes in articular cartilage. Cartilage degeneration due to immobility may result from loss of the pumping action of lubrication that occurs with joint movement. These changes are more marked and appear earlier in areas of contact but occur also in areas not subject to mechanical compression. By 3 weeks after remobilization, all biochemical, metabolic, and morphologic abnormalities in the cartilage that result from immobilization are reversed. Although cartilage atrophy is rapidly reversible with activity after a period of immobilization, impact exercise during the period of remobilization can prevent reversal of the atrophy. Slow, gradual remobilization may be important in preventing cartilage injury and has clinical implications with respect to instructions to patients concerning the recommended level of physical activity after removal of a cast.

CLINICAL MANIFESTATIONS

The manifestations of osteoarthritis may occur suddenly or insidiously. Initially, pain may be described as aching and may be somewhat difficult to localize. Pain can occur at rest, several hours after the use of the involved joints. Crepitus and grinding may be evident when the joint is moved. As the disease advances, even minimal activity may cause pain.

The most frequently affected joints are the hips, knees, lumbar and cervical vertebrae, proximal and DIP joints of the hand, the first carpometacarpal joint, and the first metatarsophalangeal joints of the feet. Table 58-2 identifies the joints that are commonly affected by osteoarthritis and the common clinical features correlated with the disease activity of each particular joint.

Other clinical features are limitations of joint motion and joint instability. Joint enlargement is usually due to new bone formation, so that the joint feels hard, in contrast with the soft, spongy feeling characteristic of the joint in RA. Sometimes mild synovitis or increased synovial fluid is present, which can also cause joint enlargement.

DIAGNOSIS AND TREATMENT

Osteoarthritis is often contrasted with RA, yet the difference is sometimes not readily apparent.[30] The diagnosis of osteoarthritis is usually determined by history and physical examination, x-ray studies, and laboratory findings that exclude other diseases. Criteria for the classification of osteoarthritis of the knee, hand, and hip have been developed.[31–33]

Some patients with significant symptoms of osteoarthritis may have surprisingly normal x-rays. Characteristic radiologic changes include first medial joint space narrowing followed by subchondral bony sclerosis, formation of spikes on the tibial eminence and osteophytes. Laboratory studies are usually normal because the disorder is not a systemic disease. The sedimentation rate may be slightly elevated in generalized osteoarthritis or erosive inflammatory variations of the disease. If inflammation is present, there may be a slight increase in cell count. The synovial fluid is also usually normal.

The treatment of osteoarthritis is directed toward the relief of pain and the maintenance of mobility and is tailored to the needs of the person. Treatment is determined by the extent of the disease, the joints involved, and the response to previous and current treatment regimens. Education about the disease and type of treatment methods is important. Treatment usually proceeds in a stepwise manner from simple to more comprehensive measures.

First, the joint should not be further abused and steps should be taken to protect and rest the involved joint. This includes weight reduction (when weight-bearing surfaces are involved) and use of a cane or walker if the hips and knees are involved. Physical therapy is directed toward pain relief, maintenance or improvement in joint range of motion, and strengthening of involved muscles.

Independent studies have shown that not all NSAIDs are the same. A drug that produces the desired clinical response but at the same time is benign to cartilage should be selected. The understanding of the effects of NSAIDs on cartilage metabolism is far from complete. A comparison study of the efficacy of ibuprofen given in either an antiinflammatory dose (high dose) or an analgesic dose (low dose) with that of the commonly used, over-the-counter analgesic, acetaminophen, showed no significant differences among the treatment groups, suggesting that acetaminophen, which is less toxic and less costly, may be a better treatment for osteoarthritis.[34]

If the patient becomes more limited or the regimen is unsuccessful in adequately relieving symptoms, corticosteroid injections may be helpful, especially for those who have an effusion of the joint. Injections are usually limited to a total of four and not more than three within 1 year because their use may accelerate joint destruction.

Surgery is considered when the person is having severe pain and joint function is severely reduced. Procedures include arthroscopic lavage and debridement, bunion resections, osteotomies to change alignment of the knee and hip joints, and decompression of the spinal roots in osteoarthritic vertebral stenosis. Total hip replacements have provided effective relief of symptoms and improved range of motion for many people, as have total knee replacements, although the latter procedure has produced less consistent results. Joint replacement is available for the first carpometacarpal joint. Arthrodesis is used in advanced disease to reduce pain; however, this results in loss of motion. Cartilage transplantation may be a form of treatment in the future.

TABLE 58-2. CLINICAL FEATURES OF OSTEOARTHRITIS

JOINT	CLINICAL FEATURES
Cervical spine	Localized stiffness; radicular or nonradicular pain; posterior osteophyte formation may cause vascular compression
Lumbar spine	Low back pain and stiffness; muscle spasm; decreased back motion; nerve root compression causing radicular pain; spinal stenosis
Hip	Most common in older male adults; characterized by insidious onset of pain, localized to groin region or inner aspect of the thigh; may be referred to buttocks, sciatic region, or knee; reduced hip motion; leg may be held in external rotation with hip flexed and adducted; limp or shuffling gait; difficulty getting in and out of chairs
First carpometacarpal joint (CMC)	Tenderness at base of thumb; squared appearance to joint
Proximal interphalangeal joint (PIP) Bouchard's nodes	Same as for distal interphalangeal joint disease
Distal interphalangeal joint (DIP) Heberden's nodes	Occurs more frequently in women; usually involves multiple DIPs, lateral flexor deviation of joint, spur formation at joint margins, pain and discomfort following joint use
Knee	Localized discomfort with pain on motion; limitation of motion; crepitus; quadriceps atrophy due to lack of use; joint instability; genu varus or valgus; joint effusion
First metatarsal phalangeal joint (MTP)	Insidious onset; irregular joint contour; pain and swelling aggravated by tight shoes

In summary, osteoarthritis, the most common form of arthritis, is a localized condition affecting primarily the weight-bearing joints. The disorder is characterized by degeneration of the articular cartilage and subchondral bone. It has been suggested that the cellular events responsible for the development of osteoarthritis begin with some type of abnormal mechanical insult or stimuli including hormones and growth factors, drugs, mechanical stresses, and the extracellular environment. Studies also implicate immunologic factors in the perpetuation and acceleration of the osteoarthritic change. As cartilage ages, biochemical events such as collagen fatigue and fracture occur with less stress. Attempts at repair by increased matrix synthesis and cellular proliferation maintain the integrity of the cartilage until failure of reparative processes allows the degenerative changes to progress. Joint enlargement is usually due to new bone formation, which causes the joint to feel hard. Pain and stiffness are primary features of the disease. Inflammatory mediators (*e.g.*, prostaglandins) may increase the inflammatory and degenerative response. The treatment is directed toward the relief of pain and maintenance of mobility while preserving the articular cartilage. The next few years will see changes in the traditional conservative attitudes in the management of this underemphasized condition.

■ METABOLIC DISEASES ASSOCIATED WITH RHEUMATIC STATES

Metabolic bone disorders result from biochemical and metabolic disorders that affect the joints. As Chart 58-1 indicates, many metabolic and endocrine diseases are associated with rheumatic disorders. The discussion in this chapter is limited to the crystal-induced arthopathies.

CRYSTAL-INDUCED ARTHROPATHIES

Crystal deposition within joints has been shown to produce arthritis. In gout, monosodium urate or uric acid crystals are found in the joint cavity; in another condition called pseudogout, calcium pyrophosphate dihydrate (CPPD) crystals are found in the joints.

GOUT

The manifestations of the heterogeneous group of diseases known as the gout syndrome include: (1) acute gouty arthritis with recurrent attacks of severe articular and periarticular inflammation; (2) tophi or the accumulation of crystalline deposits in articular surfaces, bones, soft tissue, and cartilage; (3) gouty nephropathy or renal impairment; and (4) uric acid kidney stones. Primary gout is predominantly a disease of men with peak incidence in the fourth or sixth decade. Only 3% to 7% of cases occur in women, and most of these are in postmenopausal women.[35]

URIC ACID METABOLISM AND ELIMINATION

Uric acid is a metabolite of the purines, adenine and guanine. Normally, about two thirds of the uric acid produced each day is excreted through the kidneys; the rest is eliminated through the GI tract. Normal renal handling of uric acid involves three steps: (1) filtration, (2) reabsorption, and (3) secretion. Uric acid is freely filtered across the glomerulus, completely reabsorbed in the proximal tubule, and is secreted back into the tubular fluid by another mechanism in the distal end of the proximal tubule or distal tubule (see Chapter 31). The tubular secretion and postsecretory reabsorption determine the final concentration of uric acid in the urine.

Most people with gout have a reduced urate clearance. In these people, the serum urate level becomes elevated so that a normal amount of urate can be excreted and urate homeostasis can be achieved. Most people with increased production of urate have increased excretion of uric acid. However, if kidney damage is present, an increased amount of uric acid is eliminated by the GI tract.

Small doses of uricosuric agents may preferentially reduce secretion and increase uric acid retention, whereas therapeutic doses block reabsorption and increase uric acid elimination. The salicylates reduce secretion and cause retention of uric acid when given at doses used for pain relief; very large doses are needed to block both reabsorption and secretion. Consequently, aspirin and other salicylates are not recommended for use as an analgesic in people with gout. Some of the diuretics, including the thiazides, which are weak acids, are secreted by the proximal tubular cells and can also interfere with the excretion of uric acid.

MECHANISMS OF HYPERURICEMIA

Hyperuricemia reflects a metabolic derangement in extracellular fluids. Asymptomatic hyperuricemia is a laboratory finding and not a disease. Hyperuricemia is defined as a serum urate concentration greater than 7.0 mg/dL measured by the specific uricase method.[36] Monosodium urate crystal deposition develops when hyperuricemia is present. However, most people with hyperuricemia do not develop gout. Attacks of gout seem to be related to sudden increases or decreases in serum uric acid levels. Hyperuricemia may occur because of overproduction of uric acid, underexcretion of uric acid, or a combination of the two. Primary and secondary forms of hyperuricemia exist. Primary causes are related to genetic defects in purine metabolism. Secondary forms of hyperuricemia are related to certain disease conditions and medications.

An attack of gout occurs when the monosodium urate crystals precipitate within the joint and initiate an inflammatory response. This may follow a sudden rise in the serum urate levels. The excess urate is not soluble and therefore precipitates. Gout can also occur with a sudden drop in the urate level. In either situation, crystals are released into the synovial fluid and an inflammatory response is initiated.

Phagocytosis of urate crystals by the polymorphonuclear leukocytes occurs and leads to polymorphonuclear cell death with release of lysosomal enzymes. As this process continues, the inflammation causes destruction of the cartilage and subchondral bone. Tophi are large, hard nodules that have an irregular surface and contain crystalline deposits of monosodium urate that incite an inflammatory response. They are most commonly found in the synovium, olecranon bursa, Achilles tendon, subchondral bone, and extensor surface of the forearm and may be mistaken for rheumatoid nodules. Tophi usually do not appear until an average of 10 years or more after the first gout attack. This stage of gout, called chronic tophaceous gout, is characterized by more frequent and prolonged attacks, which are often polyarticular. Crystal deposition usually occurs in peripheral areas of the body such as the great toe and the pinnae of the ear. Sodium urate is less soluble at temperatures below 37°C. The peripheral tissues are cooler than other parts of the body, and this may at least partially explain why gout occurs most frequently in peripheral joints.[37]

The typical acute attack of gout is monoarticular and usually affects the first metatarsophalangeal joint. The tarsal joints, insteps, ankles, heels, knees, wrists, fingers, and elbows may also be initial sites of involvement. Acute gout often begins at night after more than usual exercise. The onset of pain is typically abrupt with redness and swelling. The attack may last for days or weeks. Pain may be severe enough to be aggravated even by the weight of a bed sheet covering the affected area.

Attacks of gout may be precipitated by certain medications, foods, or alcohol. After the first attack, it may be months or years before another attack. The attacks usually become more frequent, and, as they do, more joints become affected.

In the early stages of gout after the initial attack has subsided, the person is asymptomatic, and joint abnormalities are not evident. This is referred to as intercritical gout. As attacks recur with increased frequency, joint changes occur and become permanent.

DIAGNOSIS AND TREATMENT

Although hyperuricemia is the biochemical hallmark of gout, the presence of hyperuricemia cannot be equated with gout, because many people with this condition never develop gout. A definitive diagnosis of gout can be made only when monosodium urate crystals are present in the synovial fluid or in tissue sections of tophaceous deposits. Synovial fluid analysis is useful in ruling out other conditions, such as septic arthritis, pseudogout, and RA.

The next step is to determine if the disorder is related to overproduction or to underexcretion of uric acid. The uric acid level is determined, and a 24-hour urine sample is collected. Ideally, the person should be on a purine-free diet during the time the urine specimen is being collected. Urate urine values above the normal range of 264 to 588 mg/day indicate an overproduction of uric acid.[13] The normal serum urate concentration is 5.0 to 5.7 mg/dL in men and 3.7 to 5.0 mg/dL in women.[38]

The objectives in the treatment of gout are: (1) termination and prevention of the acute attacks of gouty arthritis and (2) correction of hyperuricemia, with consequent inhibition of further precipitation of sodium urate and absorption of urate crystal deposits already in the tissues. Management of acute disease is directed toward reducing joint inflammation. Hyperuricemia and related problems of tophi, joint destruction, and renal problems are treated after the acute inflammatory process has subsided. NSAIDs, particularly indomethacin and ibuprofen, are used for treating acute gouty arthritis. Alternative therapies include colchicine and intraarticular corticosteroids. Treatment with colchicine is used early in the acute stage. Although the drug is usually given orally, a more rapid response is obtained when colchicine is given intravenously. The nausea and diarrhea that may occur with large oral doses are avoided when the drug is given intravenously. The acute symptoms of gout usually subside within 48 hours after treatment with oral colchicine has been instituted and within 12 hours after intravenous administration of the drug.

NSAIDs are effective during the acute stage when used at their maximum dosage and are sometimes preferred to colchicine because they have fewer toxic side effects. Phenylbutazone is usually effective but is usually only used on a short-term basis because long-term use can cause bone marrow suppression. The corticosteroid drugs are not recommended for treatment of gout unless all other medications have proved unsuccessful. Intraarticular injections of corticosteroid agents may be used when only one joint is involved and the person is unable to take colchicine or nonsteroidal drugs.

With the exception of phenylbutazone, the drugs used to treat acute gout have no effect on the serum urate level and thus are valueless in tophaceous gout and the control of hyperuricemia. After the acute attack has been relieved, the hyperuricemia is treated. One method is to reduce hyperuricemia through the use of allopurinol or a uricosuric agent (probenecid or sulfinpyrazone, a phenylbutazone derivative). These compounds are not used in the treatment of acute gouty arthritis and, if given, only tend to exacerbate and prolong the inflammation. These uricosuric medications prevent the tubular reabsorption of urate. The serum urate concentrations are monitored to determine efficacy and dosage. These drugs are usually started in small doses and gradually increased over 7 to 10 days. Aspirin should not be used with these medications because it decreases the urinary excretion of uric acid.

Allopurinol is the preferred antihyperuricemic therapy for patients with frequent attacks of gout, significant hyperuricemia (greater than 9 to 11 mg/

dL), significant hyperuricosuria (greater than 800 to 1000 mg/day, tophi, uric acid urolithiasis, or urate nephropathy. Allopurinol inhibits xanthine oxidase, an enzyme needed for the conversion of hypoxanthine to xanthine and xanthine to uric acid. There is a slight possibility that xanthine kidney stones can develop if allopurinol is used for many years. It is usually reserved for the person who does not have an adequate response or is unable to tolerate other forms of treatment.

Treatment of hyperuricemia is aimed at maintaining normal uric acid levels and requires lifelong treatment. Prophylactic colchicine or NSAIDs may be used between gout attacks. If the uric acid level is normal and the person has not had recurrent attacks of gout, these medications may be discontinued.

Gout can be effectively controlled by medical management; however, it often is not, because many people with gout have a limited understanding of the disease and therefore a low compliance with treatment.[39] Education about the disease and its management is fundamental to the treatment and management of gout. The sufferer should be made aware that the prognosis is very good and that the disease, although chronic, can be controlled in almost all cases. Some changes in lifestyle may be needed, such as maintenance of ideal weight, moderation in alcohol consumption, and avoiding purine-rich foods, such as liver, kidney, sardines, anchovies, and sweetbreads, particularly in patients with excessive tophaceous deposits. Adherence to the lifelong use of medications may be the only major lifestyle change for many people.

CALCIUM CRYSTAL DEPOSITION DISEASE

Calcium pyrophosphate dihydrate crystal deposition disease, or pseudogout, is an acute, inflammatory arthritis caused by the deposition of CPPD crystals within the joint. The inflammation can occur in one or several joints and lasts for several days. The diagnosis is confirmed by x-ray studies, synovial fluid analysis, or biopsy. The knee and wrist are the joints most commonly involved. As in gout, the person with pseudogout may be asymptomatic between attacks. Colchicine may be used to treat an acute attack. Unlike gout, there are no drugs that can remove the CPPD crystals from the joints. The degenerative changes associated with pseudogout are treated by supportive measures similar to those used in the treatment of osteoarthritis.

Other calcium phosphates, including hydroxyapatite, and calcium oxalate cause extraskeletal calcific deposits. Articular and periarticular calcifica-

tions are often of no consequence. Calcium oxalates have been identified in connective tissue disease and may be a factor in some renal-dialysis arthropathies.[1]

In summary, crystal-induced arthropathies are characterized by crystal deposition within the joint. Gout is the prototype of this group. Acute attacks of arthritis occur with gout and are characterized by the presence of monosodium urate crystals in the joint. The disorder is accompanied by hyperuricemia, which results either from overproduction of uric acid or from the reduced ability of the kidney to rid the body of excess uric acid. Management of acute disease is first directed toward the reduction of joint inflammation; then the hyperuricemia is treated. Hyperuricemia is treated with uricosuric agents, which prevent the tubular reabsorption of urate, or with medication that inhibits the production of uric acid. Although gout is chronic, in most cases it can be controlled.

■ RHEUMATIC DISEASES IN CHILDREN AND THE ELDERLY

RHEUMATIC DISEASES IN CHILDREN

Children can be affected with almost all of the rheumatic diseases. In addition to disease-specific differences, these conditions affect not only the child but the family. There is need for special attention to growth and development issues. Adherence to the treatment program requires intervention with both the child and parents. School issues have to be addressed.

Juvenile Rheumatoid Arthritis. Juvenile rheumatoid arthritis is a chronic disease that affects approximately 60,000 to 200,000 children in the United States.[1] It is characterized by synovitis and can influence epiphyseal growth by stimulating growth of the affected side. Generalized stunted growth may also occur.

Systemic onset (Still's disease) affects about 20% of children with juvenile rheumatoid arthritis (JRA).[1] The symptoms include a daily intermittent high fever, which is usually accompanied by a rash, generalized lymphadenopathy, hepatosplenomegaly, leukocytosis, and anemia. Most of these children also have joint involvement. Systemic symptoms usually subside in 6 to 12 months. This form of JRA can also make an initial appearance in adulthood. Infections, heart disease, and adrenal insufficiency may cause death.

A second subgroup of JRA, pauciarticular arthritis, affects no more than four joints.[1] This subgroup affects 40% of children with JRA. The pauciarticular arthritis affects two distinct groups. The first group generally consists of females less than 6 years of age with chronic uveitis. Antinuclear antibody testing in this group is usually positive. The second group, in whom the arthritis is of late onset, is most commonly made up of males. The HLA-B27 tests are positive in over half of this group. Sacroiliitis is present and the arthritis is usually in the lower extremities.

The third subgroup of JRA, accounting for about 40% of the total, is polyarticular onset disease. It affects more than four joints during the first 6 months of the disease. This form of arthritis more closely resembles the adult form of the disease than the other two subgroups. RF is sometimes present and may indicate a more active disease process. Systemic features include a low-grade fever, weight loss, malaise, anemia, stunted growth, slight organomegaly (*e.g.*, hepatosplenomegaly), and adenopathy.[1]

The prognosis for most children with RA is good. Aspirin is the main medication used. Although some NSAIDs are available, not all have been approved by the FDA for use in children. Intramuscular gold therapy is often used when aspirin or NSAIDs have proven ineffective. Other aspects of treatment of children with JRA are similar to those used for the adult with RA. Children are encouraged to lead as normal a life as possible.

Systemic Lupus Erythematosus. The features of SLE in children are similar to the disease in adults. The incidence in children is 10 times lower, estimated to occur in 0.6 of 100,000 children. The occurrence in sexes is almost equal until pubescence, then approaches the sex ratio seen in adults. The clinical manifestations of lupus in children reflect the extent and severity of systemic involvement. The best prognostic indicator in children is the extent of renal involvement, which is more common and more severe in children than in adults with SLE. Infectious complications are the most common cause of death (40%) in children with lupus. Children with lupus may present with constitutional symptoms including fever, malaise, anorexia, and weight loss. Symptoms of the skin, musculoskeletal, central nervous, cardiac, pulmonary, and hematopoietic systems are similar to those of adults. Endocrine abnormalities include Cushing's syndrome from long-term corticosteroid use, and autoimmune thyroiditis. Adolescents often experience menstrual disturbances, which tend to resolve with disease remission.[40] Treatment of lupus in children is similar to that of adults. NSAIDs, corticosteroids, antimalarials, and immunosuppressive agents are used depending on the symptoms. Corticosteroids may cause stunting of growth and necrosis of femoral heads and other joints. Immunization schedules should be maintained using attenuated rather than live vaccines. Rest periods should be balanced with exercise; children should be encouraged to maintain as normal a

schedule as possible.[41] The diversity of the clinical manifestations of lupus in the young requires the establishment of a comprehensive program.[42]

Juvenile Dermatomyositis. Juvenile dermatomyositis (JDMS) is an inflammatory myopathy primarily involving skin and muscle and associated with a characteristic rash. Symmetric proximal muscle weakness, elevated muscle enzymes, evidence of vasculitis, and electromyogram (EMG) changes confirming an inflammatory myopathy are diagnostic for JDMS. Generalized vasculitis is not seen in the adult form of the disease. JDMS can affect children of all ages, with a mean age at onset of 8 years. There is an increased incidence in females. The etiology is unknown. The rash may precede or follow the onset of proximal muscle weakness. Periorbital edema, erythema, and eyelid telangiectasia are common. Calcifications can occur in 30% to 50% of children with JDMS and are, by far, the most debilitating symptom.

The calcifications appear at pressure point sites or sites of previous trauma. JDMS is treated primarily with corticosteroids to reduce inflammation. Occasionally, immunosuppressives are used in cases of refractory disease.[1,43]

Juvenile Spondyloarthropathies. Ankylosing spondylitis, Reiter's syndrome, psoriatic arthritis, and spondyloarthopathies associated with ulcerative colitis and regional enteritis can present in children as well as adults. In children, spondyloarthritis presents in peripheral joints first, mimicking pauciarticular JRA, with no evidence of sacroiliac or spine involvement for months to years after onset. The spondyloarthopathies are more common in boys and commonly occur in children who have a positive family history. HLA-B27 typing is helpful in diagnosing children because of the unusual presentation of the disease. Management of the disease involves physical therapy, education, attention to school and growth and development issues. Medication treatment includes the use of salicylates or other NSAIDs such as tolmetin or indomethacin. More severe disease or symptoms may require systemic corticosteroids.[1]

RHEUMATIC DISEASES IN THE ELDERLY

Arthritis is, by far, the most common complaint of elderly people. The pain, stiffness, and muscle weakness impact on daily life, often threatening independence and quality of life. The symptomatology of the rheumatic diseases also can have an indirect, and

even threat to the duration of life for the elderly. The weakness and gait disturbance that are often a part of the rheumatic diseases can contribute to the likelihood of falls and fracture, causing suffering, health care costs, further loss of independence, and potential for decreased life span. The elderly cope less well with mild to moderately severe disease that, in younger people, is less likely to lead to serious disability for the same degree of impairment.[44]

Because arthritis is the leading cause of change in the functional status of older adults, a functional status approach to the problems of the elderly is appropriate. Inactivity is a societal expectation of the elderly.[45] What activity there is tends to be of the nature of leisurely walking. Deconditioning occurs. It has been noted that the elderly seem to lose function in a roughly predictable order (doing chores and errands, rising from a chair, picking up clothes, walking, rising from bed, and lifting a cup to the mouth). Those with self-reported arthritis tend to lose function in a more variable order, especially with regard to hand function.[46]

Older patients often have multiple diagnoses. This complicates both diagnosis and management. The diagnosis of an elderly patient with musculoskeletal syndromes can lie among a wide variety of disorders that are usually regarded as outside the range of typical rheumatic disease. Among these are metastatic malignancy, multiple myeloma, musculoskeletal disorders accompanying endocrine or metabolic disorders, orthopedic conditions, and neurologic disease.

There is a difference in the manifestations, diagnosis, and treatment of some of the rheumatic diseases in the elderly. The usual presentation of these conditions has been discussed earlier in this chapter. One form of rheumatic disease that has a predilection for the elderly is polymyalgia rheumatica. This condition is discussed here.

An increased incidence of false-positive tests for RF and antinuclear antibodies is found in the elderly population with or without rheumatic disease because older people are better producers of autoantibodies than younger people.

Rheumatoid Arthritis. The prevalence of RA increases with advancing age, at least until age 75.[47] For the majority, the manifestations are less severe, with a somewhat greater chance of remission.[48] The close resemblance of the manifestations of seronegative RA in the elderly to those of polymyalgia has led to speculation concerning the relationship of these syndromes.[49] It may be that RA in the elderly is a broad disorder that includes a number of distinct subsets with characteristic manifestations, course, and outcome.

Systemic Lupus Erythematosus. SLE is another condition with different manifestations in the elderly.[50] The disease is less frequently accompanied by renal involvement. However, pleurisy, pericarditis, arthritis, and symptoms closely resembling polymyalgia rheumatica are increased. The characteristics of lupus in the elderly closely resemble those of drug-induced lupus, thus leading to speculation that the syndrome may be due to some one of the multiple drugs that are taken by many elderly patients.

Osteoarthritis. Osteoarthritis is, by far, the most common form of arthritis among the elderly and too often is either accepted by patient or expected by physician. It has been suggested that osteoarthritis begins at a very young age, expressing itself in the elderly only after a long period of latency. Osteoarthritis presents a major management problem, but there is much that can be done.

Gout. The frequency of clinical gout increases with advancing age. This is due in part to the increased incidence of clinical involvement after years (especially after approximately 20 years) of continued hyperuricemia.[51] Serum urate levels rarely occur in women before menopause, therefore one would expect to find initial attacks of clinical gout occurring about age 70 or 20 years after menopause.[52] Furthermore, gouty attacks in elderly women may be precipitated by the use of diuretics.

The treatment of gout is more difficult in the elderly. Although colchicine may be effective in controlling the symptoms of chronic gout, it may cause diarrhea in some patients, limiting its effectiveness in maintenance therapy.

Calcium Pyrophosphate Disease. As part of the tissue-aging process, osteoarthritis develops with associated cartilage degeneration. Calcium pyrophosphate crystals are shed into the joint cavity. These crystals may produce a low-grade chronic inflammation—the chronic pseudogout syndrome. The accumulation of calcium pyrophosphate and related crystalline deposits in articular cartilage is common in the elderly. Although it may be asymptomatic, its presence may contribute to more rapid cartilage deterioration. This condition may be present with severe osteoarthritis.

Polymyalgia Rheumatica. Of the forms of arthritis affecting the elderly, polymyalgia rheumatica (PMR) is one of the more difficult to diagnose and one of the most important to identify. Elderly women are known to be especially at risk. A certain percentage of patients with polymyalgia rheumatica also have temporal arteritis (giant cell arthritis), frequently with involvement of the ophthalmic arteries. If this condition is untreated, it carries a serious threat of blindness, which can be avoided by the use of large doses of corticosteroids. It is possible that a number of patients are erroneously diagnosed as having RA or osteoarthritis. In patients with an elevated Westergren ESR (above 50 mm), diagnosis is usually with a trial dose of prednisone (10 to 15 mg/day) for 3 days.[53] Patients with polymyalgia rheumatica typically exhibit striking clinical improvement about the second day. Patients with RA also show improvement but usually days later. Treatment with NSAIDs provides relief for some patients, but most require continuing therapy with prednisone, with gradual reduction of dose over the course of 1.5 to 2 years using symptoms as the primary guide. Patients need close monitoring during the maintenance phase on the prednisone. Because their symptoms are relieved, they often quit taking the steroid and symptoms recur, or doses are missed and the decreased dosage leads to an increase in symptoms. Unless careful assessment reveals the frequency of missed doses, the physician may be misled to increasing dosage when it is not needed. Because of the side effect of the corticosteroids, the goal is to use the lowest dose of the drug necessary to control the symptomatology. Weaning patients off low-dose prednisone therapy after this length of time can be difficult and extended over a period of time. The nurse must work closely with the elderly patient to give the correct dosage as the amount is slowly decreased. Even a small error in dosage can set the tapering program back by weeks or months.

For those patients at risk for temporal arteritis, adherence to the medication program is critical with preservation of sight the goal. Because this complication can occur so quickly and is relatively asymptomatic, it is vital that the patient understands the importance of taking the correct dose regularly as prescribed. Treatment is by large doses (60 to 80 mg/day) of prednisone. The usual side effects occur, some of which (osteoporosis) are more than that normally expected. This dosage is continued for 4 to 6 weeks and then decreased gradually to 10 to 15 mg/day.

Localized Musculoskeletal Disorders. The elderly are also prone to localized musculoskeletal syndromes. Years of wear of rotator cuff against the acromion frequently lead to a range of inflammatory disorders including bursitis and tendinitis. These are known collectively as impingement syndromes.

Tennis elbow (although only 5% of people with this problem actually play tennis), or humeral epicondylitis, is also frequently seen among the elderly.

Other localized inflammatory conditions of the musculoskeletal system affecting the elderly are fibrositis/fibromyalgia and Dupuytren's contracture.

Management of Rheumatic Disease. In addition to diagnosis-specific treatment, the elderly require special consideration in treatment. Management techniques that rely on modalities other than drugs are particularly important for the elderly. These include splints, walking aids, muscle-building exercise, and local heat. Muscle-strengthening and stretching exercises are particularly effective in the elderly person with age-related losses in muscle function. Rest, the cornerstone of conservative therapy, is hazardous in the elderly in whom there can be a rapid loss of muscle strength.

A study of pain management techniques used by older adults showed they used fewer combined methods than a younger group.[54] Increasing the elderly arthritis patient's use of combined pain management modalities such as medication, rest, heat, distraction, exercise, and talking with others may be helpful.

The NSAIDs may be less well tolerated by the elderly. In addition to bleeding from the GI tract, there may be cognitive dysfunction, manifested by forgetfulness, inability to concentrate, sleeplessness, paranoid ideation, and depression.

Even such things as frequent visits to the physician's office for the laboratory monitoring that is necessary with drugs such as gold can be difficult or impossible for elderly patients who live in a cold climate during the winter.

The elderly are more apt to conceal symptoms than to elaborate on them because they either feel they are a part of the aging process or that "nothing can be done." One of the ways to enhance a person's ability to combat the symptoms of arthritis is by enforcing a greater sense of control on the part of the elderly person.[55] Therefore, the more the elderly patient can be involved in the management and treatment program, the better. Joint arthroplasty is used for pain relief and increased function. Chronologic age is not a contraindication for surgical treatment of arthritis. In appropriately selected elderly candidates, survival and functional outcome after surgery are equivalent to those in younger age groups. In fact, the more sedentary activity level of the elderly makes them even better candidates for joint replacement, because the life of a joint replacement is shortened by active lifestyles.

In summary, rheumatic diseases that affect children can be similar to the adult disease, but often there are specific manifestations unique to the younger population. In addition to disease-specific differences, children with chronic diseases have to be approached with different priorities than adults. Managing rheumatic diseases in children requires a team approach to address issues of the family, school, growth and development, and coping strategies, as well as a comprehensive disease management program.

Arthritis is the most common complaint of elderly population. The pain, stiffness, and muscle weakness impact on daily life, often threatening independence and quality of life. There is a difference in the manifestations, diagnosis, and treatment of some of the rheumatic diseases in the elderly. Osteoarthritis is the most common form of arthritis among the elderly. The prevalence of RA and gout also increases with advancing age. One form of rheumatic disease that has a predilection for the elderly is polymyalgia rheumatica. A certain percentage of patients with polymyalgia rheumatica also have temporal arteritis (giant cell arthritis), frequently with involvement of the ophthalmic arteries. If this condition is untreated, it carries a serious threat of blindness.

■ REFERENCES

1. Schumacher, H.R. (Ed.). (1988). *Primer on the rheumatic diseases* (9th ed.). Atlanta: Arthritis Foundation.
2. Harris, E.D., Jr. (1989). The clinical features of rheumatoid arthritis. In W.N. Kelley, E.D. Harris, S. Ruddy, & C.B. Sledge (Eds.). *Textbook of rheumatology* (3rd ed., pp. 943–981). Philadelphia: W.B. Saunders.
3. Collo, M.C.B., Johnson, J.L., Finch, W.R., & Felicetta, J.V. (1991). Evaluating arthritic complaints. *Nurse Practitioner, 16*(2), 9–20.
4. Harris, E. (1990). Rheumatoid arthritis: Pathophysiology and implications for therapy. *New England Journal of Medicine, 322*(18), 1277–1289.
5. Harris, E.D., Jr. (1989). The pathogenesis of rheumatoid arthritis. In W.N. Kelley, E.D. Harris, S. Ruddy, & C.B. Sledge (Eds.). *Textbook of rheumatology* (3rd ed., pp. 905–942). Philadelphia: W.B. Saunders.
6. Harris, E.D., Jr. (1989). The clinical features of rheumatoid arthritis. In W.N. Kelley, E.D. Harris, S. Ruddy, & C.B. Sledge (Eds.). *Textbook of rheumatology* (3rd ed., pp. 943–981). Philadelphia: W.B. Saunders.
7. Lotke, P.A. (1985). Knee surgery. In P.D. Utsinger, N.J. Zvaifler, & G.E. Ehrlich (Eds.), *Rheumatoid arthritis: Etiology, diagnosis, and management* (p. 783). Philadelphia: J.B. Lippincott.
8. Lightfoot, R. (1990). Clinical reasoning in the management of rheumatoid arthritis. *Journal of Musculoskeletal Medicine, 11*(11): 19–35.
9. Harkon, T.M., Lampman, R.M., Banwell, B.F., & Castor, C.W. (1986). Therapeutic value of graded aerobic exercise training in rheumatoid arthritis. *Arthritis and Rheumatism, 28*(1), 32–39.
10. Massicot, J.G. (1985). Current immunologic research on systemic lupus erythematosus. *Health Values: Achieving High Level Wellness, 9*(2), 7–14.
11. Steinberg, A.D., Gourley, M.F., Klinman, D.M., et al. (1991). Systemic lupus erythematosus. *Annals of Internal Medicine 115*(7), 548–559.
12. Stevens, M.B., & Zimminski, C. (1992). Heart disease in systemic lupus erythematosus. *Journal of Musculoskeletal Medicine, 6*(6), 41–46.
13. Berman, H.M., & Blumenfield, M. (1992). Psychiatric symptoms in systemic lupus erythematosus. *Journal of Musculoskeletal Medicine, 6*(6), 81–94.
14. Tan, E.M., Cohen, A.S., Fries, J.F., et al. (1982). The 1982 revised criteria for the classification of systemic lupus erythematosus. *Arthritis and Rheumatism, 25*(11), 1271–1277.
15. Moore, M., McGory, C., & Rosenthal, R. (1991). *Learning about lupus: A user friendly guide* (pp. 7–11). Wayne, PA: Mainline Desktop Publishing.
16. Pigg, J.S., & Bancroft, D.A. (1992). Management of patients with rheumatic diseases. In S.C. Smeltzer & B.C. Bare (Eds.). *Brunner and Suddarth's textbook of medical-surgical nursing* (7th ed., pp. 1425–1428). Philadelphia: J.B. Lippincott.
17. Plotz, P.H. (moderator). (1989). Current concepts in the idiopathic inflammatory myopathies, polymyositis, dermatomyositis, and related disorders. *Annals of Internal Medicine, 111*, 143–157.
18. Ramanujam, R., & Schumacher, H.R. (1992). Ankylosing spondylitis: Early recognition and management. *Journal of Musculoskeletal Medicine, 1*(1), 75–91.
19. Arnett, F.C., Khan, M.A., & Willkens, R.F. (1989). A new look at ankylosing spondylitis. *Patient Care, 23*(19), 82–101.
20. Arnett, F.C. (1987). Seronegative spondyloarthropathies. *Bulletin on the Rheumatic Diseases, 37*(1), 1–12.
21. Winchester, R. (1990). AIDS and the rheumatic diseases. *Bulletin on the Rheumatic Diseases, 39*(5), 1–10.
22. Aguilar, J.L., & Espinoza, L.R. (1989). Psoriatic arthritis: A current perspective. *Journal of Musculoskeletal Medicine, 6*(6), 11–28.
23. Hooker, R.S. (1992). Clinical characteristics of the seronegative spondyloarthopathies. *Journal of the American Academy of Physicians' Assistants, 5*(2), 110–120.
24. Mankin, H.J., & Treadwell, B.V. (1986). Osteoarthritis: A 1987 update. *Bulletin on the Rheumatic Diseases, 16*(5), 1–10.
25. Davison, S. (1980). Rheumatic disease in the elderly. *Mount Sinai Journal of Medicine, 47*(2), 175–178.
26. Brandt, K.D., & Radin, E. (1987, January 15). The physiology of articular stress: Osteoarthrosis. *Hospital Practice*, 103–126.
27. Ghosh, P. (1988). Articular cartilage: What it is, why it fails in osteoarthritis, and what can be done about it. *Arthritis Care Research, 1*(4), 211–221.
28. Felson, D.T., Zhang, Y., Anthony, J.M., Naimark, A., & Anderson, J.J. (1992). Weight loss reduces the risk for symptomatic knee osteoarthritis in women: The Framingham study. *Annals of Internal Medicine 116*, 535–539.
29. Hochberg, M.C. (1991). Epidemiologic considerations in the primary prevention of osteoarthritis [editorial]. *Journal of Rheumatology, 18*, 1438–1440.
30. Blechman, W.B., Roth, S.H., & Wilske, K. (1992). Osteoarthritis: Are you up-to-date? *Patient Care, 26*(5), 99–144.
31. Altman, R., Alarcon, G., Appelrouth, D., et al. (1990). The American College of Rheumatology criteria for the classification and reporting of osteoarthritis of the hand. *Arthritis and Rheumatism, 33*(11), 1601–1610.
32. Altman, R., Alarcon, G., Appelrouth, D., et al. (1991). The American College of Rheumatology criteria for the classification and reporting of osteoarthritis of the hip. *Arthritis and Rheumatism, 34*(5), 505–514.
33. Altman, R., Asch, E., Bloch, D., et al. (1986). Development of criteria for the classification and reporting of osteoarthritis: Classification of osteoarthritis of the knee. *Arthritis and Rheumatism, 29*(8), 1039–1049.
34. *Arthritis, rheumatic diseases, and related disorders: 1992 research highlights.* (1992). U.S. Department of Health and Human Services, National Institutes of Health, National

Institute of Arthritis and Musculoskeletal and Skin Diseases, NIH Publication No. 92-3413.

35. Levinson, D.J., & Becker, M.A. (1993). Clinical gout and the pathogenesis of hyperuricemia. In D.J. McCarty & W.J. Koopman (Eds.). *Arthritis and allied conditions* (12th ed., pp. 1733–1805). Philadelphia: Lea & Febiger.

36. Wortman, R.L. (1993). Management of hyperuricemia. In D.J. McCarty & W.J. Koopman (Eds.), *Arthritis and allied conditions* (12th ed., pp. 1807–1818). Philadelphia: Lea & Febiger.

37. Kelley, W.N., Fox, I.M., & Pallela, T.D. (1989). Gout and related disorders of purine metabolism. In W.N. Kelley, E.D. Harris, S. Ruddy, & C.B. Sledge (Eds.). *Textbook of rheumatology* (3rd ed., pp. 1395–1448). Philadelphia: W.B. Saunders.

38. Yeomans, A.C. (1991). Assessment and management of gouty arthritis. *Nurse Practitioner, 16*(4), 20, 21, 25, 26.

39. Murphy, B.B., & Schumacher, H.R. (1984). How does patient education affect gout? *Clin Rheum Pract, 2*(2), 77.

40. Alsaeid, K., & Ayoub, E.M. (1992). Systemic lupus erythematosus in children: Part one: Diagnosis complicated by a lengthy differential list. *Journal of Musculoskeletal Medicine, 9*(9), 29–39.

41. Fuller, C., & Hartley, B. (1991, August). Systemic lupus erythematosus in adolescents. *Journal of Pediatric Nursing,* 252–257.

42. Alsaeid, K., & Ayoub, E.M. (1992). Systemic lupus erythematosus in children: Part two: Management team acts to control symptoms. *Journal of Musculoskeletal Medicine, 10*(10), 30–39.

43. Vaughn, S.M., & Whittle, E. (1984). Caring for the child with dermatomyositis. *Issues in Comprehensive Pediatric Nursing, 7,* 255–267.

44. Moskowitz, R.W., & Haug, M.R. (Eds.). (1986). *Arthritis and the elderly.* New York: Springer.

45. Collier, I.C. (1988). Assessing functional status of the elderly. *Arthritis Care and Research, 1*(1), 45–52.

46. Daltroy, L.H., Logigian, M., Iversen, M.D., & Liang, M.H. (1992). Does musculoskeletal function deteriorate in a predictable sequence in the elderly? *Arthritis Care and Research, 5*(3), 146–150.

47. Lawrence, R.C., Hochberg, M.D., Kelsey, J.L., et al. (1989). Estimates of the prevalence of selected arthritic and musculoskeletal diseases in the United States. *Journal of Rheumatology, 16,* 427–441.

48. Deal, C.L., Meenan, R.F., Goldenberg, D.L., et al. (1985). The clinical features of elderly-onset rheumatoid arthritis: A comparison with younger-onset disease of similar duration. *Arthritis and Rheumatism, 28,* 987–994.

49. Healey, L.A., & Sheets, P.K. (1988). The relation of polymyalgia rheumatica to rheumatoid arthritis. *Journal of Rheumatology, 15,* 750–752.

50. Maddison, P.J. (1987). Systemic lupus erythematosus in the elderly. *Journal of Rheumatology, 14*(S13), 182–187.

51. Calkins, E. (1991). Arthritis in the elderly. *Bulletin on the Rheumatic Diseases, 40*(3), 3.

52. Campbell, S.M. (1988). Gout: How presentation, diagnosis, and treatment differ in the elderly. *Geriatrics, 43,* 71–77.

53. Powell, M.A. (1991). Polymyalgia rheumatica. *Journal of the American Academy of Nurse Practitioners, 3*(4), 188–189.

54. Davis, G.C., Cortez, C., & Rubin, B.R. (1990). Pain management in the older adult with rheumatoid arthritis or osteoarthritis. *Arthritis Care and Research, 3*(3), 127–131.

55. Keefe, F.J., Caldwell, D.S., Queen, K.T., et al. (1987). Pain coping strategies in osteoarthritis patients. *Journal of Consulting and Clinical Psychology, 55,* 208–212.

■ BIBLIOGRAPHY

Arnett, F.C. (1990). Revised criteria for the classification of rheumatoid arthritis. *Orthopedic Nursing, 9*(2), 58–64.

Arnett, F.C. (1991). Pathogenesis of the spondyloarthropathies. *Bulletin on the Rheumatic Diseases, 40*(6), 1–3.

Arnett, F.C. (1992). Genetic aspects of human lupus. *Clinical Immunology, 63*(1), 4–6.

Bunning, R.D., & Materson, R.S. (1991). A rational program of exercise for patients with osteoarthritis. *Seminars in Arthritis and Rheumatism, 21*(S), 3343.

Campbell, S.M. (1991). Rheumatoid arthritis. *Hospital Medicine, 27*(1), 55–62.

Ellman, M.H. (1992). Treating acute gouty arthritis. *Journal of Musculoskeletal Medicine, 3*(3), 71–77.

Hamerman, D. (1989). The biology of osteoarthritis. *New England Journal of Medicine, 320*(20), 1322–1330.

Harris, E.D. (1992). Excitement in synovium: The rapid evolution of understanding of rheumatoid arthritis and expectations for therapy. *Journal of Rheumatology, 19*(S32), 18–20.

Hess, E.V. (1991). Drug-related lupus. *Bulletin on the Rheumatic Diseases, 40*(4), 1–8.

Kale, S.A., & Raymond, M.K. (1990, August). Osteoarthritis: The patient-centered approach: Part 1—Evaluation. *Consultant,* 24–26.

Kovar, P.A., Allegrante, J.P., MacKenzier, R., Peterson, M.G.E., Gutin, B., & Charlson, M.E. (1992). Supervised fitness walking in patients with osteoarthritis of the knee. *Annals of Internal Medicine, 116*(7), 529–534.

McKeag, D.B. (1992). The relationship of osteoarthritis and exercise. *Clinics in Sports Medicine, 11*(2), 471–487.

Morrey, B.F. (1992). Primary osteoarthritis of the knee: A stepwise management plan. *Journal of Musculoskeletal Medicine, 9*(9), 79–94.

Pincus, T., & Callahan, L.F. (1992). Early mortality in RA predicted by poor clinical status. *Bulletin on the Rheumatic Diseases 41*(4), 1–5.

Ramanujam, R., & Schumacher, H.R. (1992). Ankylosing spondylitis: Early recognition and management. *Journal of Musculoskeletal Medicine, 1*(1), 75–91.

Smith, C.A., & Arnett, F.C. (1991). Epidemiologic aspects of rheumatoid arthritis. *Clinical Orthopedic Research, 265,* 23–35.

Watts, R.A., & Isaacs, J.D. (1992). Immunotherapy of rheumatoid arthritis. *Annals of the Rheumatic Diseases, 51*(5), 577–579.

INDEX

Page numbers followed by f *indicate figures; those followed by* t *indicate tabular material.*